S0-AFR-312

DATE

Haines and Taylor

Obstetrical and Gynaecological Pathology

For Churchill Livingstone

Commissioning Editor: Geoff Nuttall
Project Editor: Gavin Smith
Copy Editor: Ruth Swan
Indexer: Liza Weinkove
Project Controller: Sarah Lowe
Design Direction: Erik Bigland

Haines and Taylor
Obstetrical and Gynaecological Pathology

Edited by

H. Fox MD FRCPath FRCOG

Emeritus Professor of Reproductive Pathology, Department of Pathological Sciences, The University of Manchester, Manchester, UK

Assistant Editor

M. Wells BSc(Hons) MD FRCPath

Professor of Gynaecological Pathology, University of Leeds; Honorary Consultant Pathologist, St James's University Hospital, Leeds, UK

FOURTH EDITION
VOLUME 2

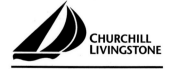
CHURCHILL
LIVINGSTONE

NEW YORK EDINBURGH LONDON MADRID MELBOURNE SAN FRANCISCO AND TOKYO 1995

CHURCHILL LIVINGSTONE
Medical Division of Pearson Professional Limited

Distributed in the United States of America by Churchill Livingstone
Inc., 650 Avenue of the Americas, New York, N.Y. 10011, and by
associated companies, branches and representatives throughout
the world.

© J. & A. Churchill Limited 1962
© Longman Group Limited 1975
© Longman Group UK Limited 1987
© Pearson Professional Limited 1995

All rights reserved. No part of this publication may be reproduced,
stored in a retrieval system, or transmitted in any form or by any means,
electronic, mechanical, photocopying, recording or otherwise, without
either the prior permission of the publishers (Churchill Livingstone,
Robert Stevenson House, 1-3 Baxter's Place, Leith Walk, Edinburgh,
EH1 3AF), or a licence permitting restricted copying in the United
Kingdom issued by the Copyright Licensing Agency Ltd, 90 Tottenham
Court Road, London, W1P 9HE.

First edition 1962
Second edition 1975
Third edition 1987
Fourth edition 1995

ISBN 0-443-04537-2

British Library Cataloguing in Publication Data
A catalogue record for this book is available from the British Library.

Library of Congress Cataloging in Publication Data
A catalog record for this book is available from the Library of Congress.

The
publisher's
policy is to use
paper manufactured
from sustainable forests

Printed in the United States of America

Contents

Contributors

Malcolm C. Anderson FRCOG FRCPath
Reader in Gynaecological Pathology, University of
Nottingham; Consultant Histopathologist, University
Hospital, Nottingham, UK

Jan P. A. Baak MD PhD FRCPath
Professor of Pathology, Free University Hospital,
Amsterdam, The Netherlands

Virginia J. Baldwin BSc MD FRCP(C)
Associate Professor, Department of Pathology, Faculty of
Medicine, University of British Columbia; Pathologist,
British Columbia's Children's Hospital, Vancouver,
British Columbia, Canada

Gillian Batcup MB BS BSc FRCPath
Consultant Paediatric/Perinatal Pathologist,
Department of Histopathology, Leeds General
Infirmary, Leeds, UK

J. A. M. Beliën MSc
Department of Pathology, University Hospital VU,
Amsterdam, The Netherlands

Debra A. Bell MD
Associate Professor, Department of Pathology, Harvard
Medical School; Associate Pathologist, Massachusetts
General Hospital; Director, Cytopathology Laboratory,
Massachusetts General Hospital, Boston, Massachusetts,
USA

Elizabeth Benjamin MB BS FRCPath
Senior Clinical Lecturer and Honorary Consultant
Pathologist, Department of Histopathology, University
College London Medical School, London, UK

Peter F. Bernhardt MD
Pathologist, Alexian Bros Medical Centre, Elk Grove
Village, Illinois, USA

Anna Berzowski MD FRCPSC
Pathology Fellow, University of Ottawa, Ottawa,
Ontario, Canada

M. Brinkhuis MD PhD
Department of Pathology, University Hospital VU,
Amsterdam, The Netherlands

M. A. M. Broeckaert MSc
Research Scientist, Department of Pathology, University
Hospital VU, Amsterdam, The Netherlands

J. Brugghe MSc
Research Scientist, Department of Pathology, University
Hospital VU, Amsterdam, The Netherlands

C. Hilary Buckley MD FRCP
Reader in Gynaecological Pathology, University of
Manchester; Consultant Histopathologist, St Mary's
Hospital, Manchester, UK

Judith N. Bulmer MB ChB PhD MRCPath
Senior Lecturer in Pathology, University of Newcastle
upon Tyne; Consultant Pathologist, Royal Victoria
Infirmary, Newcastle upon Tyne, UK

Harpal S. Buttar DVM MSc PhD
Research Scientist, Life Sciences Division, Bureau of Drug
Research, Health Protection Branch, Sir F G Banting
Research Centre, Ottawa; Adjunct Professor, University of
British Columbia, Vancouver, University of Ottawa and
Memorial University of Newfoundland, St John's, Canada

A. H. Cameron MB BS MD FRCPath
Senior Research Fellow, Department of Oncology,
Children's Hospital, Birmingham, UK

J. S. Campbell MD FRCPath FRCP(C) FCAP
Emeritus Clinical Professor, Department of Pathology,
University of Ottawa, Ottawa, Ontario, Canada

M. Castellucci MD
Professor of Human Anatomy, University of Ancona, Medical Faculty, Ancona, Italy

Philip B. Clement MD
Clinical Professor and Consultant Pathologist, Vancouver Hospital and Health Sciences Centre and the University of British Columbia, Vancouver, British Columbia, Canada

Dulcie V. Coleman MB BS MD FRCPath
Professor and Head of Department of Cytopathology and Cytogenetics, St Mary's Hospital, London, UK

Bernard Czernobilsky MD
Professor of Pathology, Medical School of the Hebrew University and Hadassah, Jerusalem, Department of Pathology, Kaplan Hospital, Rehovot, Israel

Gisela Dallenbach-Hellweg MD FIAC
Prof. Dr. med, Institut für Pathologie, Mannheim, Germany

Pierre Drouin MD FRCPSC
Chief, Gynecology and Oncology Service, Notre Dame University; Professor, Department of Obstetrics and Gynaecology, University of Montreal, Montreal, Quebec, Canada

C. W. Elston MD FRCPath
Consultant Histopathologist, Nottingham City Hospital NHS Trust; Clinical Teacher, University of Nottingham Medical School, Nottingham, UK

H. Fox MD FRCPath FRCOG
Emeritus Professor of Reproductive Pathology, Department of Pathological Sciences, The University of Manchester, Manchester, UK

N. R. Griffin BSc MD MRCPath
Consultant Histopathologist, Department of Histopathology, University Hospital, Queen's Medical Centre, Nottingham, UK

Michael R. Hendrickson MD
Professor of Pathology, Co-Director of Surgical Pathology, Department of Pathology, Stanford University Medical Center, Stanford, California, USA

Louis H. Honoré BSc MBChB FRCP(C)
Professor of Laboratory Medicine and Pathology and Honorary Professor of Obstetrics and Gynaecology, University of Alberta, Edmonton, Alberta, Canada

Peter G. Isaacson DM FRCPath DSc
Professor and Head, Department of Histopathology, University College London Medical School, London, UK

Peter M. Johnson DSc FRCPath
Professor, Department of Immunology, University of Liverpool, Liverpool, UK

Peter Kaufmann Dr Med
Professor of Anatomy, Department of Anatomy II, RWTH Aachen, Germany

A. M. Kelsey MRCPath
Consultant Paediatric Histopathologist, Royal Manchester Children's Hospital, Manchester, UK

Richard L. Kempson MD
Professor of Pathology, Co-Director of Surgical Pathology, Department of Pathology, Stanford University Medical Center, Stanford, California, USA

Hans G. Kohler Dr Med FRCPath
Formerly Consultant Pathologist, The Maternity Hospital at Leeds; Senior Clinical Lecturer, The University of Leeds, Leeds, UK

F. A. Langley MSc MD MB ChB FRCOG FRCPath
Late Emeritus Professor of Obstetrical and Gynaecological Pathology, University of Manchester, Manchester, UK

David Lowe MD FRCPath FIBiol
Reader in Histopathology, St Bartholomew's Hospital Medical College, London, UK

Teri A. Longacre MD
Assistant Professor of Pathology, Stanford University School of Medicine, Stanford, California, USA

Sebastian B. Lucas FRCP FRCPath
Professor of Histopathology, St Thomas' Hospital, London, UK

Roderick N. M. MacSween BSc MD FRCP(Edin) FRCP(Glasg) FRCPath FIBiol FRSE
Professor of Pathology, University of Glasgow; Honorary Consultant Pathologist, University Department of Pathology, Western Infirmary, Glasgow, UK

John M. McLean BSc MD
Formerly Senior Lecturer in Anatomy and Embryology, University of Manchester, Manchester, UK

G. J. Meijer MD
Department of Pathology, University Hospital VU,
Amsterdam, The Netherlands

Nadia Z. Mikhael MD FRCPC FCAP FAAP
Professor and Chairman, Department of Pathology and
Laboratory Medicine, Faculty of Medicine, University of
Ottawa; Head, Department of Pathology and Laboratory
Medicine, Ottawa General Hospital, Ottawa, Ontario,
Canada

Omar Mohamdee MBChB MRCOG MRCPath
Senior Registrar in Histopathology, Leeds General
Infirmary, Leeds, UK

Ian A. R. More BSc PhD MD FRCPath
Senior Lecturer in Pathology, University of Glasgow;
Consultant Pathologist, Western Infirmary, Glasgow, UK

E. Napke BSc MD DPH
Formerly Chief, Product Related Disease Division,
Health Canada, Ottawa, Ontario, Canada; Consultant,
WHO Drug Monitoring Program, Uppsala, Sweden

M. Newbould MRCPath
Senior Lecturer in Histopathology, King's College
School of Medicine and Dentistry, London, UK

Francisco F. Nogales MD
Professor of Pathology, Faculty of Medicine, University
of Granada, Spain

Eckhardt G. J. Olsen AKC MD FRCPath FACC
Formerly Consultant Histopathologist and Honorary
Senior Lecturer, Cardiothoracic Institute, University of
London, London, UK

Andrew G. Östör MD BS FRCPA MIAC
Chairman, Department of Pathology; Director,
Anatomical Pathology and Cytology, The Royal
Women's Hospital, Melbourne, Victoria, Australia

Jaime Prat MD FRCPath
Professor & Chairman, Department of Pathology,
Universidad Autó noma de Barcelona, Hospital de Sant
Pau, Barcelona, Spain

Helen Reid MB BS FRCPath
Lecturer in Neuropathology, University of Manchester;
Consultant Neuropathologist to the Central Manchester
Health Care Trust, Manchester, UK

C. M. Ridley MA BM FRCP
Honorary Consultant Dermatologist, St Thomas's
Hospital, London, UK

Stanley J. Robboy MD
Professor of Pathology, Obstetrics and Gynecology;
Director, Gynecologic Pathology, Duke University
Medical Center, Durham, North Carolina, USA

Terence P. Rollason BSc MBChB FRCPath
Consultant Gynaecological Pathologist, Birmingham
Women's Services Trust; Senior Clinical Lecturer,
University of Birmingham, Birmingham, UK

Lawrence M. Roth MD
Professor of Pathology, Indiana University School of
Medicine; Pathologist and Director of Surgical
Pathology, Indiana University Hospital, Indianopolis,
Indiana, USA

Paul Rowsell BSc
Biologist, Health Protection Branch, Health Canada,
Ottawa, Ontario, Canada

Ian Rushton MB ChB FRCPath
Senior Lecturer in Pathology, University of Birmingham
School of Medicine; Honorary Consultant Perinatal
Pathologist, Maternity Hospital, Birmingham, UK

Peter Russell MD BSc(Med) FRCPA
Clinical Professor of Pathology, University of Sydney;
Head, Gynaecological Pathology, King George V and
Royal Prince Alfred Hospitals, Sydney, New South
Wales, Australia

Waldemar A. Schmidt PhD MD
Chief, Anatomic Pathology, Pathology and Laboratory
Medicine Services, Veterans Affairs Medical Centre;
Professor and Director of Cytopathology, Department of
Pathology, School of Medicine, Oregon Health Sciences
University, Portland, Oregon, USA

Robert E. Scully MD
Emeritus Professor of Pathology, Massachusetts General
Hospital, Harvard Medical School, Boston,
Massachusetts, USA

Albert Singer PhD(Syd) DFIL(Oxon) FRCOG
Professor of Gynaecological Research, University of
London; Consultant Gynaecologist, Whittington and
Royal Northern Hospitals, London, UK

Gerard Slavin MB FRCPath FRCP(Glas)
Professor of Histopathology, St Bartholomew's Hospital
Medical College, London, UK

A. Talerman MD FRCPath
Peter A. Herbut Professor of Pathology, Thomas
Jefferson University, Philadelphia, USA

Andrew J. Tiltman MD MMed(Path)
Department of Anatomical Pathology, South African
Institute for Medical Research, Johannesburg, South Africa

Leander Tryphonas DVM PhD
Formerly Pathologist, Health Canada, Ottawa, Ontario,
Canada

David R. Turner MB BS PhD FRCPath
Professor of Pathology, University Hospital, Nottingham,
UK

William R. Welch MD
Associate Professor of Pathology, Brigham and Women's
Hospital, Harvard Medical School, Boston,
Massachusetts, USA

Michael Wells BSc(Hons) MD FRCPath
Professor of Gynaecological Pathology, University of
Leeds; Honorary Consultant Pathologist, St James's
University Hospital, Leeds, UK

Peter O. Yates MD FRCPath
Professor Emeritus of Neuropathology, University of
Manchester, Manchester, UK

Robert H. Young MD FRCPath
Director of Surgical Pathology, Massachusetts General
Hospital; Associate Professor of Pathology, Harvard
Medical School, Boston, Massachusetts, USA

Preface

During the years which have elapsed since the last edition of this text new information has continued to accrue, in an ever increasing flow, about all aspects of gynaecological and obstetrical pathology and this fresh material has been fully covered in the thorough updating to which every chapter of this book has been subjected.

This present edition represents, however, more than a simple updating. The aims and intent of the previous edition have been retained but there are several structural alterations, some of which have stemmed from the constructive criticism afforded that edition and some of which reflect changing pathological practice. I have, with some reluctance, excluded the contributions on perinatal pathology for with the advantage of hindsight I can appreciate that they distract from the main theme of this book and these topics are, furthermore, fully covered in the now quite numerous admirable texts devoted to peri-natal pathology. I have also reversed my stance concerning gynaecological cytopathology because I became convinced that an authorative overview of this topic could be achieved in a single chapter and would be of value. I have included chapters on immunocytochemistry, quantitative analysis and molecular biology, not simply as an obeisance to the onward march of medical technology but because such techniques have now passed from the province of the research laboratory to become routine diagnostic tools and I thought it useful to collate, into single chapters, the information about the application of these techniques to gynaecological pathology.

As before, and for reasons detailed in the Preface to the third edition, I have allowed considerable freedom to my contributors and accepted, even welcomed, some degree of overlap between chapters.

One sad event has been the death of Elizabeth Ramsey who contributed two chapters to the last edition. She was not only an embryologist of the highest international renown but also a joy and an inspiration to all those who had the privilege of knowing her.

A further, and on a personal level even sadder event, has been the death of Frederick Langley, who was my mentor and guide in the study of gynaecological pathology. He was a man of great scientific insight, allied to considerable personal kindness, and is much missed.

Manchester, 1995   H.F.

Preface to the third edition

This is the third edition of Haines and Taylor's text on Gynaecological Pathology. It is readily admitted, however, that this edition departs so radically from the format of its two predecessors that it represents a new entity rather than a simple revision and updating. Despite this lack of any evolutionary continuity, I wished to retain the names of Claude Taylor and Magnus Haines in the title as a tribute to two men who did much to establish the scientific respectability and intellectual credibility of gynaecological pathology in Great Britain.

The primary aim of this book is to give a full account of the pathology of both gynaecological and obstetrical disorders. There are, of course, many other texts devoted to this topic, but it has appeared to me that few have given sufficient attention to obstetrical pathology. The clinical chimerism of obstetrics and gynaecology should be, but is often not, reflected in pathological texts, and it is hoped that the detailed attention given in this volume will help to correct the imbalance which has tended to lead to a relative neglect of this topic.

The chapters in this multi-author book vary in length and style, and there is some repetition between the various contributions. All these features are usually considered to be defects in the format of a multi-author volume resulting from a lack of editorial control. These apparent faults are, however, the direct result of editorial decisions based upon my own concept of the strengths and weaknesses of a large and complex multi-author volume.

Thus I did not impose any minimum or maximum limits on the number of words allowed for each contribution. This decision was based on two factors, of which the first was my confidence in the ability of the invited contributors to decide for themselves the number of words required for a comprehensive consideration of their subject. A second factor was my belief that decisions as to chapter length in multi-author volumes often reflect editorial interests and thus result in an arbitrary and biased view of the relative importance of various topics: this has often resulted in certain aspects of gynaecological pathology, such as the consideration of vulvar, vaginal and tubal disease, receiving relatively inadequate attention, a fault which I hope is rectified in this volume. I have also not insisted upon any unity of style, approach or presentation from the various contributors. The major merit of literary style in a scientific text is that it allows for a lucid and easily comprehensive exposition: I therefore limited my stylistic interventions to the clarification of any obscure passages, and have not attempted to submerge the individualism or flair of my contributors by the editorial imposition of the dead hand of stylistic conformity. I have allowed, and even encouraged, some degree of repetition between chapters. This is because I felt that a book of this length is unlikely to be read in its entirely at a single sitting and that, each chapter should therefore be able to stand as a discrete entity which could be read as a review of a particular topic without the frequent necessity of following cross references to other chapters. My aim was, therefore, to ensure that each chapter was comprehensive, complete in itself and retained the authentic voice of the author.

Certain omissions and commissions in this book require comment. No chapter on gynaecological cytopathology has been included, largely because I felt this to be a subject worthy of a volume in its own right and one which could be considered only in a superficial and sketchy manner when restricted by the confines of a single chapter. By contrast I specifically asked for a rather lengthy description of the embryology and anatomy of the female genital tract; this is perhaps unusual in a textbook of pathology, but reflects my view that many gynaecological lesions can only be fully understood when placed in the context of a sound knowledge of female genital tract development and structure. Some aspects of perinatal pathology have also been included in this book, but these represent, to my mind, only those aspects of this topic which are logical extensions of obstetrical pathology. I have also included discussions of such subjects as the pathology of infertility, the pathology of contraception, the histogenesis of ovarian tumours, the immunopathology of the female genital tract and reproductive immunology: to some, these topics may appear to be out of place in a text devoted primarily to histopathology but their inclusion reflects my feeling that the pathologist must be concerned with all aspects of disorders of the female genital tract and should not be restricted by the limits of the microscope. There has also been a deliberate inclusion of two chapters on abnormalities of sexual differentiation. This was because I wished to have a general overview of this topic which could be set in apposition to chapters on normal development and on malformations of the female genital tract, together with a separate chapter devoted principally to gonadal pathology in patients with abnormal sexual development.

In most general hospitals, biopsies and surgical specimens from gynaecological and obstetrical patients constitute approximately one third of the total workload of departments of surgical pathology. It is hoped that this book will, despite its imperfections, be of assistance to the pathologist in dealing with this massive inflow of material. I hope also that this volume will indicate some of the scientific and intellectual satisfaction that can be gained from a study of this branch of pathology.

Manchester, 1987   H.F.

26. Mesenchymal tumours of the ovary

J. Prat   H. Fox

Many of the neoplasms considered in this chapter arise from those tissue elements in the ovary, such as blood vessels, nerves or lymphatics, which are not committed to the specific gonadal function of the organ. The situation is, however, complicated by the fact that such tumours, particularly those which are malignant, may have other quite different origins.

1. The tumour may arise in, and from, pre-existing foci of ovarian endometriosis: as the neoplasm grows it may destroy all evidence of the endometriotic focus from which it evolved.

2. A tissue which was originally a component of a mixed Müllerian tumour may subsequently become totally dominant and thus appear as a monomorphic tumour.

3. Mesenchymal neoplasms may arise in ovarian teratomas, either because of malignant change in a mature teratoma or as a component of an immature teratoma: in either case the mesenchymal tumour may overgrow and obliterate all other teratomatous elements.

4. A mesenchymal neoplasm may develop from heterologous elements in a Sertoli–Leydig cell tumour: again, such a neoplasm may totally obscure the sex cord components and thus masquerade as a pure mesenchymal neoplasm.

5. Mesenchymal tumours may arise in the wall of a cystic epithelial neoplasm: the theoretical possibility exists once again of progressive mesenchymal dominance.

It is thus apparent that in many examples of pure mesenchymal tumours of the ovary it is virtually impossible to reach any decision as to their original histogenesis. Consider, for example, an oncological curiosity such as a pure ovarian rhabdomyosarcoma: this could have arisen in any of the above described fashions, for whilst the most obvious tumour to develop from endometriosis is the endometrioid stromal sarcoma there is no theoretical reason why a rhabdomyosarcoma should not have a similar origin as a form of pure heterologous sarcoma. Conversely, if endometrioid adenocarcinoma can arise either from endometriotic foci or from the surface epithelium of the ovary then it is at least possible that endometrioid sarcomas, including by extrapolation pure heterologous sarcomas such as a rhabdomyosarcoma, could also originate from this site. Clearly a rhabdomyosarcoma could have developed from a mixed Müllerian neoplasm whilst a teratomatous origin for a rhabdomyosarcoma is undoubtedly possible as is an evolution from a Sertoli–Leydig cell tumour. Whether a neoplasm such as a rhabdomyosarcoma can originate directly from ovarian stroma is a debatable point but such a possibility can certainly not be excluded.

Faced with this histogenetic maze the most that a pathologist can do is to sample all apparently pure mesenchymal tumours very extensively so as to be able to exclude with some degree of confidence other tissue components. The application of common sense will, of course, suggest that mesenchymal tumours occurring in elderly women are unlikely to have originated either from ovarian endometriosis or from immature teratomas and that a similar neoplasm in a prepubertal girl may well be of teratomatous origin. Beyond that, however, the pathologist usually can not go.

In this chapter the pure mesenchymal tumours of the ovary will be discussed, as will sarcomas associated with epithelial neoplasms; sarcomas arising in teratomas (see Ch. 23) and mixed Müllerian tumours (see Ch. 16) will not be considered. Endometrioid stromal sarcomas are briefly discussed in Chapter 16 and could be considered further under the heading of Müllerian tumours or that of endometrioid neoplasms; they will be reviewed here in greater detail, partly because of their importance in the differential diagnosis of malignant mesenchymal tumours of the ovary and partly because, in some cases at least, they may arise from ovarian stromal cells.

TUMOURS OF FIBROUS TISSUE

Fibroma

The origin of fibromas is far from clear. It is possible that they arise from non-specialized ovarian tissues, such as the connective tissue of the capsule or blood vessels, in which case they merit their place in this chapter. On the other hand, there is a continuous histological spectrum between thecomas and fibromas (Scully, 1979) and it is quite legitimate to consider that many, or even most, fibromas are 'burnt out' thecomas; electronoptical studies have also supported the concept of the fibroma developing from specialized ovarian stroma (Amin et al, 1971) and hence it would be more logical to consider these neoplasms as sex cord-stromal tumours. The consideration of fibromas in this chapter is undertaken largely because they fit more tidily into a discussion of mesenchymal neoplasms and should not be taken as an implication of a belief that they should be excluded from the sex cord-stromal category.

In most series of ovarian neoplasms fibromas account for about 4% of the total: an incidence as high as 10% has been quoted (Duchini & Menegaldo, 1967) and this indicates that the reported frequency with which fibromas occur is in part dependent upon the criteria used for differentiating them from thecomas and on how 'fibrothecomas' are categorized. Between 4 and 8% of fibromas are bilateral (Dockerty & Masson, 1944; Driscoll, 1964) and most appear as moderately well defined, but not encapsulated, intraovarian nodules of variable size; a proportion totally replace the ovary and a few occur as nodules or plaques on the ovarian surface. They tend to have a smooth, lobulated or nodular outer surface and on section are usually formed of uniformly white or greyish-white solid tissue (Fig. 26.1); sometimes, however, the cut surface has a whorled or lobulated appearance. Some degree of cystic change is seen in about 20% of these neoplasms whilst calcification is not uncommon and is sometimes massive (Sengupta et al, 1979); rarely a fibroma may show ossification.

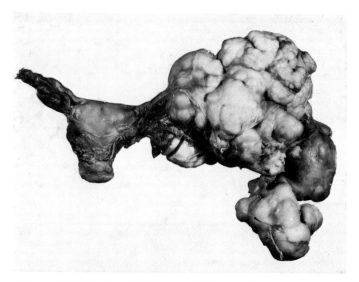

Fig. 26.2 Multiple ovarian fibromas of the type characteristically seen in women with the basal cell naevus syndrome.

Ovarian fibromas occur in a high proportion of young women with the basal cell naevus syndrome (Glendenning et al, 1963; Gorlin & Sedano, 1971; Burkett & Rauh, 1976; Raggio et al, 1983) and in these patients the fibromas are characteristically bilateral, multiple and calcified (Fig. 26.2).

Histologically (Fig. 26.3), fibromas are formed of interlacing bundles of cells which often show a 'feathertail' pattern: they are small, thin and spindle-shaped with narrow ovoid nuclei running parallel to their long axis. Nuclear palisading is sometimes seen whilst occasionally a storiform pattern, similar to that encountered in fibrous histiocytomas, is present. The cells are regular and mitotic figures are absent. The cytoplasm of the tumour cells often contains a small amount of lipid. Sharply delineated

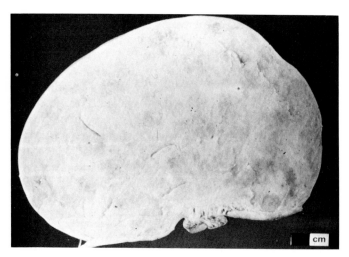

Fig. 26.1 A typical fibroma.

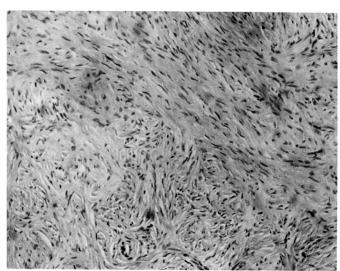

Fig. 26.3 Ovarian fibroma formed of elongated spindle-shaped cells. H & E × 125.

hyaline plaques are sometimes present whilst a more diffuse hyalinization is not uncommon: many fibromas show a variable degree of intercellular oedema or myxoid change. Occasional fibromas contain a few scattered foci of sex cord epithelial cells (Fig. 26.4) which may be represented by nests of undifferentiated cells, by small aggregates of granulosa cells or by tubules lined by Sertoli cells (Young & Scully, 1983).

Fibromas occur in women of all ages though they are most commonly found in those aged between 50 and 60 years; examples have been recorded of their occurrence in premenarchal girls (Charache, 1959; Martins & Klinger, 1964; Bower & Erikson, 1967), but it should be noted that all these cases were described before the association of these tumours with the basal cell naevus syndrome became well known. Small tumours, i.e. those measuring less than 4 cm in diameter, appear to be invariably asymptomatic, whilst many larger fibromas have also been

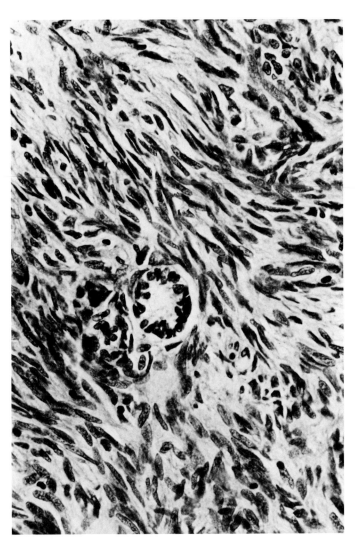

Fig. 26.4 A sex cord epithelial element in an ovarian fibroma. Tubules lined by sertoliform cells were seen in only one of 14 blocks from this tumour. H & E × 460.

incidental findings: in various series the incidence of asymptomatic tumours has ranged from 30–54% (Dockerty & Masson, 1944; Biggart & Macafee, 1955; Driscoll, 1964).

When symptoms do occur the most common are abdominal pain, abdominal enlargement or urinary disturbances; in about 5% of cases there is an acute onset of abdominal pain because of torsion of the neoplasm. It has been claimed by some that these tumours are associated with a high incidence of menstrual abnormalities, postmenopausal bleeding and infertility (Duchini & Menegaldo, 1967; Grosieux, 1970); others have suggested that although such symptoms are atypical they do occur in association with, and are apparently caused by, isolated examples of fibroma (Destro, 1958; Mazella, 1963). In most series of fibromas, however, such symptoms have either been completely absent or have been clearly due to some other factor.

Ascites is a relatively common accompaniment of fibromas, being found in between 15 and 30% of cases: it appears only to complicate those with a diameter greater than 6 cm. A typical Meigs' syndrome, though classically associated with this neoplasm, is far from common and is found in only between 1 and 2% of cases (Dockerty & Masson, 1944; Kleitsman, 1949b; Biggart & Macafee, 1955; Driscoll, 1964); very exceptionally, fluid accumulates elsewhere to produce oedema of the legs, anterior abdominal wall or vulva.

Fibromas are benign and oophorectomy will result in rapid resolution of any ascites or hydrothorax that may be present. One patient has been described in whom recurrent attacks of hypoglycaemia were permanently cured by removal of an ovarian fibroma (Michael, 1966). Although fully benign, these tumours may, in exceptional cases, seed implants on to the peritoneum (Lyday, 1952): if both these and the ovarian neoplasm appear histologically benign the prognosis is excellent and the peritoneal nodules should not be taken as evidence of malignancy.

Cellular fibroma

Prat & Scully (1981) categorized as cellular fibromas those fibromatous tumours of the ovary which are unduly cellular but contain fewer than 4 mitotic figures per 10 high power fields. These authors described 11 such neoplasms which ranged in size from 4.5–21.5 cm in diameter, with an average diameter of 12 cm. The outer surface of the tumour is generally smooth or bosselated and on section most of the neoplasms are solid throughout (Fig. 26.5), a minority being partly cystic and very occasional examples being predominantly cystic. On section these tumours have a greyish-white whorled appearance with multiple foci of haemorrhage and necrosis; the cystic areas in a minority of these tumours contain clear watery fluid.

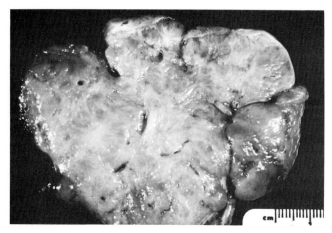

Fig. 26.5 A cellular fibroma of the ovary. This is predominantly solid but a few small cystic areas are present.

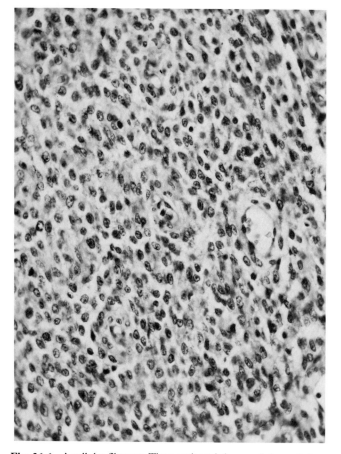

Fig. 26.6 A cellular fibroma. The neoplasm is hypercellular and there is a moderate degree of pleomorphism. There were fewer than 4 mitotic figures per 10 high power fields. H & E × 220.

Histologically (Fig. 26.6), cellular fibromas are composed largely of densely cellular tissue interspersed with a few areas of hypocellular fibrous tissue. The cells are spindle-shaped and arranged in intersecting bundles or in a storiform pattern. The cells are small and thin with ill-defined cytoplasmic borders and round to oval hyper-

chromatic nuclei; in some tumours rounded cells with abundant cytoplasm are present. The nuclei are slightly or moderately atypical, and between 1 and 3 mitotic figures per 10 high power fields are present.

Patients with cellular fibromas have ranged in age from 14–82 years with an average of 49 years. The symptoms are generally those of a pelvic mass, and follow-up of Prat & Scully's (1981) cases showed no evidence of recurrence in nine patients: one patient died seven years postoperatively of pneumonia and at autopsy recurrent tumour was found adherent to the small bowel and sigmoid colon with several smaller nodules in the small bowel mesentery; a further patient died of massive pelvic recurrence 33 months after incomplete removal of the tumour which was adherent to the pelvic wall and omentum. Because of the typically benign course and infrequent bilaterality of cellular fibromas they can justifiably be treated by unilateral salpingo-oophorectomy in a young woman desirous of retaining her fertility. If the tumour is adherent it should be removed as completely as is technically feasible. Patients with ruptured tumours should be followed carefully because of the possibility of intra-abdominal recurrence.

Fibrosarcoma

There have been sporadic reports in the literature of ovarian fibrosarcomas (Variati & Donatelli, 1966; Nieminen et al, 1969; Azoury & Woodruff, 1971; Toth et al, 1971) but it was left to Prat & Scully (1981) to render a definitive account of these neoplasms. They described six ovarian fibrosarcomas which ranged in size from 9–35 cm in diameter with a mean diameter of 17.5 cm. The tumours were soft and lobulated and completely replaced the ovary: on section they varied from greyish-white to tan and showed numerous areas of haemorrhage and necrosis.

Histologically, the neoplasms were densely cellular, the spindle-shaped cells being arranged in a herring-bone or storiform pattern: the tumour cells had indistinct borders, eosinophilic cytoplasm, and hyperchromatic nuclei with prominent nucleoli. There was a moderate to marked degree of pleomorphism and the number of mitotic figures ranged from 4–25 per 10 high power fields (Fig. 26.7).

The patients with ovarian fibrosarcomas ranged in age from 42–73 years with an average of 58 years; the principal presenting complaints were of pelvic pain, abdominal enlargement or awareness of an abdominal mass. Of the six patients, five died within four years of the initial diagnosis: in four of these cases death was due to the tumour whilst the fifth patient died of cardiac disease but had a massive pelvic recurrence. The sixth patient was lost to follow-up at 15 months but had extensive metastases at that time. The ovarian fibrosarcoma is thus seen to be a lethal neoplasm.

There is a general impression that ovarian fibrosarco-

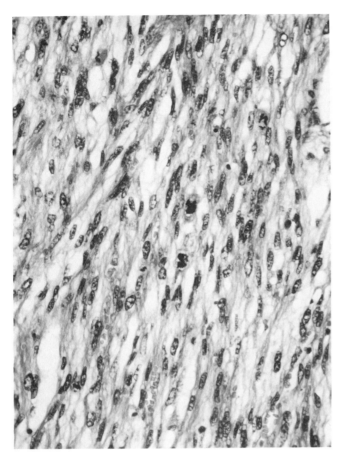

Fig. 26.7 An ovarian fibrosarcoma. There is considerable pleomorphism and many mitotic figures are present. H & E × 320.

mas develop as a result of malignant change within a fibroma rather than occurring as a malignant tumour *de novo* and strength is lent to this view by a report of a fibrosarcoma which developed in an 8-year-old girl with multiple ovarian fibromas as a component of the naevoid basal cell carcinoma syndrome (Kraemer et al, 1984); this neoplasm had a high mitotic count and a metastasis developed two years later, after removal of which, however, the patient was alive and well four years later. An ovarian fibrosarcoma has also been reported in a patient with Maffucci's syndrome (Christman & Ballon, 1990).

TUMOURS OF SMOOTH MUSCLE

Leiomyoma

Ovarian leiomyomas appear to be rare, for fewer than 60 examples have been reported (Kleitsman, 1949a; Wellman, 1961; Fallahzadeh et al, 1972; Thay et al, 1973; Kalra et al, 1981; Tsalacopoulos & Tiltman, 1981; Matamala et al, 1988; Vierhout et al, 1990; Prayson & Hart, 1992): it is highly probable, however, that most cases go unrecorded. The tumours are usually unilateral, a single bilateral case having been reported by Kandalaft

& Esteban (1992), and range in size from 1–24 cm in diameter; it has been noted that small leiomyomas appear to originate in the hilum and that the attenuated cortex is stretched over their surface but in the larger neoplasms this topographical relationship is not discernible. Leiomyomas, though lacking a true capsule, tend to be sharply delineated: they are solid and firm and on section have a white, grey or brown cut surface which often shows central bulging.

They have a whorled or multinodular structure and although commonly solid throughout may show areas of myxoid or pseudocystic change, the latter sometimes being sufficiently marked for the tumour to resemble a cystadenoma. Foci of haemorrhage, necrosis or calcification are common.

Histologically, these neoplasms show the usual features of a leiomyoma with interlacing bundles of smooth muscle fibres which are often admixed with collagenous septa. The muscle cells have elongated blunt-ended or cigar-shaped nuclei and although occasional multinucleated giant cells may be present there is otherwise no pleomorphism, and as a rule mitotic figures are either absent or extremely sparse. Two examples of 'mitotically active', but otherwise unremarkable, ovarian leiomyomas have, however, been noted (Prayson & Hart, 1992). As in uterine leiomyomas, the appearances may be altered by degenerative changes such as cystic change, hyalinization or oedema. A lipoleiomyomatous pattern has been occasionally observed (Dodd et al, 1989; Mira, 1991).

The histogenesis of ovarian leiomyomas is uncertain but they could arise from the smooth muscle fibres of the ovarian ligaments which run into the gonad, from the musculature of the ovarian blood vessels or from the smooth muscle fibres which have been demonstrated, by electronmicroscopy, in the corpus luteum and in the cortical stroma (Okamura et al, 1972).

Ovarian leiomyomas have been encountered in women aged between 20 and 65 years, with only about one-sixth of cases occurring in those who have passed their menopause. Most leiomyomas have been asymptomatic incidental findings at autopsy or surgery but about a third have produced non-specific pelvic mass symptoms such as abdominal pain or swelling. Rarely, torsion of the tumour leads to presentation with acute abdominal pain. Ascites has developed in a few patients but hydrothorax has not been noted. These tumours do not appear to cause menstrual disturbances or abnormal vaginal bleeding, for although such symptoms have often been a feature of the clinical picture of women with ovarian leiomyomas these have invariably been explicable by the presence of co-existent uterine leiomyomas, a common finding in these patients. Ovarian leiomyomas have been noted in pregnant women (Moore, 1945) but no information is available about the effects of the gravid state on the growth and vascularity of these neoplasms.

Ovarian leiomyomas are benign, including those which are 'mitotically active', and can be treated by the least radical surgery necessary for their complete removal. The only diagnostic problem they pose, not one of any great practical importance, is their differentiation from a pedunculated subserosal uterine leiomyoma which has separated off and become secondarily attached to the ovary, from which it receives its blood supply.

Leiomyosarcoma

Ovarian leiomyosarcomas of non-teratoid origin are extremely uncommon, less than 20 examples having been reported (Balazs & Lazlo, 1965; Nieminen et al, 1969; Bettendorf & Zimmermann, 1975; Mani et al, 1978; Raj-Kumar, 1982; Balaton et al, 1987; Cortes et al, 1987; Karogozov et al, 1990; Friedman & Mazur, 1991; Monk et al, 1993) though Prat & Scully (unpublished observations) have recently reviewed a series of 14 cases. The tumours usually occur in elderly women: in Prat & Scully's series the ages of the patients ranged from 30–71 years with a mean of 53 years. The presenting symptoms are usually of abdominal pain or an awareness of an abdominal mass, and a history of menstrual abnormalities is most uncommon. The tumours are nearly always unilateral (bilaterality being noted in only one of Prat & Scully's cases) and are generally large, varying in Prat & Scully's series from 7.5–20 cm in diameter with a mean of 12.4 cm. Grossly, ovarian leiomyosarcomas have a nodular outer surface and on section most are predominantly solid but with foci of cystic change; there may be extensive areas of haemorrhage and necrosis (Fig. 26.8). Their cut surface tends to be greyish-white and generally has a rather more fleshy texture than does a leiomyoma. The histological appearances (Fig. 26.9) are variable and range

from very well differentiated tumours, differing from a leiomyoma only by containing an excessive number of mitotic figures, to highly pleomorphic sarcomas with only a few small areas of recognizably smooth muscle nature. The mitotic counts in Prat & Scully's cases ranged from 4–25 mitotic figures per 10 high power fields. One of Prat & Scully's tumours had extensive myxoid change and resembled a myxoid leiomyosarcoma whilst a further neoplasm showed leiomyoblastomatous (or epithelioid) differentiation (Fig. 26.10). The former case has been recently included in a series of three myxoid leiomyosarcomas of the ovary reported by Nogales et al (1991). They were large gelatinous tumours with cystic change, necrosis and haemorrhage. Microscopically, they exhibited a reticular meshwork of elongated cells surrounded by abundant basophilic myxoid material. The use of immunohistochemical stains against smooth muscle actin demonstrated a smooth muscle type of differentiation. The differential diagnosis of this rare ovarian neoplasm in-

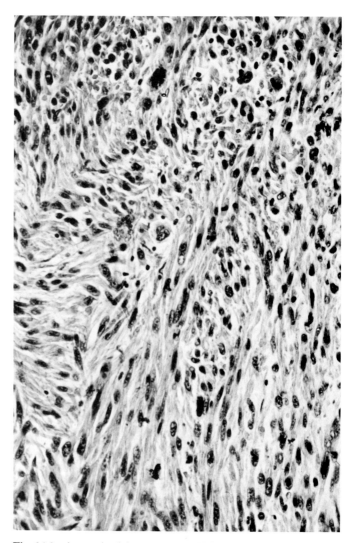

Fig. 26.9 An ovarian leiomyosarcoma. H & E × 320.

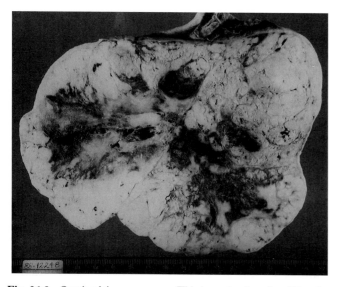

Fig. 26.8 Ovarian leiomyosarcoma. This is predominantly solid and focally haemorrhagic.

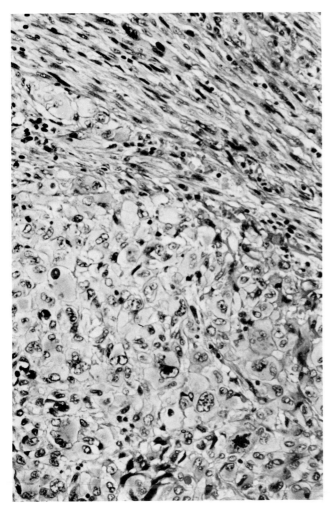

Fig. 26.10 An ovarian leiomyosarcoma which in one area (below) showed an epithelioid (or 'leiomyoblastomatous') pattern. H & E × 320.

cludes ovarian oedema, myxoma, yolk sac tumour and myxoid sarcomatous component of malignant mixed Müllerian tumour and carcinosarcoma. Due to decreased cellular density, mitotic counts are usually low; clinical stage seems to be a more reliable prognostic indicator. Like its uterine counterpart, myxoid leiomyosarcoma of the ovary is a highly aggressive tumour. Two of the three patients reported by Nogales et al died of tumour at 13 and 24 months after diagnosis.

Ovarian leiomyosarcomas are aggressive neoplasms and have commonly spread beyond the ovary at the time of initial diagnosis. Thus, in Prat & Scully's 14 cases, the tumour was confined to the ovary in only two patients whilst in the remainder there was involvement of the omentum, peritoneum, diaphragm and, in one woman, the heart and adrenal glands. The treatment of choice is probably radical surgery though radiotherapy or chemotherapy may prolong survival in some instances. All the reported cases of ovarian leiomyosarcoma have led to death within two years with only one exception, this being

the case described by Raj-Kumar (1982) in which the patient was alive and well two years after surgical therapy: there was, however, some uncertainty as to whether this particular neoplasm had arisen in the ovary or in the broad ligament. Of the eight patients in Prat & Scully's series for whom follow-up information was available, five died from widespread metastases, two were alive but with metastases one and two years postoperatively whilst one was alive and well one year after surgery.

TUMOURS OF STRIATED MUSCLE

Rhabdomyoma

A single example of an ovarian rhabdomyoma has been reported (Iizuka et al, 1992).

Rhabdomyosarcoma

Fewer than 25 acceptable cases of pure primary ovarian rhabdomyosarcoma have been recorded (Vignard, 1889; Himwich, 1920; Barris & Shaw, 1928; La Manna, 1936; Rio, 1956; Payan, 1965; Dubey & Agrawal, 1967; Srinivasa Roa & Subuadra Devi, 1967; Spies & Lorenz, 1973; Guerard et al, 1983; Kanajet & Pirkic, 1988; Chan et al, 1989). Obeisance is usually paid to Virchow (cited by Sandison, 1955) as having first described an ovarian rhabdomyosarcoma in 1850, but his report was notably lacking in both clinical and pathological documentation, whilst a reappraisal of the frequently quoted case of Sandison (1955) shows clearly that this was a mixed Müllerian tumour.

Ovarian rhabdomyosarcomas are usually unilateral and range in size from relatively small lesions of 5 cm diameter to huge masses that extend up to the umbilicus: most are, however, more than 10 cm in diameter. They are smooth and lobulated and small villiform processes may project from their surfaces. The tumours are generally solid with a firm or rubbery texture but fleshy, soft or gelatinous areas may be focally present and are sometimes dominant; the cut surface is usually greyish-white or tan. Focal cystic change is common as are areas of haemorrhage and necrosis.

Histologically, ovarian rhabdomyosarcomas in children and young adults tend to show a mixed embryonal and alveolar pattern whilst those occurring in older individuals are more commonly of the pleomorphic type; all three morphological patterns can, however, be present in a single tumour. The embryonal rhabdomyosarcomas are formed largely of small, rounded or ovoid cells with hyperchromatic nuclei and scanty cytoplasm. Intermingled with these undifferentiated cells are larger cells with ample, strongly eosinophilic, granular cytoplasm and eccentric nuclei (Fig. 26.11). Better-differentiated rhabdomyoblasts with cross striations may also be present but the finding of such striations is not a strict diagnostic

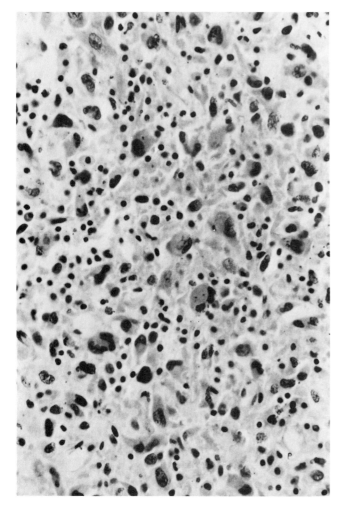

Fig. 26.11   An embryonal rhabdomyosarcoma of the ovary. Small, rounded cells are admixed with poorly-differentiated rhabdomyoblasts. H & E × 460.

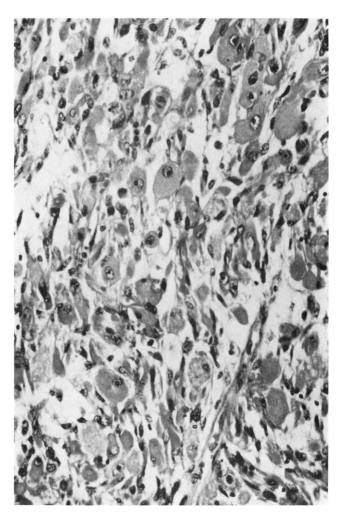

Fig. 26.12   A pleomorphic rhabdomyosarcoma of the ovary. H & E × 520.

prerequisite. The areas of typical embryonal rhabdomyo-sarcoma usually blend with alveolar areas in which the cellular elements are separated by fibrovascular septa to form alveolar lobules. The pleomorphic rhabdomyo-sarcoma is formed of spindle cells, rhabdomyoblasts in all stages of differentiation, multinucleated giant cells and racquet-shaped cells (Fig. 26.12). The diagnosis of a rhabdomyosarcoma is aided by electronmicroscopic de-tection of myofilaments and associated Z-band material, whilst immunohistological demonstration of myosin is also of great diagnostic value.

Ovarian rhabdomyosarcomas occur at any age, the youngest reported patient being 13 months and the oldest 86 years: in Prat & Scully's series of 14 ovarian rhabdo-myosarcomas the mean age was 35 years (unpublished observations). Patients usually complain of symptoms directly referable to a rapidly expanding pelvic mass but occasionally they present as an acute abdominal catastro-phe following rupture of the neoplasm: one patient, aged 16 years, presented with a leukaemia-like syndrome

(Nunez et al, 1981). The neoplasm is highly aggressive and has commonly extended beyond the ovary at the time of diagnosis: thus, in Prat & Scully's series of 14 cases, only four were confined to the ovary whilst the other 10 were either infiltrating the pelvic organs or had given rise to peritoneal implants. The prognosis is poor and all the reported patients have died within 15 months of initial diagnosis: all six patients for whom follow-up details were available in Prat & Scully's series died of tumour metastases between two and 14 months.

TUMOURS OF CARTILAGE

Chondroma

Most, probably all, ovarian chondromas which have been reported appear to have been either fibromas showing cartilaginous metaplasia or mature cystic teratomas with a prominent cartilaginous component. The lesion illus-trated in Figure 26.13 did, however, appear to be a true

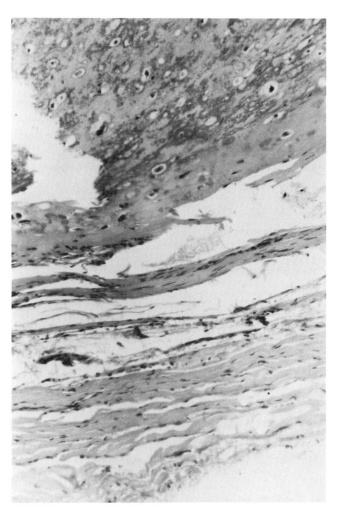

Fig. 26.13 An ovarian chondroma formed solely of mature cartilaginous tissue. H & E × 220.

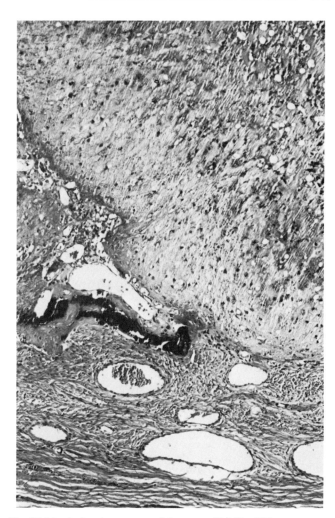

Fig. 26.14 A chondrosarcoma of the ovary. H & E × 320.

chondroma. The patient, an elderly women, presented with non-specific pelvic tumour symptoms, and an ovarian mass measuring 12 cm was removed. Histologically, this consisted solely of mature cartilaginous tissue with a thin compressed surrounding rim of ovarian cortex.

Chondrosarcoma (Fig. 26.14)

Nearly all reported ovarian chondrosarcomas have either arisen in a mature cystic teratoma or have been unusually conspicuous components of a malignant mixed Müllerian tumour. Talerman et al (1981) have, however, described an apparently pure, primary chondrosarcoma of the ovary which occurred in a 61-year-old woman who presented with a pelvic mass. The ovarian tumour was large, solid and firm; it consisted histologically of islands of cartilage containing chondrocytes in many stages of differentiation: cellular atypia and mitotic activity were manifest.

Following surgical removal the patient was alive and well four years later.

TUMOURS OF BONE

Osteoma

Occasional osteomas of the ovary have been described but all would more correctly be considered either as fibromas showing extensive osseous metaplasia or as examples of heterotopic bone formation in the ovarian stroma (Shipton & Meares, 1965).

Giant cell tumour (osteoclastoma)

Virtually all of the ovarian giant cell tumours reported in the literature have been associated with mucinous cystadenomas and would now be regarded as pseudosarcomatous mural nodules. An exception to this, however, is the neoplasm described by Lorentzen (1980). This was an asymptomatic mass in a 31-year-old woman which was discovered incidentally during investigation of infertility. The tumour was small, solid and yellow-brown: histologically, it had the characteristics of a giant cell tumour with mononuclear ovoid or spindle-shaped stromal cells interspersed with multinucleated giant cells, the latter containing up to 100 nuclei. Trabeculae of osteoid and bone were present and there was a sprinkling of mitotic figures. There was no evidence of any other tumour component and following surgery the patient was alive and well four and a half years later.

Osteogenic sarcoma

Four apparently pure primary osteogenic sarcomas of the ovary (Azoury & Woodruff, 1971; Hirakawa et al, 1988; Hines et al, 1990; Sakata et al, 1991) have been recorded. The first occurred in a 41-year-old woman, had the typical histological appearances of an osteogenic sarcoma as seen in the skeleton, contained no other tissues elements and led to the patient's death within five months. One, in a perimenopausal woman, was noted as a calcified adnexal mass on abdominal radiography: the patient was alive and well after eight courses of chemotherapy. Two other osteosarcomas, one of which had a telangiectatic pattern (Hirakawa et al, 1988), led to the death of the patients within a few months.

TUMOURS OF NEURAL ORIGIN

Neurofibroma

Only two ovarian tumours of this type have been fully documented (Smith, 1931; Hegg & Flint, 1990). The first was an incidental finding in a woman with von Recklinghausen's disease and its histological appearances were similar to neurofibromas occurring elsewhere in more conventional sites. The second, also in a patient with von Recklinghausen's syndrome, was symptomatic and simulated a malignant neoplasm.

Schwannoma

Three ovarian schwannomas have been described (Meyer, 1943; Mishura, 1963; De Franchis & Galliani, 1964). In each case the patient presented with non-specific symptoms suggestive of a pelvic mass. Histologically, the tumours showed the typical appearance of a schwannoma as seen elsewhere in the body and all the patients were alive and symptom-free after extirpation of the neoplasm.

Ganglioneuroma

A number of very small ovarian ganglioneuromas have been noted (Meyer, 1943), but these hilar clusters of ganglion cells are almost certainly hamartomatous in nature rather than neoplastic. One undoubtedly neoplastic ganglioneuroma was, however, found in a 4-year-old girl who presented with abdominal swelling (Schmeisser & Anderson, 1938); the tumour, which had almost totally replaced the ovary, was solid, weighed 200 g and was formed of well-differentiated ganglion cells.

Malignant schwannoma

Only one apparently non-teratomatous ovarian malignant schwannoma has been reported (Dover, 1950): this was in a 38-year-old woman with von Recklinghausen's disease who, whilst being treated for postabortal bleeding, was found to have a pelvic mass. The neoplasm was solid, had replaced the ovary and had the typical appearances of a malignant schwannoma with some degree of pleomorphism and mitotic activity; the patient was alive and well one year after treatment with surgery and radiotherapy.

Phaeochromocytoma

Small groups of paraganglion cells have been occasionally noted in the ovarian hilum but only one phaeochromocytoma of the ovary has been described (Fawcett & Kimbell, 1971). This was in a 15-year-old girl who presented with severe hypertension, fits and an abdominal mass. An ovarian tumour, which weighed 970 g and had undergone torsion, was removed from the left ovary: this had the typical histological appearances of a phaeochromocytoma and contained considerable quantities of adrenaline and noradrenaline. The patient was well and normotensive 15 months later.

MYXOMA

Twelve ovarian myxomas have been reported (Dutz & Stout, 1961; Masubuchi et al, 1970; Majmudar et al, 1978; Brady et al, 1987; Eichhorn & Scully, 1991; Tetu & Bonenfant, 1991; Costa et al, 1992). The patients ranged in age from 16–45 years and all presented with adnexal masses; the tumours were moderately large and partly solid and partly cystic with a gelatinous or mucinous texture. None had ruptured. Histologically, they were composed of scattered stellate or spindle-shaped cells set in a loose, abundant myxoid stroma (Fig. 26.15) which stained intensely positively with Alcian Blue due to the presence of hyaluronic acid. The tumours were richly vascularized by vessels of capillary size and contained a network of delicate reticulum fibres. The tumour cells are immunoreactive for vimentin and usually for actin, but not for desmin (Eichhorn & Scully, 1991; Costa et al, 1992). All the patients were treated by unilateral adnexectomy and none of seven tumours, with a follow-up period of 1–13 years (mean 5 years) recurred.

The histogenesis of ovarian myxoma is obscure but these neoplasms require extensive sampling to exclude other tissue components such as lipoblasts or muscle; the differential diagnosis must include massive oedema, myxoid change in a fibroma, myxoid liposarcoma (Fig. 26.16), myxoid leiomyosarcoma and sarcoma botryoides.

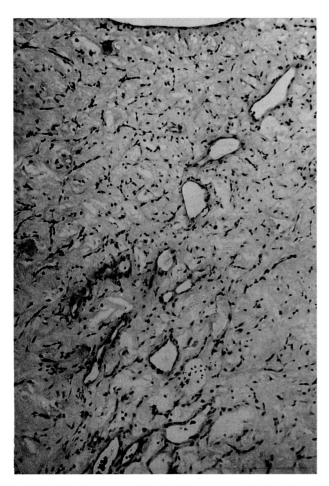

Fig. 26.15 Ovarian myxoma. Parvicellular tumour with abundant pale intercellular matrix that mimics the appearance of massive oedema of the ovary. H & E × 10 (Courtesy of Dr. Eichhorn, Boston, Ma.)

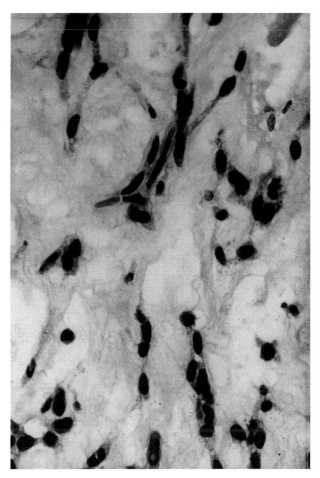

Fig. 26.16 Ovarian myxoma. Focus of capillary-sized blood vessels in a plexiform arrangement simulating myxoid liposarcoma. H & E × 100. (Courtesy of Dr. Eichhorn, Boston, Ma.)

TUMOURS OF FAT

Although a few ovarian lipomas have been described (Fahr, 1941) these seem to have been teratomas with a conspicuous adipose element, self-amputated epiploic appendages which have become adherent to the ovary or examples of the non-neoplastic accumulations of fat cells sometimes seen in the ovary and known variously as 'adipose prosoplasia' (Hart & Abell, 1970) or 'adipocytic infiltration' (Honore & O'Hara, 1980). The very occasional liposarcomas which have been reported all appear to have been ovarian metastases from extragonadal liposarcomas, though the neoplasm illustrated in Figure 26.17 was a primary ovarian neoplasm which was considered to be a pleomorphic liposarcoma.

TUMOURS OF VASCULAR ORIGIN

Haemangioma

Whether haemangiomas are hamartomas or true neoplasms is a moot point but the ovary has a complex and abundant vasculature and it is surprising that these lesions are so rare at this site, only about 40 examples having been reported (Baryluk et al, 1966; Gaal, 1967; Talerman, 1967; Gay & Janovski, 1969; Ebrahimi et al, 1971; Griffin, 1971; Caresano, 1977; Kela & Aurdra, 1980; Betta et al, 1988; Ganes et al, 1990; Pethe et al, 1991). Even this small number may, however, exaggerate the true incidence of ovarian haemangiomas, for the difficulties that may be encountered in distinguishing a small lesion of this type from dilated, congested hilar vessels do not always appear to have been taken into account and reports of small hilar haemangiomas must be regarded with some scepticism. It is difficult to define absolute criteria for the recognition of an ovarian haemangioma but it does seem reasonable to suggest that hilar lesions should only be so regarded if there is a visible and well-demarcated nodule; less strict requirements apply only to those lesions situated in the cortex.

The haemangiomas are usually unilateral, though occasional bilateral examples have been recorded (Payne, 1869; Shearer, 1935; Fundaro, 1969; Miyauchi et al, 1987). They usually have a smooth, glistening outer surface, are well demarcated from the surrounding ovarian

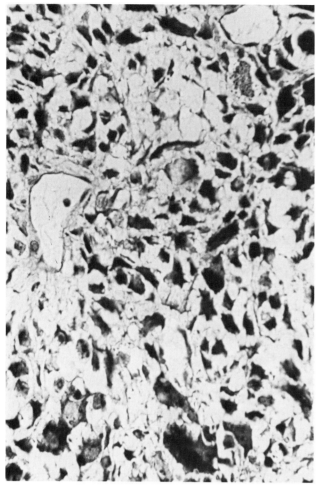

Fig. 26.17 A pleomorphic liposarcoma of the ovary. H & E × 480.

tissue and although generally small can attain a diameter of 12 cm. On section the haemangiomas tend to be of spongy texture and often have a honeycomb appearance; characteristically, they are red or purplish and not uncommonly focal calcification is noted. Nearly all ovarian haemangiomas show, histologically, a cavernous or a mixed cavernous-capillary pattern with large vascular spaces, lined by a single layer of regular endothelial cells, being separated from each other by a variable amount of fibrous tissue which is often hyalinized.

Ovarian haemangiomas have been noted in patients ranging from 4 months to 81 years in age (Rodriguez, 1979) and in approximately two-thirds of cases the tumour has been an asymptomatic incidental finding at surgery or autopsy. In the relatively few women with symptoms the principal complaints have been of abdominal pain, abdominal swelling or awareness of a mass. In these patients abdominal pain was due to torsion of a large haemangioma, this occurring chronically in one (Mann & Metrick, 1961) and acutely in two (Schaeffer & Cancelmo, 1939; Scheinman et al, 1982). Ascites has developed, and been the principal cause of symptoms, in three patients (Keller, 1927; Presno-Bastiony & Puente-

Duany, 1929; McBurney & Trumbull, 1955) whilst only in a few women have symptoms been due solely to the presence of an expanding ovarian mass unaccompanied by torsion or ascites. In one patient, bilateral ovarian haemangiomas were one component of a diffuse haemangioendotheliomatosis (Miyauchi et al, 1987). Simple oophorectomy is curative and it is followed by rapid regression of any ascites that may be present.

Haemangiopericytoma

The literature, particularly that before 1920, is replete with accounts of ovarian 'perithelioma'. These have usually been too inadequately described for their true nature to be apparent and it is probable that some were endometrioid stromal sarcomas of low-grade malignancy.

Angiosarcoma

Only a few ovarian angiosarcomas have been reported (Sovak & Carabba, 1931; Meylan, 1958; Pezullo, 1960; Patel et al, 1991; Fujii 1936). The angiosarcoma described by Ongkasuwan et al (1982) was associated with a mucinous cystadenoma and is discussed under the separate heading of 'Sarcomas associated with epithelial tumours'.

The tumours are usually unilateral and tend to be large, soft, friable and spongy; cystic change is common and can be extensive whilst foci of haemorrhage and necrosis are common. Histologically, these tumours are formed of proliferating vascular spaces of all degrees of development lined by endothelial cells showing atypia, pleomorphism and mitotic activity (Fig. 26.18). In some areas tumour cells may grow in solid cords whilst undifferentiated spindle cells may sometimes be present. In occasional cases the sarcomatous pattern predominates and any proliferating neoplastic vascular structures may be misinterpreted as being part of an inflammatory response to bleeding from the tumour.

Patients with ovarian angiosarcomas have ranged in age from 19–69 years and have presented solely with non-specific symptoms indicative of a pelvic mass; one striking feature of the clinical picture is a tendency for the tumour to rupture and cause severe intraperitoneal bleeding, this sometimes being a consequence of torsion of the tumour.

The prognosis for ovarian angiosarcomas with extra-ovarian spread is poor, but if the tumour is confined to the ovary at the time of operation the outlook appears to be reasonably good.

TUMOURS OF LYMPHATIC VESSELS

Lymphangioma

Lesions of this type, the neoplastic nature of which is debatable, occur with extreme rarity in the ovary, only

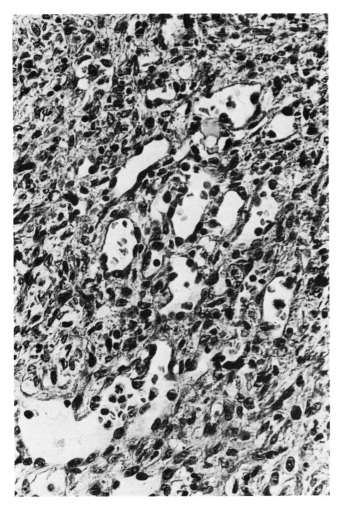

Fig. 26.18 An angiosarcoma of the ovary. H & E × 480.

a handful of cases having been described (Siddall & Clinton, 1937; Ferrari & de Angelis, 1953; Bieniasz & Sierant, 1961; Loubiere et al, 1968; Paliez et al, 1970; Khanna et al, 1979). They are usually unilateral with a smooth, grey outer surface and rarely attain a diameter of more than 6 cm; on section numerous tiny cystic spaces are seen from which clear straw-coloured fluid oozes out. They are formed of closely packed lymphatic vessels lined by a flattened layer of endothelial cells.

Lymphangiomas closely resemble an adenomatoid tumour from which, however, they can usually be distinguished by the absence of solid cords of cells between the vessels and by their lack of PAS- or Alcian Blue-positive material. Care also has to be taken not to confuse the sieve-like areas often found in mature cystic teratomas with a lymphangioma.

These tumours are usually asymptomatic incidental findings and are fully benign.

Lymphangiosarcoma

There has been only one report of an ovarian lymphangiosarcoma (Rice et al, 1943). This was a mass measuring 15 cm in diameter which was found in the ovary of a 31-year-old woman who gave a short history of abdominal enlargement. Histologically, the appearances were similar to those seen in a benign lymphangioma, but in a few areas the endothelial cells lining the lymphatic vessels showed focal proliferation with some degree of pleomorphism and nuclear hyperchromatism. The patient died within a year of widespread metastases.

ENDOMETRIOID STROMAL SARCOMA

Thirty-two cases of endometrioid stromal sarcoma of the ovary have been reported in detail (Benjamin & Campbell, 1960; Keller & Rygh, 1964; Palladino & Trousdell, 1969; Gruskin et al, 1970; Azoury & Woodruff, 1971; Silverberg & Nogales, 1981; Young et al, 1984). The neoplasms may derive from foci of ovarian endometriosis (concomitant endometriosis being present in 19 of the 32 reported cases), from foci of gland-free endometrial stroma in the ovary (ovarian stromatosis — Hughesdon, 1972, 1976) or, possibly, may arise directly from the ovarian stromal cells following metaplasia into endometrial stromal-type cells.

The tumours commonly measure less than 15 cm in diameter and were bilateral in 11 of the 23 cases described by Young et al (1984). They are predominantly solid, though foci of cystic change are present in over half; on section they usually have a homogeneous appearance, with foci of necrosis or haemorrhage being relatively uncommon. Histologically, the ovarian tumours, like their more common uterine counterparts, are composed of sheets of uniform cells resembling the stromal cells of normal proliferative endometrium (Fig. 26.19). Fibromatous areas are, however, also frequently present, this not being a feature of uterine neoplasms of this type. An important diagnostic feature is the presence of a prominent network of small arterioles, these closely resembling the spiral vessels seen in normal late secretory endometrium: this network is most clearly seen in reticulin-stained sections (Fig. 26.20). The focal intravascular growth characteristic of uterine endometrial sarcomas of low-grade malignancy is not seen within the ovarian tumours but is typically present when the neoplasm extends beyond the confines of the ovary (Fig. 26.21). The tumour cells may contain abundant intracellular lipid and, although usually growing in uniform sheets, can, like similar uterine tumours, show an epithelial or sex cord tumour-like pattern in some areas.

The nature of the cells in an endometrioid stromal sarcoma and the presence of a rich vascular network allow for the differentiation of these neoplasms from other types of ovarian sarcoma. A Müllerian adenosarcoma may, however, be mimicked if endometriotic glands are trapped within the tumour: in such circumstances the focal presence of the glands, as opposed to their uniform distribution throughout an adenosarcoma, together with the

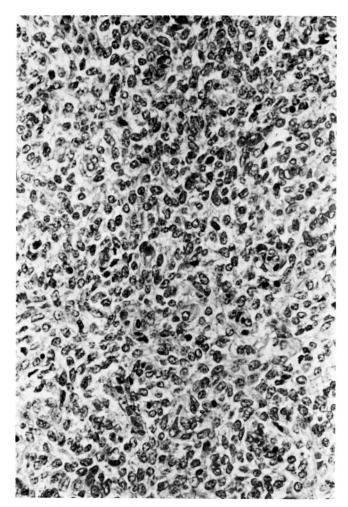

Fig. 26.19   An endometrioid stromal sarcoma of the ovary. This is composed of sheets of cells which resemble the stromal cells of normal proliferative endometrium. H & E × 360.

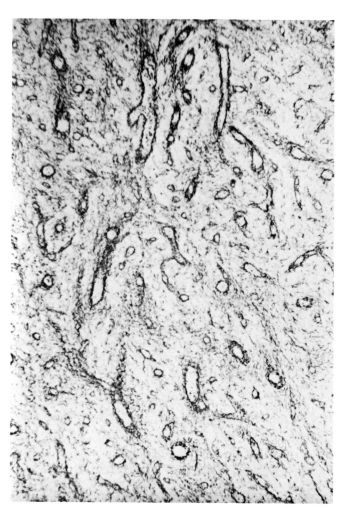

Fig. 26.20   Endometrioid stromal sarcoma of the ovary. A reticulin stain demonstrates the rich vascular network. H & E × 360.

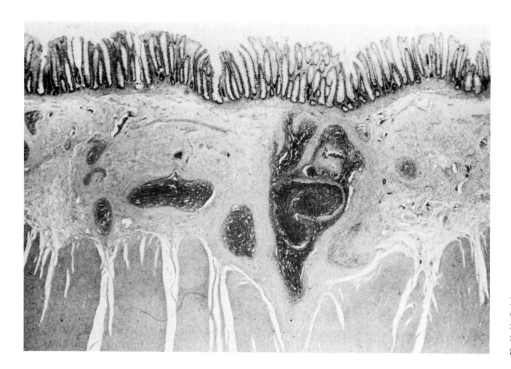

Fig. 26.21   Metastasis of ovarian endometrioid stromal sarcoma to the intestine. Metastatic deposits of this neoplasm typically show intravascular growth. H & E × 180.

absence of any stromal condensation around the glands (cambium layer), usually indicates the correct diagnosis. If a sex cord-like pattern is a prominent feature of an endometrioid stromal sarcoma this may lead to confusion with a granulosa cell tumour: the epithelial-like cells do not, however, have the nuclear features of granulosa cells.

The patients with endometrioid stromal sarcomas in the series of Young et al (1984) ranged in age from 20–76 years with a mean age at initial diagnosis of 54 years; the presenting symptoms are of a non-specific nature and are entirely related to the presence of a pelvic mass. In the series of Young et al (1984) the tumour was, at the time of operation, confined to the ovary in only four patients: in nine cases the tumour involved other pelvic structures, whilst eight tumours had spread into the abdomen and had metastasized to the lungs.

The behaviour of ovarian endometrioid stromal sarcomas is analogous to that of their uterine counterparts with the degree of mitotic activity being of major prognostic significance. Tumours with fewer than 10 mitotic figures per 10 high power fields are associated with a good prognosis, even if there is extrauterine spread: thus in Young et al's (1984) series only two of 19 patients whose neoplasms contained less than 10 mitotic figures per 10 high power fields died of their disease and nine patients with spread beyond the ovary at the time of presentation were alive one or more years postoperatively. The prognosis for those tumours containing more than 10 mitotic figures per 10 high power fields is comparable to that of other ovarian sarcomas, and three of the four women in Young et al's (1984) series with tumours showing this degree of mitotic activity were dead within four years.

It should be noted that ovarian endometrioid stromal sarcomas may be associated with a prior, synchronous or subsequent uterine endometrial stromal sarcoma, this being the case in nine of the 23 patients reported by Young et al (1984). In at least two of these cases, in which the uterine lesions preceded the ovarian neoplasm by many years, there was strong circumstantial evidence to suggest independent primary tumours of each organ. In synchronous cases it is, of course, usually impossible to exclude metastasis from one organ to the other, especially if other pelvic structures are involved. Hence, from a practical point of view, it is of value to review any prior hysterectomy specimen in a patient with an ovarian endometrioid stromal sarcoma; it is also important to recognize that if the uterus is not removed at the time of operation for an ovarian endometrioid stromal sarcoma it is possible that a uterine stromal sarcoma may have been left behind or will subsequently develop.

The primary therapeutic approach to ovarian endometrioid stromal sarcoma is surgical. If the patient is menopausal or postmenopausal, hysterectomy with bilateral salpingo-oophorectomy is the treatment of choice and, because of the high frequency of bilateral ovarian involvement and the possibility of synchronous or sub-sequent uterine endometrial stromal sarcoma, a similar approach may be optimal even for younger women. Both progesterone and radiotherapy have been used for residual or recurrent disease, but in assessing value of such therapy it has to be remembered that those tumours of low-grade malignancy (less than 10 mitotic figures per 10 high power fields) typically run a very indolent course and that patients with untreated residual disease may remain free of signs or symptoms for many years: indeed, in some cases the extraovarian lesions appear to regress spontaneously.

UNDIFFERENTIATED 'STROMAL' SARCOMA

This term has been applied to those ovarian sarcomas which appear to arise from the ovarian stromal mesenchyme but which do not show any specific differentiation (Azoury & Woodruff, 1971). How common such tumours are is a moot point: the literature is replete with reports of 'spindle cell' or 'round cell' sarcomas, most of which have clearly been examples of leiomyosarcoma, malignant lymphoma, granulosa cell tumour or endometrioid stromal sarcoma. Some quite convincing reports have appeared, however, of sarcomas which seemed to have originated in the stroma and have shown no obvious differentiation along either leiomyosarcomatous or fibrosarcomatous lines (Foda et al, 1958; Variati & Donatelli, 1966; Azoury & Woodruff, 1971) and Prat & Scully have reviewed a series of six such tumours (unpublished observations).

Azoury & Woodruff (1971) thought that these neoplasms had a predilection for relatively young girls, for five of their seven tumours occurred in patients aged less than 20 years. This was not the case, however, in Prat & Scully's series, in which age range was from 35–65 years. The tumours are generally large, measuring up to 20 cm in diameter, and may be firm, fleshy, soft or friable; histologically, they are formed of ovoid or elongated cells which have relatively large vesicular nuclei and show varying degrees of pleomorphism and mitotic activity (Fig. 26.22): there is often an admixture of multinucleated giant cells.

In Azoury & Woodruff's (1971) series four patients whose tumours were thought to be of only low-grade malignancy were alive and well at periods ranging from six to 14 years after removal of the tumour, whilst two patients with neoplasms showing considerable pleomorphism and abundant mitotic activity were dead within two years. A rather more gloomy outlook prevailed in Prat & Scully's series, for all of the five patients for whom follow-up information was available were dead from metastatic disease within two and a half years of initial diagnosis.

COMBINED SARCOMA AND EPITHELIAL TUMOUR

There have been occasional reports of ovarian sarcomas occurring in combination with an epithelial neoplasm.

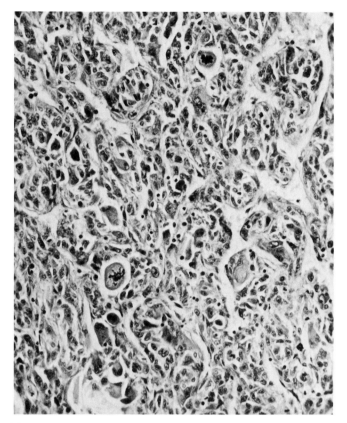

Fig. 26.22   An undifferentiated 'stromal' sarcoma of the ovary. H & E × 180.

Thus Prat & Scully (1979) described two sarcomas, each of which presented as a distinct solitary nodule in the wall of an ovarian mucinous cystic tumour: one was a fibrosarcoma in the wall of a mucinous cystadenoma and the other was an undifferentiated sarcoma in conjunction with a mucinous cystadenocarcinoma. A second example of fibrosarcoma arising as a well-circumscribed 9 cm nodule in the wall of a mucinous cystadenoma has been described by de Nictolis et al (1990). The tumour, though well-differentiated, was adherent to the omentum and contained four mitoses per 10 high power fields. The patient received radiotherapy, but she died with clinical evidence of peritoneal and hepatic metastases 18 months post-

operatively. The findings in this case support the validity of the two diagnostic criteria proposed to separate cellular fibromas from fibrosarcomas, namely, the finding of four or more mitoses per 10 high power fields and the extension of the tumour beyond the ovary (Prat & Scully, 1979). Ongkasuwan et al (1982) reported an angiosarcoma associated with a mucinous cystadenoma whilst there have been two recorded examples of leiomyosarcomas co-existing with serous tumours, one a serous cystadenoma (von Numers & Mikkonen, 1960) and the other a serous adenocarcinoma (Walts & Lichtenstein, 1977). A single case of rhabdomyosarcoma associated with a mucinous cystic tumour of the ovary has been reported (Tsujimura & Kawano, 1992). The sarcoma, a solid mass 15 cm in greatest diameter, contained pleomorphic rhabdomyoblasts with occasional cross striations. The exact nature of these apparently combined tumours is debatable: they are probably collision tumours but the possibility of malignant change in the stroma of an epithelial neoplasm can not be totally discounted.

ADENOMATOID TUMOURS

Adenomatoid tumours are virtually confined to the genital tract but the ovary is one of the least common sites for such a neoplasm to occur (Masson et al, 1942; Lee et al, 1950; Teel, 1958; Serrapiao & Serrapiao, 1964; Jones & Donova, 1965; Ferenczy et al, 1972; Boczkowski et al, 1977). Ovarian tumours of this type are nearly always small and asymptomatic incidental findings. They are usually seen as unilateral, well-delineated but non-encapsulated, firm grey-white nodules which on section are honeycombed by numerous small cystic spaces. Histologically, the tumour is formed of cystic or gland-like spaces lined by flattened or cuboidal cells having abundant vacuolated eosinophilic cytoplasm and ovoid nuclei. Cords of similar cells are also usually present and these may contain slit-like clefts. The epithelial structures are set in a variable amount of connective tissue stroma which is often hyalinized and may contain smooth muscle fibres. Alcian Blue-positive material is usually present but PAS-positive material is often absent.

REFERENCES

Amin H K, Okagaki T, Richart R M 1971 Classification of fibroma and thecoma of the ovary: an ultrastructural study. Cancer 27: 438–446.
Azoury R S, Woodruff J D 1971 Primary ovarian sarcomas: report of 43 cases from the Emil Novak ovarian tumour registry. Obstetrics and Gynecology 37: 920–941.
Balaton A, Vaury P, Imbert M C, Mussy M A 1987 Primary leiomyosarcoma of the ovary: a histological and immunocytochemical study. Gynecologic Oncology 28: 116–120.
Balazs M, Lazlo J 1965 Das Leiomyosarkome des Ovar. Zentralblatt fur Gynakologie 87: 633–638.
Barris J, Shaw W 1928 Rhabdomyosarcoma of the ovary. Proceedings of the Royal Society of Medicine 22: 320–322.

Baryluk V L, Lui H, Horn R C 1966 Hemangioma of the ovary. Henry Ford Hospital Medical Bulletin 14: 167–172.
Benjamin F, Campbell J A H 1960 Stromal "endometriosis" with possible ovarian origin. American Journal of Obstetrics and Gynecology 80: 449–453.
Betta P G, Robutti F, Spinoglio G 1988 Hemangioma of the ovary. European Journal of Gynaecological Oncology 9: 184–185.
Bettendorf U, Zimmermann H 1975 Leiomyosarkoma de Ovarium. Medizinische Welt 26: 429–430.
Bieniasz A, Sierant A 1961 A case of lymphangioma cavernosum of the ovary. Ginekologica Polska 32: 667–669.
Biggart J H, Macafee C H G 1955 Tumours of the ovarian

mesenchyme: a clinicopathological study. Journal of Obstetrics and Gynaecology of the British Empire 62: 829–837.

Boczkowski Z, Czuczwar S, Pakula H, Sikorska-Haliniare W 1977 Benign adenomatoid tumour of the ovary. Ginekologica Polska 48: 913–915.

Bower J F, Erikson E R 1967 Bilateral ovarian fibroma in a 5 year old. American Journal of Obstetrics and Gynecology 99: 880–882.

Brady K, Page D V, Benn L E, de las Morenas A, O'Brien M 1987 Ovarian myxoma. American Journal of Obstetrics and Gynecology 156: 1240–1242.

Burket R L, Rauh J L 1976 Gorlin's syndrome: ovarian fibromas at adolescence. Obstetrics and Gynecology 47: 43s–46s.

Caresano G 1977 L'emangioma cavernosa dell'ovaio: presentazione di un caso e rassegna della bibiliografia. Minerva Ginecologica 29: 103–106.

Chan Y F, Leung C S, Ma L 1989 Primary embryonal rhabdomyosarcoma of the ovary in a 4-year-old girl. Histopathology 15: 309–311.

Charache H 1959 Ovarian tumours in childhood: report of six new cases and review of the literature. Archives of Surgery 79: 573–580.

Christman J E, Ballon S C 1990 Ovarian fibrosarcoma associated with Mafucci's syndrome. Gynecologic Oncology 37: 290–291.

Cortes J, Cuartero M L, Rossello J J et al 1987 Ovarian pure leiomyosarcoma: case report. European Journal of Gynaecological Oncology 8: 19–22.

Costa M J, Thomas W, Majudar B, Hewan-Lowe K 1992 Ovarian myxoma: ultrastructural and immunohistochemical findings. Ultrastructural Pathology 16: 429–438.

De Franchis M, Galliani A 1964 Neurinoma dell ovaio. Rivista di Pathologia e Clinica 19: 567–574.

De Nictolis M, di Loreto C, Clinti S, Prat J 1990 Fibrosarcomatous mural nodule in an ovarian mucinous cystadenoma. Surgical Pathology 3: 309–315.

Destro F 1958 Contributo allo studio de fibroma ovarico in metropatia emorragica. Archivio Italiano di Pathologia 2: 329–344.

Dockerty M B, Masson J V 1944 Ovarian fibromas: a clinical and pathologic study of two hundred and eighty three cases. American Journal of Obstetrics and Gynecology 47: 741–752.

Dodd G D, Lancaster K T, Moulton J S 1989 Ovarian lipoleiomyoma: a fat-containing mass in the female pelvis. American Journal of Roentgenology 153: 1007–1008.

Dover H 1950 Malignant schwannoma of the ovary, associated with neurofibromatosis. Canadian Medical Association Journal 63: 488–490.

Driscoll J A 1964 Ovarian fibroma. Journal of the Irish Medical Association 53: 184–187.

Dubey M M, Agrawal S 1967 Rhabdomyosarcoma of ovary: a case report. Journal of Obstetrics and Gynaecology of India 17: 724–725.

Duchini L, Menegaldo R 1967 I fibroma dell'ovaio. Archivio de Vecchi per l'anatomia Patologica e la Medicina Clinica 48: 973–997.

Dutz W, Stout A P 1961 The myxoma in childhood. Cancer 14: 629–635.

Ebrahimi T, Goldsmitth J W, Okagaki J 1971 Hemangioma of the ovary: a case report. Obstetrics and Gynecology 38: 477–479.

Eichhorn J H, Scully R E 1991 Ovarian myxoma: clinicopathologic and immunocytologic analysis of five cases and a review of the literature. International Journal of Gynecological Pathology 10: 156–169.

Fahr E 1941 Eigenartige Fetgeschwulst des Ovariums. Zentralblatt fur allgemeine Pathologie and fur pathologischen Anatomie 77: 264–266.

Fallahzadeh H, Dockerty M B, Lee R A 1972 Leiomyoma of the ovary: report of five cases and review of the literature. American Journal of Obstetrics and Gynecology 113: 394–398.

Fawcett F J, Kimbell N K B 1971 Phaeochromocytoma of the ovary. Journal of Obstetrics and Gynaecology of the British Commonwealth 78: 456–459.

Ferenczy A, Fenoglio J, Richart R M 1972 Observations of benign mesothelioma of the genital tract (adenomatoid tumour): a comparative ultrastructural study. Cancer 30: 244–260.

Ferrari W, de Angelis V 1953 Linfangioma do ovario. Revista Brasileira of Cirugia 25: 329–334.

Foda M S, Shafeek M A, Hashem M 1958 Sarcoma of the ovary. Gazette of the Egyptian Society of Obstetrics and Gynecology 7: 15–37.

Friedman H D, Mazur M T 1991 Primary ovarian leiomyosarcoma: an immunohistochemical and ultrastructural study. Archives of Pathology and Laboratory Medicine 115: 941–945.

Fujii A 1936 An instance of hemangioendothelioma intravasculare of ovary, which ruptured by the pedicle torsion. Japanese Journal of Obstetrics and Gynaecology 19: 481–484.

Fundaro P 1969 Emangiomi cavernoso bilaterale dell ovaio: presentazione di un caso e rassegna della letteratura. Folia Hereditaria et Patologica 18: 45–49.

Gaal M 1967 Die Hamangiome der weiblichen Geschlectsorgane. Gynaecologia 164: 307–315.

Gay R M, Janovski N A 1969 Cavernous hemangioma of the ovary. Gynaecologia 168: 248–257.

Glendenning W E, Herdt J E, Black T B 1963 Ovarian fibromas and mesenteric cysts: their association with hereditary basal cell cancer of the skin. American Journal of Obstetrics and Gynecology 87: 1008–1012.

Gorlin R D, Sedano H O 1971 The multiple nevoid basal cell carcinoma syndrome. Birth Defects 7: 140–148.

Griffin N B 1971 Hemangiomas of the female genital tract. Southern Medical Journal 64: 104–117.

Grosieux P 1970 Les fibromes de l'ovaire. Revue Francaise de Gynecologie 65: 95–100.

Gruskin P, Osborne N G, Morley G W, Abell M R 1970 Primary endometrial stromatosis of ovary: report of a case. Obstetrics and Gynecology 36: 702–707.

Guerard M J, Arguelles M A, Ferenczy A 1983 Rhabdomyosarcoma of the ovary: ultrastructural study of a case and review of the literature. Gynecologic Oncology 15: 325–339.

Gunes H A, Egilmez R, Dulger M 1990 Ovarian haemangioma. British Journal of Clinical Practice 44: 734–735.

Hart W R, Abell M R 1970 Adipose prosoplasia of ovary. American Journal of Obstetrics and Gynecology 106: 929–931.

Hegg C A, Flint A 1990 Neurofibroma of the ovary. Gynecologic Oncology 37: 437–438.

Himwich H E 1920 Rhabdomyoma of the ovary. Journal of Cancer Research 5: 227–241.

Hines J F, Compton D M, Stacy C G, Potter M E 1990 Pure primary osteosarcoma of the ovary presenting as an extensively calcified adnexal mass: a case report and review of the literature. Gynecologic Oncology 39: 258–263.

Hirakawa T, Tsuneyoshi M, Enjoji M, Shigyo R 1988 Ovarian sarcoma with features of telangiectatic osteosarcoma of the bone. American Journal of Surgical Pathology 12: 567–572.

Honore L H, O'Hara K E 1980 Subcapsular adipocytic infiltration of the human ovary: a clinicopathological study of eight cases. European Journal of Obstetrics, Gynecology and Reproductive Biology 10: 13–20.

Hughesdon P E 1972 The origin and development of benign stromatosis of the ovary. Journal of Obstetrics and Gynaecology of the British Commonwealth 79: 348–359.

Hughesdon P E 1976 The endometrial identity of benign stromatosis of the ovary and its relation to other forms of endometriosis. Journal of Pathology 119: 201–209.

Iizuka S, Nagata J, Fukuo S, Kosaka J 1992 A case of rhabdomyoma arising from the ovary. Nippon Sanka Fujinka Gakkai Zasshi 44: 1197–2000.

Jones E G, Donova A J 1965 Adenomatoid tumor of the ovary versus mesothelial reaction. American Journal of Obstetrics and Gynecology 92: 694–698.

Kalra V B, Kalra R, Sareen P M, Lodra S K, Utreja R K 1981 Leiomyoma of ovary: case report with brief review. Journal of Obstetrics and Gynaecology of India 31: 1037–1038.

Kanajet O, Pirkic A 1988 Rhabdomiosarkom ovarija s kasnijim ispadima centrainog nervnog sistema. Jugoslavenska Ginekologija Perinatologisa (Zagreb) 28: 44–47.

Kandalaft P L, Esteban J L 1992 Bilateral massive ovarian leiomyomata in a young woman: a case report with review of the literature. Modern Pathology 5: 586–589.

Karogozov A, Chakalova G, Ganchev G 1990 Riaduk sluchai na

gigantski ovarialen leiomiosarkom. Akush Erstvo Ginekologiia (Sofia) 29: 70–72.

Kela K, Aurdra A L 1980 Haemangioma of the ovary. Journal of the Indian Medical Association 75: 201–202.

Keller O, Rygh O 1964 A case of stromal endometriosis originating from ovarian endometriosis. Acta Obstetricia et Gynecologica Scandinavica 39: 178–183.

Keller R 1927 L'hemangioma de l'ovaire. Gynecologie et Obstetrique 16: 405–407.

Khanna S, Mehrota M L, Basumallik M 1979 Lymphangioma cavernosum of the ovary. International Surgery 63: 104–105.

Kleitsman R J 1949a Ein Beitrag zur Kenntnis der Leiomyomes des Ovariums. Acta Obstetricia et Gynecologica Scandinavica 29: 161–174.

Kleitsman R J 1949b Zur Kasuistik der Eierstocksfibroma. Acta Obstetricia et Gynecologica Scandinavica 29: 234–245.

Kraemer B B, Silva E G, Sneige N 1984 Fibrosarcoma of ovary: a new component in the nevoid basal-cell carcinoma syndrome. American Journal of Surgical Pathology 8: 231–236.

La Manna D 1936 Ueber Myoblastome. Virchows Archiv A Pathological Anatomy and Histology 294: 663–691.

Lee M J, Dockerty M B, Thompson G J, Waugh J M 1950 Benign mesotheliomas (adenomatoid tumors) of the genital tract. Surgery, Gynecology and Obstetrics 91: 221–231.

Lorentzen M 1980 Giant cell tumour of the ovary. Virchows Archiv A Pathological Anatomy and Histology 388: 113–122.

Loubiere R, Ette M, Boury-Heyler G, Sangaret M, Chesney Y, Reynaud R 1968 Sur deux cas de tumeurs lymphangiomateuses de l'ovaire. Annales d'Anatomie Pathologique 16: 133–177.

Lyday R O 1952 Fibroma of the ovary with abdominal implants. American Journal of Surgery 84: 737–738.

McBurney R C, Trumbull M 1955 Hemangioma of the ovary with ascites. Mississippi Doctor 32: 271–274.

Majmudar B, Kapernick P S, Phillips R S 1978 Ovarian myxoma. Human Pathology 9: 723–725.

Mani M, Okamury H, Takenaka A et al 1975 A light and electron microscopic study of ovarian leiomyosarcoma. Acta Obstetrica et Gynecologica Japonica 30: 671–677.

Mann L S, Metrick S 1961 Hemangioma of the ovary: report of a case. Journal of International College of Surgeons 36: 500–502.

Martins S M, Klinger O J 1964 Bilateral ovarian fibromas before the menopause. American Journal of Obstetrics and Gynecology 87: 381–390.

Masson P, Riopelle J L, Simard L C 1942 Le mesotheliome benin de la sphere genital. Revue Canadienne de Biologie 1: 720–751.

Masubuchi K, Kumura M, Suzumura H 1970 Case of ovarian myxoma. Japanese Journal of Cancer Clinics 16: 156–159.

Matamala M F, Nogales F F, Aneiros J, Herraiz M A, Caracuel M D 1988 Leiomyomas of the ovary. International Journal of Gynecological Pathology 7: 190–196.

Mazella G 1963 Sul fibroma del ovaio. Rassegna Internazionale di Clinica e Terapia 43: 28–38.

Meyer R 1943 Nerve tumors of the female genitals and pelvis. Archives of Pathology 36: 437–464.

Meylan J 1958 Hemangio-endotheliome de l'ovaire (a propos des tumeurs ovariennes d'origine vasculaire). Annales d'Anatomie Pathologique 3: 558–594.

Michael C A 1966 Pelvic fibroma causing recurrent attacks of hypoglycemia in a post-menopausal patient. Proceedings of the Royal Society of Medicine 59: 835.

Mira J L 1991 Lipoleiomyoma of the ovary: report of a case and review of the English literature. International Journal of Gynecological Pathology 10: 198–202.

Mishura V I 1963 Report of large benign tumour: three cases. Voprosy Onkologii 9: 102–106.

Miyauchi J, Mukai M, Yamazaki K et al 1987 Bilateral ovarian hemangiomas associated with diffuse hemangioendotheliomatosis: a case report. Acta Pathologica Japonica 37: 1347–1355.

Monk B J, Nieberg R, Berek J S 1993 Primary leiomyosarcoma of the ovary in a perimenarchal female. Gynecologic Oncology 48: 389–393.

Moore J H 1945 Leiomyoma of the ovary complicating pregnancy. American Journal of Obstetrics and Gynecology 50: 244.

Nieminen U von, Numers C, Parola E 1969 Primary sarcoma of the ovary. Acta Obstetricia et Gynecologica Scandinavica 48: 423–432.

Nogales F F, Ayala A, Ruiz-Avila I, Sirvent J J 1991 Myxoid leiomyosarcoma of the ovary: analysis of three cases. Human Pathology 22: 1268–1273.

Nunez G, Abboud S L, Lemon N C, Kemp J A 1981 Ovarian rhabdomyosarcoma presenting as leukemia: case report. Cancer 52: 297–300.

Okamura H, Virutamasen P, Wright K H, Wallach E E 1972 Ovarian smooth muscle in the human being, rabbit and cat: histochemical and electron microscopic study. American Journal of Obstetrics and Gynecology 112: 183–191.

Ongkasuwan C, Taylor J E, Tang C K, Prempree T 1982 Angiosarcomas of the uterus and ovary: clinicopathologic report. Cancer 49: 1469–1475.

Paliez R, Delecour M, Duponi A, Monnier J C, Begueri F, Houcke M 1970 Lymphangiome ovarien: a propos d'une observation. Bulletin de la Federation des Societes de Gynecologie et d'Obstetrique de Langue Francaise 22: 51–53.

Palladino V S, Trousdell M 1969 Extra-uterine Mullerian tumors: a review of the literature and the report of a case. Cancer 23: 1413–1422.

Patel T, Ohri S K, Sundaresan M et al 1991 Metastatic angiosarcoma of the ovary. European Journal of Gynaecological Oncology 17: 295–299.

Payan H 1965 Rhabdomyosarcoma of the ovary. Obstetrics and Gynecology 26: 393–395.

Payne J F 1869 Vascular tumours of the liver, suprarenal capsule and other organs. Transactions of the Pathological Society of London 20: 203–205.

Pethe V V, Chitale S V, Godbole R N, Bidaye S V 1991 Haemangioma of the ovary: case report and review of literature. Indian Journal of Pathology and Microbiology 34: 290–292.

Pezullo G 1960 Endothelioma ovarico. Rassegna Internazionale di Clinica e Terapia 40: 481–488.

Prat J, Scully R E 1979 Sarcomas in ovarian mucinous tumors: a report of two cases. Cancer 44: 1327–1331.

Prat J, Scully R E 1981 Cellular fibromas and fibrosarcoma of the ovary: a comparative clinicopathologic analysis of seventeen cases. Cancer 47: 2663–2670.

Prayson R A, Hart W R 1992 Primary smooth-muscle tumors of the ovary: a clinicopathologic study of four leiomyomas and two mitotically active leiomyomas. Archives of Pathology and Laboratory Medicine 116: 1068–1071.

Presno-Bastiony J A, Puente-Duany S 1929 Consideraciones sobre un caso de hemangioma del ovario. Revista de Medicina v Cirugia Habana 34: 165–173.

Raggio M, Kaplan A L, Harberg J F 1983 Recurrent ovarian fibromas with basal cell nevus syndrome (Gorlin syndrome). Obstetrics and Gynecology 60: 955–965.

Raj-Kumar G 1982 Leiomyosarcoma of probable ovarian or broad ligament origin. British Journal of Obstetrics and Gynaecology 89: 327–329.

Rice M, Pearson B, Treadwell W B 1943 Malignant lymphangioma of the ovary. American Journal of Obstetrics and Gynecology 45: 884–889.

Rio F 1956 Contributo allo studio di rare neoplasie ovariche (rhabdomyosarcoma). Rivista Italiana di Ginecologia 39: 218–228.

Rodriguez M A 1979 Hemangioma of the ovary in an 81-year-old woman. Southern Medical Journal 72: 503–504.

Sakata H, Hirahara T, Ryu A et al 1991 Primary osteosarcoma of the ovary: a case report. Acta Pathologica Japonica 41: 311–317.

Sandison A T 1955 Rhabdomyosarcoma of the ovary. Journal of Pathology and Bacteriology 70: 433–438.

Schaeffer M H, Cancelmo J J 1939 Cavernous hemangioma of ovary in a girl twelve years of age. American Journal of Obstetrics and Gynecology 38: 723–772.

Scheinman H Z, McKenna A J, Rutner N 1982 Ovarian hemangioma with acute abdominal pain. Mount Sinai Journal of Medicine 49: 133–135.

Schmeisser H C, Anderson W A D 1938 Ganglioneuroma of the ovary. Journal of the American Medical Association 111: 2005–2007.

Scully R E 1979 Tumors of the ovary and abnormal gonads. Atlas of tumour pathology, second series, fascicle 16. Armed Forces Institute of Pathology, Washington, DC.

Sengupta S, Daita P, Pal A 1979 Ovarian fibroma with massive calcification. Journal of the Indian Medical Association 72: 64–65.

Serrapiao C J, Serrapiao M J 1964 "Tumour adenomatoid" de ovario. Hospital (Rio) 66: 177–182.

Shearer J P 1935 Hemangioma of the ovary: reported in a child 3½ years of age. Medical Annals of the District of Columbia 4: 223–224.

Shipton E A, Meares S D 1965 Heterotopic bone formation in the ovary. Australian and New Zealand Journal of Obstetrics and Gynaecology 5: 100–102.

Siddall R S, Clinton W R 1937 Lymphangioma of the ovary. American Journal of Obstetrics and Gynecology 34: 306–310.

Silverberg S G, Nogales F 1981 Endolymphatic stromal myosis of the ovary: a report of three cases and literature review. Gynecologic Oncology 12: 129–138.

Smith F R 1931 Neurofibroma of the ovary associated with Recklinghausen's disease. American Journal of Cancer 15: 859–862.

Sovak F W, Carabba V 1931 Hemangioendothelioma intravasculare of the ovary. American Journal of Obstetrics and Gynecology 21: 544–550.

Spies H, Lorenz G 1973 Rhabdomyosarkom bei Ovars in Kindesalter. Zentralblatt fur Gynekologie 95: 1322–1325.

Srinivasa Rao K, Subuadra Devi N 1967 Rhabdomyosarcoma of ovary. Journal of Obstetrics and Gynaecology of India 17: 93–95.

Talerman A 1967 Hemangiomas of the ovary and the uterine cervix. Obstetrics and Gynecology 30: 108–113.

Talerman A, Ayerbach W M, van Meurs A J 1981 Primary chondrosarcoma of the ovary. Histopathology 5: 319–324.

Teel P 1958 Adenomatoid tumor of the genital tract with special reference to the female. American Journal of Obstetrics and Gynecology 75: 1347–1355.

Tetu B, Bonenfant J L 1991 Ovarian myxoma: a study of two cases with long-term follow-up. American Journal of Clinical Pathology 95: 340–346.

Thay T Y, Orizaga M, Campbell J S, de Saint Victor H 1973 Leiomyoma of ovary. European Journal of Obstetrics, Gynecology and Reproductive Biology 3: 51–55.

Toth F, Csomor S, Zambo A 1971 Primares Ovarialfibrosarkome bei einer 71 jahrigen Patientin. Strahlentherapie 141: 44–46.

Tsalacopoulos G, Tiltman A T 1981 Leiomyoma of the ovary: a report of 3 cases. South African Medical Journal 59: 574–575.

Tsujimura T, Kawano K 1992 Rhabdomyosarcoma coexistent with ovarian mucinous cystadenocarcinoma: a case report. International Journal of Gynecological Pathology 11: 58–62.

Variati G, Donatelli G F 1966 Il sarcoma dell ovaio (contributo casistico anatomo-clinico) Annali di Obstetricia e Ginecologia 88: 440–453.

Vierhout H E, Pijpers L, Tham M N, Chadha-Ajwani S 1990 Leiomyoma of the ovary. Acta Obstetricia et Gynecologica Scandinavica 69: 445–447.

Vignard E 1889 Tumeur solide de l'ovaire a fibres striees chez une jeune fille de 17 ans. Bulletin de Societe d'Anatomie 64: 33–36.

von Numers C, Mikkonen R 1960 Leiomyosarcoma arising in serous cystadenoma of ovary. Annales Chirurgiae et Gynaecologiae Fenniae 49: 240–244.

Walts A E, Lichtenstein I 1977 Primary leiomyosarcoma associated with serous cystadenocarcinoma of the ovary. Gynecologic Oncology 5: 81–86.

Wellman K F 1961 Leiomyoma of the ovary: report of an unusual case and review of the literature. Canadian Medical Association Journal 85: 429–432.

Young R H, Scully R E 1983 Ovarian stromal tumors with minor sex cord elements: a report of seven cases. International Journal of Gynecological Pathology 2: 277–284.

Young R H, Prat J, Scully R E 1984 Endometrioid stromal sarcomas of the ovary: a clinicopathologic analysis of 23 cases. Cancer 53: 1143–1155.

27. Metastatic tumours of the ovary

H. Fox

The ovary shares with the liver and the lung the dubious distinction of being a common, indeed often a preferential, site of tumour metastasis. Just why this should be so is unknown for there are no obvious features of the ovary which make it such a suitable 'soil' for secondary tumour growth.

MECHANISMS OF TUMOUR SPREAD TO THE OVARY

There are four possible pathways by which extragonadal tumours may spread to the ovary:

1. Direct spread

Direct extension of tumour from a primary site to the ovary occurs most commonly in cases of carcinoma of the Fallopian tube, endometrium and colon. This form of spread is sometimes along bridges provided by adhesions.

2. Surface implantation

Transcoelomic spread with surface implantation accounts for most cases of ovarian involvement in generalized peritoneal metastases but is sometimes an isolated phenomenon, this latter being particularly true for metastatic breast carcinoma. Surface implantation also occurs when an endometrial adenocarcinoma metastasizes to the ovary via the tubal lumen.

3. Lymphatic spread

This is a common pathway of ovarian metastasis, partly because of the rich network of lymphatic channels in the pelvis. Blaustein (1982) has pointed out that metastatic breast carcinoma in the ovary may be limited to clumps of tumour cells in the lymphatic vessels of the ovarian medulla, a finding which suggests that spread of mammary carcinoma to the ovary may well be, at least partly, via the lymphatic system. It is possible that gastric carcinoma also spreads to the ovary via the lumbar lymphatics, which connect with both the lymphatic vessels of the upper gastrointestinal tract and those of the ovary.

4. Haematogenous spread

This is probably a very common mode of ovarian metastasis, for metastatic tumour is often seen within ovarian blood vessels. The high incidence of ovarian metastases in young women with cancer may well be a reflection of the rich vascularization of the gonads during the reproductive years.

INCIDENCE OF METASTATIC OVARIAN TUMOURS

The true frequency with which metastases occur in the ovary is extremely difficult to establish, for some surveys have been restricted to autopsy cases, others to tumours encountered at operation and yet others to the incidence of clinically silent metastases from breast carcinomas in ovaries removed for therapeutic purposes (Scully, 1979). In theory, autopsy studies should produce the most accurate figures but, unfortunately, data derived from many autopsy series is of little value — either because the cases studied have included both males and females without giving any indication as to the proportions of each or because they have included women dying from both malignant and non-malignant disease without stating the numbers in each group. Even some of the surveys limited solely to women with malignant disease have blurred the issue by including cases of lymphoma. In Manchester, Fox & Langley (1976) found that amongst 272 women dying of malignant disease ovarian metastases were present in 4.4%: if only women with metastatic malignant disease were included the incidence of ovarian involvement rose to just over 6%. This is a figure which is roughly comparable to that found in other autopsy studies of women dying of malignant disease (Warren & Macomber, 1935; Walther, 1948; Willis, 1952) though in none of these series were the ovaries studied histologically in all, or even most, cases. The significance of this deficiency was shown by Virieux (1962) who found ovarian metastases in 37% of women succumbing to malignant disease: in 60% of the patients with ovarian involvement the ovaries were, however, not obviously abnormal on naked-eye examination and metastatic tumour was only detectable on histological examination. Luisi (1968), in a similar study, found ovarian metastases in 29% of women dying of carcinoma and these two series suggest that the true incidence of ovarian involvement in women with malignant disease is approximately 30%. The incidence varies, of course, with the site of the primary tumour: thus ovarian metastases have been noted in 50% of women with gastric carcinoma (Virieux, 1962), in 44% of fatal cases of breast carcinoma (Turksoy, 1960; Virieux, 1962; Luisi, 1968), in 30% with colonic carcinomas (Virieux, 1962) and in 16% of women with malignant melanomas (DasGupta & Brasfield, 1964). Figures quoted for the incidence of metastasis of genital tract cancer to the ovaries are very variable, those for cervical carcinoma ranging from less than 1% to over 40% and those for endometrial carcinoma from nil to 60% (Finn, 1951; Luisi, 1968; Fox & Langley, 1976).

Of more importance both to the pathologist and the gynaecologist is the proportion of apparently primary malignant ovarian tumours which eventually turn out to be metastases. Studies from England, Scandinavia and the United States suggest that between 13 and 18% of ovarian carcinomas are metastatic rather than primary (Parnanen & Varaja, 1954; von Numers, 1960; Israel et al, 1965; Fox & Langley, 1976) though Santesson & Kottmeier (1968) quote a much lower incidence of 6%. Ulbright et al (1984) noted an incidence of 7%, this being a particularly low figure because it included a number of cases of malignant lymphoma. Metastatic tumours masquerading as primary ovarian neoplasms stem most commonly from the stomach, large intestine and breast (Johansson, 1960; Mazur et al, 1984; Ulbright et al, 1984).

PATHOLOGY AND CLINICAL ASPECTS OF METASTATIC OVARIAN NEOPLASMS

Only those neoplasms which do not show the typical and specific features of a Krukenberg tumour are discussed in this section: Krukenberg tumours are a distinctive and specific form of metastatic neoplasm which merit, and will receive, separate consideration.

Metastatic tumours are commonly bilateral (about 60% of cases) and may appear as a diffusely solid tumour, as multiple solid nodules of tumour, as a partly cystic mass or, rather uncommonly, as entirely cystic lesions; extensive areas of haemorrhage and/or necrosis are common. Histologically, the tumours show a variety of patterns which depend, to some extent, on the site of the primary

tumour: most are adenocarcinomas and the ovarian deposits may have a similar appearance to the primary tumour, may be less well differentiated or can be better differentiated. Features indicative of a metastatic tumour include extensive areas of necrosis, surface implants, a multifocal pattern and vascular invasion (Fig. 27.1), this latter feature being highly suggestive, though not pathognomonic, of secondary neoplasia. Stromal luteinization occurs much more commonly with metastatic tumours than it does with primary ovarian neoplasms.

Specific forms of metastatic ovarian neoplasia

Metastasis from mammary carcinoma

In both autopsy series and in studies of ovaries removed for therapeutic purposes in women with disseminated breast carcinoma the incidence of ovarian metastases is in the region of 24–40% (Saphir, 1951; Johansson, 1960; Brickman & Ferreira, 1967; Harris et al, 1984): in women in whom the ovaries have been removed prophylactically in the absence of overt metastatic disease the incidence of

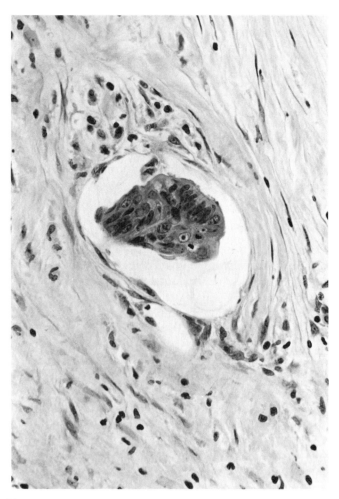

Fig. 27.1 Vascular invasion in a metastatic carcinoma of the ovary. H & E × 150.

ovarian involvement has ranged from 2–11% (Scully, 1979). Ovarian metastases are rarely the initial clinical manifestation of a mammary carcinoma, the ovarian tumours usually becoming manifest at intervals ranging from six months to 19 years after the initial diagnosis of carcinoma of the breast. Young et al (1981) have described a small series of cases of mammary cancer in which the initial manifestation was an ovarian tumour, but the very fact that such cases merit recording attests to their rarity.

Metastatic breast carcinoma in the ovary is bilateral in about 60% of cases and the involved ovary either contains multiple nodules of firm or gritty white tissue or is completely replaced by a smooth or bosselated mass; very rarely the metastatic neoplasm is predominantly cystic. Histologically, the metastatic tumour often replicates the pattern seen in the primary breast neoplasm. Lobular carcinoma of the breast has a particular tendency to metastasize to the ovary where it tends to retain its characteristic 'Indian file' pattern (Fig. 27.2), the tumour cells often being found, in early cases, in the walls of follicles or corpora lutea (Scully, 1979). Metastatic tumour of ductal origin may closely resemble an undifferentiated primary ovarian carcinoma but tends to have a more multifocal pattern. Metastatic ductal carcinoma commonly grows in nests, cords, solid tubules or diffuse sheets but glandular and microacinar patterns may also be encountered (Gagnon & Tetu, 1989; Young & Scully, 1991b). It is worth noting that ovarian metastases of breast carcinoma usually stain positively for gross cystic disease fluid protein-15 (Monteabudd et al, 1991).

Death usually ensues in less than 12 months after detection of clinically apparent ovarian metastases of mammary carcinoma (Johansson, 1960) though Osborne & Pitts (1961) noted a mean survival time of over 20 months in patients in whom metastases were diagnosed only by histological examination of therapeutic oophorectomy specimens.

Metastases from large intestinal carcinoma

The overall incidence of metastasis of colorectal cancer to the ovary is probably in the region of 30% (Virieux, 1962) and in a small proportion of cases (probably about 3%) an ovarian mass is the presenting symptom or sign of an intestinal neoplasm (Harcourt & Dennis, 1968; Herrera-Ornelas et al, 1983). The incidence of overt ovarian metastases at the time of initial surgery for an intestinal neoplasm is 3.7% but if prophylactically removed, macroscopically normal ovaries are examined histologically, metastatic deposits will be found in a further 4.5% (Graffner et al, 1983) and this has prompted the suggestion that prophylactic oophorectomy should be undertaken at the time of initial surgery in all women with intestinal carcinoma (Harcourt & Dennis, 1968; O'Brien

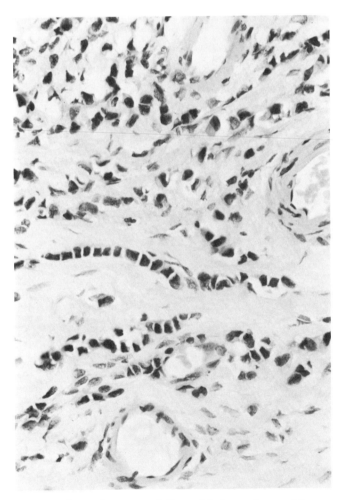

Fig. 27.2 An ovarian metastasis from a lobular carcinoma of the breast. The metastasis replicates the 'Indian file' pattern seen in primary breast neoplasms of this type. H & E × 240.

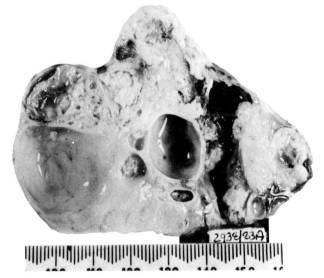

Fig. 27.3 Macroscopic appearances of an ovarian metastasis from an intestinal carcinoma.

et al, 1981; Cutait et al, 1983; Graffner et al, 1983; Morrow & Enker, 1984).

The metastatic tumours (Fig. 27.3) may be solid but are usually either partly or wholly cystic (Scully & Richardson, 1961; Scully, 1979; Ulbright et al, 1984; Lash & Hart, 1987; Daya et al, 1992); on section they are formed of soft yellowish, red or grey tissue with cystic areas that may contain necrotic material, old or fresh blood, clear fluid or mucinous fluid (Scully, 1979). The tumours are unilateral in a high proportion of cases. Histologically, the metastatic tumour tends to show either a mucinous or, more commonly, an endometrioid pattern whilst the stroma, which is usually of ovarian type, may be oedematous or show a desmoplastic reaction.

The histological distinction between a metastasis from an intestinal neoplasm showing a mucinous pattern (Fig. 27.4) and a primary ovarian mucinous adeno-carcinoma can be extremely difficult and is sometimes impossible. Ulbright et al (1984) noted that a mucus cell predominant pattern occurred at least locally in 82% of primary ovarian mucinous adenocarcinomas whereas this

pattern was found in only 11% of metastatic intestinal neoplasms: a transition from benign-appearing epithelium to atypical or frankly malignant epithelium was found in 90% of primary mucinous neoplasms but this feature does not unequivocally rule out a metastatic tumour, for a similar appearance was found in 11% of metastases from intestinal carcinomas. Other features noted by Ulbright et al (1984) as indicating a metastatic rather than a primary mucinous neoplasm were bilaterality, extensive areas of necrosis, denser more eosinophilic cytoplasm and a more frequent and prominent striated border.

The distinction between a metastatic intestinal tumour with an endometrioid pattern (Fig. 27.5) and a primary endometrioid carcinoma of the ovary can also be extremely difficult. Histological features suggestive of a metastatic neoplasm include extensive confluent necrosis, the presence (Fig. 27.6) within gland lumens and cysts of eosinophilic debris containing nuclear fragments ('dirty

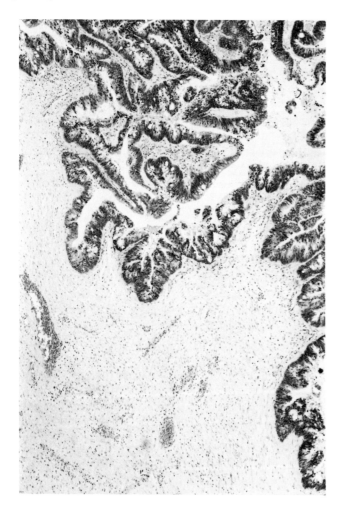

Fig. 27.4 Histological appearances of a typical ovarian metastasis from an intestinal adenocarcinoma. The pattern is virtually identical to that of a primary mucinous adenocarcinoma of the ovary. H & E × 110.

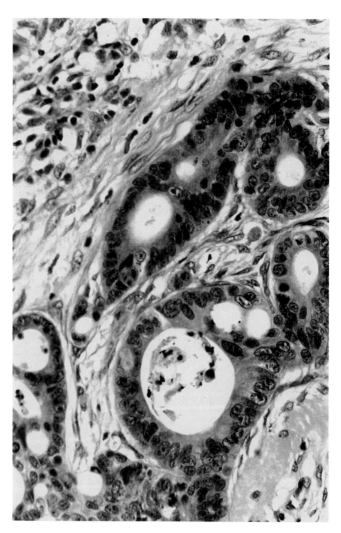

Fig. 27.5 An ovarian metastasis from an intestinal adenocarcinoma which has an 'endometrioid' pattern and resembles closely a primary endometrioid adenocarcinoma of the ovary. H & E × 190.

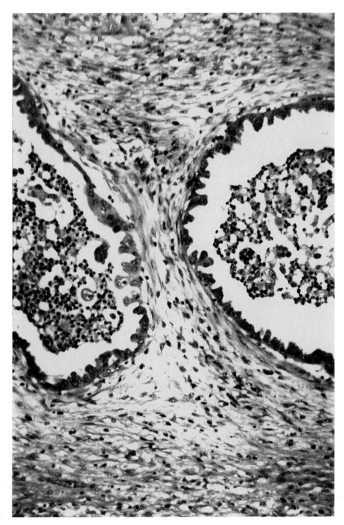

Fig. 27.6 An ovarian metastasis from an intestinal adenocarcinoma. The lumens of the neoplastic glands contain 'dirty' necrotic and inflammatory debris. H & E × 220.

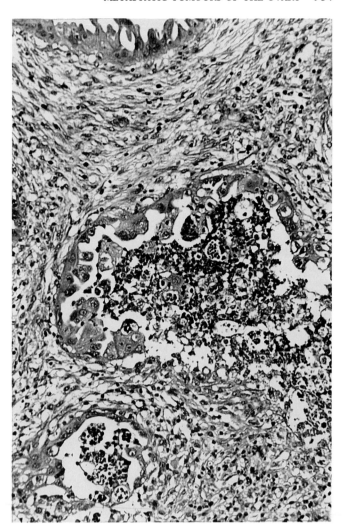

Fig. 27.7 An ovarian metastasis from an intestinal adenocarcinoma. The centrally placed gland shows segmental necrosis of its lining epithelium. H & E × 210.

necrosis'), focal segmental necrosis of glandular epithelium (Fig. 27.7) and a so-called 'garland' pattern in which there is a clustering of glands around an area of necrosis (Lash & Hart, 1987; Daya et al, 1992). In contrast, the presence of endometriosis or of squamous metaplasia will favour the diagnosis of a primary endometrioid carcinoma (Young & Scully, 1992b).

Immunohistochemical staining for CEA is of help in distinguishing metastatic intestinal cancer with an endometrioid pattern from a primary ovarian endometrioid adenocarcinoma, the former showing strong immunoreactivity and the latter either no, or only weak, focal reactivity; unfortunately, however, CEA immunostaining is of no value in the differentiation between metastatic tumours showing a mucinous pattern and primary mucinous adenocarcinomas, both showing equally strong staining (Lash & Hart, 1987).

Nearly all women with untreated ovarian metastases from an intestinal carcinoma are dead within three years of diagnosis and over 50% succumb within one year (Johansson, 1960; Richardson, 1967). These gloomy figures do not necessarily imply, however, that surgical resection of an ovarian metastasis is of no value: Morrow & Enker (1984) found that whilst the mean survival for women with non-resectable ovarian metastases from large bowel cancer was 9.8 months, that for patients with resectable tumours was 48 months. A few women (probably about 5%) survive for five or more years following simple surgical resection (Webb et al, 1975) whilst recently a 23% five-year survival rate has been achieved with aggressive surgery (Petru et al, 1992).

Metastases from appendicular carcinomas

Ovarian metastases from carcinoma of the appendix are not commonly encountered, largely because primary neoplasms at this site are relatively rare; nevertheless ovarian metastases are present in 10% of women with appendicular carcinomas and amongst such patients the ovarian lesion is the presenting feature in over 30% (Merino et al, 1985; Thorsen et al, 1991). Because small appendicular tumours, which may not be macroscopically obvious, can give rise to large ovarian metastases it has been suggested that appendicectomy should always be performed in women with apparently primary ovarian neoplasms (Merino et al, 1985).

A particular problem is posed by patients in whom a mucinous tumour is present in both the appendix and the ovary in association with pseudomyxoma peritonei. In these cases both the appendicular and ovarian neoplasms have a histological appearance which resembles either that of a mucinous cystadenoma or, more commonly, a mucinous tumour of borderline malignancy: the ovarian tumours are usually cystic whilst the appendicular neoplasms appear as mucoceles. Young & Scully (1991) have reviewed 22 such cases and concluded that the ovarian tumours were, despite their bland appearance, metastases from a low-grade mucinous adenocarcinoma of the appendix, basing this view upon the common bilaterality of the ovarian tumours, the predominance of right-sided ovarian involvement and the presence of mucin and atypical cells on the ovarian surfaces. Others have, however, refuted this concept, maintaining that the ovarian and appendicular neoplasm are usually independent of each other (Seidman et al, 1993).

Metastases from pancreatic adenocarcinoma

Ovarian metastases are rarely encountered in patients with pancreatic adenocarcinoma but Young & Hart (1989) described seven women in whom pancreatic adenocarcinomas spread to the ovary and there mimicked primary ovarian mucinous neoplasms: six of the pancreatic tumours were ductal adenocarcinomas whilst one was a mucinous adenocarcinoma. The pancreatic and ovarian neoplasms occurred synchronously in five patients whilst in two the ovarian lesion developed after diagnosis of the pancreatic adenocarcinoma: the clinical features were suggestive of a primary ovarian adenocarcinoma in four cases. The ovarian metastatic tumours were characteristically bilateral, large, cystic and multilocular and histologically usually contained areas resembling mucinous cystadenoma, mucinous tumour of borderline malignancy and mucinous adenocarcinoma. When such an ovarian neoplasm is encountered in the absence of any knowledge that the patient has a pancreatic adenocarcinoma it may be only the bilaterality that serves to raise a suspicion of metastatic tumour, a suspicion hardened if desmoplastic surface implants are present.

Young & Scully (1991b) have also described an ovarian metastasis from a pancreatic microadenocarcinoma: this closely resembled metastatic carcinoid tumour but did not contain argyrophil cells.

Metastases from carcinoma of the gallbladder and extrahepatic bile ducts

The very scanty literature on this topic suggests that between 6 and 12% of biliary neoplasms metastasize to the ovary (Brandt-Rauf et al, 1982; Albores-Saavedra & Henson, 1986; Lashgari et al, 1992). Six examples of ovarian metastases from biliary tract neoplasms were reported by Young & Scully (1990a): in one case the ovarian neoplasm was detected before the biliary tumour became clinically overt but in the other five the ovarian lesion occurred either synchronously with, or developed after, diagnosis of the primary neoplasm. Five of the metastatic ovarian tumours were bilateral and whilst most were solid one was cystic. Two of the metastatic ovarian tumours resembled mucinous neoplasms, one simulated an endometrioid adenocarcinoma and yet another bore a close resemblance to a Sertoli–Leydig cell neoplasm. The three remaining tumours showed appearances resembling closely those of a biliary adenocarcinoma.

Metastases from bronchial carcinoma

Only 5% of bronchial carcinomas metastasize to the ovaries (Galluzzi & Payne, 1955; Budinger, 1958; Warren & Gates, 1964). In most cases the ovarian metastases are an incidental unsuspected finding at autopsy and it is distinctly uncommon for a bronchial neoplasm to present initially as an ovarian tumour. Malviya et al (1982) described, however, a patient in whom an ovarian mass was the initial presentation of a small cell carcinoma of the bronchus whilst Young & Scully (1985) have reported six examples of bronchial neoplasms presenting as ovarian tumours: two of Young & Scully's patients were suffering from undifferentiated small cell carcinomas, one from an undifferentiated carcinoma, one from an adenocarcinoma and one from an atypical carcinoid tumour. Three of these patients had radiological evidence of a pulmonary neoplasm at the time of diagnosis of the ovarian lesion but in the other women evidence of a bronchial tumour did not appear until two, four and 26 months respectively after surgical removal of the ovarian metastasis. Notable features of these cases were the relatively young age of the patients (mean age 42 years) and the high incidence, unusual for ovarian metastatic disease, of unilaterality of the ovarian tumours. These two features make diagnosis difficult and in most cases only the application of the general criteria for metastatic disease, e.g. multinodularity, vascular invasion, will assist in the differential diagnosis from primary ovarian adenocarcinoma or, in the case of the metastatic undifferentiated bronchial small cell carcinoma, from the primary ovarian small cell carcinoma with hypercalcaemia: distinction from this latter entity is, however, aided by the fact that most bronchial small cell carcinomas are aneuploid whilst ovarian small cell carcinomas with hypercalcaemia are diploid (Scully, 1993).

The only histological difference between an ovarian metastasis from a pulmonary small cell carcinoma and the recently described primary ovarian small cell carcinoma of pulmonary type (Eichhorn et al, 1992) is the not infrequent presence in the latter of an epithelial component, such as endometrioid carcinoma. In the absence of this feature only a rigorous exclusion of a pulmonary neoplasm will allow for the differentiation of these two entities.

Metastasis from carcinoid tumours

Carcinoid tumours of the gastrointestinal tract, pancreas or bronchus may metastasize to the ovary (Robboy et al, 1974; Brown et al, 1980; Heisterberg et al, 1982) where they commonly present as bilateral solid tumours with smooth or bosselated surfaces; the cut surface usually shows multiple, often confluent, masses of firm white or yellow tissue though small cysts containing clear watery fluid may also be present (Robboy et al, 1974).

Histologically (Fig. 27.8), metastatic carcinoid tumours usually have either a trabecular or insular pattern but aci-

nar and solid tubular patterns may also be seen: features suggestive of a metastatic, rather than a primary lesion in such cases include bilaterality, multinodularity, the absence of other teratomatous elements and vascular invasion.

Metastatic goblet cell or mucinous carcinoids (Fig. 27.9) form rounded nests containing goblet cells and argentaffin or argyrophil cells (Zirkin et al, 1980; Heisterberg et al, 1982): this pattern may be admixed with that of a typical mucinous adenocarcinoma (Ikeda et al, 1991).

In the 25 non-autopsied cases of metastatic ovarian carcinoid tumour studied by Robboy et al (1974), one-third of the patients died within a year of diagnosis and three-quarters within five years. Six women were, however, well and free of symptoms for periods varying from six months to 29 years (mean of 5.6 years) and this has led Scully (1979) to suggest that both the metastases and the primary tumour should, if feasible, be removed: Scully further argued that menopausal or postmenopausal women

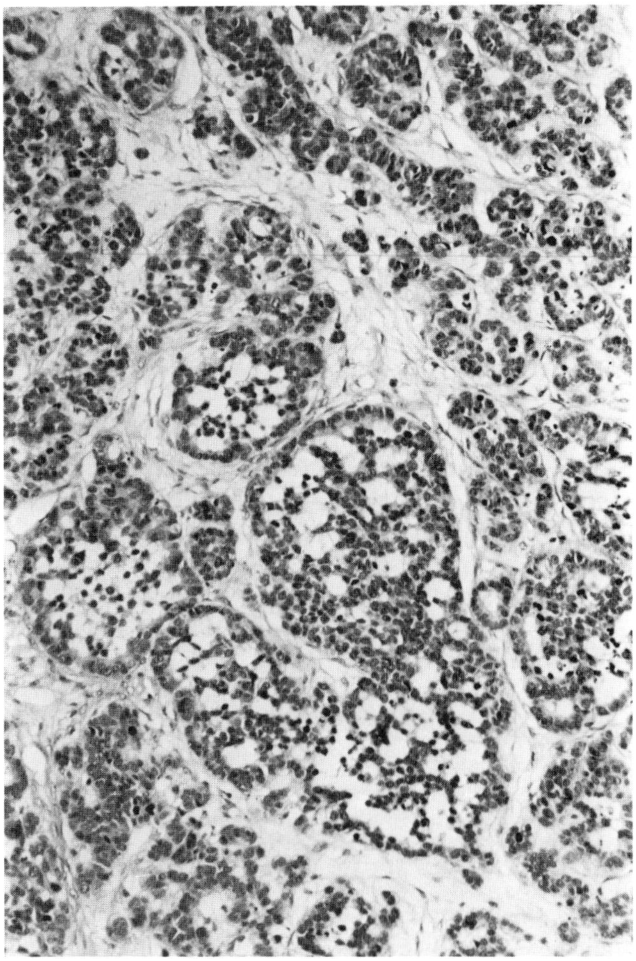

Fig. 27.8 Histological appearances of an ovarian metastasis from an intestinal carcinoid tumour. H & E × 58.

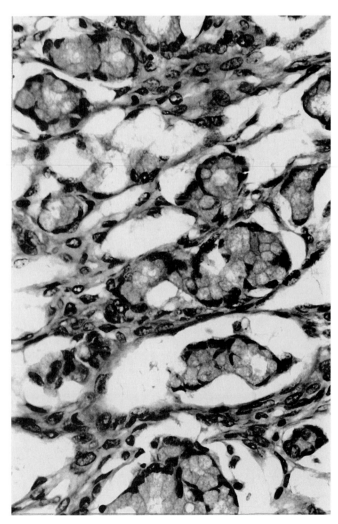

Fig. 27.9 An ovarian metastasis from a goblet cell carcinoid tumour of the terminal ileum. H & E × 320.

with intestinal carcinoid tumours should have a prophylactic bilateral salpingo-oophorectomy and that all women with bilateral ovarian carcinoid tumours should be subjected to an intensive search for an extraovarian primary lesion.

Metastases from hepatocellular carcinoma

Ovarian metastases from hepatocellular carcinoma are extremely rare but Young et al (1992) have recently reported three such cases. The ovarian tumours were bilateral in two patients and locally cystic in one case: they ranged from 4–11 cm in maximum diameter and were yellow-green or yellow on section. Histologically they were composed of cells with moderate to abundant eosinophilic cytoplasm growing diffusely or in nodules, nests or trabeculae (Fig. 27.10); cysts or glandular structures were prominent in two cases and bile was present in one tumour.

In the presence of a known hepatocellular carcinoma, which is usually the case, the diagnosis of an ovarian metastasis is straightforward. If, however, the presentation is with an ovarian tumour, a metastatic hepatocellular carcinoma has to be differentiated from, depending upon the patient's age, a yolk sac tumour showing a hepatoid pattern and from a hepatoid carcinoma. Bilaterality and the presence of bile help in the distinction from a hepatoid carcinoma whilst bilateral ovarian involvement also argues against a diagnosis of a yolk sac neoplasm.

Metastases from renal adenocarcinoma

Renal adenocarcinomas rarely metastasize to the ovary and, indeed, in one autopsy study of 324 women with renal adenocarcinoma no ovarian metastases were encountered (Saitoh, 1981). Nevertheless, there have been a number of reports of clinically apparent ovarian metastases from renal adenocarcinoma (Martzloff & Manlove, 1949; Vorder-Bruegge et al, 1957; Buller et al, 1983; Young & Hart, 1992). Most of these neoplasms have been unilateral and in over half of the patients the ovarian tumour occurred before the renal neoplasm was detected. Because of the histological similarity between metastatic renal adenocarcinoma and primary ovarian clear cell adenocarcinoma (Fig. 27.11), a diagnostic difficulty is clearly posed by such cases. Young & Hart (1992) considered that the principal features of metastatic renal adenocarcinoma that allow for its distinction from an ovarian clear cell adenocarcinoma are the presence of a striking sinusoidal vascular pattern, the absence of hobnail cells, a lack of hyaline basement membrane-like material, a negative stain for intraluminal mucin and a homogeneous clear cell pattern rather than the melange of cystic, glandular, papillary, solid, tubular and glandular patterns that characterizes ovarian clear cell adenocarcinomas.

Metastases from bladder, ureteric and urethral carcinomas

The ovary is a rare locus of tumour spread from these sites (Fetter et al, 1959; Babaian et al, 1980) but metastases have been recorded from signet-ring cell carcinomas of the bladder (Ulbright et al, 1984; Bowlby & Smith, 1986), and from transitional cell carcinomas of the bladder (Fossa et al, 1977; Svenes & Eide, 1984; Ulbright et al, 1984; Andriole et al, 1985; Young & Scully, 1988), ureter (Batata et al, 1975), renal pelvis (Hsiu et al, 1991) and urethra (Graves & Guiss, 1941).

Signet-ring cell carcinomas of the bladder metastasize to the ovary as Krukenberg tumours and do not provoke any diagnostic dilemmas. The presence, however, of simultaneous transitional cell neoplasms in the urinary tract and in the ovary raises the question as to whether there are two synchronous and independent primary neoplasms (Van der Weiden & Gratama, 1987; Young & Scully, 1988). In the absence of the general features of a metastatic ovarian tumour this distinction may be impossible.

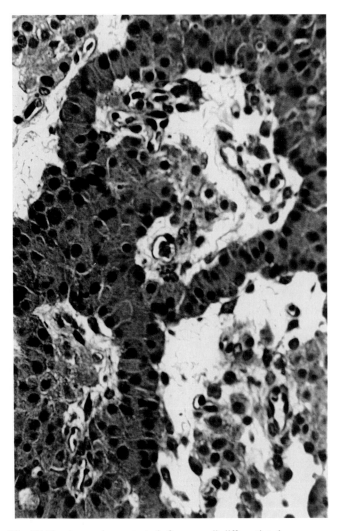

Fig. 27.10 An ovarian metastasis from a well-differentiated hepatocellular carcinoma. H & E × 360.

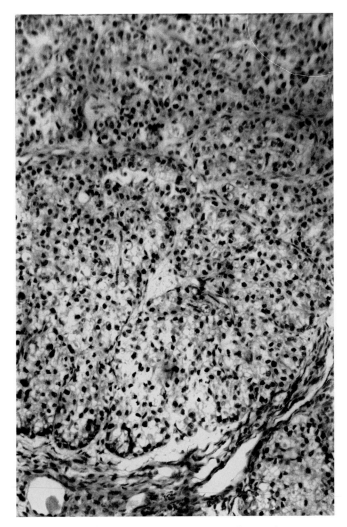

Fig. 27.11 An ovarian metastasis from a renal adenocarcinoma. H & E × 140.

Metastases from malignant melanoma

Metastases of malignant melanoma in the ovary are usually from a primary cutaneous lesion and may become apparent many years (up to 13) after removal of the skin melanoma (Fitzgibbons et al, 1987; Young & Scully, 1991a).

The tumours are usually large (10–20 cm in diameter) and are bilateral in about 45% of cases: only about one-third are obviously pigmented. Extraovarian tumour is commonly present, usually in the pelvis and upper abdomen.

Histologically a multinodular pattern is usually apparent. About 50% of the tumours are amelanotic and in most the predominant appearance is either of large cells with amphophilic or eosinophilic cytoplasm or of small cells with scanty cytoplasm; a sarcoma-like pattern is uncommon. Rounded or ovoid nests of cells having a somewhat 'naevoid' appearance are seen in some cases. Follicle-like spaces are present in about 40% of metastatic melanomas

and may lead to an erroneous diagnosis of either small cell carcinoma with hypercalcaemia or juvenile granulosa cell tumour. Specific cytological features seen in metastatic melanomas include prominent nucleoli, cytoplasmic pseudoinclusions within the nuclei and, rather uncommonly, nuclear grooving; cytoplasmic melanin granules, are, of course, a diagnostic feature when present. Metastatic malignant melanoma usually stains positively for S100 and HMB-45, the latter being the more specific.

Very often the clinical history will point strongly to a diagnosis of melanoma but in the absence of such a history the most important element in diagnosing this neoplasm is an awareness of its possibility by the pathologist. If the tumour is unilateral and there is no history of a preceding cutaneous lesion a careful search should be made for teratomatous elements.

Most patients with ovarian metastatic malignant melanoma die within a few years of diagnosis but occasional women have remained well and apparently tumour-free for as long as eight years after surgical extirpation of the ovarian metastases.

Metastases from endometrial adenocarcinoma

There is no doubt that endometrial adenocarcinomas can, and do, metastasize to the ovary and ovarian secondary deposits have been reported as occurring in between 13 and 60% of women with an endometrial neoplasm (Finn, 1951; Luisi, 1968). An endometrial adenocarcinoma with ovarian metastases would be classed as stage III and thus expected to have a gloomy prognosis; over the years it has, however, become clear that the outlook for such cases is unusually favourable (Dockerty, 1954; Woodruff et al, 1970; Bruckman et al, 1980) and this has increasingly led to the belief that many instances of endometrial adenocarcinoma with apparent ovarian metastases are in reality examples of synchronous dual primary neoplasms of the ovary and endometrium (Scully, 1979; Choo & Naylor, 1982; Zaind et al, 1984; Ulbright & Roth, 1985; Piura & Glezerman, 1989; Prat et al, 1991). This raises the question of whether the pathologist can distinguish between dual synchronous primary ovarian and endometrial neoplasms of the same histological type and endometrial adenocarcinomas with ovarian metastases. In some cases this is, as Silverberg (1984) has pointed out, relatively easy: thus if the endometrial tumour arises superficially in a polyp or is clearly seen to be emerging from a background of 'atypical hyperplasia' and the ovarian carcinoma is in direct continuity with a focus of endometriosis, it will be reasonably obvious that the ovarian lesion is not a metastasis from the endometrial neoplasm. Conversely, direct extension of a large endometrial tumour to the ovary, bilateral ovarian tumours, a multinodular ovarian tumour, extensive vascular permeation by tumour within the ovary, the presence of tumour cells in ovarian hilar lymphatics, tubal involvement with ovarian surface implantation and deep invasion of the myometrium together with involvement of vascular spaces by the endometrial tumour are all features which point to a true ovarian metastasis (Ulbright & Roth, 1985).

In some cases, however, the decision as to whether one is dealing with an ovarian metastasis or a second primary neoplasm has to be taken on grounds other than those outlined above, grounds which are of a largely circumstantial nature. Eifel et al (1982) suggested that if the tumour in both ovary and endometrium is of the endometrioid type and if the uterine neoplasm is of grade 1 differentiation and shows no, or minimal, myometrial invasion, then it is almost certain that both neoplasms are primary tumours. A similar conclusion can, according to these workers, also be drawn if the endometrial tumour is grade 2 or 3 but is not invading the myometrium: if there is deep myometrial invasion, and especially if the tumour is of grade 2 or 3 differentiation, then it would be prudent to regard the ovarian tumour as metastatic in nature, this being a view in accord with that of Zaind et al (1984). Eifel et al (1982) also thought that if both the uterine and ovarian neoplasms are of the serous papillary or clear cell types it would be reasonable to consider, for practical purposes, the ovarian lesion to be secondary to these aggressive forms of endometrial neoplasia. By contrast, Ulbright & Roth (1985) maintained that whilst all ovarian lesions found in association with a grade 3 endometrioid adenocarcinoma or an adenosquamous carcinoma of the endometrium should be regarded as metastases, independent dual primary neoplasms of papillary serous or clear cell type could be recognized and treated as such. Currently, both immunohistochemistry and flow cytometry appear to be of very limited value in resolving the problems posed by concurrent endometrial and ovarian carcinoma (Prat et al, 1991).

Metastases from tubal carcinoma

Adenocarcinoma of the Fallopian tube commonly involves the ovary, either by direct extension or via inflammatory adhesions (Scully, 1979). In many such cases, however, it may be impossible to distinguish between a tubal neoplasm invading the ovary and an ovarian serous adenocarcinoma which has spread to the tube: in the face of this dilemma the non-committal, but useful, diagnosis of 'tubo-ovarian' carcinoma is often resorted to. Perhaps the only hint in such cases of a primary tubal origin is if the contralateral tube also contains carcinoma which has not spread to the ovary, tubal carcinomas being not infrequently bilateral.

Metastases from cervical carcinoma

Ovarian metastases occur in only about 0.5% of squamous cell carcinomas of the uterine cervix (Tabata et al,

1986; Toki et al, 1991; Sutton et al, 1992), with the metastases not uncommonly being of only microscopic size and localized to the ovarian hilus (Toki et al, 1991). Somewhat rarely, however, the ovarian lesion may be not only large but also responsible for the presenting symptoms (Young et al, 1993b).

The incidence of ovarian spread is highest in patients with a cervical adenocarcinoma and has been variously estimated as between 1.3 and 7.7% (Kjorstadt & Bond, 1984; Tabata et al, 1986; Mann et al, 1987; Brown et al, 1990; Sutton et al, 1992). There appears to be a particular tendency for mucinous adenocarcinomas of the cervix to metastasize to the ovary (Kaminsky & Norris, 1984) and the co-existence of mucinous tumours in both the cervix and the ovary may give rise to difficulties in deciding whether the ovarian lesion is a metastasis or a synchronous second primary neoplasm (LiVolsi et al, 1983; Young & Scully, 1988). The finding within the ovarian tumour of areas of apparently benign or borderline epithelium is not a conclusive indication of its primary nature whilst bilaterality, the presence of desmoplastic surface implants and vascular space invasion are all suggestive of a metastatic lesion (Young & Scully, 1988).

Metastases from sarcomas

Young & Scully (1990b) described 21 sarcomas metastasizing to the ovaries and reviewed the few previous reports of sporadic examples of this phenomenon. Included in Young & Scully's series were three uterine leiomyosarcomas, eight endometrial stromal sarcomas, four extragenital leiomyosarcomas and single instances of fibrosarcoma, neural sarcoma, haemangiosarcoma, osteosarcoma, chondrosarcoma and Ewing's sarcoma. In only three cases did the ovarian tumour precede diagnosis of the primary neoplasm.

In 11 of the 21 cases the ovarian metastases were bilateral, and histologically the metastatic tumours usually recapitulated the microscopic appearances of the primary sarcoma: diagnostic difficulties were encountered only in cases of metastatic endometrial stromal sarcoma, which proved difficult to distinguish both from primary ovarian neoplasms of this type and, in a few instances, from a sex cord-stromal tumour.

Young & Scully (1989) also described two examples of alveolar rhabdomyosarcoma which had metastasized to the ovary and reviewed the previously reported six cases of ovarian metastatic rhabdomyosarcoma. Metastases from an alveolar rhabdomyosarcoma occur predominantly as small cell tumours and a distinction from the small cell carcinoma with hypercalcaemia depends upon recognition of the retained alveolar pattern in the metastasis. Young et al (1993a) have subsequently described a further three examples of rhabdomyosarcoma metastasizing to the ovaries in children.

Metastases from miscellaneous unusual sites

Tumours of any site in the body can, on occasion, meta-stasize to the ovary though often the ovarian involvement is only apparent at autopsy. Amongst such oncological exotica may be mentioned ovarian metastases from thyroid carcinoma (Luisi, 1968; Woodruff et al, 1970; Young et al, 1994), thymoma (Yoshida et al, 1981), cerebellar medulloblastoma (Paterson, 1961), Merkel cell tumour (George et al, 1985), hepatoblastoma (Green & Silva, 1989), Wilms' tumour (Jareb et al, 1977), adrenal neuro-blastoma (Sty et al, 1980; Young et al, 1993a), renal rhab-doid tumour (Young et al, 1993a), retinoblastoma (Moore et al, 1967), adenoid cystic carcinoma of the salivary gland (Young & Scully, 1991), chordoma (Zukerberg & Young, 1990) and extragenital non-pulmonary small cell carcinomas (Eichhorn et al, 1993).

Probably, with the passage of time, every known tumour will eventually have been recorded as having metastasized to the ovaries and it is a moot point whether such cases should continue to be documented.

Krukenberg tumours

The eponymous fame of Krukenberg rests upon his de-scription, in 1896, of five tumours which he thought were primary neoplasms of the ovary and to which he gave the name 'fibrosarcoma ovarii mucocellulares (carcinoma-toides)'. Schlagenhauffer (1902) recognized these tu-mours as metastases from epithelial neoplasms, but since then the term 'Krukenberg tumour' has been variously interpreted as:

1. A pathological entity in which solid, usually bilateral, ovarian tumours are formed of mucus-containing signet-ring cells set in a hyperplastic cellular stroma
2. A purely histological diagnosis which is applicable to any tumour showing the above histological characteristics irrespective of its macroscopic appearances
3. Any metastatic ovarian tumour
4. Any ovarian metastasis from a primary gastric carcinoma
5. Any ovarian metastasis from a primary tumour in any part of the gastrointestinal tract.

The diagnosis of a Krukenberg tumour should rest solely on histological grounds and although neoplasms with the characteristic histological features of a Kruken-berg tumour usually also show a typical macroscopic appearance, the absence of characteristic gross features should not be allowed to detract from the diagnosis.

Krukenberg tumours (Fig. 27.12), which account for 3–4% of all ovarian neoplasms (Soloway et al, 1956), are bilateral in over 80% of cases and range in size from 5–20 cm in diameter: they are solid with a smooth nodular

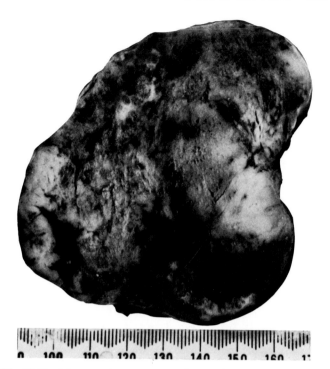

Fig. 27.12 Macroscopic appearances of an ovarian Krukenberg tumour.

or bosselated outer surface and on section are formed of firm, white, yellow or pinkish tissue which is often coarsely lobulated; the tumour is sometimes locally myxoid or mu-cinous in texture and whilst foci of necrosis are common cystic change is unusual. Occasional Krukenberg tumours are, however, predominantly cystic, the large thin-walled cysts being filled with mucinous or watery fluid.

Histologically, the Krukenberg tumour is formed of a varying number of plump, rounded epithelial cells set in dense cellular stroma. The epithelial cells occur singly or in clumps, and a proportion, sometimes small but usually considerable, contain mucus and have their nuclei displaced laterally to give a signet-ring appearance (Fig. 27.13). Poorly formed acinar structures are present in many cases and occasionally (Fig. 27.14) there is a pre-dominantly tubular pattern (Bullon et al, 1981). In some cases mucin-poor cells are arranged in trabeculae or large clumps whilst, very infrequently, cysts lined by apparently innocuous mucinous epithelium are a conspicuous com-ponent of the tumour (Scully, 1979). Carcinomatous cells may be suspended in pools of extracellular mucus.

The tumour stroma is of ovarian type and its constitu-ent cells are plump and spindle-shaped; there may be a moderate number of mitotic figures in the stromal cells and these, together with a not uncommon degree of pleo-morphism, may impart a 'pseudosarcomatous' pattern to the stromal component. The proliferating stromal cells may assume a storiform pattern in some areas and this may be associated with dense collagenization; if tumour cells are sparsely dispersed in such areas the appearances

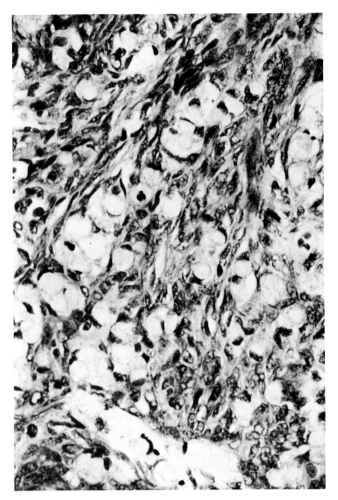

Fig. 27.13   Histological appearances of a typical ovarian Krukenberg tumour. Signet-ring, mucus-containing cells are set in a proliferating stroma. H & E × 340.

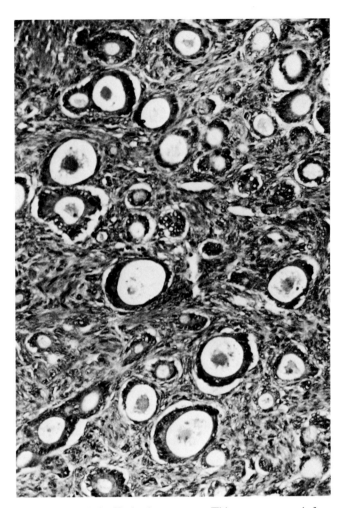

Fig. 27.14   A tubular Krukenberg tumour. This was a metastasis from a gastric adenocarcinoma and elsewhere showed a transition to a more conventional signet-ring cell appearance. H & E × 90.

may resemble those of a fibrous histiocytoma (Holtz & Hart, 1982). Foci of stromal oedema are not uncommon and stromal luteinization is often a conspicuous feature. Tumour emboli can be found in lymphatic and vascular spaces of the hilum, mesovarium, and mesosalpinx in about 50% of cases (Holtz & Hart, 1982).

The vast majority of Krukenberg tumours are metastases from a gastric carcinoma; other much less commonly encountered primary carcinomas giving rise to metastatic Krukenberg tumours occur in the large intestine, breast, gallbladder, endocervix, appendix and urinary bladder (McDuff, 1950; Karsh, 1951; Soloway et al, 1956; Woodruff & Novak, 1960; Hale, 1968; Paone et al, 1978; Scully, 1979; Kashani & Levy, 1983; Mazur et al, 1984). It should not be assumed, however, that any histological type of carcinoma can give rise to a Krukenberg tumour and that the typical signet-ring appearance of the cells in such a neoplasm represents a structural modification imposed by their ovarian environment. Krukenberg tumours are metastases of signet-ring carcinomas and such neoplasms have a particular tendency to spread to the ovary

(Saphir, 1951; Amorn & Knight, 1978; Duarte & Llanos, 1981); the reasons for this propensity are totally obscure but the predominance of the stomach as the site of origin of Krukenberg tumours simply reflects the fact that signet-ring carcinomas occur most commonly at this site and does not indicate a general tendency for all adenocarcinomas of the stomach to metastasize to the ovary.

The question arises as to whether Krukenberg tumours of the ovary are always metastatic in nature. It has been maintained that a typical Krukenberg tumour can arise as a primary neoplasm of the ovary; indeed, not only have approximately 40 such tumours been reported (Joshi, 1968), but in one series of 48 Krukenberg tumours no less than 10 were thought to have arisen *de novo* in the ovary (Woodruff & Novak, 1960). There is certainly no inherent reason why a primary signet-ring carcinoma should not occur in the ovary but extreme caution should be exercised before making such a diagnosis. The diagnosis of a primary Krukenberg tumour rests not on any special characteristics of the ovarian neoplasm but on the absence of any primary lesion elsewhere; the lack of a primary extraovarian tumour may, however, be very difficult to prove and in many of the reported cases the evidence for this has been solely that the patient survived in apparently good health for two or three years after removal of an ovarian Krukenberg tumour. This is too short a follow-up period, as is shown by the salutary case reported by McGoogan & Hatch (1972) in which a gastric carcinoma did not become apparent until four and a half years after removal of an ovarian Krukenberg tumour. Any suggested period of follow-up is, of course, arbitrary but it is widely accepted that a Krukenberg tumour should not be regarded as primary unless either the patient has lived in good health for at least five years after removal of the ovarian neoplasm or has died and been subjected to a thorough autopsy examination which has excluded a primary extraovarian lesion. Application of these criteria to the reported cases of primary Krukenberg tumours reduces their number to less than 20 (Fox & Langley, 1976) though even these are regarded with considerable scepticism by Holtz & Hart (1982), who note that some primary neoplasms may remain occult for many years and that small carcinomas of the stomach can be difficult to detect at autopsy; nevertheless, of the 27 cases of Krukenberg tumours in their series a detailed autopsy failed to identify a primary extraovarian carcinoma in two patients.

The age of women with an ovarian Krukenberg tumour tends to be unusually low for patients with metastatic carcinoma; most are between 30 and 50 years of age at the time of initial diagnosis (Diddle, 1955) and the mean age is about 45 years (Berens, 1951; Karsh, 1951; Bernier & Bonnenfant, 1955; Soloway et al, 1956; Woodruff and Novak, 1960; Hale, 1968; Holtz & Hart, 1982): these mean figures conceal, however, the fact that in some series nearly half the patients have been under the age of 40 years at initial diagnosis and that a significant proportion have been in their twenties (Linard, 1946; Holtz & Hart, 1982). The youngest patient in whom a Krukenberg tumour has been described was aged 13 years (Berens, 1951).

The symptoms of a Krukenberg tumour are generally non-specific and related solely to the presence of a pelvic mass, abdominal discomfort or pain being the most commonly encountered complaints. Accompanying ascites may cause abdominal enlargement whilst occasional Krukenberg tumours are associated with a hydrothorax which resolves after removal of the ovarian tumour (Dick et al, 1950; Bernier & Bonnenfant, 1955; Woodruff & Novak, 1960). Because of the relative youth of many of the women with this tumour it is not surprising that occasional Krukenberg tumours have occurred during pregnancy (Fox & Stamm, 1965; Spadoni et al, 1965; Ward, 1966; Connor et al, 1968; Forest et al, 1978). Menstrual disturbances and postmenopausal bleeding are common, though rarely dominant, complaints in women with a Krukenberg tumour, whilst a much smaller proportion of women with such neoplasms show evidence of virilization: the endocrine effects are regarded as being due to an associated stromal luteinization and are discussed fully in Chapter 29. It is worth noting, however, that pregnant women with a Krukenberg tumour show a particular tendency to become virilized (Fox & Langley, 1976; Bullon et al, 1981): this is thought to be due to stimulation of the luteinized cells by hCG, and the maternal virilization may be associated with partial masculinization of female children resulting from such pregnancies.

Only between 20 and 30% of patients with an ovarian Krukenberg tumour have a history of a previously removed extraovarian neoplasm (Johansson, 1960; Scully, 1979): in such cases the time interval between diagnosis of the extraovarian tumour and presentation of an ovarian metastasis is usually less than six months (Johansson, 1960), with very few cases having an apparently tumour-free interval of more than two years (Hale, 1968). Nevertheless, in occasional cases there may be a long time interval, up to 12 years, between diagnosis of an extraovarian neoplasm and the appearance of an ovarian metastasis (Hale, 1968). In most cases the extraovarian neoplasm is diagnosed at the time of presentation of the ovarian tumour, even though it may have been, until then, clinically silent. In a proportion of cases a Krukenberg tumour is the initial presentation of an extraovarian primary neoplasm and in such circumstances the extragonadal tumour may not become apparent for anything up to six years (Johansson, 1960).

The prognosis for a woman with a Krukenberg tumour is extremely poor, with most patients surviving only between three and ten months (Leffel et al, 1942; Soloway et al, 1956; Hale, 1968); only 10% of patients survive for more than two years after diagnosis of the ovarian tumour.

REFERENCES

Albores-Saavedra A, Henson D E 1986 Tumors of the gallbladder and extrahepatic bile ducts. In: Atlas of tumour pathology, second series, fascicle 22. Armed Forces Institute of Pathology, Washington, DC.

Alndriole G L, Garnick M B, Richie J P 1985 Unusual behaviour of low grade, low stage transitional cell carcinoma of bladder. Urology 25: 524–526.

Amorn Y, Knight W A 1978 Primary linitis plastica of the colon: report of two cases and review of the literature. Cancer 41: 2420–2425.

Babaian R J, Johnson D E, Llamas L, Ayala A G 1980 Metastases from transitional cell carcinoma of urinary bladder. Urology 16: 142–144.

Batata M A, Whitmore W F, Hilaris B S, Tokita N, Grabstald H 1975 Primary carcinoma of the ureter: a prognostic study. Cancer 35: 1616–1632.

Berens J J 1951 Krukenberg tumors of the ovary. American Journal of Surgery 81: 484–491.

Bernier L, Bonnenfant J L 1955 La tumeur de Krukenberg. Gynecologie et Obstetrique 54: 615–621.

Blaustein A 1982 Metastatic carcinoma in the ovary. In: Blaustein A (ed) Pathology of the female genital tract, 2nd edn. Springer Verlag, New York, ch 26, pp 705–715.

Bowlby L S, Smith M L 1986 Signet-ring cell carcinoma of the urinary bladder: presentation as a Krukenberg tumor. Gynecologic Oncology 25: 376–381.

Brandt-Rauf P W, Pincus M, Adelson S 1982 Cancer of the gallbladder: a review of forty-three cases. Human Pathology 13: 48–53.

Brickman M, Ferreira B 1967 Metastasis of breast carcinoma to the ovaries — incidence, significance and relationship to survival: a preliminary study. Grace Hospital Bulletin 45: 44–49.

Brown B L, Sharifker D A, Gordon R, Deppe G, Cohen C J 1980 Bronchial carcinoid tumor with ovarian metastasis: a light microscopic and ultrastructural study. Cancer 46: 543–546.

Brown J W, Fu Y S, Berek J S 1990 Ovarian metastases are rare in Stage 1 adenocarcinoma of the cervix. Obstetrics and Gynecology 76: 623–626.

Bruckman J E, Bloomer W D, Marck A, Ehrmann R L, Knapp R C 1980 Stage III adenocarcinoma of the endometrium: two prognostic groups. Gynecologic Oncology 9: 12–17.

Budinger J M 1958 Untreated bronchogenic carcinoma: a clinicopathological study of 250 autopsied cases. Cancer 11: 106–116.

Buller R E, Braga C A, Tanagho E A, Miller T 1983 Renal cell carcinoma metastatic to the ovary: a case report. Journal of Reproductive Medicine 28: 217–220.

Bullon A, Arseneau J, Prat J, Young R H, Scully R E 1981 Tubular Krukenberg tumor: a problem in histopathologic diagnosis. American Journal of Surgical Pathology 5: 225–232.

Choo Y C, Naylor B 1982 Multiple primary neoplasms of the ovary and uterus. International Journal of Gynaecology and Obstetrics 20: 327–334.

Connor T B, Ganis F M, Levin H S, Migeon C J, Martin L G 1968 Gonadotrophic-dependent Krukenberg tumor causing virilization during pregnancy. Journal of Clinical Endocrinology and Metabolism 28: 198–214.

Cutait R, Lesser M, Enker W E 1983 Prophylactic oophorectomy in surgery for large bowel cancer. Diseases of the Colon and Rectum 26: 6–11.

DasGupta T, Brasfield R 1964 Metastatic melanoma: a clinicopathological study. Cancer 17: 1323–1339.

Daya D, Nazerali L, Frank G L 1992 Metastatic ovarian carcinoma of large intestinal origin simulating primary ovarian carcinoma: a clinicopathologic study of 25 cases. American Journal of Clinical Pathology 27: 751–758.

Dick H J, Spire L J, Worboys C S 1950 Association of Meig's syndrome with Krukenberg tumors. New York State Journal of Medicine 50: 1842–1846.

Diddle A W 1955 Krukenberg tumors: diagnostic problem. Cancer 8: 1026–1034.

Dockerty M B 1954 Primary and secondary ovarian adenoacanthoma. Surgery, Gynecology and Obstetrics 99: 392–400.

Duarte I, Llanos O 1981 Patterns of metastasis in intestinal and diffuse types of carcinoma of the stomach. Human Pathology 12: 237–242.

Eichhorn J H, Young R H, Scully R E 1992 Primary ovarian small cell carcinoma of pulmonary type: a clinicopathologic, immunohistologic and flow cytometric analysis of 11 cases. American Journal of Surgical Pathology 16: 926–938.

Eichhorn J H, Young R H, Scully R E 1993 Non-pulmonary small cell carcinomas of extragenital origin metastatic to the ovary: a report of seven cases. Cancer 71: 177–186.

Eifel P, Hendrickson M, Ross J, Ballon S, Martinez A, Kempson R 1982 Simultaneous presentation of carcinoma involving the ovary and the uterine corpus. Cancer 50: 163–170.

Fetter T R, Bogaev J H, McCuskey B, Seres J L 1959 Carcinoma of the bladder: sites of metastases. Journal of Urology 81: 746–748.

Finn W F 1951 Diagnostic confusion of ovarian metastases from endometrial carcinoma with primary ovarian cancer. American Journal of Obstetrics and Gynecology 62: 403–408.

Fitzgibbons P L, Martin S E, Simmons T J 1987 Malignant melanoma metastatic to the ovary. American Journal of Surgical Pathology 11: 959–964.

Forest M G, Orgiazzi J, Tranchant D, Mornex R, Bertrand J 1978 Approach to the mechanism of androgen overproduction in a case of Krukenberg tumour responsible for virilization during pregnancy. Journal of Clinical Endocrinology and Metabolism 47: 428–434.

Fossa S D, Schjolseth J A, Miller A 1977 Multiple urothelial tumours with metastases to uterus and left ovary: a case report. Scandinavian Journal of Urology and Nephrology 11: 81–84.

Fox H, Langley F A 1976 Tumours of the ovary. Heinemann, London.

Fox L P, Stamm W J 1965 Krukenberg tumor complicating pregnancy: report of a case with androgenic activity. American Journal of Obstetrics and Gynecology 92: 702–709.

Gagnon Y, Tetu B 1989 Ovarian metastases of breast carcinoma: a clinicopathologic study of 59 cases. Cancer 64: 892–898.

Galluzzi S, Payne P M 1955 Bronchial carcinoma: a statistical study of 741 necropsies with special reference to the distribution of blood-borne metastases. British Journal of Cancer 9: 511–527.

George T K, di Sant'Agnese P A, Bennett J M 1985 Chemotherapy for metastatic Merkel cell carcinoma. Cancer 56: 1034–1038.

Graffner H D L, Alm P O R, Oscarson J E A 1983 Prophylactic oophorectomy in colorectal cancer. American Journal of Surgery 146: 233–235.

Graves R C, Guiss L W 1941 Tumors of the urethra. Journal of Urology 46: 925–947.

Green L K, Silva E G 1989 Hepatoblastoma in an adult with metastasis to the ovaries. American Journal of Clinical Pathology 92: 110–115.

Hale R W 1968 Krukenberg tumor of the ovary: a review of 81 records. Obstetrics and Gynecology 32: 221–225.

Harcourt K F, Dennis D L 1968 Laparotomy for 'ovarian tumors' in unsuspected carcinoma of the colon. Cancer 21: 1244–1246.

Harris M, Howell A, Chrissohou M et al 1984 A comparison of the metastatic pattern of infiltrating lobular carcinoma and infiltrating duct carcinoma of the breast. British Journal of Cancer 50: 23–30.

Heisterberg L, Wahlin A, Nieldsen K S 1982 Two cases of goblet cell carcinoid tumour of the appendix with bilateral ovarian metastases. Acta Obstetricia et Gynecologica Scandinavica 61(2): 153–156.

Herrera-Ornelas L, Natarajan N, Tsukada I et al 1983 Adenocarcinoma of the colon masquerading as primary ovarian neoplasia: an analysis of ten cases. Diseases of the Colon and Rectum 26: 377–380.

Holtz F, Hart W R 1982 Krukenberg tumors of the ovary: a clinicopathologic analysis of 27 cases. Cancer 50: 2438–2447.

Hsiu J-G, Kemp G A, Singer G A, Rawis W H, Siddiky M A 1991 Transitional cell carcinoma of the renal pelvis with ovarian metastasis. Gynecologic Oncology 41: 178–181.

Ikeda E, Tsutsumi Y, Yoshida H, Yanagi K 1991 Goblet cell carcinoid of the vermiform appendix with ovarian metastasis. Acta Pathologica Japonica 41: 455–460.

Israel S L, Helsel E W, Hausman D H 1965 The challenge of metastatic ovarian carcinoma. American Journal of Obstetrics and Gynecology 93: 1094–1101.

Jereb B, Golough R, Havlicek S 1977 Ovarian cancer in children and adolescents: a review of 15 cases. Medical Pediatric Oncology 3: 339–343.

Johansson M 1960 Clinical aspects of metastatic ovarian cancer of extragenital origin. Acta Obstetricia et Gynecologica Scandinavica 39: 681–697.

Joshi V V 1968 Primary Krukenberg tumor of the ovary: review of literature and case report. Cancer 22: 1199–1207.

Kaminski P F, Norris H J 1984 Coexistence of ovarian neoplasms and endocervical adenocarcinoma. Obstetrics and Gynecology 64: 553–556.

Karsh J 1951 Secondary malignant disease of the ovaries: a study of 72 autopsies. American Journal of Obstetrics and Gynecology 61: 154–160.

Kashani M, Levy M 1983 Primary adenocarcinoma of the appendix with bilateral Krukenberg ovarian tumors. Journal of Surgical Oncology 22: 101–105.

Kjorstad K E, Bond B 1984 Stage 1b adenocarcinoma of the cervix: metastatic potential and patterns of dissemination. American Journal of Obstetrics and Gynecology 54: 553–556.

Krukenberg F E 1896 Ueber das Fibrosarcoma ovarii mucocellulare (carcinomatides). Archiv fur Gynakologie 50: 287–321.

Lash R H, Hart W R 1987 Intestinal adenocarcinomas metastatic to the ovaries: a clinicopathologic evaluation of 22 cases. American Journal of Surgical Pathology 11: 114–121.

Lashgari M, Bemmaram B, Hoffman J S et al 1992 Primary biliary carcinoma with metastasis to the ovary. Gynecologic Oncology 47: 272–274.

Leffel J M, Masson J C, Dockerty M B 1942 Krukenberg's tumors: a survey of forty-four cases. Annals of Surgery 115: 102–113.

Linard P 1964 Carcinomes metastatiques bilateraux des ovaries du tumeurs du Krukenberg. Journal de Chirurgie 62: 15–29.

LiVolsi V A, Merino M J, Schwarz P E 1983 Coexistent endocervical adenocarcinoma and mucinous adenocarcinoma of ovary: a clinicopathological study of four cases. International Journal of Gynecological Pathology 1: 391–402.

Luisi A 1968 Metastatic ovarian tumours. In: Junqueira A C, Gentil F (eds) Ovarian cancer, UICC monograph series, vol 11. Springer Verlag, Berlin, pp 87–104.

McDuff H C 1950 Metastatic Krukenberg tumor of the ovary: primary in the breast with six-year survival. Rhode Island Medical Journal 33: 589–593.

McGoogan L S, Hatch K D 1972 Krukenberg tumor: report of two cases. Nebraska Medical Journal 57: 409–415.

Malviya V K, Baysal M, Chayiuiau P, Deppe G, Lauersen H, Gordon R E 1982 Small cell anaplastic lung cancer presenting as an ovarian metastasis. International Journal of Gynaecology and Obstetrics 20: 487–493.

Mann W J, Chumas J, Amalfitano T, Westermann C, Patsner C 1987 Ovarian metastases from Stage 1B adenocarcinoma of the cervix. Cancer 60: 1123–1126.

Martzloff K H, Manlove C H 1949 Vaginal and ovarian metastases from hypernephroma: report of a case and review of the literature. Surgery, Gynecology and Obstetrics 88: 145–154.

Mazur M T, Hsueh S, Gersell D J 1984 Patterns of metastasis to the female genital tract: analysis of 325 cases. Cancer 53: 1978–1984.

Merino M J, Edmonds P, LiVolsi V 1985 Appendiceal carcinoma metastatic to the ovaries and mimicking primary ovarian tumors. International Journal of Gynecological Pathology 4: 110–120.

Monteagodo C, Merino M J, LaPorte N, Neumann R D 1991 Value of gross cystic disease fluid protein-15 in distinguishing metastatic breast carcinomas amongst poorly differentiated neoplasms involving the ovary. Human Pathology 22: 368–372.

Moore J G, Schifrin B S, Erez S 1967 Ovarian tumors in infancy, childhood and adolescence. American Journal of Obstetrics and Gynaecology 99: 913–922.

Morrow M, Enker W E 1984 Late ovarian metastases in carcinoma of the colon and rectum. Archives of Surgery 119: 1385–1388.

O'Brien P H, Newton B B, Metcalfe J S, Rittenburg M S 1981 Oophorectomy in women with carcinoma of the colon and rectum. Surgery, Gynecology and Obstetrics 153: 827–830.

Osborne M P, Pitts R M 1961 Therapeutic oophorectomy for advanced breast cancer: the significance of metastases to the ovary and of ovarian cortical stromal hyperplasias. Cancer 14: 128–130.

Paone J F, Bixler T J, Imbembo A L 1978 Primary mucinous adenocarcinoma of appendix with bilateral ovarian Krukenberg tumors. Johns Hopkins Medical Journal 143: 43–47.

Parnanen P O, Vataja U 1954 Metastatic carcinoma of the ovary. Annales Chirurgie Fennae 43 (suppl 5): 322–331.

Paterson E 1961 Distant metastases from medulloblastoma of the cerebellum. Brain 84: 301–309.

Petru E, Pickel H, Haydarfadai M et al 1992 Nongenital cancer metastatic to the ovary. Gynecologic Oncology 44: 83–86.

Piura B, Glezerman M 1989 Synchronous carcinomas of endometrium and ovary. Gynecologic Oncology 33: 261–264.

Prat J, Matias-Guiu X, Barreto J 1991 Simultaneous carcinoma involving the endometrium and the ovary: a clinicopathologic, immunohistochemical and DNA flow cytometric study of 18 cases. Cancer 68: 2455–2459.

Richardson G S 1967 Ovariectomy in cancer of the colon. New England Journal of Medicine 276: 526.

Robboy S J, Scully R E, Norris H J 1974 Carcinoid metastatic to the ovary: a clinicopathologic analysis of 35 cases. Cancer 33: 798–811.

Santesson L, Kottmeier H L 1968 General classification of ovarian tumours. In: Junqueira A C, Gentil F (eds) Ovarian cancer, UICC monograph series, vol 11. Springer Verlag, Berlin, pp 1–8.

Saphir O 1951 Signet-ring cell carcinoma. Military Surgeon 105: 360–369.

Schlagenhauffer F 1902 Ueber das metastatiche Ovarialcarcinoma nach Krebs des Magens, Darmes und anderer Bauchorgane. Monatschrift fur Geburtshilfe und Gynakologie 15: 485–528.

Scully R E 1979 Tumors of the ovary and maldeveloped gonads. Atlas of tumor pathology, second series, fascicle 16. Armed Forces Institute of Pathology, Washington DC.

Scully R E 1993 Small cell carcinoma of hypercalcemic type. International Journal of Gynecological Pathology 12: 148–152.

Scully R E, Richardson G S 1961 Luteinization of the stroma of metastatic cancer involving the ovary and its endocrine significance. Cancer 14: 827–840.

Seidman J D, Elsayed A M, Sobin L H et al 1993 Association of mucinous tumours of the ovary and appendix: clinicopathologic study of 25 cases. American Journal of Surgical Pathology 17: 85–90.

Silverberg S G 1984 New aspects of endometrial carcinoma. Clinics in Obstetrics and Gynaecology 11: 189–208.

Soloway I, Latour J P A, Young M H V 1956 Krukenberg tumors of the ovary. Obstetrics and Gynecology 8: 636–638.

Spandoni L R, Linoberg M C, Mottet N K, Herman W L 1965 Virilization co-existing with Krukenberg tumor during pregnancy. American Journal of Obstetrics and Gynecology 92: 198–201.

Sty J R, Kum L F, Casper J T 1980 Bone scintigraphy in neuroblastoma with ovarian metastasis. Winsconsin Medical Journal 79: 28–29.

Sutton G P, Bundy B N, Delgado G et al 1992 Ovarian metastases in Stage 1b carcinoma of the cervix: a Gynecologic Oncology Group study. American Journal of Obstetrics and Gynecology 166: 50–53.

Svenes K B, Eide J 1984 Proliferative Brenner tumor or ovarian metastases? A case report. Cancer 53: 2692–2697.

Tabata M, Ichinoe K, Skuragi N et al 1986 Incidence of ovarian metastasis in patients with cancer of the uterine cervix. Gynecologic Oncology 28: 255–261.

Thorsen P, Dybdahl H, Sogaard H, Moller B R 1991 Ovarian tumors caused by metastatic tumors of the appendix: two case reports. European Journal of Obstetrics, Gynecology and Reproductive Biology 40: 67–71.

Toki N, Tsukamoto N, Kaku T et al 1991 Microscopic ovarian metastasis of uterine cervical cancer. Gynecologic Oncology 41.

Turksoy N 1960 Ovarian metastasis of breast carcinoma: a surgical surprise. Obstetrics and Gynecology 15: 573–578.

Ulbright T M, Roth L M 1985 Metastatic and independent cancers of the endometrium and ovary: a clinicopathologic study of 34 cases. Human Pathology 16: 28–34.

Ulbright T M, Roth L M, Stehman F B 1984 Secondary ovarian neoplasms: a clinicopathologic study of 35 cases. Cancer 53: 1164–1174.

Van der Weiden R M F, Gratama S 1987 Proliferative and malignant Brenner tumors (BT) and their differentiation from metastatic transitional cell carcinoma of the bladder: a case report and review of the literature. European Journal of Obstetrics, Gynecology and Reproductive Biology 26: 251–260.

Virieux C 1962 Untersuchungen uber Haufigkeit und Enstehungweise von Krebsmetastasen in den Eirstocken. Gynaecologia (Basel) 153: 209–224.

von Numers C 1960 Sind die Krukenberg Tumoren wirklich metastatiche. Eierstockgeschwulste. Geburtshilfe und Frauenheilkunde 20: 726–731.

Vorder-Bruegge C G, Hobbl J E, Weener C R, Wintemute R W 1957 Bilateral ovarian metastases from renal adenocarcinoma. Obstetrics and Gynecology 9: 198–205.

Walther H 1948 Krebsmetastasen. Schwabe Verlag, Basel.

Ward R T H 1966 Krukenberg tumours in pregnancy. Australian and New Zealand Journal of Obstetrics and Gynaecology 6: 312–315.

Warren S, Gates O 1964 Lung cancer and metastases. Archives of Pathology 78: 467–473.

Warren S, Macomber W B 1935 Tumor metastasis. VI. Ovarian metastasis of carcinoma. Archives of Pathology 19: 75–82.

Webb M G, Decker D G, Mussey E 1975 Cancer metastatic to the ovary: factors influencing survival. Obstetrics and Gynecology 45: 391–396.

Willis R A 1952 The spread of tumours in the human body, 2nd edn. Butterworths, London.

Woodruff J D, Novak E R 1960 The Krukenberg tumor: study of 48 cases from the ovarian tumor registry. Obstetrics and Gynecology 15: 356–360.

Woodruff J D, Murphy Y S, Bhaskar T N, Borobar F, Tseng S S 1970 Metastatic ovarian tumors. American Journal of Obstetrics and Gynecology 107: 202–209.

Yoshida A, Shigematsu T, Mori H, Yoshida H, Fukunishi R 1981 Non-invasive thymoma with widespread blood-borne metastasis. Virchows Archives A Pathological Anatomy 390: 121–126.

Young R H, Hart W R 1989 Metastases from carcinoma of the pancreas simulating primary mucinous tumours of the ovary: a report of seven cases. American Journal of Surgical Pathology 13: 748–756.

Young R H, Hart W R 1992 Renal cell carcinoma metastatic to the ovary: a report of three cases emphasizing possible confusion with ovarian clear cell adenocarcinoma. International Journal of Gynecological Pathology 11: 96–104.

Young R H, Scully R E 1985 Ovarian metastases from cancer of the lung: problems in interpretation: a report of seven cases. Gynecologic Oncology 21: 337–350.

Young R H, Scully R E 1988 Urothelial and ovarian carcinomas of identical cell types: problems in interpretation: a report of three cases and review of the literature. International Journal of Gynecological Pathology 7: 197–211.

Young R H, Scully R E 1989 Alveolar rhabdomyosarcoma metastatic to the ovary: a report of two cases and discussion of the differential diagnosis of small cell malignant tumors of the ovary. Cancer 64: 899–904.

Young R H, Scully R E 1990a Ovarian metastases from carcinoma of the gallbladder and extrahepatic bile ducts simulating primary tumors of the ovary: a report of six cases. International Journal of Gynecological Pathology 9: 60–72.

Young R H, Scully R E 1990b Sarcomas metastatic to the ovary; a report of 21 cases. International Journal of Gynecological Pathology 9: 231–252.

Young R H, Scully R E 1991a Malignant melanoma metastatic to the ovary: a clinicopathologic analysis of 20 cases. American Journal of Surgical Pathology 15: 849–860.

Young R H, Scully R E 1991b Metastatic tumors of the ovary: a problem-orientated approach and review of the recent literature. Seminars in Diagnostic Pathology 8: 250–276.

Young R H, Carey R W, Robboy S J 1981 Breast carcinoma masquerading as primary ovarian neoplasm. Cancer 48: 210–212.

Young R H, Gilks C B, Scully R E 1991 Mucinous tumors of the appendix associated with mucinous tumors of the ovary and pseudomyxoma peritonei: a clinicopathological analysis of 22 cases supporting an origin in the appendix. American Journal of Surgical Pathology 15: 415–429.

Young R H, Gersell D J, Clement P B, Scully R E 1992 Hepatocellular carcinoma metastatic to the ovary: a report of three cases discovered during life with discussion of the differential diagnosis of hepatoid tumors of the ovary. Human Pathology 23: 574–580.

Young R H, Kozakewich H P W, Scully R E 1993a Metastatic ovarian tumors in children: a report of 14 cases and review of the literature. International Journal of Gynecological Pathology 12: 8–19.

Young R H, Gersell D J, Roth L M, Scully R E 1993b Ovarian metastases from cervical carcinomas other than pure adenocarcinomas: a report of 12 cases. Cancer 71: 407–418.

Young R H, Jackson A, Wells M 1994 Ovarian metastasis from thyroid carcinoma twelve years after thyroidectomy mimicking struma ovarii. International Journal of Gynecological Pathology 13: 181–185.

Zaind R J, Unger E R, Whitney C 1984 Synchronous carcinomas of the uterine corpus and ovary. Gynecological Oncology 19: 329–335.

Zirkin R, Brown S, Hertz M 1980 Adenocarcinoid of appendix presenting as bilateral ovarian tumors. Diagnostic Gynecology and Obstetrics 2: 269–274.

Zukerberg L R, Young R H 1990 Chordoma metastatic to the ovary. Archives of Pathology and Laboratory Medicine 114: 208–210.

28. Ovarian tumours of uncertain origin

Andrew J. Tiltman

INTRODUCTION

This chapter gathers together a number of miscellaneous, uncommon, primary tumours of the ovary which cannot be readily classified among the major categories of ovarian neoplasms. In some the histogenesis is presumed but in others it remains unknown. They can be divided broadly into three groups.

1. Those possibly of mesonephric or displaced renal blastemic origin
   a. Tumour of probable Wolffian origin
   b. Tumours of the rete ovarii
   c. Wilms' tumour
2. Small cell tumours
   a. Small cell undifferentiated carcinoma of hypercalcaemic type
   b. Small cell carcinoma of pulmonary type
   c. Desmoplastic small round cell tumour
3. A miscellaneous group, possibly of mesothelial or epithelial origin
   a. Adenomatoid tumour
   b. Hepatoid carcinoma
   c. Oncocytoma

TUMOURS OF POSSIBLE MESONEPHRIC ORIGIN

The mesonephros and the mesonephric ducts arise within the intermediate mesoderm early in embryogenesis. The mesonephric ducts are destined to form the trigone of the urinary bladder, the posterior wall of the urethra and, in the male, the epididymis and vas deferens. In the female, the mesonephric ducts degenerate at about 75 days gestation but remnants may be found in the uterine corpus, cervix and vagina as Gartner's duct, in the broad ligament as the paroophoron and adjacent to the ovary as the epoophoron (Duthie, 1925) and the rete ovarii (Wenzel & Odend'hal, 1985). The indifferent gonad develops medial to the mesonephros and the mesonephric blastema is thought to play a rôle in the development of both the testis and ovary (Wartenberg, 1982).

a. Ovarian tumours of probable Wolffian origin

In 1973 Kariminejad & Scully described nine distinctive paraovarian tumours which they called female adnexal tumours of probable Wolffian origin. Later, Hughesdon (1982) and Young & Scully (1983) described morphologically similar tumours arising in the ovary itself. Because of this similarity, the ovarian and paraovarian tumours are regarded as of the same histogenesis.

Morphology

Both ovarian and paraovarian tumours have been described as being solid or solid with cystic areas (Fig. 28.1) and have varied in size from 2–25 cm in greatest diameter. The cysts contain clear yellow or haemorrhagic fluid. The solid areas may be lobulated and consist of white or cream-coloured tissue. Haemorrhage may be present. In some instances close inspection may show a spongy appearance produced by smaller cysts (Fig. 28.2).

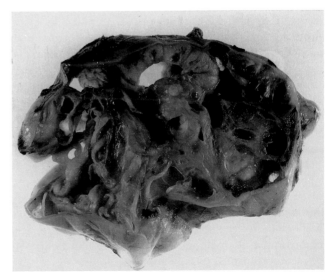

Fig. 28.1 Ovarian tumour of probable Wolffian origin which is mainly cystic with solid areas.

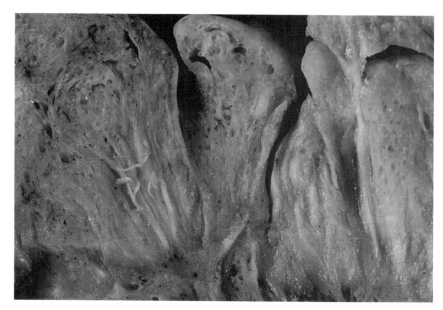

Fig. 28.2 Ovarian tumour of probable Wolffian origin showing a sponge-like appearance produced by numerous small cysts.

Microscopy shows a variety of appearances with epithelial cells arranged in tubules, as multiple dilated cysts or as diffuse sheets. All these may be present in the same tumour but one pattern often dominates.

The tubular pattern is formed by tubules or solid cords of cuboidal cells with central nuclei. The nuclei show diffuse chromatin and small nucleoli. Columnar cells and vacuolated cells have also been described. The tubules may be interwoven and branching, sometimes exhibiting a papillary or retiform appearance (Fig. 28.3), or may be so tightly packed as to resemble solid sheets on H&E-stained sections. A well-delineated PAS-positive basement membrane may be seen and reticulin stains reveal the true tubular or nested architecture (Fig. 28.4).

The cysts vary in size from very small to large and are separated by fibrous stroma or solid tumour. In places they have been described as imparting a sieve-like appearance (Fig. 28.5). In other areas, closely packed small spaces may resemble the appearance of an adenomatoid tumour (Fig. 28.6). The cells lining these spaces are flat, sometimes cuboidal and sometimes show a hobnail appearance with loss of cytoplasm. Occasionally the cells may contain coarse eosinophilic cytoplasmic granules (Fig. 28.7). The material within the cysts may stain weakly with PAS after digestion with diastase.

The solid sheets of tumour cells may be composed of polygonal cells (Fig. 28.8) or spindle cells resembling stroma. Reticulin stains usually delineate groups of cells. Small amounts of intracytoplasmic glycogen have been demonstrated. A small number of mitoses may be present but pleomorphism is usually absent.

A moderate vasculature is present throughout the tu-

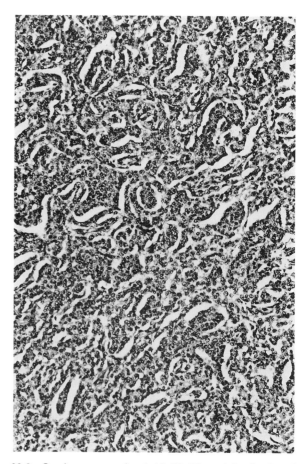

Fig. 28.3 Ovarian tumour of probable Wolffian origin. Cords and tubules with papillary formations giving a retiform appearance. H & E × 75.

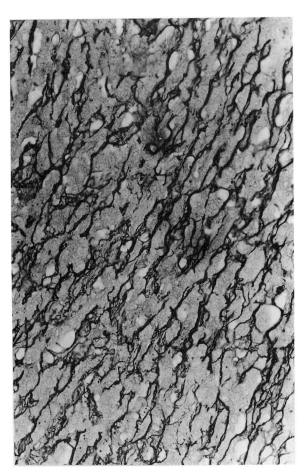

Fig. 28.4 Ovarian tumour of probable Wolffian origin. Reticulin stain showing cord-like structures. × 300.

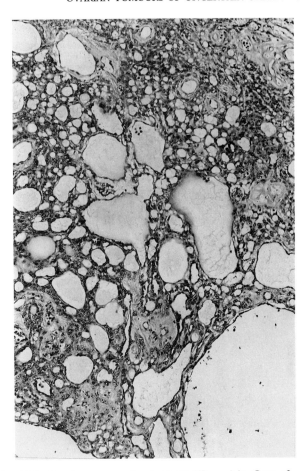

Fig. 28.5 Ovarian tumour of probable Wolffian origin. Cysts of varying sizes producing a sieve-like appearance. H & E × 75.

mour. The intervening stroma is fibrous and may become hyalinized, entrapping tumour cells within it (Fig. 28.9).

Clinical presentation and behaviour

The patients with tumours arising in the ovary have been between 28 and 79 years of age, with most patients in the sixth decade (mean 52 years). Those patients with para-ovarian tumours have been younger (18–62 years; mean 40 years) with several being less than 30 years. Presenting symptoms include lower abdominal pain, an enlarging abdomen or frequency of micturition. Most tumours are, however, discovered during pelvic examination for unrelated symptoms or are incidental findings at laparotomy. There is no evidence of any endocrine dysfunction.

Ovarian and paraovarian Wolffian tumours usually behave in a benign fashion but a small number of malignant ovarian (Hughesdon, 1982; Young & Scully, 1983) and paraovarian (Taxy & Battifora, 1976; Abbot et al, 1981) tumours have been reported. These malignant tumours have shown increased mitotic activity (> 10/10 high power

fields) or nuclear pleomorphism. One case showed areas described as undifferentiated carcinoma.

Histogenesis

The belief that these tumours are of Wolffian (meso-nephric) remnant origin is based on:

1. the observation that although epithelial in nature they do not resemble any of the ovarian tumours of Müllerian origin and have not been described in association with the common epithelial tumours
2. the fact that they are morphologically distinguishable from sex cord-stromal tumours such as Sertoli–Leydig or granulosa cell tumours
3. the finding that the extraovarian tumours occur at sites where Wolffian remnants are often found and that some of the ovarian tumours arise in the ovarian hilus where the rete ovarii could be the source
4. the presence of a prominent basement membrane around the epithelial tubules which is structurally

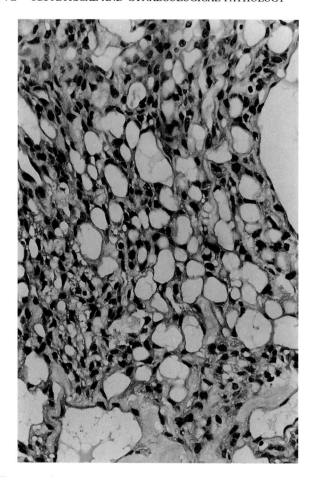

Fig. 28.6 Ovarian tumour of probable Wolffian origin. Small dilated tubules resembling an adenomatoid tumour. H & E × 300.

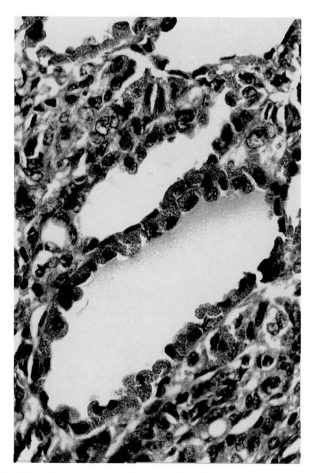

Fig. 28.7 Ovarian tumour of probable Wolffian origin. Small cystic spaces lined by cells with coarse granular cytoplasm. H & E × 500.

consistent with the Wolffian but not Müllerian ducts (Gardner et al, 1948; Lamb et al, 1960).

Ultrastructural examinations have not been helpful except that they show features compatible with a Wolffian, and do not support a Müllerian, origin (Taxy & Battifora; 1976, Demopoulos et al, 1980). Similarly, immunohistochemistry has done no more than support the compatibility between the tumour and Wolffian remnants (Tavassoli et al, 1990).

Differential diagnosis

Tumours of probable Wolffian origin need to be differentiated from Sertoli–Leydig cell tumours, granulosa cell tumours, clear cell carcinomas and adenomatoid tumours. Focal areas within the Wolffian tumours may closely mimic each of the above but if sufficient tissue is examined the variations in morphology become apparent.

Sertoli–Leydig cell tumours may show tubules, cords and solid areas composed of oval cells but the mixed composition is not as variable as that seen in the Wolffian tumour. The retiform type of Sertoli–Leydig tumour may, however, show larger spaces superficially resembling the

cystic areas in the Wolffian tumour. Sertoli–Leydig tumours usually contain luteinized stromal or Leydig cells and the patients may show endocrine manifestations.

On low power examination, the solid areas of a Wolffian tumour may resemble the diffuse form of granulosa cell tumour and, when admixed with cystic spaces, may superficially resemble the juvenile granulosa cell tumour. Granulosa cell tumours either show the typical cytological morphology of the adult type or the vacuolated cytoplasm of the juvenile form, both of which differ from the Wolffian tumour.

The cystic spaces lined by hobnail-like cells resemble those seen in the Müllerian clear cell carcinoma but the remainder of the Wolffian morphology is quite unlike that seen in the clear cell carcinoma.

The sponge-like areas and small cystic spaces may resemble the canalicular pattern of an adenomatoid tumour but the solid tubules and cords of the Wolffian tumour differ from the solid cords of the adenomatoid tumour, and solid spindle cell areas are not present in the latter. Adenomatoid tumours are generally much smaller and hyaluronic acid may be demonstrable in cytoplasmic vacuoles.

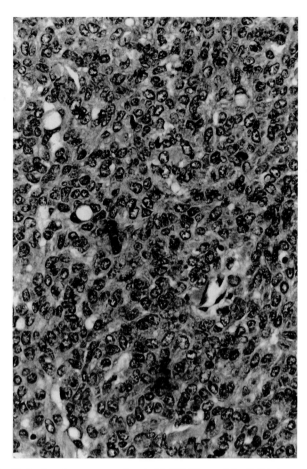

Fig. 28.8 Ovarian tumour of probable Wolffian origin. Solid sheets of polygonal cells. H & E × 300.

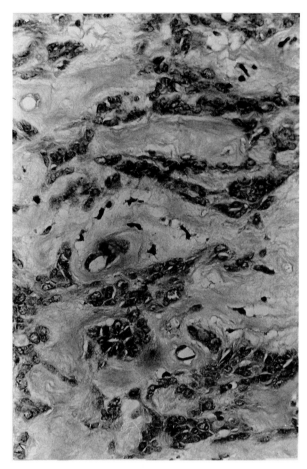

Fig. 28.9 Ovarian tumour of probable Wolffian origin. Hyalinized collagenous stroma with entrapped epithelial elements. H & E × 300.

b. Tumours of the rete ovarii

The rete ovarii is a small irregular tubular structure in the hilus of the ovary which is thought to be of mesonephric origin (Wenzel & Odend'hal, 1985). There is, therefore, a close, if not inseparable, histogenetic relationship between tumours arising from the rete and the tumours of probable Wolffian origin. In an early report a tumour arising in the ovarian hilus and later accepted as a Wolffian tumour was initially called an adenoma of the rete body (Greene & Dilts, 1965) and the review by Tavassoli et al (1990) referred to the Wolffian tumours as 'retiform' because of the close immunohistochemical and ultrastructural similarities. There are, however, a small group of morphologically distinct tumours of the rete ovarii.

Adenomas of the rete are rare, small tumours measuring up to 5 mm in diameter (Janovski & Paramanandhan, 1973). Microscopically they consist of tubules lined by a single layer of cuboidal or columnar cells morphologically resembling those of the rete (Rutgers & Scully, 1988). These tubules are separated and usually distorted by the supporting fibrous stroma and may contain intraluminal fibropapillary projections. Adenomatous hyperplasia of the rete is morphologically similar on high power exami-

nation (Fig. 28.10) but is not as well circumscribed as the adenoma. The dividing line between the two is not well defined. Cysts of the rete ovarii may measure up to 27 cm in diameter. Most of these are probably non-neoplastic but some cysts show stratification of the lining cells and have been regarded as cystadenomas (Rutgers & Scully, 1988). Adenocarcinoma of the rete is extremely rare. The case described by Rutgers & Scully (1988) showed a papillary and tubular pattern and also contained areas of urothelial-like cells.

c. Wilms' tumour

Extrarenal adult Wilms' tumours have been described in several sites including the ovary (Sahin & Benda, 1988) where they consist of blastematous tissue with tubules or glomeruloid structures surrounded by small spindle cells typical of Wilms' tumour in the kidney (Fig. 28.11). Nephroblastematous elements may be present in teratomas of the ovary (Nogales et al, 1980) and have also been described in association with a juvenile granulosa cell tumour where it was not certain whether it represented an independent tumour or was part of a mixed sex cord-stromal/germ cell neoplasm (O'Dowd & Ismail, 1990).

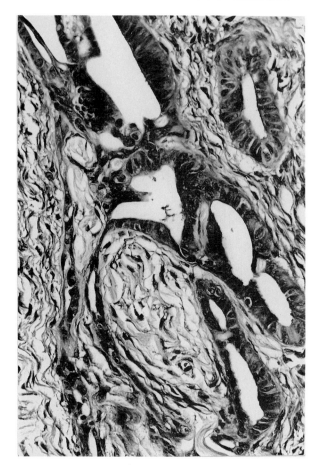

Fig. 28.10 Hyperplasia of rete ovarii. Tubules and cords lined by columnar cells within a fibrous stroma. H & E × 300.

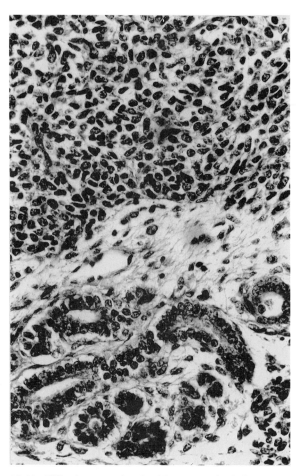

Fig. 28.11 Wilms' tumour showing blastema and tubular structures. H & E × 300.

The histogenetic theories of extrarenal Wilms' tumour include derivation from misplaced renal blastema, primitive extrarenal mesoderm or as part of a teratoma. A diagnosis of primary Wilms' tumour of the ovary requires that no teratomatous elements be present. The differential diagnosis includes other small cell tumours, Sertoli–Leydig cell tumours and malignant mixed Müllerian tumour.

SMALL CELL TUMOURS

A number of ovarian neoplasms consist of small cells with little cytoplasm. Some of these are metastatic to the ovary such as oat cell carcinoma from the lung, rhabdomyosarcoma, lobular carcinoma of the breast, melanoma, lymphomas and leukaemias. Others are primary ovarian neoplasms of known histogenesis such as primitive neuroectodermal tumour and granulosa cell tumours.

A third group of uncertain histogenesis includes:

a. Small cell undifferentiated carcinoma — hypercalcaemic type
b. Small cell carcinoma — pulmonary type
c. Desmoplastic small round cell tumour.

a. Small cell undifferentiated carcinoma — hypercalcaemic type

Small cell undifferentiated carcinoma of the ovary in young women was first described by Dickersin et al in 1982 in association with hypercalcaemia. Since then there have been several reports of morphologically similar tumours, but not always accompanied by raised serum calcium levels, and while the tumour is most frequently found in younger patients it is also described in older women.

Morphology

The tumours are generally unilateral and from 8–21 cm in greatest diameter. The cut surface shows solid tissue which is grey-white, grey-yellow or tan coloured. Haemorrhage and necrosis are frequently present and cystic degeneration or small cysts may be seen.

Microscopically the tumours are composed of small epithelial cells with little cytoplasm (Fig. 28.12). The nuclei are generally round or polygonal with some clumping of chromatin and a small nucleolus. Mitoses are easily

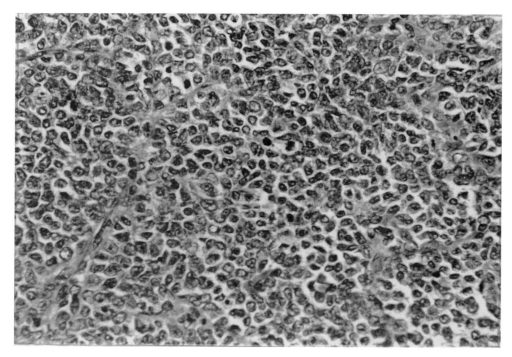

Fig. 28.12 Ovarian small cell carcinoma with hypercalcaemia. Small cells with little cytoplasm are lying in sheets. Elsewhere in the neoplasm there was extensive haemorrhage and necrosis. H & E × 860.

found but nuclear pleomorphism is not a feature and flow cytometric analysis has shown a diploid DNA content in all tumours examined (Eichhorn et al, 1992a). In about 25% of cases, larger cells with abundant cytoplasm may be seen and, in 10% of cases, cells containing intracytoplasmic mucin are present (Young et al, 1987). The cells are arranged in diffuse sheets, in smaller islands or as anastomosing cords. Small cystic, follicle-like, spaces surrounded by tumour cells are usually present. Necrosis is common.

Immunohistochemistry has shown varying results (Ulbright et al, 1987; Abeler et al, 1988; McMahon & Hart, 1988; Aguirre et al, 1989; Scully, 1993) which are summarized in Table 28.1. Tumour cells stain for both cytokeratins and vimentin. Neurone-specific enolase (NSE) is generally positive. Chromogranin may be present in some instances. Parathormone has been demonstrated in 4 of 26 patients, 11 of whom were hypercalcaemic, and alpha-antitrypsin in 3 of 6 tumours.

Electronmicroscopy confirms the epithelial nature of the cell with desmosome-like junctions and a basal lamina surrounding groups of cells (Dickersin et al, 1982; McMahon & Hart, 1988). Cells may be arranged around a central space and microvilli and cilia have been demonstrated. The cytoplasm typically contains dilated rough endoplasmic reticulum. In most studies neurosecretory granules have not been demonstrated but some workers (Abeler et al, 1988; Nesland & Abeler, 1989) have found scattered membrane-bound electron-dense granules in 3 of 6 cases examined.

Table 28.1 Immunohistochemistry of small cell carcinomas — hypercalcaemic type (SCC. HT) (Ulbright et al, 1987; Abeler et al, 1988; McMahon & Hart, 1988; Aguirre et al, 1989; Scully, 1993); small cell carcinoma — pulmonary type (SCC. PT) Eichhorn et al, 1992a) and desmoplastic small round cell tumour (DSRCT) (Young et al, 1992)

Antibody	no. positive/no. tested		
	SCC.HC	SCC.PT	DSRCT
Cytokeratin	5/6	6/9	
AE-1/AE-3	6/14		2/3
CAM 5.2	15/15		2/3
EMA	5/15	5/9	3/3
Vimentin	13/21	0/8	3/3*
NSE	15/21	6/9	1/3
Chromogranin	5/11	2/9*	0/3

AE-1/AE-3 = high molecular weight cytokeratin; CAM 5.2 = low molecular weight cytokeratin; EMA = epithelial membrane antigen; NSE = neurone-specific enolase; * = focal only

Clinical presentation and behaviour

The age at presentation ranges from 9–55 years with a mean age of 23 years. Few patients are over the age of 40 years. The presenting symptoms are typically abdominal swelling and/or pain. Hypercalcaemia, up to 4.5 mmol/l, which returns to normal after resection of the tumour and is not associated with bone involvement by tumour, occurs in about in two-thirds of the patients (Young et al, 1987).

Although tumours are frequently stage I at presentation, small cell carcinoma of the ovary has generally behaved in a very aggressive manner. In one series, 43 of

49 patients died of disease, usually within a year (Young et al, 1987). The remaining 6 were alive and disease free 4–11 years later. As with other ovarian carcinomas, spread is predominantly into the peritoneal cavity and retroperitoneal lymph nodes.

Histogenesis

Despite detailed morphological and immunohistochemical investigations the histogenesis of ovarian small cell carcinomas remains an enigma. While they are regarded as epithelial they do not resemble the common epithelial tumours of the ovary, are not seen in combination with them and generally occur at a younger age. This last factor has suggested a germ cell origin but other germ cell elements have not been seen in these tumours and the arguments presented by Ulbright et al (1987) in favour of a germ cell origin are not convincing. Neurosecretory granules have only been demonstrated by electronmicroscopy on rare occasions but chromogranin and NSE have been shown by immunohistochemistry. These have suggested a neuroendocrine cell origin but the overall morphology is not in keeping with such a conclusion.

Differential diagnosis

Small cell undifferentiated carcinoma needs to be distinguished from other small cell tumours.

Metastatic oat cell carcinoma from the lung may be recognized by the clinical history, pulmonary involvement and the widespread distribution of metastases. The cells are smaller and may show nuclear smearing. The nuclei show more diffuse chromatin and the nucleoli are generally inconspicuous. Small cell carcinomas of the oat cell type may also arise in the endometrium and cervix and metastasize to the ovary.

Other small cell tumours that may metastasize to the ovary include:

• Lobular carcinoma of the breast which may maintain its 'single file' growth pattern or show nests of small cells with central nuclei. Mucin may be demonstrable. Ovarian involvement is usually late and the presence of the breast primary obvious.
• Melanomas may present as small cell tumours but may show areas of pleomorphism. Melanin is usually demonstrable and the tumour cells are S100 positive.
• Rhabdomyosarcoma is an uncommon metastasis to the ovary (Young & Scully, 1989) and may have an alveolar growth pattern, multinucleate giant cells and bilateral involvement.
• Lymphomas and leukaemia may present as ovarian neoplasms (Osborne & Robboy, 1983; Fox et al, 1988; Monterroso et al, 1993). Their recognition may be confirmed by immunohistochemistry.

The juvenile granulosa cell tumour may be confused with small cell undifferentiated carcinoma. The follicles of the juvenile granulosa cell tumour are less regular in outline, sometimes appear to be surrounded by a collar of cells and contain weakly staining mucicarminophilic material. The cells show some pleomorphism and may contain lipid. The diffuse forms of adult granulosa cell tumour can resemble small cell carcinomas but the nuclei may show nuclear grooving and mitoses are infrequent.

Malignant neuroectodermal tumour of the ovary is of germ cell origin and may show focal glial or ependymal differentiation (Aguirre & Scully, 1982).

b. Small cell carcinoma — pulmonary type

Eichhorn et al (1992b) have recently described primary small cell carcinomas of the ovary that resemble small cell carcinomas of the lung and differ from the small cell undifferentiated carcinoma of hypercalcaemic type described above.

Morphology

As described by these authors, the tumours are bilateral in about half the cases and vary from 4.5–26 cm in greatest diameter. The cut surface shows solid tumour with cystic spaces. Microscopically the tumours are composed of small cells with little cytoplasm arranged in sheets, closely packed nests or islands. The nuclei are small, oval and generally monomorphic with evenly dispersed chromatin and small nucleoli. Flow cytometry has shown aneuploidy in five of the eight tumours investigated. The immunohistochemical findings are shown in Table 28.1. Occasional cells may demonstrate argyrophilia.

Clinical presentation and behaviour

The 11 cases reported by Eichhorn et al (1992b) presented at ages between 28 and 85 years (mean 59 years) with symptoms referable to the mass. Endocrine abnormalities were not present and no patient had hypercalcaemia. Six of the neoplasms were stage III on presentation but even the stage I tumours behaved in an aggressive fashion, with most patients either dead of disease or alive with recurrence within a year of presentation.

Histogenesis

Ovarian small cell carcinomas of pulmonary type are considered to be of neuroendocrine origin. Argyrophilic cells have been demonstrated in a range of ovarian epithelial tumours and, of the 11 cases of small cell carcinoma of pulmonary type reported by Eichhorn et al, four had an associated endometrioid carcinoma and two a benign Brenner tumour.

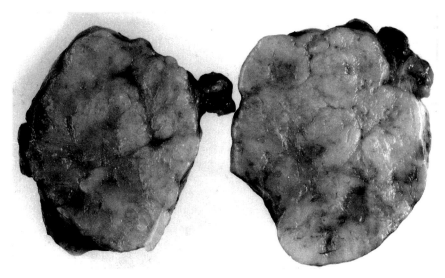

Fig. 28.13 Desmoplastic small round cell tumour. Two slices through a solid tumour showing a lobulated structure and small areas of haemorrhage.

Differential diagnosis

The differential diagnosis includes all those listed under small cell undifferentiated carcinoma — hypercalcaemic type. The small cell carcinoma of pulmonary type, which occurs at a mean age of 59 years, differs from the small cell undifferentiated carcinoma of hypercalcaemic type with a mean age of 23 years. In addition the pulmonary type is bilateral in about half the cases, may be associated with another epithelial component and is not associated with hypercalcaemia. In contrast to the hypercalcaemic type, the pulmonary type tumours may be aneuploid and are vimentin negative.

Ovarian small cell carcinoma of pulmonary type must be distinguished from metastatic carcinoma from the lung. If both lung and ovary are involved it is better regarded as a lung primary.

c. Desmoplastic small round cell tumour

The tumour designated intra-abdominal desmoplastic small round cell tumour with divergent differentiation occurs, as its name implies, within the abdominal cavity in young patients — mainly in the first and second decades but up to the age of 30 years with occasional cases in the fourth decade (Gerald et al, 1991). It is more common in males but three cases involving the ovary have been reported (Young et al, 1992) and two of these were initially regarded as primary at that site.

Morphology

Multiple tumour nodules are present within the abdominal cavity. The ovaries contain solid tan-white tumour (Fig. 28.13). Microscopically there are nests of small tumour cells separated by a fibrous stroma (Fig. 28.14).

Necrosis may be present in the centre of these islands and at the periphery there may be palisading of tumour cells. The tumour cells are small, with little cytoplasm and round to polygonal hyperchromatic nuclei with some

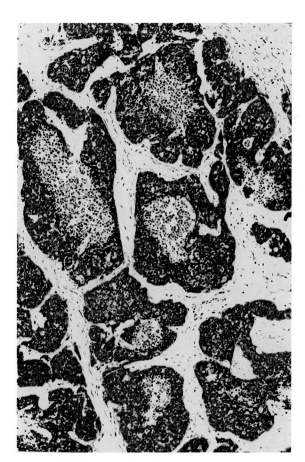

Fig. 28.14 Desmoplastic small round cell tumour. Nests of small tumour cells surrounded by fibrous stroma and showing central necrosis. H & E × 75.

chromatin clumping (Fig. 28.15). Mitoses are frequent. The fibrous stroma varies in cellularity with collagenous and occasional myxoid areas.

Immunohistochemistry shows positive staining with a wide spectrum of antibodies. Table 28.1 compares the findings to other small cell tumours of the ovary. In addition to those shown in the table, desmin characteristically stains as a paranuclear globule.

Electronmicroscopy shows cells with tight junctions, arranged in groups, sometimes with poorly formed lumina at the centre and surrounded at the periphery by a basal lamina. The cytoplasm contains numerous ribosomes, a few mitochondria and some glycogen.

Clinical presentation and behaviour

Desmoplastic small round cell tumour generally occurs in young patients. The three ovarian tumours reported by Young et al (1992) were 14, 15 and 15 years old. Other intra-abdominal cases, without ovarian involvement, have ranged in age from 3–38 years of age with a mean of about 18 years (Gonzalez-Crussi et al, 1990; Gerald et al, 1991; Variend et al, 1991). The tumours behave in a malignant fashion with death occurring within four years.

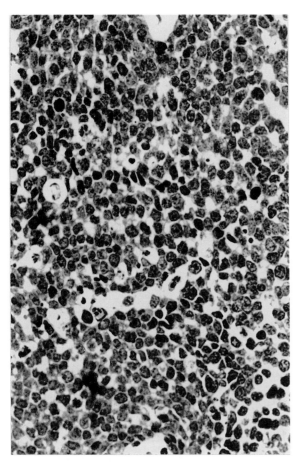

Fig. 28.15 Desmoplastic small round cell tumour. Nests consist of small cells with little cytoplasm. H & E × 500.

Histogenesis

The origin of desmoplastic small round cell tumour is not known. Some have considered a neuroectodermal (Variend et al, 1991) and others a mesothelial origin (Gerald et al, 1991).

Differential diagnosis

Desmoplastic small round cell tumour needs to be differentiated from other small cell tumours, as discussed under both hypercalcaemic and pulmonary types of small cell undifferentiated carcinoma. A striking feature of the desmoplastic tumour is the low magnification appearance of nests of cells separated by fibrous stroma.

MISCELLANEOUS TUMOURS

a. Adenomatoid tumours

Adenomatoid tumours are not infrequently found in the uterine corpus or adjacent to the Fallopian tube but are an uncommon finding in the ovary. Ovarian adenomatoid tumours have been reported in patients between 23 and 79 years of age and are usually incidental findings at surgery for some unrelated reason.

Morphology

Adenomatoid tumours of the ovary are generally small grey lesions measuring less than 1 cm in diameter and are usually present in the ovarian hilus extending into the medulla. Williamson & Moore (1964) describe a tumour measuring 3 cm in diameter occurring within the ovary, and a 5 cm juxtaovarian tumour is reported by Young et al (1991). The diffuse involvement of the ovary described by Morehead (1946) is not a convincing example of adenomatoid tumour.

Microscopically the typical features of adenomatoid tumours seen elsewhere may be present, either alone or in combination (Fig. 28.16). A plexiform pattern is produced by nests or cords of eosinophilic cuboidal cells, some of which may be vacuolated. A tubular pattern contains spaces lined by cuboidal cells. Vacuolation within the cytoplasm is usual. A canalicular pattern is produced by spaces of varying size lined by flattened cells. Scattered lymphocytes are frequently seen. Small amounts of smooth muscle may be present. Focal, intracytoplasmic positivity for Alcian Blue can be eliminated by prior digestion with hyaluronidase. Mucicarmine stain is negative.

Adenomatoid tumours are benign. It is generally held that they are of mesothelial origin but the almost exclusive occurrence within the genital tract has not been adequately explained.

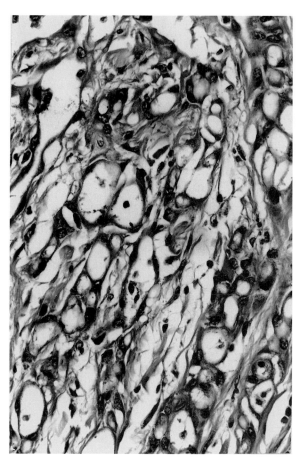

Fig. 28.16 Adenomatoid tumour showing both short cords of vacuolated cuboidal cells and dilated spaces lined by flattened cells. H & E × 300.

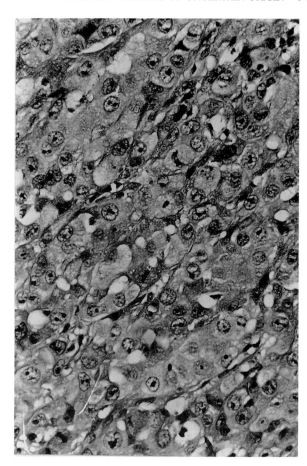

Fig. 28.17 Hepatoid carcinoma. Cells with abundant eosinophilic cytoplasm arranged in trabeculae. H & E × 300.

b. Hepatoid carcinoma

There are a small number of primary ovarian carcinomas which morphologically resemble hepatocellular carcinoma and have hence been labelled hepatoid carcinomas (Ishikura & Scully, 1987). These tumours have occurred in women between 42 and 78 years of age with no specific clinical presentation.

The tumours are solid or solid and cystic and have measured up to 20 cm in greatest diameter. Microscopically they are composed of cells with abundant eosinophilic cytoplasm and central nuclei. The cells are arranged in sheets or trabeculae (Fig. 28.17). Intra- and extracytoplasmic PAS-positive hyaline globules are present but sometimes only in small numbers (Fig. 28.18a). Variable numbers of giant cells are scattered throughout the tumour (Fig. 28.18b). Small amounts of glycogen may be demonstrated. Alphafetoprotein is present in the tumour cells and serum and is considered essential for the diagnosis.

The histogenesis of hepatoid carcinoma is unknown but it has been described in association with a 'tubular' adenocarcinoma and may possibly be the same as the common epithelial tumours of the ovary (Matsuta et al, 1991).

Hepatoid carcinoma needs to be distinguished from the hepatoid yolk sac tumour which is of germ cell origin, occurs at an earlier age and also contains areas showing more typical yolk sac features.

c. Oncocytic tumour

There have been two reports of oncocytic tumours of the ovary. One was a solid and cystic tumour measuring 15 cm in greatest diameter occurring in a 39-year-old woman (Takeda et al, 1983) and the other a solid tumour, 11 cm in diameter, in a 22-year-old woman (Yoshida et al, 1984). Microscopically, both showed cells with a granular eosinophilic cytoplasm and electronmicroscopy showed numerous mitochondria. In the first case, the cells were arranged in a tubular or papillary arrangement and in the second they were in solid sheets. The first tumour showed stromal invasion and was diagnosed as a carcinoma. The second was regarded as benign.

Ovarian oncocytoma may represent an oncocytic metaplasia within a common epithelial ovarian tumour and not a specific tumour type.

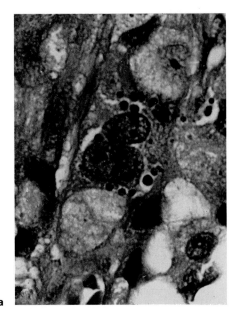
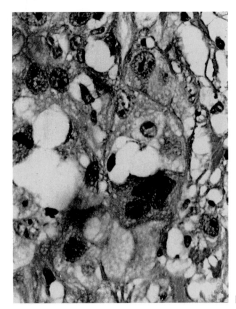

Fig. 28.18   Hepatoid carcinoma. **a** Hyaline globules. H & E × 800. **b** Giant cell. H & E × 300.

REFERENCES

Abbot R L, Barlogie B, Schmidt W A 1981 Metastasizing malignant juxtaovarian tumor with terminal hypercalcemia. Cancer 48: 860–865.

Abeler V, Kjorstad K E, Nesland J M 1988 Small cell carcinoma of the ovary. International Journal of Gynecological Pathology 7: 315–329.

Aguirre P, Scully R E 1982 Malignant neuroectodermal tumor of the ovary, a distinctive form of monodermal teratoma. American Journal of Surgical Pathology 6: 283–292.

Aguirre P, Thor A D, Scully R E 1989 Ovarian small cell carcinoma: histogenetic considerations based on immunohistochemical and other findings. American Journal of Clinical Pathology 92: 140–149.

Demopoulos R I, Sitelman A, Flotte T, Bigelow B 1980 Ultrastructural study of a female adnexal tumor of probable Wolffian origin. Cancer 46: 2273–2280.

Dickersin G R, Kline I W, Scully R E 1982 Small cell carcinoma of the ovary with hypercalcemia. Cancer 49: 188–197.

Duthie G M 1925 An investigation of the occurrence, distribution and histological structure of the embryonic remains in the human broad ligament. Journal of Anatomy 59: 410–431.

Eichhorn J H, Bell D A, Young R H et al 1992a DNA content and proliferative activity in ovarian small cell carcinomas of the hypercalcemic type: implications for diagnosis, prognosis and histogenesis. American Journal of Clinical Pathology 98: 579–586.

Eichhorn J H, Young R H, Scully R E 1992b Primary ovarian small cell carcinoma of pulmonary type: a clinicopathologic, immunohistologic and flow cytometric analysis of 11 cases. American Journal of Surgical Pathology 18: 926–938.

Fox H, Langley F A, Govan A D T, Hill A S, Bennett M H 1988 Malignant lymphoma presenting as an ovarian tumour: a clinicopathological analysis of 34 cases. British Journal of Obstetrics and Gynaecology 95: 386–390.

Gardner G H, Greene R R, Peckham B M 1948 Normal and cystic structures of the broad ligament. American Journal of Obstetrics and Gynecology 55: 917–939.

Gerald W L, Miller H K, Battifora H, Miettinen M, Silva E G, Rosai J 1991 Intra-abdominal desmoplastic small round-cell tumour. American Journal of Surgical Pathology 15: 499–513.

Gonzalez-Crussi F, Crawford S E, Sun C-C J 1990 Intra-abdominal desmoplastic small-cell tumors with divergent differentiation. American Journal of Surgical Pathology 14: 633–642.

Greene R R, Dilts P V 1965 Adenoma of the rete body. American Journal of Obstetrics and Gynecology 93: 886–888.

Hughesdon P E 1982 Ovarian tumours of Wolffian or allied nature: their place in ovarian oncology. Journal of Clinical Pathology 35: 526–535.

Ishikura H, Scully R E 1987 Hepatoid carcinoma of the ovary. Cancer 60: 2775–2784.

Janovski N A, Paramanandhan T L 1973 Ovarian tumors. In: Friedman E A (ed) Major problems in obstetrics and gynecology, vol 4. Saunders, Philadelphia, pp 104–105.

Kariminejad M H, Scully R E 1973 Female adnexal tumor of probable Wolffian origin: a distinctive pathologic entity. Cancer 31: 671–677.

Lamb E J, Fucilla I, Greene R R 1960 Basement membranes in the female genital tract. American Journal of Obstetrics and Gynecology 79: 79–85.

McMahon J T, Hart W R 1988 Ultrastructural analysis of small cell carcinomas of the ovary. American Journal of Clinical Pathology 90: 523–529.

Matsuta M, Ishikura H, Murakami K, Kagabu T, Nishiya I 1991 Hepatoid carcinoma of the ovary. International Journal of Gynecological Pathology 10: 302–310.

Monterroso V, Jaffe E S, Merino M J, Medeiros L J 1993 Malignant lymphoma involving the ovary: a clinicopathological analysis of 39 cases. American Journal of Surgical Pathology 17: 154–170.

Morehead R P 1946 Angiomatoid formations in the genital organs with and without tumor formation. Archives of Pathology and Laboratory Medicine 42: 56–63.

Nesland J M, Abeler V 1989 Response to letter by Scully R E and Dickersen G R. International Journal of Gynecological Pathology 8: 296–297.

Nogales F F, Ortega I, Rivera F, Armas J R 1980 Metanephrogenic tissue in immature ovarian teratoma. American Journal of Surgical Pathology 4: 297–299.

O'Dowd J, Ismail S M 1990 Juvenile granulosa cell tumour of the ovary containing a nodule of Wilm's tumour. Histopathology 17: 468–470.

Osborne B M, Robboy S J 1983 Lymphomas or leukemia presenting as ovarian tumors: an analysis of 42 cases. Cancer 52: 1933–1943.

Rutgers J L, Scully R E 1988 Cysts (cystadenomas) and tumors of the rete ovarii. International Journal of Gynecological Pathology 7: 330–342.

Sahin A, Benda J A 1988 Primary ovarian Wilm's tumor. Cancer 61: 1460–1463.

Scully R E 1993 Small cell carcinoma of hypercalcemic type. International Journal of Gynecological Pathology 12: 148–152.

Takeda A, Matsuyama M, Sugimoto Y et al 1983 Oncocytic adenocarcinoma of the ovary. Virchows Archiv A Pathological Anatomy and Histology 399: 345–353.

Tavassoli F A, Andrade R, Merino M 1990 Retiform Wolffian adenoma. In: Fenoglio Preizer C (ed) Progress in surgical pathology 11: 121–136.

Taxy J B, Battifora H 1976 Female adnexal tumor of probable Wolffian origin: evidence for a low grade malignancy. Cancer 37: 2349–2354.

Ulbright T M, Roth L M, Stehman F B, Talerman A, Senekjian E K 1987 Poorly differentiated (small cell) carcinoma of the ovary in young women: evidence supporting a germ cell origin. Human Pathology 18: 175–184.

Variend S, Gerrard M, Norris P D, Goepel J R 1991 Intra-abdominal neuroectodermal tumour of childhood with divergent differentiation. Histopathology 18: 45–51.

Wartenberg H 1982 Development of the early human ovary and role of the mesonephros in the differentiation of the cortex. Anatomy and Embryology 165: 253–280.

Wenzel J G, Odend'hal S 1985 The mammalian rete ovarii: a literature review. Cornell Veterinarian 75: 411–425.

Williamson H O, Moore M P 1964 Ovarian and paraovarian adenomatoid tumors. American Journal of Obstetrics and Gynecology 90: 388–394.

Yoshida Y, Tenzaki T, Ishiguro T, Kawanami D, Ohshima M 1984 Oncocytoma of the ovary: light and electron microscopic study. Gynecologic Oncology 18: 109–114.

Young R H, Scully R E 1983 Ovarian tumors of probable Wolffian origin: a report of 11 cases. American Journal of Surgical Pathology 7: 125–135.

Young R H, Dickersin G R, Scully R E 1987 Small cell carcinoma of the ovary: an analysis of 75 cases of a distinctive ovarian tumor commonly associated with hypercalcemia. Laboratory Investigation 56: 89A.

Young R H, Silva E G, Scully R E 1991 Ovarian and juxtaovarian adenomatoid tumors: a report of 6 cases. International Journal of Gynecological Pathology 10: 364–371.

Young R, Eichhorn J H, Dickersin G R, Scully R E 1992 Ovarian involvement by the intra-abdominal desmoplastic small round cell tumour with divergent differentiation: a report of three cases. Human Pathology 23: 454–464.

29. Ovarian tumours with functioning stroma

Robert E. Scully

INTRODUCTION

Although the stroma of ovarian carcinomas is often similar to that of carcinomas elsewhere in the body, being desmoplastic, hyaline, myxoid or oedematous, it, as well as the stroma of benign epithelial tumours, may resemble the specialized ovarian stroma and its derivatives. In such cases, it may be composed of intersecting fascicles of collagen-producing small spindle cells or it may exhibit a storiform pattern; occasionally, it contains plump cells reminiscent of theca externa cells, ill-defined, lipid-rich cells similar to theca interna cells, or large, rounded, polyhedral cells that contain varying amounts of lipid and resemble luteinized theca cells and luteinized stromal cells (Fig. 29.1). Exceptionally, the cells that resemble lutein cells have crystals of Reinke in their cytoplasm, identifying them as Leydig cells (Fig. 29.2). The tumour stroma that contains theca, lutein and Leydig-type cells may be seen within the neoplasm, adjacent to it, or in both locations.

When tumours other than those in the sex cord-stromal category have a stroma that is morphologically compatible with steroid hormone secretion and are associated with clinical, biochemical or pathological evidence of endocrine function, they have been categorized under the rubric 'ovarian tumours with functioning stroma' (Scully & Morris, 1957). These tumours may be benign or malignant, and if the latter, primary or metastatic; they are capable of secreting oestrogens, androgens, and progesterone as well as combinations of these hormones. Almost all types of ovarian tumour, including non-epithelial tumours, have been reported to contain functioning stroma, but with widely varying frequencies.

The 'specialized ovarian tumours', or sex cord-stromal tumours, have been excluded by convention from the category of ovarian tumours with functioning stroma even though evidence exists that the 'stromal' component of at least some of them may be stromal in the usual sense of the term rather than neoplastic. Fathalla (1968), for example, has emphasized that when a granulosa cell tumour or Sertoli–Leydig cell tumour grows outside the ovary its

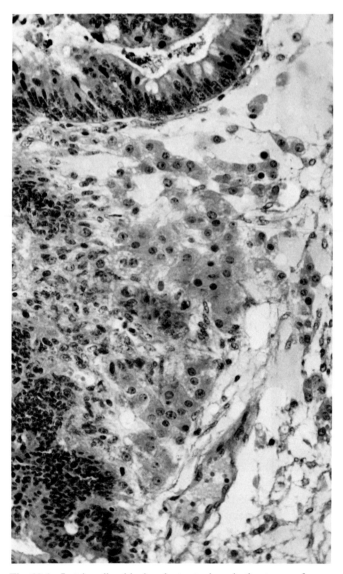

Fig. 29.1 Lutein cells with abundant cytoplasm in the stroma of a metastatic adenocarcinoma from the colon. H & E × 250. (From Scully & Richardson, 1961 [Fig. 3].)

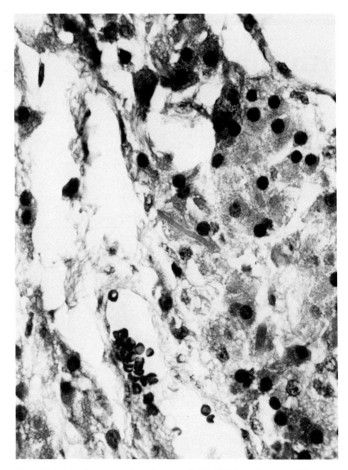

Fig. 29.2 An intracytoplasmic crystalloid of Reinke in a steroid-type cell adjacent to a strumal carcinoid. H & E × 650.

theca or Leydig cell component, respectively, is absent in most cases and endocrine effects are inapparent, suggesting that these cell types are reactive rather than neoplastic. Nevertheless, theca cells or Leydig cells are sometimes present in extraovarian tumour and are generally considered neoplastic rather than reactive for purposes of classification (Scully, 1979). Sex cord-stromal tumours are discussed in Chapter 22.

Although the major focus in cases of ovarian tumours with functioning stroma has been on their content of steroid-type lutein or Leydig cells as the source of the steroid hormone excess, the correlation between the finding of these cells and endocrine manifestations is imperfect. These cells may be present, sometimes in abundance, in the absence of endocrine manifestations, and conversely, evidence of steroid hormone production may exist in cases in which steroid-type cells cannot be found despite careful search (Fathalla, 1968; Rome et al, 1973, 1981). Several explanations are possible for these apparent discrepancies:

1. An absence of associated endocrine manifestations is not surprising since they are often absent in patients with 'functioning tumours' of other types such as granulosa cell tumours, Sertoli-stromal cell tumours and steroid cell tumours.

2. The failure to find steroid-type cells in the stroma of tumours associated with hormonal changes could be due to inadequate sampling of the tumour.

3. Immunohistochemical staining to demonstrate enzymes that take part in the interconversion of steroid hormones has disclosed in cases of stromal hyperthecosis staining of spindle-shaped cells that are transitional between unstained ovarian stromal cells and stained steroid-type lutein cells. These intermediate cells are difficult to identify in routinely stained sections and may be impossible to identify in the absence of associated steroid-type cells despite their apparent ability to secrete steroid hormones.

4. Finally, there is evidence that neoplastic ovarian epithelial cells may contribute to steroid hormone formation in tumours in the functioning stroma category. It has been known for some time that carcinoma cells, including those of ovarian cancers (Thompson et al, 1988), are capable of aromatization of androgens to oestrogens. More recently, it has been shown that ovarian epithelial cancer cells grown in culture (even from metastatic sites, where contamination by ovarian-type stroma is excluded), can secrete oestrogens and progesterone (Wimalasena et al, 1992) and that women with ovarian cancer secrete an excess of a variety of steroid hormones (Heinonen et al, 1986), with the highest levels in patients with extensive extraovarian disease (Backstrom et al, 1983; Mahlck et al, 1986, 1988, 1990). These latter findings suggest that the neoplastic epithelial cells rather than stroma derived from ovarian stroma are responsible for steroid hormone secretion in some cases and that these cells may have a similar rôle in so-called ovarian tumours with functioning stroma.

HISTORICAL ASPECTS

Moulonguet-Doleris (1924) appears to have been the first author to recognize an association of non-specialized ovarian tumours with oestrogenic manifestations, having reported reactivation of the endometrium in 19 of 74 postmenopausal women with benign and malignant ovarian tumours (26%). Five years later Esau (1929) described a Krukenberg tumour that virilized a pregnant woman. Subsequently, numerous investigators (Smith, 1937; Taylor & Millem, 1938; Grayzel & Friedman, 1941; Marwil & Beaver, 1942; Scott, 1942; Bettinger & Jacobs, 1946; Andujar et al, 1947; Teoh, 1953; Cariker & Dockerty, 1954; Biggart & MacAfee, 1955; Turunen, 1955) reported single cases or small series of cases of various types of ovarian tumour associated with either endometrial hyperplasia or virilization; some of these authors speculated that the stroma of the tumours they described was responsible for the endocrine manifestations. In 1957 Scully & Morris introduced the term 'ovarian tumours with functioning stroma' to include all types of neoplasms in this category exclusive of those in the sex cord-stromal group, and in 1986 Rutgers & Scully divided these tumours into two major groups: those in which the functioning stroma is within the neoplasm and those in which it lies adjacent to the neoplasm, so-called functioning ovarian tumours with peripheral steroid cell proliferation. The steroid cells in the latter group of tumours may be luteinized stromal cells, Leydig cells of stromal origin or hilus cells. Numerous additional clinico-pathological, histochemical and biochemical studies have greatly expanded knowledge of these tumours.

FREQUENCY

How often the stroma of an ovarian tumour is endocrinologically active is impossible to establish on the basis of currently available data. In the great majority of cases of ovarian tumours steroid hormone levels are not measured, and one has to rely on clinical manifestations, histological changes in end organs (cystic hyperplasia, secretory changes in the endometrium, or endometrial atrophy; salpingeal epithelial hyperplasia; ectopic decidua in the ovary; and squamous epithelial maturation in vaginal cytological preparations), to determine the presence or absence of an endocrine change. When a patient has become virilized recently and the androgenic manifestations disappear postoperatively, there is generally no problem relating them to the excised ovarian tumour. When, however, the clinical abnormality is of oestrogenic type, usually in the form of an abnormality of uterine bleeding, it may be impossible to ascribe it confidently to hormone secretion by the tumour, particularly if endometrium is not available for microscopical examination and menstrual function is not carefully monitored after removal of the tumour. A shift of the vaginal smear towards greater maturation than expected for the age of the patient suggests a high oestrogen level, but is not entirely reliable in this regard. Even when elevation of the oestrogen level has been demonstrated, it may be uncertain whether the stroma of the tumour was the cause of it or whether a coincidental lesion elsewhere in the ovarian tissue, such as stromal hyperthecosis or follicle cysts, or even an extraovarian factor, such as obesity, was responsible.

Cumulative evidence from the literature, however, supports the view that not only do 'non-specialized' ovarian tumours secrete stromal hormones but that this phenomenon is of frequent occurrence. Nine of 23 women with carcinoma of the ovary (39%) were reported by Rubin & Frost (1963) to have an oestrogenic type of vaginal smear, and Edwards et al (1971) recorded a similar finding in 10 of 22 postmenopausal women with ovarian cancer (45%). Wren & Frampton (1963) reported that 56% of 64 postmenopausal women with surface epithelial tumours had a moderate to marked oestrogen effect in their vaginal cytological preparations in contrast to only 28% of

570 postmenopausal women without ovarian tumours. Finally, Vesterinen and his associates (1978) found that 30% of postmenopausal women with ovarian cystadenomas had moderate to strong oestrogenic activity in their vaginal smears in contrast to only 13% of control women.

Eddie (1967) concluded that 31% of 147 postmenopausal women with surface epithelial-stromal tumours had histological evidence of definite endometrial activity indicative of abnormal oestrogenic production, Fathalla (1968) reported moderate or marked oestrogenic endometrial activity in 22% of 255 postmenopausal women with surface epithelial-stromal tumours and Rome et al (1981) found that 47% of 66 postmenopausal women with such tumours or metastatic carcinomas had a proliferative or hyperplastic endometrium. A number of authors (Smith, 1937; McNulty, 1959; Tighe, 1961; Fox, 1965; Jorgensen et al, 1970; Ehrlich & Roth, 1971; Silverberg, 1971; Fox et al, 1972) have recorded frequencies of postmenopausal endometrial proliferation and hyperplasia in the range of 10–100% in series of cases of specific subtypes of surface epithelial tumour.

The most informative studies of ovarian tumours with oestrogenic manifestations are those of Rome and his associates (1973, 1981). In their earlier publication those investigators reported that 23% of 31 postmenopausal women with surface epithelial-stromal tumours had elevated total urinary oestrogens, 45% had high urinary pregnanediol levels and 55% had high values for either one or both of these hormones. 'Stromal proliferation' within the ovarian tumour was noted in three of the six women with high oestrogen levels, but in only five of the 21 women with normal levels. In their later investigation, the authors found that 40 of 80 postmenopausal women with benign and malignant surface epithelial-stromal tumours or carcinomas metastatic to the ovary (50%) had elevated urinary oestrogen levels. 73% of those patients had luteinization of the tumour stroma, 'condensation' of the stroma, or both; a proliferative or hyperplastic endometrium was found in 68% of the patients with a high oestrogen excretion, but in only 18% of those with normal oestrogen levels. Those studies suggest that approximately half the tumours in the surface epithelial-stromal category possess a functioning stroma, as evidenced by elevated oestrogen levels.

Aiman et al (1986) found that four of 11 premenopausal females with benign and malignant epithelial and germ cell tumours had evidence of increased testosterone or androstenedione or both in their peripheral or ovarian venous blood.

FREQUENCY OF STROMAL FUNCTION AND HISTOLOGICAL VARIATIONS IN THE STROMA ACCORDING TO TUMOUR TYPE

Almost every type of ovarian tumour has been reported to

have a functioning stroma, but its histological appearance and frequency differ from one tumour type to another.

When stromal changes compatible with steroid hormone secretion are encountered in surface epithelial-stromal tumours, they are typically intraneoplastic although they may be at the periphery, particularly in cases of unilocular cystic tumours, which have no intrinsic stroma. The frequency of stromal function in benign serous neoplasms is difficult to determine because of differences in terminology and uncertainty whether simple cysts, cystadenomas and cystadenofibromas or various combinations thereof have been included in some of the series that have been analysed. For example, Eddie (1967) found that only three of 40 serous, simple, or cystadenomatous cysts (8%) were accompanied by evidence of endometrial activity after the menopause, whereas McNulty (1959) reported endometrial hyperplasia in association with 11 of 16 serous cystadenofibromas (69%) and Fox (1965) found endometrial proliferation or cystic or adenomatous hyperplasia in eight of 13 postmenopausal women with serous cystadenomas (62%). Rome and his associates (1981) reported elevated urinary oestrogens in three of four cases of serous cystadenofibroma, but in none of four cases of serous cystadenoma. The serous carcinoma, which is typically associated with a desmoplastic stroma rather than one resembling ovarian stroma, is only rarely accompanied by oestrogenic manifestations. Rome et al (1981) found elevated urinary oestrogens in only one of 20 cases of this type of tumour. Three serous cystadenomas (Fayez et al, 1974; Beauchamp et al, 1989; Okolo et al, 1990) and one serous adenocarcinoma (Plotz et al, 1966) have resulted in virilization, although the microscopic illustrations of one of the cystadenomas (Beauchamp et al, 1989) are more compatible with a rete cyst (adenoma) with adjacent hilus cell proliferation than a serous cystadenoma.

Mucinous tumours, whether benign, borderline or malignant, are associated with evidence of hyperoestrinism more often than serous tumours. Also, the former are accompanied by virilization more frequently than other primary ovarian tumours in the functioning stroma category. Eddie (1967) found an active endometrium in eight of 33 postmenopausal women with mucinous cystadenomas (24%) and in two of seven with mucinous cystadenocarcinomas (29%). Edwards and his associates (1971) reported that urinary oestriol excretion was higher in cases of mucinous cystadenoma and carcinoma than in those of serous tumours of corresponding types. Rome et al (1981) demonstrated elevated oestrogen levels in the urine in 11 of 17 postmenopausal women with mucinous cystadenomas and cystadenofibromas (65%) and in nine of 11 women in this age group with mucinous borderline tumours and carcinomas (82%). Thirteen cases of virilizing mucinous cystadenoma (Fig. 29.3), cystic tumour of borderline malignancy and low-grade cystadenocarci-

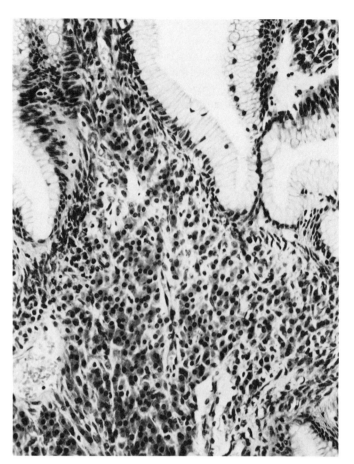

Fig. 29.3 Luteinization of the stroma in a 21-year-old woman virilized during pregnancy by a mucinous cystadenoma. H & E × 256.

noma have also been described (DaCosta, 1938; Bettinger & Jacobs, 1946; Scully, 1962; Novak et al, 1970; Chan & Prathap, 1970; Bronstein et al, 1972; Verhoeven et al, 1973; Post et al, 1978; Cotton et al, 1981; Quinn et al, 1983; Rutgers & Scully, 1986; Alvarez & Varner, 1987). In several of those cases the steroid-type cells were peripheral, and in two of them, the peripheral cells were hilus cells (Rutgers & Scully, 1986).

Isolated cases of endometrioid carcinoma of the ovary have been reported in association with postmenopausal endometrial hyperplasia (Scully & Morris, 1957; Hughesdon, 1958; Young et al, 1982); in one case the patient was virilized and had secretion in the breasts as well (Scully & Morris, 1957). The rarity of reports of oestrogenic changes accompanying endometrioid carcinomas may be related at least partly to lack of recognition of these tumours in the earlier days when most of the studies cited above were being performed. More recently, Rome and his co-workers (1981) found elevated urinary oestrogens in five of six cases of endometrioid carcinoma. Clear cell carcinomas have only rarely been documented to be accompanied by endometrial hyperplasia (Hughesdon, 1958); Rome et al (1981) found normal urinary oestrogens in four cases of this type of tumour. The latter investigators, however, reported elevated urinary oestrogen levels in two of three cases of undifferentiated carcinoma.

Brenner tumours have been associated with endometrial hyperplasia in from 10–16% of the cases in various series in the literature (Tighe, 1961; Jorgensen et al, 1970; Ehrlich & Roth, 1971; Silverberg, 1971; Fox et al, 1972; Balasa et al, 1977). One oestrogenic Brenner tumour was malignant (Kühnel et al, 1987). In another case (Hameed, 1972) Leydig cells were present in the stroma of the tumour. Three examples of virilizing Brenner tumour have also been recorded (Morris & Scully, 1958; Besch et al, 1963; Hamwi et al, 1963; Meiling et al, 1963; DeLima et al, 1989).

Germ cell tumours have been reported to have oestrogenic, androgenic and progestagenic manifestations (Herrington & Scully, 1983), but less often than surface epithelial-stromal tumours, possibly due to their relative rarity. Virilizing dysgerminomas were described occasionally in the older literature, but some of them were poorly documented and others would be reclassified as gonadoblastomas according to modern criteria. The dysgerminomas that have been most clearly associated with endocrine

function have been those containing syncytiotrophoblast cells (Fig. 29.4); cases of this type account for at least 3% of all tumours in the dysgerminoma category (Zaloudek et al, 1981). Dysgerminomas with syncytiotrophoblast cells have been accompanied by menstrual irregularities in postpubertal females (Zaloudek et al, 1981), isosexual precocity in one child (Ueda et al, 1972), and virilization in another (Case Records of the Massachusetts General Hospital, Case 11, 1972). In one patient an Arias-Stella-like reaction was found in the endometrium (Zaloudek et al, 1981). In some of the above cases lutein cells were described, particularly in the peripheral portions of the tumour and in the adjacent ovarian stroma (Fig. 29.5). Similar cells were also found in the contralateral ovary, which was uninvolved by tumour, in the case of Ueda et al (1972).

Various rare germ cell tumours — choriocarcinoma (Serment et al, 1970; DeLima & Carvalho, 1978), embryonal carcinoma (Kurman & Norris, 1976c), polyembryoma (Beck et al, 1969), and mixed germ cell tumours containing these components (Kurman & Norris, 1976a) — have also been accompanied by sexual precoc-

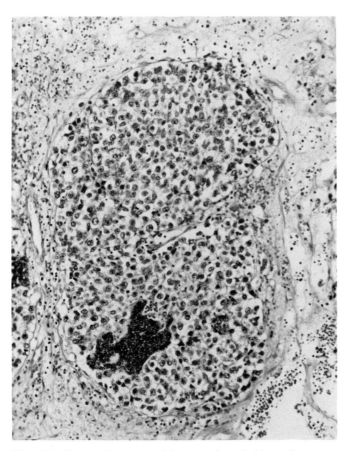

Fig. 29.4 Dysgerminoma containing syncytiotrophoblast cell. H & E × 130. (From Case Records of the Massachusetts General Hospital, Case 11, 1972 [Fig. 4].)

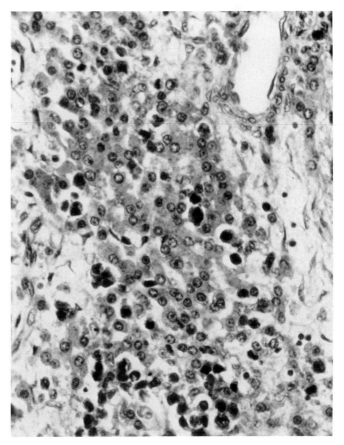

Fig. 29.5 Luteinization at the periphery of a dysgerminoma with syncytiotrophoblast cells. The tumour cells appear dark and shrunken as a result of torsion with early infarction. H & E × 375. (From Case Records of the Massachusetts General Hospital, Case 11, 1972 [Fig. 5].)

ity and by menstrual disturbances in postpubertal females. To the best of my knowledge, however, functioning stroma, as evidenced by the presence of luteinized cells, has not been described in association with these tumours. Lutein cysts have been reported frequently in the contralateral ovary, however, and their presence, as well as steroid hormone synthesis by the syncytiotrophoblast cells in these tumours may have accounted for the endocrine abnormalities observed in these cases. Four yolk sac tumours, including one of the hepatoid type, have been associated with virilizing manifestations due presumably to the presence of lutein cells in their stroma (Scully, 1962; Abell, 1968; Stewart et al, 1981; Prat et al, 1982). These cells are found much more often in yolk sac tumours, however, in the absence of clinical manifestations of steroid hormone excess (24% of the cases according to Kurman & Norris, 1967b).

Among ovarian teratomas, the solid mature form and the pure immature teratoma have not been reported to be associated with evidence of steroid hormone abnormalities. The mature cystic teratoma and several types of monodermal teratoma, at times admixed with a mature cystic teratoma, however, have been accompanied by androgenic or oestrogenic manifestations on a number of occasions. Two cases of pure mature cystic teratoma with luteinization within the peripheral portion of the tumour or in the ovarian stroma adjacent to it have been reported in virilized women (Case Records of the Massachusetts General Hospital, Case 13, 1970; Aiman et al, 1977). In the latter case it is possible that the luteinization was not directly related to the tumour, but reflected an independent stromal hyperthecosis. In another case hirsutism accompanied by a high plasma testosterone level was ascribed to hilus cell hyperplasia along the margin of a mature cystic teratoma (Rutgers & Scully, 1986). Gardneau & Cabanne (1968) described an unusual case of a virilizing mucinous cystadenoma with bile-forming hepatic cells in its wall and a peripheral hyperplasia of Leydig cells. Ober (1960) reported the case of a teratomatous struma ovarii with lutein cell hyperplasia along its rim and endometrial hyperplasia. Four other cases of struma ovarii with peripheral luteinization and evidence of hyperoestrinism (in one case accompanied by elevated androgen levels) were reported by Rutgers & Scully (1986). In some of the cases of struma rimmed by hyperplastic lutein or Leydig cells, these cells have contained large numbers of lipid vacuoles (Fig. 29.6), resulting in bright yellow streaking along the outer surface of the tumour on gross examina-

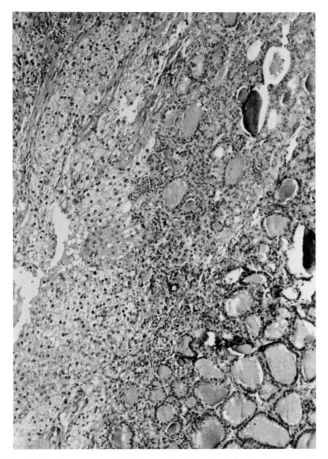

Fig. 29.6 Struma ovarii with vacuolated lutein cells along its margin. H & E × 45.

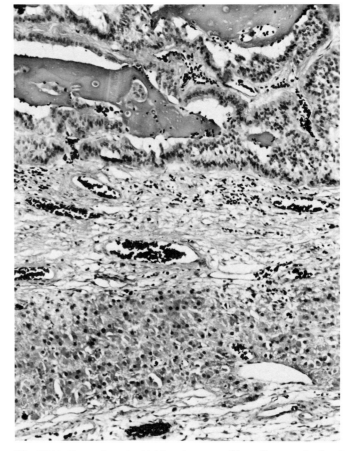

Fig. 29.7 Strumal carcinoid (above) separated by a fibrovascular band from a band of luteinized cells (below). H & E × 160.

tion. One case has been reported of a primary trabecular carcinoid of the ovary associated with both oestrogenic and androgenic manifestations (Robboy et al, 1977). In that case luteinized cells were present in the peripheral portion of the tumour and adjacent to it. Three virilizing strumal carcinoids have been recorded in the literature (Dikman & Toker, 1971; Robboy & Scully, 1980; Rutgers & Scully, 1986); in two of those cases lutein cells were present both within the tumour and at its periphery, and in the third case (Rutgers & Scully, 1986) peripheral stromal Leydig cells (Fig. 29.7) were responsible for the masculinization. Rare types of primary ovarian tumour with a functioning stroma include: rete cyst (adenomas), three and possibly four of which (Rutgers & Scully, 1986; Robinson et al, 1988; Beauchamp et al, 1989) had androgenic manifestations ascribable to peripheral hilus cell hyperplasia; a virilizing fibroma with peripheral stromal Leydig cell proliferation (Konishi et al, 1986); a virilizing leiomyoma with adjacent hilus cell hyperplasia (Parish et al, 1984); and a primary lymphoma with luteinization of its stroma and secondary amenorrhoea (Mittal et al, 1992).

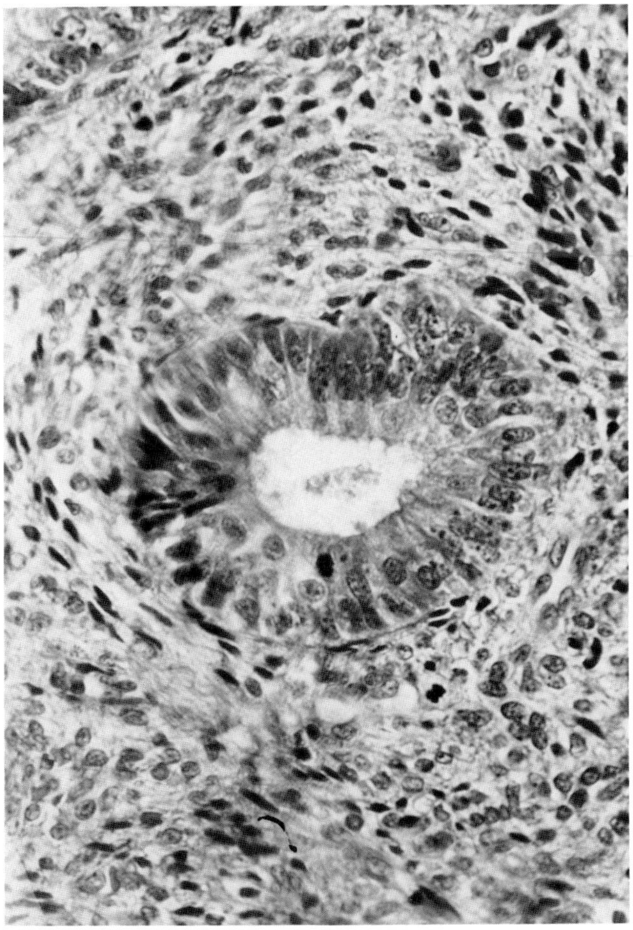

In summary, except for the very rare choriocarcinoma, embryonal carcinoma and polyembryoma, the great majority of germ cell tumours are not associated with recognized abnormalities of steroid hormone secretion. When functioning stroma is present, it is often most conspicuous within the peripheral portion of the tumour and adjacent to it instead of throughout the entire neoplasm. Leydig cell proliferation appears to be associated with neoplasms of germ cell origin more frequently than with common epithelial tumours.

The final category of ovarian tumours with functioning stroma is metastatic cancer, mostly of gastrointestinal origin, in which the stromal alterations are usually present throughout the tumour. Scully & Richardson (1961) found clinical evidence of oestrogen excess (irregular premenopausal bleeding or postmenopausal bleeding) in 13 of 53 cases of metastatic adenocarcinoma from the large intestine (Figs 29.8 and 29.9) and stomach (25%). Lutein cells (Fig. 29.9) were identified in 16 of the 31 tumours of intestinal origin (52%), but not in any of those of gastric origin. Rome and his associates (1981) reported that all eight patients with metastases to the ovary from various sites had elevated urinary oestrogens. Additional cases of metastatic intestinal adenocarcinoma have been reported with elevated oestrogen levels (Jolles et al, 1985; Brennecke et al, 1986); in the former case the patient also

Fig. 29.8 Endometrium with glandular and stromal mitotic figures from a 76-year-old woman with metastatic colonic carcinoma with functioning stroma. H & E × 338. (From Scully & Richardson, 1961 [Fig. 8].)

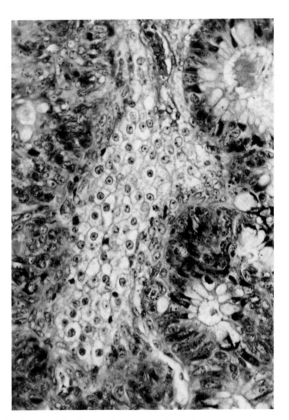

Fig. 29.9 Luteinization of the stroma of a metastatic adenocarcinoma from the colon. The lutein cells are vacuolated. H & E × 250. (From Scully & Richardson, 1961 [Fig. 4].)

had an elevated progesterone level and presented with severe breast tenderness. Nineteen Krukenberg tumours, mostly of gastric origin, but occasionally of breast (Spadoni et al, 1965) or appendiceal (Bullon et al, 1981) derivation, have been virilizing (Verhoeven et al, 1973; Salomon-Bernard et al, 1975; Bell, 1977; Forest et al, 1978; Vicens et al, 1980; Schoenfeld et al, 1982; Silva et al, 1988; Fung et al, 1991). One metastatic carcinoma from the large intestine masculinized a patient (Scully & Richardson, 1961) and another was associated with both virilizing and oestrogenic manifestations (Case Records of the Massachusetts General Hospital, Case 10, 1975); one Krukenberg tumour of gastric origin and one metastatic carcinoma that arose in the colon were accompanied by decidual changes in the endometrium (Fig. 29.10) as well as virilization (Bruno & Ober, 1959; Ober et al, 1962). Two cases have been mentioned in which hilus cell hyperplasia has been found adjacent to a virilizing Krukenberg tumour (Fox & Langley, 1976). One 57-year-old woman

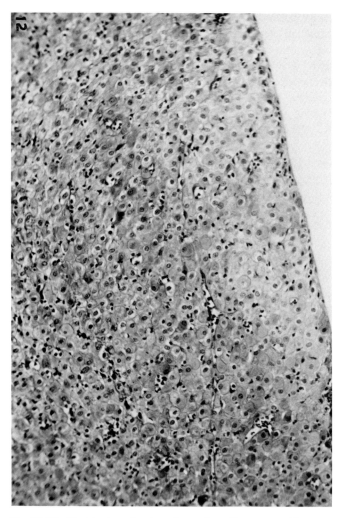

Fig. 29.10 Decidual reaction in endometrium of a woman with a functioning Krukenberg tumour of the ovary. H & E × 113. (From Scully & Richardson, 1961 [Fig. 12].)

was virilized by bilateral metastatic lobular carcinoma of the breast with luteinization of the stroma (Caron et al, 1990).

One metastatic carcinoid tumour from the colon was accompanied by peripheral stromal luteinization and was associated with endometrial hyperplasia and carcinoma (Rutgers & Scully, 1986).

CLINICAL MANIFESTATIONS AND TUMOUR TYPE

The clinical manifestations of ovarian tumours with functioning stroma depend partly on the age of the patient and partly on whether she is pregnant at the time of onset of symptoms. The only reported tumour with a functioning stroma that has resulted in isosexual precocity was the dysgerminoma with syncytiotrophoblast cells described by Ueda et al (1972). Numerous cases of surface epithelial-stromal tumors and occasional examples of germ cell and metastatic tumours with functioning stroma have been reported in postmenopausal women with oestrogenic manifestations, such as bleeding from a proliferative or hyperplastic endometrium and, rarely, swelling of the breasts, but few if any such tumours have been documented in women in the reproductive age group. This apparently lower frequency in younger women may be related to the greater difficulty in establishing a cause-and-effect relationship between the tumour and oestrogenic manifestations in the presence of a functioning contralateral ovary and the infrequency of laboratory investigation of patients in this age period. Alternatively, it may reflect a true difference in frequency, possibly related to the higher level of gonadotrophins in older women.

An extensive but incomplete review of the literature has yielded 39 well-documented examples of virilizing ovarian tumours with functioning stroma in non-pregnant patients and 23 in pregnant women. Nineteen of the 62 tumours (33%) were Krukenberg tumours (Fig. 29.11). Eight of them (Fox & Stamm, 1965; Salomon-Bernard et al, 1975; Bullon et al, 1981; Schoenfeld et al, 1982) occurred in non-pregnant patients and 11 (Verhoeven et al, 1973; Salomon-Bernard et al, 1975; Bell, 1977; Forest et al, 1978; Vicens et al, 1980; Silva et al, 1988; Fung et al, 1991) in pregnant women. Eleven of the 19 tumours were of known gastric origin, one arose from the breast (Spadoni et al, 1965), one originated in the appendix (Bullon et al, 1981), and six were of unknown derivation. Thirteen mucinous cystic tumours (nine of them benign) accounted for the second largest group of ovarian tumours with a virilizing stroma, with six occurring in non-pregnant patients (Da Costa, 1938; Bettinger & Jacobs, 1946; Cotton et al, 1981; Rutgers & Scully, 1986; Alvarez & Varner, 1987) and seven in pregnant women (Scully, 1962; Chan & Prathap, 1970; Novak et al, 1970; Bronstein et al, 1972; Verhoeven et al, 1973; Salomon-Bernard et al,

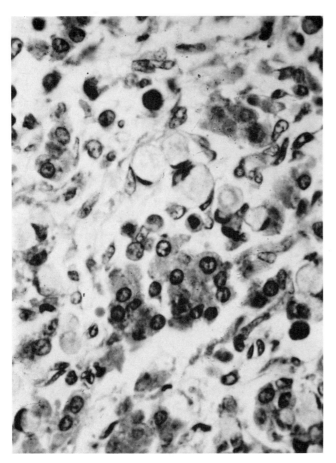

Fig. 29.11 Luteinization of the stroma of a virilizing Krukenberg tumour of gastric origin. Note the presence of signet-ring cells. H & E × 700.

1975; Post et al, 1978). The other virilizing tumours in non-pregnant women include: four rete cyst(adenoma)s (Rutgers & Scully, 1986; Robinson et al, 1988; Beauchamp et al, 1989); three metastatic carcinomas from the colon (Scully & Richardson, 1961; Ober et al, 1962; Case Records of the Massachusetts General Hospital, Case 10, 1975); three yolk sac tumours (Abell, 1968; Stewart et al, 1981; Prat et al, 1982); three strumal carcinoids (Dikman & Toker, 1971; Robboy & Scully, 1980; Rutgers & Scully, 1986); two serous cystadenomas (Fayez et al, 1974; Okolo et al, 1990); and single examples of serous papillary adenocarcinoma (Plotz et al, 1966); endometrioid carcinoma (Morris & Scully, 1958); Brenner tumour (DeLima et al, 1989); dermoid cyst (Aiman et al, 1977); dysgerminoma with syncytiotrophoblast cells (Case Records of the Massachusetts General Hospital, Case 11, 1972); trabecular carcinoid (Robboy et al, 1977); mucinous cystadenoma with bile formation and Leydig cell hyperplasia (Gardneau & Cabanne, 1968); fibroma (Konishi et al, 1986); leiomyoma (Parish et al, 1984), and metastatic lobular carcinoma of the breast (Caron et al, 1990).

The other virilizing tumours in pregnant women include: two Brenner tumours (Morris & Scully, 1958;

Besch et al, 1963; Hamwi et al, 1963; Meiling et al, 1963); and single examples of mature cystic teratoma (Case Records of the Massachusetts General Hospital, Case 13, 1970); yolk sac tumour (Scully, 1962) and serous cystadenoma (Fayez et al, 1974).

In the pregnant women the time of onset of virilization ranged from the third to the ninth month of gestation. In the 13 cases in which the endocrine status of the offspring is known, the child was a normal male in four cases, a normal female in three cases, and a virilized female in six cases. There was no correlation between the time of onset of masculinization in the mother and the presence or absence of virilization of the female offspring. Several of the non-pregnant patients with virilizing manifestations also had evidence of oestrogen excess in the form of endometrial hyperplasia or mammary symptoms. Rare tumours with functioning stroma have also been associated with progestational changes in the form of a decidual reaction of the endometrium (Krukenberg tumour) (Bruno & Ober, 1959); metastatic adenocarcinoma of the colon (Ober et al, 1962) or an endometrial Arias-Stella reaction (dysgerminoma with syncytiotrophoblast cells) (Zaloudek et al, 1981).

LABORATORY FINDINGS

Several authors have investigated various aspects of steroid hormone metabolism in cases of ovarian tumours with functioning stroma. Bhargava et al (1969) found that four of nine postmenopausal women with surface epithelial-stromal carcinomas had elevated urinary oestrogens, which fell to normal in the three cases in which the tumour was removed and postoperative measurements were done. Rome and his associates (1981) reported elevated urinary oestrogen values in 16 of 29 postmenopausal women with benign surface epithelial-stromal tumours (55%) and 16 of 43 with malignant forms of these neoplasms (37%). Thirteen of the 16 patients with high preoperative values (81%) had normal levels after removal of their tumours. Aiman et al (1986) studied the venous blood draining a variety of ovarian primary tumours outside the sex cord-stromal and steroid cell categories and found an increase in one or more androgens in three of 11 cases, but no increase in oestrogens. MacDonald and his associates (1976) concluded, on the basis of their investigation of a postmenopausal woman with a mucinous cystadenocarcinoma and endometrial hyperplasia, that the tumour produced androstenedione and that an associated elevated oestrone level, which was responsible for the endometrial hyperplasia, could be accounted for entirely by extraovarian conversion of the androstenedione. Shinada et al (1973) found that a Brenner tumour associated with oestrogenic manifestations converted androstenedione to oestrone in vitro and postulated that this conversion might explain the endocrine changes associated with tumours of this type. Quinn and his colleagues (1983), in contrast, investigated a postmenopausal woman with a mucinous cystadenoma of borderline malignancy and endometrial hyperplasia and found elevation of a wide spectrum of steroid hormones in the blood and urine with a gradient between the ovarian and peripheral blood levels. A tenfold difference between the ovarian vein and peripheral vein levels of oestradiol indicated that the tumour itself had aromatase activity. There was a marked response of the elevated steroid hormone levels to the injection of chorionic gonadotrophin (hCG), suggesting that the stroma of the tumour was responsive to this hormone. Kühnel et al (1987) found in vitro evidence of aromatase activity in a malignant Brenner tumour with oestrogenic manifestations, suggesting that it had been synthesizing oestrogens actively. Rome and his co-workers (1981) demonstrated elevated urinary oestrogens in all eight postmenopausal women with metastatic carcinoma in the ovary.

In the single reported germ cell tumour with oestrogenic manifestations that was studied most extensively from a hormonal viewpoint, a dysgerminoma with syncytiotrophoblast cells associated with sexual precocity (Ueda et al, 1972), high levels of hCG, androgens, oestrogens and pregnanediol were demonstrated in the urine. In vitro incubation studies of the tumour demonstrated the production of both androgens and oestrogens from precursors. The authors speculated that the lutein cells of the tumour might have been producing androgens, which were converted to oestrogens by the trophoblast cells. Rutgers & Scully (1986) reported an elevated oestradiol level in the ovarian vein draining an oestrogenic struma with peripheral stromal luteinization. Brennecke et al (1986) concluded that the oestrogenic manifestations of a metastatic colon adenocarcinoma were caused by peripheral conversion of androgens to oestrogens. Jolles et al (1985) reported marked elevations of oestradiol, oestrone, and progesterone in a patient with marked tenderness of the breasts associated with metastatic adenocarcinoma of the colon.

In cases of ovarian tumours with functioning stroma and virilization, high levels of various androgens have been found in the peripheral blood (Verhoeven et al, 1963; Case Records of the Massachusetts General Hospital, Case 10, 1975; Aiman et al, 1977; Post et al, 1978; Bullon et al, 1981; Cotton et al, 1981; Stewart et al, 1981; Prat et al, 1982; Schoenfeld et al, 1982; Parish et al, 1984; Konishi et al, 1986; Rutgers & Scully, 1986; Robinson et al, 1988; Silva et al, 1988, Beauchamp et al, 1989; DeLima et al, 1989; Caron et al, 1990; Okolo et al, 1990; Fung et al, 1991) and in some cases even higher values in the ovarian vein blood (Case Records of the Massachusetts General Hospital, Case 10, 1975; Bullon et al, 1981; Beauchamp et al, 1989; DeLima et al, 1989). In many of the cases a return of the high values to normal was demonstrated after removal of the tumour. Elevated levels of oestrogens (Connor et al, 1968; Novak et al, 1970; Case Records of the Massachusetts General Hospital, Case 10, 1975; Rutgers & Scully, 1986) and progesterone (Scott et al, 1967; Connor et al, 1968; Cotton et al, 1987) have also been documented in some of the cases of virilizing tumours with functioning stroma. In the case of a virilizing Brenner tumour in a 65-year-old woman (DeLima et al, 1989) and that of a virilizing metastatic breast carcinoma (Caron et al, 1990) hCG administration caused a rise in the preoperative androgen levels. In pregnant women with the tumours, a striking dependence of the abnormal steroid levels on the pregnant state, and specifically on hCG, has been demonstrated. For example, in the cases of Connor and his associates (1968) and Forest et al (1978) androgen levels fell in the postpartum period before the removal of the tumour, and subsequent administration of hCG to the patients resulted in a second rise in the androgen levels. In several cases (Morris & Scully, 1958; Fayez et al, 1974), however, androgenic manifestations progressed after the termination of the pregnancy, indicating at most only a partial dependence of the stroma on the high hCG level.

HISTOCHEMICAL AND ULTRASTRUCTURAL STUDIES

Scully & Cohen (1964) identified in the stroma of normal and pathological ovaries cells that were rich in oxidative enzymes, particularly glucose-6-phosphate dehydrogenase and isocitric dehydrogenase, which are known to be present in high concentrations in steroid hormone-producing cells. Luteinized cells in both hyperplastic stroma and the stroma of neoplasms were rich in these enzymes, but such cells accounted for only a minority of all the enzymatically active stromal cells (EASC), most of which could not be distinguished from neighbouring stromal cells by routine staining methods. EASC were found in greatest number in cases of stromal hyperthecosis and in the stroma of both primary and metastatic ovarian carcinomas (Fig. 29.12). They were not encountered in the stroma of primary extraovarian carcinomas in cases in which the ovarian metastatic tumours contained these cells. Willighagen & Thiery (1968) found EASC in 12 of 52 surface epithelial-stromal tumours and in one of three metastatic carcinomas of gastric origin; 45% of the mucinous tumours in that series were positive for these cells in contrast to only 7% of the serous tumours. Janovski & Paramanandhan (1973) tabulated, from several sources, the frequency of EASC in different types of ovarian tumour and found it to be highest in mucinous tumours (69%), endometrioid carcinomas (67%), and metastatic carcinomas (45%); the overall frequency was 34%. Pfleiderer et al (1968) reported that the occurrence of EASC in ovarian tumours was greatest in the age group

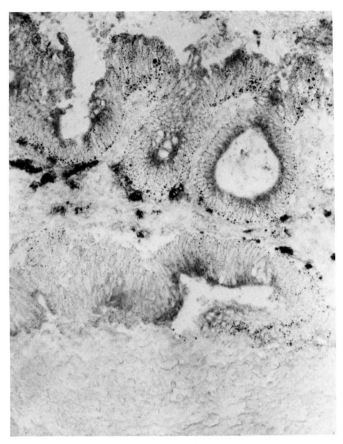

Fig. 29.12 Enzymatically active stromal cells in a case of ovarian metastatic adenocarcinoma from the colon. Glucose-6-phosphate dehydrogenase preparation × 125.

50–69 years, a period during which the stroma is subjected to the highest levels of pituitary gonadotrophins. Those authors also found that six of eight endometria of women with EASC in their surface epithelial-stromal tumours were hyperplastic, in contrast to none of 18 when EASC were absent.

Several ultrastructural studies have been done in cases of ovarian tumours with functioning stroma. Lynn and his associates (1967) found cells resembling theca cells in a non-functioning dysgerminoma from a pregnant woman; the neoplastic tissue contained oestrone and oestriol. Novak et al (1970) reported the presence of cells containing abundant smooth endoplasmic reticulum and tubular cristae, which are characteristic of steroid hormone-secreting cells, in a virilizing mucinous cystadenoma occurring during pregnancy. Cells with similar features were subsequently reported in a virilizing ovarian fibroma with stromal Leydig cell formation (Konishi et al, 1986), in a virilizing Krukenberg tumour in a pregnant woman (Silva et al, 1988), in an oestrogenic metastatic colon adenocarcinoma (Brennecke et al, 1986), and in two of 12 apparently non-functioning Krukenberg tumours (Wong et al, 1986).

MECHANISM OF STROMAL FUNCTION

The most readily explained tumours with functioning stroma are those that virilize women during pregnancy. In most cases of this type the stromal luteinization is probably largely dependent on stimulation by hCG, which is circulating at a high level. One of the most informative cases in the literature in this regard is that of Connor et al (1968), in which the patient had a unilateral Krukenberg tumour removed prior to the onset of pregnancy, but did not become virilized until a similar tumour appeared in the contralateral ovary during pregnancy. The virilism and laboratory evidence of androgen excess decreased after delivery but subsequently increased after the administration of hCG and before the removal of the tumour. A striking histological difference between the earlier non-functioning tumour and the later virilizing tumour was the presence of cells resembling lutein cells in the stroma of the latter. Another factor that may account for the apparently increased frequency of tumours with a virilizing stroma during pregnancy is the high level of circulating progesterone, which is available for conversion into androgens.

It is not surprising that dysgerminomas containing syncytiotrophoblast cells may have a functioning stroma in view of the presumed high local concentration of hCG in the presence of these cells. It is unclear, however, why a functioning stroma develops in tumours that do not contain syncytiotrophoblast cells and are not occurring during pregnancy (idiopathic group of ovarian tumours with functioning stroma). Several explanations have been offered for this phenomenon. The mechanical theory (Woodruff et al, 1963) holds that the tumour behaves like an enlarging follicle with pressure on the adjacent tissue inducing the development of theca-like cells. This explanation is most attractive for those cases in which a band of lutein or Leydig cells is found at the periphery of a tumour, a pattern that is seen primarily in association with slowly growing germ cell tumours such as struma ovarii and strumal carcinoid tumours. The mechanical theory, however, does not explain why certain tumours, such as metastatic breast carcinoma, are rarely accompanied by either luteinization of the stroma or endocrine abnormalities or why these features are more common in association with mucinous than serous tumours. A second theory (MacDonald et al, 1976) implicates both the well-known proliferative activity of the stroma of ovarian carcinomas and the high level of luteinizing hormone (LH) in postmenopausal women, in whom such tumours occur most commonly. Mitotic figures are often encountered in the stroma of an ovarian carcinoma, and cells in general are said to be most receptive to stimulation just after the completion of mitotic division. With numerous stromal cells in such a phase in the presence of a high LH level one might, therefore, expect a heightened functional activity of the stroma. There are two arguments against this theory, however. First, the stroma of benign epithelial tumours, in which mitotic activity is not conspicuous, may also function, and secondly, ovarian tumours with functioning stroma are seen in young patients with premenopausal levels of LH as well as in older women.

In view of the putative rôles of high local concentrations of hCG in some of the functioning germ cell tumours and of high circulating levels of this hormone in pregnant patients with ovarian tumours with functioning stroma, ectopic production of hCG by neoplastic cells has been postulated as another possible promoter of stromal function. Kurman (1975, personal communication), using immunohistochemical methods, demonstrated hCG in the neoplastic cells of a virilizing Krukenberg tumour and in those of an endometrioid carcinoma associated with endometrial hyperplasia. Matias-Guiu & Prat (1990) conducted the most extensive immunohistochemical investigation of hCG in ovarian tumours, using single polyclonal antibodies to the whole hormone and its beta subunit and four monoclonal antibodies to the whole hormone, its beta subunit, and two regions of the carboxyl terminal of the beta subunit. Correlating positive staining results with the presence or absence of an 'active' stroma of the tumour (luteinization and/or 'condensation') these authors found that the epithelial cells of 41% of the tumours with active stroma reacted with the polyclonal antibodies and 62% with the monoclonal antibodies; the corresponding figures for the epithelial cells of the tumours with an inactive stroma were 14% and 37%, respectively. Although a high local concentration of hCG within the neoplastic cells may explain the phenomenon of functioning stroma in some tumours within the idiopathic group, the negative staining results in other cases suggests that some other stroma-stimulating substance is also secreted by neoplastic cells.

REFERENCES

Abell M R 1968 Undifferentiated malignant germ cell neoplasm (embryonal carcinoma) of ovary with stromal luteinization and masculinization. American Journal of Obstetrics and Gynecology 101: 570–572.

Aiman J, Forney J P, Parker C R Jr 1977 The origin of androgen and estrogen in a virilized postmenopausal woman with bilateral benign cystic teratomas. Obstetrics and Gynecology 49: 695–704.

Aiman J, Forney J P, Parker C R 1986 Androgen and estrogen secretion by normal and neoplastic ovaries in premenopausal women. Obstetrics and Gynecology 68: 327–332.

Alvarez R D, Varner R E 1987 Hyperandrogenic state associated with a mucinous cystadenoma. Obstetrics and Gynecology 69: 507–510.

Andujar J J, Enloe G R, Swift W B 1947 Brenner tumor of the ovary; 2 cases associated with postmenopausal endometrial changes. Texas Journal of Medicine 43: 70–75.

Backstrom T, Mahlck C-G, Kjellgren O 1983 Progesterone as a possible tumor-marker for "non-endocrine" ovarian malignant tumors. Gynecologic Oncology 16: 129–138.

Balasa R W, Adcock L L, Prem K A, Dehner L P 1977 The Brenner tumor. Obstetrics and Gynecology 50: 120–128.

Beauchamp P J, Hughes R S, Schmidt W A 1989 Virilizing serous cystadenoma. Obstetrics and Gynecology 73: 513–517.

Beck J S, Fulman H F, Lee S T 1969 Solid malignant ovarian teratoma with 'embryoid bodies' and trophoblastic differentiation. Journal of Pathology 99: 67–73.

Bell R J M 1977 Fetal virilisation due to maternal Krukenberg tumour. Lancet 1: 1162–1163.

Besch P K, Watson D J, Verys N 1963 Testosterone synthesis by a Brenner tumor. Part II. In vitro biosynthetic steroid conversion of a Brenner tumor. American Journal of Obstetrics and Gynecology 86: 1021–1026.

Bettinger H F, Jacobs H 1946 A contribution to the problem of masculinization. Medical Journal of Australia 1: 10–13.

Bhargava V L, Beischer N A, Brown J B, Townsend L 1969 Hormonal activity of 'non-functional' ovarian tumours. Australian and New Zealand Journal of Obstetrics and Gynaecology 9: 108.

Biggart J H, MacAfee C H G 1955 Tumours of the ovarian mesenchyme: a clinico-pathological survey. Journal of Obstetrics and Gynaecology of the British Empire 62: 829–837.

Brennecke S P, McEvoy M I, Seymour A E, Bessell C K, Munday R N 1986 Caecal adenocarcinoma metastatic to ovary inducing increased oestrogen production and postmenopausal bleeding. Australian and New Zealand Journal of Obstetrics and Gynaecology 26: 158–161.

Bronstein R, Hardouin G, Henrion R 1972 Kyste mucoide virilisant au cours de la grossesse. Journal de Gynecologie, Obstetrique et Biologie de la Reproduction 1: 891–899.

Bruno M S, Ober W B 1959 Clinicopathologic conference. New York State Journal of Medicine 59: 4001–4007.

Bullon A, Arseneau J, Prat J, Young R H, Scully R E 1981 Tubular Krukenberg tumor: a problem in histopathologic diagnosis. American Journal of Surgical Pathology 5: 255–232.

Cariker M, Dockerty M 1954 Mucinous cystadenomas and mucinous cystadenocarcinomas of the ovary: a clinical and pathological study of 355 cases. Cancer 7: 302–310.

Caron P, Roche H, Gorguet B, Martel P, Bennet A, Carton M 1990 Mammary ovarian metastases with stroma cell hyperplasia and postmenopausal virilization. Cancer 66: 1221–1224.

Case Record of the Massachusetts General Hospital, Case 13, 1970. New England Journal of Medicine 282: 676–681.

Case Records of the Massachusetts General Hospital, Case 11, 1972. New England Journal of Medicine 286: 594–600.

Case Records of the Massachusetts General Hospital, Case 10, 1975. New England Journal of Medicine 292: 521–526.

Chan L K C, Prathap K 1970 Virilization in pregnancy associated with an ovarian mucinous cystadenoma. American Journal of Obstetrics and Gynecology 108: 946–949.

Connor T B, Ganis F M, Levin H S, Migeon C J, Martin L G 1968 Gonadotropin-dependent Krukenberg tumor causing virilization during pregnancy. Journal of Clinical Endocrinology and Metabolism 28: 198–214.

Cotton D B, Hanson F W, Oi R H 1981 A mucinous cystadenoma associated with testosterone production. Journal of Reproductive Medicine 26: 276–278.

Da Costa C C 1938 Tumor masculinizante. Revista de Gynecologia e d'Obstetricia 2: 3–9.

DeLima O A, Carvalho W D P 1978 Tumores funcionales do ovario. Manole, Sao Paulo.

DeLima G R, DeLima O A, Baracat E C, Vasserman J, Burnier Jr M 1989 Virilizing Brenner tumor of the ovary: case report. Obstetrics and Gynecology 73: 895–898.

Dikman S H, Toker C 1971 Strumal carcinoid of the ovary with masculinization. Cancer 27: 925–930.

Eddie D A S 1967 Hormonal activity with ovarian tumours. Journal of Obstetrics and Gynaecology of the British Commonwealth 74: 283–285.

Edwards R L, Nicholson H O, Zoidis T, Butt W R, Taylor C W 1971 Endocrine studies in postmenopausal women with ovarian tumours.

Journal of Obstetrics and Gynaecology of the British Commonwealth 78: 467–477.

Ehrlich C E, Roth L M 1971 The Brenner tumor: a clinicopathologic study of 57 cases. Cancer 27: 332–342.

Esau P 1929 Uber klimacterische Gesichtsbehaarung. Klinische Wochenschrift 8: 1670–1671.

Fathalla M F 1968 The role of the ovarian stroma in hormone production by ovarian tumours. Journal of Obstetrics and Gynaecology of the British Commonwealth 75: 78–83.

Fayez J A, Bunch T R, Miller G L 1974 Virilization in pregnancy associated with an ovarian serous cystadenoma. American Journal of Obstetrics and Gynecology 120: 341–346.

Forest M G, Orgiazzi J, Tranchant D, Morenex R, Bertrand J 1978 Approach to the mechanism of androgen overproduction in a case of Krukenberg tumor responsible for virilization during pregnancy. Journal of Clinical Endocrinology and Metabolism 47: 428–434.

Fox H 1965 Estrogenic activity of the serous cystadenoma of the ovary. Cancer 18: 1041–1047.

Fox H, Langley F A 1976 Tumours of the ovary. Year Book Medical Publishers, Chicago.

Fox L P, Stamm W J 1965 Krukenberg tumor complicating pregnancy: report of a case with androgenic activity. American Journal of Obstetrics and Gynecology 92: 702–710.

Fox H, Agrawal K, Langley F A 1972 The Brenner tumour of the ovary: a clinicopathological study of 54 cases. Journal of Obstetrics and Gynaecology of the British Commonwealth 79: 661–665.

Fung M F K, Vadas G, Lotocki R, Heywood M, Krepart G 1991 Case report: tubular Krukenberg tumor in pregnancy with virilization. Gynecologic Oncology 41: 81–84.

Gardneau R, Cabanne F 1968 Dysembryome ovarien de type enteroide et bilio-hepatoide avec hyperplasie fonctionnelle des cellules sympathicotropes de Berger: a propos d'une observation. Annales d'Anatomie Pathologique 13: 423–432.

Grayzel D M, Friedman H H 1941 Brenner tumor of the ovary. American Journal of Surgery 53: 509–511.

Hameed H 1972 Brenner tumor of the ovary with Leydig cell hyperplasia: a histologic and ultrastructural study. Cancer 30: 945–952.

Hamwi G J, Byron R C, Besch P K, Vorys N, Teteris N J, Ullery J C 1963 Testosterone synthesis by a Brenner tumor. Part I. Clinical evidence of masculinization during pregnancy. American Journal of Obstetrics and Gynecology 86: 1015–1020.

Heinonen P K, Koivula T, Rajaniemi H, Pystynen P 1986 Peripheral and ovarian venous concentrations of steroid and gonadotropin hormones in postmenopausal women with epithelial ovarian tumors. Gynecologic Oncology 25: 1–10.

Herrington J B, Scully R E 1983 Endocrine aspects of germ cell tumors. In: Damjanov I, Solter D, Knowles B (eds) Biology of human teratomas. Springer-Verlag, New York, pp 215–229.

Hughesdon P E 1958 Thecal and allied reactions in epithelial ovarian tumours. Journal of Obstetrics and Gynaecology of the British Empire 65: 702–709.

Janovski N A, Paramanandhan T L 1973 Ovarian tumors. Tumors and tumor-like conditions of the ovaries, fallopian tubes and ligaments of the uterus. Saunders, Philadelphia.

Jolles C J, Beeson J H, Abbott T 1985 Progesterone production in adenocarcinoma of the colon metastatic to the ovaries. Obstetrics and Gynecology 65: 853–857.

Jorgensen E O, Dockerty M B, Wilson R B 1970 Clinicopathologic study of 53 cases of Brenner's tumors of the ovary. American Journal of Obstetrics and Gynecology 108: 122–127.

Konishi I, Fujii S, Ishikawa Y, Suzuki A, Okamura H, Mori T 1986 Ovarian fibroma with Leydig cell hyperplasia of the adjacent stroma: a light and electron microscopic study. International Journal of Gynecological Pathology 5: 170–178.

Kühnel R, Rao B R, Stolk J G, van Kessel H, Seldenrijk C A, Willig A P 1987 Estrogen synthesizing rare malignant Brenner tumor of the ovary with the presence of progesterone and androgen receptors in the absence of estrogen receptors. Gynecologic Oncology 26: 263–269.

Kurman R 1975 Personal communication.

Kurman R J, Norris H J 1976a Malignant mixed germ cell tumors of the ovary: a clinical and pathologic analysis of 30 cases. Obstetrics and Gynecology 48: 579–589.

Kurman R J, Norris H J 1976b Endodermal sinus tumor of the ovary: a clinical and pathologic study of 71 cases. Cancer 38: 2404–2419.

Kurman R J, Norris H J 1976c Embryonal carcinoma of the ovary: a clinicopathologic entity distinct from endodermal sinus tumor resembling embryonal carcinoma of the adult testis. Cancer 38: 2420–2433.

Lynn J A, Varon H H, Kingsley W B, Martin J H 1967 Ultrastructural and biochemical studies of estrogen secretory capacity of a 'nonfunctional' ovarian neoplasm (dysgerminoma). American Journal of Pathology 51: 639–661.

MacDonald P C, Grodin J M, Edman C D, Vellios F, Siiteri P K 1976 Origin of estrogen in a postmenopausal woman with a nonendocrine tumor of the ovary and endometrial hyperplasia. Obstetrics and Gynecology 47: 644–650.

McNulty J R 1959 The ovarian serous cystadenofibroma: a report of 25 cases. American Journal of Obstetrics and Gynecology 77: 1338–1344.

Mahlck C-G, Backstrom T, Kjellgren O 1986 Androstenedione production by malignant epithelial ovarian tumors. Gynecologic Oncology 25: 217–222.

Mahlck C-G, Backstrom T, Kjellgren O 1988 Plasma level of estradiol in patients with ovarian malignant tumors. Gynecologic Oncology 30: 313–320.

Mahlck C-G, Grankvist K, Kjellgren O, Backstrom T 1990 Human chorionic gonadotropin, follicle-stimulating hormone, and luteinizing hormone in patients with epithelial ovarian carcinoma. Gynecologic Oncology 26: 219–225.

Marwil T B, Beaver D C 1942 Brenner tumor of the ovary associated with uterine bleeding. American Journal of Obstetrics and Gynecology 43: 97–102.

Matias-Guiu X, Prat J 1990 Ovarian tumors with functioning stroma: an immunohistochemical study of 100 cases with human chorionic gonadotropin monoclonal and polyclonal antibodies. Cancer 65: 2001–2005.

Meiling R L, Bouselis J G, Teteris N J, Ullery J C, George O T 1963 Histochemical observations of a Brenner cell tumor with masculinization. American Journal of Obstetrics and Gynecology 87: 463–470.

Mittal K R, Blechman A, Greco M A, Alfonso F, Demopoulos R 1992 Case report: lymphoma of ovary with stromal luteinization, presenting as secondary amenorrhea. Gynecologic Oncology 45: 69–75.

Morris J McL, Scully R E 1958 Endocrine pathology of the ovary. Mosby, St Louis.

Moulonguet-Doleris P 1924 Les metrorrhages apres la menopause causees par les tumeurs et les kystes de l'ovaire: le phenomene de la 'reactivation' uterine senile d'origine ovarienne. Gynécologie et Obstétrique 9: 493–514.

Novak D J, Lauchlan S C, McCawley J C, Faiman C 1970 Virilization during pregnancy: case report and review of literature. American Journal of Medicine 49: 281–290.

Ober W B 1960 Solid ovarian teratoma with struma ovarii, theca lutein reaction and endometrial hyperplasia. Journal of Obstetrics and Gynaecology of the British Empire 67: 451–454.

Ober W B, Pollak A, Gerstmann K E, Kupperman H S 1962 Krukenberg tumor with androgenic and progestational activity. American Journal of Obstetrics and Gynecology 84: 739–744.

Okolo S O, Darley C, Melville H A H, Kirkham N 1990 Virilizing ovarian serous cystadenoma: case report. British Journal of Obstetrics and Gynaecology 97: 269–271.

Parish J M, Lufkin E G, Lee R A, Gaffey T A 1984 Ovarian leiomyoma with hilus cell hyperplasia that caused virilization. Mayo Clinic Proceedings 59: 275–277.

Pfleiderer A Jr, Teufel G, Braun R 1968 Incidence and histochemical investigation of enzymatically active cells in stroma of ovarian tumors. American Journal of Obstetrics and Gynecology 102: 997–1003.

Plotz E J, Wiener M, Stein A A 1966 Steroid synthesis in cystadenocarcinoma of the ovaries. American Journal of Obstetrics and Gynecology 94: 189–194.

Post W D, Steele H D, Gorwill R H 1978 Mucinous cystadenoma and virilization during pregnancy. Canadian Medical Association Journal 118: 952–953.

Prat J, Bhan A K, Dickersin G R, Robboy S J, Scully R E 1982 Hepatoid yolk sac tumor of the ovary (endodermal sinus tumor with hepatoid differentiation): a light microscopic, ultrastructural and immunohistochemical study of seven cases. Cancer 50: 2344–2368.

Quinn M A, Baker H W G, Rome R, Brown J B 1983 Response of a mucinous ovarian tumor of borderline malignancy to human chorionic gonadotropin. Obstetrics and Gynecology 61: 121–126.

Robboy S J, Scully R E 1980 Strumal carcinoid of the ovary: an analysis of 50 cases of a distinctive tumor composed of thyroid tissue and carcinoid. Cancer 46: 2019–2034.

Robboy S J, Scully R E, Norris H J 1977 Primary trabecular carcinoid of the ovary. Obstetrics and Gynecology 49: 202–207.

Robinson B, Eckstein R, Stiel J N, Payne W H, Kemp J 1988 An ovarian cyst associated with virilisation. Australian and New Zealand Journal of Medicine 18: 161–163.

Rome R M, Laverty C R, Brown J B 1973 Ovarian tumours in postmenopausal women: clinicopathological features and hormonal studies. Journal of Obstetrics and Gynaecology of the British Commonwealth 80: 984–991.

Rome R M, Fortune D W, Quinn M A, Brown J B 1981 Functioning ovarian tumors in postmenopausal women. Obstetrics and Gynecology 57: 705–710.

Rubin D K, Frost J K 1963 The cytologic detection of ovarian cancer. Acta Cytologica 7: 191–195.

Rutgers J L, Scully R E 1986 Functioning ovarian tumors with peripheral steroid cell proliferation: a report of twenty-four cases. International Journal of Gynecological Pathology 5: 319–337.

Salomon-Bernard Y, Thibaud E, Vignal J, Musset R 1975 Tumeurs a stroma fonctionnel. In: Cabanne F (ed) Tumeurs de l'ovaire. Masson, Paris, ch 11, pp 309–335.

Schoenfeld A, Pistiner M, Pitlik S, Rosenfeld J B, Ovadia J 1982 Long-interval masculinizing Krukenberg tumor of the ovary. European Journal of Obstetrics Gynaecology and Reproductive Biology 14: 49–53.

Scott J S, Lumsden C E, Levell M J 1967 Ovarian endocrine activity in association with hormonally inactive neoplasia. American Journal of Obstetrics and Gynecology 97: 161–170.

Scott R B 1942 Serous adenofibromas and cystadenofibromas of the ovary. American Journal of Obstetrics and Gynecology 43: 733–737.

Scully R E 1962 Androgenic lesions of the ovary. In: Grady H G, Smith D E (eds) The ovary. International Academy of Pathology Monograph, no 3. Williams & Wilkins, Baltimore, p 143.

Scully R E 1979 Tumors of the ovary and maldeveloped gonads. Armed Forces Institute of Pathology, Washington.

Scully R E, Cohen R B 1964 Oxidative-enzyme activity in normal and pathologic human ovaries. Obstetrics and Gynecology 24: 667–681.

Scully R E, Morris J McL 1957 Functioning ovarian tumors. In: Meigs J, Sturgis S H (eds) Progress in gynecology III. Grune & Stratton, New York, p 20.

Scully R E, Richardson G S 1961 Luteinization of the stroma of metastatic cancer involving the ovary and its endocrine significance. Cancer 14: 827–840.

Serment H, Laffargue P, Piana L, Blanc B 1970 Ovarian hormone tumors of female children. International Journal of Gynaecology and Obstetrics 8: 409–456.

Shinada T, Tsukui J, Matsumoto S 1973 Estrogen synthesis by Brenner tumors. American Journal of Obstetrics and Gynecology 116: 408–411.

Silva P D, Porto M, Moyer D L, Lobo R A 1988 Clinical and ultrastructural findings of an androgenizing Krukenberg tumor in pregnancy. Obstetrics and Gynecology 71: 432–434.

Silverberg S G 1971 Brenner tumor of the ovary: a clinicopathologic study of 60 tumors in 54 women. Cancer 28: 588–596.

Smith G V S 1937 Ovarian tumors, with special reference to those having physiological activity as gauged by the endometrium after the menopause. Medical Record and Annals, Houston, Texas 31: 262–267.

Spadoni L R, Lindberg M C, Mottet N K, Herrman W L 1965 Virilization coexisting with Krukenberg tumor during pregnancy. American Journal of Obstetrics and Gynecology 92: 981–991.

Stewart K R, Casey M J, Gondos B 1981 Endodermal sinus tumor of the ovary with virilization. American Journal of Surgical Pathology 5: 385–391.

Taylor H C Jr, Millem R 1938 The causes of vaginal bleeding and the histology of the endometrium after the menopause. American Journal of Gynecology and Obstetrics 36: 22–39.

Teoh T B 1953 Histogenesis of Brenner tumours of ovary. Journal of Pathology and Bacteriology 66: 441–456.

Thompson M A, Adelson M D, Kaufaran L M, Marshall L D, Cable D A 1988 Aromatization of testosterone by epithelial tumor cells cultured from patients with ovarian carcinoma. Cancer Research 48: 6491–6497.

Tighe J R 1961 Brenner tumours of the ovary: a clinicopathological study. Journal of Obstetrics and Gynaecology of the British Empire 68: 292–296.

Turunen A 1955 Hormonal secretion of Krukenberg tumours. Acta Endocrinologica 20: 50–56.

Ueda G, Hamanaka N, Hayakawa K 1972 Clinical, histochemical, and biochemical studies of an ovarian dysgerminoma with trophoblasts and Leydig cells. American Journal of Obstetrics and Gynecology 114: 748–754.

Verhoeven A T M, Mastboom J L, Van Leusden H A I M, Van der Velden W H M 1973 Virilization in pregnancy coexisting with an (ovarian) mucinous cystadenoma: a case report and review of virilizing ovarian tumors in pregnancy. Obstetrical and Gynecological Survey 28: 597–622.

Vesterinen E, Purola E, Wahlstrom T 1978 Oestrogenic activity associated with ovarian cystadenomas after the menopause. Annales Chirurgiae et Gynaecologiae 67: 109–111.

Vicens E, Martinez-Mora J, Potau N, Sans M, Boix-Ochoa J 1980 Masculinization of a female fetus by Krukenberg tumor during pregnancy. Journal of Pediatric Surgery 15: 188–190.

Willighagen R G J, Thiery M 1968 Enzyme histochemistry of ovarian tumors. American Journal of Obstetrics and Gynecology 100: 393–404.

Wimalasena J, Dostal R, Meehan D 1992 Gonadotropins, estradiol and growth factors regulate epithelial ovarian cancer cell growth. Gynecologic Oncology 26: 1–6.

Wong P C, Ferenczy A, Fan L-D, McCaughey E 1986 Krukenberg tumors of the ovary: ultrastructural, histochemical, and immunohistochemical studies of 15 cases. Cancer 57: 751–760.

Woodruff J D, Williams T J, Goldberg B 1963 Hormone activity of the common ovarian neoplasm. American Journal of Obstetrics and Gynecology 87: 697–698.

Wren B G, Frampton J 1963 Oestrogenic activity associated with nonfeminizing ovarian tumours after the menopause. British Medical Journal 2: 842–844.

Young R H, Prat J, Scully R E 1982 Ovarian endometrioid carcinomas resembling sex cord-stromal tumors: a clinicopathological analysis of 13 cases. American Journal of Surgical Pathology 6: 513–522.

Zaloudek C J, Tavassoli F A, Norris H J 1981 Dysgerminoma with syncytiotrophoblastic giant cells: a histologically and clinically distinctive subtype of dysgerminoma. American Journal of Surgical Pathology 5: 361–367.

30. Pathology of the peritoneum and secondary Müllerian system

Debra A. Bell

LESIONS OF THE PERITONEUM

The female peritoneum is the site of a diverse group of benign and malignant lesions, many of which are seen only rarely in men. A number of these lesions maintain a peritoneal or mesothelial appearance and cellular phenotype; others show definitive Müllerian differentiation.

Mesothelial hyperplasia

Perhaps the most common lesion of the peritoneum seen in surgical pathology specimens is mesothelial hyperplasia. In general, these benign mesothelial proliferations which occur as a reaction to serosal injury cause few diagnostic problems, but occasional cases may be difficult to distinguish from diffuse malignant mesothelioma or primary or secondary carcinoma involving the peritoneum.

Mesothelial hyperplasia of the peritoneal surfaces most often is noted as an incidental finding, but in rare cases may be visible grossly as small nodules measuring up to several millimetres in diameter (McCaughey & Al-Jabi, 1986; Daya & McCaughey, 1991; Clement & Young, 1993). Microscopically, the mesothelial proliferation usually is located on the surfaces of the peritoneum but may extend for variable distances into underlying tissue. When the mesothelial surface is affected, the mesothelial cells form a single layer of enlarged polygonal cells, solid sheets of cells or papillae with delicate or prominent fibrovascular cores (Fig. 30.1). When the proliferation contains fibrosis or extends into underlying tissue, the mesothelial cells are arranged in papillae, tubulopapillary structures, tubules, cords, or trabeculae, often in linear arrays parallel to the overlying mesothelial surface (Fig. 30.2). The cells usually show minimal to moderate nuclear atypia and are polygonal or cuboidal with abundant amphophilic cytoplasm. Focally, large cytoplasmic vacuoles may be present.

Mesothelial hyperplasia must be distinguished from diffuse malignant mesothelioma and primary or secondary carcinomas involving the peritoneum. Features that aid in distinguishing mesothelial hyperplasia from diffuse malig-

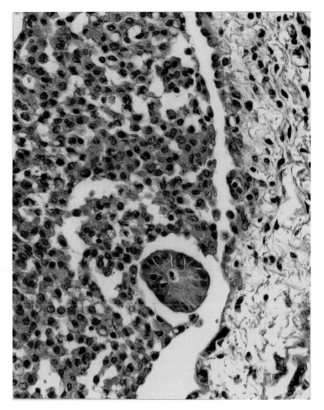

Fig. 30.1 Mesothelial hyperplasia. Bland polygonal mesothelial cells are present in sheets and a papillary cluster on the peritoneal surface. H & E × 313.

nant mesothelioma are the presence of marked cytological atypia, necrosis, prominent cytoplasmic vacuolization, and deep extension into underlying tissues in the latter. It should be noted, however, that marked cytological atypia may be present only focally in diffuse malignant mesothelioma and for this reason the absence of cytological atypia in a biopsy specimen does not exclude diffuse malignant mesothelioma absolutely (McCaughey et al, 1985; McCaughey & Al-Jabi, 1986; Daya & McCaughey, 1990). Mesothelial hyperplasia may be mistaken for primary or secondary adenocarcinoma or ovarian borderline

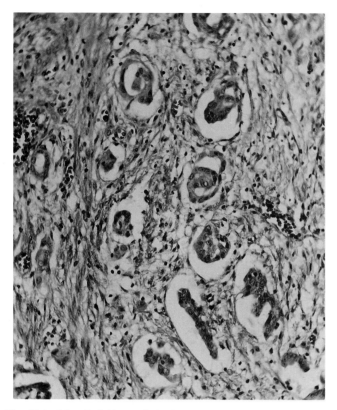

Fig. 30.2 Mesothelial hyperplasia. Tubules and papillary structures composed of polygonal mesothelial cells are present in a linear array in fibrous tissue. H & E × 200.

tumours involving the peritoneum, especially when papillae or extension into underlying tissue are present (Bell & Scully, 1989; Clement & Young, 1993). The major features that favour a diagnosis of mesothelial hyperplasia over adenocarcinoma are the absence of marked cytological atypia or deep infiltration of underlying tissue. Mesothelial hyperplasia may be especially difficult to distinguish from serous borderline tumours because both may show minimal cytological atypia. The cells of serous borderline tumours, however, usually show a greater degree of cytological atypia, and tend to be columnar with delicate cytoplasm; the cells of mesothelial hyperplasia usually have more uniform nuclei and are polygonal, with well-defined cytoplasm. Serous borderline tumours often show a greater degree of papillarity and a more haphazard arrangement of cell nests than usually is seen in mesothelial hyperplasia. Psammoma bodies may be seen in either lesion, although they are more numerous in serous borderline tumours (Bell & Scully, 1989; Clement & Young, 1993).

Multiloculated peritoneal inclusion cysts (multicystic mesothelioma)

These grossly cystic mesothelial proliferations of the peritoneum have been described by a variety of terms including, among others, peritoneal inclusion cysts (McFadden & Clement, 1986; Ross et al, 1989), cystic or multicystic mesothelioma (Mennemeyer & Smith, 1979; Moore et al, 1980; Katsube et al, 1982; Weiss & Tavassoli, 1988) and postoperative peritoneal cysts (Gussman et al, 1986), reflecting the numerous proposed theories regarding their pathogenesis.

Multiloculated peritoneal inclusion cysts occur predominantly in reproductive-aged women, although up to 17% of reported cases have been in men (Weiss & Tavassoli, 1988; Ross et al, 1989). The patients usually present with abdominal pain and the sensation of a mass; a small number have presented with symptoms of an acute abdomen. Up to 84% of patients have a history of prior abdominal surgery, endometriosis or pelvic inflammatory disease (Ross et al, 1989). On physical examination, a palpable mass is almost always present (Katsube et al, 1982; McFadden & Clement, 1986; Weiss & Tavassoli, 1988; Ross et al, 1989).

Grossly, localized aggregates or diffuse studding of the peritoneal surfaces by translucent fluid-filled cysts is usually seen. In a small number of cases, the translucent cysts are found floating free in the abdominal cavity. The cysts primarily involve the pelvic peritoneum but may involve the serosa of the intra-abdominal viscera, omentum or retroperitoneum (Weiss & Tavassoli, 1988; Ross et al, 1989). In one study, all cases with upper abdominal peritoneal or retroperitoneal involvement also had involvement of the pelvic peritoneum (Ross et al, 1989).

Microscopically, the cysts are lined by one to two layers of flattened, cuboidal, or hobnail-shaped mesothelial cells that show minimal cytological atypia. Small detached groups or papillary clusters of similar cells are often present in the cyst lumens focally. Squamous metaplasia of the lining epithelium is seen in a small number of cases. The cysts are separated by scantly to moderately cellular connective tissue that is often infiltrated by lymphocytes (Fig. 30.3). Extension of mesothelial cells into the stroma of multiple peritoneal inclusion cysts is common; this phenomenon has been termed 'mural mesothelial proliferation' (McFadden & Clement, 1986) or 'adenomatoid change' (Weiss & Tavassoli, 1988). In cases with this feature, tubules, microcysts, plexiform nests, small nests, and cords of focally vacuolated mesothelial cells are present in the stroma. These structures are often arranged in a zonal pattern or in linear arrays parallel to the mesothelial cells lining the adjacent cysts.

Although there have been no well-documented examples of fatal multiple peritoneal inclusion cysts, postoperative recurrences have been reported in up to 50% of patients (Ross et al, 1989). Thus far, neither the size of the lesion nor the presence of mural mesothelial proliferations has been predictive of recurrence (Ross et al, 1989).

The pathogenesis of multiple peritoneal inclusion cysts has yet to be determined; features favouring a reactive or neoplastic pathogenesis have been summarized in several

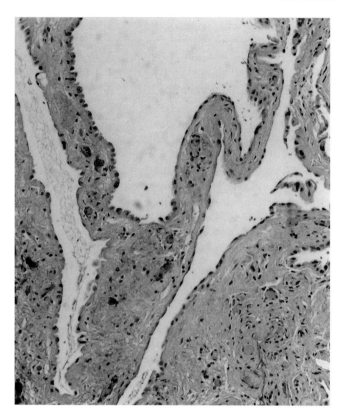

Fig. 30.3 Multiloculated peritoneal inclusion cysts. The cysts are lined by a single layer of flattened and polygonal mesothelial cells. H & E × 125.

Well-differentiated papillary mesothelioma

This mesothelial neoplasm occurs predominantly in reproductive-aged women with a smaller number occurring in men (Goepel, 1981; Addis & Fox, 1983; Daya & McCaughey, 1990, 1991) and young girls (Lovell & Cranston, 1990). The tumours are usually incidental findings; patients occasionally present with chronic pelvic pain, an acute abdomen, or ascites. Possible exposure to asbestos has been documented in rare cases (Daya & McCaughey, 1990).

On gross examination, multiple peritoneal nodules, some with a papillary appearance measuring up to several centimetres in diameter, are usually noted, although solitary nodules have also been described. The nodules may involve the omentum, pelvic and upper abdominal peritoneum (Goepel, 1981; Daya & McCaughey, 1990) or more rarely the tunica vaginalis (Chetty, 1992). Ovarian surface involvement was identified in four of 18 women with well-differentiated papillary mesotheliomas in one large study (Daya & McCaughey, 1990).

Histologically, the lesions show well-developed, often coarse, papillae lined by a single layer of uniform flattened to cuboidal mesothelial cells (Fig. 30.4). The papillary areas may be adjacent to tubules, branching cords or solid nests of similar cells. Extensive fibrosis may entrap and compress tubules, resulting in an irregular gland-like

recent publications (Weiss & Tavassoli, 1988; Ross et al, 1989). The microscopic presence of inflammation and fibrosis, the historical association with serosal injury and a benign clinical course are cited as evidence that these lesions are reactive (Ross et al, 1989), whereas the absence of a history of peritoneal injury in a substantial number of patients in many series and the microscopic association of multiple peritoneal inclusion cysts with diffuse malignant mesothelioma in one case are felt to support a neoplastic origin (Weiss & Tavassoli, 1988).

Multiple peritoneal inclusion cysts are most often confused with lymphangiomas microscopically. In contrast to multiple peritoneal inclusion cysts lymphangiomas occur in children, with a male predominance, and are located in the mesentery or retroperitoneum. Microscopically, they are lined by flattened endothelial cells and the stroma contains lymphoid aggregates or smooth muscle, features not generally present in multiple peritoneal inclusion cysts. Also, the lining cells do not form papillae or detached papillary clusters as is commonly seen in multiple peritoneal inclusion cysts (Weiss & Tavassoli, 1988; Ross et al, 1989; Daya & McCaughey, 1990). Immunohistochemical stains or ultrastructural studies are useful in establishing a definitive diagnosis of a mesothelial or endothelial origin in questionable cases (Mennemeyer & Smith, 1979; Moore et al, 1980).

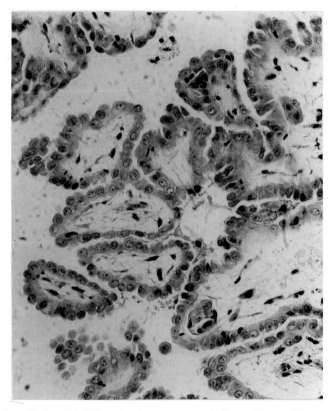

Fig. 30.4 Well-differentiated papillary mesothelioma. The papillae are lined by a single layer of cuboidal mesothelial cells. H & E × 313.

appearance. Psammoma bodies have been described in up to 25% of cases in some series (Goepel, 1981; Daya & McCaughey, 1990).

Although follow-up information is scant and in some cases is indeterminant, the majority of patients' tumours have behaved in a benign fashion. Several deaths, possibly secondary to tumour, have been reported (Burrig et al, 1990; Daya & McCaughey, 1990). The most convincing of these was in a 51-year-old man who died of extensive intra-abdominal tumour five years after the diagnosis of well-differentiated papillary mesothelioma. The recurrent tumour had the appearance of a diffuse malignant mesothelioma; however, the degree of sampling of the initial lesions was not discussed in the report (Burrig et al, 1990). Several other patients have died, but it is unclear whether their deaths resulted from intercurrent disease, complications of therapy or tumour (Daya & McCaughey, 1990). It is presently recommended that these neoplasms should be resected as completely as possible with careful clinical follow-up and that additional therapy should be withheld unless tumour progression is documented (Daya & McCaughey, 1990).

Diffuse malignant mesothelioma

Diffuse malignant mesothelioma of the peritoneum is less common than diffuse malignant mesothelioma of the pleura, accounting for 6–20% of cases in both sexes (Chahinian et al, 1982; Lerner et al, 1983; Daya & McCaughey, 1991; Sridhar et al, 1992). In our experience, peritoneal diffuse malignant mesotheliomas are rare in women; however, the percentage of female patients with such tumours varies in the literature from 7–57% (Kannerstein et al, 1977a; Casey Jones & Silver, 1979; Piccigallo et al, 1988; Plaus, 1988; Asensio et al, 1990). The great variation in incidence may reflect the erroneous classification of peritoneal serous carcinomas or well-differentiated papillary mesotheliomas as diffuse malignant mesothelioma. The frequency of asbestos exposure in patients with peritoneal diffuse malignant mesothelioma ranges from zero to 50% (Casey Jones & Silver, 1979; Chahinian et al, 1982; Piccigallo et al, 1988; Plaus, 1988). Eighty-three per cent of patients had asbestos exposure in one large series; however, most of the patients in that study were identified through records of occupational exposure to asbestos, creating substantial selection bias (Kannerstein et al, 1977a). Peritoneal diffuse malignant mesotheliomas have also been reported after radiation therapy (Babcock & Powell, 1976; Antman et al, 1983; Gilks et al, 1990) or recurrent peritonitis (Riddell et al, 1981). Peritoneal diffuse malignant mesotheliomas are most commonly diagnosed in the fifth to seventh decades of life (Kannerstein et al, 1977a; Casey Jones & Silver, 1979; Piccigallo et al, 1988; Plaus, 1988; Asensio et al, 1990), although they may occur in younger women,

especially those with childhood asbestos exposure (Kane et al, 1990). The presenting symptoms are relatively nonspecific including abdominal pain, distension and weight loss (Kannerstein et al, 1977a; Casey Jones & Silver, 1979; Piccigallo et al, 1988; Plaus, 1988; Asensio et al, 1990; Kane et al, 1990). Ascites is usually present and an abdominal or pelvic mass is often palpable (Kannerstein et al, 1977a; Casey Jones & Silver, 1979; Piccigallo et al, 1988; Plaus, 1988; Asensio et al, 1990; Kane et al, 1990).

Grossly, both the parietal and visceral peritoneal surfaces are studded with nodules or plaques of tumour measuring from several mm in diameter up to 25 cm in greatest dimension. Diffuse thickening of the peritoneum or omentum may also be seen (Kannerstein et al, 1977a). As the tumour spreads, it may encase the viscera, frequently infiltrating the bowel wall. Occasionally, the retroperitoneum, including the pancreas, may be extensively involved by tumour. Sites of metastatic tumour include lymph nodes, liver and lung; the pleura as well as peritoneum is involved in a minority of cases (Kannerstein et al, 1977a; McCaughey et al, 1985).

Microsopically, diffuse malignant mesotheliomas have a varied histological appearance and are classified as epithelial, biphasic or mixed, and sarcomatous (Kannerstein et al, 1977a; McCaughey et al, 1985; Daya & McCaughey, 1991). The majority of peritoneal diffuse malignant mesotheliomas are of epithelial type which accounted for 75% of cases, the biphasic type for 22% and the sarcomatous type for 2.4% of cases in one large detailed histological study of tumours in patients of both sexes (Kannerstein et al, 1977a).

Epithelial tumours or the epithelial component of biphasic neoplasms are characterized by tubules, branching tubules or clefts, papillae, or tubulopapillary structures lined by cuboidal, columnar, hobnail or pleomorphic cells. Sheets of round or polygonal cells may also be seen. Nuclear atypia ranges from mild to marked (Fig. 30.5). The cytoplasm is generally amphophilic; large cytoplasmic vacuoles that do not stain with PAS with diastase or mucicarmine are often present, at least focally. In rare cases the epithelial component may form nests and cords of small hyperchromatic cells similar to small cell carcinoma. In pure epithelial diffuse malignant mesothelioma, the tubules and papillae are separated by a mildly cellular, oedematous or myxoid stroma.

Pure sarcomatous diffuse malignant mesotheliomas generally have the appearance of non-specific sarcomas of spindle cell type although they may have the appearance of malignant fibrous histiocytoma, fibrosarcoma, rhabdomyosarcoma or malignant schwannoma. Focally, diffuse malignant mesotheliomas may be extensively fibrotic or desmoplastic and the tumour cells in these areas may be small, irregular, and hyperchromatic.

Diffuse malignant mesotheliomas are classified as biphasic when both the epithelial and stromal components

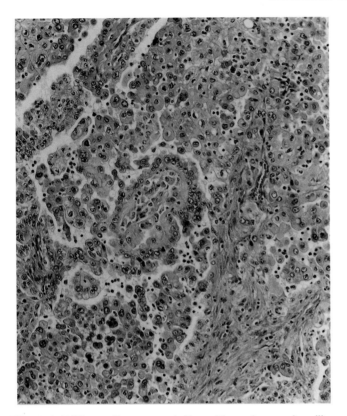

Fig. 30.5 Diffuse malignant mesothelioma. Nests, sheets and papillae are present. The cells are round or polygonal with hyperchromatic pleomorphic nuclei. H & E × 125.

are clearly malignant. The two components may be intimately intermixed or more commonly form separate areas of the neoplasm (Kannerstein et al, 1977a; McCaughey et al, 1985; Daya & McCaughey, 1991).

The histological differential diagnosis of epithelial peritoneal diffuse malignant mesothelioma generally includes mesothelial hyperplasia, multiloculated peritoneal inclusion cysts, well-differentiated papillary mesothelioma, metastatic carcinoma and primary Müllerian tumours of the peritoneum. The features that distinguish between diffuse malignant mesothelioma and other mesothelial lesions have been discussed in the previous sections. Features that favour a diagnosis of serous carcinoma over diffuse malignant mesothelioma either primarily or secondarily involving the peritoneum include the presence of columnar cells, overlapping nuclei, the presence of slit-like spaces, numerous psammoma bodies and intracytoplasmic epithelial mucin (Kannerstein et al, 1977a,b; Foyle et al, 1981; White et al, 1985; Truong et al, 1990).

Numerous studies have demonstrated that special stains, electronmicroscopy and immunohistochemical stains are valuable adjuncts in differentiating between epithelial diffuse malignant mesothelioma and adenocarcinomas involving the serosal surfaces (Dabbs & Geisinger, 1988; Bollinger et al, 1989; Tickman et al, 1990; Wick et al, 1990; Sheibani et al, 1990; Gaffey et al,

1992; Leong et al, 1992; Flynn et al, 1993; Weiss & Battifora, 1993). Adenocarcinomas often contain neutral epithelial mucin as demonstrated by mucicarmine and PAS-diastase stains, and diffuse malignant mesotheliomas frequently contain hyaluronic acid demonstrated as hyaluronidase digestible Alcian Blue or colloidal-iron positive material (McCaughey et al, 1985; Bollinger et al, 1989; Leong et al, 1992). The practical usefulness of such stains is limited, however, by the substantial proportion of tumours in both categories that do not stain for these products (Bollinger et al, 1989; Leong et al, 1992).

Ultrastructural analysis may also distinguish between diffuse malignant mesothelioma and adenocarcinoma. The epithelial elements of diffuse malignant mesothelioma have abundant, long, branching, 'bushy' circumferential microvilli and tonofilaments whereas adenocarcinomas contain gland lumens, short microvilli and mucin droplets (McCaughey et al, 1985; Bedrossian et al, 1992).

Immunohistochemical stains are the most widely used aid in distinguishing diffuse malignant mesothelioma from adenocarcinoma. Most of the immunoperoxidase studies in the literature have focused on defining the best diagnostic panel for differentiating pulmonary adenocarcinoma from pleural diffuse malignant mesothelioma, with antibodies to keratin, CEA, Leu-M1 and B72.3 having been suggested recently as the optimal diagnostic panel for these tumours (Brown et al, 1993; Weiss & Battifora, 1993).

A smaller number of studies have attempted to determine the most sensitive and specific combination of antibodies to distinguish peritoneal diffuse malignant mesothelioma from the neoplasms that commonly involve the peritoneum of women. Antibodies against CEA are not as useful in this differential diagnosis because only 6–52% of serous carcinomas of ovarian or peritoneal origin stain positively with this antibody (Dabbs & Geisinger, 1988; Bollinger et al, 1989; Tickman et al, 1990). As demonstrated in Table 30.1, antibodies against B72.3, PLAP, S100, Leu-M1 and BER-EP4 are more useful. Bollinger and co-workers (Bollinger et al, 1989) have suggested that staining with antibodies to either S100 and

Table 30.1 Antibody expression in peritoneal diffuse malignant mesothelioma (DMM) and serous carcinoma

Antibody	Percent positive	
	Peritoneal DMM	Serous carcinoma
Cytokeratin	100	100
BER-EP4	0–20★	82
Leu-M1	11–15	74–80
B72.3	0	72–100
CA-125	14	91
S100	11	87
PLAP	0	63
CEA	0	6–13

★Pleural and peritoneal diffuse malignant mesotheliomas combined (Gaffey et al, 1992)

B72.3 or S100 and PLAP may effectively separate serous carcinomas from diffuse malignant mesothelioma.

The prognosis of peritoneal diffuse malignant mesothelioma is very poor, with a median survival of 7–8 months (Chahinian et al, 1982; Piccigallo et al, 1988; Sridhar et al, 1992). Most patients die of tumour within 18 months (Casey Jones & Silver, 1979; Chahinian et al, 1982; Plaus, 1988; Spirtas et al, 1988; Asensio et al, 1990; Kane et al, 1990; Sridhar et al, 1992).

Intra-abdominal desmoplastic small round cell tumour

This recently described, distinctive small cell neoplasm appears to originate from the peritoneum and occurs in children and young adults (Gonzales-Crussi et al, 1990; Gerald et al, 1991; Layfield & Lenarsky, 1991; Young et al, 1992; Ordonez et al, 1993). Although these tumours were originally reported to have a strong predilection for adolescent males (Gerald et al, 1991), approximately 23% of reported cases in the literature have been in female patients (Ordonez et al, 1993) and ovarian involvement was prominent in several of them (Young et al, 1992). The histological and clinical features of male and female patients are similar.

A recent large series and review of the literature (Ordonez et al, 1993) found that intra-abdominal desmoplastic small round cell tumours occur in patients ranging in age from 3–38 years with a median age of 21 years. Most of the patients present with abdominal pain and distension (Gerald et al, 1991; Ordonez et al, 1993); occasional patients present with an acute abdomen (Gonzales-Crussi et al, 1990).

Macroscopic examination reveals numerous tumour nodules involving the abdominal and pelvic peritoneal surfaces. In many cases a large or dominant peritoneal mass is associated with smaller peritoneal nodules or implants. The nodules are firm with smooth or bosselated outer surfaces and are tan-white or grey on cut surface. Direct invasion of the intestinal wall or intra-abdominal viscera occasionally occurs; involvement of the retro-peritoneum as well as the peritoneum has been reported in 22–25% of cases (Gerald et al, 1991; Ordonez et al, 1993). Large ovarian masses have been reported in three female patients (Young et al, 1992).

Microscopically, desmoplastic small round cell tumour is characterized by nests or trabeculae of small cells separated by a fibrous or desmoplastic stroma that predominates, at least focally (Fig. 30.6). The cells are small with round to oval hyperchromatic nuclei and scant cytoplasm. Peripheral palisading of tumour cells is apparent focally and necrosis in the centre of tumour nests is common (Fig. 30.7). Unusual histological features which may be identified in a minority of cases include spindling of the

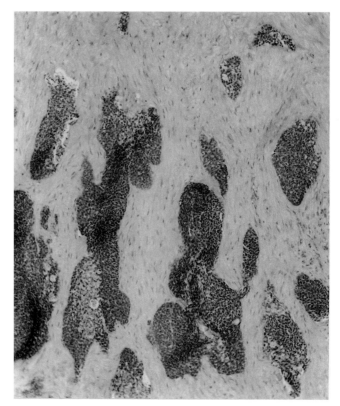

Fig. 30.6 Desmoplastic small round cell tumour. Nests of small cells are separated by a desmoplastic stroma. H & E × 31.

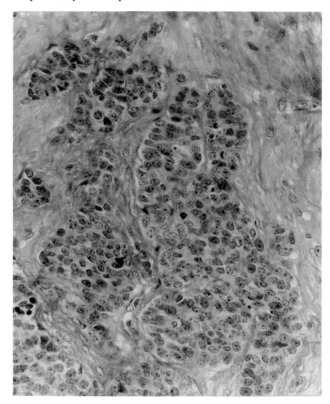

Fig. 30.7 Desmoplastic small round cell tumour. The cells are small with scant cytoplasm. Focal peripheral palisading of tumour cells is present at the periphery of the nests. H & E × 313.

neoplastic cells, formation of gland lumens or tubules, pleomorphic cells with cytological atypia, signet-ring-like cells and 'rhabdoid' cells with eosinophilic cytoplasm and eccentric nuclei (Gerald et al, 1991; Ordonez et al, 1993).

Although the histological appearance is distinctive, the diagnosis is confirmed by the unusual immunohistochemical profile expressed by these tumours. All of them show diffuse cytoplasmic positivity for antibodies against keratin; the majority of tumours also contain cells that stain for desmin. The desmin reactivity often appears as distinctive perinuclear 'dot-like' cytoplasmic staining, but may be diffuse. Stains for muscle-specific actin are generally negative (Gerald et al, 1991; Ordonez et al, 1993). The tumour cells in many cases also express neuro-endocrine markers. Most tumours that have been tested have reacted with antibodies against Leu-7 (CD57) (Layfield & Lenarsky, 1991; Young et al, 1992; Ordonez et al, 1993) and approximately one-half of them have shown staining for neurone-specific enolase. In contrast, only sporadic cases have stained with antibodies to chromogranin (Gonzales-Crussi et al, 1990) or synaptophysin (Gonzales-Crussi et al, 1990; Ordonez et al, 1993). The majority of desmoplastic small round cell tumours also stain for Leu-M1 (Young et al, 1992; Ordonez et al, 1993).

Ultrastructurally, the tumour cell nests are surrounded by basal lamina which may be discontinuous and the cells have intermediate junctions, desmosomes and, less commonly, tight junctions. A suggestion of lumens or well-developed small lumens containing microvilli has been reported in a small number of cases (Gerald et al, 1991; Ordonez et al, 1993). Many cells contain cytoplasmic aggregates of intermediate-sized filaments and cell processes have been reported infrequently (Gerald et al, 1991; Young et al, 1992; Ordonez et al, 1993). Dense core granules have been reported in only a small number of cases (Gerald et al, 1991; Young et al, 1992; Ordonez et al, 1993).

Although the clinical features support a primary peritoneal origin for this neoplasm, the histogenesis of the tumour remains uncertain. It has been postulated that the tumour is another example of a 'small round cell tumour' of childhood (Gerald et al, 1991) or that it is a primitive 'blastomatous neoplasm' of the peritoneum or mesothelium (Layfield & Lenarsky, 1991; Ordonez et al, 1993) because of the range of phenotypic expression within the neoplasm.

The differential diagnosis includes small cell neoplasms that may involve the peritoneum either primarily or secondarily. Diffuse malignant mesothelioma occurs predominantly in older individuals, but has been reported rarely in children and young adults (Grundy & Miller, 1972; Fraire et al, 1988; Kane et al, 1990). Uncommonly, the epithelial element of a diffuse malignant mesothelioma may be composed of small cells that mimic small cell carcinoma (McCaughey et al, 1985); however, further sampling of such a diffuse malignant mesothelioma usually reveals more typical areas of mesothelioma. Additionally, the immunohistochemical profiles of diffuse malignant mesothelioma and desmoplastic small round cell tumour are distinctive. Although desmoplastic small round cell tumour resembles other small cell tumours of childhood, such as Wilms' tumour, primitive neuroectodermal tumour, malignant rhabdoid tumour, and Ewing's sarcoma, these neoplasms rarely develop as diffuse peritoneal disease and have different ultrastructural and immunohistochemical characteristics. Desmoplastic small round cell tumour also must be differentiated from ovarian small cell carcinoma of the type often associated with hypercalcaemia which occurs in young females and may spread widely throughout the abdomen. Small cell carcinoma of the type associated with hypercalcaemia, in contrast to desmoplastic small round cell tumour, usually has a more diffuse growth pattern with inconspicuous stroma as well as the formation of 'follicle-like' spaces lined by tumour cells (Young et al, 1992).

The prognosis of desmoplastic small round cell tumour is very poor with a median survival of only 17 months; only very rare long-term survivors have been reported (Gonzales-Crussi et al, 1990; Gerald et al, 1991).

LESIONS OF THE SECONDARY MÜLLERIAN SYSTEM

It has been amply demonstrated that the female peritoneum is frequently the site of Müllerian epithelial lesions that exhibit the full spectrum of differentiation from benign to malignant (Lauchlan, 1984). The presence of Müllerian lesions beyond the direct derivatives of the Müllerian ducts (the cervix, endometrium and Fallopian tubes), primarily in the ovary and lower abdominal and pelvic peritoneum, has been ascribed to the existence of a 'secondary Müllerian system' of peritoneum with an increased propensity toward Müllerian differentiation. It has been speculated that the peritoneum and subperitoneal mesenchyme at these sites retains a potential for Müllerian differentiation due to its proximity to the coelomic epithelium from which the Müllerian ducts are derived. Alternatively, there may be 'nothing intrinsically specialized about peritoneum in this location' (Lauchlan, 1994). The development of Müllerian lesions may be secondary to the proximity of the pelvic peritoneum to the fimbriated end of the Fallopian tube which allows exposure of the peritoneal and ovarian surfaces to the outside environment and possible entry of a variety of external agents which may initiate Müllerian differentiation or 'mullerianosis' of the peritoneum (Lauchlan, 1972, 1984; Russell & Bannatyne, 1989; Lauchlan, 1994).

Serous lesions

Endosalpingiosis

Endosalpingiosis is defined as the presence of glandular inclusions lined by tubal-appearing epithelium located in ectopic sites. It most commonly involves the superficial layers of the peritoneum of the uterus, Fallopian tubes, ovaries or cul-de-sac (Sinykin, 1960; Schuldenfrei & Janovsky, 1962; Burmeister et al, 1969; Tutschka & Lauchlan, 1980; Holmes et al, 1981; Bryce et al, 1982; Zinsser & Wheeler, 1982; McCaughey et al, 1984; Dallenbach, 1987). Less frequent sites of involvement are the omentum (Tutschka & Lauchlan, 1980; Zinsser & Wheeler, 1982; McCaughey et al, 1984), bladder (Chen, 1981), and bowel serosa (Chen, 1981; Dallenbach, 1987; Cajigas & Axiotis, 1990), skin (Dore et al, 1980) and the pelvic or para-aortic lymph nodes (Shen et al, 1983; Ryuko et al, 1992).

Endosalpingiosis occurs in women ranging in age from 12–66 years, with a peak frequency in the third and fourth decades of life (Sinykin, 1960; Schuldenfrei & Janovsky, 1962; Burmeister et al, 1969; Dore et al, 1980; Tutschka & Lauchlan, 1980; Holmes et al, 1981; Bryce et al, 1982; Zinsser & Wheeler, 1982; Shen et al, 1983; McCaughey et al, 1984; Dallenbach, 1987; Cajigas & Axiotis, 1990; Ryuko et al, 1992). The majority of these women have clinical or pathological evidence of tubal disease such as chronic salpingitis with or without hydrosalpinx, prior tubal pregnancies, or salpingitis isthmica nodosum (Sinykin, 1960; Schuldenfrei & Janovsky, 1962; Holmes et al, 1982; Zinsser & Wheeler, 1982; Shen et al, 1983; McCaughey et al, 1984; McCaughey et al, 1985; Bell et al, 1988). Endosalpingiosis has also been identified in up to 56% of women with stage II or III ovarian serous borderline tumours (Sinykin, 1960; Burmeister et al, 1969; Zinsser & Wheeler, 1982; McCaughey et al, 1984; Bell et al, 1988; Ryuko et al, 1992); it has been noted likewise in association with benign (Sinykin, 1960; Tutschka & Lauchlan, 1980; Zinsser & Wheeler, 1982) and malignant serous tumours of the ovary (Zinsser & Wheeler, 1982).

On gross examination, endosalpingiosis usually is inapparent but can occasionally be appreciated as fine granularity or small cysts on the peritoneal surfaces (Sinykin, 1960; Schuldenfrei & Janovsky, 1962; Burmeister et al, 1969; Tutschka & Lauchlan, 1980; Holmes et al, 1981; Bryce et al, 1982; Shen et al, 1983; Dallenbach, 1987). In some cases it is associated with pelvic fibrous adhesions, which may be related to tubal inflammatory disease.

Histological examination reveals the presence of single smoothly contoured round or oval glands, or clusters of them beneath the serosa of the uterus or Fallopian tubes, the pelvic or extrapelvic parietal peritoneum, or the peritoneal surfaces of the omentum. The glands are lined by one to two layers of columnar cells that are commonly

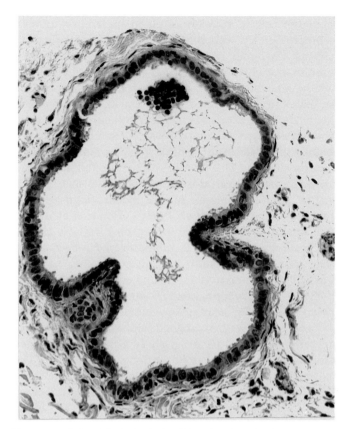

Fig. 30.8 Endosalpingiosis. A gland lined by ciliated columnar cells is present beneath the peritoneal surface. H & E × 313.

ciliated (Fig. 30.8). Less often, the lining epithelium is identical to that of the Fallopian tube, containing ciliated cells, secretory non-ciliated cells, and peg-shaped cells. The nuclei are generally round, oval or pencil-shaped, uniform, basally oriented, and show no cytological atypicality. Rarely, blunt papillae with prominent fibrovascular cores lined by similar epithelial cells are present within the glands. Mitotic figures are usually absent. Psammoma bodies are often present in the glands, in the stroma beneath the epithelium of the glands, or unassociated with epithelial cells. The glands are usually surrounded by several layers of delicate connective tissue infiltrated with scattered lymphocytes. In occasional cases, many of the glands are rimmed by a dense lymphocytic infiltrate (Sinykin, 1960; Schuldenfrei & Janovsky, 1962; Burmeister et al, 1969; Dore et al, 1980; Tutschka & Lauchlan, 1980; Holmes et al, 1981; Bryce et al, 1982; Zinsser & Wheeler, 1982; Shen et al, 1983; McCaughey et al, 1984; Dallenbach, 1987; Bell et al, 1988; Cajigas & Axiotis, 1990; Ryuko et al, 1992).

The histological differential diagnosis of endosalpingiosis includes endometriosis, mesothelial hyperplasia, peritoneal inclusion cysts, implants of ovarian serous borderline tumours, primary peritoneal serous borderline tumours, and metastatic adenocarcinoma. Although the cellular features of the glandular epithelium in endosalpingiosis and endometriosis may be similar, the obvious periglandular endometrial stroma that is usually identified in endometriosis in premenopausal women is not apparent in endosalpingiosis. It may be difficult, however, to distinguish these entities in postmenopausal women, when no endometrial stroma is discernible due to atrophy and fibrosis. The presence of stroma around some of the glands should not preclude a diagnosis of endosalpingiosis if typical endosalpingiotic glands without stroma are present as well, since endosalpingiosis and endometriosis are commonly found in continuity or in adjacent tissue (Zinsser & Wheeler, 1982). In mesothelial hyperplasia, cords, gland-like spaces and papillae may be present, although they are often arranged in rows parallel to the mesothelial surface (Rosai & Dehner, 1975; Bryce et al, 1982). The cells lining these mesothelial structures are typically not columnar and are not ciliated. Peritoneal inclusion cysts, in contrast to endosalpingiosis, are lined by one to several layers of flat-to-cuboidal mesothelial cells. Focally the cysts may be lined by columnar cells characteristic of endosalpingiosis; however, this is considered evidence of tubal metaplasia of the lining mesothelium (Ross et al, 1989). Endosalpingiosis may be differentiated from implants of ovarian serous borderline tumours and primary peritoneal serous borderline tumours by both architectural and cytological features. The papillarity, tufting, and especially detached buds of epithelial cells that are characteristic of serous borderline tumours are not seen in endosalpingiosis; also, the cells of endosalpingiosis show little or no cytological atypia. Endosalpingiosis can be distinguished from metastatic adenocarcinoma by the regular arrangement of simple glands in a non-infiltrative pattern and by the absence of cytological atypia or a significant stromal response. Cilia may be prominent in endosalpingiosis and are very rare in metastatic adenocarcinoma (Zinsser & Wheeler, 1982).

The histogenesis of endosalpingiosis remains in dispute. Theories of its origin are similar to those that have been suggested for the origin of endometriosis (Holmes et al, 1981; Zinsser & Wheeler, 1982; Shen et al, 1983). It has been suggested that endosalpingiosis results from direct extension of proliferating tubal epithelium to surrounding tissue, from implantation of sloughed tubal epithelium into the peritoneal cavity, from 'Müllerian' metaplasia of the coelomic epithelium, or from lymphatic or haematogenous spread to lymph nodes. The two most widely accepted theories currently are that of Müllerian metaplasia, which would also explain the common co-existence of endosalpingiosis and endometriosis, and that of peritoneal implantation by sloughed tubal epithelium, which would explain in part the strong association between endosalpingiosis and diseases of the Fallopian tubes (Zinsser & Wheeler, 1982).

Although endosalpingiosis is presumed to be benign, few reports with long-term follow-up are available.

Zinsser & Wheeler (1982) reported that subsequent tumour did not develop in any of their 16 patients with endosalpingiosis who were followed from 1–16 years.

Rare cases of endosalpingiosis with architectural and cytological atypia ranging in severity from mild nuclear pleomorphism and cellular stratification to moderate-to-severe nuclear atypia with prominent stratification, tufting and detachment of solid clusters of atypical epithelial cells have been reported (Zinsser & Wheeler, 1982; Fievez et al, 1983; Dallenbach, 1987). Lesions spanning this spectrum of histological appearance have been termed 'atypical endosalpingiosis' by some authors (Zinsser & Wheeler, 1982; Fievez et al, 1983; Dallenbach, 1987); we classify the former lesions as endosalpingiosis with atypia and the latter as peritoneal serous borderline tumours.

Peritoneal serous borderline tumours

In a small number of patients peritoneal lesions histologically identical to the peritoneal implants associated with ovarian serous borderline tumours are seen in the absence of ovarian involvement, in the presence of only a minimal degree of ovarian involvement, or in association with a serous cystadenoma. Two series of 25 and 17 patients each with these lesions which have been designated as 'serous borderline tumour of the peritoneum' or 'peritoneal serous micropapillomatosis of low malignant potential (serous borderline tumours of the peritoneum)' have been reported (Bell & Scully, 1990; Biscotti & Hart, 1992).

Peritoneal serous borderline tumours occur in women ranging from 16–67 (mean, 31–33) years of age. Infertility and abdominal pain are the most common presenting complaints, although many lesions are discovered as incidental findings.

Grossly, adhesions or granularity of the peritoneal surfaces is present. A mass is only rarely seen. In two-thirds of the cases, only the pelvic peritoneum is involved, with the upper abdominal peritoneum being affected as well in the remainder. Histologically, the tumours have the typical appearance of non-invasive implants of ovarian serous borderline tumours. Papillae or nests of moderately atypical columnar, cuboidal or polygonal cells are present on the peritoneal surfaces, in subperitoneal invaginations, or in crevices between omental fat lobules, either without an accompanying stromal response or compressed within a dense or reactive fibrous stroma. Invasion of underlying tissue is not seen (Fig. 30.9).

The histological differential diagnosis of peritoneal serous borderline tumour includes endosalpingiosis and florid papillary mesothelial hyperplasia. The features that differentiate between these entities have already been discussed.

Most women with peritoneal serous borderline tumour have been treated by hysterectomy with bilateral salpingo-

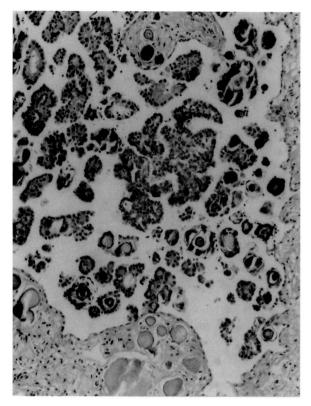

Fig. 30.9 Peritoneal serous borderline tumour. Papillae lined by cuboidal to columnar cells are present in a subperitoneal invagination. H & E × 125.

oophorectomy and omentectomy, and some also received chemotherapy. Fifteen of the patients had a limited operation to conserve fertility. Follow-up information from 37 patients revealed no clinical evidence of persistent disease in 31 of them. Borderline tumour recurred in two patients, who remained well for 1.7 and 2 years after re-excision of the recurrent tumour, and two additional patients developed small bowel obstruction and were living without progressive disease 11 and 16 years after diagnosis. Invasive low-grade serous carcinoma of the peritoneum developed in one woman, who was living with extensive intra-abdominal tumour at the last follow-up examination; another woman died of disseminated serous tumour which was diagnosed cytologically, but not confirmed by biopsy. This excellent prognosis, even with limited operative therapy, indicates that conservation of the reproductive organs may be considered in young women after careful clinical evaluation to exclude a primary ovarian serous borderline tumour.

Although most extraovarian serous borderline tumours are of the diffuse type and do not form grossly visible cysts, occasional cases in which the tumour has the typical gross features of a serous papillary cystadenoma of borderline malignancy have been reported, most frequently in the broad ligament (Aslani et al, 1988). These tumours have all been stage Ia, have been unassociated with ovarian involvement and have been cured by cystectomy.

Serous psammocarcinoma

Although it is classified separately, a tumour that shows many features similar to serous borderline tumour is the rare serous psammocarcinoma of the peritoneum (McCaughey et al, 1986; Gilks et al, 1990). This diagnosis has been proposed for serous tumours with the following microscopic features:

1. invasion of omentum, intraperitoneal viscera or their vascular spaces
2. no more than moderate nuclear atypia
3. solid epithelial nests no greater than 15 cells in diameter
4. at least 75% of the papillae or nests contain psammoma bodies (Fig. 30.10).

Except for invasion and striking calcification, these tumours are very similar in appearance to serous borderline tumours. Among the five cases reported, the patients ranged from 48–58 years of age. None of these patients developed evidence of recurrent tumour; however, only two patients had been followed for long intervals. The remaining patients had been followed for less than one year. Despite the small number of cases reported, it is felt that these tumours probably have the same prognosis as serous borderline tumours.

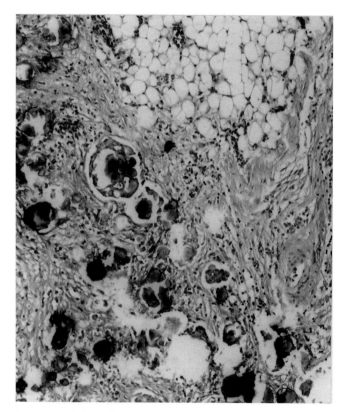

Fig. 30.10 Peritoneal serous psammocarcinoma. Papillary groups of moderately atypical epithelial cells, most associated with psammoma bodies, infiltrate the omentum. H & E × 125.

Peritoneal serous carcinoma

In the past decade, many studies have examined the clinicopathological features of this variant of serous carcinoma that extensively involves peritoneal surfaces with minimal or no ovarian parenchymal involvement (Kannerstein et al, 1977b; Foyle et al, 1981; Gooneratne et al, 1982; Tobacman et al, 1982; Hochster et al, 1984; August et al, 1985; White et al, 1985; Chen & Flam, 1986; Lele et al, 1988; Mills et al, 1988; Dalrymple et al, 1989; Raju et al, 1989; Rutledge et al, 1989; Fromm et al, 1990; Ransom et al, 1990; Truong et al, 1990; Fowler et al, 1994). The age and clinical presentation of women with serous carcinoma arising from the peritoneum are similar to those of women with advanced stage serous carcinoma of ovarian origin. On gross examination, the appearance of the peritoneal tumour is similar in both entities; the peritoneum is usually diffusely involved by small nodules or warty excrescences as well as by larger masses that often involve the omentum. In most cases the ovaries are grossly normal in size and shape but closer examination in many cases reveals fine granularity, small nodules or warty excrescences on their surfaces (Kannerstein et al, 1977b; Foyle et al, 1981; Gooneratne et al, 1982; August et al, 1985; White et al, 1985; Lele et al, 1988; Mills et al, 1988; Dalrymple et al, 1989; Fromm et al, 1990; Ransom et al, 1990). On microscopic examination, the peritoneal tumour has the typical histological appearance of serous carcinoma which, in the majority of reported cases, has been moderately or poorly differentiated (Gooneratne et al, 1982; White et al, 1985; Dalrymple et al, 1989; Rutledge et al, 1989; Ransom et al, 1990; Fowler et al, 1994). Psammoma bodies are present in most cases (Fig. 30.11).

Much of the controversy surrounding these neoplasms has focused on their biological behaviour and histogenesis. Although it has been suggested that serous surface carcinomas are highly aggressive and have a less favourable prognosis than their ovarian counterparts of similar grade and stage (Gooneratne et al, 1982; White et al, 1985; Mills et al, 1988) several recent larger studies have reported no differences in survival between these two tumours when patients were treated with standard ovarian carcinoma chemotherapeutic protocols (Lele et al, 1988; Dalrymple et al, 1989; Fromm et al, 1990; Ransom et al, 1990; Truong et al, 1990; Fowler et al, 1994); small numbers of long-term survivors have been reported after such therapy (Hochster et al, 1984; Chen & Flam, 1986). One study found a significantly longer survival in patients treated with cisplatin-containing treatment protocols compared with non-cisplatin-containing regimens, possibly accounting for the differing conclusions among various investigators (Fromm et al, 1990).

Although it has been suggested that these tumours represent massive peritoneal spread from small ovarian

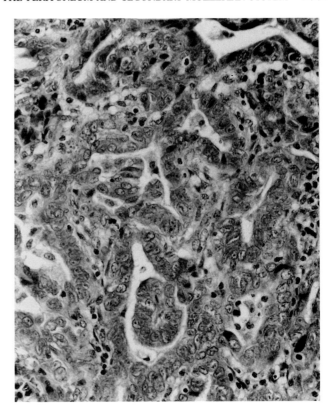

Fig. 30.11 Peritoneal serous carcinoma. Glands, papillae and slit-like spaces are lined by cuboidal to columnar cells with pleomorphic, overlapping nuclei. H & E × 313.

primary carcinomas (Gooneratne et al, 1982), the extent of peritoneal involvement, the absence of ovarian involvement in some women, and the development of these neoplasms in patients whose ovaries were normal at the time of prior bilateral oophorectomies for benign disease or family histories of ovarian carcinoma indicate that they arise from extraovarian peritoneum (Tobacman et al, 1982; Lele et al, 1988; Dalrymple et al, 1989; Fromm et al, 1990). Electronmicroscopical and immunohistochemical studies have failed to allow definitive conclusions regarding the histogenesis of these tumours. Several groups report features common to both serous carcinomas and mesotheliomas (Gooneratne et al, 1982; August et al, 1985; White et al, 1985) and other groups report features identical to those of serous carcinoma (Raju et al, 1989; Truong et al, 1990). A single study using flow cytometry has shown that 29% of serous surface carcinomas exhibit heterogeneity of DNA content at various sites (Rutledge et al, 1989), a finding that supports a multifocal peritoneal origin of these neoplasms given the high rate of agreement of DNA content, ranging from 87–100% between primary ovarian carcinomas and their peritoneal metastases (Erba et al, 1985; Volm et al, 1985; Blumenfeld et al, 1987; Iversen & Skaarland, 1987; Rodenburg et al, 1987).

Peritoneal serous carcinomas can be distinguished from peritoneal serous borderline tumours by the presence of invasion of omentum or underlying intra-abdominal viscera and the greater degree of nuclear atypicality in the former; the degree of nuclear atypicality also distinguishes serous carcinomas from the much rarer serous psammo-carcinomas of peritoneal origin. Peritoneal serous carcinomas may be differentiated from malignant mesotheliomas by the presence of columnar cells with overlapping nuclei, slit-like spaces, numerous psammoma bodies, and intra-cytoplasmic neutral mucin as demonstrated by mucicar-mine or period acid–Schiff stains after diastase digestion in the former (Kannerstein et al, 1977b; Foyle et al, 1981; White et al, 1985; Truong et al, 1990).

Mucinous lesions

Endocervicosis

Subperitoneal glandular inclusions lined by benign muci-nous epithelium have been reported only rarely involving the posterior uterine serosa, cul-de-sac (Lauchlan, 1972), subserosa of the vermiform appendix, and urinary bladder (Fig. 30.12) (Clement & Young, 1992). Similar lesions have also been reported in cutaneous scars (Lauchlan, 1965) and pelvic lymph nodes (Ferguson et al, 1969; Baird & Reddick, 1991). These lesions may be distin-guished from metastatic adenocarcinoma by the absence of cytological atypia in them.

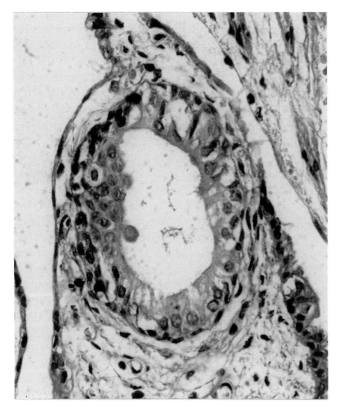

Fig. 30.12 Endocervicosis. A gland lined by mucin-containing columnar cells is present beneath the peritoneum. H & E × 500.

Mucinous neoplasms

Diffuse infiltration of the omentum or peritoneum by mucinous glands showing mild to moderately atypical epithelium has been reported in association with benign appearing mucinous lesions of the ovary and appendix (Seidman et al, 1993), but not to our knowledge in the absence of a co-existing mucinous neoplasm. Such findings have prompted the argument that some cases of pseudomyxoma peritonei are primary neoplasms of the peritoneum rather than metastatic deposits from mucinous tumours at other sites (Seidman et al, 1993).

Localized cystic mucinous tumours have been de-scribed rarely in the retroperitoneum, primarily as isolated case reports (Douglas et al, 1965; Williams et al, 1971; Lauchlan, 1972; Banerjee & Gough, 1988; Pennell & Gusdon, 1989; Park et al, 1990). These neoplasms occur in women ranging in age from 18–58 years. The spectrum of histological abnormalities in these tumours mimics that seen in primary cystic mucinous neoplasms of the ovary, ranging from benign to borderline to frankly malignant. All of the mucinous cystadenomas behaved in a benign fashion, several of the mucinous cystadenocarcinomas metastasized widely resulting in the death of the patient (Douglas et al, 1965; Roth & Ehrlich, 1977), and one tumour with a borderline histology metastasized to medi-astinal lymph nodes (Banerjee & Gough, 1988). Although it has been postulated that retroperitoneal cystic tumours may arise from teratomas or ectopic ovarian tissue (Williams et al, 1971), the absence of residual terato-matous elements or ovarian tissue in these neoplasms would support their origin from coelomic epithelium (Banerjee & Gough, 1988; Pennell & Gusdon, 1989; Park et al, 1990).

Transitional lesions

Walthard nests

Solid nests, cysts and surface plaques composed of transi-tional-like cells termed Walthard nests are common on the pelvic peritoneum. These lesions measure up to several millimetres in greatest dimension and are most frequently identified on the posterior-lateral serosa of the Fallopian tubes, on the posterior surface of the meso-salpinx and less often in the meso-ovarium or ovary (Teoh, 1953; Bransilver et al, 1974). They have also been described involving the serosa of the appendix testis and epididymis in men (Hartz, 1947; Sundarasivarao, 1953). Histologically, the nests are composed of polygonal cells with oval nuclei and scant to moderate amounts of cytoplasm that resemble urothelial cells. The nuclei focally contain longitudinal nuclear grooves; the cysts often contain eosinophilic or amorphous material (Fig. 30.13) (Teoh, 1953; Bransilver et al, 1974; Roth, 1974).

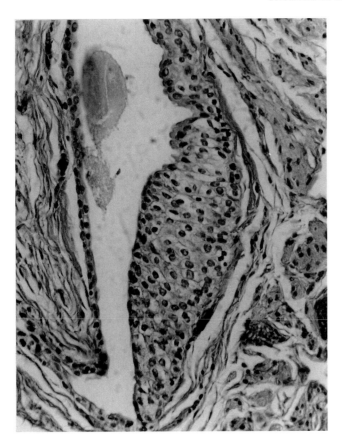

Fig. 30.13 Walthard nest. The cyst is lined by polygonal cells with bland nuclei that resemble urothelial cells. Amorphous material is present in the lumen. H & E × 313.

Because of the light- and electronmicroscopic similarities of Walthard nests to urothelium, and because of their frequently documented continuity with the surface mesothelium, these lesions are felt to arise from metaplasia of the mesothelium (Bransilver et al, 1974; Roth, 1974).

Transitional cell neoplasms

Although Walthard nests of the peritoneum are common, extraovarian Brenner tumours have been reported as individual case reports only rarely. These tumours have been identified as solid masses in older women; most have been located in the broad ligament. Borderline or malignant Brenner tumours or peritoneal transitional cell carcinomas have not been described thus far (Pschera & Wikstrom, 1991; Hampton et al, 1992).

Squamous lesions

Very few examples of squamous metaplasia of otherwise normal peritoneum have been reported (Crome, 1950; Schatz & Colgan, 1991), although squamous metaplasia of peritoneal inclusion cysts is common (Ross et al, 1989). True squamous metaplasia may be distinguished from the much more common transitional metaplasia by the

orderly maturation of the epithelial cells to superficial cells, prominent intercellular bridges and presence of cytoplasmic keratinization or keratohyaline granules in the former.

Clear cell lesions

Although focal clear cell differentiation is observed in a substantial number of peritoneal serous carcinomas (Mills et al, 1988; Truong et al, 1990), pure clear cell carcinoma of the peritoneum without co-existing evidence of endometriosis has been reported only once in a 67-year-old woman (Lee et al, 1991) and we have observed an additional case in a patient from our institution. A small number of localized clear cell carcinomas of the retroperitoneum have been reported (Brooks & Wheeler, 1977; Goldberg et al, 1979; Mostoufizadeh & Scully, 1980; Evans et al, 1990); most of them were felt to arise from endometriosis.

Ectopic decidua

Extrauterine decidua formation is common in pregnant women and occurs rarely in non-pregnant patients in association with progestational agent therapy, trophoblastic neoplasia, hormonally active lesions of the ovary and adrenal, in proximity to a corpus luteum or after radiation therapy. Occasionally ectopic decidua is observed without an apparent underlying cause in either premenopausal or postmenopausal women (Ober et al, 1957; Boss et al, 1965; Clement, 1993). Ectopic decidua has been reported in the ovary, cervix (Zaytsev & Taxy, 1987), uterine, bowel and appendiceal serosa (Suster & Moran, 1990), omentum, renal pelvis (Bettinger, 1947) and periaortic and pelvic lymph nodes (Zaytsev & Taxy, 1987; Cobb, 1988). The patients are usually asymptomatic, although a small number of women have presented with intra-abdominal haemorrhage (Sabatelle & Winger, 1973; Richter et al, 1983) or pain (Hulme-Moir & Ross, 1969; Suster & Moran, 1990).

Ectopic decidua involving peritoneal surfaces usually is not evident grossly although in a few cases the peritoneal surfaces are studded with greyish-white granules or plaques measuring up to several millimetres in diameter (O'Sullivan & Heffernan, 1960). Microscopically, single cells, nodules or ill-defined aggregates of cells are present beneath the mesothelium. The decidual cells have abundant amphophilic cytoplasm and round to oval, uniform nuclei with delicate chromatin and prominent nucleoli (Fig. 30.14). Smooth muscle cells are occasionally interspersed among the decidual cells.

Ectopic decidua can be distinguished from malignant mesothelioma, metastatic carcinoma or sarcoma by the uniformity and bland appearance of the nuclei in the former.

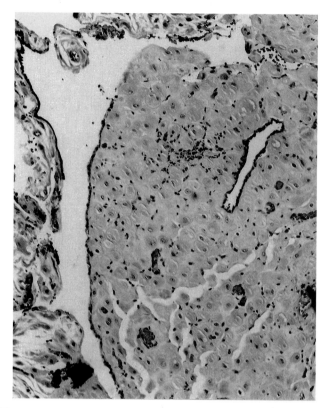

Fig. 30.14 Ectopic decidua. A nodule of decidual cells with abundant cytoplasm and uniform nuclei is present beneath the mesothelium. H & E × 125.

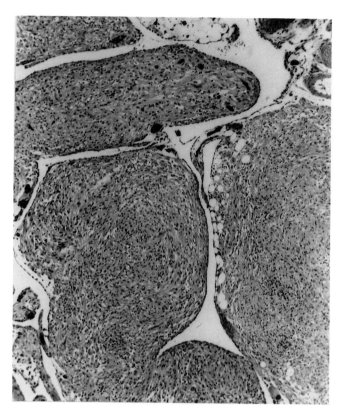

Fig. 30.15 Diffuse peritoneal leiomyomatosis. Nodules of interlacing bundles of smooth muscle cells are located beneath the mesothelium. H & E × 50.

Diffuse peritoneal leiomyomatosis

Diffuse peritoneal leiomyomatosis (DPL) is characterized by multiple subperitoneal nodules of smooth muscle that occur in reproductive-aged women (Parmley et al, 1975; Winn et al, 1976; Nogales et al, 1978; Herr et al, 1979; Pieslor et al, 1979; Kaplan et al, 1980; Kuo et al, 1980; Fujii et al, 1981; Hsu et al, 1981; Ceccacci et al, 1982; Tavassoli & Norris, 1982; Akkersdijk et al, 1990; Hales et al, 1992). The patients are usually pregnant, postpartum or on oral contraceptives, although cases have been reported in women with none of these conditions (Fujii et al, 1981; Tavassoli & Norris, 1982). Clinically, diffuse peritoneal leiomyomatosis is usually an asymptomatic incidental finding. Approximately half of the patients have abdominal pain or vaginal bleeding, which is usually attributable to co-existing uterine leiomyomas (Tavassoli & Norris, 1982).

Grossly, diffuse peritoneal leiomyomatosis is seen as numerous white or tan, firm peritoneal nodules ranging in size from less than 1 mm to 10 cm (Nogales et al, 1978; Pieslor et al, 1979; Kuo et al, 1980; Tavassoli & Norris, 1982; Akkersdijk et al, 1990; Hales et al, 1992), although the majority of lesions measure less than several centimetres in diameter. Microscopically, the nodules are located beneath the mesothelium and are composed of interlacing bundles of spindle cells with elongated, uniform nuclei (Fig. 30.15). Cytological atypia and mitotic figures are not generally identified, although Tavassoli & Norris (1982) reported up to 3 mitotic figures per 10 high power fields in two of their 20 cases. Decidual cells are often intermixed with smooth muscle cells in pregnant patients (Tavassoli & Norris, 1982). Ultrastructurally the cells in the nodules have been shown to have features of smooth muscle cells; myofibroblasts, fibroblasts and decidual cells have also been identified (Winn et al, 1976; Nogales et al, 1978; Pieslor et al, 1979; Kuo et al, 1980; Ceccacci et al, 1982; Tavassoli & Norris, 1982).

Despite the aggressive clinical appearance of diffuse peritoneal leiomyomatosis only two cases of progressive disease have been reported in which patients originally diagnosed with diffuse peritoneal leiomyomatosis subsequently developed leiomyosarcomas (Akkersdijk et al, 1990). Follow-up laparotomy or laparoscopy has documented complete or partial regression of the lesions in some patients (Tavassoli & Norris, 1982); this is the probable clinical course in most women. Persistence or recurrence in later pregnancies has been reported in a small number of women (Tavassoli & Norris, 1982; Hales et al, 1992).

It is generally accepted that diffuse peritoneal leiomyomatosis results from hormonally-related smooth muscle metaplasia of subperitoneal mesenchyme. The development of diffuse peritoneal leiomyomatosis in pregnant women or women taking oral contraceptives, the regression of the lesions postpartum or after discontinuation of exogenous hormones (Tavassoli & Norris, 1982) or after treatment with a gonadotrophin-releasing agonist (Hales et al, 1992), and the production of lesions resembling diffuse peritoneal leiomyomatosis in guinea pigs (Fujii et al, 1981) all support this hypothesis.

Diffuse peritoneal leiomyomatosis may be distinguished from metastatic leiomyosarcoma by both microscopic and gross features. Grossly, the nodules of diffuse peritoneal leiomyomatosis tend to be numerous and small whereas leiomyosarcomas usually present as one or several large masses. Histologically, diffuse peritoneal leiomyomatosis is cytologically bland with few mitotic figures; marked atypia and mitotic activity characterize metastatic leiomyosarcoma.

REFERENCES

Addis B J, Fox H 1983 Papillary mesothelioma of ovary. Histopathology 7: 287–298.

Akkersdijk G J M, Flu P K, Giard R W M et al 1990 Malignant leiomyomatosis peritonealis disseminata. American Journal of Obstetrics and Gynecology 163: 591–593.

Antman K H, Corson J M, Li F P 1983 Malignant mesothelioma following radiation exposure. Journal of Clinical Oncology 1: 695–700.

Asensio J A, Goldblatt P, Thomford N R 1990 Primary malignant peritoneal mesothelioma: a report of seven cases and a review of the literature. Archives of Surgery 125: 1477–1481.

Aslani M, Ahn G H, Scully R E 1988 Serous papillary cystadenoma of borderline malignancy of broad ligament: a report of 25 cases. International Journal of Gynecological Pathology 7: 131–138.

August C Z, Murad T M, Newton M 1985 Multiple focal extraovarian serous carcinoma. International Journal of Gynecological Pathology 4: 11–23.

Babcock T L, Powell D H 1976 Radiation induced peritoneal mesothelioma. Journal of Surgical Oncology 8: 369–372.

Baird D B, Reddick R L 1991 Extraovarian mucinous metaplasia in a patient with bilateral mucinous borderline tumors: a case report. International Journal of Gynecological Pathology 10: 96–103.

Banerjee R, Gough J 1988 Cystic mucinous tumours of the mesentery and retroperitoneum: report of three cases. Histopathology 12: 527–532.

Bedrossian C W, Bonsib S, Moran C 1992 Differential diagnosis between mesothelioma and adenocarcinoma: a multimodal approach based on ultrastructure and immunocytochemistry. Seminars in Diagnostic Pathology 9: 124–140.

Bell D A, Scully R E 1989 Benign and borderline serous lesions of the peritoneum in women. Pathology Annual 2: 1–21.

Bell D A, Scully R E 1990 Serous borderline tumors of the peritoneum. American Journal of Surgical Pathology 14: 230–239.

Bell D A, Weinstock M A, Scully R E 1988 Peritoneal implants of ovarian serous borderline tumors: histologic features and prognosis. Cancer 62: 2212–2222.

Bettinger H F 1947 Ectopic decidua in the renal pelvis. Journal of Pathology and Bacteriology 59: 686–687.

Biscotti C V, Hart W R 1992 Peritoneal serous micropapillomatosis of low malignant potential (serous borderline tumors of the peritoneum): a clinicopathologic study of 17 cases. American Journal of Surgical Pathology 16: 467–475.

Blumenfeld D, Braly P S, Ben E J et al 1987 Tumor DNA content as a prognostic feature in advanced epithelial ovarian carcinoma. Gynecologic Oncology 27: 389–402.

Bollinger D J, Wick M R, Dehner L P et al 1989 Peritoneal malignant mesothelioma versus serous papillary adenocarcinoma: a histochemical and immunohistochemical comparison. American Journal of Surgical Pathology 13: 659–670.

Boss J H, Scully R E, Wegner K H et al 1965 Structural variations in the adult ovary — clinical significance. Obstetrics and Gynecology 25: 747–763.

Bransilver B R, Ferenczy A, Richart R M 1974 Brenner tumors and Walthard cell nests. Archives of Pathology 98: 76–86.

Brooks J J, Wheeler J E 1977 Malignancy arising in extragonadal endometriosis. Cancer 40: 3065–3073.

Brown J V, Karlan B Y, Greenspoon J S et al 1993 Perioperative coagulopathy in patients undergoing primary cytoreduction. Cancer 71: 2557–2561.

Bryce R L, Barbatis C, Charnock M 1982 Endosalpingiosis in pregnancy: case report. British Journal of Obstetrics and Gynaecology 89: 166–168.

Burmeister R E, Fechner R E, Franklin R R 1969 Endosalpingiosis of the peritoneum. Obstetrics and Gynecology 34: 310–318.

Burrig K F, Pfitzer P, Hort W 1990 Well-differentiated papillary mesothelioma of the peritoneum: a borderline mesothelioma: report of two cases and review of literature. Virchows Arch A Pathological Anatomy and Histopathology 417: 443–447.

Cajigas A, Axiotis C A 1990 Endosalpingiosis of the vermiform appendix. International Journal of Gynecological Pathology 9: 291–295.

Casey Jones D E, Silver D 1979 Peritoneal mesotheliomas. Surgery 86: 556–560.

Ceccacci L, Jacobs J, Powell A 1982 Leiomyomatosis peritonealis disseminata: report of a case in a nonpregnant woman. American Journal of Obstetrics and Gynecology 144: 105–109.

Chahinian A P, Pajak T F, Holland J F et al 1982 Diffuse malignant mesothelioma: prospective evaluation of 69 patients. Annals of Internal Medicine 96: 746–755.

Chen K T 1981 Benign glandular inclusions of the peritoneum and periaortic lymph nodes. Diagnostic Gynecology and Obstetrics 3: 265–268.

Chen K T, Flam M S 1986 Peritoneal papillary serous carcinoma with long-term survival. Cancer 58: 1371–1373.

Chetty R 1992 Well differentiated (benign) papillary mesothelioma of the tunica vaginalis. Journal of Clinical Pathology 45: 1029–1030.

Clement P B 1993 Tumor-like lesions of the ovary associated with pregnancy. International Journal of Gynecological Pathology 12: 108–115.

Clement P B, Young R H 1992 Endocervicosis of the urinary bladder: a report of six cases of a benign mullerian lesion that may mimic adenocarcinoma. American Journal of Surgical Pathology 16: 533–542.

Clement P B, Young R H 1993 Florid mesothelial hyperplasia associated with ovarian tumors: a potential source of error in tumor diagnosis and staging. International Journal of Gynecological Pathology 12: 51–58.

Cobb C J 1988 Ectopic decidua and metastatic squamous carcinoma: presentation in a single pelvic lymph node. Journal of Surgical Oncology 38: 126–129.

Crome L 1950 Squamous metaplasia of the peritoneum. Journal of Pathology and Bacteriology 62: 61–68.

Dabbs D J, Geisinger K R 1988 Common epithelial ovarian tumors: immunohistochemical intermediate filament profiles. Cancer 62: 368–374.

Dallenbach H G 1987 Atypical endosalpingiosis: a case report with consideration of the differential diagnosis of glandular subperitoneal inclusions. Pathology Research and Practice 182: 180–182.

Dalrymple J C, Bannatyne P, Russell P et al 1989 Extraovarian peritoneal serous papillary carcinoma: a clinicopathologic study of 31 cases. Cancer 64: 110–115.

Daya D, McCaughey W T E 1990 Well-differentiated papillary

mesothelioma of the peritoneum: a clinicopathologic study of 22 cases. Cancer 65: 292–296.

Daya D, McCaughey W T E 1991 Pathology of the peritoneum: a review of selected topics. Seminars in Diagnostic Pathology 8: 277–289.

Dore N, Landry M, Cadotte M et al 1980 Cutaneous endosalpingiosis. Archives of Dermatology 116: 909–912.

Douglas G W, Kastin A J, Huntington R W 1965 Carcinoma arising in a retroperitoneal mullerian cyst, with widespread metastasis during pregnancy. American Journal of Obstetrics and Gynecology 91: 210–216.

Erba E, Vaghi M, Pepe S et al 1985 DNA index of ovarian carcinomas from 56 patients: in vivo and in vitro studies. British Journal of Cancer 52: 565–573.

Evans H, Yates W A, Palmer W E et al 1990 Clear cell carcinoma of the sigmoid mesocolon: a tumor of the secondary Mullerian system. American Journal of Obstetrics and Gynecology 162: 161–163.

Ferguson B R, Bennington J L, Haber S L 1969 Histochemistry of mucosubstances and histology of mixed mullerian pelvic lymph node glandular inclusions: evidence for histogenesis by mullerian metaplasia of coelomic epithelium. Obstetrics and Gynecology 33: 617–625.

Fievez M, Lambot P, Dewin B 1983 Endosalpingosis of the peritoneum and chronic salpingitis. Archives of Anatomy and Cytological Pathology 31: 355–358.

Flynn M K, Johnston W, Bigner S 1993 Carcinoma of ovarian and other origins in effusions: immunocytochemical study with a panel of monoclonal antibodies. Acta Cytologica 37: 441–447.

Fowler J M, Nieberg R K, Schooler T A, Berek J S 1994 Peritoneal adenocarcinoma (serous) of Mullerian type: a subgroup of women presenting with peritoneal carcinomatosis. International Journal of Gynecological Cancer 4: 43–51.

Foyle A, Al-Jabi M, McCaughey W T E 1981 Papillary peritoneal tumors in women. American Journal of Surgical Pathology 5: 241–249.

Fraire A E, Cooper S, Greenberg S D et al 1988 Mesothelioma of childhood. Cancer 62: 838–847.

Fromm G L, Gershenson D M, Silva E G 1990 Papillary serous carcinoma of the peritoneum. Obstetrics and Gynecology 75: 89–95.

Fujii S, Nakashima N, Okamura H et al 1981 Progesterone-induced smooth muscle-like cells in the subperitoneal nodules produced by estrogen: experimental approach to leiomyomatosis peritonealis disseminata. American Journal of Obstetrics and Gynecology 139: 164–172.

Gaffey M J, Mills S E, Swanson P E et al 1992 Immunoreactivity for BER-EP4 in adenocarcinomas, adenomatoid tumors, and malignant mesotheliomas. American Journal of Surgical Pathology 16: 593–599.

Gerald W L, Miller H K, Battifora H et al 1991 Intra-abdominal desmoplastic small round-cell tumor: report of 19 cases of a distinctive type of high-grade polyphenotypic malignancy affecting young individuals. American Journal of Surgical Pathology 15: 499–513.

Gilks C B, Bell D A, Scully R E 1990 Serous psammocarcinoma of the ovary and peritoneum. International Journal of Gynecological Pathology 9: 110–121.

Goepel J R 1981 Benign papillary mesothelioma of peritoneum: a histological, histochemical and ultrastructural study of six cases. Histopathology 5: 21–30.

Goldberg M I, Ng A B P, Belinson J L et al 1978 Clear cell adenocarcinoma arising in endometriosis of the rectosigmoid septum. Obstetrics and Gynecology (suppl) 51: 385–405.

Gonzales-Crussi F, Crawford S E, Sun C-C J 1990 Intraabdominal desmoplastic small-cell tumors with divergent differentiation: observations on three cases of childhood. American Journal of Surgical Pathology 14: 633–642.

Gooneratne S, Sassone M, Blaustein A et al 1982 Serous surface papillary carcinoma of the ovary: a clinicopathologic study of 16 cases. International Journal of Gynecological Pathology 1: 258–269.

Grundy G W, Miller R W 1972 Malignant mesothelioma in childhood: report of 13 cases. Cancer 30: 1216–1218.

Gussman D, Thickman D, Wheeler J E 1986 Postoperative peritoneal cysts. Obstetrics and Gynecology 68: 53S–55S.

Hales H A, Peterson C M, Jones K P et al 1992 Leiomyomatosis peritonealis disseminata treated with a gonadotropin-releasing hormone agonist. American Journal of Obstetrics and Gynecology 167: 515–516.

Hampton H L, Huffman H T, Meeks G R 1992 Extraovarian Brenner tumor. Obstetrics and Gynecology 79: 844–846.

Hartz P H 1947 Occurrence of Walthard cell rests in Brenner-like epithelium in the serosa of the epididymis. American Journal of Clinical Pathology 17: 654–656.

Herr J C, Platz C E, Heidger P M et al 1979 Smooth muscle within ovarian decidual nodules: a link to leiomyomatosis peritonealis disseminata? Obstetrics and Gynecology 53: 451–456.

Hochster H, Wernz J C, Muggia F M 1984 Intra-abdominal carcinomatosis with histologically normal ovaries [letter]. Cancer Treatment Reports 68: 931–932.

Holmes M D, Levin H S, Ballard L A J 1981 Endosalpingiosis. Cleveland Clinic Quarterly 48: 345–352.

Hsu Y K, Rosenshein N B, Parmley T H et al 1981 Leiomyomatosis in pelvic lymph nodes. Obstetrics and Gynecology 57: 91S–93S.

Hulme-Moir I, Ross M S 1969 A case of early postpartum abdominal pain due to haemorrhagic deciduosis peritonei. Journal of Obstetrics and Gynaecology of the British Commonwealth 76: 746–749.

Iversen O E, Skaarland E 1987 Ploidy assessment of benign and malignant ovarian tumors by flow cytometry: a clinicopathologic study. Cancer 60: 82–87.

Kane M J, Chahinian A P, Holland J F 1990 Malignant mesothelioma in young adults. Cancer 65: 1449–1455.

Kannerstein M, Churg J 1977a Peritoneal mesothelioma. Human Pathology 8: 83–94.

Kannerstein M, Churg J, McCaughey W T et al 1977b Papillary tumors of the peritoneum in women: mesothelioma or papillary carcinoma. American Journal of Obstetrics and Gynecology 127: 306–314.

Kaplan C, Benirschke K, Johnson K C 1980 Leiomyomatosis peritonealis disseminata with endometrium. Obstetrics and Gynecology 55: 119–122.

Katsube Y, Mukai K, Silverberg S G 1982 Cystic mesothelioma of the peritoneum: a report of five cases and review of the literature. Cancer 50: 1615–1622.

Kuo T, London S N, Dinh T V 1980 Endometriosis occurring in leiomyomatosis peritonealis disseminata: ultrastructural study and histogenetic consideration. American Journal of Surgical Pathology 1980: 197–204.

Lauchlan S C 1965 Two types of mullerian epithelium in an abdominal scar. American Journal of Obstetrics and Gynecology 93: 89.

Lauchlan S C 1972 The secondary mullerian system. Obstetrical and Gynecological Survey 27: 133–146.

Lauchlan S C 1984 Metaplasias and neoplasias of mullerian epithelium. Histopathology 8: 543–557.

Lauchlan S C 1994 The secondary mullerian system revisited. International Journal of Gynecological Pathology 13: 73–79.

Layfield L J, Lenarsky C 1991 Desmoplastic small cell tumors of the peritoneum coexpressing mesenchymal and epithelial markers. American Journal of Clinical Pathology 96: 536–543.

Lee K R, Verma U, Belinson J 1991 Primary clear cell carcinoma of the peritoneum. Gynecologic Oncology 41: 259–262.

Lele S B, Piver M S, Matharu J et al 1988 Peritoneal papillary carcinoma. Gynecologic Oncology 31: 315–320.

Leong A S, Stevens M W, Mukherjee T M 1992 Malignant mesothelioma: cytologic diagnosis with histologic immunohistochemical and ultrastructural correlation. Seminars in Diagnostic Pathology 9: 141–150.

Lerner H J, Schoenfeld D A, Martin A et al 1983 Malignant mesothelioma: the eastern clinical oncology group (ECOG) experience. Cancer 52: 1981–1985.

Lovell F A, Cranston P E 1990 Well-differentiated papillary mesothelioma of the peritoneum. American Journal of Radiology 155: 1245–1246.

McCaughey W T, Kirk M E, Lester W et al 1984 Peritoneal epithelial lesions associated with proliferative serous tumours of ovary. Histopathology 8: 195–208.

McCaughey W T, Schryer M J, Lin X S et al 1986 Extraovarian pelvic serous tumor with marked calcification. Archives of Pathology and Laboratory Medicine 110: 78–80.

McCaughey W T E, Al-Jabi M 1986 Differentiation of serosal hyperplasia and neoplasia in biopsies. Pathology Annual 21: 271–292.

McCaughey W T E, Kannerstein M, Churg J 1985 Tumors and pseudotumors of the serous membranes. Armed Forces Institute of Pathology, Washington, DC.

McFadden D E, Clement P B 1986 Peritoneal inclusion cysts with mural mesothelial proliferation: a clinicopathological analysis of six cases. American Journal of Surgical Pathology 10: 844–854.

Mennemeyer R, Smith M 1979 Multicystic peritoneal mesothelioma: a report with electron microscopy of a case mimicking intra-abdominal cystic hygroma (lymphangioma). Cancer 44: 692–698.

Mills S E, Andersen W A, Fechner R E et al 1988 Serous surface papillary carcinoma: a clinicopathologic study of 10 cases and comparison with stage III–IV ovarian serous carcinoma. American Journal of Surgical Pathology 12: 827–834.

Moore J H, Crum C P, Chandler J G et al 1980 Benign cystic mesothelioma. Cancer 45: 2395–2399.

Mostoufizadeh G H M, Scully R E 1980 Malignant tumors arising in endometriosis. Clinical Obstetrics and Gynecology 23: 951–963.

Nogales F F, Matilla A, Carrascal E 1978 Leiomyomatosis peritonealis disseminata: an ultrastructural study. American Journal of Clinical Pathology 69: 452–457.

Ober W B, Grady H G, Schoenbucher A K 1957 Ectopic ovarian decidua without pregnancy. American Journal of Pathology 33: 199–217.

Ordonez N G, El-Naggar A K, Ro J Y et al 1993 Intra-abdominal desmoplastic small cell tumor: a light microscopic, immunocytochemical, ultrastructural, and flow cytometric study. Human Pathology 24: 850–865.

O'Sullivan D, Heffernan C K 1960 Deciduosis peritonei in pregnancy: report of two cases respectively simulating carcinoma and tuberculosis. Journal of Obstetrics and Gynaecology of the British Empire 67: 1013–1016.

Park U, Han K C, Chang H K et al 1990 A primary mucinous cystadenocarcinoma of the retroperitoneum. Gynecologic Oncology 42: 64–67.

Parmley T H, Woodruff J D, Winn K et al 1975 Histogenesis of leiomyomatosis peritonealis disseminata (disseminated fibrosing deciduosis). Obstetrics and Gynecology 46: 511–516.

Pennell T C, Gusdon J P J 1989 Retroperitoneal mucinous cystadenoma. American Journal of Obstetrics and Gynecology 160: 1229–1231.

Piccigallo E, Jeffers L J, Reddy K R et al 1988 Malignant peritoneal mesothelioma: a clinical and laparoscopic study of ten cases. Digestive Diseases and Sciences 33: 633–639.

Pieslor P C, Orenstein J M, Hogan D L et al 1979 Ultrastructure of myofibroblasts and decidualized cells in leiomyomatosis peritonealis disseminata. American Journal of Clinical Pathology 72: 875–882.

Plaus W J 1988 Peritoneal mesothelioma. Archives of Surgery 123: 763–766.

Pschera H, Wikstrom B 1991 Extraovarian Brenner tumor coexisting with serous cystadenoma: case report. Gynecological and Obstetrical Investigation 31: 185–187.

Raju U, Fine G, Greenawald K A et al 1989 Primary papillary serous neoplasia of the peritoneum: a clinicopathologic and ultrastructural study of eight cases. Human Pathology 20: 426–436.

Ransom D T, Patel S R, Keeney G L et al 1990 Papillary serous carcinoma of the peritoneum: a review of 33 cases treated with platin-based chemotherapy. Cancer 66: 1091–1094.

Richter M A, Choudhry A, Barton J J et al 1983 Bleeding ectopic decidua as a cause of intraabdominal hemorrhage: a case report. Journal of Reproductive Medicine 28: 430–432.

Riddell R H, Goodman M J, Moose A R 1981 Peritoneal malignant mesothelioma in a patient with recurrent peritonitis. Cancer 48: 134–139.

Rodenburg C J, Cornelisse C J, Heintz P A et al 1987 Tumor ploidy as a major prognostic factor in advanced ovarian cancer. Cancer 59: 317–323.

Rosai J, Dehner L P 1975 Nodular mesothelial hyperplasia in hernia sacs: a benign reactive condition simulating a neoplastic process. Cancer 35: 165–175.

Ross M J, Welch W R, Scully R E 1989 Multilocular peritoneal inclusion cysts (so-called cystic mesotheliomas). Cancer 64: 1336–1346.

Roth L M 1974 The Brenner tumor and the Walthard cell nest: an electron microscopic study. Laboratory Investigation 31: 15–23.

Roth L M, Ehrlich C E 1977 Mucinous cystadenocarcinoma of the retroperitoneum. Obstetrics and Gynecology 49: 486–488.

Russell P, Bannatyne P 1989 Surgical pathology of the ovaries. Churchill Livingstone, London.

Rutledge M L, Silva E G, McLemore D et al 1989 Serous surface carcinoma of the ovary and peritoneum: a flow cytometric study. Pathology Annual 2: 227–235.

Ryuko K, Miura H, Abu M A et al 1992 Endosalpingiosis in association with ovarian surface papillary tumor of borderline malignancy. Gynecologic Oncology 46: 107–110.

Sabatelle R, Winger E 1973 Postpartum intraabdominal hemorrhage caused by ectopic deciduosis. Obstetrics and Gynecology 41: 873–875.

Schatz J E, Colgan T J 1991 Squamous metaplasia of the peritoneum. Archives of Pathology and Laboratory Medicine 115: 397–398.

Schuldenfrei R, Janovsky N A 1962 Disseminated endosalpingiosis associated with bilateral papillary serous cystadenocarcinoma of the ovaries: a case report. American Journal of Obstetrics and Gynecology 84: 382–389.

Seidman J D, Elsayed A M, Sobin L H et al 1993 Association of mucinous tumors of the ovary and appendix: a clinicopathologic study of 25 cases. American Journal of Surgical Pathology 17: 22–34.

Sheibani K, Shin S S, Kezirian J et al 1991 Ber-EP4 antibody as a discriminant in the differential diagnosis of malignant mesothelioma versus adenocarcinoma. American Journal of Surgical Pathology 15: 779–784.

Shen S C, Bansal M, Purrazzella R et al 1983 Benign glandular inclusions in lymph nodes, endosalpingiosis, and salpingitis isthmica nodosa in a young girl with clear cell adenocarcinoma of the cervix. American Journal of Surgical Pathology 7: 293–300.

Sinykin M B 1960 Endosalpingiosis. Minnesota Medicine 43: 759–761.

Spirtas R, Connelly R R, Tucker M A 1988 Survival patterns for malignant mesothelioma: the SEER experience. International Journal of Cancer 41: 525–530.

Sridhar K S, Doria R, Raub W A et al 1992 New strategies are needed in diffuse malignant mesothelioma. Cancer 70: 2969–2970.

Sundarasivarao D 1953 The mullerian vestiges and benign epithelial tumors of the epididymis. Journal of Pathology 66: 417–432.

Suster S, Moran C A 1990 Deciduosis of the appendix. American Journal of Gastroenterology 85: 841–845.

Tavassoli F A, Norris H J 1982 Peritoneal leiomyomatosis (leiomyomatosis peritonealis disseminata): a clinicopathologic study of 20 cases with ultrastructural observations. International Journal of Gynecological Pathology 1: 59–74.

Teoh T B 1953 The structure and development of Walthard nests. Journal of Pathology and Bacteriology 66: 433–439.

Tickman R J, Cohen C, Varma V A et al 1990 Distinction between carcinoma cells and mesothelial cells in serous effusions: usefulness of immunohistochemistry. Acta Cytologica 34: 491–496.

Tobacman J K, Greene M H, Tucker M A et al 1982 Intra-abdominal carcinomatosis after prophylactic oophorectomy in ovarian-cancer-prone families. Lancet 2: 795–797.

Truong L D, Maccato M L, Awalt H et al 1990 Serous surface carcinoma of the peritoneum: a clinicopathologic study of 22 cases. Human Pathology 21: 99–110.

Tutschka B G, Lauchlan S C 1980 Endosalpingiosis. Obstetrics and Gynecology 55: 57S–60S.

Volm M, Bruggemann A, Gunther M et al 1985 Prognostic relevance of ploidy, proliferation, and resistance-predictive tests in ovarian carcinoma. Cancer Research 45: 5180–5185.

Weiss L M, Battifora H 1993 The search for the optimal immunohistochemical panel for the diagnosis of malignant mesothelioma. Human Pathology 24: 345–346.

Weiss S W, Tavassoli F A 1988 Multicystic mesothelioma: an analysis of pathologic findings and biologic behavior in 37 cases. American Journal of Surgical Pathology 12: 737–746.

White P F, Merino M J, Barwick K W 1985 Serous surface papillary carcinoma of the ovary: a clinical, pathologic, ultrastructural, and immunohistochemical study of 11 cases. Pathology Annual 1: 403–418.

Wick M R, Mills S E, Swanson P E 1990 Expression of "myelomonocytic" antigen in mesotheliomas and adenocarcinomas involving the serosal surfaces. American Journal of Clinical Pathology 94: 18–26.

Williams P P, Gall S A, Prem K A 1971 Ectopic mucinous cystadenoma: a case report. Obstetrics and Gynecology 38: 831–837.

Winn K J, Woodruff J D, Parmley T H 1976 Electronmicroscopic studies of leiomyomatosis peritonealis disseminata. Obstetrics and Gynecology 48: 225–227.

Young R H, Eichhorn J H, Dickersin G R et al 1992 Ovarian involvement by the intra-abdominal desmoplastic small round cell tumor with divergent differentiation: a report of three cases. Human Pathology 23: 454–464.

Zaytsev P, Taxy J B 1987 Pregnancy-associated ectopic decidua. American Journal of Surgical Pathology 11: 526–530.

Zinsser K R, Wheeler J E 1982 Endosalpingiosis in the omentum: a study of autopsy and surgical material. American Journal of Surgical Pathology 6: 109–117.

31. Lymphoproliferative disease of the ovaries and female genital tract

Elizabeth Benjamin   Peter G. Isaacson

INTRODUCTION

The term lymphoproliferative disease refers to a wide variety of conditions including Hodgkin's disease, non-Hodgkin's lymphoma and conditions which may mimic lymphoma including certain non-lymphoid haematological proliferations and various florid chronic inflammatory conditions. This group of disorders uncommonly presents in the female genital tract but, when it does so, it is important that it is correctly discriminated from the more common gynaecological neoplasms and that a precise diagnosis is made since treatment, which is often curative, is closely related to the histopathological diagnosis. Because malignant lymphoma presenting as primary tumours of the female genital tract is rare, these tumours are frequently undiagnosed or misdiagnosed (Harris & Scully, 1984). From a clinical perspective extirpative surgery is the primary mode of treatment for most gynaecological malignancies whereas malignant lymphomas are usually managed with chemotherapy or radiotherapy or a combination of the two, and radical surgery is inappropriate. This assumes increased significance in young patients in whom preservation of sexual function and reproductive capacity may be a prime consideration (Sandvei et al, 1990).

It is arguable whether Hodgkin's disease ever arises primarily in the female genital tract and indeed it seldom arises or presents outside the lymph nodes. Non-Hodgkin's lymphoma, on the other hand, frequently arises or presents extranodally and may do so in the female genital tract where it may manifest as any one of its various subtypes. Presentation of lymphoma in the female genital tract is usually a manifestation of dissemination of disease from a primary nodal site and is, therefore, an indication of an advanced stage requiring systemic treatment. Careful staging is necessary before making a diagnosis of those rare cases of early stage, true primary extranodal lymphomas which may be treated more conservatively.

Advances in immunohistochemistry in recent years such as the introduction of antibodies reactive in routinely processed paraffin-embedded tissues, and of techniques for antigen retrieval (Cattoretti et al, 1993; Cuevas et al, 1994), facilitate the identification and categorization of malignant lymphomas and their separation from other neoplasms and reactive processes. Molecular biological techniques can now also be applied to routinely processed and paraffin-embedded tissues and may be of value in supporting or confirming a diagnosis of non-Hodgkin's lymphoma.

CLASSIFICATION OF NON-HODGKIN'S LYMPHOMAS

In the 1960s it became evident that the clinical behaviour and response to treatment of non-Hodgkin's lymphoma varied according to the histological features. With better understanding of the relationship between lymphocyte biology and lymphoma, several clinically relevant histological classifications of lymphoma emerged in the late 1970s and early 1980s. Despite efforts to agree on a single classification, two classifications are in common use at the present time; these are the Working Formulation for Clinical Usage, commonly used in the USA, and the recently updated Kiel classification, which is favoured in Europe.

The Working Formulation (Table 31.1) is based entirely on morphological criteria such as pattern of growth (nodular or diffuse) and cytology (small cleaved cell and large non-cleaved cell). It was flawed from the outset by the absence of immunological categorization of lymphomas. Thus, many subgroups such as diffuse, mixed small cleaved cell and large non-cleaved cell, are a heterogeneous group of lymphomas including, amongst others, tumours composed of small and large neoplastic B cells and those composed of large neoplastic B cells with a reactive population of small T cells. Such defects will inevitably lead to the phasing out of the Working Formulation.

The Kiel classification (Table 31.2) introduced in

1015

Table 31.1 A working formulation of non-Hodgkin's lymphoma for clinical usage. (From Cancer 1982, 49: 2112.)

Low grade
A. Malignant lymphoma, small lymphocytic
   consistent with CLL plasmacytoid.
B. Malignant lymphoma, follicular.
   Predominantly small cleaved cell
      diffuse areas
      sclerosis
C. Malignant lymphoma, follicular
   Mixed small cleaved and large cell
      diffuse areas
      sclerosis

Intermediate grade
D. Malignant lymphoma, follicular
   Predominantly large cell
      diffuse areas
      sclerosis
E. Malignant lymphoma, follicular
   Small cleaved cell
      sclerosis
F. Malignant lymphoma, diffuse
   Mixed, small and large cell
      sclerosis
      epithelioid cell component
G. Malignant lymphoma, diffuse
   Large cell
      cleaved cell
      non-cleaved cell
      sclerosis

High grade
H. Malignant lymphoma
   Large cell, immunoblastic
      plasmacytoid
      clear cell
      polymorphous
      epithelioid cell component
I. Malignant lymphoma
   Lymphoblastic
      convoluted cell
      non-convoluted cell
J. Malignant lymphoma
   Small non-cleaved cell
      Burkitt's
      follicular areas

Miscellaneous
   Composite
   Mycosis fungoides
   Histiocytic
   Extramedullary plasmacytoma
   Unclassifiable
   Other

Table 31.2 Updated Kiel classification of non-Hodgkin's lymphoma. (From Lancet 1988, 1: 292 corrected table p 9 603.)

B	T
Low grade	*Low grade*
*Lymphocytic — chronic lymphocytic and prolymphocytic leukaemia; hairy cell leukaemia	Lymphocytic — chronic lymphocytic and prolymphocytic leukaemia
	Small, cerebriform cell — mycosis fungoides, Sezary's syndrome
Lymphoplasmacytic/cytoid (LP immunocytoma)	Lymphoepithelioid (Lennert's lymphoma)
Plasmacytic	Angioimmunoblastic (AILD, LgX)
*Centroblastic/centrocytic — follicular +/– diffuse — diffuse	T zone
*Centrocytic	Pleomorphic, small cell (HTLV-1 +/–)
High grade	*High grade*
Centroblastic	Pleomorphic, medium and large cell (HTLV-1 +/–)
*Immunoblastic	Immunoblastic (HTLV-1 +/–)
*Large cell anaplastic (Ki-1 +)	Large cell anaplastic (Ki-1 +)
Burkitt's lymphoma	
*Lymphoblastic	Lymphoblastic
Rare types	*Rare types*

*Indicates some degree of correspondence, either in morphology or in functional expression, between categories in two columns.

More recently an international lymphoma study group composed of haematopathologists mainly from Europe and North America has put forward a proposal for an international consensus on the classification of neoplasms (Table 31.3) (Harris et al, 1994). This group has defined entities that can be recognized with currently available morphological, immunological and genetic techniques. Many of these entities are associated with distinctive clinical presentations and natural histories. Cases that do not fit into these defined categories have been left unclassified or provisionally classified. The terminology used is mainly that of the Kiel classification.

An important feature of this proposed consensus classification is that it identifies defined clinicopathological entities based on their morphological, immunological, genetic, molecular biological and clinical features. This contrasts with the Working Formulation in which morphology alone is paramount. The recognition of clinicopathological entities is important in understanding the nature and probable behaviour of malignant lymphomas at any particular site. Thus, most low-grade B-cell lymphomas are usually widespread diseases and therefore involvement of the female genital tract by, for example, follicular lymphoma, is more likely to be part of a disseminated disease process than a primary tumour. Amongst the high-grade lymphomas, lymphoblastic tumours are, similarly, part of a widespread, often leukaemic, neoplastic process and should never be interpreted as a stage I or primary tumour.

1974 (Gerard-Marchant et al, 1974), was updated in 1988 (Stansfeld et al, 1988). It is widely used in Europe but like all classifications it requires constant updating to accommodate new knowledge and changing concepts (Banks et al, 1992). In the field of T-cell lymphomas in particular, considerable confusion exists as to the exact definition and relationship of entities to each other and some authors have found the Kiel classification to be unreproducible (Hastrup et al, 1991).

Table 31.3 List of lymphoid neoplasms recognized by the International Lymphoma Study Group (Harris et al, 1994)

B-CELL NEOPLASMS
 I. **Precursor B-cell neoplasm:** Precursor B-lymphoblastic leukaemia/lymphoma
 II. **Peripheral B-cell neoplasm**
  1. B-cell chronic lymphocytic leukaemia/prolymphocytic leukaemia/small lymphocytic lymphoma
  2. Lymphoplasmacytoid lymphoma/immunocytoma
  3. Mantle cell lymphoma
  4. Follicle centre lymphoma, follicular
   Provisional cytologic grades: I (small cell), II (mixed small and large cell), III (large cell)
   Provisional subtype: diffuse, predominantly small cell type
  5. Marginal zone B-cell lymphoma
   Extranodal (MALT type +/– monocytoid B cells)
   Provisional subtype: Nodal (+/– monocytoid B cells)
  6. *Provisional entity:* Splenic marginal zone lymphoma (+/– villous lymphocytes)
  7. Hairy cell leukaemia
  8. Plasmacytoma/plasma cell myeloma
  9. Diffuse large B-cell lymphoma*
   Subtype: Primary mediastinal (thymic) B-cell lymphoma
  10. Burkitt's lymphoma
  11. *Provisional entity:* High grade B-cell lymphoma, Burkitt-like*

T-CELL AND PUTATIVE NK-CELL NEOPLASMS
 I. **Precursor T-cell neoplasm:** Precursor T-lymphoblastic lymphoma/leukaemia
 II. **Peripheral T-cell and NK-cell neoplasms**
  1. T-cell chronic lymphocytic leukaemia/prolymphocytic leukaemia
  2. Large granular lymphocyte leukaemia (LGL)
   T-cell type
   NK-cell type
  3. Mycosis fungoides/Sezary syndrome
  4. Peripheral T-cell lymphomas, unspecified*
   Provisional cytologic categories: Medium-sized cell, mixed medium and large cell, large cell, lymphoepithelial cell
   Provisional subtype: Hepatosplenic gd T-cell lymphoma
   Provisional subtype: Subcutaneous panniculitic T-cell lymphoma
  5. Angioimmunoblastic T-cell lymphoma (AILD)
  6. Angiocentric lymphoma
  7. Intestinal T-cell lymphoma (+/– enteropathy associated)
  8. Adult T-cell lymphoma/leukaemia (ATL/L)
  9. Anaplastic large cell lymphoma (ALCL), CD30+, T- and null-cell types
  10. *Provisional entity:* Anaplastic large-cell lymphoma, Hodgkin's-like

HODGKIN'S DISEASE (HD)
 I. Lymphocyte predominance
 II. Nodular sclerosis
 III. Mixed cellularity
 IV. Lymphocyte depletion
 V. *Provisional entity:* Lymphocyte-rich classical HD

* These categories are thought likely to include more than one disease entity

SUBTYPES OF MALIGNANT LYMPHOMA

Non-Hodgkin's lymphomas are categorized into systemic lymphomas and those derived from mucosa-associated lymphoid tissue (MALT lymphomas). This influences their presentation and pattern of dissemination. For a fuller account the reader is referred to Isaacson (1992) and Stansfeld & d'Ardenne (1992). Both types may in-volve the female genital tract, although systemic lymphomas are far more common.

Low-grade B-cell lymphomas

The main types of low-grade B-cell lymphomas of systemic lymphoid tissue include: lymphocytic lymphoma (which in most cases is associated with chronic lymphocytic leukaemia), lymphoplasmacytic lymphoma (in which evidence of plasma cell differentiation is present); plasmacytic lymphoma; follicular or follicular/diffuse centroblastic/centrocytic lymphoma (follicular, mixed small cleaved and large cell); and centrocytic or mantle cell lymphoma (diffuse small cleaved cell). These lymphomas tend to be widely disseminated at presentation (stages 3 and 4) but may follow an indolent course despite their widespread dissemination. They are, in the majority of cases, associated with long survival, sometimes even without treatment. They are, however, generally not as sensitive to chemotherapy as are high-grade lymphomas. Some may transform into high-grade lymphomas.

High-grade B-cell lymphomas

These may arise by transformation of low-grade lymphomas but more commonly arise *de novo*. Lymphomas in this category include centroblastic lymphoma (diffuse, large non-cleaved cell); immunoblastic lymphoma; large cell anaplastic and unclassifiable malignant lymphoma of B-cell phenotype. These lymphomas are frequently localized tumours at presentation (stages 1 and 2). They show aggressive behaviour and rapid dissemination. Many tumours, however, respond well to chemotherapy. B-lymphoblastic lymphoma (which is related to acute lymphoblastic leukaemia) and Burkitt's lymphoma (discussed later) are often included in this group although, in the Kiel classification, Burkitt's lymphoma has been assigned a separate category. The term 'Burkitt-like' is used for a type of lymphoma which resembles Burkitt's lymphoma but which does not meet the stringent histological criteria for that diagnosis.

T-cell lymphomas

T-cell lymphomas are far less common than B-cell tumours in the western world, comprising 10–15% of non-Hodgkin's lymphoma. They include lymphoblastic lymphomas (presenting as acute T-lymphoblastic leukaemia) which arise from early T-cell precursors and are well characterized. The cutaneous forms include mycosis fungoides and Sézary's syndrome and are also well defined. Those arising from mature T cells, the peripheral T-cell lymphomas, however, are a less well understood group. Their classification and definition is still a matter of debate and controversy. Tumours which are considered low grade in the Kiel classification include chronic lymphocytic leukaemia (T-CLL); mycosis fungoides and Sézary's syndrome; lymphoepithelioid lymphoma (Lennert's lymphoma); angioimmunoblastic lymphoma; T-zone lymphoma and pleomorphic, small cell lymphoma (HTLV-1 positive or negative). High-grade tumours include pleomorphic, medium and large cell lymphomas (HTLV-I positive or negative); immunoblastic (HTLV-1 positive or negative) and large cell anaplastic (Ki-1 positive). The proposed classification of T-cell lymphomas in the consensus classification is shown in Table 31.3.

Rare forms of malignant lymphoma

These include malignant lymphoma, histiocytic (ML, miscellaneous, histiocytic). These lesions have been over-diagnosed in the past. The term 'histiocytic' has also been applied to large cell lymphomas, in the older literature. True histiocytic neoplasms do occur and present either as a disseminated malignancy or as a localized lymph node tumour. Stringent immunohistochemical requirements must be fulfilled before a diagnosis of a histiocytic malignancy is made. These include immunoreactivity with one or more macrophage-specific monoclonal antibodies and the synthesis of lysozyme by tumour cells. Reactive macrophages present in both B- and T-cell lymphomas should not be mistaken for the tumour cell population.

Lymphomas of mucosa-associated lymphoid tissue (MALT)

It was noted that certain primary extranodal lymphomas did not fit into any of the established categories of systemic lymphomas. The concept of lymphomas of mucosa-associated lymphoid tissue is now widely accepted (Isaacson & Wright, 1983, 1984; Isaacson & Spencer, 1987). Such lymphomas recapitulate the properties of mucosa-associated lymphoid tissue (MALT). Unlike nodal low-grade B-cell lymphomas, MALT lymphomas tend to remain localized for long periods and have a good prognosis. The concept of lymphomas of mucosa-associated lymphoid tissue is probably of particular relevance to the understanding of primary lymphomas of the female genital tract. In rodents, migration of mucosal B lymphocytes to the lower female genital tract has been shown to occur in pregnancy (McDermott et al, 1980) and it is likely that the female genital tract is part of the mucosal immune system. MALT lymphomas are thought to be derived from marginal zone B cells and are composed of marginal zone cells that often resemble centrocytes. These centrocyte-like cells invade epithelia to form characteristic lymphoepithelial lesions. They frequently colonize pre-existing reactive germinal centres and they may show plasmacytic differentiation. The latter two features may

lead to the miscategorization of MALT lymphoma as either follicular lymphoma or as lymphoplasmacytic or plasmacytic lymphoma. The natural history of MALT lymphomas is to progress from a low-grade to a high-grade B-cell lymphoma. In the stomach, co-existent low-grade and high-grade lymphomas with the same immunoglobulin phenotype may be found (Chan et al, 1990). When transformation to a high-grade lymphoma occurs the tumours cannot be distinguished from other high-grade B-cell lymphomas, in the absence of co-existing low-grade tumour. In the stomach, stage rather than grade appears to be important in determining the good prognosis of MALT lymphomas (Cogliatti et al, 1991).

MALT lymphomas usually arise in a setting of pre-existing inflammation. Thus, thyroid MALT lymphomas arise in glands affected by Hashimoto's or lymphocytic thyroiditis, salivary MALT lymphomas arise in glands affected by autoimmune sialadenitis and gastric MALT lymphomas arise on a background of *Helicobacter pylori* gastritis. This may be of significance in determining the frequency of lymphomas arising in the cervix in comparison with other parts of the female genital tract.

STAGING

Staging is performed for most neoplastic diseases for the purpose of determining treatment regimes and of predicting survival. In gynaecological oncology, the staging system introduced by the Federation Internationale of Gynaecologists and Obstetricians, FIGO, in 1979 and in 1986 is widely used (Ulfelder, 1981). This system was, however, designed for the staging of primary epithelial neoplasms of the ovary and is therefore inappropriate for primary lymphomas at this site. The Ann Arbor system (Carbone et al, 1971) is a staging classification for Hodgkin's disease that is also used for the staging of non-Hodgkin's lymphomas (Table 31.4). Staging data must of course be interpreted in the context of the histopathology. As stated above, most low-grade B-cell lymphomas form widespread (stage 3 and 4) disease processes. This is a characteristic of the lymphoma and with few exceptions does not affect the management of the disease nor the relatively good prognosis of these neoplasms.

Ziegler (1981) found that the Ann Arbor staging system was not well suited to the management of patients with Burkitt's lymphoma. He introduced a staging scheme that reflected the poor prognosis associated with bulky abdominal tumours compared with involvement of single or multiple non-abdominal sites and the serious prognosis accompanying a combination of intra-abdominal and multiple extra-abdominal sites (Ziegler & Magrath, 1974).

In a study of 42 lymphomas and leukaemias presenting as ovarian tumours, Osborne & Robboy (1983) staged their cases using the FIGO system, stating that the Ann

Arbor staging method for non-Hodgkin's lymphoma was less sensitive and that no differentiation is made between unilateral and bilateral ovarian involvement. However, Fox et al (1988), in their study of 34 patients with lymphoma presenting as ovarian tumour, found the Ann Arbor system to be a more sensitive prognostic indicator than the FIGO system. Monterroso et al (1993) investigated the problems associated with the staging of non-Hodgkin's lymphoma of the ovary. They noted that the Ann Arbor staging system was designed for Hodgkin's disease and has inherent deficiencies in the staging of non-Hodgkin's lymphomas, particularly those neoplasms arising at extranodal sites. They noted the failure of the Ann Arbor staging system to take into account tumour bulk, which appears to be of paramount importance in the management and prognosis of Burkitt's lymphoma (Ziegler & Magrath, 1974). Finally, the Ann Arbor system does not address the issue whether patients with bilateral ovarian involvement are best considered as having stage 4 disease. To resolve these issues Monterroso et al (1993) staged 39 patients with malignant lymphomas of the ovary using the FIGO system, the Ann Arbor system and the modification proposed by Ziegler & Magrath (1974). The conclusion of this study was that the FIGO and Ziegler systems did not offer any significant advantage over the Ann Arbor system in the staging of ovarian lymphoma and that bilateral ovarian involvement indicated stage 4 disease.

OVARY

Non-Hodgkin's lymphoma

Incidence and pathogenesis

Primary ovarian lymphomas are rare. In a study of 1467 extranodal lymphomas, 47% of which were in female

Table 31.4 Ann Arbor staging system for Hodgkin's disease. (Adapted from Carbone et al, 1971.)

Stage 1
Involvement of a single lymph node region (1) or a single extralymphatic organ or site (1E).

Stage 2
Involvement of two or more lymph node regions on the same side of the diaphragm (2) or localized involvement of an extralymphatic organ or site and one or more lymph node regions on the same side of the diaphragm (2E).

Stage 3
Involvement of lymph node regions on both sides of the diaphragm (3) which may also be accompanied by localized involvement of an extralymphatic organ or site (3E) or by involvement of the spleen (3S) or both (3SE).

Stage 4
Diffuse or disseminated involvement of one or more extralymphatic organs or tissues with or without associated lymph node enlargement.

Note: Each stage is further divided into A and B categories. B is for those patients with any of (a) unexplained weight loss of more than 10% of body weight over the previous 6 months, (b) unexplained fever with temperatures 38°C and (c) night sweats.

patients, Freeman et al (1972) found only two cases. Chorlton et al (1974a) identified only 19 cases with disease localized to the ovary in a review of 9500 cases of lymphoma in female patients accessioned at the Armed Forces Institute of Pathology. It is possible that the number of cases in this series was boosted by the inclusion of cases of Burkitt's lymphoma, reflecting the referral bias of the Armed Forces Institute of Pathology. Norris & Jensen (1972), in a study of 353 ovarian tumours in females under the age of 20, found only two cases of ovarian lymphoma. Chorlton (1987) recorded 165 cases of lymphoma presenting initially in the ovary and either published or known personally to the author. The current number of documented primary ovarian lymphomas is in the region of 200 cases. This does not fully represent the prevalence of this type of lymphoma presentation since the tumour is not so rare that individual cases or small series are likely to be published.

In contrast to the rare presentation of lymphomas in the ovary, the ovaries are the most common site of involvement of the female genital tract by lymphoma found at autopsy (Lathrop, 1967). Autopsy studies of women dying of lymphomas have found an incidence of lymphoma in one or both ovaries of between 7 and 18% (Lucia et al, 1952; Woodruff et al, 1963).

There has been considerable debate in the literature as to whether ovarian lymphomas can ever be considered as primary tumours or whether they are always part of a more widespread disease process. One argument advanced against the possibility that ovarian lymphomas could be primary tumours is that lymphoid tissue is not a normal constituent of the ovary (Nelson et al, 1958). Others have argued that ovarian lymphomas could arise from hilar lymphoid tissue (Woodruff et al, 1963), from lymphocytes in an inflammatory infiltrate (Walther, 1934) or from lymphoid tissue in a teratoma (Durfee et al, 1937). With respect to the last suggestion, it is of interest that a lymphoma arising in the thyroid tissue in a mature cystic teratoma of the ovary has been reported (Seifer et al, 1986). A case of histiocytic lymphoma, transforming later to a monoblastic leukaemia, has been reported as arising in a malignant teratoma in the ovary of a patient with 46,XY gonadal dysgenesis (Koo et al, 1992). This mode of origin is, however, unlikely to account for the majority of ovarian lymphomas.

As part of their study of ovarian lymphomas, Monterroso et al (1993) reviewed the histology of 35 ovaries removed at autopsy from 24 women aged from 18–58 years. Lymphoid cells were found in the hilus or medulla of 13 individuals (54%), and in two of these formed distinct aggregates. It would appear therefore that lymphoid aggregates are not uncommon in the ovary and could provide a possible origin for primary ovarian lymphomas.

Fox & Langley (1976) proposed the following criteria for the diagnosis of primary ovarian lymphomas:

1. At the time of diagnosis the lymphoma is clinically confined to the ovary and full investigation fails to reveal evidence of lymphoma elsewhere. A lymphoma can still, however, be considered as primary if spread has occurred to immediately adjacent lymph nodes or if there has been direct spread to infiltrate immediately adjacent structures.

2. The peripheral blood and bone marrow should not contain any abnormal cells.

3. If further lymphomatous lesions occur at a site remote from the ovary, then at least several months should have elapsed between the appearance of the ovarian and extraovarian lesions.

Application of these criteria to reported cases of ovarian lymphoma (Chorlton, 1987) indicates that approximately 54 examples of primary lymphoma of the ovary had been reported up to that time. Paladugu et al (1980), however, suggested that the above criteria for the designation of primary ovarian lymphomas were insufficiently stringent and they proposed that there should be a disease-free interval of at least 60 months following treatment of the ovarian lesion by surgery alone. If this more restrictive definition had been adopted, there would have been only five acceptable reported cases of primary ovarian lymphomas up to 1987 (Chorlton, 1987). It is likely that many more cases with survival exceeding 60 months now exist.

The above arguments are, however, to some extent unrealistic since they do not take into account the nature of the lymphoma under consideration. Most low-grade B-cell lymphomas, with the exception of lymphomas of MALT, are widespread at the time of diagnosis. The findings of a stage 1, low-grade, B-cell lymphoma of the ovary should therefore raise suspicions of a MALT lymphoma. High-grade B-cell lymphomas might present with stage 1 disease but it is unlikely that they would be treated with surgery alone and it is very probable that they would receive chemotherapy. If the criteria of Paladugu et al are applied, such cases would never be diagnosed as primary ovarian lymphomas. Fox et al (1988) state, 'it would be reasonable to conclude therefore that an ovarian lymphoma should always be considered for therapeutic purposes as a local manifestation of systemic disease and that to rely upon the possibility of such a lesion being primary to the ovary is unduly optimistic'. In practical terms all ovarian lymphomas should be graded histologically and staged using the Ann Arbor system, and both histology and stage should be taken into account in determining further management.

Age

Five large series of ovarian lymphomas (Paladugu et al, 1980; Rotmensch & Woodruff, 1982; Osborne & Robboy, 1983; Fox et al, 1988; Monterroso et al, 1993), totalling 181 cases, show an age range of 3 months to 77 years with a mean of approximately 35 years. Two-thirds of the patients are under the age of 40 years (Fox et al, 1988). This contrasts with testicular lymphomas which occur predominantly in older age groups with a mean age of 64 years (Paladugu et al, 1980).

Clinical features

The common presenting features of ovarian lymphomas are as abdominal and pelvic masses causing abdominal distension. Fox et al (1988) noted three main patterns of clinical presentation: (1) acute presentation with abdominal pain and distension, sometimes accompanied by vomiting; (2) chronic onset of symptoms with abdominal pain and distension of 1–6 months duration; (3) with non-specific gynaecological symptoms such as menorrhagia and oligomenorrhoea. Those patients presenting with rapid onset of abdominal distension and pain more frequently had symptoms of fever and weight loss and had a worse prognosis than those in whom onset of symptoms was more gradual. A smaller number of patients present with symptoms of menorrhagia or oligomenorrhoea. Presentation with amenorrhoea and resumption of periods after removal of tumour occurred in a patient whose B-cell lymphoma was associated with ovarian stromal luteinization (Mittal et al, 1992). In the series of cases reported by Monterroso et al (1993), all of the tumours that were thought to be primary in the ovary were discovered incidentally on clinical examination or at surgery performed for other reasons. A number of cases have been discovered during pregnancy with presentations ranging from first-trimester abortions to full-term deliveries (Finkle & Goldman, 1974; Armon, 1976; Rotmensch & Woodruff, 1982; Monterroso et al, 1993).

Gross pathology

In most reported series of ovarian lymphomas over half the tumours have been bilateral. When unilateral they show no consistent predilection for either side. The tumours are frequently described as smooth-surfaced and bosselated. They may be associated with ascites which is sometimes blood-stained. Tumour size varies widely, from a maximum of 5280 g reported by Rotmensch & Woodruff (1982), to a tumour of only 15 g discovered as an incidental finding (Monterroso et al, 1993); tumour diameters have ranged from microscopic to 25 cm (Osborne & Robboy, 1983).

Grossly, on section the tumours have a mainly solid, creamy, white, 'fish-flesh' appearance with areas of necrosis and haemorrhage in the larger tumours. Other sites of involvement most frequently identified at operation are the Fallopian tubes and other parts of the female genital tract, the serosa, omentum and mesentery (Monterroso et al, 1993).

Histology

It is difficult to evaluate and compare the histopathology of the reported series of ovarian lymphomas because of the different classification systems used. Monterroso et al (1993) used the terminology of the Working Formulation to classify their 39 cases of non-Hodgkin's lymphoma that presented as ovarian tumours: 21 (54%) were small cleaved cell (Burkitt and Burkitt-like), 9 (23%) diffuse large cell (high-grade B-cell lymphomas, centroblastic diffuse), 3 (8%) follicular and diffuse large cell (centroblastic, follicular and diffuse), 3 (8%) diffuse, mixed small and large cell (centroblastic/centrocytic diffuse), 2 (5%) large cell immunoblastic (one Richter's syndrome, one anaplastic large cell) and 1 (2%) follicular and diffuse small cleaved cell (centroblastic/centrocytic, follicular and diffuse). There was a large number of Burkitt or Burkitt-like lymphomas in this series (54%), probably related to the referral bias at the National Cancer Institute, USA. The large majority of the lymphomas in this series were of high or intermediate grade; 25 of the 26 (96%) cases on which immunohistochemistry was performed were B-cell tumours and only one was a T-cell lymphoma.

Fox et al (1988) analysed 34 cases of ovarian non-Hodgkin's lymphoma. Twelve were diagnosed as B-cell lymphomas (6 follicle centre cell type and 6 diffuse large cell); 5 were of histiocytic type; 2 were diffuse, undifferentiated large cell lymphomas and 15 were poorly-differentiated, lymphocytic/lymphoblastic lymphomas. The latter group included 7 Burkitt's lymphoma, 2 T-cell lymphomas and 6 lymphoblastic lymphomas, 3 of which were leukaemia related.

In the series of 40 patients reported by Osborne & Robboy (1983), 11 cases (27%) were categorized as small non-cleaved cell (Burkitt or Burkitt-like) lymphomas and 6 (15%) as follicular lymphomas (small cleaved cell, mixed small cleaved and large cell, and large cell types). The majority of the cases (58%) were categorized as diffuse large cell or immunoblastic. Rotmensch & Woodruff (1982) used the terminology of the Rappaport classification. This cannot always be easily translated into Working Formulation or Kiel terminology. Among the 55 cases of ovarian lymphoma in their series 18 were categorized as nodular histiocytic; 18 as diffuse poorly-differentiated lymphocytic; 6 as diffuse well-differentiated lymphocytic; 8 as nodular, mixed lymphocytic and histiocytic; 4 as Hodgkin's disease and one as Burkitt's lymphoma. If one accepts nodularity as indicating follicle centre cell derivation, 47% of the cases in this series were follicle centre cell lymphoma. Well-differentiated lymphocytic lymphoma is usually regarded as the tissue equivalent of chronic lymphocytic leukaemia, not a neoplasm that would be expected to form tumour masses at extranodal sites and a category that does not appear in any of the other series of ovarian lymphomas.

High-grade B-cell (large cell) lymphomas show a range of morphology from centroblastic monomorphic to centroblastic polymorphic including cells that may be centrocytoid (large cleaved cells) and multilobated (Hui et al, 1988; Lennert & Feller, 1990). Admixture with variable numbers of immunoblasts with prominent central nucleoli may be seen. Residual centrocytes (small cleaved cells) may indicate the follicle centre cell origin of some of these neoplasms (Monterroso et al, 1993) as may follicular areas. Marked sclerosis may be a feature of these tumours (Monterroso et al, 1993). Although mitotic figures are usually easily found, these lymphomas do not show as high a mitotic index as Burkitt-type lymphomas. In addition to high-grade lymphomas with residual features of follicle centre cell origin, occasional ovarian lymphomas of low-grade follicle centre cell origin with a follicular growth pattern have been described (Rotmensch & Woodruff, 1982; Osborne & Robboy, 1983; Monterroso et al, 1993). Monterroso et al (1993) concluded that 10 of 39 ovarian lymphomas were of follicle centre cell origin excluding the large number of cases of Burkitt's lymphoma in their series which some authors believe to be follicle centre cell derived (Mann et al, 1976).

Ovarian lymphomas, in common with lymphomas of the female genital tract, may show prominent sclerosis ranging from collagen fibrils between groups of tumour cells to extensive collagen bands in which tumour cells are embedded. Ovarian lymphoma may grow in diffuse sheets (Fig. 31.1) but may also show areas of cord-like growth pattern, particularly in the capsule. Tumour cells tend to encircle residual corpora lutea (Fig. 31.2), corpora albicantes and Graafian follicles rather than to obliterate them. Prominent ovarian stromal luteinization may rarely occur in lymphomas (Ferry & Young, 1991; Mittal et al, 1992).

Specific subtypes of non-Hodgkin's lymphoma

Plasmacytoma (Bambira et al, 1982; Hautzer, 1984; Cook & Boylston, 1988). Ovarian tumours of this type have been up to 24 cm in diameter and may be bilateral. Some have occurred in patients with widespread myeloma and others have preceded the diagnosis of myeloma. Plasmacytic tumours, particularly the less well differentiated ones, may mimic anaplastic carcinoma. If immunohistochemistry is used to resolve this problem it should be borne in mind that plasmacytomas are usually leucocyte common antigen negative, EMA positive and may express cytokeratins (Norton & Isaacson, 1989b). The identification of monotypic immunoglobulin production by the tumour cells will establish the diagnosis of plasmacytoma.

T-cell lymphoma. Available information suggests that T-cell lymphomas are much less common than B-cell lymphomas in the ovary, but their precise incidence is not

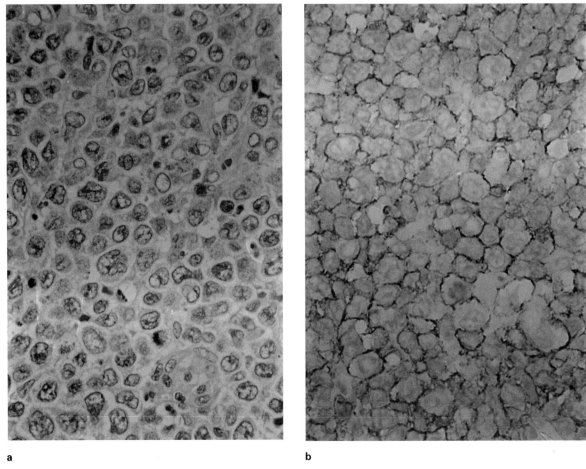

a   b

Fig. 31.1   a Ovary replaced by high-grade, centroblastic, B-cell lymphoma. H & E × 640. **b** Lymphoma cells immunostain for L26 (CD20) indicating B-cell lineage. × 640.

known. Monterroso et al (1993) recorded one case of T-cell lymphoma confirmed by immunohistochemistry (see below).

Burkitt's lymphoma. Burkitt (1958), working in Uganda, drew attention to the full clinical syndrome of jaw and abdominal tumours now known as Burkitt's lymphoma. The jaw tumours are age related and probably dependent on tooth development, so the proportion of jaw tumours in any series will be dependent on the age of the patients being studied (Burkitt, 1970). Burkitt's lymphoma has a predilection for the female genital tract with ovarian lymphomas, usually bilateral, occurring in 75–86% of patients (Fig. 31.3) (O'Conor, 1961; Wright, 1964). The histopathological features of Burkitt's lymphoma have been well described (Berard et al, 1969; Wright, 1970), the lymphoma being composed of monomorphic blast cells with a high proliferation rate. A WHO-sponsored group defined Burkitt's lymphoma on the basis of its histological features (Berard et al, 1969) and, using these histological criteria, cases of Burkitt's lymphoma have been identified outside the endemic areas of Africa and Papua New Guinea (Wright, 1966; Levine et al, 1982). These non-endemic cases may have clinical fea-

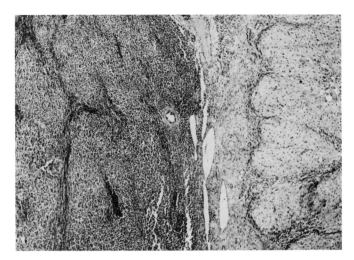

Fig. 31.2   Follicular non-Hodgkin's lymphoma of the ovary with adjacent uninvolved corpus luteum. (From Chorlton I et al, 1974a.)

tures similar to those of endemic cases but the majority of patients have abdominal tumours in the region of the terminal ileum or tumours of the oropharynx that are not characteristic of the endemic cases (Wright, 1966; Grogan

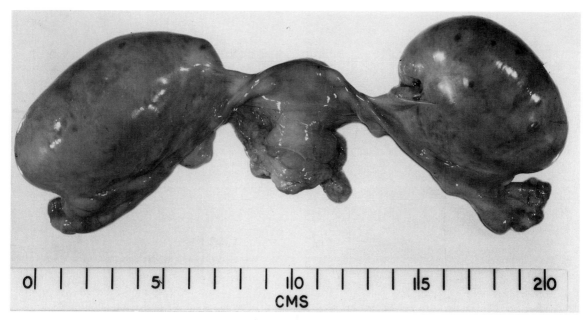

Fig. 31.3 Burkitt's lymphoma producing bilateral ovarian tumours. (From Burkitt & Wright, 1970.)

et al, 1982). Epstein–Barr virus can be found in virtually 100% of cases of endemic Burkitt's lymphoma but in only approximately one-third of non-endemic cases. In both the endemic and non-endemic cases translocations involving the immunoglobulin genes and the c-*myc* oncogene are found (Pelicci et al, 1986; Neri et al, 1988). However, the break points on the immunoglobulin genes differ between the two groups suggesting that they arise at different stages of B-cell differentiation. In both tumours disregulation of the c-*myc* oncogene is probably responsible for both the high rate of proliferation and the undifferentiated nature of the blast cells. While the exact relationship between endemic and non-endemic Burkitt's lymphomas is unclear it is apparent that ovarian and gynaecological tumours are frequent in both groups (Dorfman, 1965; Levine et al, 1982). Monterroso et al (1993) speculate that possible hormonal influences and growth factors may lead to localization in the ovaries and breasts and note the association of tumours at these sites with pregnancy. Magrath (1991) has similarly postulated that growth factors may influence the predilection of Burkitt's lymphoma for the jaws. Wright (1985), however, noting the correspondence between the distribution of Burkitt's lymphoma and lymphoid cells of MALT and the influence of pregnancy on the distribution of these cells (McDermott et al, 1980), has postulated that endemic Burkitt's lymphoma is a tumour of mucosa-associated lymphoid tissue.

The tumour cells of Burkitt's lymphoma have rounded, regular nuclei with granular chromatin and 3–4 small nucleoli. The cytoplasm forms a well-defined rim around the nucleus and is amphophilic in H & E-stained sections and deeply basophilic in Giemsa stain preparations. The cytoplasmic lipid vacuoles that form such a prominent feature in imprint preparations can be seen in well-fixed histological preparations with the aid of oil immersion. Burkitt's lymphomas always show a high mitotic index with several mitotic figures visible in a high power field. Large numbers of apoptotic nuclei are also present and they are frequently engulfed by the abundant 'starry sky' macrophages present in the tumour (Fig. 31.4a). In the ovary, the tumour forms a diffuse infiltrate that may surround and eventually infiltrate residual ovarian follicles (Monterroso et al, 1993). At the hilum of the ovary and in the capsule, the tumour cells can frequently be seen infiltrating in an Indian file or cord-like fashion (Fig. 31.4b).

Immunohistochemistry

Immunohistochemistry usually permits the characterization of non-Hodgkin's lymphoma into B- and T-cell categories. Neoplastic B-cell proliferations may be identified and separated from reactive proliferations by the presence of light chain restriction (Fig. 31.5) which marks a monoclonal proliferation. When this is not possible because of technical or other reasons, evidence for monoclonal B-cell proliferation can be obtained by analysis of tumour DNA for clonal immunoglobulin gene rearrangement using techniques such as Southern blotting and the polymerase chain reaction (Diss et al, 1994). In T-cell lymphomas, unlike B-cell lymphomas, there is no consistent method of establishing clonality using immunohistochemistry. Distinguishing between reactive and neoplastic T-cell proliferations depends on the demonstration of T-cell

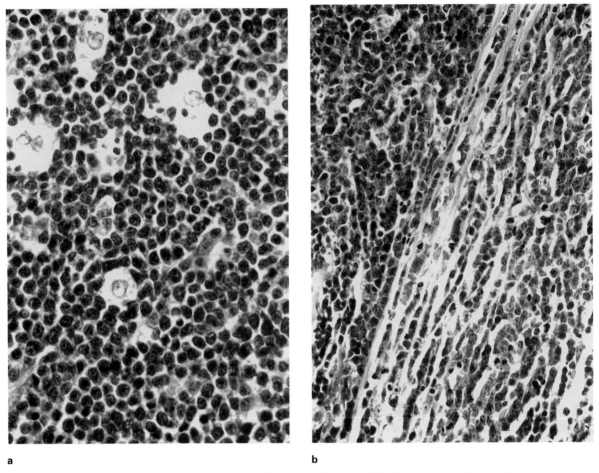

a   b

Fig. 31.4   a Burkitt's lymphoma showing a population of monomorphic lymphoid cells and scattered macrophages producing 'a starry sky' appearance. H & E × 640. **b** Burkitt's lymphoma of ovary. Tumour cells infiltrate in an 'Indian file' pattern. H & E × 300.

antigens in cells judged to be malignant on morphological grounds (Isaacson, 1992). More specific demonstration of clonal T-cell receptor gene rearrangements is also possible by analysis of tumour DNA using molecular biological techniques (McCarthy et al, 1991).

There have been few studies of immunohistochemistry of ovarian lymphomas. Linden et al (1988) performed immunohistochemistry and gene rearrangement studies using Southern blot analysis on three ovarian lymphomas. All three expressed B-cell lineage markers and showed clonal rearrangements of their immunoglobulin genes with germ line T-cell receptor genes. The most comprehensive immunohistochemical study of ovarian lymphomas is that reported by Monterroso et al (1993). They were able to undertake immunophenotypic studies on 26 of their 39 cases. In 25 of the 26 cases (96%) the neoplastic cells were of B-cell phenotype. In 23 of 24 cases studied using paraffin sections the tumour cells were positive for L26 (CD20) and negative with at least one T-associated antibody. The T-cell antibodies used in the study were UCHL1 (CD45 RO), MT1 (CD43) and Leu-

22 (CD43). Five of the B-cell lymphomas reacted with one of these antibodies, however, none of these antibodies is entirely specific for T-cells and may be expressed in cells of other lineages, including B cells (Picker et al, 1987; Linden et al, 1988; Norton & Isaacson, 1989a,b).

One case in the series of Monterroso et al (1993) is particularly instructive. The patient was aged 35 and had bilateral ovarian tumours with extensive intra-abdominal disease. Following surgery and chemotherapy the patient was reported to have no evidence of disease after six years. Histologically the tumour was diagnosed as an anaplastic large cell lymphoma of T-cell phenotype (Stein et al, 1985; Delsol et al, 1988). It was Ber H2 (CD30), epithelial membrane antigen (EMA) and UCHL1 (CD45 RO) positive and negative for leucocyte common antigen (CD45), Leu-M1 (CD15), L26 (CD20), LN1 (CDw75), KP1 (CD68) and lysozyme. In the absence of evidence of CD3 or T-cell receptor expression, this tumour should have been categorized as being of null cell or indeterminate phenotype. The importance of this tumour however is that the leucocyte common antigen negative, epithelial

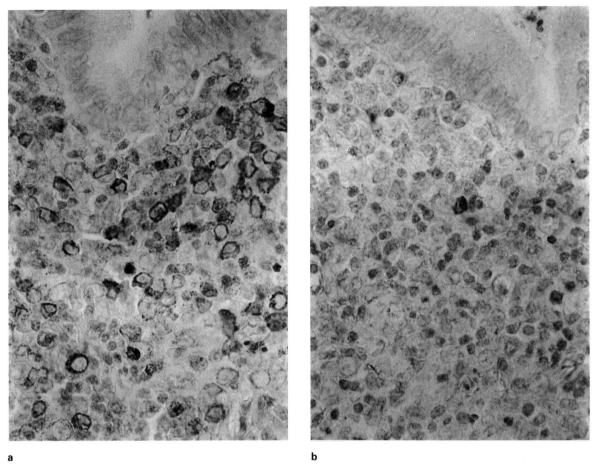

a   b

Fig. 31.5 Follicle centre cell, B-cell lymphoma. **a** Tumour cells show kappa immunoglobulin light chain restriction, confirming a monoclonal proliferation. × 640. **b** Tumour cells do not immunostain for immunoglobulin lambda light chain. × 640.

membrane antigen positive phenotype could have led the unwary pathologist into believing that this was an epithelial neoplasm, which would have resulted in inappropriate management. Occasional anaplastic large cell lymphomas can even express cytokeratins, making their distinction from an epithelial neoplasm difficult (Gustmann et al, 1991). Pathologists need to be aware of the morphological features of this lymphoma and of its histological and immunophenotypic resemblance to an epithelial neoplasm in some cases.

Differential diagnosis

The two ovarian tumours for which lymphomas are most commonly mistaken are granulosa cell tumour and dysgerminoma (Osborne & Robboy, 1983). Granulosa cell tumours account for nearly half the misdiagnoses of ovarian lymphoma at all ages; misdiagnosis was made most often when patients had Burkitt-type lymphoma. In these patients the 'starry sky' macrophages surrounded by tumour cells were frequently misinterpreted as Call–Exner bodies. Osborne & Robboy (1983) attribute these errors, in part, to poor fixation and processing of tissues, a factor aggravated by the frequent large size of the ovarian tumours and consequent slow penetration of fixative.

Clinical features may help to distinguish granulosa cell tumours from ovarian lymphomas. Endocrine manifestations such as breast enlargement, growth of pubic and axillary hair and onset of menses indicative of oestrogen secretion have been observed in three-quarters of patients with juvenile granulosa cell tumours, but were not encountered in any of the patients with lymphoma. Many patients of reproductive age with granulosa cell tumours have disturbances in their menstrual patterns due to oestrogenic effects on the endometrium. Older patients often complain of postmenopausal bleeding. In contrast Osborne & Robboy (1983) found that only two of the 19 patients aged 11–44 years with ovarian lymphomas complained of irregular menses or amenorrhoea and that only one of 16 women older than 45 years had postmenopausal bleeding, and in this patient the lymphoma infiltrated the myometrium and endometrium.

Osborne & Robboy (1983) found that large cell lymphomas were frequently misdiagnosed as dysgerminomas, despite the fact that this tumour is uncommonly bilateral. Notwithstanding the fact that dysgerminoma is uncommon after the age of 30, the diagnosis was considered in 28% of the patients above this age. The presence of stromal lymphocytes and epithelioid granulomas, together with the occasional presence of syncytiotrophoblast-like cells, are histological features that aid the diagnosis of dysgerminoma. Metastatic carcinoma, particularly from the breast, undifferentiated and primary small cell carcinomas also need to be considered in the differential diagnosis of lymphomas of the ovary (Chorlton, 1987). Fortunately these problems of differential diagnosis can usually easily be resolved by application of immunohistochemistry in difficult cases. What remains is the need for pathologists to be aware of the differential diagnosis of undifferentiated ovarian neoplasms so that the appropriate investigations are undertaken.

Prognosis and survival

The interpretation of survival data for ovarian lymphomas must take into account advances in staging and treatment that have occurred in recent years and the increasing use of chemotherapy either as first line or adjunctive therapy. In the large series of cases reported from the National Cancer Institute (Monterroso et al, 1993), 4 patients were stage 1E, 4 patients stage 2E, and 25 patients stage 4 using the Ann Arbor system. Thirty-two patients, of 39 reported cases, received chemotherapy. Forty seven per cent were alive between 15 and 16.5 years following treatment and 53% had died between one week and 9 years from the time of diagnosis. These results are less dismal than the 7% survival reported by Rotmensch & Woodruff (1982) in a series of patients, most of whom had been treated with surgery alone or in combination with radiotherapy. Osborne & Robboy (1983) reported an actuarial survival at five years of 35%; low stage and follicular growth pattern were good prognostic features. Fifteen of the 34 patients (44%) reported by Fox et al (1988) survived between one and more than five years following diagnosis. These authors found that a history of rapid onset of symptoms and advanced stage were poor prognostic features. Association with pregnancy was stated to be a bad prognostic feature (Rotmensch & Woodruff, 1982), although some long-term survivors have now been reported (Monterroso et al, 1993).

Hodgkin's disease

Hodgkin's disease has rarely been reported to involve the ovary. In three patients the disease was apparently localized to the ovaries (Bare & McCloskey, 1961; Long &

Patchefsky, 1971; Khan et al, 1986); in the others ovarian involvement was part of more widespread disease (Heller & Palin, 1946; Nelson et al, 1958). In their review of 55 ovarian lymphomas from the Ovarian Tumour Registry, Rotmensch & Woodruff (1982) include four cases of Hodgkin's disease but details of individual patients are not given. We support the scepticism expressed by Monterroso et al (1993) who noted that some of the published cases of Hodgkin's disease of the ovary were poorly documented and that most were reported before the availability of immunophenotypic analysis. Primary Hodgkin's disease of the ovary is extremely rare if it occurs at all.

Leukaemia

In the huge autopsy study of 1206 cases of acute and chronic leukaemia, Barcos et al (1987) found ovarian involvement in 11% of patients with acute granulocytic leukaemia, 9% with chronic granulocytic leukaemia, 21% with acute lymphoblastic leukaemia and 22% with chronic lymphocytic leukaemia (Fig. 31.6). Involvement of the ovary in lymphoblastic leukaemia (21%) is less frequent than involvement of the testes (40%) and the incidence of ovarian deposits fell during the period of the study (1958–1982), presumably as a result of improvements in therapy. Leukaemic relapse in the ovaries during bone marrow remission (Obeid et al, 1979; Chu et al, 1981; Cecalupo et al, 1982; Wyld & Lilleyman, 1983; Heaton & Duff, 1989) may occur several years after treatment and may produce tumours up to 15 cm in diameter. It has been postulated that ovarian and central nervous system relapse are associated (Case Records of the Massachusetts General Hospital, 1981). The tumours have the

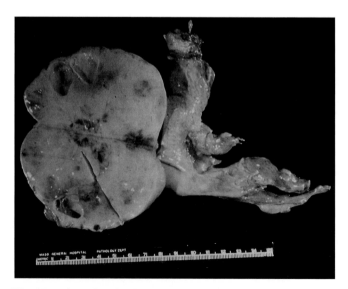

Fig. 31.6 Acute lymphoblastic leukaemia involving the ovary. (Reprinted with permission from Ferry & Young, 1991.)

typical morphology of lymphoblastic lymphomas, being composed of blast cells with delicate nuclear chromatin, small nucleoli and inconspicuous cytoplasm. These cells expand the ovarian stroma and infiltrate in an Indian file fashion. If immunohistochemistry is used to confirm the diagnosis, it should be borne in mind that lymphoblastic lymphomas may be negative for leucocyte common antigen and may not express T- or B-cell lineage markers (null or indeterminate phenotype) (Norton & Isaacson, 1989b).

Granulocytic sarcoma

The term chloroma (Hindkamp & Szanto, 1959) has been largely replaced by granulocytic sarcoma (Rappaport, 1956). Neither term is strictly appropriate since the majority of tumours do not have a green colour and many show little granulocytic differentiation. Myelosarcoma or extramedullary myeloid tumours are probably more appropriate terms. Granulocytic sarcoma may occur in patients with no leukaemia, or during remission, or may precede the diagnosis of leukaemia by months or years (Rappaport, 1966; Neiman et al, 1981; Meis et al, 1986). In the two largest published series of granulocytic sarcoma, involvement of the genital tract was observed in only one of 30 females (Neiman et al, 1981; Meis et al, 1986). Nevertheless, although rare, involvement of the ovaries does appear to be a characteristic feature of granulocytic sarcoma. In a more recent review of 29 patients with granulocytic sarcoma of the female genital tract Friedman et al (1992) noted that 13 (45%) had ovarian involvement.

Ovarian granulocytic sarcomas may be unilateral or bilateral and have been recorded as up to 19 cm in diameter. They form solid tumours though cystic degeneration or entrapped serous cysts may occur (Hindkamp & Szanto, 1959; Gralnick & Dittmark, 1969; Ballon et al, 1978; Morgan et al, 1981; PreBler et al, 1992). The tumours are composed of blastic cells with delicate nuclear chromatin and inconspicuous cytoplasm (Fig. 31.7). They are most likely to be misdiagnosed as malignant lymphomas and therefore to receive inappropriate therapy. The finding of granulated myelocytes is diagnostic of granulocytic sarcoma. However, such cells may be scanty and are unlikely to be found unless carefully sought. Eosinophilic myelocytes are the cells most easily seen in haematoxylin and eosin-stained sections, but in general granulation is best observed in Giemsa-stained preparations.

In view of the therapeutic implications of the diagnosis of granulocytic sarcoma, the diagnosis should be confirmed using immunohistochemistry. The tumour cells are leucocyte common antigen positive. They are negative with most B- and T-cell lineage markers but usually express CD43 (MT1, DFT1, Leu-22) and may express UCHL1 (CD45 RO) (PreBler et al, 1992). Among the B-cell markers, they may express MB2 and KiB3 (PreBler et al, 1992). Granulocytic sarcomas usually express muramidase and alpha-1-antitrypsin (Muller et al, 1986). The staining should be cytoplasmic, granular and accentuated in the Golgi region; diffuse non-granular staining is due to non-specific uptake and is particularly likely to be seen in poorly-fixed tissues. CD68 (KP1, PG-M1) staining is seen in most granulocytic sarcomas. KP1 stains myelomonocytic cells, although it is not a specific haematological marker. PG-M1 (Falini et al, 1993) stains cells at the monocyte end of the myelomonocyte spectrum and, in the absence of KP1 staining, is a marker of monocyte differentiation. CD15 (Leu-M1) and antibodies to neutrophil elastase identify granulocytic differentiation. The naphthol AS-D chloro-acetate esterase stain (Leder, 1964), although widely used for the identification of granulocytic sarcoma, is only of value in those cases showing granulocytic differentiation and is unhelpful in those tumours showing predominantly monocytic differentiation. Megakaryocyte differentiation can be identified by staining for factor VIII-related antigen (PreBler et al, 1992).

FALLOPIAN TUBE

The Fallopian tubes are frequently infiltrated by tumour in patients with ovarian lymphomas, particularly those of the small non-cleaved cell, i.e. Burkitt and Burkitt-like type (Osborne & Robboy, 1983; Ferry & Young, 1991). Primary lymphoma of the Fallopian tube has been reported only twice. Ferry & Young (1991) reported a 68-year-old patient who had previously undergone hysterectomy. At the time of bilateral salpingo-oophorectomy she had a left hydrosalpinx and tubo-ovarian adhesions. The tubal walls were fleshy and studded with nodules, no other abnormality was found in the abdomen. Histology showed a follicle centre cell lymphoma (follicular mixed small cleaved and large cell type) (Fig. 31.8). Isaacson & Norton (1994) reported a case of MALT lymphoma of the Fallopian tube and question whether the case reported by Ferry & Young might also be a MALT lymphoma.

UTERUS AND CERVIX

Non-Hodgkin's lymphoma

Incidence

Lymphomas presenting in the uterus are uncommon; when they do so, they more frequently involve the cervix than the uterine corpus (Ferry & Young, 1991). Only 2 malignant lymphomas were identified in a series of 25 000 primary cervical neoplasms (Carr et al, 1976). In a review of 12 447 malignant lymphomas, 1467 presented at an

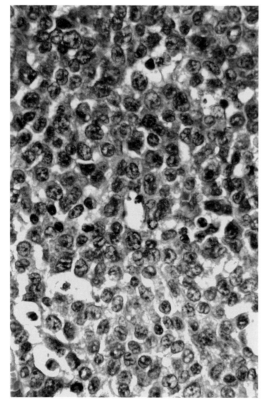

a

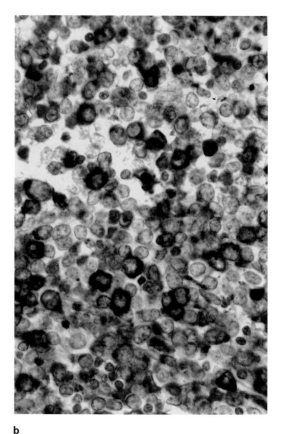

b

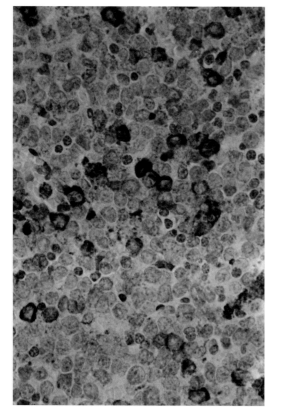

c

Fig. 31.7 **a** Granulocytic sarcoma. H & E × 575. **b** Immature myeloid cell immunostain for muramidase. × 575. **c** CD68 positivity in tumour cells. × 575.

extranodal site without evidence of disseminated disease and of these only 3 presented in the cervix, 3 in the body of the uterus and 2 in unspecified sites in the uterus (Freeman et al, 1972). In a series of 9500 women with haematological malignancies reported from the Armed Forces Institute of Pathology, 13 cases of malignant lymphoma and 2 cases of granulocytic sarcoma presented in the body of the uterus, cervix or vagina (Chorlton et al, 1974b). These tumours can present at any age and may mimic squamous cell carcinoma of the cervix clinically and histologically (Perren et al, 1992), but treatment of the two conditions is fundamentally different.

Clinical features

The reported age range for lymphoma of the uterus is 20–80 years with a median age at presentation of 43 years (Harris & Scully, 1984; Muntz et al, 1991; Perren et al, 1992). Seventy seven per cent of patients are premenopausal at presentation (Muntz et al, 1991). The most common presenting symptom is with abnormal

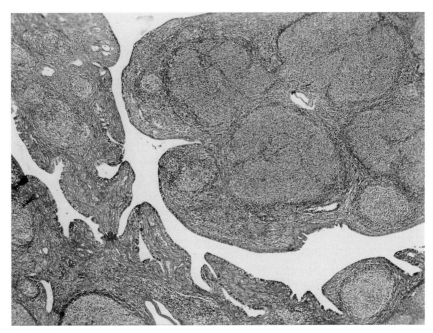

Fig. 31.8 Fallopian tube involved by a follicular lymphoma. (Reprinted with permission from Ferry & Young, 1991.)

bleeding, postcoital or postmenopausal, although 20% were asymptomatic (Muntz et al, 1991).

Variable success has been reported in the detection of uterine lymphomas and leukaemias on cervical smears (Ferry & Young, 1991). This is in part due to misinterpretation of abnormal cells found in smears (Katayama et al, 1973), a factor that may be rectified by greater awareness amongst, and improved training of, screeners and cytopathologists (Ceden & Sakurai, 1962; Colmenares & Zuker, 1965; Whittaker, 1976; Krumerman & Chung, 1978; Mikhail et al, 1989). It appears however that the failure of cervical cytology to detect leukaemia and lymphoma is partly due to the fact that only 10–40% of cervical lymphomas yield a positive smear (Andrews et al, 1988). This is because lymphomas often infiltrate beneath an intact cervical epithelium with sparing of a narrow zone deep to the squamous epithelium (Harris & Scully, 1984) in contrast to carcinoma of the cervix where the surface epithelium itself is abnormal.

Gross appearance

The most common recorded appearance of cervical lymphomas is a diffuse, barrel-shaped enlargement of the cervix without mucosal abnormality (Fig. 31.9). Other appearances recorded are of multinodular masses, polypoid masses protruding through the cervical os or discrete submucosal masses. Ulceration due to lymphoma is distinctly uncommon (Harris & Scully, 1984). Extension into the body of the uterus, the vagina, parametrium and pelvic side walls may occur (Harris & Scully, 1984; Ferry & Young, 1991; Perren et al, 1992) making the exact origin of the lymphoma difficult to ascertain in some cases. Most cervical lymphomas are large tumours, half being over 4 cm in diameter. In two patients, lymphoma originated from an endocervical polyp (Muntz et al, 1991). Of the 21 cases reported by Harris & Scully (1984) 19 presented in the cervix and 2 in the endometrium. The endometrial lymphomas formed polypoid masses within the uterus. In the case reported by Maeda et al (1988) lymphoma was only found in endometrial curettings but not in the subsequent hysterectomy specimen.

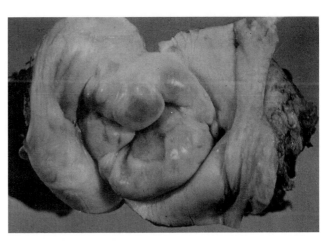

Fig. 31.9 Uterine cervix enlarged by malignant lymphoma producing a barrel-shaped cervix. The overlying mucosa is intact. (Reprinted with permission from Ferry & Young, 1991.)

Histology

Harris & Scully (1984) categorized 21 cases of lymphoma of the uterus using both the Rappaport and the Kiel classification. Using the latter, sixteen cases were considered to be of follicle centre cell derivation: 6 centroblastic/centrocytic follicular; 7 centroblastic/centrocytic diffuse and 3 centroblastic (Fig. 31.10). The remainder included immunoblastic lymphoma (2), lymphoplasmacytic lymphoma (1), Burkitt's lymphoma (1) and unclassified lymphoma (1). Muntz et al (1991) categorized 43 primary malignant lymphomas of the cervix, using the Working Formulation, and categorized 5 as low grade, 36 as intermediate grade and 2 as high grade. Eight (19%) of the patients in this pooled series of cases had tumours with a follicular growth pattern, 5 of low grade and 3 of intermediate grade. Thirty (70%) were diffuse large cell malignant lymphomas; 3 diffuse small cleaved cell lymphomas; 2 mixed small and large cell lymphomas; all of intermediate grade. The high-grade tumours included a large cell immunoblastic lymphoma and a small non-cleaved cell lymphoma.

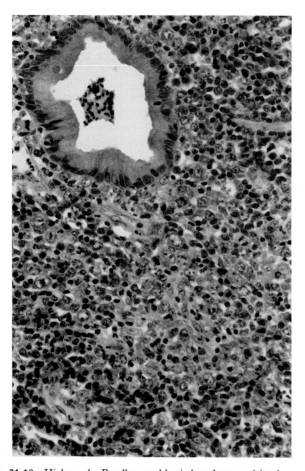

Fig. 31.10 High-grade, B-cell centroblastic lymphoma, arising in the cervix. Tumour cells infiltrate around endocervical glands. H & E × 250.

In the few cases where immunohistochemistry has been performed (Ferry & Young, 1991; Muntz et al, 1991), nearly all tumours were of B-cell lineage. However, Jack & Lee (1986), in an immunohistochemical study of T-cell lymphomas at various sites, found 2 cases involving the uterus; one was a 25-year-old female with endometrial involvement and the other had cervical involvement. In both cases there was a uniform population of tumour cells with high mitotic rate and a starry sky pattern. Both patients had stage 4 disease and died at 1 and 6 months after diagnosis.

A case of MALT lymphoma of the cervix has been reported by Pelstring et al (1991) (see below). The authors have also seen another case where a 29-year-old woman presented with complaints of a vaginal discharge; she had a total hysterectomy and bilateral salpingo-oophorectomy before the correct diagnosis of MALT lymphoma was established. Following clinical staging, it was found that the disease had been present only in the cervix (stage 1E). Phenotypically this was a B-cell tumour in which there was transformation to a high-grade lymphoma of multi-lobated type together with residual low-grade areas with infiltration of residual endocervical glands by small lymphoid cells to form the characteristic lymphoepithelial lesions (Fig. 31.11).

Sclerosis may be a prominent feature of both cervical and vaginal lymphomas. Traction artifact can present diagnostic problems with cervical biopsies, making differentiation from carcinomas or inflammatory infiltrates difficult. In such cases immunohistochemistry may be of considerable value and techniques such as polymerase chain reaction (PCR) may be used to determine the clonality of the infiltrate (McCarthy et al, 1991; Diss et al, 1994). The endometrial lymphomas reported by Harris & Scully (1984) were devoid of sclerosis and were sharply demarcated from underlying myometrium.

Stage and survival

In the series of 25 cases of malignant lymphoma of the uterus and vagina reported by Harris & Scully (1984), 21 were in Ann Arbor stage 1E. The overall actuarial survival of all patients was 73% but with stage 1E tumours it was 89%, compared with 20% for patients with lymph node or ovarian involvement. Muntz et al (1991) reported 5 patients with Ann Arbor stage 1E lymphoma of the cervix and reviewed 38 previously reported stage 1E patients. Using the FIGO system for staging cervical carcinoma, 44% were stage 1, 42% stage 2, 12% stage 3 and 2% stage 4. Most of the patients had been treated by a combination of surgery and radiotherapy. Among 28 patients so treated and followed for at least two years there was only one treatment failure. Muntz et al (1991) conclude that 'most cases of primary lymphoma of the uterine cervix are Ann

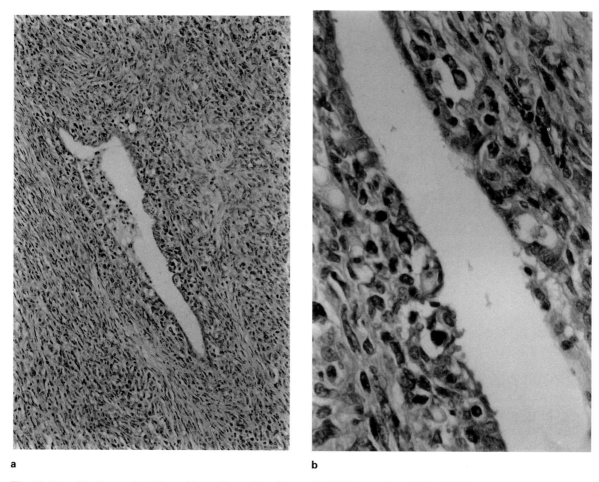

Fig. 31.11 **a** Uterine cervix infiltrated by malignant lymphoma of 'MALT' type. Lymphoid cells infiltrate endocervical gland epithelium. H & E × 100. **b** Higher magnification shows formation of lymphoepithelial lesions within the glandular epithelium. H & E × 640. (Courtesy of Dr. A. Norton, St. Bartholomew's Hospital.)

Arbor stage 1E and can be cured with traditional combination of surgery and radiation therapy after careful evaluation'. They do however acknowledge that chemotherapy may be the preferred option in young patients in whom preservation of fertility is important (Johnston et al, 1989; Sandvei et al, 1990). The patient reported by Sandvei et al (1990) was free of disease after chemotherapy for a large cell lymphoma of the cervix, having had one termination of pregnancy and one full-term pregnancy following treatment. Perren et al (1992) reported 5 patients with non-Hodgkin's lymphoma of the cervix and upper vagina seen at the Royal Marsden Hospital over a period of 20 years and they reviewed a further 72 cases reported in the literature. Seventy three per cent of patients were Ann Arbor stage 1E and 25% stage 2E. According to the FIGO stage, 40% were stage 1, 38% stage 2, 11% stage 3 and 11% stage 4. In a selected group of 37 of these patients, the survival rate was 76% with only a weak association with stage but a stronger association with grade.

It is apparent from the foregoing data that non-Hodg-kin's lymphomas of the uterus and vagina are generally of a lower grade and lower stage than ovarian lymphomas and have a better prognosis. An apparent paradox is the association of low-grade and follicular tumours with low stage and with long-term survival following surgery alone (Perren et al, 1992). This raises the possibility that some of these patients may have had MALT lymphomas, possibly showing follicular colonization. In the case of MALT lymphoma of the cervix reported by Pelstring et al (1991), the patient aged 40 years experienced dysfunctional uterine bleeding and underwent a vaginal hysterectomy for presumed uterine fibroids. A 2 cm leiomyoma was identified but sections of the cervix revealed a diffuse infiltrate of marginal zone and lymphoplasmacytoid cells forming lymphoepithelial lesions within the endocervical glands. The lymphoplasmacytic cells showed kappa light chain restriction. The resection margins were involved by lymphoma and computed tomography showed pelvic lymphadenopathy. The patient was given local radiation therapy and had no evidence of disease at three months follow-up.

Hodgkin's disease

Several cases interpreted as primary Hodgkin's disease of the cervix have been reported (Ferry & Young, 1991). All these, however, date back to the 1960s before the advent of modern immunohistochemistry and it must be questioned whether critical review would sustain these diagnoses. Hung & Kurtz (1985) reported a case of Hodgkin's disease of the endometrium in a patient who had been treated three years earlier for stage 4 Hodgkin's disease. It is possible that endometrial involvement may have resulted from retrograde lymphatic flow from involved pelvic lymph nodes. This type of spread may be equivalent to the apparent retrograde flow of Hodgkin's cells into skin, which has occurred in patients with advanced Hodgkin's disease (Benninghoff et al, 1970).

Granulocytic sarcoma (myelosarcoma)

We have already discussed the diagnosis of granulocytic sarcoma in the ovary. This tumour may accompany, precede or signal relapse of acute myelogenous leukaemia. In a recent report of a case and review of the literature, Friedman et al (1992) identified 29 cases, including their own, that involved the female genital tract. Fifteen cases occurred in the cervix (Fig. 31.12) and 2 in the vulva or vagina in patients without a history of acute myelogenous leukaemia. Grossly the tumour forms nodules, ulcers or large infiltrating masses extending into adjacent tissues (Chorlton et al, 1974b; Kapadia et al, 1978). Histologically, granulocytic precursor cells (Fig. 31.12) infiltrate the tissue and immunohistochemistry is useful in confirming the diagnosis, as discussed above.

Other uterine or vaginal tumours may occur as a manifestation of relapse of leukaemia. The importance of making the correct diagnosis in these rare cases, particularly those without overt leukaemia, is that current opinion indicates that they should be treated as for acute myelogenous leukaemia despite the absence of blood or bone marrow disease (Eshghabadi et al, 1986; Banik et al, 1989; Hutchinson et al, 1990).

Foci of extramedullary haemopoiesis have rarely been detected in the endometrium (Sirgi et al, 1994) in the absence of a known haemopoietic disorder. A full histological work-up is nevertheless desirable in these patients to exclude leukaemia.

Differential diagnosis

Undifferentiated neoplasms of the uterus and cervix might enter into the differential diagnosis of malignant lymphomas at this site. These would include lymphoepithelial-like carcinoma (lymphoepithelioma) of the cervix which resembles nasopharyngeal carcinoma (Hamazaki et al,

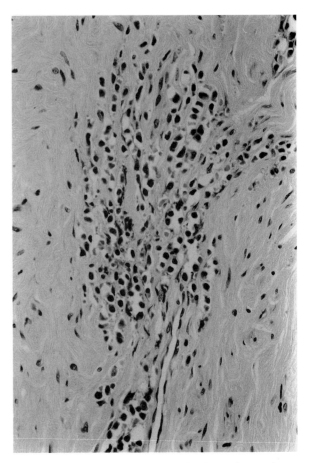

Fig. 31.12 Focus of granulocytic sarcoma in the uterine cervix. H & E × 250.

1968; Hasumi et al, 1977; Hafiz et al, 1985; Mills et al, 1985; Halpin et al, 1989), and small cell (neuroendocrine) carcinoma of the cervix (Ueda et al, 1988). However, the judicious use of lymphocyte and epithelial markers should readily identify the nature of these tumours.

A range of inflammatory lesions may be observed in the uterus and cervix (Ferry & Young 1991), sometimes associated with chlamydial infections (Winkler et al, 1984). The polymorphous nature of these reactions should make confusion with lymphomas rare. Young et al (1985) studied 16 reactive lymphoma-like lesions involving the cervix (10), endometrium (5) and vulva (1). The reactive lesions were often superficial, involving the overlying epithelium, polymorphous in nature and lacked tumour masses in contrast to lymphomas which usually spared the surface epithelium, were monomorphous and were usually associated with gross tumour masses.

Two examples of so-called inflammatory pseudotumour of the uterus have been described, in a 6-year-old girl and a 30-year-old woman (Gilks et al, 1987). A further case was described in a child (Scott et al, 1988) and more recently an inflammatory pseudotumour of the cervix has been described (Abenoza et al, 1994). These were similar to those described in the lung and elsewhere. They are composed of spindle cells with characteristics of myofibroblasts with a mixed inflammatory infiltrate rich in plasma cells. Such lesions are unlikely to be confused with malignant lymphomas.

Ferry et al (1989) described 7 patients aged 35–50 years with leiomyomas containing a lymphoid infiltrate of sufficient intensity to simulate lymphoma. The distinction from lymphoma could be made by the polymorphous nature of the infiltrate and by the fact that it was confined to the leiomyoma and present only to a minor extent in the adjacent myometrium (Fig. 31.13).

A case of Rosai–Dorfman disease (sinus histiocytosis with massive lymphadenopathy) has been reported in a 37-year-old woman (Murray & Fox, 1991). The lesion was confined to the cervix and consisted of large histiocytic cells containing engulfed lymphocytes admixed with other inflammatory cells. Apart from malignant lymphoma, this lesion also needs to be distinguished from Langerhans cell histiocytosis which may rarely affect the cervix.

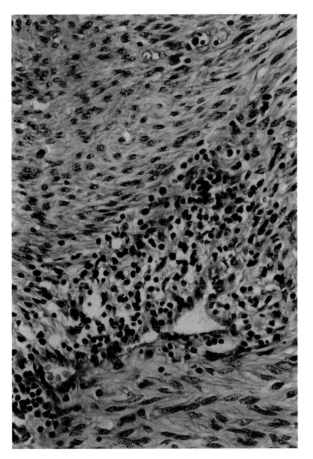

Fig. 31.13 Uterine leiomyoma showing prominent lymphoid infiltration. H & E × 300.

VAGINA

Non-Hodgkin's lymphoma

Malignant lymphoma of the vagina is rare and vaginal involvement is more commonly a manifestation of disseminated disease. In some cases, however, the vagina does appear to have been the primary site of origin (Chorlton et al, 1974b; Castaldo et al, 1979; Harris & Scully, 1984; Perren et al, 1992; Prévot et al, 1992). In the series of 9500 women with lymphoma from the Armed Forces Institute of Pathology, there were 4 cases originating in the vagina (Chorlton et al, 1974b). Prévot et al (1992) reviewed 17 cases of primary non-Hodgkin's lymphoma of the vagina, in the literature, and added 3 cases of their own. Perren et al (1992) described a further 3 primary cases of vaginal lymphoma. The tumours occurred in the fourth to sixth decades with an age range of 19–79 years. Presentation of vaginal lymphoma has been as a vaginal mass or induration, with vaginal bleeding or discharge and, occasionally, urinary symptoms such as frequency or recurrent cystitis.

A total of 23 cases of primary vaginal lymphoma (Perren et al, 1992; Prévot et al, 1992) were categorized using the Kiel classification or the Working Formulation. Using the Kiel classification, 6 were from the older literature and could only be categorized as large cell, malignant lymphoma (high grade); 2 were lymphocytic; 6 follicular or diffuse centroblastic/centrocytic; 2 immunoblastic; 5 centroblastic; 1 anaplastic large cell and 1 angiocentric, pleomorphic T-cell lymphoma. The vast majority of vaginal lymphomas are of B-cell lineage and in the 10 cases of vaginal lymphoma reported in the most recent series (Harris & Scully, 1984; Perren et al, 1992; Prévot et al, 1992) 9 were follicle centre cell-derived B-cell tumours and 1 was of T-cell lineage. We have seen a case of lymphoplasmocytic lymphoma, confirmed by immunophenotyping, in the vagina of a female aged 77 who presented with postmenopausal bleeding and had a narrow stenosed vagina (Fig. 31.14). Histologically, vaginal lymphomas, like cervical lymphomas, may show sclerosis ranging from fine fibrils to prominent dense bands of collagen. Traction or crush artifacts often obscure the histology in small biopsies.

In 19 cases of vaginal lymphomas in the literature, staging information was available (Perren et al, 1992; Prévot et al, 1992). Of those, 15 cases were Ann Arbor stage 1E, two were stage 2E (with inguinal lymph node involvement) and two were stage 4. Prognosis of primary vaginal lymphomas, although unpredictable in the individual case, is generally favourable, even with high-grade or extensive disease. Full staging is essential to avoid inappropriate treatment. Radical surgery is considered unnecessary and most localized cases have been treated by radiotherapy, combination chemotherapy and, in some cases, limited surgery. Of the 19 patients reviewed or

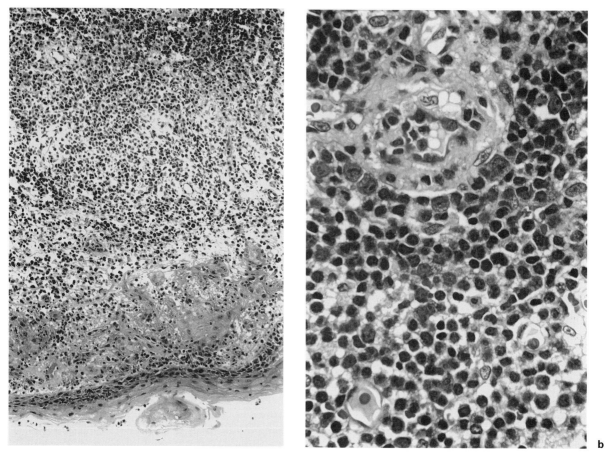

Fig. 31.14 **a** Malignant lymphoma of the vagina. H & E × 40. **b** Higher magnification showing a lymphoplasmocytic lymphoma with plasma cell differentiation. H & E × 640.

reported by Prévot et al (1992), 6 patients died of lymphoma within 17 months of diagnosis and 2 died later of unrelated causes. The remainder were alive at follow-up periods ranging from 2 months to over 11 years, the mean follow-up period being 75 months.

Other tumours

Vaginal involvement by Burkitt-type lymphoma has been reported (Castaldo et al, 1979). Six cases of plasmacytoma involving the vagina have also been described (Doss, 1978; Osanto et al, 1981) in women aged between 34 and 78 years. One patient subsequently developed lytic bone lesions but no bone involvement was noted in the others. Rare cases of granulocytic sarcoma and leukaemic vaginal deposits in patients with acute myeloid leukaemia have also been reported.

Differential diagnosis

A lymphoepithelioma-like carcinoma of the vagina has been described (Dietl et al, 1994), similar to those reported in the cervix. Immunohistochemistry of the lymphoid infiltrate within the tumour showed a predominant

T-cell and macrophage population but with scanty numbers of B lymphocytes. The polymorphous nature of the inflammatory infiltrate will aid in distinguishing this condition from a true vaginal lymphoma.

VULVA

Non-Hodgkin's lymphoma

Most lymphomas presenting in the vulva are usually a manifestation of more widespread disease (Schiller & Madge, 1970; Egwuatu et al, 1980). Lathrop (1967) noted 4% of cases of vulvar involvement among an autopsy series of lymphomas involving the female genital tract. Cases of apparent primary lymphomas of the vulva mostly pre-date the use of critical staging procedures (Taussig, 1973; Buckingham & McClure, 1955; Hahn, 1958; Iliya et al, 1968; Wishart, 1973). The reported patients have had an age range of 33–75 years and presented with indurated or ulcerated vulvar lesions. One patient treated by radical vulvectomy for a large cell lymphoma was well five years later (Iliya et al, 1968). The vulva may also be involved by Burkitt's lymphoma (Egwuatu et al, 1980). Involvement of Bartholin's gland by lymphoma

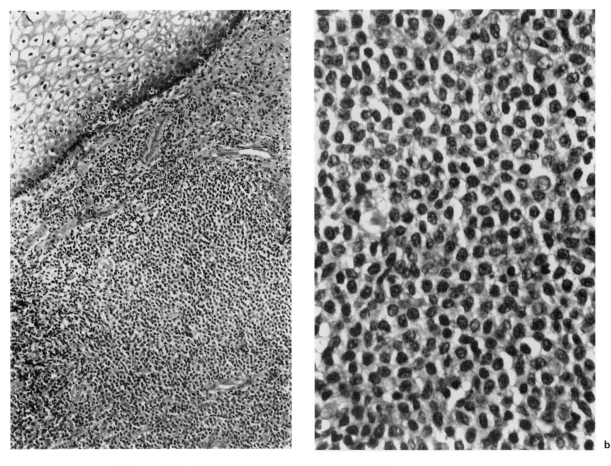

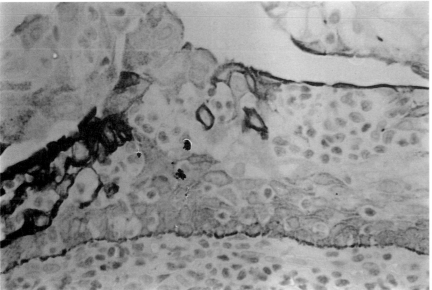

Fig. 31.15 **a** Vulva: low grade B-cell lymphoma of 'MALT' type involving the urethral meatus. H & E × 40. **b** Higher magnification showing a monomorphic population of centrocyte-like cells. H & E × 640. **c** Immunostaining for cytokeratin delineates surface epithelium, within which are collections of lymphoid cells forming a lymphoepithelial lesion. CAM 5.2 × 640.

has also been reported (Plouffe et al, 1984). We have seen a low-grade MALT lymphoma of the urethral meatus presenting as a vulvar tumour in a 23-year-old woman (Fig. 31.15).

Delayed diagnosis and inappropriate management of lymphomas in the vulva may lead to widely destructive disease of the perineum. Tuder (1992) reported two cases of vulvar lymphoma presenting as progressive non-healing vulvar ulcers. One case was a lymphoplasmacytic lymphoma which was untreated and resulted in the patient's death after four years, and the second was an angiocentric, mixed cell lymphoma, the immunopheno-

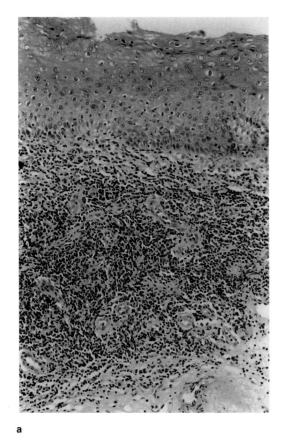

a

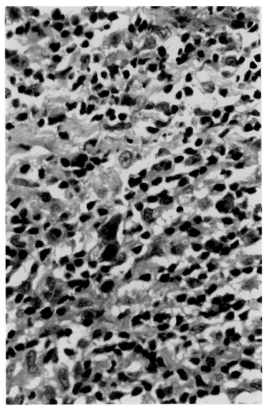

b

Fig. 31.16 **a** Vulvar, anaplastic T-cell lymphoma. H & E × 27. **b** Higher magnification shows a population of larger pleomorphic cells and smaller lymphocytes. **c** CD3 immunostaining of tumour cell indicates T-cell lineage. (× 110)

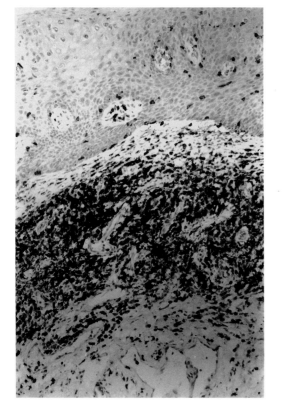

c

type of which was not characterized. The aggressive behaviour of these cases was likened to the 'midline lethal granuloma syndrome' of the upper respiratory tract.

One patient alleged to have Hodgkin's disease was treated with radical vulvectomy and nitrogen mustard and was reported to be well 22 months after presentation (Hahn, 1958). It is unlikely that Hodgkin's disease would present as a primary lesion in the vulva, although anaplastic large cell lymphoma may present as a cutaneous tumour (De Bruin et al, 1993) and may histologically resemble Hodgkin's disease. We have also seen an anaplastic (Ki1-positive) large cell lymphoma of T-cell phenotype that presented as a vulvar tumour in a 25-year-old woman with a presenting complaint of pruritis vulvae (Fig. 31.16).

Inflammatory lesions mimicking lymphoma

Inflammatory lesions of the vulva may sometimes simulate malignant lymphoma. The one condition worthy of special consideration is infectious mononucleosis which

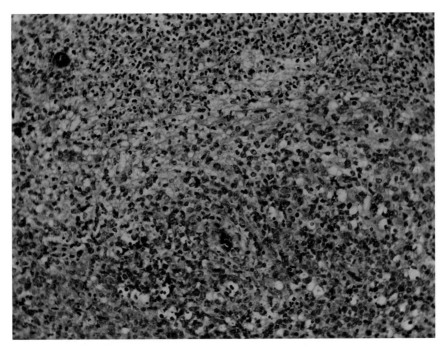

Fig. 31.17 Vulvar lesions of infectious mononucleosis. There is surface ulceration and an underlying infiltrate of large and small lymphoid cells. (Reprinted with permission from Ferry & Young, 1991.)

may cause vulvar ulceration and inguinal lymphadenopathy. The cervix is a recognized site of shedding of the EB virus and ulceration of the lower genital tract is a feature of infectious mononucleosis. It is fortunate that these lesions are rarely biopsied since the blastic proliferation can appear alarming. Biopsy of these lesions reveals a diffuse lymphoid infiltrate with a proliferation of large blastic cells (Fig. 31.17) that might well trap the unwary into making a diagnosis of high-grade lymphoma (Brown & Stenchever, 1977; Portnoy et al, 1984a; Young et al, 1985). In small biopsies it may be impossible to distinguish this blastic proliferation from high-grade lymphoma on morphology alone. Immunohistochemistry may be of help in resolving the problem by identifying both T and B blasts and showing polytypic immunoglobulin in the B cells (Young et al, 1985). In most cases, serological tests will confirm Epstein–Barr virus infection. A consideration of the histology in the context of the clinical history should, however, prevent such lesions from being diagnosed as lymphomas.

LANGERHANS CELL HISTIOCYTOSIS

The female genital tract may rarely be involved by Langerhans cell histiocytosis (histiocytosis X) (Dupree & Lee, 1973; Issa et al, 1980; Lechner et al, 1983). Lesions occur most frequently in the vagina and vulva and, rarely, in the cervix and uterus. Lesions are usually part of a more widespread disease involving the lungs and/or the skeleton. With vulvar involvement, patients usually present with one or more painful or itching papules or nodules or ulcers; the clitoris is often involved. Histologically, there is an admixture of Langerhans cells and eosinophils (Fig. 31.18). The presence of eosinophils, often in clusters, may alert the pathologist to the correct diagnosis. However, eosinophils are not always prominent in Langerhans cell histiocytosis and the diagnosis rests on the recognition of the characteristic grooved, 'coffee bean' nuclei of the Langerhans cells and their abundant pale-staining cytoplasm. In the vagina and vulva these cells infiltrate immediately below the mucosa. Langerhans cells stain weakly and patchily for many histiocyte markers but strongly express S100 protein. The lesions have been treated by local excision, radiation therapy and, rarely, chemotherapy for recurrence (Dupree & Lee, 1973; Issa et al, 1980).

LYMPHOMA AND PREGNANCY

The occurrence of genital tract lymphomas in pregnancy is well recognized (Armon, 1976; Rotmensch & Woodruff, 1982; Monterroso et al, 1993). Some of the recorded cases are Burkitt's and Burkitt-like lymphomas of the ovary (Finkle & Goldman, 1974; Armon, 1976). Lymphoma associated with pregnancy was reported to be a bad prognostic feature by Rotmensch & Woodruff (1982), although Monterroso et al (1993) recorded long-term survivors. Successful pregnancy has also been reported after treat-

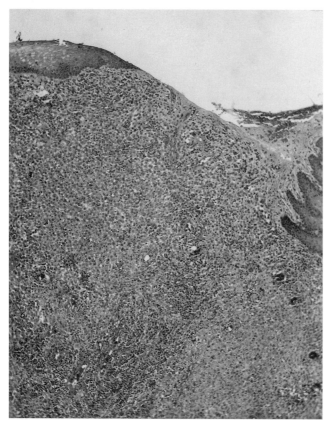

Fig. 31.18 Langerhans cell histiocytosis of vulva. Tumour cells have abundant cytoplasm and are admixed with eosinophils and lymphocytes. (Reprinted with permission from Ferry & Young, 1991.)

ment of ovarian and cervical lymphomas by chemotherapy alone or chemotherapy and surgery (Clifford, 1968; Sandvei et al, 1990).

Non-Hodgkin's lymphomas at all sites may occur during pregnancy and present clinicians with a dilemma of achieving optimum maternal survival without impairing the welfare of the fetus (Steiner-Salz et al, 1985). The use of chemotherapy in the first trimester of pregnancy, with its potential for causing congenital malformations, is a matter of particular concern. Aviles et al (1990) record the chemotherapy and obstetric care of 16 pregnant patients with non-Hodgkin's lymphomas, mostly of high grade and high stage, seen between 1975 and 1986. Of these, 8 were large cell lymphoma; 2 diffuse, mixed cell lymphoma; 3 diffuse, small non-cleaved cell; 2 lymphoblastic and 1 immunoblastic cell type. Lymphomas occurring in pregnancy are likely to be in younger rather than older women and low-grade follicular lymphomas are, therefore, less likely to be encountered. All patients received chemotherapy, including 8 patients in the first trimester. At the time of birth, 12 mothers were in remission and there were no congenital defects. Fifteen babies were alive and well 3–11 years after birth and 8 mothers who achieved complete remission were alive and free of disease 4–9 years after delivery. Pregnancy is not therefore a contraindication to the treatment of non-Hodgkin's lymphoma with chemotherapy and long-term remissions can be obtained in the mothers.

CONCLUSIONS

Malignant lymphomas of the female genital tract are rare. Their recognition is, however, important, since the treatment of these neoplasms is different from that of epithelial malignancies and may result in long-term survival. Most lymphomas that present in the female genital tract will be found to be part of more widespread disease. However, primary lymphomas at this site undoubtedly occur. These primary tumours often have a good prognosis. Their nature and their relationship to physiological or reactive lymphoid infiltrates at this site merit further study.

REFERENCES

Abenoza P, Shek Y H, Perrone T 1994 Inflammatory pseudotumors of the cervix. International Journal of Gynecological Pathology 13: 80–86.

Andrews S J, Hernandez E, Woods J, Cook B 1988 Burkitt's like lymphoma presenting as a gynecologic tumor. Gynecologic Oncology 30: 131–136.

Armon P J 1976 Burkitt's lymphoma of the ovary in association with pregnancy: two case reports. British Journal of Obstetrics and Gynaecology 83: 169–172.

Aviles A, Diaz-Maques J C, Torras V, Garcia E L, Guzman R 1990 Non-Hodgkin's lymphomas and pregnancy: presentation of 16 cases. Gynecologic Oncology 37: 335–337.

Ballon S C, Donaldson R C, Berman M L, Swanson G A, Byron R L 1978 Myeloblastoma (granulocytic sarcoma) of the ovary. Archives of Pathology and Laboratory Medicine 102: 474–476.

Bambira E A, Miranda D, Mugalhaes G M C 1982 Plasma cell myeloma simulating Krukenberg's tumor. Southern Medical Journal 75: 511–512.

Banik S, Borg Grech A, Eyden B P 1989 Granulocytic sarcomas of the cervix: an immunohistochemical histochemical and ultrastructural study. Journal of Clinical Pathology 42: 483–488.

Banks P, Chan J, Cleary M et al 1992 Mantle cell lymphoma: a proposal for unification of morphologic, immunologic and molecular data. American Journal of Surgical Pathology 16: 637–640.

Barcos M, Lane W, Gomez G A, Han T, Freeman A, Preisler H, Henderson E 1987 An autopsy study of 1206 acute and chronic leukemias (1958–1982). Cancer 60: 827–837.

Bare W W, McCloskey J F 1961 Primary Hodgkin's disease of the ovary: report of a case. Obstetrics and Gynecology 17: 477–480.

Benninghoff D L, Medina A, Alexander L L, Camiel M R 1970 The mode of spread of Hodgkin's disease to the skin. Cancer 26: 1135–1140.

Berard C, O'Conor G T, Thomas L B, Torloni H 1969 Histopathological definition of Burkitt's tumour. Bulletin of the World Health Organisation 40: 601–607.

Brown Z A, Stenchever M A 1977 Genital ulceration and infectious mononucleosis: report of a case. American Journal of Obstetrics and Gynecology 127: 673–674.

Buckingham J C, McClure J H 1955 Reticulum cell sarcoma of the vulva. Obstetrics and Gynecology 6: 138–143.

Burkitt D 1958 A sarcoma involving the jaws in African children. British Journal of Surgery 46: 218–233.

Burkitt D P 1970 General features and facial tumours in Burkitt's lymphoma. In: Burkitt D P, Wright D H (eds) Burkitt's lymphoma. Livingstone, Edinburgh, pp 6–15.

Burkitt D P, Wright D H (eds) 1980 Burkitt's lymphoma. Livingstone, Edinburgh.

Carbone P P, Kaplan H S, Musshoff K, Smithers D W, Tubiana M 1971 Report of the committee on Hodgkin's disease staging classification. Cancer Research 31: 1860–1861.

Carr I, Hill A S, Hancock B, Neal F E 1976 Malignant lymphoma of the cervix uteri: histology and ultrastructure. Journal of Clinical Pathology 29: 680–686.

Case Records of the Massachusetts General Hospital (case 45—1981) 1981 New England Journal of Medicine 305: 1135–1146.

Castaldo T W, Ballon S C, Lagasse L D, Petrilli E S 1979 Reticuloendothelial neoplasia of the female genital tract. Obstetrics and Gynecology 54: 167–170.

Cattoretti G, Pileri S, Paravicini C et al 1993 Antigen unmasking in formalin fixed paraffin embedded tissue sections. Journal of Pathology 171: 83–98.

Cecalupo A J, Frankel L S, Sullivan M P 1982 Pelvic and ovarian extramedullary leukemia relapse in young girls. Cancer 50: 587–593.

Ceden G H, Sakurai M 1962 Vaginal cytology in leukemia. Acta Cytologica 6: 379–391.

Chan J K C, Ng C S, Isaacson P G 1990 Relationship between high grade lymphoma and low grade B cell mucosa associated lymphoid tissue lymphoma (MALToma) of the stomach. American Journal of Pathology 136: 1153–1164.

Chorlton I 1987 Malignant lymphoma of the female genital tract and ovaries. In: Fox H (ed) Haines and Taylor's Textbook of obstetrical and gynaecological pathology, 3rd edn. Churchill Livingstone, Edinburgh, pp 737–762.

Chorlton I, Norris H J, King F M 1974a Malignant reticuloendothelial disease involving the ovary as a primary manifestation: a series of 19 lymphomas and 1 granulocytic sarcoma. Cancer 34: 397–407.

Chorlton I, Kamei R F, King F M, Norris H J 1974b Primary malignant reticuloendothelial disease involving the vagina, cervix and corpus uteri. Obstetrics and Gynecology 44: 735–748.

Chu J-Y, Cradock T V, Davis R K, Tennant N E 1981 Ovarian tumor as manifestation of relapse in acute lymphoblastic leukemia. Cancer 48: 377–379.

Clifford P 1968 Treatment of Burkitt's lymphoma. Lancet i: 559.

Cogliatti S B, Schusia K, Shumaacher K et al 1991 Primary B cell gastric lymphoma: a clinicopathological study of 145 patients. Gastroenterology 101: 1159–1170.

Colmenares R F, Zuker M N 1965 Significance of lymphocytic pools in the routine vaginal smear. Obstetrics and Gynecology 26: 909–912.

Cook H T, Boylston A W 1988 Plasmacytoma of the ovary. Gynecologic Oncology 29: 378–381.

Cuevas E C, Bateman A C, Wilkins B S et al 1994 Microwave antigen retrieval in immunocytochemistry: a study of 80 antibodies. Journal of Clinical Pathology 47: 448–452.

de Bruin P, Beljaards R, van Heerde P et al 1993 Differences in clinical behaviour and immunophenotype between primary cutaneous and primary nodular anaplastic large cell lymphoma of T-cell or null cell phenotype. Histopathology 23: 127–136.

Delsol G, Al Saate T, Gatter K et al 1988 Co-expression of epithelial membrane antigen (EMA), Ki-1 and interleukin 2 receptor by anaplastic large cell lymphomas: diagnostic value in so-called malignant histiocytosis. American Journal of Pathology 130: 59–70.

Dietl J, Horny H P, Kaiserling E 1994 Lymphoepithelioma-like carcinoma of the vagina: a case report with special reference to the immunophenotype of the tumour cells and tumour-infiltrating lymphoreticular cells. International Journal of Gynecological Pathology 13: 186–189.

Diss T C, Pan L, Peng H, Wotherspoon A C, Isaacson P G 1994 Sources of DNA for detecting B cell monoclonality using PCR. Journal of Clinical Pathology 47: 493–496.

Dorfman R 1965 Childhood lymphoma in St Louis, Missouri, clinically and histologically resembling Burkitt's tumour.Cancer 18: 418–430.

Doss L L 1978 Simultaneous extramedullary plasmacytomas of the vagina and vulva: a case report and review of the literature. Cancer 41: 2468–2474.

Dupree E L, Lee R A 1973 Histiocytosis X in the female genital tract. Obstetrics and Gynecology 42: 201–204.

Durfee H A, Clark B F, Peers J H 1937 Primary lymphosarcoma of the ovary: report of a case. American Journal of Cancer 30: 567–573.

Egwuatu V E, Ejeckam G C, Okaro J M 1980 Burkitt's lymphoma of the vulva: case report. British Journal of Obstetrics and Gynaecology 87: 827–830.

Eshghabadi M, Shojania A M, Carr I 1986 Isolated granulocytic sarcoma: report of a case and review of the literature. Journal of Clinical Oncology 4: 912–917.

Falini B, Flenghi L, Pileri S et al 1993 PGM-I: A new monoclonal antibody directed against a fixative-resistant epitope on the macrophage-restricted form of CD68 molecule. American Journal of Pathology 142: 1359–1372.

Federation International of Gynaecologists and Obstetricians (FIGO) Cancer Committee: Annual Report on the Results of Treatment in Gynecological Cancer, vol 17. Stockholm 1979.

Ferry J A, Young R H 1991 Malignant lymphoma, pseudolymphoma and haematopoietic disorders of the female genital tract. In: Rosen P P, Fechner R E (eds) Pathology Annual Part I 26: 227–263.

Ferry J A, Harris N L, Scully R E 1989 Uterine leiomyomas with lymphoid infiltration simulating lymphoma: a report of seven cases. International Journal of Gynecological Pathology 8: 263–270.

Finkle H I, Goldman R L 1974 Burkitt's lymphoma: gynecological considerations. Obstetrics and Gynecology 43: 281–284.

Fox H, Langley F A 1976 Tumours of the ovary. Heinemann, London.

Fox H, Langley F A, Govan A D T, Hill S A, Bennett M H 1988 Malignant lymphoma presenting as an ovarian tumour: a clinico-pathological analysis of 34 cases. British Journal of Obstetrics and Gynaecology 95: 386–390.

Freeman C, Berg J W, Cutler S J 1972 Occurrence and prognosis of extranodal lymphomas. Cancer 29: 252–260.

Friedman H D, Adelson M D, Eider R C, Lemke S M 1992 Case report. Granulocytic sarcoma of the uterine cervix — literature review of granulocytic sarcoma of the female genital tract. Gynecological Oncology 46: 128–137.

Gerard-Marchant R, Hamlin I, Lennert K, Rilke F, Stansfeld A, van Unnik J 1974 Classification of non-Hodgkin's lymphomas. Lancet ii: 406–408.

Gilks C B, Taylor G P, Clement P B 1987 Inflammatory pseudotumor of the uterus. International Journal of Gynecological Pathology 6: 275–286.

Gralnick H R, Dittmark K 1969 Development of myeloblastoma with massive breast and ovarian involvement during remission in acute leukemia. Cancer 24: 746–749.

Grogan T, Warnke R, Kaplan H 1982 A comparative study of Burkitt's and non-Burkitt's "undifferentiated" malignant lymphoma: immunological cytochemical ultrastructural, cytologic, histopathologic, clinical and cell culture features. Cancer 49: 1817–1828.

Gustmann C M A, Osborn M, Griesser H, Feller A C 1991 Cytokeratin expression and vimentin content in anaplastic large cell lymphomas and other non-Hodgkin's lymphomas. American Journal of Pathology 138: 1413–1422.

Hafiz M A, Kragel P J, Toker C 1985 Carcinoma of the uterine cervix resembling lymphoepithelioma. Obstetrics and Gynecology 66: 829–831.

Hahn G A 1958 Gynecological considerations in malignant lymphomas. American Journal of Obstetrics and Gynecology 75: 673–683.

Halpin T F, Hunter R E, Cohen M B 1989 Lymphoepithelioma of the uterine cervix. Gynecologic Oncology 34: 101–105.

Hamazaki M, Fujita H, Ara T et al 1968 Medullary carcinoma with marked lymphoid infiltration of the uterine cervix. Japanese Journal of Clinical Oncology 4: 787–790.

Harris N L, Scully R E 1984 Malignant lymphoma and granulocytic sarcoma of the uterus and vagina: a clinicopathologic analysis of 27 cases. Cancer 53: 2530–2545.

Harris N L, Jaffe E S, Stein H et al 1994 A revised European — North American classification of lymphoid neoplasms: a proposal from the International Lymphoma Study Group. Blood 84: 1361–1392.

Hastrup N, Hamilton Dutoit S, Ralfkiaer E, Palleson G 1991 Peripheral T-cell lymphomas: an evaluation of reproducibility of the updated Kiel classification. Histopathology 18: 99–105.

Hasumi K, Sugano H, Sakamoto G et al 1977 Circumscribed carcinomas of the uterine cervix with marked lymphocytic infiltration. Cancer 39: 2503–2508.

Hautzer N W 1984 Primary plasmacytoma of the ovary. Gynecologic Oncology 18: 115–118.

Heaton D C, Duff G B 1989 Ovarian relapse in a young woman with acute lymphoblastic leukemia. American Journal of Hematology 30: 42–43.

Heller E L, Palin W 1946 Ovarian involvement in Hodgkin's disease. Archives of Pathology 41: 282–289.

Hindkamp J F, Szanto P B 1959 Chloroma of the ovary. American Journal of Obstetrics and Gynecology 78: 812–816.

Hui P K, Feller A C, Lennert K 1988 High grade non-Hodgkin's lymphoma of B-cell type. I Histopathology. Histopathology 12: 127–143.

Hung L H Y, Kurtz D M 1985 Hodgkin's disease of the endometrium. Archives of Pathology and Laboratory Medicine 109: 952–953.

Hutchinson R E, Kuree A S, Davey F R 1990. Granulocytic sarcoma. Clinics in Laboratory Medicine 10: 889–901.

Iliya F A, Muggia F M, O'Leary J A, King T M 1968 Gynecologic manifestations of reticulum cell sarcoma. Obstetrics and Gynecology 31: 266–269.

Isaacson P G 1992 The non-Hodgkin's lymphomas. In: McGee J O D, Isaacson P G, Wright N A (eds) Oxford Textbook of pathology. Oxford University Press, Oxford, pp 1775–1787.

Isaacson P G, Norton A J (eds) 1994 Malignant lymphoma of the urogenital tract. In: Extranodal lymphomas. Churchill Livingstone, Edinburgh, pp 273–280.

Isaacson P, Spencer J 1987 Malignant lymphoma of mucosa associated lymphoid tissue. Histopathology 11: 445–462.

Isaacson P, Wright D H 1983 Malignant lymphoma of mucosa associated lymphoid tissue: a distinctive type of B-cell lymphoma. Cancer 52: 1410–1416.

Isaacson P, Wright D H 1984 Extranodal malignant lymphoma arising from mucosa associated lymphoid tissue. Cancer 53: 2512–2542.

Issa P Y, Salem P A, Brihi E, Azoury R S 1980 Eosinophilic granuloma with involvement of the female genitalia. American Journal of Obstetrics and Gynecology 137: 608–612.

Jack A S, Lee F D 1986 Morphological and immunohistochemical characteristics of T-cell malignant lymphomas in the West of Scotland. Histopathology 10: 223–234.

Johnston C, Senckjiam E, Ratain M, Talerman A 1989 Conservative management of primary cervical lymphoma using combination chemotherapy: a case report. Gynecologic Oncology 35: 391–394.

Kapadia S B, Krause J R, Kambour A J, Hartsock J R 1978 Granulocytic sarcoma of the uterus. Cancer 41: 687–691.

Katayama I, Hajian G, Evjy J T 1973 Cytological diagnosis of reticulum cell sarcoma of the uterine cervix. Acta Cytologica 17: 498–501.

Khan M A T, Dahill S W, Stewart K S 1986 Primary Hodgkin's disease of the ovary: case report. British Journal of Obstetrics and Gynaecology 93: 1300–1301.

Koo C H, Reifel J, Kogut N, Cove J K, Rappaport H 1992 True histiocytic malignancy associated with a malignant teratoma in a patient with 46XY gonadal dysgenesis. American Journal of Surgical Pathology 16: 175–183.

Krumerman M S, Chung A 1978 Solitary reticulum cell sarcoma of the uterine cervix with initial cytodiagnosis. Acta Cytologica 22: 46–50.

Lathrop J C 1967 Views and reviews: malignant pelvic lymphomas. Obstetrics and Gynecology 30: 137–145.

Lechner W, Ortner A, Thoni A et al 1983 Histiocytosis X in gynecology. Gynecologic Oncology 15: 253.

Leder L D 1964 Über die selektive fermentcytochemische Darstellung von neutrophilen myeloischen Zellen und Gewebmastzellen im paraffin-schmitt. Klinische Wochenschrift 42: 553.

Lennert K, Feller A (eds) 1990 Histopathology of non-Hodgkin's lymphomas, 2nd edn. Springer Verlag, New York, ch 3, pp 53–162.

Levine P H, Kamaraju L S, Connelly R P et al 1982 The American Burkitt's Lymphoma Registry: eight years experience. Cancer 49: 1016–1022.

Linden M D, Tubbs R R, Fishleder A F, Hart W R 1988 Immunotypic and genotypic characterisation of non-Hodgkin's lymphomas of the ovary. American Journal of Clinical Pathology 89: 156–162.

Linder J, Ye Y, Harrington D S, Armitage J O, Weisenberger D D 1987 Monoclonal antibodies marking T-lymphocytes in paraffin-embedded tissue. American Journal of Pathology 127: 1–8.

Long H P, Patchefsky A S 1971 Primary Hodgkin's disease of the ovary: a case report. Obstetrics and Gynecology 38: 680–681.

Lucia S P, Mills H, Lowenhaup E, Hunt M L 1952 Visceral involvement in primary neoplastic diseases of the reticuloendothelial system. Cancer 5: 1193–1200.

McCarthy K P, Sloane J P, Kabarowski J H S, Matutes E, Weidemann L M 1991 The rapid detection of clonal T-cell proliferations in patients with lymphoid disorders. American Journal of Pathology 138: 821–829.

McDermott M R, Clark D A, Bienenstock J 1980 Evidence for a common mucosal immunologic system II. Influence of the estrous cycle on B immunoblast migration into genital and intestinal tissues. Journal of Immunology 124: 2536–2539.

Maeda T, Komegai H, Mori H 1988 Malignant lymphoma presenting as initial symptom in the uterus: case report. British Journal of Obstetrics and Gynaecology 95: 1195–1197.

Magrath I T 1991 African Burkitt's lymphoma: history, biology, clinical features and treatment. American Journal of Pediatric Hematological Oncology 13: 222–246.

Mann R B, Jaffe E S, Braylan R C, Nanka K, Frank M M, Ziegler J L, Berard C W 1976 Non-endemic Burkitt's lymphoma: a B-cell tumor related to germinal centers. New England Journal of Medicine 295: 685–691.

Meis J M, Butler J J, Osborne B M, Manning J T 1986 Granulocytic sarcoma in non-leukemic patients. Cancer 58: 2697–2709.

Mikhail M S, Runowicz C D, Kadish A S, Romney S L 1989 Colposcopic and cytologic detection of chronic lymphocytic leukemia. Gynecologic Oncology 34: 106–108.

Mills S E, Austin M B, Randall M E 1985 Lymphoepithelioma-like carcinoma of the uterine cervix. American Journal of Surgical Pathology 9: 883–889.

Mittal K R, Blechman A, Alba Greco M, Alfonso F, Demopoulos R 1992 Lymphoma of ovary with stromal luteinization, presenting as secondary amenorrhoea. Gynecologic Oncology 45: 69–75.

Monterroso V, Jaffe E S, Merino M J, Medeiros J 1993 Malignant lymphoma involving the ovary: a clinicopathological analysis of 39 cases. American Journal of Surgical Pathology 17: 154–170.

Morgan E R, Labotka R J, Gonzalez-Crussi F, Niaderhold M, Sherman J O 1981 Ovarian granulocytic sarcoma as the primary manifestation of acute infantile myelomonocytic leukemia. Cancer 48: 1819–1824.

Muller S, Sangster G, Crocker J, Nar P, Burnett D, Brown G, Leyland M J 1986 An immunohistochemical and clinicopathological study of granulocytic sarcoma ("chloroma"). Hematological Oncology 4: 101–102.

Muntz H G, Ferry J A, Flynn D, Fuller A F, Tarraza H M 1991 Stage 1E primary malignant lymphomas of the uterine cervix. Cancer 66: 2023–2032.

Murray J, Fox H 1991 Rosai Dorfman disease of the uterine cervix. International Journal of Gynecological Pathology 10: 209–213.

Neiman R S, Barcos M, Berard C, Mann R, Rydell R E, Bennett J M 1981 Granulocytic sarcoma: a clinicopathologic study of 61 biopsied cases. Cancer 48: 1426–1437.

Nelson G A, Docherty M B, Pratt J H, Remine W H 1958 Malignant lymphoma involving the ovaries. American Journal of Obstetrics and Gynecology 76: 861–871.

Neri A, Barriga F, Knowles D, Magrath I, Dalla-Favera R 1988 Different regions of the immunoglobulin heavy chain locus are involved in chromosomal translocations in distinct pathogenetic forms of Burkitt's lymphoma. Proceedings of the National Academy of Sciences USA 85: 2748–2752.

Non-Hodgkin's lymphoma pathologic classification project. National Cancer Institute sponsored study of classifications of non-Hodgkin's lymphomas: summary and description of a Working Formulation for clinical usage 1982. Cancer 49: 2112–2135.

Norris H J, Jensen R D 1972 Relative frequency of ovarian neoplasms in children and adolescents. Cancer 30: 713–719.

Norton A J, Isaacson P G 1989a Lymphoma phenotyping in formalin fixed and paraffin wax embedded tissues: I. Range of antibiotics and staining patterns. Histopathology 14: 437–446.

Norton A J, Isaacson P G 1989b Lymphoma phenotyping in formalin-fixed and paraffin-wax embedded tissues: II. Profiles of reactivity in the various tumour types. Histopathology 14: 557–579.

Obeid D, Cotter P, Sturdee D W 1979 Acute leukaemia relapse presenting as ovarian tumour. British Journal of Obstetrics and Gynaecology 86: 578–580.

O'Conor G T 1961 Malignant lymphoma in African children II. A pathological entity. Cancer 14: 270–283.

Osanto S, Valk P, Meijer C J L M et al 1981 Solitary plasmacytoma of the vagina. Acta Haematologica 66: 140.

Osborne B M, Robboy S J 1983 Lymphomas and leukemia presenting as ovarian tumours: an analysis of 42 cases. Cancer 52: 1933–1943.

Paladugu R R, Bearman R M, Rappaport H 1980 Malignant lymphoma with primary manifestation in the gonad: a clinicopathological study of 38 patients. Cancer 45: 561–571.

Pelicci P, Knowles D, Magrath I, Dalla-Favera R 1986 Chromosomal breakpoints and structural alterations of the C-myc locus differ in endemic and sporadic forms of Burkitt lymphomas. Proceedings of the National Academy of Sciences USA 83: 2984–2988.

Pelstring R J, Essell J H, Kurtin P J, Cohen A R, Banks P M 1991 Diversity of organ site involvement among malignant lymphomas of mucosa associated tissues. American Journal of Clinical Pathology 93: 738–745.

Perren T, Farrant M, McCarthy K, Harper P, Wiltshaw E 1992 Lymphomas of the cervix and upper vagina: a report of five cases and a review of the literature. Gynecologic Oncology 44: 87–95.

Picker L J, Weiss L M, Medeiros C J, Wood G S, Warnke R A 1987 Immunophenotypic criteria for the diagnosis of non-Hodgkin's lymphoma. American Journal of Pathology 128: 181–201.

Plouffe L, Tulandi T, Rosenberg A, Ferenczy A 1984 Non-Hodgkin's lymphoma in Bartholin's gland: case report and review of literature. American Journal of Obstetrics and Gynecology 148: 608–609.

Portnoy J, Ahronheim G A, Ghibu F et al 1984 Recovery of Epstein Barr virus from genital ulcers. New England Journal of Medicine 311: 966–968.

PreBler H, Horny H-P, Wolf A, Kaiserling E 1992 Isolated granulocytic sarcoma of the ovary: histologic, electron microscopic and immunohistochemical findings. International Journal of Gynecological Pathology 11: 68–74.

Prévot S, Hugol D, Andouin J, Diebold J, Truc J B, Decroix Y, Poitout P 1992 Primary non-Hodgkin's malignant lymphoma of the vagina: report of 3 cases with review of the literature. Pathology Research and Practice 188: 78–85.

Rappaport H 1966 Tumors of the hematopoietic system. Atlas of tumor pathology, section III, fascicle 8. Armed Forces Institute of Pathology, Washington DC, pp 97–161.

Rotmensch J, Woodruff J D 1982 Lymphoma of the ovary: report of twenty nine cases and update of previous series. American Journal of Obstetrics and Gynecology 143: 870–875.

Sandvei R, Lote K, Svendsen E, Thunold S 1990 Case report: successful pregnancy following treatment of primary malignant lymphoma of the uterine cervix. Gynecological Oncology 38: 128–131.

Schiller H M, Madge G E 1970 Reticulum cell sarcoma presenting as a vulvar lesion. Southern Medical Journal 63: 471–472.

Scott L, Blair G, Taylor G, Dimmick J, Fraser G 1988 Inflammatory pseudotumors in children. Journal of Pediatric Surgery 23: 755–758.

Seifer D B, Weiss L M, Kempson R L 1986 Malignant lymphoma arising within thyroid tissue in a mature cystic teratoma. Cancer 58: 2459–2461.

Sirgi K E, Swanson P E, Gershell D J 1994 Extramedullary

hematopoiesis in the endometrium. American Journal of Clinical Pathology 101: 643–646.

Staging announcement: FIGO Cancer Committee 1986 Gynecologic Oncology 25: 383–385.

Stansfeld A G, D'Ardenne A J (eds) 1992 Lymph node biopsy interpretation. Churchill Livingstone, Edinburgh.

Stansfeld A, Diebold J, Kapanci Y et al 1988 Updated Kiel classification for lymphomas. Lancet i: 292–293 (corrected table as p 603).

Stein H, Mason D, Gerdes J et al 1985 The expression of the Hodgkin's disease associated antigen Ki-I in reactive and neoplastic lymphoid tissue: evidence that Reed-Steinberg cells and histiocytic malignancies are derived from activated lymphoid cells. Blood 66: 848–858.

Steiner-Salz D, Yahalom J, Samnelov A, Pollack A 1985 Non-Hodgkin's lymphoma associated with pregnancy. Cancer 56: 2087–2091.

Taussig 1937 Sarcoma of the vulva. American Journal of Obstetrics and Gynecology 33: 1017–1026.

Tuder R M 1992 Vulvar destruction by malignant lymphoma. Gynecologic Oncology 45: 52–57.

Ueda G, Shimizu C, Shimizu H et al 1988 An immunohistochemical study of small cell and poorly differentiated carcinomas of the cervix using neuroendocrine markers. Gynecologic Oncology 54: 164–169.

Ulfelder H 1981 Classification systems. International Journal of Radiation, Oncology, Biology, Physics 7: 1083–1086.

Walther G 1934 Über die lymphosarkomatose der weiblichen Genital organe. Archiv dur Gynäkologie 157: 44–64.

Whitaker D 1976 The role of cytology in the detection of malignant lymphoma of the uterine cervix. Acta Cytologica 20: 510–513.

Winkler B, Reumann W, Mitao M et al 1984 Chlamydial endometritis: histological and immunohistochemical analysis. American Journal of Surgical Pathology 8: 771–778.

Wishart J 1973 Reticulosarcoma of the vulva complicating azathioprine-treated dermatomyositis. Archives of Dermatology 108: 563–564.

Woodruff J D, Noli Castillo R D, Novak E R 1963 Lymphoma of the ovary — a study of 35 cases from the Ovarian Tumor Registry of the American Gynecological Society. American Journal of Obstetrics and Gynecology 85: 912–918.

Wright D H 1964 Burkitt' s tumour: a post-mortem study of 50 cases. British Journal of Surgery 51: 245–251.

Wright D H 1966 Burkitt's tumour in England: a comparison with childhood lymphosarcoma. International Journal of Cancer 1: 503–514.

Wright D H 1970 Microscopic features, histochemistry, histogenesis and diagnosis in Burkitt's lymphoma. In: Burkitt D P, Wright D H (eds) Burkitt's lymphoma. Livingstone, Edinburgh, pp 92–103.

Wright D H 1985 Histogenesis of Burkitt's lymphoma: a B-cell tumour of mucosa-associated lymphoid tissue. In: Lenoir G, O'Conor G, Olweny C L M (eds) Burkitt's lymphoma: a human cancer model. ARC Scientific Publications, Lyons, no. 60, pp 37–45.

Wyld P J, Lilleyman J S 1983 Ovarian disease in childhood lymphoblastic leukaemia. Acta Haematologica 69: 278–280.

Young R H, Harris N L, Scully R E 1985 Lymphoma-like lesions of the lower female genital tract: a report of 16 cases. International Journal of Gynecological Pathology 4: 289–299.

Ziegler J L 1981 Burkitt's lymphoma. New England Journal of Medicine 305: 735–745.

Ziegler J L, Magrath I T 1974 Burkitt's lymphoma. Pathobiology Annual 4: 129–142.

32. Endometriosis

Bernard Czernobilsky

INTRODUCTION

Endometriosis can be defined as the presence of ectopic foci of endometrial-type glands and stroma which tend to respond to ovarian hormones in a manner similar to that of the mucosa which lines the uterine body. This response, however, is often variable and incomplete (Metzger et al, 1988). Foci of endometrial mucosa within the myometrium, which are sometimes designated as 'internal endometriosis', do not constitute endometriosis and represent adenomyosis, which is a different entity. On the other hand, endometrial tissue situated on the uterine serosa is truly ectopic and therefore represents endometriosis. According to Ranney (1980a), the various sites of endometriosis in order of frequency are as follows: ovary, cul-de-sac, uterosacral ligaments, the anterior wall of the rectosigmoid bowel, bladder peritoneum, round ligaments, appendix, small bowel, umbilicus, abdominal scars and, rarely, pleura, lungs and extremities.

AETIOLOGY

The occurrence of endometriosis during the reproductive years and its not uncommon association with uterine leiomyomata, ovarian follicular cysts and endometrial polyps suggests that a disturbance of ovarian hormonal function may play a rôle in its aetiology (Fox, 1983). Scott & Wharton (1957) have shown that oestrogen was indeed necessary for the maintenance of endometriotic implants. On the other hand, the experimental studies of Dizerega et al (1980) indicate that ovarian steroids are not necessary for the growth of endometrial implants, a point also supported by clinical observations of endometriosis in postmenopausal women in whom there is no evidence of oestrogenic activity.

Another possible aetiological factor is a deficiency in cellular immunity in women with endometriosis (Dmowski et al, 1981). According to Dmowski et al (1990), it is possible that changes in humoral immunity are secondary to deficient cellular mechanisms in endo-metriosis. Thus endometriosis may develop if the peritoneal 'disposal system' is overwhelmed or defective and permits implantation of endometrial fragments. Investigations in this field are still in progress but recent studies have focused on the possibility that decreased natural killer (NK) cell activity may be a key factor in the development of endometriosis (Oosterlynck et al, 1991, 1992; Hill, 1992; Garzetti et al, 1993). Experiments in rhesus monkeys showed that those with endometriosis had a defective cellular response to autologous uterine endometrium injected into their skin as compared to monkeys without endometriosis.

There have been reports of familial endometriosis (Ridley, 1968) and a genetic predisposition has also been proposed (Malinak et al, 1980; Simpson et al, 1980). The risk of endometriosis appears to follow a maternal inheritance pattern of polygenetic or multifactorial type (Haney, 1991).

PATHOGENESIS

There are numerous hypotheses concerning the pathogenesis of endometriosis. These have been reviewed by, among others, Javert (1949), Gardner et al (1953), Ridley (1968), Lauchlan (1972), Ranney (1980a,b), Haney (1990, 1991) and Thomas (1993). Endometriosis was first believed to originate in either Wolffian (von Recklinghausen, 1885) or Müllerian rests (Cullen, 1925). This latter phenomenon is referred to as 'müllerianosis' and implies an embryonic origin of certain forms of endometriosis, a view which has won some recent support (Batt & Smith, 1989; Batt et al, 1990). In 1921 Sampson advanced the theory that abnormally sited endometrium in the pelvis is due to regurgitation of endometrial fragments through the Fallopian tube as a result of retrograde menstruation. The evidence in favour of this hypothesis included:

a. demonstration of tubal menstrual regurgitation when the normal exit through the cervix was blocked
b. a distribution of pelvic endometriosis which

corresponds to that which one might expect from tubal regurgitation

c. a patent tubal lumen in patients with endometriosis, and

d. animal experiments in which endometrium grew when implanted in the peritoneal cavity.

Halban (1925) and, later, Javert (1951) suggested a lymphatic pathway for the dissemination of endometriotic tissue, a view based on the finding of endometriotic tissue in lymphatic channels and in lymph nodes; Ueki (1991) has argued cogently in support of this concept. Haematogenous spread has also been suggested, especially for the rare extra-abdominal endometriosis, such as that occurring in the brain (Thibodeau et al, 1987), skin (Tidman & MacDonald, 1988; Naseman, 1990), extremities (Gupta, 1985; Giangara et al, 1987), pleura or lungs (Charles, 1957; Di Palo et al, 1989; Espaulella et al, 1991; Svendstrup & Husby, 1991) in which the haematogenous pathway appears to be the only plausible explanation. The not infrequent occurrence of endometriosis in laparotomy scars following a variety of gynaecological procedures involving the uterine lumen points to yet another possible pathogenetic mechanism, namely, that of direct transplantation of endometrial tissue (Steck & Helwig, 1965). The presence of endometrium within the scar tissue and in the actual tract made at the operation supports such a mechanism in these cases. There is also the coelomic metaplastic theory, first proposed by Robert Meyer, which now appears to be the most plausible, at least for endometriosis situated in the ovary and other pelvic organs (Novak & de Lima, 1948; Hertig & Gore, 1961; Fujii, 1991; Suginami, 1991; Nakamura et al, 1993). Finally it should be mentioned that Levander & Norman (1955) have attempted to reconcile the reflux and metaplastic theories by suggesting that the menstrual endometrium which is being regurgitated through the Fallopian tube does not itself implant and grow, but rather induces endometrial metaplasia of the serosa. This induction theory is supported by the experimental study of Merrill (1966) who introduced endometrial tissue within millipore filters into the peritoneal cavity and was able to induce endometrial metaplasia within the peritoneum by this technique.

From the above, it appears that there is probably no one single pathogenetic mechanism causing endometriosis and that some of the different theories mentioned may apply to different circumstances and locations of this disease. However, since this chapter will centre on pelvic endometriosis, which without doubt is the most common and clinically significant form of the disease, the coelomic metaplastic theory will be emphasized and elaborated upon.

The striking metaplastic potential of the pelvic mesothelium in the female is a well-known fact. This mesothe-

lium, which also covers the ovary where it is designated as 'surface epithelium', is of coelomic origin. In the embryo it gives rise to the Müllerian duct and consequently to the epithelium and stroma of the various organs derived from it such as the uterus, Fallopian tubes and, possibly, part of the vagina. It is this epithelium which is now considered to constitute the source of the common epithelial tumours of the ovary including both benign endometriosis and endometrioid carcinoma (Czernobilsky, 1982). The appearance of endometrial-type cells in ovarian surface epithelium as well as the presence of such cells in ovarian inclusion cysts is commonplace and supports the coelomic metaplastic theory of endometriosis (Fig. 32.1). It should be emphasized, however, that this theory does not only apply to ovarian endometriosis but to endometriosis of other abdominal organs and structures as well. In spite of the attractiveness of the coelomic theory, the validity of this concept has been questioned. The arguments against the metaplasia hypothesis have been summarized by Haney (1990). These include the extreme rarity of endometriosis in males and in peritoneal surfaces other than that of the pelvic cavity, its predominance in reproductive-

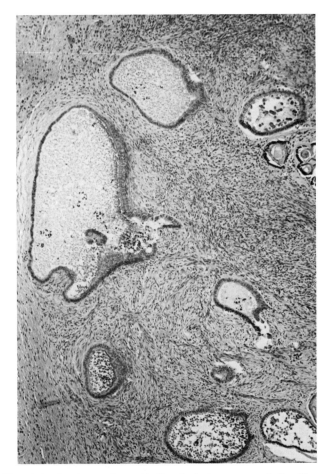

Fig. 32.1 Ovarian surface epithelium inclusion cysts partly lined by endometrial-type cells. H & E × 60.

aged women and the apparent necessity of the presence of the uterus in cases of endometriosis.

Whatever the pathogenetic mechanism or site of endometriosis might be, the ectopic areas of endometrial tissue, which contain oestrogen and progesterone receptors (Bergquist, 1991; Bergquist et al, 1993), tend to proliferate when stimulated by cyclic oestrogen while subsequent progesterone will produce a secretory response. As in normal endometrium, withdrawal of these hormones causes bleeding which, in cases of cystic endometriosis, may result in intraluminal haemorrhage (Scott & Wharton, 1957). After months of repeated haemorrhage an inflammatory reaction followed by a scar develops in the surrounding tissue which, according to Sturgis & Call (1954), may interfere with subsequent blood supply and thus gradually decrease the response of the endometriosis to hormonal stimulation.

EPIDEMIOLOGY

Incidence data on endometriosis is limited and variable. Houston et al (1987) reported an incidence ratio of 2.5 cases per 1000 woman-years based on clinically possible disease in Minnesota. When the cases were restricted to histologically confirmed or surgically visualized cases, the incidence was 1.6. Since prevalence is equal to incidence multiplied by the average duration of the disease, which is 40 years, the prevalence of endometriosis in the general United States population, based on an incidence of 2.5, would be 10% (Goldman & Cramer, 1990). Rawson (1991) has suggested that the true prevalence, even in asymptomatic fertile women, may be very much higher.

According to Houston et al (1987), the peak incidence is in women aged 35–44. In the United States the disease appears to be most common among middle-class white patients (Novak & Woodruff, 1979b). The risk of endometriosis among orientals appears to be as high or even higher than that in whites (Miyazawa, 1976). It is of interest to note that endometriosis appears to be less frequent in Jewish women in Israel as compared to other non-Jewish western populations (Brzezinki & Koren, 1962; Lancet, Rotenstreich and Czernobilsky, unpublished data), a phenomenon which remains unexplained.

Familial endometriosis has also been reported (Ridley, 1968), and in these cases the disease appears to be more severe (Malinak et al, 1980). It can be estimated that a family history of endometriosis with an affected primary relative increases the risk for the disease to about ten times that of women lacking a familial history. Another risk factor may be that of genital abnormalities, especially those related to Müllerian fusion (Shifrin et al, 1973): it is probable, however, that this only applies to those malformations in which there is obstruction to menstrual outflow (Fedele et al, 1992).

CLASSIFICATION

Endometriosis can be classified according to its location (Novak & Woodruff, 1979a), its macroscopic appearance, i.e. cystic or non-cystic, or according to its severity. The latter is a modification by Cohen (1980) from Acosta et al's (1973) classification which divided endometriosis into mild, moderate and severe. Whereas in 'mild' endometriosis the lesions are small and superficial, 'moderate' is characterized in addition by scarring, retraction and adhesions, while the hallmarks of 'severe' endometriosis are tumour-like lesions and distant organ involvement. A revised American Fertility Society classification was reported in 1985. Attention in this classification was paid to the three-dimensional volume and the depths of invasion. Different scores were assigned to ovarian and peritoneal lesions.

Another controversial classification is that of the World Health Organization (WHO) (Serov et al, 1973) which divided ovarian endometriosis into 'tumours' and 'tumour-like conditions'. Benign endometrioid 'tumours' in this classification include adenomas, cystadenoma, adenofibroma and cystadenofibroma. Scully et al (1966) also mention an endometrial polyp, a papillary mucinous adenoma originating in an endometrial cyst and an endometrioid adenofibroma as examples of benign endometrioid tumours of the ovary. The 'tumour-like' endometriosis listed in the WHO Classification (Serov et al, 1973) was not further defined. It is difficult, if not impossible, in some cases to draw a sharp line between these two categories. In addition, the occurrence of polypoid, hyperplastic and atypical changes in endometriosis (Scully et al, 1966; Cantor et al, 1979; Czernobilsky & Morris, 1979), the common association of all forms and not just the 'tumour' variety of endometriosis with various ovarian epithelial neoplasms and the not uncommon actual transformation of various types of endometriosis to carcinoma (Brooks & Wheeler, 1977; Mostoufizadeh & Scully, 1980), may favour the classification of all forms of intraabdominal endometriosis under one heading, preferably that of 'endometrioid neoplasia'. On the other hand, endometriosis within a surgical scar or tract, following intrauterine procedures, is of course most likely due to direct implantation.

GROSS AND MICROSCOPIC APPEARANCES

Endometriosis may appear as tiny foci or as large cystic masses. Because of the frequent bleeding which occurs in endometriosis, as a result of its response to the rise and fall of ovarian hormones, these foci are often dome shaped, of dark bluish colouration with tan to brownish staining of adjacent tissues. In early stages of the disease, however, the endometriotic lesions may be non-pigmented as has been pointed out by Jansen & Russell

(1986). Rupture of endometriosis and repeated haemorrhages are responsible for the fibrous adhesions and adjacent scarring which are more frequent in older lesions. Endometriotic cysts are usually well encapsulated and, as has been pointed out above, with increasing age of the lesion show a thick, fibrotic capsule with numerous adhesions (Novak, 1931). They can reach dimensions of up to 20 cm in diameter. The lumen of these cysts contains dark brown fluid ranging from watery to syrupy, hence the term 'chocolate cysts'. The cyst wall is usually shaggy with dark brown deposits (Figs 32.2 and 32.3). In addition to ample sampling for histological examination from the cyst wall, any thickened or protruding intraluminal areas should be sectioned for microscopic examination. Occasionally ovarian or extraovarian pelvic endometriosis

presents as polypoid masses of soft grey tissue which may simulate a malignant tumour and have been designated 'polypoid endometriosis' (Scully et al, 1966).

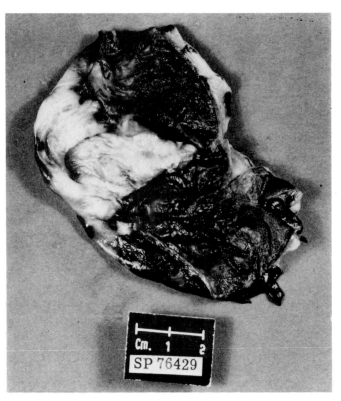

Fig. 32.3   Opened ovarian endometriotic cyst with haemorrhagic lining and thick fibrous wall. (Courtesy of Dr. L. M. Roth, Indianapolis, Indiana, USA.)

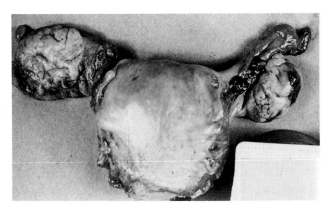

Fig. 32.2   Uterus with both adnexae showing scattered haemorrhagic foci representing endometriosis, especially on right Fallopian tube and adjacent ovary. (Courtesy of Dr. H. T. Enterline, Philadelphia, USA.)

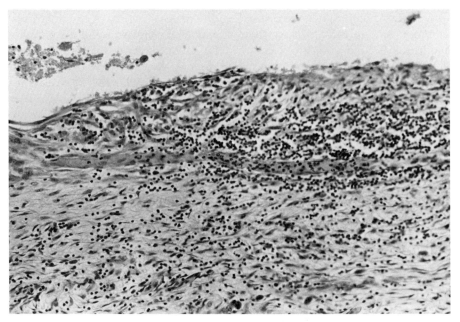

Fig. 32.4   Ovarian cyst, probably endometriosis, lined by granulation tissue. H & E × 150.

It should be emphasized that haemorrhage occurs in a variety of ovarian cysts and neoplasms, and not exclusively in endometriosis. Thus, although haemorrhagic ovarian cysts are certainly suggestive of endometriosis, the exact diagnosis of such cysts can only be established by histological examination.

The histological diagnosis of endometriosis may prove difficult because of the secondary changes occurring in the lesions due to bleeding and fibrosis. These latter may transform the areas of endometriosis, including the lining of large cysts, into granulation tissue, with numerous histiocytes, or so-called 'pseudoxanthoma' cells, and fibrosis. In such circumstances, the pathologist can only reach the diagnosis of 'consistent with endometriosis' (Figs 32.4 and 32.5).

The pseudoxanthoma cells contain degradation products of blood, especially ceroid (lipofuscin, haemofuchsin), and thus stain positively with periodic acid–Schiff, Ziehl–Neelsen and oil Red-0 stains (Clement et al, 1988). These cells also exhibit autofluorescence, which is one of the properties of ceroid (Fig. 32.6). Haemosiderin is much less conspicuous than ceroid in these cells, a fact which does not seem to be generally known (Clement, 1990). Rarely granulomatous nodules, characterized by a central zone of necrosis surrounded by pseudoxanthoma cells, often in a palisaded arrangement, referred to as 'necrotic pseudoxanthomatous nodules', have been observed in endometriosis (Clement et al, 1988) (Fig. 32.7).

A definite histological diagnosis of endometriosis can be established only when both endometrial-type glands and

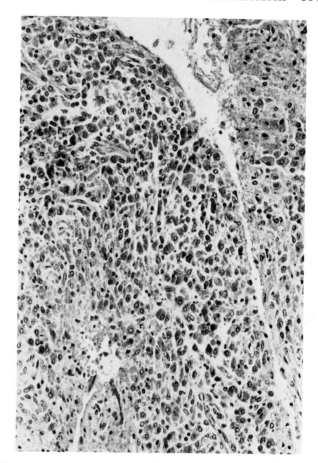

Fig. 32.5 Cyst lining, probably endometriosis, with numerous haemosiderin-laden macrophages. H & E × 240.

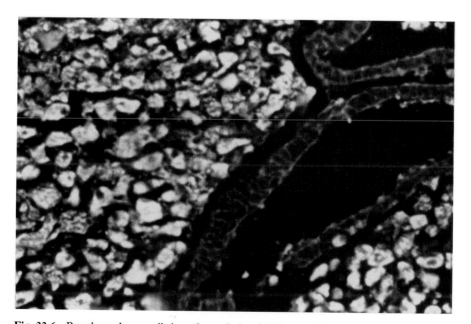

Fig. 32.6 Pseudoxanthoma cells in endometriosis exhibiting autofluorescence (unstained section photographed with fluorescent light). × 200. (Reprinted with permission from Clement, 1990.)

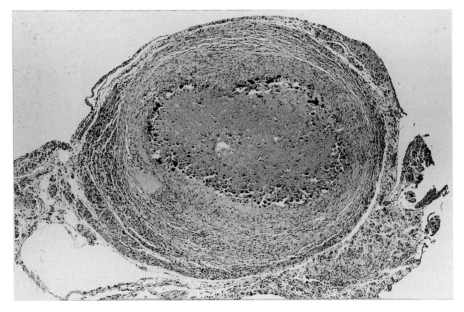

a

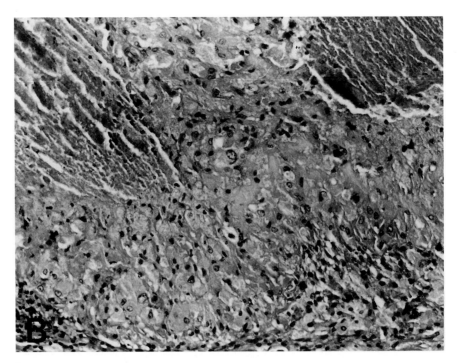

b

Fig. 32.7 Necrotic pseudoxanthomatous nodule of endometriosis. **a** Granulomatous peritoneal nodule with central necrosis and calcified material. H & E × 12. **b** The necrotic centre is surrounded by pseudoxanthoma cells. H & E × 200. (Reprinted with permission from Clement et al, 1988.)

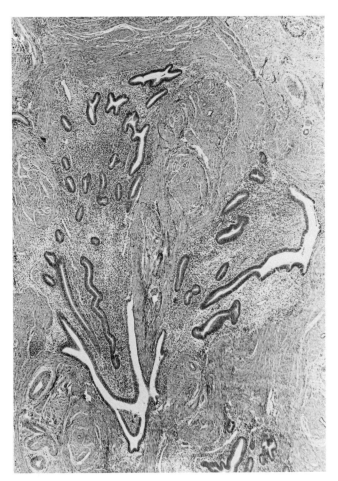

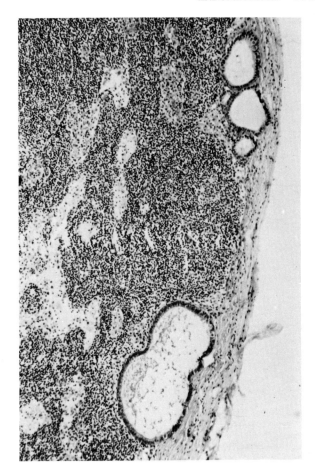

Fig. 32.8 Endometriosis in wall of Fallopian tube showing well-formed endometrial glands with surrounding endometrial stroma. H & E × 24.

Fig. 32.9 Abdominal lymph node with glandular endometrial-like inclusions in cortical portion. Note absence of surrounding endometrial stroma and of haemorrhage. H & E × 50.

stroma are evident in ectopic sites (Fig. 32.8). However, because of the great metaplastic potential of mesothelial cells capable of forming inclusions and cysts partially or completely lined by endometrial-type epithelium but lacking endometrial stroma, the latter is more characteristic of endometriosis than the mere presence of endometrial-type glands. It has also been stated that bleeding in endometriosis originates from stromal blood vessels (Hertig & Gore, 1961). Thus ovarian surface epithelial inclusion cysts lined by endometrial-type epithelium or endometrial-type glandular inclusions in pelvic lymph nodes, which also originate in mesothelial cells (Karp & Czernobilsky, 1969), do not constitute endometriosis since they are lacking endometrial-type stroma (Fig. 32.9). This is more than of semantic importance because these inclusions without stroma do not respond to ovarian hormones, do not bleed and thus are usually asymptomatic. True endometriosis within pelvic lymph nodes exists but is a rare phenomenon.

An interesting observation is the presence of mesothelial inclusions in ovaries which are the site of endometrio-

sis (Kerner et al, 1981) (Figs 32.10 and 32.11). Since the endometriosis in these cases is always located at a distance from the mesothelial inclusions, it is unlikely that the endometriotic foci act as a non-specific stimulus to the surface epithelium. It appears more likely that a common, possibly hormonal, stimulus is responsible for the development of both the endometriosis and the mesothelial inclusions in these cases.

The distinction between non-specific fibrous, ovarian and endometrial-type stroma can be difficult. The problem becomes even more complex because of the presence of haemorrhage, inflammatory cells, macrophages and fibrosis in the stroma of endometriosis. In the absence of progestational effect the stroma of endometriosis is characterized by its dense cellularity and is composed of cells with large hyperchromatic round or elongated nuclei with blunted edges and little cytoplasm. These stromal cells closely surround, and adhere to, the endometrial epithelium. By contrast, non-specific fibrous stroma or ovarian stroma in which glandular inclusions are present does not show such an intimate relationship to the epithelial com-

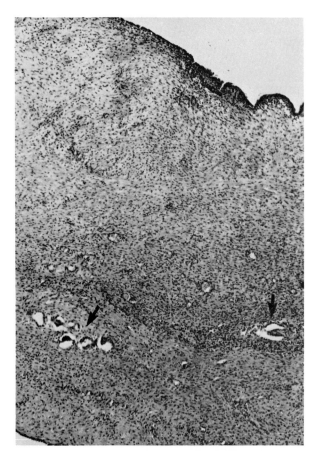

Fig. 32.10 Ovary with endometriotic cyst lining (above) and mesothelial inclusions in opposite area (arrow). H & E × 36.

ponents. In some instances the stroma of endometriosis shows a decidual change due to pregnancy. Predecidual changes have also been observed in endometriosis secondary to intrinsic or extrinsic hormonal effects (Fig. 32.12). Although, as mentioned above, the endometrial stroma constitutes the most specific element in endometriosis, it is not advisable to reach a diagnosis of endometriosis in the presence of nodules composed solely of endometrial-type stroma which lack haemorrhage and/or haemosiderin-laden macrophages (Fig. 32.13). Rather than endometriosis such foci may represent a low-grade stromal sarcoma (Kempson, 1973) which by its very nature may be present in various sites outside the uterus. Even nodules made up of decidual tissue without glandular elements cannot be safely diagnosed as endometriosis since pelvic ectopic decidual reactions also occur, probably as a result of stimulation by progesterone and, possibly, adrenal or pituitary hormones (Bassis, 1956). Thus, whilst in ectopic sites the endometrial stromal component in the presence of endometrial glands is diagnostic of endometriosis, the latter diagnosis cannot be reached when the stromal component alone is present, especially in the absence of evidence of repeated bleeding. In the presence of the latter, however, a presumptive diagnosis of endometriosis can be made.

The epithelial component of endometriosis may be part of a cyst lining, or represent glandular structures, or both (Figs 32.6 and 32.14). In a study of 194 cases of ovarian endometriosis the epithelium presented as a cyst lining in

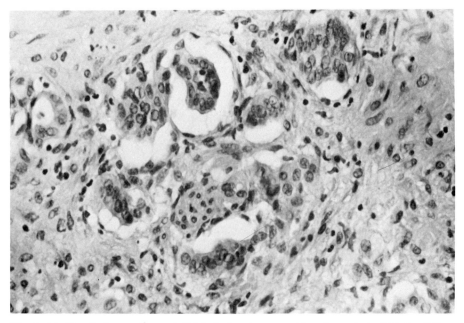

Fig. 32.11 Detail of unusual mesothelial inclusions in ovary with endometriosis. H & E × 125.

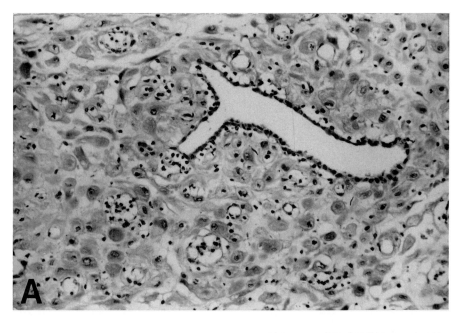

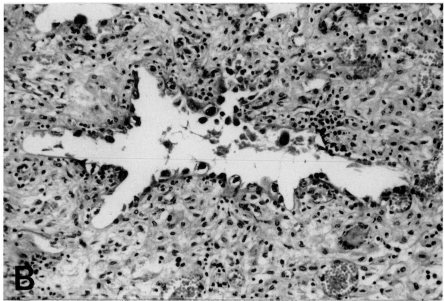

Fig. 32.12 Pregnancy-induced changes in endometriosis. **a** Decidua surrounding atrophic gland. H & E × 150. **b** Arias-Stella reaction in endometriotic gland. H & E × 180. (Reprinted with permission from Clement, 1990.)

89, as glandular structures in 28, while in 77 cases both features were evident; papillary formations lined by endometrial-type epithelium were also observed (Czernobilsky & Morris, 1979) (Fig. 32.15). Histological examination of the epithelial elements showed a variety of features such as typical endometrial glands which, although occasionally secretory, were most often of the inactive or proliferative type, as well as simple or complex hyperplasia (Fig. 32.16), hobnail cells and oviduct-type epithelium (Fig. 32.17) (Czernobilsky & Morris, 1979). Endosalpingi-

osis' which has been defined as ectopic tubal epithelium and which, according to Tutschka & Lauchlan (1980), is 'homologous' with endometriosis, is a confusing term and should not be used as synonymous with endometriosis. The appearance of tubal-type epithelium in female genital tract mesothelium, cysts and epithelial neoplasms is quite common and merely reflects the Müllerian metaplastic potential of the coelomic epithelium.

Czernobilsky & Morris (1979) described severe epithelial atypia in ovarian endometriosis in 3.6% of their cases.

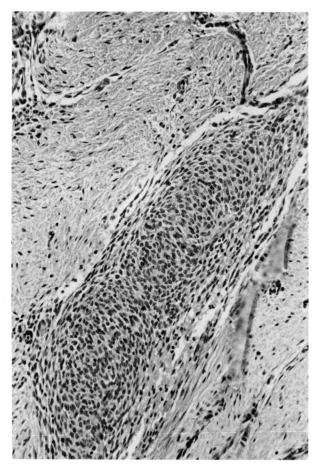

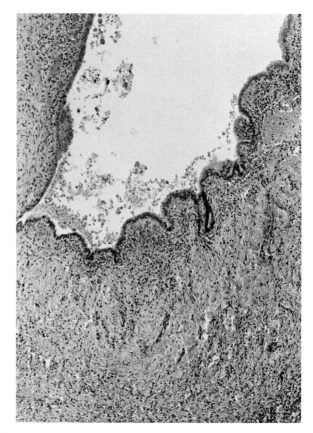

Fig. 32.14 Endometriotic cyst lined by endometrial epithelium with adjacent stromal cells. H & E × 60.

Fig. 32.13 Endometrial-type stroma in abdominal wall without haemorrhage or haemosiderin-laden cells. H & E × 60.

This was characterized by pleomorphic, often hyperchromatic nuclei, eosinophilic cytoplasm, squamoid features, tufting and stratification which were present in the lining of endometriotic cysts (Figs 32.18 and 32.19). Although some of these changes may be of reactive origin, one should also consider the possibility that, in some instances, these atypical changes may constitute a neoplastic potential. This latter hypothesis is borne out by the fact that not infrequently the epithelium of endometriotic cysts adjacent to endometrioid carcinomas shows similar changes.

Other histological features of endometriosis include the presence of smooth muscle fibres (Rolfing et al, 1981), calcifications, ossification or myxoid changes (Gerbie et al, 1958). The uterus-like masses in various pelvic sites (Clement, 1990) may constitute a special morphological form of endometriosis, although a congenital basis has also been suggested for these structures (Pueblitz-Peredo et al, 1985). A rare finding is that of acellular, ring-like structures or Liesegang rings encountered in debris or cyst wall of endometriosis. These probably represent zones of periodic precipitation of supersaturated colloid solutions and can be confused with organisms or foreign material (Clement et al, 1989) (Fig. 32.20).

In conclusion, the definite histological diagnosis of endometriosis is a difficult one. It depends on the presence of both endometrial glands and stroma, often showing evidence of repeated haemorrhage. In addition, in some instances morphological features can be traced to oestrogenic (Kapadia et al, 1984) or progestational influences (Andrews et al, 1959) as well as to pregnancy (Moller, 1959). These hormonal responses however are often incomplete and variable, a fact which is also supported by ultrastructural (Schweppe et al, 1984), histochemical (Prakash et al, 1965) and steroid receptor studies (Lyndrup et al, 1987). Ectopic endometrial-type glands without stroma, or endometrial-type stroma without glands, do not enable the pathologist to reach a diagnosis of endometriosis since these structures can be representative of other pathological entities. If, however, ectopic endometrial glands devoid of endometrial-type stroma or endometrial type stroma devoid of glands show in their respective immediate vicinity evidence of repeated haemorrhage, such as free haemosiderin pigment and pigment-laden macrophages with or without fibrosis, a

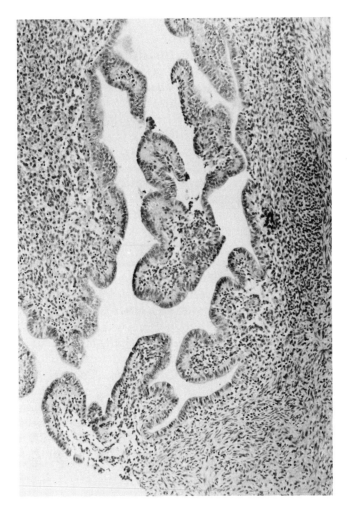

Fig. 32.15 Endometriosis showing papillary formation. H & E × 120.

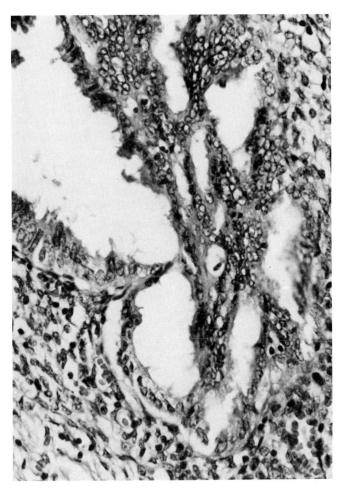

Fig. 32.16 Endometriosis showing evidence of atypical adenomatous hyperplasia. H & E × 304. (Reprinted with permission from Czernobilsky & Morris, 1979, and from the American College of Obstetricians and Gynecologists.)

presumptive diagnosis of endometriosis can be made. Such a presumptive diagnosis can also be made, although with less assurance, in cases of ovarian or pelvic haemorrhagic cysts in which, because of the haemorrhagic episodes, both epithelial and stromal elements have been destroyed.

RELATIONSHIP TO NEOPLASIA

The relationship of endometriosis to ovarian malignancy was first documented by Sampson in 1925, and was reappraised by Czernobilsky (1982). In order to prove that a tumour indeed originated in endometriosis Sampson (1925) required a demonstration of the direct origin of the carcinoma from the endometriotic tissue (Fig. 32.21). These rigid criteria have by now been abandoned and it was Sampson himself who, in his article in 1925, speculated that ovarian endometrial-type carcinomas might arise *de novo* from the surface epithelium of the ovary.

The classic example of a malignant tumour arising from endometriosis is the ovarian endometrioid carcinoma which histologically mimics adenocarcinoma or adenoacanthoma of the endometrium (Figs 32.22 and 32.23). However, since, as mentioned above, endometrioid carcinomas can arise *de novo* from the ovarian surface epithelium and since even in these cases where the tumour originates from pre-existing endometriosis, it may overgrow the benign process, an actual transition between endometriosis and endometrioid carcinoma can only be demonstrated in relatively few cases. In the series of Czernobilsky et al (1970a,b), this was demonstrated in 4% of the patients. According to Scully (1977) such a continuity between benign endometriosis and endometrioid carcinoma can be shown in 5–10% of cases. Two of four proliferating endometrioid adeno- and cystadenofibromatous tumours reported by Roth et al (1981) arose in ovarian endometriosis. As has been mentioned before, the adjacent endometriosis may show atypical changes

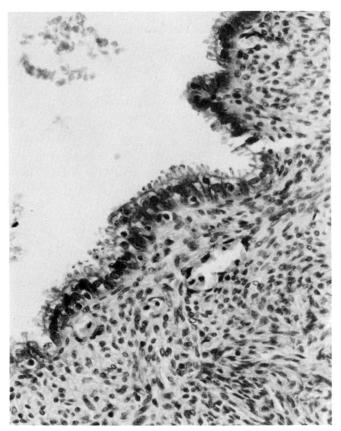

Fig. 32.17 Ovarian endometriosis lined by ciliated oviduct-like epithelium. H & E × 175. (Reprinted with permission from Czernobilsky & Morris, 1979, and from the American College of Obstetricians and Gynecologists.)

(Czernobilsky & Morris, 1979; LaGrenade & Silverberg, 1988). Endometriosis in the ipsi- or contralateral ovary not showing continuity with endometrioid carcinoma has been reported in 9–17% of cases (Czernobilsky et al, 1970a; Aure et al, 1971), whereas pelvic extraovarian endometriosis was present in 11–28% of patients with endometrioid carcinoma (Czernobilsky et al, 1970a; Kurman & Craig, 1972; Curling & Hudson, 1975; Russell, 1979). Scully et al (1966) have shown that four of 17 cases of clear cell carcinoma actually arose in endometriosis. The close relationship of endometriosis to ovarian clear cell tumours has been advanced as one of the arguments in favour of Müllerian rather than mesonephric origin of clear cell tumours (Scully & Barlow, 1967).

Although some other common epithelial tumours of the ovary have also been shown to be occasionally associated with endometriosis, the frequency of this association is much lower than that seen in endometrioid and clear cell carcinomas. According to Russell (1979), pelvic endometriosis was present in 3% of patients with serous and 4% of patients with ovarian mucinous carcinomas. In addition there have been reports of mixed mesodermal (Müllerian) tumours which arose in endometriosis (Cooper, 1978; Marchevsky & Kaneko, 1978). Well-differentiated endometrioid stroma sarcoma has also been reported to originate in ovarian endometriosis (Palladino & Trousdell, 1969; Gruskin et al, 1970; Baiocchi et al, 1990), as has, very rarely, squamous cell carcinoma (Naresh et al, 1991).

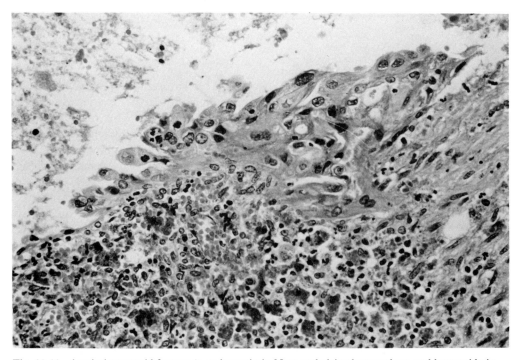

Fig. 32.18 Atypical squamoid features in endometriosis. Note underlying haemorrhage and haemosiderin-laden macrophages. H & E × 200.

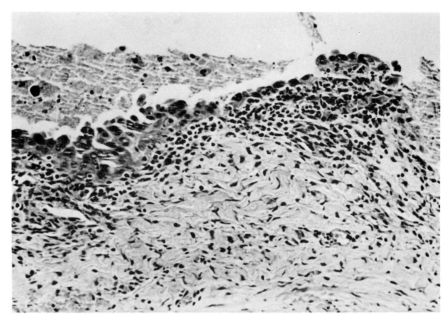

Fig. 32.19 Atypical epithelial lining of endometriotic cyst with large hyperchromatic nuclei. H & E × 150.

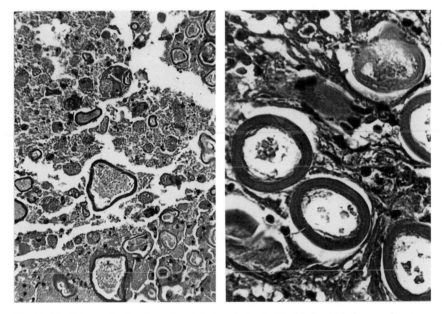

Fig. 32.20 Liesegang rings in endometriosis, admixed with debris within lumen of cyst (left; H & E × 60) and embedded within cyst wall (right; H & E × 125). (Reprinted with permission from Clement, 1990.)

Malignant tumours also arise in extraovarian endometriosis (Brooks & Wheeler, 1977; Heaps et al, 1990). Most of these consist of endometrioid carcinoma and about one-third of these are situated in the rectovaginal septum (Mostoufizadeh & Scully, 1980). Occasionally clear cell carcinomas develop in extragonadal endometriosis (Brooks & Wheeler, 1977; Goldberg et al, 1978; Hitti et al, 1990). Other types of carcinomas as well as endometrioid stroma sarcoma (Vierhout et al, 1992) have also been reported to arise in endometriosis outside the ovary. These occurred in the Fallopian tube, rectovaginal septum, vagina, the large intestine, urinary bladder, omentum and pleura (La Pava et al, 1963; Scully et al, 1966; Palladino & Trousdell, 1969; Labay & Feiner, 1971; Brooks & Wheeler, 1977; Berkowitz et al, 1978; Brunson et al, 1988; Baiocchi et al, 1990). A transition

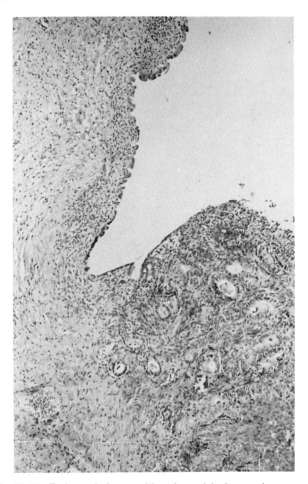

Fig. 32.21 Endometriotic cyst with endometrial adenocarcinoma directly arising from it. H & E × 36.

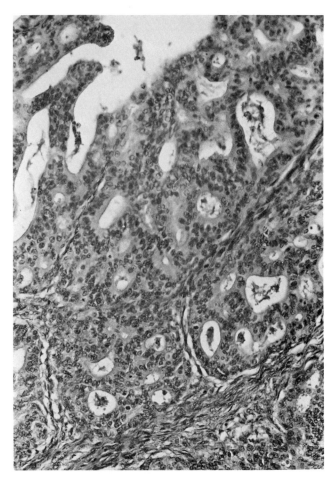

Fig. 32.22 Well-differentiated endometrioid adenocarcinoma of ovary. H & E × 150.

from benign endometriosis to the malignant neoplasms could only be demonstrated in some of these cases.

CLINICAL ASPECTS

The symptomatology of endometriosis varies considerably from patient to patient and depends, at least in some degree, on the extent of the disease as well as on the location of the endometriotic lesions. Furthermore, about 25% of patients with endometriosis have no symptoms at all (Parsons & Sommers, 1978). In the remaining patients there is, in order of decreasing frequency, pelvic pain or discomfort, dyspareunia and irregular uterine bleeding (Ranney, 1980b). In those patients in whom endometriosis involves the vagina (Fig. 32.24), uterine cervix (Fig. 32.25), intestinal tract (Fig. 32.26), urinary bladder or ureter, the symptomatology is frequently related to the specific areas involved. Thus, with endometriosis of the large intestine it is not unusual for obstruction or tenesmus to develop, whereas patients with endometriosis of the small intestine may suffer from volvulus or intussusception and can even develop a protein-losing enteropathy (Henley et al, 1993). Endometriosis of the urinary tract may result in haematuria or obstructive phenomena.

One of the most significant features of endometriosis is the often associated infertility. The true incidence of infertility in these patients is difficult to determine accurately, but it appears that about 40% of patients with endometriosis suffer from this complication (Parsons & Sommers, 1978), whereas in patients presenting with infertility, endometriosis is found in 20–50% of cases (Thomas, 1991). Although the exact mechanism of the infertility in these patients remains unknown, the relatively good results following a variety of surgical procedures indicate that mechanical factors, particularly involving ovaries and oviducts such as fibrosis, adhesions, tubal obstruction (Fig. 32.27) and a retroverted uterus, play a rôle in at least a number of these patients (Kistner, 1975; Weed & Holland, 1977). It has also been suggested that altered tubal secretion due to chronic salpingitis

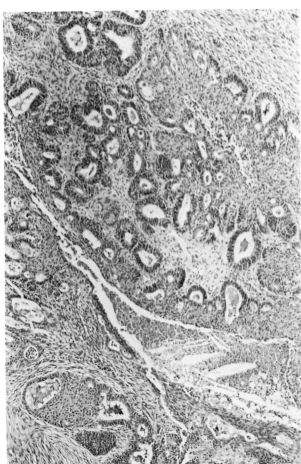

Fig. 32.23   Endometrioid adenocarcinoma with benign squamous metaplasia (adenoacanthoma). H & E × 60.

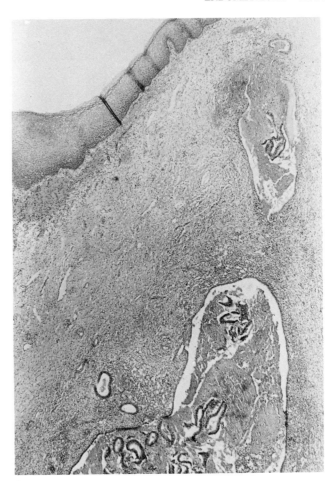

Fig. 32.24   Vagina with endometriosis in wall. H & E × 24.

may be instrumental in infertility associated with endometriosis. Some support for this may be found in the surprisingly high incidence (33%) of chronic salpingitis without obstruction in patients with ovarian endometriosis (Czernobilsky & Silverstein, 1978) (Fig. 32.28). To this should also be added other possible factors such as ovarian dysfunction, anovulatory bleeding, and an increase in the incidence of underdeveloped uteri (Parsons & Sommers, 1978). Kistner (1975) claims that if other pathological conditions such as submucous leiomyomas and endometrial polyps are excluded, the most important factor responsible for infertility in endometriosis is an inadequacy of tubo-ovarian motility secondary to fibrosis and scarring resulting in imperfect ovum acceptance by the fimbriae.

Another interesting theory which attempts to explain the infertility associated with endometriosis is an auto-immune mechanism. Weed & Arquembourg (1980) suggested that endometriosis stimulates an immune response to the host's own endometrial proteins which are recognized by the host as 'foreign' and that this immune

response may result in the rejection of early implantation of embryos or interfere with sperm passage. Anti-endometrial antibodies certainly occur in endometriosis but evidence that such antibodies are not epiphenomenal and play a rôle in the infertility associated with endometriosis is currently lacking (Halme & Surrey, 1990). Yet another hypothesis concerns the rôle of prostaglandins in the infertility of these women. Young et al (1981) demonstrated that under in vivo and in vitro conditions ectopically situated endometrium produced larger quantities of prostaglandin F, which affects tubal motility, than in normal conditions, whilst there is also evidence that prostacyclin (PGI_2), which causes relaxation of tubal musculature, is produced in excess by the peritoneal epithelium in women with endometriosis (Drake et al, 1981). Although much attention has been lavished upon the putative rôle of prostanoids in endometriosis-related infertility, their significance in this respect is currently out of favour (Hurst & Rock, 1991). It has also been shown that peritoneal macrophages in women with endometriosis are unusually numerous and have an enhanced capacity for

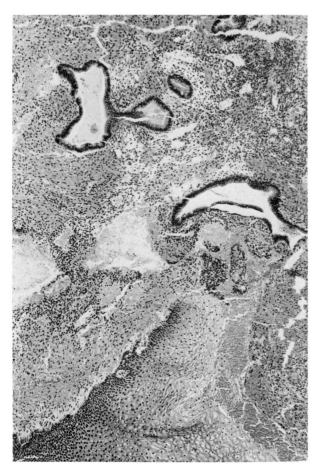

Fig. 32.25   Cervical endometriosis showing endometrial glands surrounded by stroma and haemorrhage causing ulceration of overlying exocervical epithelium. H & E × 60.

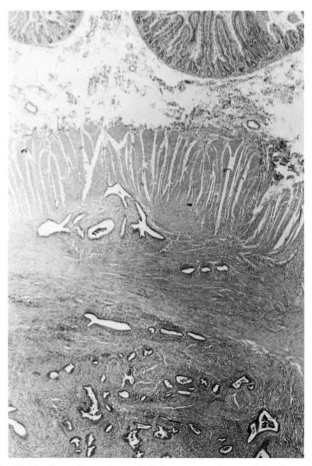

Fig. 32.26   Extensive endometriosis in serosa and muscularis of small intestine. H & E × 24.

phagocytosing sperm (Muscato et al, 1982); it has therefore been thought that entry of such cells into the tube could lead to excessive engulfment of sperm and hence to infertility. The many studies of peritoneal macrophages in endometriosis have, however, yielded inconsistent results and are open to considerable methodological criticism (Hurst & Rock, 1991).

While detailed discussion of the therapy of endometriosis is beyond the scope of this chapter, it suffices to say that in addition to surgical management, hormonal therapy plays an important rôle in the control of this disease. This includes oestrogen-progestagen or so-called pseudopregnancy therapy which transforms functioning endometriosis into decidua with subsequent necrosis and healing (Kistner, 1958), or the administration of Danazol (Danocrine) to produce a temporary menopausal state. This latter drug is an orally active gonadotrophin inhibitory agent devoid of oestrogenic and progestational activ-

ity (Dmowski et al, 1971). More recently, LH-releasing hormone analogues, which decrease pituitary sensitivity to LH-releasing hormone, have also been used successfully for the treatment of endometriosis (Shaw, 1991). While the advantages of surgical and/or medical therapy for endometriosis are being debated it appears that surgery still remains the principal means of treatment. According to Puolakka et al (1980), who evaluated the results of operative treatment of pelvic endometriosis, 30% of the patients became symptomless, 41% estimated the overall result as good, and 19% as moderate, whereas only 10% experienced deterioration or had no help from the operation. Eight per cent of the patients had recurrence of the disease that demanded re-operation. Since infertility constitutes one of the major complications of pelvic endometriosis, it is important to note that in Puolakka et al's series (1980) a 63% pregnancy rate was achieved following surgical therapy in 32 patients.

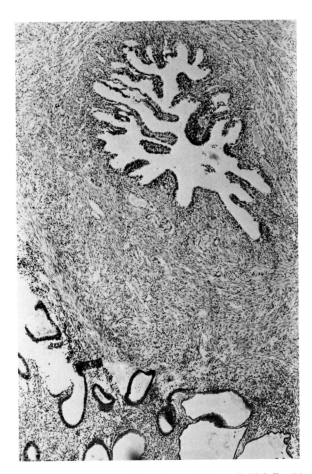

Fig. 32.27 Fallopian tube with endometriosis in wall. H & E × 24.

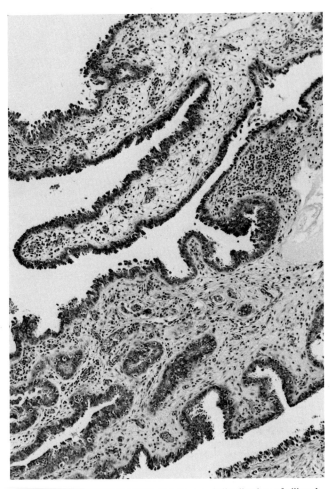

Fig. 32.28 Chronic salpingitis with abnormal distribution of ciliated and secretory cells in a case of ovarian endometriosis. H & E × 94. (Reprinted with permission from Czernobilsky & Silverstein, 1978, and from the American Fertility Society.)

REFERENCES

Acosta A A, Buttram V C Jr, Besch P K, Malinak L R, Franklin R R, Vanderheyden J D 1973 A proposed classification of pelvic endometriosis. Obstetrics and Gynecology 42: 19–25.

American Fertility Society 1985 Revised American Fertility Society classifications of endometriosis. Fertility and Sterility 43: 351–352.

Andrews M C, Andrews W C, Strauss A F 1959 Effects of progestin-induced pseudopregnancy on endometriosis: clinical and microscopic studies. American Journal of Obstetrics et Gynecolog 78: 776–785.

Aure J C, Loeg K, Kolstadt P 1971 Carcinoma of the ovary and endometriosis. Acta Obstetrica et Gynecologica Scandinavica 50: 63–67.

Baiocchi G, Kavanagh J J, Wharton J T 1990 Endometrioid stromal sarcomas arising from ovarian and extraovarian endometriosis: report of two cases and review of the literature. Gynecologic Oncology 36: 147–151.

Bassis M L 1956 Pseudodeciduosis. American Journal of Obstetrics and Gynecology 72: 1029–1037.

Batt R E, Smith R A 1989 Embryologic theory of histogenesis of endometriosis in peritoneal pockets. Obstetrical and Gynecologic Clinics of North America 16: 15–28.

Batt R E, Smith R A, Buck G M, Severino M F, Naples J D 1990 Mullerianosis. In: Chadha D R, Buttram V C (eds) Current concepts in endometriosis. Alan R Liss, New York, pp 413–426.

Bergquist A 1991 Steroid receptors in endometriosis. In: Thomas E J, Rock J A (eds) Modern approaches to endometriosis. Kluwer Academic Press, Dordecht, pp 33–55.

Bergquist A, Ljungberg O, Skoog L 1993 Immunohistochemical analysis of oestrogen and progesterone receptors in endometriotic tissue and endometrium. Human Reproduction 8: 1915–1922.

Berkowitz R S, Ehrmann R, Knapp R C 1978 Endometrial stromal sarcoma arising from vaginal endometriosis. Obstetrics and Gynecology 51: 34S–37S.

Brooks J J, Wheeler J E 1977 Malignancy arising in extragonadal endometriosis: a case report and summary of the world literature. Cancer 40: 3065–3073.

Brunson G L, Barclay D L, Sanders M, Araoz C A 1988 Malignant extraovarian endometriosis: two case reports and review of the literature. Gynecologic Oncology 30: 125–130.

Brzezinski A, Koren Z 1962 Endometriosis in Israel. American Journal of Obstetrics and Gynecology 83: 414–416.

Cantor J O, Fenoglio C M, Richart R M 1979 A case of extensive endometriosis. American Journal of Obstetrics and Gynecology 134: 846–847.

Charles D 1957 Endometriosis and hemorrhagic pleural effusion. Obstetrics and Gynecology 10: 309–312.

Clement P B 1990 Pathology of endometriosis. In: Rosen P R, Fechner R E (eds) Pathology annual, part 1, vol 25. Appleton & Lange, Norwalk, pp 245–295.

Clement P V, Young R H, Scully R E 1988 Necrotic pseudoxanthomatous nodules of ovary and peritoneum in endometriosis. American Journal of Surgical Pathology 12: 390–397.

Clement P B, Young R H, Scully R E 1989 Liesengang rings in the female genital tract: a report of three cases. International Journal of Gynecologic Pathology 8: 271–276.

Cohen M R 1980 Laparoscopic diagnosis and pseudomenopause treatment of endometriosis cysts with danazol. Clinical Obstetrics and Gynecology 23: 901–915.

Cooper P 1978 Mixed mesodermal tumour and clear cell carcinoma arising in ovarian endometriosis. Cancer 42: 2827–2831.

Cullen T S 1925 Discussion: Symposium on misplaced endometrial tissue. American Journal of Obstetrics and Gynecology 10: 732–733.

Curling O M, Hudson C N 1975 Endometrioid tumours of the ovary. British Journal of Obstetrics and Gynaecology 82: 405–411.

Czernobilsky B 1982a Primary epithelial tumors of the ovary. In: Blaustein A (ed) Pathology of the female genital tract, 3rd edn. Springer Verlag, New York, pp 550–606.

Czernobilsky B 1982b Endometrioid neoplasia of the ovary: a reappraisal. International Journal of Gynecological Pathology 1: 203–210.

Czernobilsky B, Morris W J 1979 A histologic study of ovarian endometriosis with emphasis on hyperplastic and atypical changes. Obstetrics and Gynecology 53: 318–323.

Czernobilsky B, Silverstein A 1978 Salpingitis in ovarian endometriosis. Fertility and Sterility 30: 45–49.

Czernobilsky B, Silverman B B, Mijuta J J 1970a Endometrioid carcinoma of the ovary: a clinicopathologic study of 75 cases. Cancer 26: 1141–1152.

Czernobilsky B, Silverman B B, Enterline H T 1970b Clear cell carcinoma of the ovary: a clinicopathologic analysis of pure and mixed forms and comparison with endometrioid carcinoma. Cancer 25: 762–772.

Di Palo S, Mari G, Castolda R et al 1989 Endometriosis of the lung. Respiratory Medicine 83: 255–258.

Dizerega G S, Barber D L, Hodgen G D 1980 Endometriosis: role of ovarian steroids in initiation, maintenance and suppression. Fertility and Sterility 33: 649–653.

Dmowski W P, Scholer H F, Mahesch V B, Greenblatt R B 1971 Danazol: a synthetic steroid derivative with interesting physiologic properties. Fertility and Sterility 22: 9–18.

Dmowski W P, Steele R W, Baker G F 1981 Deficient cellular immunity in endometriosis. American Journal of Obstetrics and Gynecology 141: 377–383.

Dmowski W P, Braun D, Gebel H 1990 Endometriosis: genetic and immunologic aspects. In: Chadha D R, Buttram V C (eds) Current concepts in endometriosis. Proceedings of the second international symposium on endometriosis. Alan R Liss, New York, 323: 15–31.

Drake T S, O'Brien W F, Ramwell P W, Metz S A 1981 Peritoneal fluid thromboxane B2 and 6-keto-prostaglandin FIa in endometriosis. American Journal of Obstetrics and Gynecology 140: 401–404.

Espaulella J, Armengol J, Bella F, Lain J M, Calaf J 1991 Pulmonary endometriosis: conservative treatment with GnRH agonists. Obstetrics and Gynecology 78: 535–537.

Fedele L, Bianchi S, Di-Nola G et al 1992 Endometriosis and non-obstructive mullerian anomalies. Obstetrics and Gynecology 79: 515–517.

Fox H 1983 The pathology of endometriosis. Irish Journal of Medical Sciences 152 (suppl 2): 9–13.

Fox H, Buckley C H 1984 Current concepts of endometriosis. Clinics in Obstetrics and Gynaecology 11: 279–287.

Fujii S 1991 Secondary mullerian system and endometriosis. American Journal of Obstetrics and Gynecology 165: 219–225.

Gardner G H, Greene R R, Ranney B 1953 The histogenesis of endometriosis — recent contributions. Obstetrics and Gynecology 1: 615–637.

Garzetti G G, Ciavattini A, Provincial I M et al 1993 Natural killer cell activity in endometriosis: correlation between serum estradiol levels and cytotoxicity. Obstetrics and Gynecology 81: 685–688.

Gerbie A B, Green R R, Reis R A 1958 Heteroplastic bone and cartilage in the female genital tract. Obstetrics and Gynecology 11: 573–578.

Giangarra C, Gallo G, Newman R, Dorfman H 1987 Endometriosis in the biceps femoris: a case report and review of the literature. Journal of Bone and Joint Surgery 69: 290–292.

Goldberg M I, Ng A B P, Belinson J L, Hutson E D, Nordquist S R B 1978 Clear cell adenocarcinoma arising in endometriosis of the rectovaginal septum. Obstetrics and Gynecology 51: 38S–40S.

Goldman M B, Cramer D W 1990 The epidemiology of endometriosis. In: Chadha D R, Buttram V C (eds) Current concepts in endometriosis. Proceedings of the second international symposium on endometriosis. Alan R Liss, New York 323: 15–31.

Gruskin P, Osborne N G, Morley G W, Abell M R 1970 Primary endometrial stromatosis of ovary: report of a case. Obstetrics and Gynecology 36: 702–707.

Gupta S D 1985 Endometriosis in the thumb. Journal of the Indian Medical Association 83: 122–124.

Halban Y 1925 Hysteroadenosis metastatica. Archive fur Gynakologie 124: 457–482.

Halme J, Surrey J S 1990 Endometriosis and infertility: the mechanisms involved. In: Chadha D R, Buttram V C (eds) Current concepts in endometriosis. Alan R Liss, New York, pp 157–178.

Haney A F 1990 Etiology and histogenesis of endometriosis. In: Chadha D R, Buttram V C (eds) Current concepts in endometriosis. Alan R Liss, New York.

Haney A F 1991 The pathogenesis and aetiology of endometriosis. In: Thomas E J, Rock J A (eds) Modern approaches to endometriosis. Kluwer Academic Press, Dordrecht, pp 3–19.

Heaps J M, Nieberg R K, Berek J S 1990 Malignant neoplasms arising in endometriosis. Obstetrics and Gynecology 75: 1023–1028.

Henley J D, Kratzer S S, Seo I S et al 1993 Endometriosis of the small intestine presenting as a protein-losing enteropathy. American Journal of Gastroenterology 88: 130–133.

Hertig A T, Gore H 1961 Tumors of female sex organs. Part 3 Tumors of the ovary and fallopian tube. In: Atlas of tumor pathology, section IX, fascicle 33. Armed Forces Institute of Pathology, Washington, DC, pp 106–108.

Hill J A 1992 Immunology and endometriosis. Fertility and Sterility 58: 262–264.

Hitti I F, Glasberg S S, Lubicz S 1990 Clear cell carcinoma arising in extraovarian endometriosis: report of three cases and review of the literature. Gynecologic Oncology 39: 314–320.

Houston D E, Noller K L, Melton L Y, Selwyn B J, Hardy R J 1987 Incidence of pelvic endometriosis in Rochester, Minnesota, 1970–1979. American Journal of Epidemiology 125: 959–969.

Hurst B S, Rock J A 1991 The peritoneal environment in endometriosis. In: Thomas E J, Rock J A (eds) Modern approaches to endometriosis. Kluwer Academic Press, Dordrecht, pp 79–96.

Jansen R P, Russell P 1986 Non-pigmented endometriosis: clinical, laparoscopic and pathologic definition. American Journal of Obstetrics and Gynecology 155: 1154–1159.

Javert C T 1949 Pathogenesis of endometriosis based upon endometrial homeoplasia, direct extension, exfoliation and implantation, lymphatic and hematogenous metastasis (including five case reports of endometrial tissue in pelvic lymph nodes). Cancer 2: 399–410.

Javert C T 1951 Observations on the pathology and spread of endometriosis based on the theory of benign metastases. American Journal of Obstetrics and Gynecology 62: 477–487.

Kapadia S B, Russak R R, O'Donnell W F, Harris R N, Lecky J W 1984 Postmenopausal ureteral endometriosis with atypical adenomatous hyperplasia following hysterectomy, bilateral oophorectomy and long-term estrogen therapy. Obstetrics and Gynecology 64: 60S–63S.

Karp L A, Czernobilsky B 1969 Glandular inclusions in pelvic and abdominal para-aortic lymph nodes: a study of autopsy and surgical material in males and females. American Journal of Clinical Pathology 52: 212–218.

Kempson R K 1973 Sarcomas and related neoplasms. In: Norris H G, Hertig A T, Abell M R (eds) The uterus. Williams & Wilkins, Baltimore, pp 298–319.

Kerner H, Gaton E, Czernobilsky B 1981 Unusual ovarian, tubal and pelvic mesothelial inclusions in patients with endometriosis. Histopathology 5: 277–283.

Kistner R W 1958 The use of newer progestins in the treatment of endometriosis. American Journal of Obstetrics and Gynecology 75: 264–278.

Kistner R W 1975 Management of endometriosis in the infertile patient. Fertility and Sterility 26: 1151–1166.

Kurman R J, Craig J M 1972 Endometrioid and clear cell carcinoma in the ovary. Cancer 29: 1653–1664.

Labay G R, Feiner F 1971 Malignant pleural endometriosis. American Journal of Obstetrics and Gynecology 110: 478–480.

LaGrenade A, Silverberg S G 1988 Ovarian tumor associated with atypical endometriosis. Human Pathology 19: 1080–1084.

La Pava S, Nigogosyan G, Pickren J W 1963 Sarcomatous transformation of "true" endometriosis. New York State Journal of Medicine 63: 2548–2553.

Lauchlan S C 1972 The secondary Mullerian system. Obstetrical and Gynecological Survey 27: 133–146.

Levander G, Norman P 1955 The pathogenesis of endometriosis: an experimental study. Acta Obstetrica et Gynecologica Scandinavica 34: 366–398.

Lyndrup J, Thorpe S, Glenthoj A, Obel E, Sele V 1987 Altered progesterone/estrogen receptor ratios in endometriosis: a comparative study of steroid receptors and morphology in endometriosis and endometrium. Acta Obstetrica et Gynecologica Scandinavica 66: 625–629.

Malinak L R, Buttram V C, Elias S, Simpson J L 1980 Heritable aspects of endometriosis. II. Clinical characteristics of familial endometriosis. American Journal of Obstetrics and Gynecology 137: 322–327.

Marchewsky A M, Kaneko M 1978 Bilateral ovarian endometriosis associated with carcinosarcoma of the right ovary and endometrioid carcinoma of the left ovary. American Journal of Clinical Pathology 70: 709–712.

Merrill J A 1966 Endometrial induction of endometriosis across millipore filters. American Journal of Obstetrics and Gynecology 94: 780–790.

Metzger D A, Olive D L, Haney A F 1988 Limited hormonal responsiveness of ectopic endometrium: histologic correlation with intrauterine endometrium. Human Pathology 19: 1417–1424.

Miyazawa K 1976 Incidence of endometriosis among Japanese women. Obstetrics and Gynecology 48: 407–409.

Moller N E 1959 The Arias-Stella phenomenon in endometriosis. Acta Obstetrica et Gynecologica Scandinavica 38: 271–274.

Mostoufizadeh G H M, Scully R E 1980 Malignant tumors arising in endometriosis. Clinical Obstetrics and Gynecology 23: 951–963.

Muscato J J, Haney A F, Weinberg J B 1982 Sperm phagocytosis by human peritoneal macrophages: a possible cause of infertility in endometriosis. American Journal of Obstetrics and Gynecology 144: 503–510.

Nakamura M, Katabuchi H, Tohya T et al 1993 Scanning electron microscopic and immunohistochemical studies of pelvic endometriosis. Human Reproduction 8: 2218–2226.

Naseman T R 1990 Zur Endometriose der Haut. Zeitschrift fur Hautkrangungen 65: 117–119.

Naresh K N, Ahuja V K, Rao C R, Mukherjee G, Bhargava M K 1991 Squamous cell carcinoma arising in endometriosis of the ovary. Journal of Clinical Pathology 44: 958–959.

Novak E 1931 Pelvic endometriosis: spontaneous rupture of endometrial cysts, with a report of three cases. American Journal of Obstetrics and Gynecology 22: 326–335.

Novak E, de Lima A 1948 Correlative study of adenomyosis and pelvic endometriosis, with special reference to the hormonal reaction of ectopic endometrium. American Journal of Obstetrics and Gynecology 56: 634–644.

Novak E R, Woodruff Y D 1979a Novak's Gynecologic and obstetric pathology with clinical and endocrine relations, 8th edn. WB Saunders, Philadelphia, p 578.

Novak E R, Woodruff J D 1979b Novak's Gynecologic and obstetric pathology with clinical and endocrine relations, 8th edn. WB Saunders, Philadelphia, ch 29, pp 561–584.

Oosterlynck D J, Cornillie F J, Waer M, Vanderputte M, Koninckx P R 1991 Women with endometriosis show a defect in natural killer activity resulting in a decreased cytotoxicity to autologous endometrium. Fertility and Sterility 56: 45–51.

Oosterlynck D J, Meuleman C, Waer M, Vanderputte M, Koninckx P R 1992 The natural killer activity of peritoneal fluid lymphocytes in women with endometriosis. Fertility and Sterility 58: 292–295.

Palladino V S, Trousdell M 1969 Extra-uterine Mullerian tumors. Cancer 23: 1413–1422.

Parsons L, Sommers S C 1978 Gynecology, 2nd edn. WB Saunders, Philadelphia, ch 45, pp 957–997.

Prakash S, Ulfelder H, Cohen R B 1965 Enzyme-histochemical observations on endometriosis. American Journal of Obstetrics and Gynecology 91: 990–997.

Pueblitz-Peredo S, Luevano-Flores E, Rincon-Taracena R, Ochoa-Carrillo F J 1985. Uterus like mass of the ovary: endometriosis or congenital malformation?: a case with a discussion of histogenesis. Archives of Pathology and Laboratory Medicine 109: 361–364.

Puolakka Y, Kauppila A, Ronnenberg L 1980 Results in the operative treatment of pelvic endometriosis. Acta Obstetrica et Gynecologica Scandinavica 59: 429–431.

Ranney B 1980a Endometriosis: pathogenesis, symptoms and findings. Clinical Obstetrics and Gynecology 23: 865–874.

Ranney B 1980b Etiology, prevention and inhibition of endometriosis. Clinical Obstetrics and Gynecology 23: 875–883.

Rawson J M 1991 Prevalence of endometriosis in asymptomatic women. Journal of Reproductive Medicine 36: 513–515.

Ridley J H 1968 The histogenesis of endometriosis: a review of facts and fancies. Obstetrical and Gynecological Survey 23: 1–35.

Rolfing M B, Kao K Y, Woodard B H 1981 Endomyometriosis: possible association with leiomyomatosis dissemination and endometriosis. Archives of Pathology and Laboratory Medicine 105: 556–557.

Roth L M, Czernobilsky B, Langley F A 1981 Endometrioid adenofibromatous and cystadenofibromatous tumours: benign, proliferating and malignant. Cancer 48: 1838–1845.

Russell P 1979 The pathological assessment of ovarian neoplasms: I. Introduction to the common "epithelial" tumours and analysis of benign, "epithelial" tumours. Pathology 11: 5–26.

Sampson J A 1921 Perforating hemorrhagic (chocolate) cysts of the ovary, their importance and especially their relation to pelvic adenomas of the endometrial type. Archives of Surgery 3: 245–323.

Sampson J A 1925 Endometrial carcinoma of ovary, arising in endometrial tissue in that organ. Archives of Surgery 10: 1–72.

Schweppe K W, Wynn R W, Beller F K 1984 Ultrastructure comparison of endometriotic implants and ectopic endometrium. American Journal of Obstetrics and Gynecology 148: 1024–1039.

Scott R B, Wharton L R Jr 1957 The effect of estrone and progesterone on the growth of experimental endometriosis in Rhesus monkeys. American Journal of Obstetrics and Gynecology 74: 852–865.

Scully R E 1977 Ovarian tumors: a review. American Journal of Pathology 87: 686–720.

Scully R E, Barlow J F 1967 "Mesonephroma" of ovary: tumor of Mullerian nature related to the endometrioid carcinoma. Cancer 20: 1405–1417.

Scully R E, Richardson G S, Barlow J F 1966 The development of malignancy in endometriosis. Clinical Obstetrics and Gynecology 9: 384–411.

Serov S F, Scully R E, Sobin L H 1973 International histological classification of tumours, no. 9. Histological typing of ovarian tumours. World Health Organization, Geneva, pp 17–21.

Shaw R W 1991 GnRH analogues in the treatment of endometriosis — rationale and efficacy. In: Thomas E J, Rock J A (eds) Modern approaches to endometriosis. Kluwer Academic Publishers, Dordrecht, pp 257–274.

Shifrin B S, Erez S, Moore J G 1973 Teen-age endometriosis. American Journal of Obstetrics and Gynecology 116: 973–980.

Simpson J L, Elias S, Malinak L R 1980 Heritable aspects of endometriosis. I. Genetic studies. American Journal of Obstetrics and Gynecology 137: 327–331.

Steck W D, Helwig E B 1965 Cutaneous endometriosis. Journal of the American Medical Association 191: 167–170.

Sturgis S H, Call B J 1954 Endometriosis peritonei: relationship of pain to functional activity. American Journal of Obstetrics and Gynecology 68: 1421–1431.

Suginami H 1991 A reappraisal of the coelomic metaplasia theory by reviewing endometriosis occurring in unusual sites and instances. American Journal of Obstetrics and Gynecology 165: 214–218.

Svendstrup F, Husby H 1991 Parenchymal pulmonary endometriosis. Journal of Laryngology and Otology 105: 235–236.

Thibodeau L L, Pridleau G R, Manuelidis E E, Merino M J, Heafner M D 1987 Cerebral endometriosis: case report. Journal of Neurosurgery 66: 609–610.

Tidman M J, MacDonald D M 1988 Cutaneous endometriosis: a histopathologic study. Journal of the American Academy of Dermatology 18: 373–377.

Thomas E J 1991 Endometriosis and infertility. In: Thomas E J, Rock J A (eds) Modern approaches to endometriosis. Kluwer Academic Publishers, Dordrecht, pp 113–128.

Thomas E J 1993 Endometriosis: still an enigma. British Journal of Obstetrics and Gynaecology 100: 615–617.

Tutschka B G, Lauchlan S C 1980 Endosalpingiosis. Obstetrics and Gynecology 55: 57S–60S.

Ueki M 1991 Histologic study of endometriosis and examination of lymphatic drainage in and from the uterus. American Journal of Obstetrics and Gynecology 165: 201–209.

Vierhout M E, Chadha-Ajwani S, Wijner J A et al 1992 Extra-uterine endometrial stromal sarcoma with DNA flow cytometric analysis. European Journal of Obstetrics and Gynecology and Reproductive Biology 43: 157–161.

von Recklinghausen F 1885 Uber die venose Embolie und den retrograden Transport in den Venen und in den Lymphgefassen. Virchows Archiv A 100: 503–539.

Weed J C, Arquembourg P C 1980 Endometriosis: can it produce an autoimmune response resulting in infertility? Clinical Obstetrics and Gynecology 23: 885–895.

Weed J C, Holland J B 1977 Endometriosis and infertility: an enigma. Fertility and Sterility 28: 135–140.

Young S, Moon D V M, Leung P C S, Yuen B H, Gomel V 1981 Prostaglandin F in human endometriosis tissue. American Journal of Obstetrics and Gynecology 141: 344–346.

33. Pathology of infertility

Louis H. Honoré

INTRODUCTION

Fertility is defined as the ability to procreate, i.e. to achieve a live birth following successful fusion of male and female gametes (fertilization). Human fertility is the resultant of two interacting sets of factors: behavioural and biological (Leridon, 1977).

The behavioural factors comprise:

1. Sexual behaviour, which influences the probability of conception as a result of the length of physical separation between husband and wife, coital frequency when they are living together, coital distribution within the cycle and the nature of intercourse. It is worth noting that, among married couples not using contraceptives, the peak coital rate occurs on the day of the LH surge, implying that female sex hormones can influence sexual behaviour in favour of conception (Hedricks et al, 1987).

2. The duration of postpartum infertility related to breast feeding varies from culture to culture. It has a physiological basis and in some societies it is reinforced by sexual taboos prohibiting intercourse during lactation. In the West the low frequency of breast feeding has significantly reduced the length of postpartum infertility to less than three months with the result that the mean interval between two live births has dropped to potentially just over 20 months. This increase in the duration of the fertile period is more than balanced by contraception.

3. The deliberate control of fertility by voluntary infertility, delayed child-bearing and contraception (affecting fecundability), induced abortion (affecting intrauterine mortality) and sterilization (affecting the overall level of fertility). These methods of fertility control also have negative short-term or long-term effects on fertility following cessation or reversal. Post pill usage there is short-term depression of fecundability depending on the patient's age and the oestrogen dose (Bracken et al, 1990). After removal of an intrauterine contraceptive device (IUCD) there is a definite increase in the prevalence of infertility (Eschenbach, 1992). There are conflicting data on the effects of induced abortion on subsequent fertility but the evidence argues against any significant impact (Huggins & Cullins, 1990). Fertility rates are variably reduced after reversal of tubal sterilization (Rock et al, 1987).

4. Nuptiality (marital customs), as determined socially by the types of union (stable marriage, common law and successive relationships), age at marriage, conditions or obligations of remarriage following widowhood and consequences of marital infidelity. It has been shown that the level of fertility of a population is greatly affected by these practices (Leridon, 1977) with the final number of offspring depending on the number of years a woman has lived 'in unions' and on the nature of these unions.

5. Lifestyle, especially in the affluent societies, has a considerable influence on fertility. Thus the ability to achieve and successfully carry a pregnancy is significantly reduced by exposure to smoking, alcohol and other recreational or therapeutic drugs (Stillman et al, 1986; Phipps et al, 1987; Smith & Asch, 1987; Elenbogen et al, 1991; Feichtinger, 1991; Laurent et al, 1992). Environmental and occupational exposures to toxic substances also have adverse effects on fertility (Feichtinger, 1991; Jaffe & Jewelewicz, 1991).

The biological factors include:

1. Fecundability, defined as the probability that a woman will conceive during a particular month in the absence of contraception. This parameter is conditioned by the biological potential of the subject and the quality and quantity of coital exposure. In women it decreases steadily with age, especially after the age of 35 (Gindoff & Jewelewicz, 1986; Healy et al, 1994). In men there is no conclusive evidence that, all things being equal, the probability of achieving successful fertilization decreases with age, and the finding of an age-dependent decline in overall fecundity (Anderson, 1975) is marred by the failure to control for an important age-dependent variable, i.e. coital frequency. It is worth noting that after the age of 40, despite normal seminal characteristics, there is a

significant increase in the number of abnormal sperms (Schwartz et al, 1983) but the relevance of this observation in terms of fertility is not yet established.

2. Permanent sterility secondary to the menopause and preceded by a variable period of relative infertility (Kushner, 1979). The menopause is occurring later in industrialized countries but the lengthening of the fertile period is more than compensated for by voluntary contraception.

3. Intrauterine mortality has a significant effect on fertility and in humans pregnancy loss, subclinical and clinical, is substantial (Edmonds et al, 1982). It increases with maternal age (Tsuji & Nakano, 1978; Hassold et al, 1980).

Involuntary infertility is defined as the inability to achieve a live birth after a year of regular unprotected coitus. The prevalence of infertility varies widely from 6–60% depending on the definition, the age of the couples examined and the population studied but the average figure for the West is close to 15% (Page, 1989; Jaffe & Jewelewicz, 1991). There has been an increase in infertility since the fifties and sixties when the infertility rate was estimated at 7–8% (Feichtinger, 1991) but there has been no further rise in the eighties (Mosher & Pratt, 1991; Templeton et al, 1991). Clearly, infertility is a 'couple problem' and should be conceptualized, investigated and treated as such. The 'fault' may lie with one of the partners, with both partners to a variable extent (Dunphy et al, 1990a) or with neither, at least as far as can be determined by modern methods (Jaffe & Jewelewicz, 1991). For didactic reasons the subject will be discussed under the following three headings:

1. Male infertility: for the sake of completeness the contribution of the male to human infertility will be briefly mentioned.

2. Interactive infertility: this important aspect covers the negative fertility-depressing effects of the biological, physical and psychological consequences of the coital act.

3. Female infertility: this facet of the problem will be discussed in detail.

MALE INFERTILITY

For sundry reasons, including biological and racial differences, the disparate diagnostic criteria used and the non-uniform availability of comprehensive and concerted infertility investigations, the true contribution of male infertility to overall infertility is unknown but there are estimates ranging from one-third male, one-third female, one-third both to 50/50 (Steinberger & Rodriguez-Rigau, 1983). These estimates are not derived from systematic prospective studies but reflect clinical impressions obtained from separate assessments of each member of the couple by different specialists.

Regardless of the magnitude of the problem there is no doubt that the male factor can be the dominant cause of infertility. Biologically the function of the male is to deposit in the upper vagina, close to the cervical os, 'fertile' seminal fluid with adequate numbers of normally structured, actively motile sperms able to reach the tubal ampulla and fertilize the ovum. The efficiency of this process demands perfect co-ordination of a complex set of psychological, physical and biological processes, which can fail singly or in combination. Male infertility, which can result from erectile or ejaculatory dysfunction, spermatozoal and seminal abnormalities and various forms of inherited or acquired endocrinopathy (Lipshutz & Howards, 1983; Tesarik & Testart, 1989), will not be discussed further.

INTERACTIVE INFERTILITY

This form of infertility, which can be transient or permanent, is related to the following factors acting singly or in concert:

Age

In humans fertility peaks in the third decade. 'Adolescent sterility' (Montagu, 1946) is a well-recognized entity supported by the rare occurrence of illegitimate births in the populations where premarital sex is tolerated and even encouraged. It is largely due to immaturity of the reproductive system in both sexes, reflected in the female by significantly lower fecundity (Jain, 1969). In addition there is some evidence, still inconclusive, that young maternal and paternal age predisposes to an increased incidence of lethal heteroploidy in the conceptus, i.e. monosomy X (Warburton et al, 1980) and triploidy (Hassold et al, 1980) respectively.

The reproductive capacity of the human couple is limited in time by progressive, age-dependent subfertility and eventually by the menopause, which imposes absolute sterility (Leridon, 1977). This age-dependent subfertility is multifactorial. Decreased coital frequency, especially after the age of 35 (Leridon, 1977), reduces the statistical probability of mid-cycle fertilization and increases the possibility of fusion of gametes which are defective as a result of prolonged prefertilization sojourn in the female reproductive tract (Guerrero & Rojas, 1975; Bomsel-Helmreich, 1976). In women there is a progressive drop in fecundity after the age of 30 (Gindoff & Jewelewicz, 1986) accompanied by a higher spontaneous abortion rate (Kushner, 1979) and a higher frequency of fetal trisomy (Hassold et al, 1980). There is no comparable age-dependent impairment of male fertility (Nieschlag et al, 1982) but men tend to show a variable degree of reproductive dysfunction related to social, professional and psychological pressures, chronic abuse of alcohol and nicotine and intercurrent systemic and urological diseases.

Physical factors

Since ovulation occurs once a month at mid-cycle and the shed gemetes have a short fertile life span, successful fertilization depends critically on the timing of intercourse, its frequency and its nature. Mistiming is often due to ignorance of reproductive physiology but can result from avoidance of the fertile period by collusion on the part of an infertile couple with an unconscious aversion to parenthood (Abse, 1966). A low coital frequency (Freeman et al, 1983) reduces the chance of gamete fusion and enhances the probability of fusion of defective ageing gametes; a high coital frequency gives rise to deficient seminal fluid and oligospermia (Schwartz et al, 1979). The physical effectiveness of coitus can also be impaired by:

1. The excessive practice of coital variations with the avoidance of penovaginal intercourse, essential for optimal insemination. It is possible that sperm deposition in the alimentary canal may lead to sperm isoimmunity in women, as it does in homosexual men (Witkin & Sonnabend, 1983), but a recent study has failed to support this theoretical possibility (Chacho et al, 1991).

2. Inadequate or absent vaginal penetration resulting from organic or psychogenic dyspareunia or vaginismus (Fordney, 1978) or from male erectile dysfunction (Turnbull & Weinberg, 1983).

3. Inadequate vaginal insemination may be due to ejaculatory dysfunction, i.e. premature, sham or retrograde ejaculation (Thomas, 1983). Moreover, the quantitative efficiency of the emission reflex can be impaired by feelings of guilt and anxiety (Abse, 1966) and enhanced by pleasurable foreplay, which releases oxytocin and potentiates the contractility of the excurrent ducts (Amann, 1981).

Psychological factors

Psychogenic infertility, considered as significant in 5–10% of cases (Mosley, 1976) remains controversial (Seibel & Taymor, 1982; Healy et al, 1994) and the problem revolves about the primary or secondary nature of psychological disturbances in infertile couples. Some studies claim to show the primacy of emotional factors in the causation of infertility: infertile couples are more ambivalent in their attitude towards children than fertile couples (Mai et al, 1972); infertile women are more neurotic, dependent and anxious than fertile women and experience conflict over their femininity and fear of pregnancy (Sturgis et al, 1957; Sandler, 1959); infertile men are prone to psychosexual conflicts related to unconscious incestuous desires, sadistic fantasies and incomplete male identification (Abse, 1966). Other studies have failed to support a primary relationship between psychological factors and infertility (Noyes & Chapnick, 1964; Singh & Neki, 1982; Freeman et al, 1983).

There is little doubt that infertility causes secondary psychological upsets (Menning, 1980), which become reinforced by reactive hostility developing between the two members of a couple (Abse, 1966). Emotional stress, often compounding a pre-existing problem of reproductive dysfunction, can adversely affect all levels of the reproductive system in both sexes (Seibel & Taymor, 1982). In the male the stress of an infertility investigation may cause secondary impotence when azoospermia is first detected (Berger, 1980), at the time of a postcoital test (Bullock, 1974) or at mid-cycle, when the male feels threatened about his ability to achieve conception (Drake & Grunert, 1979). Interest in the psychological aspect of infertility has been rekindled by a recent report that attendance at an infertility clinic significantly enhanced the conception rate in a subgroup of couples with prolonged infertility (> 4 years) and a 'normal' female partner (Dunphy et al, 1990b).

The rôle of psychological factors in habitual abortion leading to infertility is also unclear. Habitual aborters are characterized by an inability to plan and anticipate, poor emotional control, emphasis on conformity, stronger feelings of dependency and greater proneness to guilt and depression (Kai et al, 1969; Seibel & Graves, 1980). The psychogenic aetiology of spontaneous abortion is indirectly supported by the success of psychotherapy in preventing further pregnancy losses (Tupper & Weil, 1962) and the increased incidence of spontaneous abortion in women following a sudden infant death (Mandell & Wolfe, 1974). Careful review of the literature demonstrates an association between psychological upsets and habitual abortion but evidence for causality is lacking. It is felt that the frustration resulting from recurrent pregnancy losses is the cause of the psychological distress (Seibel & Taymor, 1982; Rock & Zacur, 1983).

Genetic factors

Genetic factors are critical in setting the fertility potential of an individual by qualitatively and/or quantitatively affecting gonadal endocrine activity and gametogenesis and conditioning the structural development of genital ducts. They also directly impact on the product of interaction, i.e. the zygote-embryo fetus and depress fertility by influencing intrauterine survival rate. Major genetic differences between mother and father, expressed as ABO (Schaap et al, 1984) and P system (Rock & Zacur, 1983) incompatibility between mother and fetus, can lead to subfertility and recurrent abortion. The controversial rôle of excessive sharing of the major histocompatibility antigens between mother and father in recurrent abortion is discussed in Chapter 61.

The prevalence of detectable chromosomal abnormalities in couples with recurrent spontaneous abortion is about 5% (Campana et al, 1986; Fortuny et al, 1988;

Smith & Gaba, 1990; Coulam, 1991) but it is much lower (< 1%) in couples experiencing only recurrent abortions without any other form of reproductive failure (Simpson et al, 1989). The chromosomal abnormalities fall into three groups:

1. Structural rearrangements. The commonest form is the non-homologous balanced reciprocal (Fortuny et al, 1988) or Robertsonian translocation. Less common forms include: inversions and polymorphisms, balanced homologous translocations (Sudha & Gopinath, 1990), intra- or inter-chromosomal insertional translocations (Abuelo et al, 1988), familial or *de novo* complex rearrangements (Timar et al, 1991) and maternal gonosomal mosaicism (Holzgreve et al, 1984). Variations in the size of the Y chromosome are not considered responsible for recurrent pregnancy loss (Verma et al, 1983).

2. Abnormal chromosomal behaviour.

- Premature or delayed centromere separation leading to non-disjunctional aneuploidy in the offspring (Mehes & Kosztolanyi, 1992)
- Increased chromosomal instability detected as increased numbers of aphidicolin-induced fragile sites (Schlegelberger et al, 1989)
- Increased chromosome breaks and acentric fragments in sperm chromosomes of male partners (Rosenbusch & Sterzik, 1991).

3. Submicroscopic genetic mutations. These are inferred from circumstantial evidence and also contribute to pregnancy wastage. They include:

- familial recessive lethal genes linked to the major histocompatibility complex (Mowbray et al, 1991).
- autosomal lethal genes apparently arising *de novo* (McDonough, 1987)
- X-linked lethal syndromes, i.e. focal dermal hypoplasia, incontinentia pigmenti, oral-facial-digital I syndrome (McDonough, 1987) and the lethal multiple pterygium syndrome (Lockwood et al, 1988).

It is worth noting that recurrent spontaneous abortion is not an absolute cause of infertility. Even after three consecutive losses the chances of having a normal pregnancy are close to 60% (Smith & Gaba, 1990) but these couples are still more prone to other forms of reproductive failures, e.g. ectopic pregnancy, stillbirth, preterm birth, congenital malformation, intrauterine growth retardation and placenta praevia (Coulam et al, 1991; Thom et al, 1992).

Immunological factors (see also Ch. 41)

Immunological infertility is now a recognized entity but the magnitude of its contribution to human infertility is unknown. Clinical estimates vary widely but it is considered to be significant in 10–20% of couples with un-explained infertility, i.e. couples with no abnormalities on routine investigation of both partners and normal semen analysis (Mandelbaum et al, 1987). Immune intervention occurs at all levels of the reproductive process, including the pituitary (Kovacs & Horvath, 1987) and the gonads (Sedmak et al, 1987; Luborsky et al, 1990).

The immunogenic potential of sperm and seminal fluid is well established and yet male autoimmunization and female isoimmunization are relatively rare. The protective mechanisms essential for successful impregnation include sharing of antigens produced by the homologous male and female genital tracts (De Fazio & Ketchel, 1971) and the presence of potent immunosuppressive agents present in semen and in the genital tracts and active at multiple levels of the immune response (Alexander & Anderson, 1987; Thaler, 1989; Quan et al, 1990).

Male autoimmunization can result from genital infections, accidental trauma, anatomical abnormalities, vasectomy and herniorrhaphy with accidental vas deferens occlusion (Haas, 1987) and from a genetic predisposition associated with the HLA-B7 antigen (Mathur et al, 1983a). Female isoimmunization correlates strongly with sperm autoimmunity in the male (Mathur et al, 1981) and in infertile couples antibody titres are higher against the husband's sperms than against sperms from controls (Mathur et al, 1983b). It can result from abnormally immunogenic sperms (Mathur et al, 1988), from excessive autoimmune sperm destruction (Mathur et al, 1981) and from deficiency of immune inhibitors (Prakash, 1981). There is also a genetic predisposition to isoimmunization, as suggested by the high frequency of HLA-BW35 in women with sperm isoantibodies and the sharing of HLA-B7, HLA-B8 and HLA-BW35 in infertile couples with sperm immunity (Mathur et al, 1983a). One mechanism of sperm immunogenicity in the female and male genital tracts is the presence of immunostimulators, e.g. autoantibodies coating the sperm surface, and the secondary induction of interferon production by T cells and the release of macrophage chemotactic factor. Normally macrophages phagocytose and display processed sperm antigens on their surfaces in the absence of Ia antigens; locally produced interferon induces Ia expression on the macrophages and the concurrent display of sperm antigens and Ia antigens leads to immune system activation (Witkin, 1988).

The causal link between sperm antibodies and human infertility is well established (Bronson, 1987) with the proviso that circulating serum antibodies are not directly linked to infertility (Critser et al, 1989); the effective antibodies must be present in the genital tract fluids and bound to the sperm surface (McClure et al, 1989). The antibodies are directed against fertility-related antigens (Naz, 1990), and the immunoglobulin idiotypes and their location of binding on the sperm surface condition their clinical significance (Haas, 1987).

Four types of immune reactions to constituents of the ejaculate may occur:

1. Allergy to seminal fluid, manifested as immediate or delayed, localized or systemic, hypersensitivity reactions (Jones, 1991) and rarely as fixed cutaneous eruptions (Best et al, 1988). In the case of reaginic immunity to seminal fluid the severe systemic anaphylactic reaction and the local painful sterile vulvovaginitis can lead to avoidance of coitus and infertility by default. These couples show a high degree of sharing of HLA antigens but the significance of this finding is unclear (Jones, 1991).

2. Cell-mediated response to sperm antigens, which is a universal response to repeated exposure to sperms without any impact on fertility (Mettler, 1980).

3. Systemic response to sperm antigens: circulating antisperm antibodies are seen in similar frequency in fertile and infertile couples and do not cause infertility (Critser et al, 1989).

4. Local immune response in the female and male genital tracts is considered to be the underlying mechanism of immunological infertility. The modes of action of antisperm antibodies (Bronson, 1987; Clarke, 1988; Mahony & Alexander, 1991; Eggert-Kruse et al, 1993) include:

(i) Disturbed interaction between sperms and cervical mucus reflected in a poor postcoital test. There is reduced penetration of the mucus, decreased migration through the mucus and loss of progressive motility due to the development of the shaking phenomenon (Kremer & Jager, 1988). Coating antibodies may reduce mucus penetration by entangling their Fc portion in the glycoprotein matrix of cervical mucus (Jager et al, 1978). Massive sperm elimination in the cervix decreases their availability for intratubal fertilization.

(ii) Reduced migration through the uterine corpus and the tubes.

(iii) Blocking of the capacitation reaction, essential for sperm hyperactivation and the acrosome reaction prior to fertilization.

(iv) Failure of hyaluronidase release required for dissolution and penetration of the cumulus oophorus.

(v) Inhibition of sperm binding to, and penetration of, the zona pellucida (de Almeida et al, 1989).

(vi) Interference with the acrosome reaction.

(vii) Inhibition of sperm-egg fusion.

(viii) Postfertilization embryotoxicity (Menge, 1988) leading to subclinical abortion. There is some evidence that sperm antibodies may be a cause of recurrent clinical abortions (Haas, 1987).

(ix) Interference with nidation: sperm immobilizing antibodies, detected in the blastocyst, block endometrial implantation (Menge, 1988); this experimental finding needs clinical confirmation.

Other immunological mechanisms of interactive infertility, unrelated to coitus, include the formation of the following autoantibodies:

1. Antibodies to the zona pellucida: at present the evidence denies any rôle for these antibodies in infertility (Bronson, 1987)

2. Anti-oocyte antibodies, which may act during follicular development or after fertilization (Bronson, 1987)

3. Anti-endometrial antibodies, which may prevent apposition of trophectoderm and endometrial surface and thus inhibit implantation (Bronson, 1987)

4. Embryotoxic serum factor (? antibody) in patients with mild to moderate endometriosis (Simon et al, 1992)

Microbiological factors

The relationship between overt or subclinical genital tract infections and infertility is well established (Weström, 1980; Rosenfeld et al, 1983; Seibel, 1986). After the epidemic of sexually transmitted diseases in the seventies and early eighties, there has been an increase in STD-related infertility and ectopic pregnancy (Seibel, 1986) but the total prevalence of infertility has not increased over the last decade (Mosher & Pratt, 1991; Templeton et al, 1991). In Africa the rate of infectious infertility is over three times that of the developed countries (World Health Organization, 1987). Since upper genital tract infections in women are mostly transmitted sexually, the resultant infertility can be considered under the rubric of interactive infertility. Male contamination of the female lower genital tract can be followed by postcoital ascending infection or may remain dormant until cervical manipulation sets the stage for ascending infection (Weström, 1980). Spermatozoa make a direct contribution by carrying 'hitchhiking' bacteria on their surfaces (Keith et al 1984; Wolner-Hanssen & Mardh, 1984). As the couple constitutes a microbiological ecosystem with recycling (the 'ping pong effect'), it follows that both partners must be cultured and treated simultaneously.

The organisms involved in these infertility-causing infections (pelvic inflammatory disease) include:

1. *Neisseria gonorrhoeae* still remains an important cause of salpingitis and tubal infertility (Shafrin et al, 1992).

2. Genital mycoplasmas have been implicated in infertility and pregnancy wastage but the evidence is so far inconclusive (Taylor-Robinson & MacCormack, 1980; Rock & Zacur, 1983; Styler & Shapiro, 1985). These organisms (especially *Ureaplasma urealyticum*) have been isolated from the vagina, cervix and endometrium of infertile women with a significantly higher frequency than from controls (Stray-Pedersen et al, 1982); others have failed to confirm this (Gump et al, 1984). Cassell et al (1983) reported that *Ureaplasma urealyticum* was associated with a

defined subpopulation of infertile couples, i.e. with male factor infertility. No study has shown a higher rate of mycoplasmal isolation from damaged tubes of infertile women despite the fact that these organisms can cause severe salpingitis (Weström, 1980). There is also no evidence that doxycycline treatment of infertile couples with mycoplasma infection improves fertility (Hinton et al, 1979; Stray-Pedersen et al, 1982), the evidence implicating *Ureaplasma urealyticum* in recurrent spontaneous abortion is also inconclusive (Quinn et al, 1983a,b; Styler & Shapiro, 1985; Naessens et al, 1987).

3. *Chlamydia trachomatis* is known to cause subclinical and clinical salpingitis followed by severe tubal damage (Wolner-Hanssen et al, 1982) and there is also good experimental support of chlamydial tubal pathogenicity (Zana et al, 1990). There is now conclusive evidence that chlamydial infection is significantly associated with infertility (Anestad et al, 1987; Hodgson et al, 1990; Ruijs et al, 1991; Wessels et al, 1991) but not with recurrent abortion (Quinn et al, 1987).

4. Viruses, e.g. *Herpes simplex* (Nahmias et al, 1971) and cytomegalovirus (Kriel et al, 1970), are transmitted sexually and may cause chronic endometritis with spontaneous abortion (Dehner & Askin, 1975).

5. *Listeria monocytogenes* is no longer considered a cause of recurrent abortion (Manganiello & Yearke, 1991).

The predisposing factors to ascending genital infection in women include: genetic susceptibility, probably linked to the major histocompatibility antigens (Kuberski, 1980); young age, due to the greater penetrability of the oestrogen-dominated mucus in adolescence (Holmes et al, 1980); coitus around the time of menstruation (Holmes et al, 1980); the use of the IUCD (Eschenbach, 1992) and therapeutic or diagnostic instrumentation of the cervix (Weström, 1980). The pathogenesis involves passive transport of bacteria by unknown mechanisms, facilitated transport by bacterial adherence to sperms and trichomonads (Keith et al, 1984) and by iatrogenic disturbance of host-microbe equilibrium in the cervix leading to microbial spread mucosally or transmurally via dilated blood vessels and lymphatics (Westrom, 1980).

The mechanisms underlying inflammatory infertility are complex. Chronic endocervicitis may cause infertility by altering the mucus and impairing sperm motility, survival and penetration (Odeblad, 1978); one is tempted to associate infertility with severe chlamydial cervicitis, which causes such dramatic changes in the cervix (Hare et al, 1982) but there is to date no convincing evidence of such an association (Paavonen et al, 1979; Battin et al, 1984). Asymptomatic chronic endometritis due to *Ureaplasma urealyticum* (Horne et al, 1973; Cumming et al, 1984) is not associated with abnormal endometrial maturation or excessive formation of pelvic adhesions (Fahmy et al, 1987); infertility may be due to infection of the implanted

conceptus or depression of sperm motility, egg recognition or egg penetration (Styler & Shapiro, 1985). Chlamydial endometritis (Winkler & Crum, 1987) may contribute to infertility by secondary damage to sperms and conceptus caused by local leucocyte release of cytokines and reactive nitrogen intermediates (Tomlinson et al, 1992).

Biophysical factors

Sperm transport, essential for intratubal fertilization, is the result of a finely tuned dynamic interaction between semen and female genital tract tissues (Barratt & Cooke, 1991). There is a high rate of loss in the vagina with only about 0.05% of ejaculated sperms entering the cervix (Fordney-Settlage et al, 1973). After cervical rescue there is an early rapid phase of transport due to contraction of the uterotubal musculature, stimulated by seminal prostaglandins (Jaszczak et al, 1980), with oxytocin released at orgasm acting as a potentiator. It is uncertain whether infertility can result from failure of this mechanism, secondary to seminal prostaglandin deficiency (Bygdeman, 1970) or stressful intercourse associated with suppression of oxytocin release and neural inhibition of uterotubal activity.

The later and more important phase of sperm transport, which may last up to two days, is due to the storage and release function of the cervix (Zinamen et al, 1989). The cervix eliminates abnormal sperms (Katz et al, 1990) and may initiate capacitation, which is a prerequisite for the acrosome reaction. There is rapid transit through the uterine cavity where massive sperm phagocytosis occurs. The survivors reaching the tubes, estimated at one per every 14 million ejaculated, are then nurtured by tubal epithelium, which has been shown in vitro to enhance sperm fertilizing capacity, and by tubal fluid, which promotes the acrosome reaction by providing progesterone and human oviductin-1 (Lippes & Waugh, 1989). Finally the cumulus oophorus produces substances that promote the acrosome reaction and 'linearize' sperm motility (Barratt & Cooke, 1991).

The dynamic interaction can be perturbed at many levels but the pathophysiology of sperm transport in humans is still poorly defined. One can speculate that infertility can result from excessive sperm loss in the vagina, reduced penetration and survival in the cervix, increased elimination in the uterus and failure of terminal support by the tube and the cumulus oophorus.

Biochemical factors

Biochemical interaction between the ejaculate and the female tract is not widely appreciated. Despite the abundance of fructose in semen, glucose is the preferential substrate and is critical for sperm viability and motility

(Martikainen et al, 1980). Because of the normally low levels of glucose in semen, an alternative source of supply is provided by cervical mucus, and infertility can result when the cervical supply of glucose is reduced (Weed & Carrera, 1970). The physiological significance of glucose and fructose in cervical mucus is still unclear, especially as peak values occur only after ovulation (van der Linden et al, 1992). The seminal fluid has a higher pH than the vaginal secretions and its buffering capacity is critical for initial sperm survival. Some patients with oligospermia have significantly depressed levels of seminal free amino acids associated with reduced buffering capacity, a factor which may contribute to their infertility (Silverstroni et al, 1979). Low levels of bicarbonate in seminal fluid contribute to infertility by decreasing buffering capacity and sperm motility (Okamura et al, 1986). Finally, sperms stimulate the endometrium by direct cell-to-cell contact causing stimulation of carbonic anhydrase (Collado et al, 1979) and increased incorporation of labelled precursors into endometrial macromolecules (Hicks et al, 1980). This increased carbonic anhydrase activity, also stimulated by progesterone (Falk & Hodgen, 1972), is important in regulating pH and bicarbonate levels, which are critical for fertilization (Stambaugh et al, 1969) and implantation (Friedley & Rosen, 1975). If sperms promote fertilization and implantation, oligospermia may cause infertility by yet another mechanism. It is possible that biochemical male-female interactions may be more important than is currently realized, as is suggested by the protective effect of semen on breast cancer (Gjorgov, 1980) and the positive effect of coitus on pregnancy rates after gamete intrafallopian transfer.

FEMALE INFERTILITY

The female contribution to human infertility varies from population to population but in the West a fair estimate would be 40–50%. Often the reproductive system is involved at multiple levels but, for didactic purposes, the infertility-producing lesions will be discussed organ by organ.

Vulva and vagina

By impeding or preventing normal penovaginal intercourse and vaginal insemination, congenital and acquired abnormalities of these structures can lead to infertility in a small proportion of potentially fertile couples. Congenital malformations interfering with coitus include rigid hymen, transverse vaginal septum (Beyth & Mor-Yosef, 1982) and vaginal aplasia, which may be associated with concurrent cervicoisthmic aplasia (Niver et al, 1980) and has a poor reproductive prognosis (Singh & Devi, 1983). Acquired lesions include:

1. Infections, e.g. chronic vulvovaginitis (Friedrich, 1976) and subacute vaginitis due to *Candida albicans*, *Gardnerella vaginalis*, Trichomonas, genital mycoplasmas and *Chlamydia trachomatis* (Fordney, 1978). Asymptomatic infections of the vaginal fornices and the adjacent exocervix, detected as cervico-vaginal leucocytosis, can also contribute to infertility by decreasing sperm survival and motility; leucocyte-derived products and enhanced phagocytosis underlie this effect (Wah et al, 1990).

2. Vulvar atrophy with introital stenosis (Friedrich, 1976).

3. Mechanical disorders, e.g. scars secondary to childbirth, episiotomy, introital injury and paravaginal lesions such as uterine prolapse, ovarian fixation to vaginal vault or cervix, endometriosis of uterosacral ligaments, broad ligament varicosities and the Allen–Masters syndrome (Fordney, 1978).

4. Drug-induced dysfunction seen with amphetamines and cocaine (Gay & Shepard, 1972).

It is worth noting that organic dyspareunia can lead to vaginismus. Despite their positive effects on the frequency and enjoyability of coitus, some vaginal lubricants may reduce fertility by their spermicidal action and their depressant effect on sperm motility (Boyers et al, 1987).

Uterine cervix

The cervix plays a critical rôle in reproduction by controlling sperm transport and by protecting the intrauterine conceptus from premature expulsion and ascending infection (Chretien, 1978). Impediment to sperm ascent can be due to mechanical or biophysical abnormalities. The mechanical lesions of the cervix constitute a rare cause of infertility and include:

1. Malposition of the cervix due to severe anteflexion of the cervix, fixed retroversion of the uterus or uterine prolapse. The significant spatial dissociation between the external os and the vaginal pool, aggravated by oligospermia, can seriously curtail upward sperm migration (Moghissi, 1979).

2. Stenosis can follow the trauma of delivery, criminal abortion and diagnostic or therapeutic instrumentation. Conization for cervical neoplasia is a rare cause of stenosis, which can be managed by dilatation (Moinian & Andersch, 1982) and there is no convincing evidence that it impairs fertility (Weber & Obel, 1979). Stenosis is not seen after cryotherapy (Hemmingson, 1982) or electrocoagulation diathermy (Hollyock et al, 1983). Congenital aplasia of the cervix (Niver et al, 1980) is rare and is often associated with absence of the vagina and/or of the uterine isthmus, i.e. the Rokitansky–Küstner–Hauser syndrome (Golan et al, 1989), which rarely may be caused by maternal galactosaemia (Cramer et al, 1987). Pure cervical

aplasia leads to haematometra with reflux menstruation and tubo-ovarian endometriosis. When combined with isthmic atresia there is reflex suppression of menstruation and no ensuing haematometra (Musset et al, 1978). As a rule, cervical aplasia presents with painful or painless amenorrhoea fairly early in adolescence but, unless successfully treated (Zarou et al, 1973), it can be a cause of permanent sterility.

Mucus is fundamental to cervical function (Nasir-ud-Dhin et al, 1982). The cervix can be viewed as a biological valve which is closed to spermatozoal penetration for most of the cycle and allows entry only in the periovulatory period. The valve is controlled by hormone-induced variations in the physical properties of cervical mucus with its highly organized infrastructure. Its glycoprotein solid phase is disposed as a meshwork of fibrils cross-linked by oblique or transverse bonds, i.e. a 'tricot-like macromolecular arrangement' (Odeblad, 1968; Cazabat et al, 1982; Barros et al, 1985). At mid-cycle, with rising oestrogen levels, endocervical secretions increase in amount with higher levels of sialomucin (Gaton et al, 1982) and a higher content of water and salt (Gould & Ansari, 1983) causing viscosity to drop, stretchability (spinnbarkeit) to increase and characteristic fern patterns to appear on air drying. This mucoid hydrogel (E-type mucus) is organized into fibrils to form a meshwork large enough to allow sperm passage and these fibrillar 'micelles' act as harmonic oscillators promoting onward progress of sperms through the intermicellar spaces by 'thermal modulations' which can cause the cavities to expand and contract rhythmically (Odeblad, 1962). With low levels of oestrogen in the early part of the cycle and after the menopause and with high levels of progesterone in the luteal phase and in pregnancy (Chretien, 1978) the glycoprotein chains assume greater autonomy and form tighter cross-linkages to produce an obstructive meshwork (G-type mucus). Postpartum mucus (Vigil et al, 1991) from amenorrhoeic breast-feeding women is predominantly of the dense obstructive pattern but some samples are of the penetrable spongy periovulatory type, which probably accounts for the occasional 'contraceptive failure' of lactational infertility.

Another important periovulatory change in cervical mucus is chemical and consists of a significant decrease in the content of C'3, immunoglobulins, proteinase inhibitors and lysozyme, substances potentially harmful to sperm viability and motility (Schumacher et al, 1977). The fertility-promoting effects of these periovulatory alterations in cervical mucus include (Moghissi, 1979):

1. rapid sequestration of viable sperms from the lethal vaginal acidic milieu
2. storage and preservation of actively motile sperms, particularly in the large and giant crypts of the endocervix (Insler et al, 1980)

3. sustained and prolonged postcoital release of sperms into the uterine cavity thus enhancing the probability of successful fertilization.

Interaction between cervical mucus and sperms is critical for their survival and ability to reach and fertilize the ovum and can be studied clinically with the use of the postcoital test (Overstreet, 1986). Abnormalities of cervical mucus, i.e. the cervical factor (Zegers et al, 1981), can be a cause of infertility in 5–10% of women and they include:

1. Inadequate mucus secretion due to surgical removal or electrical destruction of the endocervical glands, end-organ insensitivity to oestrogen due to hypoplasia or receptor deficiency (Abuzeid et al, 1987) and oestrogen deficiency (Roumen et al, 1982), which also produces viscid impenetrable mucus (Sher & Katz, 1976; Vigil et al, 1991).

2. Changes in composition resulting from chronic cervicitis or cervicovaginitis. Depending on the type, duration and severity of the inflammation the secretory cells lose their sensitivity to oestrogen and start to secrete autonomously E- or G-type mucus and a third type (Q type) of mucus, which is variable in constitution and is made up of subunits or partial components. This viscid mucus, consisting of a mixture of E, G and Q types of mucus, is impenetrable to sperms (Odeblad, 1978). Penetrability is also reduced by increasing acidity with inflammation (Ansari et al, 1980). Finally, inflammation increases cervical levels of immunoglobulins and inflammatory mediators (Wah et al, 1990), which are potentially toxic to sperms (Tomlinson et al, 1992).

3. The presence of sperm-coating autoantibodies or isoantibodies on the sperm surface (Shulman, 1986) decreases mucus penetration by entangling the Fc portion in the glycoprotein matrix of the mucus (Jager et al, 1978). The immunological reaction also causes mucus hypersecretion and intraluminal exudation of active leucocytes (Nicosia & Johnson, 1983) with acidification of the mucus (Parish & Ward, 1968).

4. Production of a hostile mucus after clomiphene citrate treatment due to abnormally high levels of testosterone in the mid-follicular and periovulatory periods; this can be reversed by adding oestrogen to the treatment schedule (Langer et al, 1990; Gelety & Buyalos, 1993).

5. Specific incompatibility of sperm and mucus in some infertile couples for unknown reasons (Overstreet, 1986).

Cervical incompetence

The cervix plays a critical rôle in pregnancy by mechanically supporting the enlarging conceptus and preventing its premature expulsion. It is not surprising therefore that cervical incompetence can lead to repeated pregnancy loss in the second trimester. An aetiological classification of cervical incompetence includes four types (Shortle & Jewelewicz, 1989):

1. Acquired: a gross defect is visible in the cervix. This follows traumatic deliveries with inadequately repaired lacerations or may be iatrogenic, i.e. produced by diagnostic and therapeutic procedures. Excessive and rapid cervical dilatation during dilatation and curettage is the commonest causative factor but there is no consensus about the rôle of the more gradual and more gentle dilatation achieved by laminaria tents during induced second-trimester abortions. Conization can cause incompetence depending on cone size and depth but cryotherapy and shallow laser surgery are harmless.

2. Congenital: the cervix is grossly normal but there is a histological defect which compromises its ability to resist pressure during pregnancy. This can be due to an abnormally high ratio of smooth muscle to collagen, a deficiency of elastin or a biochemical abnormality in the collagen, as in the Ehlers–Danlos syndrome (Leduc & Wasserstrum, 1992). Primary incompetence is also common with prenatal exposure to DES and in association with uterine anomalies.

3. Physiological or dysfunctional: early effacement and dilatation of the cervix follow subclinical inappropriate uterine irritability.

4. Anatomical: the normal cervico-isthmic region is distorted by local lesions, e.g. low-lying leiomyomas.

The diagnosis of cervical incompetence is suggested by recurrent second-trimester spontaneous abortions in the absence of uterine contractions, especially if the fetus is fresh and not macerated or survives briefly after expulsion. During pregnancy, symptoms include a sense of pressure in the lower abdomen or in the upper vagina, watery or mucoid vaginal discharge and urinary frequency and urgency without dysuria. The diagnostic sign is the palpation or visualization of bulging membranes in the second trimester without evidence of premature labour. Diagnosis is more difficult in the non-pregnant state and relies on the use of dilators, hysterosalpingography and ultrasonography (Zlatnik & Burmeister, 1993; Guzman et al, 1994). The indications for treatment and the therapeutic modalities, including cerclage, remain controversial.

Corpus uteri

The corpus uteri plays a vital rôle in reproduction by providing a free passageway to the sperms in their ascent from cervix to tube and by harbouring the conceptus from implantation to delivery. Its function depends on normal structural development, its position relative to the cervix and the structural and functional integrity of its blood supply and its two components, i.e. endometrium and myometrium. Corporeal abnormalities, causing infertility by interfering with pre- and postfertilization events, can be classified as structural, positional, vascular, endometrial, and myometrial.

Structural abnormalities

These lesions, whether arising spontaneously or after intrauterine exposure to diethylstilboestrol (DES), are an uncommon cause of female infertility by preventing conception and increasing pregnancy loss. They are discussed in Chapter 2.

Positional disturbances

There is little evidence to suggest that infertility can result from abnormal positions of the uterus per se. For instance, fixed retroversion is due to concomitant pelvic disease, e.g. endometriosis or salpingitis, which is more likely to underlie the infertility (Wallach, 1972). Uterine hyperflexion has been implicated in infertility and recurrent abortion (Liliequist & Lindgren, 1964).

Vascular abnormalities

Anatomical variations of blood vessels are usually harmless but in the uterus a simple variation of arterial supply can lead to a significant increase in the incidence of low birth weight infants and of early sporadic, but not necessarily recurrent, abortion. Normally the uterine artery gives off a single ascending branch from which all the arcuate arteries arise. In some patients the ascending artery divides into two separate branches which give rise to the anterior and posterior arcuate arteries and this arterial configuration is associated with reproductive dysfunction (Burchell et al, 1978). This suggests that an adequate uterine blood supply is essential for successful pregnancy. The rôle of uterine vascular insufficiency in infertility and early pregnancy loss is gaining support from Doppler studies of uterine blood flow (Goswany et al, 1988; Kurjak et al, 1991; Steer et al, 1994). Postpubertal uterine growth is also critically dependent on adequate perfusion and uterine hypoplasia can be produced experimentally by devascularization (Gardey et al, 1975a) or prevented by combining devascularization with beta-adrenergic drug therapy (Gardey et al, 1975b). It is likely, although unproven, that the hypoplastic or infantile uterus, seen in endocrinologically normal adults and characterized by a small uterus with a disproportionately long, narrow, poorly vascularized cervix with a pinhole os, is the result of congenital hypovascularity. The associated infertility (Field-Richards, 1954) is due to a combination of factors, i.e. the hypoplastic endometrium and myometrium, the poorly developed cervix, and the associated shallow vaginal fornix and retroflexion or acute anteflexion of the uterus.

Myometrial abnormalities

Uterine adenomyosis, except when combined with traumatic uterine synechiae (Klein & Garcia, 1973), does not cause infertility (Owalabi & Strickler, 1977) and the only relevant myometrial lesion is the leiomyoma, which clinically can be confused with an adenomatoid tumour (Honoré, unpublished observations), an adenomyoma (Honoré et al, 1988a) or the rare leiomyosarcoma (Hitti et al, 1991). This common benign tumour, much commoner in black than in white women (Sengupta et al, 1978), usually occurs in perimenopausal women and is thus an infrequent cause of infertility (Buttram & Reiter, 1981). The mechanisms underlying the infertility include:

1. Interference with sperm transport. The tumour may mechanically obstruct sperm passage through the cervix and the uterotubal junction or it may distort the uterine cavity, thus increasing the distance to be covered by the sperms (Hunt & Wallach, 1974). It may also interfere with sperm transport facilitation by rhythmic myometrial contraction induced by seminal prostaglandins (Coutinho & Maia, 1971).

2. Myometrial irritation and hyperactivity due to degeneration or torsion of the tumour.

3. Atrophy or alteration of the endometrium overlying a submucous leiomyoma (Fig. 33.1), if extensive, can prevent successful nidation.

4. Vascular disturbances in the endometrium may interfere with implantation. A leiomyoma may compress endometrial and myometrial venous plexuses to cause venous ectasia and congestion or hypoperfusion of the endometrium (Farrer-Brown et al, 1971). There is also a significant reduction in the blood flow through the leiomyoma and adjacent uterus (Forssman, 1976).

5. Failure of blastocyst retention. It has been suggested that the biological function of endometrial thickening in the luteal phase, produced by tissue increase, stromal oedema and particularly by occlusion and distension of the secretory glands, is to obliterate the lumen and retain the blastocyst. Irregularity of the lumen caused by leiomyoma(s) could prevent its complete occlusion and thus blastocycst retention (Datnow, 1973).

6. Associated salpingitis (Mitami et al, 1959).

7. Bilateral cornual obstruction by multiple leiomyomas which can be successfully treated by a GnRH agonist (Gardner & Shaw, 1989).

The rôle of myomectomy in the treatment of infertility and habitual abortion is limited (Berkeley et al, 1983) but it undoubtedly improves fertility in some patients (Garcia & Tureck, 1984). The factors determining the success of myomectomy include (Buttram & Reiter, 1981; Verkauf, 1992): uterine size at the time of surgery, tumour number, size and location, co-existence of other causes of infertility, postoperative recurrence with a 10-year cumulative rate of 27% (Candiani et al, 1991; Friedman et al, 1992)

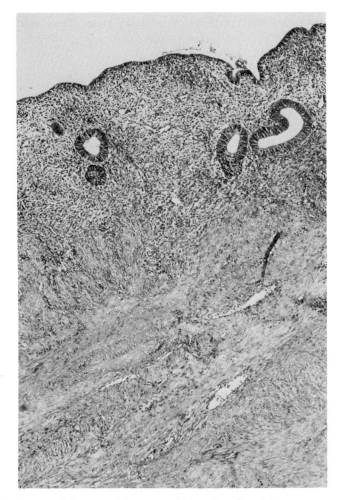

Fig. 33.1 Submucous leiomyoma with atrophy of overlying endometrium. H & E × 59.

and the surgical induction of pelvic adhesions (Berkeley et al, 1983).

Endometrial abnormalities

The endometrium, which is the site of implantation, undergoes an orderly series of hormonally controlled structural, histochemical, biochemical and vascular changes (see Ch. 10). These cyclical changes, i.e. proliferation, secretory transformation and gestational decidualization or menstruation, affect principally the anterior and posterior walls of the corpus with the isthmus and cornua exhibiting lesser degrees of proliferation (Ferenczy et al, 1979) and secretory alterations. It is tempting to suggest that such geographical disparities underlie nature's way of preventing isthmic or cornual implantation with its attendant complications.

Unlike the proliferative phase, the secretory or luteal phase is more constant in duration and the tissue changes follow a fairly uniform schedule, which allows accurate day dating of the secretory endometrium (Noyes et al, 1950). Despite early warnings (Noyes & Haman, 1954) the accuracy of endometrial dating and the ability of the endometrium to reflect corpus luteum function has been taken for granted and the clinical diagnosis of luteal phase deficiency is now based on at least two sequential endometrial biopsies showing a discrepancy of more than ± two days between histological dating and chronological dating established by the time of occurrence of post-biopsy menstruation. This simplistic equation between endometrial dating and corpus luteum dysfunction is now under attack on multiple fronts, as follows:

1. The accuracy of histological day dating is affected by subjectivity of interpretation (Scott et al, 1993) and by regional endometrial variability. The overall error (Gibson et al, 1991) is due to inconsistencies between evaluators (65%), intra-observer discrepancies (27%) and regional differences in the endometrium (8%). This lack of precision of endometrial dating (Li et al, 1989) has raised serious doubts about its value in the diagnosis of luteal phase defects and it has been estimated that a false positive diagnosis may be made in 22–39% of patients, depending on the clinical setting (Scott et al, 1988). Hence the need to devise other methods of endometrial evaluation, e.g. morphometry (Kim-Bjorklund et al, 1991; Li et al, 1991), immunocytochemistry (Self et al, 1989; Tabibzadeh, 1990), biochemistry (Klentzeris et al, 1991). It is unlikely that ultrasonographic measurement of endometrial thickness can replace endometrial biopsy (Li T-C et al, 1992).

2. The timing of the endometrial biopsy can influence the accuracy of endometrial dating. Most authors recommend a late luteal phase biopsy, i.e. about 2 days before the expected menses, but recent studies claim that accuracy of dating is better when the biopsy is taken in the first half of the luteal phase (Li et al, 1991; Castelbaum et al, 1994).

3. The criteria used for chronological dating of the cycle: the classical method uses the first day of the post-biopsy menstruation to define the length of the luteal phase (retrospective dating) but new evidence suggests that greater accuracy is achieved when the dating is prospective using the day of LH surge as the landmark (Bonhoff et al, 1990; Kim-Bjorklund et al, 1991; Li et al, 1991).

4. The type of biopsy instrument, i.e. the stainless steel Novak curette or the polypropylene cannula ('Pipelle'), can significantly affect the frequency of out of phase endometrial biopsies, raising the possibility that the diagnosis of an inadequate luteal phase can be influenced by a purely technical factor (Honoré et al, 1988b).

5. The incidence of luteal phase defect, as determined by serial endometrial biopsies, was found not to be significantly different between a fertile and an infertile population (Davis et al, 1989): this casts some doubt on the standard criteria for diagnosing luteal defect but the study was small and uncontrolled.

Despite these criticisms luteal phase deficiency is still recognized as a cause of infertility and recurrent abortion and the endometrial biopsy remains a useful, although not fully validated, test of corpus luteum function (Davidson et al, 1987; McNeely & Soules, 1988; Li & Cooke, 1991). The luteal phase defect, diagnosed by endometrial biopsy, is due to inadequate progesterone secretion following normal or deficient folliculogenesis (Grunfeld et al, 1989) or to an inappropriate response of the endometrium to normal progesterone levels (Cumming et al, 1985; McNeely & Soules, 1988). It is more common after ovulation induction by clomiphene citrate and is due to defective follicular maturation (Keenan et al, 1989) or a direct anti-oestrogenic effect without steroid receptor disruption (Fritz et al, 1991). It is usually manifested by retarded secretory maturation of the endometrium; the significance of such qualitative abnormalities as gland-stroma dissociation or persistence of oestrogenic influence remains unestablished (McNeely & Soules, 1988).

Unlike the variable proliferative phase, the secretory phase is more constant in duration and the tissue changes follow a fairly uniform schedule, which allows accurate 'dating' of the secretory endometrium (Noyes et al, 1950).

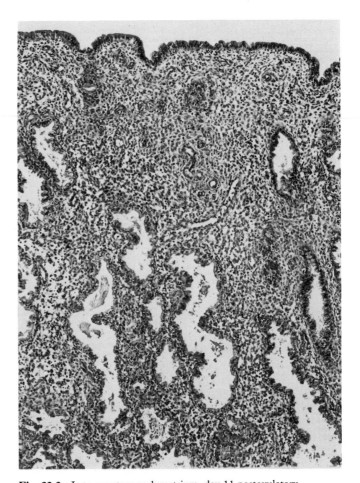

Fig. 33.2 Late secretory endometrium, day 11 postovulatory. H & E × 59.

Despite the fact that gestational hyperplasia has been beautifully described and illustrated by Hertig (1954), it regularly goes unrecognized in endometrial biopsies taken during the luteal phase of the cycle of conception (Karrow et al, 1971; Rosenfeld & Garcia, 1975; Mazur et al, 1989). In the sterile cycle the phase of active glandular secretions peaks around day 6 postovulatory and is followed by progressive epithelial exhaustion; the stromal phase, typified by condensation of stroma with loss of oedema, vascular development and stromal growth and differentiation (Fig. 33.2), starts after the ninth postovulatory day. With early pregnancy there is overlapping and exaggeration of the glandular and stromal phases (Hertig, 1954). I have found the following criteria (Honoré & Scott, 1982) useful in the diagnosis of a concurrent undisturbed pregnancy from a luteal phase endometrial biopsy:

1. Focal resurgence of subnuclear vacuolization in the surface epithelium and in the subsurface glands, seen only in early or midluteal biopsies.

2. Persistence and exaggeration of glandular secretion in the presence of well-developed arterial fields and decidualization (Fig. 33.3).

3. Co-existence of patchy oedema with well-established vascular and predecidual changes (Fig. 33.4).

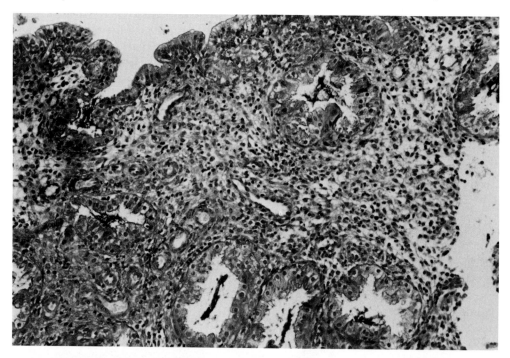

Fig. 33.3 'Secretory' endometrium with viable undisturbed intrauterine pregnancy: persistent and enhanced glandular secretion in presence of arterial fields and stromal decidualization. PAS–Alcian Blue × 147.

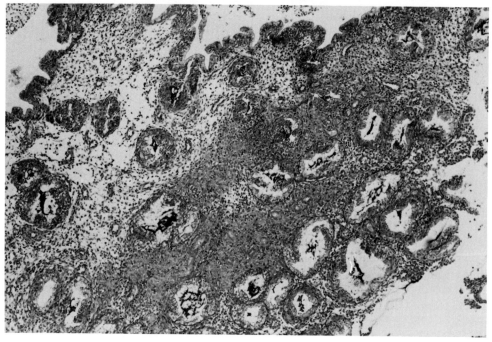

Fig. 33.4 'Secretory' endometrium with viable undisturbed intrauterine pregnancy: co-existence of stromal oedema, well-developed arterial fields, perivascular decidualization and persistent glandular secretion. PAS–Alcian Blue × 147.

4. Dilatation and congestion of the superficial blood vessels.

5. Reduced 'leucocytic' infiltration of the premenstrual stroma (Daly et al, 1982). These 'leucocytes' are stromal granulocytes, which become degranulated and apparently more prominent as the premenstrual endometrium dehydrates and the stromal cells shrink. The early gestational endometrium does not undergo premenstrual collapse and the stromal granulocytes appear less prominent, without any decrease in numbers (Mazur et al, 1989).

The diagnosis of an undisturbed concurrent pregnancy was followed in some cases by a successful pregnancy and in others by 'menstruation'. Because of the high rate of early embryonic mortality (Edmonds et al, 1982) it is hypothesized that 'menstruation' followed postimplantation failure or, in other words, the bleeding was due to a subclinical abortion. This hypothesis, which is now being tested by combined hormonal and morphological studies, is indirectly supported by the detection of a degenerating conceptus (Fig. 33.5) in curettings obtained from an infertile patient.

Endometrial disturbances often passively reflect ovarian dysfunction but there are primary endometrial lesions, which can be the dominant cause of infertility. These include:

1. Endometrial insensitivity to progesterone resulting in a proliferative pattern in the presence of normal luteal levels of progesterone (Perez et al, 1981) or in the selective persistence of proliferative stroma (Keller et al, 1979).

2. Acquired uterine adhesions (Asherman syndrome). This endometrial lesion is discussed in detail in Chapter 12.

3. Endometrial polyps have been described in patients with primary and secondary infertility (Valle, 1980) but their aetiological significance must be viewed with caution, as suggested by a study showing a 15% incidence of polyps in women with no apparent cause of infertility except voluntary tubal sterilization (Goerzen et al, 1983). There is some evidence that fertility impairment may be due to a higher propensity to spontaneous abortion (Overstreet, 1959).

4. Chronic endometritis, which can be divided into non-specific and specific forms, is a rare cause of infertility (Czernobilsky, 1978). Non-specific chronic endometritis is typically due to ascending infection from the lower tract and can be part of a generalized genital infection or can follow an abortion or delivery, usually complicated by retention of decidua and/or fetal tissue, or can result from stagnation of menstrual flow due to obstruction by isthmic or cervical stenosis, polyps or neoplasms. Rarely it can follow retention of fetal bones with secondary infertility (Dawood & Jarrett, 1982) or cause metaplastic endometrial ossification with primary infertility (Wetzels et al, 1982). The associated infertility is often due to more important associated lesions but on occasions antibiotic

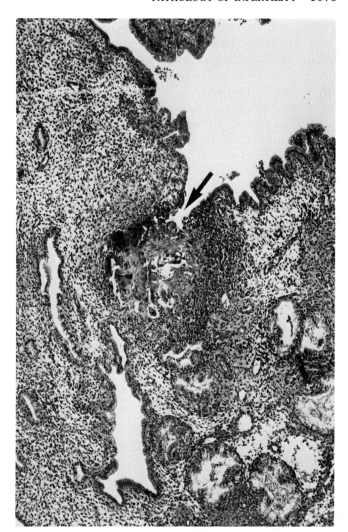

Fig. 33.5 Late 'secretory' endometrium with early postimplantation failure: 'ulceration' of endometrial surface epithelium, degenerating trophoblast and lymphoid infiltration of adjacent stroma. H & E × 147.

treatment results in successful pregnancy. The specific forms of chronic endometritis include:

(i) Tuberculous endometritis is a rare cause of infertility in the West but has a significantly higher prevalence in developing countries (Bazak-Malik et al, 1983). The lesion, typically involving the spongiosa and the compacta and less commonly the basalis and the myometrium, consists in most cases of single or coalescent granulomas with absent, minimal or rarely extensive caseation (Fig. 33.6), epithelioid cells, lymphocytes, scanty plasma cells and a variable number of Langhans giant cells. In some cases tubercles are not seen and the focal or diffuse infiltration is made up of lymphocytes, plasma cells and a few eosinophils, but the presence of dilated glands with or without intraluminal exudate or glands with microabscesses should alert the pathologist to the fact that tuberculous endometritis can masquerade as a non-specific non-granulomatous lesion (Govan, 1962; Bazak-Malik et al, 1983). Acid-fast bacilli are rarely detected in excised tissue but guinea pig inoculations are consistently positive (Nogales-Ortiz et al, 1979). Endometrial tuberculosis is usually secondary to descending infection from the infected tubes and tuberculous infertility can be due to a combination of endometrial and tubal damage. Despite intensive therapy the reproductive prognosis is poor (Schaeffer, 1976).

(ii) Mycoplasmal endometritis has been described in patients investigated for infertility (Horne et al, 1973; Stray-Pedersen et al, 1982; Cumming et al, 1984) but the actual rôle of *Ureaplasma urealyticum* in the causation of infertility is still unsettled. The lesion, as a rule asymptomatic, consists of a non-granulomatous non-necrotizing subacute inflammation featuring a variable number of small discrete clusters of lymphocytes lying under the surface epithelium or flanking the occasional gland or blood vessel (Fig. 33.7). The lymphocytes often infiltrate the glandular epithelium without causing necrosis. This inflammatory reaction, typically focal, discrete and centred on anatomical structures, differs from the commonly encountered lymphoid follicles in perimenopausal women

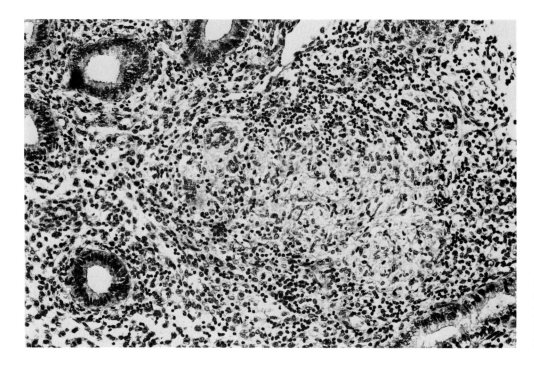

Fig. 33.6 Tuberculous endometritis: non-caseating epithelioid granuloma with Langhans giant cells. H & E × 210. (Courtesy of Dr. R. Hodkinson, Edmonton.)

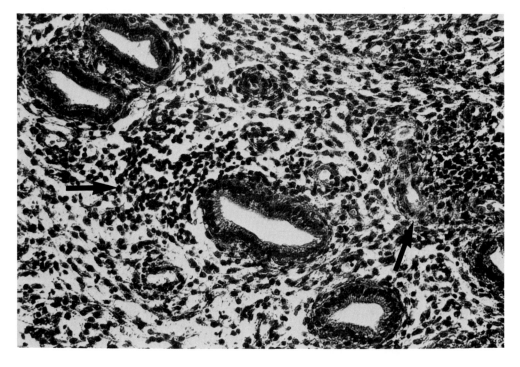

Fig. 33.7 Mycoplasmal endometritis (*Ureaplasma urealyticum* isolated from endometrial biopsy sample): patchy discrete paraglandular and paravascular lymphocytic clusters (arrows). H & E × 147.

(Sen & Fox, 1967) which lie in the deep stroma without any glandular or vascular relationship, and also from the premenstrual leucocyte infiltration of the stroma (Daly et al, 1982), which is diffuse and bears no relationship to blood vessels, glands or surface epithelium. The significance of this subacute focal endometritis is still undefined but we find it more commonly in biopsies obtained from infertile patients (Honoré, personal observations). Some authors have claimed that subacute focal endometritis is a significant indicator of pelvic adhesions and endometriosis (Burke et al, 1985); we have failed to confirm this and we have found that this lesion does not interfere with normal secretory maturation of the endometrium (Fahmy et al, 1987).

(iii) Chlamydial endometritis is an uncommon, and certainly an underdiagnosed, finding in infertility (Gump et al, 1984). It arises by direct contiguous spread from the inflamed cervix and is usually associated with a salpingitis (Wolner-Hanssen et al, 1982). Histologically the lesion resembles non-specific endometritis and is characterized by loss of glandular response to progesterone and infiltration of the superficial endometrium by plasma cells, lymphocytes and polymorphs (Winkler & Crum, 1987). Undoubtedly chlamydial endometritis contributes to infertility but it is not clear whether it can be a sole cause.

The mechanisms underlying human infertility related to chronic endometritis are unknown but they include the toxic effects of leucocytic extracts on ascending spermatozoa (Tredway et al, 1975) and on the preimplantation zygote (Parr & Shirley, 1976).

5. Biochemical defects have been sporadically identified in the endometria of infertile women but there has been no controlled systematic study of endometrial biochemistry in infertility. Hughes et al (1963) showed that endometria obtained from women with infertility and repeated abortions were deficient in RNA and DNA, glycogen, alkaline phosphatase, glucose-6-phosphatase, isocitric dehydrogenase and malic dehydrogenase; without concurrent hormone studies they were unable to determine if these deficiencies were primary or secondary. Disturbances in glycogen metabolism (Mimori et al, 1981), e.g. significantly reduced levels of glycogen, glycogen synthetase and glycogen phosphorylase, were detected in endometria of patients with unexplained infertility in the presence of normal progesterone levels; the authors could not establish whether these deficiencies were due to an abnormal endometrial response or reflected inadequate oestrogenic stimulation in the follicular phase. In some patients with unexplained infertility, there is defective biosynthesis and distribution of glycoconjugates in the glandular epithelium, as determined by lectin histochemistry; as these substances play a significant rôle in recognition and attachment (the 'sugar language'), their deficiency and maldistribution may lead to implantation failure (Klentzeris et al, 1991). Finally, a deficiency of the oestrogen and progesterone sensitive endometrial RNA polymerase has been reported in women with persistent unexplained infertility (Soutter et al, 1979). The rôle of primary biochemical or molecular aberrations of the endometrium in infertility remains uncharted territory.

6. Abnormal ciliary structure in the endometrial surface epithelium was reported in a 29-year-old woman with primary infertility and Kartagener's syndrome (Marchini et al, 1992). The cilia lacked the central pair of microtubules and one of the outer doublets was transposed, while the dynein arms were unaffected. It was suggested that ciliary immotility or dyskinesia altered the flow of endometrial secretions and interfered with the upstream migration of spermatozoa.

The Fallopian tube

The tube plays a pivotal rôle in reproduction by regulating bidirectional gamete transport, providing the site for fertilization, supporting the newly fertilized zygote and releasing it after a physiologically timed delay (Bateman et al 1987; Harper, 1988). As the tube is geographically specialized it is tempting to ascribe unique functions to these individual segments but experience with clinical and experimental ablative surgery has shown that appreciable functional compensation occurs when isolated segments are missing. Thus in rabbits selective microsurgical resection of the fimbria, ampulla, ampulloisthmic junction (AIJ) and uteroisthmic junction (UIJ) has failed to significantly impair fertility but excision of the fimbria along with the distal ampulla (Halbert & McComb, 1981) and of the entire isthmus including the AIJ and UIJ (McComb et al, 1981) causes sterility. In women successful pregnancy occurs, although at a variably reduced rate, after selective segmental loss (Gomel, 1983). Aside from patency the crucial factor for maintenance of fertility is tubal length (McComb et al, 1981); in humans, following microsurgical reversal of tubal sterilization, the critical length is 5 cm and the pregnancy rate drops from 100% to 18% as tubal length decreases to below 3 cm (Silber & Cohen, 1983; Rock et al, 1987). Experimental tubal lengthening in rabbits reduces fertility (Bateman et al, 1983) but it is not clear whether human infertility can result from excessively long tubes, as seen in some women with idiopathic infertility after intrauterine exposure to diethylstilboestrol. Dependency on the tube is not absolute as evidenced by the low but far from negligible pregnancy rate after the Estes operation, i.e. intrauterine ovarian implantation (Adams, 1979).

The tubal mechanisms ensuring gamete transport are not fully understood (Jansen, 1984). In women the ovum reaches the fimbria seven hours after ovulation, stays in the ampulla for 72 hours and traverses the isthmus rapidly to reach the uterine cavity after 80 hours (Croxatto et al, 1978; Harper, 1987). Ovum pick-up is achieved by increased periovulatory contractility of the ovary, meso-tubarium ovaricum and adnexal ligaments (Morikawa et al, 1980); as a result the fimbria sweep the ovarian surface and directly contact the ovum as it emerges through the ovulation stigma.

This contact between ovum and tubal fimbriae is enhanced by the presence of a sticky gelatinous matrix on the outer aspect of the cumulus oophorus. The fimbrial cilia, stuck to the outer cumulus, pull it out into long streamers as they move the ovum towards the tubal ostium, a process aided by rhythmic contractions of the fimbriae and adjacent broad ligament (Harper, 1987). This anatomical and functional co-operation between tube and ovary is not essential for ovum capture as pregnancy occurs after salpingoneostomy (Gomel, 1983), microsurgical dissociation of ovary and fimbria (Eddy & Laufe, 1983) and when the patient has one functional tube and ovary on opposite sides (First, 1954). In the ampulla the ovum is conveyed *ad uterum* by to-and-fro pendular motions caused by alternating peristaltic waves propagated for short distances in the tubal muscle. This random Brownian movement of the ovum has a definite aduterine bias provided for by at least three possible mechanisms, i.e. aduterine ciliary action (Verdugo et al, 1980), asymmetry of muscular contraction with statistical preponderance *ad uterum* (Chatkoff, 1975) and the peculiar tubal anatomy with a reflecting barrier at the fimbria and an absorbing barrier at the isthmus (Portnow et al, 1977). The compensatory synergism between ciliary and muscular action in the ampulla is shown by the occasional pregnancy after surgical reversal of an ampullary segment in rabbits (McComb et al, 1980) and the occurrence of fertility (Jean et al, 1979) or infertility (McComb et al, 1986) in women with defective cilia depending on the degree of ciliary dyskinesia.

The transient hold-up followed by eventual release of the ovum at the ampulloisthmic junction is a consistent phenomenon but its *modus operandi* is uncertain (Sayegh & Mastroianni, 1991). The following mechanisms have been proposed:

1. The ampulloisthmic junction, which displays periodic electrical activity, dilates for a brief period after ovulation and allows passage of the ovum (Anand & Guha, 1982). This process is probably facilitated by ovum size reduction, achieved by stripping of the cumulus and corona cells by locally secreted acid phosphatase (Gupta et al, 1970).

2. The periovulatory rise in oestrogen levels leads to the production of tenacious mucus in the isthmus and to ciliary immobilization; postovulatory progesterone disperses the mucus and frees the cilia for ovum carriage (Jansen, 1980).

3. Modulation of adrenoreceptor activity of the isthmic muscle: alpha-activity and muscle contraction are pro-moted by high periovulatory oestrogen levels: beta-activity and muscle relaxation are enhanced by rising postovulatory progesterone levels (Korenaga & Kadota, 1981). This shift in adrenoreceptor function is favoured by the higher concentration of postovulatory progesterone in isthmic than in ampullary tissues (De Voto et al, 1980) and the predominance of beta receptors in the inner longitudinal and circular coats of the isthmus (Wilhelmsson & Lindblom, 1981). Vasoactive intestinal polypeptide may also contribute to the postovulatory relaxation of the isthmic sphincter (Harper, 1987; Sayegh & Mastroianni, 1991).

Finally, isthmic transport of the ovum is rapid (Croxatto et al, 1978) and is due to ciliary action (Jansen, 1980) or, more likely, to periodic to-and-fro muscular contractions resulting in forward motion through the uteroisthmic junction (McComb et al, 1981).

Transport of the bulky immotile ovum is absolutely dependent on tubal activity but migration of sperms to and through the tube is largely contingent on their morphology and motility with only 'normal' motile sperms reaching the ampulla (Fordney-Settlage et al 1973). Sperm passage through the isthmus is facilitated around the time of ovulation by the thick intraluminal mucus, which provides a three-dimensional meshwork for upstream sperm migration and also reduces antagonistic downstream ciliary action and fluid flow. With its mucus plug the isthmus resembles the cervix and exerts an additional 'purifying' effect (Jansen, 1980). The isthmus is also critical in preventing polyspermy (Hunter & Leglise, 1971) by reducing the number of sperms entering the ampulla. Since the number of sperms reaching the tube is directly proportional to the sperm density of the ejaculate (Fordney-Settlage et al, 1973) it is possible that the isthmic filter is overwhelmed in cases of polyzoospermia (Glezerman et al, 1982) resulting in polyspermy and embryonic loss. In the ampulla the vastly reduced numbers of motile sperms, i.e. probably less than 200, swim up the tube to reach the peritoneal cavity for macrophagic disposal and they only accumulate in the ampulla when the ostium is closed (Ahlgren, 1975).

The tube plays an active rôle in supporting perifertilization events, which include (Aitken, 1979):

1. Preparation of the sperm for ovum penetration. Metabolic support of sperm viability depends on multiple factors in tubal secretion, i.e. glucose, lactate, pyruvate, amylase, LDH, glycerophosphoryl choline diesterase and an unidentified heat-labile factor found in the ewe and the rabbit. Capacitation is a prerequisite for sperms to be able to penetrate the zona pellucida and form pronuclei; with human sperms the process in vitro takes about two hours but exactly where and how it occurs in vivo is unknown. Albumin and calcium are somehow involved and the rôle of the seminal decapacitation factor is obscure (Van der

Ven et al, 1982). During capacitation there is loss of cholesterol and proteins with increased fluidity of the sperm plasma membrane and calcium permeability. This sets the stage for the spontaneous or zona-induced acrosome reaction which allows the sperm to release hyaluronidase and acrosin for zona penetration (Storey, 1991). Following capacitation the acrosome reaction sets the stage for zonal penetration by generating on the inner acrosomal membrane a trypsin-like enzyme (acrosin) essential for digesting a path for the sperms through the zona. This process, highly sensitive to protease inhibitors, is facilitated by the periovulatory drop in such inhibitors in tubal secretion.

2. Preparation of ovum for sperm penetration. Partial zona exposure is achieved by stripping the corona cells surrounding the ovum; bicarbonate, which increases in concentration after ovulation, is one of the mediators.

3. The embryotrophic rôle of the tube is indirectly supported by the failure of most mammalian preimplantation embryos to sustain prolonged normal growth and development even in the best in vitro culture media and by the higher pregnancy rate after tubal transfer and by improved pregnancy rates following transfer of embryos grown in human tubal cell coculture (Bongso et al, 1992). The factors underlying this effect are unknown but include a chemically ideal medium supplemented by appropriate levels of peptide growth factors (Sayegh & Mastroianni, 1991; Maguiness et al, 1992).

4. The tubal contribution to the immune protection of early preimplantation embryos includes the production of a glycoprotein with anticomplement activity (Sayegh & Mastroianni, 1991) and the postovulatory hormone-dependent downregulation of major histocompatibility complex class II antigen expression in the endosalpinx (Edelstam et al, 1992).

Pregnancy can occur without tubal contribution under special circumstances, i.e. in vitro fertilization and embryo transfer, and after intrauterine ovarian implantation (the Estes procedure), but in nature the tube is the physiological regulator of perifertilization events and it is not surprising that tubal disease is the single commonest cause of female infertility. Tubal lesions can be primarily functional or anatomical. Functional lesions, considered as biophysical and biochemical derangements, are probably common but have not been intensively studied because of technical problems. Three such lesions deserve comment:

1. Chronic tubal spasm, manifested as proximal obstruction seen at salpingography, is an uncommon cause of infertility (Mendel, 1964) and of ectopic pregnancy (Grant, 1962), which can resolve spontaneously or respond to antispasmodics (Smitham, 1982). It is psychogenic in origin and its pathogenesis undoubtedly involves disturbed interaction among catecholamines, prostaglan-

dins, sex steroids and substance P (Skrabanek & Powell, 1983). It has been suggested (Honoré, 1978b) that chronic tubal spasm leads to salpingitis isthmica nodosa, a lesion discussed more fully in Chapter 17. How SIN causes infertility and ectopic pregnancy remains speculative but the following mechanisms may contribute: narrowing of the isthmic lumen, resulting from spasm and secondary myohypertrophy, may accentuate the filtering effect of the isthmus and reduce the available number of sperms for fertilization; it is also possible that the sperms may be 'lost' in the diverticula. Incomplete relaxation may interfere with downstream release of the zygote, which may be trapped and implant in the ampulla or may degenerate on its way through a 'tight' isthmus.

2. Hyperactive tubal macrophages (Haney et al, 1983) compete with the ovum for sperm availability and reduce the probability of fertilization. These phagocytes, which normally come from the peritoneal cavity, are increased in numbers and activity in endometriosis, probably as a result of peritoneal irritation from recurrent menstrual reflux. This phenomenon may account for infertility in women who have normal ovaries and tubes.

3. 'Tubo-ovarian interference' across the midline. Normally the ovulating ovary is in close contact with the fimbria, ovum pick-up occurs within seven hours of ovulation (Croxatto et al, 1978) and fertilization takes place in the ampulla. In a small percentage of women one tube may be non-functional while the ipsilateral ovary and the contralateral adnexa are normal; this disturbed anatomy leads to infertility, which responds to excision of the diseased tube and the normal ipsilateral ovary, i.e. the so-called paradoxical oophorectomy (Trimbos-Kemper et al, 1982b). The mechanisms underlying the infertility are unknown but ectopic pregnancy, which can follow ovum transmigration (Honoré, 1978a), is not a major factor.

The morbid anatomy of the tube is discussed in detail in Chapter 17 and the anatomical lesions associated with infertility will be briefly reviewed. Tubal disease is the most important single factor in female infertility and is often unsuspected clinically (Rosenfeld et al, 1983); some of the lesions are endosalpingeal and undetectable by palpation or laparoscopy but can be diagnosed histologically (Cumming et al, 1988), by transvaginal falloposcopy (Kerin et al, 1992) or by transfimbrial salpingoscopy (Marconi et al, 1992). The relevant lesions include the following:

1. Congenital defects are rare and include segmental atresia (Richardson et al, 1982; Wanerman et al, 1986), hypoplasia (Aronnet et al, 1969), excessive convolution associated with elongated ovarian and tubal ligaments (Cohen & Katz, 1978), ostial phimosis, segmental sacculation or diverticula and accessory tubes or ostia (Yablonski et al, 1990). Unique structural defects, related to infertility and ectopic pregnancy, are seen in women

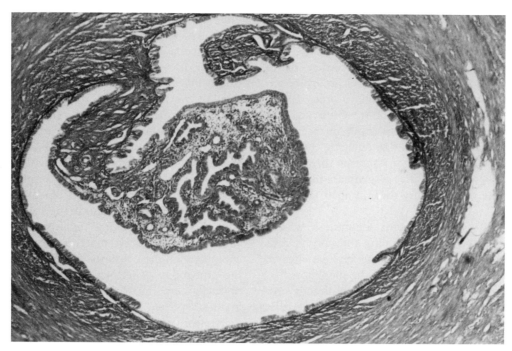

Fig. 33.8 Benign adenofibromatous polyp of the intramural segment of the Fallopian tube. H & E × 59.

exposed in utero to diethylstilboestrol, e.g. foreshortening and convolution of the tube, 'withered' fimbria and a pin-point ostium (De Cherney et al, 1981). Congenital absence of the tubes can be mimicked by autoamputation following torsion (Beyth & Bar On, 1984).

2. Mucosal polyps of the intramural portion of the tube, especially if bilateral, are a rare cause of infertility (David et al, 1981). These benign lesions of unknown causation are sessile or polypoid masses with a fibrous or a loose vascular stroma and canalicular or adenoid structures lined by tubal epithelium (Fig. 33.8).

3. Tubal infection is the single most important cause of female infertility and its incidence has risen dramatically in recent decades (Curran, 1980). Non-granulomatous salpingitis is an ascending infection and the risk factors include sexual activity, puerperal or postabortal endometritis, therapeutic or diagnostic manipulations of the cervix and the use of the intrauterine contraceptive device (Weström, 1980; Trimbos-Kemper et al, 1982a; Eschenbach, 1992). The organisms involved include: *Neisseria gonorrhoeae*, anaerobic organisms, *Mycoplasma hominis*, *Ureaplasma urealyticum* and *Chlamydia trachomatis* (Shafrin et al, 1992). In the West, the major pathogen responsible for tubal infertility is *Chlamydia trachomatis*, as demonstrated directly by cultures of tubal tissue (Shepard & Jones, 1989; Marana et al, 1990) and indirectly by serology (Sellors et al, 1988); there is also convincing experimental evidence of its rôle in causing tubal damage and infertility (Zana et al, 1990).

Salpingitis causes infertility by the following mechanisms (Frantzen & Schlosser, 1982):

(i) Fimbrial agglutination with ostial phimosis or occlusion, secondary hydrosalpinx (Fig. 33.9) and loss of the fimbria ovarica. The net result is failure of ovum pick-up (Bateman et al, 1987).

(ii) Midtubal occlusion due to tuberculosis, arrested tubal pregnancy, endometriosis or surgical damage during inguinal herniorrhaphy (Urman et al, 1992). It is now recognized that some tubal pregnancies may arrest with spontaneous subsidence of symptoms and progressive tubal damage leading to occlusion and secondary infertility (Gomel & Filmar, 1987).

(iii) Proximal cornual or isthmic occlusion (Fig. 33.10) due to interfrondal adhesions, obliterative fibrosis (Fortier & Haney, 1985; Letterie & Sakas, 1991; Honoré, unpublished observations) or dislodgeable obstructive intraluminal casts containing mucin, collagen and calcium (Sulak et al, 1987).

(iv) Mesh-like adhesions at the uterotubal ostium, visualized hysteroscopically (Daly et al, 1986).

(v) Follicular salpingitis in the ampulla.

(vi) Perisalpingeal (Fig. 33.11), tubo-ovarian, uterotubal and periovarian adhesions interfering with ovum pick-up and transport.

(vii) Constrictive perisalpingitis with obstruction of the proximal third of the tube (Resnick, 1962).

Microsurgical repair has significantly improved the reproductive outlook and the prognosis for fertility depends on the residual tubal length, the severity of mural fibrosis, the extent of epithelial deciliation (Vasquez et al, 1980) and the degree of loss of oestrogen and progesterone receptors (De Voto et al, 1984).

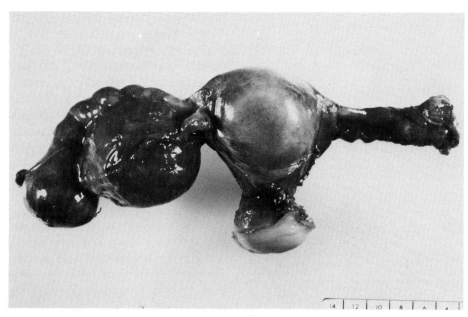

Fig. 33.9 Postinflammatory bilateral fimbrial occlusion with hydrosalpinx and tubo-ovarian adhesions (right).

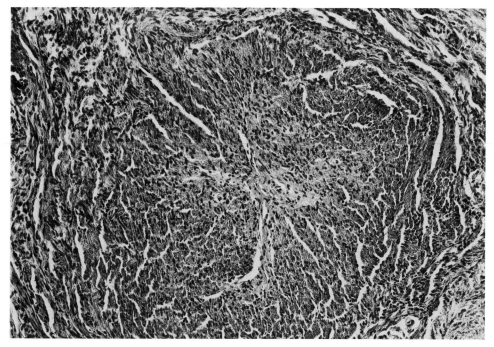

Fig. 33.10 Isthmic occlusion: loss of endosalpinx and replacement by fibrous tissue. H & E × 147.

Granulomatous salpingitis in the West is largely due to *Mycobacterium tuberculosis* and it is an uncommon cause of infertility with a particularly dismal prognosis (Schaeffer, 1976) and a significantly increased chance of ectopic nidation (Durukan et al, 1990). As a rule, the tubal lesions are typical with a diffuse infiltration of the endosalpinx in particular by lymphocytes, histiocytes and giant cells (Fig. 33.12) together with a variable degree of caseating necrosis, ulceration and fibrosis. Occasionally the pattern is atypical and may mimic a non-specific salpingitis or even sarcoidosis (De Brux & Dupre-Froment, 1965). Tuberculosis can occasionally be associated with chronic lipoid salpingitis (Fig. 33.13) secondary to salpingography. Parasitic salpingitis is dealt with in Chapter 37.

4. Postoperative adhesions (Stangel et al, 1984) are the bête noire of infertility surgery and can occur following the most meticulous operation. They result from trauma to the peritoneum resulting in a sterile inflammatory

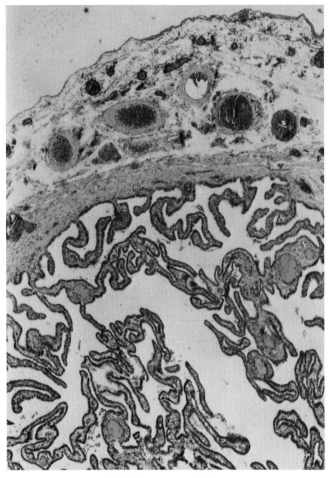

Fig. 33.11 Perisalpingeal adhesion: vascular stage. H & E × 59.

reaction with fibrin deposition, establishment of a fibrin bridge between apposed surfaces, consolidation of this bridge by organization of the exudate and finally mature fibrosis with contraction of the scar. They can also be produced by a granulomatous reaction to cornstarch powder present in surgical gloves (Yaffe et al, 1980). They can also occur after pelvic surgery, especially caesarian section (Stovall et al, 1989) or after appendectomy, even when a normal appendix is removed (Lehmann-Willenbrock et al, 1990). Such adhesions, causing mechanical infertility, are an important reason for the failure of reconstructive surgery.

5. Tubal lesions causing infertility after attempts at sterilization reversal include adhesions, reocclusion, excessively short tubes and more subtle changes in the presence of grossly normal and patent tubes, i.e. loss and distortion of mucosal folds, epithelial deciliation, intraluminal polyp formation (Vasquez et al, 1980), development of intramural epithelial inclusions and endometriosis (Donnez et al, 1984).

6. Tubointestinal fistulas are a rare cause of infertility. They arise as a complication of tuberculosis, pelvic inflammatory disease, diverticulitis, Crohn's disease, lymphogranuloma venereum and appendicitis and they can develop between the tube and the sigmoid, rectum, appendix, caecum and ileum (Locher & Maroulis, 1983).

7. Tubal endometriosis is an important cause of infertility. The lesion is discussed in Chapter 32.

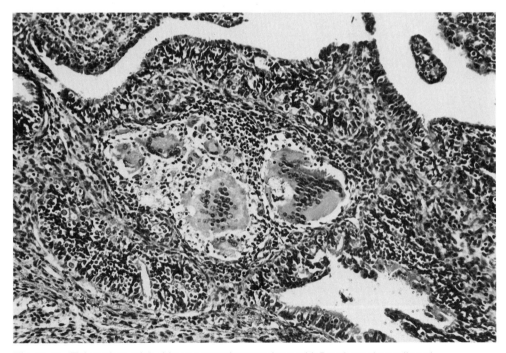

Fig. 33.12 Tuberculous salpingitis: non-caseating granuloma with Langhans giant cells and lymphocytes. H & E × 147.

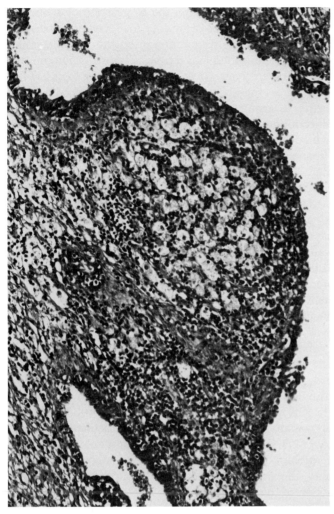

Fig. 33.13 Lipoid salpingitis following salpingography: lymphocytes and foamy macrophages. H & E × 147.

Ovary

Unlike the testis, which is continuously active in adult life, the cyclic ovary is critical in regulating the pattern and efficiency of human fertility by determining the monthly occurrence of ovulation and hence of the fertile period in women, the refractory period in pregnancy and post-partum and the onset of premenopausal subfertility and postmenopausal sterility. Ovulation integrates the endo-crine and 'exocrine' (ovum release) functions of the ovary and is thus the pivot of ovarian activity. Ovarian infertility is intimately related to ovulatory dysfunction and can only be understood in terms of disturbances of the normal process of ovulation.

Ovulation, culminating in ovum release and corpus lu-teum formation, is a complex event comprising four inter-dependent components, i.e. feedback interactions in the hypothalamus-pituitary-ovary (HPO) axis, structural and functional intraovarian events, mechanical release of the ovum and the development of the corpus luteum. These components will be discussed separately.

Feedback mechanisms (Fritz & Speroff, 1982; Sizonenko & Aubert, 1986) determine the tonic and phasic activity of the HPO axis. In primates the ovary is essential for cyclic ovulation and the 'ovarian clock' sets its timing by exerting sustained negative and acute tran-sient positive feedback effects on the hypothalamus and pituitary. Thus ovarian oestradiol (E_2) and inhibin sup-press hypothalamic GnRH release and pituitary FSH and LH secretion while the late follicular phase rise in E_2 destabilizes the system and allows the mid-cycle FSH/LH surge. The pituitary acts as an amplifier and transducer of hypothalamic signals and the activity of the gonadotroph, now considered to be a single cell type producing both FSH and LH, is cyclically modulated by changes in GnRH and sex steroid levels. The gonadotroph is ontogenically endowed with the ability to synthesize and release FSH and becomes capable of producing and secreting LH only after exposure to GnRH. Differential secretion of these hormones is achieved by external forces, including E_2 and inhibin, which preferentially block FSH release, and testosterone, which potentiates GnRH-mediated FSH release. During the menstrual cycle the gonadotroph undergoes changes in its secretory capacity, which consists of two separate secretory pools, i.e. an acute releasable pool equating with pituitary sensitivity and a slowly releasable pool equating with pituitary re-serve. In the early follicular phase both sensitivity and reserve are minimal; in the mid to late follicular phase there is a preferential increase in reserve over sensitivity; at mid-cycle there is a marked increase in sensitivity due to expansion of the acutely releasable pool; in the luteal phase there is a progressive decline in reserve and capac-ity. Thus at mid-cycle the pituitary is primed for acute gonadotrophin release and is further sensitized to GnRH by low levels of progesterone.

The hypothalamus, under the stimulatory and inhibi-tory control of noradrenaline and dopamine and opioids (Jewelewicz, 1984; Leyendecker & Wiidt, 1989; Seifer & Collins, 1990), respectively, releases GnRH in discrete pulses resulting in a pulsatile secretion of pituitary gona-dotrophins. This pulsatility, essential for the normal func-tion of the HPO axis, is modulated by ovarian steroids: hypogonadal women show high frequency and high amplitude pulses while normally cycling women exhibit a pattern of high frequency and low amplitude in the follicular phase and low frequency and high amplitude in the luteal phase. The triggering mechanism for the mid-cycle GnRH surge is unknown (Djahanbaruch et al, 1984) but is probably related to E_2 reciprocal activation and suppression of NA and DA neurones respectively and the E_2-induced increase in central catecholoestrogens, which results in competitive inhibition of catechol-O-methyltransferase with a secondary increase in NA and facilitation of GnRH release and also in direct competi-tion for E_2 receptors thus reducing the negative feedback of E_2 on the hypothalamus. Likewise, the mode of termination of the GnRH surge is unclear but may be due to high levels of pituitary gonadotrophins exerting a short loop negative feedback effect on the hypothalamus via retrograde portal blood flow. The mid-cycle GnRH surge, potentiated by the sensitizing effects of preovulatory oestrogen and progesterone on the gonadotrophs, is followed by a large LH surge and a smaller FSH surge (Corsan et al, 1990).

It is important to realize that the feedback loop of the HPO axis is not normally affected by the negligible amounts of oestrogen produced by the adrenals and by the low levels of extraglandular formation of oestrogen from ovarian and adrenal androgenic precursors.

Preovulatory intraovarian events, which occur throughout the follicular phase of the cycle, are critical for ovulation and the development of an adequate corpus luteum (Fritz & Speroff, 1982; Hodgen, 1982; Jones, 1990). In the luteal phase, follicular growth is arrested and recruitment starts after the onset of menstruation when the antifolliculogenic effects of progesterone are removed. In the early follicular phase a fresh cohort of follicles is recruited for growth and by day 5 the follicle destined to ovulate is selected by mechanisms as yet not fully understood. The process appears to be stochastic and the choice of the dominant follicle depends on a delicate balance between progressive oestrogenization or androgenization of the intrafollicular milieu. As a rule, one follicle is at the right stage to be able to establish a rapidly progressive oestrogenic environment essential for development. This dominance is due to local positive feedback synergism between E_2 and FSH, achieved by three mechanisms:

1. FSH induces and stimulates aromatase in granulosa cells thus increasing local E_2 production from thecal androgenic precursors.
2. E_2 increases FSH receptors in granulosa cells thus potentiating its stimulatory effect.
3. Thecal vascularity in the dominant follicle increases significantly causing preferential FSH delivery to the follicle with the highest density of FSH receptors.

Meanwhile, increasing levels of E_2 and inhibin produced by the developing follicles suppress FSH, which is preferentially shunted to the dominant follicle. The other follicles, deprived of FSH, show a decline in aromatase and a rise in the activity of the 5α-reductase resulting in a progressively androgenic milieu and follicular atresia. Under FSH influence the preovulatory follicle develops LH and prolactin receptors and is able to produce escalating levels of E_2 needed for the LH surge and also small sensitizing amounts of progesterone.

Mechanics of ovulation. The LH surge is essential for ovulation, which is estimated to occur 10–12 hours after the LH peak, 28–32 hours after the onset of the LH surge and 24–36 hours after the E_2 peak (Fritz & Speroff, 1982). Rising levels of LH induce the formation of cAMP, which mediates the resumption of oocyte meiosis, granulosa cell luteinization and synthesis of prostaglandins and proteolytic enzymes. At the same time these high LH levels suppress thecal steroidogenesis in other antral follicles, further asserting the dominance of the chosen follicle. The more modest concurrent FSH surge also plays a rôle in ovulation: LH receptor development in granulosa cells is enhanced, plasminogen activator is induced and detachment of the oocyte-bearing cumulus is elicited by mucification of the cumulus matrix. It is not clear whether the ovulatory follicle actively migrates to the ovarian surface or whether the ovulatory cone approaches the ovarian capsule as a result of follicular expansion due to increased wall compliance and a rapid accumulation of follicular fluid. Softening of the follicular wall and stigma formation are caused by locally generated proteolytic enzymes, such as plasmin, peptidases and a specific collagenase, which is rate-limiting (Fukumoto et al, 1981; Yoshimura & Wallach, 1987). The prostaglandins are critical in the ovulation process: they stimulate intrafollicular progesterone synthesis and they participate in ovum expulsion by promoting the activity of collagenolytic enzymes and stimulating the contraction of perifollicular smooth muscle cells in the theca externa (Kohda et al, 1983). The rôle of ovarian nerves in ovulation is still undefined (Weiner et al, 1977). The physical act of ovulation culminates in the gentle non-explosive extrusion of the oocyte *cum* cumulo onto the ovarian surface for pick-up by the sweeping action of the tubal fimbria.

Exposure to the synergistic effect of high levels of LH and steroids in the preovulatory follicle leads to co-ordinated nuclear and cytoplasmic maturation of the oocyte. Before release the oocyte completes the first meiotic division and is primed for the fertilization-induced second meiotic division and the formation of a haploid female pronucleus; the critical event in cytoplasmic maturation is the production of proteins needed for mRNA synthesis, which will help the oocyte through fertilization and the first four mitotic divisions (Jones, 1990).

Corpus luteum (CL) formation (Jones, 1990). After ovum escape the follicle collapses and the antrum fills with lymph and blood, which then stimulates the centripetal growth of blood vessels from the theca, a process enhanced by thecal cell production of an angiogenetic factor related to angiotensin II. Granulosal vascularization is essential for luteal function as progesterone synthesis (Hansen et al, 1991) is critically dependent on a supply of blood-borne cholesterol, which is avidly picked up by specific receptors induced by LH and prolactin. At the time of the LH surge and at ovulation the granulosal and thecal cells luteinize forming two functional compartments. The granulosal cells stop dividing and acquire LH neoreceptors, which when occupied do not internalize and thus limit LH sensitivity and progesterone synthesis in time. After 10 days the cells run out of stable mRNA species and they stop producing progesterone while becoming refractory to LH or hCG stimulation. In contrast, the endogenous LH receptors of luteinized thecal cells are normally internalized and these cells respond to LH by proliferation and secretion of oestrogen and progesterone. In the absence of pregnancy the corpus luteum involutes as a result of E_2-induced luteolysis, mediated by reduced LH binding capacity and sensitivity of the luteal cells and by a rise in the $PGF_{2\alpha}/PGE_2$ (Vijayakumar & Walters, 1983). If pregnancy occurs, trophoblastic hCG rescues the corpus luteum by stimulating the luteinized thecal cells to produce increasing amounts of oestrogen and progesterone. Early pregnancy, up to 7 weeks, is absolutely dependent on steroids produced by the corpus luteum and lutectomy causes abortion; thereafter a luteal placental shift takes place with corpus luteum involution and placental takeover. Recent work clashes with this classic concept of the luteal-placental shift, which implies corpus luteum failure followed by transfer of steroid production to the placenta (Nakajima et al, 1991). What happens in the first and early second trimesters is a puzzling dose-response relationship between the corpus luteum and exponentially rising hCG levels: progesterone secretion by the corpus luteum is clamped at a steady level without decline while placental secretion keeps rising and in effect takes over pregnancy maintenance. This explains why there is still hCG-dependent steroid production by the corpus luteum at term. Postpartum luteolysis occurs rapidly but at a slower rate in nursing mothers (Fritz & Speroff, 1982).

Ovulatory disorders

Ovulation is not an all-or-none event but constitutes a spectrum characterized by 'normal' ovulation at the one end and anovulation at the other with intermediate grades of suboptimal quantity and quality. Infertility can thus result from anovulation, oligo-ovulation or dysovulation. These ovulatory disturbances will be discussed under the following headings.

1. ***Absent or reduced follicular pool.*** Ovulation, a highly selective process, requires a grossly superfluous follicular pool for recruitment, and anovulation or oligo-ovulation can result from:

(i) Congenital anomalies of the ovary, which are discussed in detail in Chapter 40. Only a few relevant comments are included here. The streak gonad (Fig. 33.14), seen with chromosomal anomalies, or with a 46,XX and 46,XY constitution, is usually afollicular and absolutely sterile but rarely follicles persist into adult life (Coulam, 1982). Such patients can become pregnant but their gestational outcome is poor with an increased incidence of spontaneous abortion, stillbirth and abnormal offspring

(Reyes et al, 1976; Wray et al, 1981). Rare causes of chromosome-related ovarian failure include the triple X syndrome (Itu et al, 1990), X-autosome translocation (Katayama et al, 1991), and familial terminal deletion of the long arm of X (Veneman et al, 1991). Two other inherited conditions due to genetic mutations cause premature ovarian failure. The first is galactosaemia due to deficiency of galactose-1-phosphate uridyl transferase activity: unlike the affected males, who show normal testicular function, the affected females, despite treatment, develop progressive damage to follicles and stroma with reduced oestrogen and androgen production and hypogonadotrophic ovarian failure (Kaufman et al, 1987; Hagenfeldt et al, 1989). The second is blepharophimosis type I, which is an autosomal dominant syndrome associated with hypergonadotrophic hypogonadism due to follicular gonadotrophin resistance or premature follicular depletion (Fraser et al, 1988). Ovarian hypoplasia, associated with primary amenorrhoea, can be due to subtle abnormalities of the D chromosomes and is characterized by

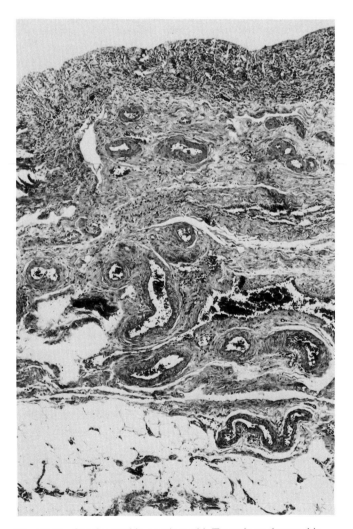

Fig. 33.14 Streak gonad in a patient with Turner's syndrome: thin ovarian cortex with wavy stromal cells and no follicles. H & E × 39.

small shrunken ovaries containing closely packed inactive primordial follicles in a fibrous cortex (Lazlo et al, 1976).

(ii) Acquired lesions resulting in severe follicular damage are relatively uncommon. Mumps oophoritis, which affects 5% of patients with mumps parotitis, can cause extensive follicular damage followed by cortical fibrosis, and pubescent females are more sensitive (Prinz & Taubert, 1968). The late sequelae include infertility, menstrual disturbances and premature menopause (Morrison et al, 1975). Ovarian failure with subfertility, infertility or premature menopause often follows abdominal irradiation and chemotherapy for the treatment of childhood or adolescent malignancy (Damewood & Grochow, 1986; Byrne et al, 1992). Chemotherapy has been shown by electronmicroscopy to damage, and thus reduce the number of, follicles and to cause diffuse stromal damage with fibrosis, hyalinization, calcification and vascular sclerosis (Marcello et al, 1990; Familiari et al, 1993). These deleterious effects depend on the dose used, the type of treatment (alkylating agents being particularly harmful) and the age of the patient (older patients being more sensitive).

(iii) Premature menopause, defined as cessation of ovarian activity before the age of 40, is characterized by loss of follicles and stromal fibrosis (Fig. 33.15) and is probably due to accelerated follicular atresia. Its aetiology and pathogenesis are unknown but in galactosaemia it appears to result from deficient germ cell migration to the primitive gonad (Coulam, 1982). It may be genetically determined (Coulam et al, 1983).

2. *Anatomical or functional folliculopathy* includes the following four unrelated conditions:

(i) The recurrent empty follicle syndrome, first described by Coulam et al (1986), is seen in cases of unexplained infertility and of infertility related to endometriosis or the tubal factor and after treatment with pure FSH preparations (Ashkenazi et al, 1987). It is diagnosed by follicular aspiration which yields only follicular fluid and granulosa cells (La Scala et al, 1991). Its aetiology and pathogenesis are unknown but it is probably due to premature atresia related to a primary abnormality in the oocyte, as suggested by oocyte studies done during IVF (Rudak et al, 1990).

(ii) Defective oocytes (Ezra et al, 1992). Diagnosis of this condition is based on circumstantial evidence provided by the significantly greater in vitro failure rates of oocytes retrieved from women with unexplained infertility as compared to those with tuboperitoneal infertility. Possible mechanisms for this oocyte defect include defective zona pellucida sperm receptor, antizona antibody and failure of maternal pronucleus formation or syngamy.

(iii) Occult ovarian failure (Healy, 1991) is a newly recognized syndrome characterized by infertility, regular menses and hypergonadotrophic hypogonadism. It represents a state of partially compensated granulosa cell failure,

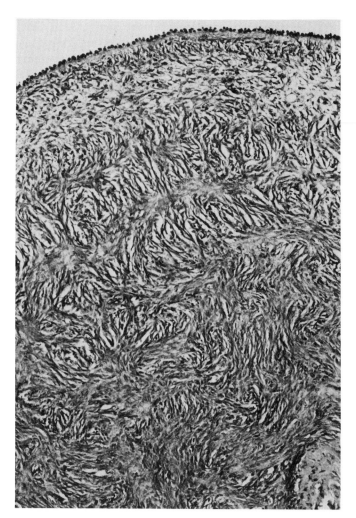

Fig. 33.15 Premature menopause: ovarian cortex with patchy stromal fibrosis and no follicles. H & E × 147.

which may be primary or secondary due to antiovarian antibodies or subclinical growth hormone deficiency.

(iv) Congenital increase in aromatase activity of ovarian follicles and peripheral tissues is associated with elevated serum oestrogen and progesterone levels, hyperprolactinaemia, menometrorrhagia due to endometrial hyperplasia and infertility (Odell & Meikle, 1986).

3. *The gonadotrophin-resistant ovary syndrome* is characterized by increased gonadotrophin levels, normally structured ovaries and complete follicular inactivity. Its diverse clinical presentations indicate a multiplicity of causes, which are largely unknown. Autoimmunity plays a rôle in some cases, as evidenced by its concurrence with other autoimmune diseases, e.g. the polyglandular syndrome and myasthenia gravis, by the presence of serum antiovarian antibodies and by a chronic oophoritis featuring lymphocytic infiltration of developing follicles (Coulam, 1982; Rebar et al, 1982). The process, which resembles the autoimmune oophoritis of thymectomized animals, involves a defect in the humoral and cell mediated arms of the immune system, as indicated by direct

studies of lymphocyte abnormalities (Rabinowe et al, 1989) and by immunotyping of the cellular infiltrate (Sedmark et al, 1987). Rarely there can be concomitant degeneration of oocytes in primary or secondary follicles with dystrophic calcification, absence of antral follicles and corpora lutea/albicantia and ovarian hypoplasia (Biberoglu et al, 1988). Gonadotrophin resistance is due in some instances to antibodies inhibiting gonadotrophin binding to the follicular cells (Escobar et al, 1982) or to the development of a non-immune receptor or post-receptor defect (Talbert et al, 1984). Another possible pathogenetic mechanism is a primary failure of oestrogen synthesis in the follicles, as suggested by the occurrence of pregnancy in some women with insensitive ovaries treated with oestrogen and also by the severe follicular disorganization observed in women with absent oestrogen as a result of 17α-hydroxylase deficiency (Coulam, 1982; Araki et al, 1987).

4. *The 'hyperresponsive' ovary* is a rare and poorly-defined entity characterized by the recurrence of painful functional ovarian cysts and reproductive difficulties in young women. There is no direct evidence of ovarian hypersensitivity to gonadotrophins (Stone & Swartz, 1979).

5. *Abnormal hypothalamo-hypophysio-ovarian relationships* will be discussed under the rubrics of hypothalamic and pituitary disturbances. To complete the picture abnormal feedback mechanisms are presented here. The normal feedback loop depends on a well-defined pattern of oestrogen and progesterone secretion by the ovary and the loop can be opened by an uncontrolled extraovarian supply of sex steroids. This can result from:

(i) The combined contraceptive pill, which suppresses tonic secretion of gonadotrophins and inhibits the mid-cycle surge. Normal ovarian function and fertility usually return after cessation of contraception but in about 1 in 1000 users postpill amenorrhoea ensues as a result of a cycle initiation defect (Hull et al, 1981). These women respond well to ovulation induction and their prognosis is excellent (Soltan & Hancock, 1982).

(ii) Excessive extraglandular oestrogen formation from androgenic precursors occurs in obesity resulting in anovulatory infertility (Bates & Whitworth, 1982).

(iii) Increased supply of androgenic precursors from extraglandular conversion to oestrogen arises from adrenal hypersecretion (Lobo et al, 1983) and/or overproduction by the ovaries as a result of polycystic ovarian disease, hyperthecosis or an androgen/oestrogen secreting tumour (Wiebe & Morris, 1983; Insler & Lunenfeld, 1991). The feedback disturbances, associated with excessive extraovarian oestrogen, often lead to the development of polycystic ovarian disease, which is discussed in Chapter 19.

6. *Dysovulation* can result from dissociation of the physical and endocrine components of ovulation, i.e. pseudo-ovulation, luteal insufficiency and disturbances in ovum pick-up.

(i) The luteinized unruptured follicle (LUF) syndrome is now a recognized cause of infertility in some women with no detectable male or female factors and may contribute to infertility in some women with endometriosis or pelvic adhesive disease (Aksel, 1987; Katz, 1988; Bateman et al, 1990). It reflects a dissociation between the mechanical (follicle rupture and ovum release) and the endocrine (luteinization of the dominant follicle) components of ovulation and may be due to disturbed prostaglandin activity, since its incidence is significantly increased in normally cycling women treated with prostaglandin synthetase inhibitors (Killick & Elstein, 1987). The unruptured luteinized follicle becomes transformed into a luteal cyst, which produces subnormal levels of progesterone (Hamilton et al, 1990).

(ii) Follicular rupture with failure of ovum release or ovum retention can be seen in spontaneous and induced ovulations (Stanger & Yovich, 1984). It may differ from the luteinized unruptured follicle only in degree (Hamilton et al, 1990); it is followed by luteal cyst formation and marginal progesterone deficiency, indicating the importance of follicular rupture for efficient progesterone synthesis. It is characterized by failure of dispersal of the cumulus oophorus and ovum release, possibly due to inhibition of LH-induced hyaluronic acid synthesis caused by excessive production of FSH-stimulated glycosaminoglycan (Katz, 1988).

(iii) Premature luteinization is diagnosed if serum progesterone levels greater than 1.5 ng/ml are associated with an LH surge before serum oestradiol levels reach 100 pg/ml and before the follicle is fully mature. It is a cause of pregnancy failure in anovulatory women treated with human menopausal gonadotrophin and clomiphene citrate and also in a small subset of untreated infertile women (Check et al, 1991; Taney et al, 1991). One mechanism underlying its antifertility effect is the production of poor quality cervical mucus (Taney et al, 1991).

(iv) Luteal phase deficiency (LPD) is now a recognized cause of infertility and early recurrent spontaneous abortion (McNeely & Soules, 1988; Jaffe & Jewelewicz, 1991; Blumenfeld & Ruach, 1992), despite the problems inherent in its diagnosis (Davis et al, 1989; Li & Cooke, 1991). It is common as a sporadic event in normal women, occurring in about 30% of random cycles but it is less common as a recurrent event, ranging in frequency from 3–14% in the infertile population. It is due to corpus luteum insufficiency with inadequate progesterone secretion or defective endometrial response to progesterone. The commonest cause of corpus luteum insufficiency is inadequate preovulatory folliculogenesis due to deficiency of FSH and intrafollicular oestrogen but it can also follow normal follicular development (Grunfeld et al, 1989). Other causes include (a) neuroendocrine dysfunction, e.g. increased LH pulse frequency, inadequate LH surge or luteal levels, follicular phase FSH deficiency, abnormal

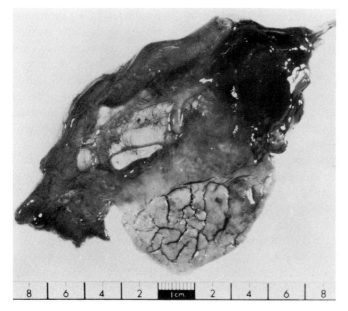

Fig. 33.16 Normal tubo-ovarian relationship: freely mobile tube and ovary with no adhesions.

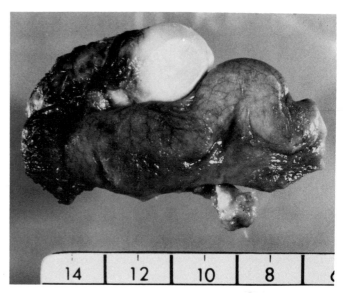

Fig. 33.17 Extensive tubo-ovarian adhesions (?postinflammatory).

follicular phase LH:FSH ratio and hyperprolactinaemia; (b) ovarian abnormalities, e.g. follicle depletion, luteinized unruptured follicle, ovum retention; (c) systemic disorders, e.g. chronic liver or kidney disease, thyroid dysfunction, significant deviations from ideal body weight, exercise and psychological stress; (d) treatment with ovulation-inducing drugs, e.g. clomiphene citrate and gonadotrophins. Defective endometrial response to progesterone may be due to inadequate receptors or endometritis (Jaffe & Jewelewicz, 1991). The endometrial patterns associated with luteal insufficiency are discussed in Chapter 11.

7. *Disturbed tubo-ovarian relationships* interfere with the passage of the ovum from ovary to tube (Fig. 33.16). In women ovum pick-up is normally achieved by direct contact of the cilia with the ovarian surface. This close apposition is brought about by coordinate movements of the fimbria ovarica, ovarian ligament, mesovarium and mesosalpinx. Such contact can be prevented by an excessively long fimbria ovarica and surgical shortening by plication leads to pregnancy in some infertile women (Cohen, 1980). This contact can also fail to occur if the ligaments are shortened and fixed by fibrosis or if the ovaries and tubes are bound down by adhesions to each other (Fig. 33.17) and to the ligaments (Fig. 33.18). Unilateral or bilateral malposition of the ovary above the pelvic brim due to an unusually long utero-ovarian ligament is a rare contributor to infertility in women with associated Müllerian and renal anomalies (Rock et al, 1986). Periovarian adhesions, which can be localized or diffuse, filmy and avascular or coarse, vascular and fibrous (Fig. 33.19), cause infertility depending on their severity (Hulka, 1982) and it is presumed that they

interfere with ovum release from the ovary. In addition these adhesions appear to block ovulation (Quan et al, 1963), as ovaries surrounded by adhesions show fewer corpora lutea and corpora albicantia and a micropolycystic pattern commonly seen with chronic anovulation.

A recent study (Bychkov, 1990) has failed to confirm ovulatory failure in chronic pelvic inflammatory disease; there was an increase in both follicular and corpus luteum cysts, presumably due to alterations in the ovarian supply.

Peritoneum

The peritoneum is critically located with respect to the female genitalia and peritoneal fluid, which is an ovarian exudate influenced by follicular activity, corpus luteum vascularity and hormone production (Syrop & Halme, 1987), conditions the microenvironment of fertilization and early embryonic development. Infertility often results from gross mechanical disturbances of the peritoneum, i.e. adhesions. It can also be caused by functional disorders of the peritoneum, associated with increases in peritoneal fluid, volume, white cell count, prostanoid concentrations and levels of acid phosphatase, lysozyme (Olive et al, 1987; Syrop & Halme, 1987) and tumour necrosis factor (Eiserman et al, 1988). The mechanisms whereby peritoneal fluid abnormalities cause infertility are speculative and include (Syrop & Halme, 1987):

1. Disturbed ovulation or corpus luteum function: peritoneal macrophages can decrease granulosal progesterone production in vitro.
2. Gamete transport or survival: oviductal and peritoneal macrophages and other unidentified factors adversely

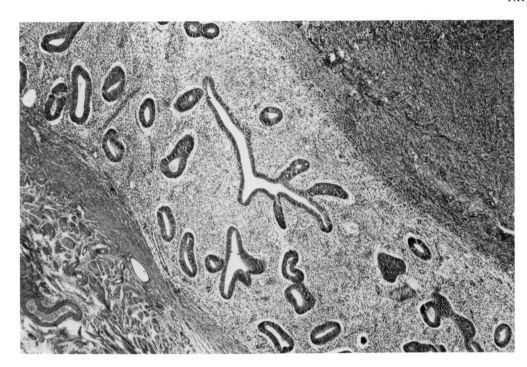

Fig. 33.18 Ovarioligamentous adhesions with a surface endometriotic bridge. H & E × 59.

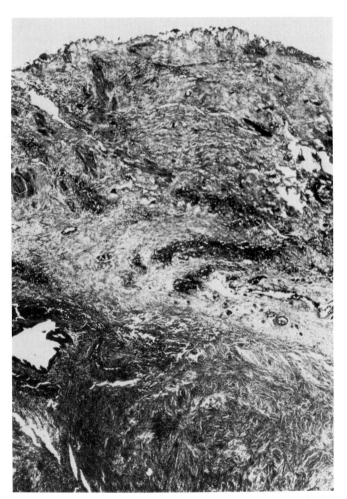

Fig. 33.19 Periovarian adhesion: coarse, vascular and fibrous. Masson trichrome × 59.

affect sperm function by direct toxicity, depression of motility and enhanced spermiophagy. Ovum capture by the fimbria is also compromised.

3. Sperm-egg interaction: a filterable heat-labile factor from peritoneal fluid of patients with endometriosis reduces fertilization rate in a mouse assay.

4. Early embryonic development: cytokines released by leucocytes adversely affect early embryonic cleavage and development.

Disturbances of the hypothalamo-hypophysial system

Despite their embryological and anatomical distinctness the hypothalamus and the anterior pituitary constitute a single functional unit crucial in reproductive control. This functional unity is largely achieved by structural contiguity and the hypothalamo-hypophysial portal venous system, which links the median eminence and the pituitary and funnels the hypophysiotrophic factors at high concentrations into the gland. The hypothalamus can thus be viewed as the noise generator in the system and the pituitary as a multichannel amplifier. The system is stabilized and integrated with the nervous system and the soma via negative or positive long, short and ultra-short feedback loops (Locke, 1978). Reproductive dysfunction can be caused by anatomical or functional lesions of the hypothalamus or pituitary and by vascular disconnection of these two elements.

Hypothalamic disorders

These can be subdivided into anatomical and functional.

Anatomical. These rare lesions consist of:

1. Intrinsic hypothalamic tumours, e.g. gliomas, especially the juvenile astrocytomas, and parahypophysial tumours which compress the hypothalamus or the portal venous system. These latter include pituitary neoplasms, ectopic pinealomas or germinomas, dural meningiomas and posterior pituitary tumours (Landholt, 1975).

2. Selective dysgenesis of the medial basal hypothalamus due to failure of migration of GnRH neurones from the olfactory placode to the arcuate nucleus whence they send their terminals to the median eminence (Schwanzel-Fukuda et al, 1989). This is the basis of the Kallman syndrome, which in humans is not caused by absence of the GnRH gene as in the murine model of the disease. This rare condition, which can be familial and affects females only rarely, is characterized by primary isolated gonadotrophin deficiency, hypogonadism and hyposmia or anosmia. The anatomical lesions are variable, and include defective development of the olfactory area, the anterior hypothalamus and the lateral tuberal nuclei (Kovacs & Sheehan, 1982). Primary gonadal dysplasia is not an integral part of the syndrome (Wortsman et al, 1982).

3. Damage to the arcuate nucleus and the GnRH neurones caused by infectious (tuberculosis) and non-infectious (sarcoidosis) granulomas, histiocytosis X and primary or secondary neoplasms (Kovacs & Horvath, 1987).

Functional. These disturbances, which can be transient or permanent, often afflict young women and arise from malfunction of the hypothalamic neurotransmitter network. They can be subdivided into the following categories:

1. Subclinical relative growth hormone (GH) deficiency has been detected in some patients with primary infertility, anovulation and regular menses (Ovesen et al, 1992). These patients have normal basal GH levels but show a significantly reduced response to an arginine challenge, which would indicate reduced GH secretory capacity and lack of synergism with gonadotrophins to induce mid-cycle ovulation. It is worth noting that GH activity is not absolutely essential for ovulation as spontaneous pregnancies can occur in women with Laron-type dwarfism which is due to lack of GH receptor activity (Menashe et al, 1991).

2. Stress-induced amenorrhoea/anovulation. These disturbances constitute a spectrum of hypothalamic response to sustained emotional stress depending on the subject's sensitivity to stressful stimuli. Initially stress inhibits only the cyclic centre causing anovulation, i.e. the responsive phase; if anovulation persists for over a year, ovarian function deteriorates by mechanisms similar to those operative in the premenopausal state, oestrogen production drops and there is a secondary rise in gonadotrophin secretion, i.e. the refractory phase (Yaginuma, 1979). Exactly how stress inhibits gonadotrophin secretion is not fully known but the following mechanisms are considered contributory (Seibel & Taymor, 1982).

(i) Increased dopaminergic and opioid activity in the hypothalamus (Quigley et al, 1980a); stress activates the corticotrophs with release of ACTH and β-endorphin and GnRH inhibition is caused by the increased levels of cortisol and β-endorphin (Seifer & Collins, 1990).

(ii) Increased production of catecholoestrogens, i.e. 2-hydroxy-oestrone, causing suppression of LH and FSH release

(iii) Hyperprolactinaemia

(iv) Adrenocortical hyperactivity causing hirsutism and acne in susceptible patients.

3. Exercise-related hypomenorrhoea/amenorrhoea, seen in women engaged in strenuous sports, appear to be variably related to young age, prior menstrual irregularities, low body weight and a strong perception of emotional stress (Baker, 1981; Galle et al, 1983; Glass et al, 1987). The hormonal changes are inconsistent and reports include normal, increased or decreased levels of oestrogen, testosterone, prolactin and gonadotrophins (Baker, 1981; Boyden et al, 1983). The mechanisms of hypothalamic suppression are probably similar to those operative in stress amenorrhoea with increased levels of hypothalamic opioids reflected in the feeling of euphoria in athletes after competition or an extensive workout (Speroff, 1981). Another mechanism that may underlie runners' amenorrhoea is the increased cardiac output and hepato-renal clearance of gonadal steroids; the chronically low oestrogen and progesterone levels may disrupt their positive and negative feedback effects (Casper et al, 1984).

4. Undernutrition and reproductive dysfunction (Warren, 1983; Reid & Van Vugt, 1987). Anorexia nervosa results from a disturbed perception of body image or a perverted attitude to food, eating and body weight and a severe self-imposed weight loss to the point of malnutrition. It is associated with multiple systemic disturbances, including amenorrhoea, anovulation and infertility (Eisenberg, 1981). Hypothalamic suppression, caused by stress and the severe weight loss, is mediated partly by increased central dopaminergic activity (Barry & Klawans, 1976) and raised levels of catecholoestrogens (Fishman et al, 1975), which inhibit catechol-O-methyltransferase, the enzyme concerned with inactivation of dopamine and noradrenaline (Adashi et al, 1979a).

5. Body weight abnormalities and ovulatory infertility (Green et al, 1988). Significant deviations from 'ideal' body weight as determined by the Metropolitan Life Insurance Tables, i.e. below 85% or above 120% of ideal, can lead to primary or secondary infertility with ovulatory dysfunction, evidenced by oligomenorrhoea and/or abnormal basal body temperature graphs.

Pituitary disorders

Mammalian reproduction is critically dependent on the hypothalamo-hypophysial complex, which is not only the vital link between the nervous system and the reproductive tract but also an indispensable controller of the tonic and phasic activity of the female gonads. The pituitary plays a key rôle as an endocrine transducer and amplifier of neural microsignals and it has an enormous reserve capacity that ensures functional compensation until over 90% of the gland is destroyed. Pituitary failure of relevance to female infertility is caused by anatomical and functional lesions interfering with the secretion of the gonadotrophins and prolactin.

Destructive anatomical lesions include:

1. Infarctive necrosis due to postpartum haemorrhage (Sheehan & Summers, 1949).

2. Inflammation, infectious and non-infectious, can rarely cause widespread pituitary damage, followed by hypofunction since the gland has a very poor regenerative capacity. Infectious processes include abscess formation or chronic infections, e.g. tuberculosis, syphilis, fungal and parasitic infestations. Non-infectious lesions include giant cell granulomas, sarcoidosis and histiocytosis X. Lymphocytic hypophysitis, which is a rare but distinct entity, is often associated with other endocrine autoimmune disorders and can lead to variable degrees of hypopituitarism, presenting as infertility, hypoprolactinaemia, hypoglycaemia or pituitary tumour (Kovacs & Horvath, 1987).

3. Systemic diseases. Secondary pituitary amyloidosis is a rare cause of hypogonadism (Las & Surks, 1983). With the progressive deposition of amyloid fibres between the pituitary cells and the blood vessels there is ischaemic atrophy, failure of delivery of GnRH to the gonadotrophs and failure of release of FSH and LH into the circulation. In haemosiderosis or haemochromatosis the excess iron is deposited in many tissues including the pituitary, and the gonadotrophs are the most prone of the pituitary cells to the effects of iron storage. Hence hypogonadotrophic hypogonadism is the earliest sign of pituitary involvement (Kovacs & Horvath, 1987; Meyer et al, 1990).

4. The empty sella mimics a pituitary adenoma radiologically and the differentiation is made by the demonstration of air entering the sella during pneumoencephalography. The cause of this peculiar anatomical aberration is unclear but theories of causation include rupture of an intra- or parasellar cyst, infarction of normal or abnormal (neoplastic) sellar contents, pituitary hypertrophy followed by atrophy and transmission of cerebrospinal fluid pressure through a congenitally deficient sellar diaphragm. As a result, the pituitary is flattened and distorted but maintains its vascular link with the hypothalamus (Neelon et al, 1973). The lesion is rarely associated with significant endocrinopathy (Futterweit et al, 1984) but occasionally it may be found with myxoedema, hypogonadotrophic hypogonadism and hyperprolactinaemia (Archer et al, 1978).

5. Neoplastic disorders of the pituitary include:

(i) Extrapituitary intrasellar and parasellar tumours can cause hypogonadotrophic hypogonadism by direct destruction of the gland, obstruction of the portal circulation with reduced GnRH delivery or ischaemic necrosis, and damage to the median eminence or hypothalamus. They include primary tumours, e.g. craniopharyngiomas, meningiomas and malignant lymphomas, and the even rarer metastatic carcinomas, especially from breast (Kovacs & Horvath, 1987). There is often associated diabetes insipidus from neurohypophysial damage.

(ii) Primary pituitary tumours, which are predominantly adenomas, can now be accurately classified into distinct morphological entities on the basis of their cellular composition, hormone content and their immunocytochemical and ultrastructural features (Kovacs & Horvath, 1987). Any pituitary adenoma can cause hypogonadism by directly or indirectly compromising FSH and LH secretion but there are two adenomas which are particularly associated with hypogonadism — the prolactinoma and the gonadotroph cell adenoma.

As with other endocrine tumours, malignant behaviour of pituitary neoplasms cannot be reliably predicted on the basis of the usual histological criteria, i.e. cellular pleomorphism, mitotic activity and nuclear atypia, and ultrastructural features do not permit differentiation between benign, locally invasive and metastasizing lesions. Locally invasive adenomas, which are mostly chromophobic, prolactin producing or hormonally inactive, are less expansive than non-invasive adenomas and thus less likely to cause pituitary destruction with hypopituitarism or visual defects by suprasellar extension; they erode the sella and the body and wings of the sphenoid and compress adjacent nerves and brain. Pituitary carcinomas with cerebrospinal and extracranial metastases are rare (Scheithauer, 1984).

Functional disorders of the pituitary include:

1. Hyperprolactinaemia is the commonest form of pituitary dysfunction (Sluijmer & Lappöan, 1992). In women it may be associated with amenorrhoea and galactorrhoea (Kleinberg et al, 1977), infertility with luteal insufficiency (St. Michel & Di Zerega, 1983), chronic anovulation (Coulam et al, 1982), polycystic ovaries (Corenblum & Taylor, 1982; Futterweit, 1984), infertility with normal ovarian function and high molecular weight prolactin (Andersen et al, 1982) and even normal reproductive activity (Tambascia et al, 1980). This condition can be seen with severe hypothyroidism, renal failure and the use of psychotropic drugs interfering with central dopamine activity (Quigley & Haney, 1980); the contraceptive pill can also cause functional galactorrhoea but it is not followed by a significantly increased incidence of prolactinoma (Pituitary Adenoma Study Group, 1983).

Hyperprolactinaemia may follow childhood exposure to an absent or violent father preventing the normal development of the oedipal triangulation. Paternal deprivation leads to inappropriate persistence of mother-child symbiosis and a 'neurotic' patterning of endocrine response to stress, e.g. with excessive prolactin release. In a small number of patients individual susceptibility conditions the appearance of pathological hyperprolactinaemia, functional or neoplastic (Sobrinho et al, 1984). Its pathogenesis is hypothalamic dopamine deficiency, quite different from the physiological alterations seen in postpartum lactation (Rao et al, 1982). One primary disturbance appears to be an abnormal pituitary vasculature with decreased dopamine delivery (Quigley et al, 1980b); this chronic pituitary hypodopaminaemia releases the lactotroph from inhibition causing functional hypersecretion and anatomical changes, i.e. diffuse hyperplasia (Stoffer et al, 1981) or, more commonly, a prolactinoma associated with defective dopamine receptors (Bression et al, 1980). Incomplete lactotroph suppression may also result from a generalized defect of peripheral metabolism of dopamine, as evidenced by a decreased metabolic clearance rate (Ho et al, 1984). The excess prolactin via short-loop feedback increases hypothalamic release of dopamine, which fails to suppress completely the overactive lactotrophs. The pathophysiology of hyperprolactinaemic reproductive dysfunction is not fully understood. McNatty et al (1974) suggested a peripheral site of action with excess prolactin depressing progesterone secretion by the corpus luteum; this suggestion has not received experimental support (Tan & Biggs, 1983). A pituitary site of action is indicated by the finding that with hyperprolactinaemia the basal levels of FSH and LH are normal while the pituitary reserves are inadequate for an LH surge (Monroe et al, 1981).

Pathologically the prolactinoma can be a microadenoma (Serri et al, 1987), a circumscribed non-encapsulated macroadenoma or a locally invasive tumour extending through the dura and the bone of the sellar floor to invade the sphenoid sinus. Usually the prolactinoma is a solitary lesion of the pituitary but rarely the microprolactinoma with hyperprolactinaemic secondary amenorrhoea can be the initial finding in patients with familial multiple endocrine neoplasia syndrome type 1 (Lucas et al, 1988). When small, the tumour is often deeply set and lies posteriorly within the lateral wing of the pituitary; when larger, it often lies in one of the lateral wings. Grossly it is soft grey, creamy white or purple and histologically it consists of solid epithelial sheets and strands often arranged concentrically around small simple capillaries (Fig. 33.20); the cells are small and polygonal with an ovoid central nucleus. Mitotic figures and multinucleated cells are rare. Depending on the degree of granule storage the cells stain poorly (chromophobe) or are acidophilic with fine discrete rosy red erythrosinophilic granules

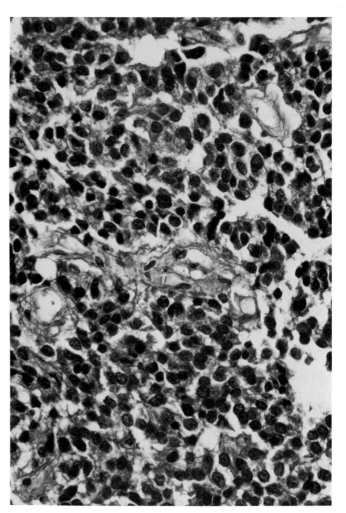

Fig. 33.20 Prolactin cell pituitary adenoma: sheets of polygonal cells with scanty granular cytoplasm and dark ovoid nuclei. H & E × 210.

(Herlant's tetrachrome) or bright red carmoisin-positive granules (Brooke's stain). The histological 'special' stains require perfect fixation and technique and are not entirely reliable for diagnosis (Robert & Hardy, 1975). The immunoperoxidase technique, using specific antisera, is far more reliable and sensitive (Mukai, 1983). The ultrastructure is the final arbiter in the morphological diagnosis of a prolactinoma (Kovacs & Horvath, 1987). Typically the well-granulated 'acidophilic' cell contains an ovoid, often pleomorphic, nucleus, parallel stacks of well-developed RER usually located at the periphery, a prominent Golgi apparatus with few dense immature secretory granules and well-formed electron-dense secretory granules with characteristic size and morphology (Fig. 33.21). The granules, averaging 600 nm in diameter, are oval or pleomorphic with a loosely arranged limiting membrane and an irregular electron-lucent halo between the membrane and the dark core. The sparsely granulated 'chromophobe' cell contains extensively-developed RER with concentric whorls and free ribosomes; a prominent Golgi

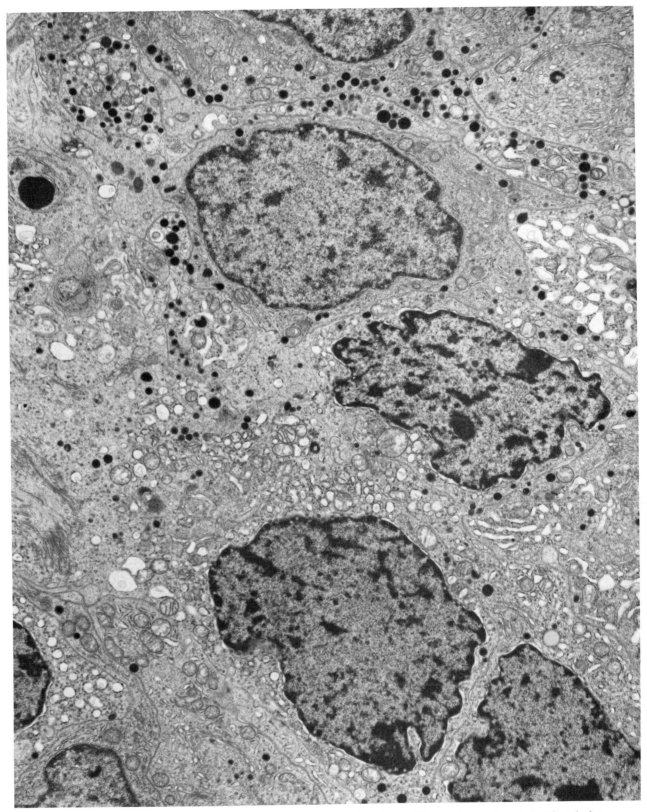

Fig. 33.21 Sparsely granulated prolactin cell pituitary adenoma. Note the irregular nuclei, extensive rough endoplasmic reticulum, scattered Golgi areas, and dense spherical or pleomorphic secretory granules, ranging in diameter from 130–400 nm. × 11 250. (Courtesy of Dr. T. K. Shnitka, Edmonton.)

complex occupying almost a third of the cytoplasmic area and variably filled with immature granules; and sparse dense spherical or pleomorphic granules with an average diameter of 250 nm. Some granules are often seen being extruded on the lateral cell membranes into the intercellular space away from the perivascular spaces and the intercellular extensions of basement membrane — a phenomenon called misplaced exocytosis (Horvath & Kovacs, 1976).

The clinical behaviour of pituitary tumours, like other endocrine neoplasms, cannot be predicted histologically. They are mostly benign despite significant aneuploidy, which correlates with secretory status. Thus aneuploid lesions are associated with higher serum hormone levels, shorter clinical histories and concomitant secretion of various hormones, e.g. growth hormone and prolactin (Anniko et al, 1984).

Macroprolactinomas respond to medical treatment. Bromocriptine, a DA agonist, directly inhibits prolactin synthesis and secretion leading to secondary cellular atrophy with reduction in cell size, nuclear shrinkage and marked involution of the rough endoplasmic reticulum and Golgi system. This cellular collapse underlies the tumour shrinkage following bromocriptine therapy (Bassetti et al, 1984).

2. Neoplastic hypersecretion of ACTH related to a benign ACTH or ACTH-MSH adenoma or rarely to a carcinoma associated with extracranial metastases. These rare tumours, comprising about 10% of all pituitary adenomas, give rise to secondary hypercorticism (Cushing's disease) and derangements of the reproductive axis (Berry & Caplan, 1979).

3. Silent corticotroph adenoma (Serri et al, 1987), without manifestations of Cushing's disease, can present with infertility, amenorrhoea, galactorrhoea and hyperprolactinaemia. These microadenomas, secreting ACTH β-lipotrophin and β-endorphin, probably cause hyperprolactinaemia either by compressing the pituitary stalk or because of the high intrahypothalamic levels of ACTH or β-endorphin.

4. The newly recognized gonadotroph cell adenomas secrete a variable excess of complete FSH or LH or of molecular fragments or subunits with apparently no biological activity. Many patients with these tumours are hypogonadal, probably as a result of inappropriate occupancy of ovarian receptors by tumour-derived inactive gonadotrophin molecules (Kovacs & Horvath, 1987).

Hypothalamo-hypophysial disconnection

This process is an uncommon cause of pituitary failure with decreased or increased prolactin secretion. It is achieved by interruption of the crucial hypothalamo-hypophysial portal system by surgery or by space-occupy-ing lesions, e.g. parahypophysial tumours, suprasellar tumours like craniopharyngioma or Rathke cleft cyst and large non-functioning pituitary adenomas (Berry & Caplan, 1979). If the disconnection is coupled with pituitary destruction progressive panhypopituitarism results; if the disconnection occurs with preservation of the pituitary cells, the lactotrophs are released from their blood-borne inhibitor (dopamine) and oversecrete prolactin, i.e. dissociated hypopituitarism (McCarty & Dobson, 1980).

Systemic and endocrine diseases and female infertility

In women reproductive function is delicately balanced and can be disrupted by many systemic and endocrine diseases. The result is a varying degree of infertility manifested as the inability to conceive and/or carry the live conceptus to term. As a rule the severity of the disease correlates with the degree of fertility impairment.

Systemic diseases tend to depress fertility by significantly increasing the rate of spontaneous abortion and stillbirth. Congenital heart disease is associated with high rates of pregnancy loss, exceeding 50% and probably secondary to chronic fetal hypoxaemia (McAnulty et al, 1982). Chronic renal disease causes fetal wastage only in the presence of hypertension; fetal well-being is not compromised by moderate renal insufficiency without hypertension (Katz et al, 1980). Clinical or subclinical autoimmune diseases (especially systemic lupus erythematosus), characterized by circulating autoantibodies, polyclonal hypergammaglobulinaemia and hypocomplementaemia, do not impair the ability to conceive but significantly increase fetal loss and pregnancy complications (Cowchock, 1991; Nicklin, 1991). The link between maternal autoimmunity and fetal loss is placental damage (Labarrere et al, 1986), evidenced by a variable combination of non-specific lesions, i.e. non-infectious chronic villitis, chronic parietal and basal deciduitis, haemorrhagic endovasculitis, villous infarction and basal arterial lesions (fibrinoid necrosis, acute atherosis and excessive intramural immunoglobulin deposition). Autoimmune thrombocytopenic purpura and myasthenia gravis are associated with increased perinatal morbidity and mortality (Levy, 1982).

Endocrine diseases depress fertility by decreasing a woman's fecundability or ability to give birth to a live infant. The effects of pituitary dysfunction have already been described and the discussion here will be confined to the peripheral endocrine organs. In the pre-insulin era, young diabetics had a 5% chance of conceiving as compared with non-diabetics and their pregnancies often came to grief. Insulin has greatly improved their prognosis but the incidence of dysovulation and infertility is still higher in diabetics. Anovulation occurs with normal prolactin levels and a reduced LH:FSH ratio. The mechanism underlying this hypothalamic defect is unknown but it may be related to an increased dopaminergic activity in the hypothalamus with a normal dopamine-prolactin system (Djursing et al, 1982). Insulin therapy and tighter metabolic control have greatly improved their prognosis. Their ability to conceive is now normal but they still have fewer pregnancies and fewer births than non-diabetics. This is due to a higher rate of voluntary infertility, pregnancy complications and late intrauterine and neonatal death (Kjaer et al, 1992). There is no evidence that well-controlled diabetics are more prone to recurrent spontaneous abortion (Crane & Wahl, 1981).

Chronic reactive hyperinsulinaemia, which is the opposite of the hypoinsulinaemia of juvenile diabetes, results from impaired peripheral insulin action caused by intrinsic abnormalities in the insulin receptor, circulating antibodies to the receptor and inappropriate levels of physiological insulin antagonists, as in acromegaly and Cushing's syndrome (Buyalos et al, 1992). While insulin action on glucose disposal is reduced, its action on the ovarian thecal and stromal cells, largely dependent on the IGF-1 receptor-effector mechanism, remains unaffected. Thus the excess insulin synergizes with LH to increase intraovarian androstenedione and testosterone production, which leads to secondary derangements in gonadotrophin secretion and the development of polycystic ovaries with anovulation and infertility (Barbieri et al, 1988). A rare but serious complication of untreated polycystic ovarian syndrome is endometrial carcinoma (Honoré & Davey, 1989).

In women and adolescents primary hypothyroidism, usually of the autoimmune type, can cause menstrual irregularities, anovulation and infertility, disturbances readily reversed by substitution therapy. The mechanism whereby decreased thyroid function disturbs the hypothalamus-pituitary-gonad axis is unclear but abnormal responses to TRH, LH and bromocriptine have been described, suggesting a central defect (Muechler & Huang, 1982). It is possible that sellar enlargement due to secondary thyrotroph hypertrophy interferes with gonadotroph function resulting in a failure of LH surge and an acyclic secretory pattern often associated with polycystic ovaries (Lindsay et al, 1983). In hypothyroidism there is also an increased rate of spontaneous abortion, stillbirth and fetal anomalies which may be related to decreased availability of maternal thyroxine to the developing embryo before fetal thyroid ontogenesis and to maternal deficiencies in some thyroxine-dependent crucial enzymes, i.e. Na^+-K^+ adenosine triphosphatase critical in the membrane transport of glucose (Potter, 1980). Occult hypothyroidism may lead to the polycystic ovarian syndrome and infertility (Insler & Lunenfeld, 1991). Hypothyroidism (Graves disease) is associated with fetal growth retardation, thrombocytopenia and a high neonatal mortality rate (Levy, 1982).

Hyperparathyroidism in pregnancy is associated with a significant increase in spontaneous abortion, fetal death, premature labour and neonatal hypocalcaemia and tetany (Ludwig, 1962; Delmonico et al, 1976). The disease can present insidiously (Shangold et al, 1982) or acutely with pancreatitis (Hess et al, 1980). A significant association between nephrolithiasis and spontaneous abortion has been noted; it is possible that these stone-formers had subclinical hyperparathyroidism (Honoré, 1980).

Severe hypofunction or hyperfunction of the adrenal cortex causes widespread systemic disturbances that reduce fertility but these problems as a rule present to the internist. There is a more subtle and selective form of adrenal dysfunction with direct reproductive impact, i.e. adrenal hyperandrogenism. This condition, often co-existing with ovarian hyperandrogenism, is associated with infertility, anovulation, oligomenorrhoea and somatic manifestations, i.e. hirsutism, acne, clitoromegaly, etc. It can be diagnosed by measurements of serum androgens including dehydroepiandrosterone sulphate, and by the dexamethasone suppression test. Excessive androgen secretion by the adrenals can result from (Maroulis, 1981):

1. Benign or malignant tumours with excessive production of adrenal androgens and/or testosterone.

2. Late-onset congenital or acquired adrenal hyperplasia due to partial deficiency of 11- or 21-hydroxylase or 3β-hydroxysteroid dehydrogenase (Bongiovanni, 1981). Late-onset 21-hydroxylase deficiency is considered to be an allelic variant of the congenital virilizing adrenal hyperplasia with an attenuated enzymatic defect (Chrousos et al, 1982) and it can mimic polycystic ovarian disease (Lobo & Goebelsmann, 1980). Late-onset congenital adrenal hyperplasia due to partial 21-hydroxylase deficiency is one of the commonest autosomal recessive disorders in humans with an overall incidence of 5% among hirsute women (Brodie & Wentz, 1987).

3. Selective androgen hypersecretion in the presence of normal levels of cortisol and ACTH and normal appearing adrenal glands with slight widening of the zona fasciculata and the zona reticularis (Benedict et al, 1962). The functional defect appears to be due to an 'exaggerated adrenarche' with a higher than normal setting for androgen secretion, resulting not from primary enzyme deficiency and feedback-related ACTH hypersecretion but from dysregulation of one critical enzyme, i.e. cytochrome P-450C 17α-hydroxylase in the adrenal cortex and ovaries (Rosenfield et al, 1990).

4. Chronic stress may activate the adrenals and account for the raised serum androgens detected in some infertile women (Lobo et al, 1983).

The mechanisms whereby hyperandrogenism causes infertility include (Maroulis, 1981):

(i) Anovulation with or without polycystic ovaries
(ii) Corpus luteum deficiency due to depression of progesterone secretion by testosterone (Rodriguez-Rigau et al, 1979)
(iii) Interference with fertilization or nidation, as indirectly suggested by the failure of pregnancy to occur despite clomiphene-induced ovulation (Dupon et al, 1973)
(iv) Possible interference with oestrogen-induced changes in the cervical mucus (Langer et al, 1990).

Rare maternal diseases causing primary or secondary infertility include:

- Neurofibromatosis (Blickstein & Lurie, 1990).
- Primary epilepsy (Bilo et al, 1991): paroxysmal discharges in the central nervous system disrupt the setting of the central GnRH generator leading to an abnormally high LH pulsatility frequency, anovulation with polycystic ovaries and primary or secondary amenorrhoea.
- Wilson's disease, an inherited disorder of copper metabolism, can cause recurrent spontaneous abortion (Van Leeuwen et al, 1991) or ovulatory disturbances due to copper toxicity exerted on follicular aromatase (Kaushansky et al, 1987).
- Coeliac disease (Joske & Martin, 1971): folate deficiency leads to recurrent abortions.
- Coagulation disorders with recurrent fetal loss due to placental infarction or abruption. These include deficiency of fibrinogen (Evron et al, 1985), factor XII (Schved et al, 1989) and factor XIII (Frydman et al, 1986) and primary thrombocythaemia (Snethlage & Ten Cate, 1986).

COMPLICATIONS OF INFERTILITY DIAGNOSIS AND TREATMENT

Infertility is now a recognized affliction that demands action and infertile couples are automatically exposed to an ever-increasing list of investigations and therapeutic modalities. It is salutary to pause and reflect that these patients can develop life-threatening, crippling or infertility-enhancing complications, which, although admittedly infrequent, arise in young healthy 'normal' people and thus assume greater clinical and personal significance. Moreover, since these patients are often emotionally distressed and frustrated (Menning, 1980), such complications can be perceived with hostility and lead to litigation. For these reasons the significant complications of infertility diagnosis and treatment in women will be briefly discussed.

Complications of infertility investigations

These are uncommon and are best discussed in relation to the four primary forms of investigation performed:

Endometrial sampling

Excepting the rare complication of uterine perforation requiring emergency hysterectomy, the time-honoured diagnostic curettage is safe and widely used in gynaecology but recent studies have cast serious doubt on its safety and advisability in infertility investigation. It can give rise to intrauterine adhesions (Taylor et al, 1981) and to chronic pelvic inflammatory disease with its usual sequelae, i.e. tubal adhesions, hydrosalpinx, proximal tubal occlusion and distal phimosis (Taylor & Graham, 1982). Hence it has been suggested that curettage be avoided and replaced by endometrial biopsy, which is less traumatic and can be performed on an outpatient basis. Its complications are minimal and include inadequate sampling due to cervical stenosis, excessive haemorrhage, excessive discomfort, fever, vasovagal reaction, uterine perforation and interruption of pregnancy. The chances of biopsying the endometrium during the cycle of conception are 3–5%; the overall risk of interrupting a pregnancy is 0.06% and about 2% if the implantation site is biopsied (Jaffe & Jewelewicz, 1991). It would appear that endometrial biopsy has a detrimental effect on pregnancies following gonadotrophin therapy (Jacobson & Marshall, 1980).

Laparoscopy

Laparoscopy is extensively used to assess ovulation, tubal patency and normalcy or otherwise of tubo-ovarian anatomy. Significant complications of gynaecological laparoscopy are rare, with an overall incidence of 7.4 per 1000 cases (Loffer & Pent, 1975). The most serious complication is death from cardiac arrest, which occurs in about one to three patients per 10 000. Other non-lethal complications include: cardiac arrest and arrhythmia with survival; vascular disturbances, i.e. deep vein thrombosis and pulmonary embolism, hypertension and gas embolism; bleeding arising at the site of abdominal puncture or at the site of biopsy; bowel burn or trauma (Loffer & Pent, 1975; Carron Brown et al, 1978); subcutaneous emphysema, gas extravasation into the mesentery, mediastinum or pleural sacs and anaesthetic complications (Loffer & Pent, 1975; Carron Brown et al, 1978; Ohlgisser et al, 1985). Rarely bowel injuries may not be recognized at the time of direct vision laparoscopy and fragments of small intestine are only detected pathologically (Gentile & Siegler, 1981); direct traumatic injury to bowel can be distinguished pathologically from injury caused by electrocoagulation (Levy et al, 1985). Small bowel obstruction due to herniation through an incisional defect following laparoscopy is a rare complication (Sauer & Jarrett, 1984). Significant infections, i.e. infection of pelvic haematoma or pelvic inflammatory disease, rarely follow investigative laparoscopy.

Hysteroscopy

Hysteroscopy is now a well-established procedure with negligible risks in experienced hands (Daly et al, 1983; Siegler & Valle, 1988). Its complications include cervical laceration, uterine perforation, especially when therapeutic manoeuvres are performed, uterine bleeding rarely needing transfusion, ascending genital infection, which so far appears to be a theoretical rather than a real danger, gas embolism, bowel burn and perforation (Sugimoto, 1978). Additional complications related to the use of dextran as a distending medium include cardiovascular overload, allergic reactions (Trimbos-Kemper & Veering, 1990) and non-cardiogenic pulmonary oedema (Leake et al, 1987). Severe haemorrhage after hysteroscopic division of a uterine septum is rare (Kazer et al, 1992).

Hysterosalpingography

Hysterosalpingography is widely used to evaluate the uterine cavity and the tubes. Adverse reactions, occurring in 2% of cases, include: mechanical complications, i.e. cervical laceration, uterine perforation, tubal rupture; chemical complications, i.e. acute allergic reactions (Schwitemaker et al, 1990), slight and transient thyroid dysfunction, and lipoid granulomas of the tube; vascular complications, i.e. pulmonary oil embolism; infective complications, i.e. usually due to exacerbation of chronic pelvic infection giving rise to acute salpingitis and peritonitis. The most serious complication is death occurring during the procedure or within two weeks as a result of peritonitis, pulmonary embolism or lipoid pneumonia (Siegler, 1983; Jaffe & Jewelewicz, 1991).

Hysterosalpingography increases the pregnancy rate in some women and its therapeutic effect is due to the bacteriostatic effect of iodine, enhancement of ciliary action, hydrotubation effect with mechanical lavage and adhesiolysis and decreased spermiophagy (Jaffe & Jewelewicz, 1991).

Complications of infertility therapy

These complications, arising from deliberate interventions in the female, are variably inherent in the methods and secondary to extraneous factors, such as patient selection, the skill of the operator and the efficiency of patient monitoring during and after treatment. A brief review is included in terms of the three major therapeutic modalities, i.e. surgery, medical therapy and transfer methods.

Surgery

Surgery plays an important rôle in infertility therapy and recent advances in anaesthesia, surgical technique, postoperative support and a better understanding of reproductive anatomy and physiology have greatly improved the success rate. The complications will be discussed in relation to the organ operated upon:

Tubal surgery has changed drastically with the introduction of microsurgery and the results are significantly better than those obtained by conventional macrosurgery (Fayez & Suliman, 1982). Lysis of tubal or tubo-ovarian adhesions, with or without associated uterine suspension, has no significant complication (Fayez & Suliman, 1982; Gomel, 1983). A higher rate of ectopic pregnancy, the major complication of tubal surgery, is associated with fimbrioplasty (the surgical correction of partial fimbrial occlusion), salpingoneostomy (the surgical repair of a totally occluded distal tube) and tubotubal or tubocornual anastomosis (De Cherney et al, 1983; Gomel, 1983). There is also an increased incidence of spontaneous abortion, especially after uterotubal implantation (Jansen, 1982). Rare complications of tuboplasty include traumatic femoral neuropathy (Hassan et al, 1986) and intercornual bridging by a swollen blocked tube showing haematosalpinx, chronic salpingitis and perisalpingeal endometriosis (Honoré & Scott, 1992).

Postoperative adhesions, leading to mechanical infertility, are still a nightmare to the infertility surgeon but the use of intraperitoneal dextran has significantly reduced their occurrence. Unfortunately, dextran can occasionally give rise to serious complications, e.g. non-cardiogenic pulmonary oedema, anaphylactoid reactions, and pelvic abscess (Siegler & Valle, 1988; King, 1989). Laparoscopic surgery has also reduced the incidence of postoperative adhesions (Lundorff et al, 1991).

Ovarian surgery, confined to bilateral wedge resection in drug-resistant cases of polycystic ovarian disease, is followed by significant pelvic adhesions in at least 8% of cases (Adashi et al, 1981). These adhesions, constituting an iatrogenically induced mechanical cause of infertility (Weinstein & Polishuk, 1975), account in large measure for the discrepancy between the rate of postoperative ovulation and the crude pregnancy rate. Microsurgery appears to reduce the chances of postoperative adhesions. Another complication is the significantly increased incidence of ectopic pregnancy after wedge resection (Adashi et al, 1981).

Uterine surgery involves intervention at the level of the cervix, myometrium and endometrium. Cervical cerclage, done for incompetence, can be associated with premature rupture of membranes, ascending membranitis, prematurity and uterine rupture requiring hysterectomy (Peters et al, 1979). Myomectomy, despite its variable success in correcting infertility (Berkeley et al, 1983), is not followed by obstetrical problems (Sengupta et al, 1978), except for the occasional rupture of the pregnant uterus (Levi, 1961). Metroplasty, performed for symptomatic uterine anomalies, is followed by a high rate of successful uncomplicated pregnancy (Daly et al, 1983; Ayhan et al, 1992). Lysis of intrauterine adhesions by conventional methods is complicated by a high rate of pregnancy loss, prematurity, placenta accreta and placenta praevia (Schenker & Margalioth, 1982); these complications are significantly reduced by hysteroscopic lysis (March & Israel, 1981).

Pituitary surgery by the trans-sphenoidal route is a safe and highly successful form of treatment for hyperprolactinaemia due to a pituitary adenoma. Mortality is nil and postoperative complications include transient diabetes insipidus, hypocorticism, visual disturbances, leakage of cerebrospinal fluid and nasal septal perforation (Post et al, 1979; Woosley et al, 1982). Postoperative partial hypopituitarism is exceptional (Dawood et al, 1982).

Laser surgery is now used for treating endometriosis, adnexal adhesions and tubal occlusions. It is a very safe procedure in trained hands and complications include inadvertent damage to adjacent non-target tissues, fires from ignition of sponges and drapes, anaesthetic gas explosions and irritation of the surgeon's lungs (Daniell, 1984).

Medical therapy

Medical therapy is widely used and its complications can be reproductive or systemic depending on the drug used. The reports of the adverse effects of clomiphene citrate, used to stimulate ovulation, are so discrepant that no meaningful conclusions can be drawn (Adashi et al, 1979b). It is still unclear whether the drug is associated with a higher incidence of spontaneous abortion, ectopic pregnancy, hydatidiform mole, prematurity and pre-eclampsia (Correy et al, 1982; Hammond & Talbert, 1982; Shoham et al, 1991; Bateman et al, 1992). There is, however, good evidence that such treatment is followed by multiple gestations including superfetation (Bsat & Seoud, 1987) but there is no increase in congenital malformations (Shoham et al, 1991). Clomiphene often causes cystic enlargement of the ovaries (Farrari et al, 1969), which is rarely symptomatic (Chow & Chou, 1984); bilateral adnexal torsion is exceptional (Bider et al, 1991).

Ovarian hyperstimulation is deliberately induced by combined human menopausal gonadotrophin (hMG) and human chorionic gonadotrophin (hCG) to provide as many retrievable oocytes as possible for in vitro fertilization and embryo transfer. Its control is delicate and mild forms of excessive hyperstimulation are common while the severe life-threatening form is less than 1%. The complications of the ovarian hyperstimulation syndrome include ovarian enlargement, adnexal torsion, ascites, hydrothorax anasarca, haemoconcentration, oliguric renal failure, liver dysfunction, adult respiratory distress syndrome, venous thrombosis and death (Asch et al, 1991; Fournet et al, 1991; Mills et al, 1992; Navot et al, 1992). There are two theories about its pathogenesis: the first implicates increased vascular permeability, especially in the enlarged ovaries, as the primary event followed by fluid leakage into the peritoneum and hypovolaemia; the second implicates arteriolar dilatation as the primary event with underfilling of the vascular bed and hypovolaemic shock (Balasch et al, 1991). The risk factors include excessive serum oestradiol levels on the day of hCG administration and a large number of oocytes retrieved (Asch et al, 1991). Gonadotrophins are also used to induce ovulation and achieve spontaneous pregnancy. Pregnancies following such treatment have a high rate of multiple gestations, fetal wastage (Ben-Rafael et al, 1983) and associated pre-eclampsia (March, 1978). The relationship between gonadotrophin treatment and complete hydatidiform mole (Altaras et al, 1992), combined uterine and ectopic pregnancy (Yovich et al, 1984), visual disturbances (Lee et al, 1983) and uterine and ovarian carcinoma (Bamford & Steele, 1982) is unclear. There are also mild androgenic effects, e.g. acne, hirsutism, clitoral hypertrophy and deepening of the voice (Mercaitis et al, 1985).

The antigonadotrophin drug, danazol, is widely used in the conservative management of endometriosis, particularly in the young infertile patient, and its side effects are relatively minor (Dmowski, 1979) including carpal tunnel syndrome (Sikka et al, 1983), sensorineural hearing loss (Ennyeart & Price, 1984), post-therapy amenorrhoea (Peress, 1984) and reversible elevation of serum enzymes (Holt & Keller, 1984). There is surprisingly little information regarding its possible effects on pregnancy. The rate of spontaneous abortion is reported as increased or unchanged after cessation of therapy (Dmowski & Cohen, 1978; Barbieri et al, 1982) and there are no teratological consequences when the drug is taken in early pregnancy. Two cases of female pseudohermaphroditism with intrauterine danazol exposure are on record (Duck & Katayama, 1981; Peress et al, 1982). A rare complication is the combination of toxic dermatitis, fulminant hepatic failure and aplastic anaemia (Nakajima et al, 1986).

Bromocriptine, a dopaminergic agonist used in the treatment of hyperprolactinaemia, has no adverse effects on the pregnancy or the fetus (Dewit et al, 1984) and the only 'complication' of bromocriptine-induced pregnancy is symptomatic growth of a prolactinoma (Dommerholt et al, 1981). Rarely, low dose treatment of infertile hyperprolactinaemic patients can cause cold-induced vasospasm or Raynaud's phenomenon (Quagliarello & Barakat, 1987).

Gonadotrophin-releasing hormone (GnRH), or its agonists (GnRH-a), used to induce ovulation in hypogonadotrophic infertility, rarely cause ovarian hyperstimulation (Schweditsch et al, 1984) and multiple pregnancy (Heineman et al, 1984) when given as pulsatile therapy. Long-acting agonists often produce asymptomatic follicular and luteal cysts (Ben-Rafael et al, 1990; Sampaio et al, 1991). Synthetic luteinizing hormone-releasing hormone can induce local or systemic anaphylactic reactions (McLeod et al, 1987).

Prednisone, used for the treatment of anovulation due to adrenal hyperandrogenism, has a variable effect on pregnancy depending on the dose and the length of administration during pregnancy. Large doses and prolonged administration can cause increased fetal wastage, adrenal atrophy, congenital malformations and intrauterine growth retardation; low dose therapy has no ill effects (Lee et al, 1982). Intramuscular injections rarely cause local complications but progesterone, administered as part of an IVF treatment schedule, can rarely provoke severe thigh myositis (Phipps et al, 1988).

Transfer methods

These include artificial insemination and in vitro fertilization and embryo transfer.

Artificial insemination is used increasingly to treat infertility due to azoospermia and severe oligospermia; its major complication is transmitted genital infection, which occurs despite bacteriological screening of donor semen and can cause secondary infertility in a previously fertile woman. There is no convincing evidence of an increased incidence of ectopic pregnancy, pregnancy loss, obstetrical complications or congenital malformations (Stone, 1980). Artificial insemination with the husband's semen is associated with a high spontaneous abortion rate (Jansen, 1982).

The complications of intrauterine insemination, alone or in combination with ovarian stimulation, include anaphylactic shock (Sonenthal et al, 1991), ascending pelvic infection and a slight increase in spontaneous abortions. Two theoretical complications, i.e. induction of sperm antibodies and congenital anomalies as a result of abnormal sperms, have not so far materialized (Dodson & Haney, 1991). The risk of HIV transmission is ever present but it would appear to be negligible. The transmission of the ubiquitous *human papilloma virus* (HPV) poses a real threat but so far its impact on the development of cervical neoplasia is unknown (Rogers et al, 1992).

Assisted reproductive technology (ART)

Over the last decade many forms of assisted technology have come into use including in vitro fertilization-embryo transfer (IVF-ET), gamete intra-Fallopian transfer (GIFT), zygote intra-Fallopian transfer (ZIFT), frozen embryo transfer and IVF with donated oocytes (Medical Research International Society for Assisted Reproductive Technology [ART], The American Fertility Society, 1992). Since these techniques are new and investigational the full range of complications is still being reported. They include:

1. Increased preclinical and clinical losses with reduced rate of successful pregnancy (Acosta et al, 1990). The cause of such a high rate of fetal loss is not known but there is conflicting evidence about the rôle of aneuploidy (Roseler et al, 1990; Zenzes & Casper, 1992).

2. Increased rate of ectopic pregnancy (Karande et al, 1991), especially the heterotopic type, i.e. combined intrauterine and extrauterine pregnancy (Dimitry et al, 1990; Li H P et al, 1992). A single case of combined intrauterine and cervical pregnancy after IVF is on record (Bayati et al, 1989). The factors underlying this increase in ectopic pregnancy include pre-existing tubal disease, high oestradiol levels following ovulation induction and internal embryo migration from uterus to tube (Peek & Graham, 1992).

3. Hydatidiform mole is not increased after ART. There is a case on record of a hydatidiform mole with co-existing twin pregnancy after GIFT (van de Geijn et al, 1992).

4. Superfetation resulting from fertilization of two or more oocytes from successive ovulations is very rare in humans. There is a single case recorded after IVF (Lefebvre et al, 1990).

5. Pelvic infection is rare after ART, with two cases recorded, one of bilateral acute salpingitis and left ovarian abscess complicating GIFT (Hickling & Killick, 1991) and one of an acute tubo-ovarian abscess after transcervical embryo transfer in an agonadal woman (Sauer & Paulson, 1992).

6. Uterine neoplasia is a potential complication due to the hormonal disturbances produced by ovulation induction. So far only a case of endometrial sarcoma has been described in a 38-year-old woman following IVF for male factor infertility (Waterstone & Parsons, 1992).

7. Mechanical complications have not been systematically reported despite the fact that they must occur. There are two cases of instrument failure with lodgement of metal pieces in the patient's abdomen (Whitman & Di Lauro, 1990).

8. Adnexal torsion associated with gonadotrophin-induced superovulation for ovum retrieval (Chin et al, 1987; Mashiach et al, 1990).

Acknowledgements

I would like to express my sincere thanks to Ms Lynda Harrison for her patience and unfailing support during the typing of the updated manuscript and to Mr Tom Turner for the excellent photographs.

REFERENCES

Abuelo D N, Barsel-Powers G, Richardson A 1988 Insertional translocations: report of two new families and review of the literature. American Journal of Medical Genetics 31: 319–329.

Abse D W 1966 Psychiatric aspects of human male infertility. Fertility and Sterility 17: 133–139.

Abuzeid M I, Weibe R H, Askel S, Shepherd J, Yeoman R R 1987 Evidence of a possible cytosol estrogen receptor deficiency in endocervical glands of infertile women with poor cervical mucus. Fertility and Sterility 47: 101–107.

Acosta A A, Oehninger S, Hammer J, Muasher S J, Liang H M, Jones D L 1990 Preclinical abortions: incidence and significance in the Norfolk in vitro fertilization program. Fertility and Sterility 53: 673–676.

Adams C E 1979 Consequences of accelerated ovum transport, including a reevaluation of Estes' operation. Journal of Reproduction and Fertility 55: 239–246.

Adashi E Y, Rakoff J, Divers W, Fishman J, Yen S S C 1979a The effect of acutely administered 2-hydroxyestrone on the release of gonadotropins and prolactin before and after estrogen priming in hypogonadal women. Life Sciences 25: 2051–2053.

Adashi E Y, Rock J A, Sapp K C, Martin E J, Wentz A C, Seegar-Jones G A 1979b Gestational outcome of clomiphene related conceptions. Fertility and Sterility 31: 620–626.

Adashi E Y, Rock J A, Guzick D, Wentz A C, Seegar-Jones G A, Jones J W Jr 1981 Fertility following bilateral ovarian wedge resection: a critical analysis of 90 consecutive cases of the polycystic ovary syndrome. Fertility and Sterility 36: 320–325.

Ahlgren M 1975 Sperm transport to and survival in the human fallopian tube. Gynecologic Investigation 6: 206–214.

Aitken R J 1979 Tubal and uterine secretion; the possibilities for contraceptive attack. Journal of Reproduction and Fertility 55: 247–254.

Aksel 1987 Thou shalt luteinize, not rupture. Fertility and Sterility 47: 762–764.

Alexander N J, Anderson D J 1987 Immunology of semen. Fertility and Sterility 47: 192–205.

Altaras M M, Rosen D J D, Ben-nun I, Aviram R, Bernheim J, Beyth Y 1992 Hydatidiform mole existing with a fetus in twin gestation following gonadotrophin induction of ovulation. Human Reproduction 7: 429–431.

Anand S, Guha S K 1982 Dynamics of the ampullary-isthmic junction in rabbit oviduct. Gynecologic and Obstetrical Investigation 14: 39–46.

Andersen A N, Pedersen H, Djursing H, Andersen B N, Friesen H G 1982 Bioactivity of prolactin in a woman with an excess of large molecular size prolactin, persistent hyperprolactinemia and spontaneous conception. Fertility and Sterility 38: 625–628.

Anderson B A 1975 Male age and fertility: results from Ireland prior to 1911. Population Index 41: 561–574.

Anestad G, Lunde O, Moen M, Dalaker K 1987 Infertility and Chlamydial infection. Fertility and Sterility 48: 787–790.

Anniko M, Tribukait B, Wersall J 1984 DNA ploidy and cell phase in human pituitary tumors. Cancer 53: 1708–1713.

Ansari A H, Gould K C, Ansari V M 1980 Sodium bicarbonate douching for improvement of the postcoital test. Fertility and Sterility 33: 608–612.

Araki S, Chikazawa K, Sekiguchi I, Yamauchi H, Motoyama M, Tamada T 1987 Arrest of follicular development in a patient with 7α-hydroxylase deficiency: folliculogenesis in association with a lack of estrogen synthesis in the ovaries. Fertility and Sterility 47: 169–172.

Archer D F, Maroon J C, Dubois P J 1978 Galactorrhoea, amenorrhoea, hyper-prolactinemia and an empty sella. Obstetrics and Gynecology 52: 23S–27S.

Aronnet G H, Eduljee S Y, O'Brien J R 1969 A nine-year survey of fallopian tube dysfunction in human infertility. Fertility and Sterility 20: 903–908.

Asch R H, Li H-P, Balmaceda J P, Weckstein L N, Stone S C 1991 Severe ovarian hyperstimulation syndrome in assisted reproduction technology: definition of high risk groups. Human Reproduction 10: 1395–1399.

Ashkenazi J, Feldberg D, Shelef M, Dicker D, Goldman J A 1987 Empty follicle syndrome: an entity in the etiology of infertility of unknown origin or a phenomenon associated with purified follicle-stimulating hormone therapy. Fertility and Sterility 48: 152–154.

Ayhan A, Yucel I, Tuncer Z S, Kisnisci 1992 Reproductive performance after conventional metroplasty: an evaluation of 102 cases. Fertility and Sterility 57: 1194–1196.

Baker E R 1981 Menstrual dysfunction and hormonal status in athletic women: a review. Fertility and Sterility 36: 691–696.

Balasch J, Arroyo V, Carmona F, Llach J, Jimenez W, Pare J C, Vanrell J A 1991 Severe ovarian hyperstimulation syndrome: role of peripheral vasodilatation. Fertility and Sterility 56: 1077–1083.

Bamford P O V, Steele S J 1982 Uterine and ovarian carcinoma in a patient receiving gonadotropin therapy: case report. British Journal of Obstetrics and Gynaecology 89: 962–964.

Barbieri R L, Evans S, Kistner R W 1982 Danazol in the treatment of endometriosis: analysis of 100 cases with a 4-year follow-up. Fertility and Sterility 37: 737–746.

Barbieri R L, Smith S, Ryan K J 1988 The role of hyperinsulinemia in the pathogenesis of ovarian hyperandrogenism. Fertility and Sterility 50: 197–212.

Barratt C L R, Cooke I D 1991 Sperm transport in the human female reproductive tract: a dynamic interaction. International Journal of Andrology 14: 394–411.

Barros C, Arguello B, Jedlicki A, Vigil P, Herrera E 1985 Scanning electron microscopy study of human cervical mucus. Gamete Research 12: 85–89.

Barry V C, Klawans H L 1976 On the role of dopamine in the pathophysiology of anorexia nervosa. Journal of Neural Transmission 38: 107–114.

Bassetti M, Spada A, Pezzo G, Giannattasio G 1984 Bromocriptine treatment reduces cell size in human macroprolactinomas: a morphometric study. Journal of Clinical Endocrinology and Metabolism 58: 268–273.

Bateman B G, Eddy C A, Kitchin J D III 1983 Effect of lengthening the fallopian tube on fertility in the rabbit. American Journal of Obstetrics and Gynecology 147: 569–573.

Bateman B G, Nunley W C Jr, Kitchen J D III 1987 Surgical management of distal tubal obstruction — are we making progress? Fertility and Sterility 48: 523–542.

Bateman B G, Kolp L A, Nunley W C Jr, Thomas T S, Milles S E 1990 Oocyte retention after follicle luteinization. Fertility and Sterility 54: 793–798.

Bateman B G, Kolp L A, Nunley W C Jr, Felder R, Burkett B 1992 Subclinical pregnancy loss in clomiphene citrate-treated women. Fertility and Sterility 57: 25–27.

Bates G W, Whitworth N S 1982 Effect of body weight reduction on plasma androgens in obese infertile women. Fertility and Sterility 38: 406–409.

Battin D A, Barnes R B, Hoffman D I, Schachter J, Di Zerega G S, Yonekura M C 1984 Chlamydia trachomatis is not an important cause of abnormal postcoital tests in ovulating women. Fertility and Sterility 42: 233–236.

Bayati J, Garcia J E, Rosey J H, Padilla S L 1989 Combined intrauterine and cervical pregnancy from in vivo fertilization and embryo transfer. Fertility and Sterility 51: 725–727.

Bazak-Malik G, Mashewari B, Lan N 1983 Tuberculous endometritis: a clinicopathological study of 100 cases. British Journal of Obstetrics and Gynaecology 90: 84–86.

Benedict P H, Cohen R, Cope O, Scully R E 1962 Ovarian and adrenal morphology in cases of hirsutism or virilism and the Stein-Leventhal syndrome. Fertility and Sterility 13: 380–395.

Ben-Rafael Z, Dor J, Mashiach S, Blankstein J, Lunenfeld B, Berr D M 1983 Abortion rate in pregnancies following ovulation induced by human menopausal gonadotropin/human chorionic gonadotropin. Fertility and Sterility 39: 157–161.

Ben-Rafael Z, Bider D, Menashe Y, Maymon R, Zolti M, Mashiach S 1990 Follicular and luteal cysts after treatment with gonadotrophin-releasing hormone analog for in vitro fertilization. Fertility and Sterility 53: 1091–1094.

Berger D M 1980 Impotence following the discovery of azoospermia. Fertility and Sterility 34: 154–157.

Berkeley A S, DeCherney A H, Polan M H 1983 Abdominal myomectomy and subsequent fertility. Surgery, Gynecology and Obstetrics 156: 319–322.

Berry R G, Caplan H J 1979 An overview of pituitary tumors. Annals of Clinical and Laboratory Science 9: 94–102.

Best C L, Walters G, Adelman D C 1988 Fixed cutaneous eruptions to seminal-plasma challenge: a case report. Fertility and Sterility 50: 532–534.

Beyth Y, Bar-On E 1984 Tubo-ovarian amputation and infertility. Fertility and Sterility 42: 932–934.

Beyth Y, Mor-Yosef S 1982 Combined medical and surgical treatment for transverse vaginal septum associated with anovulation. Fertility and Sterility 37: 704–706.

Biberglu K O, Damewood M D, Parmley T, Rock J A 1988 Insensitive ovary syndrome with a unique process of follicular degeneration. Fertility and Sterility 49: 367–369.

Bider D, Goldenberg M, Ben-Rafael Z, Oelsner G 1991 Bilateral adnexal torsion after clomiphene citrate therapy. Human Reproduction 6: 1443–1444.

Bilo L, Meo R, Valentino R, Buccaino G, Striano S, Nappi C 1991 Abnormal pattern of luteinizing hormone pulsatility in women with epilepsy. Fertility and Sterility 55: 705–711.

Blickstein I, Lurie S 1990 The gynaecological problems of neurofibromatosis. Australian and New Zealand Journal of Obstetrics and Gynaecology 30: 380–382.

Blumenfeld Z, Ruach M 1992 Early pregnancy wastage: the role of repetitive human chorionic gonadotrophin supplementation during the first 8 weeks of gestation. Fertility and Sterility 58: 19–23.

Bomsel-Helmreich O 1976 The aging of gametes, heteroploidy and embryonic death. International Journal of Gynaecology and Obstetrics 14: 98–104.

Bongiovanni A M 1981 Acquired adrenal hyperplasia: with special reference to 3β hydroxysteroid dehydrogenase. Fertility and Sterility 35: 599–608.

Bongso A, Ng S-C, Fong C Y, Anandakumar C, Marshall B, Edirisinghe R, Ratnam S 1992 Improved pregnancy rate after transfer of embryos grown in human fallopian tubal cell coculture. Fertility and Sterility 58: 569–574.

Bonhoff A, Johannison E, Bohnet H G 1990 Morphometric analysis of the endometrium of infertile patients in relation to peripheral hormone levels. Fertility and Sterility 54: 84–89.

Boothroyd C V, Lepre F 1990 Permanent voice change resulting from Danazol therapy. Australian and New Zealand Journal of Obstetrics and Gynaecology 30: 275–276.

Boyden T W, Pamenter R W, Stanforth P, Rotkis T, Wilmore J H 1983 Sex steroids and endurance running in women. Fertility and Sterility 39: 629–632.

Boyers S P, Corrales M D, Huszar G, De Cherney A H 1987 The effects of Lubrin on sperm motility in vitro. Fertility and Sterility 47: 882–884.

Bracken M B, Hellenbrand K G, Holford T R 1990 Conception delay after oral contraceptive use: the effect of estrogen dose. Fertility and Sterility 53: 21–27.

Bression D et al 1980 Dopaminergic receptors in human prolactin-secreting adenomas: a quantitative study. Journal of Clinical Endocrinology and Metabolism 51: 1037–1043.

Brodie B L, Wentz A C 1987 Late onset congenital adrenal hyperplasia: a gynecologist's perspective. Fertility and Sterility 48: 175–188.

Bronson R A 1987 Immunologic abnormalities of the female reproductive tract. In: Gondos B, Riddick D H (eds) Pathology of infertility. Thieme Medical Publlshers, New York, p 13.

Bsat F A, Seoud M A F 1987 Superfetation secondary to ovulation induction with clomiphene citrate: a case report. Fertility and Sterility 47: 516–518.

Bullock J L 1974 Iatrogenic impotence in an infertility clinic: illustrative cases. American Journal of Obstetrics and Gynecology 120: 476–480.

Burchell R C, Creed F, Rasoulpour M, Whitcomb M 1978 Vascular anatomy of the human uterus and pregnancy wastage. British Journal of Obstetrics and Gynaecology 85: 698–706.

Burke K, Hertig A T, Miele A 1985 Diagnostic value of subacute focal inflammation of the endometrium, with special reference to pelvic adhesions as observed on laparoscopic examination: an eight year review. Journal of Reproductive Medicine 30: 646–649.

Buttram V C Jr, Reiter R C 1981 Uterine leiomyomata: etiology, symptomatology and management. Fertility and Sterility 36: 433–445.

Buyalos R P, Geffner M E, Bersch N et al 1992 Insulin and insulin-like growth factor-1 responsiveness in polycystic ovarian syndrome. Fertility and Sterility 57: 796–803.

Bychkov V 1990 Ovarian pathology in chronic pelvic inflammatory disease. Gynecologic and Obstetric Investigation 30: 31–33.

Bygdeman M 1970 The relation between fertility and prostaglandin content of seminal fluid in man. Fertility and Sterility 21: 622–629.

Byrne J, Mulvihill J J, Myers M H et al 1992 Early menopause in long-term survivors of cancer during adolescence. American Journal of Obstetrics and Gynecology 166: 788–793.

Campana M, Serra A, Neri G 1986 Role of chromosome aberrations in recurrent abortion: a study of 269 balanced translocations. American Journal of Medical Genetics 24: 341–356.

Candiani G B, Fedele L, Parazzini F, Villa L 1991 Risk of recurrence after myomectomy. British Journal of Obstetrics and Gynaecology 98: 385–389.

Carron Brown J A, Chamberlain G V P, Jordan J A et al 1978 Gynaecological laparoscopy. The report of the working party of the confidential inquiry into gynaecological laparoscopy. British Journal of Obstetrics and Gynaecology 85: 401–403.

Casper R F, Wilkinson D, Cotterell M A 1984 The effect of increased cardiac output on luteal phase gonadal steroids: a hypothesis for runners' amenorrhoea. Fertility and Sterility 41: 364–368.

Cassell G H, Younger B J, Brown M B et al 1983 Microbiologic study of infertile women at the time of diagnostic laparoscopy: association of Ureaplasma urealyticum with a defined subpopulation. New England Journal of Medicine 308: 502–505.

Castelbaum A J, Wheeler J, Coutifaris C B, Mastroianni L, Lessey B A 1994 Timing of the endometrial biopsy may be critical for the accurate diagnosis of luteal phase deficiency. Fertility and Sterility 61: 443–447.

Cazabat A M, Volochine B, Kuntsmann J M, Chretien F C 1982 Human cervical mucus. Acta Obstetricia et Gynecologica Scandinavica 61: 385–392.

Chacho K J, Hage C W, Shulman S 1991 The relationship between female sexual practices and the development of antisperm antibodies. Fertility and Sterility 56: 461–464.

Chatkoff M L 1975 A biophysicist's view of ovum transport. Gynecologic Investigation 6: 105–122.

Check J H, Chase J S, Nowroozi K, Dietterich C J 1991 Premature luteinization: treatment and incidence in natural cycles. Human Reproduction 6: 190–193.

Chin N W, Friedman C I, Awaldalla S G, Miller F A, Kim M H 1987 Adnexal torsion as a complication of superovulation for ovum retrieval. Fertility and Sterility 48: 149–151.

Chow K K, Choo H T 1984 Ovarian hyperstimulation syndrome with clomiphene citrate: case report. British Journal of Obstetrics and Gynaecology 91: 1051–1052.

Chretien F C 1978 Ultrastructure and variations of human cervical mucus during pregnancy and the menopause. Acta Obstetricia et Gynecologica Scandinavica 57: 337–348.

Chrousos G P, Loriaux D L, Mann D L, Cutler B 1982 Late onset 21-hydroxylase deficiency mimicking idiopathic hirsutism or polycystic ovarian disease. Annals of Internal Medicine 96: 143–148.

Clarke G N 1988 Sperm antibodies and human fertilization. American Journal of Reproductive Immunology 17: 65–71.

Cohen B M 1980 Surgical repair and abnormal fimbrial gonadal relationships in the human female. Journal of Reproductive Medicine 25: 33–37.

Cohen B M, Katz M 1978 The significance of the convoluted oviduct in the infertile woman. Journal of Reproductive Medicine 21: 31–35.

Collado M L, Castro G, Hicks J J 1979 Effect of spermatozoa upon carbonic anhydrase activity of rabbit endometrium. Biology of Reproduction 20: 747–750.

Corenblum B, Taylor P J 1982 The hyperprolactinemic polycystic ovary syndrome may not be a distinct entity. Fertility and Sterility 38: 349–352.

Correy J F, Marsden D E, Schokman F M C 1982 The outcome of pregnancies resulting from clomiphene-induced ovulation. Australian and New Zealand Journal of Obstetrics and Gynaecology 22: 18–21.

Corsan G H, Ghazi D, Kemmann E 1990 Home urinary luteinizing hormone immunoassays: clinical applications. Fertility and Sterility 53: 591–601.

Coulam C B 1982 Premature gonadal failure. Fertility and Sterility 38: 645–655.

Coulam C B 1991 Epidemiology of recurrent spontaneous abortion. American Journal of Reproductive Immunology 26: 23–27.

Coulam C B, Annegers J F, Krantz J S 1982 The association between pituitary adenomas and chronic anovulation syndrome. American Journal of Obstetrics and Gynecology 143: 319–322.

Coulam C B, Stringfellow S, Hoefnagel D 1983 Evidence of a genetic factor in the etiology of premature ovarian failure. Fertility and Sterility 40: 693–695.

Coulam C B, Bustilloa M, Schulman J D 1986 Empty follicle syndrome. Fertility and Sterility 46: 1153–1155.

Coulam C B, Wagenknecht D, McIntyre J A, Faulk W P, Annegers J F 1991 Occurrence of other reproductive failures among women with recurrent spontaneous abortion. American Journal of Reproductive Immunology 25: 96–98.

Coutinho E M, Maia H S 1971 The contractile response of the human uterus, fallopian tubes and ovary to prostaglandins in vivo. Fertility and Sterility 15: 367–372.

Cowchock S 1991 Autoantibodies and pregnancy wastage. American Journal of Reproductive Immunology 26: 38–41.

Cramer D W, Ravnikar V A, Craighill M, Ng W G, Goldstein D P, Reilly R 1987 Mullerian aplasia associated with maternal deficiency of galactose-1-phosphate uridyl transferase. Fertility and Sterility 47: 930–934.

Crane J P, Wahl N 1981 The role of maternal diabetes in repetitive spontaneous abortion. Fertility and Sterility 36: 477–479.

Critser J K, Villines P M, Coulam C B, Critser E S 1989 Evaluation of circulating anti-sperm antibodies in fertile and infertile patient populations. American Journal of Reproductive Immunology 21: 137–142.

Croxatto H B, Ortiz M E, Diaz S, Hess R, Balmaceda J, Croxatto H-D 1978 Studies on the duration of egg transport by the human oviduct II Ovum location at various intervals following luteinizing hormone peak. American Journal of Obstetrics and Gynecology 132: 629–634.

Cumming D C, Honoré L H, Scott J Z 1984 Mycoplasmal endometritis: correlation with cervical and endometrial bacteriology. Infertility 7: 203–214.

Cumming D C, Honoré L H, Scott J Z, Williams K E 1985 The late luteal phase in infertile women: comparison of simultaneous endometrial biopsy and progesterone levels. Fertility and Sterility 43: 715–719.

Cumming D C, Honoré L H, Scott J Z, Williams K E 1988 Microscopic evidence of silent inflammation in grossly normal fallopian tubes with ectopic pregnancy. International Journal of Infertility 33: 324–328.

Curran J W 1980 Economic consequences of pelvic inflammatory disease in the United States. American Journal of Obstetrics and Gynecology 138: 848–851.

Czernobilsky B 1978 Endometritis and infertility. Fertility and Sterility 30: 119–130.

Daly D C, Tohan N, Doney T J, Masler I A, Riddick D H 1982 The significance of lymphocytic-leukocytic infiltrates in interpreting late luteal phase endometrial biopsies. Fertility and Sterility 37: 786–791.

Daly D C, Walters C A, Soto-Albors C E, Riddick D H 1983 Hysteroscopic metroplasty: surgical technique and obstetric outcome. Fertility and Sterility 39: 623–628.

Daly D G, Soto-Albers C E, Aversa M A 1986 Hysteroscopic detection and treatment of adhesions at the tubal ostium/uterine junction in infertile patients. Fertility and Sterility 46: 138–140.

Damewood M D, Grochow L B 1986 Prospects for fertility after chemotherapy or radiation for neoplastic disease. Fertility and Sterility 45: 443–459.

Daniell J F 1984 The role of lasers in infertility surgery. Fertility and Sterility 42: 815–823.

Datnow A D 1973 A reconsideration of the secretory function of the human endometrium. Journal of Obstetrics and Gynaecology of the British Commonwealth 80: 865–871.

David M P, Ben-Zwi D, Langer L 1981 Tubal intramural polyps and their relationship to infertility. Fertility and Sterility 35: 526–531.

Davidson B J, Thrasher T V, Seaji M 1987 An analysis of endometrial biopsies performed for infertility. Fertility and Sterility 48: 770–774.

Davis O K, Berkeley A S, Naus G J, Cholst I N, Freedman K S 1989 The incidence of luteal phase defect in normal fertile women determined by serial endometrial biopsies. Fertility and Sterility 51: 582–586.

Dawood M Y, Jarrett J C II 1982 Prolonged intrauterine retention of fetal bones after abortion causing infertility. American Journal of Obstetrics and Gynecology 143: 715–717.

Dawood M Y, Jarrett J C II, Choe J K 1982 Partial hypopituitarism and hyperprolactinemia: successful induction of ovulation with bromocriptine and human menopausal gonadotropins. Fertility and Sterility 38: 415–418.

De Almeida M, Gasagne I, Jeulin C et al 1989 In vitro processing of sperm with autoantibodies and in vitro fertilization results. Human Reproduction 4: 49–53.

De Brux J, Dupré-Froment J 1965 Etude anatomo-pathologique de la tuberculose génitale féminine cliniquement "latente". Revue Française de Gynécologie 60: 57–88.

De Cherney A H, Cholst I, Naftolin F 1981 Structure and function of the fallopian tubes following exposure to diethylstilbestrol (DES) during gestation. Fertility and Sterility 36: 741–745.

De Cherney A H, Mezer H C, Naftolin F 1983 Analysis of failure of microsurgical anastomosis after midsegment, non-coagulation tubal ligation. Fertility and Sterility 39: 618–622.

De Fazio S R, Ketchel M M 1971 Immuno-electrophoretic analysis of human cervical mucus and seminal plasma with an antiserum of cervical mucus. Journal of Reproduction and Fertility 25: 11–19.

Dehner L P, Askin F B 1975 Cytomegalovirus endometritis. Obstetrics and Gynecology 45: 211–213.

Delmonico F L, Neer R M, Cosimi A B, Barnes A B, Russel P S 1976 Hyperparathyroidism during pregnancy. American Journal of Surgery 131: 328–337.

De Voto L, Soto E, Majofke A M, Sierralta W 1980 Unconjugated steroids in the fallopian tube and peripheral blood during the normal menstrual cycle. Fertility and Sterility 33: 613–617.

De Voto L, Pino A M, Las Heras J, Soto E, Gunther A 1984 Estradiol and progesterone nuclear and cytosol receptors of hydrosalpinx. Fertility and Sterility 42: 594–597.

Dewit W, Bennink H J T, Gerards L J 1984 Prophylactic bromocriptine treatment during pregnancy in women with macroprolactinomas: report of 13 pregnancies. British Journal of Obstetrics and Gynaecology 91: 1059–1069.

Dimitry E S, Subak-Sharpe R, Mills M, Margara R, Winston R 1990 Nine cases of heterotopic pregnancies in 4 years of in vitro fertilization. Fertility and Sterility 53: 100–107.

Djahanbaruch O, Warner P, McNeilly A S, Baird D T 1984 Pulsatile release of LH and oestradiol during the periovulatory period in women. Clinical Endocrinology 20: 579–589.

Djursing H, Nyholm H C Chr, Hagen G, Molsted-Pedersen L 1982 Depressed prolactin levels in diabetic women with anovulation. Acta Obstetricia et Gynecologica Scandinavica 61: 403–406.

Dmowski W B 1979 Endocrine properties and clinical application of danazol. Fertility and Sterility 31: 237–251.

Dmowski W B, Cohen M R 1978 Antigonadotropin (danazol) in the treatment of endometriosis: evaluation of posttreatment fertility and three-year follow up data. American Journal of Obstetrics and Gynecology 130: 41–45.

Dodson W C, Haney A F 1991 Controlled ovarian hyperstimulation and intrauterine insemination for treatment of infertility. Fertility and Sterility 55: 457–467.

Dommerholt H B R, Assies J, Van der Werf A J M 1981 Growth of a prolactinoma during pregnancy: case report and review. British Journal of Obstetrics and Gynaecology 88: 62–70.

Donnez J, Casanas-Roux F, Ferin J, Thomas K 1984 Tubal polyps, epithelial inclusions and endometriosis after tubal sterilization. Fertility and Sterility 41: 564–568.

Drake T S, Gruner G M 1979 A cyclic pattern of sexual dysfunction in the infertility investigation. Fertility and Sterility 32: 542–546.

Duck S C, Katayama K P 1981 Danazol may cause female pseudohermaphroditism. Fertility and Sterility 35: 230–231.

Dunphy B C, Li T C, McLeod I C, Barratt C L R, Lenton E A, Cooke I D 1990a The interaction of parameters of male and female infertility in couples with previously unexplained infertility. Fertility and Sterility 54: 824–827.

Dunphy B C, Kay R, Robinson J N, Cooke I D 1990b The placebo response of subfertile couples to attending a tertiary referral centre. Fertility and Sterility 54: 1072–1075.

Dupon C, Rosenfeld R L, Cleary R E 1973 Sequential changes in total and free testosterone and androstenediol in plasma during spontaneous and clomid-induced ovulatory cycles. American Journal of Obstetrics and Gynecology 115: 478–482.

Durukan T, Urman B, Yarali H, Arikan U, Beykal O 1990 An abdominal pregnancy 10 years after treatment for pelvic tuberculosis. American Journal of Obstetrics and Gynecology 163: 594–595.

Eddy C J, Laufe L E 1983 Fertility following microsurgical dissociation of the ovary and fimbria in the rhesus monkey. Fertility and Sterility 39: 566–568.

Edelstam G A, Lundkvist O E, Klaresko G L, Larsson-Parra A 1992 Cyclic variation of major histocompatibility complex class II antigen expression in the human fallopian tube epithelium. Fertility and Sterility 57: 1225–1229.

Edmonds D K, Kindsay K S, Miller J F, Williamson E, Wood P J 1982 Early embryonic mortality in women. Fertility and Sterility 38: 447–453.

Eggert-Kruse W, Bockem-Hellweg S, Doll A et al 1993 Antisperm antibodies in cervical mucus in an unselected subfertile population. Human Reproduction 8: 1025–1031.

Eisenberg E 1981 Toward an understanding of reproductive function in anorexia nervosa. Fertility and Sterility 36: 543–550.

Eiserman J, Gast M J, Pineda J, Odem R R, Coluns J L 1988 Tumor necrosis factor in peritoneal fluid of women undergoing laparascopic surgery. Fertility and Sterility 50: 573–579.

Elenbogen A, Lipitz S, Maschiach S, Dor J, Levran O, Ben-Rafael Z 1991 The effect of smoking on the outcome of in vitro fertilization embryo transfer. Human Reproduction 6: 242–244.

Ennyeart J J, Price W A 1984 Bilateral sensorineural hearing loss from danazol therapy: a case report. Journal of Reproductive Medicine 29: 351–353.

Eschenbach D A 1992 Earth, motherhood and the intrauterine device. Fertility and Sterility 57: 1177–1179.

Escobar M E, Cigorraga S B, Chiauzzi V A, Charreau E H, Rivarola M A 1982 Development of the gonadotropic-resistant ovary syndrome in myasthenia gravis: suggestion of similar autoimmune mechanisms. Acta Endocrinologica 99: 431–436.

Evron S, Antery S O, Brzezinsky A, Samueloff A, Eldor A 1985 Congenital afibrinogenemia and recurrent early abortion: a case report. European Journal of Obstetrics, Gynecology and Reproductive Biology 19: 307–311.

Ezra Y, Simon A, Laufer N 1992 Defective oocytes: a new subgroup of unexplained infertility. Fertility and Sterility 58: 24–27.

Fahmy N W, Honoré L H, Cumming D C 1987 Subacute focal endometritis: association with cervical colonization with ureaplasma urealyticum, pelvic pathology and endometrial maturation. Journal of Reproductive Medicine 32: 685–687.

Falk R K, Hodgen G D 1972 Carbonic anhydrase isoenzymes in normal human endometrium and erythrocytes. American Journal of Obstetrics and Gynecology 112: 1047–1051.

Familiari G, Gaggiati A, Nottola S et al 1993 Ultrastructure of human ovarian primordial follicles after combination therapy for Hodgkin's disease. Human Reproduction 8: 2020–2087.

Farrari A N, Russowsky M, Wanderley C de B 1969 Morphology of ovaries treated with Clomiphene citrate. International Journal of Fertility 14: 289–294.

Farrer-Brown G, Bellby J O W, Tarbit M H 1971 Venous changes in the endometrium of myomatous uteri. Obstetrics and Gynecology 38: 743–746.

Fayez J A, Suliman S O 1982 Infertility surgery of the oviduct: comparison between macrosurgery and microsurgery. Fertility and Sterility 37: 73–78.

Feichtinger W 1991 Environmental factors and fertility. Human Reproduction 6: 1170–1175.

Ferenczy A, Bertrand G, Gelfand M M 1979. Proliferation kinetics of human endometrium during the normal menstrual cycle. American Journal of Obstetrics and Gynecology 133: 859–867.

Field-Richards S 1954 A preliminary series of cases of uterine hypoplasia treated by local injection of an oestrogenic emulsion. Journal of Obstetrics and Gynaecology of the British Empire 62: 205–213.

First A 1954 Transperitoneal migration of ovum or spermatozoon. Obstetrics and Gynecology 4: 431–433.

Fishman J, Boyar R M, Hellman L 1975 Influence of body weight on estradiol metabolism in young women. Journal of Clinical Endocrinology and Metabolism 41: 989–992.

Fordney D S 1978 Dyspareunia and vaginismus. Clinical Obstetrics and Gynecology 21: 205–221.

Fordney-Settlage D S, Motoshima M, Tredway D R 1973 Sperm transport from the external cervical os to the fallopian tubes in women: a time and quantitation study. Fertility and Sterility 24: 655–661.

Forssman L 1976 Distribution of blood flow in myomatous uteri as measured by locally injected ^{133}Xenon. Acta Obstetricia et Gynecologica Scandinavica 5: 101–105.

Fortier K J, Haney A F 1985 The pathologic spectrum of uterotubal junction obstruction. Obstetrics and Gynecology 65: 93–98.

Fortuny A, Carrio A, Soler A, Cararach J, Fuster S, Salani C 1988 Detection of balanced chromosome rearrangements in 445 couples with repeated abortion and cytogenetic prenatal testing in carriers. Fertility and Sterility 49: 774–779.

Fournet N, Surrey E, Kerin J 1991 Internal jugular vein thrombosis after ovulation induction with gonadotropins. Fertility and Sterility 56: 354–356.

Frantzen C, Schlosser H W 1982 Microsurgery and post-infectious tubal infertility. Fertility and Sterility 38: 397–402.

Fraser I S, Shearman R P, Smith A, Russell P 1988 An association among blepharophimosis, resistant ovary syndrome, and true premature menopause. Fertility and Sterility 50: 747–751.

Freeman E W, Garcia C-R, Rickels K 1983 Behavioural and emotional factors: comparisons of an ovulatory infertile woman with fertile and other infertile women. Fertility and Sterility 40: 195–201.

Friedley N J, Rosen S 1975 Carbonic anhydrase activity in mammalian ovary, fallopian tube and uterus. Histochemical and biochemical studies. Biology of Reproduction 12: 293–304.

Friedman A J, Daly M, Junea-Norcross M, Fine C, Rein M S 1992 Recurrence of myomas after myomectomy in women pretreated with leuprolide acetate depot or placebo. Fertility and Sterility 58: 205–208.

Friedrich E G Jr 1976 Vulvar disease. Major problems in obstetrics and gynecology, vol 9. Saunders, Philadelphia.

Fritz M A, Speroff L 1982 The endocrinology of menstrual cycle: the interaction of folliculogenesis and neuroendocrine mechanisms. Fertility and Sterility 38: 509–529.

Fritz M A, Holmes R T, Keenan E J 1991 Effect of clomiphene citrate on endometrial estrogen and progesterone receptor induction in women. American Journal of Obstetrics and Gynecology 165: 177–185.

Frydman M, Bonne-Tamir B, Braude E, Zamir R, Creter D 1986 Male fertility in factor XIII deficiency. Fertility and Sterility 45: 729–731.

Fukumoto M, Yajima Y, Oakamura H, Midorikawa O 1981 Collagenolytic enzyme activity in the human ovary: an ovulatory enzyme system. Fertility and Sterility 36: 746–750.

Futterweit W, Smith H Jr, Holt J E 1984 Dissociation of serum prolactin response to sequential thyrotropin-releasing hormone and chlorpromazine stimulation in patients with primary empty sella syndrome. Fertility and Sterility 42: 573–578.

Galle P C, Freeman E W, Galle M G, Huggins G R, Sendheimer S J 1983 Physiologic and psychologic profiles in a survey of women runners. Fertility and Sterility 39: 633–639.

Garcia C-R, Tureck R W 1984 Submucosal leiomyomas and infertility. Fertility and Sterility 42: 16–19.

Gardey G, Viala J L, Caderas de Kerleau J, Serrano J S, Lalaurie M, Boucard M 1975a Etude experimentale de l'hypoplasie uterine I — influence du facteur vasculaire. Journal de Gynecologie, Obstetrique et de Biologie de la Reproduction 4: 43–49.

Gardey G, Viala J L, Caderas de Kerleau J, Serrano J J, Lalaurie M, Boucard M 1975b Etude experimentale de l'hypoplasie uterine II — influence du traitement par un beta-mimetique. Journal de Gynecologie, Obstetrique et de Biologie de la Reproduction 4: 177–182.

Gardner R L, Shaw R W 1989 Cornual fibroids: a conservative approach to restoring tubal patency using a gonadotropin-releasing hormone agonist (goserelin) with successful pregnancy. Fertility and Sterility 52: 332–334.

Gaton E, Sejdel L, Bernstein D, Glezerman M, Czernobilsky B, Insler V 1982 The effects of estrogen and gestagen on the mucus production of endocervical cells: a histochemical study. Fertility and Sterility 29: 257–265.

Gay G, Shepard C 1972 Sex in the 'drug culture'. Medical Aspects of Human Sexuality 6: 28–33.

Gelety T J, Buyalos R P 1993 The effect of clomiphene citrate and menopausal gonadotropins on cervical mucus in ovulatory cycles. Fertility and Sterility 60: 471–476.

Gentile G P, Siegler A M 1981 Inadvertent intestinal biopsy during laparoscopy and hysteroscopy: a report of two cases. Fertility and Sterility 36: 402–404.

Gibson M, Badger G J, Byrn F, Lee K R, Korson R, Trainer T D 1991 Error in histologic dating of secretory endometrium: variance component analysis. Fertility and Sterility 56: 242–247.

Gindoff P R, Jewelewicz R 1986 Reproductive potential in the older woman. Fertility and Sterility 46: 989–1001.

Gjorgov A N 1980 Barrier contraception and breast cancer. Contributions to Gynecology and Obstetrics 8: 1–153.

Glass A R, Deuster P A, Kyle S B, Yahiro J A, Vigersky R A, Schoomaker E B 1987 Amenorrhea in Olympic marathon runners. Fertility and Sterility 48: 740–745.

Glezerman M, Bernstein D, Zakut C, Misgav N, Insler V 1982 Polyzoospermia: a definite pathologic entity. Fertility and Sterility 38: 605–608.

Goerzen J L, Leader A, Taylor P J 1983 Hysteroscopic findings in 100 women requesting reversal of a previously performed voluntary tubal sterilization. Fertility and Sterility 39: 103–104.

Golan, Langer R, Bukovsky I, Caspi E 1989 Congenital anomalies of the Mullerian system. Fertility and Sterility 51: 747–755.

Gomel V 1983 An odyssey through the oviduct. Fertility and Sterility 39: 144–156.

Gomel V, Filmar S 1987 Arrested tubal pregnancy. Fertility and Sterility 48: 1043–1047.

Goswany R K, Williams G, Steptoe P C 1988 Decreased uterine perfusion — a cause of infertility. Human Reproduction 3: 955–958.

Gould K G, Ansari A H 1983 Chemical alteration of cervical mucus by electrolytes. American Journal of Obstetrics and Gynecology 145: 92–99.

Govan A D T 1962 Tuberculous endometritis. Journal of Pathology and Bacteriology 83: 363–372.

Grant A 1962 The effect of ectopic pregnancy on fertility. Clinics in Obstetrics and Gynecology 5: 861–874.

Green B B, Weiss N S, Daling J R 1988 Risk of ovulatory infertility in relation to body weight. Fertility and Sterility 50: 721–726.

Grunfeld L, Sandler B, Fox J, Boyd C, Kaplan P, Navot D 1989 Luteal phase deficiency after completely normal follicular and periovulatory phases. Fertility and Sterility 52: 919–923.

Guerrero R, Rojas O I 1975 Spontaneous abortion and aging of human ova and spermatozoa. New England Journal of Medicine 293: 573–575.

Gump D W, Gibson M, Askikaga T 1984 Lack of association between genital mycoplasmas and infertility. New England Journal of Medicine 310: 937–941.

Gupta D M, Karkun J N, Kar A B 1970 Biochemical changes in different parts of the rabbit fallopian tube during passage of ova. American Journal of Obstetrics and Gynecology 106: 833–837.

Guzman E R, Rosenberg J C, Houlihan C et al 1994 A new method using vaginal ultrasound and transfundal pressure to evaluate the asymptomatic incompetent cervix. Obstetrics and Gynecology 83: 248–252.

Haas G G Jr 1987 How should sperm antibody tests be used clinically? American Journal of Reproductive Immunology 15: 106–111.

Hagenfeldt K, Den Dobeln U, Hagenfeldt L 1989 Gonadal failure in young women with galactose-1-phosphate uridyl transferase activity. Fertility and Sterility 51: 177–178.

Halbert S A, McComb P F 1981 Function and structure of the rabbit oviduct after fimbriectomy II Proximal ampullary salpingostomy. Fertility and Sterility 35: 355–358.

Hamilton M P R, Fleming R, Coutts J R T, MacNaughton M C, Whitfield C R 1990 Luteal cysts and unexplained infertility: biochemical and ultrasonic evaluation. Fertility and Sterility 54: 32–37.

Hammond M G, Talbert L M 1982 Clomiphene citrate treatment of infertile women with low luteal phase progesterone levels. Obstetrics and Gynecology 89: 675–679.

Haney A F, Musukonis M A, Weinberg J B 1983 Macrophages and infertility: oviductal macrophages as potential mediators of infertility. Fertility and Sterility 39: 310–315.

Hansen K K, Knopp R H, Soules M R 1991 Lipoprotein-cholesterol levels in infertile women with luteal phase deficiency. Fertility and Sterility 55: 916–921.

Hare M J, Taylor-Robinson D, Cooper P 1982 Evidence for an association between Chlamydia trachomatis and cervical intraepithelial neoplasia. British Journal of Obstetrics and Gynaecology 89: 489–491.

Harper M J K 1988 Gamete and zygote transport. In: Knobil E, Neill J (eds) The physiology of reproduction. Raven Press, New York, p 103.

Hassan A A, Reiff R H, Fayez J A 1986 Femoral neuropathy following microscopical tuboplasty. Fertility and Sterility 45: 889–891.

Hassold T, Jacobs P, Kline J, Stein Z, Warburton D 1980 Effect of maternal age on autosomal trisomies. Annals of Human Genetics 44: 29–36.

Healy D L 1991 Occult ovarian failure. Annals of the New York Academy of Sciences 626: 157–160.

Healy D L, Trounson A O, Anderson A N 1994 Female infertility: causes and treatment. Lancet 343: 1539–1544.

Hedricks C, Piccino L J, Udry J R, Chimbira T H K 1987 Peak coital rate coincides with onset of luteinizing hormone surge. Fertility and Sterility 48: 234–238.

Heineman M J, Bouckaert P X J M, Schellekens L A 1984 A quadruplet pregnancy following ovulation induction with pulsatile luteinizing hormone-releasing hormone. Fertility and Sterility 42: 300–302.

Hemmingson E 1982 Outcome of third trimester pregnancies after cryotherapy of the uterine cervix. British Journal of Obstetrics and Gynaecology 89: 675–679.

Hertig A T 1954 Gestational hyperplasia of endometrium. Laboratory Investigations 13: 1153–1191.

Hess H M, Dickson J, Fox H E 1980 Hyperfunctioning parathyroid carcinoma presenting as acute pancreatitis in pregnancy. Journal of Reproductive Medicine 25: 83–87.

Hickling D J, Killick S R 1991 An unusual complication of gamete intra-fallopian transfer (GIFT). Human Reproduction 6: 604.

Hicks J J, Callado M L, Castro-Osuna G 1980 Effect of rabbit spermatozoa on the incorporation of labeled precursors into endometrial macromolecules. Archives of Andrology 5: 349–354.

Hinton R A, Egdell L M, Andrews B E, Clarke S K R, Richmond S J 1979 A double-blind cross-over study of the effect of doxycycline on mycoplasma infection and infertility. British Journal of Obstetrics and Gynaecology 86: 379–383.

Hitti I F, Glasberg S S, McKenzie C, Meltzer B A 1991 Uterine leiomyosarcoma with massive necrosis diagnosed during gonadotropin-releasing hormone analog therapy for presumed uterine fibroid. Fertility and Sterility 56: 778–780.

Ho K Y, Smythe G A, Duncan M, Lazarus L 1984 Dopamine infusion studies in patients with pathological hyperprolactinemia: evidence of normal prolactin suppressibility but abnormal dopamine metabolism. Journal of Clinical Endocrinology and Metabolism 58: 128–133.

Hodgen G D 1982 The dominant follicle. Fertility and Sterility 38: 281–300.

Hodgson R, Driscoll G L, Dodd J K, Tyler J P P 1990 Chlamydia trachomatis: the prevalence, trend and importance in initial infertility management. Australian and New Zealand Journal of Obstetrics and Gynaecology 30: 251–254.

Hollyock V E, Chanen W, Wein R 1983 Cervical function following treatment of intraepithelial neoplasia by electrocoagulation diathermy. Obstetrics and Gynecology 61: 79–81.

Holmes K K, Eschenbach D A, Knapp J S 1980 Salpingitis: overview of etiology and epidemiology. American Journal of Obstetrics and Gynecology 138: 893–900.

Holt J P, Keller D 1984 Danazol treatment increases serum enzyme levels. Fertility and Sterility 41: 70–74.

Holzgreve W, Schonberg S A, Douglas R G, Golbus M S 1984 X-chromosome hyperploidy in couples with multiple spontaneous abortions. Obstetrics and Gynecology 63: 237–240.

Honoré L E 1978a Tubal ectopic pregnancy with contralateral corpus luteum: a report of 5 cases. Journal of Reproductive Medicine 21: 269–271.

Honoré L H 1978b Salpingitis isthmica nodosa in female infertility and ectopic tubal pregnancy. Fertility and Sterility 29: 164–168.

Honoré L H 1980 The increased incidence of renal stones in women with spontaneous abortion: a retrospective study. American Journal of Obstetrics and Gynecology 137: 145–146.

Honoré L H, Davey S J 1989 Endometrial carcinoma in young women: a report of four cases. Journal of Reproductive Medicine 34: 845–849.

Honoré L H, Scott J Z 1982 Human infertility: the histologic diagnosis of pregnancy from endometrial biopsies. Presented at the Poster Session of the Meeting of Canadian Investigators in Reproduction, Toronto, June 1982.

Honoré L H, Scott J Z 1992 An unusual acquired lesion: post-salpingostomy intercornual bridging with hematosalpinx, chronic salpingitis and perisalpingeal endometriosis. Journal of Reproductive Medicine 37: 221–222.

Honoré L H, Cumming D C, Scott J Z 1985 Mycoplasmal endometritis in female infertility. Infertility 7: 203–208.

Honoré L H, Cumming D C, Dunlop D L, Scott J Z 1988a Uterine adenomyoma associated with infertility: report of three cases. Journal of Reproductive Medicine 33: 331–335.

Honoré L H, Cumming D C, Fahmy N 1988b Significant difference in the frequency of out-of-phase endometrial biopsies depending on the use of the Novak curette or the flexible polypropylene endometrial biopsy cannula ("Pipelle"). Gynecologic and Obstetric Investigation 26: 338–340.

Horne H W, Hertig A T, Knudsin R B, Kosasa T S 1973 Subclinical endometrial inflammation and T-mycoplasma. International Journal of Fertility 18: 226–231.

Horvath E, Kovacs K 1976 Ultrastructural classification of pituitary adenomas. Canadian Journal of Neurological Sciences 3: 9–21.

Hughes E G, Jacobs R D, Rubulis A, Husney R M 1963 Carbohydrate pathways of the endometrium. American Journal of Obstetrics and Gynecology 85: 594–608.

Huggins G R, Cullins V E 1990 Fertility after contraception or abortion. Fertility and Sterility 54: 559–573.

Hulka J F 1982 Adnexal adhesions: a prognostic staging and classification system based on a five year survey of results at Chapel Hill, North Carolina. American Journal of Obstetrics and Gynecology 144: 141–147.

Hull M G R, Bromham D R, Savage P E, Barlow T M, Hughes A O, Jacobs H S 1981 Postpill amenorrhea: a causal study. Fertility and Sterility 36: 472–476.

Hunt J E, Wallach E E 1974 Uterine factors in infertility — an overview. Clinical Obstetrics and Gynecology 17: 44–59.

Hunter R H F, Leglise P C 1971 Polyspermic fertilization following tubal surgery in pigs, with particular reference to the role of the isthmus. Journal of Reproduction and Fertility 24: 233–246.

Insler V, Lunenfeld B 1991 Pathophysiology of polycystic ovarian disease: new insights. Human Reproduction 6: 1025–1029.

Insler V, Glezerman M, Zeidel L, Bernstein D, Misgav N 1980 Sperm storage in the human cervix: a quantitative study. Fertility and Sterility 33: 288–293.

Itu M, Neelam T, Ammini A C, Kucheria K 1990 Primary amenorrhea in a triple X female. Australian and New Zealand Journal of Obstetrics and Gynaecology 30: 286–288.

Jacobson A, Marshall J R 1980 Detrimental effect of endometrial biopsies on pregnancy rate following human menopausal gonadotropin/human chorionic gonadotropin-induced ovulation. Fertility and Sterility 33: 602–604.

Jaffe S B, Jewelewicz R 1991 The basic infertility investigation. Fertility and Sterility 56: 599–613.

Jager S, Kremer J, Van Slockteren-Draaisma T 1978 A simple method of spermatozoal surface IgG with the direct mixed antiglobulin reaction carried out on undiluted fresh human semen. International Journal of Fertility 23: 12–21.

Jain A K 1969 Fecundability and its relation to age in a sample of Taiwanese women. Population Studies 23: 69–85.

Jansen R P 1980 Cyclic changes in the human fallopian tube isthmus and their functional significance. American Journal of Obstetrics and Gynecology 136: 292–308.

Jansen R P S 1982 Spontaneous abortion incidence in the treatment of infertility. American Journal of Obstetrics and Gynecology 143: 451–473.

Jansen R P S 1984 Endocrine response in the fallopian tube. Endocrine Reviews 5: 525–551.

Jaszczak S, Moghissi K S, Hafez E S E 1980 Effect of prostaglandin Fsα on sperm transport in the reproductive tract of female macaques (Macaca fascicularis). Archives of Andrology 4: 17–27.

Jean Y, Langlais J, Roberts K D, Chapdelain A, Bleau G 1979 Fertility of a woman with nonfunctional ciliated cells in the fallopian tubes. Fertility and Sterility 31: 349–350.

Jewelewicz R 1984 The role of endogenous opioid peptides in control of the menstrual cycle. Fertility and Sterility 42: 683–685.

Jones G S 1990 Corpus luteum: composition and function. Fertility and Sterility 54: 1–18.

Jones W R 1980 Immunologic infertility — fact or fiction? Fertility and Sterility 33: 577–586.

Jones W R 1991 Allergy to coitus. Australian and New Zealand Journal of Obstetrics and Gynaecology 31: 137–141.

Joske R A, Martin J D 1971 Coeliac disease presenting as recurrent abortion. Journal of Obstetrics and Gynaecology of the British Commonwealth 78: 754–758.

Kai J, Malmquist A, Nilsson A 1969 Psychiatric aspects of spontaneous abortion II The importance of bereavement attachment and neurosis in early life. Journal of Psychosomatic Research 13: 53–58.

Karande V C, Flood J T, Heard N, Veeck L, Muasher S J 1991 Analysis of ectopic pregnancies resulting from in vitro fertilization and embryo transfer. Human Reproduction 6: 446–449.

Karrow W G, Gentry W C, Skeels R F, Payne S A 1971 Endometrial biopsy in the luteal phase of the cycle of conception. Fertility and Sterility 22: 482–495.

Katayama K P, Valencia A L, Wise L, Stehlik E 1991 Pregnancy with X-autosome translocation. Fertility and Sterility 55: 438–439.

Katz A I, Davidson J M, Hayslett J P, Singson E, Lindheimer M D 1980 Pregnancy in women with kidney disease. Kidney International 18: 192–198.

Katz D F, Morales P, Samuels S J, Overstreet J W 1990 Mechanisms of filtration of morphologically abnormal human sperm by cervical mucus. Fertility and Sterility 54: 513–516.

Katz E 1988 The luteinized unruptured follicle and other ovulatory dysfunctions. Fertility and Sterility 50: 839–850.

Kaufman F R, Donnell G N, Lobo R A 1987 Ovarian androgen secretion in patients with galactosemia and premature ovarian failure. Fertility and Sterility 47: 1033–1034.

Kaushansky A, Frydman M, Kaufman H, Homburg R 1987 Endocrine studies of the ovulatory disturbances in Wilson's disease (hepatolenticular degeneration). Fertility and Sterility 47: 270–273.

Kazer R R, Meyer K, Valle R F 1992 Late hemorrhage after transcervical division of a uterine septum: a report of two cases. Fertility and Sterility 57: 930–932.

Keenan J A, Herbert C M, Bush J R, Wentz A C 1989 Diagnosis and management of out-of-phase endometrial biopsies among patients receiving clomiphene citrate for ovulation induction. Fertility and Sterility 51: 964–967.

Keith L G, Berger G S, Edelman D A, Newton W, Fullan N, Bailey R, Friberg J 1984 On the causation of pelvic inflammatory disease. American Journal of Obstetrics and Gynecology 149: 215–224.

Keller D W, Wiest W G, Askin F B, Johnson L W, Strickler R C 1979

Pseudocorpus luteum insufficiency: a local defect of progesterone action on endometrial stroma. Journal of Clinical Endocrinology and Metabolism 48: 127–132.

Kerin J F, Williams D B, San Roman G A, Pearlstone A C, Grundfest W S, Surrey E S 1992 Falloscopic classification and treatment of fallopian tube lumen disease. Fertility and Sterility 57: 731–741.

Killick S, Elstein M 1987 Pharmacologic production of luteinized unruptured follicles by prostaglandin synthetase inhibitors. Fertility and Sterility 47: 773–777.

Kim-Bjorklund T, Landeren B M, Hamberger L, Johannison E 1991 Comparative morphometric study of the endometrium, fallopian tube and the corpus luteum during the post-ovulatory phase in normally menstruating women. Fertility and Sterility 56: 842–850.

King I R 1989 Candida albicans pelvic abscess associated with the use of 32% Dextran-70 in conservative pelvic surgery. Fertility and Sterility 51: 1050–1052.

Kjaer K, Hagen C, Sando S H, Eshoj O 1992 Infertility and pregnancy outcome in an unselected group of women with insulin-dependent diabetes mellitus. American Journal of Obstetrics and Gynecology 166: 1412–1418.

Klein S M, Garcia C R 1973 Asherman's syndrome: a critique and current review. Fertility and Sterility 24: 722–735.

Kleinberg D L, Noel G L, Frantz A G 1977 Galactorrhea: a study of 235 cases including 48 with pituitary tumors. New England Journal of Medicine 296: 589–598.

Klentzerus L D, Bulmer J N, Li T C, Morrison L, Warren A, Cooke I D 1991 Lectin binding of endometrium in women with unexplained infertility. Fertility and Sterility 56: 660–667.

Kohda H, Mori T, Nishimura T, Kambegawa A 1983 Cooperation of progesterone and prostaglandins in ovulation induced by human chorionic gonadotrophin in immature rats primed with pregnant mare serum gonadotrophin. Journal of Endocrinology 96: 387–393.

Korenaga M, Kadota T 1981 Changes in the mechanical properties of the circular muscle of the isthmus of the human fallopian tube in relation to hormonal domination and postovulatory time. Fertility and Sterility 36: 343–350.

Kovacs K, Horvath E 1987 Hypothalamic-pituitary abnormalities in ovulatory disorders. In: Gondos B, Riddick D H (eds) Pathology of infertility. Thieme Medical Publishers, New York, p 185.

Kovacs K, Sheehan H L 1982 Pituitary changes in Kallmann's syndrome: a histologic, immunocytologic, ultrastructural and immunoelectron-microscopic study. Fertility and Sterility 37: 83–89.

Kremer J, Jager S 1988 Sperm-cervical mucus interaction, in particular in the presence of antispermatozoal antibodies. Human Reproduction 3: 69–73.

Kriel R L, Gates G A, Wulff H, Powell N, Poland J D, Chin T D Y 1970 Cytomegalovirus isolations associated with pregnancy wastage. American Journal of Obstetrics and Gynecology 106: 889–891.

Kuberski T 1980 Histocompatibility antigens and the sexually transmitted diseases. Sexually Transmitted Diseases 7: 203–205.

Kurjak A S, Kupesic-Urek S, Schulman H, Zalud I 1991 Transvaginal color flow Doppler in the assessment of ovarian and uterine blood flow in infertile women. Fertility and Sterility 56: 870–873.

Kushner D H 1979 Fertility in women after age forty five. International Journal of Fertility 24: 289–293.

Labarrere C A, Catoggio L J, Mullen E G, Althabe O H 1986 Placental lesions in maternal autoimmune disease. American Journal of Reproductive Immunology 12: 78–86.

Landholt A M 1975 Ultrastructure of human sella tumors: correlation of clinical findings and morphology. Acta Neurochirurgica (Wien) 22: 1–67.

Langer R, Golan A, Ron-El R, Pansky M, Neuman M, Caspi E 1990 Hormonal changes related to impairment of cervical mucus in cycles stimulated by Clomiphene citrate. Australian and New Zealand Journal of Obstetrics and Gynaecology 30: 254–256.

Las M S, Surks M I 1983 Hypopituitarism associated with systemic amyloidosis. New York State Journal of Medicine 83: 1183–1185.

La Scala G B, Ghirardini G, Cantarelli M, Dotti C, Cavalieri S, Torelli M G 1991 Recurrent empty follicle syndrome. Human Reproduction 6: 651–652.

Laurent S L, Thompson S J, Addy C, Garrison C Z, Moore E E 1992 An epidemiologic study of smoking and primary infertility in women. Fertility and Sterility 57: 565–572.

Lazlo J, Gaal M, Bosze P 1976 Chromosome studies in ovarian hypoplasia. Clinical Genetics 9: 61–70.

Leake J F, Murphy A A, Zacur H A 1987 Noncardiogenic pulmonary edema: a complication of operative hysteroscopy. Fertility and Sterility 48: 497–499.

Leduc L, Wasserstrum N 1992 Successful treatment with the Smith-Hodge pessary of cervical incompetence due to defective connective tissue in Ehlers-Danlos syndrome. American Journal of Perinatology 9: 25–27.

Lee F, Nelson N, Faiman C, Choi N W, Reyes F I 1982 Low-dose corticoid therapy for anovulation: effect upon fetal weight. Obstetrics and Gynecology 60: 314–317.

Lee M, Fried W I, Sharifi R 1983 Ocular adverse effects of human chorionic gonadotrophin. Fertility and Sterility 40: 266–268.

Lefebvre G, Vauthier D, Gonzales J, Lesourd S 1990 Assisted reproductive technology and superfetation: a case report. Fertility and Sterility 53: 1100–1101.

Lehmann-Willenbrock E, Mecke H, Riedel H-H 1990 Sequelae of appendectomy, with special reference to intraabdominal adhesions, chronic abdominal pain and infertility. Gynecologic and Obstetric Investigation 29: 241–245.

Leridon H 1977 Human fertility. The University of Chicago Press, Chicago.

Letterie G S, Sakas E L 1991 Histology of proximal tubal obstruction in cases of unsuccessful tubal canalization. Fertility and Sterility 56: 831–835.

Levi A A 1961 Rupture of the pregnant uterus: relationship to previous myomectomy. Obstetrics and Gynecology 18: 223–229.

Levy B S, Soderstrom R M, Dail D M 1985 Bowel injuries during laparoscopy: gross anatomy and histology. Journal of Reproductive Medicine 30: 168–172.

Levy D L 1982 Fetal-neonatal involvement in maternal autoimmune disease. Obstetrical and Gynecological Survey 37: 122–127.

Leyendecker G, Wildt L 1989 Pulsatile gonadotropin-releasing hormone: physiological and clinical aspects. Contributions to Gynecology and Obstetrics 17: 18–36.

Li H P, Balmaceda J P, Zouves C, Cittadini E, Figueroa Casas P, Johnston I, Asch R H 1992 Heterotopic pregnancy associated with gamete intra-Fallopian transfer. Human Reproduction 7: 131–135.

Li T-C, Cooke I D 1991 Evaluation of the luteal phase. Human Reproduction 6: 484–499.

Li T-C, Rogers W, Dockery P, Lenton E A, Cooke I D 1988 A new method of histologic dating of human endometrium in the luteal phase. Fertility and Sterility 50: 52–60.

Li T-C, Dockery P, Rogers A W, Cooke I D 1989 How precise is histologic dating of endometrium using the standard dating criteria? Fertility and Sterility 51: 759–763.

Li T-C, Dockery P, Cooke I D 1991 Endometrial development in the luteal phase of women with various types of infertility: comparison with women of normal fertility. Human Reproduction 6: 325–330.

Li T-C, Nuttall L, Klentzeris L, Cooke I D 1992 How well does ultrasonographic measurement of endometrial thickness predict the results of histological dating? Human Reproduction 7: 1–5.

Liliequist B, Lindgren L 1964 Hyperflexion of the uterus and infertility. Acta Obstetricia et Gynecologica Scandinavica 43: 240–254.

Lindsay A H, Voorhess M L, MacGillivray M H 1983 Multicystic ovaries in primary hypothyroidism. Obstetrics and Gynecology 61: 433–437.

Lippes J, Waugh P V 1989 Human oviductal fluid (hOF) proteins. IV. Evidence of hOF proteins binding to human sperm. Fertility and Sterility 51: 89–94.

Lipshutz L I, Howards S S 1983 Infertility in the male. Churchill Livingstone, New York.

Lobo R G, Goebelsmann U 1980 Adult manifestation of congenital adrenal hyperplasia due to incomplete 21 hydroxylase deficiency mimicking polycystic ovarian disease. American Journal of Obstetrics and Gynecology 138: 720–726.

Lobo R G, Granger L R, Paul W L, Goebelsmann U, Mishell D R Jr 1983 Psychological stress and increases in urinary norepinephrine metabolites, platelet serotonin, and adrenal androgens in women with polycystic ovary syndrome. American Journal of Obstetrics and Gynecology 145: 496–503.

Locher E W, Maroulis G B 1983 Tubointestinal fistula. Fertility and Sterility 39: 235–237.

Locke W 1978 Control of anterior pituitary function. Archives of Internal Medicine 138: 1541–1545.

Lockwood C, Irons M, Troiani T, Kawada C, Chaudhury A, Cetrulo C 1988 The prenatal sonographic diagnosis of lethal multiple pterygium syndrome: a heritable cause of recurrent abortion. American Journal of Obstetrics and Gynecology 159: 474–476.

Loffer F D, Pent D 1975 Indications, contraindications and complications of laparoscopy. Obstetrical and Gynecological Survey 30: 407–427.

Luborsky J L, Visintin I, Boyers S, Asari T, Caldwell B, De Cherney A 1990 Ovarian antibodies detected by immobilized antigen immunoassay in patients with premature ovarian failure. Journal of Clinical Endocrinology and Metabolism 70: 69–75.

Lucas J A, Kahlstorf J H, Cowan B D 1988 Multiple endocrine neoplasia — type I syndrome and hyperprolactinemia. Fertility and Sterility 50: 514–515.

Ludwig G D 1962 Hyperparathyroidism in relation to pregnancy. New England Journal of Medicine 267: 637–640.

Lundorff P, Hahlin M, Kallfelt B, Thorburn J, Lindblom B 1991 Adhesion formation after laparoscopic surgery in tubal surgery: a randomized trial versus laparotomy. Fertility and Sterility 55: 911–915.

McAnulty J H, Metcalfe T, Veland K 1982 Cardiovascular disease. In: Burrow G N, Ferris T F (eds) Medical complications during pregnancy. Saunders, Philadelphia, pp 145–168.

McCarty K S Jr, Dobson C E II 1980 Pituitary pathology associated with abnormalities of prolactin secretion. Clinical Obstetrics and Gynecology 23: 367–384.

McClure R D, Tom R A, Watkins M, Murthy S 1989 Spermcheck: a simplified screening assay for immunological infertility. Fertility and Sterility 52: 650–654.

McComb P F, Halbert S A, Gomel V 1980 Pregnancy, ciliary transport and the reversed ampullary segment of the rabbit fallopian tube. Fertility and Sterility 34: 386–390.

McComb P F, Newman H, Halbert S A 1981 Reproduction in rabbits after excision of the oviductal isthmus, ampullary-isthmic junction and uteroisthmic junction. Fertility and Sterility 36: 669–677.

McComb P, Langley L, Villalon M, Verdugo P 1986 The oviductal cilia and Kartagener's syndrome. Fertility and Sterility 46: 412–416.

McDonough P G 1987 Recurrent aneuploidic and euploidic abortion. Obstetrics and Gynecology Clinics of North America 14(4): 1099–1113.

MacLeod J L, Eisen A, Sussman G L 1987 Anaphylactic reaction to synthetic luteinizing hormone-releasing hormone. Fertility and Sterility 48: 500–502.

McNatty K P, Sawers R S, McNeely A S 1974 A possible role for prolactin in control of steroid secretion by the human Graafian follicle. Nature (London) 250: 653–655.

McNeely M J, Soules M R 1988 The diagnosis of luteal phase deficiency: a critical review. Fertility and Sterility 50: 1–15.

Maguiness S D, Shrimank E R, Djahanbaruch O, Grudzinskas J G 1992 Oviduct proteins. Contemporary Review of Obstetrics and Gynecology 4: 42–50.

Mahony M C, Alexander N J 1991 Sites of antisperm antibody action. Human Reproduction 6: 1426–1430.

Mai F, Monday R, Rump E 1972 Psychiatric interview comparisons between infertile and fertile couples. Psychosomatic Medicine 34: 430–435.

Mandelbaum S L, Diamond M P, De Cherney A H 1987 The impact of antisperm antibodies on human fertility. Journal of Urology 138: 1–8.

Mandell F, Wolfe L C 1974 Sudden infant death syndrome and subsequent pregnancy. Pediatrics 56: 774–776.

Manganiello P D, Yearke R R 1991 A 10 year prospective study of women with a history of recurrent fetal losses fails to identify Listeria monocytogenes in the genital tract. Fertility and Sterility 56: 781–782.

Marana R, Lucisano A, Leone F, Sanna A, Dell'Acqua S, Mancuso S 1990 High prevalence of silent Chlamydial colonization of the tubal mucosa in infertile women. Fertility and Sterility 53: 354–356.

Marcello M F, Nuciforo G, Romeo R et al 1990 Structural and ultrastructural study of the ovary in childhood leukemia after successful treatment. Cancer 66: 2099–2104.

March C M 1978 Complications of gonadotropin therapy. Journal of Reproductive Medicine 21: 208–211.

March C M, Israel R 1981 Gestational outcome following hysteroscopic lysis of adhesions. Fertility and Sterility 36: 455–459.

Marchini M, Losa G A, Mava S, Di Nola G, Fedele L 1992 Ultrastructural aspects of endometrial surface in Kartegener's syndrome. Fertility and Sterility 57: 461–463.

Marconi G, Auge L, Sojo E, Young E, Quintana R 1992 Salpingoscopy: systematic use in diagnostic laparoscopy. Fertility and Sterility 57: 742–746.

Maroulis G H 1981 Evaluation of hirsutism and hyperandrogenemia. Fertility and Sterility 36: 273–305.

Martikainen P, Sanikaa E, Suominen J, Santti R 1980 Glucose content as a parameter of semen quality. Archives of Andrology 5: 337–343.

Mashiach S, Bider D, Moran O, Goldenberg M, Ben-Rafael Z 1990 Adnexal torsion of hyperstimulated ovaries in pregnancies after gonadotrophin therapy. Fertility and Sterility 53: 76–80.

Mathur S, Williamson H O, Baker E R, Fudenberg H H 1981 Immunoglobulin E levels and antisperm antibody titers in infertile couples. American Journal of Obstetrics and Gynecology 140: 923–930.

Mathur S, Williamson H O, Genes P V et al 1983a Association of human leukocytic antigens B7 and BW35 with sperm antibodies. Fertility and Sterility 39: 343–349.

Mathur S, Williamson H O, Genco P V, Koopmann W R, Rust P F, Fudenberg H H 1983b Sperm immunity in fertile couples: antibody titers are higher against husband's sperm than to sperm from controls. American Journal of Reproductive Immunology 3: 18–27.

Mathur S, Chao L, Goust J M et al 1988 Special antigens on sperm from autoimmune infertile men. American Journal of Reproductive Immunology 17: 5–13.

Mazur M T, Duncan D A, Younger I B 1989 Endometrial biopsy in the cycle of conception: histologic and lectin histochemical evaluation. Fertility and Sterility 51: 764–769.

Medical Research International Society for Assisted Reproductive Technology (ART), the American Fertility Society 1992 In vitro fertilization-embryo transfer (IVF-ET) in the United States: 1990 results from the IVF-ET Registry. Fertility and Sterility 57: 15–24.

Mehes K, Kosztolanyi G 1992 A possible mosaic form of delayed centromere separation and aneuploidy. Human Genetics 88: 477–478.

Menashe Y, Sack J, Mashiach S 1991 Spontaneous pregnancies in two women with Laron-type dwarfism: are growth hormone and circulating insulin-like growth factor mandatory for induction of ovulation? Human Reproduction 6: 670–671.

Mendel E B 1964 Chronic tubal spasm. International Journal of Fertility 9: 383–389.

Menge A C 1988 Immunologic reactions involving sperm cells and preimplantation embryos. American Journal of Reproductive Immunology 18: 17–20.

Menning B E 1980 The emotional needs of infertile couples. Fertility and Sterility 34: 313–319.

Mercaitis P A, Peaper R E, Schwartz P A 1985 Effect of Danazol on vocal pitch: a case study. Obstetrics and Gynecology 65: 131–134.

Mettler L 1980 Immunology and reproduction I Sterility immunology. Gynecologic and Obstetrical Investigation 11: 129–160.

Meyer A R, Hutchinson-Williams K A, Jones E E, De Cherney A H 1990 Secondary hypogonadism in hemochromatosis. Fertility and Sterility 54: 740–742.

Mills M S, Eddowes H A, Fox R, Wardle P G 1992 Subclavian vein thrombosis: a late complication of ovarian hyperstimulation syndrome. Human Reproduction 7: 370–371.

Mimori H, Fukuma K, Matsuo I, Nakahara K, Maeyama M 1981 Effect of progesterone on glycogen metabolism in the endometrium of infertile patients during the menstrual cycle. Fertility and Sterility 35: 289–295.

Mitami Y, Takaki C H, Iwasaki H 1959 Myoma of the uterus and sterility with particular reference to the tubal pathology. Journal of the Japanese Obstetrical and Gynecological Society 6: 347–352.

Moghissi K S 1979 The cervix in infertility. Clinical Obstetrics and Gynecology 22: 27–42.

Moinian M, Andersch B 1982 Does cervix conization increase the risk of complications in subsequent pregnancies? Acta Obstetricia et Gynecologica Scandinavica 61: 101–103.

Monroe S E, Levine C, Chang J, Keye W R, Yamamoto M, Jaffe R B 1981 Prolactin-secreting pituitary adenomas. V Increased gonadotroph sensitivity in hyperprolactinemic women with pituitary adenomas. Journal of Clinical Endocrinology and Metabolism 52: 1171–1178.

Montagu M F A 1946 Adolescent sterility. Thomas, Springfield, Illinois.

Morikawa H, Okamura H, Takenaka A, Morimoto K, Nishimura T 1980 Physiological study of the human mesotubarium ovarica. Obstetrics and Gynecology 55: 493–496.

Morrison J C, Givens J R, Wiser W L, Fish S A 1975 Mumps oophoritis: a cause of premature menopause. Fertility and Sterility 26: 655–659.

Mosher W D, Pratt W F 1991 Fecundity and infertility in the United States: incidence and trends. Fertility and Sterility 56: 192–193.

Mosley P D 1976 Psychophysiologic infertility: an overview. Clinical Obstetrics and Gynecology 19: 407–417.

Mowbray J F, Underwood J, Gill T J III 1991 Familial recurrent spontaneous abortions. American Journal of Reproductive Immunology 26: 17–18.

Muechler E K, Huang K-E 1982 Paradoxical pituitary hormone response in a case of primary hypothyroidism and Hashimoto's thyroiditis. Fertility and Sterility 38: 423–426.

Mukai K 1983 Pituitary adenomas: immunocytochemical study of 150 tumors with clinicopathologic correlation. Cancer 52: 648–653.

Musset R, Poitout P L, Truc J B, Paniel B J 1978 Aplasie vaginale avec uterus fonctionnel: resultats operatoires et commentaires. Journal de Gynecologie, Obstetrique et Biologie de la Reproduction 7: 316–333.

Naessens A, Foulon W, Cammu H, Goossens A, Lauwers S 1987 Epidemiology and pathogenesis of ureaplasma urealyticum in spontaneous abortion and early preterm labor. Acta Obstetricia et Gynecologica Scandinavica 66: 513–517.

Nahmias A J, Josey W E, Naib Z M, Freeman M G, Fernandez R J, Wheeler J H 1971 Perinatal risk associated with maternal herpes simplex virus infections. American Journal of Obstetrics and Gynecology 110: 825–829.

Nakajima I, Mizushima N, Matsuda H et al 1986 Fulminant hepatic failure associated with aplastic anemia after treatment with Danazol. British Journal of Obstetrics and Gynaecology 93: 1013–1015.

Nakajima S T, Nason F G, Badger G J, Gibson M 1991 Progesterone production in early pregnancy. Fertility and Sterility 55: 516–521.

Nasir-ud-Dhin, Walker-Nasir E, McArthur J W et al 1982 Immunologically induced changes in macaque cervical mucus function: inhibition of sperm penetration. Fertility and Sterility 37: 431–435.

Navot D, Bergh P A, Laufer N 1992 Ovarian hyperstimulation syndrome in novel reproductive technologies: prevention and treatment. Fertility and Sterility 58: 249–261.

Naz R K 1990 Effects of sperm-reactive antibodies present in human infertile sera on fertility of female rabbits. Journal of Reproductive Immunology 18: 161–177.

Neelon F A, Goree J A, Lebowitz H E 1973 The primary empty sella: clinical and radiographic characteristics and endocrine function. Medicine 52: 72–92.

Nicklin J L 1991 Systemic lupus erythematosus and pregnancy at the Royal Women's Hospital, Brisbane 1979–1989. Australian and New Zealand Journal of Obstetrics and Gynaecology 31: 128–133.

Nicosia S V, Johnson J H 1983 Histochemistry and ultrastructure of the rabbit endocervical mucosa after intravaginal antigen administration. Fertility and Sterility 39: 408–409.

Nieschlag E, Lammers U, Freischeem C W, Langer K, Wickings E J 1982 Reproduction in young fathers and grandfathers. Journal of Clinical Endocrinology and Metabolism 55: 676–680.

Niver D H, Barrett G, Jewelewicz R 1980 Congenital atresia of the uterine cervix and vagina: three cases. Fertility and Sterility 33: 25–29.

Nogales-Ortiz F, Tarancon I, Nogales F F Jr 1979 The pathology of female genital tuberculosis. Obstetrics and Gynecology 53: 422–428.

Noyes R W, Chapnick E M 1964 Literature on psychology and infertility: a critical analysis. Fertility and Sterility 15: 543–558.

Noyes R W, Haman J O 1954 Accuracy of endometrial dating. Fertility and Sterility 4: 504–508.

Noyes R W, Hertig A T, Rock J 1950 Dating the endometrial biopsy. Fertility and Sterility 1: 3–25.

Odeblad E 1962 Undulations of macromolecules in cervical mucus. International Journal of Fertility 7: 313–318.

Odeblad E 1968 The functional structure of human cervical mucus. Acta Obstetricia et Gynecologica Scandinavica 47 (suppl 1): 59–70.

Odeblad E 1978 Cervical factors. Contributions to Obstetrics and Gynecology 4: 132–142.

Odell W D, Meikle A W 1986 Menorrhagia, infertility, elevated serum estradiol, and hyperprolactinemia resulting from increased aromatase activity (MIEHA syndrome). Fertility and Sterility 46: 321–324.

Ohlgisser M, Sorokin Y, Heifetz M 1985 Gynecologic laparoscopy: a review article. Obstetrical and Gynecological Survey 40: 385–396.

Okamura N, Tajima Y, Ishikawa H, Yoshi I S, Koiso K, Sugita Y 1986 Lowered bicarbonate levels in seminal plasma cause the poor sperm motility in human infertile patients. Fertility and Sterility 45: 265–272.

Olive D L, Haney A F, Weinberg J B 1987 The nature of the intraperitoneal exudate associated with infertility: peritoneal fluid and serum lysozyme activity. Fertility and Sterility 48: 802–806.

Overstreet E W 1959 Endometrial polyps: their relationship to fertility and abortion. International Journal of Fertility 4: 263–267.

Overstreet J W 1986 Evaluation of sperm-cervical mucus interactions. Fertility and Sterility 45: 324–326.

Ovesen P, Moller J, Moller N, Christiansen D S, Orskov H, Jorgensen J O L 1992 Growth hormone secretory capacity and serum insulin-like growth factor I levels in primary infertile anovulatory women with regular menses. Fertility and Sterility 57: 97–101.

Owalabi T O, Strickler R C 1977 Adenomyosis: a neglected diagnosis. Obstetrics and Gynecology 50: 424–427.

Paavonen J, Saikku P, Vesterinen E, Lehtovirta P 1979 Infertility and cervical Chlamydia trachomatis infection. Acta Obstetricia et Gynecologica Scandinavica 58: 301–303.

Page H 1989 Estimation of the prevalence and incidence of infertility in a population: pilot study. Fertility and Sterility 51: 571–577.

Parish W E, Ward A 1968 Studies of cervical mucus and serum from infertile women. Journal of Obstetrics and Gynaecology of the British Commonwealth 75: 1089–1092.

Parr E L, Shirley R L 1976 Embryotoxicity of leukocyte extracts and its relationship to intrauterine contraception in humans. Fertility and Sterility 27: 1067–1077.

Peek J C, Graham F M 1992 Ectopic pregnancy in a non-patent fallopian tube following transfer of embryos to the contralateral tube. Human Reproduction 7: 136–137.

Peress M R 1984 Persistent amenorrhea following discontinuation of danazol therapy. Fertility and Sterility 41: 322–323.

Peress M R, Kreutner A K, Mathur R S, Williamson H O 1982 Female pseudohermaphroditism with somatic chromosomal anomaly in association with in utero exposure to danazol. American Journal of Obstetrics and Gynecology 142: 708–709.

Perez R J, Plurad A V, Palladino V S 1981 The relationship of the corpus luteum and the endometrium in infertile patients. Fertility and Sterility 35: 423–427.

Phipps W R, Cramer D W, Schiff I et al 1987 The association between smoking and female infertility as influenced by cause of the infertility. Fertility and Sterility 48: 377–382.

Phipps W R, Benson C B, McShane P M 1988 Severe thigh myositis following intramuscular progesterone injections in an in vitro fertilization patient. Fertility and Sterility 49: 536–537.

Pituitary Adenoma Study Group 1983 Pituitary adenomas and oral contraceptives: a multicenter case-control study. Fertility and Sterility 39: 753–760.

Portnow J, Talo A, Hodgson B J 1977 A random walk model of ovum transport. Bulletin of Mathematical Biology 39: 349–357.

Post K D, Biller B J, Adelman L S, Molitch M E, Wolpert S M, Reichlin S 1979 Selective transsphenoidal adenomectomy in women with galactorrhea-amenorrhea. Journal of the American Medical Association 242: 158–162.

Potter J D 1980 Hypothyroidism and reproductive failure. Surgery Gynecology and Obstetrics 150: 251–255.

Prakash C 1981 Etiology of immune infertility. In: Gleicher N (ed) Reproductive immunology, progress in clinical and biological research, vol 70. Liss, New York, pp 403–412.

Prinz W, Taubert H-D 1968 Mumps in pubescent females and its effect on later reproductive function. Gynaecology 167: 23–27.

Quagliarello J, Barakat R 1987 Raynaud's phenomenon in infertile women treated with bromocriptine. Fertility and Sterility 48: 877–879.

Quan A, Charles D, Craig J M 1963 Histologic and functional consequences of periovarian adhesions. Obstetrics and Gynecology 22: 96–101.

Quan C P, Roux C, Rillot J, Bouvet J-P 1990 Delineation of T and B suppressive molecules from human seminal plasma II spermine is the major suppressor of T-lymphocytes in vitro. American Journal of Reproductive Immunology 22: 64–69.

Quigley M E, Sheehan K L, Casper R F, Yen S S C 1980a Evidence for increased dopaminergic and opioid activity in patients with hypothalamic hypogonadotropic amenorrhea. Journal of Clinical Endocrinology and Metabolism 50: 949–954.

Quigley M E, Judd S J, Guilliland G B, Yen S S C 1980b Functional studies of dopamine control of prolactin secretion in normal women and women with hyperprolactinemic pituitary microadenoma. Journal of Clinical Endocrinology and Metabolism 50: 994–999.

Quigley M M, Haney A F 1980 Evaluation of hyperprolactinemia: clinical profiles. Clinical Obstetrics and Gynecology 23: 337–348.

Quinn P A, Shewchuk A B, Shuber J et al 1983a Efficacy of antibiotic therapy in preventing spontaneous pregnancy loss among couples colonized with genital Mycoplasma. American Journal of Obstetrics and Gynecology 145: 239–244.

Quinn P A et al 1983b Serologic evidence of Ureaplasma urealyticum infection in women with spontaneous pregnancy loss. American Journal of Obstetrics and Gynecology 145: 245–250.

Quinn P A, Petric M, Barkin M et al 1987 Prevalence of antibody to Chlamydia trachomatis in spontaneous abortion and infertility. American Journal of Obstetrics and Gynecology 156: 291–296.

Rabinowe S L, Ravnilcar V A, Dib S A, George K L, Dluhy R G 1989 Premature menopause: monoclonal antibody defines T-lymphocyte abnormalities and antiovarian antibodies. Fertility and Sterility 51: 450–454.

Rao R, Scommegna A, Frohman L A 1982 Integrity of central dopaminergic system in women with postpartum hyperprolactinemia. American Journal of Obstetrics and Gynecology 143: 883–887.

Rebar B W, Connolly H V 1990 Clinical features of young women with hypergonadotrophic amenorrhea. Fertility and Sterility 53: 804–810.

Rebar R W, Erickson G F, Yen S S C 1982 Idiopathic premature ovarian failure: clinical and endocrine characteristics. Fertility and Sterility 37: 35–41.

Reid R L, Van Vugt D A 1987 Weight-related changes in reproductive function. Fertility and Sterility 48: 905–913.

Resnick L 1962 Constrictive perisalpingitis. South African Journal of Medicine 2: 769–772.

Reyes F I, Kohn S, Faiman C 1976 Fertility in women with gonadal dysgenesis. American Journal of Obstetrics and Gynecology 126: 668–670.

Richardson D A, Evans M I, Talerman A, Maroulis G B 1982 Segmental absence of the mid-portion of the fallopian tube. Fertility and Sterility 37: 577–578.

Robert F, Hardy J 1975 Prolactin-secreting adenomas. Archives of Pathology 99: 625–633.

Rock J A, Zacur H A 1983 The clinical management of repeated early pregnancy wastage. Fertility and Sterility 39: 123–140.

Rock J A, Parmley T, Murphy A A, Jones H W Jr 1986 Malposition of the ovary associated with uterine anomalies. Fertility and Sterility 45: 561–563.

Rock J A, Guzick D S, Katz E, Zacur H A, King T M 1987 Tubal anastomosis: pregnancy success following reversal of Fallopian or monopolar cautery sterilization. Fertility and Sterility 48: 13–17.

Rodriguez-Rigau L J, Steinberger E, Atkins B J, Lucci J A 1979 Effect of testosterone on human corpus luteum steroidogenesis in vitro. Fertility and Sterility 31: 448–450.

Rogers R S, Ben Brook D M, Walker J L, Lord B J, Haas G G 1992 "Silent" carriers of Human Papilloma Virus (HPV) identified in sperm bank donor populations. Fertility and Sterility Annual Meeting Program, Supplement S119–S120 (abstract).

Roseler M, Wise L, Katayama K P 1990 Karyotype analysis of blighted ova in pregnancies achieved by in vitro fertilization. Fertility and Sterility 51: 1065–1066.

Rosenbusch B, Sterzik K 1991 Sperm chromosomes and habitual abortion. Fertility and Sterility 56: 370–372.

Rosenfeld D L, Garcia C-R 1975 Endometrial biopsy in the cycle of conception. Fertility and Sterility 26: 1088–1093.

Rosenfeld D L, Seidman S M, Bronson R A, Scholl G M 1983 Unsuspected chronic pelvic inflammatory disease in the infertile female. Fertility and Sterility 39: 44–48.

Rosenfield R L, Barnes R B, Cara J F, Lucky A W 1990 Dysregulation of cytochrome P450C 17α as the cause of polycystic ovarian syndrome. Fertility and Sterility 53: 785–791.

Roumen F J M E, Doesburg W H, Rolland R 1982 Hormonal patterns in infertile women with a deficient postcoital test. Fertility and Sterility 38: 42–47.

Rudak E, Dor J, Goldman B, Levren D, Mashiach S 1990 Anomalies of human oocytes from infertile women undergoing treatment by in vitro fertilization. Fertility and Sterility 53: 292–296.

Ruijs G J, Kaver F M, Jager S, Schroder F P, Schirm J, Kremer J 1991 Further details on sequelae at the cervical and tubal level of Chlamydia trachomatis infection in infertile women. Fertility and Sterility 56: 20–26.

Sampaio M, Serra V, Miro F, Calatayu D C, Castellini M, Pellicer A 1991 Development of ovarian cysts during gonadotrophin-release hormone agonist (GnRHa) administration. Human Reproduction 6: 194–197.

Sandler B 1959 Emotional stress and infertility. British Journal of Clinical Practice 13: 328–330.

Sauer M, Jarrett J C II 1984 Small bowel obstruction following diagnostic laparoscopy. Fertility and Sterility 42: 653–654.

Sauer M V, Paulson R J 1992 Pelvic abscess complicating transcervical embryo transfer. American Journal of Obstetrics and Gynecology 166: 148–149.

Sayegh R, Mastroianni L Jr 1991 Recent advances in our understanding of tubal function. Annals of the New York Academy of Sciences 626: 266–275.

Schaap T, Shemer R, Palti Z, Sharon R 1984 ABO incompatibility and reproductive failure. I. Prenatal selection. American Journal of Human Genetics 36: 143–151.

Schaeffer G 1976 Female genital tuberculosis. Clinical Obstetrics and Gynecology 19: 223–239.

Scheithauer B W 1984 Surgical pathology of the pituitary: the adenomas. Part II. Pathology Annual 19(2): 267–329.

Schenker J G, Margalioth E J 1982 Intrauterine adhesions: an updated appraisal. Fertility and Sterility 37: 593–610.

Schlegelberger B, Gripp K, Grote W 1989 Common fragile sites in couples with recurrent spontaneous abortions. American Journal of Medical Genetics 32: 45–51.

Schumacher G F B, Kim M H, Hossienian A H, Dupon C 1977 Immunoglobulins, proteinase inhibitors, albumin and lysozymes in human cervical mucus I Communication: hormonal profiles and cervical mucus changes — methods and results. American Journal of Obstetrics and Gynecology 129: 629–636.

Schved J F, Gris J C, Nereu S, Dupaigne D, Mares P 1989 Factor XII congenital deficiency and early spontaneous abortion. Fertility and Sterility 52: 335–336.

Schwanzel-Fukuda M, Bick D, Pfaff D W 1989 Luteinizing hormone-releasing hormone (LHRH)-expressing cells do not migrate normally in an inherited hypogonadal (Kallmann) syndrome. Brain Research and Molecular Brain Research 6: 311–326.

Schwartz D, Mayaux M-J, Spira A et al 1983 Semen characteristics as a function of age in 833 fertile men. Fertility and Sterility 39: 530–535.

Schweditsch M O, Keller P J, Floersheim Y, Möhr E 1984 Ovarian hyperstimulation during chronic pulsatile GnHR therapy. Gynecologic and Obstetric Investigation 17: 276–277.

Schwitemaker N W E, Helderhorst F M, Tjontham R T O, van Saase J L C 1990 Late anaphylactic shock after hysterosalpingography. Fertility and Sterility 54: 535–536.

Scott R T, Snyder R R, Strickland D M et al 1988 The effect of interobserver variation in dating endometrial biopsy on the diagnosis of luteal phase defects. Fertility and Sterility 50: 888–892.

Scott R T, Snyder R R, Bagnall J W et al 1993 Evaluation of the impact of intra-observer variability on endometrial dating and the diagnosis of luteal phase dafects. Fertility and Sterility 80: 652–657.

Sedmak D D, Hart W R, Tubbs R R 1987 Autoimmune oophoritis: a histopathologic study of involved ovaries with immunologic characterization of the mononuclear cell infiltrate. International Journal of Gynecological Pathology 6: 73–81.

Seibel M M 1986 Infection and infertility. In: De Cherney A H (ed) Reproductive failure. Churchill Livingstone, New York, pp 203–217.

Seibel M M, Graves W L 1980 The psychological implication of spontaneous abortions. Journal of Reproductive Medicine 25: 161–165.

Seibel M M, Taymor M L 1982 Emotional aspects of infertility. Fertility and Sterility 37: 137–145.

Seifer D B, Collins R L 1990 Current concepts of β-endorphin physiology in female reproduction dysfunction. Fertility and Sterility 54: 757–771.

Self M N, Aplin J D, Buckley C H 1989 Luteal phase defect: the possibility of an immunohistochemical diagnosis. Fertility and Sterility 51: 273–279.

Sellors J W, Mahony J B, Chernesky M A, Rath D J 1988 Tubal factor infertility: an association with prior Chlamydial infection and asymptomatic salpingitis. Fertility and Sterility 49: 451–457.

Sen D K, Fox H 1967 The lymphoid tissue of the endometrium. Gynaecologia 163: 371–378.

Sengupta B S, Wynter H H, Lennox M, Halfen A 1978 Myomectomy in infertile Jamaican women. International Journal of Gynaecology and Obstetrics 15: 397–399.

Serri O, Robert F, Pelletier G, Beauregard H, Hardy J 1987 Hyperprolactinemia associated with clinically silent adenomas: endocrinologic and pathologic studies; a report of two cases. Fertility and Sterility 47: 792–796.

Shafrin S, Schachter J, Dahrouge D, Sweet R L 1992 Long term sequelae of acute pelvic inflammatory disease. American Journal of Obstetrics and Gynecology 166: 1300–1305.

Shangold M M, Dor N, Welt S I, Fleischman A R, Crenshaw M C 1982 Hyperparathyroidism and pregnancy: a review. Obstetrical and Gynecological Survey 37: 217–228.

Sheehan H L, Summers V K 1949 The syndrome of hypopituitarism. Quarterly Journal of Medicine 72: 319–378.

Shepard M K, Jones R B 1989 Recovery of Chlamydia trachomatis from endometrial and fallopian tube biopsies in women with infertility of tubal origin. Fertility and Sterility 52: 232–238.

Sher G, Katz M 1976 Inadequate cervical mucus — a cause of 'idiopathic' infertility. Fertility and Sterility 27: 886–889.

Shoham Z, Zosmer A, Insler V 1991 Early miscarriage and fetal malformations after induction of ovulation (by clomiphene citrate and/or human menotropins), in vitro fertilization and gamete intrafallopian transfer. Fertility and Sterility 55: 1–11.

Shortle B, Jewelewicz R 1989 Cervical incompetence. Fertility and Sterility 52: 181–188.

Shulman S 1986 Infertility as caused by sperm antibodies. Gynecologic and Obstetric Investigation 22: 113–127.

Siegler A M 1983 Hysterosalpingography. Fertility and Sterility 40: 139–158.

Siegler A M, Valle R F 1988 Therapeutic hysteroscopic procedures. Fertility and Sterility 50: 685–701.

Sikka A, Kemmann E, Vrablik R M, Grossman L 1983 Carpal tunnel syndrome associated with danazol therapy. American Journal of Obstetrics and Gynecology 147: 102–103.

Silber S J, Cohen R S 1983 Microsurgical reversal of tubal sterilization: 5-year follow up. Fertility and Sterility 39: 398.

Silverman A Y, Greenberg E I 1983 Absence of a segment of the proximal portion of a fallopian tube. Obstetrics and Gynecology (suppl) 62: 90–91.

Silverstroni L, Morisi G, Malandrino F, Frajese G 1979 Free amino acids in semen: measurement and significance in normal and oligozoospermic men. Archives of Andrology 2: 257–261.

Simon C, Gomez E, Mir A, de Los Santos M J, Pellice R A 1992 Glucocorticoid treatment decreases sera embryo toxicity in endometriosis patients. Fertility and Sterility 58: 284–289.

Simpson J L, Meyers C M, Martin A O, Slias S, Ober C 1989 Translocations are infrequent among couples having repeated spontaneous abortions but no other abnormal pregnancies. Fertility and Sterility 51: 811–814.

Singh J, Devi Y L 1983 Pregnancy following surgical correction of nonfused Mullerian bulbs and absent vagina. Obstetrics and Gynecology 61: 267–269.

Singh J R, Neki J S 1982 Psychogenic factors in some genetic and non-genetic forms of infertility. International Journal of Gynaecology and Obstetrics 20: 119–123.

Sizonenko P C, Aubert M L 1986 Neuroendocrine changes characteristic of sexual maturation. Journal of Neural Transmission 21: 159–168.

Skrabanek P, Powell D 1983 Substance P in obstetrics and gynecology. Obstetrics and Gynecology 61: 641–646.

Sluijmer A V, Lappöhn R E 1992 Clinical history and outcome of 59 patients with idiopathic hyperprolactinemia. Fertility and Sterility 58: 72–77.

Smith A, Gaba T J 1990 Data on families of chromosome translocation carriers ascertained because of habitual spontaneous abortion. Australian and New Zealand Journal of Obstetrics and Gynaecology 30: 57–62.

Smith C G, Asch R H 1987 Drug abuse and reproduction. Fertility and Sterility 48: 355–373.

Smitham J H 1982 Radiological investigation of tubal infertility. In: Chamberlain G, Winston R (eds) Tubal infertility diagnosis and treatment. Blackwell, Oxford, ch 3, p 47.

Snethlage N, Ten Cate J W 1986 Thrombocythaemia and recurrent late abortions: normal outcome of pregnancies after anti-aggregatory treatment: case report. British Journal of Obstetrics and Gynaecology 93: 386–388.

Sobrinho L G, Nunes M C P, Calhaz-Jorge C, Afonso A M, Perira M C, Santos M A 1984 Hyperprolactinemia in women with paternal deprivation during childhood. Obstetrics and Gynecology 64: 465–468.

Solewski J, Warm S P, McGaffic W 1980 Endometrial biopsy during a cycle of conception. Fertility and Sterility 34: 538–551.

Soltan M H, Hancock K W 1982 Outcome in patients with postpill amenorrhea. British Journal of Obstetrics and Gynaecology 89: 745–748.

Sonenthal K R, McKnight T, Shaughnessy M A, Grammer L C, Jeyendran R S 1991 Anaphylaxis during intrauterine insemination secondary to bovine serum albumin. Fertility and Sterility 56: 1188–1191.

Soutter W P, Allan H, Cowan S, Aitchison T C, Leake R E 1979 A study of endometrial RNA polymerase activity in infertile women. Journal of Reproduction and Fertility 55: 45–52.

Speroff L 1981 Getting high on running. Fertility and Sterility 36: 149–151.

St. Michel P, Di Zerega G S 1983 Hyperprolactinemia and luteal phase dysfunction in infertility. Obstetrical and Gynecological Survey 38: 248–254.

Stambaugh R, Noriega C, Mastroianni L 1969 Bicarbonate ion; the coronal cell dispersing factor of rabbit tubal fluid. Journal of Reproduction and Fertility 18: 51–58.

Stangel J J, Nisbet J D II, Settles H 1984 Formation and prevention of postoperative abdominal adhesions. Journal of Reproductive Medicine 29: 143–156.

Stanger J D, Yovich J L 1984 Failure of human oocyte release at ovulation. Fertility and Sterility 41: 827–832.

Steer C V, Tan S L, Mason B A, Campbell S 1994 Midluteal phase vaginal color Doppler assessment of uterine artery impedance in a subfertile populaton. Fertility and Sterility 61: 53–58.

Steinberger E, Rodriguez-Rigau L J 1983 The infertile couple. Journal of Andrology 4: 111–118.

Stillman R J, Rosenberg M J, Sachs B P 1986 Smoking and reproduction. Fertility and Sterility 46: 545–566.

Stoffer S S, McKeel D W, Randall R V, Laws E R 1981 Pituitary prolactin cell hyperplasia with autonomous prolactin secretion and primary hypothyroidism. Fertility and Sterility 36: 682–685.

Stone S C 1980 Complications and pitfalls of artificial insemination. Clinical Obstetrics and Gynecology 23: 667–682.

Stone S G, Swartz W J 1979 A syndrome characterized by recurrent symptomatic ovarian cysts in young women. American Journal of Obstetrics and Gynecology 134: 310–314.

Storey B T 1991 Sperm capacitation and the acrosome reaction. Annals of the New York Academy of Sciences 637: 459–473.

Stovall T G, Elder R F, Ling F W 1989 Predictors of pelvic adhesions. Journal of Reproductive Medicine 34: 345–348.

Stray-Pedersen B, Brun A L, Molne K 1982 Infertility and uterine colonization with Ureaplasma urealyticum. Acta Obstetricia et Gynecologica Scandinavica 61: 21–24.

Sturgis S H, Taymor M L, Morris T 1957 Routine psychiatric interviews in a sterility investigation. Fertility and Sterility 8: 521–525.

Styler M, Shapiro S S 1985 Mollicutes (mycoplasma) in infertility. Fertility and Sterility 44: 1–11.

Sudha T, Gopinath P M 1990 Homologous Robertsonian translocation (21q21q) and abortions. Human Genetics 85: 253–255.

Sugimoto O 1978 Diagnostic and therapeutic hysteroscopy. Igaku-Shoin, Tokyo, pp 27–28.

Sulak P J, Letterie G S, Coddington C C, Hayslip C C, Woodward J E, Klein T A 1987 Histology of proximal tubal occlusion. Fertility and Sterility 48: 437–440.

Syrop C H, Halme J 1987 Peritoneal fluid environment and infertility. Fertility and Sterility 48: 1–9.

Tabibzadeh S 1990 Immunoreactivity of human endometrium: correlations with endometrial dating. Fertility and Sterility 54: 624–631.

Talbert L M, Raj M H G, Hammond M G, Greer T 1984 Endocrine and immunologic studies in a patient with resistant ovary syndrome. Fertility and Sterility 42: 741–744.

Tambascia M, Bahamondes L, Pinotti L, Collier A M, Dachs J L, Faundes A 1980 Sustained hyperprolactinemia in a normally menstruating woman with apparently normal ovarian function. Fertility and Sterility 34: 282–284.

Tan G J J, Biggs J S G 1983 Effects of prolactin on steroid production by human luteal cells in vitro. Journal of Endocrinology 96: 499–503.

Taney F H, Grazi R V, Weiss G, Schmidt C L 1991 Detection of premature luteinization with serum progesterone levels at the time of the postcoital test. Fertility and Sterility 55: 513–515.

Taylor P J, Graham G 1982 Is diagnostic curettage harmful in women with unexplained infertility? British Journal of Obstetrics and Gynaecology 89: 296–298.

Taylor P J, Cumming D C, Hill P 1981 The significance of hysteroscopically detected intrauterine adhesions in eumenorrheic infertile women and the role of antecedent curettage in their formation. American Journal of Obstetrics and Gynecology 139: 239–242.

Taylor-Robinson D, MacCormack W M 1980 The genital mycoplasmas (second of two parts). New England Journal of Medicine 302: 1063–1067.

Templeton A, Fraser C, Thompson B 1991 Infertility — epidemiology and referral practice. Human Reproduction 6: 1391–1394.

Tesarik J, Testart J 1989 Human sperm-egg interaction and their disorders: implications in the management of infertility. Human Reproduction 4: 729–741.

Thom D H, Nelson L M, Vaughan T L 1992 Spontaneous abortion and subsequent adverse birth outcomes. American Journal of Obstetrics and Gynecology 166: 111–116.

Thomas A J 1983 Ejaculatory dysfunction. Fertility and Sterility 39: 445–454.

Thompson L A, Tomlinson M J, Barratt C L R, Bolton A E, Cooke I D 1991 Positive immunoselection — a method of isolating leukocytes from leukocytic reacted human cervical mucus samples. American Journal of Reproductive Immunology 26: 58–61.

Timar L, Beres J, Kosztolanyi G, Nemeth I 1991 De novo complex chromosomal rearrangement in a woman with recurrent spontaneous abortion and one healthy daughter. Human Genetics 86: 421.

Tomlinson M J, East S J, Barratt C L R, Bolton A E, Cooke I D 1992 Preliminary communication: possible role of reactive nitrogen intermediates in leucocyte-mediated sperm dysfunction. American Journal of Reproductive Immunology 27: 89–92.

Toth A, O'Leary A M, Ladger W 1982 Evidence of microbial transfer by spermatozoa. Obstetrics and Gynecology 59: 556–559.

Tredway D R, Umezaki C U, Mishell D Jr, Germanowski J 1975 Effect of intrauterine devices on sperm transport in the human being. American Journal of Obstetrics and Gynecology 123: 734–735.

Trimbos-Kemper T C M, Veering B T 1990 Anaphylactic shock from intracavitary 32% Dextran-70 during hysteroscopy. Fertility and Sterility 51: 1053–1054.

Trimbos-Kemper T, Trimbos B, Van Hall E 1982a Etiologic factors in tubal infertility. Fertility and Sterility 37: 384–388.

Trimbos-Kemper T C M, Trimbos J V, Van Hall E 1982b Management of infertile patients with unilateral tubal pathology by paradoxical oophorectomy. Fertility and Sterility 37: 623–626.

Tsuji K, Nakano R 1978 Chromosome studies of embryos from induced abortions in pregnant women aged 35 and over. Obstetrics and Gynecology 52: 542–544.

Tupper C, Weil R J 1962 The problem of spontaneous abortion. American Journal of Obstetrics and Gynecology 83: 421–424.

Turnbull J M, Weinberg P C 1983 Psychological factors involved in impotence. Journal of Andrology 4: 59–66.

Urman B, Gomel V, McComb P, Lee N 1992 Midtubal occlusion: etiology, management and outcome. Fertility and Sterility 57: 747–750.

Valle R 1980 Hysteroscopy and evaluation of female infertility. American Journal of Obstetrics and Gynecology 137: 425–429.

Van de Geijn E J, Yedema C A, Hemrika D T, Schutte M F, ten Velden J J A M 1992 Hydatidiform mole with coexisting twin pregnancy after gamete intra-fallopian transfer. Human Reproduction 7: 568–572.

Van der Linden P J Q, Kets M, Gimpel J A, Wiegerinck M A H M 1992 Cyclic changes in the concentration of glucose and fructose in human cervical mucus. Fertility and Sterility 57: 573–577.

Van der Ven H, Bhattacharaya A K, Binor Z, Leto S, Zaneveld L J D 1982 Inhibition of human sperm capacitation by a high-molecular-weight factor from human seminal plasma. Fertility and Sterility 38: 753–755.

Van Leeuwen J H S, Christiaens G M L, Hoogenraad T U 1991 Recurrent abortion and the diagnosis of Wilson's disease. Obstetrics and Gynecology 78: 547–549.

Vasquez G, Winston R M L, Boeckx W D, Brosens I 1980 Tubal lesions subsequent to sterilization and their relationship to fertility after attempts at reversal. American Journal of Obstetrics and Gynecology 138: 86–92.

Veneman T F, Beverstock G C, Exalto N, Mollevenger P 1991 Premature menopause because of an inherited deletion of the long arm of the X-chromosome. Fertility and Sterility 55: 631–633.

Verdugo P, Lee W I, Halbert S A, Blandau R J, Tam P Y 1980 A stochastic model for oviductal egg transport. Biophysical Journal 29: 257–270.

Verkauf B S 1992 Myomectomy for fertility enhancement and preservation. Fertility and Sterility 58: 1–15.

Verma R S, Shah J V, Dosik H 1983 Size of Y chromosome not associated with abortion risk. Obstetrics and Gynecology 61: 633–634.

Vigil P, Perez A, Neira J, Morales P 1991 Postpartum cervical mucus: biological and rheological properties. Human Reproduction 6: 475–479.

Vijayakumar R, Walters W A W 1983 Human luteal tissue prostaglandins, 17β-estradiol, and progesterone in relation to the growth and senescence of the corpus luteum. Fertility and Sterility 39: 298–303.

Wah P M, Anderson D J, Hill J A 1990 Asymptomatic cervicovaginal leukocytosis in infertile women. Fertility and Sterility 54: 445–450.

Wallach E E 1972 The uterine factor in infertility. Fertility and Sterility 23: 138–158.

Wanerman J, Wolwick R, Brenner S 1986 Segmental absence of the fallopian tube. Fertility and Sterility 46: 525–527.

Warburton D, Kline J, Stein Z, Susser M 1980 Monosomy X: a chromosomal anomaly associated with young maternal age. Lancet 1: 167–169.

Warren M P 1983 Effects of undernutrition on reproductive function in the human. Endocrine Reviews 4: 363–377.

Waterstone J, Parsons J 1992 Endometrial stromal sarcoma after a successful in vitro fertilization treatment schedule. Human Reproduction 7: 72.

Weber T, Obel E 1979 Pregnancy complications following conization of the uterine cervix. Acta Obstetricia et Gynecologica Scandinavica 58: 259–263.

Weed J C, Carrera A E 1970 Glucose content of cervical mucus. Fertility and Sterility 21: 866–872.

Weiner S, Wright K H, Wallach E E 1977 The influence of ovarian denervation and nerve stimulation on ovarian contractions. American Journal of Obstetrics and Gynecology 128: 154–160.

Weinstein D, Polishuk W Z 1975 The role of wedge resection of the ovary as a cause of mechanical infertility. Surgery Gynecology and Obstetrics 141: 417–418.

Wessels P H, Viljoen G J, Maracs N F, Antonie de Beer J A, Smith M, Gericke A 1991 The prevalence, risks and management of Chlamydia trachomatis infections in fertile and infertile patients from a high socioeconomic bracket of the South African population. Fertility and Sterility 56: 485–488.

Weström L 1980 Incidence, prevalence and trends of acute pelvic inflammatory disease in industrialized countries. American Journal of Obstetrics and Gynecology 138: 880–892.

Wetzels L C G, Essed G G M, deHaan J, Van de Kar A J F, Willebrand D 1982 Endometrial ossification: unilateral manifestation in a septate uterus. Gynecologic and Obstetrical Investigation 14: 47–55.

Whitman G F, Di Lauro S 1990 Morbidity from in vitro fertilization secondary to instrument failure: a case report. Fertility and Sterility 53: 375–376.

Wiebe R H, Morris C V 1983 Testosterone/androstenedione ratio in the evaluation of women with ovarian androgen excess. Obstetrics and Gynecology 61: 279–284.

Wilhelmsson L, Lindblom B 1980 Adrenergic responses of the various smooth muscle layers at the human uterotubal junction. Fertility and Sterility 33: 280–282.

Winkler B, Crum C P 1987 Chlamydia trachomatis infection of the female genital tract: pathogenetic and clinicopathologic correlations. Pathology Annual 22(1): 193–223.

Witkin S S 1988 Production of interferon gamma by lymphocytes exposed to antibody-coated spermatozoa: a mechanism for sperm antibody production in females. Fertility and Sterility 50: 498–502.

Witkin S S, Sonabend J 1983 Immune responses to spermatozoa in homosexual men. Fertility and Sterility 39: 337–342.

Wolner-Hanssen P, Mardh P-A 1984 In vitro tests of the adherence of Chlamydia trachomatis to human spermatozoa. Fertility and Sterility 42: 102–107.

Wolner-Hanssen P, Mardh P-A, Moller B, Westrom L 1982 Endometrial infection in women with Chlamydial salpingitis. Sexually Transmitted Diseases 9: 84–88.

Woosley R E, King J S, Talbert L 1982 Prolactin-secreting pituitary adenomas: neurosurgical management of 37 patients. Fertility and Sterility 37: 54–60.

World Health Organization 1987 Infections, pregnancies and infertility: perspectives on prevention. Fertility and Sterility 47: 964–968.

Wortsman J, Hansen M, Kousseff B G, Hamidinia A 1982 Incomplete differentiation of Wolffian structures: a form of Kallmann's syndrome. Fertility and Sterility 37: 123–125.

Wray H L, Freeman M V R, Ming P M L 1981 Pregnancy in the Turner syndrome with only 45, X chromosome constitution. Fertility and Sterility 35: 509–514.

Yablonski M, Sarge T, Wild R A 1990 Subtle variations in tubal anatomy in infertile women. Fertility and Sterility 54: 455–458.

Yaffe H, Beyth J, Reinhartz T, Levi J 1980 Foreign body granulomas in peritubal and periovarian adhesions: a possible cause for unsuccessful reconstructive surgery in infertility. Fertility and Sterility 33: 277–279.

Yaginuma T 1979 Progress and therapy of stress amenorrhea. Fertility and Sterility 32: 36–39.

Yoshimura Y, Wallach E E 1987 Studies of the mechanisms of mammalian ovulation. Fertility and Sterility 47: 22–34.

Yovich J L, Stanger J D, Tuvic A, Hahnel R 1984 Combined pregnancy after gonadotropin therapy. Obstetrics and Gynecology 64: 855–858.

Zana J, Thomas D, Muffat-Joly M et al 1990 An experimental model for salpingitis due to Chlamydia trachomatis and residual tubal infertility in the mouse. Human Reproduction 5: 274–278.

Zarou G S, Esposito J M, Zarou D M 1973 Pregnancy following the surgical correction of congenital atresia of the cervix. International Journal of Gynaecology and Obstetrics 11: 143–145.

Zegers F, Lenton E A, Sulaiman R, Cooke I D 1981 The cervical factor in patients with ovulatory infertility. British Journal of Obstetrics and Gynaecology 88: 537–542.

Zenzes M T, Casper R F 1992 Cytogenetics of human oocytes, zygotes and embryos after in vitro fertilization. Human Genetics 88: 367–375.

Zinamen M et al 1989 The physiology of sperm recovered from the human cervix: acrosomal status and response to inducers of the acrosome reaction. Biology of Reproduction 41: 790–797.

Zlatnik F J, Burmeister L F 1993 Interval evaluation of the cervix for predicting pregnancy outcome and diagnosing cervical incompetence. Journal of Reproductive Medicine 38: 365–369.

34. Ectopic pregnancy

H. Fox

INTRODUCTION

An ectopic pregnancy is one in which the conceptus implants either outside the uterus or in an abnormal position within the uterus. In practice, between 95% and 98% of ectopic pregnancies occur in the Fallopian tube, other sites, in probable descending order of frequency, being the ovary, cervix and abdominal cavity with occasional instances being reported in such exotic locations as the vagina, liver or spleen.

Studies of the incidence, epidemiology and aetiology of ectopic gestation almost invariably consider all varieties of ectopic implantation as a single entity and this practice will, of necessity, be followed in this chapter even though it is recognized that this 'blunderbuss' approach may well conceal subtle differences in the aetiological factors which are of particular importance for each different site.

INCIDENCE

The incidence of ectopic pregnancies within any given institution or centre is commonly expressed as a proportion of the number of live births, e.g. from 1 ectopic pregnancy per 32 live births to 1 ectopic pregnancy per 300 live births (Douglas, 1963; Macafee, 1982; Weinstein et al, 1983). Figures such as these do not, however, yield any valid information about the proportion of conceptions which implant ectopically for they take no account of those pregnancies which are terminated by either spontaneous or induced abortion (Beral, 1975).

Optimally the incidence of ectopic gestation should be defined in terms of the population at risk and the incidence in any given area or country should be quoted as the number of ectopic pregnancies per 100 000 women in the population aged between 14 and 44 (Barnes et al, 1983). Community-based data of this type have rarely been reported but nevertheless it is clear that there has been, over the last two or three decades, at least a doubling, and in some areas a trebling or quadrupling, of the incidence of tubal pregnancies (Chow et al, 1987; Drife, 1990a; Stabile & Grudzinskas, 1990; Doyle et al,

1991; Cartwright, 1993), to the extent that the usage of the term 'epidemic' (Weinstein et al, 1983; Coupet, 1989; Maymon et al, 1992) does not appear unduly hyperbolic. There is some evidence that the incidence is now stabilizing at a plateau (Centers for Disease Control, 1992) but the level of this plateau remains disturbingly high, probably at between 14 and 17 per 1000 reported pregnancies in North America and Western Europe. The reasons for this increased incidence are debatable and possible factors will be considered later: it is of interest to note, however, that it has not been universal for there was no change in the incidence of ectopic pregnancies in Jamaica between 1963 and 1986 (Turner, 1989).

DEMOGRAPHY

It is usually stated that ectopic pregnancies occur more commonly in urban than in rural populations, are encountered most often in women of low socio-economic status and occur more frequently in black than in white women (Douglas, 1963; Breen, 1970; Dow et al, 1975; Gilstrap & Harris, 1976; Tatum & Schmidt, 1977; Kallenberger et al, 1978; Helvacioglu et al, 1979; Gonzalez & Waxman, 1981). These factors are, rather obviously, interrelated but there has been no real attempt to determine which is the key one or whether these social and ethnic differences are independent of confounding factors, such as the incidence of pelvic inflammatory disease or the rate of cigarette smoking.

The increased frequency of ectopic pregnancy in women of African descent in North America mirrors the high incidence of this condition in the West Indies and in many African countries (Douglas, 1963; Van Iddekinge, 1972; Dow et al, 1975) and it is of note that in Trinidad ectopic gestations occur much more frequently in women of African descent than in those of Indian origin (Daisley, 1989). Any assumption that international variations in the incidence of ectopic pregnancy are related principally to the proportion of the population that are of African origin is, however, dispelled by the high incidence of this condition in Spain (Cagliero, 1961) and, most strikingly, in Greenland (Johnsen & Becker-Christensen, 1990); there is, interestingly and in contrast, an unusually low incidence of ectopic pregnancy in Malaysia (Sambhi, 1967) and a relatively low incidence in both Nigeria (Makinde & Oguniyi, 1990) and Ethiopia (Yoseph, 1990).

There has, over the years, been a remarkable consistency in the reported mean age of women with ectopic pregnancies, this being between 25 and 28 years (Franklin et al, 1973; Brenner et al, 1975; Helvacioglu et al, 1979; De Cherney et al, 1981a; Gonzalez & Waxman, 1981; Cole & Corlett, 1982; Dudley & Arnold, 1982). Although the mean age at which an ectopic pregnancy occurs has remained constant the actual incidence increases with advancing maternal age (Breen, 1970; Beral, 1975; Westrom et al, 1981; Rubin et al, 1983; Skjeldestad & Backe, 1990; Doyle et al, 1991), the highest incidence being in women aged between 35 and 44 years. In view of this age distribution it is not surprising that most women suffering an ectopic gestation are parous, the highest incidence being in those having two or three children (Johnson, 1952; Kleiner & Roberts, 1967; Hlavin et al, 1978; De Cherney et al, 1981a). The reported proportion of primigravida amongst women with an ectopic pregnancy has ranged from 11–32% (Johnson, 1952; Kleiner & Roberts, 1967; Breen, 1970; Franklin et al, 1973; Schoen & Nowak, 1975; Kitchin et al, 1979; Helvacioglu et al, 1979; Randall, 1983) with the figure, in most series, being towards the lower, rather than the higher, extreme of this range.

Despite the fact that women with an ectopic gestation are generally parous, many have a history of diminished reproductive capacity. The incidence of antecedent infertility has been quoted as being between 19% and 37% (Swolin & Fall, 1972; Hughes, 1980; De Cherney et al, 1981a; Sherman et al, 1982; Li et al, 1990; Parazzini et al, 1992) but these figures do not adequately take into account the rather high frequency of one child infertility, or the incidence of three or more years preceding infertility, often either unrecognized or not complained of, in multiparous women. If all these patients are grouped together the incidence of antecedent infertility in patients with an ectopic pregnancy is very high, probably between 55% and 80% (Bobrow & Bell, 1962; Tancer et al, 1981). It should be noted that infertility persists as a strong independent risk factor for ectopic pregnancy even after elimination of confounding factors such as pelvic inflammatory disease, anovulation, drug therapy and pelvic surgery (Marchbanks et al, 1988; Coulam & Wells, 1992). Furthermore, a high proportion of patients have suffered one or more spontaneous abortions (Honoré, 1979; Hughes, 1980; Eskes & van Oppen, 1984; Fedele et al, 1989; Coulam et al, 1988, 1989), many give a history of pelvic inflammatory disease (see later) and a significant proportion, between 6% and 16%, have had a previous ectopic pregnancy (Halpin, 1970; Brenner et al, 1975; De Cherney et al, 1981a; Alsuleiman & Grimes, 1982; Coste et al, 1991a; Nlome-Nze et al, 1992).

The overall picture which emerges is that the women most likely to have an ectopic pregnancy are those who are relatively elderly and who, despite being parous, have a poor reproductive history, women of African descent being particularly at risk.

AETIOLOGY AND PATHOGENESIS

It is certain that no single factor is responsible for all ectopic gestations and probable that most cases are multifactorial in origin. Nevertheless, each proposed aetiological factor is dealt with here independently and it will be appreciated that most apply principally, and often only, to tubal pregnancies though some are of equal importance in ovarian gestations.

Tubal factors

Congenital abnormalities

A number of congenital abnormalities of the tube have been implicated in the causation of tubal pregnancy: these include diverticula, accessory ostia, hypoplasia and focal aplasia (Oscakina-Rojdestvenskaia, 1935; Kurcz & Sharp, 1948; Szlachter & Weiss, 1979; Beyth & Kopolovic, 1982) but claims that such abnormalities account for approximately 20% of tubal gestations (Oscakina-Rojdestvenskaia, 1935) would be generally considered as exaggerated.

The incidence and significance of congenital tubal diverticula is a matter of some dispute. Niles & Clark (1969) found such lesions to be extremely rare in tubes harbouring a gestation but Persaud (1970) is often quoted as having demonstrated that diverticula are present in 49% of gravid tubes: it is in fact clear that the vast majority of the lesions described by Persaud were examples of salpingitis isthmica nodosa and were not spatially related to the site of implantation.

Women who have been prenatally exposed to diethylstilboestrol suffer a considerable excess of ectopic pregnancies (Barnes et al, 1980; Schmidt et al, 1980; Pons et al, 1988) and this may be related to the fact that a proportion of such women have foreshortened, convoluted, 'withered' tubes with minimal fimbrial tissue and a pin-hole os (De Cherney et al, 1981b).

Tubal neoplasms

These are commonly listed as a possible cause of an ectopic pregnancy but, in reality, there have been only a few recorded instances of a tubal gestation complicating either an intrinsic tubal neoplasm or an extrinsic paraovarian tumour (Zelinger et al, 1960; Honoré & Korn, 1976; Casapeto et al, 1978; Moore et al, 1979; Gray et al, 1983; Kutteh & Albert, 1991).

Salpingitis isthmica nodosa

There is a probable, though not fully proven, association between this condition and ectopic pregnancy (Honoré, 1978b; Green & Kott, 1989; Saracoglu et al, 1992). Gonzalez & Waxman (1981), studying a largely black population, noted salpingitis isthmica nodosa in 9.9% of patients with an ectopic pregnancy but in our own series in Manchester, in which a careful search was made for this lesion, it was found in only 3.3% of gravid tubes (Randall, 1983). Persaud (1970) and Majmudar et al (1983) have, by contrast, quoted incidences of 49% and 57% respectively of salpingitis isthmica nodosa in tubal pregnancies. Two points require note, however, about these latter studies: firstly, the populations studied were almost entirely black and, secondly, both have broadened the concept of salpingitis isthmica nodosa in so far as over a third of the diverticular lesions were ampullary rather than isthmic and were not necessarily associated with visible nodularity. There is a consensus that salpingitis isthmica nodosa is found unduly commonly in black women but there would be less agreement as to whether all the lesions described in these two studies as salpingitis isthmica nodosa truly merit this designation.

Even the strongest proponents of the association between salpingitis isthmica nodosa and tubal pregnancy admit that implantation of the conceptus is rarely into a diverticulum in such cases and have noted the discrepancy between the site of the diverticula and that of tubal pregnancy. It has been suggested that the hypertrophied muscle which is a characteristic feature of salpingitis isthmica nodosa may either undergo spasm and thus obstruct the tubal lumen or, by its presence, disturb tubal motility.

Tubal endometriosis

Endometriosis of the tube is often cited as a risk factor for tubal pregnancy, it being argued that endometrial tissue in this site confers an increased 'receptivity' of the tube for a fertilized ovum (Eastman & Hellman, 1966). Nevertheless, Gonzalez & Waxman (1981) found endometriosis in only 1.2% of gravid tubes, a figure virtually identical to that (1.1%) in our own series (Randall, 1983) and very similar to the incidence (1.5%) noted by Kleiner & Roberts (1967). Women with endometriosis do not, as a group, have any excess risk of suffering an ectopic gestation (Marchbanks et al, 1988).

Tubal sterilization

A significant proportion, variously estimated as between 10% and 15%, of pregnancies which occur after a failed tubal sterilization are ectopic (Chakravarti & Shardlow, 1975; Tatum & Schmidt, 1977; Athari & Ravengard, 1978; Wright & Stadel, 1981; WHO, 1985; Makar et al,

1990; Falfoul et al, 1993). The proportion of pregnancies which are ectopic varies with the type of procedure employed, being 4.4% after clipping, 19.5% after ligation, 43–51% following laparoscopic diathermy and 60% after application of Falope rings (Tatum & Schmidt, 1977; McCausland, 1982). If laparoscopic diathermy is accompanied by tubal transection the proportion of ectopic pregnancies falls to 14.5% (McCausland, 1982) whilst if Haulker clips are used instead of Falope rings only 4.4% of subsequent gestations are ectopically sited (Hughes, 1980). It is possible that these differing rates of ectopic pregnancy following different forms of tubal sterilization are simply a reflection, in part at least, of the efficiency of each particular technique in preventing *intrauterine* pregnancies (Chow et al, 1987). It has been claimed that there is a particularly high risk of later ectopic implantation if sterilization is performed during the postpartum or postabortal period (Sivanesaratnam & Ng, 1975; Honoré & O'Hara, 1978) but in more recent carefully controlled studies it has been shown that postpartum sterilization is associated with a lower risk of subsequent tubal gestation than is interval sterilization (Holt et al, 1991).

The actual mechanisms by which tubal implantation occurs following tubal sterilization are somewhat uncertain but both recanalization and the formation of tuboperitoneal fistulas, of sufficient size to allow for the passage of a sperm but not of an embryo, have been proposed as possible factors (Chakravarti & Shardlow, 1975; McCausland, 1982). The ability of tubal epithelium to recanalize an occluded segment has not, however, been conclusively established.

With the increasing number of women being subjected to tubal sterilization this factor is of increasing importance in the aetiology of ectopic pregnancy. Badawy et al (1979) noted that in the United States between 1947 and 1967 only 0.6% of patients with an ectopic pregnancy had been previously sterilized but that this proportion had risen to 4.2% by 1972 and to 7% by 1977. In Canada the proportion of patients who had been previously sterilized was 7.6% in a study of cases of tubal pregnancy reported in 1991 (Greisman, 1991).

It should be noted that although a greater proportion of pregnancies after failed sterilization are ectopic, tubal sterilization actually decreases the absolute risk of ectopic implantations and diminishes an individual woman's risk of future ectopic pregnancy when compared with all women who have not undergone sterilization or women using no contraceptives (de Stefano et al, 1982; WHO, 1985; Kjer & Knudsen, 1989).

Reconstructive tubal surgery

Approximately 5–10% of pregnancies which follow reconstructive operations, of all types and including reversal of sterilization, on the tube are ectopically sited (Gomel, 1978; Rock et al, 1979; Lauritsen et al, 1982; Hulka &

Halme, 1988; Singhal et al, 1991; Tomazevic & Ribic-Pucelj, 1992); the incidence of tubal pregnancy is strikingly high after repeated tuboplasties (Lauritsen et al, 1982).

Tubal deciliation

Vasquez et al (1983) have shown, with the aid of the scanning electronmicroscope, a marked deficiency of epithelial cilia in the tubes of women currently suffering from, or having a history of, a tubal pregnancy. They suggest that diminished ampullary cilial action lessens the efficiency of ovum transport and that delayed entry into the isthmus will result in tubal implantation.

Granulomatous salpingitis

Women with tubal tuberculosis rarely conceive but patients treated for this disease have a high risk of an ectopic pregnancy (Halbrecht, 1957; Varela-Nunez, 1961) this being attributed to residual tubal scarring with narrowing and distortion of the lumen.

Bilharzial salpingitis, relatively common in some areas of the world, results in marked tubal deformity and is associated with a significant risk of an ectopic gestation (Rosen & Kim, 1974; Okonofua et al, 1990; Picaud et al, 1990; Ville et al, 1991a).

Non-granulomatous salpingitis

It is usually taken as axiomatic that pelvic inflammatory disease and tubal infection are major risk factors for tubal pregnancy, it being assumed that postinflammatory damage, in the form of scarring together with deciliation and plical fusion, predisposes to arrest of the fertilized ovum in the tube. It has, however, been rather difficult to establish the true rôle of tubal inflammatory disease in the aetiology of tubal pregnancy for the following reasons:

1. In most studies of ectopic pregnancy there has been a very poor correlation between a history of pelvic inflammatory disease, macroscopic evidence of postinflammatory damage and histological evidence of a tubal inflammatory process (Kleiner & Roberts, 1967; Helvacioglu et al, 1979; Gonzalez & Waxman, 1981; Cumming et al, 1988).

2. Amongst women with a tubal pregnancy the reported incidence of a history of previous pelvic inflammatory disease has varied from 6% to 58%, that of macroscopically evident postinflammatory damage from 21% to 72% and that of histologically proven salpingitis from 18% to 55% (Bone & Greene, 1961; Kleiner & Roberts, 1967; Brenner et al, 1975; Helvacioglu et al, 1979; Gonzalez & Waxman, 1981; Alsuleiman & Grimes, 1982; Cole & Corlett, 1982; Weinstein et al, 1983; Krantz et al, 1990).

3. Case-control studies showing an association between ectopic pregnancy and a history of either pelvic inflammatory disease or sexually transmitted disease (World Health Organization, 1985; Coste et al, 1991a) have used control groups consisting of women with normal pregnancies; this latter group may have been less likely than the general population to have had pelvic infections since their fertility was unimpaired.

Quite apart from the methodological difficulties encountered in trying to prove an association between tubal inflammatory disease and ectopic pregnancy it has to be pointed out that there is only a weak association between the incidences of hospitalization for ectopic gestations and pelvic inflammatory disease (Beral, 1975; Westrom et al, 1981; Shiono et al, 1982) and that during a decade when, in the United States, there was a huge increase in the incidence of tubal pregnancies the annual rate of pelvic inflammatory disease increased only moderately (Chow et al, 1987).

Despite these discrepancies and inconsistencies it remains true that inflammation is present in areas remote from the implantation site in nearly 40% of tubes containing an ectopic gestation (Bone & Greene, 1961; Randall, 1983). Even, however, if it is accepted that about 40% of tubes in which a conceptus is lodged show evidence of salpingitis this does not, in itself, prove an association unless the incidence of tubal inflammation in the overall population of women of reproductive age is known. This particular difficulty has, to some extent, been overcome by a prospective cohort study which has shown that women with laparoscopically proven salpingitis have a much greater risk of eventually having an ectopic gestation than do those with laparoscopically normal tubes (Westrom, 1975, 1985; Westrom et al, 1992).

It is now recognized that *Chlamydia trachomatis* is the most important cause of pelvic inflammatory disease and that infection of this type is often asymptomatic. It is therefore of particular note that there has been, during the last decade, a considerable number of reports that women who are seropositive for antibodies to Chlamydia have a markedly increased risk of ectopic pregnancy and that patients with such antibodies form a high proportion (40–50%) of cases of tubal pregnancy (Svensson et al, 1985; Brunham et al, 1986; Robertson et al, 1988; Chaim et al, 1989; Chow et al, 1990; De Muylder et al, 1990; Hodgson et al, 1990; Kihlstrom et al, 1990; Miettinen et al, 1990; Sherman et al, 1990; Tu et al, 1990; Coste et al, 1991a; Picaud et al, 1991; Ville et al, 1991b; Chrysostomou et al, 1992). The particular importance of this observation, which has admittedly not been totally unanimous (Phillips et al, 1992), is that it circumvents the discrepancies between clinical history and pathological findings and provides an objective criterion of past or current tubal infection. In fact, plasma cell infiltration of tubes harbouring a gestation in women seropositive for

Chlamydia is not always present (Brunham et al, 1992) whilst cultures for the organism are usually negative (Berenson et al, 1991; Neiger & Croom, 1991; Maccato et al, 1992) and chlamydial DNA cannot be detected with the polymerase chain reaction (Osser & Persson, 1992).

Women with antibodies to *Mycoplasma hominis* also are at increased risk for suffering an ectopic gestation and are well represented amongst patients with tubal pregnancies (Miettinen et al, 1990) but the proportion of women with a tubal pregnancy who are seropositive for antibodies to *Neisseria gonorrhoea* is low (Miettinen et al, 1990; Ville et al, 1991b).

Extratubal factors

Ovulatory dysfunction

Iffy (1961, 1963) noted that the fetus in a tubal gestation often appeared to be three to four weeks older than would be expected from the period of amenorrhoea, this suggesting that conception had actually occurred before the bleeding episode which the patient considered as her last menstrual period. He therefore proposed that a conception leading to a tubal pregnancy occurred during a cycle in which there was delayed ovulation and a short, inadequate luteal phase. Hence, at the time of corpus luteum decay the conceptus would not have reached the stage when it was producing sufficient human chorionic gonadotrophin to prevent luteolysis and subsequent menstruation. During the subsequent menstrual bleeding the fertilized ovum could be arrested in its transit through the tube by a reflux of menstrual blood or, if it had already reached the uterine cavity, be flushed back into the tube by menstrual regurgitation. Iffy's hypothesis is supported by the frequency, between 10% and 50% of cases, with which the corpus luteum of pregnancy is on the opposite side to a tube containing a gestation (Berlind, 1960; Kleiner & Roberts, 1967; Halpin, 1970; Honoré, 1978a; Kitchin et al, 1979; Pauerstein et al, 1986) and by the fact that ectopic pregnancy is virtually confined to humans and those primates which menstruate (McElin & Iffy, 1976).

The presence of a corpus luteum of pregnancy in the gonad contralateral to the gravid tube could, of course, also be due to transuterine migration of the fertilized ovum into the opposite tube (Honoré, 1978a).

Contraceptive factors

Intrauterine contraceptive device. If a pregnancy occurs in a woman wearing an intrauterine contraceptive device (IUCD) it will be ectopically sited in about 4–8% of cases, an incidence much in excess of that found in non-contraceptive users (Tatum & Schmidt, 1977; Savolainen & Saksela, 1978; Vessey et al, 1979; Paavonen

et al, 1985; Skjeldestad et al, 1988): furthermore, about 10% of the ectopic pregnancies will be ovarian (Herbertsson et al, 1987; Sandvei et al, 1987). It should not, however, be thought that IUCDs actually *cause* ectopic implantation for the absolute risk of an ectopic pregnancy is, with one exception, reduced in women wearing an IUCD relative to that for women using no contraception (Ory, 1981; Sivin, 1991): the one exception to this general rule are those devices which are progesterone coated and releasing 65 micrograms, or more, of progesterone per day (Sivin, 1991).

The cause of the high incidence of ectopic pregnancies in IUCD users is far from being fully understood. It is tempting to attribute the high proportion of such pregnancies to IUCD-induced tubal inflammation but this appears unlikely as there is now wide, though perhaps not universal, agreement that, with the exception of those who had used a Dalkon shield, former IUCD wearers are not at any increased risk of suffering a tubal pregnancy (Vessey et al, 1979; WHO, 1985; Chow et al, 1986; Marchbanks et al, 1988; Edelman & Van-Os, 1990; Pouly et al, 1991a,b; Randic & Haller, 1992): further, tubal damage could not account for the high proportion of ovarian pregnancies. A more plausible explanation is that IUCDs are much more effective in inhibiting uterine implantation than they are in inhibiting either tubal or ovarian implantation (Lehfeldt et al, 1970; Savolainen & Saksela, 1978). A further possibility is that IUCDs reduce the number of ciliated cells in the tube and thus hamper ovum transport (Vasquez et al, 1983; Wollen et al, 1984), a view supported by the much lower incidence of ectopic gestations in the proximal third of the tube in IUCD users than in non-users (WHO, 1985; Pouly et al, 1991a,b).

Oral steroid contraception. Prior use of combined oral steroid contraception is not associated with either an excess or a deficit of ectopic pregnancies (Vessey et al, 1979) and there is no tendency for pregnancies occurring in current users of combined oral steroid contraceptives to be ectopically sited (Vessey et al, 1976, 1979); indeed, as would perhaps be expected, combined oral contraceptive usage reduces the absolute risk of an ectopic pregnancy in any individual woman (WHO, 1985; Drife, 1990b), largely by preventing pregnancy in the first place. An increased incidence of tubal gestation has, however, been noted in women who became pregnant whilst using low-dose progestagen-only oral contraception (Bonnar, 1974; Smith et al, 1974; Liukko & Erkkola, 1976; Tatum & Schmidt, 1977), possibly because of the inhibitory effect of progesterone on tubal peristalsis.

Pregnancy continuing despite postcoital oestrogen contraception appears to occur unduly frequently in an ectopic site (Morris & van Wagenen, 1973): this may be a reflection of the fact that high oestrogen levels inhibit endometrial implantation whilst having no influence on tubal nidation.

Barrier contraception.   Condom usage is associated with a reduced risk of ectopic pregnancy (Li et al, 1990), this probably being due to the decreased risk of pelvic inflammatory disease.

Ovulatory agents

It has been claimed that pregnancies resulting from ovulation induction, by either clomiphene or gonadotrophins, are more likely to be ectopic than are those derived from a spontaneous ovulation (McBain et al, 1980; Marchbanks et al, 1985; Chow et al, 1987), though Grab et al (1992) found that this risk is confined to the use of gonadotrophins. The reasons for this association are far from clear for many of the ectopic pregnancies have occurred in patients without any evidence of pelvic disease and with normal hysterosalpingograms (Cartwright, 1993).

Prior abortion

As already noted, there are many reports of an increased incidence of ectopic pregnancy in women who have suffered a spontaneous abortion, especially amongst those with a history of recurrent abortion (Coulam et al, 1989; Fedele et al, 1989): it is only fair to note, however, that not all studies have confirmed this finding (Chow et al, 1987; Holt et al, 1989; Coste et al, 1991a; Kalandidi et al, 1991).

Whether or not a history of induced abortion is a risk factor for ectopic pregnancy is a debatable point. Reports noting an increased incidence of ectopic gestation after induced abortion (Panayotou et al, 1977; Levin et al, 1982; Marchbanks et al, 1988; Orhue et al, 1989; Kalandidi et al, 1991) have been countered by others which failed to detect any such association (Beric et al, 1973; Chung et al, 1982; Burkman et al, 1988; Holt et al, 1989; Atrash & Hogue, 1990; Nordenskjold & Ahlgren, 1991). Daling et al (1985) took an equivocal position on this point, noting that the relative risk of an ectopic pregnancy was modestly increased after an induced abortion but not being able to exclude their findings being attributable to chance; this is perhaps an accurate summary of the present position.

Abdominal surgery

In most studies of patients with ectopic pregnancies it has been noted that 25–30% had undergone previous abdominal surgery, most commonly an appendectomy (Kallenberger et al, 1978; De Cherney et al, 1981a; Chow et al, 1987; Marchbanks et al, 1988; Coste et al, 1991a; Michalas et al, 1992) but in only a few of these studies was the incidence considered, in the population studied, of previous abdominal surgery in women of similar age having an intrauterine pregnancy.

In one case-control study there was no increased risk of ectopic gestation after removal of an unruptured appendix and only a slight increase in risk after removal of a ruptured appendix (Ni et al, 1990). It is, in fact, probable that uncomplicated abdominal surgery not directly involving the adnexa has little or no influence on the subsequent risk of tubal pregnancy (Cartwright, 1993).

Assisted reproduction

Between 2% and 10% of pregnancies resulting from assisted reproductive techniques occur in the tube (Yuzpe et al, 1989; Formigli et al, 1990; Jansen et al, 1990, Rizk et al, 1990; Dubuisson et al, 1991; Herman et al, 1991; Karande et al, 1991; Nygren et al, 1991; Wennerholm et al, 1991; Yang et al, 1992), the incidence being somewhat higher with in vitro fertilization and embryo transfer (IVF) than with gamete intra-Fallopian transfer (GIFT). Amongst women undergoing IVF the incidence of ectopic gestation is much higher in those with tubal infertility than in those who are infertile from other causes. A possible explanation for this is that many transferred embryos reflux into the tube and are then later regurgitated to the uterus: it has been suggested that the embryos may fail to be returned to the uterus if there is tubal dysfunction (Cartwright, 1993).

Cigarette smoking

It has been claimed that women who smoke cigarettes during pregnancy are at increased risk of a tubal gestation, smoking appearing to act as an independent risk factor which is dose related (Chow et al, 1989; Handler et al, 1989; Coste et al, 1991b; Lochen, 1992; Phillips et al, 1992): in one case-control study, however, smoking did not persist as a risk factor after adjusting for confounding factors (Parazzini et al, 1992). Proffered explanations for any association between smoking and ectopic gestation include impaired tubal motility, decreased ciliary action and abnormal blastocyst implantation, all possibly related to the reduced oestrogen levels found in smokers (Cartwright, 1993).

Abnormal conceptus

It has intermittently been suggested that an abnormal conceptus is more likely to implant in the tube than is a normal one (Carr, 1969; Emmrich & Kopping, 1981). Phillipe et al (1970) and Elias et al (1981) examined the chromosomal constitution of ectopic embryos, the latter combining their results with those of two other studies (Busch & Benirschke, 1974; Poland et al, 1976): it was clearly shown that ectopic conceptuses do not have a higher frequency of chromosomal abnormalities than do intrauterine embryos of comparable gestational age (Stabile & Grudzinkas, 1994). Nevertheless, hypothetical embryonic chromosomal abnormalities have recently been invoked to explain the increased frequency of ectopic gestations in nurses who handle anti-neoplastic drugs (Saurel-Cubizolles et al, 1993) whilst flow cytometric analysis of tissue from tubal conceptuses has shown a very high incidence of fetal aneuploidy (Karikoski et al, 1993).

Cause of increasing incidence

The increased incidence of ectopic pregnancy during the last three decades is usually attributed principally to an increased incidence of sexually transmitted disease and the introduction of the IUCD. Other factors do, however, need to be considered such as the fact that attempts to preserve, or restore, fertility may well increase the incidence of ectopic gestations; thus antibiotic treatment of salpingitis will result in a scarred, rather than a blocked, tube, as will many instances of tubal surgery, whilst the use of ovulatory agents and of assisted reproductive techniques also increases the risk of an ectopic pregnancy. Quite apart from these iatrogenic factors is the change in life style amongst many women: increased cigarette smoking will increase the incidence of ectopic pregnancies whilst it has been suggested that both dieting and exercise may have a similar effect (James, 1989), the common factor linking these activities being reduced oestrogen levels with possible consequent impairment of tubal motility. None of these factors appears, however, to afford a complete answer and it has been suggested that the increasing incidence of ectopic pregnancies is largely a cohort phenomenon (Makinen, 1989).

TUBAL PREGNANCY

Over 50% of tubal pregnancies are situated in the ampulla whilst approximately 20% occur in the isthmus: around 12% are fimbrial whilst about 10% are interstitial. The pregnancy is usually unilateral and singleton but bilateral tubal pregnancies (Falk & Lackritz, 1977; Robertson, 1980; Sherman et al, 1991) and twins within a single tube (Storch & Petrie, 1976; Misra et al, 1992) can occur, albeit rarely. In bilateral tubal pregnancies the two fetuses may be of the same or different age (Hakim-Elahi, 1965) whilst tubal twin pregnancies, though usually monozygotic, may be dizygotic (Neuman et al, 1990). Triplet tubal pregnancies have been recorded (Forbes & Natale, 1968; Singhal & Chin, 1992).

Combined tubal and intrauterine (heterotopic) pregnancies are distinctly uncommon, though probably less rare than was previously thought (Keskes et al, 1989). Such pregnancies have been noted with increased frequency after administration of ovulatory agents (Berger & Taymor, 1972; Paldi et al, 1975; Eckshtein et al, 1978; Glassner et al, 1990; Dietz et al, 1993) and after both IVF and GIFT (Lower & Tyack, 1989; Dimitry et al, 1990;

Guirgis, 1990; Molloy et al, 1990; Dor et al, 1991; Lewin et al, 1991; Rizk et al, 1991; Tanbo et al, 1991; Chang et al, 1992; Goldman et al, 1992; Svare et al, 1993): whether this is simply a reflection of the high incidence of multiple gestations following these procedures is a moot point.

Implantation and placentation in the tube

Implantation in the tube may be fimbrial, plical, mural or muro-plical (Schumann, 1921). In a plical implantation the conceptus implants on the tip of a mucosal fold and although it may subsequently embed into the plical tissues it does not establish contact with the wall of the tube (Fig. 34.1). This is a rare form of tubal implantation and, indeed, doubts have been expressed as to its existence: scepticism on this point has, however, been dispelled by Falk et al (1975) who described and fully illustrated an undoubted example of plical implantation, and this form of implantation was noted in 11% of our cases (Randall et al, 1987).

Mural implantation occurs when the conceptus is in

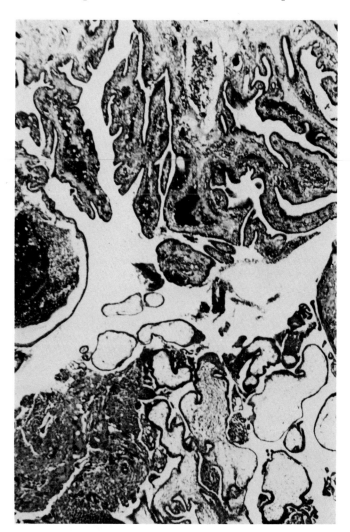

Fig. 34.1 Plical implantation in the tube. H & E × 100.

direct contact with the lumenal surface of the tubal wall between the plicae whilst in a muro-plical implantation the fertilized ovum embeds between adjacent plical folds and trophoblast invades both the plicae and the tubal wall. Fimbrial implantation occurs in about 7% of cases and in these it may be difficult to know whether one is dealing with a tubal or an ovarian pregnancy, it not uncommonly being necessary to resort to the somewhat non-committal and unsatisfactory diagnosis of 'tubo-ovarian pregnancy'.

In mural implantations the process is very similar to that which occurs in an intrauterine gestation for the conceptus penetrates the tubal mucosa and becomes embedded in the tissues of the tubal wall. In a plical implantation the situation is different for here there is, of course, little volume of tissue in which the conceptus can embed; early rupture of the involved plical fold, usually after its almost complete replacement by trophoblast, is the rule. It is not known if, after implantation, the trophoblast becomes ori-

entated at one pole of the conceptus to form a definitive placenta: certainly in some tubal pregnancies the trophoblast does appear to penetrate a localized area of the tubal wall to form an approximation of a discoid placenta but in most cases all the trophoblast surrounding the blastocyst develops to form a circumferential placental attachment, one almost akin to a placenta membranacea in an intra-uterine pregnancy.

Following implantation the two layers of trophoblast, the inner cytotrophoblast and the outer syncytiotrophoblast, can be identified and if implantation has occurred into a site which offers a sufficient area for placentation to occur, as in mural and muro-plical implantations, then the process of placentation will ensue in a manner which is virtually identical to that occurring in an intrauterine site (Randall et al, 1987). Thus, anchoring villi, cytotrophoblastic cell columns and a trophoblastic shell all develop (Fig. 34.2) and extravillous cytotrophoblast streams out from the tips of the cytotrophoblastic cell columns to infiltrate, and extensively colonize, the adjacent tubal tissues. Extravillous interstitial trophoblast, sometimes known as intermediate trophoblast, grows into the mural tissue in a fashion akin to that seen in the penetration of the decidua and inner myometrium in an intrauterine gestation (Fig. 34.3) and infiltrates between the muscle cells of the tubal wall as it does between the myometrial fibres (Fig. 34.4). The invading interstitial cytotrophoblast fans out towards the serosal surface, not infrequently penetrating the full thickness of the muscular layer to reach the subserosa. There may be relatively little lateral spread of these interstitial cytotrophoblastic cells but in some tubes there is a considerable spread laterally, in the longitudinal axis of the tube, either in the muscle coat (Fig. 34.5) or in the subserosa. Overall, the degree and extent of invasion of the muscle coat of the tube is often more exuberant than is the similar invasion of the myometrium in an intrauterine pregnancy and this may be indicative of an absence of regulating factors at this site. Very few multi-nucleated cells are seen in this interstitial population but the invading trophoblastic cells do tend to aggregate around vessels in the tubal wall.

Extravillous cytotrophoblast, from the cytotrophoblastic cell columns, also grows directly into the lumens of the arteries of the tube (Fig. 34.6), destroys the endothelium, invades the vessel wall and destroys the medial musculo-elastic tissue, the wall being eventually replaced by fibrinoid material (Fig. 34.7). Changes in the tubal vessels usually extend through the full thickness of the muscular coat of the tubal wall and, exceptionally, may extend into vessels outside the serosa.

Although it is true that tubal placentation occurs in a less consistent and more erratic pattern than it does in the uterus the overall pattern of placentation is the same in the two sites and, in particular, the vascular changes are identical to those which occur in an intrauterine preg-

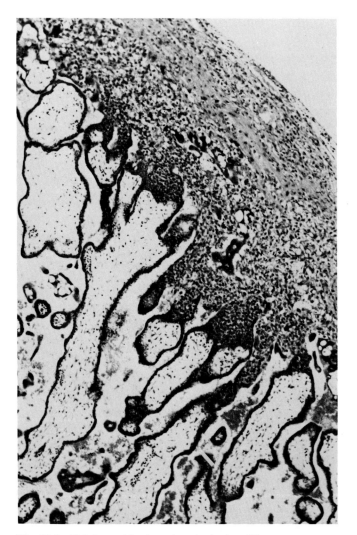

Fig. 34.2 Tubal mural implantation. Anchoring villi, cytotrophoblastic cell columns and trophoblastic shell are all apparent. H & E × 240.

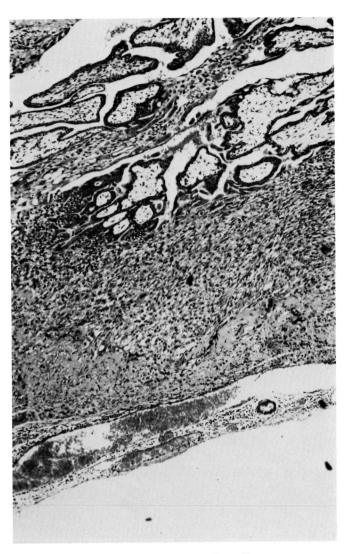

Fig. 34.3 Mural implantation in the tube. Extravillous cytotrophoblast is colonizing the 'decidua' at the site of placental attachment. H & E × 140.

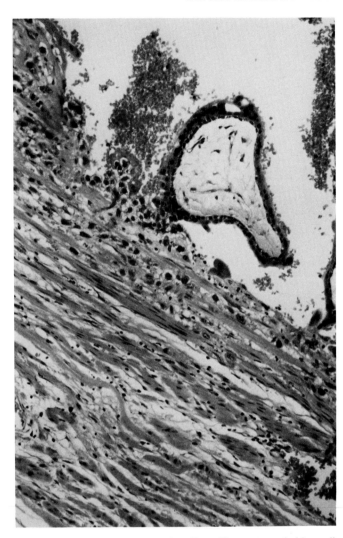

Fig. 34.4 Tubal mural implantation. Extravillous cytotrophoblast cells are infiltrating between muscle fibres in the tubal wall at a point immediately adjacent to the site of placental attachment. H & E × 380.

nancy during the transformation of the spiral arteries into uteroplacental vessels.

This description of tubal placentation is based on our own observations (Randall et al, 1987) which are broadly in accord with those of Stock (1991, 1993). A different version was, however, suggested by Budowick et al (1980) who maintained that trophoblast rapidly penetrates the tube wall to grow principally, together with the embryo, in an extratubal site, invading the retroperitoneal space and growing circumferentially around the outside of the tube. Stock (1993) has, however, provided good evidence that this concept of primary extratubal growth is based upon misinterpretation of an artifact caused by convolution of the tube.

Morphology of placental villi in tubal pregnancy

The appearances of the placental villi in tubal gestations have received little attention. Laufer et al (1962) found that in most cases the placental villous morphology resembled that found in an intrauterine abortion but noted that in 12% of cases the villous appearances were suggestive of a 'blighted ovum'. Emmrich & Kopping (1981) thought that the placental villi showed changes suggestive of a 'blighted ovum' in a very high proportion of tubal pregnancies, attributing this phenomenon to the effects of the unfavourable environment on the fertilized ovum. When considering these reports it is necessary to bear in mind that these authors are equating hydropic change in the villi with a 'blighted ovum' (by which is presumably meant an anembryonic pregnancy); in reality, hydropic change can occur in abortions of any type after longstanding fetal death and is by no means an absolute indication of an anembryonic gestation.

In our experience approximately a third of placentas from tubal pregnancies have a fully normal first-trimester

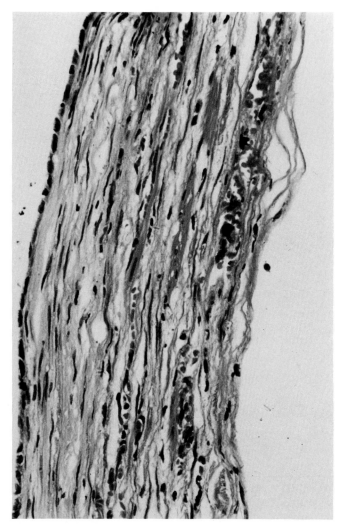

Fig. 34.5 Tubal pregnancy. At a site some distance from the area of placental attachment there is longitudinal spread of extravillous cytotrophoblast between the muscle fibres of the tubal wall. H & E × 380.

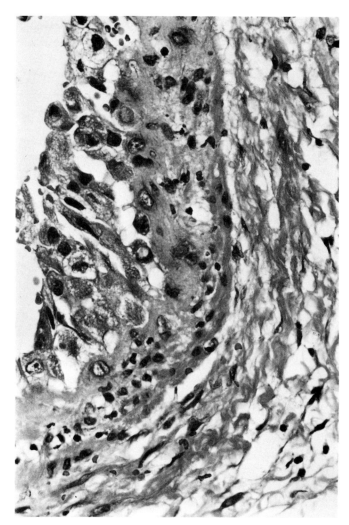

Fig. 34.6 Tubal pregnancy. Extravillous trophoblastic cells in the lumen of a mural artery at the site of placental implantation. H & E × 600.

appearance (Fig. 34.8), this usually being in cases in which tubal rupture has been rapidly followed by operative removal. In the remaining two-thirds of cases the villi show no abnormality apart from those changes which normally follow fetal death, whether this be in an intrauterine or extrauterine site, i.e. stromal fibrosis and sclerosis of the villous fetal vessels. Amongst the placentas showing post mortem changes a minor degree of hydropic change is common (Fig. 34.9) but this is rarely a conspicuous feature. The placental tissue may show areas of infarction or perivillous fibrin deposition as may placentas of similar gestational age from intrauterine pregnancies.

Immunological and immunohistochemical features of trophoblast in tubal pregnancy

The distribution of major histocompatibility antigens in the villous and extravillous trophoblast in tubal gestations

is identical to that noted in the trophoblast populations of an intrauterine pregnancy (Earl et al, 1986). Similarly, the distribution of trophoblastic membrane antigens, hCG, human placental lactogen (hPL) and Schwangerschafts protein 1 (SP1) in a tubal pregnancy is similar to that described in normal early intrauterine placentas (Earl et al, 1985). Immunohistochemical studies have also shown that the distribution of proteinases and proteinase inhibitors in trophoblast is identical in intrauterine and tubal pregnancies (Earl et al, 1989). The only disparity that has been shown between intrauterine and extrauterine trophoblast is that pregnancy-associated plasma protein A (PAPP-A) can be demonstrated in the former but not in the latter (Chemnitz et al, 1984).

Tubal response to pregnancy

The tube can show a decidual response in a tubal preg-

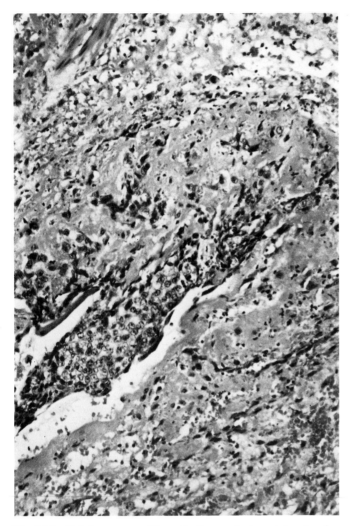

Fig. 34.7 Tubal pregnancy. The wall of a mural artery at the site of placental implantation is infiltrated by trophoblastic cells and shows fibrinoid necrosis. H & E × 480.

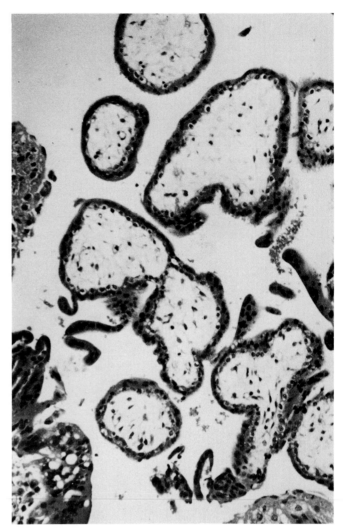

Fig. 34.8 Normal first-trimester villi in a placenta from a tubal pregnancy. H & E × 510.

nancy (Randall et al, 1987; Green & Kott, 1989): whether this is, in fact, a direct response to the tubal implantation is a moot point for a degree of decidual change is not uncommonly seen in tubes removed during the immediate postpartum period following an intrauterine gestation and there is little or no information as to whether the degree of decidual change in a gravid tube exceeds that normally occurring in association with an intrauterine gestation. Be that as it may, any decidual response seen in a tube containing a pregnancy tends to be patchy and relatively inconspicuous, possibly because gravid tubes appear to lack progesterone receptors (Land & Arends, 1992): in our own series a decidual change was, in fact, seen in only 25% of gravid tubes (Fig. 34.10) and this was patchy in 11%, involved only scattered cells in 10% and was extensive in only 4%. The degree and extent of decidual change in the tube is unrelated to the site of implantation, the duration of the pregnancy or the size of the implantation site; even in those few tubes showing extensive decidual

change the 'decidua' is, of course, very much thinner than that found in the gravid uterus. A non-specific mixed acute and chronic inflammatory cell infiltration, which includes T lymphocytes and macrophages but not large granular lymphocytes (Earl et al, 1987), of the tubal wall and plicae at the site of implantation is a common, but not invariable, feature (Fig. 34.11); this localized inflammatory response is sometimes mistakenly considered as evidence of prior tubal inflammatory disease.

Focal endosalpingeal hyperplasia has been noted in association with a tubal pregnancy and the hyperplastic epithelium can occasionally show, in some areas, appearances reminiscent of an Arias-Stella reaction (Mikhael et al, 1977).

Uterine response to tubal pregnancy

In an ectopic gestation the endometrium usually, though far from invariably, responds to the hormonal changes of

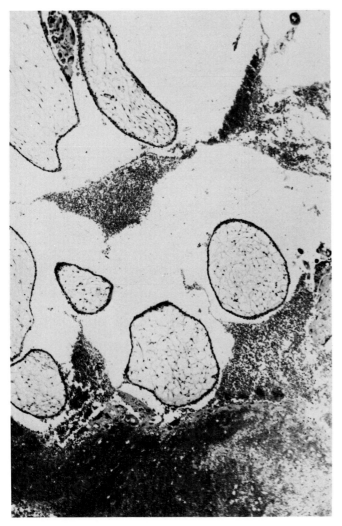

Fig. 34.9   A minor degree of placental villous hydropic change following fetal death in a tubal pregnancy. H & E × 420.

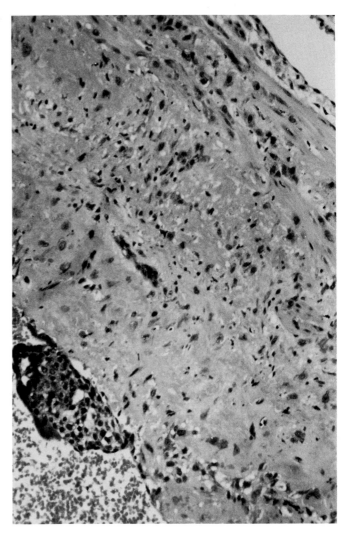

Fig. 34.10   Tubal pregnancy. A decidual reaction in the wall of the tube. H & E × 240.

pregnancy and undergoes decidual change (Fig. 34.12); the degree and extent of the decidual change is somewhat variable but is not uncommonly quantitatively comparable to that found in an intrauterine gestation. The endometrial glands also commonly undergo a typical pregnancy change and are hypersecretory with a markedly scalloped outline. An Arias-Stella reaction (Fig. 34.13) is seen focally in a proportion, variably reported as between 2.9% and 100% of cases, with a majority of authors agreeing that this change can be found in between 60% and 70% of endometria from women with a tubal pregnancy (Birch & Collins, 1961; Charles, 1962; Laluppa & Cavanagh, 1963; Lloyd & Feinberg, 1965; Bernhardt et al, 1966; Ollendorff et al, 1987): our own experience would be that this figure is too high. The Arias-Stella reaction is invariably focal and involves only one gland or a group of glands which show a variable degree of epithelial multilayering and papillary infolding: the cells in these glands lose their polarity, have enlarged, pleomorphic, hyperchromatic nu-

clei and vacuolated clear cytoplasm (Arias-Stella, 1954). This change is not specific to an ectopic pregnancy and can occur in association with any pregnancy, either normal and abnormal, in either an intrauterine or an extrauterine site: there is no doubt that an Arias-Stella reaction can occur in a normal, fully viable intrauterine gestation (Silverberg, 1972; Oertel, 1978).

If the ectopically sited fetus dies the uterine decidua may slough off as a cast (Fig. 34.14) but more commonly crumbles, fragments and is irregularly shed. If there is a long interval between fetal death and endometrial sampling the original decidua may be completely lost and replaced by a proliferative endometrium which, because the first few cycles after an ectopic gestation tend to be anovulatory, may be mildly hyperplastic (Robertson, 1981).

The findings in uterine curettings from a woman with a tubal pregnancy vary considerably, therefore, with the progestational response of the endometrium, the viability or otherwise of the conceptus and with the time interval

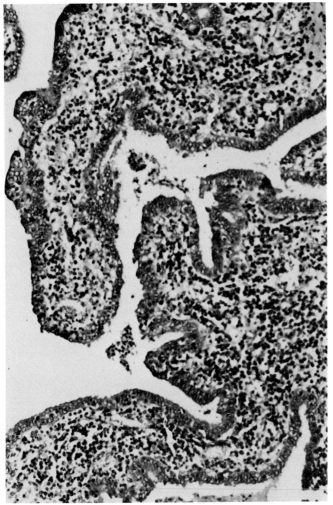

Fig. 34.11 Tubal pregnancy. A non-specific chronic inflammatory cell infiltration in plicae immediately adjacent to the site of placental implantation. H & E × 240.

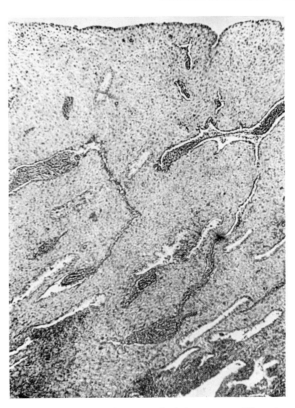

Fig. 34.12 Endometrium in a case of tubal pregnancy. There is a well-marked decidual change but no placental site reaction is seen. H & E × 80.

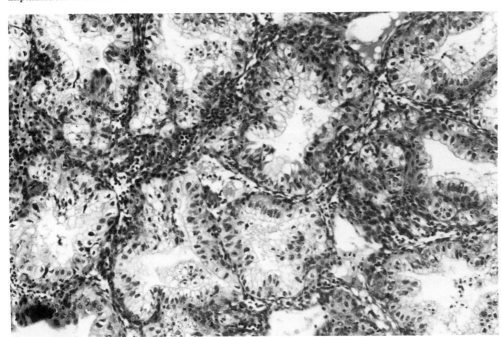

Fig. 34.13 Arias-Stella change in the endometrium. From a case of tubal pregnancy. H & E × 280.

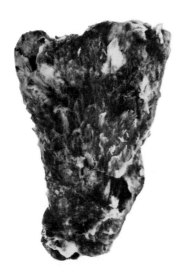

Fig. 34.14 A uterine decidual cast in a case of ectopic pregnancy.

between fetal demise and endometrial sampling. In some instances the endometrium may show no pregnancy-related changes and a normal secretory or proliferative endometrium is found (Ollendorf et al, 1987). The most characteristic appearances are, however, seen in a continuing viable gestation when curettage produces decidua and pregnancy-type endometrial glands, with or without an Arias-Stella change: there is typically little necrosis or inflammation and, most importantly, there is an absence not only of placental villi but also of a placental site reaction in the decidual tissue. The mere absence of placental villi does not necessarily indicate an ectopic pregnancy for they may be lacking in samples obtained after an abortion from an undoubted intrauterine site. Conversely, the presence of placental villi does not invalidate completely a diagnosis of tubal pregnancy for a tubal gestation may abort into the uterine cavity; only the finding of a placental site reaction offers absolute proof of an intrauterine gestation. If the clinical picture of an ectopic pregnancy is associated with clear-cut histological evidence of an intrauterine gestation the possibility of a heterotopic pregnancy should be borne in mind.

Natural history of tubal pregnancies

Tubal pregnancies may terminate in a number of ways:

1. Abortion without tubal rupture

A high proportion of tubal pregnancies spontaneously abort during the early stages of gestation. This is invariably the rule in cases of plical and fimbrial implantation, simply because these sites offer insufficient tissue to allow for adequate placentation, but is also common with mural implantations. There is usually intramural and intralumenal haemorrhage with subsequent fetal death and it

is assumed that this bleeding is largely a consequence of trophoblastic invasion of the tubal wall and vasculature. It has to be borne in mind that the haemostatic mechanisms which are operative in the uterus are lacking in the tube and that minor degrees of bleeding from eroded vessels, during the process of placentation, which are easily controlled in the uterus may, in the tube, assume a magnitude sufficient to endanger the continuing viability of the fetus.

Following abortion the products of conception may persist for a considerable period of time within the tube as one form of 'chronic ectopic pregnancy', or be gradually absorbed, this latter event probably occurring with a greater frequency than is realized (Atri et al, 1993) and often escaping clinical diagnosis. Alternatively the dead fetus, with or without associated blood clot, may be expelled into the abdominal cavity via the ostium or can pass through the isthmus to enter the uterus from whence it is expelled via the cervix.

It is assumed that the rare primary hydatidiform moles and choriocarcinomas of the tube follow a 'silent' tubal abortion.

2. Tubal rupture

At least 60% of tubal pregnancies result in rupture of the tube. This is due largely to the limited distensibility of the tube which is unable to dilate adequately to accommodate the developing conceptus; whether the deep trophoblastic penetration of the wall contributes to a liability to rupture is a debatable point but Stock (1991, 1993) has pointed out that the site of rupture does not necessarily correspond with the site of mural implantation. In at least some cases the tubal rupture appears to be a consequence of the intratubal placental tissue acting as a placenta percreta: we have observed a number of examples of deep villous penetration of the wall (Randall et al, 1987) with the villous tissue penetrating the tubal wall in the same fashion as an intrauterine placenta percreta penetrates the myometrium. This invasiveness may be secondary to the failure of the tube to mount a decidual reaction, for lack of decidualization is considered as an aetiological factor for intrauterine placenta percreta.

Tubal rupture is usually acute, macroscopically obvious and associated with a dramatic clinical picture. Less commonly, however, there is a slow leakage of tubal contents and blood into the abdominal cavity. The clinical features are, in these circumstances, far less striking and the slow seepage of blood results in a gradually enlarging haematoma and causes dense adhesions between the ruptured tube and adjacent structures: not uncommonly the tube is bound down to omentum, small and large bowel, pelvic wall and, occasionally, the contralateral adnexa (Johnson, 1952; Parker & Parker, 1957; Cole & Corlett, 1982). The ureters may be obstructed as a result of entrapment in this paratubal mass (Hovadhanakul et al, 1971).

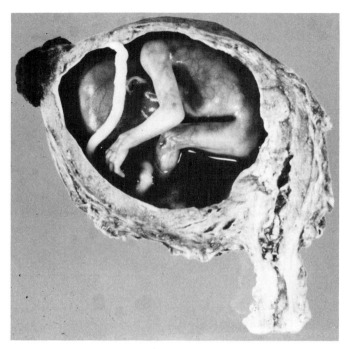

Fig. 34.15 An advanced tubal pregnancy.

Although tubal rupture is usually accompanied by fetal death it is occasionally the case that the fetus, following the rupture, retains sufficient attachment to its blood supply to maintain its viability: the trophoblast grows out from the rupture site and forms a secondary placental site on the tubal serosa, in the broad ligament or in the abdomen (Pauerstein et al, 1986; Randall et al, 1987). A secondary abdominal pregnancy of this type can proceed to term (Clark & Jones, 1975; Paterson & Grant, 1975).

3. Unruptured term pregnancy

There have been many reports of term, or third-trimester, pregnancies (Fig. 34.15) in unruptured tubes (Deopuria, 1970; Clark & Jones, 1975; Augensen, 1983). In theory the following criteria, suggested by McElin & Randall (1951), should be met for the establishment of a diagnosis of term tubal pregnancy:

a. Complete extirpation of the fetal sac and products of conception is achieved by salpingectomy.
b. There is no evidence of tubal rupture.
c. Ciliated columnar epithelium is demonstrable at some point in the inner lining of the sac.
d. Smooth muscle is present in the cyst wall.

In practice the meeting of the first of these criteria is usually accepted as sufficient proof of a tubal gestation at term. The reasons why some tubal pregnancies are capable of progressing to term without rupture of the tube are unknown and no studies have been made of the vascular supply of the placenta and fetus in such pregnancies.

Pathological findings

From what has been said above it will be clear that the operative specimen received by the pathologist after surgical treatment of a tubal pregnancy, usually a salpingectomy specimen, will show a range of appearances which vary with the site of nidation within the tube, the viability or otherwise of the fetus, the duration of the pregnancy and whether or not tubal rupture has occurred. In a 'typical' case the tube is focally or generally distended to a variable degree whilst the peritoneal surface is congested

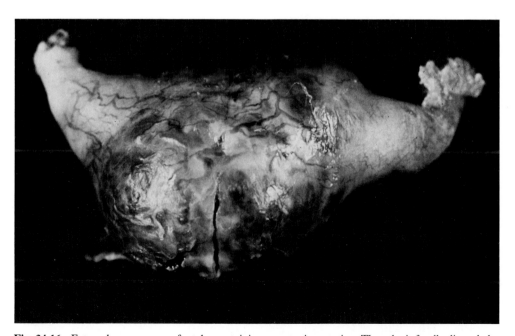

Fig. 34.16 External appearances of a tube containing an ectopic gestation. The tube is focally distended and congested.

and sometimes inflamed (Fig. 34.16). The fimbrial ostium may be occluded by blood clot but if it is still patent blood may be seen oozing from the fimbrial end of the tube. If rupture has occurred blood clot and placental tissue may be seen protruding through the rupture site and blood clot may envelop the tube. On opening the tube a complete amniotic sac and fetus is sometimes seen (Fig. 34.17) but more commonly the lumen appears to contain only fresh and old blood clot: the accumulation of blood clot may be sausage shaped and sufficiently large to distend the tube (Fig. 34.18).

If a recognizable fetus is not present the diagnosis of a tubal gestation can only be confirmed by histological examination. Usually a few placental villi will be found, either embedded within the blood clot or attached to the tubal wall, whilst, occasionally, fragments of fetal tissue are seen. In some cases many sections have to be examined before placental tissue is detected whilst in some cases of abortion or tubal rupture no residual fetal or placental tissue is present: even in such circumstances, however, an implantation site can often be identified by the presence of extravillous trophoblastic tissue which is infiltrating the wall and invading its vessels.

OVARIAN PREGNANCY

Less than 1% of ectopic pregnancies in women not using an IUCD are found in an ovarian site (Lehfeldt et al, 1970); in women using an IUCD the proportion of ovarian to tubal gestations is much higher and has been variously reported as 1 to 9 (Lehfeldt et al, 1970), 1 to 7 (Tietze, 1968) and 1 to 3 (Gray & Ruffolo, 1978). There is, however, some evidence that the incidence of ovarian pregnancy is increasing both in IUCD wearers and non-wearers (Grimes et al, 1983; Schwartz et al, 1993).

Criteria for the recognition of an ovarian pregnancy (Fig. 34.19) were first formulated by Spiegelberg in 1878 and have not been improved on since that date (Speigelberg, 1878):

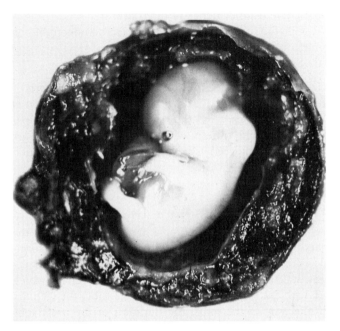

Fig. 34.17   A tube containing a clearly recognizable fetus.

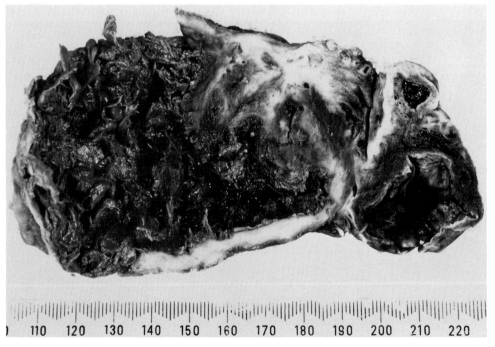

Fig. 34.18   A tubal pregnancy. The tube is distended with old and fresh blood clot.

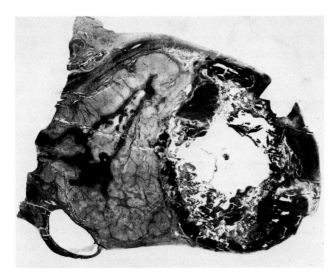

Fig. 34.19 Ovarian pregnancy. Chorionic villi can be seen in the blood clot (right) attached to a corpus luteum.

1. The Fallopian tube on the affected side must be morphologically normal, clearly separated from the ovary and devoid of any evidence of a tubal gestation.

2. The gestational sac must occupy the normal position of the ovary.

3. The gestational sac must be connected to the uterus by the ovarian ligament.

4. Ovarian tissue must be histologically demonstrable in the wall of the gestational sac.

Ovarian pregnancy may be primary or secondary. A primary ovarian pregnancy occurs if the ovum is fertilized whilst still within the follicle or if an ovum, fertilized outside the tube, primarily implants in the ovary. A secondary ovarian pregnancy occurs when fertilization takes place in the tube and the conceptus is regurgitated to implant on the ovary: a secondary ovarian pregnancy may also occur as a consequence of tubal rupture though this is distinctly uncommon. An ovarian gestation may be intrafollicular or extrafollicular and it will be appreciated that Spiegelberg's criteria apply particularly to an intrafollicular pregnancy, which is presumed to be invariably primary. Many extra-follicular ovarian pregnancies, whether they be primary or secondary, do not fulfil the criteria in so far as ovarian tissue is not necessarily present in the wall of the gesta-tional sac.

It is assumed that an intrafollicular ovarian pregnancy is due to fertilization of the ovum whilst it is still retained within the follicle, and this phenomenon is postulated to be a consequence of ovulatory dysfunction (Boronow et al, 1965; Procope & Vesanto, 1966). There is a clear association between ovarian pregnancy and IUCD usage (Lehfeldt et al, 1970; Hallatt, 1976; Grimes et al, 1983; Rivera et al, 1988; Raziel et al, 1990; Xie et al, 1991) but, as previously pointed out, this does not mean that an IUCD causes an ovarian pregnancy but that it simply fails

to prevent such a gestation: hence IUCD usage is not associated with any absolute increase in the incidence of ovarian pregnancy. There have been several reports of ovarian pregnancy following in vitro fertilization and em-bryo transfer (Carter & Jacobson, 1986; Rizk et al, 1990) and GIFT (Lehmann et al, 1991), whilst ovarian preg-nancy combined with an intrauterine gestation (hetero-topic pregnancy) has occurred following the use of an ovulatory agent (McLain & Kirkwood, 1987).

Ovarian pregnancies usually abort during the first tri-mester but there have been a number of such gestations which have proceeded to term or into the third trimester (Nicholls, 1941; Pratt-Thomas et al, 1974; Williams et al, 1982; Belfar et al, 1991; Kosovski et al, 1992).

CERVICAL PREGNANCY

Ectopic pregnancies located in the uterine cervix are rare, probably accounting for only 1% of ectopic gestations (Kouyoundjian, 1984). The aetiology and pathogenesis of cervical pregnancy clearly differ from those of a tubal pregnancy and Studdiford (1945) suggested that unusu-ally rapid transport of the fertilized ovum was an impor-tant aetiological factor, this resulting in it having reached the endocervical canal before reaching a stage of develop-ment compatible with nidation. Schneider & Dreizin (1957) suggested, as an alternative view that, whilst ovum transport was normal, maturation of the conceptus was delayed, this again allowing it to enter the endocervical canal before having reached a stage at which it could implant. These are, however, hypothetical concepts and, in more practical terms, a correlation has been reported between induction of abortion by sharp curettage and subsequent cervical pregnancy (Shinagawa & Nagayama, 1969; Parente et al, 1983) whilst Dicker et al (1985) noted an association of cervical pregnancy with Asherman's syndrome. It is reports such as these that have led to a growing agreement that adverse endometrial factors ('endometrial hostility') are probably the most important aetiological factors in cervical implantation (Yankowitz et al, 1990; Casson, 1993).

Cervical pregnancy has also been reported after IVF (Weyerman et al, 1989), possibly because of unusually low placement of the embryo within the endocervical canal.

Women with a cervical pregnancy usually present as an apparent spontaneous abortion and a clinical suspicion of a cervical pregnancy may be raised by the finding of an expanded cervix in association with a normally-sized uter-ine body. Proof of a cervical pregnancy, as distinct from the cervical stage of an abortion from an intrauterine site, rests solely, however, on pathological examination; the criteria (Rubin, 1911) are:

1. Cervical crypts must be in close approximation to placental tissue.

2. There must be an intimate attachment between the placenta and the cervix.

3. The entire placenta must lie below the entry point of the uterine vessels or below the site of peritoneal reflection on the anterior and posterior uterine surfaces.

4. Fetal tissue must not be present in the uterine cavity.

It is rare for cervical pregnancies to progress beyond the first trimester though occasional third-trimester live births have been documented (Pisarki, 1960; Mitrani, 1973; Jelsema & Zuidema, 1992; Casson, 1993). Abortion of a cervical pregnancy is often accompanied by severe bleeding which has, in the past, led to a high maternal mortality rate. With current therapeutic measures, however, the maternal death rate is now extremely low.

ABDOMINAL PREGNANCY

The incidence of abdominal pregnancy in the United States has been estimated to be just over 1 in 10 000 deliveries (Atrash et al, 1987), a figure that probably applies to other western countries. Abdominal implantation may be either primary or secondary and it is highly probable that most cases are of the secondary type and are a consequence of tubal rupture: even those which are apparently primary probably result from regurgitation of an ovum which has been fertilized in the tube. The criteria for the diagnosis of a primary abdominal pregnancy (Studdiford, 1942) are:

1. Both tubes and ovaries must be normal.

2. There must be no evidence of a uteroperitoneal fistula.

3. The pregnancy must be related principally to the peritoneum.

An abdominal gestation may implant anywhere within the peritoneal cavity and reported sites include the broad ligament, colonic mesentery, lumbar gutter, mesentery of the small bowel, omentum, ileum and lesser peritoneal cavity (Friedrich, 1968). Cases have also been described in which the conceptus has implanted onto the liver (Mear et al, 1965; Kirkby, 1969; Harris et al, 1989), spleen (Yackel et al, 1988; Kahn et al, 1989) or diaphragm (Norenberg et al, 1977). A particular form of abdominal pregnancy is an intraligamentous gestation

(Cordero et al, 1994): this may be due to rupture of a tubal pregnancy at the mesosalpingeal margin of the tube or to burrowing into the ligament of a gestation primarily implanted on the surface of the broad ligament.

Despite this availability of possible sites most early abdominal pregnancies are located in the cul-de-sac and involve either the posterior surface of the uterus or the anterior aspect of the rectosigmoid colon. In advanced gestations the placenta has a broad base of attachment and it may be extremely difficult to localize the site of implantation (Dehner, 1972).

A gestation situated within the abdominal cavity is not subject to the same restraints of space as is a pregnancy within a tube and the limiting factor determining whether the pregnancy aborts or continues is the ability of the placenta to establish an adequate blood supply. Surprisingly, as many as 25% of abdominal pregnancies do achieve adequate placentation and progress to an advanced stage (Hlavin et al, 1978; Golan et al, 1985; White, 1989). It has to be said, however, that the mechanism of placentation within the abdominal cavity remains obscure.

The term abdominal pregnancy presents a surgical challenge for attempts at removing the placenta, though often successful, may be complicated by severe haemorrhage. The placenta can, however, be left in the abdominal cavity and its presence there does not usually appear to cause any signs or symptoms (Petrie & Duchin, 1980) though instances have been noted of sepsis, abscess formation, intestinal obstruction and fistula formation (Casson, 1993).

POST-HYSTERECTOMY PREGNANCY

There have been a considerable number of reports of post-hysterectomy ectopic pregnancy (Cooks, 1980; Zolli & Rocko, 1982; Nehra & Loginsky, 1984; Salmi et al, 1984; Reese et al, 1989). In most cases the woman had conceived immediately prior to the hysterectomy and the fertilized ovum had been trapped in the tube. Some gestations have, however, occurred many years after removal of the uterus and it is thought that under such circumstances fertilization had occurred as a result of sperm passage through a fistulous track in the vaginal vault.

REFERENCES

Alsuleiman S A, Grimes T 1982 Ectopic pregnancy: a review of 147 cases. Journal of Reproductive Medicine 27: 101–106.
Arias-Stella J 1954 Atypical endometrial changes associated with the presence of chorionic tissue. Archives of Pathology 58: 112–128.
Athari T A, Ravengard F 1978 Ectopic pregnancy following tubal sterilization. West Virginia Medical Journal 74: 229–232.
Atrash H K, Hogue C J 1990 The effect of pregnancy termination on future reproduction. Baillieres Clinical Obstetrics and Gynaecology 4: 391–405.

Atrash H K, Friede A, Hogue C J R 1987 Abdominal pregnancy in the United States: frequency and maternal mortality. Obstetrics and Gynecology 69: 333–337.
Atri M, Bret P M, Tulandi T 1993 Spontaneous resolution of ectopic pregnancy: initial appearance and evolution of transvaginal US. Radiology 186: 83–86.
Augensen K 1983 Unruptured tubal pregnancy at term with survival of mother and child. Obstetrics and Gynecology 61: 259–261.

Badawy S, Gilman T, Mroziewicz E 1979 The role of recanalization in tubal pregnancy after sterilization. International Surgery 64: 49–51.

Barnes A B, Colton T, Gunderson J et al 1980 Fertility and outcome of pregnancy in women exposed in utero to diethylstilbestrol. New England Journal of Medicine 302: 609–613.

Barnes A B, Wennberg C N, Barnes B A 1983 Ectopic pregnancy: incidence and review of determinant factors. Obstetrical and Gynecological Survey 38: 345–356.

Belfar H, Heller K, Edelstone D I, Hill L M, Martin J G 1991 Ovarian pregnancy resulting in a surviving neonate: ultrasound findings. Journal of Ultrasound Medicine 10: 465–467.

Beral V 1975 An epidemiological study of recent trends in ectopic pregnancy. British Journal of Obstetrics and Gynaecology 82: 775–782.

Berenson A, Hammill H, Martens M, Faro S 1991 Bacteriologic findings with ectopic pregnancy. Journal of Reproductive Medicine 36: 118–120.

Berger M J, Taymor M L 1972 Simultaneous intrauterine and tubal pregnancies following ovulation induction. American Journal of Obstetrics and Gynecology 113: 812–813.

Beric B, Kupresanin N, Kapor-Stanulovic N A 1973 Accidents and sequelae of medical abortions. American Journal of Obstetrics and Gynecology 116: 813–821.

Berlind M 1960 The contralateral corpus luteum: an important factor in ectopic pregnancies. Obstetrics and Gynecology 16: 51–57.

Bernhardt R N, Bruns P D, Drose V E 1966 Atypical endometrium associated with ectopic pregnancy. Obstetrics and Gynecology 28: 849–853.

Beyth Y, Kopolovic J 1982 Accessory tubes: a possible contributing factor in infertility. Fertility and Sterility 38: 382–383.

Birch H W, Collins C G 1961 Atypical changes in genital epithelium associated with ectopic pregnancy. American Journal of Obstetrics and Gynecology 82: 1198–1208.

Bobrow M L, Bell H G 1962 Ectopic pregnancy: a 16 year survey of 905 cases. Obstetrics and Gynecology 60: 500–502.

Bone N L, Greene R R 1961 Histologic study of uterine tubes with tubal pregnancy. American Journal of Obstetrics and Gynecology 82: 1166–1171.

Bonnar J 1974 Progestagen-only contraception and tubal pregnancies. Lancet i: 170–171.

Boronow R C, McElin T W, West R H, Buckingham J C 1965 Ovarian pregnancy. American Journal of Obstetrics and Gynecology 91: 1095–1106.

Breen J L 1970 A 21 year survey of 654 ectopic pregnancies. American Journal of Obstetrics and Gynecology 106: 1104–1019.

Brenner P F, Roy S, Mishell D R 1975 Ectopic pregnancy: a study of 300 surgically treated cases. Journal of the American Medical Association 243: 673–676.

Brunham R C, Binns B, McDowell J, Paraskevas M 1986 Chlamydia trachomatis infection in women with ectopic pregnancy. Obstetrics and Gynecology 67: 722–736.

Brunham R C, Peeling R, McLean I, Kosseim M L, Oaraskevas M 1992 Chlamydia trachomatis-associated ectopic pregnancy: serologic and histological correlates. Journal of Infectious Diseases 165: 1076–1081.

Budowick M, Johnson T R B, Genadry R, Parmley T H, Woodruff J D 1980 The histopathology of the developing tubal ectopic pregnancy. Fertility and Sterility 34: 1169–1171.

Burkman R T, Mason K J, Gold E B 1988 Ectopic pregnancy and prior induced abortion. Contraception 37: 21–27.

Busch D H, Benirschke K 1974 Cytogenetic studies of ectopic pregnancies. Virchows Archiv B Cell Pathology 16: 319–330.

Cagliero L 1961 Fertilita nelle donne gravidanza extra uterina. Minerva Ginecologica 13: 10–13.

Carr D H 1969 Cytogenetics and the pathology of hydatidiform degeneration. Obstetrics and Gynecology 33: 333–341.

Carter J E, Jacobsen A 1986 Reimplantation of a human embryo with subsequent ovarian pregnancy. American Journal of Obstetrics and Gynecology 155: 282–283.

Cartwright P S 1993 Incidence, epidemiology, risk factors, and etiology. In: Stovall, T G, Ling F W (eds) Extrauterine pregnancy. McGraw-Hill, New York, pp 27–63.

Casapeto R, Nogales F F, Matilla A 1978 Ectopic pregnancy coexisting with a primary carcinoma of the Fallopian tube: a case report. International Journal of Gynecology and Obstetrics 16: 263–264.

Casson P R 1993 The non-tubal ectopic pregnancy: cervical, abdominal, and ovarian. In: Stovall T G, Ling F W (eds) Extrauterine pregnancy. McGraw-Hill, New York, pp 287–303.

Centers For Disease Control 1992 Ectopic pregnancy in the USA. CDC surveillance summary.

Chaim W, Sarov B, Sarov I et al 1989 Serum IgG and IgA antibodies to chlamydia in ectopic pregnancies. Contraception 40: 59–71.

Chakravarti S, Shardlow J 1975 Tubal pregnancy after sterilization. British Journal of Obstetrics and Gynaecology 82: 58–60.

Chang J C, Sun T T, Li Y C 1992 Simultaneous ectopic pregnancy with intrauterine gestation after in vitro fertilization and embryo transfer. European Journal of Obstetrics and Gynecology and Reproductive Biology 44: 157–160.

Charles D 1962 The Arias-Stella reaction. Journal of Obstetrics and Gynaecology of the British Commonwealth 69: 1006–1010.

Chemnitz J, Tornehave D, Teisner B, Poulsen H K, Westergaard J G 1984 The localization of pregnancy proteins (hPL, SP1 and PAPP-A) in intra- and extrauterine pregnancies. Placenta 5: 489–494.

Chow J M, Yonekura M L, Richwald G A, Greenland S, Sweet R L, Schachter J 1990 The association between Chlamydia trachomatis and ectopic pregnancy: a matched pair, case control study. Journal of the American Medical Association 263: 3164–3167.

Chow W H, Daling J R, Weiss N S et al 1986 IUD use and subsequent ectopic pregnancy. American Journal of Public Health 76: 536–539.

Chow W H, Daling J R, Cates W Jr, Greenberg R S 1987 Epidemiology of ectopic pregnancy. Epidemiologic Reviews 9: 70–94.

Chow W H, Daling J R, Weiss N S, Voigt L F 1989 Smoking and tubal pregnancy. Obstetrics and Gynecology 71: 167–170.

Chrysostomou M, Karafyllidi P, Papadimitriou V, Bassiotou V, Mayakos G 1992 Serum antibodies to Chlamydia trachomatis in women with ectopic pregnancy, normal pregnancy or salpingitis. European Journal of Obstetrics and Gynecology and Reproductive Biology 44: 101–105.

Chung C S, Smith R G, Steinhoff P G, Mim P 1982 Induced abortion and ectopic pregnancy in subsequent pregnancies. American Journal of Epidemiology 115: 879–887.

Clark J F, Jones S A 1975 Advanced ectopic pregnancy. Journal of Reproductive Medicine 14: 30–33.

Cole T, Corlett R C 1982 Chronic ectopic pregnancy. Obstetrics and Gynecology 59: 63–68.

Cooks P S 1980 Ectopic pregnancy after vaginal hysterectomy. British Journal of Obstetrics and Gynaecology 87: 363–365.

Cordero D R, Adra A, Yasin S, O'Sullivan M J 1994 Intraligamentous pregnancy. Obstetrical and Gynecological Survey 49: 206–209.

Coste J, Job-Spira N, Fernandez H, Papiernik E, Spira A 1991a Risk factors for ectopic pregnancy: a case control study in France with special focus on infectious factors. American Journal of Epidemiology 133: 839–849.

Coste J, Job-Spira N, Fernandez H 1991b Increased risk of ectopic pregnancy with maternal cigarette smoking. American Journal of Public Health 81: 199–201.

Coulam C B, Wells M 1992 Ectopic pregnancy loss. In: Coulam C B, Faulk W P, McIntyre J A (eds) Immunological obstetrics. Norton, New York, pp 464–478.

Coulam C B, Wagenknecht D R, Faulk W P, McIntyre J A 1988 Prevalence of ectopic pregnancies among women with recurrent spontaneous abortion. American Journal of Reproductive Immunology and Microbiology 16: 100.

Coulam C B, Johnson P M, Ramsden P H et al 1989 Occurrence of ectopic pregnancy among women with recurrent spontaneous abortion. American Journal of Reproductive Immunology 21: 105–107.

Coupet E 1989 Ectopic pregnancy: the surgical epidemic. Journal of the National Medical Association 81: 567–572.

Cumming D C, Honore L E, Scott J Z, Williams K E 1988 Microscopic evidence of silent inflammation in grossly normal fallopian tubes with ectopic pregnancies. International Journal of Fertility 33: 324–328.

Daisley H 1989 Ectopic pregnancies in Trinidad: a clinico-pathological study of 154 consecutive surgically treated cases. West Indian Medical Journal 38: 222–227.

Daling J R, Chow W H, Weiss N S, Metch B J, Soderstrom R 1985 Ectopic pregnancy in relation to previous induced abortion. Journal of the American Medical Association 253: 1005–1008.

De Cherney A H, Minkin M J, Spangler S 1981a Contemporary management of ectopic pregnancy. Journal of Reproductive Medicine 26: 519–523.

De Cherney A H, Cholst I, Naftolin F 1981b Structure and functions of the Fallopian tubes following exposure to diethylstilbestrol (DES) during gestation. Fertility and Sterility 36: 741–745.

Dehner L P 1972 Advanced extra-uterine pregnancy and the fetal death syndrome. Obstetrics and Gynecology 40: 525–534.

De Muylder X, Laga M, Tennstedt C, Van Dyck E, Aelbers G H, Plot P 1990 The role of Neisseria gonorrhoeae and Chlamydia trachomatis in pelvic inflammatory disease and its sequelae in Zimbabwe. Journal of Infectious Diseases 162: 501–505.

Deopuria R H 1970 Full term, unruptured, intra-tubal pregnancy. Journal of Obstetrics and Gynaecology of India: 566–571.

De Stefano F, Peterson H B, Layde P, Rubin G L 1982 Risk of ectopic pregnancy following tubal sterilization. Obstetrics and Gynecology 60: 326–330.

Dicker D, Feldberg D, Samuel N, Goldman J 1985 Etiology of cervical pregnancy: association with abortion, pelvic pathology, IUDs and Asherman's syndrome. Journal of Reproductive Medicine 30: 25–27.

Dietz T U, Haenggi W, Birkhaeuser M, Gyr T, Dreher T 1993 Combined bilateral tubal and multiple intrauterine pregnancy after ovulation induction. European Journal of Obstetrics and Gynecology and Reproductive Biology 48: 69–71.

Dimitry E S, Subak-Sharpe R, Mills M, Margara R, Winston R 1990 Nine cases of heterotopic pregnancies in 4 years of in vitro fertilization. Fertility and Sterility 53: 107–110.

Dor J, Seidman D S, Levran D, Ben-Rafael Z, Ben-Shilomo I, Mashiach S 1991 The incidence of combined intrauterine and extrauterine pregnancy after in vitro fertilization and embryo transfer. Fertility and Sterility 55: 833–834.

Douglas C P 1963 Tubal ectopic pregnancy. British Medical Journal 2: 838–841.

Dow E K, Wilson J B, Klufio C A 1975 Tubal pregnancy: a review of 404 cases. Ghana Medical Journal 14: 232–237.

Doyle M B, DeCherney A H, Diamond M P 1991 Epidemiology and etiology of ectopic pregnancy. Obstetrics and Gynecology Clinics of North America 18: 1–17.

Drife J 1991a Tubal pregnancy. British Medical Journal 301: 1057–1058.

Drife J 1990b Benefits and risks of oral contraceptives. Advances in Contraception 6 (suppl): 15–25.

Dubuisson J B, Aubriot F X, Mathieu L, Foulot H, Mandelbrot L, De Joliere J B 1991 Risk factors for ectopic pregnancy in 556 pregnancies after in vitro fertilization: implications for preventive management. Fertility and Sterility 56: 686–690.

Dudley A G, Arnold F W 1982 Ectopic pregnancy in a rural environment: a 10 year review of 79 cases. Journal of the Medical Association of Georgia 71: 339–341.

Earl U, Wells M, Bulmer J N 1985 The expression of major histocompatibility antigens by trophoblast in ectopic tubal pregnancy. Journal of Reproductive Immunology 8: 13–24.

Earl U, Wells M, Bulmer J N 1986 Immunohistochemical characterization of trophoblast antigens and secretory products in ectopic tubal pregnancy. International Journal of Gynecological Pathology 5: 132–142.

Earl U, Lunny D P, Bulmer J N 1987 Leukocyte populations in ectopic tubal pregnancy. Journal of Clinical Pathology 40: 901–910.

Earl U, Morrison L, Gray C, Bulmer J N 1989 Proteinase and proteinase inhibitor localization in the human placenta. International Journal of Gynecological Pathology 8: 114–124.

Eastman N J, Hellman L M 1966 William's Obstetrics, 13th edn. Appleton-Century-Crofts, New York.

Eckshtein N, Ismajowich B, Yedwab G, David M P 1978 Combined tubal and multiple intrauterine pregnancies following ovulation induction. Fertility and Sterility 30: 707–709.

Edelman D A, Van-Os W A 1990 Safety of intrauterine contraception. Advances in Contraception 6: 207–217.

Elias S, LeBeau M, Simpson J L, Martin A D 1981 Chromosome analysis of ectopic human conceptuses. American Journal of Obstetrics and Gynecology 141: 698–703.

Emmrich P, Kopping H 1981 A study of placental villi in extrauterine gestation: a guide to the frequency of blighted ova. Placenta 2: 63–70.

Eskes T K, van Oppen A C 1984 Ectopic pregnancy: not only a tubal disease. European Journal of Obstetrics, Gynecology and Reproductive Biology 18: 391–394.

Falfoul A, Friaa R, Chelli M, Kharouf M 1993 Grossesses survenues apres sterilisation chirurgicale feminine: etude apropos de 30 cas. Journal de Gynecologie, Obstetrique et Biologie de Reproduction (Paris) 22: 23–25.

Falk R J, Lackritz R M 1977 Bilateral simultaneous tubal pregnancies after ovulation induction with clomiphene-menotrophin combination. Fertility and Sterility 28: 32–34.

Falk H C, Hassid R, Dazo E P 1975 Tubal pregnancy: a report of a very early luminal form of imbedding. Obstetrics and Gynecology 45: 215–216.

Fedele L, Acaia B, Parazzini F, Ricciardiello O, Candiani G B 1989 Ectopic pregnancy and recurrent spontaneous abortion: two associated reproductive failures. Obstetrics and Gynecology 73: 206–208.

Forbes D A, Natale A 1968 Unilateral tubal triplet pregnancy: report of a case. Obstetrics and Gynecology 31: 360–362.

Formigli L, Coglitore M T, Roccio C, Belotti G, Stangalini A, Formigli G 1990 One-hundred-and-six gamete intra-fallopian transfer procedures with donor semen. Human Reproduction 5: 549–552.

Franklin E W, Zeiderman A M, Laemmle P 1973 Tubal ectopic pregnancy: etiology and obstetric and gynecologic sequelae. American Journal of Obstetrics and Gynecology 117: 220–225.

Friedrich M A 1968 Primary omental pregnancy: 2 cases of primary peritoneal pregnancy. Obstetrics and Gynecology 31: 104–109.

Gilstrap L C III, Harris R E 1976 Ectopic pregnancy: a review of 122 cases. Southern Medical Journal 69: 23–24.

Glassner M J, Aron E, Eskin B A 1990 Ovulation induction with clomiphene and the rise in heterotopic pregnancies: a report of two cases. Journal of Reproductive Medicine 35: 175–178.

Golan A, Sandbank O, Adronikou A, Rubin A 1985 Advanced extrauterine pregnancy. Acta Obstetricia et Gynecologica Scandinavica 64: 21–25.

Goldman G A, Fisch B, Ovadia J, Tadir Y 1992 Heterotopic pregnancy after assisted reproductive technologies. Obstetrical and Gynecological Survey 47: 217–221.

Gomel V 1978 Profile of women requesting sterilization reversal. Fertility and Sterility 30: 39–46.

Gonzalez F A, Waxman M 1981 Ectopic pregnancy: a retrospective study of 501 consecutive patients. Diagnostic Gynecology and Obstetrics 3: 181–186.

Grab D, Wolf A, Kunzel H, Sterzik K 1992 Die ovarielle Stimulation mit climifen stelt keinen Riskfaktor fur eine Extrauteringravidatat dar. Zentralblatt fur Gynakologie 114: 289–291.

Gray C L, Ruffolo E H 1978 Ovarian pregnancy associated with intrauterine contraceptive devices. American Journal of Obstetrics and Gynecology 132: 134–139.

Gray C, Wells M, Kingston R 1983 Tubal pregnancy associated with a papillary serous neoplasm arising in a paraovarian cyst. Journal of Obstetrics and Gynaecology 4: 61–62.

Green L K, Kott M L 1989 Histopathologic findings in ectopic tubal pregnancy. International Journal of Gynecological Pathology 8: 255–262.

Greisman B 1991 Ectopic pregnancy in women with previous tubal sterilization at a Canadian community hospital. Journal of Reproductive Medicine 36: 206–209.

Grimes H C, Nosal R A, Gallagher J C 1983 Ovarian pregnancy: a review of 24 cases. Obstetrics and Gynecology 61: 174–180.

Guirgis R R 1990 Simultaneous intrauterine and ectopic pregnancies following in-vitro fertilization and gamete intra-fallopian transfer: a review of nine cases. Human Reproduction 5: 484–486.

Hakim-Elahi E 1965 Unruptured bilateral tubal pregnancy: report of a case. Obstetrics and Gynecology 26: 763–766.

Halbrecht 1957 Healed genital tuberculosis. Obstetrics and Gynecology 10: 73–76.

Hallatt J G 1976 Ectopic pregnancy associated with the intrauterine device: a study of seventy cases. American Journal of Obstetrics and Gynecology 125: 754–758.

Halpin T F 1970 Ectopic pregnancy: the problem of diagnosis. American Journal of Obstetrics and Gynecology 106: 227–236.

Handler A, Davis F, Ferre C, Yeko T 1989 The relationship of smoking and ectopic pregnancy. American Journal of Public Health 79: 1239–1242.

Harris G J, Al-Jurf A S, Yuh W T, Abu-Yousef M M 1989 Intrahepatic pregnancy: a unique opportunity for evaluation with sonography, computed tomography, and magnetic resonance imaging. Journal of the American Medical Association 261: 902–904.

Helvacioglu A, Long E M Jr, Yang S 1979 Ectopic pregnancy: an eight-year review. Journal of Reproductive Medicine 22: 87–92.

Herbertsson G, Magnusson S S, Benediktsdottir K 1987 Ovarian pregnancy and IUCD use in a defined complete population. Acta Obstetrica et Gynecologica Scandinavica 66: 607–610.

Herman A, Ron-El R, Golan A, Weinraub Z, Bukovsky I, Caspi E 1991 Role of tubal pathology and other parameters in ectopic pregnancies occurring in in-vitro fertilization and embryo transfer. Fertility and Sterility 54: 864–868.

Hlavin G E, Ladoski L T, Breen J L 1978 Ectopic pregnancy: an analysis of 153 patients. International Journal of Gynecology and Obstetrics 16: 42–47.

Hodgson R, Driscoll G I, Dodd J K, Tyler J P 1990 Chlamydia trachomatis: the prevalence, trend and importance in initial infertility management. Australian and New Zealand Journal of Obstetrics and Gynaecology 30: 251–254.

Holt V L, Daling J R, Voigt L F et al 1989 Induced abortion and the risk of subsequent ectopic pregnancy. American Journal of Public Health 79: 1234–1238.

Holt V L, Chu J, Daling J R, Stergachis A S, Weiss N S 1991 Tubal sterilization and subsequent ectopic pregnancy: a case control study. Journal of the American Medical Association 266: 242–246.

Honoré L H 1978a Tubal ectopic pregnancy with contralateral corpus luteum: a report of five cases. Journal of Reproductive Medicine 21: 269–271.

Honoré L H 1978b Salpingitis isthmica nodosa in female fertility and ectopic tubal pregnancy. Fertility and Sterility 29: 164–168.

Honoré L H 1979 A significant association between spontaneous abortion and tubal pregnancy. Fertility and Sterility 32: 401–402.

Honoré L H, Korn G W 1976 Coexistence of tubal ectopic pregnancy and adenomatoid tumor. Journal of Reproductive Medicine 17: 342–344.

Honoré L H, O'Hara K E 1978 Failed tubal sterilization as an etiologic factor in ectopic pregnancy. Fertility and Sterility 29: 509–511.

Hovadhanakul P, Eachempati U, Cavanagh D 1971 Ureteral obstruction in chronic ectopic pregnancy. American Journal of Obstetrics and Gynecology 110: 311–313.

Hughes G J 1980 Fertility and ectopic pregnancy. European Journal of Obstetrics, Gynecology and Reproductive Biology 10: 361–365.

Hulka J F, Halme J 1988 Sterilization reversal: results of 101 attempts. American-Journal of Obstetrics and Gynecology 159: 767–774.

Iffy L 1961 Contribution to the aetiology of ectopic pregnancy. Journal of Obstetrics and Gynaecology of the British Commonwealth 68: 441–450.

Iffy L 1963 The role of premenstrual, post-mid cycle conception in the aetiology of ectopic gestation. Journal of Obstetrics and Gynaecology of the British Commonwealth 70: 996–1000.

James W H 1989 A hypothesis on the increasing rates of ectopic pregnancy. Paediatric and Perinatal Epidemiology 3: 189–193.

Jansen R P, Anderson J C, Birrell W A et al 1990 Outpatient gamete intrafallopian transfer: a clinical analysis of 710 cases. Medical Journal of Australia 153: 182–188.

Jelsema R D, Zuidema L 1992 First-trimester diagnosed cervico-isthmic pregnancy resulting in term delivery. Obstetrics and Gynecology 80: 517–519.

Johnsen H M, Becker-Christensen F 1990 Ectopic pregnancy in Greenland: an epidemiological study. Arctic Medical Research 49: 43–47.

Johnson W O 1952 A study of 245 cases of ruptured ectopic pregnancy. American Journal of Obstetrics and Gynecology 64: 1102–1110.

Kahn J A, Skjeldestad F E, During V et al 1989 A spleen pregnancy. Acta Obstetricia et Gynecologica Scandinavica 68: 83–84.

Kalandidi A, Doulgerakis M, Tzonou A, Hsieh C C, Aravandinos D, Trichopoulos D 1991 Induced abortions, contraceptive practices, and tobacco smoking as risk factors for ectopic pregnancy in Athens, Greece. British Journal of Obstetrics and Gynaecology 98: 207–213.

Kallenberger D A, Ronk D A, Kimerson G K 1978 Ectopic pregnancy: 15-year review of 160 cases. Southern Medical Journal 71: 758–765.

Karande V C, Flood J T, Heard N, Veeck L, Muasher S J 1991 Analysis of ectopic pregnancies resulting from in-vitro fertilization and embryo transfer. Human Reproduction 6: 446–449.

Karikoski P, Aine R, Heinonen P K 1993 Abnormal embryogenesis in the etiology of ectopic pregnancy. Gynecologic and Obstetric Investigation 36: 158–162.

Keskes J, Ben-Siad A, Khairi H, Hidar M 1989 Simultaneous intra- and extra-uterine pregnancy: a report of six cases. Journal de Gynecologie, d'Obstetrique et de la Biologie de Reproduction 18: 181–184.

Kihlstrom E, Lindgren R, Ryden G 1990 Antibodies to Chlamydia trachomatis in women with infertility, pelvic inflammatory disease and ectopic pregnancy. European Journal of Obstetrics and Gynecology and Reproductive Biology 35: 199–204.

Kirkby N G 1969 Primary hepatic pregnancy. British Medical Journal 1: 296.

Kitchin J D, Wein R M, Nunley W C, Thiagarajah S, Thornton W N 1979 Ectopic pregnancy: current clinical trends. American Journal of Obstetrics and Gynecology 134: 870–876.

Kjer J J, Knudsen L B 1989 Ectopic pregnancy subsequent to laparoscopic sterilization. American Journal of Obstetrics and Gynecology 160: 1202–1204.

Kleiner G J, Roberts T W 1967 Current factors in causation of tubal pregnancy: a prospective clinicopathologic study. American Journal of Obstetrics and Gynecology 99: 21–28.

Kosovski I, Schopova P, Skotschev S 1992 Ein Fall einer austgetragenen Ovarialschwangerschaft. Zentralblatt fur Gynakologie 114: 316–317.

Kouyoundjian A J 1984 Cervical pregnancy: case report and literature review. Journal of the National Medical Association 76: 791–796.

Krantz S G, Gray R H, Damewood M D, Wallach E E 1990 Time trends in risk factors and clinical outcome of ectopic pregnancy. Fertility and Sterility 54: 42–46.

Kurcz J A, Sharp M S 1948 Congenital absence of one ovary associated with contra-lateral tubal pregnancy. American Journal of Obstetrics and Gynecology 55: 1065.

Kutteh W H, Albert T 1991 Mature cystic teratoma of the fallopian tube associated with an ectopic pregnancy. Obstetrics and Gynecology 78: 984–986.

Laluppa M A, Cavanagh D 1963 The endometrium in ectopic pregnancy: a study based on 35 patients by hysterectomy. Obstetrics and Gynecology 21: 155–164.

Land J A, Arends J W 1992 Immunohistochemical analysis of estrogen and progesterone receptors in fallopian tubes during ectopic pregnancy. Fertility and Sterility 58: 335–337.

Laufer A, Sadovsky A, Sadovsky E 1962 Histologic appearance of the placenta in ectopic pregnancy. Obstetrics and Gynecology 20: 350–353.

Lauritsen J G, Pagel J D, Vangsted P, Starup J 1982 Results of repeated tuboplasties. Fertility and Sterility 37: 68–72.

Lehfeldt H, Tietze C, Gorstein F 1970 Ovarian pregnancy and the intrauterine device. American Journal of Obstetrics and Gynecology 108: 1005–1009.

Lehmann F, Baban N, Harms B, Gethmann U, Krech R 1991 Ovargraviditat nach Gametentransfer (GIFT); ein Fallbericht. Geburtshilfe und Frauenheilkunde 51: 945–947.

Levin A A, Schoenbaum S C, Stubblesfield P G, Zimicki S, Morison R R, Ryan K J 1982 Ectopic pregnancy and prior induced abortion. American Journal of Public Health 72: 253–255.

Lewin A, Simon A, Rabinowitz R, Schenker J G 1991 Second trimester heterotopic pregnancy after in-vitro fertilization and embryo transfer:

a case report and review of the literature. International Journal of Fertility 36: 227–230.

Li D K, Daling J P, Stergachis A S, Chu J, Weiss N S 1990 Prior condom use and the risk of tubal pregnancy. American Journal of Public Health 80: 964–966.

Liukko P, Erkkola R 1976 Low dose progestogens and ectopic pregnancy. British Medical Journal 2: 1257–1258.

Lloyd H E D, Feinberg R 1965 The Arias-Stella reaction: a nonspecific involutional phenomenon in intra- as well as extrauterine pregnancy. American Journal of Clinical Pathology 43: 428–432.

Lochen M L 1992 Royking og eskstrauterine svangerskap. Tidsskrift Norwege Laegeforen 112: 1479–1480.

Lower A M, Tyack A J 1989 Heterotopic pregnancy following in-vitro fertilization and embryo transfer: two case reports and a review of the literature. Human Reproduction 4: 126–128.

Macafee C A J 1982 Ectopic pregnancy. British Journal of Hospital Medicine 28: 246–249.

McBain J C, Evans J H, Pepperell R J, Robinson H P, Smith M A, Brown J B 1980 An unexpectedly high rate of ectopic pregnancy following the induction of ovulation with human pituitary and chorionic gonadotrophin. British Journal of Obstetrics and Gynaecology 87: 5–9.

Maccato M, Estrada H, Hammill H, Faro S 1992 Prevalence of active Chlamydia trachomatis at the time of exploratory laparotomy for ectopic pregnancy. Obstetrics and Gynecology 79: 211–213.

McCausland A 1982 Endosalpingosis ('endosalpingoblastosis') following laparoscopic tubal coagulation as an etiologic factor of ectopic pregnancy. American Journal of Obstetrics and Gynecology 143: 12–21.

McElin T W, Iffy L 1976 Ectopic gestation: a consideration of new and controversial issues relating to pathogenesis and management. Obstetrics and Gynecology Annual 5: 241–291.

McElin T W, Randall L M 1951 Intratubal term pregnancy without rupture: review of the literature and presentation of diagnostic criteria. American Journal of Obstetrics and Gynecology 61: 130–138.

McLain P L, Kirkwood C R 1987 Ovarian and intrauterine heterotopic pregnancy following clomiphene ovulation induction: report of a healthy live birth. Journal of Family Practice 24: 76–79.

Majmudar B, Henderson P H, Semple E 1983 Salpingitis isthmica nodosa: a high risk factor for tubal pregnancy. Obstetrics and Gynecology 62: 73–78.

Makar A P, Vanderheyden J S, Schatteman E A, Albertyn G P, Verkinderen J J, Van Marck E A 1990 Female sterilization failure after bipolar electrocoagulation: a 6 year retrospective study. European Journal of Obstetrics and Gynecology and Reproductive Biology 37: 237–246.

Makinde O O, Ogunniyi S O 1990 Ectopic pregnancy in a defined Nigerian population. International Journal of Gynaecology and Obstetrics 33: 239–241.

Makinen J I 1989 Increase of ectopic pregnancy in Finland— combination of time and cohort effects. Obstetrics and Gynecology 73: 21–24.

Marchbanks P A, Annegers J F, Coulam C B, Strathy J H, Kurland L T 1988 Risk factors for ectopic pregnancy: a population based study. Journal of the American Medical Association 259: 1823–1827.

Maymon R, Shulman A, Maymon B B, Bar-Levy F, Lotan M, Bahary C 1992 Ectopic pregnancy, the new gynecological epidemic disease: review of the modern work-up and the non-surgical treatment option. International Journal of Fertility 37: 146–164.

Mear Y, Ekra J B, Raoelison S 1965 Un cas de grossesse a implantation hepatique avec enfant. Semaine des Hopitaux de Paris 41: 1430–1433.

Michalas S, Minaretzis D, Tsiomou C, Maos G, Kioses G, Aravantinos D 1992 Pelvic surgery, reproductive factors and risk of ectopic pregnancy: a case controlled study. International Journal of Gynaecology and Obstetrics 38: 101–105.

Miettinen A, Heinonen P K, Teisala K, Hakkarainen K, Punnonen R 1990 Serologic evidence for the role of Chlamydia trachomatis Neisseria gonorrhoeae, and Mycoplasma hominis in the etiology of tubal factor infertility and ectopic pregnancy. Sexually Transmitted Diseases 17: 10–14.

Mikhael N Z, Campbell J S, Lee S Y, Acharya V C, Hurteau G D 1977 Tubal Arias-Stella atypia. European Journal of Obstetrics, Gynecology and Reproductive Biology 7: 13–15.

Misra R, Misra K, Agrawal D 1992 Bilateral ectopic pregnancy. International Journal of Fertility 37: 24–25.

Mitrani A 1973 Cervical pregnancy ending in a live birth. Journal of Obstetrics and Gynaecology of the British Commonwealth 80: 761–763.

Molloy D, Deambrosis W, Keeping D, Hynes J, Harrison K, Hennessy J 1990 Multiple-sited (heterotopic) pregnancy after in-vitro fertilization and gamete intrafallopian transfer. Fertility and Sterility 53: 1068–1071.

Morris J M, van Wagenen G 1973 Interception: the use of post-ovulatory estrogens to prevent implantation. American Journal of Obstetrics and Gynecology 115: 101–106.

Nehra P C, Loginsky S J 1984 Pregnancy after vaginal hysterectomy. Obstetrics and Gynecology 64: 735–737.

Neiger R, Croom C S 1991 Culturing tubal pregnancies for Chlamydia trachomatis: is it beneficial? International Journal of Fertility 36: 215–218.

Neuman W L, Ponto K, Farber R A, Shangold G A 1990 DNA analysis of unilateral twin ectopic gestation. Obstetrics and Gynecology 75: 479–483.

Ni H, Daling J R, Chu J et al 1990 Previous abdominal surgery and tubal pregnancy. Obstetrics and Gynecology 75: 919–922.

Nicholls R R 1941 Ovarian pregnancy with living child and mother. American Journal of Obstetrics and Gynecology 42: 341.

Niles J H, Clark J J 1969 Pathogenesis of tubal pregnancy. American Journal of Obstetrics and Gynecology 105: 1230–1234.

Nlome-Nzear A R, Picaud A, Ogowet-Igumu N, Faye A, Ella-Ekogha R 1992 Recurrent extra-uterine pregnancies: 63 cases treated at the Hospital Center Libreville from 1985 to 1989. Revue Francaise de Gynecologie et d'Obstetrique 87: 12–16.

Nordenskjolo F, Ahlgren M 1991 Risk factors in ectopic pregnancy: results from a population-based case-control study. Acta Obstetricia et Gynecologia Scandinavica 70: 575–579.

Norenberg D D, Gundersson J H, Janis J F et al 1977 Early pregnancy on the diaphragm with endometriosis. Obstetrics and Gynecology 49: 620–624.

Nygren K G, Bergh T, Nylund L, Wramsby H 1991 Nordic in-vitro fertilization embryo transfer (IVF/ET) treatment outcomes 1982–1989. Acta Obstetricia et Gynecologica Scandinavica 70: 561–563.

Oertel Y C 1978 The Arias-Stella reaction revisited. Archives of Pathology and Laboratory Medicine 102: 651–654.

Okonofua F E, Ojo O S, Odunsi O A, Odesanmi W O 1990 Ectopic pregnancy associated with schistosomiasis in a Nigerian woman. International Journal of Gynaecology and Obstetrics 32: 281–284.

Ollendorf D A, Fejgin M D, Barzilai M, Ben-Noon I, Gerbie A B 1987 The value of curettage in the diagnosis of ectopic pregnancy. American Journal of Obstetrics and Gynecology 157: 71–72.

Orhue A A, Unuigbe J A, Ogbeide W E 1989 The contribution of previous induced abortion to tubal ectopic pregnancy. West African Medical Journal 8: 257–263.

Ory H W 1981 Ectopic pregnancy and intrauterine contraceptive devices: new perspectives. Obstetrics and Gynecology 57: 137–143.

Oscakina-Rojdestvenskaia A J 1935 Etiology of extrauterine pregnancy. Surgery, Gynecology and Obstetrics 67: 308–311.

Osser S, Persson K 1992 Chlamydial antibodies and deoxyribonucleic acid in patients with ectopic pregnancy. Fertility and Sterility 57: 578–582.

Paavonen J, Varjonen-Toivonen M, Komulaine M, Heinomen P K 1985 Diagnosis and management of tubal pregnancy: effect on fertility outcome. International Journal of Gynecology and Obstetrics 23: 129–133.

Paldi E, Gergely R Z, Abramavici H, Rimor-Tritsch I 1975 Clomiphene-citrate induced simultaneous intra- and extrauterine pregnancy: case report. Fertility and Sterility 26: 1140.

Panayotou P P, Kaskarelis D B, Miettinen O, Trichopoulos D B, Kalandidi A K 1977 Induced abortion and ectopic pregnancy. American Journal of Obstetrics and Gynecology 114: 507–510.

Parazzini F, Tozzi L, Ferraroni M, Bocciolone L, La Vecchia C, Fedele L 1992 Risk factors for ectopic pregnancy: an Italian case control study. Obstetrics and Gynecology 80: 821–826.

Parente J T, Ou C, Levy J, Legatt E 1983 Cervical pregnancy analysis: a review and report of five cases. Obstetrics and Gynecology 62: 79–82.

Parker S L, Parker R T 1957 'Chronic' ectopic tubal pregnancy. American Journal of Obstetrics and Gynecology 74: 1174–1179.

Paterson W G, Grant K A 1975 Advanced intraligamentous pregnancy: report of a case, review of the literature and a discussion of the biological implications. Obstetrical and Gynecological Survey 30: 715–726.

Pauerstein C J, Croxatto H B, Eddy C A, Ramzy I, Walters M P 1986 Anatomy and pathology of tubal pregnancy. Obstetrics and Gynecology 67: 301–308.

Persaud V 1970 Etiology of tubal ectopic pregnancy. Radiologic and pathologic studies. Obstetrics and Gynecology 36: 257–263.

Petrie R H, Duchin S 1980 Diagnosis and placental management of a viable term abdominal gestation. Diagnostic Gynecology and Obstetrics 2: 299–301.

Phillipe E, Ritter J, Lefakis D 1970 Grossesse tubaire, ovulation tardive et anomalie de nidation. Gynecologie et Obstetrique 69: 617–621.

Phillips R S, Tuomala R E, Feldblum P J, Schachter J, Rosenberg M J, Aronson M D 1992 The effect of cigarette smoking, Chlamydia trachomatis infection, and vaginal douching on ectopic pregnancy. Obstetrics and Gynecology 79: 85–90.

Picaud A, Walter P, Bennani S, Minko-Mi-Etoua D, Nlome-Nze A R 1990 Bilharziose tubaire a Schistosoma intercalatum revelee par un hemoperitonia. Archives d'Anatomie, Cytologie et Pathologie 38: 208–211.

Picaud A, Berthonneau J P, Nlome-Nze A R, Ogowet-Igumu H, Engomgah-Beka T 1991 Serologie des Chlamydiae et grossesse extra-uterine; frequence du syndrome Fitz-Hugh-Curtis, Journal de Gynecologie, Obstetrique et Biologie de la Reproduction (Paris) 20: 209–215.

Pisarki T S 1960 Cervical pregnancy. Journal of Obstetrics and Gynaecology of the British Empire 67: 759–762.

Poland B J, Dill F J, Styblo C 1976 Embryonic development in ectopic human pregnancy. Teratology 14: 315–321.

Pons J C, Goujard J, Derbanne C, Tournaire M 1988 Devenir des grossesses des patientes exposees in utero au diethylstiboestrol. Journal de Gynecologie, Obstetrique et Biologie de la Reproduction (Paris) 17: 307–316.

Pouly J L, Chapron C, Canis M et al 1991a Grossesses extra-uterines sur sterilet: caracteristiques et fertilite ulterieurs. Journal de Gynecologie, Obstetrique et Biologie de la Reproduction (Paris) 20: 1069–1073.

Pouly J L, Chapron C, Canis M, Mage G et al 1991b Subsequent fertility for patients presenting with an ectopic pregnancy and having an intra-uterine device in situ. Human Reproduction 6: 999–1001 .

Pratt-Thomas H R, White L, Messka H H 1974 Primary ovarian pregnancy: presentations of the cases including one full term pregnancy. Southern Medical Journal 67: 920–925.

Procope B-J, Vesanto T 1966 Primary ovarian pregnancy. Acta Obstetricia et Gynecologica Scandinavica 44: 534–542.

Randall S 1983 A clinico-pathological study of ectopic pregnancy. MD Thesis, University of Manchester.

Randall S, Buckley C H, Fox H 1987 Placentation in the Fallopian tube. International Journal of Gynecological Pathology 6: 132–139.

Randic L, Haller H 1992 Ectopic pregnancy amongst past IUD users. International Journal of Gynaecology and Obstetrics 58: 299–304.

Raziel A, Golan A, Neuman M, Ron-El R, Bukovsky I, Caspi E 1990 Ovarian pregnancy: a report of twenty cases in one institution. American Journal of Obstetrics and Gynecology 163: 1182–1185.

Reese W A, O'Connor R, Bouzoukis J K, Sutherland S F 1989 Tubal pregnancy after total vaginal hysterectomy. Annals of Emergency Medicine 18: 1107–1110.

Rivera F H, Torres F J, Rodreguez A F 1988 Ovarian pregnancy: a clinicopathological study of eight cases. European Journal of Obstetrics and Gynecology and Reproductive Biology 29: 339–345.

Rizk B, Lachelin G C, Davies M C, Hartshorne G M, Edwards R G 1990 Ovarian pregnancy following in vitro fertilization and embryo transfer. Human Reproduction 5: 763–764.

Rizk B, Tan S I, Morcos S et al 1991 Heterotopic pregnancies after in-vitro fertilization and embryo transfer. American Journal of Obstetrics and Gynecology 164: 161–164.

Robertson J N, Hogston P, Ward H E 1988 Gonococcal and Chlamydial antibodies in ectopic and intrauterine pregnancy. British Journal of Obstetrics and Gynaecology 95: 711–716.

Robertson W B 1981 The endometrium. Butterworths, London.

Robertson W H 1980 Bilateral Fallopian tube pregnancy. Fertility and Sterility 33: 86–87.

Rock J A, Katayama K P, Martin E J, Rock B M, Woodruff J D, Jones H W 1979 Pregnancy outcome following uterotubal implantation: a comparison of the reamer and sharp conual wedge excision techniques. Fertility and Sterility 31: 634–640.

Rosen Y, Kim B 1974 Tubal gestation associated with Schistosoma mansoni salpingitis. Obstetrics and Gynecology 43: 413–417.

Rubin G L, Peterson H B, Dorfman S F et al 1983 Ectopic pregnancy in the United States: 1970–1978. Journal of the American Medical Association 249: 1725–1729.

Rubin I C 1911 Cervical pregnancy. Surgery, Gynecology and Obstetrics 13: 625–627.

Salmi T, Punnonen R, Gronroos M 1984 Tubal pregnancy after vaginal hysterectomy. Obstetrics and Gynecology 64: 826.

Sambhi J S 1967 Ectopic pregnancy in Malaya. Medical Journal of Malaya 21: 344–351.

Sandvei R, Sandstad E, Steier J A, Ulstein M 1987 Ovarian pregnancy associated with the intra-uterine contraceptive device. Acta Obstetricia et Gynecologica Scandinavica 66: 137–141.

Saracoglu F O, Mungan T, Tanzer F 1992 Salpingitis isthmica nodosa in infertility and ectopic pregnancy. Gynecologic and Obstetric Investigation 34: 202–205.

Saurel-Cubizolles M J, Job-Spira N, Estryn-Behar M 1993 Ectopic pregnancy and occupational exposure to antineoplastic drugs. Lancet 341: 1169–1171.

Savolainen E, Saksela A 1978 Ectopic pregnancy associated to the preceding contraception. Annales Chirurgiae et Gynaecologica Fennae 67: 198–202.

Schmidt G, Fowler W C, Talbert L M, Edelman D A 1980 Reproductive history of women exposed to diethylstilbestrol in utero. Fertility and Sterility 33: 21–24.

Schneider P, Dreizin D H 1957 Cervical pregnancy. American Journal of Surgery 93: 27.

Schoen J A, Nowak R J 1975 Repeat ectopic pregnancy: a 16 year clinical survey. Obstetrics and Gynecology 45: 542–546.

Schumann E A 1921 Extra-uterine pregnancy. Appleton, New York.

Schwartz L B, Carcangiu M L, DeCherney A H 1993 Primary ovarian pregnancy: a case report. Journal of Reproductive Medicine 38: 155–158.

Sherman D, Langer R, Sadovsky G, Bukovsky I, Caspi E 1982 Improved fertility following ectopic pregnancy. Fertility and Sterility 37: 497–502.

Sherman K J, Daling J R, Stergachis A et al 1990 Sexually transmitted diseases and tubal pregnancy. Sexually Transmitted Diseases 17: 115–121.

Sherman S J, Werner H, Husain M 1991 Bilateral ectopic gestations. International Journal of Gynaecology and Obstetrics 35: 255–257.

Shinagawa S, Nagayama M 1969 Cervical pregnancy as a possible sequela of abortion: report of 19 cases. American Journal of Obstetrics and Gynecology 105: 282–284.

Shiono P H, Harlap S, Pellegrin F 1982 Ectopic pregnancies: rising incidence rates in northern California. American Journal of Public Health 72: 173–175.

Silverberg S G 1972 Arias-Stella phenomenon in spontaneous and therapeutic abortion. American Journal of Obstetrics and Gynecology 112: 777–780.

Singhal A M, Chin V P 1992 Unilateral triplet ectopic pregnancy: a case report. Journal of Reproductive Medicine 37: 187–188.

Singhal V, Li T C, Cooke I D 1991 An analysis of factors influencing the outcome of 232 consecutive tubal microsurgery cases. British Journal of Obstetrics and Gynaecology 98: 628–636.

Sivanesaratnam V, Ng K H 1975 Tubal pregnancies following postpartum sterilization. Fertility and Sterility 26: 945–946.

Sivin J 1991 Dose- and age-dependent ectopic pregnancy risks with intrauterine contraception. Obstetrics and Gynecology 78: 291–298.

Skjeltdestad F E, Backe B 1990 Incidence of extrauterine pregnancy in Norway in 1986: a population based overview from 15 countries. Tidsskrift Norwege for Laegeforen 110: 470–473.

Smith M, Vessey M, Bounds W, Warn J 1974 Progestagen only oral contraception and ectopic gestation. British Medical Journal 3: 104–105.

Spiegelberg O 1878 Zur Casuistik der Ovarialschwangerschaft. Archiv fur Gynakologie 13: 73–79.

Stabile I, Grudzinskas J G 1990 Ectopic pregnancy: a review of incidence, etiology and diagnostic aspects. Obstetrical and Gynecological Survey 45: 335–347.

Stabilo I, Grudzinskas J G 1994 Ectopic pregnancy: what's new? In: Studd J (ed) Progress in Obstetrics and Gynaecology 11. Churchill Livingstone, Edinburgh, pp 281–307.

Stock R J 1991 Tubal pregnancy: associated histopathology. Obstetrics and Gynecology Clinics of North America 18: 73–94.

Stock R J 1993 Gross pathology and microscopic histopathology. In: Stovall T G, Ling F W (eds) Extrauterine pregnancy. McGraw-Hill, New York, pp 65–96.

Storch M P, Petrie R H 1976 Unilateral tubal twin gestation. American Journal of Obstetrics and Gynecology 125: 1148.

Studdiford W E 1942 Primary peritoneal pregnancy. American Journal of Obstetrics and Gynecology 44: 487–491.

Studdiford W E 1945 Cervical pregnancy. American Journal of Obstetrics and Gynecology 49: 169–174.

Svare J, Norup P, Grove-Thomsen S et al 1993 Heterotopic pregnancies after in-vitro fertilization and embryo transfer—a Danish survey. Human Reproduction 8: 116–118.

Svensson L, Mardh P A, Ahlgren M et al 1985 Ectopic pregnancy and antibodies to Chlamydia trachomatis. Fertility and Sterility 44: 313–317.

Swolin K, Fall M 1972 Ectopic pregnancy: recurrence, postoperative fertility and aspects of treatment based on 192 patients. Acta Europaea Fertilitatis 3: 147–157.

Szlachter N, Weiss G 1979 Distal tubal pregnancy in a patient with a bicornuate uterus and segmental absence of the Fallopian tube. Fertility and Sterility 32: 602–603.

Tanbo T, Dale P O, Lunde O, Abyholme T 1991 Heterotopic pregnancy following in vitro fertilization. Acta Obstetricia et Gynecologica Scandinavica 70: 335–338.

Tancer M L, Delke I, Veridiano 1981 A fifteen year experience with ectopic pregnancy. Surgery, Gynecology and Obstetrics 152: 179–182.

Tatum H J, Schmidt F H 1977 Contraceptive and sterilization practices and extrauterine pregnancy: a realistic perspective. Fertility and Sterility 28: 407–421.

Tietze C 1968 Wanted: ovarian pregnancies. American Journal of Obstetrics and Gynecology 101: 275.

Tomazevic T, Ribic-Pucelj M 1992 Ectopic pregnancy following the treatment of tubal infertility. Journal of Reproductive Medicine 37: 611–614.

Tu F C, Sun L S, Chen P C, Tsui M S, Li Y T, Hau K P 1990 Chlamydia trachomatis infection in women with ectopic pregnancy. Chung Hua I Hsueh Tsa Chih 46: 220–224.

Van Iddekinge B 1972 Ectopic pregnancy: a review. South African Medical Journal 46: 1844.

Varela-Nunez A 1961 Tubal pregnancy following treated genital tuberculosis: report of 2 cases and review of literature. American Journal of Obstetrics and Gynecology 82: 1162–1165.

Vasquez G, Winston R M L, Brosens I A 1983 Tubal mucosa and ectopic pregnancy. British Journal of Obstetrics and Gynaecology 90: 468–474.

Vessey M P, Doll R, Peto R, Johnson B, Wiggins P 1976 A long-term follow-up study of women using different methods of contraception. Journal of Biosocial Science 8: 373–427.

Vessey M P, Yeates D, Flavel R 1979 Risk of ectopic pregnancy and duration of use of an intrauterine device. Lancet i: 501–502.

Ville Y, Leruez M, Picaud A, Walter P, Fernandez H 1991a Tubal schistosomiasis as a cause of ectopic pregnancy in endemic areas: a report of three cases. European Journal of Obstetrics and Gynecology and Reproductive Biology 42: 77–79.

Ville Y, Leruez M, Glowaczower E, Robertson J N, Ward M E 1991b The role of Chlamydia trachomatis and Neisseria gonorrhoeae in the aetiology of ectopic pregnancy in Gabon. British Journal of Obstetrics and Gynaecology 98: 1260–1266.

Weinstein L, Morris M B, Dotters D, Christian C D 1983 Ectopic pregnancy: a new surgical epidemic. Obstetrics and Gynecology 61: 698–701.

Wennerholm U B, Janson P O, Wennergren M, Kjellmer I 1991 Pregnancy complications and short term follow up of infants born after in vitro fertilization and embryo transfer (IVF/ET). Acta Obstetricia et Gynecologica Scandinavica 70: 565–573.

Westrom L 1975 Effect of pelvic inflammatory disease on fertility. American Journal of Obstetrics and Gynecology 121: 707–713.

Westrom L 1985 Influence of sexually transmitted diseases on sterility and ectopic pregnancy. Acta Europaea Fertilitatis 16: 21–24.

Westrom L, Bengtsson L P H, Mardh P-A 1981 Incidence, trends and risks of ectopic pregnancy in a population of women. British Medical Journal 282: 15–18.

Westrom L, Joesoef R, Reynolds G, Hagdu A, Thompson S E 1992 Pelvic inflammatory disease and fertility: a cohort study of 1,844 women with laparoscopically verified disease and 657 control women with normal laparoscopic results. Sexually Transmitted Diseases 19: 185–192.

Weyerman P C, Verhoeven A T M, Alberda A T 1989 Cervical pregnancy after in vitro fertilization and embryo transfer. American Journal of Obstetrics and Gynecology 161: 1145–1146.

White R G 1989 Advanced abdominal pregnancy: a review of 23 cases. Irish Journal of Medical Sciences 158: 77–78.

Williams P C, Malvar T C, Kraft J R 1982 Term ovarian pregnancy with delivery of a live female infant. American Journal of Obstetrics and Gynecology 142: 589–591.

Wollen A L, Flood P R, Sandvei R et al 1984 Morphological changes in tubal mucosa associated with the use of intrauterine contraceptive devices. British Journal of Obstetrics and Gynaecology 91: 1123–1128.

World Health Organization 1985 WHO Task Force on Intrauterine Devices for Fertility Regulation. A multinational case control study of ectopic pregnancy. Clinical Reproduction and Fertility 3: 131–143.

Wright N H, Stadel B V 1981 Ectopic pregnancy and tubal ligation. American Journal of Obstetrics and Gynecology 139: 611–612.

Xie P Z, Feng Y Z, Zhao B H 1991 Primary ovarian pregnancy: report of fifteen cases. Chinese Medical Journal 104: 217–220.

Yackel D B, Panton O M N, Martin D J, Lee D 1988 Splenic pregnancy—case report. Obstetrics and Gynecology 71: 471–473.

Yang M H, Ng S C, Ratnam S S et al 1992 Outcome of 143 pregnancies conceived by assisted reproductive techniques. Asia Oceania Journal of Obstetrics and Gynaecology 18: 299–307.

Yankowitz J, Leake J, Huggins G, Gazaway P, Gates E 1990 Cervical ectopic pregnancy: review of the literature and report of a case treated by single-dose methotrexate therapy. Obstetrical and Gynecological Survey 45: 405–414.

Yoseph S 1990 Ectopic pregnancy at Tikur Anbessa Hospital, Addis Ababa, Ethiopia, 1981–1987: a review of 176 cases. Ethiopian Medical Journal 28: 113–118.

Yuzpe A A, Brown S E, Casper R F, Nisker J A, Graves G 1989 Rates and outcomes of pregnancies achieved in the first 4 years of an in-vitro fertilization program. Canadian Medical Association Journal 140: 167–172.

Zelinger B B, Grinvalsky H T, Fields C 1960 Simultaneous dermoid cyst of the tube and ectopic pregnancy. Obstetrics and Gynecology 15: 340–343.

Zolli A, Rocko J M 1982 Ectopic pregnancy months and years after hysterectomy. Archives of Surgery 117: 962–964.

35. Pathology of contraception and of hormonal therapy

C. Hilary Buckley

INTRODUCTION

A wide variety of progestational and oestrogenic compounds is used for therapeutic and contraceptive purposes in gynaecological practice, synthetic products often being preferred to their natural counterparts because of their potency and efficacy. The hormones may be given orally, vaginally, systemically, by means of depot injections or implants, topically or by skin patches. The therapeutic effects are, to a large extent, independent of their mode of administration.

A range of other drugs, such as goserelin, tamoxifen and tibolone, is also used therapeutically to suppress ovulatory function, to modulate oestrogen-induced activity and to act as hormone replacement respectively. In addition to their desired clinical effect these products too may induce changes in both the target organs and other tissues.

THE PATHOLOGY OF HORMONAL THERAPY

Oestrogens

The oestrogens used therapeutically are of three main types, the conjugated and esterified naturally occurring hormone, such as that found in mare's urine, the non-steroidal stereochemical mimics of oestrogen, such as diethylstilboestrol, and non-conjugated steroids derived from oestrogen, such as ethinyloestradiol and its 3-methyl ether mestranol.

Oestrogens may be given alone, but it is more usual and prudent to use a regimen combining them with a progestagen, particularly in those women retaining their uterus. They have a wide variety of therapeutic indications which, broadly, include replacement or supplement of an endogenous deficit or correction of an endogenous imbalance.

Effects on the endometrium

Oestrogens are responsible, in the normal proliferative phase, for the synchronous growth of the glands, stroma and vasculature of the endometrium and the induction of progesterone receptors. Following ovulation, they cause the oedema characteristic of the mid-secretory phase and promote the growth of the spiral arteries in the late secretory phase, following their differentiation by progesterone.

Withdrawal of oestrogen after prolonged use results in withdrawal bleeding, but this can be distinguished, in curettings, from menstruation by the absence of secretory glands. Bleeding may also occur spontaneously if small doses of oestrogen are given continuously.

If oestrogens are given to a patient early in the normal proliferative phase, endometrial growth is prolonged and the endometrium may exhibit features of a prolonged proliferative phase: ovulation is suppressed due to gonadotrophin inhibition and the secretory phase is delayed or absent (Dallenbach-Hellweg, 1981). If oestrogen is given to a patient already in the secretory phase, there may be severe stromal oedema, a delay in the secretory transformation of the glands and retarded maturation of the stroma (Egger & Kindermann, 1980).

More commonly, however, oestrogens are used in patients in whom there is a paucity of endogenous hormone and thus an absence of normal cyclical changes. The appearance of the endometrium in these women is due, therefore, entirely to the exogenous hormone. The morphological pattern most commonly encountered in the postmenopausal patient receiving small doses of oestrogen, or absorbing oestrogen from vaginal pessaries given to relieve dryness and soreness, is that of a weakly proliferative endometrium (Fig. 35.1). This is characterized by the presence of glands lined by single-layered or, occasionally, focally multilayered, epithelium containing only infrequent mitoses, and a densely cellular inactive stroma. There is little thickening of the endometrium and the functionalis is poorly defined. In some patients, the appearances, at least initially, may resemble those seen in the normal proliferative phase. Gradually, however, or sometimes *ab initio*, the picture becomes that of 'disordered proliferative endometrium' (Hendrickson & Kempson, 1980) (Fig. 35.2) or mild complex hyperplasia.

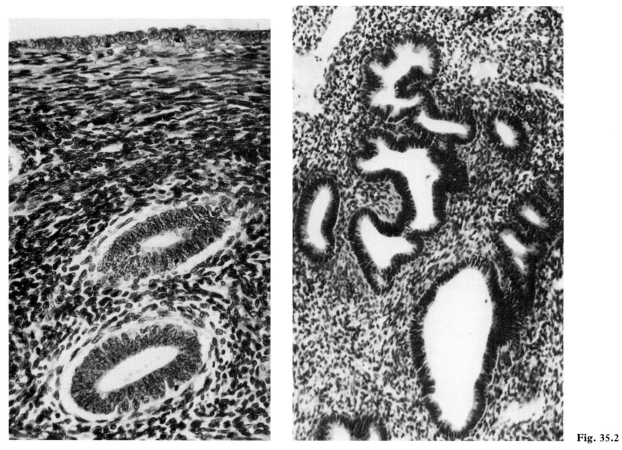

Fig. 35.1

Fig. 35.2

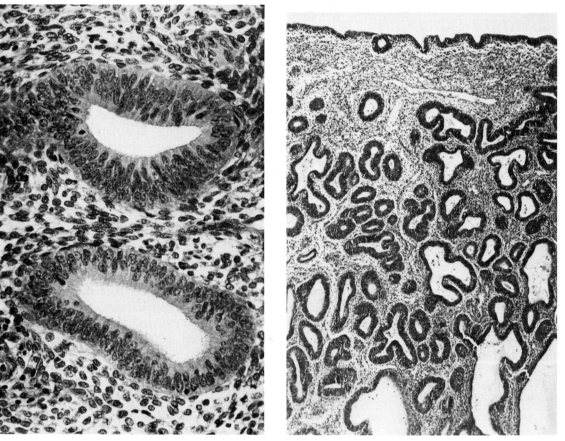

Fig. 35.3

Fig. 35.4

Fig. 35.1 The endometrium from a postmenopausal patient who has been using oestrogens. The glandular epithelium is multilayered but the stroma is compact. H & E × 450.

Fig. 35.2 The endometrium from a postmenopausal woman who had been given small cyclical doses of oestrogen. There is a minor degree of complex hyperplasia characterized by invaginations and outpouchings of the glands. The epithelium lining the glands is multilayered but there is no evidence of cytological atypia. H & E × 205.

Fig. 35.3 Simple endometrial hyperplasia. The glands are smooth contoured and their epithelium multilayered but there is no loss of nuclear polarity. H & E × 450.

Fig. 35.4 Complex endometrial hyperplasia. Variably sized, irregularly shaped glands lined by a multilayered epithelium lie closely packed; the intervening stroma is rather sparse. H & E × 75.

The endometrial stroma is abundant and of normal structure whilst the glands show varying degrees of architectural atypia and dilatation; there is no evidence of cytological atypia.

Squamous metaplasia has been reported in the endometrium of experimental animals given large doses of oestrogen (Baggish & Woodruff, 1967) and is not uncommonly seen in the endometrium of postmenopausal women receiving oestrogen-only hormone replacement therapy (Hendrickson & Kempson, 1980). Tubal (serous) metaplasia is also common under such circumstances and mucinous metaplasia is occasionally seen.

A significant proportion of women who are given continuous or cyclical unopposed oestrogen for menopausal symptoms (Schiff et al, 1982) or for primary hypo-oestrogenic amenorrhoea (Van Campenhout et al, 1980) develop a hyperplastic endometrium. Whilst this may have a simple pattern (Fig. 35.3), in some cases it may be complex (Fig. 35.4) or atypical (Fig. 35.5) (Whitehead et al, 1977; Fox & Buckley, 1982; Buckley & Fox, 1989). Hyperplasia may occur soon after therapy commences or be delayed for up to two years. The administration of progestagens alone or in combination with an oestrogen in sequential or continuous pattern has been observed to reverse hyperplasia (Whitehead et al, 1977) or protect against its development (Sturdee et al, 1978; Whitehead et al, 1981).

It is widely accepted that the use of unopposed oestrogens is an important aetiological factor in the development of endometrial carcinoma (Antunes et al, 1979; Brinton & Hoover, 1993) both in postmenopausal women and in younger women with dysgenetic gonads (McCarty et al, 1978). It makes no difference whether the oestrogen used is conjugated or unconjugated nor whether it is used continuously or cyclically (Shapiro et al, 1980) and this form of therapy is, therefore, seldom recommended. There is also some evidence that the risk of developing carcinoma persists after the cessation of therapy and that it may be related to the total dose of oestrogen given (Rosenwaks et al, 1979; Brinton & Hoover, 1993). The

tumours which arise following oestrogen therapy are generally lower staged, better differentiated and occur in younger women than do those occurring in non-hormone users (Robboy & Bradley, 1979; Elwood & Boyes, 1980) (Fig. 35.6). Histologically, they comprise a greater proportion of well-differentiated endometrioid adenocarcinomas with squamous metaplasia than do tumours from oestrogen non-users, whilst the proportion of prognostically unfavourable subtypes, such as adenosquamous carcinoma and clear cell carcinoma, occur less frequently (Silverberg et al, 1982). The use of a progestagen for at least ten days per month (Paterson et al, 1980) or, alternatively, the use of a combined oestrogen/progestagen preparation, in no way appears to affect adversely the therapeutic effect of the oestrogen but does appear to protect the patient from the risk of carcinoma.

A rare association between atypical polypoid adenomyoma of the uterus and oestrogen therapy has also been described (Clement & Young, 1987).

Effect on other tissues

The cervical smear of women using oestrogens characteristically has a superficial pattern whilst histologically the

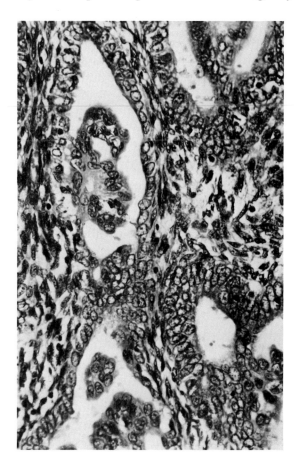

Fig. 35.5 Atypical endometrial hyperplasia in a woman receiving oestrogens. The glandular epithelium is irregularly invaginated and there is loss of nuclear polarity. H & E × 450.

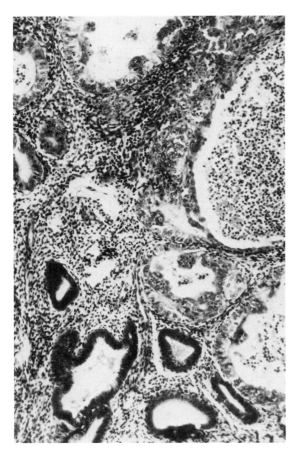

Fig. 35.6 Well-differentiated endometrioid endometrial adenocarcinoma in the right of the field arising in a patient with endometrial hyperplasia. H & E × 180.

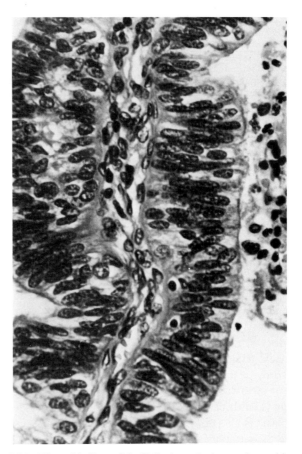

Fig. 35.7 The epithelium of the Fallopian tube in a patient subjected to prolonged high levels of oestrogenic stimulation from a granulosa cell tumour. The epithelium is multilayered and contains few secretory cells. H & E × 720.

squamous epithelium is mature, thickened and contains glycogen (Hammond & Maxson, 1982).

The epithelium of the Fallopian tube is hormone responsive (Fig. 35.7) and there may be general hyperplasia or multiple hyperplastic foci which may be remarkably localized (Fox & Buckley, 1983).

Hypercellular leiomyomas, which also grow rapidly, are encountered in some women receiving oestrogens (Dallenbach-Hellweg, 1980a).

Foci of endometriosis, being sensitive to oestrogenic stimulation, may undergo proliferative activity or become hyperplastic when oestrogen therapy is given.

The risk of breast carcinoma does not appear to be increased when unopposed oestrogen is used for hormone replacement (Kaufman et al, 1991).

Diethylstilboestrol.   Twenty per cent of the women exposed to diethylstilboestrol (DES) in utero exhibit a range of genital tract abnormalities rarely encountered in non-exposed women (Herbst et al, 1975). The features are also discussed in Chapter 36 and will be only summarized here.

Between 34% and 45% of such women have vaginal adenosis (Kurman & Scully, 1974; Hart et al, 1976;

Robboy et al, 1979; Ostergard, 1981). The condition affects 73% of the women who were exposed before the eighth week of gestation (Herbst et al, 1975), but after the twentieth week of intrauterine life the effect is much reduced (Robboy et al, 1979), although there is some evidence that the total dose of DES that the fetus receives may be significant (Robboy et al, 1982).

Vaginal adenosis is not limited to women exposed to DES; it also occurs in 4% of fetuses and neonates exposed in utero to progestagens and oestrogens other than DES (Johnson et al, 1979) and in women with no history of exposure to hormone therapy.

Cervical and vaginal deformities are also described (Herbst et al, 1972; O'Brien et al, 1979; Antonioli et al, 1980). In addition, hysterosalpingograms may demonstrate small T-shaped uterine cavities with dilatation of the interstitial and proximal isthmic portions of the Fallopian tubes (Kaufman et al, 1977; Haney et al, 1979; DeCherney et al, 1981). The tubes may also be foreshortened and convoluted and have 'withered' fimbria (DeCherney et al, 1981).

Functional uterine problems arise as a consequence of these structural anomalies. These women have an increased number of spontaneous abortions, ectopic pregnancies and premature deliveries and their children are more likely to die in the perinatal period than are children of normal women (Herbst, 1981a; Stillman, 1982).

Probably the most serious complication developing in the DES-exposed woman is clear cell carcinoma of the cervix or vagina (Herbst & Scully, 1970; Herbst et al, 1974; Herbst, 1981b). Fortunately, it occurs in only 0.014–0.14% of affected women (Herbst et al, 1977), a much lower incidence than was originally feared. Very few cases have occurred in the United Kingdom (Buckley et al, 1982). The pathology of these tumours is described in Chapter 36.

Cytological surveillance has accurately predicted the development of clear cell carcinoma in patients with DES-associated adenosis (Taft et al, 1974; Anderson et al, 1979; Kaufman et al, 1982; Ghosh & Cera, 1983). Cytological atypia, in the areas of adenosis, has been described and almost certainly represents a precursor of the carcinoma (Antonioli et al, 1979).

Fowler et al (1981) hold the view that there is an increased risk of squamous intraepithelial neoplasia in the large metaplastic transformation zone of women with cervical ectopy and adenosis but Herbst (1981b) and Robboy et al (1981) could find no evidence to support this and, indeed, intraepithelial neoplasia may be less frequent in DES-exposed individuals than in matched controls (Robboy et al, 1982).

Invasive neoplasms other than clear cell carcinoma appear to be very rare; as the cohort of DES-exposed women ages, however, the position may change. A single case of cervical adenosquamous carcinoma has been reported (Vandrie et al, 1983) but its occurrence may have been a coincidence.

Tamoxifen

Tamoxifen is a triphenylethylene non-steroidal synthetic oestrogen usually regarded as an anti-oestrogen. Its behaviour is, however, more typical of a partial agonist (MacNab et al, 1984), exhibiting oestrogen agonistic or antagonistic effects depending upon the relative concentrations of oestrogen and tamoxifen. In experimental conditions, the drug has an antagonistic effect when endogenous oestrogen levels are high and an agonistic effect when oestrogen levels are low. Its use, therefore, particularly in the premenopausal patient, usually results in a reduction in the effect of endogenous oestrogen and it is widely used, for this purpose, in the treatment of oestrogen receptor-rich breast carcinoma. The drug is considered separately here, however, as the extent of the oestrogenic effect of tamoxifen on hormone-responsive tissues is not yet fully established and the size of the problem, in patients receiving tamoxifen for the treatment of breast carcinoma, remains to be determined. An evaluation of the relative advantages and disadvantages of the therapy must also be completed.

In patients in whom the drug exerts an anti-oestrogenic effect, the endometrium is inactive, but in those in whom tamoxifen acts as an oestrogen agonist, the endometrial appearances are similar to those seen with other oestrogens. There is endometrial growth, proliferation and the induction of progesterone receptors; there may be hyperplasia (Buckley & Fox, 1989; Neven et al, 1989; Cross & Ismail, 1990), the development of carcinoma (Killackey et al, 1985; Hardell, 1988; Fornander et al, 1989) or carcinosarcoma (Altaras et al, 1993; Seoud et al, 1993), and, in certain circumstances, stimulation of the growth of endometrial carcinoma (Gottardis et al, 1988). Amongst the carcinomas there seems to be an unusually high incidence of clear cell tumours (Silva et al, 1994). Endometrial and endocervical polyps are also reported more often in tamoxifen users (Neven et al, 1989, 1990).

The oestrogenic effects of tamoxifen are not limited to the endometrium. Oestrogenization of the vaginal mucosa (Ferrazzi et al, 1977) and the induction of hyperplasia in endometriosis of the ovary in a postmenopausal woman (Buckley, 1990) have also been recorded.

Progestagens

The synthetic progestagens used therapeutically, which are preferred to their natural counterparts for their more sustained action when given orally, are derived either from 17α-hydroxy-progesterone or 19-nortestosterone. A variety of progestagens which have fewer undesirable side effects have been developed in recent years.

Progestagens may be given alone for the treatment of dysfunctional uterine bleeding, endometriosis or neoplasms and as contraceptives. They are, however, more commonly used in combination with oestrogens for contraception and as part of the programme of hormone replacement therapy at, or after, the menopause.

Effects on the endometrium

Progestagens will act only upon an endometrium in which progesterone receptors have been induced by prior exposure to oestrogen. They cause cellular differentiation and inhibit the effects of oestrogen. When they are given in the proliferative phase, ovarian follicular development is depressed, ovulation is postponed or prevented and endometrial growth ceases (Dallenbach-Hellweg, 1980b). Even if given only briefly, the cycle will be prolonged (Carter et al, 1964). Withdrawal of the hormone will produce bleeding in a few days and if it is given continuously irregular spontaneous breakthrough bleeding will occur.

The effect which high doses of progestagen have depends upon the extent to which the endometrium has been previously stimulated by endogenous or exogenous

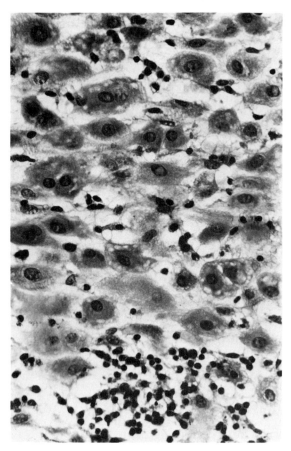

Fig. 35.8   The stroma of the functional layer of the endometrium in a patient given norethisterone. The individual cells have copious densely staining cytoplasm and are interspersed with granulated lymphocytes. H & E × 450.

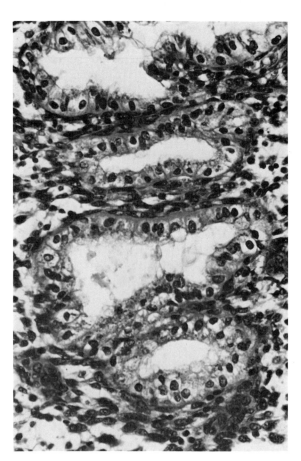

Fig. 35.9   An endometrial gland in a patient given norethisterone. This particular gland has a hypersecretory appearance. Elsewhere secretion was less well developed. H & E × 510.

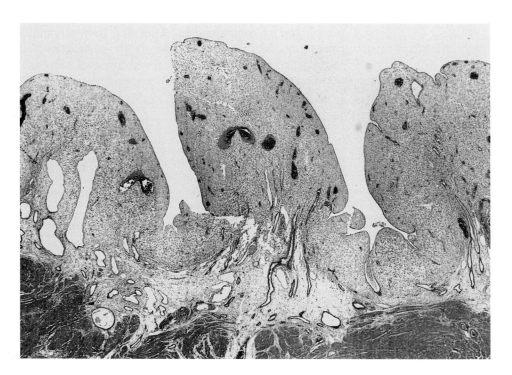

Fig. 35.10   Progestagen therapy: the polypoidal appearance which the endometrium assumes following treatment with norethisterone. The superficial part of the stroma is markedly pseudodecidualized and contains congested, thin-walled blood vessels: there is no spiral artery development. The glands are sparse and inactive. H & E × 18.5. (From Buckley & Fox, 1989. By courtesy of Chapman & Hall Ltd.)

oestrogen and upon the properties of the particular hormone.

If the hormone is given early in the proliferative phase, there is little stromal pseudodecidualization and there may be only minimal abortive glandular secretory change. Spiral artery differentiation does not occur. Similar doses of hormone given in the late secretory phase induce marked stromal pseudodecidualization (Fig. 35.8), a granulated lymphocytic (K-cell) infiltrate and transitory glandular secretory activity. As the glands are more sensitive to progestagens than is the stroma, however, they rapidly become refractory to stimulation and cease functioning (Dallenbach-Hellweg, 1980b), becoming small and inactive, though occasional glands may retain a secretory, or even hypersecretory appearance (Fig. 35.9). The picture of small, inactive glands set in a pseudodecidualized stroma with little or no spiral artery growth (Fig. 35.10) contrasts with the well-developed spiral arteries and glandular hypersecretion seen in both early intrauterine and ectopic pregnancy.

The prolonged use of progestagens produces an atrophic endometrium with sparse, uncoiled glands set in a shallow, compact, sometimes weakly pseudodecidualized stroma (Fig. 35.11). Although the glands are inactive their epithelium may remain columnar rather than becoming cuboidal. It is usual for the granulated lymphocytic infiltrate to persist, whilst thin-walled vascular channels are a conspicuous feature (Fig. 35.10). Spiral artery growth is absent. In some cases more marked atrophy may develop (Fig. 35.12). Atrophy of this type, which is due to the anti-oestrogenic effect of the progestagen, persists as long as the therapy continues but usually recovers rapidly after withdrawal of the exogenous hormone. An irreversible atrophy with stromal hyalinization has also been

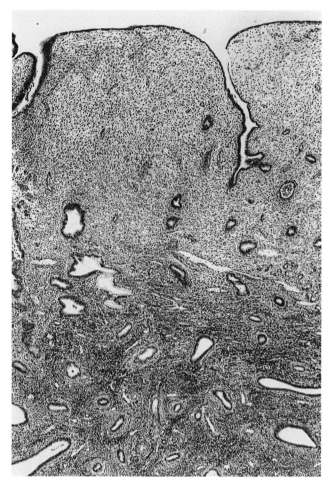

Fig. 35.11 Moderate endometrial atrophy, the result of prolonged progestagen therapy. The endometrial depth is reduced, there is weak stromal pseudodecidualization and the glands are uncoiled and inactive. H & E × 47. (From Buckley & Fox, 1989. By courtesy of Chapman & Hall Ltd.)

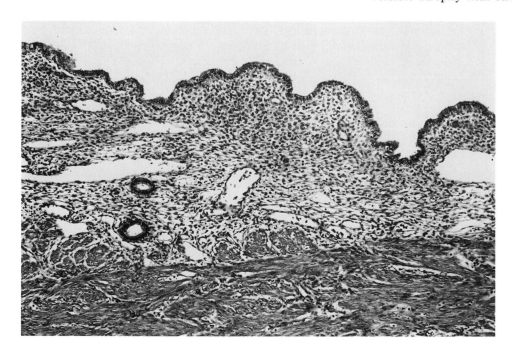

Fig. 35.12 Endometrial atrophy resulting from prolonged progestagen therapy. H & E × 93. (From Buckley & Fox, 1989. By courtesy of Chapman & Hall Ltd.)

described (Dallenbach-Hellweg, 1980b) but is rarely encountered in practice.

The appearances described above are seen most markedly in women receiving 19-nortestosterone-derived progestagens. In women using some of the modern progestagens and the weakly progestagenic, synthetic anti-gonadotrophic androgen danazol (Fig. 35.13), a moderately atrophic endometrium, lacking stromal decidualization and secretory activity, develops rapidly *ab initio*.

The appearance of the endometrium in patients given progestagens for the treatment of dysfunctional uterine bleeding is extremely varied and depends upon the nature of the underlying hormonal abnormality and the stage of the cycle at which therapy was commenced. Commonly, the appearances resemble those which have already been described. When the patient is anovulatory, however, secretory changes may be superimposed upon a hyperplastic endometrium (Fig. 35.14). This is indistinguishable from the appearance which is seen if such a patient ovulates. With continued therapy simple and mild complex hyperplasia may regress completely, but atypical hyperplasia may regress only partly, leaving islands of architecturally atypical glands set in an endometrium which is otherwise normal in appearance, pseudodecidualized or atrophic. The failure of an atypical hyperplasia to respond to progestagen therapy is usually regarded as an indication for surgical therapy.

Hormonally-responsive endometrial adenocarcinomas, which are usually well differentiated, may also show glandular secretory changes within 10–14 days of administering progestagens (Figs 35.15 and 35.16), and the stromal cells may resemble those of the late secretory phase, normal pregnancy, or those seen in the endometrium of other exogenous hormone users (Ferenczy, 1980). In addition, there is often focal cellular degeneration, growth of the tumour may be suppressed and the tumour may regress (Anderson, 1972; Rozsier & Underwood, 1974; Dallenbach-Hellweg, 1980b; Ferenczy, 1980).

There is evidence that progestagens protect against the development of endometrial carcinoma in women who receive oestrogen replacement therapy (see above). This is thought to be due to their interrupting endometrial growth by lowering the concentration of oestradiol receptors, promoting endometrial shedding and inducing the formation of endometrial 17β-dehydrogenase which converts oestradiol to the less potent oestrone (Judd, 1980).

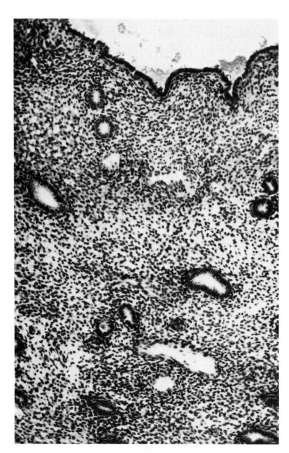

Fig. 35.13 Endometrium after the administration of danazol. The glands are small and there is neither secretory nor proliferative activity. The stroma is immature. H & E × 180.

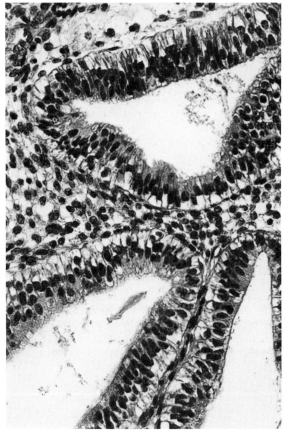

Fig. 35.14 Secretory changes, seen here as subnuclear vacuolation of the glandular epithelium, superimposed upon a simple endometrial hyperplasia by the administration of norethisterone. H & E × 450.

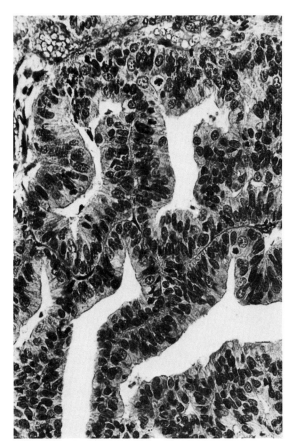

Fig. 35.15   An endometrial biopsy from a woman with a well-differentiated endometrioid adenocarcinoma of the corpus uteri. H & E × 450.

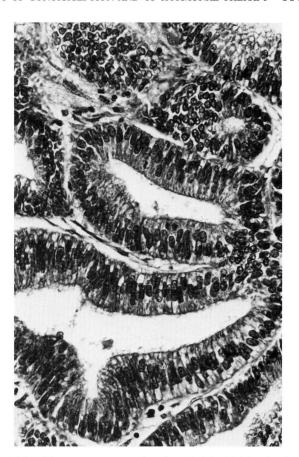

Fig. 35.16   The same tumour as that shown in Fig. 35.15 at the time of the hysterectomy when progestagens had been given for three weeks. Vacuolation of the epithelium is indicative of secretory change. H & E × 450.

Effects on the myometrium

Leiomyomas may enlarge and show mitotic activity, increased cellularity and cellular atypia (Prakash & Scully, 1964; Fechner, 1968) when large doses of progestagen are given continuously for a prolonged period, but there is no risk of malignant change. Occasionally, leiomyomas may undergo degeneration, such as that seen in pregnancy, or may shrink and become highly cellular.

Effects on the cervix

Distension of the cervical crypts by mucus and microglandular hyperplasia of the cervix are concomitants of progestagen therapy. Microglandular hyperplasia is described more fully below.

Effects on the ovary

With high doses of exogenous progestagen, just as in normal pregnancy, there may be multifocal decidualization of the subepithelial stroma of the ovary (Figs 35.17 and 35.18).

Effects on endometriosis

In the treatment of endometriosis, the inhibition of proliferation and induction of atrophy in the endometrium consequent to progestagen therapy is used to advantage. The progestagen acts both directly on the endometriotic foci and indirectly by suppression of ovulation. Initially, the stroma of the endometriotic foci may become pseudo-decidualized (Fig. 35.19) and increasingly vascular but, later, focal necrobiosis of the individual cells indicates the commencement of degeneration (Gunning & Moyer, 1967). Eventually, the foci may consist only of inactive glands set in an atrophic stroma and care should be taken to distinguish such foci histologically from endosalpingiosis.

Effects in other extragenital sites

A progestagenic effect may also be manifest as decidualized foci in subperitoneal stroma, in the great omentum and in pelvic lymph nodes.

Goserelin

Goserelin is a luteinizing hormone-releasing hormone

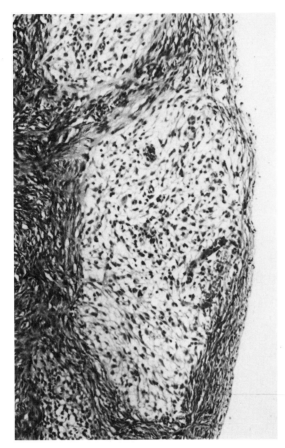

Fig. 35.17   The surface of the ovary in a patient given norethisterone. Many nodules of similar decidua-like tissue were present in both ovaries. H & E × 180.

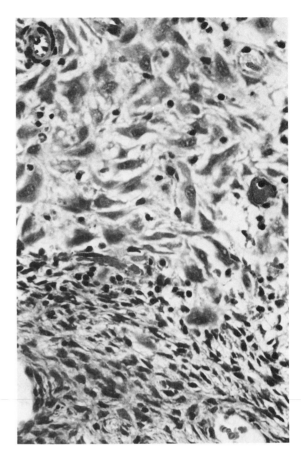

Fig. 35.18   A detail from an area similar to those seen in Fig. 35.17, showing the somewhat spindle-celled shape of the individually decidualized cells. H & E × 510.

(LHRH) agonist, the prolonged use of which has the effect of suppressing ovulatory function. It is used for this purpose prior to the induction of superovulation in women being treated by in vitro fertilization (IVF) or gamete intra-Fallopian transfer (GIFT). It is also used to treat menorrhagia and endometriosis. Its administration in women with uterine leiomyomas has the effect of causing leiomyomas to shrink and to assume a markedly cellular appearance.

THE PATHOLOGY OF HORMONE REPLACEMENT THERAPY

Hormone replacement therapy is used in young women who are hypogonadal, such as those with gonadal dysgenesis, and in postmenopausal women. It is also used, in a more precise way, to provide a suitable environment in which to replace donated pre-embryos in infertile women (Critchley et al, 1990).

It is generally considered unwise to use oestrogen alone as hormone replacement therapy when the uterus is in situ. Nonetheless, this sometimes occurs and the appearance of the endometrium varies according to the dose and duration of therapy (see above).

More commonly, oestrogen is given in combination with progestagen. This may be in a sequential pattern, with, for example, oestrogen alone being given for between 10 and 15 days, on average, and then a progestagen being added to the regimen for the next 5–10 days, followed by a hormone-free interval to allow bleeding. Alternatively, an oestrogen and progestagen may be given in combination every day. The combined hormone may be given continuously or may be interrupted to allow hormone withdrawal bleeding. These patterns of treatment eliminate the risk that iatrogenic endometrial carcinoma may be induced (Whitehead et al, 1981). This does not, however, mean that carcinoma cannot develop spontaneously in the endometrium of a woman taking hormone replacement therapy.

Effects on the endometrium

In women receiving a sequential pattern of hormonal therapy, the oestrogen in the first part of the cycle causes endometrial growth and, after the introduction of progestagen, there is a brief, poorly developed, delayed secretory phase which may not appear until shortly before hormone withdrawal bleeding. There is little or no stro-

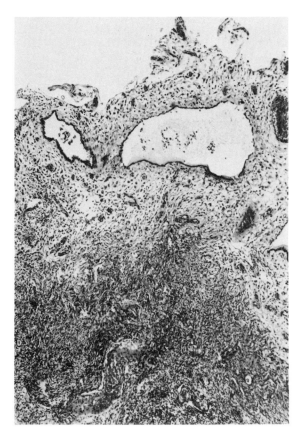

Fig. 35.19 An endometriotic focus from the ovary of a patient treated with norethisterone. The glands are dilated and there is neither secretory nor proliferative activity: the stroma is pseudodecidualized. H & E × 75.

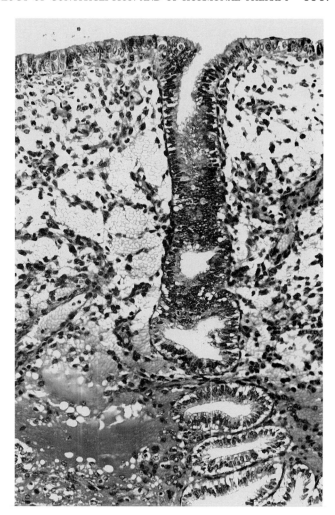

Fig. 35.20 Hormone replacement therapy, sequential pattern. The sample was taken on the 23rd day of an artificial 28-day cycle. The endometrium is well grown and there is subnuclear vacuolation of the glandular epithelium. Stromal oedema is marked and spiral artery differentiation has not yet occurred. H & E × 186. (From Buckley & Fox, 1989. By courtesy of Chapman & Hall Ltd.)

mal pseudodecidualization, though there may be marked stromal oedema, a reflection of the dominant oestrogenic activity (Fig. 35.20): granulated lymphocytes are sparse or absent. In some women, particularly those being prepared for pre-embryo transfer, an endometrial appearance approximating to the normal may be achieved (Fig. 35.21) (Critchley et al, 1990), although the induction of an endometrium of normal appearance is not a necessary prerequisite to successful pregnancy.

Prolonged, balanced hormone replacement therapy has, as far as is known, no adverse effect on the endometrium and endometrial atrophy does not occur.

Systemic effects

Hormone replacement therapy protects, to some extent, against osteoporosis and myocardial ischaemia (Knopp, 1990; La Vecchia, 1992) and it may suppress disease activity in rheumatoid arthritis.

Tibolone

Tibolone is a modern drug combining oestrogenic and progestagenic activity with weak androgenic activity. It is used for the treatment of the vasomotor symptoms of the menopause and is given continuously. We have not had the opportunity of examining large series of cases but its effect on the endometrium may vary. It may be predominantly oestrogenic and it is not uncommon to find proliferative activity in the endometrium in women using the drug. Alternatively, the endometrium may be moderately well grown with the development of a shallow functionalis in which there is weak, irregular secretory activity.

HORMONES IN THE TREATMENT OF INFERTILITY

Downregulation of the ovulatory cycle, by an LHRH agonist, is frequently used prior to the harvesting of ova in assisted reproduction, that is, in vitro fertilization (IVF) and gamete intra-Fallopian transfer (GIFT) (see above).

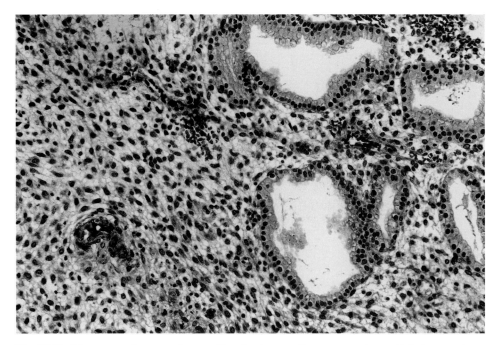

Fig. 35.21   Hormone replacement therapy. The glands are well grown, secretory activity is present, spiral artery differentiation has occurred and mild stromal pseudodecidualization has developed. H & E × 186. (From Buckley & Fox, 1989. By courtesy of Chapman & Hall Ltd.)

Ovulation is subsequently induced by the administration of human chorionic gonadotrophin (hCG). Studies of the endometrial changes following ovulation in such patients reveal glandular maturation which corresponds with that which would have been expected had ovulation occurred naturally, but there is premature differentiation of the spiral arteries (Seif et al, 1992).

THE PATHOLOGY OF CONTRACEPTION

Introduction

In any reasoned account of the pathology of contraceptive methods, the morbidity, mortality and minor pathological manifestations resulting from their use must be compared with the morbidity and mortality of the 80 pregnancies per 100 woman years, and their sequelae, which it is estimated would have occurred had contraception not been practised. Examined in these terms, the majority of modern contraceptives are not only highly effective, but are also extremely safe. Furthermore, in addition to their prime purpose, the prevention of unwanted pregnancy, a number of desirable 'side effects' result from the use of steroid contraceptives and these must be considered in any balanced view of the pros and cons of this form of contraception. Nonetheless, such lesions and complications that do develop, occur, for the most part, in a population of healthy women and an understanding and recognition of the more serious side effects is a prerequisite to the identification of the individuals at greatest risk.

The majority of simple contraceptives are virtually

devoid of risk although occasionally local irritation and eczematous lesions may accompany the use of spermicides, whilst cystitis may occur if, in addition, a diaphragm is used (Vessey et al, 1976). Problems most commonly occur with steroid contraceptives and intrauterine contraceptive devices (IUCDs) and whilst the undesirable effects of the IUCD usually remain local, widespread systemic disturbances may accompany steroid contraception.

Steroid contraception

Steroid contraceptives fall into two main groups, those in which an oestrogen and progestagen are given in combination and those composed entirely of a progestagen. The term 'pill' is often used colloquially to encompass all such preparations.

The majority of women follow a regimen in which a combination of between 20 and 50 µg of oestrogen, usually ethinyloestradiol, and a progestagen is given for 21 days out of 28 with seven hormone-free days which are either pill-free or on which a placebo is taken. The active preparation commences on the first day of the first cycle as it has been shown that by postponing the commencement to the 5th day, as was previously recommended, ovulation may not be inhibited in the first cycle. This is the biphasic pattern. Alternatively a phased formulation is given in which the proportions of hormone differ in different phases of the cycle. A small number of women also use combined, monthly injectable steroid contraceptives (Thomas et al, 1989).

The quantity of hormone in the early steroid contraceptives is now known to have been unnecessarily high, simply to inhibit ovulation. As a consequence, there were many undesirable systemic side effects such as thromboembolic disease (Vessey & Doll, 1969) and bizarre morphological abnormalities in the target organs. The present low dose steroid contraceptives, with a new generation of synthetic gestagens, produce fewer systemic side effects and the changes in the target organs are less dramatic. Patients included in the current follow-up series may, however, in their early days, have taken high doses of hormones and data collected from these women may not be applicable to patients who have used only the more modern low dose preparations.

Not only have the quantities of hormone in the preparations been altered in the light of experience, but so too have the patterns of administration. It was recognized some time ago, for example, that some of the sequential patterns of administration, in which relatively large doses of oestrogen alone were given from day 5 to day 15–20 of the cycle followed by a progestagen-oestrogen combination for the following 10 or 5 days, were associated with the development of endometrial carcinoma in some women.

The reporting of abnormalities identified in steroid contraceptive users has also followed trends, and anecdotal case reports have created the impression that certain problems may be more common than they in fact are. This is clearly seen in the clustering of reports concerning certain topics which is apparent in this review. It is important, therefore, that when we consider the pathology of contraception we allow sufficient time to permit placing of the problems in perspective.

Combined steroid contraceptives prevent ovulation by their negative feedback effect on pituitary gonadotrophin secretion, acting via the hypothalamus (Bye, 1982; Fay, 1982) to diminish FSH secretion and the mid-cycle LH surge (Mishell, 1976).

The progestagen-only 'mini-pill', which is taken every day, suppresses ovulation in only about 50% of cycles. It depends for its contraceptive effect not only upon the suppression of ovulation but also upon changes in the quality of cervical mucus which impedes sperm transport, upon modification of endometrial maturation rendering it unsuitable for nidation (Hawkins & Elder, 1979), and upon alterations in tubal motility and secretions. It is used by a smaller proportion of women, particularly those over the age of 35 years, heavy smokers and those in whom oestrogen induces severe side effects.

Combined steroid contraceptives have a very low failure rate, estimated as 0.2%, if they are taken regularly, though poor patient compliance reduces this considerably (Hillard, 1992).

Their efficacy may also be diminished, or even abolished, if they are taken simultaneously with a wide variety of commonly used drugs such as barbiturates, phenytoin, rifampicin, ampicillin and phenylbutazone, which accelerate their metabolism. Rifampicin also accelerates the metabolism of progestagen-only contraceptives.

Steroid contraceptives are sometimes accompanied by a number of undesirable local and systemic effects such as breakthrough bleeding, headache, nausea, hirsutes, acne, chloasma and increases in body weight (Berger & Talwar, 1978; Speroff, 1982; London, 1992; Rosenberg & Long, 1992). These are, however, less common with the modern generation of low dose preparations and the newer gestagens. Progestagen-only regimens are particularly associated with disturbances of the bleeding pattern (Chi, 1993) but are the treatment of choice for women who are breastfeeding.

Impairment of the glucose tolerance test was a fairly constant finding when older high dose oral contraceptives were in vogue but the introduction of the newer low dose pill and new gestagens have reduced this risk. These newer contraceptives are even regarded as suitable for women at high risk of developing diabetes mellitus, for example, those with a history of gestational diabetes and those having a first-degree relative with diabetes (Harvengt, 1992).

It has been reported that persistent trophoblastic disease is more common in women using contraceptive steroids than in those using other forms of contraception (Stone et al, 1976; Palmer, 1991).

Effects on the endometrium

The appearance of the endometrium depends upon the potency, quantity and proportion of the constituent hormones in the pill and their pattern of administration. The changes currently seen are far more subtle than those which related to high dose hormone preparations.

Combined steroid contraceptives. In the first few months of use, a discernible cyclical pattern can be recognized and with the newer low dose preparations this may persist for as long as the product is used. With the higher dose formulations the regenerative capacity of the endometrium may be diminished due to progestagen predominance and there is variable, though rarely profound, atrophy.

The morphological effects of combined steroid contraceptives, whilst being generally similar whatever the precise hormone combination and dosage, show sufficient variation for the relative importance of the oestrogen and progestagen in the combination to be recognized (Buckley & Fox, 1989). Following withdrawal bleeding (Fig. 35.22), at the end of each cycle, the endometrium proliferates. This phase is short because of the inhibiting effect of the progestagen on the oestrogen-stimulated growth, and the endometrium, therefore, remains shallow. The glands at this stage are narrow, tubular and lined by a single layer of cubo-columnar cells or, much less commonly, by

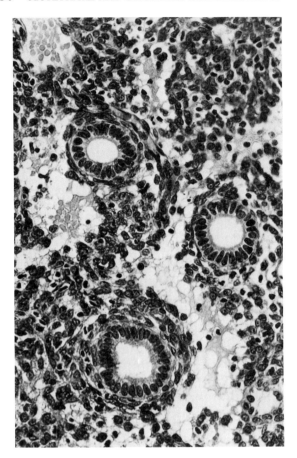

Fig. 35.22 Hormone withdrawal bleeding in a patient using a combined steroid contraceptive containing 50 μg ethinyloestradiol and 1 mg norethisterone acetate. The glands are small and inactive and there is no stromal decidualization — contrast with menstrual endometrium. H & E × 450.

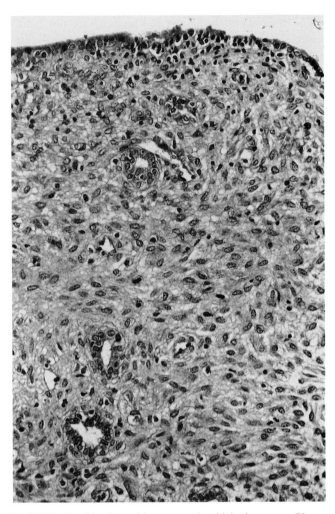

Fig. 35.23 Combined steroid contraceptive, bipbasic pattern, 50 mg ethinyloestradiol, 250 mg levonorgestrel, 26th day of the cycle. The glands are extremely narrow and inactive, the stroma is markedly pseudodecidualized, forming a compacta, and there is a granulated lymphocyte infiltrate. H & E × 232. (From Buckley & Fox, 1989. By courtesy of Chapman & Hall Ltd.)

pseudostratified epithelium. Scanty mitoses can be seen in both the stroma and epithelium. The stromal cells remain spindled and have the so-called 'bare-nucleus' appearance.

At about the eighth day of the cycle, the progestagen effect becomes apparent, with the appearance, in the glandular epithelium, of subnuclear vacuoles. However, because of the brief, inadequate oestrogenic priming in the early part of the cycle, progesterone receptors are few and glandular secretory changes are weak and poorly developed. By day 10, the subnuclear vacuoles move into the supranuclear cytoplasm and there is a brief, premature secretory phase lasting only until day 14 or 15. The glands remain narrow, or only minimally dilated, and straight or only gently convoluted. The apices of the cells remain, for the most part, intact and there is only a trace of secretion within the lumina. There may be a little stromal oedema. In the latter half of the cycle there is regression of the secretory changes and the endometrium becomes inactive. The degree of spiral artery differentiation and growth, the quality of the stromal pseudodecidualization and the extent of the glandular secretory transformation vary

according to the relative potency of the oestrogen and progestagen in the combination (Figs 35.23–26).

With high doses of progestagen and oestrogen there is stromal pseudodecidualization and the glands are narrow and inactive (Fig. 35.23). When the same dose of progestagen is combined with a lower dose of oestrogen there is no stromal decidualization, the glands are atrophic and the stroma is immature (Fig. 35.24). In other cases the stroma contains many thin-walled vascular channels (Fig. 35.25) and in yet other cases the endometrium may contain well-developed secretory glands and the stroma may contain differentiated spiral arteries (Fig. 35.26).

The effects of phased steroid contraceptives are very variable even in women using the same hormone preparation. Sometimes the appearances, in the later part of the cycle, are indistinguishable from those seen in the biphasic contraceptive users whilst in others the appearances

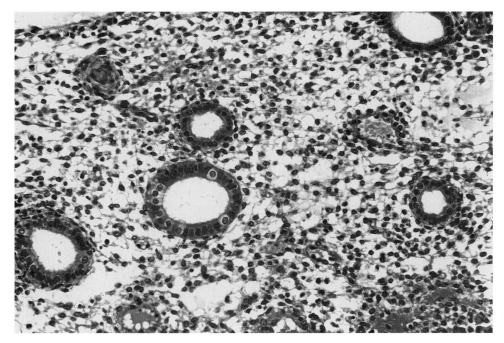

Fig. 35.24 Combined steroid contraceptive, biphasic pattern, 30 mg ethinyloestradiol, 250 mg levonorgestrel, three weeks since hormone withdrawal bleed. In comparison with Fig. 35.23, the glands are less atrophic and the stroma is immature; there is no decidualization. H & E × 232. (From Buckley & Fox, 1989. By courtesy of Chapman & Hall Ltd.)

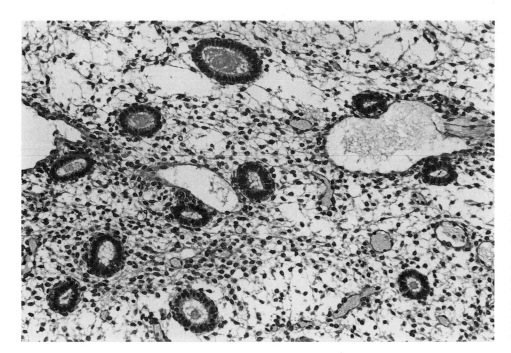

Fig. 35.25 Combined steroid contraceptive, biphasic pattern, 35 mg ethinyloestradiol, 1 mg norethisterone. The glands are small and inactive, the stroma is immature and there is no spiral artery differentiation; thin-walled vascular channels are present. The appearances are similar to those seen in Fig. 35.24. H & E × 186. (From Buckley & Fox, 1989. By courtesy of Chapman & Hall Ltd.)

are those of a weakly secretory endometrium (Figs 35.27 and 35.28) which persists to the time of hormone withdrawal bleeding. In those preparations with increased mid-cycle oestrogen, perhaps as a consequence of more adequate progesterone receptor induction, there is better growth and muscularization of the spiral arteries (Buckley & Fox, 1989). This correlates well with the clinical observation of a reduced incidence of mid-cycle breakthrough bleeding (Elder, 1982).

The alternating nodules of stromal hyperplasia and oedema described by Dallenbach-Hellweg (1981) are not,

in our experience, a feature of modern steroid contraceptives, nor are the bizarre stromal pseudosarcomatous changes described by Dockerty et al (1959). It is most important to note that profound irreversible endometrial atrophy (Fig. 35.29) resulting from prolonged high dose contraception no longer appears to occur.

In a proportion of women who have stopped taking steroid contraceptives in the previous month or so, there is a mild to moderate, non-specific chronic endometritis which is probably due to a low-grade infection (Buckley & Fox, 1989). Alterations in the quality of the cervical mu-

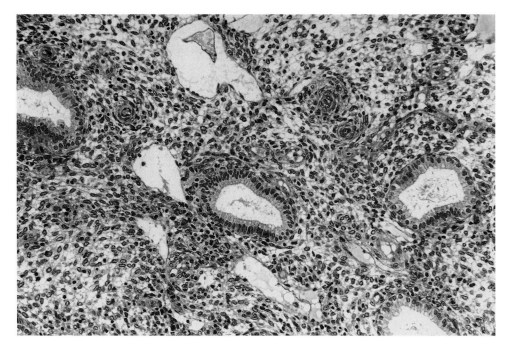

Fig. 35.26 Combined steroid contraceptive, biphasic pattern, 30 mg ethinyloestradiol, 150 mg levonorgestrel, three weeks since hormone withdrawal bleed. In contrast to the three preceding illustrations, the glands are moderately well grown, they exhibit secretory activity and spiral artery differentiation has occurred. A granulated lymphocyte infiltrate is present. H & E × 186. (From Buckley & Fox, 1989. By courtesy of Chapman & Hall Ltd.)

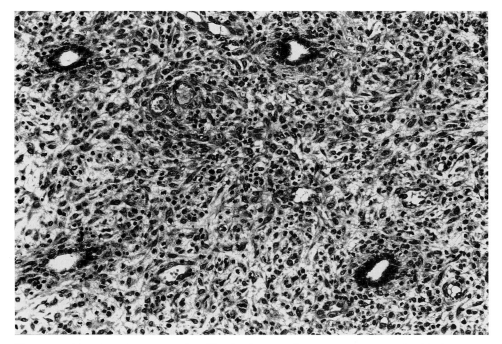

Fig. 35.27 Phased steroid contraceptive. The glands are small, narrow, tubular and devoid of secretion. The stroma is pseudodecidualized and infiltrated by granulated lymphocytes. The degree of glandular regression is similar to that seen in Fig. 35.23. H & E × 186. (From Buckley & Fox, 1989. By courtesy of Chapman & Hall Ltd.)

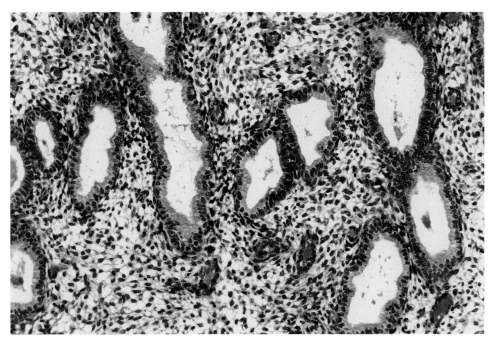

Fig. 35.28   Phased steroid contraceptive. This biopsy was from a patient receiving a hormone combination identical to that given to the woman whose biopsy appears in Fig. 35.27. In striking contrast, glandular growth and secretion are much better developed, there is a minor degree of spiral artery differentiation and granulated lymphocyte infiltration is absent. H & E × 186. (From Buckley & Fox, 1989. By courtesy of Chapman & Hall Ltd.)

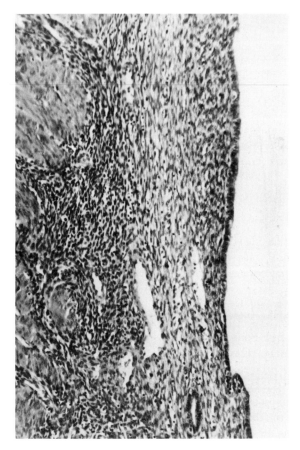

Fig. 35.29   Endometrial atrophy following the prolonged use of high dose steroid contraceptives. H & E × 180.

cus may render it less able to provide a satisfactory barrier to ascending infection and shedding of the endometrium may have been inadequate when the pill was used.

Early reports of an increased risk of endometrial adenocarcinoma in women using steroid contraceptives are now known to have been limited, almost entirely, to a particular 100 μg oestrogen pill (Cohen & Deppe, 1977; Blythe & Ali, 1979; Weiss & Sayvetz, 1980). More recent studies show that the current, low dose combined steroid contraceptives halve the risk of endometrial carcinoma (Huggins & Giuntoli, 1979; Kaufman et al, 1980; Hulka et al, 1982). In the WHO Collaborative Study (WHO, 1988a), ever-users of combined steroid contraceptives had a relative risk of developing endometrial carcinoma of 0.55, which represents a significant reduction in risk. Maximum protection is obtained by those who are nulliparous and have used the pill for more than one year. There is also, as might be expected, a negative correlation between the use of depot medroxyprogesterone acetate and the development of endometrial carcinoma (WHO, 1991a).

The beneficial effect of the use of steroid contraception persists after the menopause providing that the woman is not subsequently given sequential or unopposed oestrogen hormone replacement therapy.

Progestagen-only contraceptives.   The so-called 'mini-pill' or progestagen-only pill produces a much more variable picture in the endometrium than that which is seen in patients using combined regimens, the appearances resembling those seen in spontaneously occurring

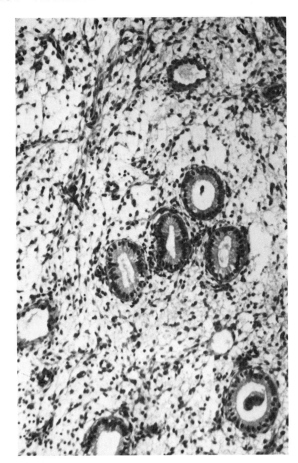

Fig. 35.30 Endometrium from a woman using a continuous progestagen contraceptive (0.35 mg norethisterone daily). The glands are small and there is variable secretory activity. Vascular and stromal development is poor. H & E × 205.

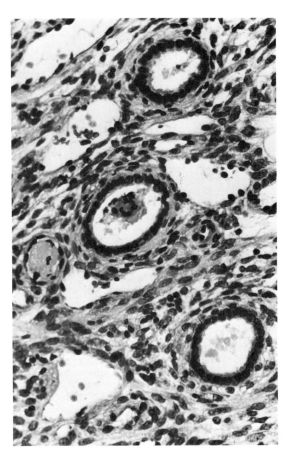

Fig. 35.31 Endometrium from a patient with a renal transplant, given 0.35 mg norethisterone daily as a contraceptive. Her clinical complaint of repeated, prolonged bleeding can possibly be explained on the basis of the numerous thin-walled blood vessels in the endometrial stroma. H & E × 450.

luteal phase defect (Fig. 35.30) following an inadequate follicular phase. The variability of the appearance depends on a number of factors. Firstly, ovulation is not consistently inhibited. Secondly, bleeding occurs somewhat erratically and is followed by a healing rather than a true proliferative phase, unless there is ovarian follicular activity, when a more adequate proliferative phase may be observed. Most commonly the endometrium is shallow, proliferative activity somewhat limited and occasional mitoses may be observed at almost any time, whilst mature glands or glands showing variable secretory activity coexist. Stromal decidualization is poorly developed because of the low oestrogen levels and the failure of progesterone receptor induction. Occasional granulated lymphocytes may be seen. In some women numerous thin-walled capillary-like stromal vascular channels are seen (Fig. 35.31) though spiral artery growth is absent or diminished (Hourihan et al, 1991). There are also larger numbers of blood vessels with endothelial gaps and haemostatic plugs than normal (Hourihan et al, 1991). Taken over a long period of time, the preparation leads to atrophy because of the absence of both endogenous and exogenous oestro-

gen. A marked degree of atrophy is often seen in patients who have been given depot progestagens for contraceptive purposes and this may take many months to recover (Dallenbach-Hellweg, 1980b).

Effects on the cervix

The older high dose combined hormone preparations were frequently associated with the development of cervical oedema, congestion and, in the majority of cases, a large ectopy. An ectopy is still common but generally less florid. Reserve cell hyperplasia is observed more frequently in the cervices of pill users (Schaude et al, 1980), probably a natural consequence of squamous metaplasia of the columnar epithelium of the ectopy.

The progestagen in the combined pill, or in the minipill, induces minor degrees of microglandular hyperplasia (Kyriakos et al, 1968), often detectable only microscopically, on the surface of the endocervical canal or on an ectopy. Less commonly, it forms a sessile or polypoidal mass in the endocervix (Govan et al, 1969; Tsukada et al, 1977), on an ectopy or in areas of vaginal adenosis

(Robboy & Welch, 1977). There is no evidence that microglandular hyperplasia is associated with, or is a precursor of, adenocarcinoma of the cervix (Jones & Silverberg, 1989).

Histologically it consists of closely packed glandular acini lined by flattened or cuboidal epithelium poor in mucin (Fig. 35.32). Foci of reserve cell hyperplasia, squamous metaplasia and an inflammatory cell infiltrate are often present. Usually the cells lining the acini are regular, and their nuclear chromatin uniformly dispersed. Sometimes, however, the lesion is particularly florid (Fig. 35.33) and the glandular component arranged in a reticulated or solid pattern (Taylor et al, 1967). In these cases the cells may have pleomorphic, hyperchromatic nuclei and the solid areas appear vacuolated due to cystic dilatation of the intercellular spaces: there can therefore be a resemblance to clear cell carcinoma (Fox & Buckley, 1983) whilst microglandular hyperplasia of this type may be mimicked by carcinoma (Young & Scully, 1992).

Arguments have been put forward linking the use of steroid contraceptives with the development of intraepithelial neoplasia of the cervix (Joswig-Priewe & Schlüster, 1980) and invasive carcinoma. Doubts have been ex-

pressed, however, as to whether this is a cause and effect relationship (Boyce et al, 1977) or might not be explained simply by taking sexual factors (Swan & Brown, 1981), the pattern of sexual activity, the time since the last cervical smear and the absence of a barrier contraceptive into consideration (Vessey, 1979). Further analyses, taking these confounding factors into consideration, have failed to provide incontrovertible evidence concerning the relationship of intraepithelial neoplasia and the use of steroid contraceptives (Ebeling et al, 1987; Cuzick et al, 1990; Coker et al, 1992; Delgado-Rodriguez et al, 1992; Gram et al, 1992).

The positive relationship between steroid contraceptive use and the development of invasive cervical carcinoma does, however, become statistically significant when steroid contraceptives have been used for more than seven years and use commenced under the age of 24 years, the relative risks being 1.8 and 3.0 respectively (Ebeling et al, 1987). The WHO Collaborative Study (WHO, 1985a) found similar results with ever-users having a relative risk of developing cervical carcinoma of 1.19 compared with non-users, the relative risk rising to 1.53 after five years of use. The Royal College of General Practitioners' Study

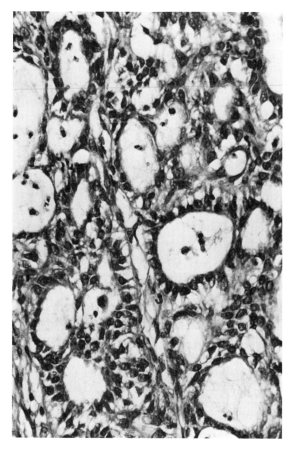

Fig. 35.32 Microglandular hyperplasia of the cervix in a combined steroid contraceptive user. H & E × 450.

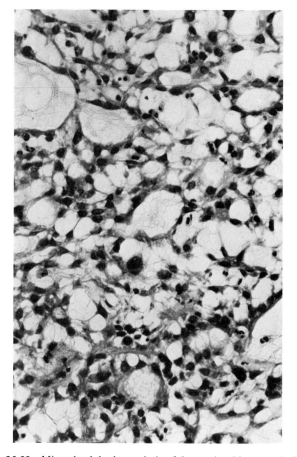

Fig. 35.33 Microglandular hyperplasia of the cervix with an atypical reticulated pattern. H & E × 510.

(Hannaford, 1991) also reports a possible increased risk of cervical carcinoma in women using steroid contraceptives. The risk of developing carcinoma does not appear to apply to women who have used depot medroxy-progesterone acetate (WHO, 1992). A suggestion that the risk of developing adenocarcinoma may be even greater than that of developing squamous carcinoma (relative risk 2.2 compared with 1.1) has been made (Brinton et al, 1990) although this has been refuted by others (Honoré et al, 1991). A possible association with, in particular, well-differentiated villoglandular adenocarcinoma, has been described (Jones et al, 1993).

The Oxford Study (Vessey et al, 1989a) examined the risk that pill users have of dying from cervical carcinoma and found a relative risk of 4.9 for those who had used the pill for more than eight years. The numbers in this latter study are, however, small and, because the study commenced in the 1960s, include women who took the early high dose contraceptives. The risk may not, therefore, be so high for users of modern, low dose formulations.

These reports suggest that there may well be a causal relationship between the use of steroid contraceptives and the development of invasive cervical carcinoma and that the effect of steroid contraceptives on the risk of developing cervical carcinoma is not limited simply to the absence of a mechanical barrier. The relationship of intraepithelial neoplasia and the use of steroid contraceptives, however, remains less clear.

Effects on the vagina

In women who have used a combined contraceptive with a low oestrogen content or a relatively potent progestagen, the vaginal epithelium may be atrophic (Joswig-Priewe & Schlüster, 1980) and this may be of sufficient severity to produce symptoms.

There is also some evidence that women using steroid contraceptives have almost twice the risk of developing chlamydial infection (Cottingham & Hunter, 1992) but are at decreased risk of developing bacterial vaginosis and trichomonal infection compared with users of other forms of contraception (Roy, 1991).

Effects on the ovary

Steroid contraceptives do not inhibit ovulation in every cycle (Hawkins & Elder, 1979) nor do they alter the process of normal follicular atresia. Indeed, tertiary follicles, varying greatly in size and development, can be found even after many years of combined steroid contraceptive use (Mestwerdt & Kranzfelder, 1980), although with prolonged use there is usually a reduction in the number of developing follicles and the cortex may become narrowed and fibrosed (Mishell, 1976). A feature not usually observed in the normal ovary is a thickening of the basement membrane of primary follicles which may be seen on lightmicroscopy (Mestwerdt & Kranzfelder, 1980).

The Boston Collaborative Drug Surveillance Program (Ory, 1974) revealed a reduction in the number of functional ovarian cysts, presumably a reflection of the general diminution in follicular activity. More recent studies on the effects of the modern lower dose preparations, however, suggest that these do not substantially reduce the risk of a woman's developing functional ovarian cysts (Holt et al, 1992).

Studies have shown a reduced incidence of malignant epithelial tumours of the ovary in steroid contraceptive users (McGowan et al, 1979; Weiss et al, 1981; Cramer et al, 1982; Rosenberg et al, 1982; WHO, 1988b). Protection appears to increase with duration of use, starting after three years (Weiss et al, 1981; Cramer et al, 1982; Rosenberg et al, 1982) and persisting for at least 10 years after cessation of use (Rosenberg et al, 1982). The greatest reduction is variously quoted as occurring in women between the ages of 35 years and 55 years (Weiss et al, 1981) and between 40 and 59 years (Cramer et al, 1982). This advantageous effect can still be demonstrated even when allowances are made for age and parity. An explanation of these findings has been provided by observations that ovarian carcinoma occurs most frequently in those women who ovulate incessantly (Casagrande et al, 1979), the implication being either that the surface epithelium, which is in a constant state of repair, is particularly susceptible to carcinogens, a finding corresponding with the finding of a reduced number of epithelial tumours in parous patients (Newhouse et al, 1977; McGowan et al, 1979), or that there is more chance of surface epithelial cysts forming from which carcinomas may develop (Fathalla, 1972). A retrospective, case-control study of the occurrence of benign epithelial tumours in the ovary in steroid contraceptive users, however, found that there was no reduction in their incidence, a finding that tends to refute the view that benign epithelial tumours are the precursors of carcinomas (Fox, personal communication — data from Manchester Ovarian Tumour Registry).

The relative risk of an ever-user of steroid contraceptives developing carcinoma of the ovary is 0.75 (WHO, 1988b) after allowing for the confounding effect of pregnancy. The reduction of risk is most marked in nulliparous women and is reduced for all epithelial types except mucinous. This last observation may, perhaps, be explained by the fact that some mucinous tumours are of germ cell origin and the aetiological factors may differ from those which are of surface epithelial origin.

There is also, as would be expected, a reduced risk of steroid contraceptive users dying of ovarian carcinoma. The Oxford Study found that the relative risk was only 0.4 compared with never-users of steroid contraceptives (Vessey et al, 1989a).

An as yet unexplained finding has been that of Cramer

et al (1982), who observed that pill users under the age of 40 years had an increased risk of developing epithelial tumours of borderline malignancy.

Effects on the breast

It is generally accepted that steroid contraceptives are associated with a decreased risk of benign breast disease (Ory et al, 1976; LiVolsi et al, 1978; Huggins & Giuntoli, 1979; Brinton et al, 1981; Huggins & Zucker, 1987; Vessey, 1989) and that the overall risk of a woman developing breast carcinoma is not increased by the use of combined or progestagen-only steroid contraceptives (Royal College of General Practitioners' Study, 1981a; Olsson, 1989; Paul et al, 1989; Romieu et al, 1989; Stanford et al, 1989; UK National Case-Control Study Group, 1989; WHO, 1991b). More specifically, there is no increased risk for the woman over the age of 40 years (Vessey et al, 1989b; Harlap, 1991) or for those taking contraceptives around the time of the menopause (Romieu et al, 1990; Thomas & Noonan, 1991).

Many studies, however, report an increased risk of breast carcinoma in younger women (Chilvers & Deacon, 1990; Rosenberg et al, 1992; Wingo et al, 1993). The increased risk is variably reported as affecting those who have used steroid contraceptives for a long time (Miller et al, 1989a; UK National Case-Control Study Group, 1989), those who started the pill at an early age (Johnson, 1989; Olsson et al, 1989), those who are nulliparous (Meirik et al, 1989; Rushton & Jones, 1992) and those who used the pill before the first pregnancy (Lund et al, 1989). A similar, but not statistically significant trend was reported by the WHO (WHO, 1990), in which study 2116 cases of newly diagnosed carcinoma of the breast were compared with 12 077 controls. Ever-users of combined steroid contraceptives were found to have a relative risk of 1.15 of developing carcinoma. Women under the age of 35 years had a relative risk of 1.26 and those over 35 years had a relative risk of 1.12 but neither of these figures reached statistical significance. The highest risk was in recent and current users and declined with time since last use, regardless of the duration of use. The risk was not found to increase with use of the pill before the age of 25 years or before the first pregnancy but there was a borderline statistically significant relative risk of 1.5 in women who had used the pill for more than two years before the age of 25 years.

Carcinoma developing at any time before the menopause is linked, in some studies, to the use of steroid contraceptives (Olsson et al, 1991; Ursin et al, 1992).

An explanation of the apparently contradictory evidence that cases of breast carcinoma may be increased in younger women whilst the total number of cases has not increased is provided by the evidence from the UK National Case-Control Study Group (1989). This found that there was marginally significant evidence that oral contraceptives with less than 50 µg of oestrogen had a lower risk of causing carcinoma and that progestagen-only contraceptives may even be protective. A second possible explanation is that the pill may accelerate the presentation of carcinoma rather than cause it because fewer cases are found as the cohort ages (Schlesselman, 1990).

The relative risk of dying from breast carcinoma in steroid contraceptive users is 0.9 (Vessey et al, 1989a). The histological type of carcinoma is not affected by the use of oral contraceptives (Miller et al, 1989b).

Effects on the liver

A variety of functional and morphological changes have been described in the livers of hormone contraceptive users. Transient small rises in serum bilirubin (Orellana-Alcade & Dominguez, 1966) and transaminases are recorded in the first few cycles of usage. Women who have a pre-existing hepatic disorder, such as Dubin–Johnson or Rotor syndrome, or who have had idiopathic jaundice of pregnancy may become jaundiced on the pill and should not use this form of contraception. The histological features are of a bland hepatocellular and canalicular cholestasis with no evident liver cell necrosis or inflammation (Fig. 35.34). Steroid contraceptives are also contraindicated in patients with acute or severe chronic hepatocellular disease because occasionally severe cholestatic jaundice may develop in these patients also. Generally, cholestasis resolves when the hormone is stopped but occasionally the condition may persist (Weden et al, 1992).

Sinusoidal dilatation occurring in periportal areas (Figs 35.35 and 35.36) and producing hepatomegaly which recedes after withdrawal of the steroids, has been reported with both contraceptive steroids and also with androgenic steroids (Winkler & Poulsen, 1975; Spellberg et al, 1979). The liver function tests show only minor changes and electronmicroscopic studies show dilatation of the endoplasmic reticulum in the liver cells (Spellberg et al, 1979). Peliosis, an extreme form of vascular dilatation with the formation of large blood-filled cysts or lacunae, may also develop in these patients; sinusoidal dilatation is often present elsewhere in the liver (Wight, 1982). Peliosis also occurs within and around steroid contraceptive-induced hepatic neoplasms (Taxy, 1978; Williams & Neuberger, 1981) and is believed to be due to a direct effect of the steroids (Editorial, 1973).

Rarely, Budd–Chiari syndrome has been described after prolonged use of contraceptive steroids with a latent period of about 20 months (Wu et al, 1977). It may be due to obliteration of the central and sublobular hepatic veins by a process of intimal cell proliferation and fibrosis (Alpert, 1976) or hepatic vein thrombosis which appears to develop over a period of time and may or may not extend into the inferior vena cava (Ecker et al, 1966;

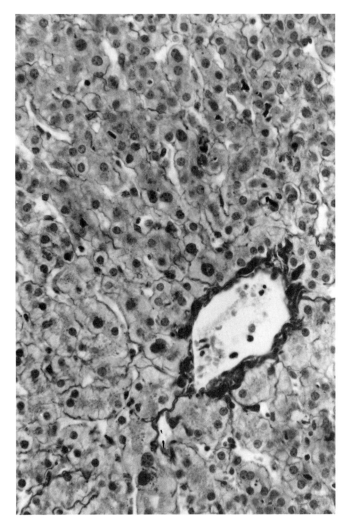

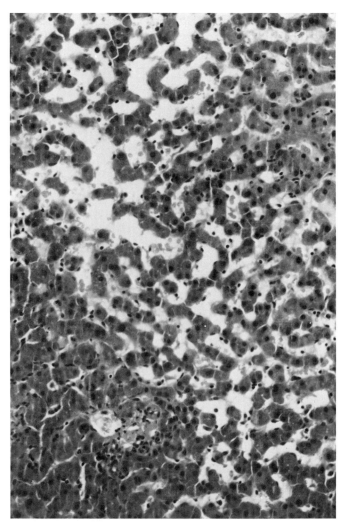

Fig. 35.34 Intrahepatic cholestasis in a steroid contraceptive user: canalicular bile retention is present but no liver cell swelling and no inflammatory reaction. Van Gieson × 220. (Courtesy of Professor R. N. M. MacSween.)

Fig. 35.35 Contraceptive steroid-induced hepatic sinusoidal dilatation: this is periportal in distribution and of a mild degree — compare with Fig. 35.36. H & E × 136. (Courtesy of Professor R. N. M. MacSween.)

Sterup & Mosbech, 1967; Irey et al, 1970; Hoyumpa et al, 1971; Barnet & Joffe, 1991). In many cases the condition has been fatal but recovery may occur after stopping the steroids (Hoyumpa et al, 1971). It is difficult to place this information in context as it appears likely that the problem was another aspect of the high oestrogen content of the earlier pills although occasional cases are still reported, perhaps in women in whom there is already some defect of the clotting mechanism.

Earlier reports that the development of hepatic adenoma was causally related to the use of steroid contraceptives have, to some extent, been substantiated (Horvath et al, 1972; Baum et al, 1973; Contostavlos, 1973; Edmondson et al, 1976; Fechner, 1977; Klatskin, 1977; Christopherson & Mays, 1979; Rooks et al, 1979; Kerlin et al, 1983). Reports of an association continue to appear in the literature (Tao, 1992) and case-control studies provide evidence that the risk is greatest in, but not limited to, those

who have used steroid contraceptives for a long time (Rosenberg, 1991; Shortell & Schwartz, 1991). There have also been reports that adenomas in which there is dysplasia may be the precursors of hepatocellular carcinoma in some steroid contraceptive users (Tao, 1991).

Hepatocellular carcinoma (Christopherson & Mays, 1979; Ishak, 1979; Neuberger et al, 1980), hepatoblastoma (Klatskin, 1977), rhabdomyosarcoma (Coté & Urmacher, 1990) and cholangiocarcinoma (Klatskin, 1977; Ellis et al, 1978) have been reported in steroid contraceptive users. There has been considerable debate as to whether there is a causal relationship or not, and opinions differ. A positive association between oral contraceptive use and hepatocellular carcinoma (Palmer et al, 1989; Prentice, 1991; Rosenberg, 1991; Hsing et al, 1992; Tavani et al, 1993) is reported in countries where hepatocellular carcinoma is uncommon. Steroid contraceptive ever-users are reported to have a relative risk of develop-

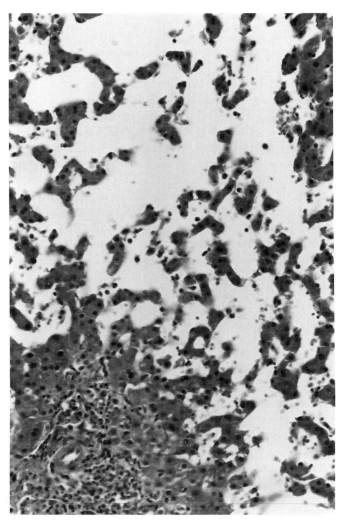

Fig. 35.36 Contraceptive steroid-induced hepatic sinusoidal dilatation: there is more marked atrophy and disruption of the liver cell plates than in Fig. 35.35. H & E × 136. (Courtesy of Professor R. N. M. MacSween.)

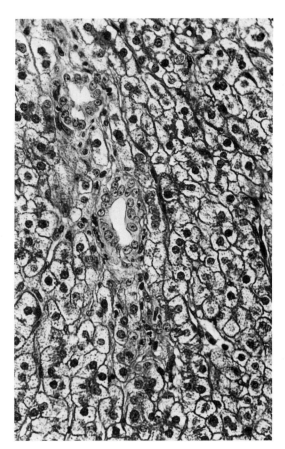

Fig. 35.37 Focal nodular hyperplasia of the liver showing hepatocytes and bile ducts of normal form. Masson trichrome × 450.

ing hepatocellular carcinoma of 1.6 compared with never-users and, for those who had used steroid contraceptives for more than 10 years, the odds ratio was 2.0 (Hsing et al, 1992). The WHO Collaborative Study of Neoplasia and Steroid Contraceptives (WHO, 1989a), on the other hand, based upon the examination of 122 newly reported cases of hepatocellular carcinoma and 802 controls from countries in which hepatitis B is endemic, found no evidence that short-term use of combined steroid contraceptives increases the risk of either hepatocellular carcinoma or cholangiocarcinoma: the relative risk in ever-users was 0.71. In addition, depot medroxyprogesterone acetate, when used as a contraceptive in a population in which hepatitis B is endemic (WHO, 1991c), did not increase the risk of hepatoma or cholangiocarcinoma.

Focal nodular hyperplasia of the liver occurs in the absence of steroid contraceptive use (Ishak & Rabin, 1975; Kerlin et al, 1983; Shortell & Schwartz, 1991) but case reports indicate that following the use of steroid contra-

ceptives, and in pregnancy, focal nodular hyperplasia and, more commonly, hepatic adenoma may enlarge, undergo necrosis and rupture (Mays et al, 1974; Knowles & Wolff, 1976; Kent et al, 1977; Kinch & Lough, 1978; Buckley & Lewis, 1982; Leborgne et al, 1990). The mortality associated with rupture of such hepatic lesions is around 5–10% (Brady & Coit, 1990). The behaviour of focal nodular hyperplasia in pregnancy is considered in Chapter 57.

Focal nodular hyperplasia forms a well-circumscribed, often lobulated mass of morphologically normal hepatocytes. A fibrous core may be present from which bands radiate between the lobules; bile ducts and thick-walled arteries within fibrous septa (Fig. 35.37) help to distinguish the lesion from an adenoma (Knowles & Wolff, 1976). An adenoma is a completely or partially encapsulated cellular mass of hepatocytes showing only minimal cellular atypia and lacking a normal lobular architecture and bile ducts (Fig. 35.38). These lesions may be multiple (Mdel et al, 1975). Hepatocellular carcinoma occurring in pill takers is similar to that seen under other conditions.

Steroid contraceptives are not a significant aetiological factor in the development of gallstones (Kay, 1984; van Beek et al, 1991; La Vecchia et al, 1992). There is no evidence that steroid contraceptives affect the risk of indi-

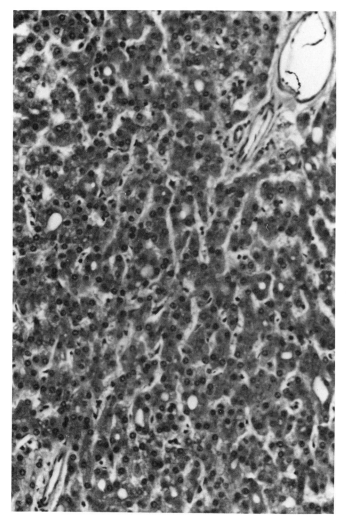

Fig. 35.38 A liver cell adenoma in a steroid contraceptive user. The tumour cells resemble normal hepatocytes but with irregular plate formation and some acinar development. There are no portal tracts: two thin-walled vessels are seen. H & E × 104. (Courtesy of Professor R. N. M. MacSween.)

viduals developing carcinoma of the gallbladder (WHO, 1989b).

Effects on the cardiovascular system

The oestrogen in combined steroid contraceptives is responsible for a dose-related increase in serum levels of fibrinogen (Ernst, 1992), factors VIIc and XIIc (Kelleher, 1990), triglycerides and HDL-cholesterol (HDL-C) and a decrease in LDL-cholesterol (LDL-C). The progestagen is associated with a decrease in HDL-cholesterol and an increase in LDL-cholesterol (Mishell, 1992). Modifications in the hormone content of the pill and the production of new progestagens have, however, diminished these changes (Janaud et al, 1992). The formulation of the oral contraceptive, the relative potency of the progestagen and the oestrogen/progestagen balance, nonetheless, continue

to have an impact on cardiovascular disease (Godsland et al, 1991).

The majority of early studies found that combined steroid contraceptive users had an increased risk of death from a variety of cardiovascular diseases when compared with non-users (Inman et al, 1970; Collaborative Group for the Study of Stroke, 1973; Royal College of General Practitioners, 1981b; Vessey et al, 1981a; Wingrave, 1982). The early report from the Royal College of General Practitioners' Study (Beral, 1977), however, suggesting that death rate from circulatory disease increased with duration of pill use, was later shown to have been fallacious (Royal College of General Practitioners, 1981b).

Deaths due to coronary artery disease (Inman et al, 1970) were found to occur more frequently in current contraceptive users (Royal College of General Practitioners, 1981b, 1983) (relative risk 4.2) and were related to the dose of oestrogen in the combination (Meade et al, 1980).

In 1981, the relative risk of a pill user dying from myocardial infarction was 4.2 (Royal College of General Practitioners, 1981b) but by 1991 it had fallen to between 1.5 (Vessey et al, 1989a) and 1.9 (Thorogood et al, 1991) for current and past users of oral contraceptives, and previous use of steroid contraceptives carried no increased risk of myocardial infarction (Stampfer et al, 1990). This was almost certainly a reflection of the reduction in the oestrogen content of the pill because in those women who continued to use preparations with 50 µg of oestrogen the relative risk remained at 4.2 (Thorogood et al, 1991). In heavy smokers the relative risk of dying from a myocardial infarct, in the Royal College of General Practitioners' Study, remained very high (relative risk 20.8) if they continued to use the pill (Croft & Hannaford, 1989). Progestagen-only contraceptives are, therefore, now recommended for women over the age of 35 years who continue to smoke.

The mechanism by which the combined steroid contraceptives affect the incidence of ischaemic heart disease is believed to be related to the effect of the progestagen component in lowering HDL-C (Kremer et al, 1980) a reduction in which, it is generally accepted, is associated with an increased incidence of arterial disease, especially ischaemic heart disease (Miller et al, 1977; Yaari et al, 1981; Kay, 1982). The newer progestagens used in many of the current combined steroid contraceptives have, however, much less effect on the HDL-C (Janaud et al, 1992) and it might be expected, therefore, that the incidence of ischaemic heart disease might fall even further in women who have used only these newer preparations.

Cerebrovascular disease. The Royal College of General Practitioners' Study (1981b) found a statistically significant risk of subarachnoid haemorrhage in women using the pill. Vessey et al (1981a), reporting data from the Oxford Study, found only a slight increase which was not of statistical significance and was confined to women with systemic hypertension. The most recent report from the Oxford Study, however, confirms that there is a slightly increased risk of subarachnoid haemorrhage (Thorogood et al, 1992) in women using steroid contraceptives.

The 1983 report of the Royal College of General Practitioners' Study (Royal College of General Practitioners' Study, 1983) described a significantly increased risk of cerebrovascular disease in both current users and former steroid contraceptive users, particularly for cerebral thrombosis and transient ischaemic attacks. The risk remained elevated for more than six years after stopping the pill and may have been related to the duration of oral contraceptive use. More recent analysis of the Oxford data (Thorogood et al, 1992) confirms that there is a substantial risk of veno-occlusive stroke.

Thromboembolic disease. In 1978, the Royal College of General Practitioners' Study (1978) reported an increased risk of both superficial and deep vein thrombosis in pill users, but whilst thrombosis in the superficial veins was related to both the oestrogen and progestagen content of the pill and occurred more frequently in patients with varicose veins, the incidence of deep vein thrombosis was unrelated to these factors. High doses of oestrogen had already been linked to thromboembolic disease (Vessey & Doll, 1969), possibly due to their effect on vascular endothelium, a reduction in the rate of venous blood flow and increased coagulability of the blood (Stadel, 1981). A decrease in the oestrogen content of the pill was associated with a reduction in the number of general thromboembolic episodes (Böttiger et al, 1980) but combined oral contraceptive users are still at risk of developing venous thromboembolic disease (WHO, 1989c; Katerndahl et al, 1992) and cerebral thrombosis (Thorogood et al, 1992).

Protein C normally inhibits coagulation and promotes fibrinolysis. Attention has been drawn to the increased risk of thrombosis which may be present in women who use steroid contraceptives and who have a congenital deficiency of protein C (Trauscht van Horn et al, 1992).

In 1970, Irey et al reported 20 deaths which had occurred during the years 1966–1968 and in which proliferative endothelial lesions with intravascular thrombosis in both arteries and veins were present. In some cases the pulmonary vasculature was affected and in others the hepatic veins: other authors described mesenteric vascular occlusion (Nothmann et al, 1973). The severity of the lesions was almost certainly a reflection of the high dose hormone therapy used at that time and is no longer encountered.

Hypertension. The 1974 report of the Royal College of General Practitioners' Oral Contraceptive Study noted a small reversible elevation in the systemic blood pressure of oral contraceptive users. This amounted to between 3.6 and 5.0 mm of mercury in systolic pressure and between 1.9 and 2.7 mm of mercury in diastolic pressure (WHO, 1989d; Leaf et al, 1991). This may be due to an increase in renin substrate through increased generation of either angiotensin (Laragh, 1976) or an unusually potent renin substrate (Eggena et al, 1978). The report further suggests that hypertensive changes might be related to the potency of the progestagen (Royal College of General Practitioners, 1974). These observations have been confirmed (Meade et al, 1977; Andrew, 1979; Kay, 1982; Khaw & Peart, 1982), but it is apparent that the effect depends not only on the progestagen content of the pill, but also upon the oestrogen/progestagen balance (Edgren & Sturtevant, 1975) and on the duration of contraceptive use (Khaw & Peart, 1982).

Effects on other tissues

The Royal College of General Practitioners' Oral Contraception Study has shown that, contrary to earlier reports that the use of steroid contraceptives might reduce the risk of fracture from osteoporosis later in life, they significantly increase the risk (Cooper et al, 1993). Depot medroxyprogesterone acetate, used as a contraceptive, has also been shown to reduce bone densities because of the associated reduction in oestrogen levels (Cundy et al, 1991).

Earlier reports that women using steroid contraceptives were at increased risk of developing malignant melanoma have not been substantiated (Grimes, 1991; Hannaford et al, 1991).

There are differences of opinion as to whether the use of combined steroid contraceptives improves or worsens Crohn's disease and ulcerative colitis. Lashner et al in the USA found no increased risk in either Crohn's disease (Lashner et al, 1989) or ulcerative colitis (Lashner et al, 1990) whilst Logan & Kay (1989), using data from the Royal College of General Practitioners' Study, found that both Crohn's disease and ulcerative colitis were more common in oral contraceptive users.

Intrauterine contraceptive devices

The composition and structure of intrauterine contraceptive devices (IUCDs) has changed over the years and thus data relating to women in the 1970s or early 1980s is almost certainly inapplicable to current users.

Current IUCDs are made of plastic partly covered by coils of closely wound copper wire or are made of plastic impregnated by progestagen. Although inert, non-medicated plastic devices are no longer inserted, women who have worn them for many years still have them in situ and it is appropriate, when considering the pathology of IUCD usage, to include data relating to these devices.

The uterus may be perforated or lacerated when the IUCD is inserted. Perforation of the uterus is said to occur, at the time of insertion, in between 0.012% and 0.29% of insertions (Key & Kreutner, 1980; Van Os & Edelman, 1989), the variation being mainly due to differences in operative skill and training (Craig, 1975). The hazard of perforation is said to be greatest in the postpartum and postabortive states when the tissues are soft (Heinonen et al, 1984; Kiilholma et al, 1990) but this claim has not always been substantiated (Mishell & Roy, 1982) unless the patient is lactating (Heartwell & Schlesselman, 1983). Cervical laceration is a rare complication of IUCD insertion which happens most commonly in nulliparous women. The accident occurs in 1.8% of insertions (Chi et al, 1989) and is more common with a copper or multiload device than with a loop.

Studies of the forces required to perforate the uterus suggest that the majority of perforations may, initially, be partial (Goldstuck, 1987) and that the device gradually works its way through the uterine wall. Perforation may occur in the corpus uteri or in the cervix (Rienprayura et al, 1973). If the perforation is partial, the tail of the IUCD may remain palpable at the external cervical os and the operator may not be aware of the fact that the uterus has been perforated unless the patient complains of abnormal bleeding (Tadesse & Wamsteker, 1985) or until attempts are made to remove the device, when great difficulty may be encountered.

When the perforation is partial, the IUCD is usually found lying malaligned partly within the uterine cavity and partly embedded in the myometrium. When a complete perforation has occurred, or a partial perforation has become complete due to migration of the IUCD through the uterine wall, a complication perhaps more likely to occur if the patient is breastfeeding (Mittal et al, 1986), the device may be found in the broad ligament, peritoneal cavity (Gorsline & Osborne, 1985), bladder (Hefnawi et al, 1975; Thomalla, 1986; Kiilholma et al, 1989; Khan & Wilkinson, 1990; Dietrick et al, 1992), adjacent to the ureter (Timonen & Kurppa, 1987), in the large bowel (Key & Kreutner, 1980; Hays et al, 1986; Browning & Bigrigg, 1988) or in the rectum (Sepulveda, 1990; Ramsewak et al, 1991; Sogaard, 1993). A vesico-uterine fistula has also been reported in association with an ectopic IUCD (Schwartzwald et al, 1986). Those devices containing copper are a particular hazard as the copper may elicit a brisk inflammatory response (Fig. 35.39) and if this occurs in the peritoneal cavity it may cause adhesions leading to intestinal obstruction (Osborne & Bennett, 1978; Mittal et al, 1986; Adoni & Ben Chetrit, 1991).

Multiple device insertion has been described when a woman believes, erroneously, that her previous device has been expelled (Porges, 1973; Nanda & Rathee, 1992) and a complaint of infertility may be made when the presence of a device has been forgotten (Olson & Jones, 1967; Abramovici et al, 1987).

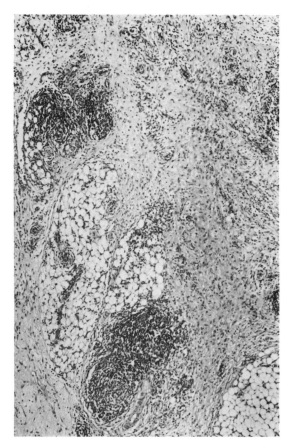

Fig. 35.39   The omentum from a patient in whom a copper-containing IUCD had perforated the uterus and entered the peritoneal cavity. There is extensive fibrosis and a non-specific chronic inflammatory cell infiltrate. H & E × 75.

A transient bacteraemia can be detected in 13% of women within a few minutes of replacing an IUCD (Murray et al, 1987). This clearly has implications for the patient at risk of developing endocarditis (Smith et al, 1983).

Some devices are spontaneously expelled, the proportion depending upon the type of device, the duration of the study and on the patient. The expulsion rate for copper devices ranges from approximately 5.0% (19 821 treatment cycles) within 36 months of use (Fylling, 1987) to 1.8% (1038 women, 66% of whom were in the postpartum or postabortive state) within two years (Tsalikis et al, 1986). Expulsion rates are not affected by the timing of insertion in relation to the menstrual cycle (Otolorin & Ladipo, 1985). There is, however, an increased rate of expulsion if the device is fitted immediately following delivery of the placenta (Thiery et al, 1985) and this risk can be reduced if insertion is delayed for between 2 and 72 hours (Chi et al, 1985).

On rare occasions the device may fracture in utero and this may hinder removal (Custo et al, 1986; Blaauwhof

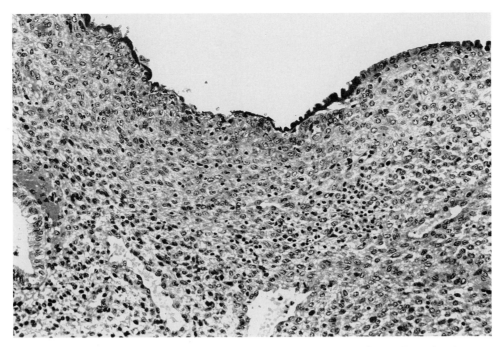

Fig. 35.40 Inert intrauterine contraceptive device contact site. The surface of the endometrium is depressed, the epithelium flattened and the underlying stroma pseudodecidualized and infiltrated by a round cell population. H & E × 186. (From Buckley & Fox, 1989. By courtesy of Chapman & Hall Ltd.)

& Goldstuck, 1988). Fragmentation of the copper on the device increases with duration of use but in only 0.1% of cases is this of sufficient degree as to impair future fertility (Edelman & van Os, 1990).

Death seldom occurs as a direct consequence of IUCD use but deaths from septic abortion are well documented (Christian, 1974; Preston et al, 1975; Cates et al, 1976; Foreman et al, 1981). These were almost entirely confined to one particular device, a fact that prompted its withdrawal from the market (Cates et al, 1976) (see below).

Effects on the endometrium

Morphological changes in the endometrium, although often subtle, are an almost invariable accompaniment of the IUCD. In most IUCD wearers, the changes are limited to the contact sites of the IUCD, are relatively minor, and are the result of irritation and pressure. In the majority of cases, the changes affect only the superficial layers of the endometrium and, on removal of the device, the abnormal tissue is shed in the next menstrual cycle (Badrawi et al, 1988).

At the contact sites, there is compression of the tissue, pseudodecidualization of the stroma and, almost invariably, an inflammatory cell response (Fig. 35.40). Although the inflammatory infiltrate may persist for some time after removal of the device (Moyer & Mishell, 1971) there is little doubt that it is the consequence of irritation and not infection, as an infiltrate is seen in experimental animals kept in a germ-free environment (Davis, 1972). An inflammatory infiltrate extending beyond the contact site, however, suggests an infectious rather than an irritative aetiology.

In the period immediately following insertion of the device, the inflammatory infiltrate is composed entirely of polymorphonuclear leucocytes but with time, in the absence of infection, polymorphs become scanty and limited to the surface epithelium, to the immediate subepithelial stroma and to the lumina of the superficial stromal capillaries. Gradually, the infiltrate, which is most marked with copper-covered devices (Moyer et al, 1970; Sheppard, 1987), becomes plasma-lymphocytic (Figs 35.41 and 35.42). Lymphocytes are generally increased throughout the tissue, beyond the contact sites, but this may not be apparent on routine histological examination (Mishell & Moyer, 1969).

At the contact sites of the IUCD, the compression artifact may accurately reflect the surface contours of the device (Fig. 35.43). The surface epithelium may be flattened or there may be reactive cellular atypia (Fig. 35.44) with some loss of nuclear polarity, mild nuclear pleomorphism, increased nucleo-cytoplasmic ratios, the development of nucleoli and cytoplasmic vacuolation. Much less commonly these days, there is ulceration of the surface epithelium (Moyer & Mishell, 1971), sometimes with preservation of the underlying basement membrane, the formation of non-specific granulation tissue and stromal

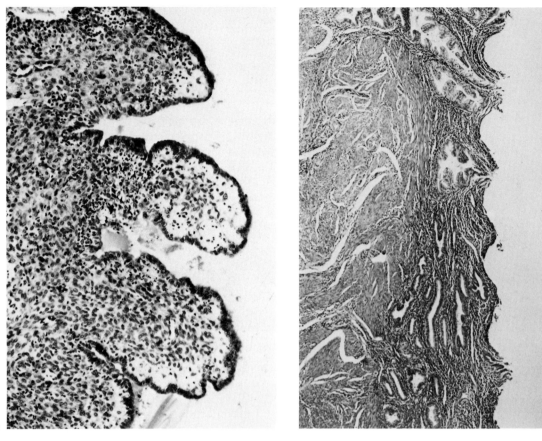

Fig. 35.41

Fig. 35.43

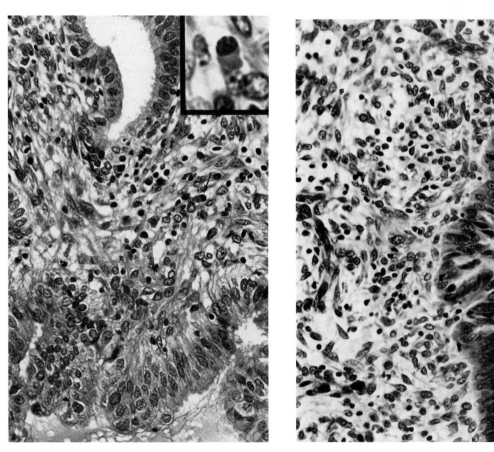

Fig. 35.42

Fig. 35.44

Fig. 35.41 An endometrial IUCD contact site. In addition to the copper wire imprint, there is a scattering of intrastromal and intraepithelial inflammatory cells. H & E × 180.

Fig. 35.42 A detail from the endometrium shown in Fig. 35.41, showing the scanty nature of the inflammatory cell infiltrate. H & E × 205. Insert of cell group indicated by the arrow.

Fig. 35.43 The endometrium in a copper IUCD wearer. The imprint of the copper wire can be clearly seen on the endometrial surface. Loss of surface epithelium is artifactual, having occurred as the device was removed after tissue fixation. H & E × 75.

Fig. 35.44 The endometrial surface epithelium at an IUCD contact site. There is irregularity of the epithelium with nuclear enlargement, an increase in nucleo-cytoplasmic ratios and some loss of cellular polarity. Nuclear chromatin dispersion is, however, normal. H & E × 450.

fibrosis (Fig. 35.45) (Bonney et al, 1966; Shaw et al, 1979a). These features are more typically associated with the presence of an inert IUCD. Rarely there is squamous metaplasia (Tamada et al, 1967) or the development of foreign body granulomas (Fig. 35.46) (Ragni et al, 1977).

In addition to the local irritative effects, there are, with progestagen-impregnated devices, changes which are attributable to the progestagen and are dose dependent.

Initially, in the tissue immediately adjacent to the device (Dallenbach-Hellweg, 1981; Ermini et al, 1989), there is pseudodecidualization of the stroma and the cells in the glandular and surface epithelium gradually become cuboidal. The glands become fewer, smaller in calibre and inactive whilst the stroma becomes less mature, losing its decidualized appearance and appearing spindle-celled. Over a period, which may be as long as 6–12 months if the amount of progestagen liberated is sufficient, these appearances may spread to the whole of the endometrium. The functionalis thus becomes thin and there are no cyclical changes (El-Mahgoub, 1980; Silverberg et al, 1986). The appearances may closely resemble those seen in systemic progestagen users (Buckley & Fox, 1989). With devices delivering only a small dose, the changes may remain limited to the tissue adjacent to the contact site and the stroma may remain locally pseudodecidualized (Shaw, 1985). With devices delivering 20–30 µg of progestagen (Sheppard, 1987) profound atrophy develops within a month of insertion of the device. Stromal calcification, microscopic polyps and thick-walled fibrotic blood vessels, similar to those seen in endometrial polyps, may develop after several years of use (Silverberg et al, 1986). Ulceration of the surface epithelium is less common with

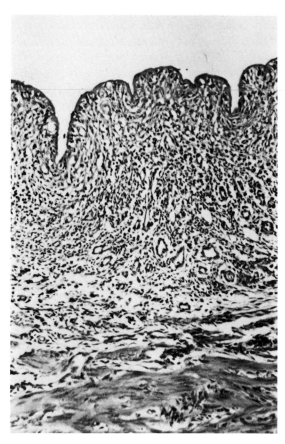

Fig. 35.45 Postinflammatory fibrosis in an endometrium from a patient wearing an inert IUCD and in whom there had been sepsis. H & E × 180.

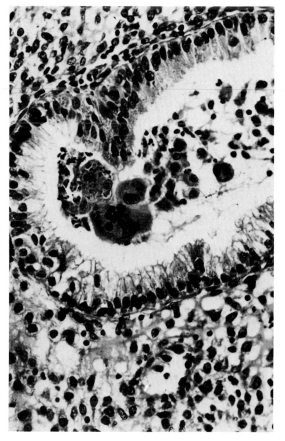

Fig. 35.46 Intraglandular giant cells in an endometrium from an IUCD wearer. H & E × 450.

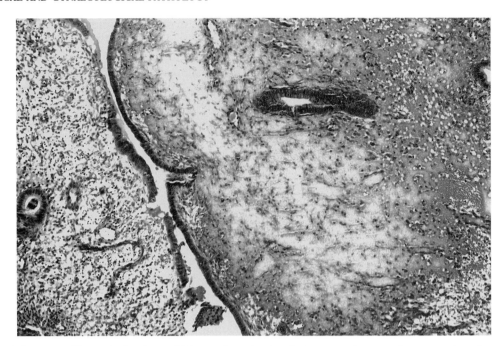

Fig. 35.47   The marked oedema which sometimes develops in the stroma between the contact sites of an IUCD is seen in the fragment of endometrium to the right; the endometrium on the left is of more normal appearance. H & E × 93. (From Buckley & Fox, 1989. By courtesy of Chapman & Hall Ltd.)

progestagen-impregnated devices than with either inert or copper-covered devices (Sheppard & Bonnar, 1985).

Between the contact sites, particularly of inert and large devices, there is oedema (Fig. 35.47) and vascular congestion whilst at the contact sites there is vascular blanching (Shaw, 1985). Both beneath and adjacent to the device there are microvascular defects with endothelial damage. With progestagen-impregnated devices vascular damage also occurs but there is a reduction in the vascularity of the tissues commensurate with the reduction in bleeding experienced by these women (Shaw et al, 1979b, 1981). Oestrogen and progesterone receptors are decreased in proportion to the amount of copper in the device (de Castro et al, 1986). However, as copper concentration becomes lower towards the end of the first year, the endometrium, more consistently, shows secretory changes indicating a return of steroid receptors. With devices having a surface area of 375 mm², and hence delivering a larger concentration of copper, however, the endometrium remains shallow.

Sometimes, the glands immediately deep to the contact site have a pattern of maturation which differs slightly from that in the adjacent areas: there may be delayed maturation, premature secretory maturation or, rarely, the glands may be inactive (Buckley & Fox, 1989). Even when the endometrium is of apparently normal morphology, and ovarian function is normal, there is a reduction in the binding of D9B1, a monoclonal antibody binding to a polypeptide-associated oligosaccharide epitope that is secreted by endometrial epithelium in the luteal phase (Seif et al, 1989).

Infection is less common with modern copper-covered than with earlier inert devices. When it occurs, it is associated with a widespread inflammatory cell infiltrate which may extend into the myometrium and persist after removal of the device. When it is severe, it interferes with the development or function of hormone receptors and the endometrium fails to show normal cyclical changes. It is characterized by intraglandular polymorphonuclear leucocytes and a stromal infiltrate of polymorphonuclear leucocytes, plasma cells and lymphocytes (Fig. 35.48). The plasma cells are often predominantly periglandular whilst the lymphocytes may be diffuse or form aggregates or lymphoid follicles. The irritative cytological atypia in the epithelial cells (Fig. 35.49) may be so severe that the detection of these cells in a cervical smear may give rise to a suspicion of malignancy (Gupta et al, 1978a). Low-grade inflammation (Fig. 35.50) does not significantly disturb the cyclical changes.

Uterine malignancy has developed in association with long-term use of an IUCD but no causal relationship has been demonstrated (Hsu et al, 1989). On the contrary, Pike (1990) has suggested that a progestagen-containing IUCD could reduce the incidence of endometrial carcinoma.

Effects on the cervix and vagina

Non-specific, non-infectious cervicitis occurs more often in wearers of both copper-containing and progestagen-releasing IUCDs (Winkler & Richart, 1985; Fahmy et al, 1990) than in women using other forms of contraception. This is associated with cytological atypia in both the squa-

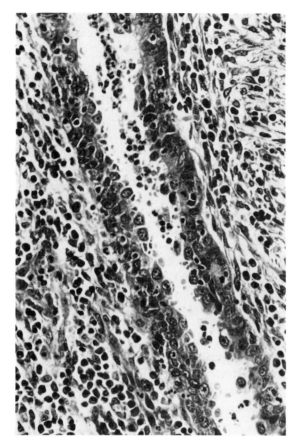

Fig. 35.48 Intrauterine infection in an inert IUCD wearer. The glands contain polymorphonuclear leucocytes and cellular debris and the stroma is infiltrated by plasma cells and lymphocytes. Note the reactive cellular atypia and the absence of hormonal changes in the epithelium. H & E × 450.

mous and the columnar epithelium of the cervix (Gupta et al, 1978a) and is more severe with copper than inert devices (Misra et al, 1977). In the squamous epithelium the nuclear atypia is usually mild, but in the columnar epithelium it may be so severe as to suggest the presence of an adenocarcinoma or adenocarcinoma in situ.

In asymptomatic, sexually active, healthy women using an IUCD or steroid contraceptives, the vaginal flora is more likely to contain anaerobes than is that from a barrier contraceptive user (Haukkamaa et al, 1986) and IUCD wearers are more likely to develop bacterial vaginosis than are steroid contraceptive users (Roy, 1991). There are no significant differences between users of copper-containing devices and users of progestagen-containing devices (Ulstein et al, 1987).

Fig. 35.49 A cluster of highly atypical endometrial epithelial cells from an IUCD wearer with endometritis. There is nuclear pleomorphism, cytoplasmic vacuolation, an increased nucleo-cytoplasmic ratio in many cells and a complete loss of cellular polarity. H & E × 720.

Fig. 35.50 Intraglandular polymorphonuclear leucocytes and cellular debris in an endometrium from an IUCD wearer. H & E × 450.

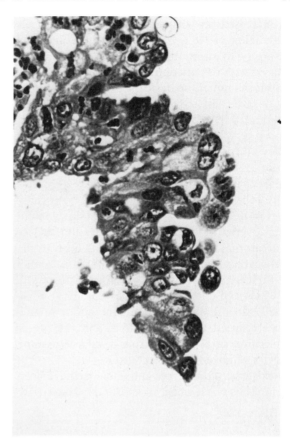

Fig. 35.49

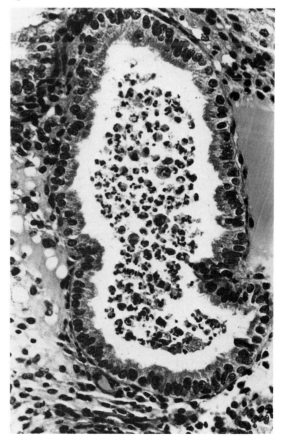

Fig. 35.50

An increased prevalence of various strains of Candida in the vagina of women, in whom there are no factors predisposing to infection, occurs in 20% of IUCD wearers compared with 6% of controls. In some the fungus is also found on the tail of the device (Parewijck et al, 1988).

Actinomyces-like organisms are reported in between 11.6% and 2.8% (Nayar et al, 1985; Mali et al, 1986; Cleghorn & Wilkinson, 1989) of cervical smears and the majority of these women are asymptomatic. Indeed many of these organisms have neither the immunological nor cultural characteristics of Actinomyces (Gupta et al, 1978b; Valicenti et al, 1982) (Fig. 35.51). Proven *Actinomyces israelii* may, however, be found in women using copper-covered or inert plastic devices and they tend to be more common when the device has been in place for several years (Cleghorn & Wilkinson, 1989). Actinomycosis of the cervix may result in the formation of a cervical mass which can mimic a cervical carcinoma (Snowman et al, 1989). In the absence of inflammation, Actinomyces can be regarded as saprophytic but in the presence of inflammation an aetiological rôle should be assumed and the device removed (Grimes, 1981).

Co-existent Actinomyces and amoebae have been identified in the cervical smear of an IUCD wearer (Arroyo & Quinn, 1989). Colonization of the uterus by *Entamoeba gingivalis*, usually an inhabitant of the mouth (Clark & Diamond, 1992), has also led to its detection in the cervical smear.

Over a period of time, material collects on the surface of IUCDs of all types and is amorphous or filamentous, eosinophilic, often partly calcified and resembles dental plaque. It is composed of a mixture of leucocytes, erythrocytes, epithelial cells, sperm and bacteria, fibrillary material, which is mainly fibrin, and amorphous acellular material consisting of calcite, calcium phosphate (Khan & Wilkinson, 1985) and magnesium (Rizk et al, 1990). In patients in whom there has been heavy bleeding there is often a very thick layer of amorphous deposits. In a histological or cytological preparation it forms so-called 'pseudo-sulphur granules' (O'Brien et al, 1981, 1985) which may be confused with bacterial colonies (Fig. 35.52).

In women wearing copper-covered devices, immunoglobulin levels (IgG, IgA and IgM) in the serum and in the mucus on the tail of the device are significantly higher than in women using steroid contraception or no contraceptive (Eissa et al, 1985). It is uncertain whether this represents a response to the bacteria that are present in

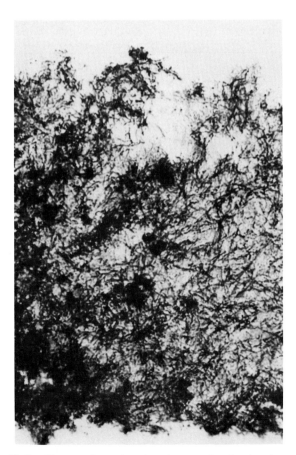

Fig. 35.51   Clusters of organisms in a tissue section showing the pseudofilamentous arrangement that may be mistaken for *Actinomyces*. Gram stain × 815.

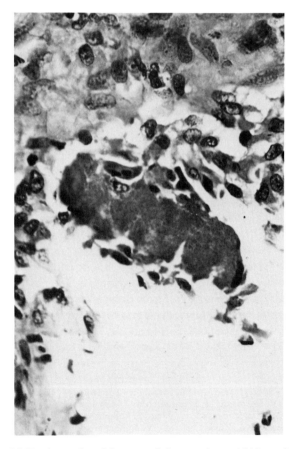

Fig. 35.52   A pseudo-sulphur granule in an endometrial biopsy from a patient wearing an inert intrauterine device. H & E × 815.

these patients or is a form of foreign body response to the device.

Changes in the fatty acid composition of mid-cycle lecithin in the cervical mucus, which is similar to that detected in women with unexplained primary infertility, suggest that part of the contraceptive effect of copper IUCDs may be due to changes in the cervical mucus (Pschera et al, 1988).

In a comparison between IUCD users and combined steroid contraceptive users, Fiore (1986) found that mild dyskaryosis was more likely to be found in the cervical smears from IUCD users (17.6%) when compared with steroid contraceptive users (10.53%).

Effects on the Fallopian tube, ovary and pelvic organs

The incidence of pelvic inflammatory disease (PID) in IUCD wearers, that is, infection centred on the Fallopian tube and adjacent structures, varies according to the population studied and the criteria used for its diagnosis. Early reports indicated that IUCD wearers had a 1.6 to 3 times increased risk of developing pelvic inflammatory disease when compared with an otherwise similar group of non-users (Flesh et al, 1979; Burkman, 1981). More recent reports (Lee et al, 1988; Kessel, 1989; Kronmal et al, 1991) have questioned the interpretation of the original data and have evaluated the more modern copper-covered and progestagen-releasing devices.

Case-control studies which have been widely used to evaluate the risk of pelvic inflammatory disease are vulnerable to bias even when carefully conducted (Edelman & Porter 1986a; Mumford & Kessel, 1992). Firstly, most series are hospital based, and as women with acute pelvic inflammatory disease who use an IUCD are more likely to be admitted to hospital than are women with pelvic inflammatory disease who are not wearing an IUCD, the apparent risk of acute pelvic inflammatory disease in IUCD wearers may appear higher than it really is. Secondly, case-control studies only provide a comparison between the two chosen groups of women so that if there is a reduced risk of pelvic inflammatory disease in women forming the control group, the risk of pelvic inflammatory disease in IUCD wearers will appear relatively higher though the rate of infection may actually be similar to that of the general population. Most case-control studies have not considered the contraceptive methods of their control patients (Edelman, 1985) yet there is evidence that methods of contraception other than the IUCD, in particular steroid contraceptives and barrier methods, provide some protection against pelvic inflammatory disease (Keith & Berger, 1985; Wolner-Hanssen et al, 1985; Buchan et al, 1990). Finally, whilst case-control studies almost invariably reveal an increased risk of pelvic inflammatory disease in IUCD wearers, cohort studies usually reveal an increase in only certain groups of IUCD wearers (Edelman & Porter, 1986a).

Undoubtedly, certain groups of IUCD wearers are at increased risk of developing pelvic inflammatory disease (Daling et al, 1985). There is, for example, a transient increased risk in the first few months after insertion (Mishell et al, 1966; Vessey et al, 1981b; Wright & Aisien, 1989; Lovset, 1990). The incidence then declines the longer the device remains in place (Vessey et al, 1981b). Cautious interpretation of these data is required, however, as it is only in asymptomatic women that the device is left, whilst in women with pelvic inflammatory disease the device has often been removed. The risk of pelvic inflammatory disease is also computed to be greater for IUCD-wearing women with multiple sexual partners who would have been at risk of contracting sexually transmitted disease whether they used an IUCD or not (Burkman, 1981; Cramer et al, 1985; Huggins & Cullins, 1990; Farley et al, 1992). The Oxford Family Planning Study (Buchan et al, 1990) also identified an increased risk of pelvic inflammatory disease for non-medicated (inert) IUCD users (with 95% CI) of 3.3 (2.3–5.0). This compares with those wearing medicated devices where the relative risk is 1.8 (0.8–4.0) and for ex-users 1.3 (0.7–2.3). In considering these data, however, it should be remembered that inert devices are no longer inserted. Nowadays, many believe that there is little risk of infection for women in a monogamous relationship who are not at risk of sexually transmitted disease and who are parous at the time of insertion (Cramer et al, 1985; Lee et al, 1988; Burkman, 1990; Lovset, 1990).

Some of this change in opinion may be the result of the changes in the composition of IUCDs. Toivonen and colleagues (1991), for example, found that pelvic inflammatory disease is less likely to develop with a device releasing 20 µg of levonorgestrel per day than with a standard copper device.

In fact, the presence of an intrauterine device of any type may compromise the sterility of the uterine cavity (Hill et al, 1986). Bacteria are introduced into the uterus when the device is inserted (Mishell et al, 1966) and small numbers of bacteria ascend from the vagina and cervix into the cavity of both mono- and multi-filamentous tailed device wearers (Sparks et al, 1977, 1981). In contrast, devices which are tailless or ones in which the tail no longer lies in the endocervical canal will be sterile in 50% of cases (Wolf & Kriegler, 1986). Infection may also be reduced by placing the tail of the device within the uterine cavity at the time of insertion (Akeson et al, 1992).

Pelvic inflammatory disease in IUCD users may be caused by a variety of organisms, including Pneumococcus (Goldman et al, 1986), but is frequently polymicrobiol with a preponderance of anaerobic organisms (Landers & Sweet, 1985). Pelvic inflammatory disease can range from minor, asymptomatic episodes of endosalpingitis to major pelvic sepsis with tubo-ovarian abscess, which may be unilateral or bilateral (Landers & Sweet, 1985), and has been reported as leading to rectal stenosis (Girardot et al, 1990), local or generalized peritonitis

(Brinson et al, 1986), hepatic phlebitis and intrahepatic or subphrenic abscess formation. Such complications are, however, rare and reports frequently pre-date the introduction of copper-containing devices.

Tubal damage, as determined histologically, may be minimal but often, in those patients in whom pelvic infection requires surgery, it is extensive and severe. The histopathologist's view is, therefore, somewhat biased. Smith Soderstrom (1976), for example, reported a 47% incidence of salpingitis in tubal sterilization specimens from IUCD users, and in our own series an incidence of approximately 30% was seen. The majority of women included in these data, however, wore only inert devices and the current figures can be expected to be lower.

The endosalpingitis which occurs in IUCD wearers is histologically characteristic of infection ascending from the uterine cavity. In the acute stage there is a polymorphonuclear leucocyte infiltrate in the tubal mucosa and with more severe infection this may extend through the tube wall with the subsequent development of local peritonitis. Active chronic inflammation is characterized by the presence of an infiltrate of polymorphonuclear leucocytes, plasma cells and lymphocytes which may be limited to the mucosa or involve the deeper tissues (Fig. 35.53); there may be collections of macrophages in the mucosal stroma. More commonly, at the time of surgery, the tubes show evidence of chronic inflammation, previous inflammatory episodes or acute on chronic inflammation. There may, therefore, be active chronic endosalpingitis, hydrosalpinx follicularis, salpingitis isthmica nodosa (diverticular disease of the tube), mural scarring, local chronic peritonitis with peritoneal adhesions or a pyosalpinx lined only by non-specific granulation tissue. Inflammation may be limited to the tube but more commonly there is also evidence of inflammation of the ovary. This may take the form of an acute on chronic peri-oophoritis, an intraovarian abscess or a tubo-ovarian abscess.

Exceptionally, infection may be due to Actinomyces and there may be an endometritis, endocervicitis, salpingitis (Hansen, 1989), ovarian abscess (Maroni & Genton, 1986; de Clercq et al, 1987), tubo-ovarian abscess (Schmidt et al, 1980), abdomino-pelvic abscess (O'Brien, 1975; Yoonessi et al, 1985; Maenpaa et al, 1988), which may extend to the bladder (Franz et al, 1992), acute peritonitis (Dawson et al, 1992) or an abdominal wall abscess (Adachi et al, 1985). On rare occasions disseminated infection (Fisher, 1980) or hepatic abscess has occurred secondary to the pelvic infection (Shurbaji et al, 1987).

Inflammation, sufficient to cause structural or functional damage to the Fallopian tubes, may occur in the absence of symptoms. Asymptomatic sterile, histologically proven endosalpingitis may also be detected more often in IUCD wearers than never-wearers or former wearers during hysterectomy for non-IUCD-associated disease (Kajanoja et al, 1987; Vanlancker et al, 1987; Ghosh

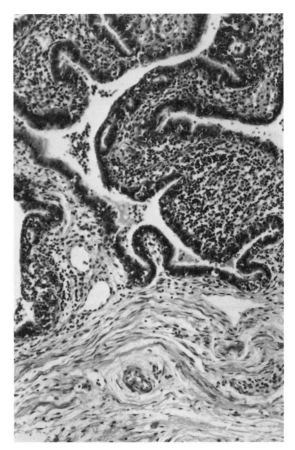

Fig. 35.53 An active chronic endosalpingitis from a patient wearing an IUCD. Inflammation is almost entirely limited to the mucosa in this example with minimal mural involvement. H & E × 205.

et al, 1989) and is more frequent in copper device users (Vanlancker et al, 1987). At an ultrastructural level, in a small series, Wollen et al (1990) have described a reduction in tubal epithelial cilial length, less well orientated cilia and a reduction in the proportion of cilia with a ciliary crown.

Pregnancy and the IUCD

Pregnancy may occur in an intrauterine or ectopic site in an IUCD user and occasionally it occurs in both simultaneously (Clausen et al, 1990). Between 5% and 7.8% of accidental pregnancies in IUCD wearers are ectopic compared with 0.5% to 1.3% in non-users (Dommisse, 1977; Snowden et al, 1977; Tatum & Schmidt, 1977; WHO, 1985b; Skjeldestad et al, 1988).

Intrauterine pregnancy occurs in less than 1 woman per 100 wearing a copper-impregnated device in the first year of use (Sivin, 1985a). The risk is similar with inert and low dose copper devices but is lower with both modern high dose copper devices and those delivering 20 µg/day of levonorgestrel (Sivin & Schmidt, 1987; Lovset, 1990; Toivonen et al, 1991). The cumulative gross pregnancy rate at five years of use is 1.1 ± 0.5 with levonorgestrel-releasing devices and 1.4 ± 0.4 for copper device users (Sivin et al, 1990). The reason for the lower rate with progestagen-releasing devices is that they act not only locally but that the amount of progestagen absorbed, although small, may be sufficient to impair ovarian follicular development by disturbing the pituitary-ovarian axis (Barbosa et al, 1990).

Up to 50% of pregnancies that occur in IUCD wearers end in spontaneous abortion (Dommisse, 1977) although this figure has been modified in recent years by termination of pregnancy on request. It is said that, of women who conceive with an IUCD in situ, up to three-quarters will request a termination of pregnancy (Tews et al, 1988) and of the patients reported to the University of Exeter Family Planning Research Unit, in whom the outcome of the pregnancy was known, 41% were terminated and 26% aborted spontaneously (Snowden et al, 1977).

Early removal of the device can reduce the spontaneous abortion rate to approximately 25% (Alvior, 1973), although abortion during removal may occur if the device lies lateral to the fetus or nearer the uterine fundus than the implantation site (Serr & Shalev, 1985). A comparison of women with and without IUCDs who presented for termination of pregnancy in Trondheim, Norway, (n = 962) (Skjeldestad et al, 1988) revealed that, despite removal of the device in the first trimester, women who had an IUCD in place when they became pregnant were more likely to experience a spontaneous abortion (15.6% compared with 7.0%, p = 0.05). In the 1970s, mid-trimester abortion accompanied by pyrexia was frequently reported (Kim-Farley et al, 1978). This seems to have been a hazard with a particular inert device and is no longer a problem. The adverse publicity associated with this was largely responsible for the withdrawal of the IUCD from the American market.

In pregnancies going to term, 28% of those reported to the Exeter Family Planning Research Unit (Snowden et al, 1977), there is no evidence of an increased risk of fetal abnormality and the device is usually found embedded in the placenta where, if copper-covered, it elicits a minor degree of focal inflammation: occasionally, intrauterine monilial infection of the fetus and placenta have occurred (Spaun & Klunder, 1986; Smith et al, 1988; Michaud et al, 1989). There have, however, been reports that women with an IUCD in situ have an increased risk of preterm labour (Chaim & Mazor, 1992).

There is a statistically significant negative relationship between the IUCD and complete molar pregnancies (Honoré, 1986) and a reduced risk of having a spontaneous abortion with morphological evidence suggestive of heteroploidy (Honoré, 1985). It has been suggested that the IUCD may selectively inhibit chromosomally abnormal conceptuses.

The reason that some women with an IUCD become pregnant whilst others do not has led to speculation as to the reason but few data are available. It is known, however, that in women who become pregnant the percentage of CD3+ mature T lymphocytes is fewer in the cells adherent to the device than in non-pregnant women. CD4+ cells are increased and CD8+ cells are decreased. This raises the possibility that immunological factors may play a part. The percentage of B lymphocytes is similar in pregnant and non-pregnant IUCD wearers (Randic et al, 1990).

Ectopic pregnancy. It is generally reported that the proportion of ectopic pregnancies occurring in the Fallopian tube and ovary is greater in IUCD wearers than in women using other forms of contraception (Paavonen et al, 1985). A statistically insignificant number also occur in other sites (Muzsnai et al, 1980; Goldman et al, 1988). This view is not, however, universally held.

The WHO (WHO, 1985b) multinational case-control study describes an increased relative risk of ectopic pregnancy of 6.4 for IUCD wearers compared with pregnant non-users matched for parity and marital status. Edelman & Porter (1986b), on the other hand, analysing published data, reached the conclusion that there is no increased risk of ectopic pregnancy in current and past users of the IUCD. Those reporting an increased risk, however, find that the risk is different for different types of device and the series examined by Edelman & Porter may not be comparing like with like.

The lowest rate of ectopic pregnancy is found in copper device users and the highest rate in those using low dose (2 µg/24 h) progestagen-releasing devices (WHO, 1987; Sivin, 1991). There is also some evidence of an increased risk of ectopic pregnancy for users of progestagen-impregnated devices delivering high doses, up to 65 µg per day (Fylling & Fagerhol, 1979; Larsen et al, 1981), but the risk for those using devices delivering between 20 and 30 µg of progestagen daily (Sivin, 1985b) is similar to that found in wearers of copper-covered or inert devices.

Sivin (1991) analysed randomized trials of copper IUCDs and confirmed that the ectopic pregnancy rate varied, not only according to the dose of progestagen, but also inversely with the surface area of the copper on the device.

The incidence of ectopic pregnancy doubled between the eighth and ninth decades of this century and there is a consensus that the increase is related to the increased incidence of tubal damage secondary to sexually transmitted disease (Sivin, 1985b). This increase has coincided with a time when the IUCD has been more widely used (Tuomivaara et al, 1986; Thorburn et al, 1987). It is important, therefore, to distinguish between an increased incidence of ectopic pregnancy in the population as a whole and that which might be attributable to the use of the IUCD. Evaluation of the rôle of the IUCD in the increased reporting of ectopic gestation is complex, although multivariate analysis (Makinen et al, 1989) indicates that it plays an aetiological rôle.

Tubal damage is a potent and well-recognized cause of tubal ectopic pregnancy and this may be a factor in the development of ectopic pregnancy in IUCD wearers. This presupposes, however, that conception regularly occurs in IUCD users, that there is sufficient tubal damage in IUCD users to account for the increased incidence of tubal ectopic pregnancy and that it is the tubal damage, together with the greater protection against intrauterine compared with extrauterine pregnancy afforded to IUCD wearers, which determines the tubal implantation site. This is not, however, supported by the evidence.

Firstly, in women wearing the newer, high dose copper and progestagen-releasing IUCDs, monitoring of hCG in the latter part of the menstrual cycle indicates that covert pregnancies do not routinely occur (Segal et al, 1985; Wilcox et al, 1987; Sivin, 1989). Indeed recovery of ova flushed from the Fallopian tubes also shows that conception rates are lower than would be expected in normally ovulating women having unprotected coitus (Alvarez et al, 1988). It may be, however, that in the past, frequent conception did play an important part in the development of ectopic pregnancies because, in women wearing an inert IUCD, conception occurs in about 20% of cycles (Videla-Rivero et al, 1987) and in those wearing the older copper-containing devices in up to 50% of cycles (Capitanio et al, 1978).

Secondly, the ratio of ovarian to all ectopic pregnancies in IUCD wearers lies between 1:10 and 1:13 compared with 1:78 to 1:111 in a group of non-IUCD wearers (Herbertsson et al, 1987; Sandvei et al, 1987) and it seems unlikely that tubal damage alone would cause this.

Thirdly, it is only in women who are at risk of developing sexually transmitted pelvic inflammatory disease that the tubes are likely to be damaged and they constitute a small proportion of wearers (see above).

The single most important clinical correlate remains the history of pelvic inflammatory disease which increases the risk of subsequent ectopic pregnancy in both pregnant and non-pregnant controls (2.8 and 2.0 relative risk respectively) and the risk may be increased with multiple episodes of pelvic inflammatory disease (Herbertsson et al, 1987). It may be that the reported incidence of ectopic gestation in IUCD wearers represents simply a combination of an increased risk, in certain users, of tubal damage secondary to pelvic inflammatory disease, the device's somewhat reduced efficiency in preventing tubal implantation and its inefficiency in preventing ovarian implantation.

Systemic effects

Systemic effects are much less common in women wearing IUCDs than they are in women using steroid contraceptives.

Menstrual blood loss tends to be increased in women wearing an IUCD (Christiaens et al, 1981) and this may be sufficient to require removal of the device. Rarely does haemorrhage, in the presence of an IUCD, reach life-threatening proportions (Glew & Singh, 1989). In contrast, amenorrhoea, scanty menstrual loss and intermenstrual spotting occurs with the progestagen-impregnated devices and this may also be grounds for removal (Sivin, 1985a; Scholten et al, 1987; Sivin et al, 1990). Whilst prolonged menstrual bleeding may lead to depletion of body iron stores, the scanty menstrual loss caused by most progestagen-releasing devices enhances the body's iron stores (Haukkamaa et al, 1985; Andrade & Pizarro-Orchard, 1987; Luukkainen et al, 1987; Faundes et al, 1988). This advantageous effect does not however, apply to devices delivering only 2 µg levonorgestrel which are less effective in reducing bleeding (WHO, 1987).

There is no evidence that copper absorbed from the device results in increased serum copper levels even after 12 months of continuous use (Arowojolu et al, 1989), although there has been a report of interstitial nephritis which resolved when a copper-containing IUCD was removed (Hocher et al, 1992).

Effects on fertility

In the absence of significant pelvic inflammatory disease, removal of the device, in asymptomatic women, is accompanied by the return of normal fertility, as measured by the pregnancy rate, and this is independent of the type of device (Rioux et al, 1986). Within three months of removal, in women wishing to conceive, Randic et al (1985) found that 55.9% of women became pregnant and, in longer term follow-up, 94.3% conceived. In India, Gupta et al (1989) reported a pregnancy rate of 96.7% in the 18 months following the removal of an IUCD. The duration of use, the type of IUCD, and the timing of insertion have no influence on the return to fertility. Pregnancy rates are similar even for the progestagen-impregnated devices delivering 20 µg of levonorgestrel which are associated with a marked degree of endometrial atrophy (Andersson et al, 1992). Older age at removal is, however, associated with a reduced conception rate which is probably a consequence of the natural decline in fecundity with age.

The relative risk of primary tubal infertility in nulligravid women who have ever used an IUCD lies between 2.0 and 2.6 times that in women who have never used one (Cramer et al, 1985; Daling et al, 1985). In an examination of the results following the use of inert devices, the risk was greater for those using the Dalkon Shield (6.8 to 3.3) and lower for Lippes loop and Saf-T-coil (3.2 to 2.9). The smallest risk is for those using copper-covered devices (1.9 to 1.6) and if they have used only a copper-covered device it is 1.3. These latter figures are the ones that are applicable nowadays to women using only medicated devices.

REFERENCES

Abramovici H, Faktor J H, Bornstein J, Sorokin Y 1987 The "forgotten" intrauterine device. Fertility and Sterility 47: 519–521.

Adachi A, Kleiner G J, Bezahler G H, Greston W M, Friedland G H 1985 Abdominal wall actinomycosis with an IUD: a case report. Journal of Reproductive Medicine 30: 145–148.

Adoni A, Ben Chetrit A 1991 The management of intrauterine devices following uterine perforation. Contraception 43: 77–81.

Akeson M, Solheim F, Thorbert G, Akerlund M 1992 Genital tract infections associated with the intrauterine contraceptive device can be reduced by inserting the threads into the uterine cavity. British Journal of Obstetrics and Gynaecology 99: 676–679.

Alpert L I 1976 Veno-occlusive disease of the liver associated with oral contraceptives: case report and review of the literature. Human Pathology 7: 709–718.

Altaras M M, Aviram R, Cohen I et al 1993 Role of prolonged stimulation of Tamoxifen therapy in the etiology of endometrial sarcomas. Gynecologic Oncology 49: 255–258.

Alvarez F, Brache V, Fernandez E et al 1988 New insights on the mode of action of intrauterine contraceptive devices in women. Fertility and Sterility 49: 768–773.

Alvior G T Jr 1973 Pregnancy outcome with removal of intrauterine device. Obstetrics and Gynecology 41: 894–896.

Anderson B, Watring W G, Edinger D D Jr, Small E C, Netland A T, Safaii H 1979 Development of DES-associated clear-cell carcinoma: the importance of regular screening. Obstetrics and Gynecology 53: 293–299.

Anderson D G 1972 The possible mechanisms of action of progestins on endometrial adenocarcinoma. American Journal of Obstetrics and Gynecology 113: 195–211.

Andersson K, Batar I, Rybo G 1992 Return to fertility after removal of a levonorgesterel-releasing intrauterine device and Nova-T. Contraception 46: 575–584.

Andrade A T, Pizarro-Orchard E 1987 Quantitative studies on menstrual blood loss in IUD users. Contraception 36: 129–144.

Andrew W C 1979 Oral contraception. Clinics in Obstetrics and Gynaecology 6: 3–26.

Antonioli D A, Rosen S, Burke L, Donahue V 1979 Glandular dysplasia in diethylstilbestrol-associated vaginal adenosis: a case report and review of the literature. American Journal of Clinical Pathology 71: 715–721.

Antonioli D A, Burke L, Friedman E A 1980 Natural history of diethylstilbestrol-associated genital tract lesions: cervical ectopy and cervicovaginal hood. American Journal of Obstetrics and Gynecology 137: 847–853.

Antunes C M F, Strolley P D, Rosenshein N B et al 1979 Endometrial cancer and estrogen use: report of a large case-control study. New England Journal of Medicine 300: 9–13.

Arowojolu A O, Otolorin E O, Ladipo O A 1989 Serum copper levels in users of multiload intra-uterine contraceptive devices. African Journal of Medical Science 18: 295–299.

Arroyo G, Quinn J A Jr 1989 Association of amoebae and actinomyces in an intrauterine contraceptive device user. Acta Cytologica 33: 298–300.

Badrawi H H, van Os W A, Edelman D A, Rhemrev P E 1988 Effects of intrauterine devices on the surface ultrastructure of human endometrium before and after removal. Advances in Contraception 4: 295–305.

Baggish M S, Woodruff J D 1967 The occurrence of squamous epithelium in the endometrium. Obstetrical and Gynecological Survey 22: 69–115.

Barbosa I, Bakos O, Olsson S E, Odlind V, Johansson E D 1990 Ovarian function during use of a levonorgestrel-releasing IUD. Contraception 42: 51–66.

Barnet B, Joffe A 1991 Hepatic vein thrombosis in a teenager: a case report. Journal of Adolescent Health 12: 60–62.

Baum J K, Bookstein J J, Holtz F, Klein E W 1973 Possible association between benign hepatomas and oral contraceptives. Lancet 2: 926–929.

Beral V 1977 Royal College of General Practitioners Oral Contraception Study. Mortality among oral-contraceptive users. Lancet ii: 727–731.

Berger G S, Talwar P P 1978 Oral contraceptive potencies and side effects. Obstetrics and Gynecology 51: 545–547.

Blaauwhof P C, Goldstuck N D 1988 Intrauterine breakage of a Multiload Cu250 intrauterine device: report of a case. Advances in Contraception 4: 217–220.

Blythe J G, Ali Z 1979 Endometrial adenocarcinoma: in estrogen, oral contraceptive and non-hormone users. Gynecologic Oncology 7: 199–205.

Bonney W A Jr, Glasser S R, Clewe T H, Noyes R W, Cooper C L 1966 Endometrial response to the intrauterine device. American Journal of Obstetrics and Gynecology 96: 101–113.

Böttiger L E, Boman G, Eklund G, Westerholm B 1980 Oral contraceptives and thromboembolic disease: effects of lowering oestrogen content. Lancet 1: 1097–1101.

Boyce J G, Lu T, Nelson J H Jr, Fruchter R G 1977 Oral contraceptives and cervical carcinoma. American Journal of Obstetrics and Gynecology 128: 761–766.

Brady M S, Coit D G 1990 Focal nodular hyperplasia of the liver. Surgery Gynecology and Obstetrics 171: 377–381.

Brinson R R, Kolts B E, Monif G R 1986 Spontaneous bacterial peritonitis associated with an intrauterine device. Journal of Clinical Gastroenterology 8: 82–84.

Brinton L A, Hoover R N 1993 Estrogen replacement therapy and endometrial cancer risk: unresolved issues. Obstetrics and Gynecology 81: 265–271.

Brinton L A, Vessey M P, Flavel R, Yeates D 1981 Risk factors for benign breast disease. American Journal of Epidemiology 113: 203–214.

Brinton L A, Reeves W C, Brenes M M et al 1990. Oral contraceptive use and risk of invasive cervical cancer. International Journal of Epidemiology 19: 4–11.

Browning J J, Bigrigg M A 1988 Recovery of the intrauterine contraceptive device from the sigmoid colon: three case reports. British Journal of Obstetrics and Gynaecology 95: 530–532.

Buchan H, Villard-Mackintosh L, Vessey M, Yeates D, McPherson K 1990 Epidemiology of pelvic inflammatory disease in parous women with special reference to intrauterine device use. British Journal of Obstetrics and Gynaecology 97: 780–788.

Buckley C H 1990 Tamoxifen and endometriosis: case report. British Journal of Obstetrics and Gynaecology 97: 645–646.

Buckley C H, Fox H 1989 Biopsy pathology of the endometrium. Chapman & Hall, London.

Buckley C H, Lewis G J 1982 Focal nodular hyperplasia of the liver presenting as a postpartum abdominal mass. Journal of Obstetrics and Gynaecology 2: 173–174.

Buckley C H, Butler E B, Donnai P et al 1982 A fatal case of DES-associated clear cell adenocarcinoma of the vagina. Journal of Obstetrics and Gynaecology 3: 126–127.

Burkman R T and the Women's Health Study 1981 Association between intrauterine device and pelvic inflammatory disease. Obstetrics and Gynecology 57: 269–276.

Burkman R T 1990 Modern trends in contraception. Obstetrics and Gynecology Clinics of North America 17: 759–774.

Bye P 1982 Failure with the new triphasic oral contraceptive Logynon. British Medical Journal 284: 422–423.

Capitanio G L, Conte N, Ragni N, Rossato P, Pedretti E 1978 Demonstration of human chorionic gonadotropin during the second half of the menstrual cycle in plasma of regularly menstruating women users of copper IUDs. Acta Europaea Fertilitatis 9: 11–19.

Carter E R, Faucher G L, Greenblatt R B 1964 Evaluation of a new progestational agent, 6, 17alpha-dimethyl-6-dehydro-progesterone. American Journal of Obstetrics and Gynecology 89: 635–641.

Casagrande J T, Louie E W, Pike M C et al 1979 "Incessant ovulation" and ovarian cancer. Lancet 2: 170–173.

Cates W Jr, Ory H W, Rochat R W, Tyler C W Jr 1976 The intrauterine device and deaths from spontaneous abortion. New England Journal of Medicine 295: 1155–1159.

Chaim W, Mazor M 1992 Pregnancy with an intrauterine device in situ and preterm delivery. Archives of Gynecology and Obstetrics 252: 21–24.

Chi I 1993 The safety and efficacy issues of progestin-only

contraceptives — an epidemiological perspective. Contraception 47: 1–21.

Chi I C, Wilkens L, Rogers S 1985 Expulsions in immediate postpartum insertions of Lippes Loop D and Copper T IUDs and their counterpart Delta devices — an epidemiological analysis. Contraception 32: 119–134.

Chi I C, Wilkens L R, Robinson N, Dominik R 1989 Cervical laceration at IUD insertion — incidence and risk factors. Contraception 39: 507–518.

Chilvers C E D, Deacon J M 1990 Oral contraceptives and breast cancer. British Journal of Cancer 61: 1–4.

Christiaens G C M L, Sixma J J, Haspels A A 1981 Haemostasis in menstrual endometrium in the presence of an intrauterine device. British Journal of Obstetrics and Gynaecology 88: 825–837.

Christian C D 1974 Maternal deaths associated with an intrauterine device. American Journal of Obstetrics and Gynecology 119: 441–444.

Christopherson W M, Mays E T 1979 Relation of steroids to liver oncogenesis. In: Lupis W, Johanessen J (eds) Liver carcinogenesis. Hemisphere Publishing Corporation, Washington, p 207.

Clark C G, Diamond L S 1992 Colonization of the uterus by the oral protozoan Entamoeba gingivalis. American Journal of Tropical Medicine and Hygiene 46: 158–160.

Clausen I, Borium K G, Frost L 1990 Heterotopic pregnancy: the first case with an IUD in situ. Zentralblatt für Gynäkologie 112: 45–47.

Cleghorn A G, Wilkinson R G 1989 The IUCD-associated incidence of Actinomyces israelii in the female genital tract. Australian and New Zealand Journal of Obstetrics and Gynaecology 29: 445–449.

Clement P B, Young R H 1987 Atypical polypoid adenomyoma of the uterus associated with Turner's syndrome: a report of three cases, including a review of estrogen-associated neoplasms and neoplasms associated with Turner's syndrome. International Journal of Gynecological Pathology 6: 104–113.

Cohen C J, Deppe G 1977 Endometrial carcinoma and oral contraceptive agents. Obstetrics and Gynecology 49: 390–392.

Coker A L, McCann M F, Hulka B S, Walton L A 1992 Oral contraceptive use and cervical intraepithelial neoplasia. Journal of Clinical Epidemiology 45: 1111–1118.

Collaborative Group for the Study of Stroke in Young Women 1973 Oral contraception and increased risk of cerebral ischemia or thrombosis. New England Journal of Medicine 288: 871–878.

Contostavlos D L 1973 Benign hepatomas and oral contraceptives. Lancet 2: 1200.

Cooper C, Hannaford P, Croft P, Kat C R 1993 Oral contraceptive pill use and fractures in women: a prospective study. Bone 14: 41–45.

Coté R J, Urmacher C 1990 Rhabdomyosarcoma of the liver associated with long-term oral contraceptive use: possible role of estrogens in the genesis of embryologically distinct liver tumors. American Journal of Surgical Pathology 14: 784–790.

Cottingham J, Hunter D 1992 Chlamydia trachomatis and oral contraceptive use: a quantitative review. Genitourinary Medicine 68: 209–216.

Craig J M 1975 The pathology of birth control. Archives of Pathology 99: 233–236.

Cramer D W, Hutchison G B, Welch W R, Scully R E, Knapp R C 1982 Factors affecting the association of oral contraceptives and ovarian cancer. New England Journal of Medicine 307: 1047–1051.

Cramer D W, Schiff I, Schoenbaum S C et al 1985 Tubal infertility and the intrauterine contraceptive device. New England Journal of Medicine 312: 941–947.

Critchley H O D, Buckley C H, Anderson D C 1990 Experience with a "physiological" steroid replacement regimen for the establishment of a receptive endometrium in women with premature ovarian failure. British Journal of Obstetrics and Gynaecology 97: 804–810.

Croft P, Hannaford P C 1989 Risk factors for acute myocardial infarction in women: evidence from the Royal College of General Practitioners' oral contraception study. British Medical Journal 298: 165–168.

Cross S S, Ismail S M 1990 Endometrial hyperplasia in an oophorectomized woman receiving tamoxifen therapy: case report. British Journal of Obstetrics and Gynaecology 97: 190–192.

Cundy T, Evans M, Roberts H, Wattie D, Ames R, Reid I R 1991 Bone density in women receiving depot medroxyprogesterone acetate for contraception. British Medical Journal 303: 13–16.

Custo G, Saitto C, Cerza S, Cosmi E V 1986 Intrauterine rupture of the intrauterine device "ML Cu 250": an uncommon complication: presentation of a case. Fertility and Sterility 45: 130–131.

Cuzick J, Singer A, De Stavola B L, Chomet J 1990 Case-control study of risk factors for cervical intraepithelial neoplasia in young women. European Journal of Cancer 26: 684–690.

Daling J R, Weiss N S, Metch B J et al 1985 Primary tubal infertility in relation to the use of an intrauterine device. New England Journal of Medicine 312: 937–941.

Dallenbach-Hellweg G 1980a Morphological changes induced in the human uterus and Fallopian tube by exogenous estrogens. In: Dallenbach-Hellweg G (ed) Functional morphologic changes in the female sex organs induced by exogenous hormones. Springer Verlag, Berlin, pp 39–44.

Dallenbach-Hellweg G 1980b Morphological changes induced by exogenous gestagens in normal human endometrium. In: Dallenbach-Hellweg G (ed) Functional morphologic changes in the female sex organs induced by exogenous hormones. Springer Verlag, Berlin, pp 95–100.

Dallenbach-Hellweg G 1981 Histopathology of the endometrium, 3rd edn. Springer Verlag, Berlin, pp 126–256.

Davis H J 1972 Intrauterine contraceptive devices: present status and future prospects. American Journal of Obstetrics and Gynecology 114: 134–151.

Dawson J M, O'Riordan B, Chopra S 1992 Ovarian actinomycosis presenting as acute peritonitis. Australian and New Zealand Journal of Surgery 62: 161–163.

de Castro A, Gonzalez-Gancedo P, Contreras F, Lapena G 1986 The effect of copper ions in vivo on specific hormonal endometrial receptors. Advances in Contraception 2: 399–404.

DeCherney A H, Cholst I, Naftolin F 1981 Structure and function of the fallopian tubes following exposure to diethylstilbestrol (DES) during gestation. Fertility and Sterility 36: 741–745.

de Clercq A G, Bogaerts J, Thiery M, Claeys G 1987 Ovarian actinomycosis during first-trimester pregnancy. Advances in Contraception 3: 167–171.

Delgado-Rodriguez M, Sillero-Arenas M, Martin-Moreno J M, Galvez-Vargas R 1992 Oral contraceptives and cancer of the cervix uteri: a meta-analysis. Acta Obstetricia et Gynecologica Scandinavica 71: 368–376.

Dietrick D D, Issa M M, Kabalin J N, Bassett J B 1992 Intravesical migration of intrauterine device. Journal of Urology 147: 132–134.

Dockerty M B, Smith R A, Symmonds R E 1959 Pseudomalignant endometrial changes induced by administration of new synthetic progestins. Proceedings of the Mayo Clinic 34: 321–328.

Dommisse J 1977 Intra-uterine contraceptive devices. South African Medical Journal 52: 495–496.

Ebeling K, Nischan P, Schwindler C 1987 Use of contraceptives and risk of invasive cervical cancer in previously screened women. International Journal of Cancer 39: 427–430.

Ecker J A, McKittrick J E, Failing R M 1966 Thrombosis of the hepatic veins: "the Budd–Chiari syndrome" — a possible link between oral contraceptives and thrombosis formation. American Journal of Gastroenterology 45: 429–443.

Edelman D A 1985 Selection of appropriate comparison groups to evaluate PID risk in IUD users. In: Zatuchni G I, Goldsmith A, Sciarra J J (eds) Intrauterine contraception: advances and future prospects. Harper & Row, Philadelphia, pp 412–419.

Edelman D A, Porter C W Jr 1986a Pelvic inflammatory disease and the IUD. Advances in Contraception 2: 313–325.

Edelman D A, Porter C W Jr 1986b The intrauterine device and ectopic pregnancy. Advances in Contraception 2: 55–63.

Edelman D A, van Os W A 1990 Duration of use of copper releasing IUDs and the incidence of copper wire breakage. European Journal of Obstetrics, Gynecology and Reproductive Biology 34: 267–272.

Edgren R A, Sturtevant F M 1976 Potencies of oral contraceptives. American Journal of Obstetrics and Gynecology 125: 1029–1038.

Editorial 1973 Liver tumours and steroid hormones. Lancet 2: 1481.

Edmondson H A, Henderson B, Benton B 1976 Liver cell adenomas associated with use of oral contraceptives. New England Journal of Medicine 294: 470–472.

Eggena P, Hidaka H, Barrett J D, Sambhi M P 1978 Multiple forms of human plasma renin substrate. Journal of Clinical Investigation 26: 367–372.

Egger H, Kindermann G 1980 Effects of high estrogen doses on the endometrium. In: Dallenbach-Hellweg G (ed) Functional morphologic changes in the female sex organs induced by exogenous hormones. Springer Verlag, Berlin, pp 51–53.

Eissa M K, Sparks R A, Newton J R 1985 Immunoglobulin levels in the serum and cervical mucus of tailed copper IUD users. Contraception 32: 87–95.

Elder M G 1982 New hormone contraceptives: injectable preparations. Journal of Obstetrics and Gynaecology 3 (suppl): s21–s24.

Ellis E F, Gordon P R, Gottlieb L S 1978 Oral contraceptives and cholangiocarcinoma. Lancet 1: 207.

El-Mahgoub S 1980 The Norgestrel-T IUD. Contraception 22: 271–286.

Elwood J M, Boyes D A 1980 Clinical and pathological features and survival of endometrial cancer patients in relation to prior use of estrogens. Gynecologic Oncology 10: 173–187.

Ermini M, Carpino F, Petrozza V, Benagiano G 1989 Distribution and effect on the endometrium of progesterone released from a progestasert device. Human Reproduction 4: 221–228.

Ernst E 1992 Oral contraceptives, fibrinogen and cardiovascular risk. Atherosclerosis 93: 1–5.

Fahmy K, Ismail H, Sammour M, el Tawil A, Ibrahim M 1990 Cervical pathology with intrauterine contraceptive devices — a cyto-colpo-pathological study. Contraception 41: 317–322.

Farley T M, Rosenberg M J, Rowe P J, Chen J H, Meirik O 1992 Intrauterine devices and pelvic inflammatory disease: an international perspective. Special Programme of Research, Development, and Research Training in Human Reproduction, World Health Organization. Lancet 339: 785–788.

Fathalla M F 1972 Factors in the causation and incidence of ovarian cancer. Obstetrical and Gynecological Survey 27: 751–768.

Faundes A, Alvarez F, Brache V, Tejada A S 1988 The role of the levonorgestrel intrauterine device in the prevention and treatment of iron deficiency anemia during fertility regulation. International Journal of Gynaecology and Obstetrics 26: 429–433.

Fay R A 1982 Failure with the new triphasic oral contraceptive Logynon. British Medical Journal 284: 17–18.

Fechner R E 1968 Atypical leiomyomas and synthetic progestin therapy. American Journal of Clinical Pathology 49: 697–703.

Fechner R E 1977 Benign hepatic lesions and orally administered contraceptives: a report of seven cases and a critical analysis of the literature. Human Pathology 8: 255–268.

Ferenczy A 1980 Morphological effects of exogenous gestagens on abnormal human endometrium. In: Dallenbach-Hellweg G (ed) Functional morphologic changes in the female sex organs induced by exogenous hormones. Springer Verlag, Berlin, pp 101–110.

Ferrazzi E, Cartei G, Mattarazzo R, Fiorentino M 1977 Oestrogen-like effect of tamoxifen on vaginal epithelium. British Medical Journal i: 1351–1352.

Fiore N 1986 Epidemiological data, cytology and colposcopy in IUD (intrauterine device), E-P (estro-progestogens) and diaphragm users: studies of cytological changes of endometrium IUD related. Clinical and Experimental Obstetrics and Gynecology 13: 34–42.

Fisher M S 1980 "Miliary" actinomycosis. Journal of the Canadian Radiology Association 31: 149–150.

Flesh G, Weiner J M, Corlett R C, Boice C, Mishell D R Jr, Wolf R M 1979 The intrauterine contraceptive device and acute salpingitis: a multifactor analysis. American Journal of Obstetrics and Gynecology 135: 402–408.

Foreman H, Stadel B V, Schlesselman S 1981 Intrauterine device usage and fetal loss. Obstetrics and Gynecology 58: 669–677.

Fornander T, Rutqvist L E, Cedermark B et al 1989 Adjuvant tamoxifen in early breast cancer: occurrence of new primary cancers. Lancet i: 117–120.

Fowler W C Jr, Schmidt G, Edelman D A, Kaufman D G, Fenoglio C M 1981 Risks of cervical intraepithelial neoplasia among DES-exposed women. Obstetrics and Gynecology 58: 720–724.

Fox H, Buckley C H 1982 The endometrial hyperplasias and their relationship to neoplasia. Histopathology 6: 493–510.

Fox H, Buckley C H 1983 Atlas of gynaecological pathology. MTP Press, Lancaster.

Franz H B, Strohmaier W L, Geppert M, Wechsel H 1992 Infiltrierender Tuboovarialabszess bei IUP-assoziierter Aktinomykose. Geburtshilfe und Frauenheilkunde 52: 496–498.

Fylling P 1987 Clinical performance of Copper T 200, Multiload 250 and Nova–T: a comparative multicentre study. Contraception 35: 439–446.

Fylling P, Fagerhol M 1979 Experience with two different medicated intrauterine devices: a comparative study of the Progestasert and Nova T. Fertility and Sterility 31: 138–141.

Ghosh T K, Cera P J 1983 Transition of benign vaginal adenosis to clear cell carcinoma. Obstetrics and Gynecology 61: 126–130.

Ghosh K, Gupta I, Gupta S K 1989 Asymptomatic salpingitis in intrauterine contraceptive device users. Asia-Oceania Journal of Obstetrics and Gynaecology 15: 37–40.

Girardot C, Legman P, Le Goff J Y 1990 La stenose rectale: une complication rare des salpingites chroniques sur dispositifs intra-uterins. Journal de Radiologie 71: 23–26.

Glew S, Singh A 1989 Uterine bleeding with an IUD requiring emergency hysterectomy. Advances in Contraception 5: 51–53.

Godsland I F, Crook D, Wynn V 1991 Coronary heart disease risk markers in users of low-dose oral contraceptives. Journal of Reproductive Medicine 36(3 suppl): 226–237.

Goldman G A, Dicker D, Ovadia J 1988 Primary abdominal pregnancy: can artificial abortion, endometriosis and IUD be etiological factors. European Journal of Obstetrics, Gynecology and Reproductive Biology 27: 139–143.

Goldman J A, Yeshaya A, Peleg D, Dekel A, Dicker D 1986 Severe pneumococcal peritonitis complicating IUD: case report and review of the literature. Obstetrics and Gynecology 41: 672–674.

Goldstuck N D 1987 Insertion forces with intrauterine devices: implications for uterine perforation. European Journal of Obstetrics, Gynecology and Reproductive Biology 25: 315–323.

Gorsline J C, Osborne N G 1985 Management of the missing intrauterine contraceptive device: report of a case. American Journal of Obstetrics and Gynecology 153: 228–229.

Gottardis M M, Robinson S P, Satyaswaroop P G, Jordan V C 1988 Contrasting actions of tamoxifen on endometrial and breast tumor growth in the athymic mouse. Cancer Research 48: 812–815.

Govan A D T, Black W P, Sharp J L 1969 Aberrant glandular polypi of the uterine cervix associated with contraceptive pills: pathology and pathogenesis. Journal of Clinical Pathology 22: 84–89.

Gram I T, Macaluso M, Stalsberg H 1992 Oral contraceptive use and the incidence of cervical intraepithelial neoplasia. American Journal of Obstetrics and Gynecology 167: 40–44.

Grimes D A 1981 Nongonococcal pelvic inflammatory disease. Clinical Obstetrics and Gynecology 24: 1227–1243.

Grimes D A 1991 Neoplastic effects of oral contraceptives. International Journal of Fertility 36 (suppl 1): 19–24.

Gunning J E, Moyer D 1967 The effect of medroxyprogesterone acetate on endometriosis in the human female. Fertility and Sterility 18: 759–774.

Gupta B K, Gupta A N, Lyall S 1989 Return of fertility in various types of IUD users. International Journal of Fertility 34: 123–125.

Gupta P K, Burroughs F, Luff R D, Frost J K, Erozan Y S 1978a Epithelial atypias associated with intrauterine contraceptive devices (IUD). Acta Cytologica 22: 286–291.

Gupta P K, Erozan Y S, Frost J K 1978b Actinomycetes and the IUD: an update. Acta Cytologica 22: 281–282.

Hammond C B, Maxson W S 1982 Current status of estrogen therapy for the menopause. Fertility and Sterility 37: 5–25.

Haney A F, Hammond C B, Soules M R, Creasman W T 1979 Diethylstilbestrol-induced upper genital tract abnormalities. Fertility and Sterility 31: 142–146.

Hannaford P C 1991 Cervical cancer and methods of contraception. Advances in Contraception 7: 317–324.

Hannaford P C, Villard-Mackintosh L, Vessey M P, Kay C R 1991 Oral contraceptives and malignant melanoma. British Journal of Cancer 63: 430–433.

Hansen L K 1989 Bilateral female pelvic actinomycosis. Acta Obstetricia et Gynecologica Scandinavica 68: 189–190.

Hardell L 1988 Tamoxifen as a risk factor for carcinoma of the corpus uteri. Lancet 2: 563.

Harlap S 1991 Oral contraceptives and breast cancer: cause and effect? Journal of Reproductive Medicine 36: 374–395.

Hart W R, Townsend D E, Aldrich J O et al 1976 Histopathologic spectrum of vaginal adenosis and related changes in stilbestrol-exposed females. Cancer 37: 763–775.

Harvengt C 1992 Effect of oral contraceptive use on the incidence of impaired glucose tolerance and diabetes mellitus. Diabetes/Metabolism Reviews 18: 71–77.

Haukkamaa M, Allonen H, Heikkilä M et al 1985 Long-term clinical experience with Levonorgestrel-releasing IUD. In: Zatuchni G I, Goldsmith A, Sciarra J J (eds) Intrauterine contraception: advances and future prospects. Harper & Row, Philadelphia, pp 232–237.

Haukkamaa M, Stranden P, Jousimies-Somer H, Siitonen A 1986 Bacterial flora of the cervix in women using different methods of contraception. American Journal of Obstetrics and Gynecology 154: 520–524.

Hawkins D F, Elder M G 1979 Human fertility control. Butterworth, London.

Hays D, Edelstein J A, Ahmad M M 1986 Perforation of the sigmoid colon by an intrauterine contraceptive device. Contraception 34: 413–416.

Heartwell S F, Schlesselman S 1983 Risk of uterine perforation among users of intrauterine devices. Obstetrics and Gynecology 61: 31–36.

Hefnawi F, Hosni M, El-Shiekha Z, Serour G I, Hasseeb F 1975 Perforation of the uterine wall by Lippes loop in postpartum women. In: Hefnawi F, Segal S J (eds) Analysis of intrauterine contraception. North-Holland, Amsterdam, pp 469–476.

Heinonen P K, Merikari M, Paavonen J 1984 Uterine perforation by copper intrauterine device. European Journal of Obstetrics, Gynecology and Reproductive Biology 17: 257–261.

Hendrickson M R, Kempson R L 1980 Surgical pathology of the uterine corpus. W.B. Saunders, Philadelphia.

Herbertsson G, Magnusson S S, Benediktsdottir K 1987 Ovarian pregnancy and IUCD use in a defined complete population. Acta Obstetricia et Gynecologica Scandinavica 66: 607–610.

Herbst A L 1981a Diethylstilbestrol and other sex hormones during pregnancy. Obstetrics and Gynecology 58 (suppl): 35s–40s.

Herbst A L 1981b Clear cell adenocarcinoma and the current status of DES-exposed females. Cancer 48 (suppl): 484–488.

Herbst A L, Scully R E 1970 Adenocarcinoma of the vagina in adolescence: a report of 7 cases including 6 clear-cell carcinomas (so-called mesonephromas). Cancer 25: 745–757.

Herbst A L, Kurman R J, Scully R E 1972 Vaginal and cervical abnormalities after exposure to stilbestrol in utero. Obstetrics and Gynecology 40: 287–298.

Herbst A L, Robboy S J, Scully R E, Poskanzer D C 1974 Clear-cell adenocarcinoma of the vagina and cervix in girls: analysis of 170 reported cases. American Journal of Obstetrics and Gynecology 119: 713–724.

Herbst A L, Poskanzer D C, Robboy S J, Friedlander L, Scully R E 1975 Prenatal exposure to stilbestrol: a prospective comparison of exposed female offspring with unexposed control. New England Journal of Medicine 292: 334–339.

Herbst A L, Cole P, Colton T, Robboy S J, Scully R E 1977 Age-incidence and risk of diethylstilbestrol-related clear cell adenocarcinoma of the vagina and cervix. American Journal of Obstetrics and Gynecology 128: 43–50.

Hill J A, Talledo E, Steele J 1986 Quantitative transcervical uterine cultures in asymptomatic women using an intrauterine contraceptive device. Obstetrics and Gynecology 68: 700–704.

Hillard P J 1992 Oral contraceptive noncompliance: the extent of the problem. Advances in Contraception 8 (suppl): 13–20.

Hocher B, Keller F, Krause P H, Gollnick H, Oelkers W 1992 Interstitial nephritis with reversible renal failure due to a copper-containing intrauterine contraceptive device. Nephron 61: 111–113.

Holt V L, Daling J R, McKnight B et al 1992 Functional ovarian cysts in relation to the use of monophasic and triphasic oral contraceptives. Obstetrics and Gynecology 79: 529–533.

Honoré L H 1985 The negative effect of the IUCD on the occurrence of heteroploidy-correlated abnormalities in spontaneous abortions: an update. Contraception 31: 253–260.

Honoré L H 1986 The intrauterine contraceptive device and hydatidiform mole: a negative association. Contraception 34: 213–219.

Honoré L H, Koch M, Brown L B 1991 Comparison of oral contraceptive use in women with adenocarcinoma and squamous cell carcinoma of the uterine cervix. Gynecologic and Obstetric Investigation 32: 98–101.

Horvath E, Kovacs K, Ross R C 1972 Ultrastructural findings in a well-differentiated hepatoma. Digestion 7: 74–82.

Hourihan H M, Sheppard B L, Belsey E M, Brosens I A 1991 Endometrial vascular features prior to and following exposure to levonorgestrel. Contraception 43: 375–385.

Hoyumpa A M Jr, Schiff L, Helfman E L 1971 Budd-Chiari syndrome in women taking oral contraceptives. American Journal of Medicine 50: 137–140.

Hsing A W, Hoover R N, McLaughlin J K et al 1992 Oral contraceptives and primary liver cancer among young women. Cancer Causes and Control 3: 43–48.

Hsu C T, Hsu M L, Hsieh T M et al 1989 Uterine malignancy developing after long term use of IUCD additional report of 2 cases: endometrial stromal sarcoma and leiomyosarcoma. Asia-Oceania Journal of Obstetrics and Gynaecology 15: 237–243.

Huggins G R, Cullins V E 1990 Fertility after contraception or abortion. Fertility and Sterility 54: 559–573.

Huggins G R, Giuntoli R L 1979 Oral contraceptives and neoplasia. Fertility and Sterility 32: 1–23.

Huggins G R, Zucker P K 1987 Oral contraceptives and neoplasia: 1987 update. Fertility and Sterility 47: 733–761.

Hulka B S, Chainbless L E, Kaufman D G, Fowler W C Jr, Greenberg B G 1982 Protection against endometrial carcinoma by combination-product oral contraceptives. Journal of the American Medical Association 247: 475–477.

Inman W H W, Vessey M P, Westerholm B, Engelund A 1970 Thromboembolic disease and the steroidal content of oral contraceptives: a report to the Committee on Safety of Drugs. British Medical Journal 2: 203–209.

Irey N S, Manion W C, Taylor H B 1970 Vascular lesions in women taking oral contraceptives. Archives of Pathology 89: 1–8.

Ishak K G 1979 Morphologic hepatic lesions associated with oral contraceptives (OC) and anabolic steroids (AS). In: Olive G (ed) Advances in pharmacology and therapeutics, vol 8. Pergamon Press, Oxford, p 185.

Ishak K G, Rabin L 1975 Benign tumors of the liver. Medical Clinics of North America 59: 995–1013.

Janaud A, Rouffy J, Upmalis D, Dain M P 1992 A comparison study of lipid and androgen metabolism with triphasic oral contraceptive formulations containing norgestimate or levonorgestrel. Acta Obstetricia et Gynecologica Scandinavica 156 (suppl): 33–38.

Johnson J H 1989 Weighing the evidence on the pill and breast cancer. Family Planning Perspectives 21: 89–92.

Johnson L D, Driscoll S G, Hertig A T, Cole P T, Nickerson R J 1979 Vaginal adenosis in stillborns and neonates exposed to diethylstilbestrol and steroidal estrogens and progestins. Obstetrical and Gynecological Survey 34: 845–846.

Jones M W, Silverberg S G 1989 Cervical adenocarcinoma in young women: possible relationship to microglandular hyperplasia and use of oral contraceptives. Obstetrics and Gynecology 73: 984–989.

Jones M W, Silverberg S G, Kurman R J 1993 Well-differentiated villoglandular adenocarcinoma of the uterine cervix: a clinicopathological study of 24 cases. International Journal of Gynecological Pathology 12: 1–7.

Joswig-Priewe H, Schlüster K 1980 Comparative study of vaginal cytology involving controls and patients receiving oral contraceptive agents. In: Dallenbach-Hellweg G (ed) Functional morphologic changes in female sex organs induced by exogenous hormones. Springer Verlag, Berlin, p 199.

Judd H L 1980 Menopause and postmenopause. In: Benson R C (ed) Current obstetrics and gynecologic diagnosis and treatment. Large Medical Publications, Los Altos, Cal, pp 510–529.

Kajanoja P, Lang B, Wahlstrom T 1987 Intra-uterine contraceptive devices (IUDs) in relation to uterine histology and microbiology. Acta Obstetricia et Gynecologica Scandinavica 66: 445–449.

Katerndahl D A, Realini J P, Cohen P A 1992 Oral contraceptive use and cardiovascular disease: is the relationship real or due to study bias? Journal of Family Practice 35: 147–157.

Kaufman R H, Binder G L, Gray P M Jr, Adam E 1977 Upper genital tract changes associated with exposure in utero to diethylstilbestrol. American Journal of Obstetrics and Gynecology 128: 51–59.

Kaufman D W, Shapiro S, Slone D et al 1980 Decreased risk of endometrial cancer among oral contraceptive users. New England Journal of Medicine 303: 1045–1047.

Kaufman R H, Korhonen M O, Strama T, Adam E, Kaplan A 1982 Development of clear cell adenocarcinoma in DES-exposed offspring under observation. Obstetrics and Gynecology 59 (suppl): 68s–72s.

Kaufman D W, Palmer J R, de Mouzon J et al 1991 Estrogen replacement therapy and the risk of breast cancer: results from the case-control surveillance study. American Journal of Epidemiology 134: 1375–1385.

Kay C R 1982 Progestogens and arterial disease — evidence from the Royal College of General Practitioners' Study. American Journal of Obstetrics and Gynecology 142: 762–765.

Kay C R 1984 The Royal College of General Practitioners' Oral Contraception Study: some recent observations. Clinics in Obstetrics and Gynaecology 11: 759–786.

Keith L G, Berger G S 1985 The pathogenic mechanisms of pelvic infection. In: Zatuchni G I, Goldsmith A, Sciarra J J (eds) Intrauterine contraception: advances and future prospects. Harper & Row, Philadelphia, pp 232–237.

Kelleher C C 1990 Clinical aspects of the relationship between oral contraceptives and abnormalities of the hemostatic system: relation to the development of cardiovascular disease. American Journal of Obstetrics and Gynecology 163: 392–395.

Kent D R, Nissen E D, Nissen S E, Chambers C 1977 Maternal death resulting from rupture of liver adenoma associated with oral contraceptives. Obstetrics and Gynecology 50 (suppl): 5s–6s.

Kerlin P, Davis G L, McGill D B et al 1983 Hepatic adenoma and focal nodular hyperplasia: clinical, pathologic, and radiologic features. Gastroenterology 84: 994–1002.

Kessel E 1989 Pelvic inflammatory disease with intrauterine device use: a reassessment. Fertility and Sterility 51: 1–11.

Key T C, Kreutner A K 1980 Gastrointestinal complications of modern intrauterine devices. Obstetrics and Gynecology 55: 239–244.

Khan S R, Wilkinson E J 1985 Scanning electron microscopy, X-ray diffraction, and electron microprobe analysis of calcific deposits on intrauterine contraceptive devices. Human Pathology 16: 732–738.

Khan S R, Wilkinson E J 1990 Bladder stone in a human female: the case of an abnormally located intrauterine contraceptive device. Scanning Microscopy 4: 395–398.

Khaw K T, Peart W S 1982 Blood pressure and contraceptive use. British Medical Journal 285: 403–407.

Kiilholma P, Makinen J, Vuori J 1989 Bladder perforation: uncommon complication with a misplaced IUD. Advances in Contraception 5: 47–49.

Kiilholma P, Makinen J, Maenpaa J 1990 Perforation of the uterus following IUD insertion in the puerperium. Advances in Contraception 6: 57–61.

Killackey M A, Hakes T B, Pierce V K 1985 Endometrial adenocarcinoma in breast cancer patients receiving antiestrogens. Cancer Treatment Reviews 69: 237–238.

Kim-Farley R J, Cates W Jr, Ory H W, Hatcher R A 1978 Febrile spontaneous abortion and the IUD. Contraception 18: 561–570.

Kinch R, Lough J 1978 Focal nodular hyperplasia of the liver and oral contraceptives. American Journal of Obstetrics and Gynecology 132: 717–727.

Klatskin G 1977 Hepatic tumors: possible relationship to use of oral contraceptives. Gastroenterology 73: 386–394.

Knopp R H 1990 Effects of sex steroid hormones on lipoprotein levels in pre- and post menopausal women. Canadian Journal of Cardiology 6 (suppl B): 31B–35B.

Knowles D M, Wolff M 1976 Focal nodular hyperplasia of the liver. Human Pathology 7: 533–545.

Kremer J, de Bruijn H W A, Hindriks F R 1980 Serum high density lipoprotein cholesterol levels in women using a contraceptive injection of depot-medroxy-progesterone acetate. Contraception 22: 359–367.

Kronmal R A, Whitney C W, Mumford S D 1991 The intrauterine device and pelvic inflammatory disease: the Women's Health Study reanalysed. Journal of Clinical Epidemiology 44: 109–122.

Kurman R J, Scully R E 1974 The incidence and histogenesis of vaginal adenosis: an autopsy study. Human Pathology 5: 265–276.

Kyriakos M, Kempson R L, Konikov N F 1968 A clinical and pathologic study of endocervical lesions associated with oral contraceptives. Cancer 22: 99–110.

Landers D V, Sweet R L 1985 Current trends in the diagnosis and treatment of tuboovarian abscess. American Journal of Obstetrics and Gynecology 151: 1098–1110.

Laragh J H 1976 Oral contraceptives — induced hypertension — nine years later. American Journal of Obstetrics and Gynecology 126: 141–147.

Larsen S, Hansen M K, Jacobsen J C, Ladehoff P, Sorensen T, Westergaard J G 1981 Comparison between two IUDs: Progestasert and CuT 200. Contraception Delivery Systems 2: 281–286.

Lashner B A, Kane S V, Hanauer S B 1989 Lack of association between oral contraceptive use and Crohn's disease: a community-based matched case-control study. Gastroenterology 97: 1442–1447.

Lashner B A, Kane S V, Hanauer S B 1990 Lack of association between oral contraceptive use and ulcerative colitis. Gastroenterology 99: 1032–1036.

La Vecchia C 1992 Sex hormones and cardiovascular risk. Human Reproduction 7: 162–167.

La Vecchia C, Negri E, D'Avanzo B et al 1992 Oral contraceptives and non-contraceptive oestrogens in the risk of gallstone disease requiring surgery. Journal of Epidemiology and Community Health 46: 234–236.

Leaf D A, Bland D, Schaad D, Neighbor W E, Scott C S 1991 Oral contraceptive use and coronary risk factors in women. American Journal of the Medical Sciences 301: 365–368.

Leborgne J, Lehur P A, Horeau J M et al 1990 Problemes therapeutiques lies aux ruptures de volumineux adenomes hepatiques de siege central: a propos de 3 observations. Chirurgie 116: 454–460.

Lee N C, Rubin G L, Borucki R 1988 The intrauterine device and pelvic inflammatory disease revisited: new results from the Women's Health Study. Obstetrics and Gynecology 72: 1–6.

LiVolsi V A, Stadel B V, Kelsey J L, Holford T R, White C 1978 Fibrocystic breast disease in oral contraceptive users: a histopathological evaluation of epithelial atypia. New England Journal of Medicine 299: 381–385.

Logan R F, Kay C R 1989 Oral contraception, smoking and inflammatory bowel disease — findings in the Royal College of General Practitioners' Oral Contraception Study. International Journal of Epidemiology 18: 105–107.

London R S 1992 The new era in oral contraception: pills containing gestodene, norgestimate and desogestrel. Obstetrical and Gynecological Survey 47: 777–782.

Lovset T 1990 A comparative evaluation of the Multiload 250 and Multiload 375 intra-uterine devices. Acta Obstetricia et Gynecologica Scandinavica 69: 521–526.

Lund E, Meirik O, Adami H O, Bergstrom R, Christoffersen T, Bergsjo P 1989 Oral contraceptive use and premenopausal breast cancer in Sweden and Norway: possible effects of different pattern of use. International Journal of Epidemiology 18: 527–532.

Luukkainen T, Allonen H, Haukkamaa M et al 1987 Effective contraception with the levonorgestrel-releasing intrauterine device: 12-month report of a European multicenter study. Contraception 36: 169–179.

McCarty K S Jr, Barton T K, Peete C H Jr, Creasman W T 1978 Gonadal dysgenesis with adenocarcinoma of the endometrium: an electron microscopic and steroid receptor analysis with a review of the literature. Cancer 42: 512–520.

MacNab M W, Tallarida R J, Joseph R 1984 An evaluation of tamoxifen as a partial agonist by classical receptor theory — an explanation of the dual action of tamoxifen. European Journal of Pharmacology 103: 321–326.

McGowan L, Parent L, Lednar W, Norris H J 1979 The woman at risk for developing ovarian cancer. Gynecologic Oncology 7: 325–344.

Maenpaa J, Taina E, Gronroos M, Soderstrom K O, Ristmaki T, Narhinen L 1988 Abdominopelvic actinomycosis associated with intrauterine devices: two case reports. Archives of Gynecology and Obstetrics 243: 237–241.

Makinen J I, Erkkola R U, Laippala P J 1989 Causes of the increase in the incidence of ectopic pregnancy: a study on 1017 patients from 1966 to 1985 in Turku, Finland. American Journal of Obstetrics and Gynecology 160: 642–646.

Mali B, Joshi J V, Wagle U et al 1986 Actinomyces in cervical smears of women using intrauterine contraceptive devices. Acta Cytologica 30: 367–371.

Maroni E S, Genton C Y 1986 IUD-associated ovarian actinomycosis causing bowel obstruction. Archives of Gynecology and Obstetrics 239: 59–62.

Mays E T, Christopherson W M, Barrows G H 1974 Focal nodular hyperplasia of the liver: possible relationship to oral contraceptives. American Journal of Clinical Pathology. 61: 735–746.

Mdel D G, Fox J A, Jones R W 1975 Multiple hepatic adenomas associated with an oral contraceptive. Lancet 1: 865.

Meade T W, Haines A P, North W R S et al 1977 Haemostatic, lipid, and blood pressure profiles of women on oral contraceptives, containing 50 μg or 30 μg oestrogen. Lancet 2: 948–951.

Meade T W, Greenberg G, Thompson S G 1980 Progestogens and cardiovascular reactions associated with oral contraceptives and a comparison of the safety of 50 and 30 μg oestrogen preparations. British Medical Journal 280: 1157–1161.

Meirik O, Farley T M, Lund E et al 1989 Breast cancer and oral contraceptives: patterns of risk among parous and nulliparous women — further analysis of the Swedish-Norwegian material. Contraception 39: 471–475.

Mestwerdt W, Kranzfelder D 1980 Morphological findings in the human ovary under physiologic conditions and after contraceptive use. In: Dallenbach-Hellweg G (ed) Functional and morphologic changes in female sex organs induced by exogenous hormones. Springer Verlag, Berlin, pp 168–179.

Michaud P, Lemaire B, Tescher M 1989 Avortement spontane d'une grossesse sur DIU par chorioamniotite a Candida. Revue Francaise de Gynecologie et d'Obstetrique 84: 45–46.

Miller D R, Rosenberg L, Kaufman D W et al 1989a Breast cancer before age 45 and oral contraceptive use: new findings. American Journal of Epidemiology 129: 269–280.

Miller N, McPherson K, Jones L, Vessey M 1989b Histopathology of breast cancer in young women in relation to use of oral contraceptives. Journal of Clinical Pathology 42: 387–390.

Miller N E, Thelle D S, Førde O H, Mjøs O D 1977 The Tromso heart-study: high density lipoprotein and coronary heart disease: a prospective case control study. Lancet 1: 965–968.

Mishell D R Jr 1976 Current status of oral contraceptive steroids. Clinical Obstetrics and Gynecoloy 19: 743–764.

Mishell D R Jr 1992 Oral contraception: past, present, and future perspectives. International Journal of Fertility 37 (suppl 1): 7–18.

Mishell D R Jr, Moyer D L 1969 Association of pelvic inflammatory disease with the intrauterine device. Clinical Obstetrics and Gynecology 12: 179–197.

Mishell D R Jr, Roy S 1982 Copper intrauterine contraceptive device event rates following insertion 4 to 8 weeks post partum. Obstetrics and Gynecology 143: 29–35.

Mishell D R Jr, Bell J H, Good R G, Moyer D L 1966 The intrauterine device: a bacteriologic study of the endometrial cavity. American Journal of Obstetrics and Gynecology 96: 119–126.

Misra J S, Engineer A D, Tandon P 1977 Cytological studies in women using copper intrauterine devices. Acta Cytologica 21: 514–518.

Mittal S, Gupta I, Lata P, Mahajan U, Gupta A N 1986 Management of translocated and incarcerated intrauterine contraceptive devices. Australian and New Zealand Journal of Obstetrics and Gynaecology 26: 232–234.

Moyer D L, Mishell D R Jr 1971 Reactions of human endometrium to the intrauterine foreign body. II. Long term effects on the endometrial histology and cytology. American Journal of Obstetrics and Gynecology 111: 66–80.

Moyer D L, Mishell D R Jr, Bell J 1970 Reactions of human endometrium to the intrauterine device. I. Correlation of the endometrial histology with the bacterial environment of the uterus following short-term insertion of the IUD. American Journal of Obstetrics and Gynecology 106: 799–809.

Mumford S D, Kessel E 1992 Was the Dalkon Shield a safe and effective intrauterine device? The conflict between the case-control and clinical trial study findings. Fertility and Sterility 57: 1151–1176.

Murray S, Hickey J B, Houang E 1987 Significant bacteremia associated with replacement of intrauterine contraceptive device. American Journal of Obstetrics and Gynecology 156: 698–700.

Muzsnai D, Hughes T, Price M, Bruksch L 1980 Primary abdominal pregnancy associated with the IUD (2 case reports). European Journal of Obstetrics, Gynecology and Reproductive Biology 10: 275–278.

Nanda S, Rathee S 1992 Three intrauterine contraceptive devices in a single uterus. Tropical Doctor 22: 33–44.

Nayar M, Chandra M, Chitraratha K, Kumari-Das S, Rai-Chowdhary G 1985 Incidence of actinomycetes infection in women using intrauterine contraceptive devices. Acta Cytologica 29: 111–116.

Neuberger J, Portmann B, Nunnerley H B et al 1980 Oral contraceptive-associated liver tumours: occurrence of malignancy and difficulties in diagnosis. Lancet i: 273–276.

Neven P, De Muylder X, Van Belle Y, Vanderick G, De Muylder E 1989 Tamoxifen and the uterus and endometrium. Lancet i: 375.

Neven P, De Muylder X, Van Belle Y, Vanderick G, De Muylder E 1990 Hysteroscopic follow-up during tamoxifen treatment. European Journal of Obstetrics, Gynecology and Reproductive Biology 35: 235–238.

Newhouse M L, Pearson R M, Fullerton J M, Boesen E A M, Shannon H S 1977 A case control study of carcinoma of the ovary. British Journal of Preventative and Social Medicine 31: 148–153.

Nothmann B J, Chittinand S, Schuster M M 1973 Reversible mesenteric vascular occlusion associated with oral contraceptives. American Journal of Digestive Diseases 18: 361–368.

O'Brien P C, Noller K L, Robboy S J et al 1979 Vaginal epithelial changes in young women enrolled in the National Comparative Diethylstilbestrol Adenosis (DESAD) Project. Obstetrics and Gynecology 53: 300–308.

O'Brien P K 1975 Abdominal and endometrial actinomycosis associated with an intrauterine device. Canadian Medical Association Journal 112: 596–597.

O'Brien P K, Roth-Moyo L A, Davis B A 1981 Pseudo-sulfur granules associated with intrauterine contraceptive devices. American Journal of Clinical Pathology 75: 822–825.

O'Brien P K, Lea P J, Roth-Moyo L A 1985 Structure of a radiate pseudocolony associated with an intrauterine contraceptive device. Human Pathology 16: 1153–1156.

Olson R O, Jones S 1967 The forgotten IUD as a cause of infertility: review of world literature and report of a case. Obstetrics and Gynecology 29: 579–580.

Olsson H 1989 Oral contraceptives and breast cancer: a review. Acta Oncologica 28: 849–863.

Olsson H, Moller T R, Ranstam J 1989 Early oral contraceptive use and breast cancer among premenopausal women: final report from a study in southern Sweden. Journal of the National Cancer Institute 81: 1000–1004.

Olsson H, Borg A, Ferno M, Moller T R, Ranstam J 1991 Early oral contraceptive use and premenopausal breast cancer — a review of studies performed in southern Sweden. Cancer Detection and Prevention 15: 265–271.

Orellana-Alcalde J M, Dominguez J P 1966 Jaundice and oral contraceptives. Lancet 2: 1279–1280.

Ory H W, Boston Collaborative Drug Surveillance Program 1974 Functional ovarian cysts and oral contraceptives: negative association confirmed surgically. Journal of American Medical Association 228: 68–69.

Ory H W, Cole P, MacMahon B, Hoover R 1976 Oral contraceptives and reduced risk of benign breast diseases. New England Journal of Medicine 294: 419–422.

Osborne J L, Bennett M J 1978 Removal of intra-abdominal intrauterine contraceptive devices. British Journal of Obstetrics and Gynaecology 85: 868–871.

Ostergard D R 1981 DES-related vaginal lesions. Clinical Obstetrics and Gynecology 24: 379–394.

Otolorin E O, Ladipo O A 1985 Comparison of intramenstrual IUD insertion with insertion following menstrual regulation. Advances in Contraception 1: 45–49.

Paavonen J, Varjonen-Toivonen M, Komulainen M, Heinonen P K

1985 Diagnosis and management of tubal pregnancy: effect on fertility. International Journal of Gynaecology and Obstetrics 23: 129–133.

Palmer J R 1991 Oral contraceptive use and gestational choriocarcinoma. Cancer Detection and Prevention 15: 45–48.

Palmer J R, Rosenberg L, Kaufman D W et al 1989 Oral contraceptive use and liver cancer. American Journal of Epidemiology 130: 878–882.

Parewijck W, Claeys G, Thiery M, van Kets H 1988 Candidiasis in women fitted with an intrauterine contraceptive device. British Journal of Obstetrics and Gynaecology 95: 408–410.

Paterson M E L, Wade-Evans T, Sturdee D W, Thom M H, Studd J W W 1980 Endometrial disease after treatment with oestrogens and progestogens in the climacteric. British Medical Journal 1: 822–824.

Paul C, Skegg D C, Spears G F 1989 Depot medroxyprogesterone (Depo-Provera) and risk of breast cancer. British Medical Journal 299: 759–762.

Pike M C 1990 Reducing cancer risk in women through lifestyle-mediated changes in hormone levels. Cancer Detection and Prevention 14: 595–607.

Porges R F 1973 Complications associated with the unsuspected presence of intrauterine contraceptive devices. American Journal of Obstetrics and Gynecology 116: 579–580.

Prakash S, Scully R E 1964 Sarcoma-like pseudopregnancy changes in uterine leiomyomas. Obstetrics and Gynecology 24: 106–110.

Prentice R L 1991 Epidemiologic data on exogenous hormones and hepatocellular carcinoma and selected other cancers. Preventive Medicine 20: 38–46.

Preston E J, Ervin D K, McMichael A O, Preston L W 197S Septic spontaneous abortion associated with the Dalkon Shield. In: Hefnawi F, Segal S J (eds) Analysis of intrauterine contraception. North Holland, Biomedical Press, Amsterdam, pp 417–428.

Pschera H, Larsson B, Lindhe B A, Kjaeldgaard A 1988 The influence of copper intrauterine device on fatty acid composition of cervical mucus lecithin. Contraception 38: 341–348.

Ragni N, Rugiati S, Rossato P et al 1977 Modificazioni istologiche ed ultrastrutturali dell' endometrio in portatrici di iud e di iud potenziati al rame. Acta Europaea Fertilitatis 18: 193–210.

Ramsewak S, Rahaman J, Persad P, Narayansingh G 1991 Missing intrauterine contraceptive device presenting with strings at the anus. West Indian Medical Journal 40: 185–186.

Randic L, Vlasic S, Matrljan I, Waszak C S 1985 Return to fertility after IUCD removal for planned pregnancy. Contraception 32: 253–259.

Randic L, Haller H, Susa M, Rukavina D 1990 Cells adherent to copper-bearing intrauterine contraceptive devices determined by monoclonal antibodies. Contraception 42: 35–42.

Rienprayura D, Phaosavasdi S, Semboonsuk S 1973 Cervical perforation by the copper-T intrauterine device. Contraception 7: 515–521.

Rioux J E, Cloutier D, Dupont P, Lamonde D 1986 Pregnancy after IUD use. Advances in Contraception 2: 185–192.

Rizk M, Shaban N, Medhat I, Moby el Dien Y, Ollo M A 1990 Electron microscopic and chemical study of the deposits formed on the copper and inert IUCDs. Contraception 42: 643–653.

Robboy S J, Bradley R 1979 Changing trends and prognostic features in endometrial cancer associated with exogenous estrogen therapy. Obstetrics and Gynecology 54: 269–277.

Robboy S J, Welch W R 1977 Microglandular hyperplasia in vaginal adenosis associated with oral contraceptives and prenatal diethylstilbestrol exposure. Obstetrics and Gynecology 49: 430–434.

Robboy S J, Kaufman R H, Prat J et al 1979 Pathologic findings in young women enrolled in the National Cooperative Diethylstilbestrol Adenosis (DESAD) Project. Obstetrics and Gynecology 53: 309–317.

Robboy S J, Truslow G Y, Anton J, Richart R M 1981 Roles of hormones including diethylstilbestrol (DES) in the pathogenesis of cervical and vaginal intraepithelial neoplasia. Gynecologic Oncology 12: 98–110.

Robboy S J, Young R H, Herbst A L 1982 Female genital tract changes related to prenatal diethylstilbestrol exposure. In: Blaustein A (ed) Pathology of the female genital tract, 2nd edn. Springer Verlag, New York, pp 99–118.

Romieu I, Willett W C, Colditz G A 1989 Prospective study of oral contraceptive use and risk of breast cancer in women. Journal of the National Cancer Institute 81: 1313–1321.

Romieu I, Berlin J A, Colditz G 1990 Oral contraceptives and breast cancer: review and meta-analysis. Cancer 66: 2253–2263.

Rooks J B, Oray H W, Ishak K G et al 1979 Epidemiology of hepatocellular adenoma: the role of oral contraceptive use. Journal of the American Medical Association 242: 644–648.

Rosenberg L 1991 The risk of liver neoplasia in relation to combined oral contraceptive use. Contraception 43: 643–652.

Rosenberg L, Shapiro S, Slone D et al 1982 Epithelial ovarian cancer and combination oral contraceptives. Journal of the American Medical Association 247: 3210–3212.

Rosenberg L, Palmer J R, Clarke E A, Shapiro S 1992 A case-control study of the risk of breast cancer in relation to oral contraceptive use. American Journal of Epidemiology 136: 1437–1444.

Rosenberg M J, Long S C 1992 Oral contraceptives and cycle control: a critical review of the literature. Advances in Contraception 8 (suppl) 1: 35–45.

Rosenwaks Z, Wentz A C, Jones G S et al 1979 Endometrial pathology and estrogens. Obstetrics and Gynecology 53: 403–410.

Rozsier J G Jr, Underwood P B 1974 Use of progestational agents in endometrial adenocarcinoma. Obstetrics and Gynecology 44: 60–64.

Roy S 1991 Nonbarrier contraceptives and vaginitis and vaginosis. American Journal of Obstetrics and Gynecology 165: 1240–1244.

Royal College of General Practitioners 1974 Oral contraceptives and health. Pitman Medical, London.

Royal College of General Practitioners' Oral Contraceptive Study 1978 Oral contraceptives, venous thrombosis and varicose veins. Journal of the Royal College of General Practitioners 28: 393–399.

Royal College of General Practitioners' Oral Contraceptive Study 1981a Breast cancer and oral contraceptives: findings in Royal College of General Practitioners' Study. British Medical Journal 282: 2089–2093.

Royal College of General Practitioners' Oral Contraceptive Study 1981b Further analyses of mortality in oral contraceptive users. Lancet 1: 541–546.

Royal College of General Practitioners' Oral Contraception Study 1983 Incidence of arterial disease among oral contraceptive users. Journal of the Royal College of General Practitioners 33: 75–82.

Rushton L, Jones D R 1992 Oral contraceptive use and breast cancer risk: a meta-analysis of variations with age at diagnosis, parity and total duration of oral contraceptive use. British Journal of Obstetrics and Gynaecology 99: 239–246.

Sandvei R, Sandstad E, Steier J A, Ulstein M 1987 Ovarian pregnancy associated with the intra-uterine contraceptive device: a survey of two decades. Acta Obstetricia et Gynecologica Scandinavica 66: 137–141.

Schaude H, Dallenbach-Hellweg G, Schlaefer K 1980 Histologic changes of the cervix uteri following contraceptive use. In: Dallenbach-Hellweg G (ed) Functional morphologic changes in the female sex organs induced by exogenous hormones. Springer Verlag, Berlin, pp 191–198.

Schiff I, Sela H K, Cramer D, Tulchinsky D, Ryan K J 1982 Endometrial hyperplasia in women on cyclic or continuous estrogen regimens. Fertility and Sterility 37: 79–82.

Schlesselman J J 1990 Oral contraceptives and breast cancer. American Journal of Obstetrics and Gynecology 163: 1379–1387.

Schmidt W A, Bedrossian C W, Ali V, Webb J A, Bastian F O 1980 Actinomyosis and intrauterine contraceptive devices — the clinicopathologic entity. Diagnostic Gynecology and Obstetrics 2: 165–177.

Scholten P C, Christaens G C, Haspels A A 1987 Intrauterine steroid contraceptives. Wiener Medizinische Wochenschrift 137: 479–483.

Schwartzwald D, Mooppan U M, Tancer M L, Gomez-Leon G, Kim H 1986 Vesicouterine fistula with menouria: a complication from an intrauterine contraceptive device. Journal of Urology 136: 1066–1067.

Segal S J, Alvarez-Sanchez F, Adejuwon C A, Brache-de-Mejia V, Leon P, Faundes A 1985 Absence of chorionic gonadotropin in sera of women who use intrauterine devices. Fertility and Sterility 44: 214–218.

Seif M W, Aplin J D, Awad H, Wells D 1989 The effect of the intrauterine contraceptive device on endometrial secretory function: a possible mode of action. Contraception 40: 81–89.

Seif M W, Pearson J M, Ibrahim Z H Z et al 1992 Endometrium in in-vitro fertilization cycles: morphological and functional differentiation in the implantation phase. Human Reproduction 7: 6–11.

Seoud M A, Johnson J, Weed J C Jr 1993 Gynecologic tumors in Tamoxifen-treated women with breast cancer. Obstetrics and Gynecology 82: 165–169.

Sepulveda W H 1990 Perforation of the rectum by a Copper-T intra-uterine contraceptive device: a case report. European Journal of Obstetrics, Gynecology and Reproductive Biology 35: 275–278.

Serr D M, Shalev J 1985 Ultrasound guidance for IUD removal in pregnancy. In: Zatuchni G I, Goldsmith A, Sciarra J J (eds) Intrauterine contraception: advances and future prospects. Harper & Row, Philadelphia, pp 194–197.

Shapiro S, Kaufman D W, Slone D et al 1980 Recent and past use of conjugated estrogens in relation to adenocarcinoma of the endometrium. New England Journal of Medicine 303: 485–489.

Shaw S T 1985 Endometrial histopathology and ultrastructural changes with IUD use. In: Zatuchni G I, Goldsmith A, Sciarra J J (eds) Intrauterine contraception: advances and future prospects. Harper & Row, Philadelphia, pp 276–296.

Shaw S T Jr, Macaulay L K, Hohman W R 1979a Vessel density in endometrium of women with and without intrauterine contraceptive devices: a morphometric evaluation. American Journal of Obstetrics and Gynecology 135: 202–206.

Shaw S T Jr, Macaulay L K, Hohman W R 1979b Morphologic studies on IUD-induced metrorrhagia. I. Endometrial changes and clinical correlations. Contraception 19: 47–61.

Shaw S T Jr, Macaulay L K, Aznar R, Gonzalez-Angulo A, Roy S 1981 Effects of a progesterone-releasing intrauterine contraceptive device on the endometrial blood vessels: a morphometric study. American Journal of Obstetrics and Gynecology 141: 821–827.

Sheppard B L 1987 Endometrial morphological changes in IUD users: a review. Contraception 36: 1–10.

Sheppard B L, Bonnar J 1985 Endometrial morphology and IUD-induced bleeding. In: Zatuchni G I, Goldsmith A, Sciarra J J (eds) Intrauterine contraception: advances and future prospects. Harper & Row, Philadelphia, pp 297–306.

Shortell C K, Schwartz S I 1991 Hepatic adenoma and focal nodular hyperplasia. Surgery Gynecology and Obstetrics 173: 426–431.

Shurbaji M S, Gupta P K, Newman M M 1987 Hepatic actinomycosis diagnosed by fine needle aspiration: a case report. Acta Cytologica 31: 751–755.

Silva E G, Tornos C S, Follen-Mitchell M 1994 Malignant neoplasms of the uterine corpus in patients treated for breast carcinoma: the effects of Tamoxifen. International Journal of Gynecological Pathology 13: 248–258.

Silverberg S G, Mullen D, Faraci J A et al 1982 Endometrial carcinoma: clinical-pathologic comparison of cases in post-menopausal women receiving and not receiving exogenous estrogens. Cancer 45: 3018–3026.

Silverberg S G, Haukkamaa M, Arko H, Nilsson C G, Luukkainen T 1986 Endometrial morphology during long-term use of Levonorgestrel-releasing intrauterine devices. International Journal of Gynecological Pathology 5: 235–241.

Sivin I 1985a Recent studies of more effective copper-T devices. In: Zatuchni G I, Goldsmith A, Sciarra J J (eds) Intrauterine contraception: advances and future prospects. Harper & Row, Philadelphia, pp 70–78.

Sivin I 1985b IUD-associated ectopic pregnancies, 1974 to 1984. In: Zatuchni G I, Goldsmith A, Sciarra J J (eds) Intrauterine contraception: advances and future prospects. Harper & Row, Philadelphia, pp 340–353.

Sivin I 1989 IUDs are contraceptives, not abortifacients: a comment on research and belief. Studies in Family Planning 20: 355–359.

Sivin I 1991 Dose- and age-dependent ectopic pregnancy risks with intrauterine contraception. Obstetrics and Gynecology 78: 291–298.

Sivin I, Schmidt F 1987 Effectiveness of IUDs: a review. Contraception 36: 55–84.

Sivin I, el Mahgoub S, McCarthy T, Mishell D R Jr, Shoupe D, Alvarez F 1990 Long-term contraception with the levonorgestrel 20 mcg/day (LNg 20) and the copper T 380Ag intrauterine devices: a five-year randomized study. Contraception 42: 361–378.

Skjeldestad F E, Hammervold R, Peterson D R 1988 Outcomes of pregnancy with an IUD in situ — a population based case-control study. Advances in Contraception 4: 265–270.

Smith C V, Horenstein J, Platt L D 1988 Intraamniotic infection with Candida albicans associated with a retained intrauterine contraceptive device: a case report. American Journal of Obstetrics and Gynecology 159: 123–124.

Smith M R, Soderstrom R 1976 Salpingitis: a frequent response to intrauterine contraception. Journal of Reproductive Medicine 16: 159–162.

Smith P A, Ellis C J, Sparks R A, Guillebaud J 1983 Deaths associated with intrauterine contraceptive devices in the United Kingdom between 1973 and 1983. British Medical Journal 287: 1537–1538.

Snowden R, Williams M, Hawkins D 1977 The IUD: a practical guide. Croom Helm, London, p 38.

Snowman B A, Malviya V K, Brown W, Malone J M Jr, Deppe G 1989 Actinomycosis mimicking pelvic malignancy. International Journal of Gynaecology and Obstetrics 30: 283–286.

Sogaard K 1993 Unrecognized perforation of the uterine and rectal walls by an intrauterine contraceptive device. Acta Obstetricia et Gynecologica Scandinavica 72: 55–56.

Sparks R A, Purrier B G A, Watt P J, Elstein M 1977 The bacteriology of the cervix and uterus. British Journal of Obstetrics and Gynaecology 84: 701–704.

Sparks R A, Purrier B G A, Watt P J, Elstein M 1981 Bacteriological colonisation of the uterine cavity: role of tailed intrauterine contraceptive device. British Medical Journal 282: 1189–1191.

Spaun E, Klunder K 1986 Candida chorioamnionitis and intra-uterine contraceptive device. Acta Obstetricia et Gynecologica Scandinavica 65: 183–184.

Spellberg M A, Mirro J, Chowdhury L 1979 Hepatic sinusoidal dilatation related to oral contraceptives. A study of two patients showing ultrastructural changes. American Journal of Gastroenterology 72: 248–252.

Speroff L 1982 The formulation of oral contraceptives: does the amount of estrogen make any clinical difference? Johns Hopkins Medical Journal 150: 170–176.

Stadel B V 1981 Oral contraceptives and cardiovascular disease. New England Journal of Medicine 305: 612–618 and 305: 672–677.

Stampfer M J, Willett W C, Colditz G A, Speizer F E, Hennekens C H 1990 Past use of oral contraceptives and cardiovascular disease: a meta-analysis in the context of the Nurses' Health Study. American Journal of Obstetrics and Gynecology 163: 285–291.

Stanford J L, Brinton L A, Hoover R N 1989 Oral contraceptives and breast cancer: results from an expanded case-control study. British Journal of Cancer 60: 375–381.

Sterup K, Mosbech J 1967 Budd-Chiari syndrome after taking oral contraceptives. British Medical Journal 4: 660.

Stillman R J 1982 In utero exposure to diethylstilbestrol: adverse effects on the reproductive tract and reproductive performance in male and female offspring. American Journal of Obstetrics and Gynecology 142: 905–921.

Stone M, Dent J, Kardana A, Bagshawe K D 1976 Relationship of oral contraception to development of trophoblastic tumour after evacuation of a hydatidiform mole. British Journal of Obstetrics and Gynaecology 83: 913–916.

Sturdee D W, Wade-Evans T, Paterson M E L, Thom M, Studd J W 1978 Relations between the bleeding pattern, endometrial histology and oestrogen treatment in menopausal women. British Medical Journal 1: 1575–1577.

Swan S H, Brown W L 1981 Oral contraceptive use, sexual activity, and cervical carcinoma. American Journal of Obstetrics and Gynecology 139: 52–57.

Tadesse E, Wamsteker K 1985 Evaluation of 24 patients with IUD-related problems: hysteroscopic findings. European Journal of Obstetrics, Gynecology and Reproductive Biology 19: 37–41.

Taft P D, Robboy S J, Herbst A L, Scully R E 1974 Cytology of clear cell adenocarcinoma of genital tract in young females: review of 95 cases from the registry. Acta Cytologica 19: 279–290.

Tamada T, Okagaki T, Maruyama M, Matsumoto S 1967 Endometrial histology associated with an intrauterine contraceptive device. American Journal of Obstetrics and Gynecology 98: 811–817.

Tao L C 1991 Oral contraceptive-associated liver cell adenoma and hepatocellular carcinoma: cytomorphology and mechanism of malignant transformation. Cancer 68: 341–347.

Tao L C 1992 Are oral contraceptive-associated liver cell adenomas premalignant? Acta Cytologica 36: 338–344.

Tatum H J, Schmidt F H 1977 Contraceptive and sterilization practices and extrauterine pregnancy: realistic perspective. Fertility and Sterility 28: 407–421.

Tavani A, Negri E, Parazzini F, Franceschi S, La Vecchia C 1993 Female hormone utilization and risk of hepatocellular carcinoma. British Journal of Cancer 67: 635–637.

Taxy J B 1978 Peliosis: a morphologic curiosity becomes an iatrogenic problem. Human Pathology 9: 331–340.

Taylor H B, Irey N S, Norris H J 1967 Atypical endocervical hyperplasia in women taking oral contraceptives. Journal of the American Medical Association 202: 637–639.

Tews G, Arzi W, Stoger H 1988 74 Schwangerschaften trotz liegendem IUD. Geburtshilfe und Frauenheilkunde 48: 349–351.

Thiery M, Van Kets H, Van der Pas H 1985 Immediate post-placental IUD insertion: the expulsion problem. Contraception 31: 331–349.

Thomalla J V 1986 Perforation of urinary bladder by intrauterine device. Urology 27: 260–264.

Thomas D B, Noonan E A 1991 Risk of breast cancer in relation to use of combined oral contraceptives near the age of menopause: WHO Collaborative Study of Neoplasia and Steroid Contraceptives. Cancer Causes and Control 2: 389–394.

Thomas D B, Molina R, Rodriguez-Cuevas H et al 1989 Monthly injectable steroid contraceptives and cervical carcinoma. American Journal of Epidemiology 130: 237–247.

Thorburn J, Friberg B, Schubert W, Wassen A C, Lindblom B 1987 Background factors and management of ectopic pregnancy in Sweden: changes over a decade. Acta Obstetricia et Gynecologica Scandinavica 66: 597–602.

Thorogood M, Mann J, Murphy M, Vessey M 1991 Is oral contraceptive use still associated with an increased risk of fatal myocardial infarction? Report of a case-control study. British Journal of Obstetrics and Gynaecology 98: 1245–1253.

Thorogood M, Mann J, Murphy M, Vessey M 1992 Fatal stroke and use of oral contraceptives: findings from a case-control study. American Journal of Epidemiology 136: 35–45.

Timonen H, Kurppa K 1987 IUD perforation leading to obstructive nephropathy necessitating nephrectomy: a rare complication. Advances in Contraception 3: 71–75.

Toivonen J, Luukkainen T, Allonen H 1991 Protective effect of intrauterine release of levonorgestrel on pelvic infection: three years' comparative experience of levonorgestrel- and copper-releasing intrauterine devices. Obstetrics and Gynecology 77: 261–264.

Trauscht Van Horn J J, Capeless E L, Easterling T R, Bovill E G 1992 Pregnancy loss and thrombosis with protein C deficiency. American Journal of Obstetrics and Gynecology 167: 968–972.

Tsalikis T, Stamatopoulos P, Kalachanis J, Mantalenakis S 1986 Experience with the MLCu250 IUD. Advances in Contraception 2: 393–398.

Tsukada Y, Piver M S, Barlow J J 1977 Microglandular hyperplasia of the endocervix following long-term estrogen treatment. American Journal of Obstetrics and Gynecology 127: 888–889.

Tuomivaara L, Kauppila A, Puolakka J 1986 Ectopic pregnancy — an analysis of the etiology, diagnosis and treatment in 552 cases. Archives of Gynecology and Obstetrics 237: 135–147.

UK National Case-Control Study Group 1989 Oral contraceptive use and breast cancer risk in young women. Lancet 1: 973–982.

Ulstein M, Steier A J, Hofstad T, Digranes A, Sandvei R 1987 Microflora of cervical and vaginal secretion in women using copper- and norgestrel-releasing IUCDs. Acta Obstetricia et Gynecologica Scandinavica 66: 321–322.

Ursin G, Aragaki C C, Paganini Hill A, Siemiatycki J, Thompson W D, Haile R W 1992 Oral contraceptives and premenopausal bilateral breast cancer: a case-control study. Epidemiology 3: 414–419.

Valicenti J F, Pappas A A, Graber C D, Williamson H O, Willis N F 1982 Detection and prevalence of IUD-associated *Actinomyces* colonization and related morbidity: a prospective study of 69,925 cervical smears. Journal of the American Medical Association 247: 1149–1152.

van Beek E J, Farmer K C, Millar D M, Brummelkamp W H 1991 Gallstone disease in women younger than 30 years. Netherlands Journal of Surgery 43: 60–62.

Van Campenhout J, Choquette P, Vauclair R 1980 Endometrial pattern in patients with primary hypoestrogenic amenorrhoea receiving estrogen replacement therapy. Obstetrics and Gynecology 56: 349–355.

Vandrie D M, Puri S, Upton R T, DeMeester L J 1983 Adenosquamous carcinoma of the cervix in a woman exposed to diethylstilbestrol in utero. Obstetrics and Gynecology 61 (suppl): 84s–87s.

Vanlancker M, Dierick A M, Thiery M, Claeys G 1987 Histologic and microbiologic findings in the fallopian tubes of IUD users. Advances in Contraception 3: 147–157.

Van Os W A, Edelman D A 1989 Uterine perforation and use of the Multiload IUD. Advances in Contraception 5: 121–126.

Vessey M P 1979 Oral contraception and neoplasia. British Journal of Family Planning 4: 65–71.

Vessey M P 1989 Epidemiologic studies of oral contraception. International Journal of Fertility 34 (suppl): 64–70.

Vessey M P, Doll R 1969 Investigation of relation between use of oral contraceptives and thromboembolic disease: a further report. British Medical Journal ii: 651–657.

Vessey M P, Doll R, Peto R, Johnson B, Wiggins P 1976 Long-term follow-up of women using different methods of contraception — an interim report. Journal of Biosocial Science 8: 373–427.

Vessey M P, McPherson K, Yeates D 1981a Mortality in oral contraceptive users. Lancet 1: 549–550.

Vessey M P, Yeates D, Flavel R, McPherson K 1981b Pelvic inflammatory disease and the intrauterine device: findings in a large cohort study. British Medical Journal 282: 855–857.

Vessey M P, Viilard-Mackintosh L, McPherson K, Yeates D 1989a Mortality among oral contraceptive users: 20 year follow up of women in a cohort study. British Medical Journal 299: 1487–1491.

Vessey M P, McPherson K, Villard-Mackintosh L, Yeates D 1989b Oral contraceptives and breast cancer: latest findings in a large cohort study. British Journal of Cancer 59: 613–617.

Videla-Rivero L, Etcheparreborda J J, Kesseru E 1987 Early chorionic activity in women bearing inert IUD, copper IUD and levonorgestrel-releasing IUD. Contraception 36: 217–226.

Weden M, Glaumann H, Einarsson K 1992 Protracted cholestasis probably induced by oral contraceptive. Journal of Internal Medicine 231: 561–565.

Weiss N S, Sayvetz T A 1980 Incidence of endometrial cancer in relation to the use of oral contraceptives. New England Journal of Medicine 302: 551–554.

Weiss N S, Lyon J L, Liff J M, Vollmer W M, Daling J R 1981 Incidence of ovarian cancer in relation to the use of oral contraceptives. International Journal of Cancer 28: 669–671.

Whitehead M I, McQueen J, Beard R J, Minardi J, Campbell S 1977 The effects of cyclical oestrogen therapy and sequential oestrogen/progestogen therapy on the endometrium of post-menopausal women. Acta Obstetricia et Gynecologica Scandinavica (suppl) 65: 91–101.

Whitehead M I, Townsend P T, Pryse-Davies J, Ryder T A, King R J B 1981 Effects of estrogens and progestins on the biochemistry and morphology of the post-menopausal endometrium. New England Journal of Medicine 305: 1599–1605.

Wight D G D 1982 Atlas of liver pathology. MTP Press, Lancaster.

Wilcox A J, Weinberg C R, Armstrong E G, Canfield R E 1987 Urinary human chorionic gonadotropin among intrauterine device users: detection with a highly specific and sensitive assay. Fertility and Sterility 47: 265–269.

Williams R, Neuberger J 1981 Occurrence, frequency and management of oral contraceptive associated liver tumours. British Journal of Family Planning 7: 35–41.

Wingo P A, Lee N C, Ory H W, Beral V, Peterson H B, Rhodes P 1993 Age-specific differences in the relationship between oral contraceptive use and breast cancer. Cancer 71 (4 suppl): 1506–1517.

Wingrave S 1982 Progestogen effects and their relationship to lipoprotein changes: a report from the Oral Contraception Study of the Royal College of General Practitioners. Acta Obstetricia et Gynecologica Scandinavica 105(suppl): 33–36.

Winkler B, Richart R M 1985 Cervical/uterine pathologic considerations in pelvic infection. In: Zatuchni G I, Goldsmith A, Sciarra J J (eds) Intrauterine contraception: advances and future prospects. Harper & Row, Philadelphia, pp 438–449.

Winkler K, Poulsen H 1975 Liver disease with periportal sinusoidal dilatation: a possible complication to contraceptive steroids. Scandinavian Journal of Gastroenterology 10: 699–704.

Wolf A S, Kriegler D 1986 Bacterial colonization of intrauterine devices (IUDs). Archives of Gynecology and Obstetrics 239: 31–37.

Wollen A L, Flood P R, Sanvei R 1990 Altered ciliary substructure in the endosalpinx in women using an IUCD. Acta Obstetricia et Gynecologica Scandinavica 69: 307–312.

Wolner-Hanssen P, Svensson L, Mårdh P A, Westrom L 1985 Laparoscopic findings and contraceptive use in women with signs and symptoms suggestive of acute salpingitis. Obstetrics and Gynecology 66: 233–238.

World Health Organization Collaborative Study of Neoplasia and Steroid Contraceptives 1985a Invasice cervical cancer and combined oral contraceptives. British Medical Journal 290: 961–965.

World Health Organization's Special Programme of Research, Development and Research Training in Human Reproduction 1985b Task Force on Intrauterine Devices for Fertility Regulation: a multinational case-control study of ectopic pregnancy. Clinical Reproduction and Fertility 3: 131–143.

World Health Organization Special Programme of Research, Development and Research Training in Human Reproduction 1987 Task Force on Intrauterine Devices for Fertility Regulation: microdose intrauterine levonorgestrel for contraception. Contraception 35: 363–379.

World Health Organization Collaborative Study of Neoplasia and Steroid Contraceptives 1988a Endometrial cancer and combined oral contraceptives. International Journal of Epidemiology 17: 263–269.

World Health Organization Collaborative Study of Neoplasia and Steroid Contraceptives 1988b Epithelial ovarian cancer and combined oral contraceptives. International Journal of Epidemiology 18: 538–545.

World Health Organization Collaborative Study of Neoplasia and Steroid Contraceptives 1989a Combined oral contraceptives and liver cancer. International Journal of Cancer 43: 254–259.

World Health Organization Collaborative Study of Neoplasia and Steroid Contraceptives 1989b Combined oral contraceptives and gallbladder cancer. International Journal of Epidemiology 18: 309–314.

World Health Organization Collaborative Study of Cardiovascular Disease and Use of Oral Contraceptives 1989c Bulletin of the World Health Organization 67: 417–423.

World Health Organization Multicentre Trial of the Vasopressor Effects of Combined Oral Contraceptives: 1. Comparisons with IUD. Task Force on Oral Contraceptives 1989d WHO Special Programme of Research, Development and Research Training in Human Reproduction. Contraception 40: 129–145.

World Health Organization Collaborative Study of Neoplasia and Steroid Contraceptives 1990 Breast cancer and combined oral contraceptives: results from a multinational study. British Journal of Cancer 61: 110–119.

World Health Organization Collaborative Study of Neoplasia and Steroid Contraceptives 1991a Depot-medroxyprogesterone acetate (DMPA) and risk of endometrial cancer. International Journal of Cancer 49: 186–190.

World Health Organization Collaborative Study of Neoplasia and Steroid Contraceptives 1991b Breast cancer and depot-medroxyprogesterone acetate: a multinational study. Lancet 338: 833–838.

World Health Organization Collaborative Study of Neoplasia and Steroid Contraceptives 1991c Depot-medroxyprogesterone acetate (DMPA) and risk of liver cancer. International Journal of Cancer 49: 182–185.

World Health Organization Collaborative Study of Neoplasia and Steroid Contraceptives 1992 Depot-medroxyprogesterone acetate (DMPA) and risk of invasive squamous cell cervical cancer. Contraception 45: 299–312.

Wright E A, Aisien A O 1989 Pelvic inflammatory disease and the intrauterine contraceptive device. International Journal of Gynaecology and Obstetrics 28: 133–136.

Wu S M, Spurny O M, Klotz A P 1977 Budd-Chiari syndrome after taking oral contraceptives: a case report and review of 14 reported cases. American Journal of Digestive Disease 22: 623–628.

Yaari S, Goldbourt U, Even-Zohar S, Neufeld H N 1981 Associations of serum high density lipoprotein and total cholesterol with total, cardiovascular, and cancer mortality in a 7-year prospective study of 10,000 men. Lancet 1: 1001–1015.

Yoonessi M, Crickard K, Cellino I S, Satchidanand S K, Fett W 1985 Association of actinomyces and intrauterine contraceptive devices. Journal of Reproductive Medicine 30: 48–52.

Young R H, Scully R E 1992 Uterine carcinomas simulating microglandular hyperplasia: a report of six cases. American Journal of Surgical Pathology 16: 1092–1097.

36. Iatrogenic disease of the female genital tract

James S. Campbell   E. Napke   N. Z. Mikhael   Harpal S. Buttar
Anna Berzowski   Leander Tryphonas   Pierre Drouin   Paul Rowsell

OBJECTIVES AND STRATEGIES

The objectives and strategies of this chapter are:

1. To provide information selected from case material of the authors and from the literature, emphasis being placed upon the pitfalls that the diagnostic anatomical pathologist may expect to encounter in day-to-day gynaecological pathology. The literature review concentrates mainly on the major North American and Western European journals on obstetrics and gynaecology.

2. To help develop sensitivity, habitual suspicion and apprehension for presently unapprehended conditions, e.g. lesions due to new drugs or new procedures or new uses for old drugs and old procedures or, more often, for adverse responses to familiar standard drug products, medicines and therapy.

No attempt is made here to provide encyclopaedic and comprehensive documentation, for such an aim would be self-defeating by reason of bulk. On the contrary, the selection of topics has been rigorous — excluded conditions include toxicity related to cancer chemotherapy, irradiation and antibiotic therapy; irradiation-induced inflammation and necrosis; postoperative infections; technical errors in major surgical operations; transplacental passage (except diethylstilboestrol); most fetal lesions, e.g. neoplasia due to maternal irradiation; and placental lesions.

DEFINITION OF ADVERSE IATROGENIC CONDITIONS

An adverse iatrogenic condition is deemed to exist when the results obtained from investigative, therapeutic or prophylactic measures are undesirable and harmful, or lack bearing upon management of the patient's illness. Or conversely, when such measures are appropriate and clearly indicated, *nothing* happens. Negative results can set the stage for complications arising from physicians' lack of response or lack of initiative. Such a definition should include misadventure prevailing because of: (a) errors or omissions in standard diagnostic, therapeutic or prophylactic procedures or in their interpretation; (b) the procedures themselves being faulty or inappropriate; or (c) malfunction in equipment (Campbell et al, 1981). Not all such adverse events lie within the province of the pathologist who may, however, become enmeshed in iatrogenic errors of communication, some of which may be of his own doing.

Even in these days of automation, not all messages can be taped, coded, computerized, stored and retrieved by foolproof systems. Some very important information must be conveyed under pressure, verbally or in brief handwritten notes, or in typewritten reports transcribed from dictation. Not all of these 'messages' are conveyed accurately (Campbell, 1972). Verbal communication remains quite essential but is often misunderstood, e.g. through lack of common vocabularies amongst the various persons involved; written confirmation with much the same shortcomings in vocabulary may be slow to overtake, and be ineffective in clearing up, earlier oral, and perhaps imprecise, exercises in 'thinking out loud'. In the meantime, proliferating jargon compounds existing linguistic hazards, thus far without adequate recompense from proliferating computer codes.

Access to literature: legal implications

A recent British Columbia court ruling awarded $883 000 Cdn against a gynaecologist whose artificial insemination by donor programme resulted in infection by human immunodeficiency virus (Godley, 1992). Two patients and one donor — also a defendant — were involved. The exposure in question took place on January 21st, 1985. A letter had been published on the 27th of October, 1983, in the New England Journal of Medicine (Mascola et al 1983) under the title 'Should sperm donors be screened for STD'. The text of the letter referred to 'at least 10 anecdotal reports' and various pathogens, including 'possibly the agent responsible for the autoimmune deficiency syndrome'. Available on line by January, 1984, the indices recorded for this letter did not include HIV transmission, nor would entry in current contents have included citation from the text. Such detail as is presently available has been recorded by Godley (1992) and by Waugh (1992a,b). The case is presently under appeal. However, a precedent has been set whereby even anecdotal reporting may be considered in evidence and lead to judgement adverse to a medical defendant unaware of such anecdotal reports. The literature may therefore be searched for purely defensive rather than informative intent, thus provoking anxiety on the part of physicians who by reason of urgency or distance from appropriately equipped libraries must act without precautionary literature searches. Foster (1992), commenting upon Godley and Waugh (op cit), noted 'ongoing current awareness mechanisms' as safeguards, e.g. using Medline or the Dialogue system to help ensure that subjects such as artificial insemination by donor are automatically indexed for the clinician's attention.

Other definitions

Simple things such as the definitions of a drug, drug product and medicine, need to be clearly defined. Unfortunately, in law, in the literature, and in verbal usage such terms are freely interchanged to the detriment of the scientific literature and our understanding of efficacy, safety, adverse reactions, risk/benefit, and epidemiological methods used in 'active ingredient' and 'medicine' studies. The term 'drug' in Canada's Food and Drug Regulations can mean both or either, i.e. an 'active ingredient' or a drug product containing an active ingredient plus a number of other chemicals, e.g. excipients and additives. Patients receive complex medicines/drug products and rarely, if ever, a single chemical called the 'active ingredient'. The products that patients are given consist of a large number of chemicals, any one of which, alone or in combination, can cause a permanent or reversible toxic effect. One must consider the patient as a walking test tube. Unfortunately, the past and current literature ascribes adverse reactions to active ingredients. It took unusual circumstances epidemiologically to discover adverse reactions caused by excipients such as metabisulphites, monosodium glutamate, tartrazine, etc. In North America the excipients and additives in drug products are not usually known to the clinician or researchers. Leachates, such as mercaptobenzolthiazides, a catalytic agent in rubber products, can also cause adverse reactions and perhaps death; again, such chemicals are not usually taken into consideration when investigating a pathological problem.

The case of the drug product Dilantin is a classic example of the importance of the excipient/additive factor in pathology. The authorities in New Zealand and Australia were convinced that the Dilantin product used in these countries should be reformulated to be similar to that product as used in the USA. The reformulation consisted simply of replacing the lactose in the New Zealand products by calcium sulphate, as in the American product. According to Tyrer et al (1970), this change caused an outbreak of anticonvulsant intoxication in an Australian city. These differences in formulation of a product having the same trade name in different countries and sometimes within the same country, makes it very hazardous and misleading to attempt to make country-to-country comparisons for safety and efficacy, considering only the 'active ingredient' of the product and not the product as a whole. Researchers and regulators cannot assume that, because the trade name is the same in different countries, the entire formulation is the same and hence presents the same toxicity, safety and efficacy factors (Repmeyer & Juhl, 1983; Napke & Stevens, 1984; Hamilton, 1987).

PREVALENCE OF ADVERSE IATROGENIC CONDITIONS

The prevalence of adverse iatrogenic reactions has been much disputed. In a post-1974 undated, but in other respects excellent, pamphlet entitled *Adverse drug reaction in the United States* (published by Medicine in the Public Interest, Inc.) a statement appears that 'Extrapolation of the available data cannot provide a valid estimate of the adverse drug reaction problem in the United States. Adequate data for valid extrapolation are simply not available.' The pathologist can not abandon the question of the prevalence of iatrogenic disease affecting patients but, unfortunately, constraints are met with in three main spheres: autopsy studies, surgical pathology examination and the limitations of light microscopy.

Autopsy cases

Adequately studied autopsy cases have provided estimates of prevalence of DAR (drug product-related adverse reactions); e.g. in Gotti's study (1974), an incidence of 8.3% of DAR was found in 2168 autopsy cases. Considering reports of DAR in 10–40% of hospitalized patients, Gotti concludes that 'the [discrepancy] reflects two essential points: (1) those reactions that were primarily functional in nature are either not given attention by the pathologist or are not noted in clinical records; and (2) the interest and awareness of the pathologist concerning adverse drug reactions is generally not yet at a reliable level'. Mikhael & Kacew (1984) found 467 adverse reactions to drugs and alcohol in 1938 autopsies (an incidence of 24%), in which 216 of the reactions had contributed to death. Roberts (1978) noted that 'the autopsy nearly always provides additional diagnoses and occasionally (in about 25% of cases) it alters completely the prevailing major clinical diagnoses'. In the same article attention is drawn to a decline from 41% in 1964 to 22% in 1975 in autopsy rates in the United States at a time when reliance upon drug therapy is on the increase. Such a decline must have an adverse impact upon efforts to control DAR.

Referral to New England Journal of Medicine case records of the Massachusetts General Hospital provides a continuing way to monitor, week by week, contributions of necropsies to clinical studies by experts in selected cases, including some problems in obstetrics and gynaecology. Unfortunately, the aggregate autopsy rate was only 12.4% of 10 003 diagnostic face sheets recently reviewed from 418 participating institutions, including pathology resident teaching institutions (Baker & Zarbo, 1991). Moreover, data collection among participating institutions varied. It is idle to suggest that, from such surveys, useful estimates of the frequency of iatrogenic events can be reached.

Surgical pathology examinations

Mikhael (1985) studied 57 881 surgical pathology cases and encountered 841 instances of DAR, of which 78.72% were in females. This sort of surgical pathology data is generally an underestimate of iatrogenic conditions and the lack of an adequate history is unquestionably the greatest shortcoming (Irey, 1972; 1976), though light microscopy is also intrinsically imprecise (Campbell & Tryphonas, 1983).

Light microscopy limitations

It is an obvious and dangerous fallacy to ascribe complete confidence to histopathological diagnoses, as in the phrase 'proven by biopsy'. Perhaps 5% of histopathological diagnoses of human cancer are inconclusive or wrong. Ninety five per cent confidence limits are laudable enough in statistics but, in this instance, this seemingly innocent 5% figure is not a statistic, it is a guess and, educated or otherwise, cold comfort to the 5% of patients whose diagnoses lie beyond the 95% limit (Campbell & Tryphonas, 1983). One simply can not say what proportion of the disputable 5% is in whole or in part iatrogenic. One must conclude that light microscopy solves more problems than it creates and that iatrogenic catastrophes arising thereby are not common, certainly so if only those related to DAR are taken into account. However, Roberts' 1978 findings remain very disquieting.

Multiple factors and interactions

Postulates for recognizing DAR have been detailed elsewhere (Irey, 1976). 'Eligibility' of any incident, or drug or other chemical to be considered as a factor responsible for an adverse reaction rests upon (a) consideration of time ('temporal eligibility'), and (b) upon the dynamics of the factors involved, e.g. pharmacodynamics, known toxicity, and known capacity to excite tissue reaction (Tryphonas et al, 1983). Where drugs are concerned, it is unusual to find that only one has been administered. Out of many, one may be responsible, as may be indicated by time-flow studies and considerations of pharmacokinetics. However, interactions are commonplace and should never be dismissed from any review of diagnostic data merely because it may appear, at first sight, that some drug alone could be responsible, e.g. anticoagulant alone versus anticoagulant plus acetylsalicylic acid. This subject has been dealt with elsewhere (Irey, 1976; Campbell et al, 1981).

CATEGORIES OF ERROR

Pitfalls and safeguards are main leitmotifs in studies of iatrogenic conditions, which arise in varied unsuspected ways and circumstances. Some classes and sources of error of particular concern to histopathologists are:

1. Procedural error reflected in tissue specimens. Some iatrogenic findings are straightforward, and recognizing their iatrogenic origin offers no difficulty. Not so easy is the working out of safeguards to prevent them.

2. Failure to recognize iatrogenic factors. Some iatrogenic lesions, such as talc granulomas, may closely mimic naturally occurring diseases, e.g. tuberculosis.

3. Histopathological error. The hazard may be wholly created by the histopathologist alone, through diagnostic misinterpretation.

4. Complications and misadventures related to clinically unsuspected lesions. Situations may arise which reflect some shortcoming or omission in clinical management and a chain of events is set up which can lead to some unexpected and surprising ultimate event, e.g. haemorrhage in unsuspected ovarian masses in pregnancy.

5. Idleness in calling attention to preventive measures may contribute to iatrogenic disease (e.g. alleged association between talc use and ovarian cancer).

6. Error related to unawareness of the literature.

Workloads

The Royal College of Pathologists (1992) workload norms for district community hospitals are that 4000 surgical pathology specimens per pathologist per annum is acceptable, and that each pathologist ought not to perform more than 300 autopsies per year. For teaching hospitals these numbers should be halved. Dawson's (1992) survey of Canadian hospitals reveals figures for surgical pathology specimens that are consistently higher and for autopsies consistently lower than those recommended by the Royal College for the United Kingdom. Dawson also cites deviant figures from California, e.g. 7500 surgical pathology cases per pathologist per annum. For higher workload figures alarm was expressed, i.e. 'don't know how (they) manage'. Clearly, under such conditions the risk of error is increased.

Duty hours

Duty hours for house staff are of concern in the context of the clinical team concept outlined below. House officers faced with averages of 110 duty hours per week, with as much as 36 consecutive hours on duty, cannot maintain consistently high standards of patient care and certainly not consistent receptivity of data or performance in clinical teaching rounds and conferences. Accordingly a New York grand jury ruled that house officer duty hours should not exceed 80 hours per week. Long-term effects upon patient care and resident education await further appraisal but improved patient care is not apparent (Kelly et al, 1991).

Strategic planning, etc.

The general references at the end of this chapter pertain to medico-legal aspects, quality assurance, strategic planning for health care education as touching upon iatrogenic problems and the changing economic and social climates in which these occur, e.g. 'if we fail to eradicate mass illiteracy, all the indications are that even the small initial gains in reducing maternal mortality... will slip away, and ... hardly anything will be left to show for our efforts' (Harrison, 1989).

ORGANIZATION: SAFEGUARDS AGAINST ERROR, 'TASK FORCE' CONCEPT AND RELEVANCE TO IATROGENIC CONDITIONS

It seems obvious that advantages accrue by way of efficient service and practical clinical investigation, basic research and education at all levels when gynaecological and obstetrical pathology becomes the province of a specific team, representing both laboratory and clinical colleagues, i.e. a 'task force'.

The advantages of this approach to iatrogenic conditions are twofold:

1. Concentration upon a well-defined field permits the laboratory diagnostician to become familiar in depth with clinical methods and their pitfalls, and the clinical practitioner to become au fait with laboratory pitfalls.

2. With the improved communications within the task force, the pathologist is more likely to be informed of historical and other clinical data in puzzling problems, including their iatrogenic possibilities.

Case referral should include routine referrals to adverse reaction programmes, whether drug or medical devices or other factors appear to be involved; all relevant circumstances relating to adverse reactions of whatever cause should in confidence be retrievable.

That some such programmes are underutilized is clear from the Canadian experience in reporting adverse effects relating to intrauterine contraceptive devices (IUDs). Intensive monitoring of IUD use in St. Clare's Mercy Hospital, St. John's, Newfoundland, quickly accounted for almost as many reports as did general voluntary reporting for a longer period in all of Canada (Table 36.1).

Within hospitals, adverse reaction teams may focus upon DAR much in the manner of infection control teams upon their object (Westwood et al, 1974, 1976). Unfortunately, adverse reaction teams are still exceptional — perhaps because clinical pharmacologists, clinical toxicologists and clinical pharmacists are few and pharmacological or toxicological pathologists with clinical rather than industrial or governmental leanings are rare. Departments of laboratory medicine, even those capable of therapeutic drug monitoring, are almost invariably without an identifiable section specifically dedicated to pharmacological pathology. In such settings iatrogenic hazards may flourish without giving rise to much attention. The mind set, or how we are programmed, is perhaps the biggest impediment to forming a post-marketing surveillance team in a hospital or in a regional setting.

Table 36.1 Comparative incidence of intrauterine contraceptive device (IUD)-related adverse events, with and without intensive monitoring.

A. Reporting of IUD-related complications (Wilansky et al, 1978) St. Clare's Mercy Hospital, St. John's, Nfld: intensive monitoring of IUD use

Survey period	1972–1978
No. active treatment gynaecological beds	31
No. patients with reported adverse reaction to IUD	161
No. gyn. admissions	6859
2.34% gyn. admissions IUD-related	

B. Product-Related Diseases Division (Health and Welfare, Canada) General voluntary reporting

Survey period	1967–1978
No. reported adverse reactions to IUD	167
No. postoperative gyn. discharges Canada	2 568 987

C. Statistics Canada recording of data relevant to IUD-related adverse reactions

No. postoperative gyn. discharges reported in Canada 04/79–03/80	229 131
No. IUD-related op. procedures reported in Canada 04/79–03/80	527

0.23% discharges were related to IUD removal in Canada for 12-month period following 31/03/79: these are standard hospital statistics; compare with results of intensive monitoring in A above

Attention has been drawn to under-reporting of adverse reaction to IUDs in Canada. Figures from Devon suggest this problem may be more widespread, with 7% of gynaecological admissions to Plymouth General Hospital being IUD related, 1.6% of 2250 deliveries resulting from IUD failure (Fraundorfer, 1983). Pitkin (1988) remarks that 'The IUD has had a long and somewhat checkered career'. Panda (1990), in describing an instance of primary ovarian twin pregnancy in a progesterone-only oral contraceptive user, noted that among IUD users a ratio of one ovarian in 9 ectopic pregnancies had been reported (Lehfeldt et al 1970), while Veress & Wallmander (1987) report an instance of primary hepatic pregnancy in an IUD user. In view of under-reporting it can hardly be held with complete assurance that such events are truly extraordinary.

REACTIONS TO FOREIGN MATERIALS

Starch granulomas

Starch glove powder-induced peritoneal granulomas may mimic tuberculosis (Fig. 36.1) even to the extent of producing 'tuberculoid necrosis' (Davies & Neely, 1972). In one personally studied case an erroneous diagnosis of pelvic tuberculosis had been made and treatment with para-aminosalicylic acid and isoniazid begun. In due course, cultures proved to be negative. The use of polarizers had initially been omitted and resort to polarized light led to a revised histopathological diagnosis of starch granuloma. The source of the starch was previous pelvic surgery, no history of which had reached the laboratory (Acharya et al, 1973; Campbell et al, 1981). Peritonitis due to starch powder may cause adhesions and intestinal obstruction (Cooke & Hamilton, 1977). Evidence suggesting immunological factors in the production of such granulomas has been reviewed by Grant et al (1976).

Mineral oil granulomas

These lesions are still being encountered (Ghosh, 1976), are not uncommonly misdiagnosed microscopically as malignant and are probably either incompletely reported or going unrecognized.

Pelvic mineral oil granulomas appear likely to be sequelae of uterine dilatation and curettage when, mistakenly

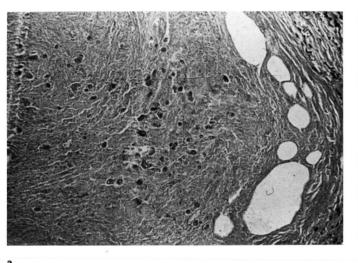

a

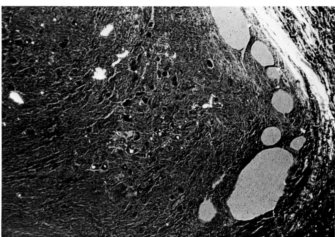

b

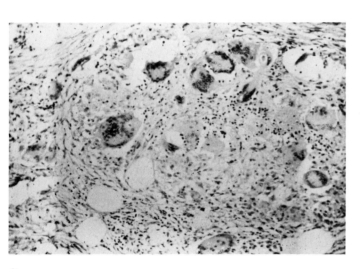

c

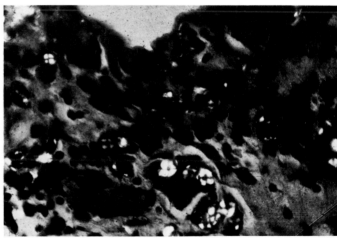

d

Fig. 36.1 **a**. Starch granuloma. Lesion integral with fibrous adhesions involving uterus and adnexa. Zone of structureless debris appeared as caseation, bordered by crescentic zone of fibrosis. Little attention was paid initially to eosinophilic, rounded, rather irregular structures in the necrotic zone. **b**. Starch granuloma. On review with polarized light, doubly refractile fragments were seen within and exterior to structures taken to represent phagocytes, now deemed defunct. Some doubly refractile fragments conformed to Maltese cross pattern of starch particles. Other fragments resembled lint, as from sponges or towels. Diagnosis changed from granulomatous pelvic inflammatory disease consistent with tuberculosis to pelvic inflammatory disease consistent with foreign body reaction following caesarean section, with subsequent clinical symptoms of pelvic inflammatory disease. **c**. More typical granulomatous reaction to starch. Langhans-type and foreign body giant cells are conspicuous. **d**. Starch granuloma. Polarized light reveals characteristic 'Maltese cross of surgery' of Acharya et al (1973). Haematoxylin, phloxine and saffron: **a–c**. × 100 approx; **d**. × 450 approx.

or unwittingly, mineral oil is used as a lubricant for the instruments. Possibly, however, a paraffin coital lubricant (e.g. vaseline) may be involved in some cases (Fig. 36.2) (Campbell et al, 1981).

Transuterine passage of douche contaminants and condom emulsion

Instances of pelvic peritoneal granulomas have been attributed to douching and condom emulsion (Saxén et al, 1963; Hidvegi et al, 1978). Such lesions exemplify the transuterine passage of foreign materials.

Pseudoneoplastic reactions to silica and talc

Xanthogranulomatous vaginal pseudotumour

The presence of magnesium and silica 'in quantities similar to that of standard talc examined by the same

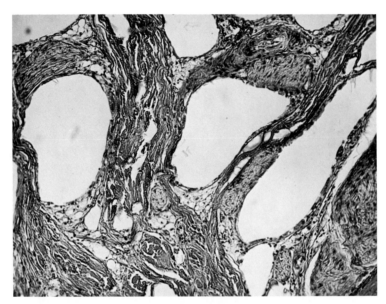

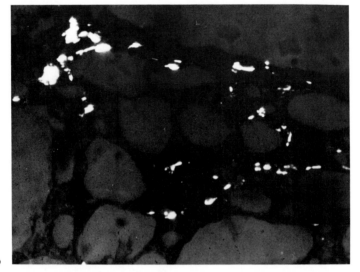

Fig. 36.2 **a**. Canadian Tumour Reference Centre (CRCCP Canadian Reference Centre for Cancer Pathology) 2068. Granuloma of parametrial and retroperitoneal pelvic connective tissues. Note distension of perineural spaces and focal accumulations of foamy histiocytes. Originally misdiagnosed as neoplastic but unclassified process. Mineral oil was subsequently extracted from this lesion. H & E × 70. **b**. Same lesion seen by polarized light. Concentrated mineral acids did not dissolve these doubly refractile crystals, deemed therefore to be an additional, silicious contaminant. H & E × 100. (Reproduced from Campbell et al, 1964, with permission of the publisher, the American Fertility Society, and of the Editors of the Canadian Journal of Surgery. See Campbell et al, 1981.)

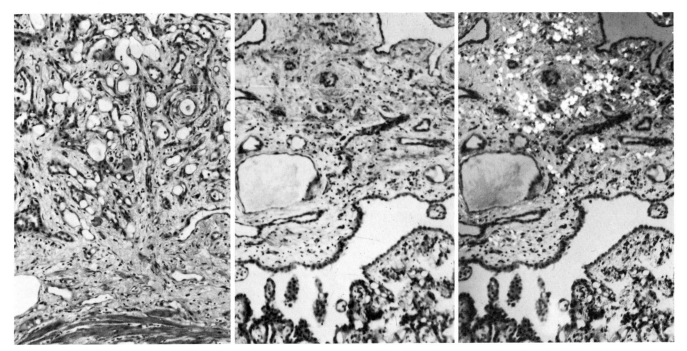

Fig. 36.3 Talc-induced pseudoadenomatoid tumour. Adenomatoid zones and spaces with partly papillary linings are deemed to be made up of mesothelium displaced at surgery. The field on the right represents the middle field as seen in polarized light; here and there are interstitial deposits of talc-like particles, deemed to represent glove-dusting powder. H & E × 100 approx. (Reproduced by permission of S. Karger, Basel: see Campbell et al 1981.)

technique' in the xanthogranulomatous pseudotumour of the vagina reported by Strate et al (1983) suggests that a pseudoneoplastic reaction to talc could possibly be a factor in inciting such a lesion. In this particular case a hysterectomy had been performed at the age of 56 and the lesion appeared at the age of 81. It was greeted by a gamut of histological opinions, including alveolar soft part sarcoma and malacoplakia. For a thorough description of the techniques involved in dealing with this sort of lesion the report of Strate et al (1983) should be consulted.

Pseudoadenomatoid tumour

In a personally studied case a tumour was found on the surface of the fundus uteri. Microscopically, there were fields of fibrosis penetrated by islands of mesothelial-like cells; the lesion was riddled with talc-like crystals which resisted digestion by concentrated mineral acid (Fig. 36.3). There had been a previous exploratory laparotomy and, almost certainly, a grasping of the fundus with a talc-ridden tenaculum. Similar lesions have more recently been found in old caesarean scars (Campbell et al, 1981).

Pseudofibrous histiocytomas

Weiss et al (1978) have described abdominal wall and inguinal reactions to injected silica which simulated fibrous histiocytomas. Five of the seven patients were female. The silica was usually from sclerosing agents, in-

jected for non-operative repair of hernias. In five of the patients, 10–41 years had elapsed since an injection in the site. Figure 36.4 has been deemed by some to represent such a process. Proppe et al (1984) described silica-free postoperative pseudosarcomas of the vagina, prostate, bladder and urethra, noting that 'the similar clinical background' could link these lesions with the pseudofibrous histiocytoma described by Weiss et al (1978).

Talc and asbestos in carcinoma of uterus and ovary

Cramer et al (1982) published an epidemiological study implicating talc as a possible factor in producing 'malignant' epithelial tumours of the ovary, the putative source of talc being perineal dusting powder on sanitary napkins. These authors note 'the chemical relation of talc to asbestos', the latter being notorious for causing mesotheliomas.

Henderson et al (1971) recovered talc from squamous cell carcinomas of cervix uteri, papillary adenocarcinomas of endometrium and papillary serous cystadenocarcinomas of the ovary. Their extraction replication procedure required extensive high magnification electronmicroscopic study to detect talc particles. Warning was given of the 'unreliability of polarized light for identifying asbestos; however, asbestos was not found in the ovarian tumours but there was good evidence for the presence of talc, often indistinguishable from anthrophylite asbestos . . .'. Shugar (1979) noted that 'asbestos is often a natural contaminant of talc — in 22 talcum products the mineral fibre content

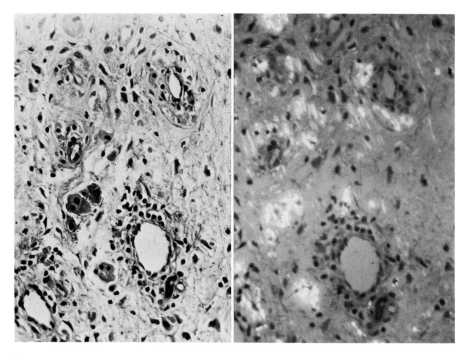

Fig. 36.4 Vaginal mass with content of talc-like particles, seen only on the right by using polarized light. Present also in lesional borders, this material was not abundant. H & E × 250 approx. (Courtesy of S. Karger, Basel.)

represented 8–30% of the total talcum particulates: most of the fibres were thought to be fibrous talc with minor amounts of asbestos fibres'.

Anteby et al (1983) noted ovarian cancer death rates in female asbestos workers *seven times* greater than those of women in a control group, but the number of asbestos-exposed females so afflicted was only four.

In the interim, the alleged association between ovarian cancer and asbestos exposure has dissolved into controversy (reflected in the bibliography of Cramer et al, 1982). During this time, Parmley & Woodruff (1974) postulated that neoplasms derived from the surface cells of ovary are actually mesotheliomas: these authors speculated upon the transuterine route from vagina to pelvis by which 'environmental substances' could contaminate the ovaries (Fig. 36.5), there to be entrapped in ovarian inclusion cysts. Entrapment of talc forms a piece of the jigsaw puzzle which Cramer et al (1982) have noted in drawing attention to the implantation of foreign materials into epithelial-lined lumens as a factor favouring ovarian carcinogenesis.

The last word on this subject may not be heard for quite some time (see Ch. 20), but a question of possible prophylaxis is posed and rests squarely upon the medical practitioner (among others): is the use of talc worth *any* finite risk of ovarian cancer? If not, what should be done about it?

Pseudosulphur granules associated with intrauterine contraceptive devices

O'Brien et al (1981) call attention to synthetic material from IUDs simulating actinomyces, thus possibly confounding diagnosis and treatment. Such objects are distinguishable from true mycetoma by Gram staining.

Barium enema with barium embolization and barium 'deportation'

David et al (1983) drew attention to the unusual but arresting, indeed lethal, outcome of introducing barium, intended for barium enema, into atrophic vaginas of elderly patients. Mucosal laceration from the catheters and contrast media under pressure lead to venous intravasation and pulmonary embolization by barium with extraperitoneal barium infiltration or some combination of these untoward effects.

Barium escaping from the gut may contribute to pelvic inflammation. Benirschke et al (1984) describe granulomatous oophoritis with inclusions of barium and *Phaseolus vulgaris*, i.e. red bean cells. An IUD user, the 28-year-old patient had suffered a tubo-ovarian abscess eight years earlier when, at barium enema, the gut had evidently been perforated to release barium and bean tissues into the pelvis. No pelvic operation had earlier been performed.

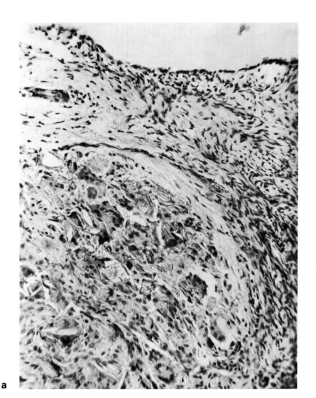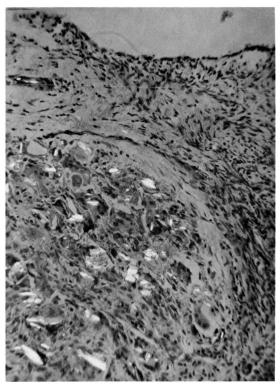

a   b

Fig. 36.5 a. Granuloma close beneath cortical surface of ovary, non-polarized light. **b**. Polarized light reveals doubly refractile talc-like crystals. In the lower left-hand field crystals are deemed to be in histiocytes. It cannot be shown here that these crystals are entrapped in inclusion cysts. H & E × 165. (Courtesy of the Editor of Fertility and Sterility and reproduced by permission of the publisher, the American Fertility Society.)

NECROTIZING VASCULITIS (POSSIBLY DRUG-INDUCED)

Necrotizing vasculitis, having a pattern resembling that seen in periarteritis nodosa (PAN), has been described in cervices and uterine adnexa (Fig. 36.6) removed during gynaecological surgery (Ansell et al, 1974; Wilansky et al, 1980; Womak, 1987). Some such lesions were in part exudative, some partly proliferative and some partly fibrotic, as though of varying duration. In Wilansky's report some lesions were associated with penicillin hypersensitivity, which would militate against a view that vasculitides of this sort are necessarily isolated (Ansell et al, 1974).

The lesions described in Wilansky's report were reviewed by Mullick et al (1979) who regarded them as consistent with drug- or chemical-induced vasculitis although in several of Wilansky's cases clinical data was insufficient to give additional support to such a view. Mullick et al (1979) established that drug-induced vasculitis is typically productive, but the gamut of drug-induced vasculitides includes necrotizing and exudative forms (McCombs et al, 1956; McCombs, 1965; Wilansky et al, 1980). Mullick's study and the earlier work of Irey & Norris (1973) on drug- and chemical-induced vasculitides do not focus upon the female genital tract.

It should be noted, however, that virus-associated necrotizing arteritis in mice has been found in ovaries and uterus.

Were a necrotizing vasculitis generalized and widely distributed, serious results would almost assuredly occur, but none appeared in Wilansky's or Ansell's cases. One must infer that these lesions, if generalized, must be sparse and patchily distributed. Only one such patient came to autopsy, having succumbed during surgery for carcinoma of the urinary bladder: here, the distal colon and kidneys as well as the uterus and adnexa were involved, but the patient had received irradiation for her cancer.

What action is called for when necrotizing vasculitis is an unsuspected finding in cervical biopsy tissues? Follow-up studies in most of Wilansky's cases have provided no suggestion of progressive systemic vascular disease, and the optimal policy is one of hopeful watching. If the patient has polyarteritis nodosa or some related systemic vascular disease this will announce itself soon enough to the alert observer.

THE DIETHYLSTILBOESTROL (DES) SYNDROME

Both male and female offspring of DES-treated mothers may display an array of genital lesions and the DES

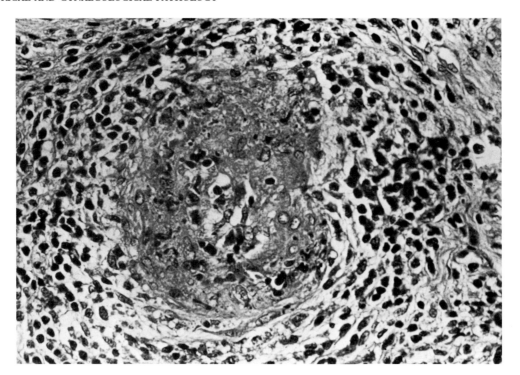

Fig. 36.6   Necrotizing vasculitis in cervix uteri of patient with history of penicillin reactions. Haematoxylin, phloxine and saffron × 400 approx.

syndrome provides a model for studying the diverse consequences of transplacental transfer of various oestrogenic substances upon both sexes.

Robboy (1983) notes that (a) differentiation of Müllerian epithelium appears to be determined by adjacent Müllerian duct mesenchyme, being destined according to level to produce endocervical (mucinous) or tuboendometrial epithelial types and (b) after the tenth week of gestation, the squamous epithelium of the urogenital sinus ordinarily grows upwards to replace the primitive Müllerian epithelium of the developing vagina to the level of the maternal cervical os.

Robboy (1983) has proposed a fourfold hypothesis, postulating a sequence of events which could explain the early effects of DES upon the fetal lower genital tract in females:

1. abnormal distribution of mesenchymal layers destined to form cervix and corpus uteri, leading to:
   a. a heaping up of stroma into hyperplastic ridges, or
   b. a converse failure of mesenchyme to develop into the contours of cervix and vaginal fornices, with loss of definition of these structures, and
   c. abnormal contours of the uterine fundus
2. a spreading out of stroma destined to become cervical, with the result that an abnormally wide zone of mucinous epithelium comes to cover the future portio vaginalis and upper vagina
3. DES-exposed mesenchyme of exocervix and vagina then opposes and blocks the upward migration of urogenital sinus squamous epithelium
4. the vaginal wall mesenchyme thereupon induces residual 'native' embryonic Müllerian epithelium to differentiate into adult-type tuboendometrial epithelium with glandular components, i.e. adenosis.

In such a milieu classical clear cell adenocarcinomas of vagina and cervix occur in offspring of mothers treated for threatened abortion by DES. Although notorious, this carcinoma is uncommon, affecting 0.14–1.4 per 1000 DES-exposed daughters by the age of 24 (Herbst, 1981; Herbst & Bern, 1981): even so, more than 400 such cases of vaginal clear cell adenocarcinoma have been described (Herbst, 1981). There appears not to have been an increase in epidermoid carcinoma in the lower genital tract of females exposed to DES, a point disputed, however, by Veridiano et al (1978). The incidence of non-neoplastic malformations of the genital tract is much greater than that of the DES-related neoplasms. Non-neoplastic structural anomalies related to DES exposure may affect substantially more than half of the individuals at risk (Goldstein, 1978); transverse cervico-vaginal ridges appear in about 25% of these patients (Kaufman et al, 1980; Herbst, 1981; Herbst et al, 1981) (Fig. 36.7). Jeffries et al (1984), also reporting DES-related cervical and vaginal structural anomalies in 25% of 1655 DES-exposed patients, noted that these anomalies disappeared over periods of one to five years in 41% of a group of 361 patients,

NORMAL   DES

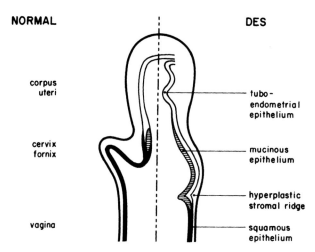

corpus
uteri

cervix
fornix

vagina

tubo-
endometrial
epithelium

mucinous
epithelium

hyperplastic
stromal ridge

squamous
epithelium

Fig. 36.7   Gross vaginal and uterine abnormalities in DES-exposed girls. Note uterine corpus deformities as visualized from hysterosalpingograms. (Adapted from Kaufman et al, 1980; Robboy, 1983; Herbst & Bern, 1981.)

particularly among those experiencing pregnancy, i.e. 33 of 60 patients.

Classical DES-related juvenile clear cell adenocarcinomas of vagina and cervix (Fig. 36.8) have been found in intimate association with atypical adenosis, thus giving rise to the hypothesis that adenosis may be a harbinger of the clear cell neoplasm. However, histories of maternal DES use have been negative in as many as 37% of young women with adenocarcinoma or, counting those whose mothers received unidentified medication, about 25% of these patients have no history of relevant maternal drug use. Adenosis can be observed at vaginal examination in somewhat less than 1% of females *not* exposed to DES, where the lesions take the form of minute symptomless cysts, but as many as 50% of such individuals may be found with clinically inapparent adenosis when at necropsy many vaginal tissue blocks are examined microscopically (Robboy, 1983). Observations of vaginal adenosis antedate the use of DES (Abell, 1969) and 23 cases of clear cell adenocarcinoma of cervix unrelated to DES exposure have been reported (Kaminski & Maier, 1983). Seven of these patients were 24 years of age or younger.

Returning to Robboy's (1983) postulates, one may feel stirrings of concern lest oncogenic exposure other than to DES may be responsible for some instances of clear cell adenocarcinoma of the lower genital tract. Kaminsi & Maier (1983) speculate upon such a possibility, noting the view of Herbst et al (1977) that DES is probably not a complete carcinogen and that other factors, e.g. changes associated with puberty, may be involved in the DES carcinogenic process. Kaminski & Maier's group of seven younger patients were free from adenosis or DES-associated non-neoplastic structural anomalies of the vagina or cervix but, plainly, another local tissue target and other

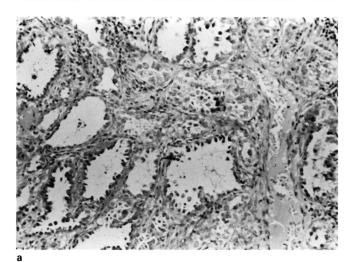

a

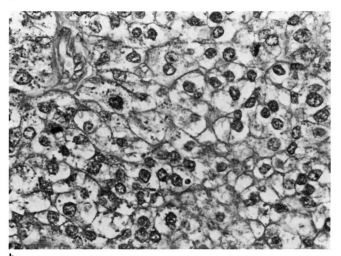

b

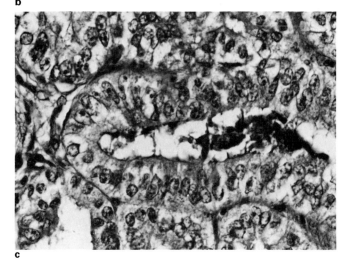

c

Fig. 36.8   **a**. Tubulocystic pattern in vaginal adenocarcinoma attributed to diethylstilboestrol (DES). Clear cells are not conspicuous in this lesion. H & E × 120. **b**. Clear cell carcinoma, solid pattern. This pattern is common to clear cell carcinoma of endometrium, oviduct and ovary. Such patterns are not at all specific to DES-related vaginal adenocarcinomas. Haematoxylin, phloxine and saffron × 500 approx. **c**. Endometrioid-appearing carcinoma; variant pattern that may occur in DES-related vaginal carcinoma. Haematoxylin, phloxine and saffron × 500 approx.

mechanism could be involved with other carcinogenic exposures.

Observers who hew to the line that clear cells are necessary as markers for the diagnosis of DES-induced vaginal neoplasms when positive drug histories are lacking will, logically enough, exclude non-clear cell tumours from full membership in the DES syndrome, while not excluding them from retrieval in the event that rethinking should at some future time become advisable. This is rational because some bona fide juvenile DES-associated vaginal adenocarcinomas are not conspicuously clear celled (Herbst & Bern, 1981). One might surmise, for the present, that the likelihood of forgotten or misleading drug histories exceeds the likelihood of finding authentic DES-unassociated vaginal adenocarcinomas in young women.

For the future, Kaminski & Maier (citing Herbst et al, 1979) comment that 'if other factors acting in a manner similar to DES are involved in (this) carcinogenesis, a second peak in DES-related clear adenocarcinomas may occur after age 45'. Indeed, Kaminski & Maier's DES-unassociated cases show such a peak and one senses clear warnings of a 'tip of the iceberg' syndrome.

A detailed description of the DES syndrome requires a monograph of its own, fortunately provided by Herbst & Bern (1981).

Findings additional to those already noted are uterine hypoplasia, constrictions of uterine lumens, T-shaped uterine lumens, bulbous uterotubal junctions and oviduct deformities detected in hysterosalpingograms (Kaufman et al, 1980). 'Withered' oviducts, where fimbriae are small, few or none and ostial lumens reduced to pinpoints, have been found to characterize DES transplacental effects on oviduct development (De Cherney et al, 1981).

Also of concern to the pathologist are the relatively high levels of infertility, so-called 'spontaneous' abortion, cervical incompetence and fetal loss, preterm delivery and ectopic pregnancy (Goldstein, 1978; De Cherney et al, 1981; Herbst et al, 1981), for the latter a four- to fivefold increase (De Cherney et al, 1981). One could infer a concomitant increase in maternal mortality, particularly in respect to ectopic pregnancy, the commonest cause of first-trimester maternal death (Schenker & Evron, 1983; Wolfman & Holtz, 1983). A liability to pelvic inflammatory disease and unexplained pelvic masses has also been described; hirsutism and menstrual irregularities have been attributed to transplacental DES transfer (Peress et al, 1982).

Transplacentally-induced lesions in male offspring of mothers treated with DES for threatened abortion include testicular seminomas, hypoplasia, maldescent of the testes, oligospermia, morphological abnormalities of spermatozoa, microphallus, epididymal cysts and varicocele (Stillman, 1982; Conley et al, 1983).

A history regarding DES exposure should routinely be sought in all patients of appropriate age with suspect lesions and no work-ups should be regarded as adequate without an assiduous inquiry for such data. Characterization of DES-related oviduct abnormalities is probably incomplete, e.g. in terms of electronmicroscopy and morphometry. Searching histories with regard to DES exposure, together with meticulous histopathological examination of resected oviducts with known hysterosalpingographic deformities as well as those from ectopic pregnancy cases are mandatory.

Fortunately, the DES syndrome has been cut off, so to speak, by elimination of DES from clinical use where transplacental transfer could occur. Nevertheless the former use of DES still continues to produce further unwelcome vistas, e.g. the prospect from mouse studies of an increased incidence of mammary cancer in ageing human populations exposed to DES by transplacental transfer (Bern & Talamentes, 1981).

In the interim, Senekjian et al (1988) have confirmed 'an estimated cumulative rate . . . of first pregnancy of 16% for the (DES) exposed group and 30% for the unexposed group . . . one year after . . . primary infertility (was diagnosed)'. Ludmir et al (1987) described the advantages of prophylactic cerclage in the management of DES-exposed pregnant patients, thus inciting controversy (Harger, 1989). Sharp et al (1990) point out that most mothers of daughters with vaginal and vaginal/exocervical clear cell adenocarcinomas who denied DES intake were 'positive by written records', and in ageing DES-exposed offspring, cases may continue to occur or recur, as emphasized by Herbst & Anderson (1990), both for vaginal and cervical lesions, where recurrent clear cell adenocarcinomas have been found 20 years after 'primary therapy'. For DES-related clear cell adenocarcinoma development Herbst et al (1986) reviewed risk factors, e.g. DES intake prior to week 12 of pregnancy, winter conception, and prior miscarriage. Adams et al (1989) suspect in utero DES exposure to be a possible cause of intrapartum uterine rupture in a multiparous patient displaying no predisposing events or factors.

IATROGENIC CARCINOGENESIS

Irradiation-induced malignancy

Irradiation-induced carcinogenesis has been reviewed by Sadove et al (1981) who included two cases in which radiation therapy for pelvic carcinomas (one tubal, one ovarian) induced malignancy (one fibrosarcoma of sacrum, one carcinosarcoma of uterus). The latter case (Williamson & Christopherson, 1972) occurred 11 years after radiation for abdominal and pelvic carcinomatosis for an 'unspecified primary ovarian tumour'. Paik & Komorowski (1976) reported an instance of haemangiosarcoma of the abdominal wall following radiation therapy of endometrial carcinoma.

While noting that uterine leiomyosarcoma has been attributed to pelvic irradiation, Taylor & Norris (1966) were unable to confirm such an association. Previous irradiation was, however, recorded in 12% of uterine sarcomas, not including leiomyosarcoma. In a study of 64 instances of postirradiation pelvic malignancies, Rodriguez & Hart (1982) confirmed a negative correlation regarding uterine leiomyosarcoma, but associated five uterine carcinosarcomas with prior irradiation. In this study, 17.2 years represented the mean interval between irradiation and the diagnosis of subsequent malignancy; 13 initial tumours were squamous cell cervical carcinomas and 10 of the subsequent ones were endometrial adenocarcinomas.

Kleinerman et al (1982) reported on 5997 women followed for up to 38 years (mean 8.9) after radiotherapy for cervical cancer, noting after 15 years an excess incidence of subsequent malignancies in bladder, kidneys, rectum, ovaries and corpus uteri.

Anteby et al (1983) found no apparent correlation between irradiation and ovarian cancer in humans.

Lowell et al (1983) reported seven cases of genital condyloma virus infection following pelvic irradiation. Patients' ages ranged from 25–68 years, median 42 years. The youngest patient developed invasive squamous cell carcinoma in a condyloma acuminatum 11 years after irradiation for Hodgkin's disease.

Fujimura et al (1991) investigated the implication of human papillomavirus in postirradiation dysplasia. They examined biopsy tissue of cervix and/or vagina from 17 patients who previously had radiation therapy for gynaecological malignancy and found that persistent or repeated HPV infection was the most likely aetiological factor for postirradiation dysplasia. They concluded that HPV infection might be facilitated by immunosuppression due to pelvic irradiation.

Gynaecological cancer and immunosuppression

There is strong evidence that human papillomavirus is a co-factor in the development of cervical neoplasia (Zur Hansen, 1987). Clinical experience indicates that there is an increase in the incidence of cervical carcinoma in situ (CIN 3) in immunosuppressed women (Cordiner et al, 1980; Penn, 1980; Schneider et al, 1982). Schafer et al (1991) studied cytological smears of the uterine cervix of 111 human immunodeficiency virus infected women and found that cervical neoplasia, including invasive carcinoma, was seen in 41% of patients compared to 9% in an HIV-negative intravenous drug user control group and 4% in a sample from outpatients. Studies of lymphocytes were performed and showed that the frequency and severity of neoplasia was inversely related to the number of CD4 T lymphocytes. They concluded that an increased risk for the development of cervical neoplasia in HIV-infected women is related to the degree of immunosup-

pression. Similar associations were reported by Vermund et al (1991), Henry et al (1989) and Johnson et al (1992).

Matorras et al (1991) found that HIV-positive women have a greater relative risk for HPV infection and that these infections are recurrent and resistant to treatment. Maiman et al (1991) suggested that abnormal cervical pathology is common among HIV-positive women and recommended that cervical colposcopy be part of the routine management.

Women who are immunosuppressed from causes other than HIV are also at increased risk for cervical neoplasia. Alloub et al (1989) reported a significantly increased incidence of HPV infection and cervical intraepithelial neoplasia in 49 women with renal allografts and emphasized the need for regular colposcopic examination.

A case of endometrial carcinoma in a premenopausal woman with systemic lupus erythematosus was reported by Sekiya et al (1988). She had received both prednisolone and an immunosuppressive agent for more than 10 years.

For other immunosuppressant effects related to neoplasia, e.g. non-lymphoid leukaemia following treatment of ovarian cancer by alkylating agents, the reviews of Clayson (1972, 1981) dealing with therapy and subsequent cancer are especially helpful.

Transplacental carcinogenesis

The relationship between clear cell adenocarcinoma of the vagina and prenatal exposure to DES has already been discussed.

Oestrogens and endometrial carcinoma

Endometrial adenocarcinoma and exogenous oestrogens have long been considered a classic example of iatrogenic carcinogenesis. Thus increased usage of oestrogens is paralleled by a rise in the incidence of endometrial adenocarcinoma and case-control studies have demonstrated that oestrogen therapy is associated with a considerably increased risk of endometrial carcinoma, the magnitude of the risk being both time- and dose-related (Fox, 1984). Many objections have, however, been raised to these studies, these including the retrospective nature of case-control studies, the effect of women receiving oestrogens having greater access to medical care and increased medical surveillance, the overdiagnosis of atypical hyperplasia as adenocarcinoma, the wrong choice of control groups in case-control studies and the possibility that oestrogens simply unmask an otherwise clinically silent endometrial adenocarcinoma. All these objections have now been countered and a World Health Organization Scientific Group (1981) stated that 'The magnitude of the association is such that the factors by which large doses (certainly as little as 1.25 mg a day for five years and perhaps less) increase the risk from endometrial cancer is comparable to the factor by which heavy smoking increases the risk from lung cancer'.

Tamoxifen and uterine neoplasia

Tamoxifen is an anti-oestrogen which, whilst being widely used as adjuvant therapy in women with carcinoma of the breast, also has, under certain conditions, an oestrogenic effect. A wide range of uterine neoplasms has been reported as occurring in women receiving tamoxifen therapy (Killackey et al, 1985; Hardell, 1988; Malfetano, 1990; Fornander et al, 1991; Magriples et al, 1993; Silva et al, 1994). Tamoxifen usage has been linked to the development not only of endometrial carcinomas but also of uterine sarcomas and mixed tumours; whether, however, there is a true causal relationship between tamoxifen and the development of these neoplasms and, if so, the magnitude of the risk is currently uncertain.

Iatrogenic malignant change in endometriosis

Brooks & Wheeler (1977) reviewed the literature on malignant change in endometriosis and noted, among 45 cases, three with histories of previous pelvic irradiation and four having 'exogenous oestrogens or oestrogen secreting ovarian tumours'. Czernobilsky & Morris (1979) reviewed 194 instances of ovarian endometriosis, noting 'severe epithelial atypism' in seven and atypical hyperplasia in four of them. Although citing the reports of Brooks & Wheeler (1977) and Hyman (1977), Czernobilsky & Morris do not cite histories of oestrogen use or prior irradiation but Reimnitz et al (1988) note prior and unopposed oestrogen replacement.

IATROGENIC ATYPIAS

Irradiation

Two kinds of radiation are responsible for cellular injury: particular rays and electromagnetic waves.

Radiation induces intracellular chemical changes through generation of free radicals, very unstable, reactive molecules. Most vulnerable to radiation is DNA, therefore cells with high DNA content and frequent mitoses are particularly affected. The cellular injury related to radiation can be reversible or irreversible. The reversible injury can be acute or chronic.

Graham (1947) first described the effects of radiation on squamous epithelia of the vagina and cervix. The acute radiation changes consist of: cellular and nuclear enlargement with cytoplasmic and sometimes nuclear vacuolization. In addition, nuclei show degenerative changes ranging from pyknosis and karyorrhexis to homogeneous finely granular chromatin. Sometimes multinucleated forms are present. An acute inflammation completes the picture of the acute radiation changes. Chronic radiation changes may be seen many years after radiotherapy within the epithelial cells and stroma. There is cellular and nuclear enlargement, and nuclear chromatin is hyperchromatic but homogeneous (Patten et al, 1963; Little, 1968; Patten, 1976; Koss, 1979). Multinucleated cells can persist. The inflammatory background is replaced by hyalinized stroma.

Podophyllin-induced atypias

Podophyllin-induced atypias may ensue following application of this chemical to condylomas of the lower genital tract. The view that mitotic activity is inconsistent with this diagnosis is not tenable. Indeed, because of metaphase arrest, mitoses may appear numerous (Ferenczy, 1977) and nuclear atypia may persist after cells resume complete mitotic division. A history of podophyllin use may ward off the disaster of misinterpretation and should always be sought in any questionable lesion.

Steroid hormones

Bizarre, confusing and sometimes hazardous are the capacities of leiomyomas to respond with atypias to oral contraceptive use, as noted by Prakash & Scully as early as 1964. Goldzieher et al (1966) related such atypias to progestagen therapy. A drug history is required when assessing uterine leiomyomas in patients receiving progestagen-containing oral contraceptives. Goldzieher et al (1966) found that, in some instances, infarction may be responsible for enlargement in such lesions. Mitoses are rare in progestagen-provoked atypias in uterine leiomyomas (Prakash & Scully, 1964).

Norris et al (1988) reported clinical and pathological findings in 22 women with haemorrhagic cellular leiomyomas ('apoplectic leiomyoma'). Seventeen women were taking oral contraceptives, four were pregnant or postpartum, and only one woman was using hydrochlorothiazide.

DRUG-INDUCED LESIONS — MISCELLANEOUS

Spermatocide-induced inflammation

Nonoxynol-9 (n-9) spermatocide preparations produce, at dosage levels only 10–20 times greater than those approved for human subjects, hyperacute vaginitis and endometritis in rats (Tryphonas & Buttar, 1982) (Fig. 36.9). These lesions heal by fibrosis which can cause complete obliteration of vaginal or uterine lumens. Embryotoxic effects have also been noted in rats (Tryphonas & Buttar, 1983). Cynomolgus monkeys suffer lesser degrees of acute inflammation and fibrosis (Tryphonas et al 1983). An epidemiological inquiry is currently being designed to settle the obvious question, how frequently is n-9 responsible for appreciable lower genital tract inflammation in

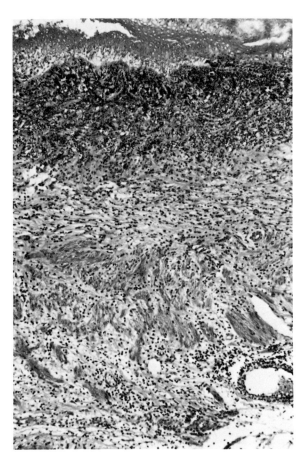

Fig. 36.9 Vagina of rat 12 hours following instillation of nonoxynol-9 spermatocide. Note extensive ulceration and widespread inflammatory infiltration. H & E × 100 approx.

Table 36.2 Adverse effects reported following per vaginam application of various agents. This list excludes agents causing adverse effects unlikely to come to the attention of the laboratory physician. n.b. Review of a sample of five spermatocide manufacturers' package inserts reveals warnings to patients of vaginitis-related symptoms in terms of 'burning', 'itching', 'irritation', 'discharge'.

Agent	Adverse effects	References
Benzalkonium chloride	Heat or burning sensation Itching and increased vaginal discharge	Interpharm Pharmaceutical Inc. Product monograph (1982)
Douching products	Vaginal haemorrhage Chemical peritonitis Endometritis Allergic reactions	Hoag (1979)
Hexachlorophene* vaginal packs	Lethargy, confusion, convulsions, death	Lockhart (1972)
Non-ionic spermicides (incl. nonoxynol-9 containing formulations)	Vaginitis or soreness Burning or irritation Allergic reactions, cystitis Cervico-vaginitis Endometritis	Huff & Hernandez (1979) McKinnon (1980) Gottesman (1980) Melchior & Hamann (1980) Tryphonas & Buttar (1982, 1984)
Phenylmercuric acetate	Increase in blood urea Nephrotoxicity	Al-Jobori (1975)
Potassium permanganate tablets	Vaginal bleeding, vaginal and cervical burns	Shull (1941) McDonough (1945) Johnson (1949) Abd-El-Salam (1977)
Povidone-iodine	Hyperthyroidism Allergy and dermatitis Burning vaginal sensation	Jacobson et al (1981) Reybrouck (1983)

* A potential for fetotoxicity from use of hexachlorophene-containing surgical soaps in vaginal examinations during labour has been reported by Strickland et al (1983).

humans? n-9 and other spermatocides, including vaginal douching products, have been incriminated in a variety of urogenital inflammations encountered in clinical practice (see Table 36.2).

Recently observed following a single intravaginal application of the spermatocide benzalkonium chloride in Wistar rats, was an acute necrotizing vaginitis with arteritis, polymorphonuclear leucocytic infiltrations, fibrinoid necrosis, perimural and mural fibrosis, mural thickening and luminal stenosis. Similar treatment in rhesus monkeys evoked a necrotizing vaginitis without vasculopathy. No such lesions were found in untreated tissues (Tryphonas & Buttar, unpublished data). We suggest that, should such lesions be observed in human vaginal biopsy specimens, a history of spermatocide use be sought for prior to invasive and expensive investigation for systemic vascular disease. Lauritzen & Meineke (1987) reported two cases of isolated arteritis in the human cervix, also supporting a conservative, expectant approach in follow-up studies (see also Necrotizing vasculitis).

The morphological effects of benzalkonium chloride on the female genital tract were investigated in adult female rhesus monkeys (*Macaca mulatta*) given a single per vaginam application (100 mg/kg) of a fresh 40% (w/v) solution of benzalkonium chloride. The vagina of control females, given intravaginal instillates of an equal volume (0.25 ml/kg) of physiological saline, had a normal appearance (Fig. 36.10a,c). Treated females developed acute necrotizing vaginitis which at 24 hours was characterized by necrosis of the vaginal epithelium and oedema with diapedesis of polymorphonuclear leucocytes into the lamina propria. At 48 hours this process was complicated by extensive sloughing of the vaginal epithelium and intravaginal accumulation of necrotic debris, and was accompanied by early reparative activation of surviving basal epithelial cells (Fig. 36.10b,d) (Tryphonas & Buttar, unpublished observations).

Venereal drug adverse reaction

Little attention seems to have been paid to reactions to drugs, drug metabolites or other chemicals transmitted by semen. Nevertheless, to produce an adverse reaction to penicillin, it is enough for a sensitized female to receive benzylpenicillin-rich ejaculate from a penicillin-treated partner (Hennigar, 1971). Propranolol as a novel sperma-

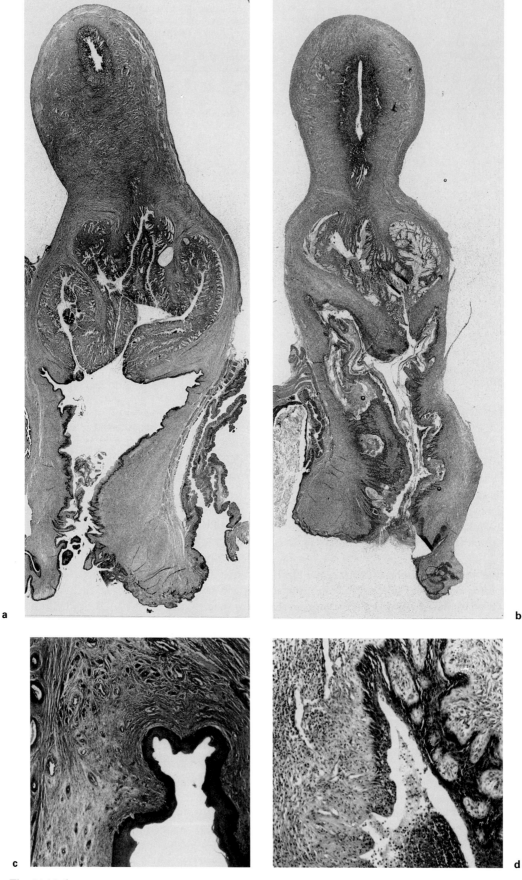

Fig. 36.10–d

Fig. 36.10 **a.** Gross longitudinal section of vagina, cervix, and uterus of a control rhesus monkey 48 h following intravaginal administration of physiological saline (0.25 ml/kg). The vaginal epithelium has a normal appearance. **b.** A similar section from a rhesus monkey 48 h after a single intravaginal application of benzalkonium chloride (100 mg/kg). Note sloughing of the vaginal mucosa. **c.** Higher magnification of fornix from control rhesus shown in **a**. The vaginal epithelium has a normal appearance. **d.** Higher magnification of fornix from **b** above. There is diffuse accumulation of polymorphonuclear leucocytes at the lamina propria, reparative activation of surviving basal layer cells, and sloughing of necrotic epithelium.

tocide is absorbed so readily per vaginam as to produce plasma concentrations about double that obtained by the oral route (Patel et al, 1983). No adverse effects were observed, but Zipper et al (1983) suggest systemic modes of action. No comment was made about systemic spermicidal action in propranolol-treated males, nor about venereal transfer of propranolol to susceptible or sensitized female partners.

Steroid hormones

Oestrogens and progestagens are the commonest cause of drug-induced abnormalities of the female genital tract: these are considered at length in Chapter 35 (n.b. Young & Scully, 1989).

Digitalis

Digitalis has an oestrogenic effect and long-term administration can be associated with endometrial proliferation and vaginal keratinization in postmenopausal women (Britsch & Azar, 1963; Winkler et al, 1982).

Gold

This drug, used in the treatment of rheumatoid arthritis, has been reported as causing acute vaginitis (Webster & Guden, 1979).

Anticoagulants

The administration of anticoagulants to premenopausal women may cause ovarian haemorrhage from a corpus luteum, follicular cyst or Graafian follicle (Wong & Gillett, 1977; Winkler et al, 1982).

Chemotherapy and fertility

Impaired fertility and premature menopause following mustine, vinblastine, procarbazine and prednisolone therapy for Hodgkin's disease are common. Fertility in males is more severely affected (King et al, 1985).

Chemotherapy and atypical proliferation in endometrial polyps

Atypical proliferations including borderline neoplastic appearances have been observed in endometrial polyps following tamoxifen therapy for breast carcinoma (Nuovo et al, 1989), emphasizing a need for a history of drug use when contemplating diagnoses of malignancy.

Toxicity of vaginally administered drugs

Buttar (1993) has reviewed this topic, noting a human fatality from a benzalkonium chloride-containing douche to secure abortion and an instance of erythema multiforme in a penicillin-sensitive female following intercourse with a penicillin-treated male (Goette & Odom, 1980; see also Hennigar, 1971; Jacobson et al, 1981). Buttar also cites the forensic classic of Macht (1918), who described 'arsenic administered per vaginam to (a first) wife . . . to get rid of her and repeating the . . . procedure to get rid of a . . . second (wife)'.

SURGICALLY-INDUCED IATROGENIC DISEASE — MISCELLANEOUS

Endometriosis

Heterotopia of endometrium may ensue following invasive procedures on the uterus, e.g. abdominal wall endometriosis following amniocentesis, as in the case of Kaunitz & DiSant'Agnese (1979), and a case of uterine wall endometriosis at the site of ovarian implantation in a uterine window (Estes procedure) (Szlachter et al, 1980). Kaunitz & Di Sant'Agnese also refer to a report of abdominal wall endometriosis following hysterotomy. We have not seen endometrial heterotopia related to caesarian section.

Post dilatation and curettage salpingitis

Mild but acute tubal inflammation may follow uterine curerttage, this possibly being induced by debris forced into the oviducts at the time of the uterine surgery (Kraus, 1967). Such lesions should, by referral to clinical notes, be distinguished from physiological salpingitis and from pyogenic disease.

Asherman's syndrome

Uterine curettings occasionally contain a considerable depth of myometrium. This observation is most likely to be made in specimens obtained following miscarriage, especially when the myometrium is extensively involved by organizing placental bed inflammation. This finding should always be reported as a warning of possible secondary amenorrhoea and fertility problems to come in the form of Asherman's syndrome (Asherman, 1960), and as a precaution to the operator lest, in the future, he come to penetrate the entire myometrium. Asherman comments that 'this type of amenorrhoea is a trying sequel to uterine curettage, especially post-partum curettage, the lesions being 'stricture or obliteration of the cervical canal . . . the uterine cavity [being] diminished and deformed by adhesions but (in regard to 'total atresia') some crumbs of tissue . . . were microscopically identified as endometrium'.

Uterine perforation

Very rarely an endometrial curetting contains fields of fat consistent with that of omentum (Fig. 36.11). At elective hysterectomy performed three weeks after such an incident, a tract of healthy granulation tissue was found leading in a straight line from near the cornu through the fundic myometrium to the serosa. This perforation, like the others, was without sequelae. It has been suggested that contractility of the myometrium seals off the deficit and stifles bleeding promptly. With infection, graver results are predictable.

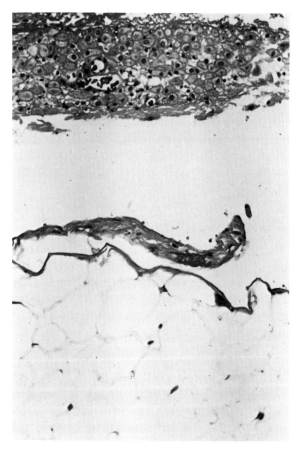

Fig. 36.11 Fat in endometrial curettings. Fat deemed to have been derived from some extrauterine source such as omentum, adherent or otherwise, is present. Haematoxylin, phloxine and saffron × 150 approx.

Uterine rupture

Rupture of the uterus following classical caesarean section haunts the memory, recalling that mural scars provide for defective decidua, favouring deep ingrowth of the placenta; and scars can stretch. Seemingly for the same reasons, uterine rupture has been reported following curettage (Nuyens & Campbell, 1957; Fox, 1972).

Oviduct prolapse (see Ch. 4)

In the vaginal vault small raspberry-like structures in the line of closure of a previous hysterectomy often prove to be a prolapse of the fimbriated end of the oviduct (Bilodeau, 1982). This entity is now well recognized and confusion with an adenocarcinoma should not arise.

Anastasiades & Majmudar (1983) have, however, documented an instance of Fallopian tube prolapse into the urinary bladder — a lesion originally diagnosed as a papillary bladder carcinoma.

The 'tube-tied' syndrome

Menstrual changes encountered after tubal sterilization procedures have included irregular and more frequent menstrual periods, prolonged and increased flow, intermenstrual spotting, reduced menstrual flow and dysmenorrhoeas. Such symptoms have been attributed to a reduced ovarian blood supply as a result of mesosalpingeal damage, and mastodynia and fibrocystic breast disease have also been attributed to consequent ovarian malfunction. In the long term about half of the patients do well following such procedures, but as many as 50% of 'tubal sterilization' patients may require (further) gynaecological surgery (Vorherr et al, 1983). DeStefano et al (1983) followed 2456 patients for two years after tubal sterilization: 50% of such patients with prior menstrual dysfunction were improved, and these investigators conclude that an association between menstrual dysfunction and prior tubal sterilization is denied by epidemiological findings. Claims that prior sterilization may be a precipitating cause of hysterectomy should therefore be treated with some caution.

Ovarian remnant syndrome (see also Ch. 19)

This condition is considered to be present whenever ovarian function persists after surgery in which attempts to remove both ovaries *in toto* have failed. It is usual to find that oophorectomy had been difficult because of periovarian scars and adhesions from endometriosis or other sources of pelvic inflammatory disease. Illustrative cases (Muram & Drouin, 1982) were found with (a) pelvic pain, (b) pelvic mass, (c) urinary frequency, and (d) abnormal uterine bleeding. Treatment required removal of the pelvic masses, which were cystic or multicystic, varying from 4–20 cm in diameter. By histopathological examination of these masses, ovarian cortical remnants and corpora lutea were found, along with endometriosis. These cystic masses may, in the authors' experience, be confused with primary ovarian neoplasms and, indeed, the latter may be present and malignant (Shemwell & Weed, 1970). Ureteral obstruction was not a feature of these cases but has repeatedly been recorded elsewhere, as noted in Muram & Drouin's (1982) references.

Cabanne & Bonenfant (1980) draw attention to accessory, supernumerary and ectopic ovaries. Ectopic ovaries in a lumbosacral location, or redundant accessory or supernumerary ovaries in ectopic sites, may perhaps be overlooked when unsuspected at oophorectomy.

IATROGENIC LESIONS DUE TO ERRORS IN HISTOLOGICAL DIAGNOSIS

Errors of overdiagnosis

Arias-Stella atypia (Fig. 36.12)

Arias-Stella atypia may well be misdiagnosed as an endometrial carcinoma, but a diagnosis of well-differentiated clear cell carcinoma of endometrium should not be considered unequivocal unless pregnancy and the use of progestagens have been excluded. It should be noted that Arias-Stella atypia may also occur in endometriosis (Campbell et al, 1974) and in the tube, particularly in tubal pregnancies (Mikhael et al, 1977).

Atypical microglandular endocervical hyperplasia

This lesion, occurring in oral contraceptive users, is now well known, but may perhaps still sometimes be misdiagnosed as an adenocarcinoma (Young & Scully, 1989). One might remark that such lesions are *not* limited to oral contraceptive users (Nichols & Fidler, 1971) and, in the presence of mucoviscidosis, the proportion of mucus should be expected to increase and the lesions to assume polypoid forms (Dooley et al, 1974).

Menstrual endometrium and carcinoma

It occasionally happens in curettings of menstrual endometrium that fields of glands, crowded together amidst polymorphonuclear leucocytes and remnants of dissociated stroma, are mistakenly interpreted as adenocarcinoma.

Experience soon accustoms the observer to recognize this pitfall, but the rule of thumb regarding inflammation in curettings as a clue to endometrial carcinomas is here misleading.

Postoperative spindle cell nodules

These reactive proliferative spindle cell lesions that develop shortly after surgery (Proppe et al, 1984; Kay

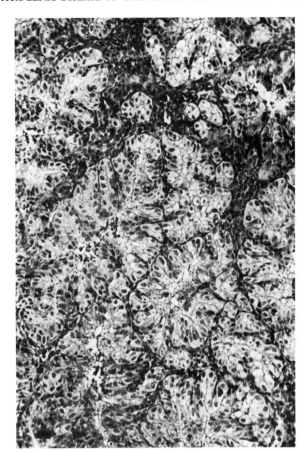

Fig. 36.12 Arias-Stella atypia of endometrium from intrauterine pregnancy which aborted. Haematoxylin, saffron and eosin × 150 approx.

& Schneider, 1985) can easily be overdiagnosed as sarcomas.

Endosalpingeal proliferations

Pseudoneoplastic hyperplasia of the endosalpinx is characteristic of tuberculous inflammation, although far from constant in that condition.

This sort of lesion may also occur as a feature of chronic pyogenic inflammation in the course of resolution, as an exaggeration of a repair process. Marked examples are fortunately rare, since individual fields of a carcinoma may be indistinguishable from pseudocarcinomatous hyperplasia of the endosalpinx. Populations of lymphocytes may only serve to confuse the issue, since their presence may, on one hand, represent a part of resolving inflammation or, on the other, a reaction to tumour antigen. A past history suggestive of inflammatory disease, consideration of age and thorough histological evaluation may still fail to provide a final solution, even where the suspect proliferation is, in multiple sections, clearly non-invasive. If total hysterectomy and bilateral salpingo-oophorectomy have been performed, the presence of ovarian and endometrial neoplasia might help settle the question in favour of tubal cancer, on the basis of a Müllerian field change; otherwise the conundrum may remain.

Obviously the problem will usually arise in examining oviducts removed from putative cases of inflammatory disease where isolated in situ proliferative endosalpingeal lesions are almost assuredly benign.

Mesothelial cystic lesions

Particularly around the uterine adnexa, complexes of spaces and entanglements of fibrous adhesions may form multiple small- to medium-sized cysts up to several centimetres in greatest diameter, or form sponge-like serosal thickenings. When such lesions are found to be lined by serosal cells, a diagnosis of mesothelioma is tempting and, indeed, may well be made (Katsube et al, 1982), but findings of lint, starch or talc-like particles point to previous surgery.

Peritoneal gliomatosis (see Ch. 23)

The association of ovarian teratomas containing glial or neural elements with widely scattered peritoneal implants has long been recognized as a pitfall in diagnosis. If such peritoneal lesions are misdiagnosed as malignant, the stage is set for catastrophic therapeutic 'overkill'.

Errors of underdiagnosis

These occur particularly in the case of unusually well-differentiated neoplasms such as verrucous carcinoma of the vulva, cervix and vagina or the 'adenoma malignum' of the endocervix: these are fully discussed in Chapters 3, 4 and 7.

Errors may also arise because the pathologist is presented with an inadequate biopsy. Punch biopsy cervical specimens, initially colposcopically directed, failed to reveal unsuspected severe lesions, e.g. adenocarcinoma in situ, which appeared in loop excision specimens of cervical transformation zones (Buxton et al, 1991) and hence are inadequate for establishing end points. The revelance of such considerations is reflected upon in a review of the events which took place in New Zealand (Flagler & Winkler, 1992).

REFERENCES

General

Argent V 1988 Failed sterilization and the law. British Journal of Obstetrics and Gynaecology 95: 113–115.

Benirschke K 1990 The placenta in the litigation process. British Journal of Obstetrics and Gynaecology 162: 1445–1450.

Bibbo M 1979 Transplacental effects of diethylstilbestrol. Current Topics in Pathology 66: 191–211.

Brand K G, Johnson K H, Buoen L C 1976 Foreign body tumorigenesis. CRC Critical Reviews in Toxicology 4: 353–394.

Brennan M 1992 Err on side of caution when prescribing to the elderly, physician advises. Canadian Medical Association Journal 146: 1605.

Buttar H S 1993 Absorption and toxicity of drugs intended for vaginal administration. Canadian Pharmaceutical Journal 126: 27–33.

Clayson D B, Shubik P 1976 The carcinogenic action of drugs. Cancer Detection and Prevention 1: 43–77.

Clements R V 1991 Litigation in obstetrics and gynecology. British Journal of Obstetrics and Gynaecology 98: 423–426.

Cook D C, Dent O, Hewitt D 1974 Breast cancer following multiple chest fluoroscopy: the Ontario experience. Canadian Medical Association Journal 111: 406–412.

Craighead J E 1992 The pathologist as an expert witness. Archives of Pathology and Laboratory Medicine 118: 488–489.

Cuniff C, Jones K L, Phillipson J, Benirschke K, Short S, Wuje K J 1990 Oligohydramnios sequence and renal tubular malformation associated with enalapril use. American Journal of Obstetrics and Gynecology 162: 187–189.

Dankwa E K, Davies J D 1985 Frozen section diagnosis: an audit. Journal of Clinical Pathology 38: 1235–1240.

Ford M R W, Turner M F, Wood C, Soutter W P 1988 Endometriosis developing during tamoxifen therapy. American Journal of Obstetrics and Gynecology 158: 1119.

Grossman, The Honorable Larry, Minister of Health 1983 Data from Ontario Ministry of Health, hospital statistics. In: Remarks to launch a fund-raising drive for Metro women's groups, Toronto, 24th May.

Herbst A L 1990 Medical professional liability and obstetric care: The Institute of Medicine report and recommendations. Obstetrics and Gynecology 75: 705–709.

Kubinski M, Kubinski Z O, Javid M 1982 Suspected cancer-causing agents in the hospital environment. Ecotoxicology and Environmental Safety 6: 9–18.

Last J 1980 The hazards of medical care. In: Sartwell P E (ed) Maxcy Roseneau public health and preventive medicine. Appleton-Century-Crofts, New York, pp 1787–1799.

Last J 1992 The Barer-Stoddart Report. Annals of the Royal College of Physicians and Surgeons of Canada 25: 94–95.

Lewkonia R M 1991 Quality assurance training in graduate clinical education. Annals of The Royal College of Physicians and Surgeons of Canada 24: 49–50.

McLachlan J A, Dixon R L 1976 Transplacental toxicity of diethylstilbestrol: a special problem in safety evaluation. In: Melmon M A, Shapiro R E, Blumental H (eds) Advances in modern toxicology, vol 1, part 1. New concepts in safety evaluation. Hemisphere Publishing, Washington. Wiley, New York, pp 423–448.

Messerti M, Parmley T, Woodruff J D et al 1987 Inter- and intra-pathologist variability in the diagnosis of gestational trophoblastic neoplasia. Obstetrics and Gynecology 89: 622–626.

Metheny W P, Bloun T H, Holzman C B 1991 Considering obstetrics and gynecology as a speciality: current attractors and detractors. Obstetrics and Gynecology 78: 308–312.

Napke E 1983 Adverse reactions: some pitfalls and postules. In: Side effects of drugs annual 7. Excerpta Medica, Amsterdam, pp xv–xxv.

Newbold R R, Bullock B C, McLachlan J A 1983 Exposure to diethylstilbestrol during pregnancy permanently alters the ovary and oviduct. Biology of Reproduction 28: 735–744.

Perucca E, Richers A 1982 In: Gundermann E (ed) The pathophysiological basis of drug toxicity in drug-induced pathology. Springer Verlag, Berlin, pp 18–68.

Prichard J R S et al 1990 Liability and compensation in health care, Appendix B vol 1, vol 2, vol 3. University of Toronto Press. Vide Appendix A 1.10 Future Trends and Uncertainties p 169 through 2.1 Reform Agenda To p 191. Health Policy Directorate. Health and Welfare Canada, Ottawa.

Repacholi M H 1981 Ultrasound: characteristics and biological action. National Research Council of Canada (criteria document), publication no. NRCC 19244.

Robertson A J et al 1989 Observer variability in histopathologic reporting of cervical biopsy specimens. Journal of Clinical Pathology 42: 231–238.

Rosendaal G M A 1992 Quality assurance and academic medicine. Annals of The Royal College of Physicians and Surgeons of Canada 25: 98.

Sandmire H F 1989 Malpractice — the syndrome of the 80s. Obstetrics and Gynecology 73: 145.

Shertine D M, Metheny W P 1988 A comparison of resident and program director views on the effects of subspecialty fellowships on residency training in obstetrics and gynecology. American Journal of Obstetrics and Gynecology 158: 625.

Vincent C A, Martin T, Ennis M 1991 Obstetric accidents: the patient's perspective. British Journal of Obstetrics and Gynaecology 98: 390–395.

Waugh D 1992 Royal College symposium offers plethora of opinions on future of academic medicine. Canadian Medical Association Journal 146: 267–268.

Weinstein L 1988 Malpractice — the syndrome of the 80s. Obstetrics and Gynecology 72: 130–135.

Whitehead M E, Fitzwater J E, Lindley S K, Kern S B, Ulinsch R C, Winecoff W F 1984 Quality assurance of histopathologic diagnoses: a prospective audit of three thousand cases. American Journal of Clinical Pathology 81: 487–491.

Whitelaw J M 1990 Hysterectomy: A medico-legal perspective 1975–1985. American Journal of Obstetrics and Gynecology 162: 1451–1458.

Zarbo R J, Hoffman G G, Howanitz P J 1991 Interinstitutional comparison of frozen-section consultation. Archives of Pathology and Laboratory Medicine 115: 1187–1194.

Specific

Abd-El-Salam A F 1977 The use of potassium permanganate as an abortifacient amongst Egyptian rural communities. Ain Shams Medical Journal 28: 201–205.

Abell M R 1969 The Reynold L. Mass Memorial Lecture: gynecologic curiosities and concepts. University of Michigan Medical Centre Journal 35: 1–9.

Acharya V, Tolnai G, Campbell J S, Hooper D 1973 Maltese cross surgery. Canadian Medical Association Journal 109: 1183–1186.

Adams D M, Druzin M L, Cederovist L L 1989 Intrapartum uterine rupture. Obstetrics and Gynecology 73: 471–473.

Al-Jobori I M 1975 Mercury levels in females exposed to phenyl mercuric acetate. Baghdad College of Pharmacy, University of Baghdad, pp 10–110. (Cited in Federal Register 45: 82014–82049, 1980.)

Alloub M I, Borr B B, McLorier K M, Smith I H, Bunry M H, Smart G E 1989 Human papilloma virus infections and cervical intraepithelial neoplasia in women with renal allografts. British Medical Journal 298: 153–156.

Anastasiades K D, Majmudar B 1983 Prolapse of Fallopian tube into urinary bladder, mimicking bladder carcinoma. Archives of Pathology and Laboratory Medicine 107: 613–614.

Ansell I D, Evans D J, Wight D G D 1974 Asymptomatic arteritis of the uterine cervix. Journal of Clinical Pathology 27: 664–668.

Anteby S O, Mor-Yosef S, Schenker J G 1983 Ovarian cancer: geographical host and environmental factors: an overview. Archives of Gynecology 234: 137–148.

Argent V 1988 Failed sterilization and the law. British Journal of Obstetrics and Gynaecology 95: 113–115.

Asherman J G 1960 The myth of tubal and endometrial transplantation. Journal of Obstetrics and Gynaecology of the British Empire 67: 228–233.

Baker P B, Zarbo R J 1991 Interinstitutional comparison of data reporting in current autopsy front sheets: a Q-probes study. Laboratory Investigation 64: 120.

Benirschke K, Bonin M L, Rost T 1984 Plant material in ovary following barium enema. Archives of Pathology and Laboratory Medicine 108: 359–360.

Bern H A, Talamentes F J 1981 Neonatal mouse models and their relation to disease in the human female mammary gland. In: Herbst A L, Bern H A (eds) Developmental effects of diethylstilbestrol (DES) in pregnancy. Thieme Stratton, New York, p 139.

Bilodeau B 1982 Intravaginal prolapse of the Fallopian tube following vaginal hysterectomy. American Journal of Obstetrics and Gynecology 143: 970–971.

Britsch C J, Azar H A 1963 Estrogen effect in exfoliated vaginal cells following treatment with digitalis: a case report with experimental observations in mice. American Journal of Obstetrics and Gynecology 85: 989–993.

Brooks J J, Wheeler J E 1977 Malignancy arising in extragonadal endometriosis: a case report and summary of the world literature. Cancer 40: 3065–3073.

Buttar H S 1993 Absorption and toxicity of drugs intended for vaginal administration. Canadian Pharmaceutical Journal 126: 27–33.

Buxton E J, Luesley D M, Shafi M I, Rollason M 1991 Colposcopically directed punch biopsy: a potentially misleading investigation. British Journal of Obstetrics and Gynaecology 98: 1273–1276.

Cabanne F, Bonenfant J L (eds) 1980 Anatomie pathologique: principes de pathologie generale et speciale. Presses de l'Université Laval, Quebec.

Campbell J S 1972 Mangled and missed messages. Canadian Medical Association Journal 106: 219.

Campbell J S, Tryphonas L 1983 Interface between pathology and epidemiology in carcinogenesis. Toxicologic Pathology 11: 69–73.

Campbell J S, Nigam S, Hurtig A, Sahasrabudhe M R, Marino I 1964 Mineral oil granulomas of the uterus and parametrium and granulomatous salpingitis with Schaumann bodies and oxalate deposits. Fertility and Sterility 15: 278–289.

Campbell J S, Hacquebard S, Mitton D M, Hurteau G D, Bobra S T, Sirois J 1974 Acute hemoperitoneum, IUD, and occult ovarian pregnancy. Obstetrics and Gynecology 43: 438–442.

Campbell J S, Mikhael N Z, Napke E 1981 Evidence and appraisal of adverse reactions to drugs and other preparations used in hospital practice. In: Jasmin G, Cantin M (eds) Methods and achievements in experimental pathology vol 10. Karger, Basel, pp 221–243.

Clayson D B 1972 Carcinogenic hazards due to drugs. Drug Induced Disease 4: 91–109.

Clayson D B 1981 Therapeutic agents and procedures in cancer induction. In: Sontag J M (ed) Carcinogens in industry and the environment. Marcel Dekker, New York, pp 535–571.

Clayson D B, Shubik P 1976 The carcinogenic action of drugs. Cancer Detection and Prevention 1: 43–77.

Conley G R, Sant G R, Ucci A A, Mitcheson H D 1983 Seminoma and epididymal cysts in a young man with known diethylstilbestrol exposure in utero. Journal of the American Medical Association 249: 1325–1326.

Cooke S A R, Hamilton D G 1977 The significance of starch powder contamination in the aetiology of peritoneal adhesions. British Journal of Surgery 64: 410–412.

Cordiner J W, Sharp F, Briggs J D 1980 Cervical intraepithelial neoplasia in immunosuppressed women after renal transplantation. Scottish Medical Journal 25: 275–277.

Cramer D W, Welch W R, Scully R E, Wojciechowski C A 1982 Ovarian cancer and talc: a case-control study. Cancer 50: 372–376.

Cuniff C, Jones K L, Phillipson J et al 1990 Oligohydramnios sequence and renal tubular malformation associated with enalapril use. American Journal of Obstetrics and Gynecology 162: 187–189.

Czernobilsky B, Morris W J 1979 A histologic study of ovarian endometriosis with emphasis on hyperplastic and atypical changes. Obstetrics and Gynecology 53: 318–323.

David R, Berezesky I K, Bohlman M et al 1983 Fatal barium embolization due to incorrect vaginal rather than colonic insertion: an ultrastructural and x-ray microanalysis study. Archives of Pathology and Laboratory Medicine 107: 548–551.

Davies J D, Neely J 1972 Histopathology of peritoneal starch granulomas. Journal of Pathology 107: 265.

Dawson D 1992 Report of pathologist workload survey results.

De Cherney A H, Cholst I, Naftolin F 1981 Structure and function of the Fallopian tubes following exposure to diethylstilbestrol (DES) during gestation. Fertility and Sterility 36: 741–745.

De Stefano F, Huezo C M, Peterson H B, Rubin G L, Layde P M, Ory H W 1983 Menstrual changes after tubal sterilization. Obstetrics and Gynecology 62: 673–681.

Dooley R R, Braunstein H, Osher A B 1974 Polypoid cervicitis in cystic fibrosis patients receiving oral contraceptives. American Journal of Obstetrics and Gynecology 118: 971–974.

Elliot C B, Reynolds H H, Fidler H K 1968 Pseudosarcoma botryoides of cervix and vagina in pregnancy. Journal of Obstetrics and Gynaecology of the British Commonwealth 74: 728–733.

Ezra Y, Fields S, Kopolovic, Anteby S O 1988 Benign uterine leiomyoma suspected of sarcomatous change on an ultrasound scan and computerized tomography. Archives of Gynecology and Obstetrics 241: 255–258.

Ferenczy A 1977 In: Blaustein A (ed) Pathology of the female genital tract. Springer Verlag, Berlin, p 139.

Flagler E A, Winkler E R 1992 An unfortunate experiment: the New Zealand study of cancer of the cervix. Annals of the Royal College of Physicians and Surgeons of Canada 25: 124–130.

Ford M R W, Turner M F, Wood C, Soutter W P 1988 Endometriosis developing during tamoxifen therapy. American Journal of Obstetrics and Gynecology 158: 1119.

Fornander T, Rutqvist L E, Wilking N 1991 Effects of tamoxifen on the female genital tract. New York Academy of Sciences 622: 468–475.

Foster D 1992 Personal communication to the Authors.

Fox H 1972 Placenta accreta 1945–1969. Obstetrical and Gynecological Survey 27: 475–490.

Fox H 1984 Endometrial carcinogenesis and its relation to oestrogens. Pathology Research and Practice 179: 13–19.

Fraundorfer M R 1983 The intra-uterine device and hospital admission. British Journal of Family Planning 9: 79–85.

Fujimura M, Ostrow R S, Okagaki T 1991 Replication of human papillomavirus in postirradiation dysplasia. Cancer 68: 2181–2185.

Ghosh A 1976 Lipogranuloma of the uterine parametrium. British Journal of Obstetrics and Gynaecology 83: 409–410.

Godley E 1992 AIDS court case could lead to higher costs, CMA spokesman warns. Canadian Medical Association Journal 146: 227–231.

Goette D K, Odom R B 1980 Vaginal medications as a cause for varied widespread dermatitides. Cutis 26: 406–409.

Goldstein D P 1978 Incompetent cervix in offspring exposed to diethylstilbestrol in utero. Obstetrics and Gynecology 52: 73s–75s.

Goldzieher J W, Magyeo M, Ricaud L, Aguilar J A, Canales E 1966 Induction of degenerative changes in uterine myomas by high-dosage progestin therapy. American Journal of Obstetrics and Gynecology 96: 1078–1087.

Gottesman J E 1980 Contraceptive-induced cystitis. New England Journal of Medicine 302: 633.

Gotti E W 1974 Adverse drug reactions and the autopsy: prevalence and perspective. Archives of Pathology 97: 201–204.

Graham R M 1947 Effect of radiation on vaginal cells in cervical carcinoma. I. Description of cellular changes. II. Prognostic significance. Surgery, Gynecology and Obstetrics 84: 153–173.

Graham R M, Graham J B 1953 Cellular index of sensitivity to ionizing radiation, sensitization response. Cancer 6: 215–223.

Grant J B F, Davies J D, Jones J V, Espiner H J, Elleringham W K 1976 The immunogenicity of starch glove powder and talc. British Journal of Surgery 63: 864–866.

Haapasio H, Collan Y 1989 Volume corrected mitotic index (M/V-index): the standard of mitotic activity in neoplasms. Pathology Research and Practice 185: 551–554.

Hamilton G 1987 Contamination of contrast agents by MBT in rubber seals. Canadian Medical Association Journal 136: 1020–1021.

Hardell L 1988 Tamoxifen as risk factor for carcinoma of corpus uteri. Lancet 2: 563.

Harger J H 1989 Management of pregnancy in diethylstilbestrol-exposed patients. American Journal of Obstetrics and Gynecology 160: 273.

Harrison K A 1989 Maternal mortality in developing countries. British Journal of Obstetrics and Gynaecology 96: 1–3.

Henderson W J, Joslin C A F, Turnbull A C, Griffiths K 1971 Talc and carcinoma of the ovary and cervix. Journal of Obstetrics and Gynaecology of the British Commonwealth 78: 266–272.

Hennigar G R 1971 Drugs and chemical injury. In: Anderson W A D (ed) Pathology, 6th edn. Mosby, St Louis, pp 174–241.

Henry M J, Stanley M W, Cruikshank S, Carson L 1990 Association of human immunodeficiency virus induced immunosuppression with human papillomavirus infection and cervical intraepithelial neoplasia. American Journal of Obstetrics and Gynecology 160: 352–353.

Herbst A L 1981 Clear cell adenocarcinoma and the current status of DES-exposed females. Cancer 48: 484–488.

Herbst A L, Anderson. D 1990 Clear cell adenocarcinoma of the vagina and cervix secondary to exposure to diethylstilbestrol. Seminars in Surgical Oncology 6: 343–346.

Herbst A L, Bern H A (eds) 1981 Developmental effects of diethylstilbestrol (DES) in pregnancy. Thieme, Stuttgart.

Herbst A L, Cole P, Colton T, Robboy S J, Scully R E 1977 Age-incidence and risk of diethylstilbestrol-related clear cell adenocarcinoma of the vagina and cervix. American Journal of Obstetrics and Gynecology 128: 43–50.

Herbst A L, Cole P, Norusis M J, Welch W R, Scully R E 1979 Epidemiologic aspects and factors related to survival in 384 Registry cases of clear cell adenocarcinoma of the vagina and cervix. American Journal of Obstetrics and Gynecology 135: 876–886.

Herbst A L, Hubby M M, Azizi F, Makii M M 1981 Reproductive and gynecologic surgical experience in diethylstilbestrol-exposed daughters. American Journal of Obstetrics and Gynecology 141: 1019–1028.

Herbst A L, Anderson S, Hubby M M et al 1986 Risk factors for the development of diethylstilbestrol-associated clear cell adenocarcinoma: a case-control study. American Journal of Obstetrics and Gynecology 154: 814–822

Hidvegi D, Hidvegi I, Barrett J 1978 Douche-induced pelvic peritoneal starch granuloma. Obstetrics and Gynecology 52: 15s–18s.

Hoag S G 1979 Feminine cleansing and deodorant products. In: Penna R P (ed) Handbook of non-prescription drugs, 6th edn. American Pharmaceutical Association, Washington DC, pp 259–267.

Huff J, Hernandez L 1979 Contraceptive methods and products. In: Penna R P (ed) Handbook of non-prescription drugs, 6th edn. American Pharmaceutical Association, Washington DC, pp 247–257.

Hyman M P 1977 Extraovarian endometrioid carcinoma: review of the literature and report of two cases with unusual features. American Journal of Clinical Pathology 68: 522–527.

Interpharm Pharmaceutical Inc 1982 Product monograph. Laval, Quebec.

Irey N S 1972 Diagnostic problems drug induced diseases. In: Meyer L, Peek H M (eds) Drug induced diseases, vol 4. Excerpta Medica, Amsterdam, pp 1–4.

Irey N S 1976 Tissue reactions to drugs. American Journal of Pathology 82: 617–648.

Irey N S, Norris H J 1973 Intimal vascular lesions associated with female reproductive steroids. Archives of Pathology 96: 227–234.

Jacobson J M, Hankins G V, Murray J M, Young R L 1981 Self-limited hyperthyroidism following intravaginal iodine administration. American Journal of Obstetrics and Gynecology 140: 472–473.

Jeffries J A, Robboy S J, O'Brien P et al 1984 Structural anomalies of the cervix and vagina in women enrolled in the diethylstilbestrol adenosis (DESAD) project. American Journal of Obstetrics and Gynecology 148: 59–66.

Johnson C M 1949 Vaginal bleeding from the use of potassium permanganate. New Orleans Medical and Surgical Journal 102: 68–70.

Johnson J C, Burnett A F, Willet G D, Young M A, Doniger J 1992 The frequency of latent and clinical papillomavirus cervical lesions in immunocompromised human immunodeficiency virus-infected women. Obstetrics and Gynecology 79: 321–327.

Kaminski P F, Maier R C 1983 Clear cell adenocarcinoma of the cervix unrelated to diethylstilbestrol exposure. Obstetrics and Gynecology 62: 720–727.

Katsube Y, Mukai K, Silverberg S G 1982 Cystic mesothelioma of the peritoneum: a report of five cases and review of the literature. Cancer 50: 1615–1622.

Kaufman R H, Adam E, Bindes G L, Gerthoffer E 1980 Upper genital tract changes and pregnancy outcome in offspring exposed in utero to diethylstilbestrol. American Journal of Obstetrics and Gynecology 137: 299–308.

Kaunitz A, DiSant'Agnese P A 1979 Needle tract endometriosis: an unusual complication of amniocentesis. Obstetrics and Gynecology 54: 753–755.

Kay S, Schneider V 1985 Reactive spindle cell nodule of the endocervix simulating uterine sarcoma. International Journal of Gynecological Pathology 4: 255–257.

Kelly A, Marks F, Westhoff C, Raren M 1991 The effect of the New York State restrictions on resident work hours. Obstetrics and Gynecology 78: 468–473.

Killackey M A, Hakes T B, Pierce V K 1985 Endometrial adenocarcinoma in breast cancer patients receiving antiestrogens. Cancer Treatment Reports 69: 237–238.

King D J, Ratcliffe M A, Dawson A A, Bennett B, MacGregor J E 1985 Fertility in young men and women after treatment for lymphoma: a study of a population. Journal of Clinical Pathology 38: 1247–1251.

Kleinerman R A, Curtis R E, Boice J D Jr, Flannery J T, Fraumeni J F 1982 Second cancers following radiotherapy for cervical cancer. Journal of the National Cancer Institute 69: 1027–1033.

Koss L G 1979 The effects of some therapeutic procedures and drugs on the epithelia of the female genital tract. In: Diagnostic cytology and its histopathologic basis. Lippincott, Philadelphia, pp 510–528.

Kraus F T 1967 Gynecologic pathology. Mosby, St Louis.

Lauritzen A F, Meineke B 1987 Isolated arteritis of the uterine cervix. Acta Obstetricia et Gynecologica Scandinavica 66: 659–660.

Lehfeldt H, Tietze C, Gorstein F 1970 Ovarian pregnancy and intrauterine device. American Journal of Obstetrics and Gynecology 108: 1005–1009.

Little J B 1968 Cellular effects of ionizing radiation. New England Journal of Medicine 278: 369–376.

Lockhart J D 1972 How toxic is hexachlorophene. Pediatrics 50: 229–235.

Lowell D M, LiVolsi V A, Ludwig M E 1983 Genital condyloma virus infection following pelvic radiation therapy: report of seven cases. International Journal of Gynecological Pathology 2: 294–302.

Ludmir J et al 1960 To the Editors (in reply to Harger J H). American Journal of Obstetrics and Gynecology 160: 273–274.

Ludmir J, Landon M B, Gabbe S E, Samuels P, Mennuti M 1987 Management of the diethylstilbestrol-exposed pregnant patient: a prospective study. American Journal of Obstetrics and Gynecology 157: 665–669.

Luxman D, Bergman A, Sagi J, David M P 1991 The postmenopausal adnexal mass: correlation between ultrasonic and pathologic findings. Obstetrics and Gynecology 77: 726–731.

McCombs R P, Patterson J F, MacMahon H E 1956 Syndromes associated with 'allergic' vasculitis. New England Journal of Medicine 255: 251–261.

McCombs R P 1965 Systemic 'allergic' vasculitis: clinical and pathological relationships. Journal of the American Medical Association 194: 1059–1064.

McDonough J F 1945 Vaginal bleeding from potassium permanganate as an abortifacient. New England Journal of Medicine 232: 189–190.

Macht D I 1918 On the absorption of drugs and poisons through the vagina. Journal of Pharmacology and Experimental Therapeutics 10: 509–552.

McKinnon S 1980 Contraceptives and feminine care products. In: Chiles V K (ed) Canadian self-medication. A reference for the health professions. Canadian Pharmaceutical Association, Ottawa, pp 77–84.

Magriples U, Naftolin F, Schwartz P E, Carcangiu M L 1993 High grade endometrial carcinoma in tamoxifen-treated breast cancer patients. Journal of Clinical Oncology 11: 485–490.

Maiman M, Tarricone N, Vieirra J et al 1991 Colposcopic evaluation of human immunodeficiency virus-positive women. Obstetrics and Gynecology 78: 84–88.

Malfetano J H 1990 Tamoxifen-associated endometrial carcinoma in postmenopausal breast cancer patients. Gynecologic Oncology 44: 104–109.

Mascola L, Colwell B Y, Couch J A 1983 Should sperm donors be screened for sexually transmitted diseases? New England Journal of Medicine 309: 1058.

Matorras R, Ariceta J M, Montoya F et al 1991 Human immunodeficiency virus-induced immunodeficiency: a risk factor for human papillomavirus infection. American Journal of Obstetrics and Gynecology 164: 42–44.

Melchior H, Hamann F 1980 Abakterielle Zystitis durch lokal wirksame Spermicide. Helvetica Chirurgica Acta 47: 323–324.

Mikhael N Z 1985 Adverse reactions to drugs in the hospital milieu. Annals of the Royal College of Physicians and Surgeons of Canada 18: 477–483.

Mikhael N Z, Kacew S 1984 Monitoring of adverse drug reactions by means of autopsy tissue examination. Human Toxicology 3: 133–140.

Mikhael N Z, Campbell J S, Lee W H, Acharya V C, Hurteau G D 1977 Tubal Arias-Stella atypia. European Journal of Obstetrics, Gynecology and Reproductive Biology 7: 13–15.

Moore S W, Enterline H T 1975 Significance of proliferative epithelial lesions of the uterine tube. Obstetrics and Gynecology 45: 385–390.

Mullick F G, McAllister H A, Wagner B M, Fenoglio J J Jr 1979 Drug related vasculitis: clinicopathologic correlations in 30 patients. Human Pathology 10: 313–325.

Muram D, Drouin P 1982 Ovarian remnant syndrome. Journal of the Canadian Medical Association 127: 399–400.

Napke E, Stevens D G H 1984 Excipients and additives: hidden hazards in drug products and in product substitution. Canadian Medical Association Journal 131: 1449–1452.

Nichols T M, Fidler H K 1971 Microglandular hyperplasia in cervical cone biopsies taken for suspicious and positive cytology. American Journal of Clinical Pathology 56: 424–429.

Norris H J, Hilliard G D, Irey N S 1988 Hemorrhagic cellular leiomyomas ("apoplectic leiomyoma") of the uterus associated with pregnancy and oral contraceptives. International Journal of Gynecological Pathology 7: 212–224.

Nuovo M A, Nuovo G J, McCaffrey R M et al 1989 Endometrial polyps in postmenopausal patients receiving tamoxifen. International Journal of Gynecological Pathology 8: 125–131.

Nuyens A J J, Campbell J S 1957 Spontaneous rupture of uterus in second trimester of pregnancy. Canadian Medical Association Journal 77: 789–792.

O'Brien P K, Roth-Moyo L, Davies B A 1981 Pseudo-sulfur granules associated with intra uterine contraception devices. American Journal of Clinical Pathology 75: 822–825.

Paik H H, Komorowski R 1976 Hemangiosarcoma of the abdominal wall following irradiation therapy of endometrial carcinoma. American Journal of Clinical Pathology 66: 810–814.

Panda J K 1990 Primary ovarian twin pregnancy: case report. British Journal of Obstetrics and Gynaecology 97: 540–541.

Parmley T H, Woodruff J D 1974 The ovarian mesothelioma. American Journal of Obstetrics and Gynecology 120: 234–241.

Patel L G, Warrington S J, Pearson R M 1983 Propanolol concentrations in plasma after insertion into the vagina. British Medical Journal 287: 1247–1248.

Patten S F Jr 1976 Postradiation dysplasia of the uterine cervix: cytopathology and clinical significance. In: Wied G L, Koss L G, Reagan J (eds) Compendium on diagnostic cytology. University of Chicago, Chicago, pp 268–274.

Patten S F Jr, Reagan J W, Obenauf M, Ballard L A 1963 Post irradiation dysplasia of uterine cervix and vagina: an analytical study of the cells. Cancer 16: 173–182.

Penn I 1980 Some contributions of transplantation to our knowledge of cancer. Transplantation Proceedings 12: 676–680.

Peress M R, Tsai C C, Mathur R S, Williamson H O 1982 Hirsutism and menstrual patterns in women exposed to diethylstilbestrol in utero. American Journal of Obstetrics and Gynecology 144: 135–140.

Pettit P D, Lee R A 1988 Ovarian remnant syndrome: dilemma and surgical challenge. Obstetrics and Gynecology 71: 580–583.

Pitkin R M 1988 The return of the IUD. Obstetrics and Gynecology 72: 119.

Prakash S, Scully R E 1964 Sarcoma-like pseudopregnancy changes in uterine leiomyomas: report of a case resulting from prolonged norethindrone therapy. Obstetrics and Gynecology 24: 106–109.

Proppe K H, Scully R E, Rosai J 1984 Post operative spindle cell nodules of genitourinary tract resembling sarcomas — a report of 8 cases. American Journal of Surgical Pathology 8: 101–108.

Reimnitz C, Brand E, Nieberg R K, Hacker N F 1988 Malignancy arising in endometriosis associated with unopposed estrogen replacement. Obstetrics and Gynecology 71: 444–447.

Repmeyer J C, Juhl Y H 1983 Contamination of injectable solutions with 2-mercaptobenzothiazole leached from rubber closures. Journal of Pharmaceutical Sciences 72: 1302–1305.

Reybrouck G 1983 Antiseptic drugs and disinfectants. In: Dukes M N G, Elis J (eds) Side effects of drugs annual 7. Excerpta Medica, Amsterdam, pp 265–270.

Robboy S J 1983 A hypothetic mechanism of diethylstilbestrol (DES)-induced anomalies in exposed progeny. Human Pathology 14: 831–833.

Roberts W C 1978 The autopsy: its decline and a suggestion for its revival. New England Journal of Medicine 299: 332–338.

Rodriguez J, Hart W R 1982 Endometrial cancers occurring 10 or more years after pelvic irradiation for carcinoma. International Journal of Gynecological Pathology 1: 135–144.

Royal College of Pathologists 1992 Medical and Scientific Staffing of National Health Service Pathology Departments (Histopathology) pp 5–6.

Sadan O, Kruger S, van Iddekinge 1987 Vaginal tumors in pregnancy: case report and review of the literature. Acta Obstetricia et Gynecologica Scandinavica 66: 559–562.

Sadove A M, Block M, Rossof A H et al 1981 Radiation carcinogenesis in man: new primary neoplasms in fields of prior therapeutic radiation. Cancer 48: 1139–1143.

Saxén L, Kassinen A, Saxén E 1963 Peritoneal foreign-body reaction caused by condom emulsion. Lancet 1: 1295–1296.

Schafer A, Friedmann W, Mielke M, Schwartlander B, Koch M A 1991 The increased frequency of cervical dysplasia-neoplasia in women infected with the human immunodeficiency virus is related to the degree of immunosuppression. American Journal of Obstetrics and Gynecology 164: 543–547.

Schenker J G, Evron S 1983 New concepts in the surgical management of tubal pregnancy and the consequent postoperative results. Fertility and Sterility 40: 709–723.

Schneider V, Lee H M, Kay S 1982 Immune suppression: high risk factor for the development of cervical neoplasia. Acta Cytologica 25: 71–72.

Schneider V, Partridge J R, Gutierrez F, Hurt W G, Maizels M S, De May R M 1983 Benign cystic mesothelioma involving the female genital tract: report of four cases. American Journal of Obstetrics and Gynecology 145: 355–359.

Sekiya S, Iwaseki H, Takeda B, Takamizawa H 1988 Endometrial carcinoma following chronic anovulation and immunosuppressive therapy for systemic lupus erythematosus. Acta Obstetrica et Gynecologica Scandinavica 67: 653–656.

Senekjian E K et al 1988 Infertility among daughters either exposed or not exposed to diethylstilbestrol. American Journal of Obstetrics and Gynecology 158: 493–498.

Sharp G B, Cole P, Anderson D, Herbst A L 1990 Clear cell adenocarcinoma of the lower genital tract: correlation of mother's recall of diethylstilbestrol history with obstetrical records. Cancer 66: 2215–2220.

Shemwell R E, Weed J C 1970 Ovarian remnant syndrome. Obstetrics and Gynecology 32: 748–753.

Shugar S 1979 Effects of asbestos in the Canadian environment. National Research Council of Canada, publication no 16452.

Shull J C 1941 Vaginal bleeding from potassium permanganate burns. American Journal of Obstetrics and Gynecology 41: 161–162.

Silva E G, Tornos C S, Follen-Mitchell M 1994 Malignant neoplasms of the uterine corpus in patients treated for breast carcinoma: the effects of tamoxifen. International Journal of Gynecological Pathology 13: 248–258.

Smith R D 1983 Acquired immunodeficiency syndrome: summary of recent information. College of American Pathologists AIDS Task Force Report.

Stewart G J, Cunningham A L, Driscoll G L, Lamont B J, Gold J, Barr J A, Tyler J P P 1985 Transmission of human T-cell lymphotrophic virus type III (HTLV-III) by artificial insemination by donor. Lancet 2: 581–585.

Stillman R J 1982 In utero exposure to diethylstilbestrol: adverse effects on the reproductive tract and reproductive performance in male and female offspring. American Journal of Obstetrics and Gynecology 142: 905–921.

Strate S M, Taylor W E, Forney J P, Silva F G 1983 Xanthogranulomatous pseudotumor of the vagina: evidence of a local response to an unusual bacterium (mucoid Escherichia coli). Journal of Clinical Pathology 79: 637–643.

Strickland D M, Leonard R G, Stavchansky S, Benoit T, Wilson R T 1983 Vaginal absorption of hexachlorophene during labour. American Journal of Obstetrics and Gynecology 147: 769–772.

Stutman O 1977 Immunological surveillance mechanisms of carcinogenesis. In: Hiatt H H, Watson J D, Winston J A (eds) Origins of human cancer. Proceedings of the Cold Spring Harbor Conferences on Cell Proliferation 48: 729–750.

Szlachter N B, Mokowitz J, Bigelow B, Weiss G 1980 Iatrogenic endometriosis: substantiation of the Sampson hypothesis. Obstetrics and Gynecology 55: 52s–53s.

Taylor H B, Norris H J 1966 Mesenchymal tumors of the uterus. IV. Diagnosis and prognosis of leiomyosarcomas. Archives of Pathology 82: 40–44.

Tepper R, Goldberaer S, Beyth Y 1991 The post menopausal mass: correlation between ultrasonic and pathologic findings. Obstetrics and Gynecology 78: 726.

Tryphonas L, Buttar H S 1982 Genital tract toxicity of nonoxynol-9 in female rats: temporal development, reversibility and sequelae of the induced lesions. Fundamental and Applied Toxicology 2: 211–219.

Tryphonas L, Buttar H S 1983 Nonoxynol-9 effects on the uterus and the conceptus in the rat. Seminar at the Reproductive Biology Workshop Ottawa Civic Hospital.

Tryphonas L, Buttar H S 1984 Morphologic evidence for vaginal toxicity of Delfen contraceptive cream in the rat. Toxicology Letters 20: 289–295.

Tryphonas L, Campbell J S, Munro I C 1983 The need to 'read' 40 or more tissues. Winter Toxicology Forum, Arlington, Virginia.

Tyrer J H, Dadie M J, Sutherland M J, Sutherland J M, Hooper W D 1970 Outbreak of anticonvulsant intoxication in an Australian city. British Medical Journal 4: 271–273.

Veress B, Wallmander 1987 Primary hepatic pregnancy. Acta Obstetricia et Gynecologica Scandinavica 66: 563–564.

Veridiano N P, Tancer M L, Weiner E A 1978 Squamous cell carcinoma in situ of the vagina and cervix after intrauterine DES exposure. Obstetrics and Gynecology 52: 30s–33s.

Vermund S H, Kelley K F, Klein R S et al 1991 High risk of human papilloma virus infection and cervical squamous intraepithelial lesions among women with concomitant human immunodeficiency virus infection. American Journal of Obstetrics and Gynecology 165: 393–400.

Vorherr H, Messer R H, Reid D 1983 Complications of tubal sterilization: menstrual abnormalities and fibrocystic breast disease. American Journal of Obstetrics and Gynecology 145: 644–645.

Waugh D 1992a Royal College symposium offers plethora of opinions on future of academic medicine. Canadian Medical Association Journal 146: 267–268.

Waugh D 1992b There but for the grace ... Canadian Medical Association Journal 146: 62.

Webster J C, Guden A G 1979 Vaginitis complicating gold therapy for rheumatoid arthritis. American Journal of Obstetrics and Gynecology 131: 700.

Weiss S W, Enzinger F M, Johnson F B 1978 Silica reaction simulating fibrous histiocytoma. Cancer 42: 2738–2743.

Westwood J C N, Legacé S, Mitchell M A 1974 Hospital-acquired infection: present and future impact and need for future action. Canadian Medical Association Journal 110: 769–774.

Westwood J C N, Legacé S, Mitchell M A 1976 Infection surveillance on a shoe-string budget. Dimensions in Health Service 53: 42–44.

Whitehead M E, Fitzwater J E, Lindley S K et al 1984 Quality assurance of histopathologic diagnosis: a prospective audit of three thousand cases. American Journal of Clinical Pathology 81: 487–491.

WHO Scientific Group 1981 Research on the menopause. World Health Organization, Geneva.

Wilansky R, Corrigan R, Campbell J S 1978 IUD-related complications. Seminar for Health and Welfare, Canada Laboratory Centre for Disease Control, Ottawa.

Wilansky R, Maclean J N, Miro R et al 1980 Necrotizing vasculitis in gynecological surgery. European Journal of Obstetrics, Gynecology and Reproductive Biology 10: 401–406.

Williamson E D, Christopherson W M 1972 Malignant mixed Müllerian tumors of the uterus. Cancer 29: 585–592.

Winkler B, Norris H J, Fenoglio C M 1982 The female genital tract. In: Riddell R H (ed) Pathology of drug-induced and toxic diseases. Churchill Livingstone, New York, pp 297–324.

Wolfman W, Holtz G 1983 Update on ectopic pregnancy. Canadian Medical Association Journal 129: 1265–1269.

Womak K C 1987 Isolated arteritis of the ovarian hilum. Journal of Clinical Pathology 40: 1484–1487.

Wong K P, Gillett P G 1977 Recurrent hemorrhage from corpus luteum during anticoagulant therapy. Canadian Medical Association Journal 116: 388–390.

Woodruff J D, Pauerstein C J 1969 The Fallopian tube: structure, function, pathology and management. Williams & Wilkins, Baltimore.

Young R H, Scully R E 1989 Atypical forms of microglandular hyperplasia of the cervix simulating carcinoma: a report of five cases and review of the literature. American Journal of Surgical Pathology 13: 50–56.

Zarbo R J, Hoffman G G, Howanitz P J 1991 Interinstitutional comparison of frozen-section consultation. Archives of Pathology and Laboratory Medicine 115: 1187–1194.

Zipper J, Wheeler R G, Potts D M, Rivers M 1983 Propranolol as a novel, effective spermatocide: preliminary findings. British Medical Journal 287: 1245–1246.

Zur Hansen H 1987 Papillomaviruses in human cancer. Cancer 15: 1692–1696.

37. Tropical pathology of the female genital tract and ovaries

S. B. Lucas

INTRODUCTION

By tradition, 'tropical pathology' implies exotic parasitic diseases (protozoal and helminthic) endemic in poor countries in hot climates. In practice, two overlapping topics are included. First, 'developing countries in the tropics' are those in warm climates where health is affected by mass poverty, poor sanitation, poor provision of clean water, poor access to medical care, poor provision of pathology services, and low per capita expenditure on health (World Bank, 1993): in other words, resource-poor countries. Such countries are characterized by high transmission rates of infectious diseases, high infant and maternal mortalities, and by having up to half the population under 16 years of age (Mahler, 1987; Parkin et al, 1988a). Secondly, there is the vast range of infectious diseases. Some are ecologically restricted to warm climates (such as filariasis and schistosomiasis), some are global but more common in warm climates. However, with modern international travel, a patient with any infectious disease may present anywhere in the world.

Since the previous edition of this book, a major change in world health has been the pandemic of infection with human immunodeficiency virus (HIV) and consequent acquired immunodeficiency syndrome (AIDS). The impact of HIV on gynaecological disease is summarized.

A large part of the histopathologist's work in the tropics — in the post-mortem room as in the biopsy reporting room — is concerned with gynaecological and obstetric pathology. In this chapter, the emphasis is on gynaecological conditions that pathologists encounter in resource-poor countries, plus some unusual infections that are not covered elsewhere in this book. The standard encyclopaedia of infectious disease, particularly microbial, is by Mandell et al (1990). For the parasitic infections discussed, no details of life cycles are given: these can be found in Lucas (1992). A comprehensive account of all parasitic infections, including rarities occurring in the female genital tract, is by Gutierrez (1990).

INFECTIONS

Bacterial infections

Pelvic inflammatory disease

Acute and chronic inflammatory disease is common in the lower socio-economic groups of the tropics not only because of the high prevalence of sexually transmitted diseases and post-abortion or postpartum sepsis but also because therapy is often delayed (Muir & Belsey, 1980; Bang et al, 1989). Early age of first intercourse — in some regions, before the menarche — is associated with increased risk of sexually transmitted diseases (Duncan et al, 1990). The sequelae of criminal abortion, a common practice in many developing countries, are particularly demanding of hospital resources (Liskin, 1980) and are a major septic cause of maternal mortality in the tropics (Graham, 1991). An analysis of gynaecological admissions to a major hospital in Uganda showed that 30% were for pelvic inflammatory disease. This is associated with a high rate of sterility (26%) and ectopic gestation (Grech et al, 1973).

For the practising histopathologist, acute and chronic salpingitis, tubo-ovarian abscess, ectopic pregnancy and 'non-specific chronic endometritis' account for a large proportion of gynaecological pathology. In the main pathology laboratory in Nairobi in the early 1980s, receiving specimens from all around Kenya, one-quarter of submitted histology specimens were endometrial curettings with a clinical label of infertility (personal observations). This comes as an initial surprise considering the high population growth rate, but reflects the social pressures to bear children, coupled with the high prevalence of pelvic inflammatory disease. The logistical consequence for resource-poor laboratories is that unless a clinical indication of ?carcinoma, ?tuberculosis, or ?trophoblastic disease in the lower genital tract is present, analysis of endometrial curettings is not productive of clinically useful results (personal observations).

The late effects of untreated pelvic sepsis present problems to both clinicians and pathologists. The pelvis may be filled with a mass of proliferating vascular fibrous tissue — the 'plaster of Paris' pelvis — which is often mistaken for a diffusely invasive cancer. Proliferation of entrapped mesothelial cells may also mimic carcinoma.

Chronic endometritis and tuberculosis

Plasma cell infiltration of the endometrial stroma is the morphological hallmark of chronic endometritis, and may be focal or diffuse (see also Ch. 12). In many resource-poor countries, 'routinely' submitted endometrial curettings show this in up to 20% of specimens (Farooki, 1967; Liomba et al, 1982), associated with infertility in up to one-third of patients. The distribution of the main aetiological agents — chlamydial infection and gonorrhoea — is partly documented for poor tropical countries (Muir & Belsey, 1980; Laga et al, 1991), and the histological appearances are non-specific. Identifiable chronic endometritis histology includes donovanosis and tuberculosis (see below). Endometrial actinomycete infections,

associated with intrauterine contraceptive devices, and artefactual pseudoactinomycotic granules occur globally (Bhagavan et al, 1982; Arroyo & Quinn, 1989).

Infection by *Mycobacterium tuberculosis* has always been one of the most important causes of morbidity and mortality in the tropics. In a typical resource-poor country in the tropics, the annual rate of acquisition of tuberculous infection is 1–2.5% per annum from birth, so that the majority of adults harbour infection which can reactivate to produce disease. The incidence of female genital tract tuberculosis parallels closely the overall prevalence of tuberculosis. Its spread to the genital tract is predominantly haematogenous from a pulmonary lesion. In a large series from India of non-pregnant endometrial curettings examined up to 1980, tuberculosis was diagnosed in 2.3% (Bazaz-Malik et al, 1983). During an 11-year period of routine diagnostic histopathology from Malawi, female genital tuberculosis was found in 90 patients: 59 endometrial curettings, 17 tubes, 9 cervical biopsies, and two cases of ovarian tuberculosis (Liomba & Chiphangwi, 1982). Up to 6% of infertility has been attributed to pelvic tuberculosis in resource-poor countries (Muir & Belsey, 1980).

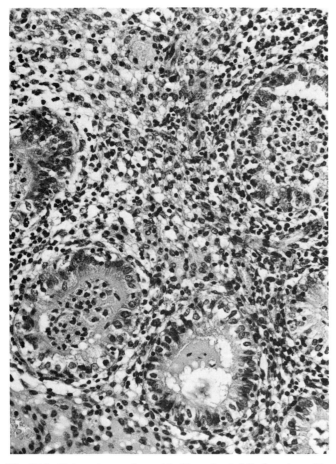

Fig. 37.1 Tuberculous endometritis. Note glands full of exudate with blurring of epithelial outlines. No granulomas are seen. H & E × 100.

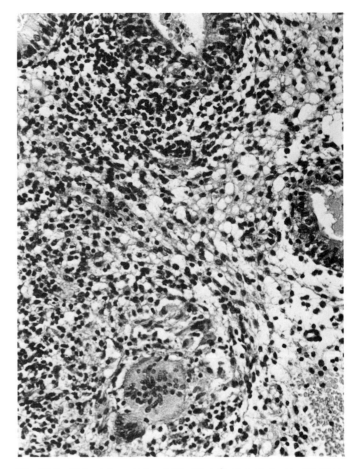

Fig. 37.2 Tuberculous endometritis. Ill-defined granuloma with giant cell (bottom), non-specific infiltrate of stroma and extension of these cells (lymphocytes) into glandular epithelium. H & E × 250.

The histological diagnosis of genital tuberculosis presents no problems when the typical caseating epithelioid and giant cell granulomas are present in tissues from any site. However, in curettings this well-developed picture is often lacking and the lesions are focal and scanty. Tuberculous endometritis has to be diagnosed as an occasional finding in a sea of non-specific endometritis. Focal lymphocytic and plasma cell infiltration are seen in both. Most tuberculous granulomas start in the stroma adjacent to a gland. The early lesions are mainly composed of lymphocytes with only an occasional macrophage, and necrosis may be minimal (Fig. 37.1). The wall of the gland is involved and the lumen filled with exudate, often eosinophilic, and inflammatory cells including polymorphs, lymphocytes and macrophages. The residual epithelial lining of these glands may be stratified with some papillary infoldings and show nuclear pleomorphism. Dissociation between the glandular and stromal appearances causes difficulty in dating the endometrium (Liomba & Chiphangwi, 1982). In proliferative endometrium, the glands are often angulated, and in the secretory phase the affected glands may be non-secretory. In more advanced cases, granulomas are seen in the stroma although caseation is usually minimal unless the patient has amenorrhoea (Fig. 37.2). Glands may then be very scanty. In such advanced disease, cervical, vaginal and vulvar tuberculous lesions occur (Fig. 37.3). Acid-fast bacilli are usually difficult to detect in endometrial tuberculosis. The exception to this is non-reactive tuberculosis in immunosuppressed patients where abundant bacilli are seen in necrotic tissue that has a poor cellular reaction and no giant cells.

Although tuberculosis of the Fallopian tubes is almost always the primary site of infection of the female genital tract, tuberculous salpingitis will not commonly be encountered by the pathologist (see also Ch. 17). The macroscopic appearances may be indistinguishable from those of chronic non-specific salpingitis, unless there is extensive caseation or a tuberculous pyosalpinx. In advanced cases, typical coalescing granulomas are present in the tubal folds and may involve the muscularis and serosa (Fig. 37.4). In early cases the diagnosis may be more difficult. The appearances are those of chronic salpingitis, often the follicular type, with only occasional non-necrotic

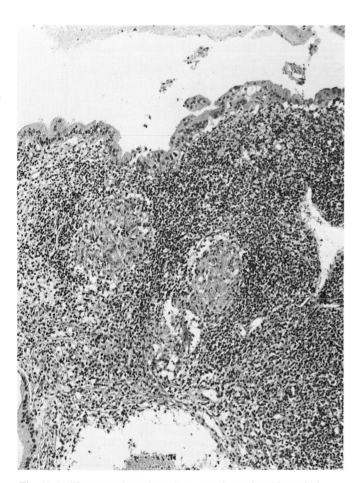

Fig. 37.3 Non-caseating tuberculous granulomas in endocervical tissues. H & E × 100.

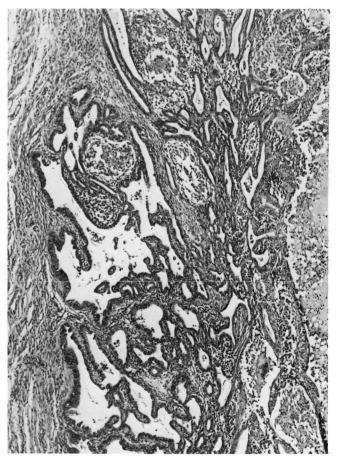

Fig. 37.4 Tuberculous salpingitis with plical adhesions giving appearance of follicular salpingitis and scattered epithelioid cell granulomas. H & E × 100.

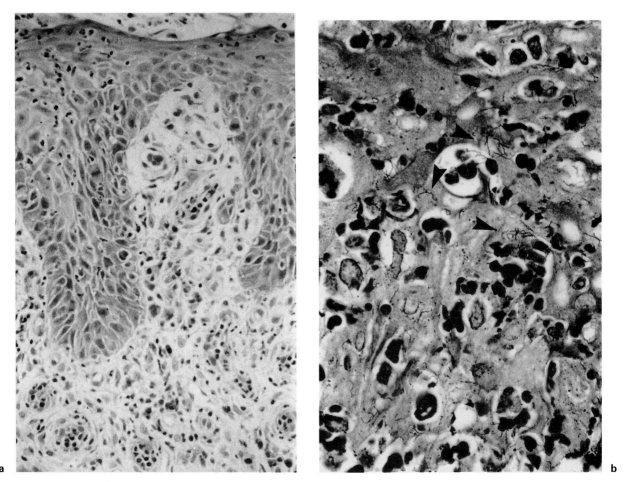

Fig. 37.5 Secondary syphilis of the vulva. **a** Hyperplastic oedematous epithelium containing scattered polymorphs; the dermis is vascular and the endothelial cells are hypertrophied. H & E × 200. **b** Warthin–Starry stain of the epithelium with several spirochaetes (arrowheads). × 1000.

granulomas. In tubes containing predominantly non-caseating granulomas, laminated haematoxyphilic bodies indistinguishable from Schaumann bodies of sarcoidosis may be seen. Superficially these resemble dead and calcified schistosome eggs.

Syphilis

Infection with *Treponema pallidum* is widely associated with poverty. Within Africa, prevalence rates of positive syphilis serology among pregnant women range from 1–17%, and among female prostitutes from 18–38% (Laga et al, 1991). Consequently congenital syphilis is an important cause of perinatal death (Lucas et al, 1983).

Primary and secondary syphilis lesions (see also Ch. 4) are not always easy to specify amidst the inflow of vulvar inflammatory lesions that are biopsied. The condyloma latum of secondary syphilis has an oedematous hyperplastic epithelium diffusely infiltrated by polymorphs, and underlying chronic inflammatory infiltrate that includes variable numbers of plasma cells. The oft-mentioned hypertrophy of endothelial cells in small vessels ('endarteritis obliterans') may not be seen. However, a silver stain such as Dieterle or Warthin–Starry usually demonstrates spirochaetes within the epithelium (Fig. 37.5) (Freinkel, 1987). Serological evidence and empirical chemotherapy may be required to prove syphilis.

Granuloma inguinale (donovanosis)

Donovanosis is a sexually transmitted disease caused by the Gram-negative bacillus *Calymmatobacterium granulomatis*, and is found throughout the tropics.

In the female the initial lesion is a papule which then ulcerates. The vulva and perineum are the commonest sites, but vaginal and cervical ulcers also occur (Fig. 37.6). The ulcer enlarges, has a thick rolled edge and a beefy, red granulation tissue base. Satellite lesions are frequent, but inguinal node involvement is uncommon (Freinkel, 1988). Left untreated, donovanosis has a relapsing course and may heal with an atrophic scar. It may spread upwards to involve the endometrium, tubes, ovaries and adnexae,

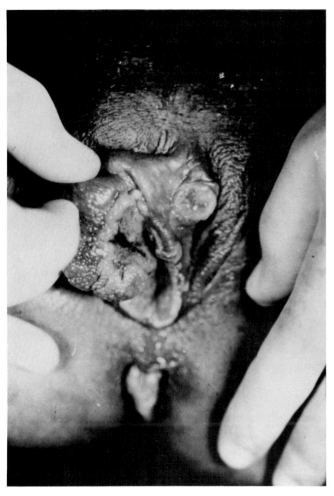

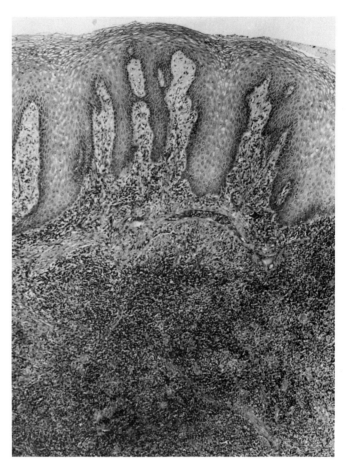

Fig. 37.7 Granuloma inguinale of the vagina. Granulation tissue beneath acanthotic epithelium. H & E × 63.

Fig. 37.6 Granuloma inguinale. Ulceration of the labia, resembling carcinoma. (Reproduced by kind permission of Mr. J. B. Lawson.)

causing a frozen pelvis (Bhagwandeen & Mottiar, 1972; Sengupta & Das, 1984). Secondary fusospirochaetal infection of the ulcer produces widespread mutilation of the external genitalia. Occasionally the inflammation with fibrosis results in vulvar elephantiasis and urethral stricture. Clinically the ulcerated lesion resembles diverse other conditions such as carcinoma and amoebiasis (Bhagwandeen & Naik, 1977).

Histologically, donovanosis may seem non-specific. The overlying epithelium may be hyperplastic (Fig. 37.7). The inflammatory tissue comprises microabscesses, vascular proliferation and variable numbers of macrophages and plasma cells (Fig. 37.8). The characteristic feature is large macrophages with clear or foamy cytoplasm; these may be so numerous as to produce a starry-sky appearance. In their cytoplasm are the Donovan bodies (Fig. 37.9); these are the bacilli of *C. granulomatis* which, faintly seen on H & E and PAS stains, are well shown by the Giemsa, Dieterle or Warthin–Starry method. They measure 1–1.5 × 0.6 μm, and are also seen within polymorphs and in extracellular matrix. This histology is similar to that of rhinoscleroma. A smear of fresh tissue, air-dried and stained with a Romanovsky stain, will demonstrate the typical macrophages and organisms. The term 'Donovan body' should not be confused with 'Leishman–Donovan body' which is a *Leishmania* amastigote.

Lymphogranuloma venereum (LGV)

This disease is distinct from granuloma inguinale. It is caused by *Chlamydia trachomatis*, is transmitted sexually, and is most prevalent in the tropics.

The vulva, vagina and cervix are the sites of infection and the earliest lesion is a vesicle which breaks down to form a punched-out painless ulcer. This may heal and the primary lesion is often unnoticed. Histologically, it has a non-specific appearance of granulation tissue.

Instead of healing, the primary lesion may become secondarily infected and persist. Involvement of the inguinal lymph nodes is less common in females than in males. It occurs within a month of the primary lesion and buboes may develop. Their histology shows the familiar stellate abscess with surrounding epithelioid cell reaction (Fig. 37.10). This is similar to the node lesions of cat

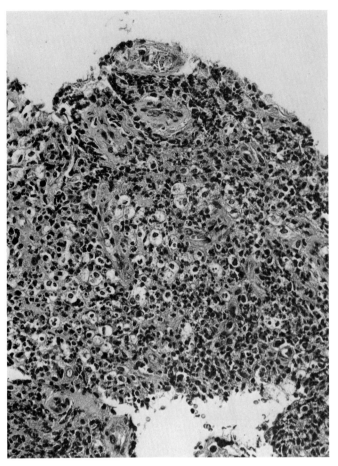

Fig. 37.8   Granuloma inguinale. Within the granulation tissue are large, empty-looking macrophages. H & E × 250.

scratch disease and of *Yersinia enterocolitica* intestinal infection. The bubo may discharge with sinus formation.

The later response to LGV infection is abundant granulation tissue with scarring. This cicatrization around both an unhealed primary lesion and pelvic nodes causes the chronic form of the disease. The urethra may be destroyed (Fig. 37.11) or undergo stricture (as occurs in the rectum). Multiple labial ulcers, recto-vaginal fistula and vaginal fibrosis can occur. Lymphatic obstruction may result in vulvar swelling or elephantiasis (so-called 'esthiomène'). At this stage, the histology is non-specific. Serology and culture of tissue are important aids to the diagnosis.

Clinically, LGV can mimic vulvar carcinoma; subsequent development of vulvar and anal malignancy is held to be a true aetiological association.

Other bacterial genital ulcer diseases

The prevalence of sexually transmitted diseases (STD) relates to poverty, and the highest rates are found in the tropics (Bang et al, 1989; Laga et al, 1991). In Africa, chancroid, caused by *Haemophilus ducreyi*, is the commonest identifiable genital ulcer disease, and gonorrhoea is ubiquitous (Muir & Belsey, 1980). The histological features of gonorrhoeal ulcers are non-specific — acute inflammation and much exudate. Chancroid may show a characteristic vertical pattern of three zones: superficial necrotic exudate (in which short Gram-negative bacilli

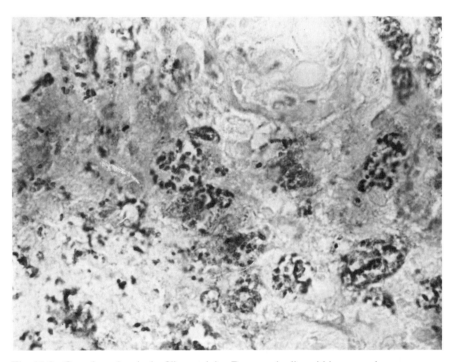

Fig. 37.9   Granuloma inguinale. Silver-staining Donovan bodies within macrophages. Dieterle × 1000.

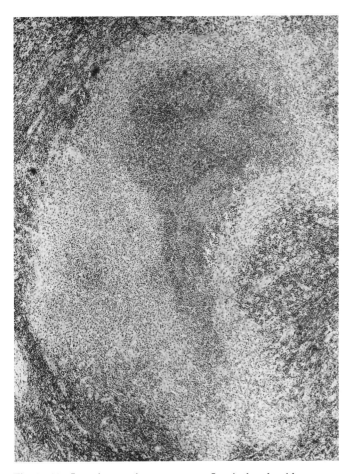

Fig. 37.10 Lymphogranuloma venereum. Inguinal node with a necrotic granuloma. H & E × 63.

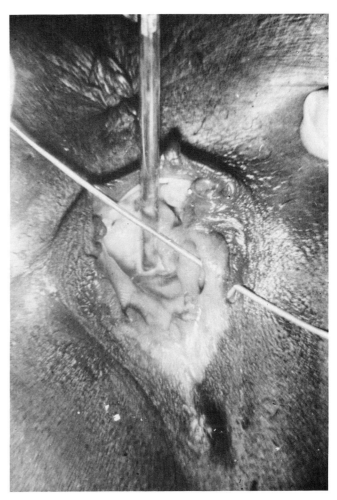

Fig. 37.11 Lymphogranuloma venereum. Gross vulval damage with ulceration and destruction of the urethra — the catheter is entering the base of the bladder. (Reproduced by kind permission of Mr. J. B. Lawson).

may be visible on Gram stain), a broad layer of oedematous granulation tissue and a deep zone with many plasma cells and lymphocytes (Freinkel, 1987).

Fungal infections

Candida infections of the vagina are ubiquitous (see also below in 'HIV and AIDS'). Disseminated fungal infections in immunocompromised patients (e.g. systemic candidiasis and aspergillosis) or apparently immunocompetent patients (e.g. coccidioidomycosis and histoplasmosis) may involve the female genital tract, but are unlikely to present a primary diagnostic problem (Chandler et al, 1980). In contrast, subcutaneous zygomycosis (ex 'phycomycosis') may present as a vulvar lesion, although it usually affects the thighs and buttocks. Seen in Central America, Africa and Asia, this disease follows traumatic implantation of *Basidiobolus haptosporus*. It causes a diffuse subcutaneous panniculitis which forms a woody-hard plaque and may ulcerate. Histologically, the fungal hyphae are seen as circular holes or clefts on H & E stain (Fig. 37.12). A PAS or Grocott stain demonstrates non-septate, irregularly branching hyphae of variable width —

up to 30 μm. Initially the host reaction is granulomatous with abundant eosinophils, and a Hoeppli–Splendore reaction around the hyphae is typical. With chronicity, extensive fibrosis develops.

Protozoal infections

Amoebiasis

Carriage of *Entamoeba histolytica* infection in the large bowel is ubiquitous, with about 10% of the global population infected. *Entamoeba* cysts may be encountered as faecal contaminants in cervical smears. However, invasive amoebic disease is more common in the tropics with poor socio-economic conditions and sanitation. Also it is now clear that only certain strains of *E. histolytica* are ever pathogenic (Spice & Ackers, 1992). Whilst the classical patterns of amoebiasis are of colo-rectal ulceration and liver abscess, amoebiasis of the perineum and male and female genitalia may occur. This follows either direct

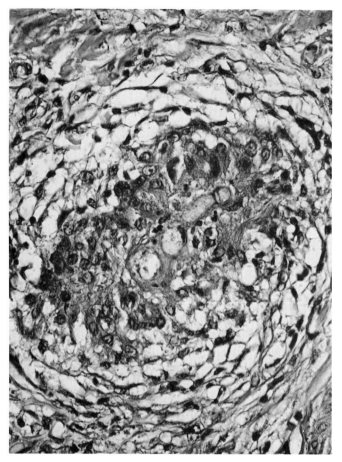

Fig. 37.12 Zygomycosis. Within the granuloma are broad hyphae, seen in cross and longitudinal section. H & E × 400.

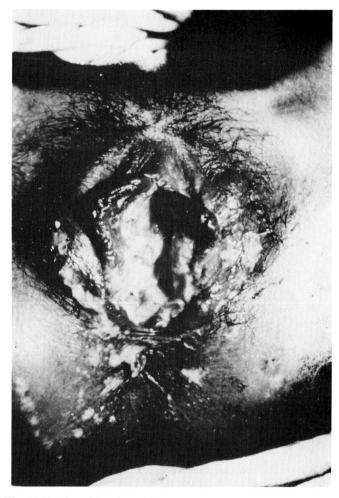

Fig. 37.13 Amoebic vulvo-vaginitis with extensive tissue destruction. (Reproduced by kind permission of Mr. J. B. Lawson.)

spread from rectal lesions or is due to homosexual or heterosexual intercourse (Mylius & Ten Seldam, 1962; Phillips et al, 1981).

Perianal amoebiasis presents with raised irregularly ulcerated lesions. As shown in Figure 37.13, similar ulcerated destructive lesions may occur on the clitoris, urethra, labia, vagina and cervix following sexual transmission (Agranal & Bausal, 1981). In all these sites, the clinical impression is frequently that of carcinoma; there are also occasional reports of carcinoma of the cervix associated with concurrent or treated amoebic cervicitis (Haibach et al, 1985; Arroyo & Elgueta, 1989).

Histopathologically, these lesions are characterized by epithelial necrosis, reactive epithelial hyperplasia, which may simulate carcinoma, and a variable inflammatory response. Amoebic trophozoites are seen on the superficial parts of the epithelium as well as in the ulcer slough (Figs 37.14–16). In H & E stains they are large cells (15–30 μm in diameter) with pale grey to mauve cytoplasm, a well-defined round purple nucleus, and, often, phagocytosed erythrocytes. Viable amoebae are strongly PAS positive. Once secondary infection has occurred, widespread non-

specific inflammatory changes may complicate the lesion and dominate the overall picture.

Leishmaniasis

Cutaneous leishmaniasis due to various species of *Leishmania* is endemic in the tropics, Mediterranean basin, the Middle East and Indian subcontinent. Transmission is via the bite of an infected sandfly, hence genital lesions are rare. A case of vulvar leishmaniasis by sexual transmission from a man with visceral leishmaniasis is recorded (Symmers, 1960). The histopathology showed the typical amastigotes within macrophages in the dermis.

Mucocutaneous leishmaniasis is caused by *L. brasiliensis* infection in South America. Lesions at mucocuteanous junctions ('espundia') occasionally involve the vulva as well as the more frequent facial and pharyngeal locations. They are ulcerative and widely destructive; histopathology usually does not reveal parasites (Binford & Connor, 1976).

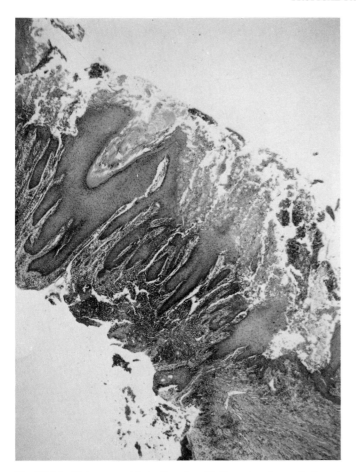

Fig. 37.14 Vulvar amoebiasis. Pseudoepitheliomatous hyperplasia and necrotic inflammatory slough. H & E × 40.

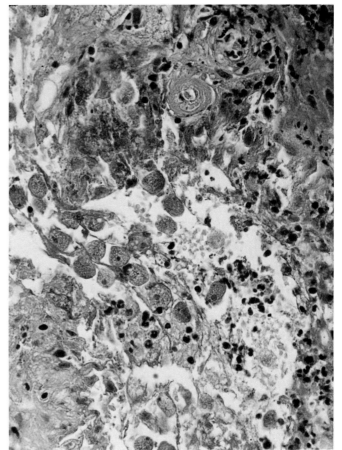

Fig. 37.15 Numerous amoebae in slough over perianal lesions. H & E × 400.

Helminth infections

Nematode infections

Filariasis. Chronic lymphoedema of the vulva, usually associated with elephantiasis of the legs, may be due to filariasis. *Wuchereria bancrofti* is endemic in South and Central America and Africa. Filariasis in south-east Asia is caused by *Brugia malayi*: both worms cause similar clinical features.

Adult male and female worms inhabit the large lymphatic vessels, most frequently adjacent to the large lymph nodes in the inguinal region.

Clinical disease usually develops months or years after infection and is due to repeated episodes of lymphangitis caused by the reaction to worms in the lymphatics. Blockage of lymphatics may lead to lymphoedema of the vulva. The vulva may be grossly distorted by warty fibrous masses with a crusted surface. There may be associated chyluria and ascites. Histologically the features in vulvar skin are of chronic lymphoedema: epithelial hyperplasia, dermal oedema and fibrosis, and dilated lymphatics. The amount of inflammation is variable. A specific histological diagnosis can only be made if a worm or fragments of worm are found in the deeper tissues. They are easily recognizable when viable, and the gravid female contains embryonic microfilariae in the uterine cavity (Figs 37.17 and 37.18). More frequently the worms are degenerate with some loss of internal structures, and may calcify. Later a giant cell granulomatous reaction develops. An aetiological association of filariasis with pelvic inflammatory disease and tubal occlusion is unlikely (Muir & Belsey, 1980).

Enterobiasis. This is a common large bowel and appendiceal infection by the nematode *Enterobius vermicularis* (the pin-worm). It is usually found in younger people and is more a disease of temperate than tropical zones (Sinniah et al, 1991). That there may be an ethnic susceptibility to infection is suggested by studies in the USA which detected a lower infection prevalence in Puerto Rican and black children compared with caucasian controls (Most et al, 1963).

Usually symptoms arise from deposition of eggs on the perineum. During their nocturnal perineal perambulations, the gravid female worms may enter the vagina and

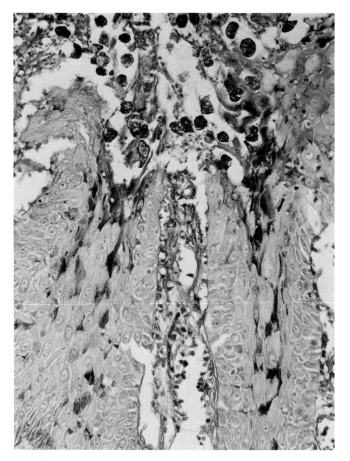

Fig. 37.16   Amoebae in slough over vulvar skin. PAS × 250.

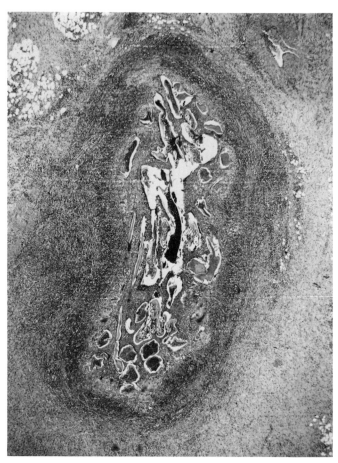

Fig. 37.17   Bancroftian filariasis. A degenerating female worm; the inflammation has obliterated the lymph node and there is surrounding fibrosis. H & E × 25.

ascend the female genital tract. A worm lodging on the hymen may cause pain. Both deposited eggs, and the worm as it degenerates, elicit a host reaction, resulting in inflammatory lesions of the vulva, vagina, endometrium, myometrium, tubes, ovaries and peritoneum (Sinniah et al, 1991; Sun et al, 1991). The commonest lesions are serosal nodules on the uterus and mesosalpinx. Pyosalpinx and tubo-ovarian abscess may occur. One patient with a tubo-ovarian abscess that had ruptured and caused generalized peritonitis had had a hysterectomy four years earlier (Khan & Stell, 1981). Despite the abscess formation evident in *Enterobius* lesions, cultures for bacteria are negative. Rarely, an adult worm may be found solely within the ovarian parenchyma, suggesting an entry through a recently ruptured Graafian follicle. An *Enterobius* granuloma within serosal endometriosis has also been described (Lansman et al, 1960).

The lesion around a worm is characteristically a 1–3 cm nodule with central yellow necrotic core. Histologically, within a fibrous capsule there is granulation tissue and variable amounts of eosinophilic necrosis, admixed with tuberculoid granulomas. In lesions with no worm residue evident, eggs are seen within non-necrotic granulomas.

Occasionally, the eggs have a Hoeppli–Splendore reaction around the shells. The eggs are unilaterally flat, measure 50–60 × 20–30 μm and have a thick shell (Fig. 37.19); recently laid specimens contain a coiled larva. A degenerate *Enterobius* worm is 0.5 mm in diameter and, apart from the characteristic internal structure of uterine tubes and gut, the lateral paired triangular alae on the cuticle are distinctive (Fig. 37.20).

Other nematode infections.   Calcospherites are to be distinguished from helminth eggs. The main differential diagnosis of invasive female genital enterobiasis is schistosomiasis (see below). *Ascaris* eggs are occasionally found in granulomatous peritoneal and adnexal lesions. *Gnathostoma* is a cause of visceral larva migrans, and may result in abscesses in the upper female genital tract, containing a larval worm.

Cestode infections

Hydatid disease of the female genital tract.
Hydatid disease is acquired by ingestion of eggs of *Echino-*

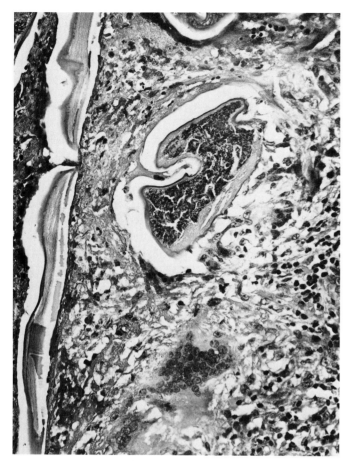

Fig. 37.18 Bancroftian filariasis. Parts of a degenerating female adult worm. Note the dark-staining microfilariae within a uterus, and the giant cell inflammatory reaction. H & E × 250.

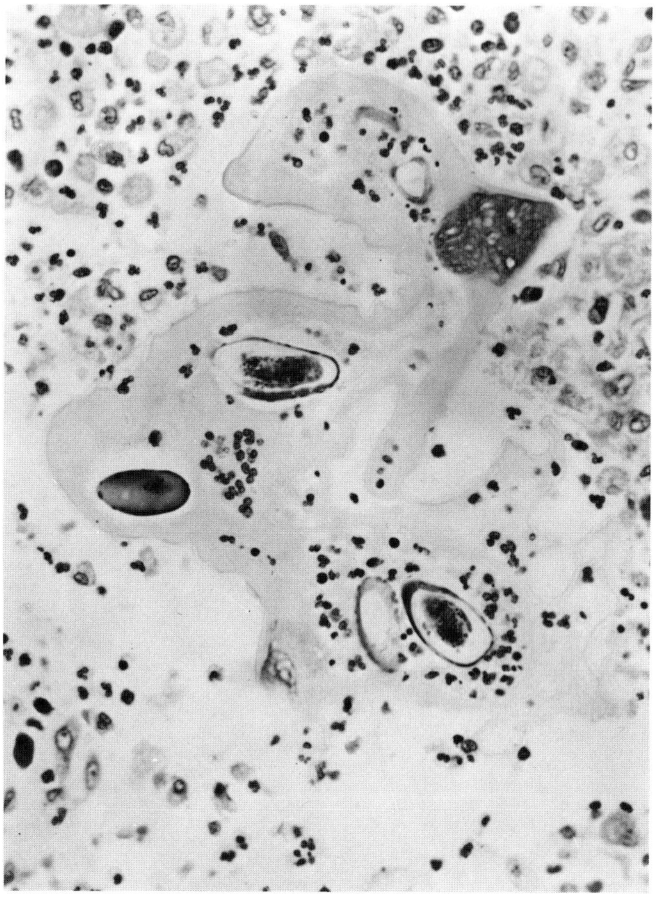

Fig. 37.19 Ova of *Enterobius vermicularis* within a degenerate adult. H & E × 400.

coccus granulosus tapeworm in the faeces of infected canines. It is prevalent in the Middle East and Africa, but is also endemic in South America, Australia and Europe. The liver and peritoneal cavity are the most frequent locations of cysts. The female genital tract thus becomes involved secondarily; primary uterine cysts are very rare. A study in Lebanon of 532 patients with hydatidosis found ovarian involvement in 0.75% and uterine cysts in 0.4% (Bickers, 1970). Cysts may be located in the pouch of Douglas and adnexae (Rahman et al, 1982), and there are frequently adhesions between the cyst and adjacent omentum, bowel, bladder and other pelvic structures. Cyst size may reach 15 cm.

Histologically, gynaecological hydatid cysts have the usual structure of laminated membrane and germinal layer with internal daughter cysts containing protoscolices. Externally there is a host fibrous capsule of variable thickness, which may calcify. Clinical effects include a pelvic mass and obstructed labour. Occasionally cysts are passed per vaginam from the uterus.

Other cestode infections. *Spirometra* is a cause of visceral larva migrans and may present as an abscess, containing a worm, in the upper female genital tract and adnexae.

Trematode infections

Schistosomiasis. Some 200 million people in tropical zones of Asia, Africa and South America are infected with schistosome worms. The major species affecting the female genital tract is *Schistosoma haematobium*, but *S. mansoni* is also found in some lesions. *S. haematobium* is endemic in 54 countries in Africa and the Middle East (WHO, 1993). Prevalence of infection varies widely, but in some communities in Africa nearly 100% of children and adolescent females are infected, infection rates declining thereafter.

The dioecious *S. haematobium* worms locate and move in the pelvic veins, and cause no direct pathology. The main exit for their eggs — laid at the rate of 200–400 per worm pair per day — is the bladder mucosa and urine. The inflammatory reaction around eggs deposited in the

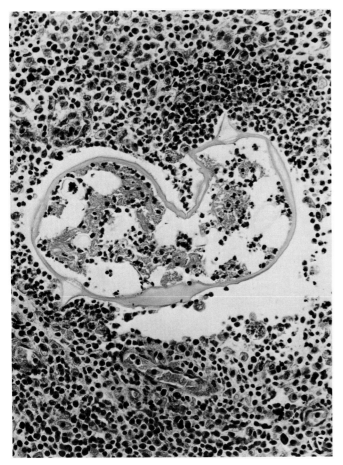

Fig. 37.20 *Enterobius* abscess in adnexae. Transverse section of an adult female showing the paired, pyramidal lateral alae. H & E × 250.

small veins disrupts the vessels, enabling the eggs to enter tissues. There they induce a mixed eosinophil and granulomatous host response, with ensuing fibrosis. About half of the eggs deposited in the bladder are excreted; the rest remain, die, and calcify or are destroyed by macrophages. Eggs deposited in extravesical organs thus form chronic inflammatory masses. Often a worm pair remains in one location and cumulatively lays vast numbers of eggs to produce a large tumour mass ('bilharzioma'). Autopsy studies find that about 10% of eggs are deposited in the internal genitalia (Cheever et al, 1977).

The prevalence of schistosomal lesions of the genitalia reflects the prevalence of urinary schistosomiasis in the population. The lower female organs — vagina, vulva and cervix — are involved more often than the uterus, ovary and tubes. Cervical lesions are most commonly encountered in all series (Table 37.1), though a distinction is to be made as to whether the schistosomal pathology is an incidental finding or is the prime cause of the clinical lesion and hence of the biopsy. For example, blind biopsy of the vagina in a population heavily infected with *S. haematobium* found a 75% prevalence of eggs in the vagina among women with proven urinary schistosomiasis, but most of the lesions were subclinical (Renaud et al, 1989).

Vulvar lesions are typically encountered in girls and adults under 20 years. They are warty or nodular masses on any part such as the clitoris, labia minora and majora (Fig. 37.21). They may be ulcerated or have an intact surface, and sizes up to 5 cm are noted (Attili et al, 1983; Mawad et al, 1992). Histologically, paired worms may be seen in veins (Fig. 37.22). In the earlier stages of infection large numbers of eggs are present in subepidermal tissues. These are viable, with brown chitinous shells, and have an internal miracidium with haematoxyphilic nuclei and deeply eosinophilic cytoplasm. The eggs are surrounded by a granulomatous reaction with giant cells, and eosinophils and plasma cells (Fig. 37.23). Sometimes eggs are seen within an eosinophil abscess. *S. haematobium* eggs have a terminal spine (those of *S. mansoni* have a lateral spine), but malorientation within the section and the crushing effect of the microtome blade often preclude precise speciation of *Schistosoma* on histology. The eggs die after three weeks, the internal nuclei shrink, the cytoplasm vanishes, and the eggshell becomes distorted. The tissue eosinophilia diminishes and fibrosis increases. Finally the shells disintegrate and many are engulfed by macrophage giant cells (Fig. 37.24). These stages are common to the natural history of all schistosomal urinary and gynaecological lesions, but the early stage is more frequently seen in vulvar lesions, probably because the clinical features are external and therefore biopsies are taken early in the course of infection. Because reinfection is common in endemic areas, the different stages often co-exist in the same tissue. In vulvar lesions, the majority of eggs are deposited near the surface, and this induces pseudoepitheliomatous hyperplasia of the epidermis (Fig. 37.25). Florid lesions are to be distinguished from condylomata acuminata which coincidentally contain a few eggs. There is no indication that vulvar schistosomiasis is a premalignant condition.

Table 37.1 The distribution of lesions in gynaecological schistosomiasis in three countries

Country	Vulva	Vagina	Cervix	Endometrium	Tube	Ovary	Total specimens	Reference
South Africa	15	5	120	6	12	7	165	(Frost, 1975)
Iraq	3	4	7	1	14		29	(Al-Adnani & Saleh, 1982)
Malawi	16	17	106	4	28	17	198	(Wright et al, 1982)

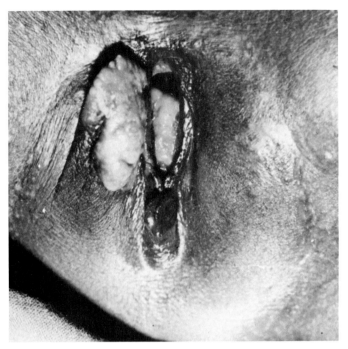

Fig. 37.21 Polypoid vulval lesions due to schistosomiasis in an 11-year-old girl. (Reproduced by kind permission of Mr. J. B. Lawson.)

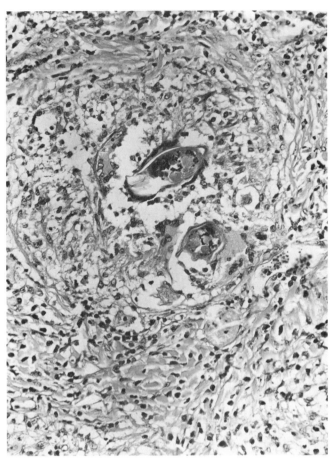

Fig. 37.23 Warty lesion of left labium. Granulomatous reaction around schistosomal ova in subepidermal tissues. Non-specific inflammation and fibrosis around the granuloma. H & E × 250.

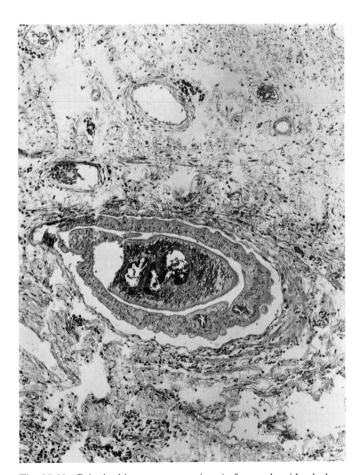

Fig. 37.22 Paired schistosome worms in vein from polypoid vulval lesion. The female is embraced by the male. H & E × 100.

Vaginal and cervical schistosomiasis may present clinically as nodules, polyps or warty tumours. These may be mistaken for neoplasms. Large numbers of eggs are deposited in the immediate subepithelial tissues and associated, as in the vulva, with a diffuse and granulomatous inflammatory reaction (Figs 37.26 and 37.27). There is no epidemiological evidence that cancer of the cervix is associated with schistosomiasis. In Malawi, 25 of the 793 cases of squamous cervical carcinoma had associated schistosomal eggs (Lowe et al, 1981).

Endometrial and myometrial schistosomiasis is uncommon, fewer than 1% of specimens received from Malawi being affected (Wright et al, 1982). This is possibly because the tortuous venules of the uterine wall prevent access by the worms, and the endometrium is regularly shed. Occasionally, ova are seen in endometrial curettings with little or no inflammatory reaction but in postmenopausal women the characteristic tissue histology is present. Eggs are sometimes found in leiomyomas.

Schistosomiasis of the ovary and tube often co-exist, sometimes with involvement of the adnexae. Ovarian schistosomiasis is comprehensively reviewed by Tiboldi

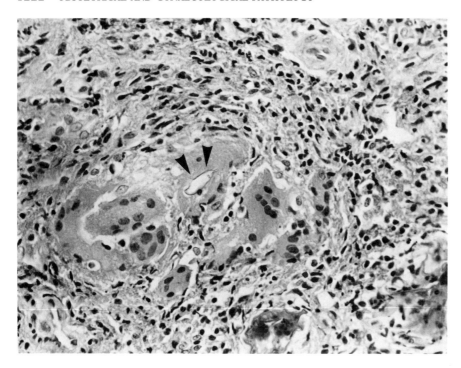

Fig. 37.24 Foreign body giant cell reaction around degenerate and distorted schistosomal ova (arrow) from biopsy of cervix. H & E × 400.

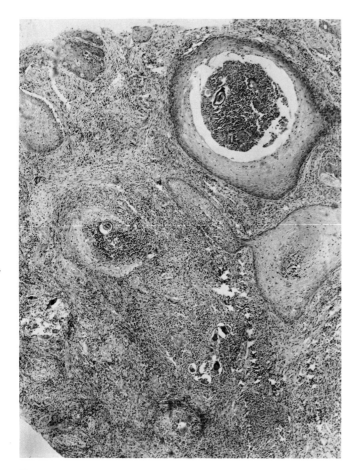

Fig. 37.25 Warty polyp of vulva. Widespread inflammation and pseudoepitheliomatous hyperplasia are present. Schistosomal ova (black) are scattered through the tissues. H & E × 63.

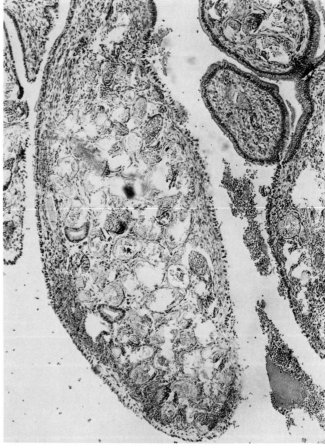

Fig. 37.26 Endocervical schistosomal polyp containing large numbers of dead ova, many of which are 'empty' and only recognizable by their shells. H & E × 100.

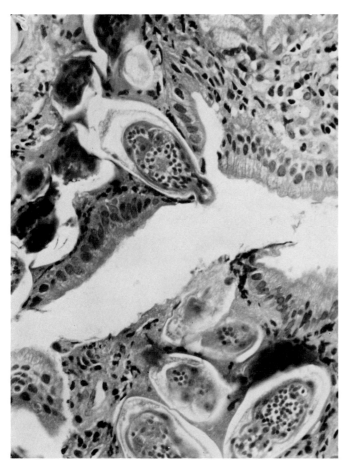

Fig. 37.27 Schistosomal cervicitis with many ova in the tissues. Most of these ova are viable with well-developed internal structure (miracidium). One is being extruded through a cervical gland. H & E × 400.

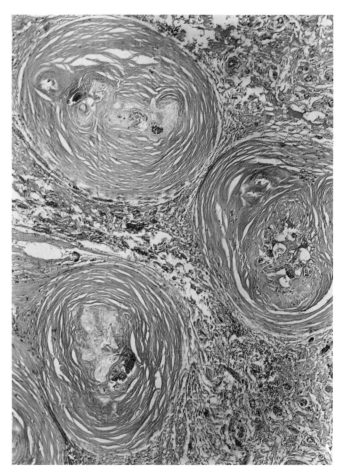

Fig. 37.28 Schistosomal hyaline nodules found on the external aspects of a Fallopian tube. A few degenerate ova are present in the centre of each nodule. H & E × 63.

(1978), and its prevalence varies widely. In spite of case reports, there is no good evidence of hormonal dysfunction of the ovaries (Chen & Mott, 1989). Eggs are usually an incidental finding, as for example in resected cystic teratomas which can also contain adult worms. Adnexal lesions, fibrous 'sandy patches' and nodules less than 1 cm in size are seen (El-Mahgoub, 1982). Larger bilharziomas in the pelvis may mimic neoplasms because of the fibrous tissue that develops around the egg-granulomas (Fig. 37.28). A 10 cm diameter parauterine inflammatory mass of schistosomiasis that also contained the tube and ovary is reported (Bac et al, 1987).

Tubal schistosomiasis has been implicated in infertility and tubal pregnancy (El-Mahgoub, 1982). Given that an inflammatory mass may obstruct the lumen this is reasonable, but again, there is no good epidemiological evidence of an aetiological association (Chen & Mott, 1989) and bacterial pelvic inflammatory disease is far more important. Egg densities in tubal resections for infertility are generally small when estimated by histology. However systematic evaluation of autopsy and surgical biopsy material using the more sensitive technique of tissue di-

gestion for schistosome eggs has shown that 10–30% of female genital organs can contain eggs without any being identified in standard tissue sections (Edington et al, 1975; Frost, 1975).

The eggshell of *S. haematobium* is not acid-fast with carbol fuchsin stains whereas that of *S. mansoni* is. This is a useful empirical method of distinguishing species in histological sections and can highlight mixed infections.

Schistosomiasis may rarely affect the placenta. Worms are seen in decidual vessels and lying free in the maternal sinus. The eggs may be found in the intervillous space and also within villi, accompanied by a variable inflammatory reaction. Fetal infection does not occur and the functional effect of the schistosomal infection on the placental unit appears to be minimal (Bittencourt et al, 1980).

Cytology.   As might be expected (Fig. 37.27), schistosome eggs emerge from cervical glands and may be detected in cervical smears. High numbers, up to 250 per smear, may be encountered although the usual is 1–2 per smear (Fig. 37.29) (Berry, 1966). If the egg is orientated appropriately, the terminal spine of *S. haematobium* is visible.

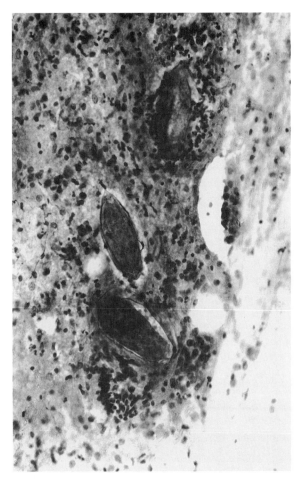

Fig. 37.29 Cervical smear with three schistosome eggs. A terminal spine is barely visible in the central egg. Papanicolaou stain × 400.

Other trematode infections. Extrapulmonary *Paragonimus* and ectopic *Fasciola* worms are uncommon; they may be found within abscesses in the uterus and Fallopian tube. Pentastomiasis, caused by worm-like parasites *(Armillifer)* in Africa and the Far East, can also involve the upper female genital tract with inflammatory lesions containing nymphs (Ong, 1974).

Parasites in cervical smears

Cervical smears may contain parasites. In addition to schistosomiasis, discussed above, eggs of *Enterobius* are noted from invasive infection. *Ascaris* eggs in smears arise from faecal contamination rather than genital tract infection. Larvae of *Strongyloides* (a rare occurrence) must be distinguished from free-living nematodes that contaminate laboratory water supplies. Various protozoa are encountered in smears. *Trichomonas* is well known. *Entamoeba histolytica* trophozoites are uncommon but can be confused with a variety of contaminant free-living protozoa and the commensal *Entamoeba gingivalis*.

NEOPLASTIC DISEASES

The world over, there is an approximately fourfold variation in estimated female mortality rates due to all non-skin cancers, the highest rates occurring in industrialized countries, the lowest in poor countries in the tropics (Parkin et al, 1988a). These differences may in reality be less, given the difficulties of accurate diagnosis and consequent under-registration in poor countries, and it is unfortunate that the cancer registries in Africa that, in the past, provided excellent data for epidemiological studies have found it nearly impossible to continue (Wabinga et al, 1993). Gynaecological malignancies, particularly cancer of the cervix, contribute importantly to cancer in the tropics (Table 37.2).

Carcinoma of the cervix

In most populations in the tropics, cervical carcinoma is the commonest malignant tumour of women (Parkin et al, 1988). Clinically, cervical carcinoma tends to present at a relatively early age in the tropics, though many cases are seen at a late stage because medical facilities are scarce, particularly in rural and poor urban areas (Rogo & Kavoo-Linge, 1990). In Malawi and Kenya, over 55% of newly diagnosed patients are stage 3 or 4. The histopathological features of cervical carcinoma are similar to those reported from other parts of the world, and massive eosinophilia is occasionally seen, as elsewhere (Ojwang & Mati, 1978; Lowe et al, 1981). Adenocarcinoma accounts for 4–5% of cases in Africa as it does in India (Kushtagi & Rao, 1991).

The types of human papillomavirus (HPV) associated with carcinoma of the cervix in industrialized countries — HPV 16 and 18 — are also found infecting patients in Africa, South America and India (Das et al, 1989; Reeves et el, 1989; Schmauz et al, 1989). Early age at onset of sexual activity is also a risk factor for cervical cancer (Duncan et el, 1990). The association of HIV infection with cervical neoplasia is discussed below.

Table 37.2 Incidences of cancer of cervix, endometrium (corpus uteri) and ovary in various regions of the world: estimated crude rates in 1980, per 100 000 women. Data from Parkin et al (1988a).

Region	Cervix	Corpus uteri	Ovary
Western Europe	19	20	16
North America	11	26	14
Japan	16	3	5
Tropical South America	32	7	6
East Africa	23	2	4
Caribbean	24	5	5
China	27	3	4
India	20	1	4

Carcinoma of the endometrium

In industrialized countries, the ratio of endometrial carcinoma to cervical carcinoma has changed greatly in the last 60 years. In earlier times cervical cancer was 6–8 times more frequent than endometrial cancer, but now the ratios approach unity or are even inverted (Table 37.2). By contrast, in tropical countries the cervical/endometrial cancer ratios are 5–15 to 1. In many African countries, choriocarcinoma is more frequent than endometrial cancer (James et al, 1973). These differences are not mainly attributable to age since they remain after age-standardization of incidence rates. Overall in 'developing countries', whilst cancer of the cervix is the commonest non-skin malignancy, endometrial cancer ranks sixteenth; in 'developed countries' the respective rankings are tenth and ninth (Parkin et al, 1988a).

As might be expected from the age structure of populations in poor countries, with many fewer old people, patients with endometrial cancer present at a lower mean age than elsewhere. In India, the mean age at presentation is 51 years, with postmenopausal bleeding in 56% of patients (Kapila & Verma, 1981). Infertility was not a major factor.

In industrialized countries, many studies have noted the association of endometrial cancer with diabetes, hypertension and obesity. This elderly archetype is less common in the tropics, though hypertension is common among some black populations. The important rôle of dietary factors, particularly the consumption of fats, in predisposing to endometrial cancer is suggested by the low incidence in Japan (Table 37.2) (Gusberg & Mulvihill, 1986).

Tumours of the ovary

In resource-poor countries in the tropics the whole range of ovarian tumours is seen, but the frequency and patterns differ from those in Europe and North America. The incidence of primary ovarian cancer is less, as is the total proportion of cancer among women that is ovarian (Table 37.2). This also applies to metastatic tumours, because of the lower incidence of gastrointestinal tract and breast cancers in these populations.

Ovarian tumours in blacks in Africa present a distinctive spectrum. Compared with the USA and Europe, epithelial tumours form a smaller proportion overall. Of these the proportion that are malignant (i.e. invasive plus borderline tumours) is greater, at around half of cases. Sex cord and stromal tumours are more frequent (Dennis et al, 1980; Lucas & Vella, 1983). Germ cell tumours are more frequent, the great majority being mature cystic teratomas (Akang et al, 1992). This frequency of cystic teratomas is probably a reflection of demography. Everywhere they are the commonest ovarian tumour in children and adolescents. Thus in African countries where half the population is 15 years or younger, their reported prevalence of about 40% of all ovarian tumours is hardly surprising.

In Asian countries, the data suggests that the patterns of ovarian tumours more resemble those found in industrialized countries (Ramachandran et al 1972; Verma and Bhatia, 1980; Gatphoh & Darnal, 1990) although the overall incidence of ovarian cancer is significantly less (Parkin et al, 1988a).

The aetiological factors for ovarian tumours are still being determined (Parazzini et al, 1991). In the USA, caucasian females have a higher incidence of ovarian cancer than blacks, and reproductive factors do not account for this difference, suggesting there may be genetic factors (John et al, 1993). Certain risk factors for ovarian cancer may explain some of the geographical variation: multiple pregnancies and interventions to reduce the number of ovulations protect against cancer, and everywhere the age-specific incidence increases to a peak in the sixth to eighth decades. Regarding the apparently different histogenetic patterns, the age-specific decline in incidence of sex cord-stromal and germ cell tumours with increasing age may be important (Yancik, 1993). However, we await studies of ovarian tumours from different geographical centres, which stratify according to histological type as well as for age, to provide further epidemiological evidence.

Burkitt's lymphoma (see also Ch. 31 for pathological description)

Prior to the classical account of Burkitt's lymphoma which described ovarian involvement as a common clinical feature (Burkitt, 1958), there had been many reports of children with ovarian lymphosarcoma in several countries in Africa; in retrospect these were recognized to be the same tumour. Aetiologically, the predisposing factors for endemic Burkitt's lymphoma are early infection with Epstein–Barr virus and holoendemic falciparum malaria.

This lymphoma accounts for 68% of all childhood malignancies in the West Nile District of Uganda and for 47% in Ibadan, Nigeria (Parkin et al, 1988b). Clinically, ovarian tumours are the commonest presenting feature in girls over the age of five years in endemic areas (Burkitt, 1970). In Nigeria, of females under 20 years, Burkitt's lymphoma is the commonest neoplasm (55%) of the ovary (Junaid, 1981).

Gestational trophoblastic tumours

The received wisdom is that the incidence of trophoblastic tumours — hydatidiform mole and choriocarcinoma — is greater in Africa and Asia (particularly among the Chinese) than in caucasian populations. For example, choriocarcinoma comprised 2% of female cancers in Uganda (James et al, 1973). However, there are considerable methodological problems in determining the population incidences of these tumours (Grimes, 1984) (and see Ch. 52) and it is currently unclear whether there really are large regional differences. What is undoubted is that pathologists in resource-poor countries see more trophoblastic tumours than their counterparts in industrialized countries; their submitted specimens come from a larger population base and women there have more pregnancies.

Histologically these tumours are no different from those in industrialized countries, except that the host inflammatory reaction to choriocarcinoma may be less marked. The types of pregnancy antecedent to choriocarcinoma and the time intervals before presentation with it appear to be similar everywhere. However, the mode of presentation of choriocarcinoma is more varied than in industrialized countries. Although vaginal bleeding is the commonest presenting sign (Makokha & Mati, 1982), a tumour nodule in the vagina or vulva, or a haemorrhagic carcinoma anywhere in the body of a woman during reproductive life should be considered a choriocarcinoma until proved otherwise.

Autopsy series indicate the wide distribution of choriocarcinoma metastases, with lung, liver and brain as the commonest sites (Ch. 52). However, in the tropics, a metastasis is often the presenting feature. A clinical stroke, meningoencephalitis or cauda equina lesion may result from a deposit (Bahemuka, 1981). Haematemesis and melaena from gastric or ileal metastases may be the first indication of tumour (Villet et al, 1979). Other unusual presentations include a polyp in the finger (Fig. 37.30) and ejection of a tooth from the mandible by a deposit of choriocarcinoma (personal observations).

It is an impression that tubal mole and choriocarcinoma, very rare tumours in industrialized countries, are more common in the tropics, probably due to the high incidence of ectopic pregnancy.

OTHER DISEASES OF THE FEMALE GENITAL TRACT

Ectopic pregnancy

The incidence of ectopic pregnancy — whether expressed per total deliveries or pregnancies or per gynaecological admissions or per female surgical emergencies — is higher (up to threefold) in resource-poor countries than in industrialized countries (Muir & Belsey, 1980; Oronsaye & Odiase, 1981). Over 95% of these ectopic pregnancies are tubal; the proportion of abdominal pregnancies amongst total ectopic pregnancies appears to be similar in the USA and Africa at 1.5%. Thus 1 in 4000–5000 pregnancies in African women is abdominal (Paes, 1981). Patients in the tropics with ectopic pregnancy are half as likely to be

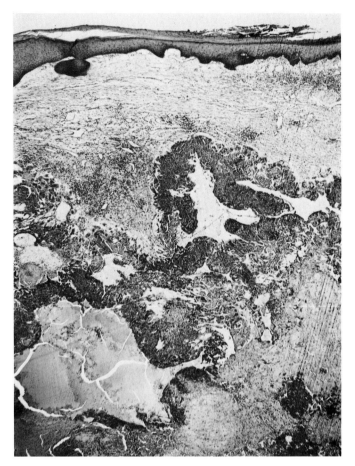

Fig. 37.30 Part of a metastatic choriocarcinoma on the finger of a 19-year-old female; it formed a polyp 4 cm in diameter. H & E × 25.

nulliparous compared with their sisters in industrialized countries. Tubal obstruction from previous salpingitis is the most popular hypothesis to explain the high frequency of tubal pregnancy (Muir & Belsey, 1980).

Female circumcision

The major form of female circumcision — infibulation — is practised in some Islamic cultures, and has many late complications in addition to the immediate sequelae of an unhygienically practised mutilating operation. Keloid scarring, abscess formation, implantation dermoid cysts and traumatic neuroma of the vulva are common. Haematocolpos and chronic urinary fistula also occur (McLean & Graham, 1983; Dirie & Lindmark, 1992).

Adenomyosis and endometriosis

Adenomyosis is only diagnosable after hysterectomy. Its prevalence among hysterectomy specimens in resource-poor countries (11–57%) appears similar to that in industrialized countries (Pendse, 1981; Daisley, 1987; Shaikh & Khan, 1990).

For endometriosis, on the other hand, there are held to be significant ethnic and regional differences in its frequency. Reports from Jamaica, India and Nigeria all indicate that the prevalence of endometriosis at gynaecological laparoscopic or operative procedures is considerably less than that seen in industrialized countries (Pendse, 1981; Rao & Persaud, 1984; Osefo & Okele, 1989). Personal experience of gynaecological material from Africa supports this impression, although rare cases of skin endometriosis are reported (Fahal & Yagi, 1987). In contrast, endometriosis is more common in Asian women in Kuala Lumpur than in caucasian women in the UK (Arumugam & Templeton, 1992).

In fact, the descriptive epidemiology of endometriosis is unclear, due to the methodological problems of case definition and study populations (Mangtani & Booth, 1993). Whether black women are genuinely less prone to endometriosis than caucasian (a phenomenon not observed in private practice in the USA) or whether socio-economic conditions may account for any real observed differences remain to be proved. The implication of immunological factors in the pathogenesis of endometriosis (Rock & Markham, 1992), may also help to explain the apparent infrequency of the disease in Africa and other areas where the populations are subject to multiple chronic infections.

HIV, AIDS and gynaecological diseases

Of the global total of more than 10 million adults infected with the human immunodeficiency viruses (HIV-1 and/or HIV-2), half are women, and most of them are of reproductive age. The modes of HIV transmission vary from country to country, but in poor countries in the tropics, it is overwhelmingly by heterosexual intercourse (Ancelle-Park & De Vincenzi, 1993). Africa has borne the major brunt of this pandemic, and in some cities HIV prevalence among women of reproductive age is up to 32% (Allen et al, 1991). Countries in Asia such as India and Thailand are now experiencing increasing transmission of HIV (Mann et al, 1992). In addition to predisposing to certain diseases of the female genital tract (Table 37.3), through AIDS, HIV contributes to premature mortality in women. Combined with the already high rate of maternal mortality in poor countries, it means that disease related to sexual behaviour is by far the major cause of adult female

mortality in many tropical countries (De Cock et al, 1990).

In Africa, women acquire HIV infection earlier than men, and the modal age at presentation with AIDS is the third decade (Mann et al, 1992). Epidemiological studies have shown that in asymptomatic women who are not significantly immunocompromised, HIV infection has no consistent effect on the menstrual cycle or on fertility (Carpenter et al, 1991; Ryder et al, 1991). There appears to be a slight effect on the outcome of pregnancy, with increased frequency of spontaneous abortion, preterm labour and low birth weight among HIV-positive compared with HIV-negative women (Gichangi et al, 1993; Johnstone, 1993). Some of this may relate to the increased frequency of chorioamnionitis in HIV-positive women; this lesion is also associated with a greater likelihood of HIV-1 transmission to the fetus (St Louis et al, 1993). There is no good evidence that pregnancy per se accelerates the course of HIV disease (Mandlebrot & Henrion, 1993).

Pelvic inflammatory disease is expected to be more frequent and more severe in HIV-positive women, given the bidirectional positive interactions of STDs and HIV infection (Laga et al, 1991). Studies to prove this are still awaited (McCarthy & Norman, 1993). Genital ulcer diseases are more prevalent among HIV-positive than HIV-negative women. This is mainly due to herpes simplex and chancroid; in Africa, granuloma inguinale and lymphogranuloma venereum do not appear to contribute to the increase. HIV itself has been demonstrated in endometrial macrophages in an HIV-positive woman with chronic endometritis (Peuchmaur et al, 1989). HIV infection is the most significant risk factor for the development of tuberculosis (De Cock et al, 1992), and in countries in Africa where both infections are endemic, tuberculosis is the cause of death in more than 30% of HIV-positive adults (Lucas et al, 1993). The adnexae are involved as part of miliary tuberculosis in HIV-positive women (personal observations), but there is no data demonstrating an increase in clinically significant gynaecological tuberculosis because of HIV infection.

Herpes zoster is reactivated by HIV infection, usually before an AIDS-defining diagnosis has occurred. It often affects multiple dermatomes and can involve the female genital area, producing painful ulceration which heals with a scar. Herpes simplex ulceration of more than one month's duration is an AIDS-defining disease and vulvar ulceration is seen among older children and adults with HIV infection (Fig. 37.31).

Vulvo-vaginal candidiasis is more frequent among HIV-positive women compared with HIV-negative, and may be more refractory to treatment. The severity appears to be inversely related to the patient's degree of immunocompetence as measured by blood CD4+ T-lymphocyte count (McCarthy & Norman, 1993).

Table 37.3 Associations of gynaecological disease with HIV infection; lesions known to be, or probably, more prevalent and severe in HIV-infected than in non-infected women

1. Fungal infections: vulvo-vaginal candidiasis
2. Viral infections: herpes simplex and zoster virus; human papillomaviruses
3. Bacterial infections: pelvic inflammatory disease; chorioamnionitis
4. Tumours: Kaposi's sarcoma; lymphoma; cervical neoplasia

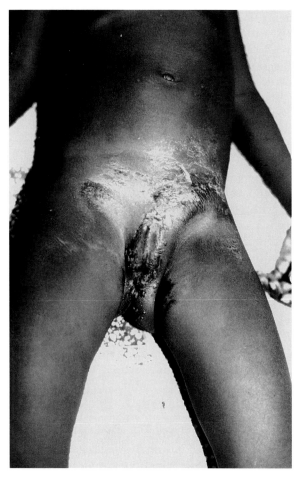

Fig. 37.31 Ulcerating herpes simplex infection of the vulva in a 6-year-old girl who died of HIV-associated disseminated herpes infection.

Although non-Hodgkin's lymphoma has a greatly augmented incidence in HIV-positive patients and tends to be extranodal, pelvic lymphoma has only occasionally been reported in HIV-positive women (Fineberg & Schinella, 1990). In Africa, Burkitt's lymphoma of the ovary is not more frequent in HIV-positive children than in HIV-negative, probably because children who are infected with HIV perinatally do not usually survive beyond five years (Lucas et al, 1994). Kaposi's sarcoma can involve the epithelium of the lower genital tract and the adnexal surfaces.

HIV, HPV and cervical neoplasia

In 1993 the Centers for Disease Control and Prevention modified the surveillance case definition for AIDS in adolescents and adults. For HIV-positive women, the criteria for AIDS now include invasive carcinoma of the cervix. It should be noted that HIV-infected women who are asymptomatic, or who have persistent vulvo-vaginal candidiasis or pelvic inflammatory disease or cervical dysplasia, are also counted as having AIDS if the CD4+ T-lymphocyte count in the blood is $< 200 \times 10^6/l$ (Centers for Disease Control and Prevention, 1992). In the USA the addition of cervical cancer resulted in less than 1% of extra reported cases of AIDS in 1993 (Centers for Disease Control and Prevention, 1993).

The associations of HIV with cervical neoplasia and HPVs are complex and are still being evaluated. There is no doubt that both in industrialized nations and in countries in Africa, HIV seropositivity is associated with an increased prevalence of HPV infection (Kreiss et al, 1992; Hankins et al, 1994). The prevalence of HPV infection increases as the CD4+ T-lymphocyte count declines. In most, but not all, studies HIV-positive women have a higher prevalence of cervical intraepithelial neoplasia (CIN), with odds ratios of up to 14 (Laga et al, 1992; Mandelblatt et al, 1992). The prevalence of CIN also increases as CD4+ T-lymphocyte counts drop (LaGuardia, 1993). Cases of carcinoma of the cervix that progress with greater rapidity in HIV-positive patients are reported (Maiman et al, 1990; Schwartz et al, 1991). What is not yet clear is whether HIV-positive women have a higher incidence of invasive carcinoma compared with HIV-negative women; the epidemiological problem is that many of the risk factors for CIN are also risk factors for HIV infection. If the incidence of invasive disease is not greatly increased by HIV infection, it may be because the patients with CIN tend to die of other HIV-related disease before the tumour spreads.

A recent autopsy study in Côte d'Ivoire found no invasive cervical cancer in HIV-positive or HIV-negative women (Lucas et al, 1993). Available cancer registry data from Uganda shows a progressive increase in the incidence of cancer of the cervix since the 1950s, but a causative association with HIV infection is not known (Wabinga et al, 1993). Conversely, in Zambia, where HIV infection is also epidemic, there has been no change in the incidence or age distribution of cervical cancer over the decade since 1980 (Rabkin & Blattner, 1991). A study of cervical cancer patients in Kenya, performed early on in the epidemic, found no increased prevalence of HIV infection compared with the non-cancer female population (Rogo & Kavoo-Linge, 1990). Natural history studies of HIV infection and cervical neoplasia in tropical resource-poor countries are being done, and if the length of survival with HIV infection increases, cervical cancer may become more prominent. At present, however, there seems little prospect of the universal availability of cervical smear screening that is advocated for HIV-positive women in industrialized countries (Hankins et al, 1994).

Acknowledgements

Professor Michael Hutt co-authored the previous edition of this chapter. Much of his years of experience of pathology in Africa and his wisdom has been retained in this new version.

REFERENCES

Agranal S, Bausal M P 1981 Amoebiasis of the uterine cervix and vagina mimicking carcinoma. Journal of Obstetrics and Gynaecology of India 31: 153–154.

Akang E E, Odunfa A O, Aghadiuno P U 1992 Childhood teratomas in Ibadan, Nigeria. Human Pathology 23: 449–453.

Al-Adnani M S, Saleh K M 1982 Extraurinary schistosomiasis in Southern Iraq. Histopathology 6: 747–752.

Allen S, Lindan C P, Serufilira A et al 1991 Human immunodeficiency virus infection in urban Rwanda. Journal of the American Medical Association 266: 1657–1663.

Ancelle-Park R, De Vincenzi I 1993 Epidemiology and natural history of HIV/AIDS in women. In: Johnson M A, Johnstone F D (eds) HIV infection in women. Churchill Livingstone, Edinburgh, pp 1–15.

Arroyo G, Elgueta R 1989 Squamous cell carcinoma associated with amoebic cervicitis. Acta Cytologica 33: 301–304.

Arroyo G, Quinn J A 1989 Association of amoebae and *Actinomyces* in an intrauterine contraceptive device user. Acta Cytologica 3: 298–300.

Arumugam K, Templeton A A 1992 Endometriosis and race. Australia and New Zealand Journal of Obstetrics and Gynaecology 32: 164–165.

Attili V R, Hira S K, Dube M K 1983 Schistosomal genital granulomas: a report of 10 cases. British Journal of Venereal Diseases 59: 269–272.

Bac D J, Teichler M J, Jonker L C, van der Merwe C F 1987 Schistosomiasis in ectopic or unusual sites, a report of 5 cases. South African Medical Journal 72: 717–718.

Bahemuka M 1981 Neurological complications of choriocarcinoma at Kenyatta National Hospital. East African Medical Journal 58: 117–123.

Bang R A, Bang A T, Baitule M, Choudhary Y, Sarmukaddam S, Tale O 1989 High prevalence of gynaecological diseases in rural Indian women. Lancet 1: 85–88.

Bazaz-Malik G, Maheshwari B, Lal N 1983 Tuberculous endometritis: a clinicopathological study of 1000 cases. British Journal of Obstetrics and Gynaecology 90: 84–86.

Berry A 1966 A cytopathological and histopathological study of bilharziasis of the female genital tract. Journal of Pathology and Bacteriology 91: 325–338.

Bhagavan B S, Ruffier J, Shinn B 1982 Pseudoactinomycotic radiate granules in the lower female genital tract: relationship to Splendore-Hoeppli phenomenon. Human Pathology 13: 898–904.

Bhagwandeen S B, Mottiar Y A 1972 Granuloma venereum. Journal of Clinical Pathology 25: 812–816.

Bhagwandeen S B, Naik K G 1977 Granuloma venereum (granuloma inguinale) in Zambia. East African Medical Journal 54: 637–642.

Bickers W M 1970 Hydatid disease of the female pelvis. American Journal of Obstetrics and Gynecology 107: 477–483.

Binford C H, Connor D H 1976 Pathology of tropical and extraordinary diseases. Armed Forces Institute of Pathology, Washington, DC.

Bittencourt A L, de Almeida M A C, Junes M A F, da Motta L D C 1980 Placental involvement in schistosomiasis mansoni: report of four cases. American Journal of Tropical Medicine and Hygiene 29: 571–575.

Burkitt D P 1958 A sarcoma involving the jaws in African children. British Journal of Surgery 46: 218–223.

Burkitt D P 1970 General features and facial tumours: lesions outside the jaws. In: Burkitt D P, Wright D H (eds) Burkitt's lymphoma. Livingstone, Edinburgh, pp 6–16.

Carpenter C C J, Mayer K H, Stein M D, Leibman B D, Fisher A, Fiore T C 1991 Human immunodeficiency virus infection in north American women: experience with 200 cases and a review of the literature. Medicine 70: 307–325.

Centers for Disease Control and Prevention 1992 1993 revised classification system for HIV infection and expanded surveillance case definition for AIDS among adolescents and adults. Morbidity and Mortality Weekly Report 41 [RR-17]: 1–19.

Centers for Disease Control and Prevention 1993 Impact of the expanded AIDS surveillance case definition on AIDS case reporting — United States, First Quarter, 1993. Morbidity and Mortality Weekly Report 42: 308–310.

Chandler F W, Kaplan W, Ajello L 1980 A color atlas and text of the histopathology of mycotic diseases. Wolfe Medical, London.

Cheever A W, Kamel I A, Elwi A M, Mosimann J E, Danner R 1977 *Schistosoma mansoni* and *Schistosoma haematobium* infections in Egypt. II. Quantitative parasitological findings at necropsy. American Journal of Tropical Medicine and Hygiene 26: 702–716.

Chen M G, Mott K E 1989 Progress in assessment of morbidity due to *Schistosoma haematobium* infection: a review of recent literature. Tropical Diseases Bulletin 86 (no 4): R1–R36.

Daisley H 1987 Adenomyosis uteri: a prospective study in Trinidad & Tobago (January – May 1986). West Indian Medical Journal 36: 166–173.

Das B C, Murthy N S, Sharma J K et al 1989 Human papillomavirus and cervical cancer in Indian women. Lancet 2: 1271.

De Cock K M, Barrere B, Diaby et al 1990 AIDS — the leading cause of adult death in the West African city of Abidjan, Cote d'Ivoire. Science 249: 793–796.

De Cock K M, Soro B, Coulibaly I-M, Lucas S B 1992 Tuberculosis and HIV infection in sub-Saharan Africa. Journal of the American Medical Association 268: 1581–1587.

Dennis P M, Coode P E, Hulewicz B S F, Kung'u A 1980 Comparative study of ovarian neoplasms in Kenya and Britain. East African Medical Journal 57: 562–565.

Dirie M A, Lindmark G 1992 The risk of medical complications after female circumcision. East African Medical Journal 69: 479–482.

Duncan M E, Tibaux G, Pelzer A et al 1990 First coitus before menarche and risk of sexually transmitted disease. Lancet 335: 338–340.

Edington G M, Nwabuebo I, Junaid T A 1975 The pathology of schistosomiasis in Ibadan, Nigeria with special reference to the appendix, brain, pancreas and genital organs. Transactions of the Royal Society of Tropical Medicine and Hygiene 69: 153–162.

El-Mahgoub S 1982 Pelvic schistosomiasis and infertility. International Journal of Gynaecology and Obstetrics 20: 201–206.

Fahal A H, Yagi K I 1987 Skin endometriosis in Sudan. Tropical and Geographical Medicine 39: 383–384.

Farooki M A 1967 Epidemiology and pathology of chronic endometritis. International Surgery 48: 566–573.

Fineberg S A, Schinella R 1990 Human immunodeficiency virus infection in women: report of 102 cases. Modern Pathology 3: 575–580.

Freinkel A L 1987 Histological aspects of sexually transmitted genital lesions. Histopathology 11: 819–831.

Freinkel A L 1988 Granuloma inguinale of cervical lymph nodes simulating tuberculous lymphadenitis: two case reports and review of the literature. Genitourinary Medicine 64: 339–343.

Frost O 1975 Bilharziasis of the Fallopian tube. South African Medical Journal 49: 1201–1203.

Gatphoh E D, Darnal H K 1990 Pattern of ovarian neoplasm in Manipur. Journal of the Indian Medical Association 88: 338–339.

Gichangi P B, Nyongo A O, Temmerman M 1993 Pregnancy outcome and placental weights: their relationship to HIV-1 infection. East African Medical Journal 70: 85–89.

Graham W J 1991 Maternal mortality: levels, trends, and data deficiencies. In: Feachem R G, Jamison D T (eds) Disease and mortality in sub-Saharan Africa. World Bank/OUP, Oxford, pp 101–116.

Grech E S, Everett J V, Mukasa F 1973 Epidemiological aspects of acute pelvic inflammatory disease in Uganda. Tropical Doctor 3: 123–127.

Grimes D A 1984 Epidemiology of gestational trophoblastic disease. American Journal of Obstetrics and Gynecology 150: 309–318.

Gusberg S B, Mulvihill M N 1986 Epidemiology [endometrial cancer]. Clinics in Obstetrics and Gynecology 13: 665–672.

Gutierrez Y 1990 Diagnostic pathology of parasitic infections with clinical correlations. Lea & Febiger, Philadelphia.

Haibach H, Bickel J T, Podrecca G I, Llorens A S 1985 Squamous cell carcinoma of the uterine cervix subsequent to amebiasis. Archives of Pathology and Laboratory Medicine 109: 1121–1123.

Hankins C A, Lamont J A, Handley M A 1994 Cervicovaginal screening in women with HIV infection: a need for increased vigilance? Canadian Medical Association Journal 150: 681–686.

James P D, Taylor C W, Templeton A C 1973 Tumours of the female genitalia. In: Templeton A C (ed) Tumours in a tropical country. Heinemann, London, pp 101–131.

John E M, Whittemore A S, Harris R, Itnyre J, Collaborative Ovarian Cancer Group 1993 Characteristics relating to ovarian cancer risk: collaborative analysis of seven US case control studies. Epithelial cancer in black women. Journal of the National Cancer Institute 85: 142–146.

Johnstone F D 1993 Pregnancy outcome and pregnancy management in HIV-infected women. In: Johnson M A, Johnstone F D (eds) HIV infection in women. Churchill Livingstone, Edinburgh, pp 187–199.

Junaid T A 1981 Ovarian neoplasms in children and adolescents in Ibadan. Cancer 47: 610–614.

Kapila K, Verma K 1981 Adenocarcinoma of the endometrium — a clinicopathological study. Journal of Obstetrics and Gynaecology of India 31: 538–542.

Khan J S, Stell R J C 1981 Enterobius vermicularis infestation of the female genital tract causing generalised peritonitis. British Journal of Obstetrics and Gynaecology 88: 681–683.

Kreiss J K, Kiviat N B, Plummer F A et al 1992 Human immunodeficiency virus, human papilloma virus, and cervical intraepithelial neoplasia in Nairobi prostitutes. Sexually Transmitted Diseases 19: 54–59.

Kushtagi P, Rao K 1991 Primary adenocarcinoma of the uterine cervix: changing clinical profile. Australia and New Zealand Journal of Obstetrics and Gynaecology 31: 86.

Laga M, Nzila N, Goeman J 1991 The interrelationship of sexually transmitted diseases and HIV infection: implications for the control of both epidemics in Africa. AIDS 5 (suppl 1): S55–S63.

Laga M, Icenogle J P, Marsella R et al 1992 Genital papillomavirus infection and cervical dysplasia — opportunistic complications of HIV infection. International Journal of Cancer 50: 45–48.

LaGuardia K D 1993 Other sexually transmitted disease: cervical intraepithelial neoplasia. In: Johnson M A, Johnstone F D (eds) HIV infection in women. Churchill Livingstone, Edinburgh, pp 247–261.

Lansman H H, Lapin A, Blaustein A 1960 Pelvic Oxyuris granuloma associated with endometriosis. American Journal of Obstetrics and Gynecology 79: 1178–1180.

Liomba N G, Chiphangwi J D 1982 Female genital tuberculosis in Malawi: a report of 90 cases. Journal of Obstetrics and Gynaecology of Eastern and Central Africa 1: 69–72.

Liomba N G, Castro F, Chiphangwi J D 1982 Chronic endometritis in Malawi: a report of 112 cases. Journal of Obstetrics and Gynaecology of Eastern and Central Africa 1: 117–120.

Liskin L S 1980 Complications of abortion in developing countries. Population Reports 8. Johns Hopkins University, Boston, pp 105–155.

Lowe D, Jorizzo J, Chiphangwi J D, Hutt M S R 1981 Cervical carcinoma in Malawi: a histopathologic study of 460 cases. Cancer 47: 2493–2495.

Lucas S B 1992 Pathology of tropical infections. In: McGee J O'D, Isaacson P G, Wright N A (eds) Oxford textbook of pathology. OUP, Oxford, pp 2187–2266.

Lucas S B, Vella E J 1983 Ovarian tumours in Malawi — a histopathological study. Journal of Obstetrics and Gynaecology of Eastern and Central Africa 2: 97–101.

Lucas S B, Mati J K G, Aggarwal V P, Sanghvi H C G 1983 The pathology of perinatal mortality in Nairobi, Kenya. Bulletin de la Societe de Pathologie Exotique 76: 579–583.

Lucas S B, Hounnou A, Peacock C S et al 1993 The mortality and pathology of HIV disease in a West African city. AIDS 7: 1569–1579.

Lucas S B, Diomande M, Hounnou A et al 1994 HIV-associated lymphoma in Africa: an autopsy study in Côte d'Ivoire. International Journal of Cancer 59: 20–24.

McCarthy K H, Norman S G 1993 Gynaecological problems in women infected with the human immunodeficiency virus. In:

Johnson M A, Johnstone F D (eds) HIV infection in women. Churchill Livingstone, Edinburgh, pp 263–268.

McLean S, Graham S E 1983 Female circumcision, excision and infibulation: the facts and proposals for change. Report No. 47, Minority Rights Group Ltd, London.

Mahler H 1987 The safe motherhood initiative: a call to action. Lancet 1: 668–670.

Maiman M, Fruchter R G, Serur E, Remy J C, Feuer G, Boyce J 1990 Human immunodeficiency virus infection and cervical neoplasia. Gynecologic Oncology 38: 377–382.

Makokha A E, Mati J K G 1982 Choriocarcinoma at Kenyatta National Hospital 1973–79. Journal of Obstetrics and Gynaecology of Eastern and Central Africa 1: 27–31.

Mandelblatt J S, Fahs M, Garibaldi K, Senie R T, Peterson H B 1992 Association between HIV infection and cervical neoplasia: implications for clinical care of women at risk for both conditions. AIDS 6: 173–178.

Mandell G L, Douglas R G, Bennett J E 1990 Principles and practice of infectious diseases, 3rd edn. Churchill Livingstone, New York.

Mandlebrot L, Henrion R 1993 Does pregnancy accelerate disease progression in HIV-infected women? In: Johnson M A, Johnstone F D (eds) HIV infection in women. Churchill Livingstone, Edinburgh, pp 157–171.

Mangtani P, Booth M 1993 Epidemiology of endometriosis. Journal of Epidemiology and Community Health 47: 84–88.

Mann J M, Tarantola D J M, Netter T W 1992 AIDS in the world. Harvard University Press, Cambridge, Mass.

Mawad N M, Hassanein O M, Mahmoud O M, Taylor M G 1992 Schistosomal vulval granuloma in a 12 years old Sudanese girl. Transactions of the Royal Society of Tropical Medicine and Hygiene 86: 644.

Most H, Gellin G A, Yager R, Aron B, Friedlander M, Quarfordt S 1963 Enterobiasis (pinworm infection): a study of 951 Puerto Rican and 315 non-Puerto Rican children in New York City. American Journal of Tropical Medicine and Hygiene 12: 65–68.

Muir D G, Belsey M A 1980 Pelvic inflammatory disease and its consequences in the developing world. American Journal of Obstetrics and Gynecology 138: 913–928.

Mylius R E, Ten Seldam R E 1962 Venereal infection by Entamoeba histolytica in a New Guinea native couple. Tropical and Geographical Medicine 14: 20–26.

Ojwang S B O, Mati J K G 1978 Carcinoma of the cervix in Kenya. East African Medical Journal 55: 194–198.

Ong H C 1974 An unusual case of pentastomiasis of the Fallopian tube in an Aborigine woman. Journal of Tropical Medicine and Hygiene 77: 187–189.

Oronsaye A U, Odiase G I 1981 Incidence of ectopic pregnancy in Benin City, Nigeria. Tropical Doctor 11: 160–163.

Osefo N J, Okele B C 1989 Endometriosis: incidence among the Igbos of Nigeria. International Journal of Gynecology and Obstetrics 30: 349–353.

Paes E H J 1981 Advanced abdominal pregnancy: case report and review of the recent literature. East African Medical Journal 58: 142–147.

Parazzini F, Franceschi S, La Vecchia C, Fasoli M 1991 The epidemiology of ovarian cancer. Gynecologic Oncology 43: 9–23.

Parkin D M, Läärä E, Muir C S 1988a Estimates of the worldwide frequency of sixteen major cancers in 1980. International Journal of Cancer 41: 184–197.

Parkin D M, Stiller C A, Draper G J, Bieber C A 1988b The international incidence of childhood cancer. International Journal of Cancer 42: 511–520.

Pendse V 1981 Adenomyosis uteri. Journal of the Indian Medical Association 76: 75–77.

Peuchmaur M, Emilie D, Vazeux R et al 1989 HIV-associated endometritis. AIDS 3: 239–241.

Phillips S C, Mildran D, William D C 1981 Sexual transmission of enteric protozoa and helminths in a venereal disease clinic population. New England Journal of Medicine 305: 603–605.

Rabkin C S, Blattner W A 1991 HIV infection and cancers other than non-Hodgkin lymphoma and Kaposi's sarcoma. In: Beral V, Jaffe H W, Weiss R A (eds) Cancer, HIV and AIDS. Cold Spring Harbour Laboratory Press, New York, pp 151–160.

Rahman M S, Rahman J, Lysikiewicz A 1982 Obstetric and gynaecological presentations of hydatid disease. British Journal of Obstetrics and Gynaecology 89: 665–670.

Ramachandran G, Harilal K R, Chinnamma K K, Thangavelu H 1972 Ovarian neoplasms — a study of 903 cases. Journal of Obstetrics and Gynaecology of India 22: 309–315.

Rao B N, Persaud V 1984 Endometriosis in Jamaica: report on a 15-year study at the University Hospital of the West Indies (1968–1982). West Indian Medical Journal 33: 36–44.

Reeves W C, Brinton L A, García M et al 1989 Human papilloma virus infection and cervical cancer in Latin America. New England Journal of Medicine 320: 1437–1441.

Renaud G, Devidas A, Develoux M, Lamothe F, Bianchi G 1989 Prevalence of vaginal schistosomiasis caused by *Schistosoma haematobium* in an endemic village in Niger. Transactions of the Royal Society of Tropical Medicine and Hygiene 83: 797.

Rock J A, Markham S M 1992 Pathogenesis of endometriosis. Lancet 340: 1264–1267.

Rogo K O, Kavoo-Linge 1990 Human immunodeficiency virus seroprevalence among cervical cancer patients. Gynecologic Oncology 37: 87–92.

Ryder R W, Batter V L, Nsuami M et al 1991 Fertility rates in 238 HIV-1-seropositive women in Zaire followed for 3 years post-partum. AIDS 5: 1521–1527.

Schmauz R, Okong R, de Villiers E-M et al 1989 Multiple infections in cases of cervical cancer from a high incidence area in tropical Africa. International Journal of Cancer 43: 805–809.

Schwartz L B, Carcangiu M L, Bradham L, Schwartz P E 1991 Rapidly progressive squamous cell carcinoma of the cervix coexisting with human immunodeficiency virus infection: clinical opinion. Gynecologic Oncology 41: 255–258.

Sengupta S K, Das N 1984 Donovanosis affected cervix, uterus, and adnexae. American Journal of Tropical Medicine and Hygiene 33: 632–636.

Shaikh H, Khan K S 1990 Adenomyosis in Pakistani women: four year experience at the Aga Khan University Medical Centre, Karachi. Journal of Clinical Pathology 43: 817–819.

Sinniah B, Leopairut J, Neafie R C, Connor D H, Voge M 1991 Enterobiasis: a histopathological study of 259 patients. Annals of Tropical Medicine and Parasitology 85: 625–635.

Spice W M, Ackers J P 1992 The amoeba enigma. Parasitology Today 8: 402–406.

St Louis M E, Kamenga M, Brown C et al 1993 Risk for perinatal HIV-1 transmission according to maternal, immunologic, virologic, and placental factors. Journal of the American Medical Association 269: 2853–2859.

Sun T, Schwartz N S, Sewell C, Lieberman P, Gross S 1991 Enterobius egg granuloma of the vulva and peritoneum; review of the literature. American Journal of Tropical Medicine and Hygiene 45: 249–253.

Symmers W St C 1960 Leishmaniasis acquired by contagion: a case of marital infection in Britain. Lancet i: 127–132.

Tiboldi T 1978 Involvement of human and primate ovaries in schistosomiasis: a review of the literature. Annales de la Societe Belge de Medecine Tropicale 58: 9–20.

Verma K, Bhatia A 1980 Ovarian neoplasm: a study of 403 tumours. Journal of Obstetrics and Gynaecology of India 30: 106–111.

Villet W T, du Toit D F, Conroy C 1979 Unusual presentation of choriocarcinoma. South African Medical Journal 55: 96–98.

Wabinga H R, Parkin D M, Wabwire-Mangen F, Mugerwa J W 1993 Cancer in Kampala, Uganda, in 1989–91; changes in incidence in the era of AIDS. International Journal of Cancer 54: 26–36.

WHO 1993 The control of schistosomiasis. Second report of the WHO expert committee. WHO, Geneva.

World Bank 1993 World development report 1993. Investing in Health. Oxford University Press, Oxford.

Wright E D, Chiphangwi J D, Hutt M S R 1982 Schistosomiasis of the female genital tract: a histopathological study of 176 cases from Malawi. Transactions of the Royal Society of Tropical Medicine and Hygiene 76: 822–829.

Yancik R 1993 Ovarian cancer: age contrasts in incidence, histology, disease stage at diagnosis, and mortality. Cancer 71 (suppl 2): 517–523.

38. Pathology of the female genital tract and ovaries in childhood and adolescence

Anna M. Kelsey   Melanie J. Newbould

INTRODUCTION

Most of the information in this chapter can be found scattered throughout the rest of this volume. The aim of this chapter is, however, to collect together these widely disseminated pieces of information so as to give an indication of how gynaecological disorders present to pathologists working in a children's hospital and to give non-paediatric pathologists, who may well encounter a gynaecological lesion in an unexpectedly young patient, a concise overview of gynaecological disease in childhood and adolescence.

DEVELOPMENTAL DISORDERS OF THE GONADS AND GENITAL TRACT

Development of the gonads, urogenital tract and perineum

Ovarian development requires the presence of two intact X chromosomes and the absence of a Y chromosome. The latter contains a gene which determines testis development, the testis-determining factor (TDF): this has now been shown to be the SRY gene which encodes a testis-specific transcript (Berta et al, 1990; Gubbay et al, 1990; Sinclair et al, 1990). The Müllerian ducts differentiate autonomously into Fallopian tubes, uterus and, possibly, the upper portion of the vagina in the absence of specific developmental factors. Development of the testis depends on the presence of the testis-determining factor (Scully, 1991), but also on other less well defined factors such as rate of gonadal growth (Blyth & Duckett, 1991). The testis-determining factor stimulates the gonadal stromal cells to differentiate into Sertoli cells, which secrete Müllerian inhibitory factor (MIF), which in turn promotes the regression of Müllerian structures. Leydig cells, stimulated initially by human chorionic gonadotrophin (hCG) and subsequently by pituitary luteinizing hormone (LH), produce testosterone which, providing its receptor is intact, results in development of male secondary sex organs (Scully, 1991).

The influence of androgens leads to the formation of male external genitalia at 58–63 days gestation and in their absence the female phenotype develops (Lauchlan, 1991). In the absence of androgens and Müllerian inhibitory factor (MIF) paired structures, the paramesonephric (Müllerian) ducts, form the lining of the Fallopian tubes, the endometrium, the endocervical epithelium and possibly part of the vagina. By the eighth to ninth week, the caudal parts of the ducts lie in close apposition and fuse to form a uterovaginal canal. The fusion is initially partial with a dividing septum. The smooth muscle of these structures differentiates from the urogenital ridge and the serosa from the coelomic epithelium. The vagina develops as a solid cord initially, and results from the fusion of cells growing downwards from the tip of the uterovaginal canal with a cord of endodermal cells growing upwards from the urogenital sinus. The cord is canalized, with the hymen representing the site of fusion between the two cell cords (Huffman et al, 1981; Risdon, 1987; Lauchlan, 1991).

Many of the Müllerian anomalies encountered can be explained in terms of different degrees of failure of fusion or canalization of the Mullerian ducts. For example, persistence of the septum between the ducts or atresia of the lower part of one or other ducts or of the urogenital endoderm results in duplications, unilateral or bilateral developmental failure respectively.

In early embryonic development, the ducts from the primitive kidney and the hindgut open into a common channel, the cloaca. Further development requires septation of the cloaca into an anterior urogenital sinus and a posterior anorectum. Caudally, the fusion of endoderm and ectoderm without the interposition of mesoderm results in the formation of the cloacal membrane which later perforates to form the perineum and anal openings. A wide range of malformations are possible given the complicated nature of this process.

Anomalies of the genital tract and perineum

Many of these present during the reproductive years with

obstetric problems. Disorders presenting during the perinatal period or childhood are amongst the more severe or form one part of a lethal malformation syndrome or sequence.

Imperforate hymen

This may present in the neonate with hydrometrocolpos, in which the vagina above the obstruction and the uterus become severely distended due to the presence of mucoid secretions or it may present during adolescence with haematocolpos (Huffman et al, 1981).

Vaginal atresia

This occurs in one in approximately 4000–5000 births (Lauchlan, 1991). It can present in a similar way to imperforate hymen, but may also be one of a lethal constellation of malformations.

Perineal abnormalities

The most severe of these is agenesis of the cloacal membrane in which the usual fusion of endoderm and ectoderm at the caudal end of the embryo is prevented by the interposition of mesoderm. In its most complete form there is a complete absence of anal, genital and urinary orifices in the perineum. This results in dilatation of the viscera which usually open into the perineum and there may be megacolon, hydrometrocolpos, megacystis, megaureter renal dysplasia, prune belly and also features of the oligohydramnios sequence, including pulmonary hypoplasia (Lauchlan, 1991).

There are a large number of possible varieties of malformations which represent lesser degrees of cloacal membrane and cloacal anomalies; anovestibular fistula in which the anal opening is absent but the distal large bowel opens into the lower vagina is said to be the commonest of these in the female (DeSa, 1991).

The vagina and uterus may also be the site into which an ectopic ureter drains and this anomaly may present during childhood with incontinence (Huffman et al, 1981).

Genital tract anomalies associated with malformation syndromes

Genital tract abnormalities are closely associated with anomalies of the renal tract. Any form of complete lower renal tract obstruction, which, as explained above, can often be associated with generalized perineal anomalies, will almost certainly be associated with renal dysplasia. There is a familial form of renal agenesis, inherited as an autosomal dominant, in which Müllerian abnormalities form an integral part (Biedel et al, 1984). However, geni-

tal tract malformations may also be seen in non-familial renal agenesis (Duncan et al, 1979) so that family studies are often required to distinguish the familial form.

Vaginal atresia and hydrometrocolpos may be seen in association with cryptophthalmos, syndactyly and multiple organ atresia in the autosomal recessive Fraser's syndrome (Gilbert-Barness & Opitz, 1991a).

Chromosomal anomalies, such as trisomy 18 or trisomy 13, often include Müllerian abnormalities as one of the features (Gilbert-Barness & Opitz, 1991b).

Sexual ambiguity in the newborn child

The commonest cause in the newborn is congenital adrenal hyperplasia. In this condition, the genotype is, of course, 46,XX and the gonads are ovaries. There is a deficiency of one of the several enzymes involved in cortisol synthesis with resulting accumulation of androgenic intermediate metabolites. In the female the increased androgen to which the fetus is exposed results in varying degrees of masculinization of the external genitalia, though not the internal organs (Scully, 1991). Several functional maternal ovarian lesions, such as pregnancy luteoma, may also lead to masculinization of a female fetus (Scully, 1991). Other disorders associated with sexual ambiguity are considered below with other developmental disorders of the gonads.

Developmental abnormalities of the ovary

Very rarely, there may be bilateral or unilateral agonadism or accessory gonads due to abnormalities of germ cell migration (Lauchlan, 1991).

Turner's syndrome

This condition results from a variety of abnormalities in one or more areas on the X chromosome which are necessary for the development and function of normal ovaries. The most common karyotype is 45,XO (Fig. 38.1), but some cases are mosaics, for example 45,XO/46,XX or other forms with additional X chromosomes or ring and dicentric chromosomes. The majority of 45,XO fetuses, probably more than 95%, are aborted early in pregnancy and only 1 in 2500 female live births have this karyotype (Machin, 1991). Only 50% of patients with Turner's syndrome surviving beyond infancy have a 45,XO genotype. These patients have no increased risk of gonadal germ cell neoplasia, but any genotype which includes Y chromosome material confers a 15–20% risk of developing a gonadoblastoma. The availability of specific DNA probes allows identification of these individuals (Cooper et al, 1991).

In those fetuses which survive, the ovaries are normal until the second trimester in utero when ova begin to

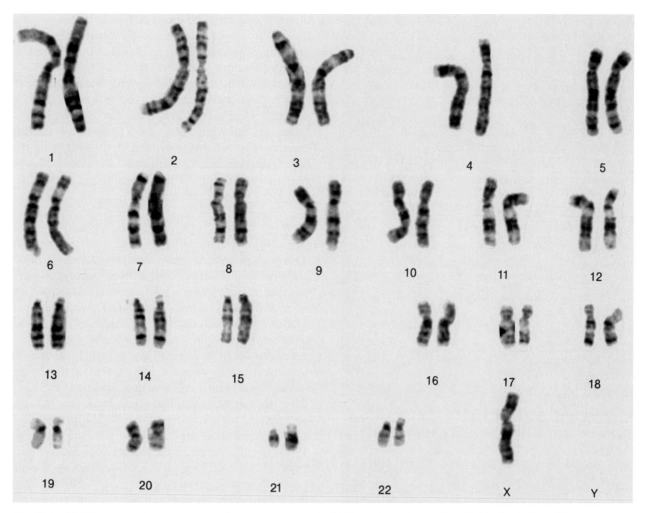

Fig. 38.1   45,X karyotype: the most common karyotype associated with Turner's syndrome. (Supplied by Dr. J. Fennell.)

undergo atresia, a process which is commonly complete before puberty so that primary amenorrhoea is a common finding (Scully, 1991). However, cases are reported in which girls with Turner's syndrome, usually those with a mosaic genotype, have borne normal children.

The phenotype is characterized by short stature, broad chest, lymphoedema with puffy fingers and toes, anomalous ears, webbed posterior neck, cubitus valgus and an excessive number of pigmented naevi (Gilbert-Barnes & Opitz, 1991b). Marked nuchal oedema is common in fetuses (Fig. 38.2), probably due to a partial agenesis of the lymphatic system. Renal tract anomalies are found in three-quarters of cases and include horseshoe kidney, duplex systems, agenesis or hypoplasia (Gilbert-Barnes & Opitz, 1991b). Common cardiac malformations include atrial septal defect, patent ductus, transposition and coarctation of the aorta (Gilbert-Barnes & Opitz, 1991b).

The mature gonads are streak-shaped structures composed entirely of ovarian-type stroma in which the hilar areas are normal, with a normal rete ovarii and hilar cells (Scully, 1991).

Streak gonads may also be seen in isolation from abnormalities of other organ systems (pure gonadal dysgenesis). The genotype of these patients may be 46,XX, in which case there is no association with an increased incidence of gonadal germ cell neoplasia.

Mixed gonadal dysgenesis and other intersex disorders with abnormal gonads

Mixed gonadal dysgenesis (MGD) is characterized by a unilateral testis, usually abdominal, with a contralateral streak gonad and persistent Müllerian structures (Davidoff & Federman, 1973); in some cases there may be bilateral abdominal streak-testes. It is the second commonest cause of ambiguous genitalia in the newborn (Scully, 1991). Phenotypic sex is commonly female (Wallace & Levin, 1990) but there is always some degree of masculinization and one-third are phenotypic males. Most individuals are genotypically 45,XO/46,XY mosaics and stigmata of Turner's syndrome, such as congenital heart disease, may be present (Wallace & Levin, 1990).

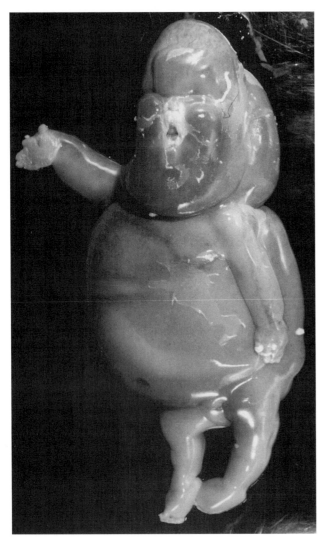

Fig. 38.2 Fetus with nuchal and generalized oedema: Turner's syndrome.

However, most individuals with a 45,XO/46,XY genotype are phenotypically normal males (Scully, 1991). In one series one-third of patients with mixed gonadal dysgenesis had a gonadoblastoma (discussed below) and this was bilateral in over half of them (Wallace & Levin, 1990). The dysgenetic testes in this condition may be involved in other forms of neoplasia including intratubular germ cell neoplasia (Müller et al, 1985; Wallace & Levin, 1990), sex cord-stromal tumour of undefined type (Wallace & Levin, 1990) and juvenile granulosa cell tumour (Young et al, 1985). Clear cell adenocarcinoma of the cervix and vagina has been recorded in mixed gonadal dysgenesis (Resnik et al, 1989) and there are a few reports of endometrial adenocarcinoma (Wallace & Levin, 1990). There is also an association with Wilms' tumour and abnormalities of renal function (Scully, 1991).

46,XY pure gonadal dysgenesis (Swyer syndrome) is characterized by persistent internal Müllerian structures, bilateral streak gonads and a female phenotype (Olsen et al, 1988; Wallace & Levin, 1990). In at least some cases the Y chromosome has been demonstrated to lack TDF (Scully, 1991). Approximately 30% of patients develop a gonadoblastoma (Rutgers & Scully, 1987).

In dysgenetic male pseudohermaphroditism the characteristic features are bilateral cryptorchid testes accompanied by persistent Müllerian structures and a 46,XY genotype (Mandell et al, 1977). There is considerable clinical and pathological overlap between this disorder and mixed gonadal dysgenesis and it may well represent one variant (Scully, 1991). Again, approximately 30% develop a gonadoblastoma.

Male pseudohermaphroditism

This may present to gynaecologists as a cause of primary amenorrhoea. Patients have a 46,XY genotype and testes but due to failure to produce active androgens or a failure to respond to them they fail to develop a male phenotype. In the absence of androgen stimulation the human sex phenotype reverts to its default type, which is female. The androgen receptor is a nuclear protein, the gene coding for which is located on the short arm of the X chromosome. Both point mutations and deletions in this region have been demonstrated to result in the complete androgen insensitivity syndrome, which is therefore in these cases inherited as an X-linked disorder (French et al, 1990). In the presence of defects in androgen synthesis, such as 5α-reductase deficiency, which is the enzyme involved in the conversion of testosterone to dihydrotestosterone, the complete male phenotype may also fail to develop. In this case the condition has an autosomal recessive inheritance (Scully, 1991). In its fully expressed form, male pseudohermaphroditism is characterized by unambiguously female external genitalia, breast development at puberty, poorly formed Wolffian structures and the persistence of Müllerian structures. The Fallopian tubes may be well developed (Rutgers & Scully, 1987). The testes can be sited anywhere along the normal path of testicular descent.

The microscopic appearance of the testes is characteristic. There are immature seminiferous tubules containing only a few germ cells, abundant Leydig cells and multiple hamartomatous nodules. The latter are more common in adults and, microscopically, nodules consist of tightly packed tubules containing Sertoli cells with only a few germ cells (Fig. 38.3); other elements, such as Leydig cells, ovarian stroma and smooth muscle may be present (Rutgers & Scully, 1987).

Five to 10 per cent of cases of male pseudohermaphroditism develop malignant germ cell tumours, almost always post-pubertally, in contrast to mixed gonadal dysgenesis and related conditions. Seminoma is the most common malignant neoplasm (Rutgers & Scully, 1987). There may be associated intratubular germ cell neoplasia

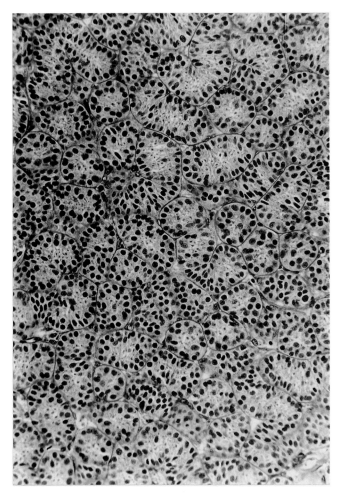

Fig. 38.3 Testis in male pseudohermaphroditism: hamartomatous nodule. H & E × 225.

(ITGCN) (Müller & Skakkebaek, 1984) (Fig. 38.4a). Placental alkaline phosphatase can be of great assistance in diagnosing this lesion (Fig. 38.4b). Though it can be demonstrated in normal fetal germ cells, this marker is largely lost by eight months of age in both normal boys and patients with testicular feminization and therefore provides a specific marker of ITGCN beyond this age (Armstrong et al, 1991). In one series, two of 14 patients with male pseudohermaphroditism had evidence of ITGCN (Armstrong et al, 1991).

There are a few reports of sex cord-stromal tumours occurring in testes in patients with the androgen insensitivity syndrome, some of which have the appearance of large cell calcifying Sertoli cell tumours (Scully, 1991). In some patients malignant sex cord-stromal tumours of the testes have been recorded (O'Dowd et al, 1990; Scully, 1991).

True hermaphroditism

In this condition, both ovarian and testicular tissue is present, either contralaterally or joined in the form of bilateral or unilateral ovotestes. The phenotype ranges from normal female to normal male but there is commonly sexual ambiguity. Most commonly the genotype is 46,XX but 46,XY and mosaics have been recorded (Scully, 1991). Epithelial neoplasms of both ovary and breast, in addition to gonadoblastoma and germ cell neoplasms have been reported in true hermaphrodites (Talerman et al, 1990; Scully, 1991). However, germ cell neoplasia is much less common than in mixed gonadal dysgenesis and has a slightly higher incidence in those patients whose genotype includes a Y chromosome (Talerman et al, 1990).

The 46,XX true hermaphrodites do not appear to have TDF. It has been suggested that in these cases the gonadal differentiation may be controlled by a more primitive evolutionary mechanism whereby the direction of differentiation is controlled by gonadal growth rate. When a certain threshold is exceeded, a testis results even in the absence of TDF (Blyth & Duckett, 1991).

NON-NEOPLASTIC LESIONS OF THE OVARY IN CHILDHOOD

Multiple cysts of follicular origin are extremely common in the neonate and in the immediate postmenarchal years. These lesions commonly regress and are asymptomatic. Marked enlargement of both ovaries due to massive multiple follicular cysts has been reported in an infant with the autosomal recessive Donahue syndrome (Lauchlan, 1991). This condition is associated with a defect in the insulin receptor (Gilbert-Barness & Opitz, 1991a). Large follicular cysts have also been noted in the infants of diabetic mothers (Huffman et al, 1981).

Symptomatic follicular cysts are less common. They are often solitary and form a substantial proportion of surgically treated ovarian lesions in infants and prepubertal children, accounting for 36% of such cases in one review (Breen & Maxson, 1977). Cysts may become symptomatic because of hormone production, usually resulting in isosexual precocious puberty, or because of abdominal pain resulting from torsion or haemoperitoneum consequent upon bleeding (Breen & Maxson, 1977; Schwöbel & Stauffer, 1991). Multiple luteinized follicular cysts are found in the ovaries of girls with the McCune–Albright syndrome, where they are functional and associated with sexual precocity. This disorder is characterized by polyostotic fibrous dysplasia of bone, cafe-au-lait spots and sexual precocity. Hyperthyroidism, acromegaly, hyperparathyroidism and Cushing's syndrome are other recorded associations. It appears therefore that there is hyperplasia of multiple endocrine organs (Danon et al, 1975).

Cysts originating in the corpus luteum may be found in postmenarchal girls, though rarely female neonates may have this type of lesion. Paraovarian cysts are also re-

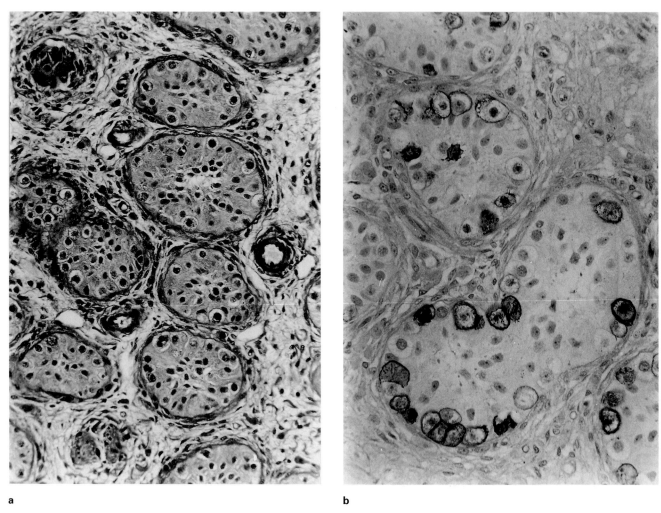

a   b

Fig. 38.4   Testis in male pseudohermaphroditism: intratubular germ cell neoplasia. **a** Characteristic large atypical germ cells within seminiferous tubules. H & E × 225. **b** Abnormal germ cells stain positively with immunostains for PLAP. × 360.

ported and are more commonly found in young women after the menarche.

Ovarian fibromatosis, described by Young & Scully, affects women from the teenage years to the fourth decade. Patients present with menstrual irregularities, excessive bleeding or androgenic symptoms. The condition may involve both ovaries and microscopically part or all of the ovary may be expanded by a spindle cell stroma with varying amounts of associated collagen. Nests of cells of sex cord type may be found within the stroma (Young & Scully, 1984). Massive ovarian oedema involves a similar age group and may also involve both ovaries. It is, according to the World Health Organization definition, a tumour-like condition in which there is ovarian enlargement due to accumulation of oedema fluid. Modes of presentation are similar to those for fibromatosis and in the prepubertal girl there may be sexual precocity. In some cases there is acute abdominal pain due to torsion, and one theory as to its cause is that fluid accumulates as a result of intermittent torsion. It has been suggested that the two

conditions may be related and that massive oedema results when the stroma in fibromatosis accumulates a large amount of tissue fluid (Young & Scully, 1984).

Torsion of the uterine adnexa where there is no tumour

This uncommon condition, which more usually involves the right side, clinically very closely mimics acute appendicitis (Huffman et al, 1981). It may occur prenatally (Mordehai et al, 1991). The involved ovary may be completely normal or follicular cysts may be present.

MISCELLANEOUS, NON-NEOPLASTIC DISEASE OF THE GENITAL TRACT IN CHILDHOOD AND ADOLESCENCE

The vulva may be involved in inflammatory conditions not specific to childhood or to this site, such as, for example, lichen sclerosus, Behçet's syndrome or ulceration associated with malnutrition (Huffman et al, 1981).

Vulvovaginitis may be associated with poor perineal hygiene, it may be secondary to intestinal parasites such as *Enterobius vermicularis*, to foreign bodies or it may be caused by an infection usually transmitted venereally in the sexually active. The latter include gonorrhoea, herpes simplex and Trichomonas. Gonorrhoeal vulvovaginitis was formerly a very common infection in children brought up in crowded conditions and, though some cases were sexually transmitted, others appear to have been infected by close non-sexual family contact and via fomites (Huffman et al, 1981).

Epithelial inclusion cysts, paraurethral cysts, and cysts of the canal of Nuck may all rarely occur during childhood. Cysts of the mesonephric (Gartner's) duct remnants are the commonest benign vaginal swellings in infancy and childhood. Cystic remnants of unfused segments of Müllerian ducts may also be found at any age and if lined with endometrial-type epithelium they may become blood filled at the menarche (Huffman et al, 1981).

PREGNANCY IN CHILDHOOD AND ADOLESCENCE

Pregnancies have been well documented in girls as young as five years, though this is clearly a most exceptional occurrence (Huffman et al, 1981). Teenage pregnancies are associated with an increased incidence of complications such as pre-eclampsia and eclampsia, anaemia, low birthweight babies, perinatal mortality, cephalopelvic disproportion and prolonged labour (Huffman et al, 1981).

NEOPLASMS OF THE FEMALE GENITAL TRACT AND OVARIES IN CHILDHOOD AND ADOLESCENCE

The pattern of disease

Considering childhood to span an age range of 0–14 years, childhood cancers comprise only 0.5–3% of all neoplastic disease, depending on population structure (Parkin et al, 1988). In the Manchester series this amounts to a total incidence of 102 tumours per 10^6 child-years, of which leukaemia, lymphoma and central nervous system tumours account for almost 80%. In the same series, germ cell and other gonadal neoplasms have a total incidence of only 2.3 per 10^6 years (Birch, 1990). Of all ovarian tumours, only 0.2–0.3% occur in girls aged less than 15 years (La Vecchia et al, 1983) and the proportion of genital tract neoplasms occurring in this age group is very much lower.

Since its foundation in 1953, the Manchester Children's Tumour registry has recorded all cases of malignant neoplasms and all germ cell neoplasms occurring in children aged 15 years or less from a defined geographical area. Data regarding the occurrence of non-germ cell benign neoplasms, which are not commonly subject to registration, are unavailable. Statistics collected by the registry are population based and avoid the bias introduced by patterns of referral which are inherent in data generated from hospitals. It originally drew from a child population of one million but boundary and demographic changes (Birch, 1988) have since resulted in a fall so that the population served is now 777 000. Over the 36 years between 1954 and 1990 less than 80 neoplasms of the ovary and female genital tract were recorded in this population, that is approximately two cases each year. Table 38.1 illustrates the tumour types, site and relative frequency. The ovary is the most common site and germ cell tumours form the most common type of neoplasm. Other studies, which were concerned with only ovarian tumours, have generated similar data regarding the relative frequency of tumour types (Norris & Jensen, 1972; Breen & Maxson, 1977; La Vecchia et al, 1983; Gribbon et al, 1992).

It is evident from Table 38.1 that genital tract neoplasms are largely tumours of the first decade, that mature ovarian teratomas and sex cord-stromal tumours occur

Table 38.1 Gynaecological tumours collected by Manchester Children's Tumour Registry, 1954–1990

Ovarian tumours (n = 67)	Number	Age range (years) in this series
Germ cell tumours	56	
Mature teratomas	31	2–15
Malignant germ cell tumours comprising:	25	6–14
dysgerminoma	10	6–13
immature teratoma	6	10–14
endodermal sinus tumour	6	6–14
embryonal carcinoma	2	12–14
choriocarcinoma	1	10
Sex cord-stromal tumours comprising:	7	2–14
juvenile granulosa cell tumour	2	2–10
Sertoli–Leydig cell tumour	2	9–13
sex cord tumour with annular tubules	2	6–12
fibroma	1	14
Other ovarian tumours comprising:	4	
small cell carcinoma	1	12
malignant neoplasm, not otherwise specified	3	2–13
Genital tract tumours (n = 9)		
Malignant germ cell tumours comprising:	5	1–8
vaginal endodermal sinus tumour	4	1–3
embryonal carcinoma of the uterine corpus	1	8
Sarcomas comprising:	3	
vaginal rhabdomyosarcoma	2	2
cervical rhabdomyosarcoma	1	2
Others		
small cell malignant tumour of the vulva	1	6

throughout childhood and that malignant ovarian germ cell neoplasms increase in frequency from the end of the first decade. There are few tumours which occur exclusively in the paediatric age group. In almost all cases, the age range of neoplasms listed in Table 38.1 extends into the second, third or subsequent decades.

Germ cell tumours

Epidemiology

Over the past 30 years the incidence of germ cell tumours has risen. This has been noted in series which have examined all germ cell neoplasms (Birch et al, 1982) and also more specifically in studies examining the incidence of malignant gonadal neoplasms (Walker et al, 1984; Senturia, 1987). This is particularly due to a rising incidence of testicular cancer, but there is evidence that at least some groups of ovarian malignant germ cell neoplasms may be subject to a similar trend (Walker et al, 1984), for example yolk sac tumours (La Vecchia, 1983).

Recently, it has been suggested that there is an increased (though very low) risk of germ cell neoplasia in both male and female offspring following maternal exposure to oestrogens, including oral contraceptives, in early pregnancy (Walker et al, 1988; Senturia, 1987).

Ovarian germ cell tumours

The ovary is usually considered to be the second commonest site of origin in the paediatric age group after the sacrococcygeal region (Dehner, 1983). However, in one population-based study (Marsden et al, 1981) and in one large series from a children's hospital (Malogolowkin et al, 1990), ovarian tumours were the most common.

Mature teratomas

Overall, at least 90% of ovarian germ cell tumours are mature teratomas and two types are described: the mature cystic teratoma (dermoid cyst) and the mature solid teratoma. The former accounts for over 20% of all ovarian neoplasms, affects women in all age groups from childhood to old age and forms over half of all ovarian tumours in the first two decades (Scully, 1979). In the Manchester series (Table 38.1), 53% of tumours in girls aged 15 years or less were mature cystic teratomas. This could represent an underestimate; whilst it is probable that all malignant neoplasms are recorded, it is possible that some benign tumours escape registration.

Mature solid teratoma is a tumour of the first two decades. In the Manchester series, there were no examples of fully mature teratoma over the 36 years. The diagnosis should be made only after careful sampling to exclude the presence of immature tissues or other malignant germ cell

elements. At least one block per centimetre of tumour is recommended (Norris et al, 1976).

Dysgerminoma

Germinoma is the general designation for the neoplasm which is known as seminoma in the testis and dysgerminoma in the ovary (Fig. 38.5). It is the commonest malignant germ cell tumour, comprising almost half of those collected in Manchester. Overall survival is high. In one series, no patient had died since the introduction of megavoltage radiotherapy in 1963 (Björkholm et al, 1990), though this treatment almost invariably results in the loss of fertility (Mitchell et al, 1991). In the series of children aged 15 years or less from Manchester, all 10 patients with dysgerminoma (three of whom had bilateral disease) have survived for more than 10 years to date.

Immature teratoma

This is the third most common malignant germ cell neoplasm and accounted for 8% of all ovarian tumours in

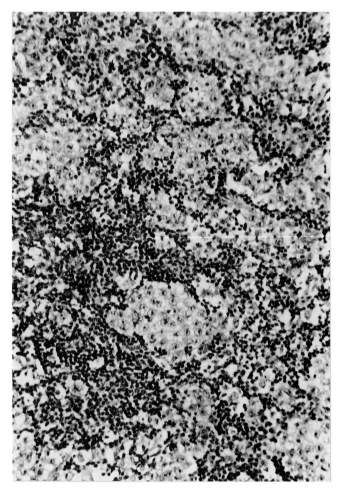

Fig. 38.5 Dysgerminoma: groups of neoplastic germ cells within a sea of lymphocytes. H & E × 225.

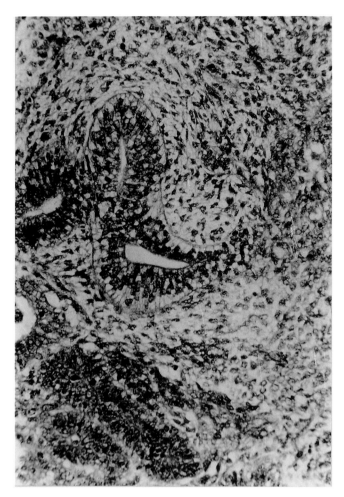

Fig. 38.6 Ovarian immature teratoma. H & E × 225.

patients aged less than 15 years in Manchester (Fig. 38.6). Grading is determined by the proportion of immature tissue present though the exact criteria used have varied from series to series (Thurlbeck & Scully, 1960; Nogales et al, 1976; Norris et al, 1976). It should be noted that this does apply specifically to ovarian teratomas. Tumours at other sites, such as the sacrococcygeal region or the mediastinum, frequently contain immature elements which are of no prognostic significance in neoplasms occurring in children in the first three months of life (Dehner, 1983; Carter et al, 1982), though they may indicate malignancy beyond infancy.

A high proportion of immature and mature solid ovarian teratomas, a third in one series (Norris et al, 1976), are associated with extraovarian disease. However, the factors determining prognosis are the grade of the primary tumour and the grade of tumour deposits in extraovarian sites rather than the stage per se. The presence of fully mature glial implants on the peritoneum increases stage but is not an adverse prognostic factor (Nogales et al, 1976; Truong et al, 1982). Therefore, pathological assessment demands adequate sampling of both the primary

tumour and extraovarian deposits to disclose the extent of immature tissues or the presence of other malignant germ cell elements. Tumours containing a small proportion of immature tissue have always been associated with an excellent prognosis, but, prior to the advent of modern combination chemotherapy in the 1970s, only 30% of patients with high-grade neoplasms survived (Norris et al, 1976). Therapeutic advances have resulted in significant improvements (Taylor et al, 1985).

Yolk sac tumour

This is the second most frequent form of malignant ovarian germ cell tumour in many series (Kurman & Norris, 1977). Numerous histological patterns have been described (Fig. 38.7a–c). Patients commonly present with an abdominal mass, fever and pain rather than with hormonal effects (Kurman & Norris, 1976a). Though yolk sac tumour was originally regarded as a highly malignant neoplasm with a 13% three-year survival (Kurman & Norris, 1976a), modern chemotherapy has reduced mortality considerably and now over 80% of patients have a long-term survival (Gershenson et al, 1983; Taylor et al, 1985). One series, considering yolk sac tumours at all sites, found a survival rate of 99% (Mann et al, 1989). Furthermore, the combination of conservative surgery and chemotherapy offers the option of preservation of fertility (Wu et al, 1991).

The introduction of serum tumour markers, such as alphafetoprotein (and hCG in the case of certain other germ cell neoplasms) and the development of better imaging techniques have also considerably facilitated follow-up of patients with malignant germ cell neoplasms (Mann et al, 1989; Gribbon et al, 1992).

Other malignant germ cell tumours of the ovary

Embryonal carcinoma resembles the tumour of the same name in the adult testis, but it is much less common in the ovary. Its distinct clinicopathological features were described by Kurman & Norris (1976b). Unlike yolk sac tumours, 60% of embryonal carcinomas present with hormonal manifestations (Kurman & Norris, 1976b).

Pure non-gestational choriocarcinoma is very rare in the ovary (Fig. 38.8). In an infant with multiple visceral lesions or in a post-pubertal female, the possibility of metastatic gestational choriocarcinoma should be considered (Kurman & Norris, 1977; Dehner, 1983; Flam et al, 1989).

Malignant neuroectodermal tumours resembling those of the central nervous system have been described in the ovary of teenage patients (Aguirre & Scully, 1982). Since some of these neoplasms contained areas of mature teratoma, it seems probable that these are germ cell neoplasms.

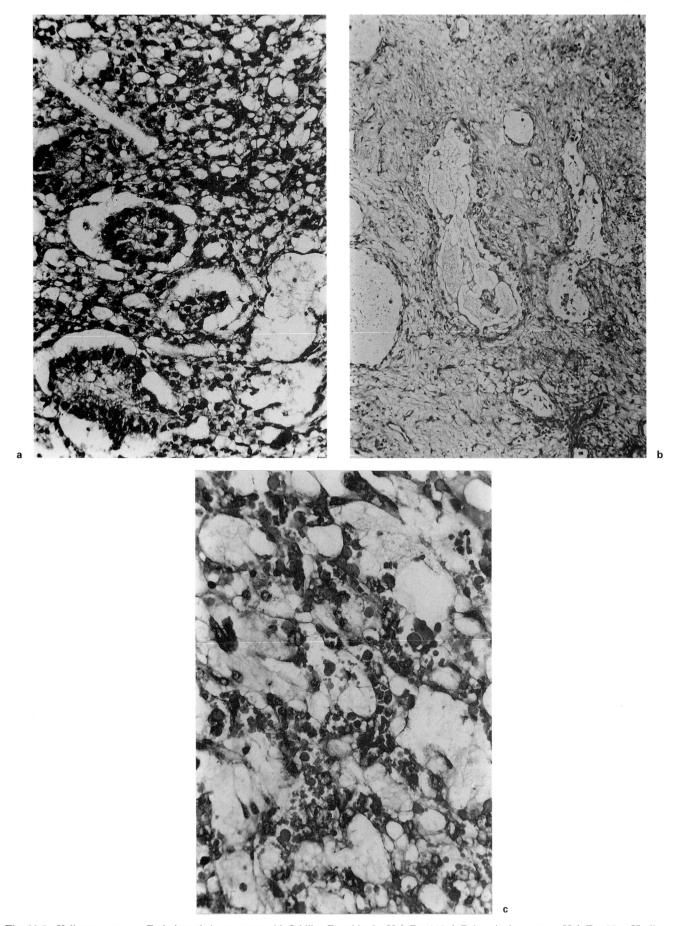

Fig. 38.7 Yolk sac tumour. **a** Endodermal sinus pattern with Schiller–Duval body. H & E × 210. **b** Polyvesicular pattern. H & E × 85. **c** Hyaline globules, both intracellular and extracellular. H & E × 340.

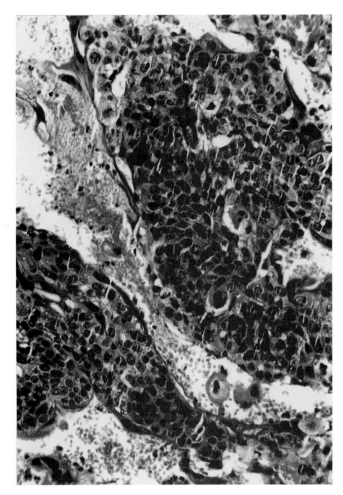

Fig. 38.8 Choriocarcinoma: solid islands of cytotrophoblast covered by a layer of syncytiotrophoblast. H & E × 360.

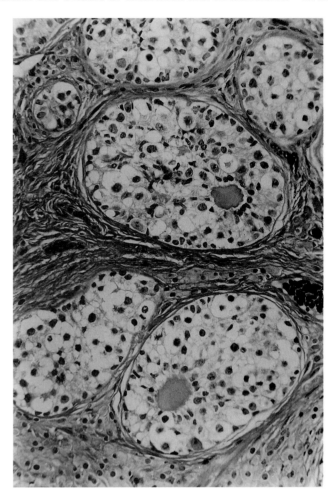

Fig. 38.9 Gonadoblastoma: islands of cells composed of both sex cord and germ cell elements. H & E × 225. (Case provided by Dr. D. L. Bisset.)

Cytogenetics

There is currently little information available on the cytogenetics of malignant ovarian germ cell tumours. Isochromosome i(12p) is a karyotypic anomaly particularly associated with testicular germ cell tumours (Atkin & Baker, 1983). It appears to be present in more than 80% of cases and can be found in neoplasms of all histological types (Geurts van Kessel et al, 1991). Though this anomaly does not appear to be observed consistently in ovarian germ cell tumours, the presence of one or more copies of this isochromosome has been reported in two dysgerminomas, a yolk sac tumour and one mixed Mullerian tumour (Dal Cin & Van Den Berghe, 1991).

Lesions associated with the development of germ cell neoplasms

Gonadoblastoma

This is one tumour within the group of mixed germ cell sex cord-stromal neoplasms. Gonadoblastoma is reported in patients aged from infancy through to the fourth decade (Rutgers & Scully, 1987).

In 50% of cases an associated malignant germ cell tumour develops either in the same or the contralateral gonad. This is most commonly a germinoma but in some cases another malignant neoplasm such as a yolk sac tumour, embryonal carcinoma, choriocarcinoma or immature teratoma may develop (Rutgers & Scully, 1987). Gonadoblastoma has a characteristic insular structure (Fig. 38.9). The lesions are frequently calcified and may be visible radiologically (Rutgers & Scully, 1987). They can be microscopic in size or may form a sizable ovarian mass.

Ninety five per cent of tumours occur in patients with a Y chromosome, though 80% of them are phenotypic females (Scully, 1970). Usually, the tumour occurs within the dysgenetic gonads of one of three syndromes, discussed earlier: mixed gonadal dysgenesis, pure XY gonadal dysgenesis or dysgenetic male pseudohermaphroditism. The risk of prepubertal germ cell malignancy is sufficiently high in these disorders to warrant gonadectomy at diagnosis. Twenty per cent of gonadoblastomas occur in a streak gonad, 20% in a testis and in most of the other cases the underlying gonad is of indeterminate type. There are a very few instances of the tumour occurring in the ovary of an apparently normal fertile women (Scully, 1970). One example has been recorded in a 46,XX infant with the autosomal recessive Fraser (cryptophthalmos) syndrome (Greenberg et al, 1986).

Family cancer syndromes

Family cancer syndromes are characterized by malignancies in more than two generations of one family. Often, age at presentation is young, the pattern of organ involvement is distinctive and a high proportion of siblings are affected.

There are several recorded instances of germ cell neoplasms occurring in several members of one family (La Vecchia et al, 1983; Dahl et al, 1990) in the absence of other types of tumour. In other examples, germ cell neoplasms have been recorded in association with tumours of different histogenesis. For example, there is a report of one kindred in which ovarian germ cell neoplasms occurred in patients from two generations and one sibling in the second generation developed a rhabdomyosarcoma (Weinblatt & Kochen, 1991).

It has been suggested that the incidence of gonadal germ cell tumours may be increased in the Li–Fraumeni cancer family syndrome (Hartley et al, 1989). The syndrome was first described in 1969 on the basis of familial clusters of cancers in association with childhood soft tissue sarcomas in other family members (Li & Fraumeni, 1969) (Fig. 38.10a, b). Germ line mutations in the p53 gene have been reported in these families (Malkin et al, 1990; Srivastava et al, 1990). As the p53 gene product, a 53 000 dalton nuclear protein, appears to play a rôle in regulation of the cell cycle and also may act as a tumour suppressor gene (Seruca et al, 1992; Toguchida et al, 1992), this mutation may have a causal association with the syndrome.

Germ cell tumours occurring in the female genital tract

Endodermal sinus tumour of the vagina is the only neoplasm to occur with any frequency in the female genital tract. It characteristically involves a younger age group than its ovarian counterpart and patients are usually in the first decade of life (Brown & Langley, 1976; Kohorn et al, 1985; Clement & Young, 1993). Classically, it was described as an aggressive neoplasm metastasizing to lymph nodes, liver and lungs (Kohorn et al, 1985) with a mean survival of less than a year (Dehner, 1987). Most series include only a few cases so that the impact of modern chemotherapy is somewhat difficult to assess. However, it is notable that in the Manchester series there have been

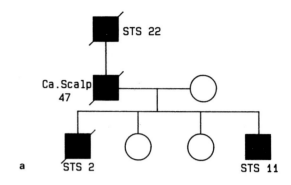

Li-Fraumeni Family C 1969

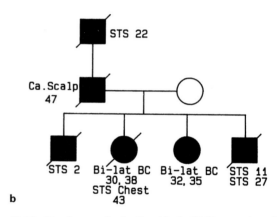

Li-Fraumeni Family C 1982

Fig. 38.10 Family tree of a family with the Li–Fraumeni syndrome. **a** 1969 — Soft tissue sarcoma (STS) in members of the first and third generations, with carcinoma of the scalp in a member of the middle generation. **b** The same family in 1982. All the members of the third generation have now developed neoplasia, either soft tissue sarcomas, bilateral breast carcinoma or both.

no deaths in the children with ovarian or genital tract malignant germ cell neoplasms who received combination chemotherapy since the mid 1970s.

Sex cord-stromal tumours of the ovary

Juvenile granulosa cell tumour

Less than 5% of all granulosa cell tumours occur in premenarchal girls but approximately 90% of those that do have distinct clinicopathological and microscopic features. The characteristic appearance of the juvenile granulosa cell tumour is well documented (Young et al, 1984) (Fig. 38.11). In the prepubertal girl presentation is typically with isosexual precocious pseudopuberty (Lack et al, 1981; Young et al, 1984; Biscotti & Hart, 1989). In one large series survival was 92% with an average of five years follow-up; extraovarian disease at diagnosis was the most significant factor in predicting an adverse prognosis (Young et al, 1984). In contrast to adult-type granulosa

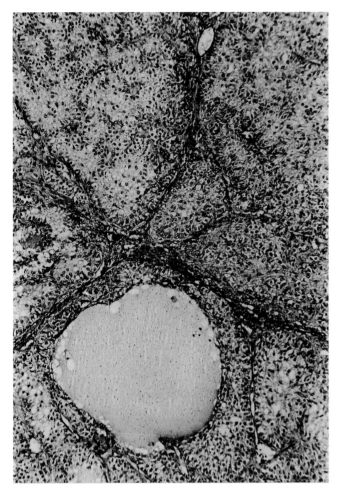

Fig. 38.11 Juvenile granulosa cell tumour. Typical lobular pattern with luteinized granulosa cells surrounding follicular spaces. H & E × 90.

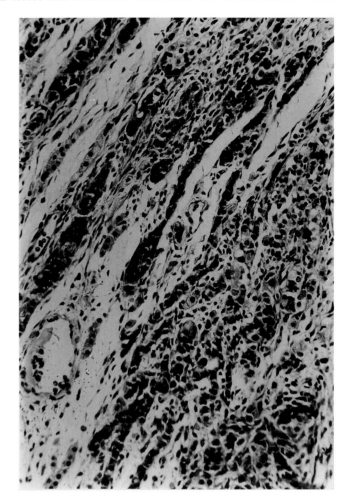

Fig. 38.12 Sertoli–Leydig cell tumour of intermediate differentiation. H & E × 225.

cell tumour, in which late recurrences occur (Young & Scully, 1982), the patients succumbing to juvenile granulosa cell tumour do so within three years of diagnosis (Young et al, 1984).

Sertoli–Leydig cell tumours

The histological and clinical features of these neoplasms are well documented (Young & Scully, 1982). Approximately half of all Sertoli–Leydig cell tumours (SLCT) (Fig. 38.12) are hormonally active with patients showing virilization, hirsutism, menstrual irregularities or occasionally oestrogenic effects (Young & Scully, 1982). Other patients present with non-specific features such as an abdominal mass (Zaloudek & Norris, 1984). These tumours do occur during the paediatric years (Young & Scully, 1985) with the exception of the well-differentiated subtype which is more commonly seen in patients aged 35 years or older. Ten to fifteen per cent of Sertoli–Leydig cell tumours contain a prominent retiform component

(Young & Scully, 1983) (Fig. 38.13). This subtype has a particular propensity to affect adolescents and young adults, with a mean age at diagnosis of 15 years, 10 years younger than the mean for Sertoli–Leydig cell tumours in general (Young & Scully, 1983). This histological variant is open to misinterpretation, particularly if it is the predominant feature in a tumour.

Prognosis depends upon stage and differentiation (Young & Scully, 1985). Overall, 12% of tumours behave in a malignant fashion and approximately 20% of those with a prominent retiform component are malignant, reflecting the fact that retiform areas are commonly associated with the less well-differentiated neoplasms (Young & Scully, 1983).

Ovarian sex cord tumour with annular tubules

This sex cord tumour has a distinctive microscopic appearance (Fig. 38.14) and up to 40% may present with symptoms of oestrogen excess (Young & Scully, 1982).

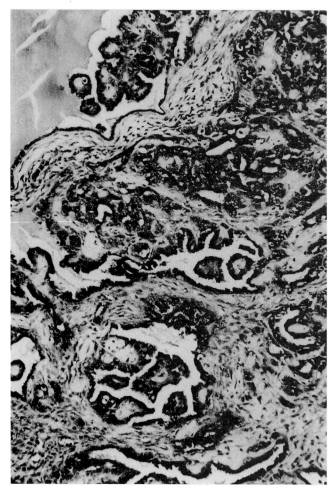

Fig. 38.13   Retiform differentiation in a Sertoli–Leydig cell tumour; blunt papillae are covered by low cuboidal epithelium. H & E × 90.

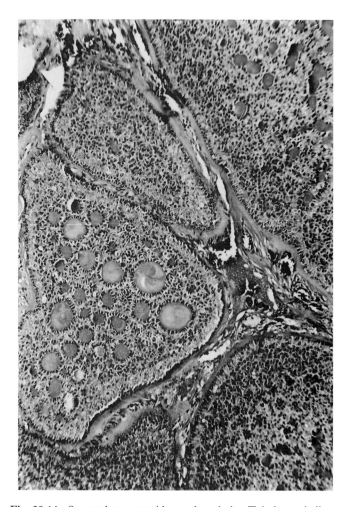

Fig. 38.14   Sex cord tumour with annular tubules. Tubules encircling nodules of hyaline material. H & E × 90.

A third of the cases are associated with the rare Peutz–Jeghers syndrome (PJS). This condition, inherited as an autosomal dominant with variable penetrance, is characterized by mucocutaneous pigmentation and hamartomas of the gastrointestinal tract. It is associated with a significantly increased risk of death from cancer at an early age (Spigelman et al, 1989). The principal sites affected are: breast, where bilateral tumours are characteristic (Trau et al, 1982); cervix, in which the well-differentiated adenocarcinoma, adenoma malignum, is the distinctive associated tumour (Young et al, 1982); and the gastro-intestinal tract, where there is evidence for a hamartoma–carcinoma sequence (Spigelman et al, 1989).

Probably all females with the syndrome have ovarian SCTAT and the tumours are characteristically small, often microscopic, multifocal, bilateral, calcified and benign (Young et al, 1982). Other, unclassified sex cord tumours may also occur in prepubertal girls with PJS (Young et al, 1983). Sertoli cell tumours have been reported in affected boys (Cantu et al, 1980).

The gene responsible remains unidentified but it appears to control growth and development of the gastrointestinal tract.

The remaining two-thirds of cases of sex cord tumour with annular tubules (SCTAT) are unassociated with PJS. Here the tumours are large and unilateral, and up to 20% are clinically malignant (Young & Scully, 1982). Rarely SCTAT has been reported in streak gonads, associated with germinoma in the same or contralateral gonad (Young et al, 1982).

Other disorders associated with sex cord-stromal tumours

Gorlin's syndrome.   The disorder is characterized by multicentric, early-appearing basal cell carcinomas (Fig. 38.15), often involving non-sun-exposed skin, odon-togenic keratocysts, pits of the palms and soles, strabismus, dysgenesis of the corpus callosum, spina bifida occulta, ectopic calcifications, hypogonadism and bifid ribs. It is inherited as an autosomal dominant disorder with variable to high penetrance. In addition to basal cell carcinomas, cerebellar medulloblastomas are also associated neo-

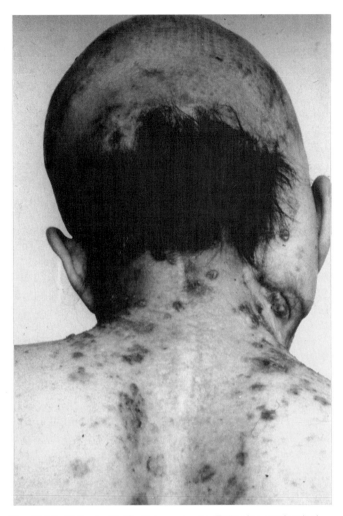

Fig. 38.15 Patient with Gorlin's syndrome. Following craniospinal irradiation for medulloblastoma, multiple basal cell carcinomas developed in the radiation field.

plasms (Kraemer et al, 1984). Female patients with the syndrome are prone to develop bilateral calcified multinodular fibromas (Young & Scully, 1982) and these tumours may form the first stigmata of the syndrome. Similar ovarian tumours have rarely been recorded in children showing no other evidence of the syndrome (Howell et al, 1990). In some cases the tumours show metaplastic stromal bone formation (Bosch-Banyeras et al, 1989). In Gorlin's syndrome, recurrences of the ovarian tumours have been recorded (Howell et al, 1990) and in one case, in which the presence of focal mitotically active areas in the tumour was in keeping with a diagnosis of low-grade fibrosarcoma, an adnexal metastasis developed two years following initial salpingo-oophorectomy (Kraemer et al, 1984).

Studies of DNA in some patients with Gorlin's syndrome have revealed loss of heterozygosity on the long arm of chromosome 9, leading to speculation that a tumour suppressor gene may be implicated (Gailani et al, 1992).

Ollier's disease.   Ollier's disease is a non-hereditary mesodermal dysplasia affecting the metaphyseal ends of long bones which predisposes to the formation of multiple enchondromas. There is often an asymmetrical hemi-skeletal distribution (Velasco-Oses et al, 1988). Maffucci's syndrome is the association of subcutaneous haemangiomas with enchondromas (Weyl-Ben & Oslander, 1991). The development of chondrosarcoma is a well-recognized complication of both disorders. Juvenile granulosa cell tumour of the ovary may also occur in both conditions (Tamimi & Bolen, 1984; Young et al, 1984; Velasco-Oses et al, 1988) and, interestingly, the ovarian tumours appear to involve the same side as the skeletal lesions (Velasco-Oses et al, 1988). There is one report of a poorly-differentiated Sertoli–Leydig cell tumour in a girl with Ollier's disease (Weyl-Ben & Oslander, 1991).

Juvenile granulosa cell tumour in dysmorphic infants.   Bilateral juvenile granulosa cell tumours have occurred in a female infant with bilateral renal agenesis and other features of the oligohydramnios sequence (Roth et al, 1979). In another case an infant, also with bilateral tumours, was the product of a consanguineous (brother-sister) pregnancy and manifested poor growth, microcephaly, facial asymmetry and a malformed left ear (Pysher et al, 1981). On the evidence of these cases, bilateral tumours appear to represent a distinct subset of this neoplasm.

Other stromal neoplasms

Less than 10% of fibrothecomas occur in patients below 30 years of age (Young & Scully, 1982). Steroid cell neoplasms, previously called lipid cell tumours, are predominantly neoplasms of the reproductive years (Scully, 1979), but cases have occurred in prepubertal girls in association with virilization (Harris et al, 1991).

The sclerosing stromal tumour is a neoplasm with a characteristic pseudolobular pattern on microscopic examination. They tend to occur in women in the third and fourth decades but have been recorded in patients under 15 years (Chalvardjian & Scully, 1973). Interestingly, bilateral tumours with this histological appearance have been reported in a pregnant adult female with Gorlin's syndrome, raising the possibility that this type of tumour and the fibroma may have a common pathogenesis (Ismail & Walker, 1990).

The ovarian myxoma is a neoplasm which mainly affects women in the reproductive years, but it has occurred in teenage patients (Eichorn & Scully, 1991).

Bilateral thecomatous ovarian neoplasms have been reported in children taking anticonvulsant therapy. Though usually benign (Faber, 1962; Schweisguth et al, 1971), at least one case of bilateral clinically and pathologically malignant thecomatous tumours has been noted in a child on anticonvulsants (Dudzinski et al, 1989).

Mixed germ cell sex cord-stromal tumours

Gonadoblastoma, described above, is the best-known neoplasm in this group. In contrast to gonadoblastoma, the other tumour types tend to occur in the normal gonads of genotypically normal individuals of both sexes; affected females are most commonly in the prepubertal years but in males the tumours are more common in adults (Talerman, 1972; Bolen, 1981). A mixed tumour which included epithelial elements in addition to germ cells and sex cord structures has been described in a female infant (Tavassoli, 1983). Mixed germ cell sex cord-stromal neoplasms are usually benign, but malignant tumours are described (Lacson et al, 1988).

Mesenchymal neoplasms

Rhabdomyosarcoma is the most common soft tissue sarcoma of childhood (Miller, 1969). Thirty to thirty five per cent are sited in the genitourinary tract or pelvic region (Clatworthy et al, 1973; Kilman et al, 1973).

Historically survival has been poor, but it has improved significantly with the implementation of combined modality therapy employing surgery, radiotherapy and chemotherapy (Pizzo & Triche, 1987). There are striking differences in outcome, however, between the two major forms of childhood rhabdomyosarcoma — embryonal and alveolar — which also show differences in their site of origin and mean age of patient at presentation. There have been several attempts to demonstrate biological differences between the tumour types, focusing on degree of differentiation (Schmidt et al, 1986) and cytogenetic abnormalities (Turc-Carel et al, 1986; Douglass et al, 1987). It has been shown that a number of alveolar rhabdomyosarcomas have a translocation involving chromosome 2 and 13, t(2;13)(q37;q14) and some embryonal rhabdomyosarcomas show a loss of heterozygosity on chromosome 11 (Scrable et al, 1989).

Rhabdomyosarcoma in the female genital tract occurs most commonly in the vagina (Hildgers et al, 1970; Davos & Abell, 1976). Grossly, most tumours originate in the anterior vaginal wall and may extend into the introitus and bladder (Fig. 38.16a,b). The Intergroup Rhabdomyosarcoma Study (IRS I–II), the results of which were published in 1988 (Hays et al, 1988), revealed that children with primary vaginal tumours were, on average, less than two years of age and histology was uniformly of embryonal type. Vulval neoplasms occurred over a wider age range (from one to 19 years) and both embryonal and alveolar patterns occurred. Uterine sarcomas involved patients in the teenage years and often, but not always, consisted of a single polyp.

In the IRS study, overall survival following a combination of surgery and chemotherapy was over 80%, though the number of patients studied was small (only 47 collected over 12 years).

The entity called sarcoma botryoides of the uterine cervix by Daya & Scully appears to be a different tumour to classical rhabdomyosarcoma. The patients are older, with a mean of 18 years, loci of cartilage are often present within the tumour and prognosis appears to be good (Daya & Scully, 1988).

Primary rhabdomyosarcoma of the ovary is rare but there are occasional case reports (Nunez et al, 1983; Aktar et al, 1989; Chan et al, 1989).

Other soft tissue tumours

Rare cases of neurofibroma of the clitoral region have been described in children with neurofibromatosis (Schepel & Tolhurst, 1981; Ravikumar & Lakshwanan, 1983; Rink & Mitchell, 1983). Malignant nerve sheath tumour of the clitoris has been reported in an infant (Thomas et al, 1989). A few examples of leiomyomas of the uterine corpus have been recorded during childhood (Huffman et al, 1981).

Aggressive angiomyxoma is a soft tissue tumour in which the bland histological appearance (Fig. 38.17) belies a tendency towards multiple local recurrences (Steeper & Rosai, 1983). Cases have been reported in the teenage years (Begin et al, 1985).

Though mixed Müllerian tumours occur almost exclusively in postmenopausal women, occasional examples have been described in children (Chumas et al, 1983; Amr et al, 1986).

Epithelial tumours

In the 36-year series from the Manchester Children's Tumour Registry there were no cases of malignant epithelial tumours at any site within the female genital tract (Table 38.1), but this is probably not unexpected in view of the upper age limit of 15 years.

Epithelial neoplasms of the ovary, both benign and malignant, are rare below 15 years of age (Norris & Jensen, 1972; La Vecchia, 1983). Occasional cases of epithelial tumours of borderline malignancy have been reported in girls under 17 years of age (Gribbon et al, 1992). In prepubertal children malignant epithelial tumours are virtually unknown, though isolated case reports do exist (Blom & Torkildsen, 1982; Akinola et al, 1988).

In the world literature there are no undisputed examples of endometrial carcinoma occurring in patients less than 15 years of age. An extensive review covering the period 1929–1976 identified five possible cases (Huffman et al, 1981) but their validity has been questioned (Lee & Scully, 1989). A recent study included ten patients under 21 years of age with complex endometrial hyperplasia or well-differentiated adenocarcinoma but there were none aged less than 15 years (Lee & Scully, 1989).

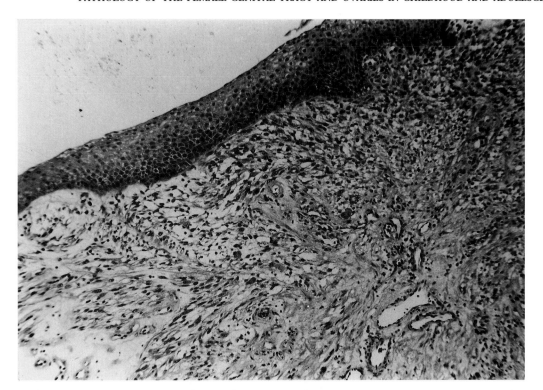

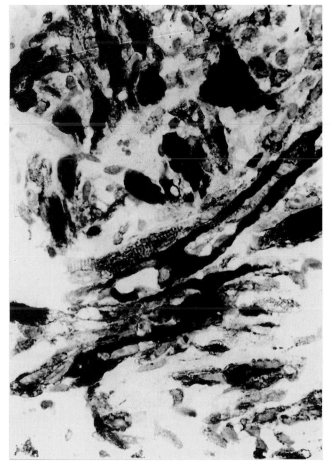

Fig. 38.16   Vaginal rhabdomyosarcoma. **a** Band of tumour cells beneath surface epithelium. H & E × 100. **b** Tumour cells showing cross striations. Immunostain for desmin × 360.

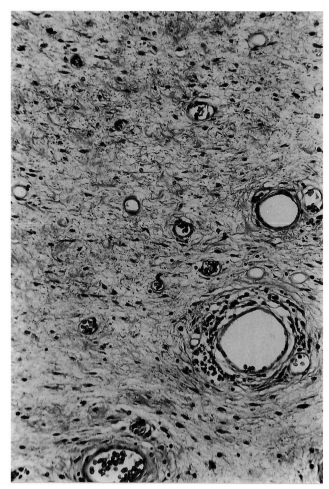

Fig. 38.17 Aggressive angiomyxoma. Prominent blood vessels within hypocellular tissue composed of spindle cells. H & E × 90. (Case supplied by Dr. M. Harris.)

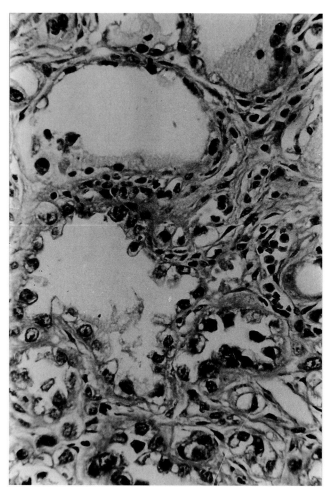

Fig. 38.18 Clear cell adenocarcinoma of the cervix. H & E × 360. (Case supplied by Dr. C. H. Buckley.)

Cervical and vaginal adenocarcinoma

Spontaneous vaginal adenocarcinoma is primarily a disease of women in the late reproductive and perimenopausal years (Herbst et al, 1970) but cases have been reported in teenage patients and infants (Drogemueller et al, 1970; Norris et al, 1970; Kaminski & Maier, 1983).

Consequences of intrauterine diethylstilboestrol (DES) exposure. DES was introduced in the late 1940s as a treatment for habitual abortion (Herbst & Anderson, 1990) and several million women received it before it was officially banned for use during pregnancy by the US Food and Drug Administration. By this time the association between intrauterine DES exposure and subsequent development of clear cell adenocarcinoma of the vagina and cervix had been recognized (Herbst et al, 1971). However, this is a very infrequent consequence of exposure; the risk is of the order of 1 in 1000 (Herbst, 1981; Herbst & Anderson, 1990). Furthermore, in the registry set up in 1971 to study the outcome, histopathology and epidemiology of clear cell adenocarcinoma

in women born after 1940, in only 60% of the cases was there definite evidence of DES exposure (Herbst & Anderson, 1990). DES-associated adenocarcinoma is predominantly a disease of the late teens and twenties, with a few cases occurring in the latter half of the first decade (Dehner, 1987; Herbst & Anderson, 1990) and some women presenting during their thirties (Herbst & Anderson, 1990). Histologically, the tumour is predominantly clear celled and is composed of cells with a characteristic 'hobnail' appearance which form papillae, cysts and tubules (Fig. 38.18).

Factors commensurate with a good prognosis are low stage, small size, predominant tubulocystic pattern and a low grade of nuclear atypia (Herbst & Anderson, 1990; Hanselaar et al, 1991). Overall, between 80% and 90% of patients survive five years (Dehner, 1987; Hanselaar et al, 1991), but most patients have low-stage disease at diagnosis. Late recurrences, up to 20 years after initial therapy, are reported and metastases seem frequently to involve the lungs and supraclavicular lymph nodes (Herbst & Anderson, 1990).

Developmental abnormalities of the cervix and vagina are far more commonly associated with maternal DES exposure. An extensive cervical ectropion is the most common finding, occurring in 95%. Though a few glands may be found in the vaginas of normal women, extensive adenosis is very rare in unexposed women, but occurs in at least one-third of young women who were exposed to DES in utero (Scully & Welch, 1981). Clear cell adenocarcinoma is often found in close apposition to vaginal adenosis (Scully & Welch, 1981). Gross anomalies of the cervix, such as cervical peaks, collars and hoods, are found in at least 20% of exposed girls (Scully & Welch, 1981; Coleman & Evans, 1988).

Squamous neoplasia of the genital tract and related lesions

Condyloma acuminata and human papillomavirus (HPV) infection. Genital warts are caused mostly by HPV types 6 and 11 and have increased in incidence in all age groups, including children, over the past two decades (Bender, 1986; Cripe, 1990). In patients aged less than 20 years the clinical incidence in females is between three and ten times that in males. In sexually active adolescent girls estimates of the incidence of genital HPV infection are between 29% and 60% (Cripe, 1990).

In prepubertal children, the infection implies the possibility of sexual abuse (Bender, 1986; Rock et al, 1986; Hanson et al, 1989; Cripe, 1990). Not surprisingly, however, in view of the controversial nature of this subject, estimates as to the proportion of cases transmitted venereally vary from virtually all (Gutman, 1990), to less than one-third of cases (Cripe, 1990). However, there are reports of congenital condylomata acuminata (Shelton et al, 1986) and in a high proportion of cases of affected infants maternal condylomata are present (Shelton et al, 1986; Cripe, 1990) so that at least some infantile lesions may be transmitted vertically or during close physical contact.

The long-term sequelae of childhood condylomata acuminata are not yet known, particularly where they involve HPV types associated with oncogenesis such as 16, which has been detected by one means or another in about 50% of all cervical carcinomas examined (Cripe, 1990).

Cervical intraepithelial neoplasia undoubtedly occurs in the mid-teenage years (Sadeghi et al, 1988) and there are a few reports of teenagers with invasive squamous carcinoma of the vulva and cervix (Cario et al, 1984; Dehner, 1987). At least one case of vulvar carcinoma in a teenager was associated with a history of anogenital warts since infancy (Bender, 1986).

Miscellaneous neoplasms

Ovarian small cell carcinoma

This neoplasm was originally described in 1982 as a tumour frequently, though not invariably, associated with

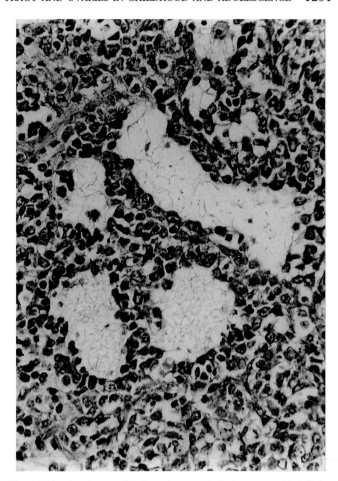

Fig. 38.19 Ovarian small cell carcinoma. Typical pattern with follicle-like spaces. H & E × 225. (Case supplied by Dr. R. Williams.)

hypercalcaemia (Dickersin et al, 1982) (Fig. 38.19). The age range is very similar to that of malignant germ cell tumours of the ovary. Published cases range in age from nine years (Malfetano et al, 1990) to 42 years with a mean of 22–23 years (Dickersin et al, 1982; Young et al, 1987). The tumour characteristically has an aggressive clinical course. In one series mortality was 88%, with most fatalities occurring in the first year. Only 12% were free of disease after four years follow-up (Young et al, 1987). Extensive intra-abdominal spread is characteristic (Dickersin et al, 1982).

The histogenesis of this tumour is unknown (Scully, 1993), but in view of the age range and histological and ultrastructural similarities to endodermal sinus tumour a poorly-differentiated germ cell neoplasm is one possibility (Ulbright et al, 1987).

Lymphoma and leukaemia

Though ovarian infiltration is present at 35–50% of autopsies performed on girls dying of acute lymphoblastic leukaemia, clinical ovarian disease is rare (Heaton & Duff, 1989; Pais et al, 1991). It can be bilateral and is most frequently seen as recurrent disease with relapse occurring some years after initial diagnosis. Treatment is with systemic chemotherapy rather than surgery (Pais et al, 1991).

Primary lymphoma of the female genital tract presenting in childhood is rare, but has been reported (Egwuata, 1989).

Non-lymphomatous, non-leukaemic metastatic ovarian tumours in childhood

These are rare, partly because the common neoplasms which spread to the ovary, such as carcinomas of breast and gastrointestinal tract, are unusual in children, but also because the ovary of the child lacks the vascularity of the adult structure. Occasional cases do occur, however, and may prove difficult diagnostically. A recent review cites examples of neuroblastoma, rhabdomyosarcoma, Ewing's sarcoma, renal rhabdoid tumour and carcinoid tumour, all of which presented initially as ovarian neoplasms and some of which were initially misdiagnosed as primary ovarian tumours (Young et al, 1993).

Müllerian papilloma

This is a benign neoplasm which occurs exclusively in children. It involves the cervix or, more rarely, the vagina. Patients are usually aged between two and five years and present with vaginal bleeding. The tumour is a small polypoid or papillary lesion involving the cervical lip or the endocervical canal. Microscopically, it consists of oedematous fibrovascular papillae, in which there may be metaplastic bone (Ulbright et al, 1981). The overlying epithelium is single-layered and varies from flat to columnar (Fig. 38.20). Some cases have recurred locally (Clement, 1990). The stroma is uniformly banal in appearance, so that the lesion is easily distinguished from embryonal rhabdomyosarcoma (Lawrence, 1991).

Other neoplasms

Extrarenal Wilms' tumours are uncommon, and appear to be least rare in the retroperitoneal site (Wakely et al, 1989) but examples have occurred adjacent to the ovary or within the female genital tract (Bell et al, 1985; Wakely

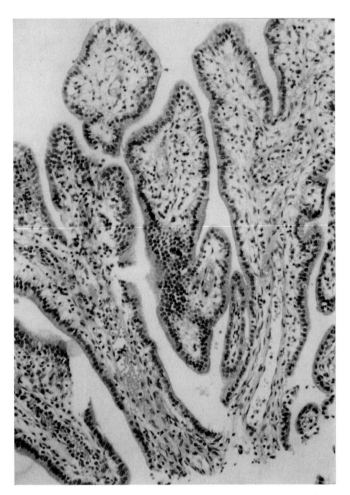

Fig. 38.20 Müllerian papilloma. Fibrovascular cores composed of bland spindle cells covered by a single layer of cuboidal epithelium. H & E × 70. (Photograph supplied by Dr. W. D. Lawrence and reproduced with kind permission from WB Saunders Company.)

et al, 1989). Cases reported in the literature have closely resembled the more common renal tumours, giving rise to the theory that they originate from heterotopic rests of renal tissue.

The vulva may be the site of several entities presenting during childhood which are not specific to this region or age group, including haemangioma (Levin & Selbst, 1988), granular cell tumour (Brooks, 1985), Langherhans cell histiocytosis (Otis et al, 1990), lymphangioma, lipoma and teratoma (Huffman et al, 1981).

REFERENCES

Aguirre P, Scully R E 1982 Malignant neuroectodermal tumor of the ovary: a distinctive form of monodermal teratoma: report of five cases. American Journal of Surgical Pathology 6: 283–292.

Akhtar M, Bakri Y, Rank F 1989 Dysgerminoma of the ovary with rhabdomyosarcoma. Cancer 64: 2309–2312.

Akinola O, Okonofua F E, Odesanmi W O, Oshinaike A I 1988 Serous papillary adenocarcinoma of the ovary in a Nigerian child. Tropical and Geographical Medicine 40: 251–253.

Amr S S, Tavassoli F A, Hassan A A, Issa A A, Madanat F F 1986 Mixed mesodermal tumor of the uterus in a 4 year old girl. International Journal of Gynecological Pathology 5: 371–378.

Armstrong G R, Buckley C H, Kelsey A M 1991 Germ cell expression of placental alkaline phosphatase in male pseudohermaphroditism. Histopathology 18: 541–547.

Atkin N B, Baker M C 1983 i(12p): specific chromosomal marker in seminoma and malignant teratoma of the testis? Cancer Genetics and Cytogenetics 10: 199–204.

Begin L R, Clement P B, Kirk M E et al 1985 Aggressive angiomyxoma of pelvic soft parts: a clinicopathologic study of nine cases. Human Pathology 16: 621–628.

Bell D A, Shimm D S, Gang D L 1985 Wilms' tumor of the endocervix. Archives of Pathology and Laboratory Medicine 109: 371–373.

Bender M E 1986 New concepts of condyloma acuminata in children. Archives of Dermatology 122: 1121–1124.

Berta P, Hawkins J R, Sinclair A H et al 1990 Genetic evidence equating SRY and the testis-determining factor. Nature 348: 448–450.

Biedel C W, Pagon R A, Zapata J O 1984 Müllerian anomalies and renal agenesis: autosomal dominant urogenital adysplasia. Journal of Pediatrics 104: 861–864.

Birch J M 1988 Manchester Children's Tumour Registry 1954–1970 and 1971–1983. In: Parkin D M, Stiller C A, Draper G J, Bieber C A, Terracini B, Young J L (eds) International agency for incidence of childhood cancer. International Agency for Research on Cancer Publications, no 87, Lyon, pp 299–304.

Birch J M 1990 Epidemiology of childhood cancer. Annales Nestlé 3 (Childhood oncology), Nestec Ltd, Vevey, Switzerland, pp 105–116.

Birch J M, Marsden H B, Swindell R 1982 Pre-natal factors in the origin of germ cell tumours of children. Carcinogenesis 3: 75–80.

Biscotti C V, Hart W R 1989 Juvenile granulosa cell tumors of the ovary. Archives of Pathology and Laboratory Medicine 113: 40–46.

Björkholm E, Lundell M, Gyftodimas A, Silfverswärd C 1990 Dysgerminoma: the Radiumhemmet series 1927–1984. Cancer 65: 38–44.

Blom G P, Torkildsen E M 1982 Ovarian cystadenocarcinoma in a 4-year-old girl: report of a case and review of the literature. Gynecologic Oncology 13: 242–246.

Blyth B, Duckett J W 1991 Gonadal differentiation: a review of the physiological process and influencing factors based on recent experimental evidence. Journal of Urology 145: 689–694.

Bolen J W 1981 Mixed germ cell-sex cord-stromal tumor: a gonadal tumor distinct from gonadoblastoma. American Journal of Clinical Pathology 75: 565–573.

Bosch-Banyeras J M, Lucaya X, Bernet M et al 1989 Calcified ovarian fibromas in prepubertal girls. European Journal of Pediatrics 148: 749–750.

Breen J L, Maxson W S 1977 Ovarian tumors in children and adolescents. Clinical Obstetrics and Gynecology 20: 607–623.

Brooks G G 1985 Granular cell myoblastoma of the vulva in a 6-year-old girl. American Journal of Obstetrics and Gynecology 153: 897–898.

Brown N J, Langley F A 1976 Teratomas and other genital tumours. In: Marsden H B, Steward J K (eds) Tumours in children. Springer-Verlag, Berlin, pp 362–402.

Cantu J M, Rivera H, Ocampo-Campos R et al 1980 Peutz-Jeghers syndrome with feminizing Sertoli cell tumor. Cancer 46: 223–228.

Cario G M, House M J, Paradinas F J 1984 Squamous cell carcinoma of the vulva in association with mixed vulval dystrophy in an 18-year-old girl. British Journal of Obstetrics and Gynaecology 91: 87–90.

Carter D, Bibro M C, Touloukin R J 1982 Benign clinical behaviour of immature mediastinal teratoma in infancy and childhood: report of two cases and review of the literature. Cancer 49: 398–402.

Chalvardjian A, Scully R E 1973 Sclerosing stromal tumors of the ovary. Cancer 31: 664–670.

Chan Y F, Leung C S, Ma L 1989 Primary embryonal rhabdomyosarcoma of the ovary in a 4-year-old girl. Histopathology 15: 309–311.

Chumas J C, Mann W J, Tseng L 1983 Malignant mixed Müllerian tumor of the endometrium in a young woman with polycystic ovaries. Cancer 52: 1478–1481.

Clatworthy H W, Braden M, Smith J P 1973 Surgery of bladder and prostatic neoplasms in children. Cancer 32: 1157–1160.

Clement P B 1990 Miscellaneous primary and metastatic tumors of the uterine cervix. Seminars in Diagnostic Pathology 7: 228–247.

Clement P B, Young R H 1993 Pathology of extragonadal yolk sac tumors. In: Nogales F F (ed) The human yolk sac and yolk sac tumors. Springer, Berlin, pp 295–308.

Coleman D V, Evans D M D 1988 Biopsy pathology and cytology of the cervix. Chapman & Hall Medical, London, pp 181–188.

Cooper C, Crolla J A, Laister C, Johnson D I, Cooke P 1991 An investigation of ring and dicentric chromosomes found in three Turner's syndrome patients using DNA analysis and in situ hybridisation with X and Y chromosome specific probes. Journal of Medical Genetics 28: 6–9.

Cripe T P 1990 Human papillomaviruses: pediatric perspectives on a family of multifaceted tumorigenic pathogens. Pediatric Infectious Disease Journal 9: 836–844.

Dahl N, Gustav K-H, Rune C, Gustavsson I, Pettersson U 1990 Benign ovarian teratomas: an analysis of their cellular origin. Cancer Genetics and Cytogenetics 46: 115–123.

Dal Cin P, Van Den Berghe H 1991 Isochromosome (12p) in germ cell tumors. In: Oosterhuis J W, Walt H, Damjanov I (eds) Pathobiology of germ cell neoplasia. Springer-Verlag, Berlin, pp 105–111.

Danon M, Robboy S J, Kim S, Scully R, Crawford J D 1975 Cushing syndrome, sexual precosity and polyostotic fibrous dysplasia (Albright syndrome) in infancy. Journal of Pediatrics 87: 917–921.

Davidoff F, Federman D D 1973 Mixed gonadal dysgenesis. Pediatrics 52: 725–742.

Davos I, Abell M R 1976 Sarcomas of the vagina. Obstetrics and Gynecology 47: 342–350.

Daya D A, Scully R E 1988 Sarcoma botryoides of the uterine cervix in young women: a clinicopathological study of 13 cases. Gynecologic Oncology 29: 290–304.

Dehner L P 1983 Gonadal and extragonadal germ cell neoplasia of childhood. Human Pathology 14: 493–511.

Dehner L P 1987 Female reproductive system. In: Dehner L P (ed) Pediatric surgical pathology. Williams & Wilkins, Baltimore, pp 743–791.

DeSa D J 1991 The alimentary tract. In: Wigglesworth J S, Singer D B (eds) Textbook of fetal and perinatal pathology. Blackwell Scientific Publications, Boston, pp 903–979.

Dickersin G R, Kline I W, Scully R E 1982 Small cell carcinoma of the ovary with hypercalcemia: a report of 11 cases. Cancer 49: 188–197.

Douglass E C, Valentine M, Etcubanas E et al 1987 A specific abnormality in rhabdomyosarcoma. Cytogenetics and Cell Genetics 45: 148–155.

Drogemueller W, Makowski E L, Taylor E S 1970 Vaginal mesonephric adenocarcinoma in two prepubertal children. American Journal of Diseases of Children 119: 168–170.

Dudzinski M, Cohen M, Ducatman B 1989 Ovarian malignant luteinized thecoma — an unusual tumor in an adolescent. Gynecologic Oncology 35: 104–109.

Duncan P A, Shapiro L R, Stangel J J, Klein R M, Addonizio 1979 The MURCS association: Müllerian duct aplasia, renal aplasia and cervicothoracic somite dysplasia. Journal of Pediatrics 95: 399–402.

Egwuata V E 1989 Non-Hodgkin's lymphoma of the uterus in a child. Journal of Pediatric Surgery 24: 220–222.

Eichorn J H, Scully R E 1991 Ovarian myxoma: clinicopathologic and immunocytologic analysis of five cases and a review of the literature. International Journal of Gynecological Pathology 10: 156–169.

Faber H K 1962 Meig's syndrome with thecomas of both ovaries in a 4 year old girl. Journal of Pediatrics 61: 769–773.

Flam F, Lundstrom V, Silfersward C 1989 Choriocarcinoma in mother and child: case report. British Journal of Obstetrics and Gynaecology 96: 241–244.

French F S, Lubahn D B, Brown T R et al 1990 Molecular basis of androgen insensitivity. Recent Progress in Hormone Research 46: 1–42.

Gailani M R, Bale S J, Leffell D J et al 1992 Developmental defects in Gorlin syndrome related to a putative tumour suppressor gene on chromosome 9. Cell 69: 111–117.

Gershenson D M, Del Junco G, Herson J, Rutledge F N 1983 Endodermal sinus tumor of the ovary: the M D Anderson experience. Obstetrics and Gynecology 61: 194–202.

Geurts van Kessel A, Suijkerbuijk R, de Jong B, Oosterhuis J W 1991 Molecular analysis of isochromosome 12p in testicular germ cell tumors. In: Oosterhuis J W, Walt H, Damjanov I (eds) Pathobiology of germ cell neoplasia. Springer-Verlag, Berlin, pp 105–111.

Gilbert-Barnes E F, Opitz J M 1991a Congenital anomalies — malformation syndromes. In: Wigglesworth J S, Singer D B (eds) Textbook of fetal and perinatal pathology. Blackwell Scientific Publications, Boston, pp 381–427.

Gilbert-Barnes E F, Opitz J M 1991b Chromosomal abnormalities. In: Wigglesworth J S, Singer D B (eds) Textbook of fetal and perinatal pathology. Blackwell Scientific Publications, Boston, pp 339–379.

Greenberg F, Keenan B, DeYanis V, Finegold M 1986 Gonadal dysgenesis and gonadoblastoma in situ in a female with Fraser (cryptophthalmos) syndrome. Journal of Pediatrics 108: 952–954.

Gribbon M, Ein S H, Mancer K 1992 Pediatric malignant ovarian tumors: a 43-year review. Journal of Pediatric Surgery 27: 480–484.

Gubbay A, Collignon J, Koopman P et al 1990 A gene mapping to the sex determining region of the mouse Y chromosome is a member of a novel family of embryonically expressed genes. Nature 346: 345–350.

Gutman L T 1990 Sexual abuse and human papilloma virus infection. Journal of Pediatrics 116: 495–496.

Hanselaar A G J M, Van Leusen N D M, De Wilde P C M, Vooijs G P 1991 Clear cell adenocarcinoma of the vagina and cervix: a report of the central Netherlands with emphasis on early detection and prognosis. Cancer 67: 1971–1978.

Hanson R M, Glasson M, McCrssin I, Rogers M 1989 Anogenital warts in childhood. Child Abuse and Neglect 13: 225–233.

Harris A C, Wakely P E, Kaplowitz P B, Loringer R D 1991 Steroid cell tumor of the ovary in a child. Archives of Pathology and Laboratory Medicine 115: 150–154.

Hartley A L, Birch J M, Kelsey A M, Marsden H B, Harris M, Teare M D 1989 Are germ cell tumors part of the Li-Fraumeni Cancer Family syndrome? Cancer Genetics and Cytogenetics 42: 221–226.

Hays D M, Shimada H, Raney R B et al 1988 Clinical staging and treatment results in rhabdomyosarcoma of the female genital tract among children and adolescents. Cancer 61: 1893–1903.

Heaton D C, Duff G B 1989 Ovarian relapse in a young woman with acute lymphoblastic leukemia. American Journal of Hematology 30: 42–43.

Herbst A L 1981 Clear cell adenocarcinoma and current status of DES exposed females. Cancer 48: 484–488.

Herbst A L, Anderson D 1990 Clear cell adenocarcinoma of the vagina and cervix secondary to intrauterine exposure to stilbestrol. Seminars in Surgical Oncology 6: 343–346.

Herbst A L, Green T H, Ulfelder R H 1970 Primary carcinoma of the vagina: an analysis of 68 cases. American Journal of Obstetrics and Gynecology 106: 210–218.

Herbst A L, Ulfelder R H, Poskanzer D C 1971 Adenocarcinoma of the vagina: association of maternal stilbestrol therapy with tumor appearance in young women. New England Journal of Medicine 284: 878–881.

Hilgers R D, Malkasian G D, Soule E D 1970 Embryonal rhabdomyosarcoma (botryoid type) of the vagina: a clinicopathological review. American Journal of Obstetrics and Gynecology 107: 484–502.

Howell C G, Rogers D A, Gable D S, Falls G D 1990 Bilateral ovarian fibromas in children. Journal of Pediatric Surgery 25: 690–691.

Huffman J W, Dewhurst J C, Copraro V J 1981 The gynecology of childhood and adolescence, 2nd edn. WB Saunders, Philadelphia, pp 270–272.

Ismail S M, Walker S M 1990 Bilateral virilizing sclerosing stromal tumours of the ovary in a pregnant woman with Gorlin's syndrome: implications for pathogenesis of ovarian stromal neoplasms. Histopathology 17: 159–163.

Kaminski P F, Maier R C 1983 Clear cell adenocarcinoma of cervix unrelated to diethylstilbestrol exposure. Obstetrics and Gynecology 62: 720–727.

Kilman J W, Clatworthy H W, Newton W A, Grosfield J L 1973 Reasonable surgery for rhabdomyosarcoma. Annals of Surgery 178: 346–351.

Kohorn E I, McIntosh S, Lytton B, Knowlton A H, Merino M 1985 Endodermal sinus tumor of the infant vagina. Gynecologic Oncology 20: 196–203.

Kraemer B B, Silva E G, Sneige N 1984 Fibrosarcoma of ovary: a new component in the nevoid basal-cell carcinoma syndrome. American Journal of Surgical Pathology 8: 231–236.

Kurman R J, Norris H J 1976a Endodermal sinus tumor of the ovary: a clinical and pathological analysis of 71 cases. Cancer 38: 2402–2419.

Kurman R J, Norris H J 1976b Embryonal carcinoma of the ovary: a clinicopathological entity distinct from endodermal sinus tumor resembling embryonal carcinoma of the adult testis. Cancer 38: 2420–2433.

Kurman R J, Norris H J 1977 Malignant germ cell tumors of the ovary. Human Pathology 8: 551–562.

Lack E E, Perez-Atayde A R, Murthy A S K, Goldstein D P, Crigler J F, Vawter G F 1981 Granulosa theca cell tumors in premenarchal girls: a clinical and pathological study of 10 cases. Cancer 48: 1846–1854.

Lacson A G, Gillis D A, Shawwa A 1988 Malignant mixed germ cell-sex cord-stromal tumors of the ovary associated with isosexual precocious puberty. Cancer 61: 2122–2133.

Lauchlan S C 1991 The reproductive system. In: Wigglesworth J S, Singer D B (eds) Text book of fetal and perinatal pathology. Blackwell Scientific Publications, Boston, pp 1145–1170.

La Vecchia C, Morris H B, Draper G J 1983 Malignant ovarian tumours in childhood in Britain, 1962–78. British Journal of Cancer 48: 363–374.

Lawrence W D 1991 Advances in the pathology of the uterine cervix. Human Pathology 22: 792–806.

Lee K R, Scully R E 1989 Complex endometrial hyperplasia and carcinoma in adolescents and young women 15–20 years of age. International Journal of Gynecological Pathology 8: 201–213.

Levin A V, Selbst S M 1988 Vulvar hemangioma simulating child abuse. Clinical Pediatrics 27: 213–215.

Li F P, Fraumeni J F 1969 Soft tissue sarcomas, breast cancer and other neoplasms. Annals of Internal Medicine 71: 747–752.

Machin G A 1991 The causes of malformations. In: Wigglesworth J S, Singer D B (eds) Textbook of fetal and perinatal pathology. Blackwell Scientific Publications, Boston, pp 307–338.

Malfetano J H, Degnan E, Florentin R 1990 Para-endocrine hypercalcemia and ovarian small cell carcinoma. New York State Journal of Medicine 90: 206–207.

Malkin D, Li F P, Strong L C et al 1990 Germline p53 mutations in a familial syndrome of breast cancer, sarcomas, and other neoplasms. Science 250: 1233–1238.

Malogolowkin M H, Mahour G H, Krailo M, Ortega J A 1990 Germ cell tumors in infancy and childhood: a 45 year experience. In: Jaffe R, Dahms B B, Krous H F, Lieberman E, Triche T J (eds) Forefront of pediatric pathology. Hemisphere Publishing Corporation, New York, pp 231–241.

Mandell J, Stevens P S, Fried F A 1977 Childhood gonadoblastoma and seminoma in a dysgenetic cryptorchid gonad. Journal of Urology 117: 674–675.

Mann J R, Pearson D, Barrett A, Raafat F, Barnes J M, Wallendszus K R 1989 Results of the United Kingdom Children's Cancer Study Group's malignant germ cell tumor studies. Cancer 63: 1657–1667.

Marsden H B, Birch J M, Swindell R 1981 Germ cell tumours of childhood: A review of 137 cases. Journal of Clinical Pathology 34: 879–883.

Miller R W 1969 Fifty-two forms of childhood cancer: United States mortality experience 1960–1966. Journal of Pediatrics 75: 685–689.

Mitchell M F, Gershenson D M, Soeters R P, Eifel P J, Delclos L, Wharton J T 1991 The long-term effects of radiotherapy on patients with ovarian dysgerminoma. Cancer 67: 1084–1090.

Mordehai J, Mares A J, Barki R, Finaly R, Meizner I 1991 Torsion of uterine adnexa in neonates and children: a report of 20 cases. Journal of Pediatric Surgery 26: 1195–1199.

Müller J, Skakkebaek N E 1984 Testicular carcinoma in situ in children with the androgen insensitivity syndrome. British Medical Journal 288: 1419–1420.

Müller J, Skakkebaek N E, Ritzen M, Plöen L, Petersen K E 1985 Carcinoma in situ of the testis in children with 45X/46XY gonadal dysgenesis. Journal of Pediatrics 106: 431–436.

Nogales F F, Favara B E, Major F J, Silverberg S G 1976 Immature teratoma of the ovary with a neural component ('solid' teratoma): a clinicopathologic study of 20 cases. Human Pathology 7: 625–642.

Norris H J, Jensen R D 1972 Relative frequency of ovarian neoplasms in children and adolescents. Cancer 30: 713–719.

Norris H J, Bagley G P, Taylor H B 1970 Carcinoma of the infant vagina: a distinctive tumor. Archives of Pathology 90: 473–479.

Norris H J, Zirkin H J, Benson W L 1976 Immature (malignant) teratoma of the ovary: a clinical and pathological study of 58 cases. Cancer 37: 2359–2372.

Nunez C, Abboud S L, Lemon N C, Kemp J A 1983 Ovarian rhabdomyosarcoma presenting as leukemia. Cancer 52: 297–300.

O'Dowd J, Gaffney E F, Young R H 1990 Malignant sex cord-stromal tumour in a patient with the androgen insensitivity syndrome. Histopathology 16: 279–282.

Olsen M M, Caldamone A A, Jackson C L, Zinn A 1988 Gonadoblastoma in infancy: indications for early gonadectomy in 46,XY gonadal dysgenesis. Journal of Pediatric Surgery 23: 270–271.

Otis C N, Fischer R A, Johnson N, Kelleher J F, Powell J L 1990 Histiocytosis X of the vulva: a case report and review of the literature. Obstetrics and Gynecology 75: 555–558.

Pais R C, Kim T H, Zwiren G T, Ragab A H 1991 Ovarian tumors in relapsing acute lymphoblastic leukemia: a review of 23 cases. Journal of Pediatric Surgery 26: 70–74.

Parkin D M, Stiller C A, Draper G J, Bieber C A, Terracini B, Young J L 1988 International incidence of childhood cancer. International Agency for Research on Cancer Publications, no 87, Lyon.

Pizzo P A, Triche T J 1987 Clinical staging in rhabdomyosarcoma: current limitations and future prospects. Journal of Clinical Oncology 5: 8–9.

Pysher T J, Hitch D C, Krous H F 1981 Bilateral juvenile granulosa cell tumors in a 4-month-old dysmorphic infant: a clinical, histologic and ultrastructural study. American Journal of Surgical Pathology 5: 789–794.

Ravikumar V R, Lakshanan D 1983 Solitary neurofibroma of the clitoris masquerading as intersex. Journal of Pediatric Surgery 18: 617.

Resnik E, Christopherson W A, Stock R 1989 Clear cell adenocarcinoma of the cervix and vagina in a woman with mixed gonadal dysgenesis: a case report. Journal of Reproductive Medicine 34: 981–984.

Rink R C, Mitchell M E 1983 Genitourinary neurofibromatosis in childhood. Journal of Urology 130: 1176–1179.

Risdon R A 1987 The urogenital system. In: Keeling J W (ed) Fetal and neonatal pathology. Springer-Verlag, London, pp 407–428.

Rock B, Naghashfar Z, Barnett N, Buscema J, Woodruff J D, Shah K 1986 Genital tract papillomavirus infection in children. Archives of Dermatology 122: 1129–1132.

Roth L M, Nicholas T R, Ehrlich C E 1979 Juvenile granulosa cell tumor: a clinicopathologic study of three cases with ultrastructural observations. Cancer 44: 2194–2205.

Rutgers J L, Scully R E 1987 Pathology of the testis in intersex syndromes. Seminars in Diagnostic Pathology 4: 275–291.

Sadeghi S B, Sadeghi A, Cosby M, Olincy A, Robboy S J 1988 Human papillomavirus infection: frequency and association with cervical neoplasia in a young population. Acta Cytologica 33: 319–323.

Schepel S J, Tolhurst D E 1981 Neurofibroma of clitoris and labium majus simulating a penis and testicle. British Journal of Plastic Surgery 34: 221–223.

Schmidt D, Reimann O, Treuner J, Harms D 1986 Cellular differentiation and prognosis in embryonal rhabdomyosarcoma. Virchow's Archiv 409: 183–194.

Schweisguth O, Gerard-Marchant R, Plainfosse B, Lemerle J, Watchi J M, Seringe P 1971 Bilateral non-functioning thecoma of the ovary in epileptic children under anticonvulsant therapy. Acta Paediatrica Scandinavica 60: 6–10.

Schwöbel M G, Stauffer U G 1991 Surgical treatment of ovarian tumors in childhood. Progress in Pediatric Surgery 26: 112–123.

Scrable H, Witte D, Shimada H et al 1989 Molecular differential pathology of rhabdomyosarcoma. Genes, Chromosomes and Cancer 1: 23–35.

Scully R E 1970 Gonadoblastoma; a review of 74 cases. Cancer 25: 1340–1356.

Scully R E 1979 Tumors of the ovary and maldeveloped gonads. Atlas of tumor pathology, fascicle 16. Armed Forces Institute of Pathology, Washington, DC.

Scully R E 1991 Gonadal pathology of genetically determined disease. In: Kraus F T, Damjanov I, Kaufman N (eds) Pathology of reproductive failure. Williams & Wilkins, Baltimore, pp 257–285.

Scully R E 1993 Small cell carcinoma of hypercalcemic type. International Journal of Gynecological Pathology 12: 148–152.

Scully R E, Welch W R 1981 Pathology of the female genital tract after prenatal exposure to diethylstilbestrol. In: Herbst A L, Bern H A (eds) Developmental effects of diethylstilbestrol (DES) in pregnancy. Thieme-Stratton, New York, pp 26–45.

Senturia Y D 1987 The epidemiology of testicular cancer. British Journal of Urology 60: 285–291.

Seruca R, David L, Holm R et al 1992 p53 mutations in gastric carcinomas. British Journal of Cancer 65: 708–710.

Shelton T B, Jerkins G R, Noe H N 1986 Condylomata acuminata in the pediatric patient. Journal of Urology 135: 548–549.

Sinclair A H, Berta P, Palmer M S et al 1990 A gene for the human sex determining region encodes a protein with homology to a conserved DNA binding motif. Nature 346: 240–244.

Spigelman A D, Muriday V, Philips R K S 1989 Cancer and the Peutz-Jeghers syndrome. Gut 30: 1588–1590.

Sivastava S, Zou Z, Pirollo K, Blattner W, Chang E H 1990 Germline transmission of a mutated p53 gene in a cancer prone family with Li-Fraumeni syndrome. Nature 348: 747–749.

Steeper T A, Rosai J 1983 Aggressive angiomyxoma of the female pelvis and perineum: report of nine cases of a distinctive type of gynecologic soft-tissue neoplasm. American Journal of Surgical Pathology 7: 463–475.

Talerman A A 1972 A mixed germ cell-sex cord tumor of the ovary in a normal female infant. Obstetrics and Gynecology 40: 473–478.

Talerman A, Verp M S, Senekjian E, Gilewski T, Vogelzang N 1990 True hermaphrodite with bilateral ovotestes, bilateral gonadoblastomas and dysgerminomas, 46,XX/46,XY karyotype and a successful pregnancy. Cancer 66: 2668–2672.

Tamimi H K, Bolen J W 1984 Enchondromatosis (Ollier's disease) and ovarian juvenile granulosa cell tumor: a case report and review of the literature. Cancer 53: 1605–1608.

Tavassoli F A 1983 A combined germ cell-gonadal stromal-epithelial tumor of the ovary. American Journal of Surgical Pathology 7: 73–84.

Taylor M H, DePetrillo A D, Turner A R 1985 Vinblastine, bleomycin and cisplatin in malignant germ cell tumors of the ovary. Cancer 56: 1341–1349.

Thomas W J, Bevan H E, Hooper D G, Downey E J 1989 Malignant schwannoma of the clitoris in a 1-year-old child. Cancer 63: 2216–2219.

Thurlbeck W M, Scully R E 1960 Solid teratoma of the ovary: a clinicopathological analysis of 9 cases. Cancer 13: 804–811.

Toguchida J, Yamaguchi T, Dayton S R et al 1992 Prevalence and spectrum of germline p53 gene mutations among patients with sarcoma. New England Journal of Medicine 326: 1301–1308.

Trau H, Schewach-Millet M, Fisher B K, Tsur H 1982 Peutz-Jeghers Syndrome and bilateral breast carcinoma. Cancer 50: 788–792.

Truong L D, Jurco S, McGavran M H 1982 Gliomatosis peritonei: report of two cases and review of the literature. American Journal of Surgical Pathology 6: 443–449.

Turc-Carel C, Lizard-Nacol S, Justrabo E et al 1986 Consistent chromosomal translocation in alveolar rhabdomyosarcoma. Cancer Genetics and Cytogenetics 19: 361–362.

Ulbright T M, Alexander R W, Kraus F T 1981 Intramural papilloma of the vagina: evidence of Müllerian histogenesis. Cancer 48: 2260–2266.

Ulbright T M, Roth L M, Stehman F B, Talerman A, Senekjian E K 1987 Poorly differentiated (small cell) carcinoma of the ovary in young women: evidence supporting a germ cell origin. Human Pathology 18: 175–184.

Velasco-Oses A, Alanso-Alvaro A, Blanco-Pozo A, Nogales F F 1988 Ollier's disease associated with ovarian juvenile granulosa cell tumor. Cancer 62: 222–225.

Wakely P E, Sprague R I, Kornstein M J 1989 Extrarenal Wilms' tumor: an analysis of four cases. Human Pathology 20: 691–695.

Walker A H, Ross R K, Pike M C, Henderson B E 1984 A possible rising incidence of malignant germ cell tumours in young women. British Journal of Cancer 49: 669–672.

Walker A H, Ross R K, Haile R W C, Henderson B E 1988 Hormonal factors and risk of ovarian germ cell cancer in young women. British Journal of Cancer 57: 418–422.

Wallace T M, Levin H S 1990 Mixed gonadal dysgenesis: a review of

15 patients reporting single cases of malignant intratubular germ cell neoplasia of the testis, endometrial adenocarcinoma and a complex vascular anomaly. Archives of Pathology and Laboratory Medicine 114: 679–688.

Weinblatt M, Kochen J 1991 An unusual family cancer syndrome manifested in young siblings. Cancer 68: 1068–1070.

Weyl-Ben M, Oslander L 1991 Ollier's disease associated with ovarian Sertoli-Leydig cell tumor and breast adenoma. American Journal of Pediatric Hematology/Oncology 13: 49–51.

Wu P O, Huang R L, Lang J H et al 1991 Treatment of malignant ovarian germ cell tumors with preservation of fertility: a report of 28 cases. Gynecologic Oncology 40: 2–6.

Young R H, Scully R E 1982 Ovarian sex cord-stromal tumors: recent progress. International Journal of Gynecological Pathology 1: 101–123.

Young R H, Scully R E 1983 Sertoli-Leydig tumors with a retiform pattern: a problem in histopathologic diagnosis. American Journal of Surgical Pathology 7: 755–771.

Young R H, Scully R E 1984 Fibromatosis and massive edema of the ovary; possibly related entities: a report of 14 cases of fibromatosis and 11 cases of massive edema. International Journal of Gynecological Pathology 3: 153–178.

Young R H, Scully R E 1985 Ovarian Sertoli-Leydig cell tumors: a clinicopathologic study of 207 cases. American Journal of Surgical Pathology 9: 543–569.

Young R H, Welch W R, Dickerson G R, Scully R E 1982 Ovarian sex cord tumor with annular tubules: review of 74 cases including 27 with Peutz-Jeghers syndrome and four with adenoma malignum of the cervix. Cancer 50: 1384–1402.

Young R H, Dickersin G R, Scully R E 1983 A distinctive ovarian sex cord-stromal tumor causing sexual precocity in the Peutz-Jeghers syndrome. American Journal of Surgical Pathology 7: 233–243.

Young R H, Dickersin G R, Scully R E 1984 Juvenile granulosa cell tumor of the ovary: a clinicopathological analysis of 125 cases. American Journal of Surgical Pathology 8: 575–596.

Young R H, Lawrence W D, Scully R E 1985 Juvenile granulosa cell tumor — another neoplasm associated with abnormal chromosomes and ambiguous genitalia: a report of three cases. American Journal of Surgical Pathology 10: 737–743.

Young R H, Dickersin G R, Scully R E 1987 Small cell carcinoma: an analysis of 75 cases of a distinctive ovarian tumor commonly associated with hypercalcemia. Laboratory Investigation 56: 89A.

Young R H, Kozakewich H P W, Scully R E 1993 Metastatic ovarian tumors in children: a report of 14 cases and review of the literature. International Journal of Gynecological Pathology 12: 8–19.

Zaloudek C, Norris H J 1984 Sertoli-Leydig tumors of the ovary: a clinicopathological study of 64 intermediate and poorly differentiated neoplasms. American Journal of Surgical Pathology 8: 405–418.

39. Interrelationships of non-gynaecological and gynaecological disease

C. Hilary Buckley

INTRODUCTION

It is important in specialized texts such as this, not to overlook the impact which systemic disease may have on the practice of gynaecology, and to see gynaecological disorders in their wider context. The gynaecologist or gynaecological pathologist may encounter systemic disease in a variety of guises and should also be aware of the systemic impact of gynaecological disease.

The relationship between gynaecological practice and non-gynaecological disease has many facets. There are congenital and acquired biochemical and haematological conditions which may affect case management, systemic or local non-gynaecological abnormalities which may present as gynaecological problems or affect the genital tract fortuitously, non-gynaecological disease which may affect the morphology and function of the genital tract and, finally, gynaecological disorders which may have local or systemic non-gynaecological complications.

NON-GYNAECOLOGICAL CONDITIONS PRESENTING AS A GYNAECOLOGICAL PROBLEM OR ASSOCIATED WITH GYNAECOLOGICAL DISORDERS

In some instances a patient with a non-gynaecological disease may present with symptoms referable to the genital tract, or histopathological examination of biopsy or surgical resection material from the female genital tract may reveal a systemic disorder.

Achlorhydria

Some patients with achlorhydria are found to have a vulvar dermatosis (Jeffcoate, 1962) and a possible causal relationship between the two has been postulated (Lavery, 1984).

Amyloidosis

Systemic amyloid has, rarely, presented as a vulvar nodule (Taylor et al, 1991).

Ataxia-telangiectasia

Ataxia-telangiectasia is an autosomal recessive inherited disorder characterized by immunodeficiency, progressive cerebellar ataxia and cutaneous telangiectases. Malignant neoplasms develop in 10–15% of patients (Gatti & Good, 1971) and in a small proportion the tumour is a dysgerminoma of the ovary (Goldsmith & Hart, 1975; Narita & Takagi, 1984), which may be bilateral (Dunn et al, 1964). Gonadoblastoma (Goldsmith & Hart, 1975) and yolk sac tumour of the ovary have also been described (Pecorelli et al, 1988). Care should be taken in interpreting a raised alphafetoprotein in these latter patients as it may also be raised as a consequence of chronic hepatitis, vascular abnormalities and an embryonic thymus.

Neoplasms are not limited to the ovary, for uterine leiomyoma, smooth muscle tumour of uncertain malignancy and leiomyosarcoma have also been recorded (Gatti et al, 1989).

Cowden's disease

Cowden's disease (multiple hamartoma syndrome) is a rare autosomal dominant condition first described by Lloyd & Dennis (1963). It is characterized by the presence of facial trichilemmomas, acral keratoses, cutaneous horns, oral mucosal papillomas, colorectal polyposis, thyroid tumours, diffuse nodular goitre, lipomas, punctate keratoses on palms and soles and angiomas: in some patients malignant changes have been reported in the hamartomatous lesions (Carlson et al, 1984; Starink, 1984). Breast lesions, including carcinoma and fibrocystic disease, are reported in 76% of female patients (Starink, 1984).

In addition, endometrial and ovarian carcinoma has been described at a somewhat earlier age than would usually be expected, in a 35-year-old woman (Carlson et al, 1984). Carcinoma of the cervix has also been recorded. A further series of gynaecological neoplasms and developmental cysts have also been reported in patients with this condition: they include benign ovarian cysts of unspecified type (Walton et al, 1986), serous cystadenoma of the ovary, immature ovarian teratoma, uterine leiomyomas, Gartner's cyst of the vagina, apocrine hydrocytoma of the vulva, sebaceous cyst of the vulva and urethral polyps (Starink, 1984; Grattan & Hamburger, 1987; Neumann, 1991). In some instances the association could be fortuitous but some of these lesions may represent further potential problems for these patients.

Cytogenetic disorders

Cytogenetic disorders affecting the sex chromosomes (Ch. 40) may be manifest as gynaecological disorders but more commonly it is their systemic features which are first identified, although, as for example in ovarian dysgenesis, some of those systemic abnormalities such as the failure of secondary sexual characteristics are secondary to the failure of ovarian development and are not primary components of the disorder. There is, however, an association between Hashimoto's thyroiditis and Turner's syndrome and a case has been reported in which there was, in addition, sarcoidosis (Tsuji et al, 1992).

Dermatological disorders

Dermatological diseases that affect the vulva are described in detail in Chapter 3 but it is important to recognize that gynaecological problems may be the first indication that the patient has a systemic dermatological problem and that the presentation may not be typical of that seen elsewhere in the body.

Pemphigus vulgaris, for example, may persist or recur in the vagina even when the skin lesions have responded to treatment (Zosmer et al, 1992).

Diabetes mellitus

The first indication of diabetes mellitus, particularly in the elderly patient, may be the development of a vulvovaginitis due to infection with *Candida albicans*. It is also a problem in the poorly controlled diabetic whilst pyogenic infection of the perineum may follow a more aggressive course than in the non-diabetic.

Delayed menarche or, more commonly, secondary amenorrhoea may also occur in diabetics. There are also well-documented problems associated with pregnancy in the diabetic patient which are outside the remit of this chapter.

Enchondromatosis (Ollier's disease)

Ollier's disease is a non-hereditary mesodermal dysplasia which affects the metaphyses of long bones. When there are, in addition, subcutaneous haemangiomas, it is known as Maffucci's syndrome. Both syndromes may be complicated by the development of ovarian neoplasms. Kuzma & King (1948) first described this association and reported an atypical granulosa cell tumour of the ovary in a patient with Maffucci's syndrome. Lewis & Ketcham (1973) subsequently described a malignant tumour of sex cord origin. When Tamimi & Bolen (1984) described a further case, they took the opportunity of re-examining the data from the previous descriptions and suggested that all three were similar and were in fact examples of juvenile granulosa cell tumours.

It should not, however, be assumed that the development of a juvenile granulosa cell tumour necessarily indicates the presence of Ollier's disease, bilateral juvenile granulosa cell tumours having also been described in patients with other abnormalities. They have been found, for example, in a poorly growing 4-month-old dysmorphic infant (Pysher et al, 1981), in a newborn with Potter's syndrome (Roth et al, 1979) and in a 14-week-old child with poor weight gain (Zemke & Herrel, 1941).

Langerhans cell histiocytosis

Langerhans cell histiocytosis, previously included under the generic designation 'histiocytosis X' to indicate its unknown aetiology, may occur as a single osteolytic lesion in bone which has a relatively benign course. It may also be multifocal with a more variable and generally less favourable outcome; in such patients, the lower genital tract may be affected (McKay et al, 1953; Borglin et al, 1966; Lieberman, 1979). For a fuller review of vulvar involvement see Chapter 3.

Patients complain of vulvar itching, irritation and pain, and may develop ulcers (Otis et al, 1990). Within the vagina, elevated dark yellow-brown mucosal papular lesions are found and similar, though paler, lesions are seen in the cervix (Issa et al, 1980).

Histologically, the papular and ulcerated lesions are characterized by sheets of histiocytes interspersed with eosinophils, lymphocytes and plasma cells. When there are areas of necrosis they are often surrounded by a rim of polymorphonuclear leucocytes. Within the endometrium there may be an eosinophilic infiltrate.

The prognosis is worst in children, particularly neonates, when the lesions are widespread and the histiocytes less well differentiated. The multifocal form of the condition is often associated with diabetes insipidus (Issa et al, 1980), and in adults the disease tends to be progressive over a period of time and may recur after treatment.

The aetiology is uncertain although in some cases it is thought to represent an abnormal immunological response to an infective agent; atypical mycobacteria have been isolated in some cases, but in others no agent has been detected. It would appear that there is some genetic predisposition to the condition (Zinkham, 1976).

Galactosaemia

Galactosaemia results in premature ovarian failure (Kaufman et al, 1986; Cramer et al, 1987; Hagenfeldt et al, 1989). Despite a low galactose diet, the follicles are damaged. This contrasts with the condition in males in whom normal gonadal function is preserved.

Müllerian aplasia has also been described in the offspring of a woman with galactose-1-phosphate uridyl transferase levels below the normal range (Cramer et al, 1987).

Gaucher's disease

The association of Gaucher's disease and malignant tumours is very rare, but Kojiro et al (1983) reviewed the literature and described an example of dysgerminoma developing in a 22-year-old woman with Gaucher's disease; it is thought likely that the association was fortuitous.

Gorlin's syndrome (basal cell naevus syndrome)

Gorlin's syndrome is an autosomal dominant inherited disorder characterized by the presence of basal cell naevi and carcinomas, dental cysts, dural calcification, ocular hypertelorism, and various skeletal abnormalities. Ovarian fibromas have been described in many adults (Clendenning et al, 1963; Raggio et al, 1983) and indeed are said to occur in 75% of female patients (Gorlin & Sedano, 1971). They are, however, rare in adolescents (Burket & Rauh, 1976) and children (Rarer et al, 1968; Raggio et al, 1983). Bilateral sclerosing stromal tumours have also been described (Ismail & Walker, 1990).

Grzybowski's generalized eruptive keratoacanthoma

Grzybowski's generalized eruptive keratoacanthoma is a disorder in which pruritic papules appear as crops which heal leaving pitted scars. They have, rarely, been described on the vulva (Yell, 1991) and in association with carcinoma of the Fallopian tube (Weber et al, 1970).

Intestinal inflammatory disease

The intrapelvic location of the genital tract renders it inevitable that it will become involved in any inflammatory process which affects the other pelvic organs or pelvic peritoneum whether this is a pyogenic infection, such as that seen following non-specific appendicitis, or a specific infection.

Diverticular disease. Diverticular disease of the large bowel, particularly if complicated by infection, may result in the formation of intestino-vaginal fistula and the patient may pass flatus per vaginam; the passage of faeces is, however, uncommon because the fistula is usually small and the contents of the bowel solid at this level.

Tubo-intestinal fistula (Rohatgi & Mukherjee, 1973) may also complicate diverticular disease of the large intestine and intestinal tuberculosis. Lymphogranuloma venereum and endometriosis should be considered in the differential diagnosis.

Crohn's disease. Crohn's disease is a chronic non-caseating granulomatous disease of unknown aetiology which typically involves one or more segments of the gastrointestinal tract but which may also affect other organs. It is characterized in the gastrointestinal tract by a transmural inflammatory process in which segments of affected bowel alternate with intestine of apparently normal appearance. There is a marked tendency for internal and external fistulae to form and the disease is often progressive.

The suspicion of Crohn's disease may be raised by the finding in patients with anal disease, both adults and children (Tuffnell & Buchan, 1991), of perineal and perianal oedema, fissures, fistulae, fenestrations or ulcers (Parks et al, 1965; Lockart-Mummery, 1972; Morson, 1972; Kao et al, 1975; Levine et al, 1982) although more commonly such lesions occur in patients in whom the condition has already been recognized. Crohn's disease may also affect the vulva and the resulting lesions (Ansell & Hogbin, 1973; Ridley, 1975; Levine et al, 1982; Kremer et al, 1984; Schulman et al, 1987; Kingsland & Alderman, 1991; Tuffnell & Buchan, 1991) may present as diffuse reddening of the skin or 'metastatic' ulcers, that is, normal skin lies between the ulcers and the gastrointestinal lesions and there is no fistulous communication. These ulcers are often secondarily infected and surrounded by a marked granulomatous response. Prezyna & Kalyanaraman (1977) described a patient in whom 'Bowen's carcinoma' complicated vulvo-vaginal Crohn's disease.

Crohn's disease may also affect other areas of the genital tract, for example, presenting rarely as an ileo-vaginal fistula (Crohn & Yarnis, 1958; Atwell et al, 1965; Kyle & Sinclair, 1969; Hudson, 1970; Geurkink et al, 1983), ileo-uterine fistula (Crohn & Yarnis, 1958), ileo-tubal fistula (Crohn & Yarnis, 1958), recto-vaginal fistula (Cornes & Stecher, 1961; Beecham, 1972; Steinberg et al, 1973; Levine et al, 1982), oophorovesicular-colonic fistula (Goldberg et al, 1988) or as disease in the Fallopian tube (Atwell et al, 1965; Brooks & Wheeler, 1977) where it may, rarely, produce bilateral obstruction (Zetzel, 1980): granulomas can be found in the tubal mucosa or muscularis (Fig. 39.1) and the tubal epithelium may show severe, non-specific reactive changes (Wheeler, 1982). A granulomatous tubo-ovarian mass may result when tubo-ovarian adhesions are dense and granulomas may be seen within the ovarian substance (Fig. 39.2), these indicating the presence of a granulomatous oophoritis (Wlodarski & Trainer, 1975).

As with any granulomatous disorder, the condition must be distinguished from tuberculosis, a complicating

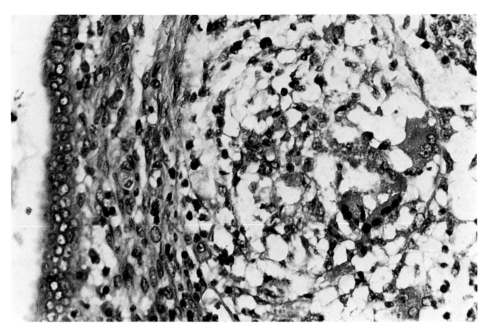

Fig. 39.1 Crohn's disease. A non-caseating tuberculoid granuloma is seen within the mucosa of the Fallopian tube: the lumen lies to the left. H & E × 450.

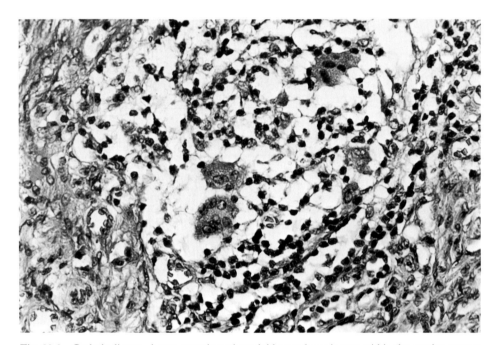

Fig. 39.2 Crohn's disease. A non-caseating tuberculoid granuloma is seen within the ovarian stroma. H & E × 450.

factor in this distinction being the occurrence within the female genital tract of non-caseating tuberculosis (Haines & Stallworthy, 1952).

The fistulae of Crohn's disease are lined by non-specific granulation tissue and contain pus, but often, deep to the tract wall, it may be possible to identify the non-caseating granulomas which are typical of the condition. The granulomas may be set in fibrous tissue and, not uncom-

monly, lie adjacent to a lymphatic channel into which they may protrude. In the absence of fistulae the granulomas may be associated with remarkably little tissue destruction and this, in itself, should raise the possibility of Crohn's disease. In vulvar lesions, particularly when the skin is ulcerated, there may also be pseudoepitheliomatous hyperplasia of the epidermis (Kingsland & Alderman, 1991).

It has been suggested that steroid contraceptives

may play an aetiological rôle in intestinal Crohn's disease (Sandler et al, 1992) but other workers have found no evidence that this is so (Lashner et al, 1989). On the other hand, there is some agreement that smoking and steroid contraceptives may act synergistically to exacerbate the activity of intestinal Crohn's disease (Wakefield et al, 1991; Sandler et al, 1992; Wright, 1992).

Ulcerative colitis. Unlike Crohn's disease, ulcerative colitis does not directly affect the genital tract but, rarely, may be complicated by the development in the groins of a pustular vegetating lesion which resembles pemphigus vegetans (Ridley, 1975).

Complications may also arise as a consequence of the necessity for surgical intervention in severe episodes of ulcerative colitis. Wittich et al (1982) reported the occurrence of a tubo-cutaneous fistula between the right Fallopian tube and the perineum in a young woman six months after a panproctocolectomy which had been carried out for the treatment of 'toxic megacolon'. It was thought probable that a drainage track in the perineal wound had provided the basis of the fistula.

Tuberculosis. Tuberculosis may spread to the genital tract, usually the Fallopian tube, via the lymphatics from an intestinal primary site (Wheeler, 1982) or may spread directly from the intestine or bladder (Rohatgi & Mukherjee, 1973).

Actinomycosis. Actinomycosis may spread directly from the intestine to the genital tract although this mode of transmission is rare.

Haemochromatosis

Selective impairment of anterior pituitary function due to the deposition of iron in the gonadotrophs of the anterior pituitary is typical of haemochromatosis in young females who present with hypogonadotrophic hypogonadism (Herick et al, 1989). Amenorrhoea persists despite the lowering of body iron.

Hydatid disease

Hydatid cysts of the ovary are rare lesions which usually develop secondary to the rupture of a hepatic cyst. They may remain asymptomatic for long periods of time and may be discovered incidentally or cause irritation or compression symptoms (Solidoro & Del Gaudio, 1991).

Klippel–Trenaunay–Weber syndrome

In Klippel–Trenaunay–Weber syndrome there are cutaneous vascular naevi extending in a segmental distribution with associated varicosities limited to the same side of the body. It is usually recognized in infancy and is associated with hypertrophy of both soft tissue and bones (Klippel & Trenaunay, 1900). Arterial abnormalities range from small malformations to large arterio-vascular fistulae.

Uterine haemangiomas with multiple feeding arteries have been described in a 25-year-old woman with this syndrome who had experienced catastrophic bleeding, requiring transfusion, since the onset of menstruation (Lawlor & Charles-Holmes, 1988).

Ligneous conjunctivitis

Ligneous conjunctivitis is a rare form of idiopathic chronic membranous conjunctivitis which is refractory to all forms of therapy. In the chronic phase there may be associated lesions in the cervix or vagina which give rise to an abnormal cervical smear (Hidayat & Riddle, 1987). Histologically, these lesions are similar to those in the conjunctiva. That is, there are subepithelial deposits of amorphous eosinophilic material superficially resembling amyloid and containing albumin, fibrin and immunoglobulin which is thought to have leaked from the local blood vessels. The amount of this material is very variable and small loci of granulation tissue, which in some cases may be a major feature, may also be present. The surface of the epithelium may ulcerate or may be hyperplastic.

Lynch syndrome II

Endometrial and ovarian carcinomas are reported in women suffering from the Lynch type II syndrome, one of the cancer family syndromes (Lynch et al, 1989; Hakala et al, 1991), and small intestinal carcinoma has been recorded.

Megaloblastic anaemia

In patients with both vitamin B_{12} and folate deficiency, there may be changes in the squamous epithelium of the cervix which are characterized by the formation of 'megaloblasts' (see Ch. 6).

Metastatic tumour in the female genital tract

Gastrointestinal neoplasms. The genital tract may be involved directly by the spread of carcinoma from an adjacent segment of the large intestine, particularly the rectum and sigmoid, as a consequence of which the patient may develop an intestino-vaginal fistula (Peterson, 1971). Tumour may also spread from the gastrointestinal tract, across the peritoneal cavity to the ovaries giving rise to the formation of Krukenberg tumours (Krukenberg, 1896; Schlagenhaufer, 1902; Burt, 1957; Woodruff & Novak, 1960; Bullon et al, 1981; Holtz & Hart, 1982; De Graaff et al, 1984) (Ch. 27). The ovary seems to be a site of predilection for such metastases, particularly those which arise from primary carcinoma of the stomach. The ovarian tumours are usually bilateral and the patient may develop menstrual irregularities or postmenopausal bleeding. The finding of a typical Krukenberg tumour should not, however, lead to an automatic assumption that the primary tumour is in the gastrointestinal tract for similar, signet-ring carcinomas, from which metastasis to the ovaries may occur, may also arise in the urinary bladder (Bowlby & Smith, 1986).

Gastrointestinal carcinomas may also metastasize to the cervix (Atobe et al, 1987) and it is important that they be distinguished from primary carcinoma of the cervix, which they may closely resemble.

Other extragenital neoplasms. Metastases may also spread to the genital tract from organs outside the abdomen, for example pulmonary carcinoma (Young & Scully, 1985) and breast carcinoma, particularly the infiltrating lobular type, may result in ovarian metastases (Woodruff & Novak, 1960; Lee & Hori, 1971) and may, on occasions, produce widespread diffusely infiltrating metastatic disease throughout the genital tract. Vulvar metastases may present as apparently primary tumours and the primary lesions should, in the first instance, be sought elsewhere in the genital tract (Buckley & Fox, 1988). If that proves negative, then kidney, urethra, breast (Mader & Friedrich, 1982), lung (Dehner, 1973) and bladder (Powell & Jones, 1983) should be considered. Vulvar metastases from the kidney may be limited to Bartholin's gland (Leiman et al, 1986) and metastatic tumour may be confined to episiotomy sites (Van Dam et al, 1992). Vaginal bleeding has been reported as a consequence of malignant rhabdoid tumour of the pelvis (Frierson et al, 1985). Cervical metastases from extragenital carcinoma are unusual (Lemoine & Hall, 1986) but rarely tumours in the kidney, stomach (Atobe et al, 1987), gallbladder (Hall et al, 1986), rectosigmoid, pancreas, breast and thyroid (Twombley & Di Palma, 1951) may metastasize to the cervix. Malignant melanoma may also metastasize to the cervix (Ferenczy, 1982; Mordel et al, 1989) or ovary (Young & Scully, 1991) and should be carefully distinguished from primary disease. When thyroid carcinoma metastasizes to the ovary (Young et al, 1994) it may mimic struma ovarii.

Lymphomas and leukaemia. All areas of the female genital tract may be involved by Hodgkin's and non-Hodgkin's lymphoma, by far and away the most common site being the ovary; less commonly the uterus, Fallopian tube, cervix, vagina and, least frequently, the vulva may be affected (Lathrop, 1967; Schiller & Madge, 1970; Egwuatu et al, 1980). Primary lymphoma of the ovary and genital tract is, however, extremely rare (Chorlton et al, 1974).

The lesion may form a mass in the vulva, vagina or cervix, and in the vulva, perineum and vagina may be extensively ulcerated (Castaldo et al, 1979; Andrews et al, 1988; Tuder, 1992). Vaginal bleeding may be the first indication of its presence. Also, rarely, a lymphoma may present as an ovarian neoplasm (Talerman, 1982) or a retroperitoneal lymphoma may clinically mimic an ovarian tumour. Involvement of the Fallopian tube by lymphomatous infiltration is also rare and when it occurs, it is almost always associated with involvement of the ipsilateral ovary (Abrams et al, 1958). Leukaemic infiltration of the cervix (Lathrop, 1967; Ferenczy, 1982) and ovary (Talerman, 1982) may be detected histologically but very rarely does it create a clinically detectable mass. The antemortem diagnosis of ovarian acute lymphoblastic leukaemia is exceptionally rare but Cecalupo et al (1982) described four such cases in which the relapse of the leukaemia produced a palpable pelvic mass. Subsequent histological examination confirmed the diagnosis and also revealed involvement of the endometrium, Fallopian tubes, broad ligaments, vagina and cervix in some patients. The development of breast and vaginal masses is also reported coincident with the development of acute myeloblastic leukaemia (Socinski et al, 1983; Harris & Scully, 1984; Banik et al, 1989).

The monotonous cellular character of an infiltrating lymphoma or leukaemic infiltration is in sharp contrast to the pleomorphism of an inflammatory infiltrate. There is also an absence of fibrosis and granulation tissue, features which would be expected in an inflammatory process and, whilst the cellular infiltrate of lymphoma obscures the normal tissue morphology, it does not interrupt it as does an inflammatory, destructive process.

Ovarian cortical necrosis has occurred when acute lymphatic leukaemia was complicated by *Cytomegalovirus* oophoritis (Iwasaki et al, 1988; Ribaux & Gloor, 1988).

Plasmacytoma. Involvement of the ovary by plasmacytoma is rare. The ovary may be involved during the course of myelomatosis or, exceptionally rarely, the ovary may be the site of a primary extranodal plasmacytoma presenting as a large, lower abdominal mass (Talerman, 1982; Hautzer, 1984). Rarely myelomatosis has been reported to form masses in the vulva and vagina (Doss, 1978).

The histological features and immunological characteristics are identical to those occurring in myelomatosis. The prognosis is uncertain.

Multiple endocrine neoplasia type I

Very rarely, multiple endocrine neoplasia type I syndrome may present with amenorrhoea (Lucas et al, 1988).

Organ transplantation

There is an increased incidence of ano-rectal and vulvar intraepithelial and invasive neoplasia in patients in receipt of immunosuppressive treatment following organ transplantation (Penn, 1986). Some women develop a field change in the lower genital tract involving the vulva, vagina and cervix; this is usually HPV-associated and may represent a considerable clinical problem. Other neoplasms, such as endometrial carcinoma, have also been reported following a successful renal transplant (Husslein et al, 1978) and infections, such as tuberculosis, may present an atypical picture — for example, vulvar tuberculosis has been reported (Tham & Choong, 1992).

Peutz–Jeghers' syndrome

Peutz–Jeghers' syndrome is a non-sex-linked, autosomal dominant inherited disorder characterized by hamartomatous polyposis of the entire gastrointestinal tract (Bartholomew et al, 1957) and melanin pigmentation of the buccal mucosa, lips and digits. It may come to the attention of the gynaecological pathologist because some patients develop ovarian sex cord-stromal tumours with annular tubules (Scully, 1970; Young et al, 1982). Such neoplasms are not limited to patients with Peutz–Jeghers' syndrome, but when they are associated with the syndrome they tend to be in the form of tumourlets which undergo calcification rather than in the form of a single large mass (Scully, 1982) which suggests that they too may represent hamartomatous malformations in these patients rather than true neoplasms. A second, as yet incompletely understood, ovarian sex cord-stromal neoplasm has also been described (Young et al, 1983) in two young girls with Peutz–Jeghers' syndrome. Its microscopic appearance suggests that it may well be a Sertoli cell neoplasm. A feminizing Sertoli cell tumour has also been described by Cantu et al (1980). Peutz–Jeghers' syndrome is also associated with the rare, well-differentiated minimal deviation adenocarcinoma of the endocervix, so-called adenoma malignum (McGowan et al, 1980; Young et al, 1982; Young & Scully, 1988; Gilks et al, 1989). Tumour in the Fallopian tube has also been documented (Spigelman et al, 1989).

An association between minimal deviation adenocarcinoma of the cervix and mucinous tumours of the ovary has also been reported (Young & Scully, 1988).

Pituitary disease

Normal fertility may be impaired in patients who have ovarian dysfunction secondary to pituitary neoplasms (Fisken et al, 1989), pituitary infarction (McAlpine & Thomson, 1989) or pituitary ablation (Ch. 33), and in those suffering from anorexia nervosa and organic endocrine disorders such as myxoedema and thyrotoxicosis. The latter probably exert their effects via disturbances to the hypothalamic-pituitary-ovarian axis.

Prader–Willi syndrome

Individuals with Prader–Willi syndrome suffer from neo-natal hypotonia and feeding difficulties, excessive appetite and obesity in early childhood, short stature and cognitive impairment. Dysmorphic features include small hands and feet, almond-shaped eyes and a triangular mouth. The syndrome may be complicated by diabetes, scoliosis and cor pulmonale. There is hypogonadism but approximately half the females with the condition menstruate although menstruation is usually of short duration or irregular (Clarke et al, 1989).

Precocious puberty

Precocious puberty has been reported in association with hepatoblastoma (Navarro et al, 1985) and as a consequence of the hCG produced by an ectopic pinealoma (Kubo et al, 1977).

Retroperitoneal fibrosis

Retroperitoneal fibrosis is an infiltrative fibromatosis characterized by ill-defined masses of fibrous tissue which encircle the lower abdominal aorta and the ureters, giving rise to ureteric narrowing or obstruction. Histologically, the fibrous tissue is infiltrated by lymphocytes, plasma cells and eosinophils and there may be foci of necrosis, phlebitis and arteritis (Mitchinson, 1970; Simon et al, 1985). It is this appearance which has led to the suggestion that the process is inflammatory rather than neoplastic, although its aetiology is uncertain.

The process may, in rare circumstances, extend down to the bladder and vagina (Heah, 1979; Manetta et al, 1987) where it may cause dysuria and abnormal bleeding per vaginam. Fibromatosis has also been reported to form a mass on the posterior wall of the uterus (Tamaya et al, 1986).

Sarcoidosis

Non-caseating epithelioid granulomas of the female genital tract are, as a matter or course, regarded as tuberculous until otherwise proven but, on rare occasions, sarcoidosis of the uterus and Fallopian tubes has been described in the course of systemic disease (Garland & Thomson, 1933; Longcope & Freiman, 1952; Cowdell, 1954; Altchek et al, 1955; Castolidi & Giudici, 1955; Kay, 1956; Zachwiej et al, 1956; Taylor, 1960; Maycock et al, 1963; Ho, 1979; Rosenfeld et al, 1989).

Occasionally the histological diagnosis of sarcoidosis in endometrial curettings has pre-dated the development of systemic disease (Elstein et al, 1994). Disease has also sometimes been limited to the endometrium (Sandvei & Bang, 1991).

Endometrial biopsy in such patients may reveal a picture quite indistinguishable from non-caseating tuberculosis (Taylor, 1960). Whilst caseation is absent in the granulomas of sarcoidosis, the central area may develop acellular fibrinoid necrosis in which Schaumann bodies, asteroids and irregular crystals may be identified. Microbiological investigations fail to reveal *Mycobacterium tuberculosis* and unlike women with pelvic tuberculosis, the patients are often parous. Sarcoidosis of the Fallopian tube (Kay, 1956) and ovary (Winslow & Funkhouser, 1968) are described but the disease in the pelvis is self-limiting (Blaustein, 1982) and does not cause the degree of tubal damage seen in tuberculosis which results in a high incidence of infertility.

Smith–Lemli–Opitz syndrome

This is a rare autosomal recessive disorder with a mixture of neurological and somatic disorders including mental and growth retardation, hypotonia, seizures, abnormalities of the face, palate, torso and extremities. A malignant mixed ovarian germ cell tumour with elements of yolk sac tumour, embryonal carcinoma and dysgerminoma has been described in a 19-year-old patient who had a contralateral streak gonad (Patsner et al, 1989).

Systemic lupus erythematosus

Menses are frequently heavy and irregular in patients with systemic lupus, in whom there are circulating anticoagulants; bleeding may be profound (Schur, 1979). In contrast, there is a tendency to vascular thrombosis, including arterial thrombosis, and high titres of antiphospholipid antibody reflect a high risk for spontaneous abortion (Harris et al, 1988). Remission of systemic lupus erythematosus has been reported (Kahn et al, 1966) following the removal of an ovarian dysgerminoma.

Thyroid adenoma and ovarian neoplasms

A familial association between thyroid adenomas and Sertoli–Leydig cell tumours (Jensen et al, 1974; O'Brien & Wilansky, 1981) has been described and there is a possibility that other ovarian neoplasms may also arise in these families as both a sex cord-stromal tumour and a mucinous cystoma were removed from a sibling of one of the patients with a Sertoli–Leydig cell tumour.

Torre–Muir syndrome

Endometrial carcinoma has been reported in 7 of 17 women with Torre–Muir syndrome (Bitran & Pellettiere, 1974; Leonard & Deaton, 1974; Tschang et al, 1976; Householder & Zeligman, 1980; Lynch et al, 1981; Graham et al, 1985), a condition characterized by multiple cutaneous sebaceous neoplasms, keratoacanthomas and visceral neoplasms. Similar cutaneous manifestations are found in some members of families exhibiting 'cancer family syndrome'; in such cases an autosomal dominant mode of inheritance is found (Lynch et al, 1981). The most common visceral neoplasms are colonic, but tumours in other areas of the gastrointestinal tract and tumours of the urinary tract also occur. Female patients are prone to develop endometrial carcinomas but tumours of the vulva and ovary have also been described (Bitran & Pellettiere, 1974; Rulon & Helwig, 1974; Graham et al, 1985).

Vasculitis

Granulomatous vasculitis. Granulomatous vasculitis may be a local, asymptomatic condition limited to the vasculature of part or all of the genital tract (Pirozynski, 1976; Summers et al, 1991), a local asymptomatic condition (Crow & McWhinney, 1979), or may be part of a systemic disease. In the latter case, an association with polymyalgia rheumatica and temporal arteritis (Polasky et al, 1965; Petrides et al, 1979) is well recognized.

The affected vessels, usually small muscular arteries, are cuffed by lymphocytes and epithelioid macrophages with or without giant cells (Fig. 39.3). The vessel wall may show signs of necrosis but even when the destructive process is well advanced, elastic stains will usually reveal fragments of elastin in the inflammatory focus (Fig. 39.4) and, in minimally affected vessels, small defects may be revealed in the elastic lamina.

The presence of epithelioid granulomas related to spiral arteries in the endometrium may give rise to a suspicion of tuberculosis but the total absence of caseation together with negative cultures and the presence of vascular damage should be sufficient to confirm the diagnosis. The morphological changes are consistent with an immunological response to a vascular wall component and this concept is supported by the finding of cell-mediated immunity to the arterial antigen in some people (Hazleman et al, 1975) and the rapid response to corticosteroids.

Necrotizing arteritis. The medium and small arteries of the uterus may be involved by an intramural non-specific inflammatory infiltrate associated with vessel necrosis (Pirozynski, 1976); an isolated arteritis of the cervix, which is identical histologically with polyarteritis nodosa, has also been reported (Crow & McWhinney, 1979; Padwell, 1986). This latter arteritis may be asymptomatic but can also be associated with bleeding. Involvement of the ovaries in polyarteritis nodosa is frequent but usually asymptomatic (Austen, 1971) and vasculitis in the uterus and cervix is usually overshadowed by the systemic component of the disease.

A somewhat similar necrotizing vasculitis, which caused massive intra-abdominal haemorrhage, has also been described in the ovary of a woman undergoing in vitro fertilization (Ilbery et al, 1991).

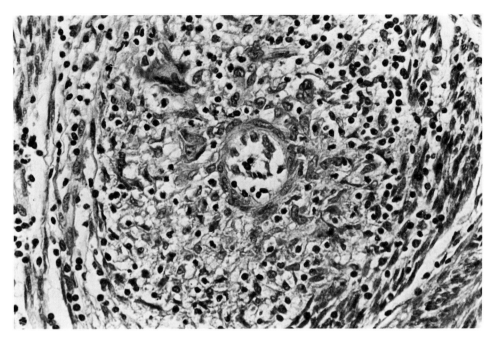

Fig. 39.3 Granulomatous arteritis. The wall of a small muscular uterine artery is infiltrated by epithelioid macrophages and lymphocytes: a giant cell lies in the upper left of the field. H & E × 450.

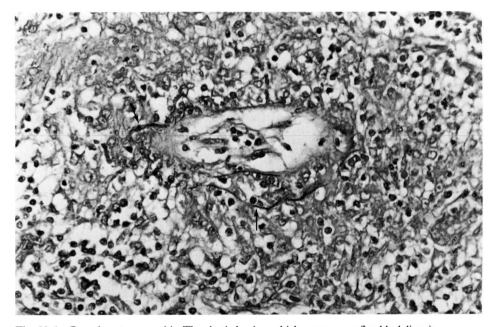

Fig. 39.4 Granulomatous arteritis. The elastic lamina, which appears as a fine black line, is fragmented and disrupted by the inflammatory infiltrate. Elastic van Gieson × 450.

Von Hippel–Lindau disease

This is a rare autosomal disorder characterized by the development of benign and malignant neoplasms widely dispersed throughout the body. Many of these are angiomatous, the most serious being the haemangioblastomas of the central nervous system. Of much less significance is the almost incidental but common occurrence of intraovarian haemangiomas (Horton et al, 1976).

A papillary cystadenoma of the mesosalpinx which was multicystic, and in which the walls were locally calcified has also been described. It was believed to be of mesonephric origin and the epithelium was cuboidal with central round nuclei and clear cytoplasm: ciliated and secretory cells were not seen. Electronoptically the cells were said to be similar to those of the adnexal tumour of Wolffian origin (Gersell & King, 1988).

Von Recklinghausen's syndrome

Von Recklinghausen's disease (neurofibromatosis) is characterized by the presence of multiple neural tumours and pigmented skin lesions, some of which are *café au lait* spots. In about half the patients there is a family history consistent with an autosomal dominant pattern of inheritance but, in the other half, there is no family history. Eighteen per cent of women with the disorder have vulvar neurofibromas (Schreiber, 1963) and an ovarian neurofibroma has been reported in an affected individual (Smith, 1931).

NON-GYNAECOLOGICAL CONDITIONS INCIDENTALLY AFFECTING THE GENITAL TRACT

In many cases the involvement of the genital tract is largely fortuitous and in fact may be detected only if it is specifically sought. This applies to the situation in which the vulva may be involved in the systemic rashes of chickenpox, scarlet fever, drug eruptions and the prodroma of measles. It also applies to a large number of dermatological disorders such as pellagra, vitiligo, albinism and alopecia and to the petechial rashes which are found in patients with bleeding disorders. There are, however, a number of circumstances when the systemic disorder shows a predilection for the genital tract or ovary, such as the ovary in mumps or the vulva in psoriasis and cicatricial pemphigoid (Ch. 3).

THE GYNAECOLOGICAL CONSEQUENCES OF THE TREATMENT OF NON-GYNAECOLOGICAL DISEASE

Whether or not a non-gynaecological disease affects the genital tract, its treatment may have a profound effect on the morphology or function of the genital tract and ovary. Such changes may be perplexing for the histopathologist or cytopathologist, particularly if the history of the systemic disease has not been provided.

In patients receiving hormone therapy for the treatment of non-gynaecological disease, for example, for the treatment of breast carcinoma, both the cervical cytology and the endometrial appearances may be abnormal. Tamoxifen, a partial oestrogen agonist, is widely used in the treatment of breast carcinoma and its oestrogenic effect may be manifest in the form of vaginal bleeding from proliferative or hyperplastic endometrium, occasionally from endometrial carcinoma and in the recrudescence of endometriotic foci (Buckley, 1990) (see Ch. 36). If progestagens are used the endometrium may show inappropriate secretory activity and pseudodecidualization (Ch. 35) or there may be endometrial atrophy. In the cervix, there may be a degree of cervical microglandular hyperplasia

and the cervical smear may show inappropriate progestational effects.

There is a large number of drugs which need to be avoided in pregnancy because of their potential teratogenic or abortifacient properties. It is also well-recognized that the metabolism of steroid contraceptives is accelerated by a variety of commonly used drugs such as, for example, antimicrobial agents and antiepileptics. Other drugs, such as Misoprostol (Cytotec), a selective orally active prostaglandin which has been used in women with peptic ulceration, may cause menorrhagia, intermenstrual bleeding, postmenopausal bleeding and, in the young woman, abortion (Committee on Safety of Medicines, 1989). It also increases uterine tone and should be avoided in pregnancy.

The use of some non-hormone preparations such as the antidepressive and anti-inflammatory drugs may exert an influence on the ovary by virtue of their interference with the control of prolactin secretion. There may subsequently be sequential changes in the Fallopian tube, cervix, vagina and endometrium.

Problems may be encountered in the interpretation of cervical and vaginal smear material in patients who have been treated either by radiotherapy locally or have received chemotherapy. It may be difficult to distinguish the observed changes from those which are the result of a neoplastic process. Opportunistic infections too may afflict patients receiving cytotoxic drugs or immunosuppressives, and those patients in whom immunosuppression is part of the disease process. They may thus present to the gynaecologist with Candida infection or condylomas. Disseminated granulomatous disease (BCGosis) has also been reported following chemoimmunotherapy for ovarian carcinoma (Kelleher et al, 1988).

THE NON-GYNAECOLOGICAL CONSEQUENCES OF GYNAECOLOGICAL DISEASE AND TREATMENT

In patients using steroid contraceptives there may be widespread systemic consequences and abnormalities may develop in the cardiovascular system, liver, breast or nervous systems (Ch. 35). Patients wearing an intrauterine contraceptive device may, in the first instance, develop pelvic sepsis and subsequently develop pelvic and subphrenic abscess, portal pyaemia or thoracic actinomycosis (Witwer et al, 1977; Anteby et al, 1991) although fortunately such occurrences are nowadays rare. As the patient will often present not to the gynaecologist but to the general surgeon, the possibility must always be borne in mind.

A further, rare, complication of the use of steroid contraceptives has been reported in a woman with McCune–Albright syndrome who suffered a pathological fracture (Maccari et al, 1989). In this syndrome the bone lesions contain oestrogen and progesterone receptors and their progression in pregnancy is also well recognized.

On the positive side, it has been suggested that women who use hormone replacement therapy after the menopause are at reduced risk of developing colonic carcinoma (Gerhardsson de Verdier & London, 1992).

The patient who presents with acute arthritis may have gonorrhoea and this may the first indication that something is wrong because the local disease in the cervix may be entirely asymptomatic.

Neoplasms of the genital tract and ovary may involve the adjacent bowel and intestinal obstruction may herald residual carcinoma (Christopherson et al, 1985).

A necrotizing vasculitis causing major intra-abdominal haemorrhage has complicated ovarian superovulation carried out for in vitro fertilization (IVF) (Ilbery et al, 1991). Intra-abdominal haemorrhage is an infrequent but well-recognized complication of IVF. In the immediate postoperative days it is usually the result of trauma to the ovary or periovarian tissues whilst, in the weeks following the procedure, it is usually due to rupture of a corpus luteum cyst or an ectopic pregnancy.

The association of congenital anomalies of the Müllerian system with systemic structural abnormalities

The most common non-gynaecological anomalies associated with Müllerian tract anomalies lie in the renal tract, and of these renal agenesis is the most common (Golan et al, 1989), being most frequently associated with unicornuate uterus (70–80% of cases). Rarely duplication of the whole urinary collecting system has been reported. Between 10% and 12% of women with Müllerian malformations also have anomalies in the musculo-skeletal system (Siegler, 1983; Bernhisel et al, 1985), 12% have imperforate anus and 6% have cardiac abnormalities and anomalies of the ear and eye (Pinsonneault & Goldstein, 1985).

Dermatological disorders

Acanthosis nigricans. Acanthosis nigricans may be the first intimation that a patient has ovarian carcinoma (Dingley & Marten, 1957). It is particularly mentioned in relation to serous carcinoma (Curth et al, 1962) and mature cystic teratoma of the ovary (Imperato-McGinley et al, 1978). In the latter case, it was associated with primary amenorrhoea, hirsutism and insulin resistance.

Linear IgA disease. Linear IgA disease is an uncommon autoimmune dermatosis with subepidermal blistering, diagnosed by demonstrating a band-like deposition of IgA in the basement membrane of non-blistered areas. Circulating IgA autoantibodies are thought to be pathogenic. It has been described in a woman with a molar pregnancy and it is suggested that the mole triggered the abnormal immune response by expressing the linear IgA antigen (Kelly & Wojnarowska, 1989).

Pemphigoid gestationis. Pemphigoid gestationis may occur in normal pregnancy (Kelly et al, 1988), where the placenta expresses a pemphigoid gestationis related antigen, and in association with hydatidiform mole (Tindall et al, 1981).

Dermatomyositis

Dermatomyositis/polymyositis may affect the vulva (Lavery et al, 1985) and may be associated with serous carcinoma of the ovary (Peters et al, 1983; Verducci et al, 1984) dysgerminoma (Solomon & Maurer, 1983) and with other ovarian carcinomas (Cortes et al, 1962; Chamberlain & Whittaker, 1963).

Endocrine disorders

A variety of systemic endocrine disturbances accompany gynaecological disorders (Shane & Naftolin, 1975).

Carcinoid syndrome. Carcinoid syndrome develops in approximately one-third of patients with an ovarian carcinoid tumour even in the absence of metastases (Qizilbash et al, 1974; Robboy et al, 1975) because secretions from such neoplasms pass, via the venous drainage, directly into the systemic circulation and are not inactivated by the liver. Carcinoid syndrome has also been reported in association with carcinoid tumour (small cell carcinoma) of the uterine cervix (Brown & Lane, 1965; Stockdale et al, 1986).

Cushing's syndrome. Cushing's syndrome has been reported as resulting from the ectopic production of cortisol in patients with lipid cell tumours of the ovary (Kepler et al, 1944; Deaton & Freedman, 1957; Rosner et al, 1964; Osborn et al, 1969; Motlik & Starka, 1973; Marieb et al, 1983; Adeyemi et al, 1986; Hayes & Scully, 1987; Young & Scully, 1987), by a pituitary cell adenoma within an ovarian teratoma (Axiotis et al, 1987) and due to the ectopic production of ACTH by a Sertoli cell tumour of the ovary (Nichols et al, 1962), by Sertoli–Leydig cell tumour (Canelo & Lisser, 1939), by a carcinoid tumour of the ovary (Brown & Lane, 1965), by other ovarian neoplasms (Parsons & Rigby, 1958; Lipsett et al, 1964; Odell et al, 1977; Baylin & Mendelsohn, 1980) and small cell endocrine tumours of the uterine cervix (Berthelot et al, 1961; Jones et al, 1976; Matsuyama et al, 1979; Lojek et al, 1980; Iemura et al, 1991).

Hyperaldosteronism. Hyperaldosteronism associated with isosexual precocious puberty has been reported in a 9-year-old girl who had a Sertoli cell tumour of the ovary (Erlich et al, 1963). The child had an elevated systemic blood pressure, hypokalaemia and a high urinary secretion of aldosterone.

Hyperaldosteronism has also been recorded in other

patients with Sertoli–Leydig cell tumours (Todesco et al, 1975) and treatment-resistant systemic hypertension has been described in association with a renin-producing ovarian Sertoli cell tumour (Korzets et al, 1986).

Hypercalcaemia. Hypercalcaemia may develop in patients with a variety of gynaecological tumours, probably due to the production of more than one humoral substance; in some cases, a parathyroid hormone-like substance has been identified (Allan et al, 1984). Hypercalcaemia has been reported, for example, in association with a variety of ovarian neoplasms, in patients with squamous carcinoma arising in ovarian teratomas (Kim et al, 1981; Ribeiro et al, 1988), papillary serous cystadenocarcinoma (Ferenczy et al, 1971; Rivett & Robinson, 1972; Josse et al, 1981), clear cell carcinoma (Powell et al, 1973; Biron et al, 1977; Skrabanck et al, 1980), endometrioid carcinoma (Stewart et al, 1982), mucinous adenocarcinoma (Boyer et al, 1989), lipid cell tumour (Abouav et al, 1959), small cell carcinoma (Dickersin et al, 1982; Taraszewski et al, 1991), undifferentiated sex cord-stromal tumour (Holtz et al, 1979) and dysgerminoma of the ovary (Stewart et al, 1982). Hypercalcaemia has also been described in a patient with a malignant paraovarian tumour of probable Wolffian origin (Abbot et al, 1981) and may also develop in patients with adenocarcinoma or adenosquamous carcinoma of the endometrium (Stewart et al, 1982), squamous carcinoma of the vulva (Shane & Naftolin, 1975; Stewart et al, 1982) and squamous carcinoma of the cervix uteri (Lacey & Morrow, 1979).

Hyperchorionic gonadotrophinism. It is well recognized that a very large concentration of hCG has a thyroid-stimulating effect (Cave & Dunn, 1976; Davies et al, 1979) and thus symptoms of thyrotoxicosis or high output cardiac failure (French et al, 1977; Twiggs et al, 1979; Soutter et al, 1981) may occur in patients with trophoblastic disease (Higgins & Herschman, 1978). It is seen in both patients with choriocarcinoma (Cohen & Utiger, 1970; Cave & Dunn, 1976; Morley et al, 1976) and in those with hydatidiform mole (Herschman & Higgins, 1971; Kim et al, 1976; Osathanondh et al, 1976; French et al, 1977). Thyrotoxicosis may also develop in patients in whom there is a struma ovarii (Fox & Langley, 1976).

Human chorionic gonadotrophin may also be secreted by other ovarian carcinomas without the development of clinical symptoms (Montiero et al, 1983; Vaitukaitis, 1974), and more specifically by serous carcinoma of the ovary (Civantos & Rywlin, 1972; Samaan et al, 1976), mucinous carcinoma (Civantos & Rywlin, 1972; Samaan et al, 1976), endometrioid carcinoma (Samaan et al, 1976) and dysgerminoma (Gough, 1939; Kapp et al, 1985). In some cases, human placental lactogen can also be identified (Samaan et al, 1976; Montiero et al, 1983).

Hypoglycaemia. Hypoglycaemia has been described as a consequence of ectopic insulin production by a primary ovarian carcinoid (Morgello et al, 1988) and as a consequence of the production of an insulin-like substance by an ovarian serous cystadenocarcinoma of the ovary (O'Neill & Mikuta, 1970), an ovarian fibroma (Michael, 1967), a dysgerminoma (Von Meyer-Hofmann et al, 1960) and a malignant schwannoma (Shetty et al, 1982).

Inappropriate antidiuretic hormone (ADH) secretion. Inappropriate antidiuretic hormone secretion has been described in a patient with an endometrial adenocarcinoma (Fung & Lee, 1985).

Masculinization. Masculinization may occur as a consequence of hormones secreted by a variety of ovarian neoplasms. These include Leydig cell tumours and other lipid cell tumours, granulosa cell tumour, thecoma, Sertoli–Leydig cell tumours and non-neoplastic conditions such as polycystic ovary syndrome, luteoma of pregnancy and massive oedema of the ovary (see Chs 19, 22 and 25).

Resistant ovary syndrome. Resistant ovary syndrome is associated in a small number of cases with blepharophimosis (Fraser et al, 1988).

Zollinger–Ellison syndrome. Zollinger–Ellison syndrome may develop in patients with gastrin-secreting mucinous cystadenomas (Julkunen et al, 1983; Morgan et al, 1985), ovarian mucinous tumours of borderline malignancy (Bollen et al, 1981) and mucinous cystadenocarcinoma (Cocco & Conway, 1975; Long et al, 1980).

Endometriosis

Endometriosis is discussed fully in Chapter 32 and it is only its non-gynaecological aspects that will be mentioned here. Pelvic endometriosis not uncommonly affects the serosa of the bowel where its tendency to undergo cyclical breakdown and bleeding may cause symptoms referable to the gastrointestinal tract. Endometriosis of the vermiform appendix may present as right iliac fossa pain mimicking acute appendicitis, whilst in the sigmoid colon its presence may elicit a fibroblastic and muscular hypertrophic response which may be so severe as to produce a segmental stenosis. The symptoms of large bowel obstruction may then closely mimic carcinoma, inflammatory bowel disease or diverticular disease. The resected specimen usually reveals an excentric mural thickening which has a dense, grey-white fibrous appearance and within which small haemorrhagic foci may be apparent. Histological examination demonstrates functional endometriotic foci set in fibrous tissue in which there are haemosiderin-containing macrophages, surrounded by hypertrophied smooth muscle. Occasionally the overlying bowel mucosa may become ulcerated, but more commonly it is of normal appearance and the lesion is limited to the serosa, subserosa and musculature of the bowel wall. These foci of endometriosis may, in rare circumstances, undergo a range of neoplastic changes similar to those which occur in the endometrium.

Haematological disorders

Erythrocytosis. The development of erythrocytosis in patients with uterine leiomyomas (Menzies, 1965; Fried et al, 1968; Wrigley et al, 1971; Ossias et al, 1973; Weiss et al, 1975), mature cystic teratoma (Ghio et al, 1981), mucinous adenocarcinoma (Hudson et al, 1993) and lipid cell tumour of the ovary (Montag et al, 1984) is attributed to the production of erythropoietin, or factors that stimulate erythropoietin production (Fried et al, 1968), by these tumours.

Haemolytic anaemia. Autoimmune haemolytic anaemia has been reported in patients with ovarian teratomas (Barry & Crosby, 1957; McAndrew, 1964; Davidsohn et al, 1968; Bernstein et al, 1974; Payne et al, 1981), with granulosa-theca cell tumour (Dawson et al, 1971), serous cystadenoma (Blau & Kaplinsky, 1982) and mucinous carcinoma of the ovary (André et al, 1969) and with uterine non-Hodgkin's lymphoma (Bär et al, 1986).

Hypercoagulability. In common with other systemic neoplasms, ovarian carcinoma may be associated with thrombophlebitis migrans (Henderson, 1955; Lieberman et al, 1961) or deep vein thrombosis (Adamson et al, 1988). Reports have also been published giving further evidence of a state of hypercoagulability in women with a variety of ovarian malignancies including serous carcinoma, mucinous carcinoma and endometrioid carcinoma (Mosesson et al, 1968; Siegman-Igra et al, 1977; Scully et al, 1978; Landolfi et al, 1984). The reports have included non-bacterial thrombotic endocarditis (Delgado & Smith, 1975).

Pancytopenia. Pancytopenia is an unusual finding in gynaecological malignancy but it has been described in association with granulosa cell tumour (Napoli & Wallach, 1976).

Thrombocytopenia. Thrombocytopenia may occur in patients with haemangiomas but the association of bilateral ovarian haemangiomas and diffuse abdominopelvic haemangiomatosis is exceptionally rare (Lawhead et al, 1985).

Hyperamylasaemia

A raised serum amylase has been described in many patients with ovarian neoplasms. They include a patient with a mucinous tumour which had benign, borderline and malignant areas (Teshima et al, 1988), a patient with a low-grade serous papillary neoplasm (Cramer & Bruns, 1979), women with serous surface papillary carcinoma and conventional serous carcinoma (Hayakawa et al, 1984; Hodes et al, 1985; O'Riordan et al, 1990), endometrioid carcinoma (Yagi et al, 1986) and adenosquamous carcinoma (Norwood et al, 1981).

Hypertrophic pulmonary osteoarthropathy

Hypertrophic pulmonary osteoarthropathy may develop in association with ovarian carcinoma (Lester & Robertson, 1981).

Malacoplakia

Malacoplakia rarely affects the female genital tract but a case has been described in which primary malacoplakia of the female genital tract led to urethral and ureteral obstruction (Bessim et al, 1991).

Meigs' syndrome

The association of ascites and hydrothorax (Meigs' syndrome) with ovarian fibromata is well-recognized and familiar (Salmon, 1934; Meigs & Cass, 1937; Rhoads & Terrell, 1937). Perhaps less familiar is the association of ascites and hydrothorax, so-called Meigs-like or pseudo-Meigs' syndrome, with uterine leiomyomas (O'Flanagan et al, 1987) and with other ovarian tumours and non-neoplastic conditions including serous tumours (Fox & Langley, 1976), benign mucinous tumours (Brenner & Scott, 1986; Jimerson, 1973), Brenner tumour (Pratt-Thomas et al, 1976), granulosa cell tumour (Meigs, 1954), thecoma (Faber, 1962), fibrothecoma (Koussidis et al, 1984), dysgerminoma (Simon & Delavierre, 1981), mature cystic teratoma (Mantouvalos et al, 1982), lymphoma (Yutani et al, 1982) and massive oedema of the ovary (Slotky et al, 1982; Fukuda et al, 1984). The combination of chylous and serous pleural effusions with ovarian cancer is sometimes termed Contarini's syndrome (Lawton et al, 1985).

Metastatic gynaecological cancer

Metastases from gynaecological neoplasms may produce symptoms which may be clinically 'misleading'. Amin (1986) described a case of classical Horner's syndrome and Pancoast's syndrome in a woman with metastatic cervical carcinoma in the lung apex. She also had ipsilateral vocal cord and phrenic nerve palsies. This particular combination of symptoms has been described as a syndrome (Rowland Payne, 1981). Superior vena cava syndrome has been reported secondary to mediastinal metastases from endometrial carcinoma and uterine leiomyosarcoma (Puleo et al, 1986). A malignant pericardial effusion has been described in a woman with metastatic squamous cell carcinoma of the uterine cervix (Rieke & Kapp, 1988). Cervical carcinoma is an important cause of cavitating metastases in the lung and these have a tendency to give rise to pneumothorax (Lane et al, 1986).

Nephrotic syndrome

Nephrotic syndrome, which is attributed to the glomerular deposition of immune complexes, has been described in women with metastatic epithelial malignancy of the ovary (Hoyt & Hamilton, 1987) and is a not uncommon feature in patients with a placental site tumour.

Neuropathy and neuromyopathy

Paraneoplastic neuropathies and neuromyopathies are not uncommon in patients with malignant disease and these have been reported in patients with gynaecological malignancy (Croft & Wilkinson, 1965). Reflex sympathetic dystrophy (shoulder-hand syndrome) has been reported to pre-date the clinical recognition of endometrial carcinoma (Hudson et al, 1993). It has also been described in patients with tubo-ovarian carcinoma (Taggart et al, 1984).

Palmar fasciitis and polyarthritis

Palmar fasciitis and polyarthritis have been described in patients with serous carcinoma of the ovary, endometrioid carcinoma of the ovary and in patients with ovarian cancer of unspecified types (Medsger et al, 1982; Shiel et al, 1985).

Premature menopause

Rosenberg et al (1981) have shown that a premature menopause, in particular removal of the ovaries during a gynaecological procedure in a woman under the age of 35 years, significantly increases the risk of non-fatal myocardial infarct, the factor being 7.2 times. After the menopause too, at whatever age it occurs, a woman is susceptible to osteoporosis, its subsequent deformities and the increased risk of fracture.

Pyrexia of unknown origin

Pyrexia may accompany the presence of many neoplasms and ovarian tumours are no exception. They may, in some instances, present with a fever for which there is no apparent cause (Maestu et al, 1979; Schofield et al, 1985).

Subacute cerebellar degeneration

A description of the paraneoplastic syndromes in women with ovarian neoplasms is provided by Russell & Bannatyne (1989) and by Hudson et al (1993). One of the most striking examples of this is subacute cerebellar degeneration associated with serous carcinoma of the ovary (Steven et al, 1982; Greenlee & Brashear, 1983; Cocconi et al, 1985; Hall et al, 1985) and in which a Purkinje cell antibody can be identified.

Miscellaneous disorders

Mature cystic teratomas may rupture not only into the peritoneum, giving rise to shock and peritonitis, but may also rupture into the bladder or rectum creating a fistula (Dandia, 1967). Fistulae may also develop should carcinoma of the vulva, vagina, cervix or endometrium spread directly to the urethra, a site in which fistulous communications are not uncommon.

Systemic sclerosis and polyarteritis have also been reported in women with ovarian neoplasms (Hudson et al, 1993).

Occasionally a gynaecological disease may simulate a systemic disorder. An unusual case is recorded by Nunez et al (1983) in which the disseminated cells from an embryonal rhabdomyosarcoma were mistaken for those of acute lymphoblastic leukaemia in both the blood and bone marrow. After death, bilateral ovarian embryonal rhabdomyosarcomas were discovered and the cellular infiltrate, previously thought to be leukaemic, was correctly identified.

Infectious pneumoperitoneum due to gas-forming organisms has been described as an uncommon presentation of endometrial carcinoma (Douvier et al, 1989).

REFERENCES

Abbot R L, Barlogie B, Schmidt W A 1981 Metastasizing malignant juxtaovarian tumor with terminal hypercalcemia: a case report. Cancer 48: 860–865.

Abouav J, Berkowitz S B, Kolb F O 1959 Reversible hypercalcemia in masculinizing hypernephroid tumor of the ovary: report of a case. New England Journal of Medicine 260: 1057–1062.

Abrams J, Kazal H L, Hobbs R E 1958 Primary sarcoma of the Fallopian tube. American Journal of Obstetrics and Gynecology 260: 180–182.

Adamson A S, Littlewood T J, Poston G J, Hows J M, Wolfe J N 1988 Malignancy presenting as peripheral venous gangrene. Journal of the Royal Society of Medicine 8: 609–610.

Adeyemi S D, Grange A O, Giwa-Osagie O F, Elesha S O 1986 Adrenal rest tumor of the ovary associated with isosexual precocious pseudopuberty and cushingoid features. European Journal of Paediatrics 145: 236–238.

Allan S G, Lockhart S P, Leonard R C, Smyth J F 1984 Paraneoplastic hypercalcaemia in ovarian carcinoma. British Medical Journal 228: 1714–1715.

Altchek A, Gaines J A, Siltzbach L E 1955 Sarcoidosis of the uterus. American Journal of Obstetrics and Gynecology 70: 540–547

Amin R 1986 Bilateral Pancoast's syndrome in a patient with carcinoma of the cervix. Gynecologic Oncology 24: 126–128.

André R, Duhamel G, Najman A, Homberg J C, Mawas C, Armangol R 1969 Anemie hemolytique auto-immune et tumeur maligne de l'ovarie. Presse Médicale 77: 2133–2136.

Andrews S J, Hernandez E, Woods J, Cook B 1988 Burkitt's-like lymphoma presenting as a gynecologic tumor. Gynecologic Oncology 30: 131–136.

Ansell I D, Hogbin B 1973 Crohn's disease of the vulva. Journal of Obstetrics and Gynaecology of the British Commonwealth 80: 376–378.

Anteby E, Milvidsky A, Goshen R, Ben Chetrit A, Ron M 1991

IUD-associated abdominopelvic actinomycosis. Harefuah 121: 150–153.

Atobe Y, Yoshmura T, Kako H, Misumi A, Akagi M 1987 Gastric cancer diagnosed by biopsy of the uterine cervix. Gynecologic Oncology 26: 135–139.

Atwell J D, Duthie H L, Goligher J C 1965 The outcome of Crohn's disease. British Journal of Surgery 52: 966–972.

Austen K F 1971 Periarteritis nodosa (polyarteritis nodosa) In: Beeson P B, McDermott W (eds) Cecil Loeb Textbook of medicine, 13th edn. Saunders, Philadelphia.

Axiotis C A, Lippes H A, Merino M J, deLanerolle N C, Stewart A F, Kinder B 1987 Corticotroph cell pituitary adenoma within an ovarian teratoma: a new cause of Cushing's syndrome. The American Journal of Surgical Pathology 11: 218–224.

Banik S, Borg Grech A B, Eyden B P 1989 Granulocytic sarcoma of the cervix: an immunohistochemical and ultrastructural study. Journal of Clinical Pathology 42: 483–488.

Bär B M, Reijinders F J, Keuning J J, Bal H, van Beek M 1986 Primary malignant lymphoma of the uterine cervix associated with cold-reacting autoantibody-mediated hemolytic anemia. Acta Haematologica (Basel) 75: 232–235.

Barry K G, Crosby W H 1957 Autoimmune hemolytic anemia arrested by removal of ovarian teratoma: review of the literature and report of a case. Annals of Internal Medicine 47: 1002–1007.

Bartholomew L G, Dahlin D C, Waugh J M 1957 Intestinal polyposis: association with mucocutaneous melanin pigmentation (Peutz–Jeghers' syndrome). Gastroenterology 32: 434–451.

Baylin S B, Mendelsohn G 1980 Ectopic (inappropriate) hormone production by tumors: mechanisms involved and the biological and clinical implications. Endocrine Reviews 1: 45–77.

Beecham C T 1972 Recurring rectovaginal fistulas. Obstetrics and Gynecology 40: 323–326.

Bernhisel M A, London S N, Haney A F 1985 Unusual Müllerian anomalies associated with distal extremity abnormalities. Obstetrics and Gynecology 65: 291–294.

Bernstein D, Naor S, Rokover M, Manahem H 1974 Hemolytic anemia related to ovarian tumor. Obstetrics and Gynecology 43: 276–280.

Berthelot P, Benhamou J P, Fauvert R 1961 Hypercorticisme et cancer de l'uterus. Presse Médicale 69: 1899–1902.

Bessim S, Heller D S, Dottino P, Deligdisch L, Gordon R E 1991 Malakoplakia of the female genital tract causing urethral and ureteral obstruction: a case report. Journal of Reproductive Medicine 36: 691–694.

Biron S, Bercovici B, Brufman G 1977 Paraneoplastic hypercalcemic syndrome associated with ovarian cancer. European Journal of Obstetrics Gynecology and Reproductive Biology 7: 239–242.

Bitran J, Pellettiere E V 1974 Multiple sebaceous gland tumors and internal carcinoma: Torre's syndrome. Cancer 33: 835–836.

Blau A, Kaplinsky J 1982 Microangiopathic haemolytic anaemia associated with recurrent pulmonary emboli and benign pelvic tumours. Postgraduate Medical Journal 58: 362–363.

Blaustein A 1982 Inflammatory diseases of the ovary. In: Blaustein A (ed) Pathology of the female genital tract, 2nd edn. Springer Verlag, New York, p 445.

Borglin N E, Söderstrom J, Wehlin L 1966 Eosinophilic granuloma (histiocytosis X) of the vulva. Journal of Obstetrics and Gynaecology of the British Commonwealth 73: 478–486.

Bollen E C, Lamers C B, Jansen J B, Larsson L I, Joosten H J 1981 Zollinger-Ellison syndrome due to gastrin producing ovarian cystadenocarcinoma. British Journal of Surgery 68: 776–777.

Bowlby L S, Smith McM L 1986 Signet-ring carcinoma of the urinary bladder: primary presentation as a Krukenberg tumor. Gynecologic Oncology 25: 376–381.

Boyer M, Friedlander M, Bannatyne P, Atkinson K 1989 Hypercalcemia in association with mucinous adenocarcinoma of the ovary: a case report. Gynecologic Oncology 35: 387–390.

Brenner W E, Scott R B 1968 Meigs-like syndrome secondary to Krukenberg's tumour. Obstetrics and Gynecology 31: 40–44.

Brooks J J, Wheeler J E 1977 Granulomatous salpingitis secondary to Crohn's disease. Obstetrics and Gynecology 49 (suppl): 31s–33s.

Brown H, Lane M 1965 Cushing's and malignant carcinoid syndromes from ovarian neoplasm. Archives of Internal Medicine 115: 490–494.

Buckley C H 1990 Tamoxifen and endometriosis: case report. British Journal of Obstetrics and Gynaecology 97: 645–646.

Buckley C H, Fox H 1988 Epithelial tumours. In: Ridley C M (ed) The vulva. Churchill Livingstone, Edinburgh, pp 263–333.

Bullon A Jr, Arseneau J, Prat J, Young R H, Scully R E 1981 Tubular Krukenberg tumor: a problem in histopathologic diagnosis. American Journal of Surgical Pathology 5: 225–232.

Burket R L, Rauh J L 1976 Gorlin's syndrome: ovarian fibromas at adolescence. Obstetrics and Gynecology 47: 43s–46s.

Burt C A V 1957 Prophylactic oophorectomy with resection of the large bowel for cancer. American Journal of Surgery 93: 77–81.

Canelo C K, Lisser H 1939 A case of arrhenoblastoma which simulated Cushing's disease. Endocrinology 24: 838–847.

Cantu J M, Rivera H, Ocampo-Campos R et al 1980 Peutz–Jeghers syndrome with feminizing Sertoli cell tumor. Cancer 46: 223–228.

Carlson G J, Nivatvongs S, Snover D C 1984 Colorectal polyps in Cowden's disease (multiple hamartoma syndrome). American Journal of Surgical Pathology 8: 763–770.

Castaldo T W, Ballon S C, Lagasse L D, Petrilli E S 1979 Reticuloendothelial neoplasia of the female genital tract. Obstetrics and Gynecology 54: 167–170.

Castolidi P, Giudici E 1955 Granuloma di Besnier-Boeck-Schaumann con localizzazioni alle salpingi. Minerva Ginecologica 7: 627–630.

Cave W T, Dunn J T 1976 Choriocarcinoma with hyperthyroidism: probable identity of the thyrotropin with human chorionic gonadotropin. Annals of Internal Medicine 85: 60–63.

Cecalupo A J, Frankel L S, Sullivan M P 1982 Pelvic and ovarian extramedullary leukemic relapse in young girls: a report of four cases and review of the literature. Cancer 50: 587–593.

Chamberlain M J, Whittaker S R F 1963 Hashimoto's disease, dermatomyositis and ovarian carcinoma. Lancet 1: 1398–1400.

Chorlton I, Karnei R F Jr, King F M, Norris H J 1974 Primary malignant reticuloendothelial disease involving the vagina, cervix and corpus uteri. Obstetrics and Gynecology 44: 735–748.

Christopherson W, Voet R, Buchsbaum H J 1985 Recurrent cervical cancer presenting as small bowel obstruction. Gynecologic Oncology 22: 109–114.

Civantos F, Rywlin A M 1972 Carcinomas with trophoblastic differentiation and secretion of chorionic gonadotrophins. Cancer 29: 789–798.

Clarke D J, Waters J, Corbett J A 1989 Adults with Prader-Willi syndrome: abnormalities of sleep and behaviour. Journal of the Royal Society of Medicine 82: 21–24.

Clendenning W E, Herdt J R, Block J B 1963 Ovarian fibromas and mesenteric cysts: their association with hereditary basal cell cancer of the skin. American Journal of Obstetrics and Gynecology 87: 1008.

Cocco A E, Conway S J 1975 Zollinger-Ellison syndrome associated with ovarian mucinous cystadenocarcinoma. New England Journal of Medicine 293: 485–486.

Cocconi G, Ceci G, Juvarra G et al 1985 Successful treatment of subacute cerebellar degeneration in ovarian carcinoma with plasmapheresis: a case report. Cancer 56: 2318–2320.

Cohen J D, Utiger R D 1970 Metastatic choriocarcinoma associated with hyperthyroidism. Journal of Endocrinology and Metabolism 30: 423–429.

Committee on Safety of Medicines 1989 Current Problems, no. 27.

Cornes J S, Stecher M 1961 Primary Crohn's disease of the colon and rectum. Gut 2: 189–201.

Cortes F M, Morris C E, Hunter R V P 1962 Polymyositis: observations in three cases. American Journal of Medical Science 243: 77–85.

Cowdell R H 1954 Sarcoidosis: with special reference to diagnosis and prognosis. Quarterly Journal of Medicine 23: 29–55.

Cramer D W, Ravnikar V A, Craighill M, Ng W G, Goldstein D P, Reilly R 1987 Müllerian aplasia associated with maternal deficiency of galactose-1-phosphate uridyl transferase. Fertility and Sterility 47: 930–934.

Cramer S F, Bruns D E 1979 Amylase producing ovarian neoplasm with pseudo-Meigs' syndrome and elevated pleural fluid amylase: case report and ultrastructure. Cancer 44: 1715–1721.

Croft P B, Wilkinson M 1965 The incidence of carcinomatous neuromyopathy in patients with various types of carcinoma. Brain 88: 427–434.

Crohn B B, Yarnis H 1958 Regional ileitis, 2nd edn. Grune & Stratton, New York, ch 5.

Crow J, McWhinney N 1979 Isolated arteritis of the cervix uteri. British Journal of Obstetrics and Gynaecology 86: 393–398.

Curth H O, Hilberg A W, Machacek G F 1962 The site and histology of the cancer associated with malignant acanthosis nigricans. Cancer 15: 364–382.

Dandia S D 1967 Rectovesical fistula following an ovarian dermoid with recurrent vesical calculus: a case report. Journal of Urology 97: 85–87.

Davidsohn I, Kovarik S, Stejskal R 1968 Immunological aspects. Influence of prognosis and treatment. In: Gentil F, Junqueira A C (eds) Ovarian cancer. UICC monograph series, vol 11. Springer Verlag, New York, pp 105–121.

Davies T F, Taliadouros G S, Catt K J, Nisula B C 1979 Assessment of urinary thyrotropin-competing activity in choriocarcinoma and thyroid disease: further evidence for human chorionic gonadotropin interacting at the thyroid cell membrane. Journal of Endocrinology and Metabolism 49: 353–357.

Dawson M A, Talbert W, Yarbro J W 1971 Hemolytic anemia associated with an ovarian tumor. American Journal of Medicine 50: 552–556.

Deaton W R, Freedman A 1957 Cushing's syndrome due to masculinovoblastoma. North Carolina Medical Journal 18: 101–105.

De Graaff J, Puyenbroek J I, Van Der Harten J J 1984 Primary mucinous adenocarcinoma of the appendix with bilateral Krukenberg tumors of the ovary and primary adenocarcinoma of the endometrium. Gynecologic Oncology 19: 358–364

Dehner L P 1973 Metastatic and secondary tumors of the vulva. Obstetrics and Gynecology 42: 47–57.

Delgado G, Smith J P 1975 Gynecological malignancy associated with nonbacterial thrombotic endocarditis (NBTE). Gynecologic Oncology 3: 205–209.

Dickersin G R, Kline I W, Scully R E 1982 Small cell carcinoma of the ovary with hypercalcemia: a report of eleven cases. Cancer 49: 188–197.

Dingley E R, Marten R H 1957 Adenocarcinoma of the ovary presenting as acanthosis nigricans. Journal of Obstetrics and Gynaecology of the British Commonwealth 64: 898–900.

Doss L L 1978 Simultaneous extramedullary plasmacytomas of the vagina and vulva: a case report and review of the literature. Cancer 41: 2468–2474.

Douvier S, Nabholtz J-M, Friedman S, Cougard P, Ferry C, Aupecle P 1989 Infectious pneumoperitoneum as an uncommon presentation of endometrial carcinoma: report of two cases. Gynecologic Oncology 33: 392–394.

Dunn H G, Meuwissen H, Livingstone C S, Pump K K 1964 Ataxia telangiectasia. Canadian Medical Association Journal 91: 1106–1118.

Egwuatu V E, Ejeckam G C, Okaro J M 1980 Burkitt's lymphoma of the vulva: case report. British Journal of Obstetrics and Gynaecology 87: 827–830.

Elstein M, Woodcock A, Buckley C H 1994 An unusual case of sarcoidosis. British Journal of Obstetrics and Gynaecology 101: 452–453.

Erlich E N, Dominguez O V, Samuels L T, Lynch D, Oberhelman H, Warner N E 1963 Aldosteronism and precocious puberty due to an ovarian androblastoma (Sertoli cell tumor). Journal of Clinical Endocrinology and Metabolism 23: 358–367.

Faber H K 1962 Meigs' syndrome with thecoma of both ovaries in a 4-year-old girl. Journal of Pediatrics 61: 769–773.

Ferenczy A 1982 Carcinoma and other malignant tumors of the cervix. In: Blaustein A (ed) Pathology of the female genital tract, 2nd edn. Springer Verlag, New York, pp 218–219.

Ferenczy A, Okagaki T, Richart R M 1971 Para-endocrine hypercalcemia in ovarian neoplasms: report of mesonephroma with hypercalcemia and review of the literature. Cancer 27: 427–433.

Fisken R A, Walker B A, Buxton P H, Jeffreys R V, Hipkin L J, White M C 1989 A pituitary thyrotrophinoma causing thyrotoxicosis and amenorrhoea: studies of α-subunit in the tumour and in blood. Journal of the Royal Society of Medicine 82: 298–299.

Fox H, Langley F A 1976 Tumours of the ovary. Heinemann, London.

Fraser I S, Shearman R P, Smith A, Russell P 1988 An association among blepharophimosis, resistant ovary syndrome, and true premature menopause. Fertility and Sterility 50: 747–751.

French W, Freund U, Carlson R W, Weil M H 1977 High output heart failure associated with pulmonary edema complicating hydatidiform mole. Archives of Internal Medicine 137: 367–369.

Fried W, Ward H P, Hopeman A R 1968 Leiomyoma and erythrocytosis: a tumor producing a factor which increases erythropoietin production. Report of a case. Blood 31: 813–816.

Frierson H F Jr, Mills S E, Innes D J Jr 1985 Malignant rhabdoid tumor of the pelvis. Cancer 55: 1963–1967.

Fukuda O, Munemura M, Tohya T, Maeyama M, Iwamasa T 1984 Massive edema of the ovary associated with hydrothorax and ascites. Gynecologic Oncology 17: 231–237.

Fung S Y, Lee K W 1985 Inappropriate antidiuretic hormone secretion associated with adenocarcinoma of the endometrium: case report. British Journal of Obstetrics and Gynaecology 92: 423–425.

Garland H G, Thomson J G 1933 Uveo-parotid tuberculosis (febris uveo-parotidea of Heerfordt). Quarterly Journal of Medicine 2: 157–177.

Gatti R A, Good R A 1971 Occurrence of malignancy in immunodeficiency diseases: a literature review, Cancer 28: 89–98.

Gatti R A, Nieberg R, Boder E 1989 Uterine tumors in ataxia-telangiectasia. Gynecologic Oncology 32: 257–260.

Gerhardsson de Verdier M, London S 1992 Reproductive factors, exogenous female hormones, and colorectal cancer by subsite. Cancer Causes and Control 3: 355–360.

Gersell D J, King T C 1988 Papillary cystadenoma of the mesosalpinx in von Hippel-Lindau disease. American Journal of Surgical Pathology 12: 145–149.

Geurkink R E, Rauter M, Bayly M A 1983 Spontaneous ileovaginal fistula caused by Crohn's disease: a case report. American Journal of Obstetrics and Gynecology 145: 107–108.

Ghio R, Haupt E, Ratti M, Boccaccio P 1981 Erythrocytosis associated with a dermoid cyst of the ovary and erythropoietic activity of the tumour fluid. Scandinavian Journal of Haematology 27: 70–74.

Gilks C B, Young R H, Aguirre P, DeLellis R A, Scully R E 1989 Adenoma malignum (minimal deviation adenocarcinoma) of the uterine cervix: a clinicopathological and immunohistochemical analysis of 26 cases. American Journal of Surgical Pathology 13: 717–729.

Golan A, Langer R, Bukovsky I, Caspi E 1989 Congenital anomalies of the Müllerian system. Fertility and Sterility 51: 747–755.

Goldberg S D, Gray R R, Cadesky K I, Mackenzie R L 1988 Oophorovesicular-colonic fistula: a rare complication of Crohn's disease. Canadian Journal of Surgery 31: 427–428.

Goldsmith C I, Hart W R 1975 Ataxia telangiectasia with ovarian gonadoblastoma and contralateral dysgerminoma. Cancer 36: 1838–1842.

Gorlin R J, Sedano H O 1971 The multiple nevoid basal cell carcinoma syndrome revisited. Birth Defects 7: 140–148.

Gough A 1938 A case of dysgerminoma of the ovary associated with masculinity. Journal of Obstetrics and Gynaecology of the British Empire 45: 799–801.

Graham R, McKee P, McGibbon D, Heyderman E 1985 Torre-Muir syndrome: an association with isolated sebaceous carcinoma. Cancer 55: 2868–2873.

Grattan C E, Hamburger J 1987 Cowden's disease in two sisters, one showing partial expression. Clinical and Experimental Dermatology 12: 360–363.

Greenlee J E, Brashear H R 1983 Antibodies to cerebellar Purkinje cells in patients with paraneoplastic cerebellar degeneration and ovarian carcinoma. Annals of Neurology 14: 609–613.

Hagenfeldt K, von Dobeln U, Hagenfeldt L 1989 Gonadal failure in young women and galactose-1-phosphate uridyl transferase activity. Fertility and Sterility 51: 177–178.

Haines M, Stallworthy J A 1952 Genital tuberculosis in the female. Journal of Obstetrics and Gynaecology of the British Empire 59: 721–747.

Hakala T, Mecklin J P, Forss M, Jarvinen H, Lehtovirta P 1991 Endometrial carcinoma in cancer family syndrome. Cancer 68: 1656–1659.

Hall D J, Dyer M L, Parker J C Jr 1985 Ovarian cancer complicated by cerebellar degeneration: a paraneoplastic syndrome. Gynecologic Oncology 21: 240–246.

Hall P A, Lemoine N R, Ryan J F 1986 Carcinoma of the gall bladder metastatic to the cervix. British Journal of Obstetrics and Gynaecology 93: 1187–1190.

Harris E N, Asherson R A, Hughes G R 1988 Antiphospholipid antibodies — autoantibodies with a difference. Annual Review of Medicine 39: 261–271.

Harris N L, Scully R E 1984 Malignant lymphoma and granulocytic sarcoma of the uterus and vagina: a clinicopathologic analysis of 27 cases. Cancer 53: 2530–2545.

Hautzer N W 1984 Primary plasmacytoma of the ovary. Gynecologic Oncology 18: 115–118.

Hayakawa T, Kameya A, Mizuno R, Noda A, Kondo T, Hirabayashi N 1984 Hyperamylasemia with papillary serous cystadenocarcinoma of the ovary. Cancer 54: 1662–1665.

Hayes M C, Scully R E 1987 Ovarian steroid cell tumors (not otherwise specified): a clinicopathological analysis of 63 cases. American Journal of Surgical Pathology 11: 835–845.

Hazleman B L, Maclennan I C, Esiri M M 1975 Lymphocyte proliferation to artery antigen as a positive diagnostic test in polymyalgia rheumatica. Annals of the Rheumatic Diseases 34: 122–127.

Heah J T 1979 Idiopathic retroperitoneal fibrosis involving the vagina: case report. British Journal of Obstetrics and Gynaecology 86: 407–410.

Henderson P H Jr 1955 Multiple migratory thrombophlebitis associated with ovarian carcinoma. American Journal of Obstetrics and Gynecology 70: 452–453.

Herick A L, McInnes G T, MacSween R N M, Goldberg A 1989 Idiopathic haemochromatosis in a young female with amenorrhoea. Journal of the Royal Society of Medicine 82: 556–558.

Herschman J M, Higgins H P 1971 Hydatidiform mole — a cause of clinical hyperthyroidism: report of two cases with evidence that the molar tissue secreted a thyroid stimulator. New England Journal of Medicine 284: 573–577.

Hidayat A A, Riddle P J 1987 Ligneous conjunctivitis: a clinicopathologic study of 17 cases. Ophthalmology 94: 949–959.

Higgins H P, Herschman J M 1978 The hyperthyroidism due to trophoblastic hormone. Clinics in Endocrinology and Metabolism 7: 167–175.

Ho K L 1979 Sarcoidosis of the uterus. Human Pathology 10: 219–222.

Hodes M E, Sisk C J, Karn R C et al 1985 An amylase producing serous cystadenocarcinoma of the ovary. Oncology 42: 242–247.

Holtz F, Hart W R 1982 Krukenberg tumors of the ovary: a clinicopathologic analysis of 27 cases. Cancer 50: 2438–2447.

Holtz G, Johnson T R Jr, Schrock M E 1979 Paraneoplastic hypercalcemia in ovarian tumors. Obstetrics and Gynecology 5: 483–487.

Horton W A, Wong V, Eldridge R 1976 Von Hippel-Lindau disease: clinical and pathological manifestations in nine families with 50 affected members. Archives of Internal Medicine 136: 769–777.

Householder M S, Zeligman I 1980 Sebaceous neoplasms associated with visceral carcinomas. Archives of Dermatology 116: 61–64.

Hoyt R E, Hamilton J F 1987 Ovarian cancer associated with the nephrotic syndrome. Obstetrics and Gynecology 70: 513–514.

Hudson C N 1970 Acquired fistulae between the intestine and the vagina. Annals of the Royal College of Surgeons of England 46: 20–40.

Hudson C N, Curling M, Potsides P, Lowe D G 1993 Paraneoplastic syndromes in patients with ovarian neoplasia. Journal of the Royal Society of Medicine 86: 202–204.

Husslein H, Breitenecker G, Tatra G 1978 Premalignant and malignant uterine changes in immunosuppressed renal transplant recipients. Acta Obstetricia et Gynecologica Scandinavica 57: 73.

Iemura K, Sonoda T, Hayakawa A et al 1991 Small cell carcinoma of the uterine cervix showing Cushing's syndrome caused by ectopic adrenocorticotropin hormone production. Japanese Journal of Clinical Oncology 21: 293–298.

Ilbery M, Lyons B, Sundaresan V 1991 Ovarian necrotizing vasculitis causing major intra-abdominal haemorrhage after IVF: case report

and literature review. British Journal of Obstetrics and Gynaecology 98: 596–599.

Imperato-McGinley J, Peterson R E, Sturla E, Dawood Y, Bar R S 1978 Primary amenorrhea associated with hirsutism, acanthosis nigricans, dermoid cysts of the ovaries and a new type of insulin resistance. American Journal of Medicine 65: 389–395.

Ismail S, Walker S M 1990 Bilateral virilizing sclerosing stromal tumours of the ovary in a pregnant woman with Gorlin's syndrome: implications for pathogenesis of ovarian stromal neoplasms. Histopathology 17: 159–163.

Issa P Y, Salem P A, Brihi E, Azoury R S 1980 Eosinophilic granuloma with involvement of the female genitalia. American Journal of Obstetrics and Gynecology 137: 608–612.

Iwasaki T, Sakuma T, Satodate R, Takano N, Sata T, Kurata T 1988 Cytomegalovirus oophoritis with cortical necrosis during remission of acute lymphatic leukemia. Acta Pathologica Japonica 38: 1069–1076.

Jeffcoate T N A 1962 The dermatology of the vulva. Journal of Obstetrics and Gynaecology of the British Commonwealth 69: 889–890.

Jensen R D, Norris H J, Fraumeni J F Jr 1974 Familial arrhenoblastoma and thyroid adenoma. Cancer 33: 218–223.

Jimerson S D 1973 Pseudo-Meigs' syndrome: an unusual case with analysis of the effusion. Obstetrics and Gynecology 42: 535–537.

Jones H W, Plymate S, Gluck F B, Miles P A, Green J F 1976 Small cell nonkeratinising carcinoma of the cervix associated with ACTH production. Cancer 38: 1629–1635.

Josse R G, Wilson D R, Heersche J N M, Mills J R F, Murray T M 1981 Hypercalcemia with ovarian carcinoma: evidence of a pathogenetic role for prostaglandins. Cancer 48: 1233–1241.

Julkunen R, Partanen S, Salaspuro M et al 1983 Gastrin-producing ovarian mucinous cystadenoma. Journal of Clinical Gastroenterology 5: 67–70.

Kahn M F, Ryckewaert A, Cannat A, Solnica J, de Seze S 1966 Systemic lupus erythematosus and ovarian dysgerminoma: remission of the systemic lupus erythematosus after extirpation of the tumour. Clinical and Experimental Immunology 1: 355–359.

Kao M S, Paulson J D, Askin F B 1975 Crohn's disease of the vulva. Obstetrics and Gynecology 46: 329–333.

Kapp D S, Kohorn E I, Merino M J, LiVolsi V A 1985 Pure dysgerminoma of the ovary with elevated serum human chorionic gonadotropin: diagnostic and therapeutic considerations. Gynecologic Oncology 20: 234–244.

Kaufman F R, Donnell G N, Roe T F, Kogut M D 1986 Gonadal function in patients with galactosemia. Journal of Inherited Metabolic Disease 9: 140–146.

Kay S 1956 Sarcoidosis of the Fallopian tubes: report of a case. Journal of Obstetrics and Gynaecology of the British Empire 63: 871–874.

Kelleher M B, Christopherson W A, Macpherson T A 1988 Disseminated granulomatous disease (BCGosis) following chemoimmunotherapy for ovarian carcinoma. Gynecologic Oncology 31: 321–326.

Kelly S E, Wojnarowska F 1989 Linear IgA disease in association with hydatidiform mole. Journal of the Royal Society of Medicine 82: 438–439.

Kelly S E, Bhogal B S, Wojnarowska F, Black M M 1988 Expression of a pemphigoid gestationis related antigen by human placenta. British Journal of Dermatology 118: 605–611.

Kepler E J, Dockerty M B, Priestley J T 1944 Adrenal-like ovarian tumor associated with Cushing's syndrome (so-called masculinovoblastoma, luteoma, hypernephroma, adrenal cortical carcinoma of the ovary). American Journal of Obstetrics and Gynecology 47: 43–62.

Kim J M, Arakawa K, McCann V 1976 Severe hyperthyroidism associated with hydatidiform mole. Anesthesiology 44: 445–448.

Kim W, Bockman R, Lemos L, Lewis J L Jr 1981 Hypercalcemia associated with epidermoid carcinoma in ovarian cystic teratoma. Obstetrics and Gynecology 57: 81s–85s.

Kingsland C R, Alderman B 1991 Crohn's disease of the vulva. Journal of the Royal Society of Medicine 84: 236–237.

Klippel M, Trenaunay P 1900 Du naevus variqueux osteo hypertrophique. Archive de General Medicine Paris 185: 641–671.

Kojiro M, Kage M, Abe H, Imamura M, Shiraisha K, Mizoguchi M 1983 Association of dysgerminoma and Gaucher's disease. Cancer 51: 712–715.

Korzets A, Nouriel H, Steiner Z, Griffel B, Kraus L, Freund U, Klajman A 1986 Resistant hypertension associated with a renin-producing ovarian Sertoli cell tumor. American Journal of Clinical Pathology 85: 242–247.

Koussidis A, Koussidou M, Dounabis A, Kiriakou K 1984 Ein Fibrothekom des Ovars mit typischem Meigs Syndrom und tumoroser Kachexie. Zentralblatt für Gynäkologie 106: 341–344.

Kremer M, Nussenson E, Steinfeld M, Zuckerman P 1984 Crohn's disease of the vulva. American Journal of Gastroenterology 79: 376–378.

Krukenberg P 1896 Ueben das Fibrosacoma Ovarii Mucocellulari (carcinomases). Archiv für Gynäkologie 50: 287–321.

Kubo O, Yamasaki N, Kamijo Y, Amano K, Kitamura K 1977 A case of HCG-producing ectopic pinealoma in a girl with precocious puberty. Neurological Surgery 5: 363–369.

Kuzma J F, King J M 1948 Dyschondroplasia with hemangiomatosis (Maffucci's syndrome) and teratoid tumor of the ovary. Archives of Pathology 46: 74–82.

Kyle J, Sinclair W Y 1969 Ileovaginal fistula complicating regional enteritis. British Journal of Surgery 56: 474–475.

Lacey C G, Morrow C P 1979 Hypercalcemia in patients with squamous cell carcinoma of the cervix. Gynecologic Oncology 7: 215–222.

Landolfi R, Storti S, Sacco F, Scribano D, Cudillo L, Leone G 1984 Platelet activation in patients with benign and malignant ovarian diseases. Tumori 70: 459–462.

Lane S, Fasano J B, Levitt A B, Brandstetter R D 1986 (letter) Spontaneous bilateral pneumothorax due to metastatic cervical carcinoma. Chest 91: 151–152.

Lashner B A, Kane S V, Hanauer S B 1989 Lack of association between oral contraceptive use and Crohn's disease: a community-based matched case-control study. Gastroenterology 97: 1442–1447.

Lathrop J C 1967 Views and reviews: malignant pelvic lymphomas. Obstetrics and Gynecology 30: 137–145.

Lavery H A 1984 Vulval dystrophies: new approaches. Clinics in Obstetrics and Gynaecology 11: 155–169.

Lavery H A, Pinkerton J H, Roberts S D, Sloan J, Walsh M 1985 Dermatomyositis of the vulva — first reported case. British Journal of Dermatology 113: 349–352.

Lawhead R A, Copeland L J, Edwards C L 1985 Bilateral ovarian hemangiomas associated with diffuse abdominopelvic hemangiomatosis. Obstetrics and Gynecology 65: 597–599.

Lawlor F, Charles-Holmes S 1988 Uterine haemangioma in Klippel-Trenaunay-Weber syndrome. Journal of the Royal Society of Medicine 81: 665–666.

Lawton F, Blackledge G, Johnson R 1985 Co-existent chylous and serous pleural effusions associated with ovarian cancer: a case report of Contarini's syndrome. European Journal of Surgical Oncology 11: 177–178.

Lee Y T, Hori J M 1971 Significance of ovarian metastasis in therapeutic oophorectomy for advanced breast cancer. Cancer 27: 1374–1378.

Leiman G, Markowitz S, Veiga-Ferreira M M, Margolius K A 1986 Renal adenocarcinoma presenting with bilateral metastases to Bartholin's glands: primary diagnosis by aspiration cytology. Diagnostic Cytopathology 2: 252–255.

Lemoine N R, Hall P A 1986 Epithelial tumors metastatic to the uterine cervix: a study of 33 cases and review of the literature. Cancer 57: 2002–2005.

Leonard D D, Deaton W R Jr 1974 Multiple sebaceous gland tumors and visceral carcinomas. Archives of Dermatology 110: 917–920.

Lester W M, Robertson D I 1981 Hypertrophic osteoarthropathy complicating metastatic ovarian adenocarcinoma. Canadian Journal of Surgery 24: 520–521, 523.

Levine E M, Barton J J, Grier E A 1982 Metastatic Crohn disease of the vulva. Obstetrics and Gynecology 60: 395–397.

Lewis R J, Ketcham A S 1973 Maffucci's syndrome: functional and neoplastic significance: case report and review of the literature. Journal of Bone and Joint Surgery American Volume 55(A): 1465–1479.

Lieberman J S, Borrero J, Urdaneta E, Wright I S 1961 Thrombophlebitis and cancer. Journal of the American Medical Association 177: 542–545.

Lieberman P H 1979 Eosinophilic granuloma and related syndromes. In: Beeson P B, McDermott W, Wyngaarden J B (eds) Cecil-Loeb Textbook of medicine, 15th edn. Saunders, Philadelphia, pp 1848–1851.

Lipsett M B, Odell W D, Rosenberg L E, Waldman T A 1964 Humoral syndromes associated with nonendocrine tumors. Annals of Internal Medicine 61: 733–756.

Lloyd K M, Dennis M 1963 Cowden's disease: a possible new syndrome complex with multiple system involvement. Annals of Internal Medicine 58: 136–142.

Lockart-Mummery H E 1972 Anal lesions of Crohn's disease. In: Clinics in gastroenterology. Saunders, Philadelphia, pp 377–382.

Lojek M A, Fer M F, Kasselberg A G et al 1980 Cushing's syndrome with small cell carcinoma of the uterine cervix. American Journal of Medicine 69: 140–144.

Long T T III, Barton T K, Draffin R, Reeves W J, McCarty K S Jr 1980 Conservative management of the Zollinger-Ellison syndrome: ectopic gastrin production by an ovarian cystadenoma. Journal of the American Medical Association 243: 1837–1839.

Longcope W T, Freiman D G 1952 A study of sarcoidosis. Medicine 31: 1–132.

Lucas J A, Kahlstorf J H, Cowan B D 1988 Multiple endocrine neoplasia — type I syndrome and hyperprolactinemia. Fertility and Sterility 50: 514–515.

Lynch H T, Lynch P M, Pester J, Fusaro R M 1981 The cancer family syndrome: rare cutaneous phenotypic linkage of Torre's syndrome. Archives of Internal Medicine 141: 607–611.

Lynch H T, Smyrk T C, Lynch P M et al 1989 Adenocarcinoma of the small bowel in Lynch syndrome II. Cancer 64: 2178–2183.

McAlpine J K, Thomson J E 1989 Hypopituitarism and empty sella due to endocarditis. Journal of the Royal Society of Medicine 82: 769–770.

McAndrew G M 1964 Haemolytic anaemia associated with ovarian teratoma. British Medical Journal 2: 1307–1308.

Maccari S, Fornaciari G, Bassi C, Beltrami M, Tinterri N, Plancher A C 1989 Contraceptive methods in the McCune-Albright syndrome. Clinical and Experimental Obstetrics and Gynecology 16: 129–130.

McGowan L, Young R H, Scully R E 1980 Peutz-Jeghers syndrome with "adenoma malignum" of the cervix: a report of two cases. Gynecologic Oncology 10: 125–133.

McKay D G, Street R B Jr, Benirschke K, Duncan C J 1953 Eosinophilic granuloma of the vulva. Surgery, Gynecology and Obstetrics 96: 437–447.

Mader M H, Friedrich E G Jr 1982 Vulvar metastasis of breast carcinoma: a case report. Journal of Reproductive Medicine 27: 169–171.

Maestu R P, Buzon L M, Fraile L et al 1979 Carcinoma de ovario como causa de fiebre de origen desconocido: a proposito de un caso. Revista Clinica Espanola 153: 65–67.

Manetta A, Abt A B, Mamourian A C et al 1987 Pelvic fibromatosis: case report and review of the literature. Gynecologic Oncology 32: 91–94.

Mantouvalos C, Metallinos C, Gouskos A 1982 Struma ovarii with Meigs' syndrome. Australian and New Zealand Journal of Obstetrics and Gynaecology 22: 101–102.

Marieb N J, Spangler S, Kashgarian M et al 1983 Cushing's syndrome secondary to ectopic cortisol production by an ovarian carcinoma. Journal of Clinical Endocrinology and Metabolism 57: 737–740.

Matsuyama M, Inoue T, Ariyoshi Y et al 1979 Argyrophil cell carcinoma of the uterine cervix with ectopic production of ACTH, beta-MSH, serotonin, histamine and amylase. Cancer 44: 1813–1823.

Maycock R L, Bertrand P, Morrison C E, Scott J H 1963 Manifestations of sarcoidosis: analysis of 145 patients with a review of nine series selected from the literature. American Journal of Medicine 35: 67–89.

Medsger T A, Dixon J A, Garwood V F 1982 Palmar fasciitis and polyarthritis associated with ovarian carcinoma. Annals of Internal Medicine 96: 424–431.

Meigs J V 1954 Pelvic tumors other than fibromas of the ovary with ascites and hydrothorax. Obstetrics and Gynecology 3: 471–486.

Meigs J V, Cass J W 1937 Fibroma of the ovary with ascites and hydrothorax. American Journal of Obstetrics and Gynecology 33: 249–267.

Menzies D N 1965 Two further cases of erythrocytosis secondary to fibromyomata. Proceedings of the Royal Society of Medicine 58: 239.

Michael C A 1967 Pelvic fibroma causing recurrent attacks of hypoglycaemia. Journal of Obstetrics and Gynaecology of the British Commonwealth 74: 301–303.

Mitchinson M J 1970 The pathology of idiopathic retroperitoneal fibrosis. Journal of Clinical Pathology 23: 681–689.

Montag T W, Murphy R E, Belinson J L 1984 Virilizing malignant lipid cell tumor producing erythropoietin. Gynecologic Oncology 19: 98–103.

Montiero J C M P, Baker G, Ferguson K M, Wiltshaw E, Munro-Neville A 1983 Ectopic production of human chorionic gonadotrophin (HCG) and human placental lactogen (HPL) by ovarian carcinoma. European Journal of Cancer and Clinical Oncology 19: 173–178.

Mordel N, Mor-Yosef S, Ben-Baruch N, Anteby S O 1989 Malignant melanoma of the uterine cervix: case report and review of the literature. Gynecologic Oncology 32: 375–380.

Morgan D R, Wells M, MacDonald R C, Johnston D 1985 Zollinger-Ellison syndrome due to a gastrin secreting ovarian mucinous cystadenoma: case report. British Journal of Obstetrics and Gynaecology 92: 867–869.

Morgello S, Schwartz E, Horwith M et al 1988 Ectopic insulin production by a primary ovarian carcinoid. Cancer 61: 800–805.

Morley J E, Jacobson R J, Melamed J, Hershman J M 1976 Choriocarcinoma as a cause of thyrotoxicosis. American Journal of Medicine 60: 1036–1040.

Morson B C 1972 Pathology of Crohn's disease. In: Clinics in gastroenterology. Saunders, Philadelphia, pp 265–277.

Mosesson M W, Colman R W, Sherry S 1968 Chronic intravascular coagulation syndrome: report of a case with special studies of an associated plasma cryoprecipitate ('cryofibrinogen'). New England Journal of Medicine 278: 815–821.

Motlik K, Starka L 1973 Adrenocortical tumor of the ovary (a case report with particular stress upon the morphological and biochemical findings). Neoplasma 20: 97–110.

Napoli V M, Wallach H 1976 Pancytopenia associated with a granulosa-cell tumor of the ovary: report of a case. American Journal of Clinical Pathology 65: 344–350.

Narita T, Takagi K 1984 Ataxia-telangiectasia with dysgerminoma of right ovary, papillary carcinoma of thyroid and adenocarcinoma of pancreas. Cancer 54: 1113–1116.

Navarro C, Corretger J M, Sancho A, Rovira J, Morales L 1985 Paraneoplastic precocious puberty: report of a new case with hepatoblastoma and review of the literature. Cancer 56: 1725–1729.

Neumann S 1991 Cowden-Syndrom mit einem Ovarialtumor (Multiple-Hamartome-Syndrom). Chirurgie 62: 629–630.

Nichols J, Warren J C, Mantz F A 1962 ACTH-Like excretion from carcinoma of the ovary. Journal of the American Medical Association 182: 713–718.

Norwood S H, Torma M J, Fontenelle L J 1981 Hyperamylasemia due to poorly differentiated carcinoma of the ovary. Archives of Surgery 116: 225–226.

Nunez C, Abboud S L, Lemon N C, Kemp J A 1983 Ovarian rhabdomyosarcoma presenting as leukemia: case report. Cancer 52: 297–300.

O'Brien P K, Wilansky D L 1981 Familial thyroid nodulation and arrhenoblastoma. American Journal of Clinical Pathology 75: 578–581.

Odell W D, Wolfsen A, Yoshimoto Y, Weitzman R, Fisher D, Hirose F 1977 Ectopic peptide synthesis: a universal concomitant of neoplasia. Transactions of the Association of American Physicians 90: 204–227.

O'Flanagan S J, Tighe B F, Egan T J, Delaney P V 1987 Meig's syndrome and pseudo-Meig's syndrome. Journal of the Royal Society of Medicine 80: 252–253.

O'Neill R T, Mikuta J J 1970 Hypoglycemia associated with serous cystadenocarcinoma of the ovary. Obstetrics and Gynecology 35: 287–289.

O'Riordan T, Gaffney E, Tormey V, Daly P 1990 Hyperamylasemia associated with progression of a serous surface papillary carcinoma. Gynecologic Oncology 36: 432–434.

Osathanondh R, Tulchinsky D, Chopra I J 1976 Total and free thyroxine and tri-iodothyronine in normal and complicated pregnancy. Journal of Clinical Endocrinology and Metabolism 42: 98–104.

Osborn R H, Bradbury J T, Yannone M E 1969 Androgen studies in a patient with lipoid-cell tumor of the ovary. Obstetrics and Gynecology 33: 666–672.

Ossias A L, Zanjani E D, Zalusky R, Estren S, Wasserman L R 1973 Case report: studies on the mechanism of erythrocytosis associated with a uterine fibromyoma. British Journal of Haematology 25: 179–185.

Otis C N, Fischer R A, Johnson N, Kelleher J F, Powell J L 1990 Histiocytosis X of the vulva: a case report and review of the literature. Obstetrics and Gynecology 75: 555–558.

Padwell A 1986 Isolated arteritis of the uterine cervix: three case reports. British Journal of Obstetrics and Gynaecology 93: 1176–1180.

Parks A G, Morson B C, Pegum J S 1965 Crohn's disease with cutaneous involvement. Proceedings of the Royal Society of Medicine 58: 241–242.

Parsons V, Rigby B 1958 Cushing's syndrome associated with adenocarcinoma of the ovary. Lancet 2: 992–994.

Patsner B, Mann W J, Chumas J 1989 Malignant mixed germ cell tumor of the ovary in a young woman with Smith-Lemli-Opitz syndrome. Gynecologic Oncology 33: 386–388.

Payne D, Muss H B, Homesley H D, Jobson V W, Baird F G 1981 Autoimmune hemolytic anemia and ovarian dermoid cysts: case report and review of the literature. Cancer 48: 721–724.

Pecorelli S, Sartori E, Favalli G, Ugazio A G, Gastaldi A 1988 Ataxia-telangiectasia and endodermal sinus tumor of the ovary: report of a case. Gynecologic Oncology 29: 240–244.

Penn I 1986 Cancers of the anogenital region in renal transplant recipients: analysis of 65 cases. Cancer 58: 611–616.

Peters W A, Andersen W A, Thornton W N Jr 1983 Dermatomyositis and co-existent ovarian cancer: a review of the compounding clinical problems. Gynecologic Oncology 15: 440–446.

Peterson M L 1971 Neoplastic diseases of the alimentary tract. In: Beeson P B, McDermott W (eds) Cecil-Loeb Textbook of medicine, 13th edn. Saunders, Philadelphia, p 1372.

Petrides M, Robertson I G, Fox H 1979 Giant cell arteritis of the female genital tract. British Journal of Obstetrics and Gynecology 86: 148–151.

Pinsonneault O, Goldstein D P 1985 Obstructing malformations of the uterus and vagina. Fertility and Sterility 44: 241–247.

Pirozynski W J 1976 Giant-cell arteritis of the uterus: report of two cases. American Journal of Clinical Pathology 65: 308–313.

Polasky N, Polasky S H, Magenheim H, Abrams N R 1965 Giant-cell arteritis: review and report of a case. Journal of the American Medical Association 191: 341–343.

Powell C S, Jones P A 1983 Carcinoma of the bladder with a metastasis in the clitoris. British Journal of Obstetrics and Gynaecology 90: 380–381.

Powell D, Singer F R, Murray T M, Minkin C, Potts T J Jr 1973 Nonparathyroid humoral hypercalcemia in patients with neoplastic diseases. New England Journal of Medicine 289: 176–181.

Pratt-Thomas H R, Kreutner A Jr, Underwood P B, Dowdeswell R H 1976 Proliferative and malignant Brenner tumors of the ovary: report of two cases, one with Meigs' syndrome, review of literature and ultrastructural comparisons. Gynecologic Oncology 4: 176–193.

Prezyna A P, Kalyanaraman U 1977 Bowen's carcinoma in vulvovaginal Crohn's disease (regional enterocolitis): report of first case. American Journal of Obstetrics and Gynecology 128: 914–916.

Puleo J G, Clarke-Pearson D L, Smith E B, Barnard D E, Creasman W T 1986 Superior vena cava syndrome associated with gynecologic malignancy. Gynecologic Oncology 23: 59–64.

Pysher T J, Hitch D C, Krous H F 1981 Bilateral juvenile granulosa cell tumors in a 4-month-old dysmorphic infant: a clinical, histologic, and ultrastructural study. American Journal of Surgical Pathology 5: 789–794.

Qizilbash A H, Trebilcock R G, Patterson M C, Lamont K G 1974 Functioning primary carcinoid tumor of the ovary: a light- and electron-microscopic study with review of the literature. American Journal of Clinical Pathology 62: 629–638.

Raggio M, Kaplan A L, Harberg J F 1983 Recurrent ovarian fibromas with basal cell nevus syndrome (Gorlin syndrome). Obstetrics and Gynecology 61: 95s–96s.

Rater C J, Selke A C, Van Epps E F 1968 Basal cell nevus syndrome. American Journal of Roentgenology Radium Therapy and Nuclear Medicine 103: 589–594.

Rhoads J E, Terrell A W 1937 Ovarian fibroma with ascites and hydrothorax (Meig's syndrome). Journal of the American Medical Association 109: 1684–1687.

Ribaux C, Gloor E 1988 Ovarite necrosante a cytomegalovirus. Schweiz Medizinische Wochenschrift 119: 160–163.

Ribeiro G, Hughesdon P, Wiltshaw E 1988 Squamous carcinoma arising in dermoid cysts and associated with hypercalcemia: a clinicopathologic study of six cases. Gynecologic Oncology 29: 222–230.

Ridley C M 1975 The vulva. Saunders, Philadelphia.

Rieke J W, Kapp D S 1988 Successful management of malignant pericardial effusion in metastatic squamous cell carcinoma of the uterine cervix. Gynecologic Oncology 31: 338–351.

Rivett J D, Robinson J M 1972 Hypercalcaemia associated with an ovarian carcinoma of mesonephromatous type. Journal of Obstetrics and Gynaecology of the British Commonwealth 79: 1047–1052.

Robboy S J, Norris H J, Scully R E 1975 Insular carcinoid primary in the ovary: a clinicopathologic analysis of 48 cases. Cancer 36: 404–418.

Rohatgi M, Mukherjee A K 1973 Tubo-intestinal fistula. Journal of Obstetrics and Gynaecology of the British Commonwealth 80: 379–380.

Rosenberg L, Hennekens C H, Rosner B, Belanger C, Rothman K J, Speizer F E 1981 Early menopause and the risk of myocardial infarction. American Journal of Obstetrics and Gynecology 139: 47–51.

Rosenfeld S I, Steck W, Breen J L 1989 Sarcoidosis of the female genital tract: a case presentation and survey of the world literature. International Journal of Gynaecology and Obstetrics 28: 373–380.

Rosner J M, Conte M F, Horita S, Forsham P H 1964 In vivo and in vitro production of testosterone by a lipid cell ovarian tumour. American Journal of Medicine 37: 638–642.

Roth L M, Nicholas T R, Ehrlich C E 1979 Juvenile granulosa cell tumor: a clinicopathologic study of three cases with ultrastructural observations. Cancer 44: 2194–2205.

Rowland Payne C M E 1981 Newly recognized syndrome in the neck: Horner's syndrome with ipsilateral vocal cord and phrenic nerve. Journal of the Royal Society of Medicine 74: 814–818.

Rulon D B, Helwig E B 1974 Cutaneous sebaceous neoplasms. Cancer 33: 82–102.

Russell P, Bannatyne P 1989 Surgical pathology of the ovaries. Churchill Livingstone, Edinburgh.

Salmon U J 1934 Benign pelvic tumors associated with ascites and pleural effusion. Journal of the Mount Sinai Hospital 1: 169–172.

Samaan N A, Smith J P, Rutledge F N, Schultz P N 1976 The significance of measurement of human placental lactogen, human chorionic gonadotropin, and carcinoembryonic antigen in patients with ovarian carcinoma. American Journal of Obstetrics and Gynecology 126: 186–189.

Sandler R S, Wurzelmann J I, Lyles C M 1992 Oral contraceptive use and the risk of inflammatory bowel disease. Epidemiology 3: 374–378.

Sandvei R, Bang G 1991 Sarcoidosis of the uterus. Acta Obstetricia et Gynecologica Scandinavica 70: 165–167.

Schiller H M, Madge G E 1970 Reticulum cell sarcoma presenting as a vulvar lesion. Southern Medical Journal 63: 471–472.

Schlagenhaufer F 1902 Uber das metastatische Ovarialkarzinom nach Krebs das Magens, Darmes und anderer Bachorgane. Wochenschrift Geburtshilfe und Gynäkologie 15: 485 (cited by Blaustein, 1982).

Schofield P M, Kirsop B A, Reginald P, Harington M 1985 Ovarian carcinoma presenting as pyrexia of unknown origin. Postgraduate Medical Journal 61: 177–178.

Schreiber M M 1963 Vulvar von Recklinghausen's disease. Archives of Dermatology 88: 320–321.

Schulman D, Beck L S, Roberts I M, Schwartz A M 1987 Crohn's disease of the vulva. American Journal of Gastroenterology 82: 1328–1330.

Schur P H 1979 Systemic lupus erythematosus. In: Beeson P B, McDermott W Y, Wyngaarden J B (eds) Cecil-Loeb Textbook of medicine, 15th edn. Saunders, Philadelphia, pp 174–180.

Scully R E 1970 Sex cord tumor with annular tubules: a distinctive ovarian tumor of the Peutz–Jeghers syndrome. Cancer 25: 1107–1121.

Scully R E 1982 Sex cord stromal tumors. In: Blaustein A (ed) Pathology of the female genital tract, 2nd edn. Springer Verlag, New York, pp 598–599.

Scully R E, Galdabini J J, McNeely B U 1978 Case records of the Massachusetts General Hospital. Case 13 — 1978. Disseminated intravascular coagulation with endometrioid carcinoma of the ovary. New England Journal of Medicine 298: 786–792.

Shane J M, Naftolin F 1975 Aberrant hormone activity by tumors of gynaecologic importance. American Journal of Obstetrics and Gynecology 121: 133–143.

Shiel W C Jr, Prete P E, Jason M, Andrews B S 1985 Palmar fasciitis and arthritis with ovarian and non-ovarian carcinomas: new syndrome. American Journal of Medicine 79: 640–644.

Sherry M R, Boghossian H M, Duffell D, Freel R, Gonzales J C 1982 Tumor-induced hypoglycemia: a result of ectopic insulin production. Cancer 49: 1920–1923.

Siegler A M 1983 Hysterosalpingography. Fertility and Sterility 40: 139–158.

Siegman-Igra Y, Flatau E, Deligdish L 1977 Chronic diffuse intravascular coagulation (DIC) in nonmetastatic ovarian cancer: report of a case and review of the literature. Gynecologic Oncology 5: 92–100.

Simon G C, Delavierre P 1981 Demons-Meigs' syndrome associated with a seminoma of the ovary (Syndrome de Demons-Meigs au cours d'un seminome ovarien). Semaine des Hopitaux de Paris 57: 653–656.

Simon N L, Mazur M T, Shingleton H M 1985 Pelvic fibromatosis: an unusual gynecologic tumor. Obstetrics and Gynecology 65: 767–769.

Skrabanck P, McParthin J, Powell D 1980 Tumor hypercalcemia and "ectopic hyperparathyroidism". Medicine 59: 262–282.

Slotky B, Shrivastav R, Lee B M 1982 Massive edema of the ovary. Obstetrics and Gynecology 59: 92s–94s.

Smith F R 1931 Neurofibroma of the ovary associated with von Recklinghausen's disease. American Journal of Cancer 15: 859–862.

Socinski M A, Ershler W B, Belinson J L 1983 Coexistent breast and vaginal granulocytic sarcoma. Gynecologic Oncology 16: 299–304.

Solidoro G, Del Gaudio G A 1991 Le cisti di echinococco dell'ovario. Descrizione di un caso. Minerva Chirurgica (Torino) 46: 571–575.

Solomon S D, Maurer K H 1983 Association of dermatomyositis and dysgerminoma in a 16-year-old patient. Arthritis and Rheumatology 26: 572–573.

Soutter W P, Norman R, Green-Thompson R W 1981 The management of choriocarcinoma causing severe thyrotoxicosis: two case reports. British Journal of Obstetrics and Gynaecology 88: 938–943.

Spigelman A D, Murday V, Phillips R K 1989 Cancer and the Peutz-Jeghers syndrome. Gut 30: 1588–1590.

Starink T M 1984 Cowden's disease: analysis of fourteen new cases. Journal of the American Academy of Dermatology 11: 1127–1141.

Steinberg D M, Cooke W T, Alexander-Williams J 1973 Abscess and fistulae in Crohn's disease. Gut 14: 865–869.

Steven M M, Mackay I R, Carnegie P R, Bhathal P S, Anderson R M 1982 Cerebellar cortical degeneration with ovarian carcinoma. Postgraduate Medical Journal 58: 47–51.

Stewart A F, Romero R, Schwartz P E, Kohorn E I, Broadus A E 1982 Hypercalcemia associated with gynaecologic malignancies: biochemical characterization. Cancer 49: 2389–2394.

Stockdale A D, Leader M, Phillips R H, Henry K 1986 The carcinoid syndrome and multiple hormone secretion associated with a carcinoid tumour of the uterine cervix: case report. British Journal of Obstetrics and Gynaecology 93: 397–401.

Summers P R, Biswas M K, Boulware D W, Green L, Herrera E H, O'Quinn A G 1991 A case report of giant cell arteritis of the uterus and adnexa. American Journal of Obstetrics and Gynecology 164: 540–542.

Taggart A J, Iveson J M, Wright V 1984 Shoulder-hand syndrome and symmetrical arthralgia in patients with tubo-ovarian carcinoma. Annals of the Rheumatic Diseases 43: 391–393.

Talerman A 1982 Mesenchymal tumors and malignant lymphoma of the ovary. In: Blaustein A (ed) Pathology of the female genital tract, 2nd edn. Springer Verlag, New York, pp 561–580.

Tamaya T, Ohno Y, Fujimoto J, Nakata Y, Sato S, Okada H 1986 Huge intraabdominal fibromatosis on the posterior wall of uterus: a case report. Gynecologic Oncology 24: 129–134.

Tamimi H K, Bolen J W 1984 Enchondromatosis (Ollier's disease) and ovarian juvenile granulosa cell tumor: a case report and review of the literature. Cancer 53: 1605–1608.

Taraszewski R, Rosman P M, Knight C A, Cloney D J 1991 Small cell carcinoma of the ovary. Gynecologic Oncology 41: 149–151.

Taylor A B 1960 Sarcoidosis of the uterus. Journal of Obstetrics and Gynaecology of the British Empire 67: 32–35.

Taylor S C, Baker E, Grossman M E 1991 Nodular vulvar amyloid as a presentation of systemic amyloidosis. Journal of the American Academy of Dermatology 24: 139.

Teshima H, Kitamura H, Mizoguchi Y et al 1988 Immunohistochemical and immunoelectron microscopic study of an amylase-producing, CA19–9 positive ovarian mucinous cystadenocarcinoma. Gynecologic Oncology 30: 372–380.

Tham S N, Choong H L 1992 Primary tuberculous chancre in a renal transplant patient. Journal of the American Academy of Dermatology 26: 342–344.

Tindall J G, Rea T H, Shulman I, Quismorio F P Jr 1981 Herpes gestationis with hydatidiform mole: immunologic studies. Archives of Dermatology 117: 510–512.

Todesco S, Terribile V, Borsatti A, Mantero F 1975 Primary aldosteronism due to a malignant ovarian tumor. Journal of Clinical Endocrinology and Metabolism 41: 809–819.

Tschang T P, Poulos P, Ho C K, Kuo T T 1976 Multiple sebaceous adenomas and internal malignant disease: a case report with chromosomal analysis. Human Pathology 7: 589–594.

Tsuji S, Matsuoka Y, Suzuki Y et al 1992 Turner's syndrome associated with Hashimoto's thyroiditis and sarcoidosis: a case report. Annals of Internal Medicine 31: 131–133.

Tuder R M 1992 Vulvar destruction by malignant lymphoma. Gynecologic Oncology 45: 52–57.

Tuffnell D, Buchan P C 1991 Crohn's disease of the vulva in childhood. British Journal of Clinical Practice 45: 159–160.

Twiggs L B, Morrow C P, Schlaerth J B 1979 Acute pulmonary complications of molar pregnancy. American Journal of Obstetrics and Gynecology 135: 189–194.

Twombley G H, Di Palma S 1951 Growth and spread of cancer of cervix uteri. American Journal of Roentgenology 65: 691–697.

Vaitukaitis J L 1974 Human chorionic gonadotropin as a tumor marker. Annals of Clinical and Laboratory Science 4: 276–280.

Van Dam P A, Irvine L, Lowe D G et al 1992 Carcinoma in episiotomy scars. Gynecologic Oncology 44: 96–100.

Verducci M A, Malkasian G D Jr, Friedman S J, Winkelmann R K 1984 Gynecologic carcinoma associated with dermatomyositis-polymyositis. Obstetrics and Gynecology 64: 695–698.

Von Meyer-Hofmann G, Schwarzhopf W, Hartmann H 1960 Spontaneous hypoglycaemia with extrapancreatic tumours. Deutsche Medizinische Wochenschrift 85: 2106–2112.

Wakefield A J, Sawyerr A M, Hudson M, Dhillon A P, Pounder R E 1991 Smoking, the oral contraceptive pill, and Crohn's disease. Digestive Diseases and Sciences 36: 1147–1150.

Walton B J, Morain W D, Baughman R D, Jordan A, Crichlow R W 1986 Cowden's disease: a further indication for prophylactic mastectomy. Surgery 99: 82–86.

Weber G, Stetter H, Pliess G, Stickl H 1970 Assoziiertes Vorkommen von eruptiven Keratoacanthomen, Tuben carcinom und Paramyeloblastenleukemie. Archiv für Klinische und Experimentelle Dermatologie 238: 107–119.

Weiss D B, Aldor A, Aboulafia Y 1975 Erythrocytosis due to erythropoietin-producing uterine fibromyoma. American Journal of Obstetrics and Gynecology 122: 358–360.

Wheeler J E 1982 Pathology of the Fallopian tube. In: Blaustein A (ed) Pathology of the female genital tract, 2nd edn. Springer Verlag, New York, pp 401–403.

Winslow R C, Funkhouser J W 1968 Views and reviews: sarcoidosis of the female reproductive organs: report of a case. Obstetrics and Gynecology 32: 285–289.

Wittich A C, Morales H, Braeuer N R 1982 Tubocutaneous fistula. American Journal of Obstetrics and Gynecology 144: 109–110.

Witwer M W, Farmer M F, Wand J S, Solomon L S 1977 Extensive actinomycosis associated with an intrauterine contraceptive device. American Journal of Obstetrics and Gynecology 128: 913–914.

Wlodarski F M, Trainer T D 1975 Granulomatous oophoritis and salpingitis associated with Crohn's disease of the appendix. American Journal of Obstetrics and Gynecology 122: 527–528.

Woodruff J D, Novak E R 1960 The Krukenberg tumor: study of 48 cases from the ovarian tumor registry. Obstetrics and Gynecology 15: 351–360.

Wright J P 1992 Factors influencing first relapse in patients with Crohn's disease. Journal of Clinical Gastroenterology 15: 12–16.

Wrigley P F, Malpas J S, Turnbull A L, Jenkins G C, McArt A 1971 Secondary polycythaemia due to a uterine fibromyoma producing erythropoietin. British Journal of Haematology 21: 551–555.

Yagi C, Miyata J, Hanai J, Ogawa M, Ueda G 1986 Hyperamylasemia associated with endometrioid carcinoma of the ovary: case report and immunohistochemical study. Gynecologic Oncology 25: 250–255.

Yell J A 1991 Grzybowski's generalized eruptive keratoacanthoma. Journal of the Royal Society of Medicine 84: 170–171.

Young R E, Welch W R, Dickersin G R, Scully R E 1982 Ovarian sex cord tumor with annular tubules: review of 74 cases including 27 with Peutz-Jeghers syndrome and 4 with adenoma malignum of the cervix. Cancer 50: 1384–1402.

Young R H, Scully R E 1985 Ovarian metastases from cancer of the lung: problems in interpretation — a report of seven cases. Gynecologic Oncology 21: 337–350.

Young R H, Scully R E 1987 Ovarian steroid cell tumors associated with Cushing's syndrome: a report of three cases. International Journal of Gynecological Pathology 6: 40–48.

Young R H, Scully R E 1988 Mucinous ovarian tumors associated with mucinous adenocarcinomas of the cervix: a clinicopathological analysis of 16 cases. International Journal of Gynecological Pathology 7: 99–111.

Young R H, Scully R E 1991 Malignant melanoma metastatic to the ovary: a clinicopathologic analysis of 20 cases. American Journal of Surgical Pathology 15: 849–860.

Young R H, Dickersin G R, Scully R E 1983 A distinctive ovarian sex cord-stromal tumor causing sexual precosity in the Peutz-Jeghers syndrome. American Journal of Surgical Pathology 7: 233–243.

Young R H, Jackson A, Wells M 1994 Ovarian metastasis from thyroid carcinoma 12 years after partial thyroidectomy mimicking struma ovarii: report of a case. International Journal of Gynecological Pathology 13: 181–185.

Yutani C, Maeda H, Nakajima H, Takeuchi N, Kimura M, Kitamura H 1982 Primary ovarian lymphomas associated with Meigs' syndrome: a case report. Acta Cytologica 26: 44–48.

Zachwiej E, Hatys-Skirzynska H, Szamborski J 1956 Sarkoioza macicy. Ginekologia Polska 28: 655 (cited by Ho, 1979).

Zemke E E, Herrel W E 1941 Bilateral granulosa cell tumors: successful removal from a child of fourteen weeks of age. American Journal of Obstetrics and Gynecology 41: 704–707.

Zetzel L 1980 Fertility, pregnancy and idiopathic inflammatory bowel disease. In: Kirsner J B, Shorter R G (eds) Inflammatory bowel disease, 2nd edn. Lea & Febiger, Philadelphia, pp 241–253.

Zinkham W H 1976 Multifocal eosinophilic granuloma: natural history, etiology and management. American Journal of Medicine 60: 457–463.

Zosmer A, Kogan S, Frumkin A, Dagni R, Lifschitz-Mercer B 1992 Unsuspected involvement of the female genitalia in pemphigus vulgaris. European Journal of Obstetrics Gynecology and Reproductive Biology 47: 260–263.

40. Pathology of abnormal sexual development

Stanley J. Robboy   Peter F. Bernhardt   William R. Welch

INTRODUCTION

New insights into the biology of sexual development and advances in chromosome analysis have led to early identification and prompt treatment of the intersexual patient which permit the individual to lead a more normal life. Based on these advances, a classification of abnormal sexual development has been developed which correlates the gonadal and genital anatomy with the chromosomal findings and specific genetic or metabolic defects (Welch & Robboy, 1981; Scully, 1991) (Table 40.1). This permits an integrated approach to this complex group of disorders according to the manner by which patients present as well as on the pathophysiological basis of the defect. The classification also groups patients who are at high risk for development of gonadal neoplasia.

OVERVIEW OF EMBRYOLOGY IN ABNORMAL SEXUAL DEVELOPMENT

In humans and other mammals, the karyotype 'XY' genetically defines the sex as male, while 'XX' defines the female sex. Sex is determined by the presence or absence of a signal from a substance called the testis-determining factor (TDF) found on the Y chromosome. Testes are formed if this gene is expressed by the embryo prior to the differentiation of the urogenital ridge. Further male development occurs under the influence of hormones secreted later by the testes (Fig. 40.1). In the absence of testis-determining factor, the gonads differentiate as ovaries and the embryo develops as a female. The timely expression of testis-determining factor is critical to the development of male sex; in the absence of timely expression of this factor, the embryo develops a female phenotype by 'default', regardless of genetic sex (McLaren, 1991).

Extensive efforts have been expended during the past two decades to identify the testis-determining factor and its products. Several candidates, such as H-Y antigen, have been proposed and later discarded. The current can-

Table 40.1 Classification of intersexual disorders

Disorders associated with a normal chromosome constitution
Female pseudohermaphroditism
  Adrenogenital syndrome (testosterone overproduction due to adrenocorticoid insufficiency)
    21α-hydroxylase deficiency
    11β-hydroxylase deficiency
  Maternal ingestion of progestins or androgens
  Maternal virilizing tumour
Male pseudohermaphroditism
  Gonadal defects
    Testicular regression syndrome (gonadal destruction)
    Leydig cell agenesis
      Defective hCG-LH receptor
    Defects in testosterone synthesis
      Testosterone and adrenocorticoid insufficiency
        20,22-desmolase deficiency
        3β-hydroxylase dehydrogenase deficiency
        17α-hydroxylase deficiency
      Testosterone insufficiency only
        17,20-desmolase deficiency
        17β-hydroxysteroid (17-ketosteroid reductase) dehydrogenase deficiency
    Persistent Müllerian duct syndrome (defect in Müllerian inhibiting system)
  End-organ defects
    Disordered androgen receptor binding
      Androgen insensitivity syndrome (testicular feminization)
      Incomplete androgen insensitivity syndrome (Reifenstein's syndrome)
    Disordered testosterone metabolism
      5α-reductase deficiency

Disorders associated with an abnormal sex chromosome constitution
Sexual ambiguity infrequent
  Klinefelter's syndrome
  Turner's syndrome
  XX male syndrome
  Pure gonadal dysgenesis (some forms)
Sexual ambiguity frequent
  Mixed gonadal dysgenesis (MGD), including:
    Pure gonadal dysgenesis (some forms)
    Dysgenetic male pseudohermaphroditism
  True hermaphroditism

'Idiopathic' or 'unclassified' conditions exist within each major category. We assume that each category of male pseudohermaphroditism with defects in specific protein products or receptors has forms where the abnormality is total or partial, or where the defect results from a qualitatively abnormal structure.

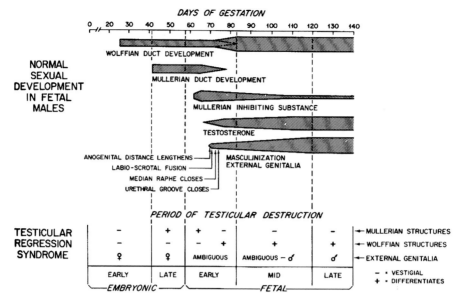

Fig. 40.1 Normal sexual development in the male and application in testicular regression syndrome. (Reprinted from Welch & Robboy, 1981, with permission of Pediatric Andrology.)

didate is a gene called SRY (sex-determining region Y), located in region 1A1 adjacent to the pseudoautosomal pairing region at the distal end of the short arm of the Y chromosome (Sinclair et al, 1990). It encodes for a DNA binding protein, the binding activity product of which is believed to regulate sexual differentiation (Harley et al, 1992). Evidence supporting this thesis includes:

- the SRY gene is absent from the normal X chromosome
- the SRY gene is present on the X chromosome of 'sex reversed' XX human males (Sinclair et al, 1990)
- the homologous gene in the mouse is initially expressed just before sexual differentiation normally occurs (Gubbay et al, 1990)
- genetic splicing of the SRY gene into the chromosomally female embryo causes it to develop as a male (Koopman et al, 1991).

During the development of both male and female human embryos, the primordial germ cells, characterized by large clear cells with vesicular nuclei, migrate from the yolk sac to the urogenital ridges via the hindgut approximately three weeks after fertilization. The mesodermal epithelium on the medial surface of the urogenital ridge begins to proliferate, resulting in the epithelium of the eventual gonad, while the gonads themselves begin to differentiate. In males, the testis is anatomically distinct with early tubular formation and immature Sertoli cells by day 44. In females, ovarian differentiation, characterized by the development of primordial follicles, begins some five weeks later. The initial stages of both testicular and ovarian development appear independent of whether the

primordial germ cells are present or absent in the gonad or have proliferated normally (McCoshen, 1982).

Once the male pathway of development has begun, two hormones produced by the fetal testis then control the differentiation of the male phenotype. The first is Müllerian inhibiting substance, a large glycoprotein which the Sertoli cells produce early in fetal life (Donahoe & Berkowitz, 1987; Kuroda et al, 1991). The gene responsible for this substance is on chromosome 19. The primary function of Müllerian inhibiting substance is to cause regression of the Müllerian (paramesonephric) ducts in the male fetus. In the female, Müllerian inhibiting substance is produced in insignificant amounts during fetal life (as there are no testes) and in the absence of this substance the Müllerian ducts develop passively to form the Fallopian tubes, uterus and wall of the vagina. Müllerian inhibiting substance is first secreted in effective amounts 56–62 days after fertilization, and the process of Müllerian regression is normally completed by about day 77, after which time the Müllerian tissue is no longer sensitive to Müllerian inhibiting substance. The Müllerian inhibiting substance receptor in Müllerian tissue appears to reside in stromal cells (Tsuji et al, 1992) and the mechanism by which Müllerian tissue loses its sensitivity to Müllerian inhibiting substance is not yet understood. Müllerian inhibiting substance has a local action, and inhibits development of the ipsilateral Fallopian tube. To prevent development of both the uterus and vagina, both testes must secrete adequate amounts of Müllerian inhibiting substance. Thus, a patient with a testis and a contralateral streak, ovary or ovotestis generally has a uterus and vagina and a single Fallopian tube on the side with the streak or ovary.

Additional functions of Müllerian inhibiting substance have recently been discovered. In the female, ovarian granulosa cells begin producing Müllerian inhibiting substance only after the Müllerian-derived tissues (Fallopian tubes, uterus and vagina) are well developed and no longer susceptible to the regressive effects of Müllerian inhibiting substance. Serum levels of Müllerian inhibiting substance in girls rise slowly after birth from nearly undetectable levels until they reach a plateau after 10 years of life equivalent to the adult male serum concentration. In contrast, the male serum Müllerian inhibiting substance concentration is relatively high at birth, peaks at 4–12 months of age, and then falls progressively to a baseline low adult level by about 10 years of age (Hudson et al, 1990). A major action of Müllerian inhibiting substance in the young female may be to inhibit oocyte meiosis in the developing follicle (Coutilainen & Miller, 1989). Dramatically high levels of Müllerian inhibiting substance have been found in women with ovarian sex cord tumours (Gustafson et al, 1992). Secondary actions of Müllerian inhibiting substance in males may be to initiate testicular descent (Yamanaka et al, 1991) and to regulate germ cell maturation (Taketo et al, 1991).

The second hormone the fetal testis secretes is testosterone. This androgenic steroid, which is critical for male development, is required for the Wolffian (mesonephric) duct to differentiate into epididymis, vas deferens and seminal vesicle. Leydig cells appear in the testis circa day 54–64 and shortly thereafter begin to produce testosterone. Leydig cell activity is probably stimulated by increased production of chorionic gonadotrophin by the placenta at that time. Testosterone acts locally on the ipsilateral Wolffian duct by binding to a specific high affinity intracellular receptor protein. This receptor hormone complex binds DNA to regulate transcription of specific genes which govern further development. In the absence of a testis or inability of a testis to produce testosterone in adequate amounts by 10–12 weeks, or insensitivity of the Wolffian duct anlage to testosterone, the epididymis, vas deferens and seminal vesicle do not differentiate. Only rarely are abnormally elevated testosterone levels reached sufficiently early during embryogenesis in a female fetus to cause the Wolffian duct to differentiate into definitive male organs (androgen administration to the mother during pregnancy, or congenital adrenogenital syndrome).

Testosterone also acts as a prohormone for dihydrotestosterone, the substance ultimately responsible for initiating masculinization of the external genitalia and differentiation of the prostate. The enzyme 5α-reductase, found in the tissues of the external genitalia and urogenital sinus, mediates the conversion of testosterone to dihydrotestosterone. Dihydrotestosterone causes:

1. the genital tubercle to enlarge and form the glans penis

2. the genital folds to enlarge and fuse to form the penile shaft with migration of the urethral orifice along the lower border of the shaft to the tip of the glans
3. the genital swellings to fuse and form a scrotum
4. the urogenital sinus tissues to differentiate into prostate.

Failure of the external genitalia to develop in males in the presence of testes may be due to a lack of adequate testosterone secretion into the systemic circulation, deficient enzyme (5α-reductase) at the end-organ level to convert testosterone to dihydrotestosterone, or complete end-organ insensitivity (testicular feminization). Lesser degrees of deficiency or end-organ insensitivity may result in partial male development characterized by a small penis, hypospadias, deficient formation of the scrotum, or a persistent urogenital sinus (vaginal opening into urethra). The effects of dihydrotestosterone begin about day 70, with fusion of the labioscrotal folds and closure of the median raphe, and continue at day 74 with closure of the urethral groove. External genital development is complete by day 120–140 (18th–20th week).

Finally, female internal organs and external genitalia develop in the absence of hormones secreted by the fetal ovary, and differentiate even when gonads are absent. Unless interrupted by the regressive influence of Müllerian inhibiting substance, differentiation of the Müllerian ducts proceeds cephalocaudally to form Fallopian tubes, a uterus and a vagina. In the absence of the masculinizing effect of dihydrotestosterone, the undifferentiated external genital anlage develops into the vulva. The genital tubercle develops into the clitoris, the genital folds into the labia minora, and the genital swellings into the labia majora. Thus, the infant with ovaries or streak gonads has female internal and external genitalia at birth. Only if a female fetus has systemically elevated levels of androgens prior to the 10th–12th week of gestation does any degree of internal male development occur. In such cases the external genitalia may appear ambiguous or may resemble that of a normal phenotypic male; the vagina in these instances opens into the membranous portion of the urethra. If the androgens are not elevated until after the 20th week, by which time the external genitalia have fully formed, the only virilizing effect is an enlarged clitoris.

GENDER IDENTIFICATION DISORDERS WITH A NORMAL CHROMOSOME CONSTITUTION

Female pseudohermaphroditism

Female pseudohermaphroditism occurs as a result of relative androgen excess in utero in an individual with two ovaries and two X chromosomes (46,XX). The elevated level of androgen present during embryogenesis usually results in genital ambiguity and may result in the appearance of a phenotypic male.

Adrenogenital syndrome

Congenital adrenal hyperplasia, unlike all other conditions responsible for the appearance of ambiguous genitalia in the newborn, may be life threatening because of a lack of synthesis of specific adrenal steroids. Prompt diagnosis and institution of appropriate therapy are therefore essential. With early treatment normal external genitalia and fertility can be achieved. The manifestations of the adrenogenital syndrome in the XX individual are most easily summarized through an understanding of the biosynthetic pathways of mineralocorticoid, glucocorticoid, and sex steroids (Fig. 40.2). Two enzymes, 21-hydroxylase and 11β-hydroxylase, participate in the formation of the glucocorticoids, desoxycorticosterone and cortisol, and the mineralocorticoid, aldosterone, but not of testosterone or the oestrogens, oestrone or oestradiol. Deficiency of either enzyme in the 46,XX female leads to elevated ACTH products and hence elevated levels of testosterone and other strongly androgenic intermediates, which may result in sexual ambiguity or marked virilization of the newborn's external genitalia (New, 1992). 3β-hydroxysteroid dehydrogenase is required for testosterone formation. In its absence, the principal androgen to form is the weak androgen, dehydroepiandrosterone (DHEA), which has one-twentieth the potency of testosterone. Patients with deficiency of this enzyme, therefore, show only signs of mild virilization, usually clitoral hypertrophy but with no labial fusion or anterior displacement of the urethral orifice.

21-hydroxylase deficiency is inherited as an autosomal recessive trait due to a lesion of the gene coding for cytochrome P-450c21. It accounts for more than 95% of cases of congenital adrenal hyperplasia, occurring once in 50 000 births. Heterozygote carriers can be identified through use of ACTH stimulation. Present data suggests that a series of allelic genes on the short arm of chromosome 6, between the HLA-B and -DR loci, code for the 21-hydroxylase enzyme and that these allelic variants, including rearrangements, deletions or point mutations, explain the occurrence of the wide variation in symptomatology observed in these patients (Morel, 1991; Strachan & White, 1991). The extent to which signs of virilization evolve depends upon at which time during fetal life the disease began. If the onset was after the 16th week of gestation, the clitoris may be enlarged; if androgen excess occurs earlier, the vagina and urethra may open into a common urogenital sinus. More marked clitoral enlargement and an opening of the urogenital sinus at the clitoral base may mimic penile hypospadias and suggest an even earlier temporal effect. On occasion the changes have been of such severity that the female infants have been misdiagnosed as cryptorchid males with or without hypospadias.

Males have no evidence of genital ambiguity but may have an enlarged phallus and a hyperpigmented rugated scrotum. Bilateral testicular nodules, composed of interstitial cells resembling Leydig cells or cells of adrenal rest origin, occasionally develop (Fig. 40.3).

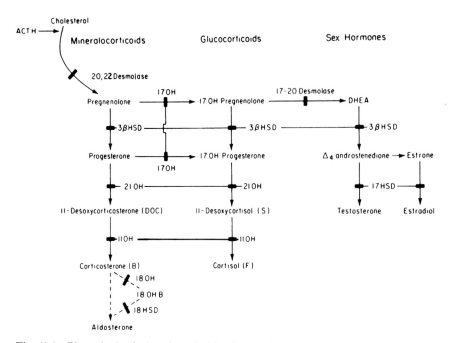

Fig. 40.2 Biosynthesis of mineralocorticoids, glucocorticoids and sex steroids. (Reprinted from Saenger et al, 1981, with permission of Pediatric Andrology)

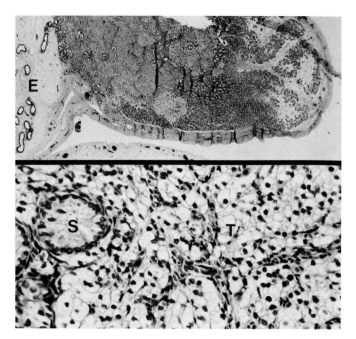

Fig. 40.3 Interstitial cell tumour of the testis in a 4-year-old infant with adrenogenital syndrome. The tumour cells (T), which are illustrated at high magnification adjacent to immature seminiferous tubules (S) in the inset, resemble adrenocortical cells more closely than Leydig cells. The epididymis (E) is adjacent to the testis. (H & E × 16, × 350). (Reprinted from Welch & Robboy, 1981, with permission of Pediatric Andrology.)

Maternal ingestion of progestins or androgens

Maternal ingestion of synthetic progestins was implicated as a cause of female pseudohermaphroditism in the late 1950s when such treatment was employed for threatened or habitual abortion; subsequently, progestins have also been implicated in the development of hypospadias in male offspring. Most cases of female pseudohermaphroditism in this category developed after maternal ingestion of Ethisterone (17α-ethinyl-testosterone) or Norlution (17α-ethinyl-19-nortestosterone), but occasionally after the ingestion of Enovid, diethylstilboestrol, androgens, or after the intramuscular administration of progesterone. Masculinization usually consists of phallic enlargement and variable degrees of labioscrotal fusion, depending on the time during gestation when the therapy was administered. Although the degree of masculinization is usually less than that associated with the adrenogenital syndrome, the sexual ambiguity in female infants has been of such severity in some instances as to result in male sex assignment. The degree of virilization does not progress with age. The gonads and internal genital organs are unaffected, and ovulation, menstruation and normal secondary female characteristics appear at puberty.

Maternal virilizing tumours

A variety of benign and malignant tumours, primary as well as metastatic to the ovary have been associated with virilization of the mother and her female offspring. The luteoma of pregnancy is the most common lesion that causes maternal virilization during pregnancy. The pregnancy luteoma is a benign hyperplastic lesion of the ovary that is most often encountered as an incidental finding at the time of caesarean section or postpartum sterilization, usually in women who are multiparous (Clement, 1993). Elevated levels of hCG are thought to induce hyperplasia of theca-lutein or stroma-lutein cells. A small percentage of the female infants have become masculinized, with mild enlargement of the clitoris and occasionally minimal degrees of labioscrotal fusion or rugate, hyperpigmented ('scrotal') labia. The nature of these changes indicates that the ovarian nodules do not function until the second half of gestation, which is in accord with the occasional onset of masculinization in the mother during the third trimester.

At operation, one and often both maternal ovaries are enlarged by one or more soft, yellow-brown nodules that are well circumscribed but not encapsulated. Although most are less than 2 cm in diameter, they may be as large as 20 cm in greatest dimension. On microscopical examination, the nodules consist of large, polygonal cells with granular, eosinophilic cytoplasm, which are smaller and more eosinophilic than the luteinized granulosa cells of the corpus luteum but larger than the theca-lutein cells. Intracellular lipid is sparse, if at all present. Mitoses may be observed, but only rarely are they numerous.

Elevated plasma and tissue levels of testosterone, dihydrotestosterone, androstenedione and DHEA have been detected in virilized patients; the plasma levels return to normal once the tumour is extirpated. Even without treatment, the nodules regress and disappear shortly after delivery. Rarely, a functional luteoma may reoccur during a subsequent pregnancy (Van Slooten et al, 1992). Other primary functioning tumours of the ovary that may lead to virilization of the female offspring as well as metastatic tumours to the ovary that induce the stroma to function during pregnancy are discussed elsewhere in this book.

Male pseudohermaphroditism

Male pseudohermaphroditism defines a heterogeneous group of intersex conditions which are characterized by an intrauterine state of relative functional androgen deficiency, an apparently normal 46,XY karyotype and either identifiable testes or evidence that testes were present during fetal development. The external genitalia are usually female or ambiguous, although in certain categories (e.g. testicular regression syndrome) they may appear as phenotypically male. The responsible defect may be in the gonad, leading to deficiency in androgens, Müllerian inhibiting substance, or both. Alternatively, end organ defects in which developing tissues are unresponsive to androgens or Müllerian inhibiting substance may lead to the abnormal phenotype.

Primary gonadal defects

A primary defect of the gonad in an XY karyotype individual may lead to male pseudohermaphroditism by any one of the following mechanisms: regression (destruction) of the gonads or their anlage during intrauterine life, agenesis of the Leydig cells, a specific enzymatic defect in testosterone synthesis, or a defect in elaboration or action of Müllerian inhibiting substance.

Testicular regression syndrome. Testicular regression follows the irreparable destruction of the testes at a critical stage of fetal development in an XY individual (Coulam, 1979). The phenotype of the affected individual reflects the specific stage of fetal development during which the testes were damaged. In general, gonadal regression which occurs during embryonic life, prior to the elaboration of Müllerian inhibiting substance and/or androgenic steroids by the testes, leads to a female phenotype. Regression of the testes during late embryonic through mid-fetal life permits a masculine phenotype (Fig. 40.1). The testicular regression syndrome has a variety of aetiologies, some possibly as diverse as inherited genetic defect, intrauterine infection, or infarction. The heterogeneity of presentation of this syndrome and its relative rarity have led to numerous and sometimes confusing terms for this disorder, including: true agonadism, testicular dysgenesis, rudimentary testis, vanishing testis, and complete bilateral anorchia. The terms pure gonadal dysgenesis and Swyer's syndrome have been used for the testicular regression syndrome by some authors. We avoid these terms so as not to confuse them with other conditions similarly named and discussed below.

At one end of the spectrum of the testicular regression syndrome, the internal genitalia and gonads are absent and the external genitalia are female. Presumably, the urogenital ridge was destroyed in its entirety during early embryonic life, even before the Müllerian ducts began to differentiate (prior to day 42).

At the other end of the spectrum, which approximates to the end point of normal genital development, the patients are phenotypic males with infantile to nearly normal male external genitalia, normally-differentiated Wolffian duct structures and completely-inhibited Müllerian duct development. Often in these cases no genital tissue is identified, but an area of fibrosis, haemorrhage or haemosiderin deposition is found at the expected site of the gonad near residual vas deferens or epididymis. Occasionally, atrophic seminiferous tubules may be found amidst a fibrous stroma. Testicular regression presumably occurred during the late fetal period (after 120 days) when Müllerian structures had already atrophied under the in-

fluence of Müllerian inhibiting substance and testosterone and dihydrotestosterone had exerted a major influence on the normal development of internal and external genitalia. Torsion and infarction of improperly descended testes has been suggested (Smith et al, 1991).

Intermediate in the spectrum of these disorders are patients with ambiguous genitalia and various combinations of Wolffian and/or Müllerian duct development. Testes that regressed during the late embryonic period (day 43–59) will have secreted insufficient testosterone to affect the Wolffian duct. The production of Müllerian inhibiting substance will have been variable, resulting in poorly-differentiated or rudimentary Müllerian structures (incomplete inhibition). In the absence of systemic androgens, the external genitalia appear female.

Regression of the testes during the early fetal period (day 59–84) after Sertoli cell Müllerian inhibiting substance and Leydig cell (testosterone) function have begun or are about to begin results in an individual with ambiguous external genitalia and various combinations of Wolffian and Müllerian development depending on the duration of androgen secretion and Müllerian inhibition.

Regression of the testes during the mid-fetal period (day 84–120) results in more advanced masculinization of the external genitalia, although degrees of ambiguity are usually present. Since Müllerian duct inhibition is normally completed by day 80, the Müllerian structures will have been suppressed and Wolffian structures are developed.

Leydig cell agenesis. Leydig cell agenesis is a very rare cause of male pseudohermaphroditism (Martinez-Mora et al, 1991). Affected individuals have a 46,XY karyotype and testes with interstitial fibrosis, but no mature Leydig cells. Tubules with Sertoli cells and, sometimes, immature spermatogonia are found. The Müllerian structures are absent, indicating appropriate testicular production of Müllerian inhibiting substance during fetal life. The Wolffian duct system is either partially or fully developed so that identifiable vasa deferentia and epididymides are present. The phenotype varies and is usually female with unremarkable or ambiguous external genitalia, although unambiguous males with evidence of primary hypogonadism have been reported. The presence of Wolffian duct development, and the variable degrees of masculinization of the external genitalia indicate that some Leydig cells must have differentiated and functioned during early fetal life. Luteinizing hormone levels are elevated in affected individuals. The underlying defect in this disorder is believed to be an absence or defect of the LH-hCG receptor on the Leydig cell or some other, unknown, factor arresting Leydig cell development.

Defects in testosterone synthesis. Congenital deficiency of any enzyme involved in the production of testosterone in the testis or adrenal gland results in a state of androgen deficiency (relative oestrogen excess) (Fig. 40.2) (Mastroyannis & Wallach, 1987). The histological appearance of the testicular tissue is variable. It has been described occasionally as 'normal', but the photomicrographs in some reports have disclosed large clusters of Leydig cells surrounding tubules lined only by Sertoli cells. In general, the number of gonads studied for any of the conditions and the range of ages studied (infancy, childhood, adulthood) have been limited. Müllerian structures are absent, but Wolffian duct structures may be present. The degree to which the external genitalia develop depends upon the type and severity of the defect.

Three inherited enzymatic defects involve both the synthesis of adrenal mineralocorticoid and glucocorticoid hormones as well as adrenal and testicular sex hormones. The most severe defect, which involves the conversion of cholesterol intermediates to pregnenolone (20,22-desmolase), almost always ends lethally from a salt-wasting crisis if untreated during infancy (Saenger et al, 1981). Although the external genitalia in the male are ambiguous or female, sufficient testosterone must be secreted during embryogenesis since the internal genitalia are male. The testes in the infant disclose immature seminiferous tubules with spermatogonia. The germ cells disappear by several years of age.

A deficiency of 3β-hydroxylase dehydrogenase, like a 20,22-desmolase deficiency, results in decreased synthesis of mineralocorticoid and glucocorticoid hormones as well as adrenal and testicular sex hormones, and may lead to life-threatening salt wasting in infancy. DHEA, which is a weak androgen secreted in high amounts, results in slight clitoral enlargement in the female, but rarely completely masculinizes the external genitalia in males. Hence, the male may be born with ambiguous genitalia and may resemble a virilized female. Males in whom the defect is partial may be born with hypospadias, but at puberty develop gynaecomastia. The testes in older boys generally are immature, exhibiting seminiferous tubules with spermatogenic arrest and diminished numbers of Leydig cells.

In contrast to the early age of diagnosis in the above two syndromes, the diagnosis in most patients with 17α-hydroxylase deficiency is not suspected until the anticipated time of puberty or later. Detailed steroid analysis of the urine of a newborn male presenting with ambiguous genitalia has, however, shown that the correct diagnosis can be made in the young (Dean et al, 1984).

Deficiencies of two enzymes, 17,20-desmolase and 17-hydroxysteroid dehydrogenase (17-ketosteroid reductase), result in deficient testosterone synthesis but do not affect the production of either mineralocorticoids or glucocorticoids. The former defect (conversion of 17-hydroxy-pregnenolone to DHEA) is extremely rare. The patients reported presented with ambiguous external genitalia and inguinal or intra-abdominal testes. Spermatogonia were present in the testis of infants but were absent in the biopsies of their older teenage relatives. All had third-degree hypospadias, but normal male internal ductal differentiation.

Genetic males with 17-hydroxysteroid dehydrogenase (17-ketosteroid reductase) deficiency have almost all been raised as females because of incomplete masculinization. Most are diagnosed at or after puberty when signs of virilization, such as clitoromegaly and hirsutism, become apparent. Müllerian duct derivatives are absent, consistent with normal anti-Müllerian hormone action. Wolffian duct differentiation, indicative of testosterone secretion during embryogenesis, is normal. The testes present in the inguinal canal or labia majora, contain rare to no spermatogonia, and may exhibit numerous Leydig cells.

Defect in Müllerian inhibiting system. The persistent Müllerian duct syndrome, also known as 'hernia uteri inguinalis' is a rare form of male pseudohermaphroditism characterized by the presence of Müllerian duct structures in 46,XY phenotypic males. These patients usually present when young with unilateral or bilateral cryptorchid testes, normal or almost normal male external genitalia and an inguinal hernia into which prolapses an infantile uterus and Fallopian tubes. The testes are histologically normal, Wolffian duct structures are developed, the pubertal development is normal and a rare patient has been fertile. Treatment is surgical, consisting of orchiopexy and herniorrhaphy with hysterectomy and bilateral salpingectomy. If at operation any patient has a streak gonad or a tumour rather than bilateral testes, the diagnosis of mixed gonadal dysgenesis should be considered (Robboy et al, 1982). In most cases of persistent Müllerian duct syndrome, the vas deferens is tightly adherent to the residual uterus or upper vagina and in some cases the Müllerian structures must be left intact to preserve the vas (Fernandes et al 1990). Malignant testicular tumours have been reported in the very rare cases of adult patients with persistent Müllerian duct syndrome and uncorrected cryptorchid testes (van Haarhoven et al, 1991). The persistent Müllerian duct syndrome seems to be a heterogeneous group of disorders, caused by different defects in the Müllerian inhibiting system. Familial cases have been reported. Some patients produce no Müllerian inhibiting substance, while others produce normal amounts of biologically active Müllerian inhibiting substance, suggesting either end-organ insensitivity to Müllerian inhibiting substance or an abnormality of the timing of Müllerian inhibiting substance secretion (Guerrier et al, 1989). Some patients may produce a biologically inactive form of Müllerian inhibiting substance.

End-organ defects

The normal development of the Wolffian duct derivatives and the external genitalia requires that these structures be responsive to androgen and that the enzyme, 5α-reductase, be present in the anlage of the prostate and external genitalia to convert testosterone to dihydrotestosterone (DHT). A molecular defect of the androgen receptor system (e.g. unstable androgen receptor or lack of androgen receptor) leads to impaired development of both Wolffian duct structures and external genitalia in 46,XY individuals. If only 5α-reductase is absent or defective, the abnormalities in the reproductive tract are confined to the external genitalia and prostate.

Androgen receptor disorders (androgen insensitivity syndromes). Disorders of androgen receptor function result in a variety of phenotypes ranging from phenotypic women with intra-abdominal testes to individuals with ambiguous genitalia to phenotypic men with minimal clinical abnormalities. Because androgen receptor defects lead to such a variety of different clinical disorders, much nosological confusion exists in the literature regarding subclassification of the androgen resistance syndromes. In Griffin's classification scheme (Griffin, 1992), the five categories in order of increasing virilization (decreasing feminization) are: complete and incomplete testicular feminization, Reifenstein's syndrome, infertile male syndrome, and undervirilized male syndrome. All share an X-linked recessive inheritance, the result of a defect in the androgen receptor gene, which has been localized to the long arm of the X chromosome, position Xq11.2–q12 (Mandel et al, 1992). A variety of different mutations of this gene have been characterized, most of which are limited to individual families. These mutations may lead to absence of the androgen receptor due to deletion of the gene. Alternatively, only the hormone binding region of the receptor may be deleted or altered such that testosterone binding is absent or impaired. Finally, some mutations alter the DNA binding region of the receptor, leaving testosterone binding intact while rendering the receptor unable to carry out its function as a regulatory protein (Griffin, 1992).

Complete testicular feminization. Complete testicular feminization is the most common form of male pseudohermaphroditism. The external genitalia are phenotypically female and, for this reason, the condition is rarely diagnosed before puberty unless an inguinal hernia or labial mass is encountered or unless the disease is known to be familial. Primary amenorrhoea is the most common complaint leading to evaluation and subsequent diagnosis. The medical history usually reveals that breast development occurred as expected at puberty. Pubic and axillary hair are scant, the vagina is shortened, and the epididymides, vasa deferentia, seminal vesicles and prostate are absent. As a rule, both the cervix and the body of the uterine corpus are absent. A fragment of Fallopian tube may be found in up to one-third of cases (Rutgers & Scully, 1991). The testes are cryptorchid and may be located in the inguinal canal, the pelvis or rarely the labia. In the complete or almost complete form of the syndrome, the individual exhibits a truly female conscious-

ness gender identity with normal extragenital erotogenic sensitivity and a normal maternal attitude.

The gonads in infants and young children are relatively normal but by age 5 years they show abnormalities (Muller, 1984). By young adulthood, the gonad is often involved with benign or malignant tumours as described below. If tumours are not present by this age, the gonad is usually small and on section is tan to brown and traversed by thin white bands. A 1–2 cm firm, white nodule of hyalinized smooth muscle is usually present at one pole of the testes. Theories regarding what this nodule might represent include an abnormally hypertrophied gubernaculum or rudimentary uterine structure. Microscopical examination of the testicular parenchyma discloses immature seminiferous tubules usually sparsely distributed or clustered in small aggregates. Spermatogonia may be present, but spermatogenesis is absent. The number of spermatogonia that are found is age dependent, diminishing as the patient ages (Muller, 1984). The interstitium is usually abundant and often resembles ovarian stroma (Fig. 40.4). Fetal-type Leydig cells may be abundant. The findings indicate that Leydig cells are active hormone producers. The Leydig cells in individuals with testicular feminization have an ultrastructure typical of cells involved in active hormone synthesis (Pierre-Louis et al, 1983) and the systemic androgen levels in these individuals are characteristically elevated. These findings indicate that the pathological defect in the testicular feminization syndrome is an end-organ defect and not lack of hormone production by the testes.

Most testes of affected individuals contain multiple benign nodules that are discrete, firm, yellow to brown and bulge above the sectioned surface (Fig. 40.4). Hamartomatous nodules have been present, usually bilaterally, in virtually every case the authors have personally examined. The typical size varies from 1 mm to 1 cm, and to 4 cm in the series of Rutgers & Scully (1991). The bulk of the nodule is usually composed of seminiferous tubules lacking lumina; spermatogonia may be present. Sertoli cell adenomas are hamartomas composed predominantly or exclusively of closely packed immature seminiferous tubules lacking lumina and lined by immature, uniform Sertoli cells. The adenomas average 3 cm in diameter, ranging up to 25 cm. The interstitium in the testes of affected patients often resembles ovarian stroma, and frequently contains Leydig cells. On rare occasions, Leydig cell nodules form, and have been considered benign tumours. In summary, the name applied to each type of nodule is somewhat arbitrary and depends largely upon the types of components present as well as their number and size. Most nodules are classified as hamartomas, Sertoli cell adenomas or, rarely, as Leydig cell tumours.

Malignant gonadal tumours develop with increasing frequency with age in patients with testicular feminization. Seminoma is the most commonly encountered gonadal

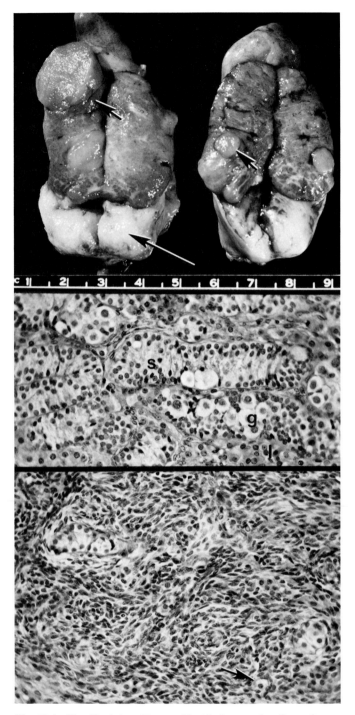

Fig. 40.4 Top Testis in a 17-year-old with the complete form of androgen insensitivity (testicular feminization) syndrome. Numerous Sertoli cell adenomas (short arrows) are present in the parenchyma. The mass near one pole (long arrow) may represent an abnormally hypertrophied gubernaculum. **Middle** Hamartoma with immature seminiferous tubules (s), numerous germ cells (g), and numerous Leydig cells (l) in the interstitium. H & E × 175. **Bottom** Contralateral testis with scattered immature seminiferous tubules embedded in a dense ovarian-type cortical stroma. Occasional interstitial cells (arrows) are present. H & E × 175. (Reprinted from Welch & Robboy, 1981, with permission of Pediatric Andrology.)

malignancy in this syndrome. Intratubular germ cell neoplasia is sometimes seen, either independently or in association with seminoma. Other malignant germ cell tumours and malignant sex cord tumours are also rarely encountered. Unlike mixed gonadal dysgenesis, in which tumours develop in young individuals, the risk of malignancy in patients with testicular feminization is only 4% by the age of 25 years (Manuel et al, 1976), but reaches 33% by 50 years. Since malignant tumours rarely develop before completion of puberty, castration can usually be delayed until after adolescence, thus permitting the patient to undergo a normal pubertal spurt and develop female secondary sex characteristics.

Incomplete testicular feminization. About 10% of patients with an androgen insensitivity syndrome have incomplete testicular feminization. This resembles complete testicular feminization except that there is partial fusion of the labioscrotal folds and usually some clitoromegaly at birth. Also, underdeveloped Wolffian duct derivatives are often present. If the diagnosis is established during childhood, gonadectomy should be performed before puberty, since disfiguring virilization may accompany breast development at puberty. Oestrogen therapy should be given at the appropriate time to initiate feminization. The pathological findings are similar to those described for the complete form of testicular feminization (Muller, 1984).

Other forms. Reifenstein's syndrome, infertile male syndrome, and undervirilized male syndrome are other forms of incomplete androgen insensitivity in which the phenotype is male. There are few reports describing the microscopic findings of the gonads.

Men with Reifenstein's syndrome usually present with gynaecomastia and severe hypospadias, and children or teenagers with perineoscrotal hypospadias. However, the phenotypic spectrum is wide, even within the same affected family with a single androgen receptor abnormality in all affected family members. The usual abnormalities include: hypospadias, breast development at puberty, female habitus, azoospermia, cryptorchidism, and hypoplasia or absence of Wolffian duct structures. The 'infertile male syndrome' is a rare androgen receptor defect characterized by a phenotypically normal man with infertility caused by azoospermia. Finally, in the 'undervirilized male syndrome' the individual is a male with gynaecomastia, a small penis, decreased beard and body hair, a normal male urethra, a normal sperm density and an identifiable androgen receptor defect. The majority of affected individuals are infertile.

Disordered testosterone metabolism

5α-reductase deficiency. Deficiency of the enzyme 5α-reductase impairs the conversion of testosterone to dihydrotestosterone, the hormone which masculinizes the indifferent urogenital sinus and induces development of the prostate (Imperato-McGinley et al, 1991; Griffin, 1992; Thigpen et al, 1992). The disorder has an autosomal recessive inheritance and is rare. The majority of reported cases come from family clusters found in three relatively isolated geographical locations in the Dominican Republic, southern Turkey and Papua New Guinea.

Affected males are typically phenotypically female with female to ambiguous external genitalia at birth (pseudovaginal perineoscrotal hypospadias). The small clitoris-like phallus lacks a urethral orifice. In most affected individuals the urogenital sinus opens on the perineum and within the sinus an anterior orifice leads to the urethra and a posterior orifice to a blind vaginal pouch. The testes are in the inguinal canals or labia. The Müllerian-derived structures are absent whereas Wolffian-derived structures (vas deferens, epididymis and seminal vesicle), the anlage of which respond to testosterone, are normal.

At puberty, virilization occurs and the breasts fail to develop. The penis lengthens, the bifid scrotum grows, becomes rugated and hyperpigmented, and the testes enlarge and descend. Testicular biopsy specimens reveal spermatogenesis and tubular atrophy in some individuals, complete spermatogenic arrest and Leydig cell hyperplasia in others. The prostate fails to develop and remains impalpable. Erection, ejaculation and orgasm are possible in some affected individuals; these individuals are not, however, fertile.

Neonates with this disorder frequently go unrecognized and are raised as females. After the virilization that accompanies puberty, individuals raised as girls sometimes reverse their sex rôles and function as men, often with a stormy period of adjustment. Individuals with a male gender identity benefit from surgical correction of hypospadias and cryptorchidism. High doses of testosterone enhance virilization. Persons raised as females who elect to continue to function as females into adulthood benefit from orchiectomy prior to the onset of puberty to avoid the accompanying virilization. Oestrogen therapy is useful to promote feminization.

GENDER IDENTIFICATION DISORDERS WITH AN ABNORMAL SEX CHROMOSOME CONSTITUTION

Additions, deletions or mosaicism of the sex chromosomes characterize individuals in this category. The appearance of the gonads is variable and ranges from the presence of a streak gonad to a nearly normal female or male gonad on both gross and microscopic examination. These disorders are subdivided into two broad categories depending on the frequency with which sexual ambiguity occurs.

Sexual ambiguity infrequent

Klinefelter's syndrome

Klinefelter's syndrome occurs in about one of every 1000 live newborn males (Schwartz & Root, 1991). The karyotype is usually 47,XXY which, in most cases, results from non-dysjunction occurring during meiosis of either paternal or maternal gametes. Less frequently, a 47,XXY/46,XY mosaic karyotype is found, caused by non-dysjunction during mitosis of the developing zygote. The diagnosis is usually first suspected at adolescence when the patient presents with gynaecomastia, obesity or signs of eunuchism. The testes are small. The beard and body hair are frequently sparse. Most patients are tall with long legs, resulting in a diminished upper to lower body segment ratio. Laboratory tests reveal low testosterone levels, elevated gonadotrophic levels (postpuberty) and azoospermia. Frequently associated clinical findings include learning disabilities, behavioural disorders, reduced economic striving and limited sexual drive. The diagnosis may also be established at other stages of life due to evaluation of age-related clinical concerns. Genetic screening programmes identify the fetus with Klinefelter's syndrome. Although infants with Klinefelter's syndrome usually have normal external male genitalia at birth, the syndrome is sometimes discovered during evaluations of newborns with hypospadias, micropenis, and small soft testes or cryptorchidism. In adults, Klinefelter's syndrome may be discovered during an evaluation for infertility or malignancy.

The Klinefelter's testis is morphologically normal at birth in most cases. Primary spermatogonia are already greatly reduced in number by late childhood. Shortly before the expected time of puberty, the seminiferous tubules begin to degenerate. The absence of elastic fibres in the tubular wall indicates that the process of atrophy began prepubertally. The testes in adult 47,XXY individuals are small and rarely exceed 2 cm in maximal dimension (Fig 40.5). On microscopical examination, they are largely atrophic, have hyalinized seminiferous tubules, and a relative increase in the number of Leydig cells. Some tubules may be preserved, but are lined only by Sertoli cells. Rarely, an occasional seminiferous tubule of the adult testis contains germ cells in varying stages of maturation. If sperm are detected, mosaicism, most likely of the 46,XY/47,XXY pattern, should be suspected. Patients with this mosaic karyotype are sometimes fertile.

The Leydig cells become pronounced in number some time after puberty. Although they appear hyperplastic relative to the atrophic appearance of the other elements, it is uncertain whether the absolute volume is greater than in normal testes. Functionally, the Leydig cells are abnormal as evidenced by low levels of serum testosterone in the setting of elevated levels of serum LH and FSH and subnormal increase in response to administration of hCG.

A variety of neoplasms have been associated with Klinefelter's syndrome. Both gonadal and extragonadal germ cell tumours develop with increased frequency. Most extragonadal tumours occur in the mediastinum as teratoma and embryonal cell carcinoma (teratocarcin-

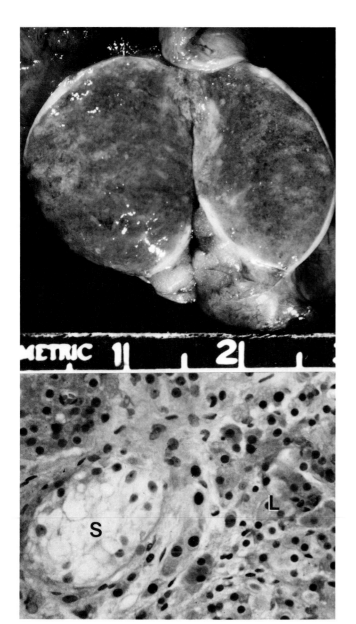

Fig. 40.5 Klinefelter's syndrome. **Top** The parenchyma of the 2 cm testis is golden-yellow to slightly brown. **Bottom** Clusters of Leydig cells (L) surround a seminiferous tubule (S). H & E × 275. (Reprinted from Welch & Robboy, 1981, with permission of Pediatric Andrology.)

oma) or choriocarcinoma (Lee & Stephens, 1987). In the testis, seminoma, teratoma and embryonal cell carcinoma have been encountered. The risk of breast carcinoma in men with Klinefelter's syndrome may be 20% higher than in normal men. Haematological malignancies have also been reported, including acute leukaemia, Hodgkin's disease, malignant lymphoma, and chronic myelogenous leukaemia.

Turner's syndrome

In the classic form, Turner's syndrome is a disorder in which sexually immature phenotypic females of short stature have various congenital anomalies and streak gonads. The cytogenetic hallmark is the 45,X karyotype with a sporadic, non-familial pattern of inheritance. Other karyotypes identified less frequently in this syndrome include mosaic 45,X/46,XX and 46,XX with isochrome X (duplication of one arm of the X chromosomes with the loss of the other arm). Patients with a 45,X/46,XY mosaic karyotype (considered in Mixed gonadal dysgenesis) usually present with obvious sexual ambiguity, but sometimes present as phenotypic females with the clinical stigmata of Turner's syndrome. A significant difference between patients with 45,X/46,XY mosaic karyotype and those with classic 45,X Turner's syndrome is that gonadoblastoma and malignant germ cell tumours are common in patients with the former and rare in those with the latter. Thus, all patients who are being evaluated for Turner's syndrome and who have a negative buccal smear should have karyotypic analysis to rule out the presence of a Y chromosome.

About 98% of fetuses with a 45,X karyotype abort; the frequency of Turner's syndrome is about 1:3000 liveborn females. In the newborn, the overt findings are related to lymph stasis, which manifests itself as oedema of the dorsum of the hands or feet or, less frequently, as swellings of the nape of the neck (cystic hygroma). Later in childhood and in adult life, webbing of the neck or elevation of the distal portion of the nails are residua of more marked swellings present during fetal life and may still provide a clue to the correct diagnosis. A rare, but important, major presentation is hydronephrosis due to ureteropelvic stenosis; all female neonates with a ureteropelvic obstruction should have a buccal smear. Congenital anomalies of other organ systems are associated with Turner's syndrome and include a short fourth metacarpal, hypoplastic nails, multiple pigmented naevi and coarctation of the aorta. The full range of somatic anomalies (more than 40) associated with this condition is presented elsewhere (Hall & Gilchrist, 1990; Lippe, 1991).

Patients who reach adolescence undiagnosed often present with primary amenorrhoea. Examination reveals underdeveloped secondary sex characteristics and a small uterus. Urinary gonadotrophins are always elevated and the vaginal smear lacks cornified cells. The buccal smear in a 45,X individual reveals few if any Barr bodies; in those 20% of patients with a mosaic karyotype (usually 45,X/46,XX or 45,X/47,XXX, the smear discloses a subnormal number of chromatin-positive cells (about 5–15% for a female). Only rare patients with Turner's syndrome have become pregnant and the majority of these have a 46,XX cell line.

At laparotomy, the internal genitalia are female and, although small, are in normal relation to one another. The adult gonads appear as white fibrous streaks, 2–3 cm long and 0.5 cm in diameter and are located ·in the position normally occupied by the ovary (Fig. 40.6). On micro-

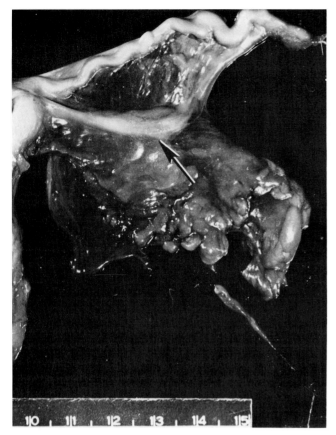

Fig. 40.6 Streak ovary (arrow) in Turner's syndrome. (Reprinted from Welch & Robboy, 1981, with permission of Pediatric Andrology.)

scopical examination a streak consists of an attenuated cortex, a medulla and a hilus. The cortex is composed of characteristic ovarian stroma in which the cells are elongate, wavy and are composed of conspicuous nuclei and scant cytoplasm. Rete tubules (rete ovarii) and hilar cells are typically present in the hilus region. Oocytes are almost always absent in adults with Turner's syndrome. Oocytes are present in normal numbers in 45,X embryos prior to the 12th week of gestation. In older fetuses and young children, the number of oocytes falls progressively relative to the normal number for the age until the number reaches zero, usually before the time of normal menarche, thus leading to primary amenorrhoea. These findings suggest that the second X chromosome is necessary for granulosa cell development and primary follicular formation; in the absence of this X chromosome, granulosa cells fail to differentiate and, as a result, the oocytes degenerate.

Gonadal tumours are exceedingly rare. Tumours of germ cell origin are undoubtedly rare due to the paucity of germ cells. Development of neoplasms of the so-called 'common epithelial type' suggests that the coelomic epithelium encapsulating the gonad can undergo malignant change even if the gonad is a streak (Murphy et al, 1979).

Endometrial carcinoma may develop occasionally in those patients who have had long-term exogenous oestrogen therapy to foster the appearance of the female secondary sex characteristics. Both natural oestrogens and synthetic non-steroidal oestrogens have been implicated. The duration of usage usually exceeds 3 years. Extragonadal tumours, most often of neurogenic origin, have been reported in children and young adults (Wertelecki et al, 1970).

XX male syndrome

The XX male syndrome is a disorder characterized by a nearly normal but infertile phenotypic male with a 46,XX karyotype (de la Chapelle et al, 1990). This syndrome, one of the rarest of all sex chromosome anomalies, occurs in about 1 of 24 000 newborn males (Zakharia & Krauss, 1990). XX males share many characteristics of men with Klinefelter's syndrome. Both have a generally masculine appearance, normal or near normal external genitalia, male psychosexual orientation, normal to weak secondary sexual characteristics, normal to low androgen levels and azoospermia. The testes are small with prominent Leydig cells and tubules lined only by Sertoli cells. The most common reasons for referral are similar to those with Klinefelter's syndrome, namely infertility or abnormal secondary sexual characteristics. XX males also tend to differ clinically from men with Klinefelter's syndrome: the former are generally shorter in height, and the frequency of hypospadias and gynaecomastia is higher. The frequency of impaired intelligence is not increased in XX males relative to the general population.

The XX male syndrome potentially results from at least three distinctly different mechanisms (Abbas et al, 1990; de la Chapelle et al, 1990; Furguson-Smith et al, 1990; Zakharia & Krauss, 1990; Fuse et al, 1991). About 70% of these patients have a small portion of paternally derived Y chromosome which contains the SRY (sex-determining region Y) gene, the testis-determining factor present abnormally on the X chromosome. These patients are called Y(+) by some. The SRY gene is normally found on the short arm of the Y chromosome adjacent to the pseudoautosomal pairing region. During meiosis in the father, an abnormal exchange sometimes leads to the transfer onto the X chromosome of the entire pseudoautosomal region plus the adjacent portion of the Y chromosome with the SRY gene. Inheritance of such an X chromosome from the father leads to the Y(+) XX male syndrome. The inheritance pattern of this form of the syndrome is sporadic. These patients have normal male external genitalia. Hypospadias and ambiguous genitalia are virtually never found. Apparently, the presence of the SRY gene is adequate to lead to normal male phenotype. Azoospermia in these patients results from the lack of other genes normally found on the Y chromosome necessary for sperm development.

Some patients with the XX male syndrome lack Y-derived DNA. Such Y(−) XX males might result from two different mechanisms. The first accounts for the familial transmission of an autosomal dominant or X-linked inheritance of XX maleness. These patients usually have ambiguous genitalia. This indicates that genes exist, probably downstream from the testis-determining factor, that can trigger testis determination when mutated. Nothing specific is known about these putative genes, but their phenotypic effect seems slightly different from that of testis determining factor. A second potential mechanism which might lead to the Y(−) condition is chromosomal mosaicism with a prevalent XX lineage. In such patients, the Y-containing cell line might simply be technically too difficult to identify due to the small number of such cells. Alternatively, a 47,XXY zygote might lose its Y chromosome by non-dysjunction early in ontogeny allowing a 46,XX cell line to persist; the 47,XXY cell line may have persisted long enough to induce male gonadal development. Such patients, just as patients with familial Y(−) XX maleness, often present with sexual ambiguity suggesting that patients with Y(−) XX male syndrome are closely related both phenotypically and aetiologically to XX true hermaphrodites, who present with both testicular and ovarian tissue.

Pure gonadal dysgenesis

Pure gonadal dysgenesis is a term that has historically been encompassed in a number of diverse conditions, including testicular regression syndrome. In the context defined herein, pure gonadal dysgenesis refers to a phenotypic female without genetic ambiguity where the internal genitalia include Müllerian structures (uterus and Fallopian tubes) and generally streak gonads, a constellation which still probably encompasses a multitude of diverse conditions. The patients may appear phenotypically normal or have hypoplastic external genitalia. The pure gonadal dysgenesis syndrome occurs with both 46,XX and 46,XY karyotypes and has both familial and sporadic patterns of inheritance.

The 46,XX type pure gonadal dysgenesis is either an autosomal recessive disorder or, less frequently, an abnormality of the X chromosome. Such patients have greater ovarian development than those with 46,XY pure gonadal dysgenesis or Turner's syndrome and present more often with signs of ovarian dysfunction (secondary amenorrhoea or infertility) rather than primary gonadal failure (primary amenorrhoea). Deletions of either the short or long arm of an X chromosome have been identified in 46,XX pure gonadal dysgenesis (Krauss et al, 1987; Scully, 1991).

The 46,XY type pure gonadal dysgenesis is more common than the 46,XX form of the disorder. The 46,XY type may be caused by: deletion of the testis-determining factor gene (Disteche et al, 1986), an inactive testis-deter-

mining factor or a defect in some testis-determining factor co-factor (Fil & Scully, 1990). The syndrome may be sporadic or familiar with either X-linked recessive or autosomal recessive patterns of inheritance (Scully, 1991). Some patients have a mosaic 45,X/46,XY karyotype.

Patients with 46,XX pure gonadal dysgenesis, like those with Turner's syndrome, very rarely develop gonadal tumours. Hilus cell hyperplasia and hilus cell tumours with the usual associated virilizing effects have been reported (Scully, 1991). Patients with 46,XY pure gonadal dysgenesis are at high risk for gonadoblastoma and other germ cell tumours, as is true of all patients with streak gonads and a Y chromosome.

Sexual ambiguity frequent

Patients in this category exhibit a wide range of phenotypic appearances and internal genitalia. A 'Y' chromosome is often present, usually as part of a mosaic complement. Sexual ambiguity is a common finding.

Mixed gonadal dysgenesis

Mixed gonadal dysgenesis is a heterogeneous syndrome characterized usually by a 45,X/46,XY or 46,XY karyotype, persistent Müllerian duct structures, an abnormal testis and a contralateral streak gonad. The functional deficit imposed by the abnormal testis is expressed as incomplete inhibition of Müllerian development, incomplete differentiation of Wolffian duct structures and incomplete male development of the external genitalia. Often, incomplete mediation of the testicular descent occurs, resulting in both internal and external asymmetry of the genitalia and a mixture of male and female features in an individual in whom neither gonad is normal. About two-thirds of the affected individuals are raised as females and the remainder as males. Some patients with mixed gonadal dysgenesis exhibit phenotypic features of Turner's syndrome. Elsewhere, we have suggested that the syndrome of mixed gonadal dysgenesis should be enlarged to incorporate some patients with bilateral streak gonads (described above as 46,XY type pure gonadal dysgenesis) or bilateral abnormal testes with mosaic 45,X/46,XY karyotype (dysgenetic male pseudohermaphroditism), since the clinical, pathological and chromosomal features of these syndromes closely resemble each other (Robboy et al, 1982).

The underlying genetic and karyotype abnormalities leading to the syndrome of mixed gonadal dysgenesis are currently under investigation. A variety of different genetic abnormalities appear to result in mixed gonadal dysgenesis, thus leading to the phenotypic heterogeneity of mixed gonadal dysgenesis. Partial deletions of both the short and long arms of chromosome Y have been detected in these individuals (Cantrell et al, 1989; Shinobara et al, 1991). Cases of dicentric Y and no detectable Y chromosomal anomaly have also been observed (Weckworth et al, 1988; Shinobara et al, 1991).

Clinically, mixed gonadal dysgenesis is usually detected in the neonate because of ambiguity of the external genitalia. Frequently, a palpable testis bulges through an indirect inguinal hernia or descends completely into the labioscrotal fold, resulting in asymmetry of the genital swellings. This clinical appearance has prompted some investigators to name the syndrome 'asymmetric gonadal dysgenesis'. If the gonads are intra-abdominal, the labioscrotal folds may appear as normal labia or as empty scrotal sacs. The condition is likely to go unrecognized unless the clitoris is sufficiently enlarged to mandate investigation, which is common. The gonad that descends is almost always a testis, and the streak gonads are always intra-abdominal unless dragged into a 'hernia uteri inguinale'.

Organs derived from the Müllerian duct persist in 95%

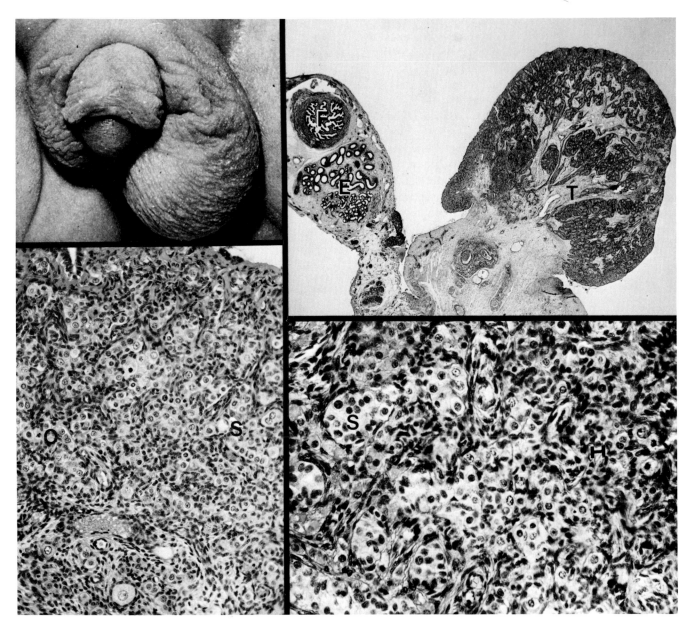

Fig. 40.7 Mixed gonadal dysgenesis. **Top left** External genitalia in MGD. The left testis had descended into the scrotum; the right streak was in the abdominal cavity. Because of this characteristic appearance, some investigators prefer the name 'asymmetric gonadal dysgenesis' rather than mixed gonadal dysgenesis. **Top right** Testis (T) and adjacent Fallopian tube (F) and epididymis (E). The medulla contains immature seminiferous tubules with germ cells and interstitial cells while the region nearer the cortex resembles fetal ovary with immature sex cords and rare primordial follicles. H & E × 9. **Bottom left** Cortex of gonad in which testicular seminiferous tubules (S) merge into fetal-type ovary (O). H & E × 190. **Bottom right** The medullary parenchyma of the testis is composed of normal immature seminiferous tubules (S) with germ cells and occasional interstitial cells, while the parenchyma in the region of the hilus (H) near the rete testis appears less committed as testis and is characterized by abnormal, pleomorphic seminiferous tubules. The photograph is taken at the junction of the two zones. H & E × 112. (Reprinted from Robboy et al, 1982, with permission of Human Pathology.)

of cases (Fig. 40.7). The uterus is usually infantile or rudimentary. The Fallopian tubes are frequently bilateral. If a testis is grossly near normal size and well differentiated, the fimbriated end of the ipsilateral tube may be absent, but in only one-third of cases is the ipsilateral tube entirely absent. Organs of Wolffian duct derivation may also be present, but their frequency is variable. The epididymis is identified in two-thirds of cases and is usually present on the side where there is a testis. The vas deferens is encountered less frequently. The seminal vesicle is only rarely identified, probably because tissue near the bladder/prostate region is not usually removed.

The gonad may be a testis or a streak. Streak gonads may be partially differentiated towards ovary or testis. Bilateral gross testes, frequently of an asynchronous degree of maturity, are found in about 15% of cases while a unilateral gross testis is found in 60%. The testis is consistently abnormal architecturally, its organization being divided into three zones, each of which reflects the quantity and type of cellular components present. The three zones, which are described below in detail, include:

1. the region of the tunica albuginea or cortex, which exhibits widely spaced seminiferous tubules or differentiation towards ovary
2. the medulla, which is composed of normal or near-normal seminiferous tubules and interstitium
3. a hilar region with poorly-differentiated seminiferous tubules that are only partly differentiated towards testis.

The superficial cortex may contain seminiferous tubules that are often widely separated by oedematous, undifferentiated stroma. Sometimes the tubules penetrate the incompletely formed tunica albuginea and open onto the serosa. Occasionally, broad zones of cortex differentiate slightly towards ovary, even displaying rare primordial follicles. Mice that spontaneously develop chromosomal mosaicism as a result of non-dysjunction often show gonads with ovarian tissue at the periphery and seminiferous cords centrally (Eicher et al, 1980).

The central zone (medulla) of the macroscopic infant testis is architecturally and cytologically normal. Narrow closed seminiferous tubules are lined by Sertoli cells with abundant cytoplasm. The number of spermatogonia varies; advanced forms of spermatogenic maturation are not observed. Leydig cells are present in small clusters of varying size. The nuclei of the Leydig cells contain finely dispersed chromatin, and the cytoplasm varies from minimal and amphophilic or slightly basophilic to abundant and eosinophilic. In older patients, the medulla is atrophic and the tubules are lined only by Sertoli cells (Fig. 40.8). The basement membranes are often thickened. Prominent clusters of Leydig cells fill the interstitium.

The architecturally disorganized hilar region discloses seminiferous tubules that are swollen by increased num-

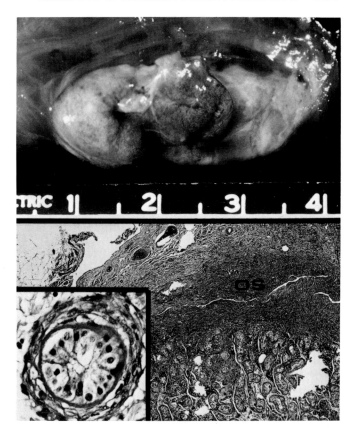

Fig. 40.8 Testis in a 35-year-old phenotypic male with mixed gonadal dysgenesis. **Upper left** The tunica albuginea is tan and maximally 1 mm thick; the parenchyma is golden yellow. **Lower** Cross section of tunica albuginea which is composed of stroma resembling the stroma of ovarian cortex (OS) and medulla with seminiferous tubules. H & E × 27. **Upper right** Detail of seminiferous tubules lined only by Sertoli cells. The interstitium is filled with Leydig cells. H & E × 400. (Reprinted from Robboy et al, 1982, with permission of Human Pathology.)

bers of Sertoli cells and are lined by indistinct basement membranes. These tubules also merge with the surrounding stroma, imparting the appearance of a homogeneous blend of Leydig cells, germ cells, Sertoli cells, and an indeterminate type of interstitial stroma. The region resembles neither fetal ovary nor testis.

The streak gonads appear similar to those found in Turner's syndrome. We have not observed a gonad that has been identifiable grossly as an ovary or has been shown microscopically to contain Graafian follicles, corpora lutea or corpora albicantia. The presence of rare primordial follicles or, as in the fetal ovary, aggregates of germ cells partially surrounded by immature granulosa cells, is evidence that a streak gonad can differentiate towards ovary. Morphological changes may occur over time in the streak gonads. Myriads of germ cells present in a streak of an infant may degenerate and disappear by puberty, resulting in a gonad composed exclusively of fibrous tissue and a few rete tubules (Fig. 40.9); similar changes occur in the streak gonads of Turner's syndrome (45,X karyotype).

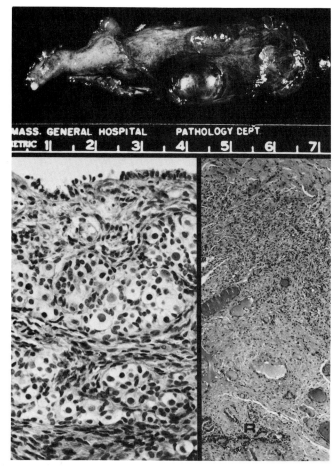

Fig. 40.9 Mixed gonadal dysgenesis. When the patient was an infant the streak gonad resembled a fetal ovary with germ cells and immature sex cords (left lower, H & E × 320). When the streak gonad was removed in entirety 13 years later (top — arrows), it existed only as several microscopical areas of whispy ovarian-type cortical stroma and rete ovarii (R) (right lower, H & E × 100). (Reprinted from Robboy et al, 1982, with permission of Human Pathology.)

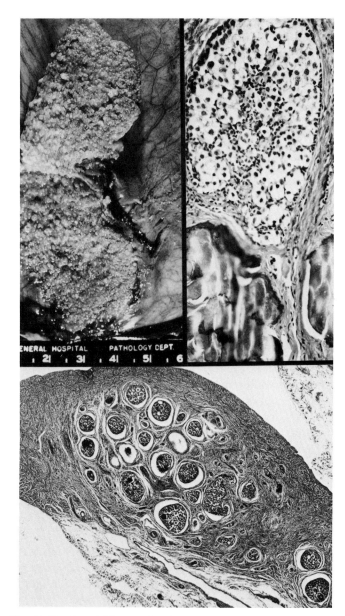

Fig. 40.10 Gonadoblastoma in mixed gonadal dysgenesis. **Top left** 15 cm gonadal tumour composed largely of dysgerminoma. At one pole is a 5 × 2 × 0.5 cm calcified gonadoblastoma. **Top right** Gonadoblastoma. Multiple mulberry-like calcific masses partially replace the tumour nests composed of germ cells surrounded by sex cord derivatives. H & E × 117. **Bottom** Gonadoblastoma occupying a gonadal streak. H & E × 16. (Reprinted from Welch & Robboy, 1981, with permission of Pediatric Andrology [XX06] and Scully, 1970, with permission of Cancer.)

Approximately one-third of patients with mixed gonadal dysgenesis develop gonadoblastoma, a tumour found almost exclusively in patients with an intersex syndrome and a Y chromosome (Page, 1987; Scully, 1991). Gonadoblastoma accounts for three-quarters of the gonadal tumours arising in dysgenetic gonads and is usually discovered during the first to fourth decades of life. Many of the isolated reports of gonadoblastoma associated with other forms of hermaphroditism described clinically and pathologically may in actuality be examples of mixed gonadal dysgenesis.

About 20% of gonadoblastomas arise in a streak gonad and another 20% arise in a dysgenetic testis; in the remaining cases, the nature of the underlying gonad cannot be determined with certainty because it is replaced by tumour. The gross appearance of the gonad with gonadoblastoma varies according to the size of the neoplasm, the presence of calcification and whether the gonadoblastoma has been overgrown by a malignant form of germ cell

tumour (usually germinoma) (Fig. 40.10). Approximately one-fifth of gonadoblastomas are discovered solely because a streak gonad was examined microscopically. The contralateral gonad also contains a gonadoblastoma in over one-third of patients (Rutgers, 1991; Scully, 1991).

On microscopical examination, the gonadoblastoma appears as circumscribed nests of neoplastic germ cells having the cytological properties of germinoma (dysgerminoma and seminoma) and which are encompassed individually or in groups by sex cord derivatives with inconspicuous cytoplasm and small round to oval nuclei resembling immature Sertoli cells (Roth & Eglen, 1989). Hyaline, composed of basement membrane material, is found along the margin or as nodules within the nests of cells. In four-fifths of cases the hyaline material is calcified, initially appearing as small, laminated spheres, which eventually fuse and coalesce into large mulberry-like masses. Not infrequently, the only evidence that a dysgerminoma originated in a gonadoblastoma is the presence focally of mulberry-like calcifications. Hormonally active cells that resemble lutein and Leydig cells are found interspersed among the nests of tumour in about two-thirds of cases. These hormonally active cells are found least frequently in non-virilized phenotypic females, more often in virilized females, and most frequently in phenotypic males. To some degree, their appearance may be related to the postpubertal age of the patient when the gonad is examined.

Approximately 30% of gonadoblastomas are overgrown by a malignant germ cell tumour, usually a germinoma; 8% are overgrown by endodermal sinus tumour, immature teratoma, embryonal carcinoma, or choriocarcinoma. Although the gonadoblastoma itself does not metastasize and therefore can be considered as an in situ malignancy, the typically malignant behaviour of the other tumours makes early prophylactic removal of the gonads in all patients advisable. Also, to avoid the consequences of onset of virilization if the patient is to be raised as a female, it is important that gonadectomy be performed before the patient reaches puberty. Patients who have been treated with long-term administration of oestrogen may on occasion develop endometrial carcinoma. Congenital cardiovascular anomalies have also been reported in patients with mixed gonadal dysgenesis (Wallace & Levin, 1990).

TRUE HERMAPHRODITISM

True hermaphroditism is defined as the presence of both testicular and ovarian tissue in a patient. Affected individuals may have either a female or male phenotype with a variable degree of sexual ambiguity. Because the wavy, cortical-type stroma typically seen in the female gonad can be found in both female and male gonads and therefore is non-specific, follicular structures must be identified to classify gonadal tissue as ovarian and seminiferous tubules to classify the tissue as testicular. In true hermaphrodites, the gonads may be ovary and testis separately or combined in an ovotestis.

The ovotestis is the most frequently encountered gonad in true hermaphroditism. In four-fifths of cases the ovarian and testicular tissues are arranged in an end-to-end fashion. The ovarian portion of an ovotestis has a convoluted surface while the testicular portion is smooth and glistening. Frequently, a distinct line demarcates the two tissues. The firm nature of the palpable ovarian tissue and the soft texture of the testis are valuable clinical signs when evaluating the nature of a gonad in an infant with ambisexual external genitalia (van Niekerk & Retief, 1981).

An ovary, which preferentially develops on the left side, is the second most common gonad in true hermaphrodites. Every patient over 15 years of age in the series of van Niekerk & Retief (1981) had either a corpus luteum or a corpus albicans. The testis, which is the gonad least often encountered, develops preferentially on the right.

The location of the gonad is influenced by the type and quantity of gonadal tissue present. Increasing amounts of ovarian tissue increase the probability that the gonad will be in an ovarian position. When a gonad with the macroscopic features of an ovary is situated in the inguinal canal or in the labioscrotal fold, the possibility of it being an ovotestis should be seriously considered. The position of the testis is less constant. The majority (63%) reside in the scrotum, 14% in the inguinal region, 1% in the internal inguinal ring, and 22% in a normal ovarian position.

The nature of the genital organ adjacent to a gonad in true hermaphroditism is dependent upon the nature of the gonad, which is in contrast to mixed gonadal dysgenesis, where a Fallopian tube is often adjacent to the gonad, regardless of whether it is a testis or streak. In true hermaphroditism a Fallopian tube is adjacent to an ovary and an epididymis or vas deferens is adjacent to a testis. Either a Müllerian or a Wolffian structure, but not both, is adjacent to an ovotestis. Müllerian inhibiting substance appears to be functional. Ninety five per cent of Fallopian tubes adjacent to ovotestes have closed ostia. Only 10% of uteri are normal; the other patients have absent uteri (13%), unicornuate uteri (10%), absent cervix (14%) or uterine hypoplasia (46%).

The most common karyotypes in true hermaphroditism are 46,XX (60%), 46,XY (12%), and mosaic (28%), usually 46,XX/46,XY, 46,XY/47,XXY, or least frequently 45,X/46,XY. Patients with a 'Y' chromosome have a 2–3-fold increased frequency of having a testis as opposed to an ovotestis. Nearly 75% of true hermaphrodites with an ovary and ovotestis have a 46,XX karyotype.

As in other subclasses of intersex, the causes of true hermaphroditism at the genetic level are under investigation. Chromosome Y specific genes (e.g. SRY) have been detected in some but not all 46,XX true hermaphrodites, suggesting several potential mechanisms for the development of XX true hermaphroditism, similar to individuals with XX male syndrome (Jager et al, 1990; Nakagome et al, 1991; Pereira et al, 1991).

The clinical presentations of true hermaphrodites vary to some extent depending upon the patient's age at the time of diagnosis. Until recently, the condition often went undetected until adolescence when phenotypic male patients were evaluated for gynaecomastia and phenotypic female patients were evaluated for amenorrhoea or failure to develop secondary sex changes. Thus, in the series of van Niekerk & Retief (1981), three-quarters of patients were raised as males and one-quarter as females. Many patients, however, menstruated and a few became pregnant. Phenotypic males may experience monthly haematuria due to menstruation into a persistent urogenital sinus. With an increased awareness of intersex states, the condition is more often recognized in infants because of ambiguous genitalia, usually in the form of a small phallus (enlarged clitoris). As in mixed gonadal dysgenesis, the scrotum may be asymmetrical, with the larger, more normal-appearing hemiscrotum containing a testis. Among 160 patients the external genitalia were asymmetrical in three-quarters (labioscrotal folds in 63% and hemiscrotums in 13%).

On microscopical examination, the gonadal tissue often appears normal if the patient is young. In infants the ovarian tissue contains numerous follicles, while the testicular parenchyma discloses normal-appearing seminiferous tubules with spermatogonia. Patients in the reproductive years may have ovarian tissue with structures indicative of ovulation, e.g. follicles, corpora lutea, and corpora albicantia, but spermatogenesis is rare in the testicular portion. The testicular portion of an ovotestis is usually abnormal with incomplete development, loss of germ cells, and tubular sclerosis. Scrotal testes in these patients show less severe changes, sometimes showing faulty spermatogenesis (Scully, 1991).

At times, distinction between true hermaphroditism and mixed gonadal dysgenesis can be difficult. In the newborn, asymmetric ambiguous genitalia may be observed in both conditions. If a streak gonad from a patient with mixed gonadal dysgenesis is serially sectioned, a rare primordial follicle may be encountered in what otherwise appears to be a fetal-type ovary admixed with testis with well-developed seminiferous tubules (Robboy et al, 1982). If the term 'true hermaphroditism' is restricted to those patients in whom the ovarian and testicular tissue are both apparent grossly, it should be possible to segregate more clearly those individuals in whom the ovarian tissue may be functional.

Gonadal tumours occur in less than 3% of affected individuals. Germinoma is the most common type of tumour, but gonadoblastomas and a variety of other tumours have been reported (Talerman et al, 1990; Rutgers, 1991).

REFERENCES

Abbas N E, Toublanc J E, Boucekkine C et al 1990 A possible common origin of "Y-negative" human XX males and XX true hermaphrodites. Human Genetics 84: 356–360.

Cantrell M A, Bicknell J N, Pagon R A et al 1989 Molecular analysis of 46,XY females and regional assignment of a new Y chromosome specific probe. Human Genetics 83: 88–92.

Clement P B 1993 Tumor-like lesions of the ovary associated with pregnancy. International Journal of Gynecological Pathology 12: 108–115.

Coulam C B 1979 Testicular regression syndrome. Obstetrics and Gynecology 53: 44–49.

Coutilainen R, Miller W L 1989 Potential relevance of mullerian inhibiting substance to ovarian physiology. Seminars in Reproductive Endocrinology 7: 88–93.

Dean H J, Shackleton C H L, Winter J S D 1984 Diagnosis and natural history of 17-hydroxylase deficiency in a newborn male. Journal of Clinical Endocrinology and Metabolism 59: 513–520.

de la Chapelle A, Hastbacka J, Korhonen T, Maenpaa J 1990 The etiology of XX sex reversal. Reproduction, Nutrition and Development Suppl 1: 39s–49s.

Disteche C M, Casanova M, Saal H et al 1986 Small deletions of the short arm of the Y chromosome in 46,XY females. Proceedings of the National Academy of Sciences 83: 7841–7844.

Donahoe P A, Berkovitz G D 1987 Female pseudohermaphroditism. Seminars in Reproductive Endocrinology 5: 233–242.

Eicher E M, Beamer W G, Washburn L L, Whitten W K 1980 A cytogenetic investigation of inherited true hermaphroditism in BALB/cWt mice. Cytogenetics and Cell Genetics 28: 104–115.

Fernandes E T, Hollabaugh R S, Young J A, Wilroy S R, Schriock E A 1990 Persistent mullerian duct syndrome. Urology 36: 516–518.

Fil C, Scully R E 1990 Case records of the Massachusetts General Hospital, case 13–1990. New England Journal of Medicine 322: 917–925.

Furguson-Smith M A, Cooke A, Affara N A, Boyd E, Tomlie J L 1990 Genotype–phenotype correlations in XX males and their bearing on current theories of sex determination. Human Genetics 84: 198–202.

Fuse H, Satomi S, Kazama T et al 1991 DNA hybridization study using Y-specific probes in an XX-male. Andrologia 23: 237–239.

Griffin J E 1992 Androgen resistance — the clinical and molecular spectrum. New England Journal of Medicine 326: 611–618.

Gubbay J, Collignon J, Koopman P et al 1990 A gene mapping to the sex determining region of the mouse Y chromosome is a member of a novel family of embryonically expressed genes. Nature 346: 245–250.

Guerrier D, Tran D, Vanderwinden J M et al 1989 The persistent mullerian duct syndrome: a molecular approach. Journal of Clinical Endocrinology and Metabolism 68: 46–52.

Gustafson M L, Lee M M, Scully R E et al 1992 Mullerian inhibiting substance as a marker for ovarian sex cord tumor. New England Journal of Medicine 326: 466–471.

Hall J C, Gilchrist D M 1990 Turner syndrome and its variants. Pediatric Clinics of North America 37: 1421–1440.

Harley V R, Jackson D I, Hextall P J et al 1992 DNA binding activity of recombinant SRY from normal males and XY females. Science 255: 453–456.

Hudson P L, Dougas I, Donahoe P K et al 1990 An immunoassay to detect human mullerian inhibiting substance in males and females during normal development. Journal of Clinical Endocrinology and Metabolism 70: 16–22.

Imperato-McGinley J, Miller M, Wilson J D, Peterson R E, Schackleton C, Gajdusek D C 1991 A cluster of male pseudohermaphrodites with 5 alpha-reductase deficiency in Papua New Guinea. Clinical Endocrinology 34: 293–298.

Jager R J, Epensperger C, Fraccaro M, Scherer G 1990 A ZFY negative 46,XX true hermaphrodite is positive for the Y pseudoautosomal boundary. Human Genetics 85: 666–668.

Koopman P, Gubbay J, Vivian N, Goodfellow P, Lovell-Badge R 1991 Male development of chromosomally female mice transgenic for Sry. Nature 351: 117–121.

Krauss C M, Turksoy R N, Atkins L, McLaughlin C, Brown L G, Page D C 1987 Familial premature ovarian failure due to an interstitial deletion of the long arm of the X chromosome. New England Journal of Medicine 317: 125–131.

Kuroda T, Lee M M, Ragin R C, Hirobe S, Donahoe P K 1991 Mullerian inhibiting substance production and cleavage is modulated by gonadotropins and steroids. Endocrinology 129: 2985–2992.

Lee M W, Stephens R L 1987 Klinefelter's syndrome and extragonadal germ cell tumors. Cancer 60: 1053–1055.

Lippe B 1991 Turner syndrome. Endocrinology and Metabolism Clinics of North America 20: 121–152.

McCoshen J A 1982 In vivo sex differentiation of congeneic germinal cell aplastic gonads. American Journal of Obstetrics and Gynecology 142: 83–88.

McLaren A 1991 Development of the mammalian gonad: the fate of the supporting cell lineage. Bioessays 13: 151–156.

Mandel J L, Monaco A P, Nelson D L, Schlessinger D, Willard H F 1992 Genome maps III (X Chromosome). Science 258: 87–102.

Manuel M, Katayama K P, Jones H W Jr 1976 The age of occurrence of gonadal tumors in intersex patients with a Y chromosome. American Journal of Obstetrics and Gynecology 124: 293–300.

Martinez-Mora J, Saey J M, Toran N et al 1991 Male pseudohermaphroditism due to Leydig cell agnesia and absence of testicular LH receptors. Clinical Endocrinology 34: 485–491.

Mastroyannis C, Wallach E E 1987 Male pseudohermaphroditism: inborn errors in testosterone biosynthesis. Seminars in Reproductive Endocrinology 5: 261–276.

Morel Y 1991 Gene heterogeneity in adrenal 21-hydroxylase deficiency. Presse Medicine 20: 945–949.

Muller J 1984 Morphometry and histology of gonads from 12 children and adolescents with the androgen insensitivity (testicular feminization) syndrome. Journal of Clinical Endocrinology and Metabolism 59: 785–789.

Murphy G F, Welch W R, Urcuyo R 1979 Brenner tumor and mucinous cystadenoma of borderline malignancy in a patient with Turner's syndrome. Obstetrics and Gynecology 54: 660–663.

Nakagome Y, Seki S, Fukutani K, Nagafuchi S, Nakahori Y, Tamura T 1991 PCR detection of distal Yp sequences in an XX true hermaphrodite. American Journal of Medical Genetics 41: 112–114.

New M I 1992 Genetic disorders of adrenal hormone synthesis. Hormone Research 37 (suppl 3): 22–33.

Page D C 1987 Hypothesis: a Y-chromosomal gene causes gonadoblastoma in dysgenetic gonads. Development 101 (suppl): 151–155.

Pereira E T, Cabal de Almeida J C, Gunha A C Y R G, Patton M, Taylor R, Jeffery S 1991 Use of probes for ZFY, SRY, and the Y pseudoautosomal boundary in XX males, XX true hermaphrodites and an XX female. Journal of Medical Genetics 28: 591–595.

Pierre-Louis M L, Kovi J, Sampson C C, Worrell R G, Rosser S B 1983 Ultrastructure of the gonads in the testicular feminization syndrome. Journal of the National Medical Association 75: 1177–1184.

Robboy S J, Miller T, Donahoe P K et al 1982 Dysgenesis of testicular and streak gonads in the syndrome of mixed gonadal dysgenesis: perspective derived from a clinicopathologic analysis of twenty-one cases. Human Pathology 13: 700–716.

Roth L M, Eglen D E 1989 Gonadoblastoma: immunohistochemical and ultrastructural observations. International Journal of Gynecological Pathology 8: 72–81.

Rutgers J L 1991 Advances in the pathology of intersex conditions. Human Pathology 22: 884–891.

Rutgers J L, Scully R E 1991 The androgen insensitivity syndrome (testicular feminization): a clinicopathologic study of 43 cases. International Journal of Gynecological Pathology 10: 126–144.

Saenger P, Levine L S, New M I 1981 Male pseudohermaphroditism due to abnormal testosterone biosynthesis and metabolism. Clinical Andrology 7: 87–97.

Schwartz I D, Root A W 1991 The Klinefelter syndrome of testicular dysgenesis. Endocrinology and Metabolism Clinics of North America 20: 153–163.

Scully R E 1970 Gonadoblastoma. A review of 74 cases. Cancer 25: 1340–1356.

Scully R E 1991 Gonadal pathology of genetically determined diseases. In: Kraus F T, Damjanov I (eds) The pathology of reproductive failure (International Academy of Pathology Monograph, no. 33). Williams & Wilkins, Baltimore, pp 257–285.

Shinobara M, Minowada S, Aso Y et al 1991 A t(Y;15) translocation with a deletion of the proximal Yq in a boy with mixed gonadal dysgenesis. Human Genetics 86: 422–444.

Simpson J L, Golbus M S 1992 Genetics in obstetrics and gynecology, 2nd edn. WB Saunders, Philadelphia, p 350.

Sinclair A H, Berta P, Palmer M S et al 1990 A gene for the human sex determining region encodes a protein with homology to a conserved DNA binding motif. Nature 346: 240–244.

Smith N M, Byard R W, Bourne A J 1991 Testicular regression syndrome — a pathological study of 77 cases. Histopathology 19: 269–272.

Strachan T, White P C 1991 Molecular pathology of steroid 21-hydroxylase deficiency. Journal of Steroid Biochemistry and Molecular Biology 40: 537–543.

Taketo T, Saeed J, Nishioka Y, Donahoe P K 1991 Delay of testicular maturation in the B6.Y (Dom) ovotestis demonstrated by immunohistochemical staining for mullerian inhibiting substance. Developmental Biology 146: 386–395.

Talerman A, Verp M S, Senekjian E, Gilewski T, Vogelzang N 1990 True hermaphrodite with bilateral ovotestes, bilateral gonadoblastomas and dysgerminomas, 46 XX/46 XY karyotype, and a successful pregnancy. Cancer 66: 2668–2672.

Thigpen A E, Davis D L, Gautier T, Imperato-McGinley J, Russell D W 1992 The molecular basis of steroid 5 alpha-reductase deficiency in a large Dominican kindred. New England Journal of Medicine 327: 1216–1219.

Tsuji M, Shima H, Yonemura C Y, Brody J, Donahoe P K, Cunha G R 1992 Effect of human recombinant mullerian inhibiting substance on isolated epithelial and mesenchymal cells during mullerian duct regression in the rat. Endocrinology 131: 1481–1488.

van Haarhoven C J H M, Juttmaran J R, Pypers P M, Roukema J A 1991 A testicular tumor in the left adnexa: the persistent mullerian duct syndrome with testicular malignancy. European Journal of Surgical Oncology 17: 97–98.

van Niekerk W A, Retief A E 1981 The gonads of human true hermaphrodites. Human Genetics 58: 117–122.

van Slooten A J, Rechner S F, Dodds W G 1992 Recurrent maternal virilization during pregnancy caused by benign androgen-producing ovarian lesions. American Journal of Obstetrics and Gynecology 167: 1342–1344.

Wallace T M, Levin H S 1990 Mixed gonadal dysgenesis. Archives of Pathology and Laboratory Medicine 114: 679–688.

Weckworth P F, Johnson H W, Pantzar J T, Coleman G U, Masterson J S T, McGillivray B, Tze W J 1988 Dicentric Y chromosome and mixed dysgenesis. Journal of Urology 139: 91–94.

Welch W R, Robboy S J 1981 Abnormal sexual development: a classification with emphasis on pathology and neoplastic conditions. Pediatric Andrology 7: 71–85.

Wertelecki W, Fraumeni J F, Mulvihill J J 1970 Nongonadal neoplasia in Turner's syndrome. Cancer 26: 485–488.

Yamanaka J, Baker M, Metcalfe S, Hutson J M 1991 Serum levels of mullerian inhibiting substance in boys with cryptorchidism. Journal of Pediatric Surgery 26: 621–623.

Zakharia G, Krauss D J 1990 Sex reversal syndrome (XX male). Urology 36: 322–324.

41. Immunopathology of the female genital tract

Judith N. Bulmer   H. Fox

INTRODUCTION

Considerable advances have recently been made in our understanding of the immunological mechanisms operative in the female genital tract. Immunological factors are important in the response of the female genital tract to infections, in gynaecological neoplasia and in infertility whilst immunopathological mechanisms may play a rôle in the aetiology of some female genital tract diseases. Despite the enormous advances made in the last twenty years it is unlikely that the full range of immunopathological abnormalities in the female genital tract has yet been defined and it is likely that further immunopathological aspects of gynaecological disease will emerge in the near future. This short review will, of necessity, consider only selected facets of this complex and often contradictory topic.

LOCAL IMMUNOLOGICAL DEFENCE MECHANISMS IN THE FEMALE GENITAL TRACT

Humoral (secretory) immunity

There is now good evidence that a local secretory immune system, qualitatively similar to that in other mucosal sites such as the intestine and upper respiratory tract, exists in the human female genital tract (Kutteh et al, 1993; Kutteh & Mestecky, 1994).

Local secretory mucosal immunity is characterized by the presence of immunoglobulin-secreting plasma cells in the submucosa, which react to a local antigenic stimulus by the production of antibodies which are subsequently secreted, via the overlying epithelium, onto the mucosal surface and into the covering mucus layer (Brandtzaeg et al, 1993). Locally secreted mucosal antibodies are predominantly of the IgA class: in contrast with circulating IgA, which is a 7S monomer, secretory IgA is an 11S dimer composed of two 7S monomers linked by J chain. J chain is a glycopeptide which is synthesized by plasma cells and incorporated into IgA immediately prior to se-cretion of the dimeric molecule; J chain is linked to IgA by disulphide bonds and may induce correct polymerization of the IgA subunits (Tomasi & McNabb, 1980). Larger IgA polymers are also secreted. During its passage across the epithelium, secretory IgA is linked with secretory component (SC), a glycoprotein synthesized by epithelial cells. SC acts as a poly-immunoglobulin transport receptor (Brandtzaeg & Prydz, 1984), facilitates transepithelial IgA transport in vesicular form across the cytoplasm, and plays a vital but poorly defined rôle in the resistance of secretory IgA to enzymatic digestion.

Secretory IgA has virus-neutralizing properties, causes bacterial agglutination, inhibits the adhesiveness of organisms to mucosal surfaces, is bactericidal in the presence of lysosome and complement, causes opsonization of bacteria for phagocytosis and blocks entry of antigens by forming non-absorbable complexes with antigenic macromolecules (Doe, 1982). The role of locally produced and secreted antibodies in protection of mucosal surfaces is thus readily apparent and the female genital tract, which is frequently exposed to a wide variety of foreign antigenic material, is an obvious candidate for possession of a local secretory immune system. Such a system has been demonstrated in the vagina, cervix and Fallopian tube but the endometrium does not possess a classical mucosal immune system as described above.

Although early reports suggested that IgA-synthesizing plasma cells were not a major component of the cervical lymphoid population (Tourville et al, 1970), subsequent studies have clearly demonstrated that such cells are the major immunocyte in endocervical tissue (Vaerman & Ferin, 1974; Rebello et al, 1975; Hurlimann et al, 1978; Arends et al, 1983; Kutteh et al, 1988). General agreement has also emerged that SC is present in endocervical epithelial cells and the cervix thus possesses all the components of a local secretory immune system (Fox, 1993). The functional significance of this is indicated by the high content of secretory IgA in cervical mucus (Waldman et al, 1971; Kutteh et al, 1993) and by the detection of secretory IgA antibodies in cervical mucus after local immunization with *Candida albicans* or poliovirus (Waldman et al, 1972; Ogra & Ogra, 1973). IgA-containing plasma cells have also recently been reported to predominate in the vagina and ectocervix, although secretory component was not detected in the cervical squamous epithelium (Kutteh et al, 1988, 1993).

Early studies of the human Fallopian tube (Forrest, 1983) failed to detect the features of a local secretory immune system in this site but more recently immunoglobulin-containing cells have been reported to be present in Fallopian tubes with IgA-secreting cells accounting for over two-thirds of the immunocytes in all segments of the tube (Kutteh et al, 1988, 1990): tubal epithelial cells were shown to be strongly positive for secretory component and the tube lumen contained IgA, SC and J chain. T cells outnumbered plasma cells in normal Fallopian tube, with low numbers of natural killer (NK) cells; plasma cells were greatly increased in number in acute and chronic salpingitis. No menstrual cycle specific changes in numbers of plasma cells, T cells or NK cells were noted in normal Fallopian tube (Kutteh et al, 1990).

Constitutive expression of class II MHC antigens by Fallopian tube epithelium has also been reported: surface expression of HLA-DR antigens by tube epithelium in the proliferative phase, with decreased reactivity in the secretory phase, may reflect variable requirements for local immunocompetence at different menstrual cycle phases (Bulmer & Earl, 1987; Edelstam et al, 1992). The regulatory mechanisms and function of expression of class II MHC antigens by tubal epithelium in normal intrauterine and ectopic tubal pregnancy are unknown (Bulmer & Earl, 1987).

Thus, evidence for the existence of a functional local secretory immune system in the uterine cervix appears unequivocal with increasing evidence for a similar system in the Fallopian tube. The situation within the endometrium is, however, more complex. Although some authors have noted small numbers of immunoglobulin-containing cells in human endometrial stroma (Tourville et al, 1970; Vaerman & Ferin, 1974; Rebello et al, 1975; Bulmer et al, 1986; Kutteh et al, 1988; Bjercke & Brandtzaeg, 1993), IgG-containing cells have sometimes predominated (Tourville et al, 1970; Bulmer et al, 1986; Bjercke & Brandtzaeg, 1993) and reactivity for kappa and lambda light chains has suggested absorption rather than synthesis of immunoglobulins (Bulmer et al, 1986). In most studies, immunoglobulin-containing cells have not been detected in human endometrial stroma at any stage of the menstrual cycle or in postmenopausal women (Yaneva, 1974; Hurlimann et al, 1978; Kelly & Fox, 1979; Arends et al, 1983). Rare IgA-containing and secretory component-positive cells have been detected in endometrial glands (Kutteh et al, 1988), particularly in secretory phase samples. The most striking feature, however, has been the localization of IgA, secretory component and J chain in surface and glandular endometrial epithelial cells, particularly in the basal glands. The IgA, SC and J chain content of endometrial epithelial cells is scanty in postmenopausal women and in proliferative endometrium but increases in the mid and late secretory phases (Kelly & Fox, 1979; Kutteh et al, 1988; Bjercke & Brandtzaeg, 1993).

IgG, IgA, and IgM have been detected in the stromal interstitium of secretory phase endometrium and are most probably derived passively from the plasma in association with stromal oedema, although not always confined to oedematous zones (Bulmer et al, 1986). IgA, IgM, SC and J chain are strongly expressed in apical glandular epithelium and in the luminal contents, reactivity for SC being mirrored by staining for IgA and IgM and, in turn, for J chain. Monomeric IgA and IgG may enter the epithelium in the secretory phase by passive diffusion from the stroma but most immunoglobulin A in endometrial epithelial cells must be polymeric for SC specifically binds J chain. In the absence of any substantial site of local polymeric IgA synthesis in endometrial stroma, it is highly probable that there is active transport of polymeric IgA and, to a lesser extent, pentameric IgM, from the bloodstream, this being mediated by secretory component within the epithelium (Kelly & Fox, 1979; Bjercke & Brandtzaeg, 1993). Stromal oedema in the secretory phase of the cycle is likely to enhance the influx of serum proteins into epithelium (Suzuki et al, 1984) and raised levels of secretory component have been noted in uterine fluid during the secretory phase (Sullivan et al, 1984). Circulating polymeric IgA can enter secretions from the peripheral blood, in which approximately 10% of IgA is polymeric (Neukirk et al, 1983), and SC appears to be unable to distinguish between locally and systemically synthesized polymeric IgA. However, at most mucosal sites the SC receptor system is normally fully loaded with locally secreted IgA, this blockage being absent in endometrium where there is a lack of local IgA synthesis.

Secretory component can persist even in cystically dilated glands in atrophic postmenopausal endometrium with preservation of its capacity for selective uptake of J chain-positive IgA (Brandtzaeg et al, 1993). Secretory component may be upregulated by T-cell and macrophage-derived cytokines including interferon-γ (IFNγ), interleukin 4 (IL4) and tumour necrosis factor α (TNF) (Sollid et al, 1987; Kvale et al, 1988; Phillips et al, 1990). Endometrial stroma contains abundant T lymphocytes, granulated lymphocytes and macrophages which vary in number according to menstrual cycle stage (see below): by cytokine production these cells may contribute to the phase-related expression of SC and IgA in human endometrium.

Endometrial epithelial cells may also express class II MHC antigens (Natali et al, 1981; Morris et al, 1985; Bulmer et al, 1988a; Bjercke & Brandtzaeg, 1993). Variation of such antigens according to menstrual cycle stage and site is inconsistent, although HLA-DR antigen expression appears to be downregulated in pregnancy (Johnson & Bulmer, 1984). Endometrial epithelial expression of class II MHC antigens can be upregulated by IFNγ, potentially produced by adjacent aggregates of T lymphocytes (Tabibzadeh et al, 1986). Distribution of class II MHC antigens and SC in human endometrial epithelium appears unrelated, suggesting different regulatory mechanisms (Bjercke & Brandtzaeg, 1993). The function of class II MHC expression by endometrial epithelial cells is not known.

Thus, the vagina, cervix and Fallopian tube possess a local mucosal immune system but there are low numbers of immunoglobulin-producing cells in endometrium. This distribution may be important for protection of both lower and upper ends of the genital tract from microorganisms while allowing implantation and development of the semi-allogeneic fetoplacental unit in the specialized endometrial environment.

Cellular immunity

Leucocytes account for a substantial proportion of the stromal cell population in normal non-pregnant endometrium (Loke et al, 1993). In the stratum basalis leucocytes are found scattered individually and in aggregates, often adjacent to glands: occasional lymphoid follicles are present. Leucocytes in the stratum basalis are macrophages and T lymphocytes with B cells detected within lymphoid aggregates (Morris et al, 1985; Bulmer et al, 1988b). In the stratum functionalis, the number of stromal leucocytes varies according to menstrual cycle stage: leucocytes account for less than 10% of stromal cells in proliferative and early secretory phase endometrium, increasing to over 20% in the late secretory phase (Bulmer et al, 1991a). Most leucocytes in the stratum functionalis are macrophages, T lymphocytes and phenotypically unusual granulated lymphocytes. T cells are scattered throughout the endometrial stroma, sometimes forming small aggregates. In contrast with peripheral blood, most endometrial stromal T cells are of the CD8-positive suppressor/cytotoxic subset. The great majority also express the αβ heterodimeric form of the T-cell receptor (Bulmer et al, 1991b). There is essentially no variation in the numbers of CD3-positive T cells with menstrual cycle stage (Morris et al, 1985; Marshall & Jones, 1988; Kamat & Isaacson, 1987; Bulmer et al, 1991a; Starkey et al, 1991; Klentzeris et al, 1992) and their function is not known. Expression of activation markers such as HLA-DR and VLA-1 has led to the suggestion that endometrial stromal T cells may induce class II MHC antigen expression on glandular epithelium by secretion of interferon-γ (Tabibzadeh, 1990).

Macrophages are scattered throughout the endo-

metrium and increase in numbers premenstrually (Kamat & Isaacson, 1987; Bulmer et al, 1991a; Klentzeris et al, 1992). They are detectable by expression of CD14 and class II MHC antigens; a proportion express the $β_2$ integrin CD11c (Starkey et al, 1991). The function of macrophages in non-pregnant endometrium has not been investigated in detail, although considerable attention has been focused on potential immunosuppressive, accessory cell, secretory and phagocytic rôles in pregnancy (see Ch. 62).

The third major leucocyte population in endometrial stroma consists of granulated lymphocytes; these cells account for most of the increase in leucocyte numbers in the late secretory phase of the menstrual cycle (Marshall & Jones, 1988; King et al, 1989; Bulmer et al, 1991a; Starkey et al, 1991; Klentzeris et al, 1992). Immunohistochemical studies have shown that these granulated lymphocytes are the so-called endometrial stromal granulocytes (Bulmer et al, 1987). The cells have an unusual antigenic phenotype, expressing some antigens characteristic of natural killer cells (CD56-positive, CD69-positive, variably CD2-positive) but lacking other natural killer (NK) cell and T-cell antigens (CD16, CD57, CD11b, CD3, CD4, CD8-negative) (Ritson & Bulmer, 1987; Bulmer et al, 1991a). The function of these unusual granulated lymphocytes is not known. Their dramatic increase in the late secretory phase of the menstrual cycle and persistence in the first trimester of pregnancy, together with the presence of granulated cells in decidua and endometrium from a number of other species, has suggested a specific rôle in implantation and early development of the fetoplacental unit (see Ch. 62). Consequently, in vitro functional studies have focused on cells separated from early pregnancy decidua and their rôle in non-pregnant endometrium has been largely overlooked.

B lymphocytes, classical CD16-positive NK cells and granulocytes are rare in normal stratum functionalis at all stages of the menstrual cycle. In common with other mucosal sites, intraepithelial lymphocytes can be detected in human endometrium, although they are scanty compared with their counterparts in the gastrointestinal tract. Endometrial intraepithelial lymphocytes consist of CD3-positive, CD8-positive cells and CD56-positive granulated lymphocytes, the latter population increasing in frequency in the late secretory phase (Pace et al, 1991). The function of endometrial intraepithelial lymphocytes is unknown and their distribution in pathological conditions of the endometrium has not been documented.

Analysis of leucocytes in the uterine cervix has focused primarily on changes associated with human papillomavirus infection and cervical intraepithelial neoplasia. Langerhans cells are present within normal cervical squamous epithelium together with both CD4- and CD8-positive T cells. CD56-positive granulated lymphocytes may also be detected in normal ectocervical epithelium, the proposed phenotype being CD2, CD3, CD8, CD56-positive and CD16-negative. CD16-positive NK cells are only present in the underlying stroma (McKenzie et al, 1991) where CD4- and CD8-positive T cells, in variable proportions, are also found, these being aggregated particularly in the transformation zone (Fox, 1993).

Immunoglobulin-containing cells have been identified in tube mucosa but B cells, identified with anti-CD22, are uncommon (Boehme & Donat, 1992). T cells are the predominant lymphocyte, with CD8-positive cells in the epithelium and both CD4-positive and CD8-positive T cells in the underlying lamina propria (Morris et al, 1986; Peters, 1986; Cooper et al, 1987; Boehme & Donat, 1992), although the relative proportion of the two T-cell subsets is disputed. NK cells are also occasionally present in the lamina propria. Most studies have not reported consistent alterations in tubal leucocytes according to menstrual cycle stage, although further studies using tubes removed at sterilization rather than from hysterectomy specimens may be worthwhile.

Hormonal control of local immunological defence systems

The amount of polymeric IgA in cervical secretions falls around the time of ovulation, rising progressively to reach a peak towards the end of secretory phase and subsequently declining during the proliferative phase (Coughlan & Skinner, 1977; Schumacher & Yang, 1977; Saha et al, 1981). These fluctuations in the IgA content of cervical secretions reflect variations in the cervical secretory immune system: immunohistochemical studies have shown that both the cervical content of IgA-producing plasma cells and the number of secretory-component-containing endocervical epithelial cells increased markedly in the secretory phase of the menstrual cycle (Murdoch et al, 1982).

These changes suggest hormonal control of the cervical secretory immune system. Studies under both physiological and pathological conditions have indicated that both the epithelial SC content and the number of subepithelial IgA-synthesizing cells are increased by progesterone and that oestrogens have no effect on SC synthesis but decrease the number of IgA immunocytes in the cervix (Murdoch et al, 1982). It is possible that a regulatory mechanism similar to that described for the breast (Weisz-Carrington et al, 1978) operates in the cervix. Thus, migration of IgA-secreting cells into the cervix may be mediated by a specific receptor, possibly localized on the endothelium of postcapillary vessels, which interacts with a counter-receptor on IgA immunoblasts. Expression of this receptor appears to be under hormonal control, being upregulated by progesterone and downregulated by oestrogen. However, it should be noted that in normal pregnancy IgA levels in cervical secretions fall in the first trimester and rise again towards term (Trnka et al, 1964; Prozorovskaya et al, 1977), raising the possibility that hCG may downregulate the IgA immunoblast receptor; an analogous rôle for LH would explain the striking decrease in IgA-containing cells at the time of ovulation.

The endometrial expression of SC and epithelial IgA uptake also varies during the menstrual cycle, increasing from proliferative to secretory phases (Kelly & Fox, 1979; Arends et al, 1983; Suzuki et al, 1984; Bjercke & Brandtzaeg, 1993). Raised SC levels have also been reported in uterine fluid during the secretory phase, with a significant reduction in proliferative endometrium and lowest levels during menstruation. Limited studies of pathological endometria have demonstrated low SC levels in simple hyperplasia, atrophic endometrium and atypical hyperplasia, but high levels in one patient with endometrial adenocarcinoma (Sullivan et al, 1984). These results suggest that progesterone also has a positive rôle in regulation of the endometrial secretory immune system. It is interesting to note that levels of SC in rat uterine secretions rise during pro-oestrus and are stimulated by oestrogen and inhibited by progesterone (Sullivan et al, 1983). Endocrine control of the human menstrual cycle is complex and the specific hormone which controls the secretory immune system in the human reproductive tract remains uncertain. Regulation may be mediated indirectly by alterations in the number and function of the endometrial stromal leucocyte populations; cytokines such as IFNγ, TNF and IL4 may upregulate secretory component (Sollid et al, 1987; Kvale et al, 1988; Phillips et al, 1990); a variety of cytokines can be produced by macrophages, T cells and granulated lymphocytes in human endometrium.

The cellular immune system in the female genital tract may also be under hormonal control. Both macrophages and granulated lymphocytes increase in number in the late secretory phase of the menstrual cycle. The dramatic increase of the latter cell type can be accounted for largely by proliferation in situ within the endometrium. Hormonal regulation may be indirect, mediated by soluble products of stromal cells or epithelial cells, rather than via specific hormone receptors on the leucocytes themselves. Adhesion molecules may also play a rôle in recruitment and localization of leucocytes in endometrial stroma. The endometrial content and distribution of extracellular matrix molecules such as fibronectin, laminin and collagen varies according to menstrual cycle stage (Kisalus et al, 1987; Aplin et al, 1988). Endometrial stromal cells and endothelial cells may express adhesion molecules such as ICAM-1, VCAM and LFA-3, although the few reports to date of their distribution within the tissue and during the menstrual cycle are inconsistent (Tabibzadeh & Poubouridis, 1990; Bulmer et al, 1991b; Lessey et al, 1992; Marzusch et al, 1993). Nevertheless, expression of counter-receptors on endometrial leucocytes may account for recruitment of leucocytes to endometrium and their distribution in scattered stromal aggregates and around glands and vessels.

CYTOKINES IN THE FEMALE REPRODUCTIVE TRACT

Cytokines are small regulatory peptides or glycoproteins which are synthesized and secreted by activated immune and mesenchymal cells. They function as intercellular signals between various cells of the immune system; most cytokine responses are local and they act in an autocrine or paracrine manner. Although studies of cytokine function have focused predominantly on immune interactions, it has become clear that cytokines play an important rôle in reproduction (Ben-Rafael & Orvieto, 1992; Hill, 1992a, 1993). Cytokines have been shown to interact with pituitary and hypothalamic hormones: for example, ACTH can suppress IFNγ production (Johnson et al, 1984) and both tumour necrosis factor (TNF) and interleukin 1 beta (IL1β) are potent ACTH secretagogues (Sharp et al, 1989). Such hormone-cytokine interactions may influence the neuroendocrine events of reproduction and hence alter fertility.

Cytokines can also mediate ovarian function. Studies in murine corpora lutea have indicated that macrophages secrete substances which stimulate luteal cell progesterone production (Kirsch et al, 1981); TNFα production by regressing rabbit corpora lutea has also been demonstrated (Bagavandoss et al, 1988). Macrophages and class II MHC-positive cells have been reported to be the most abundant immune cell type in the human menstrual corpus luteum with only small numbers of T cells being noted (Petrovska et al, 1992). Thus, by their cytokine secretion, macrophages may be involved in the growth, differentiation, functional development and eventual regression of luteal cells.

Human granulosa cells can produce TNF and production is increased by addition of FSH or hCG and macrophage colony stimulating factor (M-CSF) (Zolti et al, 1990). The effect of TNF on prostaglandin $F_{2\alpha}$ ($PGF_{2\alpha}$) production is biphasic, possibly explaining why FSH increased TNF production, while decreasing $PGF_{2\alpha}$ production. Before ovulation, TNF has been reported to increase prostaglandin production by both bovine granulosa cells and theca cells (Shemesh et al, 1990). These observations suggest that by increasing synthesis of prostaglandins by granulosa cells TNF may play a rôle in the initiation of ovulation. IL1 has been shown to modulate the function of cultured porcine and rat granulosa cells by inhibiting progesterone secretion (Gottschall et al, 1987; Fukuoka et al, 1988). IL1 can also stimulate proliferation of cultured granulosa cells from immature or developing follicles, this proliferative response being lost as the cells mature into luteal cells (Fukuoka et al, 1989).

Although studies of endometrial cytokine production have primarily focused on pregnancy (see Ch. 62) several cytokines have been localized in non-pregnant endometrium of both humans and experimental animal species. TNF has been detected both in the wall of coiled arteries and in epithelial cells in secretory phase endometrium (Philippeaux & Piguet, 1993) and in stromal cells (Tabibzadeh, 1991), and a rôle in menstruation has been proposed. Production of IL6 by cultured endometrial stromal cells has been reported (Tabibzadeh et al, 1989) and epithelial cells and macrophages can produce M-CSF (Daiter et al, 1992). Gamma-interferon (IFNγ) has been localized to T-cell aggregates in the stratum basalis (Stewart et al, 1992). Production of a wide variety of cytokines by various cell types in decidualized endometrium in pregnancy has been reported: to date there have been fewer studies of non-pregnant endometrium and cytokines will undoubtedly emerge as increasingly important regulatory molecules in endometrial growth and function.

SENSITIZATION OF THE LOCAL IMMUNE SYSTEM IN THE FEMALE GENITAL TRACT

Sensitization to organisms

Local immunization with organisms such as poliovirus or *Candida albicans* results in the appearance within cervical mucus of specific secretory IgA antibodies (Waldman et al, 1972; Ogra & Ogra, 1973). In chlamydial infections of the female genital tract: anti-chlamydial secretory IgA antibodies can be detected in cervical mucus (Terho & Meurman, 1981) and there is an inverse relationship between the titre of these antibodies and the ability to isolate organisms from the cervix (Brunham et al, 1983). A similar situation occurs in herpes simplex infections of the genital tract: women with specific secretory IgA antibodies in cervical mucus have a shorter duration of virus shedding than those women who fail to produce such antibodies, the antibody titre and frequency of positive culture again varying inversely (Merriman et al, 1984).

Neisseria gonorrhoeae appears to flourish in the cervix and sometimes appears to activate a chlamydial infection. The gonococcus is able to synthesize a protease capable of cleaving secretory IgA (Blake et al, 1979): gonococcal infections may therefore restrict the protective activity of locally secreted antibodies, allowing other infections to become established.

The local cervical immune response to human papillomavirus (HPV) is a focus for current research effort: the effectiveness of host cell-mediated immune responses and hence the local immune response in the cervix appears to be an important factor in determining the clinical outcome following HPV infection of cervical keratinocytes (Roche & Crum, 1991). Several studies have documented altered populations of immunocompetent cells in the cervix in HPV infections. Depletion of Langerhans cells, the principal intraepithelial antigen-presenting cell, has been described in both HPV infection and CIN (Morris et al, 1983; McArdle & Muller, 1986; Tay et al, 1987a). Intraepithelial T lymphocytes, predominantly the CD4-positive helper/inducer subset, have been reported to be depleted in HPV infection and all grades of CIN (Castello et al, 1986; Tay et al, 1987b), although others have noted an increase in intraepithelial T cells in high-grade CIN (Viac et al, 1990). Small increases in the number of non-specific effector cells such as macrophages (Tay et al, 1987c) and large granular lymphocytes (McKenzie et al, 1991) have also been reported in cervical HPV infection.

Cytokines can recruit and activate immunocompetent cells at infection sites. Normal endocervical and ecto-cervical cells can secrete IL1α, IL1β, IL1 receptor antagonist, IL6, IL8, TNF and granulocyte macrophage colony stimulating factor (GM-CSF) in vitro, but cervical cell lines immortalized with HPV DNAs and cervical squamous cell carcinoma cell lines secreted significantly reduced levels of cytokines. Furthermore, IFNγ consistently upregulated expression of ICAM-1 in normal cervical cells but had a variable effect on HPV-infected cells (Woodworth & Simpson, 1993). Others, however, have noted induction of ICAM-1 in high-grade CIN and a sensitive response to IFNγ by fully transformed cell lines with a lower response in immortalized non-transformed lines (Coleman et al, 1993). Thus, ectocervical and endocervical epithelial cells are potentially able to influence inflammation and immunity in cervical mucosa. Alterations in cytokine and adhesion molecule expression may influence the local host immune response to cervical HPV infection.

The cervical immune response to human immunodeficiency virus (HIV) infection has stimulated interest with regard to the mechanisms of heterosexual transmission of HIV. Heterosexual transmission is a major risk factor and women are more at risk of such transmission than men. HIV-1 related antigens have been detected in cervical lymphocytes, macrophages and endothelial cells but not epithelial cells in women with AIDS (Vande Perre et al, 1988; Pomerantz et al 1988). However, using in situ detection of polymerase chain reaction (PCR)-amplified nucleic acids, amplified HIV-1 DNA and complementary DNA was detected in the cervix of 21 women suffering from AIDS: HIV-1 nucleic acids were detected in the endocervix in stromal cells near the base of the endocervical glands, and in scattered cells in the deep mucosa around microvessels; many infected cells reacted for leucocyte common antigen, the Mac 387 macrophage marker and TNF, suggesting infection of activated macrophages (Nuovo et al 1993). The detection rate of HIV-1 by standard in situ hybridization and p24 immunohistochemistry in the same samples was much lower, probably because of low copy numbers in infected cells. Further studies are required to determine whether the HIV-1

infected macrophages in the cervix represent primary infection or result from systemic spread of virus to the cervix. If they represent primary infection, the rôle of infected cervical cells in the transport of virus to regional lymph nodes and hence in initiation of systemic infection requires further study. Cervical HIV infection may impair lymphocyte function locally, thus increasing the risk of intraepithelial and invasive cervical neoplasia, as well as potentially modifying the natural history of other gynaecological infections (Priolo & Minkoff, 1992).

The effect of infection on female genital tract sites other than the cervix has been little studied. Endometritis is often recognized by the presence of plasma cells which are normally virtually absent. However, histopathological diagnosis of endometritis in the absence of plasma cells is difficult and the leucocytic infiltrate has not been characterized in detail. The number of plasma cells in the Fallopian tubes has been shown to be increased in active salpingitis (Kutteh et al, 1990) but the responses to various infectious agents have not been studied in detail.

Sensitization to spermatozoa

Attempts to correlate female infertility with serum anti-spermatozoal antibodies have been inconclusive (Faulk & Fox, 1982). It is unlikely that serum antibodies would come into direct contact with spermatozoa and more recent studies have searched for antibodies in cervical mucus. Anti-spermatozoal antibodies have been detected in cervical mucus of infertile women, the incidence varying according to the technique used: the incidence of sperm agglutinating or immobilizing antibodies ranged from 21–62% (Cantuaria, 1977; Menge et al, 1977; Wong, 1978; Chen and Jones, 1981; Moghissi et al, 1980; Etribi et al, 1982; Menge et al, 1982) while that of antibodies detected by immunofluorescence has ranged from 17–35% (Menge et al, 1977; Harrison, 1978; Wong, 1978; Almeida & Jouannet, 1982).

Anti-spermatozoal antibodies in cervical mucus could be derived by transudation from the serum but the weight of evidence favours local synthesis of anti-spermatozoal antibodies by the cervical secretory immune system. The number of IgA-synthesizing plasma cells in the cervix is increased in many infertile women (Hutcheson et al, 1974; Sinha et al, 1977), the antibodies are predominantly secretory IgA in type (Jager et al, 1981; Ingerslev et al, 1982; Clarke et al, 1984a) and there is no correlation between the presence of serum anti-spermatozoal antibodies and detection of similar antibodies in cervical mucus (Moghissi et al, 1980; Almeida & Jouannet, 1982; Stanislavov et al, 1983).

Anti-spermatozoal antibodies are rare in cervical mucus in normally fertile women, their presence correlating well with a history of infertility and a poor postcoital test (Teland et al, 1978; Wong, 1978; Bronson et al, 1984a).

When spermatozoa come into contact with cervical mucus which contains anti-spermatozoal antibodies, their forward movement is altered to a shaking or vibrating pattern (Kremer et al, 1978): this has been attributed to the formation by the antibodies of crosslinks between the spermatozoa and the relatively rigid glycoprotein micelles of cervical mucus, effectively immobilizing the spermatozoa. These immobilizing antibodies, however, are usually of IgG type; locally secreted IgA spermatozoal agglutinating antibodies are likely to be functionally more important (Jager et al, 1981).

Although normal fertile women do not form antibodies to spermatozoa, a leucocytic reaction to spermatozoa appears to be a normal response in the cervix (Pandya & Cohen, 1985; Thompson et al, 1991). An infiltrate predominantly composed of neutrophil polymorphs and including small numbers of macrophages, T-helper and T-suppressor lymphocytes was detected in both cervical mucus and cervical smear samples 20 minutes, 4 and 24 hours after donor insemination; similar leucocytic responses were observed with 'pure' sperm but not with seminal plasma, indicating that the cervical leucocytic response is initiated by spermatozoa (Thompson et al, 1992). Three of 10 women became pregnant following extraction of mucus 20 minutes after insemination, suggesting that fertilizing spermatozoa penetrate the cervical os quickly and bypass the leucocytic response. The response of human endometrium to spermatozoa is unknown: studies of endometrial leucocytes have focused on menstrual cycle changes and have not addressed the possibility of an effect mediated by spermatozoa.

IMMUNOLOGICAL ASPECTS OF CONTRACEPTION

Immunological effects of contraceptives

Both oestrogen and progesterone have immunomodulatory activity, raising the possibility that oral contraceptive steroids may influence immune status. Some studies have indicated that cell-mediated immunity, measured by mitogen-induced lymphoproliferation, is reduced in women using oral contraceptives (Irvine et al, 1974; Keller et al, 1977) but others have not confirmed these findings (Gerretsen et al, 1980). It has been noted, however, that women taking oral contraceptives may show increased or decreased reactivity to skin testing with dinitrochlorobenzene; oestrogens appeared immunosuppressive whilst progestagens stimulated immune reactivity (Gerretsen et al, 1979). It has also been suggested that the increased tendency towards vascular thrombosis in oral contraceptive users may be immunologically mediated: Beaumont et al (1982) suggested that generation of specific antibodies to administered ethinyloestradiol leads to formation of immune complexes which damage vessel walls and predispose to thrombus. Fotherby & Hamawi (1984) did not confirm these findings, suggested that steroid binding to immunoglobulins was non-specific and found no excess of immune complexes in oral contraceptive users. Despite past controversy, it is unlikely that current low dosage oral contraceptives have any significant immunopathological effect.

Immunological contraception

The principle of a vaccine to control fertility is both physiologically and clinically attractive and has major implications for fertility regulation in both the developing and developed world. Stages of the human reproductive process up to and including implantation are potential targets for immunological fertility control, various components being both antigenically unique and immunogenic (Ada & Griffin, 1991; Jones, 1992). Advantages of an immunological contraceptive include long-lasting but reversible contraceptive effect and relatively low cost. Target antigens should be specific to the reproductive process and preferably present only transiently. Immunizations should prevent or disrupt fertilization or implantation without side effects. Potential target antigens which meet logistic and safety considerations include those in gametes, the zygote and the placenta: trophoblastic and sperm antigens are attractive targets in the female (Jones, 1992).

Progress in development of an anti-sperm vaccine has been slow. In females immunity would operate against foreign antigens introduced at coitus, whereas males would require an autoimmune reaction against antigens continually present. A target sperm antigen must be accessible on the cell surface: various potential antigens have been identified and their antifertility effects described in laboratory animals (Naz & Menge, 1990) but most are species specific. It should be noted that the possibility exists for local immunity in the female reproductive tract to sperm-specific antigens to be induced by an oral vaccine; antigens taken up by the gut-associated lymphoid tissue produce sensitized IgA immunocytes which migrate to other mucosal surfaces, including the reproductive tract (Suri et al, 1993).

The zona pellucida (ZP) is the most extensively studied potential oocyte target antigen. ZP encases the oocyte and zygote and is highly immunogenic with apparently species-specific antigens. Immunization of rodents against ZP antigens reduces fertility and antisera to ZP block sperm penetration, coating the zona surface. Furthermore, sera from infertile women with anti-ZP antibodies block in vitro fertilization with human gametes, and ova from these women are incapable of in vitro fertilization. However, although immunization of experimental animal species with ZP antigens inhibits fertility, these effects have been accompanied by altered ovarian function and/

or autoimmune ovarian pathology (Henderson et al, 1988). Efforts have thus been focused on developing a ZP immunogen with only B-cell epitopes: this approach has been successful in inducing long-term but reversible anti-fertility effects in female mice (Dean & Millar, 1990).

Antigens on the surface of placental trophoblast cells are expressed at only one anatomical site after fertilization and are in direct contact with maternal blood. Despite the development of numerous trophoblast-reactive monoclonal antibodies, few have had the desired widespread reactivity with trophoblast populations in early pregnancy together with specificity for this cell type (Anderson et al, 1987). To date, the greatest interest in anti-placental antigens has been focused on anti-hCG vaccines. hCG can be detected on trophectoderm as early as the blastocyst stage, prior to implantation; an anti-hCG vaccine would interrupt pregnancy at a very early stage either by neutralizing the luteotrophic effect of hCG or by destroying trophoblast cells. Several anti-hCG vaccines have entered clinical trials, of which the most refined is directed against the unique C-terminal peptide on the beta subunit of hCG. This vaccine produces specific anti-hCG antibodies which do not cross-react with luteinizing hormone. Preclinical studies in baboons and data from a phase I human trial indicate that this method is safe and potentially effective for up to 12 months (Stevens et al, 1981; Jones et al, 1988). Future research will be directed towards optimizing hCG vaccines but also broadening the spectrum of target antigens available for contraceptive vaccine development.

IMMUNOLOGICAL ASPECTS OF ENDOMETRIOSIS

It has been suggested that immunological factors are important both in the pathogenesis of endometriosis and in the infertility which is often a feature of this disease (Dmowski et al, 1991). Retrograde transtubal menstrual flow of endometrial cells is well established as a probable factor in the pathogenesis of endometriosis but this appears to be a physiological event in most menstruating women with patent Fallopian tubes (Liu & Hitchcock, 1986). This has led to the suggestion that it is only women with defective immunity who develop endometriosis, this defect allowing viable endometrial tissue to survive more readily in the peritoneal cavity.

ALTERED HUMORAL IMMUNITY IN ENDOMETRIOSIS

Weed & Arquembourg (1980) proposed that infertility in endometriosis has an autoimmune basis due to an abnormal antigen-antibody reaction. They demonstrated deposits of both the complement factor C3 and IgG in endometrium with a corresponding reduction in total serum complement levels of women with endometriosis and

suggested that this was an expression of an autoimmune reaction to endometrial antigens provoked by release of antigens during 'menstruation' from endometriotic foci. This hypothesis was extended to suggest that the resulting immunological reaction within endometrium could lead to infertility. The possibility of an autoimmune reaction to endometrial antigens was confirmed indirectly by the demonstration of excess IgG and IgA in the uterine endometrium of women with endometriosis (Saifuddin et al, 1983).

Mathur et al (1982) broadened the concept of autoimmunity in endometriosis by the demonstration that women with this disease not only have autoantibodies against endometrial antigens but also IgG and IgA autoantibodies against thecal and granulosa cell antigens in their sera, cervical and vaginal secretions. Subsequent studies showed low levels of circulating and peritoneal fluid antibodies to various endometrial antigens in both normally fertile women and women with endometriosis, with additional serum and peritoneal fluid antibodies to endometrial antigens of molecular weight 26 kD and 34 kD in women with endometriosis (Mathur et al, 1988). Others have also demonstrated a high frequency of anti-endometrial antibodies in the sera and peritoneal fluid of women with endometriosis (Badawy et al, 1984; Wild & Shivers, 1985; Kreiner et al, 1986) and Wild & Shivers (1985) demonstrated anti-endometrial antibodies in 85% of infertile women suffering from endometriosis, such antibodies being rare in other groups of infertile patients. However, Saifuddin et al (1983) noted no difference in the content of endometrial immunoglobulins between normally fertile women with endometriosis and those whose reproductive capacity was diminished. Furthermore, no evidence of endometrial damage has been noted, raising the possibility that anti-endometrial antibodies are not cytotoxic and may be an epiphenomenon.

Antibodies to subcellular elements or to cell structure components such as antinuclear, anti-DNA or anti-cardiolipin antibodies have also been detected in women with endometriosis, particularly IgG autoantibodies to phospholipids (Gleicher et al, 1987; El-Roeiy et al, 1988). Autoimmune diseases are characterized by increased total immunoglobulin and decreased complement levels but the findings in endometriosis have been conflicting, C3, C4 and total immunoglobulin levels having been variously reported as increased, unchanged or decreased (Weed & Arquembourg, 1980; Badawy et al, 1984; Steele et al, 1984; Gleicher et al, 1987; Meek et al, 1988).

Despite the numerous studies of humoral immunity and autoantibodies in endometriosis, doubt still remains as to whether these alterations precede or are a consequence of the disease.

Altered cell-mediated immunity in endometriosis

Support for the concept that altered cell-mediated immunity plays a rôle in endometriosis by allowing transplanted endometrial cells to survive was provided by studies in Rhesus monkeys with spontaneously occurring endometriosis: whilst there was no generalized impairment of cell-mediated immunity, specific diminished lymphocyte reactivity to autologous endometrial antigens was noted (Dmowski et al, 1981). In women with endometriosis, peripheral blood total lymphocytes and subsets have been reported to be normal (Gleicher et al, 1984), although others have noted increased peripheral blood T cells, B cells and CD4:CD8 ratios (Badawy et al, 1987). However, reduced lymphocyte-mediated cytotoxicity to autologous endometrial cells and decreased lymphocyte reactivity to endometrial antigens has been reported in women with endometriosis, all other tests of cell-mediated immune function being comparable between subjects and controls (Steele et al, 1984). Specific defects in the response to endometrial antigens may explain the development of endometrial implants (Dmowski et al, 1981) but the immunological findings could also reflect specific tolerance resulting from chronic low-grade exposure to endometrial antigens released from endometriotic foci; thus they may result from, rather than cause, the disease.

Altered local immunity in endometriosis

Several recent studies of immune function in endometriosis have focused on leucocyte function locally within the peritoneal cavity (Hurst & Rock, 1991). There have been several reports that in endometriosis peritoneal macrophages are increased in concentration, total number and activation status (Haney et al, 1981; Halme et al, 1984; Zeller et al, 1987) and also have an enhanced capacity for phagocytosing spermatozoa (Muscato et al, 1982; Halme et al, 1983), changes which have been thought to play a rôle in preventing conception. Peritoneal macrophages from women with endometriosis also produce more IL1, TNF and fibronectin than do those from women without this disease (Fakih et al, 1987; Kauma et al, 1988; Halme, 1989). Macrophages have a regulatory rôle in the function of other cell types in the peritoneal cavity by release of cytokines, prostaglandins, growth factors, complement components and hydrolytic enzymes, and the activation status of peritoneal macrophages in endometriosis had led to the suggestion that cytokine secretion by macrophages may facilitate implantation and growth of endometrial tissue at ectopic locations (Halme et al, 1987).

Many studies reporting increased numbers of peritoneal macrophages in endometriosis have been based solely on morphology but Hill et al (1988) characterized leucocytes in peripheral blood and peritoneal fluid of women with endometriosis, women with unexplained infertility and normal fertile controls using immunohistochemistry. Peripheral blood leucocytes in all groups were within normal limits but the peritoneal fluid of women with stage I and II endometriosis contained increased numbers of macrophages, CD4-positive helper T lymphocytes and NK cells: elevated levels of peritoneal macrophages, CD4 and CD8-positive T cells were also noted in cases of unexplained infertility. Altered peritoneal leucocytes could therefore contribute to infertility in mild endometriosis by secretion of cytokines which are detrimental to fertilization and implantation.

The possibility of altered local NK-cell function in endometriosis has also been suggested. NK cells are large granular lymphocytes which are defined by their ability to mediate MHC-unrestricted cytotoxicity. Defective anti-endometrial lytic activity would allow ectopic endometrial cells to survive and develop into endometriotic foci. Decreased peripheral blood and peritoneal fluid NK-cell lytic activity has been reported in patients with endometriosis (Oosterlynck et al, 1991, 1992, 1994; Garzetti et al, 1993) and it has been suggested that this is a primary defect present before development of the disease. These reports are, however, difficult to reconcile with reports of a peritoneal inflammatory response in endometriosis which would be expected to result in enhanced NK-cell activity, and with the lack of evidence of increased susceptibility to infection and malignancy in women with endometriosis. Furthermore, others have reported impaired local peritoneal NK-cell activity but normal peripheral blood NK-cell lysis (Vigano et al, 1991). There are further reports that NK-cell lysis is regulated by sera from patients with endometriosis (Kanzaki et al, 1992). The rôle of NK cells in the pathogenesis of endometriosis thus remains uncertain: altered NK-cell activity may be an epiphenomenon (Hill, 1992b) and it is noteworthy that danazol, which is used for treatment of endometriosis, appears to suppress NK-cell activity (Vigano et al, 1992) an observation which causes doubt that endometriosis is caused by suppressed NK-cell function.

The rôle of immunological factors in the pathogenesis of endometriosis therefore remains uncertain. Studies are now focusing on both local immune responses within peritoneal fluid and on comparison of eutopic and ectopic endometrium in women with endometriosis with the endometrium of normal women: abnormalities in complement deposition in eutopic endometrium in endometriosis have been reported and raise the possibility that inherent endometrial abnormalities may allow implantation and growth of ectopic endometrial foci (Isaacson et al, 1990). Future developments in analysis of adhesion molecules and cytokines may provide further clues to the enigma of endometriosis.

IMMUNOLOGICAL FACTORS IN FEMALE INFERTILITY

Approximately 15% of couples desiring children are infertile and for 10–20% of these the cause is unknown.

Immunological factors have, however, been estimated to account for up to 20% of couples with unexplained infertility (Mosher, 1982). Introduction of seminal, microbial or embryonic and trophoblast antigens into the female genital tract can evoke humoral and cellular immune responses both locally and systemically. The effect of such immune responses would include interruption of oocyte development; inhibition of ovulation; immobilization, agglutination or autolysis of spermatozoa; interference with sperm-ovum contact and transport; and early embryonic mortality (Hill & Anderson, 1988).

Sensitization to spermatozoa

Humoral immunity

A proportion of women become sensitized to spermatozoal antigens and develop antibodies which may contribute to, or cause, infertility (Mathur et al, 1981a). Anti-sperm antibodies can be detected in the serum of approximately 13% and in the cervical mucus in 8% of infertile women (Moghissi et al, 1980). It is assumed that antigen exposure occurs during coitus and that antigen recognition occurs after phagocytosis of spermatozoa by genital tract macrophages. An exaggerated antibody response to spermatozoa can occur in association with bacterial or viral genital tract infections (Friburg & Gnarpe, 1973; Rizov et al, 1973; Witkin & Toth, 1983) and in women with cervical bilharziasis (El-Mahgoub, 1972) whilst a significant correlation between anti-sperm and anti-chlamydial antibodies has been described in oral contraceptive users (Blum et al, 1989). In a study of multigravid women with primary upper genital tract infections, anti-sperm antibodies were detected in 56% of women with a clinical episode of pelvic inflammatory disease and in 69% of those who, whilst giving no history, had laparoscopic evidence of past pelvic infection (Cunningham et al, 1991). Genital tract infections may lead to immunopotentiation of anti-sperm antibodies which could affect fertility; whether this is due to an adjuvant effect or to greater antigen entry as a result of local tissue damage is not known.

In sensitized women, anti-spermatozoal antibodies may occur in serum, peritoneal fluid or cervical mucus, and serum anti-sperm antibody levels frequently do not correlate with those in peritoneal fluid or cervical mucus (Clarke et al, 1984b; Shai et al, 1990; Stern et al, 1992). Anti-spermatozoal antibodies may interfere with sperm transport, gamete interaction, embryo development, implantation or trophoblast outgrowth (Hill & Anderson, 1988). Anti-sperm antibodies are often measured in serum but no clear-cut association has been consistently established between infertility and the presence of serum anti-sperm antibodies, there being a better correlation between the finding of locally secreted antibodies in cervical mucus and impaired reproductive capacity. Thus, whilst

Isojima (1969) and Jones et al (1973) reported clear correlations between serum sperm-immobilizing antibodies and infertility, Ingerslev & Hjort (1979) detected sperm-agglutinating antibodies in both infertile and presumed normal fertile women, though there was, admittedly, a higher frequency of active sera and higher antibody titres in the sera from infertile women. The prospects for eventual fertility are lower for women with systemic immunity to sperm than in those without such responses (Moghissi et al, 1980). Furthermore, various sperm autoantibodies have been shown to interfere with human fertilization in vitro and women with humoral immunity to spermatozoa are more likely to fail in vitro fertilization if their embryos are cultured in the presence of their anti-sperm antibody-rich serum (Clarke et al, 1985a, b).

Binding of locally secreted anti-sperm antibodies to the sperm surface can cause immobilization or agglutination and can impair their ability to penetrate cervical mucus (Menge et al, 1982), thus inhibiting access of sperm to the fertilization site. Anti-sperm antibodies can also render spermatozoa susceptible to complement-mediated lysis (Beer & Neaves, 1978) whilst tail-directed IgG and IgM antibodies can fix complement and render sperm immotile (Bronson et al, 1982a). Binding of complement components to antibody-coated spermatozoa could also cause opsonization, thus increasing sperm phagocytosis by resident macrophages in female reproductive tract tissues (London et al, 1985). Sperm antibodies may also inhibit sperm-ovum reactions in the Fallopian tube (Russo & Metz, 1974; Dor et al, 1981): antibodies directed against the sperm head could interfere with the acrosome reaction or other enzyme-dependent mechanisms of sperm penetration of the oocyte (Bronson et al, 1982b) or could occlude binding sites for the zone pellucida or ovum, thus preventing sperm-oocyte attachment.

Anti-sperm antibodies may also cause early embryonic mortality for the zona pellucida is permeable to both antibody and complement (Shivers & Dunbar, 1977) and sperm antigens are present on the fertilized ovum and early embryo as a result of sperm plasma membrane fusing with that of the ovum at fertilization (Menge & Fleming, 1978). Cross-reactive antigens between sperm and trophoblast have also been documented (Anderson et al, 1987), providing an additional mechanism by which anti-sperm antibodies could disrupt implantation or trophoblast proliferation and function (Hill & Anderson, 1988). However, anti-sperm antibody titres do not necessarily correlate with inhibition of sperm-egg fusion, sperm motility or fertilization (Aitken et al, 1988; Clarke, 1988) and some antibodies can actually increase sperm motility or stimulate sperm-egg interactions (Aitken et al, 1988).

Although sperm antibodies have been reported in both male and female partners of normally fertile couples (Bronson et al, 1984b), most women do not mount a recognizable immune response following exposure to antigenically alien spermatozoa, despite repeated exposure. The extent of sperm exposure may be a factor: an increased frequency of sperm immunity has been reported in prostitutes as compared with controls (Schwimmer et al, 1967) and prevention of contact with sperm may result in a decrease or loss of anti-sperm antibodies (Kay, 1977). Female reproductive tract pathology may be a co-factor in the development of anti-sperm immunity (Boettcher, 1974): antibodies are common in association with pelvic inflammatory disease and women with cervical cancer have a higher incidence of anti-sperm antibodies than women with other gynaecological malignancies (Jones et al, 1973). The immunosuppressive properties of seminal plasma (Alexander & Anderson, 1987) may account for the lack of anti-sperm immune reactivity in normal women whilst masking of spermatozoal antigens by seminal plasma components (Johnson & Hunter, 1972) and the presence of blocking antibodies (Hancock, 1978; Bronson et al, 1984b) are alternative, but far from complete, explanations. Mathur et al (1983) suggested a rôle for genetic factors, reporting that a high proportion of immunized women are of HLA-B$_w$35 group.

There is, then, evidence that anti-sperm antibodies play a rôle in female infertility, though the precise details and nature of this rôle are uncertain. Some of the difficulties encountered in assessing the significance of anti-sperm antibodies may be due to differences in methodology which may affect results (Boettcher, 1979), and questions have been raised about the sensitivity, specificity and subjective interpretation of assays such as sperm immobilization or agglutination (Bronson et al, 1984b; Mandelbaum et al, 1987). Newer indirect techniques may provide more reproducible results (Clarke et al, 1985c; Bronson et al, 1986; Hinting et al, 1988; McClure et al, 1989; Khoo et al, 1991) and attempts are being made to determine the precise sperm antigens detected by the various anti-spermatozoal antibodies in infertile patients (Snow & Ball, 1992; Tsuji et al, 1992). Anti-spermatozoal antibodies in cervical mucus almost certainly relate more directly to infertility than serum antibodies, although the latter are much easier to detect, and there is a need to develop simplified, reproducible techniques to detect anti-sperm antibodies in small volumes of cervical mucus (Shulman & Hu, 1992).

Cell-mediated immunity

Cell-mediated immunity involves both cell–cell interactions and the effects of cytokines. Evidence for a cell-mediated immune response to spermatozoa in infertile women is fragmentary and inconclusive. Mettler & Schirwani (1975) tested leucocytes from various groups of women against pooled, washed spermatozoa and noted positive leucocyte migration inhibition in most sexually active women: no evidence of cellular sensitization was detected in virgins and it was concluded that exposure to spermatozoal antigens normally resulted in cellular sensitization. Others have documented evidence of cell-mediated immunity to spermatozoa, detected by in vitro macrophage migration inhibition or lymphocyte transformation, in significant numbers of infertile women both with and without associated anti-sperm antibodies (Marcus et al, 1973; Soffer et al, 1976; Dor et al, 1979; McShane et al, 1985).

Early studies in mice suggested that cell-mediated immunity may be less important than humoral immunity to spermatozoa in the pathogenesis of infertility for passive immunization produced greater effects than adoptive immunization (Boettcher, 1979). There is increasing evidence, however, that cytokine products of activated lymphocytes and macrophages can adversely affect reproductive functions. TNF and IFNγ cause decreased sperm motility (Hill et al, 1987; Eisermann et al, 1989) and impaired sperm-egg interactions (Maruyama et al, 1985; Hill et al, 1989) and exert negative effects on embryo viability (Hill et al, 1987; Tartakovsky & Ben-Yair, 1991), mouse trophoblast outgrowth (Haimovici et al, 1991) and choriocarcinoma cell proliferation in vitro (Berkowitz et al, 1988). Thus, cell-mediated immunity may adversely affect sperm function by cytokine secretion. Haimovici et al (1992) have demonstrated a reduced pregnancy rate on day 15 of pregnancy and a significant increase in fetal resorption sites in mice receiving T lymphocytes from sperm-immunized mice.

Cytokine effects may also explain persistently poor postcoital tests in infertile women despite abundant cervical mucus and no detectable anti-sperm antibodies. Lymphocytes and monocytes have been identified in the normal ejaculate, entering the male reproductive tract through the epididymis and efferent ducts (Olsen & Shields, 1984; Wang & Holstein, 1983; Harrison et al, 1991). Examination of lymphocyte and macrophage numbers in semen in both normal and infertile men has, however, produced conflicting results. El-Demiry et al (1986) reported significantly more leucocytes in semen from fertile men as compared with a subfertile group, although data were semiquantitative. In contrast, Wolff & Anderson (1988) using similar antibodies reported significantly more leucocytes in semen from subfertile men and subsequently demonstrated that leucocytospermia (more than 10^6 leucocytes per ml semen) was associated with poor semen quality with significant reductions in sperm number, motility, velocity, motility index, and total numbers of motile sperm (Wolff et al, 1990); high concentrations of macrophages and T lymphocytes and high levels of granulocyte elastase had different specific effects on sperm function.

Leucocytes in cervical mucus may also secrete cytokines which may adversely affect sperm function. Introduction of spermatozoa causes a leucocytic reaction in the human uterine cervix with neutrophil polymorphs predominating (Pandya & Cohen, 1985; Thompson et al, 1991, 1992). Wah et al (1990) reported high leucocyte counts (more than 2×10^5 leucocytes per ml) in cervico-vaginal cells from the ectocervix and cervico-vaginal fornices (termed asymptomatic cervico-vaginal leucocytosis) in 22% of 114 infertile women undergoing intrauterine insemination, and in none of 21 women undergoing donor insemination. Furthermore, women with cervical factor infertility had a significantly higher incidence of asymptomatic cervico-vaginal leucocytosis than those with either male factor or unexplained infertility. Antibiotic treatment of women with an abnormal postcoital test and asymptomatic cervical leucocytosis diagnosed by a Papanicolaou smear resulted in six pregnancies within 3 months in 10 treated women compared with none in eight untreated women (Matilsky et al, 1993).

Sensitization to seminal plasma antigens

Serum antibodies to seminal plasma fluid antigens have been detected in some infertile women (Carretti, 1974) and it has been claimed from absorption studies that such antibodies may be sperm-immobilizing (Isojima et al, 1972). Attempts have been made to raise a monoclonal antibody to a human seminal plasma-specific component in sperm-immobilizing antibodies; the resulting hybridoma immunostained epididymis and seminal vesicle but not testis (Kameda et al, 1991). Other studies, however, have suggested that antibodies to surface coating antigen or any other seminal plasma antigen do not have spermatozoal immobilizing or agglutinating activity (Li & Beling, 1974; Li et al, 1978). Nevertheless, Chen (1979) has maintained that antibodies to a specific fraction of seminal plasma are absent from fertile women and present in the sera of 16% of infertile women. Although rare, IgE-mediated allergic reactions to seminal plasma components have been demonstrated, and increased total levels of circulating IgE have been associated with infertility (Mathur et al, 1981a).

Sensitization to zona pellucida antigens

The zona pellucida contains ovary-specific antigens and immunization of animals with heterologous ovarian tissue results in the production of antibodies which localize principally on the zona pellucida (Porter et al, 1970; Sacco & Shivers, 1973). Shivers & Dunbar (1977) demonstrated cross-reactivity of antibodies to human zona pellucida with the zona of the pig's ovum and exploited this cross-reactivity to show that antibodies directed against pig zona pellucida were present in the sera of a high proportion of infertile women. Although the results were confirmed by others (Mori et al, 1978; Sotsiou et al, 1980; Bousquet et al, 1982), Boettcher et al (1977) observed that two women with high titres of anti-zona pellucida antibodies became pregnant within weeks of the test. Doubts about

their significance grew when anti-zona pellucida antibodies were detected in the sera of both normally fertile women and males as well as in infertile women (Sacco & Moghissi, 1979). Similarly, using a specific radio-immunoassay, Kurachi et al (1984) detected anti-zona antibodies in the sera of 27% of infertile women, 33% of normally fertile women and 30% of males, the antibody titres being no higher in infertile women than in their fertile counterparts.

Urry et al (1985) have, however, demonstrated anti-zona antibodies not only in 15% of women suffering otherwise unexplained infertility but also in 25% of women suffering recurrent miscarriage. Anti-zona pellucida antibodies have been detected in human ovarian follicular fluid and can apparently coat the ovum in situ; high titres of such antibodies can inhibit human in vitro fertilization. The presence of anti-zona antibodies does not correlate with production of other autoantibodies (Urry et al, 1985). Zona pellucida non-specifically traps proteins, including immunoglobulins, and false positives could therefore occur due to non-specific binding. Furthermore, many studies have used porcine zona pellucida as the target tissue; heteroagglutinin in human serum against porcine red blood cells may also give rise to false positive results (Mori et al, 1979, 1985; Caudle et al, 1987). A recent study of over 1800 infertile women (Kamada et al, 1992) re-examined the implication of anti-zona pellucida autoantibodies by a passive haemagglutinin reaction using bovine red blood cells sensitized with porcine zona antigen: positive anti-zona activities were detected in 5.6% of women with unexplained infertility compared with 1.7% of those with infertility of known cause and 1.5% of non-pregnant fertile and pregnant controls. Anti-zona antibodies were not detected in age-matched adult males or in children. Furthermore, in two-year follow-up studies, no pregnancies occurred in 11 women with a consistently positive passive haemagglutinin reaction with only three pregnancies in 19 women with fluctuating positive antibodies. Three of seven positive sera produced strong positive immunofluorescence reactions on human zona pellucida even after absorption with porcine and human AB blood cells. Pre-exposure of human zona pellucida to these positive sera greatly reduced the number of normal quality spermatozoa which bound to, and penetrated across, human zona pellucida. Thus, anti-zona pellucida antibodies may play a rôle in infertility: the increased availability of human zona components resulting from advances in molecular technology may allow development of more accurate and specific techniques for detection of autoantibodies to zona pellucida which will finally clarify their still somewhat confused rôle in the pathogenesis of female infertility.

Endometrial factors in infertility

The endometrium of women with unexplained infertility

may appear morphologically normal on light-microscopy but morphometric analysis of biopsies precisely timed from the luteinizing hormone (LH) surge has demonstrated subtle abnormalities in the luteal phase (Li et al, 1990). Endometrial glands in similar timed biopsies also show an abnormal distribution and secretion of glycoconjugates in unexplained infertility compared with normal fertile women (Graham et al, 1990; Klentzeris et al, 1991a). Changes in stromal morphology have not been documented. However, Lint (1980) reported high levels of T-helper cells in the endometrium of women with unexplained infertility. In contrast, Soffer et al (1983) reported a deficiency of E-rosette-bearing cells in suspensions prepared from luteal phase endometrium from infertile women; these were presumed to be T lymphocytes but could also represent endometrial granulated lymphocytes which may express CD2.

Many immunohistochemical studies of endometrial leucocytes lack precise histological dating and the definition of normal subjects is not always clear. Klentzeris et al (1991b) compared stromal leucocytes between normal fertile women and women with unexplained infertility in endometrial biopsies at 4, 7, 10 and 13 days following the LH surge. Throughout the luteal phase, endometrium from infertile women contained significantly lower numbers of CD8-positive suppressor/cytotoxic T cells and increased numbers of CD4-positive helper T cells; CD56-positive endometrial granulated lymphocytes were also decreased in number throughout the luteal phase and a lower proportion of them co-expressed CD2. Since total T-cell numbers did not change significantly, the deficiency of CD2-positive cells noted previously (Soffer et al, 1983) may reflect decreased CD2-positive endometrial granulated lymphocytes. The functional significance of the alterations in CD4, CD8 and CD56-positive cells in unexplained infertility is uncertain but a rôle for these cells in implantation and early placentation is suggested. Abnormal numbers of both T and granulated lymphocytes may affect endometrial cytokine secretion, creating a cytokine environment unfavourable for implantation or placental development.

Expression of molecules which mediate intercellular and cell-matrix adhesion may determine the influx and distribution of leucocytes within the endometrium and decidua. Endometrial granulated lymphocytes can express CD11a, VLA-4 and CD2, which can react with their respective counter-receptors ICAM-1, VCAM and LFA-3 expressed on endometrial endothelial cells (Bulmer et al, 1991b; Burrows et al, 1993; Marzusch et al, 1993). Expression of ICAM-1 by scattered stromal cells and LFA-3 by glands may stimulate formation of periglandular and stromal eGL aggregates (Bulmer et al, 1991b; Marzusch et al, 1993). Comprehensive studies of adhesion molecules in precisely timed biopsies from a well-characterized group of infertile women have yet to be reported but Lessey et al (1992) have noted deficient expression of

β_3 integrin (CD61) on epithelial cells in secretory phase endometrium in a small sample of infertile women whose endometrial biopsies were more than three days out of phase.

Adhesion molecules may also play a rôle in the implantation process itself. Klentzeris et al (1993) noted a consistent deficiency in expression of the β_1 integrin VLA-4 by endometrial glandular and surface epithelium throughout the luteal phase in infertile women. Oncofetal fibronectin is produced by the blastocyst (Feinberg et al, 1991) and deficiency of its counter-receptor VLA-4 in endometrial epithelium could result in lack of adhesion and hence failure of implantation.

An additional observation with potential immune-mediated effects on implantation is deficient serum and uterine pregnancy protein 14 (PP14) in infertile women with retarded endometrial development (Klentzeris et al, 1994). PP14 suppresses decidual lymphocyte NK-cell activity (Okamoto et al, 1992); deficiency could thus result in inappropriate cytotoxic activity directed against the implanting blastocyst or early placenta. The factors which stimulate recruitment and proliferation of endometrial granulated lymphocytes in the late luteal phase are unknown. The relationship with progesterone appears to be indirect, progesterone receptors being absent on endometrial granulated lymphocytes. However, progesterone could stimulate production of other factors by endometrial stromal or epithelial cells which in turn could affect endometrial granulated lymphocytes. The response of endometrial granulated lymphocytes to endometrial soluble products has not been studied in detail; deficiency of a luteal phase product such as PP14 could lead to deficient stimulation of and hence to decreased numbers of endometrial granulated lymphocytes within endometrium.

Further studies of endometrial leucocyte function, adhesion molecules and secretory products will cast light on the pathogenesis of some cases of hitherto unexplained infertility. Evaluation of the rôle of endometrial leucocytes in normal implantation and placentation will enhance our understanding of pathological processes but, conversely, studies of conditions such as unexplained infertility may shed light on the normal in vivo rôle of these cells.

PREMATURE OVARIAN FAILURE

The development of ovarian quiescence, together with the onset of menopausal symptoms, under the age of 35 years is referred to as premature menopause or premature ovarian failure. A subgroup of these patients can be defined by lack of response to exogenous gonadotrophin stimulation, despite the presence of ovarian follicles; immune system abnormalities may play a rôle in the pathogenesis of premature ovarian failure in this group.

Autoimmune oophoritis

A proportion of women with autoimmune adrenal failure

also suffer premature ovarian failure; such patients have circulating antibodies which are directed against steroid-synthesizing cells in the adrenal cortex and cross-react with those in the ovary (Anderson et al, 1968; Irvine et al, 1968, 1969; Irvine & Barnes, 1975). This type of ovarian failure is a clearly defined clinical and immunopathological entity which can, quite legitimately, be extended to include polyendocrinopathies in which both adrenal and ovarian failure are components (Golonka & Goodman, 1968; Edmonds et al, 1973; Vasquez & Kenny, 1973; Dempsey et al, 1981). The concept of autoimmune oophoritis has, however, been more controversially extended to explain premature ovarian failure in autoimmune disorders lacking clinical or serological evidence of adrenal disease, including hypothyroidism, rheumatoid arthritis, pernicious anaemia, hypoparathyroidism and myasthenia gravis (Vasquez & Kenny, 1973; Kleerekoper et al, 1974; Appel & Holub, 1976; Ayala et al, 1979; Collen et al, 1979; Williamson et al, 1980; Coulam & Lufkin, 1981; LaBarbera et al, 1988). However, some cases amongst these appear to be examples of non-immunological premature menopause occurring coincidentally in patients with an autoimmune disorder: thus, anti-ovarian antibodies were absent in some cases, whilst in others histological examination of the ovaries revealed total follicle loss, fibrosis and no lymphocytic infiltration.

Claims that idiopathic premature menopause in otherwise healthy women with no evidence of autoimmune disease has an autoimmune pathogenesis associated with anti-ovary antibodies have been controversial. Clearly defined anti-steroid cell antibodies are associated with ovarian failure: Moraes-Ruehsen et al (1972) detected anti-ovarian antibodies reactive with thecal cells in only eight of 55 cases of premature menopause and all of these were associated with either Addison's disease or anti-adrenal antibodies. Claims that anti-ovarian antibodies not clearly shown to be anti-steroid cell antibodies can cause premature menopause (Coulam & Ryan, 1979; Coulam et al, 1981) must be viewed in the context that such antibodies have also been detected in Addison's disease due to tuberculosis (Kamp et al, 1974), in neoplastic disease of the endometrium, kidney and bladder (Forbes et al, 1976), in 45,X0 and 46,XX gonadal dysgenesis (Mathur et al, 1980a) and in women with inflammatory or neoplastic ovarian disease (Zbroja-Sontag et al, 1982). Thus, anti-ovarian antibodies may be epiphenomenal and should not be considered as the cause of ovarian failure without stringent and detailed immunopathological studies. Occasional cases of autoimmune oophoritis have been diagnosed solely on the basis of ovarian histology in the absence of detectable anti-ovarian antibodies (Gloor & Hurlimann, 1984): it is probably unwise to make a diagnosis of autoimmune oophoritis without supporting immunological findings, no matter how apparently convincing are the histological features.

Analysis of immune mechanisms in premature ovarian failure has been based on detection of anti-ovary antibodies. These studies have been hampered by the range of ovarian tissues used, which included rat, rabbit, monkey, guinea pig, cow and human; by their degree of sexual maturation, which ranged from virgin to menopausal; and by the different patterns of antibody binding (Moncayo & Moncayo, 1992). Enzyme-linked immunosorbent assays (ELISA) have recently been used to isolate antigens recognized by the autoantibodies (Moncayo et al, 1989). Most are 'steroid cell antibodies' which bind to mature follicles and corpus luteum (Irvine et al, 1968). Antibodies to zona pellucida have been detected and, most recently, autoantibodies have been shown to bind protein complexes of 2–36 kD as well as a 70 kD complex which may correspond to the unoccupied hCG receptor (Moncayo et al, 1989). Apart from the steroid cell antibodies, the rôle of these antibody categories in the induction and maintenance of ovarian disease remains uncertain.

In vitro studies of cell-mediated immunity in patients with premature ovarian failure have yielded inconsistent results: CD4:CD8 ratios may be decreased, increased or normal (LaBarbera et al, 1988); cell-mediated immunity has been reported to be decreased (Mathur et al, 1980a) but T-cell activation and production of migration inhibition factor are increased (Edmonds et al, 1973; Rabinowe et al, 1989). These conflicting findings may reflect patient heterogeneity and the fact that peripheral blood T cells may be inappropriate for study of ovarian disease (Moncayo & Moncayo, 1992).

Various animal models of premature ovarian failure exist, including natural diseases and those induced by immunization (reviewed in Moncayo & Moncayo, 1992). Active immunization with crude ovarian extracts induces oophoritis characterized by massive follicular atresia and perivascular mononuclear cell inflammation (Ivanova et al, 1984). It remains uncertain how closely studies in experimental animals mirror premature ovarian failure in humans, in whom impairment of ovarian function is usually unrecognized until its late stages. Lymphocytic infiltration around developing follicles has been noted (Irvine et al, 1968) whilst lymphocyte and plasma cell infiltration of ovaries containing multiple macroscopic cysts has been reported (Gloor & Hurlimann, 1984; Biscotti et al, 1989). Sedmak et al (1986) found infiltration of developing cystic and atretic follicles by B cells and CD4 and CD8-positive T cells with sparing of primordial follicles whilst in a study of 12 cases of auto-immune oophoritis, lymphoplasmohistiocytic infiltrate of early and late pre-ovulatory follicles was identified in all but one, again with sparing of primordial follicles (Bannatyne et al, 1990). Anti-steroid cell antibodies are of IgG type and in immunofluorescence studies localize in the ovary to the hilar cells, to the cells of the developing follicle and to the thecal cells of the corpus luteum, although the pattern of localization is variable (Irvine & Barnes, 1975, Sotsiou et al, 1980). The pathogenetic rôle of anti-steroid cell antibodies is indicated by their complement-dependent cytotoxicity to cultured granulosa cells (McNatty et al, 1975). The histological features of oophoritis with a T-cell infiltrate suggest involvement of cell-mediated immunity, although in vitro studies have produced conflicting results as discussed above.

Ovarian granulosa cells in women with premature ovarian failure may express high levels of class II MHC antigens (Hill & Anderson, 1988): aberrant expression of these antigens by thyroid and pancreatic epithelium is associated with autoimmune disorders. Hence, expression of class II MHC antigens in the ovary, induced by IFNγ, may be a mechanism of reproductive failure. Oophoritis has also been linked with systemic lupus erythematosus (SLE). Before immunosuppressive agents became available, oophoritis was described in patients with SLE (Rose & Pillsbury, 1944) and an association between active SLE and anti-ovarian antibodies has been described (Moncayo-Naveda et al, 1989). More recently, anti-ovarian antibodies have been identified in women treated with exogenous gonadotrophins to induce superovulation for in vitro fertilization, a significant incidence of seroconversion occurring during hormonal stimulation (Moncayo et al, 1990). Following observations that primordial follicles appeared to be less antigenic than developing follicular epithelium (Irvine et al, 1968), it was suggested that antigenicity may be influenced by elevated gonadotrophin levels: autoimmunity may thus arise as a result of supraphysiological stimulation of the ovaries. A form of autoimmuine oophoritis may also complicate some cases of chronic mucocutaneous and vaginal candidiasis (Mathur et al, 1980b). Anti-candida antibodies in the patients appear to cross-react with thymocytes, T lymphocytes and with ovarian follicular cells, resulting in ovarian failure. Thus, several studies indicate that immune oophoritis is a factor in premature ovarian failure, although the precise pathogenetic mechanisms of this disease remain to be fully clarified.

Resistant ovary syndrome

A proportion of cases of the resistant ovary syndrome, in which a premature menopause occurs because the ovaries are insensitive to gonadotrophins, may have an immunological basis for there have been reports of women with both myasthenia gravis and resistant ovary syndrome who have a substance in their serum which inhibits in vitro binding of FSH to its receptor (Escobar et al, 1982); further, a patient has been described who had systemic lupus erythematosus, resistant ovary syndrome and a serum antibody specifically directed against the FSH receptor (Case Records of the Massachusetts General Hospital,

1986). Finally, in some women with the resistant ovary syndrome an IgG antibody is present which, in an in vitro system, blocks FSH-induced DNA synthesis by granulosa cells (van Weissenbruch et al, 1991).

IMMUNOLOGICAL ASPECTS OF GYNAECOLOGICAL CANCER

Immune status of women with gynaecological cancer

There is a widespread belief that many women suffering from gynaecological cancer are relatively immunodeficient, particularly in their ability to mount a cell-mediated immune response; however, the evidence is far from conclusive with mutually incompatible findings in the literature. Khoo & Mackay (1974) showed that a high proportion of women with ovarian, endometrial or cervical cancer were either anergic or showed markedly reduced reactivity in skin tests to primary antigens, such as dinitrochlorobenzene (DNCB), or to recall antigens, such as Candida or purified protein derivative (PPD); the more advanced the malignant disease, the more likely was the patient to be anergic and the authors concluded that there was a clear relationship between an inability to mount a cell-mediated immune response, as detected by skin testing, and poor prognosis. Nalick et al (1974a, 1974b) also reported diminished responses on skin testing with DNCB in many patients with ovarian or cervical carcinoma (but not in patients with endometrial adenocarcinoma or CIN) and noted a correlation between poor reactivity and a gloomy prognosis. Levin et al (1976) reported decreased skin responses to PPD in many women with ovarian carcinoma and decreased sensitivity to both primary and recall antigens has been noted in advanced, but not early, invasive cervical carcinoma (Micksche et al, 1978; Hancock et al, 1979; Alsabti, 1980).

Attempts to explain this apparent defect in cell-mediated immunity in gynaecological cancer in terms of altered numbers or reactivity of T lymphocytes have given conflicting results. There have been several reports of decreased numbers of circulating T cells in women with invasive cervical carcinoma (Rand et al, 1977; Levy et al, 1978; Ishiguro et al, 1980; Satam et al, 1981; Kietlinska, 1984; Balaram et al, 1988; Jain et al, 1990) but opinions differ between the majority, who consider this deficiency to be limited to those with advanced disease (Hancock et al, 1979; Satam et al, 1981), and others who have detected decreased T-cell levels in patients with stage I tumours (Kietlinska, 1984). In contrast, Bonneterre et al (1981) reported normal T-cell numbers in women with invasive cervical carcinoma at all stages, including 42 patients with stage III or IV disease. Findings in women with CIN also vary, some noting normal T-cell levels in all patients with CIN (Rand et al, 1977; Bonneterre et al,

1981) and others detecting a significant decrease in T-cell numbers in many cases of CIN 2 and 3 (Sawonabar et al, 1977; Ishiguro et al, 1980; Jain et al, 1990). Ashman et al (1975) also noted decreased peripheral T-cell counts in CIN but claimed an increased proportion and absolute numbers of 'active' T cells, in direct contrast with the findings of Bashford & Gough (1981). Reduction in the CD4:CD8 ratio has also been reported in women with CIN and invasive cervical carcinoma, the degree of reduction being significantly correlated with disease severity (Jain et al, 1990; Kesic et al, 1990).

Decreased lymphocyte responses to mitogens such as phytohaemagglutinin (PHA), concanavalin-A (Con-A) and pokeweed mitogen (PWM) have been reported in patients with ovarian or cervical carcinoma (Jenkins et al, 1975; Levy et al, 1978; Daunter et al, 1979; Hancock et al, 1979; Bonneterre et al, 1981; Satam et al, 1981; Stratton & DiSaia, 1982), this diminished responsiveness being usually, but not invariably, confined to or most marked in women with advanced malignant disease. However, van der Linde et al (1983) reported normal lymphocyte responses to PHA in cervical carcinoma and CIN, while Kietlinska (1984) detected exaggerated blastogenesis in some patients with stage I cervical cancer. More recently, studies of large groups of Indian women with cervical carcinoma have identified various immunodeficiencies (Balaram et al, 1988; Radhakrishna Pillai et al, 1990). Increased levels of Con-A-induced suppressor cell activity by peripheral blood lymphocytes were noted in all patients with cervical carcinoma, the levels rising progressively with stage and hence with tumour load. Suppressor activity was further increased by radiotherapy but returned to pretreatment levels within six months in women who remained disease free, whilst those who developed recurrent disease maintained high suppression levels. Reduced NK and antibody-dependent cellular cytotoxicity (ADCC) has been reported in women suffering from disseminated cervical carcinoma with recovery after radiotherapy: the number of large granular lymphocytes in peripheral blood did not differ between patients and controls (Satam et al, 1986; Balaram et al, 1988). In contrast, Siklos et al (1992) reported a significant increase in anti-D ADCC in cases of early stage cervical carcinoma, as compared with healthy controls, with a further increase after radiotherapy.

Levels of peripheral blood T cells in women with ovarian carcinoma have been variously reported as normal (Mandell et al, 1979) and decreased (Wolff & De Oliveira, 1975; Zbroja-Sontag, 1983; Lukomska et al, 1983). Similarly, both relatively normal (Chatterjee et al, 1975; Mitchell & Kohorn, 1976; Kohorn et al, 1978; Ueda et al, 1978, 1979; Mandell et al, 1979; Daunter et al, 1982) and decreased (Levin et al, 1976) lymphocyte reactivity has been described. Patients with advanced ovarian cancer have been reported to have low peripheral blood NK-cell activity (Mantovani et al, 1981), sometimes associated with a concomitant reduction in the number of circulating mononuclear cells (Lukomska et al, 1983). In contrast, Kikuchi et al (1990) have noted increased numbers of certain NK-cell subsets in ovarian carcinoma patients whilst Siklos et al (1992) have also reported increased ADCC in some cases of ovarian carcinoma.

The cell-mediated immune system is controlled by cytokines. A recent study of cytokine production by peripheral blood lymphocytes and monocytes in a whole blood culture system after initial mitogenic stimulation reported significantly reduced production of IFNγ, IL1α and IL2 in 239 patients with untreated breast, cervical, endometrial or ovarian cancer as compared with 191 healthy female controls; levels of TNFα did not differ significantly between the two groups (Elsässer-Beile et al, 1993). Levels of IFNγ, IL2 and IL1α showed a gradual decrease with increasing tumour load, particularly for breast and cervical carcinoma, and IFNγ was the best parameter for evaluating the cellular immunological competence of patients, being produced only by T cells and NK cells. Lymphocyte numbers did not differ between patients and controls. This gradual depression in cell-mediated immunity, detected by decreased cytokine production, may be due to circulating immunosuppressive factors or induction of suppressor cell populations in patients with gynaecological neoplasia (Elsässer-Beile et al, 1993). Yron et al (1986) reported reduced lymphocyte responses to PHA and decreased IL2 production in stage I endometrial carcinoma patients compared with healthy controls. Patients with postmenopausal bleeding formed a second 'high risk' control group and showed varying levels of IL2 production which did not differ significantly from those in healthy female controls.

Although there have been fewer reports of abnormalities of the humoral immune system associated with gynaecological malignancy, their inconclusiveness parallels that for studies of T cells. Thus, circulating B-cell numbers in women with cervical carcinoma have been reported to be normal (Rand et al, 1977; Levy et al, 1978; Hancock et al, 1979; Bonneterre et al, 1981; Satam et al, 1981), decreased (Ishiguro et al, 1980; Kietlinska, 1984; Jain et al, 1990) or increased (Balaram et al, 1988). Similarly, reports of serum immunoglobulin levels in cervical carcinoma are contradictory. Increased levels of serum IgG have been reported (Vasudevan et al, 1971; Adelusi & Salimonu, 1981), the values increasing with advancing disease stage (Vijayakumar et al, 1986): this increase may be due to production of anti-viral antibodies (see below). Serum IgA levels are also elevated in patients with cervical cancer (Vasudevan et al, 1971; Lee, 1977; Adelusi & Salimonu, 1981; Gupta et al, 1981), the values increasing with advanced clinical stage and returning to normal in clinically cured patients (Vijayakumar et al, 1986). Increased IgD and IgE levels have also been reported, particularly in late stage disease, but IgM levels do not differ significantly from those of healthy controls (Adelusi & Salimonu, 1981; Lee, 1977; Vijayakumar et al, 1986).

Thus, there is no clear evidence of generalized immunodeficiency in women with gynaecological cancer. Conflicting results may be due to methodology but other factors, such as the immunosuppressive effect of impaired nutritional status in advanced malignant disease or the presence of cancer-associated serum suppressor factors, have often not been considered and patient-associated immunodeficiency and tumour-associated immunosuppression have not been distinguished. Nevertheless, studies of female genital tract cancer in immunosuppressed women suggest that impaired cell-mediated immunity may play a rôle in allowing the development or progression of invasive neoplasia. An increased incidence of cervical neoplasia has been reported in women receiving immunosuppressive therapy following renal transplantations (Alloub et al, 1989) and the effectiveness of the host immune response appears to be important for determining the clinical outcome following infection of cervical keratinocytes by HPV (Roche & Crum, 1991). Further, women with HIV infection have an increased risk of developing lower genital tract intraepithelial neoplasia (Bradbeer, 1987; Spurrett et al, 1988; Byrne et al, 1989; Smith & Barton, 1992), this being particularly the case for those who are seropositive and have low CD4 counts (Chiphangwi et al, 1991; Conti et al, 1991; Fahs et al, 1991; LaGuardia et al, 1991; Smith et al, 1991).

Immunological response to gynaecological neoplasms

Humoral immune response

Antibodies reactive with tumour antigens can be detected in both serum and ascitic fluid of many women with ovarian carcinoma (DiSaia et al, 1973; DiSaia 1975; Dorsett et al, 1975; Forbes et al, 1976; Gerber et al, 1977; Hill et al, 1978; Zbroja-Sontag et al, 1983; Silburn et al, 1984) and bound immunoglobulins have been retrieved from circulating immune complexes, from surface membranes of ovarian carcinoma cells and from membrane fragments in cyst or ascitic fluid (Dawson et al, 1983; Hill et al, 1983; Taylor et al, 1983). However, these antibodies are generally not directed specifically against ovarian cancer antigens: some are autoantibodies against normal ovarian components but most are anti-nuclear, anti-mitochondrial, anti-smooth muscle or anti-gastric parietal cell antibodies (Dawson et al, 1983), whilst others have been characterized as antibodies to CEA (Hill et al, 1982).

Although the humoral response to ovarian cancer appears to be non-specific, the resulting antibodies cannot be ignored for they may act as blocking factors, either alone or by forming immune complexes. Disagreement regarding the presence of elevated levels of immune complexes in women with ovarian carcinoma appears to have been due to technical factors: those using assays based on immune complex binding to complement components have failed to detect raised levels of immune complexes in ovarian carcinoma patients (Teshima et al, 1977; Clarke et al, 1982), whilst those employing a polyethylene glycol precipitation technique have found a marked excess of immune complexes in both serum and ascites fluid of a majority of women with malignant ovarian disease (Poulton et al, 1978, 1982; Dodd et al, 1983; Mooney et al, 1983a, b; Silburn et al, 1983, 1984). This disparity, which has led some to doubt that true immune complexes occur in ovarian carcinoma (Witkin et al, 1984), appears to reflect the fact that the immune complexes associated with ovarian carcinoma differ from those in other diseases, such as rheumatoid arthritis, having altered proportions of immunoglobulins and complement components (Mooney et al, 1983b). Immune complex levels are related directly to tumour bulk, being highest in those with extensive disease and often reverting to normal during tumour remissions (Poulton et al, 1982; Smith & Oi, 1984); these complexes may represent the serum blocking factor noted in many women with progressive ovarian carcinoma (Mitchell & Kohorn, 1976; Patillo et al, 1979a). This serum blocking factor suppresses tumour-specific cell-mediated cytotoxicity and NK-cell activity; blocking factor activity is most marked in patients with advanced disease and is often absent from those in remission (Patillo et al, 1979b).

Antibodies reactive with tumour-derived antigens have been detected in cervical carcinoma (Weintraub et al, 1972; DiSaia et al, 1973; DiSaia, 1975; Chiang et al, 1976) and Vos et al (1972) were able to retrieve a cytotoxic antibody from tumour cells. There is, however, little evidence that these antibodies are directed against tumour-specific antigens since they were also detected in low titre in healthy controls. Van der Linde et al (1981) detected antibodies which appeared to react specifically with an antigen in cervical squamous cell carcinoma in 82% of women with invasive cervical neoplasms: such antibodies were not detected in women with CIN or microinvasive carcinoma. Whether these antibodies contribute to the immune complexes commonly found in patients with cervical carcinoma (Seth et al, 1979; Bonneterre et al, 1981) and whether such complexes represent the blocking factor present in many of these women (Dini & Faiferman, 1980) is not known; however, in contrast with ovarian carcinoma, both immune complexes and blocking factor can be detected at all stages of cervical cancer and are unrelated to tumour progression.

Antibodies in women with cervical carcinoma may be directed against viral antigens (Kumari et al, 1982). Various HPV epitopes may act as antigens: antibodies directed against the E7 open reading frame protein of HPV 16 have been detected in the serum of around 20% of patients with HPV16-associated cervical lesions (Jochmus-Kudielka et al, 1989) and HPV16 E7 can act as a tumour rejection antigen (Chen et al, 1991). In contrast, serum IgG and IgA antibodies directed against a synthetic peptide derived from HPV 18 open reading frame E2 are associated with a significantly increased risk for cervical adenocarcinoma, HPV 16 E2 being linked, though not to a statistically significant degree, with an increased risk of cervical squamous cell carcinoma (Lehtinen et al, 1992).

Local antibody responses in gynaecological neoplasms have been little studied. Indeed, despite the frequency of HPV infection in association with cervical intraepithelial and invasive neoplasia, little is known about the local host immune response to this virus. IgA antibodies reactive with bovine papilloma virion proteins have been detected in the cervical mucus of a proportion of women with abnormal cervical smears (Dillner et al, 1989) whilst in women with CIN associated with HPV 16 infection immunoglobulins in cervical secretions showed reactivity to HPV 16 E4 or L1, or both, but not to E7 (Snyder et al, 1991). Thus, it is possible to identify specific determinants encoded by HPV DNA which elicit a host immune response.

Cell-mediated immune responses

Systemic responses There have been several reports of in vitro toxicity to autologous or allogeneic tumour cells by lymphocytes from ovarian or cervical carcinoma patients (DiSaia et al, 1971; Chen et al, 1975; DiSaia, 1975; Mitchell & Kohorn, 1976; Patillo et al, 1979a); however, the observed cytotoxicity may be due to NK cells rather than T cells or may be induced by MHC antigens on allogeneic cells (Smith & Oi, 1984). Peripheral blood lymphocytes from 21 of 43 women with ovarian cancer proliferated when stimulated with purified autologous tumour cells (Allavena et al, 1988), indicating that some of these patients develop an immunological response to their tumour, although peripheral blood lymphocytes from these women are usually not cytotoxic to autologous tumour cells in vitro (Mantovani et al, 1980; Allavena et al, 1982). The ability of autologous ovarian tumour cells to elicit a blastogenic response in the mixed lymphocyte-tumour culture (MLTC) assay does not correlate with expression of class II MHC antigens by the tumour cells, suggesting recognition of distinct tumour-associated antigens (Di Bello et al, 1988). Lymphocyte sensitization to autologous or allogeneic tumour antigens has been detected by leucocyte migration inhibition in patients with ovarian or cervical carcinoma (Chen et al, 1973, 1975; Melnick & Barber, 1975; Faiferman et al, 1977; Goldstein et al, 1977; Cerni et al, 1979; Rivera et al, 1979; Sekiguchi

et al, 1982), but similar findings have been reported when testing lymphocytes against normal tissue antigens (Tosner & Fixa, 1979).

Although autologous tumour cells may elicit a blastogenic response in peripheral blood lymphocytes in some ovarian carcinoma patients, in others tumour cells suppress spontaneous lymphocyte proliferation in a dose-dependent manner (Akiyama et al, 1983; Allavena et al, 1988): this may be due to activation of tumour suppressor lymphocytes or to release of soluble suppressor factors. Examination of the stimulatory effects of soluble extracts of ovarian or cervical carcinoma on peripheral blood lymphocytes has produced inconsistent results. Levin et al (1975, 1976) reported blastogenic activity in most ovarian cancer patients in remission but in only a small proportion of those with progressive disease, whereas Chatterjee et al (1975) failed to detect any such responses. Van der Linde et al (1983) detected a lymphoproliferative response to antigens derived from a cervical carcinoma cell line in 70% of women with CIN but in only 42% of those with invasive neoplasm. Soluble tumour extracts may elicit lymphoproliferation by their cytokine content. Despite the conflicting data regarding T-cell activation in gynaecological cancers, high levels of soluble IL2 receptor in both serum and ascitic fluid of ovarian carcinoma patients provide evidence of T-cell activation: soluble IL2-receptor may negatively modulate the local host immune response (Barton et al, 1993).

NK cells can mediate a direct cytotoxic effect on autologous, allogeneic or xenogeneic cells and NK-cell lysis is unrestricted by MHC antigens. Low peripheral blood NK-cell lysis has been reported in patients with advanced ovarian cancer (Mantovani et al, 1981; Lotzova et al, 1984, 1988), and Berek et al (1984) noted decreased peripheral blood NK activity in 9 of 13 patients with stage III ovarian cancer. Others have noted normal peripheral blood NK-cell activity in patients with untreated ovarian cancer (Lukomska et al, 1983; Shau et al, 1983) but Lukomska et al (1983) noted reduced numbers of circulating NK cells following either surgery or chemotherapy though failing to detect any correlation between depressed NK-cell activity and advancement of the neoplastic disease.

NK-cell activity is depressed in women with invasive cervical carcinoma (Pulay et al, 1982) at all clinical stages despite normal numbers of large granular lymphocytes (Satam et al, 1986). Normal NK-cell activity has been reported in patients with CIN (Neill & Norval, 1984) but others have claimed that there is a significant defect in NK-cell immune surveillance, correctable by IFN, in women with preinvasive cervical lesions (Seltzer et al, 1983). Pulay et al (1982) noted no effect of radiotherapy on peripheral blood NK-cell activity in women treated for cervical carcinoma, whereas Satam et al (1986) reported recovery in both NK-cell activity and ADCC after radiation treatment, although not to normal levels.

Culture of NK cells in high doses of IL2 produces lymphokine-activated killer (LAK) cells. Peripheral blood mononuclear cells from both normal donors and ovarian carcinoma patients generally cannot lyse ovarian cell lines or autologous tumour cells but a high proportion are capable of lysis after incubation for 3–5 days in IL2 (Crimm et al, 1982; Allavena et al, 1986, 1989; Lotzova et al, 1988; Boyer et al, 1989). Peripheral blood mononuclear cells from patients with endometrial carcinoma show weak cytotoxicity against autologous tumour cells with increased cytotoxicity after incubation in IL2. Normal autologous endometrial epithelium was generally insensitive to lysis even after IL2 incubation. IL2-activated killer cells in this system were thus able to distinguish between normal and malignant endometrial cells and were derived from CD16-positive CD3-negative NK-cell precursors (Timonen et al, 1987).

Local responses Studies of circulating mononuclear cells in women with gynaecological cancer have yielded equivocal results and it is probably more relevant to study the host response in terms of those lymphocytes present in the stroma of many tumours (tumour-infiltrating lymphocytes: TIL) and those in the ascitic fluid of patients with advanced disease (tumour-associated lymphocytes: TAL). The majority of lymphocytes within and associated with epithelial ovarian carcinoma are T lymphocytes, both CD4-positive and CD8-positive populations being present (Haskill et al, 1982a; Kabawat et al, 1983b; Ferguson et al, 1985; Heo et al, 1988). In flow cytometric studies of lymphocytes isolated from ovarian tumours, CD3-positive T cells consistently accounted for more than 50% and often more than 70% of the leucocytes present (Heo et al, 1988). Although the ratio of CD4 to CD8-positive cells is variable in solid tumours, it tends to be higher in tumour-infiltrating lymphocytes than in peripheral blood. TIL may be enriched in CD8-positive cytolytic cells with anti-tumour activity (Cardi et al, 1989) but despite expression of IL2-receptor, suggesting in situ activation, lymphocytes freshly isolated from ovarian carcinomas do not show cytotoxicity against autologous tumour targets before prior expansion in IL2 (Heo et al, 1988).

NK cells are relatively sparse in ovarian carcinomas and associated ascitic fluid (Mantovani et al, 1980; Introna et al, 1983; Kabawat et al, 1983c; Berek et al, 1984; Ferguson et al, 1985; Heo et al, 1988; Vaccarello et al, 1990) but this paucity of NK cells is a characteristic of most solid human tumours (Moore, 1984), although the explanation for this is disputed. Vaccarello et al (1990) examined TIL in ovarian tumours of borderline malignancy and found significantly fewer infiltrating leucocytes and fewer activated (class II MHC-positive or CD25-positive) lymphocytes than in TIL from ovarian carcinomas. The proportion of CD3-negative CD56-positive NK cells was higher in borderline tumours than in inva-

sive carcinomas and it was suggested that NK cells may be associated with local anti-tumour responses in the early stages of tumour growth.

Freshly isolated lymphocytes from ovarian carcinomas show a markedly reduced response to PHA (Haskill et al, 1982b) and are usually unable to lyse autologous tumour cells (Tötterman et al, 1978; Heo et al, 1988). This relative immunological non-responsiveness could be partly due to the presence of suppressor T cells (Moore, 1984) but may also be explained by the presence of macrophages with suppressor activity within the tumours (Haskill et al, 1982c) or by cytokine secretion. Soluble factors isolated from the ascitic fluid of women with advanced ovarian cancer can inhibit T and B lymphocyte proliferation (Hess et al, 1979, 1980) and appear to be produced by macrophages (Sheid & Boyce, 1984); ascitic fluid from ovarian carcinoma patients also inhibits generation of LAK cells, apparently mediated by the suppressor activity of transforming growth factor beta (TGFβ) (Hirte & Clark, 1991a, b). Tumour-associated macrophages may exert non-specific cytotoxicity towards ovarian tumour cells but can also stimulate neoplastic cell growth, presumably by secretion of cytokines (Peri et al, 1986).

Functional studies of T and NK cells within ovarian carcinomas have primarily focused on their cytotoxic activity. Freshly isolated TIL are generally unable to lyse tumour cells but after incubation in IL2, to form LAK cells, they usually develop non-MHC-restricted cytotoxicity against autologous ovarian carcinoma cells (Apiranthitou-Drogan et al, 1992) which has been attributed to CD56-positive effectors (Heo et al, 1988). TIL cultured in both IL2 and TNF showed higher cytotoxicity against autologous tumour targets, the lytic population expressing CD8; autologous tumour lysis was, however, short-lived being replaced by non-MHC-restricted LAK activity mediated by CD3-negative CD56-positive cells (Li et al, 1989).

T cells form the major lymphoid population in ascitic fluid from ovarian carcinoma patients (Berek et al, 1984) and freshly isolated TAL from ascitic fluid do not mediate NK-cell activity or ADCC (Berek et al, 1984; Lotzova et al, 1988; Boyer et al, 1989). Although some authors have been unable to generate LAK cells from peritoneal fluid lymphocytes (Boyer et al, 1989) others have produced cells with non-MHC-restricted and autologous anti-tumour cytotoxicity by incubation in IL2 (Allavena et al, 1986, 1989; Lotzova et al, 1988; Ioannides et al, 1991; Apiranthitou-Drogan et al, 1992). Ascitic fluid may, however, contain soluble factors, such as TGFβ, which can suppress lytic activity.

Altered populations of immunocompetent cells have been reported in cervical HPV infection and CIN. Several studies have shown depletion of Langerhans cells (Morris et al, 1983; McArdle & Muller, 1986; Tay et al, 1987a; Hawthorn et al, 1988; Hughes et al, 1988), increased expression of HLA-DR and HLA-DQ by Langerhans cells (Hughes et al, 1988), increased numbers of CD56-positive granulated lymphocytes (McKenzie et al, 1991) and, with one exception (Viac et al, 1990), depletion of intraepithelial T cells, particularly CD4-positive cells (Castello et al, 1986; Tay et al, 1987b). Invasive carcinomas of the cervix are infiltrated with T cells and small numbers of NK cells (Ferguson et al, 1985); CD8-positive predominate over CD4-positive lymphocytes, only a small proportion being activated (Ghosh & Moore, 1992). Cultures of TIL expanded in IL2 exhibited NK and LAK activity and comprised predominantly CD8-positive cells with varying numbers of CD56- and CD25-positive cells: low autologous anti-tumour cytotoxocity was demonstrated (Ghosh & Moore, 1992).

The clinical significance of the in situ leucocytic infiltrate in gynaecological neoplasms remains uncertain. Several authors have reported that ovarian and cervical neoplasms with a heavy cellular infiltrate have a somewhat better prognosis than those with a sparse infiltrate (Sidhu et al, 1970; Gusberg et al, 1971; Hassumi et al, 1977; Deligdisch, 1982; Deligdisch et al, 1982) but Barber et al (1975) were unable to demonstrate any prognostic significance of the stromal infiltrate in ovarian carcinoma.

Cytokines in gynaecological malignancies

Cytokines are low molecular weight peptide regulatory factors with wide ranging effects on a variety of cell types (Balkwill & Burke, 1991). Some cytokines can directly or indirectly inhibit tumour growth and have been used in cancer therapy but there is now increasing evidence that cytokines can contribute to the development and spread of various tumours. The rôle of cytokines in the pathogenesis of gynaecological neoplasia has stimulated considerable recent interest, particularly for ovarian cancer (Malik & Balkwill, 1991). Ascitic fluid from ovarian cancer patients contains growth-promoting factors selectively mitogenic for ovarian cancer cells (Mills et al, 1988).

Constitutive production of several cytokines by human ovarian cancer cell lines and fresh tumour biopsies has been reported. Tumour necrosis factor (TNF) is cytotoxic for some tumour cell lines and causes necrosis of certain human tumour xenografts (Creasey et al, 1986; Jones & Selby, 1989) but can also promote tumour growth and invasion (Fiers, 1991). TNF stimulates fibroblast growth, contributing to generation of tumour stroma, and up-regulates certain metalloproteinase genes (Ito et al, 1990). In xenograft models, intraperitoneal TNF caused human ovarian cancer cells in ascites to clump and form solid peritoneal tumours (Malik et al, 1989). Cells transfected with TNF exhibited enhanced invasive capacity in nude mice which was neutralized with anti-TNF (Malik et al, 1990).

In the normal ovary TNF mRNA is only very occasion-ally expressed in cells of the external theca of the corpus luteum but TNF mRNA and protein are expressed by a significant proportion of tumour cells in both primary and metastatic lesions from patients with ovarian carcinoma (Naylor et al, 1990; Takayama et al, 1991) as well as in ovarian cancer cell lines (Spriggs et al, 1988; Wu et al, 1993). TNF mRNA is detectable in both neoplastic epithelial cells and infiltrating macrophages, while TNF protein is localized primarily to macrophages within the tumour stroma and at the epithelial/stromal borders (Naylor et al, 1993). Expression of the TNF p55 receptor is confined to the epithelial tumour cells whereas the p75 TNF receptor is localized to infiltrating macrophages (Naylor et al, 1993). TNF gene expression is detected more commonly in serous than in mucinous tumours, with up to 65% of neoplastic epithelial cells in serous tumours expressing TNF message (mean of 13%). The level and frequency of TNF expression increases with progression from borderline to poorly-differentiated tumours (Naylor et al, 1993). The co-expression of TNF and its receptors in ovarian epithelial neoplasms suggests that this cytokine may function as both an autocrine and paracrine growth factor in ovarian cancer (Naylor et al, 1993) whilst TNF production by ovarian carcinoma cells could result in resistance to the cytotoxic action of either endogenous or exogenous TNF.

Constitutive expression of macrophage colony stimulating factor (M-CSF) and its receptor, encoded by the c-fms oncogene, has been demonstrated in human ovarian cancer tissues and cell lines (Ramakrishnan et al, 1989; Kacinski et al, 1990; Baiocchi et al, 1991; Kacinski et al, 1989) but not in normal ovarian epithelium. A monocyte chemotactic factor produced by ovarian cancer cell lines (Bottazzi et al, 1985) has been shown to be monocyte chemotactic protein (MCP-1), which is inducible by TNF and interleukin 1 (IL1) (Bottazzi et al, 1990). Interleukin 6 (IL6) production is transiently induced in gonadotrophin-primed hyperstimulated ovaries (Motro et al, 1990), can be detected in the ascitic fluid of ovarian cancer patients (Erroi et al, 1989) and is constitutively produced by ovarian cancer tissues and cell lines (Watson et al, 1990). IL1α and IL1β genes have been detected in ovarian cancer cell lines and in tumour cells isolated from ascitic fluid from ovarian cancer patients (Li et al, 1992); however, in ovarian carcinoma tissue biopsies, IL1α and β were localized to the boundaries between stroma and epithelium by in situ hybridization, raising the possibility of production by infiltrating macrophages (Naylor et al, 1993). Interleukin 10 (IL10), gamma-interferon (IFNγ) and granulocyte macrophage colony stimulating factor (GM-CSF) mRNA have also been detected in biopsies from ovarian carcinomas; IL10 and GM-CSF were unique to tumour biopsies while IFNγ was more frequent in tumour biopsies but was also present in normal ovaries. mRNA for these cytokines is likely, however, to have been derived from infiltrating lymphocytes and macrophages incorporated in the biopsies (Pisa et al, 1992). Recent studies have also indicated that transforming growth factor alpha (TGFα) is an autocrine growth factor for an ovarian cancer cell line both in vivo and in vitro (Kurachi et al, 1991; Morishige et al, 1991).

TNF, IL1, IL6 and MCP-1 are closely related in the cytokine network (Balkwill & Burke, 1991). IL1 and M-CSF induce TNF in monocytes and mesenchymal cells, while TNF induces production of TNF, M-CSF, IL1, IL6 and MCP-1 in several cell types. The rôle of cytokines in the pathogenesis of ovarian cancer remains uncertain but could affect several levels of the neoplastic process. Tissue damage during ovulation may lead to local release of cytokines, such as TNF or TGFβ, both of which can induce metalloproteinase production by tumour cells, increasing their invasive potential (Ito et al, 1990; Welch et al, 1990). TNF can also activate putative oncogenes, and modulation of oncogene expression represents a possible mechanism of cytokine-induced effects on tumour cell growth or inhibition.

Since normal ovarian epithelium does not express the cytokines detected in ovarian epithelial tumours, cytokine production following transformation may lead to autocrine growth stimulation or metastatic potential (Malik & Balkwill, 1991). IL1, IL6 and TNF can stimulate proliferation of ovarian carcinoma cell lines (Wu et al, 1992), although IL1 has exerted an antiproliferative effect on one ovarian carcinoma cell line (Kilian et al, 1991). Expression of M-CSF and TNF with their appropriate receptors suggests autocrine growth regulation of some ovarian carcinomas. M-CSF production is high during pregnancy and can be increased by gonadotrophins (Bartocci et al, 1986): this cytokine therefore may participate in the tumour promoting rôle of gonadotrophins. Interactions between reproductive hormones and cytokines may also explain the reported inhibitory effects of oestrogens on TNF secretion (Ralston et al, 1990). The increasing incidence of ovarian carcinomas with age could conceivably be explained by loss of oestrogen secretion and high gonadotrophin levels causing induction of ovarian TNF via M-CSF.

Hormone-cytokine interactions may also be important in other gynaecological neoplasms. Growth of an endometrial adenocarcinoma cell line was modulated by TNF, the effect differing according to dose, and culture with oestrogen upregulated expression of the p75 TNF receptor (Innins et al, 1992). Similarly, culture with a synthetic progestin increased expression of M-CSF mRNA by the Ishikawa endometrial adenocarcinoma cell line (Kimura et al, 1991).

Thus, there is accumulating evidence that ovarian carcinoma can produce and respond to a variety of cytokines. Potential rôles for cytokines include autocrine growth regulation and potentiation of metastasis. Interactions between hormones and cytokines may explain hormonal modulations of tumours (Scambia et al, 1991). Understanding of cytokine actions within individual neoplasms will be crucial for the future therapeutic use of cytokines which may include inhibition of cytokine secretion, prevention of recruitment of cytokine-producing cells or treatment with cytokine antagonists (Malik & Balkwill, 1991).

Antigens associated with gynaecological cancer

The search for cancer-associated antigens specific for a particular neoplasm, which would be of great value in immunodiagnosis, has been intense. Tumour-associated antigens form three groups. Class 1 antigens are unique to an individual neoplasm and are not shared by other tumours of the same histological type. Class 2 antigens are expressed by many or most tumours of a specific histological type and by tumours of other histological types but are not widely expressed in normal adult tissues. Class 3 antigens are expressed both by cancer cells and by a wide range of normal adult tissues. Currently, no antigen has been described which is specific for a particular neoplasm but is not expressed by normal tissues. Class 2 antigens are currently the most useful, but thorough screening is required to distinguish these from class 3 antigens which are more widely expressed by normal and non-neoplastic adult tissues. The oncodevelopmental antigens, such as CEA and alphafetoprotein, and oncoplacental antigens such as hCG and placental alkaline phosphatase are a subgroup of class 2 antigens.

To date the search for cancer-associated antigens in gynaecological cancer has been focused primarily on ovarian adenocarcinoma. Prior to the development of monoclonal antibodies, detection of ovarian cancer-associated antigens was dependent on the use of polyclonal heterologous antisera, which contained a wide range of antibodies and required extensive absorption with normal tissue and biochemical separation procedures before a 'pure' antibody was obtained. Antigens dating from this period, and which are of limited value in the immunodiagnosis of ovarian carcinoma, include CEA (Rubin & Lewis, 1986), placental alkaline phosphatase (Sunderland et al, 1984; McDicken et al, 1985; Critchley et al, 1986), ovarian carcinoma-associated antigen (OCAA) (Bhattacharya & Barlow, 1973, 1978, 1979; Piver et al, 1979) and ovarian carcinoma antigen (OCA) (Knauf & Urbach, 1977, 1978, 1980).

The introduction of monoclonal antibodies has led to the production of many antibodies reactive with ovarian tumours, of which a few show restricted tissue distribution. The most intensively studied of this new range of ovarian carcinoma-associated antigens is CA125, a glycoprotein antigen recognized by the OC125 monoclonal antibody raised by immunization with a serous papillary adenocarcinoma cell line (Bast et al, 1981). Initial results with OC125 indicated a high degree of specificity, reacting with six of six epithelial ovarian carcinoma cell lines, with 12 of 20 ovarian cancers in cryostat sections, but with only one of 14 non-ovarian tumour cell lines and none of 12 non-ovarian carcinomas. Further studies, however, showed a wider antigen distribution with expression in coelomic epithelium during embryogenesis and amnion as well as with normal tissues derived from coelomic epithelium (Kabawat et al, 1983a). CA125 is not found in normal adult ovary but is expressed by over 80% of non-mucinous ovarian malignant epithelial tumours; it is present in trace quantities in endometrium, tubal epithelium and endocervical epithelium (Kabawat et al, 1983b). High serum levels of CA125 have been detected by radio-immunoassay in 0.2% of apparently healthy blood donors, up to 1% of normal healthy women, up to 5% of patients with benign gynaecological disorders, 16% of women in the first trimester of pregnancy and 25% of patients with non-gynaecological cancer (Bast et al, 1983; Canney et al, 1984; Klug et al, 1984; Niloff et al, 1984). High levels are also found in association with advanced adenocarcinoma of the cervix, endometrium and Fallopian tube. Hence, CA125 is of limited value for the diagnosis of ovarian carcinoma. Furthermore, although serum levels are frequently high in advanced ovarian cancer, raised CA125 levels are less common in early tumours. The high rate of false positives in normal women and in benign gynecological disorders, particularly endometriosis, renders serum CA125 levels of very limited value as a screening test to detect early ovarian cancer and currently CA125 is principally used for monitoring the patient's response to therapy and for detection of tumour recurrence (Bast et al, 1983; Niloff et al, 1985).

Several other monoclonal antibodies reactive with ovarian adenocarcinomas have been described (Battachary et al, 1982, 1984; Ohkawa et al, 1989, 1991; Chang et al, 1992a, b) but the only ones which appear to be of clinical value are those, 130–22 and 145–9, which react with a glycoprotein known as CA130. Serum CA130 and CA125 levels in gynaecological disease correlate closely and the epitopes recognized by 130–22 and 145–9, though differing from the CA125 epitope, are apparently on the molecule bearing CA125 (Yu et al, 1991). Increased serum CA130 was detected in 91.3% of women with epithelial ovarian cancer and levels correlated with disease progression or regression (Kobayashi et al, 1993).

The monoclonal antibodies described above are of limited individual value for diagnosis of ovarian tumours and antibody panels have been employed in an attempt to distinguish benign and malignant ovarian disease and to improve early diagnosis of ovarian cancer. Inoue et al (1992) measured serum levels of sialyl-Tn, sialyl-Lewis Xi, CA-19-9, CA125, CEA and tissue polypeptide antigen in 65 women with stage I or II ovarian cancer and 317 women with benign pelvic masses. As a single assay sialyl-Tn had the best sensitivity and specificity at 46% and 92%, respectively; CA 19–9 detected the greatest number of cancer patients but had the lowest specificity; the combination sialyl-Tn, CA125, tissue polypeptide antigen and CEA performed best with a specificity of 71% and a sensitivity of 76%. Nevertheless, even with six markers used in combination, one-fifth of the patients with early stage cancer still showed up as false negatives. Van Niekerk et al (1991) used a wide panel of 51 monoclonal antibodies against cytokeratins, tumour markers and MHC antigens to define phenotypic changes in the transition from normal human ovarian epithelium, through benign neoplasms to ovarian carcinomas.

Antigen expression by other gynaecological tumours has been less intensively studied. Yuan et al (1992) produced a monoclonal antibody (Cx-99) reactive with most cervical squamous cell carcinomas and with undifferentiated basal cells in normal cervix.

REFERENCES

Ada G L, Griffin P D 1991 The process of reproduction in humans: antigens for vaccine development. In: Ada G L, Griffin P D (eds) Vaccines for fertility regulation; the assessment of their safety and efficacy. Cambridge University Press, Cambridge, pp 13–26.

Adelusi B, Salimonu L S 1981 Serum immunoglobulin concentrations in serum of patients with carcinoma of the cervix. Gynecologic Oncology 11: 75–81.

Aitken R J, Parslow J M, Hargreave T B, Hendry W F 1988 Influence of antisperm antibodies on human sperm function. British Journal of Urology 62: 367–373.

Akiyama M, Bean M S, Sadamoto K, Takahashi Y, Brankovan V 1983 Suppression of the responsiveness of lymphocytes from cancer patients triggered by co-culture with autologous tumor-derived cells. Journal of Immunology 131: 3085–3090.

Alexander N J, Anderson D J 1987 Immunology of semen. Fertility and Sterility 47: 192–205.

Allavena P, Introna M, Sessa C, Mangioni C, Mantovani A 1982 Interferon effect on cytotoxicity of peripheral blood and tumor-associated lymphocytes against human ovarian cancer cells. Journal of the National Cancer Institute 68: 555–562.

Allavena P, Zanaboni R, Rossini S et al 1986 Lymphokine-activated killer activity of tumor-associated and peripheral blood lymphocytes isolated from patients with ascites ovarian tumors. Journal of the National Cancer Institute 77: 863–868.

Allavena P, Damia G, Colombo T, Maggioni D, D'Incalci M, Mantovani A 1989 Lymphokine-activated killer (LAK) and monocyte-mediated cytotoxicity on tumor cell lines resistant to antitumor agents. Cellular Immunology 120: 250–258.

Alloub M I, Barr B B, McLaren K M, Smith I W, Bunney M H, Smart G E 1989 Human papilloma virus infection and cervical neoplasia in women with renal allografts. British Medical Journal 298: 153–156.

Almeida M D, Jouannet P 1982 Sperm antibodies in cervical mucus. In: Shulman S, Dondero F, Nicotra M (eds) Immunological factors in human reproduction. pp 19–27.

Alsabti E A K 1980 The immunostatus of untreated cervical carcinoma. Gynecologic Oncology 9: 6–11.

Anderson D J, Johnson P M, Alexander N J, Jones W R, Griffin P D 1987 Monoclonal antibodies to human trophoblast and sperm antigens: report of two WHO-sponsored workshops. Journal of Reproductive Immunology 10: 231–257.

Anderson J R, Goudie R B, Gray K, Stuart-Smith D A 1968 Immunological aspects of idiopathic Addison's disease: an antibody to cells producing adrenal hormones. Clinical and Experimental Immunology 3: 107–117.

Apiranthitou-Drogan M, Paganin C, Bernasoni S et al 1992 In search of specific cytotoxic T lymphocytes infiltrating or accompanying human ovarian carcinoma. Cancer Immunology and Immunotherapy 35: 289–295.

Aplin J D, Charlton A K, Ayad S 1988 An immunohistochemical study of human endometrial extracellular matrix during the menstrual cycle and first trimester of pregnancy. Cell and Tissue Research 253: 231–240.

Appel G B, Holub D A 1976 The syndrome of multiple endocrine gland insufficiency. American Journal of Medicine 61: 129–132.

Arends J W, Groniowski M M, De Koning Gans H J, Bosman F T 1983 Immunohistochemical study of the distribution of secretory component and IgA in the normal and diseased uterine mucosa. International Journal of Gynecological Pathology 2: 171–181.

Ashman R, Johnson K, Nahmias A 1975 Rosette-forming lymphocytes in cervical in-situ carcinoma. Lancet 2: 1212.

Ayala A, Canales E S, Karchmer S, Alarcon D, Zarate A 1979 Premature ovarian failure and hypothyroidism associated with sicca syndrome. Obstetrics and Gynecology 53: 98s–101s.

Badawy S Z, Cuenca V, Stitzel A, Jacobs R D, Tomar R H 1984 Autoimmune phenomena in infertile patients with endometriosis. Obstetrics and Gynecology 63: 271–275.

Badawy S Z, Cuenca V, Stitzel A, Tice D 1987 Immune rosettes of T and B lymphocytes in infertile women with endometriosis. Journal of Reproductive Medicine 32: 194–197.

Bagavandoss P, Kunkel S L, Wiggins R C, Keyes P L 1988 Tumour necrosis factor-α (TNF-α) production and localization of macrophages and T lymphocytes in the rabbit corpus luteum. Endocrinology 122: 1185–1187.

Baiocchi G, Kavanagh J J, Talpaz M, Wharton J T, Gutterman J U, Kurzrock R 1991 Expression of the macrophage colony-stimulating factor and its receptor in gynecologic malignancies. Cancer 67: 990–996.

Balaram P, Radhakrishna Pillai M, Padmanabhan R K, Abraham R, Hareendran N K, Nair M K 1988 Immune function in malignant cervical neoplasia: a multiparameter analysis. Gynecologic Oncology 31: 409–423.

Balkwill F R 1989 Cytokines in cancer therapy. Oxford University Press, Oxford.

Balkwill F, Burke F 1991 The cytokine network. Immunology Today 10: 299–304.

Bannatyne P, Russell P, Shearman R P 1990 Autoimmune oophoritis: a clinicopathologic assessment of 12 cases. International Journal of Gynecological Pathology 9: 91–207.

Barber H R K, Sommers S C, Snyder R, Kwon T H 1975 Histologic and nuclear grading and stromal reactions as indices for prognosis in ovarian cancer. American Journal of Obstetrics and Gynecology 121: 795–805.

Bartocci A, Pollard J W, Stanley E R 1986 Regulation of colony stimulating factor 1 during pregnancy. Journal of Experimental Medicine 164: 956–961.

Barton D P J, Blanchard D K, Michelini-Norris B, Nicosia S V, Cavanagh D, Djeu J Y 1993 High serum and ascitic soluble interleukin-2 receptor α levels in advanced epithelial ovarian cancer. Blood 81: 424–429.

Bashford J, Gough I R 1981 High affinity erythrocyte rosette formation and inhibition in premalignant disease of the uterine cervix. Cancer Research 43: 3955–3958.

Bast R C, Feeney M, Lazarus M, Nadler L M, Colvin R B, Knapp R C 1981 Reactivity of a monoclonal antibody with human ovarian carcinoma. Journal of Clinical Investigation 68: 1331–1337.

Bast R C, Klug T L, St John E et al 1983 A radioimmunoassay using a monoclonal antibody to monitor the course of epithelial ovarian cancer. New England Journal of Medicine 309: 883–887.

Beaumont V, Lemort N, Beaumont J L 1982 Oral contraception, circulating immune complexes, antiethinylestradiol antibodies and thrombosis. American Journal of Reproductive Immunology 2: 8–12.

Beer A E, Neaves W B 1978 Antigenic status of semen from the viewpoints of the female and male. Fertility and Sterility 29: 3–22.

Ben-Rafael Z, Orvieto R 1992 Cytokines — involvement in reproduction. Fertility and Sterility 58: 1093–1099.

Berek J S, Bast R C Jr, Lichtenstein A et al 1984 Lymphocyte cytotoxicity in the peritoneal cavity and blood of patients with ovarian cancer. Obstetrics and Gynecology 64: 708–714.

Berkowitz R S, Hill J A, Kurtz C B, Anderson D J 1988 Effects of products of activated leukocytes (lymphokines and monokines) on the growth of malignant trophoblast cells in vitro. American Journal of Obstetrics and Gynecology 158: 199–203.

Bhattacharya M, Barlow J J 1973 Immunologic studies of human serous cystoadenocarcinoma of the ovary: demonstration of tumor-associated antigens. Cancer 31: 588–595.

Bhattacharya M, Barlow J J 1978 Ovarian tumor antigens. Cancer 42: 1616–1620.

Bhattacharya M, Barlow J J 1979 Ovarian cystadenocarcinoma-associated antigen (OCAA). In: Herbeman R B (ed) Compendium of assays for immunodiagnosis of human cancer. Elsevier North-Holland Biomedical Press, Amsterdam, pp 427–431.

Bhattacharya M, Chatterjee S K, Barlow J J, Fuji H 1982 Monoclonal antibodies recognising tumor associated antigen of human ovarian mucinous cystadenocarcinomas. Cancer Research 42: 1650–1654.

Bhattacharya M, Chatterjee S K, Barlow J J 1984 Identification of human cancer-associated antigen defined with monoclonal antibody. Cancer Research 44: 4528–4534.

Biscotti C V, Hart W R, Lucas J G 1989 Cystic ovarian enlargement resulting from autoimmune oophoritis. Obstetrics and Gynecology 74: 492–495.

Bjercke S, Brandtzaeg P 1993 Glandular distribution of immunoglobulins, J chain secretory component, and HLA-DR in the human endometrium throughout the menstrual cycle. Human Reproduction 8: 1420–1425.

Blake M, Holmes K K, Swanson J 1979 Studies in gonococcus infection. XVII. IgA-cleaving protease in vaginal washings from women with gonorrhoea. Journal of Infectious Diseases 139: 89–92.

Blum M, Pery J, Blum I 1989 Antisperm antibodies in young oral contraceptive users. Advances in Contraception 5: 41–46.

Boehme M, Donat H 1992 Identification of lymphocyte subsets in the human fallopian tube. American Journal of Reproductive Immunology 28: 81–84.

Boettcher B 1974 The molecular nature of sperm agglutinins and sperm antibodies in human sera. Journal of Reproduction and Fertility 21 (suppl): 151–167.

Boettcher B 1979 Immunity to spermatozoa. Clinics in Obstetrics and Gynaecology 6: 385–402.

Boettcher B, Hjort T, Rümke P, Shulman S, Vyazou O 1977 Auto and isoantibodies to antigens of the human reproductive system. I. Results of an international collaborative study. Acta Pathologica et Microbiologica Scandinavica 258: 1–69, 30: 173–180.

Bonneterre J, Santoro F, Wattre P, Beuscart R, Adenis L, Capron A 1981 Étude de la compétance immunitaire chez les malades présentant un cancer du col utérin. Gynecologie 32: 257–266.

Bottazzi B, Ghezzi P, Tarabolletti G et al 1985 Tumour-derived chemotactic factors from human ovarian carcinoma: evidence for a role in the regulation of macrophage content of neoplastic tissues. International Journal of Cancer 36: 167–173.

Bottazzi B, Collotta F, Sica A, Nobili N, Mantovani A 1990 A chemoattractant expressed in human sarcoma cells (tumour derived chemotactic factor, TDCF) is identical to monocyte chemoattractant protein 1/monocyte chemotactic and activating factor (MCP-1/MCAF). International Journal of Cancer 45: 795–797.

Bousquet D, St Jaques S, Roberts K D, Chappelaire M, Bleath G 1982 Zona pellucida antibodies in a group of women with idiopathic infertility. American Journal of Reproductive Immunology 2: 73–76.

Boyer P J, Berek J S, Zighelboim J 1989 Lymphocyte activation by recombinant interleukin-2 in ovarian cancer patients. Obstetrics and Gynecology 73: 793–797.

Bradbeer C 1987 Is infection with HIV a risk factor for CIN? Lancet ii: 1277–1278.

Brandtzaeg P, Prydz H 1984 Direct evidence for an integrated function of J chain and secretory component in epithelial transport of immunoglobulins. Nature 311: 71–73.

Brandtzaeg P, Christiansen E, Muller F, Purvis K 1993 Humoral immune response patterns of human mucosae, including the reproductive tracts. In: Griffin P D, Johnson P M (eds) Local immunity in reproductive tract tissues. Oxford University Press, Delhi, pp 97–130.

Bronson R A, Cooper G W, Rosenfeld D L 1982a Correlation between regional specificity of antisperm antibodies to the spermatozoa surface and complement-mediated sperm immobilization. American Journal of Reproductive Immunology 2: 222–224.

Bronson R A, Cooper G W, Rosenfeld D L 1982b Sperm-specific isoantibodies and autoantibodies inhibit the binding of human sperm to the human zona pellicida. Fertility and Sterility 38: 724–729.

Bronson R A, Cooper G W, Rosenfeld D L 1984a Autoimmunity to spermatozoa: effect on sperm penetration of cervical mucus as reflected by postcoital testing. Fertility and Sterility 41: 609–614.

Bronson R, Cooper G, Rosenfeld D 1984b Sperm antibodies: their role in infertility. Fertility and Sterility 42: 171–183.

Bronson R, Cooper G, Hjort T et al 1986 Antisperm antibodies detected by agglutination, immobilization, microcytotoxicity and immunobead binding assays. American Journal of Reproductive Immunology 8: 279–300.

Brunham R C, Kuo C-C, Cles L, Holmes K K 1983 Correlations of host immune response with quantitative recovery of Chlamydia trachomatis from the human endocervix. Infection and Immunity 39: 1491–1494.

Bulmer J N, Earl U 1987 The expression of class II MHC gene products by fallopian tube epithelium in pregnancy and throughout the menstrual cycle. Immunology 61: 207–213.

Bulmer J N, Hagin S V, Browne C M, Billington W D 1986 Localization of immunoglobulin-containing cells in human endometrium in the first trimester of pregnancy and throughout the menstrual cycle. European Journal of Obstetrics, Gynecology and Reproductive Biology 23: 31–44.

Bulmer J N, Hollings D, Ritson A 1987 Immunocytochemical evidence that endometrial stromal granulocytes are granulated lymphocytes. Journal of Pathology 153: 281–288.

Bulmer J N, Morrison L, Smith J C 1988a Expression of class II MHC gene products by macrophages in human uteroplacental tissues. Immunology 63: 707–714.

Bulmer J N, Lunny D P, Hagin S V 1988b Immunohistochemical characterization of stromal leukocytes in nonpregnant human endometrium. American Journal of Reproductive Immunology and Microbiology 17: 83–90.

Bulmer J N, Morrison L, Longfellow M, Ritson A, Pace D 1991a Granulated lymphocytes in human endometrium: histochemical and immunohistochemical studies. Human Reproduction 6: 791–798.

Bulmer J N, Morrison L, Longfellow M, Ritson A 1991b Leucocyte markers in human decidua: investigation of surface markers and function. Colloque INSERM 212: 189–196.

Burrows T D, King A, Loke Y W 1993 Expression of adhesion molecules by human decidual large granular lymphocytes. Cellular Immunology 147: 81–94.

Byrne M, Taylor-Robinson D, Munday P E, Harris J R W 1989 The common occurrence of human papilloma virus infection and intraepithelial neoplasia in women infected by HIV. AIDS 3: 379–382.

Canney P A, Moore M, Wilkinson P M, James R D 1984 Ovarian cancer antigen CA125: a prospective clinical assessment of its role as a tumour marker. British Journal of Cancer 50: 765–769.

Cantuaria A A 1977 Sperm immobilizing antibodies in the serum and cervico-vaginal secretions of fertile and normal women. British Journal of Obstetrics and Gynaecology 84: 865–868.

Cardi G, Mastrangelo M, Berd D 1989 Depletion of T-cells with the CD4+ CD45R+ phenotype in lymphocytes that infiltrate subcutaneous metastases of human melanoma. Cancer Research 49: 6562–6565.

Carretti N 1974 The passive haemolysis reaction for the identification of antiseminal plasma antibodies in the serum of women with unexplained sterility. In: Centara A, Carretti N (eds) Immunology in obstetrics and gynaecology. Excerpta Medica, Amsterdam, pp 71–77.

Case Records of the Massachusetts General Hospital: case 46–1986 1986 New England Journal of Medicine 315: 1336–1343.

Castello G, Esposito G, Giovanni S, Mora L D, Abate G, Germano A 1986 Immunological abnormalities in patients with cervical carcinoma. Gynecologic Oncology 25: 61–64.

Caudle M R, Shivers C A, Wild R A 1987 Clinical significance of naturally occurring anti-zona pellucida antibodies in infertile women. American Journal of Reproductive Immunology 15: 119–121.

Cerni C, Tatra G, Berger R, Micksche M 1979 Cell mediated immunity in patients with cervical cancer. Oncology 36: 144–170.

Chang K, Pastan I, Willingham M C 1992a Isolation and characterization of a monoclonal antibody, K1, reactive with ovarian cancers and normal mesothelium. International Journal of Cancer 50: 373–381.

Chang K, Pai L H, Batra J K, Pastan I, Willingham M C 1992b Characterization of the antigen (CAK1) recognised by monoclonal antibody K1 present on ovarian cancers and normal mesothelium. Cancer Research 52: 181–186.

Chatterjee M, Barlow J J, Allen H J, Chung W S, Piver M S 1975 Lymphocyte response to autologous tumor antigen(s) and phytohemagglutinin in ovarian cancer patients. Cancer 36: 956–962.

Chen C 1979 Immunological infertility: management and prognosis. Clinics in Obstetrics and Gynaecology 6: 403–423.

Chen C, Jones W R 1981 Application of a sperm micro-immobilization test to cervical mucus in the investigation of immunologic infertility. Fertility and Sterility 35: 542–545.

Chen L, Thomas E K, Hu S-L, Hellström I, Hellström K E 1991 Human papillomavirus type 16 nucleoprotein E7 is a tumor rejection antigen. Proceedings of the National Academy of Sciences of the USA 88: 110–114.

Chen S Y, Koffler D, Cohen C J 1973 Cell mediated immunity in patients with ovarian carcinoma. American Journal of Obstetrics and Gynecology 115: 467–470.

Chen S S, Koffler D, Cohen C J 1975 Cellular hypersensitivity in patients with squamous cell carcinoma of the cervix. American Journal of Obstetrics and Gynecology 121: 91–95.

Chiang W T, Wei P Y, Alexander E R 1976 Circulatory and cellular immune responses to squamous cell carcinoma of the uterine cervix. American Journal of Obstetrics and Gynecology 126: 116–121.

Chiphangwi J, Dallabetta G, Miotti P, Liomba G, Wangel A-M, Saah A 1991 Cervical squamous intraepithelial lesions (CSIL) and HIV-1 infection in Malawian women. Seventh International Conference on AIDS, Florence, p 47.

Clarke A G, Vasey D P, Symonds E M et al 1982 Levels of circulating immune complexes in patients with ovarian cancer. British Journal of Obstetrics and Gynaecology 89: 231–237.

Clarke G N 1988 Sperm antibodies and human fertilization. American Journal of Reproductive Immunology and Microbiology 17: 65–71.

Clarke G N, Stojanoff A, Cauchi M N, McBain J C, Speirs A L, Johnston W I H 1984a Detection of antispermatozoal antibodies of IgA class in cervical mucus. American Journal of Reproductive Immunology 5: 61–65.

Clarke G N, Heieh C, Koh S H, Cauchi M N 1984b Sperm antibodies, immunoglobulins and complement in human follicular fluid. American Journal of Reproductive Immunology 5: 179–181.

Clarke G N, Lopata A, McBain J C, Baker H W G, Johnston W I H 1985a Effect of sperm antibodies in males on human in vitro fertilisation. American Journal of Reproductive Immunology and Microbiology 8: 62–66.

Clarke G N, McBain J C, Lopata A, Johnston W I H 1985b In vitro fertilization results for women with sperm antibodies in plasma and follicular fluid. American Journal of Reproductive Immunology and Microbiology 8: 130–131.

Clarke G N, Elliott P J, Smaila C 1985c Detection of sperm antibodies in semen using the immunobead test: a survey of 813 consecutive patients. American Journal of Reproductive Immunology 7: 118–123.

Coleman N, Greenfield I M, Hare J, Kruger-Gray H, Chain B M, Stanley M A 1993 Characterization and functional analysis of the expression of intercellular adhesion molecule-1 in human papilloma virus-related disease of cervical keratinocytes. American Journal of Pathology 14: 355–367.

Collen R J, Lippe B M, Kaplan S A 1979 Ovarian failure, juvenile rheumatoid arthritis and vitiligo. American Journal of Diseases of Childhood 136: 353–356.

Conti M, Agarossi A, Muggiasca L, Casolati E, Ravasi L 1991 Risk of genital HPVi and CIN in HIV positive women. Seventh International Conference on AIDS, Florence, p 284.

Cooper M D, Dever C, Tempel K, Moticka E J, Hindman T, Stephens D S 1987 Characterization of lymphoid cells from the human fallopian tube mucosa. Advances in Experimental and Medical Biology 216: 387–394.

Coughlan B M, Skinner G R B 1977 Immunoglobulin concentrations in cervical mucus in patients with normal and abnormal cervical cytology. British Journal of Obstetrics and Gynaecology 84: 129–134.

Coulam C B, Lufkin E G 1981 Absence of adrenal failure in the polyglandular failure syndrome with primary ovarian failure. Fertility and Sterility 35: 365–366.

Coulam C B, Ryan R J 1979 Premature menopause I. Etiology. American Journal of Obstetrics and Gynecology 133: 639–643.

Coulam C B, Kempers R D, Randall R V 1981 Premature ovarian failure: evidence for the autoimmune mechanism. Fertility and Sterility 36: 238–242.

Creasey A A, Reynolds M T, Laird W 1986 Cures and partial regression of murine and human tumors by recombinant human tumor necrosis factor. Cancer Research 46: 5687–5690.

Critchley M, Brownless S, Patten M et al 1986 Radionuclide imaging of epithelial ovarian tumours with ^{123}I-labelled monoclonal antibody (H317) specific for placental-type alkaline phosphatase. Clinical Radiology 37: 107–112.

Cunningham D S, Fulgham D L, Rayl D L, Hansen K A, Alexander N J 1991 Antisperm antibodies to sperm surface antigens in women with genital tract infection. American Journal of Obstetrics and Gynecology 164: 791–796.

Daiter E, Pampfer S, Yeung Y G, Barad D, Stanley E R, Pollard J W 1992 Expression of colony-stimulating factor-1 in the human uterus and placenta. Journal of Clinical Endocrinology and Metabolism 74: 850–858.

Daunter B, Khoo S K, McKay E V 1979 Lymphocyte response to plant mitogens. II. The response of lymphocytes from women with carcinoma of the cervix to phytohaemagglutinin P, concanavilin A and pokeweed. Gynecologic Oncology 7: 314–317.

Daunter B, Khoo S K, Mackay E V 1982 Monocyte chemostasis in patients with cervical or ovarian cancer. Gynecologic Oncology 13: 152–157.

Dawson J R, Lutz P M, Shau H 1983 The humoral response to gynecologic neoplasms and its role in the regulation of tumor growth: a review. American Journal of Reproductive Immunology 3: 12–17.

Dean J, Millar S E 1990 Zona pellucida: target for a contraceptive vaccine. In: Alexander N J, Griffin P D, Spieler J M, Waites G M H (eds) Gamete interaction: prospects for immunocontraception. Wiley-Liss, New York, pp 313–326.

Deligdisch L 1982 Morphological correlates of host response in endometrial carcinoma. American Journal of Reproductive Immunology 2: 54–57.

Deligdisch L, Jacobs A J, Cohen C J 1982 Histologic correlates of virulence in ovarian adenocarcinoma. II. Morphologic correlates of host response. American Journal of Obstetrics and Gynecology 144: 885–889.

Dempsey A T, De Sweit M, Dewhurst C J 1981 Premature ovarian failure associated with the candida endocrinopathy syndrome. British Journal of Obstetrics and Gynaecology 88: 563–565.

Di Bello M, Lucchini V, Chiari S et al 1988 DR antigen expression on ovarian carcinoma cells does not correlate with their capacity to elicit an autologous proliferating response. Cancer Immunology and Immunotherapy 27: 63–68.

Dillner L, Bekassy Z, Jonsson N, Moreno-Lopez J, Blomberg J 1989 Detection of IgA antibodies against human papillomavirus in cervical secretions from patients with cervical intraepithelial neoplasia. International Journal of Cancer 43: 36–40.

Dini M M, Faiferman I 1980 Cytotoxic blocking activity in invasive squamous cell carcinoma of the human uterine cervix. Cancer 64: 2573–2576.

DiSaia P J 1975 Immunological aspects of gynecological malignancies. Journal of Reproductive Medicine 14: 17–20.

DiSaia P J, Rutledge F W, Smith J P, Sinkovics J J 1971 Cell mediated immune reaction to two gynecologic malignant tumors. Cancer 28: 1129–1137.

DiSaia P J, Nalick R H, Townsend D E 1973 Antibody cytotoxicity studies in ovarian and cervical malignancies. Obstetrics and Gynecology 42: 646–650.

Dmowski W P, Steele R W, Baker G F 1981 Deficient cellular immunity in endometriosis. American Journal of Obstetrics and Gynecology 141: 377–383.

Dmowski W P, Braun D, Gebel H 1991 The immune system in endometriosis. In: Thomas E J, Rock J A (eds) Modern approaches to endometriosis. Kluwer, Dordrecht, pp 97–110.

Dodd J K, Hicks L J, Tyler J P, Crandon A J, Hudson C N 1983 Circulating IgG specific immune complexes as a potential tumor marker in gynecological malignancies. Gynecologic Oncology 16: 232–239.

Doe W F 1982 Immunological aspects of the gut. In: Lachmann P J, Peters D K (eds) Clinical aspects of immunology. Blackwell Scientific Publications, Oxford, pp 985–1010.

Dor J, Neiel L A, Soffer Y, Nashiach S, Serr D 1979 Cell mediated and local immunity to spermatozoa in infertility. International Journal of Fertility 24: 94–100.

Dor J, Ruoak E, Aitken R J 1981 Antisperm antibodies: their effect on the process of fertilization studied in vitro. Fertility and Sterility 35: 535–541.

Dorsett B H, Ioachim H L, Stolbach L, Walker J, Barber H R K 1975 Isolation of tumor-specific antibodies from effusions of ovarian carcinoma. International Journal of Cancer 16: 779–786.

Edelstam G A B, Lundkvist O E, Klareskog L, Karlsson-Parra A 1992 Cyclic variation of major histocompatibility complex class II antigen expression in the human fallopian tube epithelium. Fertility and Sterility 57: 1225–1229.

Edmonds M, Lanki C, Killinger D W, Volpé R 1973 Autoimmune thyroiditis, adrenalitis and oophoritis. American Journal of Medicine 54: 782–787.

Eisermann J, Register K D, Strickler R C, Collins J L 1989 The effect of tumor necrosis factor on human sperm motility in vitro. Journal of Andrology 10: 270–274.

El-Demiry M I M, Hargreave T B, Busuttil A, James K, Chisholm G D 1986 Identifying leucocytes and leucocyte subpopulations in semen using monoclonal antibody probes. Urology 28: 492–496.

El-Mahgoub S 1972 Antispermatozoal antibodies in infertile women with cervicovaginal schistosomiasis. American Journal of Obstetrics and Gynecology 112: 781–784.

El-Roeiy A, Dmowski W P, Gleicher N et al 1988 Danazol but not gonadotrophin-releasing hormone agonist suppresses autoantibodies in endometriosis. Fertility and Sterility 50: 864–871.

Elsässer-Beile U, von Kleist S, Sauther W, Gallati H, Schulte Mönting J 1993 Impaired cytokine production in whole blood cell cultures of patients with gynaecological carcinomas in different clinical stages. British Journal of Cancer 68: 32–36.

Erroi A, Sironi M, Chiaffarino F, Zhen-Guo C, Mengozzi M, Mantovani A 1989 IL-1 and IL-6 release by tumor-associated macrophages from human ovarian carcinoma. International Journal of Cancer 44: 795–801.

Escobar M E, Cigorraga S B, Chiauzzi V A, Charreau E H, Rivarola M A 1982 Development of the gonadotropic resistant ovary syndrome in myasthenia gravis: suggestion of similar autoimmune mechanisms. Acta Endocrinologica 99: 431–436.

Etribi A, Ibrahim A, Mahmoud K, El-Haggar S, Hamada T, El-Ahmadi I 1982 Antisperm antibodies and human infertility. Fertility and Sterility 37: 236–239.

Fahs M, Mandelblatt J, Garibaldi K, Senie R, Peterson H 1991 The association between human immunodeficiency virus infection and cervical neoplasia: implications for the clinical care of women at risk of both conditions. Seventh International Conference on AIDS, Florence, p 330.

Faiferman I, Gleicher N, Cohen C J, Koffler D 1977 Leukocyte migration in ovarian carcinoma: comparison of inhibitory activity of tumor extracts. Journal of the National Cancer Institute 59: 1593–1597.

Fakih H, Baggett B, Holtz G, Tsang K Y, Lee J C, Williamson H O 1987 Interleukin-1: a possible role in the infertility associated with endometriosis. Fertility and Sterility 47: 213–217.

Faulk W P, Fox H 1982 Reproductive immunology. In: Lachman P J, Peters D K (eds) Clinical aspects of immunology. Blackwell Scientific Publications, Oxford, pp 1104–1150.

Feinberg F R, Kliman H J, Lockwood C J 1991 Is oncofetal fibronectin trophoblast glue for human implantation. American Journal of Pathology 138: 537–543.

Ferguson A, Moore M, Fox H 1985 Expression of MHC products and leucocyte differentiation antigens in gynaecological neoplasms: an immunohistological study of the tumour cells and infiltrating leucocytes. British Journal of Cancer 52: 551–563.

Fiers W 1991 Tumor necrosis factor: characterization at the molecular, cellular and in vivo level. Federation of European Biochemical Societies Letters 285: 199–212.

Forbes A P, Luke J R, Block K J 1976 Clinical significance of antibodies to ovarian antigens associated with cancer of the genitourinary tract. Clinical and Experimental Immunology 23: 436–443.

Forrest J 1983 A histological study of salpingitis in various groups of patients. BSc Thesis, University of Manchester.

Fotherby K, Hamawi A 1984 Immunological aspects of contraceptive steroids. Journal of Obstetrics and Gynaecology 4 (suppl 1): 557–561.

Fox H 1993 Immunocompetent cells in the cervix and vagina. In: Griffin P D, Johnson P M (eds) Local immunity in reproductive tract tissues. Oxford University Press, Delhi, pp 177–186.

Friberg J, Gnarpe H 1973 Mycoplasmas and human reproductive failure. II. Pregnancies in 'infertile' couples treated with deoxycline for T-mycoplasmas. American Journal of Obstetrics and Gynecology 116: 23–26.

Fukuoka M, Mori T, Taii S, Yasuda K 1988 Interleukin-1 inhibits luteinization of porcine granulosa cells in culture. Endocrinology 122: 367–369.

Fukuoka M, Yasuda K, Taii S, Takakura K, Mori T 1989 Interleukin-1 stimulates growth and inhibits progesterone secretion in cultures of porcine granulosa cells. Endocrinology 124: 884–890.

Garzetti G G, Ciavattini A, Provincial A M et al 1993 Natural killer cell activity in endometriosis: correlation between serum estradiol levels and cytotoxicity. Obstetrics and Gynecology 81: 685–688.

Gerber M A, Koffler D, Cohen C J 1977 Circulating antibodies in patients with ovarian carcinoma. Gynecologic Oncology 5: 228–232.

Gerretsen G, Kremer J, Nater J P, Bleumink E, De Gast G C, The T H 1979 Immune reactivity of women on oral contraceptives: dinitrochlorobenzene sensitization test and skin reactivity to irritants. Contraception 19: 83–89.

Gerretsen G, Kremer J, Bleumink E, Nater J P, De Gast G C, The T H 1980 Immune reactivity in women on hormonal contraceptives. Contraception 22: 25–29.

Ghosh A K, Moore M 1992 Tumour-infiltrating lymphocytes in cervical carcinoma. European Journal of Cancer 28A: 1910–1916.

Gleicher N, Dmowski W P, Siegel I et al 1984 Lymphocyte subsets in endometriosis. Obstetrics and Gynecology 63: 463–466.

Gleicher N, El-Roeiy A, Confino E, Friberg J 1987 Abnormal autoantibodies in endometriosis: is endometriosis an autoimmune disease? Obstetrics and Gynecology 70: 115–122.

Gloor E, Hurlimann J 1984 Autoimmune oophoritis. American Journal of Clinical Pathology 81: 105–109.

Goldstein M S, Shore B, Gusberg S B 1977 Cellular immunity as a host response to squamous carcinoma of the cervix. American Journal of Obstetrics and Gynecology 111: 751–755.

Golonka J E, Goodman A D 1968 Co-existence of primary ovarian insufficiency, primary adrenocortical insufficiency and idiopathic hypoparathyroidism. Journal of Clinical Endocrinology and Metabolism 28: 79–82.

Gottschall P E, Uehara A, Hoffmann S T, Arimura A 1987 Interleukin-1 inhibits follicle stimulating hormone-induced differentiation in rat granulosa cells in vitro. Biochemical and Biophysical Research Communications 149: 502–509.

Graham R A, Seif M W, Aplin J et al 1990 An endometrial factor in unexplained infertility. British Medical Journal 300: 1428–1431.

Grimm E A, Mazumder A, Zhang H Z, Rosenberg S A 1982 Lymphokine-activated killer cell phenomenon: lysis of fresh solid tumour cells by interleukin-2 activated autologous peripheral blood lymphocytes. Journal of Experimental Medicine 155: 1823–1841.

Gupta S C, Singh P A, Shukla H S, Sinha S N, Mehrotra T N, Kumar S 1981 Serum immunoglobulins in carcinoma of various organs. Indian Journal of Cancer 18: 277–281.

Gusberg S B, Yannopoulos A, Cohen C J 1971 Virulence indices and lymph nodes in cancer of the cervix. American Journal of Roentgenology 111: 273–277.

Haimovici F, Hill J A, Anderson D J 1991 The effects of soluble products of activated lymphocytes and macrophages on blastocyst implantation events in vitro. Biology of Reproduction 44: 69–75.

Haimovici F, Takahashi K, Anderson D J 1992 Antifertility effects of antisperm cell-mediated immunity in mice. Journal of Reproductive Immunology 22: 281–298.

Halme J 1989 Release of tumor necrosis factor by human peritoneal macrophages in vivo and in vitro. American Journal of Obstetrics and Gynecology 161: 1718–1725.

Halme J, Becker S, Hammond M E et al 1983 Increased activity of pelvic macrophages in infertile women with mild endometriosis. American Journal of Obstetrics and Gynecology 145: 333–337.

Halme J, Becker S, Wing R 1984 Accentuated cyclic activation of peritoneal macrophages in patients with endometriosis. American Journal of Obstetrics and Gynecology 148: 85–90.

Halme J, Becker S, Haskill S 1987 Altered maturation and function of peritoneal macrophages: possible role in the pathogenesis of endometriosis. American Journal of Obstetrics and Gynecology 156: 783–789.

Hancock B W, Bauer L, Heath J, Sugden P, Ward A M 1979 The effects of radiotherapy on immunity in patients with localised carcinoma of the cervix uteri. Cancer 43: 118–123.

Hancock R J T 1978 Sperm antigens and sperm immunogenicity. In: Cohen J, Hendry W F (eds) Spermatozoa, antibodies and infertility. Blackwell Scientific Publications, Oxford, pp 1–9.

Haney A F, Muscato J J, Weinberg J B 1981 Peritoneal fluid cell populations in infertility patients. Fertility and Sterility 35: 696–698.

Harrison R F 1978 Significance of sperm antibodies in human fertility. International Journal of Fertility 23: 288–293.

Haskill S, Becker S, Fowler W, Walton L 1982a Mononuclear cell infiltration in ovarian cancer. I. Inflammatory cell infiltrates from tumour and ascites material. British Journal of Cancer 45: 728–736.

Haskill S, Koren H, Becker S, Fowler W, Walton L 1982b Mononuclear cell infiltration in ovarian cancer. II. Immune function of tumour and ascites derived cells. British Journal of Cancer 45: 737–746.

Haskill S, Koren H, Becker S, Fowler W, Walton L 1982c Mononuclear cell infiltration in ovarian cancer. III. Suppressor cell and ADCC activity of macrophages from ascitic and solid ovarian tumours. British Journal of Cancer 45: 747–753.

Hassumi K, Sugano H, Sakamoth G, Masubuchi K, Kubo H 1977 Circumscribed carcinoma of the uterine cervix, with marked lymphocytic infiltration. Cancer 39: 2503–2507.

Hawthorn R J S, Murdoch J B, MacLean A B, Mackie R M 1988 Langerhan's cells and subtypes of human papilloma virus in cervical intraepithelial neoplasia. British Medical Journal 297: 643–646.

Henderson C J, Hulme M J, Aitken R J 1988 Contraceptive potential of antibodies to the zona pellucida. Journal of Reproduction and Fertility 83: 325–343.

Heo D S, Whiteside T L, Kanbour A, Herberman R B 1988 Lymphocytes infiltrating human ovarian tumours. I. Role of Leu-19 (NKH1) positive recombinant IL-2-activated cultures of lymphocytes infiltrating human ovarian tumours. Journal of Immunology 140: 4042–4049.

Hess A D, Gall S A, Dawson J R 1979 Inhibition of in vitro lymphocyte function by cystic and ascitic fluids from ovarian cancer patients. Cancer Research 39: 2381–2389.

Hess A D, Gall S A, Dawson J R 1980 Partial purification and characterization of a lymphocyte-inhibiting factor(s) in ascitic fluids from ovarian cancer patients. Cancer Research 40: 1842–1851.

Hill J A 1992a Cytokines considered critical in pregnancy. American Journal of Reproductive Immunology 28: 123–126.

Hill J A 1992b Immunology and endometriosis. Fertility and Sterility 58: 262–264.

Hill J A 1993 Production and effect of cytokines on local immuno-endocrine reproductive events in the female reproductive tract. In: Griffin P D, Johnson P M (eds) Local immunity in reproductive tract tissues. Oxford University Press, Delhi, pp 245–254.

Hill J A, Anderson D J 1988 Immunological mechanisms of female infertility. Baillière's Clinical Immunology and Allergy 2: 551–575.

Hill J A, Haimovici F, Politch J A, Anderson D J 1987 Effects of soluble products of activated lymphocytes and macrophages (lymphokines and monokines) on human sperm motion parameters. Fertility and Sterility 47: 460–465.

Hill J A, Faris H M P, Schiff I, Anderson D J 1988 Characterization of leukocyte subpopulations in the peritoneal fluid of women with endometriosis. Fertility and Sterility 50: 216–222.

Hill J A, Cohen J, Anderson D J 1989 The effects of lymphokines and monokines on human sperm fertilizing ability in the zona-free hamster egg penetration test. American Journal of Obstetrics and Gynecology 160: 1154–1159.

Hill R, Daunter B, Khoo S K, McKay E G 1978 Isolation of tumour associated immunoglobulins from ascites fluid. British Journal of Cancer 38: 154–157.

Hill R, Khoo S K, Daunter B, Silburn P A, Mackay E V 1982 Immunoglobulins reactive to carcinoembryonic antigen and their relationship to the antigen in malignant ascites fluid of ovarian carcinoma. International Journal of Cancer 30: 587–592.

Hill R, Daunter B, Silburn P A, Khoo S K, Mackay E V 1983 Affinity chromatography separation of tumor associated antigens from ascitic fluid of ovarian cancer patients. Gynecologic Oncology 15: 428–433.

Hinting A, Vermeulen L, Comhaire F 1988 The indirect mixed antiglobulin reaction test using a commercially available kit for the detection of antisperm antibodies in serum. Fertility and Sterility 49: 1039–1044.

Hirte H, Clark D A 1991a Generation of lymphokine-activated killer cells in human ovarian carcinoma ascitic fluid: identification of transforming growth factor β as a suppressive factor. Cancer Immunology and Immunotherapy 32: 296–302.

Hirte H W, Clark D A 1991b Factors determining the ability of cytokine-activated killer cells to lyse human ovarian carcinoma targets. Cellular Immunology 136: 122–132.

Hughes R G, Norval M, Howie S E M 1988 Expression of major histocompatibility class II antigens by Langerhans' cells in cervical intraepithelial neoplasia. Journal of Clinical Pathology 41: 253–259.

Hurlimann J, Dayal R, Gloor E 1978 Immunoglobulins and secretory component in endometrium and cervix: influence of inflammation and carcinoma. Virchows Archiv A Pathological Anatomy and Histology 337: 211–223.

Hurst B S, Rock J A 1991 The peritoneal environment in endometriosis. In: Thomas E J, Rock J A (eds) Modern approaches to endometriosis. Kluwer, Dordrecht, pp 79–86.

Hutcheson R B, Anderson T D, Holborow E J 1974 Cervical plasma cell population in infertile patients. British Medical Journal 3: 783–786.

Ingerslev H J, Hjort T 1979 Spermagglutinin antibodies and β-sperm agglutinin in sera from infertile and fertile women. Fertility and Sterility 31: 496–503.

Ingerslev H J, Moller N P M, Jager S, Kremer J 1982 Immunoglobulin class of sperm antibodies in cervical mucus from infertile women. American Journal of Reproductive Immunology 2: 296–300.

Innins E K, Gatanaga M, Cappuccini F et al 1992 Growth of the endometrial adenocarcinoma cell line AN3 CA is modulated by tumor necrosis factor and its receptor is upregulated by estrogen in vitro. Endocrinology 130: 1852–1856.

Inoue M, Fujita M, Nakazawa A, Ogawa H, Tanizawa O 1992 Sialyl-Tn, Sialyl-Lewis Xi, CA 19–9, CA125, carcinoembryonic antigen and tissue polypeptide antigen in differentiating ovarian cancer from benign tumors. Obstetrics and Gynecology 79: 434–440.

Introna M, Allavena P, Biondi A, Colombo N, Villa A, Mantovani A 1983 Defective natural killer activity within human ovarian tumors: low numbers of morphologically defined effectors present in situ. Journal of the National Cancer Institute 70: 21–26.

Ioannides C G, Platsoucas C D, Rashed S, Wharton J T, Edwards C L, Freedman R S 1991 Tumor cytolysis by lymphocytes infiltrating ovarian malignant ascites. Cancer Research 51: 4257–4265.

Irvine W J, Barnes E W 1975 Addison's disease, ovarian failure and hypoparathyroidism. Clinics in Endocrinology and Metabolism 4: 379–434.

Irvine W J, Chan M W, Scarth L et al 1968 Immunological aspects of premature ovarian failure associated with idiopathic Addison's disease. Lancet 2: 883–887.

Irvine W J, Chan M W, Scarth L 1969 The further characterization of autoantibodies reactive with extra-adrenal steroid-producing cells in patients with adrenal disorders. Clinical and Experimental Immunology 4: 489–503.

Irvine W J, MacCash A C, Barnes E W, Loudon N B 1974 Immunological function in oral contraceptive users. Journal of Reproduction and Fertility 2 (suppl): 33–41.

Isaacson K B, Galman M, Coutifaris C, Lyttle C R 1990 Endometrial synthesis and secretion of complement component-3 by patients with and without endometriosis. Fertility and Sterility 53: 836–841.

Ishiguro T, Sugutachi I, Katoh K 1980 T and B lymphocytes in patients with squamous cell carcinoma of the uterine cervix. Gynecologic Oncology 9: 80–85.

Isojima S 1969 Relationship between antibodies to spermatozoa and sterility in females. In: Edwards R G (ed) Immunology and reproduction. International Planned Parenthood Federation, London, pp 267–283.

Isojima S, Tsuchiya K, Koyama K, Tanaka C, Nako O, Adachi M 1972 Further studies on sperm-immobilizing antibody found in sera of unexplained cases of sterility in women. American Journal of Obstetrics and Gynecology 112: 199–207.

Ito A, Sato T, Iga T, Mori Y 1990 Tumor necrosis factor bifunctionally regulates matrix metalloproteinases and tissue inhibitor of metalloproteinases (TIMP) production by human fibroblasts. Federation of European Biochemical Societies Letters 269: 93–95.

Ivanova M, Bourneva V, Gitsov L, Angelova Z 1984 Experimental immune oophoritis as a model for studying the thymus-ovary interaction: 1. Morphological studies. American Journal of Reproductive Immunology 6: 99–106.

Jager S, Kremer J, Kuiken J, Schlockteren-Draaisma T 1981 In: Jager S (ed) Immunoglobulin class of antispermatozoal antibodies and inhibition of sperm penetration into cervical mucus. Veenstra Visser Offset, Groningen, pp 117–124.

Jain R, Gupta M M, Parashari A, Kaur S, Luthra U K 1990 Peripheral blood lymphocyte subpopulations in Indian women with cervical intraepithelial neoplasia and invasive cancer — an immunocytochemical study using monoclonal antibodies. Cancer Letters 54: 17–20.

Jenkins V K, Olson M H, Ellis H N, Dilland E A 1975 In vitro lymphocyte response of patients with uterine cancer as related to clinical stage and radiotherapy. Gynecologic Oncology 3: 191–200.

Jochmus-Kudielka I, Schneider A, Braun R et al 1989 Antibodies against the human papilloma virus type 16 early proteins in human sera: correlation of anti-E7 reactivity with cervical cancer. Journal of the National Cancer Institute 81: 1698–1704.

Johnson H M, Torres B A, Smith E M, Dion L D, Blalock J E 1984 Regulation of lymphokine (γ-interferon) production by corticotrophin. Journal of Immunology 132: 246–250.

Johnson P M, Bulmer J N 1984 Uterine gland epithelium in human pregnancy often lacks maternal MHC antigens but does express fetal trophoblast antigens. Journal of Immunology 132: 1608–1610.

Johnson W C, Hunter A G 1972 Seminal antigens: their alteration in the genital tract of female rabbits and during partial in vitro capacitation with beta amylase and beta glucuronidase. Biology of Reproduction 7: 332–340.

Jones A L, Selby P 1989 Tumour necrosis factor: clinical relevance. Cancer Surveys 8: 817–836.

Jones W R 1992 Contraception. Baillière's Clinical Obstetrics and Gynaecology 6: 629–640.

Jones W R, Ing R M Y, Kaye M D 1973 A comparison of screening tests for antisperm activity in the serum of infertile women. Journal of Reproduction and Fertility 32: 357–364.

Jones W R, Bradley J, Judd S J et al 1988 Phase I clinical trial of a World Health Organisation birth control vaccine. Lancet i: 1295–1298.

Kabawat S E, Bast R C, Welch W R, Knapp R C, Colvin R B 1983a Immunopathologic characterization of a monoclonal antibody that recognizes common surface antigens of human ovarian tumors of serous, endometrioid and clear cell type. American Journal of Clinical Pathology 79: 98–104.

Kabawat S E, Bast R C, Welch W R, Knapp R C, Bhan A K 1983b Expression of major histocompatibility antigens and nature of inflammatory infiltrate in ovarian neoplasms. International Journal of Cancer 32: 547–554.

Kabawat S E, Bast R C, Welch W R, Knapp R C, Bhan A K 1983c Expression of major histocompatibility antigens and nature of inflammatory infiltrate in ovarian neoplasms. International Journal of Cancer 32: 547–554.

Kacinski B M, Stanley E R, Carter D et al 1989 Circulating levels of CSF-1 (M-CSF) a lymphohaemopoietic cytokine may be a useful marker of disease status in patients with malignant ovarian neoplasms. International Journal of Radiation Oncology, Biology, Physics 17: 159–164.

Kacinski B M, Carter D, Mittal K et al 1990 Ovarian adenocarcinomas express fms-complementary transcripts and fms antigen, often with co-expression of CSF-1. American Journal of Pathology 137: 135–147.

Kamada M, Daiteh T, Mori K et al 1992 Etiological implication of autoantibodies to zona pellucida in human female infertility. American Journal of Reproductive Immunology 28: 104–109.

Kamat B R, Isaacson P G 1987 The immunocytochemical distribution of leukocytic subpopulations in human endometrium. American Journal of Pathology 127: 66–73.

Kameda K, Takada Y, Hasegawa A, Tsuji Y, Koyama K, Isojima S 1991 Sperm immobilizing and fertilization-blocking monoclonal antibody 2C6 to human seminal plasma antigen and characterization of the antigen epitope corresponding to the monoclonal antibody. Journal of Reproductive Immunology 20: 27–41.

Kamp P, Platz P, Nerup J 1974 'Steroid cell' antibody in Addison's disease. Acta Endocrinologica 76: 729–740.

Kanzaki H, Wang H-S, Kariya M, Mori T 1992 Suppression of natural killer cell activity by sera from patients with endometriosis. American Journal of Obstetrics and Gynecology 167: 257–261.

Kauma S, Clark M R, White C, Halme J 1988 Production of fibronectin by peritoneal macrophages and concentration of fibronectin in peritoneal fluid from patients with or without endometriosis. Obstetrics and Gynecology 72: 13–18.

Kay D Y 1977 Clinical significance of antibodies to antigens of the reproductive tract. In: Boettcher B (ed) Immunological influence on human fertility. Academic Press, Sydney, p 119.

Keller A J, Irvine W J, Jordan J, Loudon N B 1977 Phytohemagglutinin-induced lymphocyte transformation in oral contraceptive users. Obstetrics and Gynecology 49: 83–91.

Kelly J K, Fox H 1979 The local immunological defence system of human endometrium. Journal of Reproductive Immunology 1: 39–45.

Kesic V, Sulovic V, Bujko M, Dotlic R 1990 T lymphocytes in non-malignant, pre-malignant and malignant changes of the cervix. European Journal of Gynecological Oncology 11: 191–194.

Khoo D, Feigenbaum S L, McClure R D 1991 Screening assays for immunologic infertility: a comparison study. American Journal of Reproductive Immunology 26: 11–16.

Khoo S K, Mackay E 1974 Relation of cell mediated immunity in women with genital tract cancer to origin, histology, clinical stage and subsequent behaviour of neoplasm. Journal of Obstetrics and Gynecology of the British Commonwealth 81: 229–235.

Kietlinska Z 1984 T and B lymphocyte counts and blast transformation in patients with Stage I cervical cancer. Gynecologic Oncology 18: 247–256.

Kikuchi Y, Iwano I, Kita T et al 1990 Changes of lymphocyte subsets in peripheral blood before and after operation of patients with advanced ovarian carcinoma. Journal of Cancer Research and Clinical Oncology 116: 283–287.

Kilian P L, Kaffka K L, Biondi D A et al 1991 Antiproliferative effect of interleukin-1 on human ovarian carcinoma cell line (NIH:OVCAR-3). Cancer Research 51: 1823–1828.

Kimura T, Azuma C, Sagi F et al 1991 The biological effects of macrophage-colony-stimulating factor induced by progestin on growth and differentiation of endometrial adenocarcinoma cells. International Journal of Cancer 49: 229–233.

King A, Wellings V, Gardner L, Loke L W 1989 Immunocytochemical characterization of the unusual large granular lymphocytes in human endometrium throughout the menstrual cycle. Human Immunology 24: 195–205.

Kirsch T M, Friedman A C, Vogel R L, Flickinger G L 1981 Macrophages in the corpora lutea of mice: characterization and effects of steroid secretion. Biology of Reproduction 25: 629–632.

Kisalus L L, Herr J C, Little C D 1987 Immunolocalisation of extracellular matrix proteins and collagen synthesis in first-trimester human decidua. Anatomical Record 218: 402–415.

Kleerekoper M, Basten A, Penny R, Rosen S 1974 Idiopathic hypoparathyroidism with primary ovarian failure. Archives of Internal Medicine 134: 944–947.

Klentzeris L D, Bulmer J N, Li T C, Morrison L, Warren A, Cooke I D 1991a Lectin binding of endometrium in women with unexplained infertility. Fertility and Sterility 56: 660–667.

Klentzeris L D, Bulmer J N, Morrison L, Warren A, Li T C, Cooke I D 1991b The endometrial lymphoid tissue in women with unexplained infertility. Human Reproduction 6 (suppl 1): 8.

Klentzeris L D, Bulmer J N, Warren A, Morrison L, Li T-C, Cooke I D 1992 Endometrial lymphoid tissue in the timed endometrial biopsy: morphometric and immunohistochemical aspects. American Journal of Obstetrics and Gynaecology 167: 667–674.

Klentzeris L D, Bulmer J N, Trejdosiewicz L K, Morrison L, Cooke I D 1993 Beta-1 integrin cell adhesion molecules in the endometrium of fertile and infertile women. Human Reproduction 8: 1223–1230.

Klentzeris L D, Bulmer J N, Seppala M, Li T C, Warren M A, Cooke I D 1994 Placental protein 14 in cycles with normal and retained endometrial differentiation. Human Reproduction 9: 394–398

Klug T L, Bast R C, Niloff J, Knapp R C, Zurawaki V R 1984 A monoclonal antibody immunoradiometric assay for an antigenic determinant (CA 125) associated with human epithelial ovarian carcinomas. Cancer Research 44: 1048–1053.

Knauf S, Urbach G I 1977 Purification of human tumor-associated antigen and demonstration of circulating tumor antigen in patients with advanced ovarian malignancy. American Journal of Obstetrics and Gynecology 127: 705–711.

Knauf S, Urbach G I 1978 The development of a durable antibody radioimmunoassay in detecting ovarian tumor-associated antigen fraction OCA in plasma. American Journal of Obstetrics and Gynecology 131: 780–787.

Knauf S, Urbach G I 1980 A study of ovarian cancer patients using a radioimmunoassay for human ovarian tumor associated antigen OCA. American Journal of Obstetrics and Gynecology 138: 1222–1223.

Kobayashi H, Ohi H, Fujii T, Terao T 1993 Characterization and clinical usefulness of CA130 antigen recognised by monoclonal antibodies, 130–22 and 145–9 in ovarian cancers. British Journal of Cancer 67: 237–243.

Kohorn E I, Mitchell M S, Dwyer J M, Knowlton A H, Klein-Angerer S 1978 Effect of radiation on cell-mediated cytotoxicity and lymphocyte subpopulations in patients with ovarian carcinoma. Cancer 41: 1040–1048.

Kreiner D, Fromowitz F B, Richardson D A, Kenigsberg D 1986 Endometrial immunofluorescence associated with endometriosis and pelvic inflammatory disease. Fertility and Sterility 46: 243–245.

Kremer J, Jager S, Kuiken J, van Slochteren-Draaismat 1978 Recent advances in diagnosis and treatment of infertility due to antisperm antibodies. In: Cohen J, Hendry W F (eds) Spermatozoa, antibodies and infertility. Blackwell Scientific Publishers, Oxford, pp 117–127.

Kumari S, Bhatia R, Agarwal D S, Mitra A B, Luthra U K 1982 Microbiology of the female genital tract in cervical dysplasia and carcinoma. Indian Journal of Medical Research 75: 83–88.

Kurachi H, Wakimoto H, Sakumoto T, Anno T, Kurachi K 1984 Specific antibodies to porcine zona pellucida detected by quantitative radioimmunoassay in both fertile and infertile women. Fertility and Sterility 41: 265–269.

Kurachi H, Morishige K, Amemiya K et al 1991 Importance of transforming growth factor α/epidermal growth factor receptor autocrine growth mechanism in an ovarian cancer cell line in vivo. Cancer Research 51: 5956–5959.

Kutteh W H, Mestecky J 1994 Secretory immunity in the female genital tract. American Journal of Reproductive Immunology 31: 40–46.

Kutteh W H, Hatch K D, Blackwell R E, Mestecky J 1988 Secretory immune system of the female reproductive tract. I. Immunoglobulin and secretory component-containing cells. Obstetrics and Gynecology 71: 56–60.

Kutteh W H, Blackwell R E, Gore H, Kutteh C C, Carr B R, Mestecky J 1990 Secretory immune system of the female reproductive tract. II. Local immune system in normal and infected fallopian tube. Fertility and Sterility 54: 51–55.

Kutteh W H, Edwards R P, Menge A C, Mestecky J 1993 IgA immunity in female reproductive tract secretions. In: Griffin P D, Johnson P M (eds) Local immunity in reproductive tract tissues. Oxford University Press, Delhi, pp 229–243.

Kvale D, Brandtzaeg P, Lövhaug D 1988 Upregulation of secretory component and HLA molecules in human colonic cell line by tumor necrosis factor-α and gamma interferon. Scandinavian Journal of Immunology 61: 409–413.

LaBarbera A R, Miller M B, Ober C, Rebar R M 1988 Autoimmune etiology in premature ovarian failure. American Journal of Reproductive Immunology and Microbiology 16: 115–122.

LaGuardia K, McGuiness K, Hunter D 1991 Cervical disease among HIV infected women by immune status. Seventh International Conference on AIDS, Florence, p 47.

Lee N Y 1977 Quantitative changes of serum proteins and immunoglobulins in patients with solid cancer. Journal of Surgical Oncology 9: 179–187.

Lehtinin M, Leminen A, Paavonen J, Lehtovirta P, Hyöty H, Vesterinen E, Dillner J 1992 Predominance of serum antibodies to synthetic peptide stemming from HPV 18 open reading frame E2 in cervical adenocarcinoma. Journal of Clinical Pathology 45: 494–497.

Lessey B A, Damjanovich L, Coutifaris C, Castelbaum A, Albelda S M, Buck C A 1992 Integrin adhesion molecules in human endometrium: correlation with the normal and abnormal menstrual cycle. Journal of Clinical Investigation 90: 188–195.

Levin L, McHardy J E, Curling O M, Hudson C N 1975 Tumour antigenicity in ovarian cancer. British Journal of Cancer 32: 152–159.

Levin L, McHardy J E, Curling O M, Hudson C N 1976 Tumour associated immunity and immunocompetence in ovarian cancer. British Journal of Obstetrics and Gynaecology 83: 393–399.

Levy S, Kopersztych S, Mysatti C C, Sohen J S, Salvatorre C A, Mendes N F 1978 Cellular immunity in squamous cell carcinoma of the uterine cervix. American Journal of Obstetrics and Gynecology 130: 160–164.

Li B-Y, Mohanraj D, Olson M C, Moradi M, Twiggs L, Carson L F, Ramakrishnan S 1992 Human ovarian epithelial cancer cells cultured in vitro express both interleukin 1α and β genes. Cancer Research 52: 2248–2252.

Li T C, Dockery P, Rogers A W, Cooke I D 1990 A quantitative study of endometrial development in the luteal phase: comparison between women with unexplained infertility and normal fertility. British Journal of Obstetrics and Gynaecology 97: 576–582.

Li T S, Beling C G 1974 The effect of antibodies to the human seminal plasma-specific antigens on human sperm. Fertility and Sterility 25: 851–856.

Li T S, Pelosi M A, Gowan V W, Caterini H, Kaminetzky H A 1978 The effect of antibody against a purfied sperm-coating antigen on human sperm. International Journal of Fertility 23: 38–44.

Li W Y, Lusheng S, Kanbour A, Herberman R B, Whiteside T L 1989 Lymphocytes infiltrating human ovarian tumors: synergy between tumor necrosis factor α and interleukin 2 in the generation of CD8+ effectors from tumour infiltrating lymphocytes. Cancer Research 49: 5979–5985.

Lint T F 1980 Complement. In: Dhindsa D S, Schumacher G F B (eds) Immunological aspects of infertility and fertility regulation. Elsevier-North Holland, New York, p 13.

Liu D T Y, Hitchcock A 1986 Endometriosis: its association with retrograde menstruation, dysmenorrhoea and tubal pathology. British Journal of Obstetrics and Gynaecology 93: 859–862.

Loke Y W, King A, Drake B L 1993 Leucocytic organization in the endometrium and fallopian tube. In: Griffin P D, Johnson P M (eds) Local immunity in reproductive tract tissues. Oxford University Press, Delhi, pp 187–204.

London S N, Haney A F, Weinberg J B 1985 Macrophages and infertility: enhancement of human macrophage mediated sperm killing by antisperm antibodies. Fertility and Sterility 43: 274–278.

Lotzova E, Savary C A, Freedman R S, Bowen J M 1984 Natural killer cell cytotoxic potential of patients with ovarian cancer and its modulation with virus-modified tumour cell extract. Cancer Immunology and Immunotherapy 17: 124–129.

Lotzova E, Savary C A, Freedman R S, Edwards C L, Wharton J T 1988 Recombinant IL2-activated NK cells mediate LAK activity against ovarian cancer. International Journal of Cancer 42: 225–231.

Lukomska B, Olszewski W L, Engeset A, Kolstad P 1983 The effect of surgery and chemotherapy on blood NK cell activity in patients with ovarian cancer. Cancer 51: 465–469.

McArdle J P, Muller H K 1986 Quantitative assessment of Langerhans' cells in human cervical intraepithelial neoplasia and wart virus infection. American Journal of Obstetrics and Gynecology 154: 509–515.

McClure R D, Tom R A, Watkins M, Murthy H M S 1989 Sperm check: a simplified screening assay for immunologic infertility. Fertility and Sterility 52: 650–654.

McDicken I W, McLaughlin P J, Tromans P M, Luesley D M, Johnson P M 1985 Detection of placental type alkaline phosphatase in ovarian cancer. British Journal of Cancer 52: 59–64.

McKenzie J, King A, Hare J, Fulford T, Wilson B, Stanley M 1991 Immunocytochemical characterization of large granular lymphocytes in normal cervix and HPV associated disease. Journal of Pathology 165: 75–80.

McNatty K P, Short R V, Barnes E W, Irvine W J 1975 The cytotoxic effect of serum from patients with Addison's disease on human granulosa cells in culture. Clinical and Experimental Immunology 22: 378–384.

McShane P M, Schiff I, Trentham D 1985 Cellular immunity to sperm in infertile women. Journal of the American Medical Association 253: 3555–3559.

Malik S, Balkwill F 1991 Epithelial ovarian cancer: a cytokine propelled disease? British Journal of Cancer 64: 617–620.

Malik S T A, Griffin D B, Fiers W, Balkwill F R 1989 Paradoxical effects of tumor necrosis factor in experimental ovarian cancer. International Journal of Cancer 44: 918–925.

Malik S T A, Naylor M S, East N, Oliff A, Balkwill F R 1990 Cells secreting tumour necrosis factor show enhanced metastasis in nude mice. European Journal of Cancer 26: 1031–1034.

Mandelbaum S L, Diamond M P, DeCherney A H 1987 The impact of antisperm antibodies on human infertility. Journal of Urology 138: 1–8.

Mandell G L, Fisher R I, Bostick F, Young R C 1979 Ovarian cancer: a solid tumor with evidence of normal cellular immune function but abnormal B cell function. American Journal of Medicine 66: 621–624.

Mantovani A, Allavena P, Sessa C, Bolis G, Mangioni C 1980 Natural killer activity of lymphoid cells isolated from human ascitic ovarian tumors. International Journal of Cancer 25: 573–582.

Mantovani A, Sessa C, Peri G et al 1981 Intraperitoneal administration of Corynebacterium parvum in patients with ascitic ovarian tumors resistant to chemotherapy: effects on cytotoxicity of tumor-associated macrophages and NK cells. International Journal of Cancer 27: 437–446.

Marcus Z H, Soffer Y, Ben-David A, Peleg S, Nebel L 1973 Studies on sperm antigenicity. I. Delayed hypersensitivity to spermatozoa. European Journal of Immunology 3: 75–78.

Marshall R J, Jones D B 1988 An immunohistochemical study of lymphoid tissue in human endometrium. International Journal of Gynecological Pathology 7: 225–235.

Maruyama D K, Hale R W, Rogers B J 1985 Effects of white blood cells on the in vitro penetration of zona-free hamster eggs by human spermatozoa. Journal of Andrology 6: 127–135.

Marzusch K, Ruck P, Geiselhart A et al 1993 Distribution of cell adhesion molecules on CD56++ CD3– CD16– large granular lymphocytes and endothelial cells in first-trimester human decidua. Human Reproduction 8: 1203–1208.

Mathur S, Jerath R S, Mather R S, Williamson H O, Fudenberg H H 1980a Serum immunoglobulin levels, autoimmunity and cell-mediated immunity in primary ovarian failure. Journal of Reproductive Immunology 2: 83–92.

Mathur S, Melchers J T, Ades E W, Williamson H O, Fudenberg H H 1980b Antiovarian and antilymphocyte antibodies in patients with chronic vaginal candidiasis. Journal of Reproductive Immunology 2: 247–262.

Mathur S, Baker W R, Williamson H O, Derrick F, Teaque K J, Fudenberg H H 1981a Clinical significance of sperm antibodies in infertility. Fertility and Sterility 136: 486–495.

Mathur S, Williamson H O, Baker E R, Fudenberg H H 1981b Immunoglobulin E levels and antisperm antibody titres in infertile couples. American Journal of Obstetrics and Gynecology 40: 923–930.

Mathur S, Peress M R, Williamson H O et al 1982 Autoimmunity to endometrium and ovary in endometriosis. Clinical and Experimental Immunology 50: 259–266.

Mathur S, Genlo P V, Williamson H O et al 1983 Association of human leucocyte antigens A7 and BW35 with sperm antibodies. Fertility and Sterility 39: 343–349.

Mathur S, Chihal H J, Homm R J, Garza D E, Rust P F, Williamson H O 1988 Endometrial antigens involved in the autoimmunity of endometriosis. Fertility and Sterility 50: 860–863.

Matilsky M, Ben-Ami M, Geslevich Y, Eyali V, Shalev E 1993 Cervical leukocytosis and abnormal postcoital test: a diagnostic and therapeutic approach. Human Reproduction 8: 244–246.

Meek S C, Hodge D D, Musich J R 1988 Autoimmunity in infertile patients with endometriosis. American Journal of Obstetrics and Gynecology 158: 1365–1373.

Melnick H, Barber H R K 1975 Cellular immunologic responsiveness to extracts of ovarian epithelial tumors. Gynecologic Oncology 3: 77–86.

Menge A C, Fleming C H 1978 Detection of sperm antigen on mouse ova and early embryos. Developmental Biology 63: 111–117.

Menge A C, Schwarz M I, Riolo R L, Greenberg V N, Neda T 1977 The role of the cervix and cervical secretions in immunologic infertility. In: Insler V, Bettendorf G (eds) The uterine cervix in reproduction. Georg Thieme, Stuttgart, pp 221–230.

Menge A C, Medley N E, Mangione C M, Dietrich J W 1982 The incidence and influence of antisperm antibodies in infertile human couples on sperm–cervical mucus interactions and subsequent fertility. Fertility and Sterility 38: 439–446.

Merriman H, Woods S, Winter C, Fahnlander A, Corey L 1984 Secretory IgA antibody in cervicovaginal secretions from women with genital infections due to Herpes simplex virus. Journal of Infectious Diseases 149: 505–510.

Mettler L, Schirwani D 1975 Macrophage migration inhibitory factor in female sterility. American Journal of Obstetrics and Gynecology 121: 117–120.

Micksche M, Luger T, Michalica W, Tatra G 1978 Investigations on general immune reactivity in untreated cervical cancer patients. Oncology 35: 206–210.

Mills G B, May C, McGill M, Roifman C M, Mellors A 1988 A putative growth factor in ascitic fluid from ovarian cancer patients: identification, characterization and mechanisms of action. Cancer Research 48: 1066–1071.

Mitchell M S, Kohorn E I 1976 Cell mediated immunity and blocking factors in ovarian carcinoma. Obstetrics and Gynecology 48: 590–597.

Moghissi K S, Sacco A G, Borin K 1980 Immunologic infertility. I. Cervical mucus antibodies and post coital test. American Journal of Obstetrics and Gynecology 136: 941–948.

Moncayo R, Moncayo H E 1992 Autoimmunity and the ovary. Immunology Today 13: 255–258.

Moncayo H E, Moncayo R, Benz R, Wolf A, Lauritzen C 1989 Ovarian failure and autoimmunity: detection of autoantibodies directed against both the unoccupied luteinizing hormone/human chorionic gonadotrophin receptor and the hormone receptor of complex bovine corpus luteum. Journal of Clinical Investigation 84: 1857–1865.

Moncayo-Naveda H E, Moncayo R, Benz R, Wolf A, Lauritzen C 1989 Organ-specific antibodies against ovary in patients with systemic lupus erythematosus. American Journal of Obstetrics and Gynecology 160: 1227–1229.

Moncayo R, Moncayo H E, Dapunt O 1990 Immunological risks of IVF. Lancet 335: 180.

Mooney N A, Townsend P A, Wiltshaw E, Evans D G, Shantiraju K, Poulton T A 1983a An assessment of sequential measurements of immune complex levels in ovarian cancer patients with respect to clinical progress. Gynecologic Oncology 15: 207–213.

Mooney N A, Hay F C, Poulton A 1983b A comparative study of complement components in polyethylene glycol precipitated immune complexes from patients with ovarian cancer and patients with rheumatoid arthritis. Clinical and Experimental Immunology 52: 561–568.

Moore M 1984 Tumour resistance and the phenomenon of inflammatory cell infiltration. In: Fox B W, Fox M (eds) Handbook of experimental pharmacology, vol 72. Springer Verlag, Berlin, pp 143–185.

Moraes-Ruehsen M de, Blizzard R M, Garcia-Bunuel R, Jones G S 1972 Autoimmunity and ovarian failure. American Journal of Obstetrics and Gynecology 112: 693–703.

Mori T, Nishimoto T, Kitagawa M, Noda Y, Nisuimura T, Oikawa T 1978 Possible presence of autoantibodies to zona pellucida in infertile women. Experientia 34: 797–798.

Mori T, Nishimoto T, Kohda H, Takai I, Nishimura T 1979 A method for specific detection of autoantibodies to the zona pellucida in infertile women. Fertility and Sterility 32: 67–72.

Mori T, Kameda M, Hasebe H et al 1985 Antibody reactivity with porcine zona pellucida. Journal of Reproductive Immunology 8: 337–345.

Morishige K, Hirohisa K, Amemiya K et al 1991 Involvement of transforming growth factor α/epidermal growth factor receptor autocrine growth mechanism in an ovarian cancer cell line in vitro. Cancer Research 51: 5951–5955.

Morris H H B, Gatter K C, Sykes G, Casemore V, Mason D Y 1983 Langerhans' cells in human cervical epithelium: effects of wart virus infection and intraepithelial neoplasia. British Journal of Obstetrics and Gynaecology 90: 412–420.

Morris H, Edwards J, Tiltman A, Emms M 1985 Endometrial lymphoid tissue: an immunohistological study. Journal of Clinical Pathology 38: 644–652.

Morris H, Emms M, Visser T, Timme A 1986 Lymphoid tissue of the normal fallopian tube — a form of mucosal associated lymphoid tissue (MALT)? International Journal of Gynaecological Pathology 5: 11–22.

Mosher W D 1982 Infertility trends among US couples: 1965–1976. Family Planning Perspective 14: 22–27.

Motro B, Itin A, Sachs L, Keshet E 1990 Pattern of interleukin 6 gene expression in vivo suggests a role for this cytokine in angiogenesis. Proceedings of the National Academy of Sciences of the USA 87: 3092–3096.

Murdoch A J M, Buckley C H, Fox H 1982 Hormonal control of the secretory immune system of the human uterine cervix. Journal of Reproductive Immunology 4: 23–30.

Muscato J J, Haney A F, Weinberg J B 1982 Sperm phagocytosis by human peritoneal macrophages: a possible cause of infertility in endometriosis. American Journal of Obstetrics and Gynecology 144: 503–512.

Nalick R H, DiSaia P J, Rea T H, Morrow C P 1974a Immunocompetence and prognosis in patients with gynecologic cancer. Gynecologic Oncology 2: 81–92.

Nalick R H, DiSaia P J, Rea T H, Morrow M H 1974b Immunologic defect in gynecological malignancy as demonstrated by the delayed hypersensitivity reaction: clinical considerations. American Journal of Obstetrics and Gynecology 118: 393–405.

Natali P G, DeMartino C, Quaranta V et al 1981 Expression of Ia-like antigens in normal human nonlymphoid tissues. Transplantation 31: 75–78.

Naylor M S, Malik S T A, Stamp G W H, Jobling T, Balkwill F R 1990 In situ detection of tumour necrosis factor in human ovarian cancer specimens. European Journal of Cancer 26: 1027–1030.

Naylor M S, Stamp G W H, Foulkes W D, Eccles D, Balkwill F R 1993 Tumor necrosis factor and its receptors in human ovarian cancer. Journal of Clinical Investigation 91: 2194–2206.

Naz R, Menge A 1990 Development of antisperm contraceptive vaccine for humans: why and how? Human Reproduction 5: 511–518.

Neill W, Norval M 1984 Natural killer cell activity in patients with abnormalities of the uterine cervix. Gynecologic and Obstetric Investigation 18: 122–128.

Neukirk M M, Klein M H, Katz A, Fisher M M, Underdown B J 1983

Estimation of polymeric IgA in human serum: an assay based on binding of radiolabelled human secretory component with application in the study of IgA nephropathy, IgA monoclonal gammopathy and liver disease. Journal of Immunology 130: 1176–1181.

Niloff J M, Knapp R C, Schaetzl E, Reynolds C, Bast R C Jr 1984 CA 125 antigen levels in obstetric and gynecologic patients. Obstetrics and Gynecology 64: 703–707.

Niloff J M, Bast R C Jr, Schaetzl E, Knapp R C 1985 Predictive values of CA125 antigen levels in second-look procedures for ovarian cancer. American Journal of Obstetrics and Gynecology 151: 981–986.

Nuovo G J, Forde A, MacConnell P, Fahrenwald R 1993 In situ detection of PCR-amplified HIV-1 nucleic acids and tumor necrosis factor cDNA cervical tissues. American Journal of Pathology 143: 40–48.

Ogra P L, Ogra S S 1973 Local antibody response to polio vaccine in the human female genital tract. Journal of Immunology 110: 1307–1311.

Ohkawa K, Tsukada Y, Murae M et al 1989 Serum levels and biochemical characteristics of human ovarian carcinoma-associated antigen defined by murine monoclonal antibody CF 511. British Journal of Cancer 60: 953–960.

Ohkawa K, Takada K, Hatano T et al 1991 An evaluation of ovarian carcinoma-associated antigen defined by murine monoclonal antibody CF511 in sera from patients with ovarian carcinoma. British Journal of Cancer 64: 259–262.

Okamoto N, Uchida A, Takakura K et al 1992 Suppression by human placental protein 14 of natural killer cell activity. American Journal of Reproductive Immunology 26: 137–142.

Olsen G P, Shields J W 1984 Seminal lymphocytes, plasma and AIDS. Nature 309: 116–117.

Oosterlynk D J, Cornillie F J, Waer M, Vandeputte M, Koninckx P R 1991 Women with endometriosis show a defect in natural killer activity resulting in decreased cytotoxicity to autologous endometrium. Fertility and Sterility 56: 45–51.

Oosterlynk D J, Meuleman C, Waer M, Vandeputte M, Koninckx P R 1992 The natural killer activity of peritoneal fluid lymphocytes is decreased in women with endometriosis. Fertility and Sterility 58: 290–295.

Oosterlynk D J, Meuleman C, Lacquet F A, Waer M, Koninckx P R 1994 Flow cytometry analysis of lymphocyte subpopulations in peritoneal fluid of women with endometriosis. American Journal of Reproductive Immunology 31: 25–31.

Pace D, Longfellow M, Bulmer J N 1991 Intraepithelial lymphocytes in human endometrium. Journal of Reproduction and Fertility 91: 165–174.

Pandya I J, Cohen J 1985 The leukocytic reaction of the human uterine cervix to spermatozoa. Fertility and Sterility 70: 71–77.

Patillo R A, Story M T, Ruckert A C F 1979a Expression of cell mediated immunity and blocking factors using a new line of ovarian cancer cells in vitro. Cancer Research 39: 1185–1191.

Patillo R A, Ruckert A C F, Story M T, Mattingly R F 1979b Immunodiagnosis in ovarian cancer: blocking factor activity. American Journal of Obstetrics and Gynecology 133: 791–799.

Peri G, Zanaboni F, Rossini S et al 1986 Evaluation of the interaction of mononuclear phagocytes with ovarian carcinoma cells in a colony assay. British Journal of Cancer 53: 47–52.

Peters W M 1986 Nature of 'basal' and 'reserve' cells in oviductal and cervical epithelium in man. Journal of Clinical Pathology 39: 306–312.

Petrovska M, Sedlak R, Nouza K, Presl J, Kinsky R 1992 Development and distribution of white blood cells within various structures of the human menstrual corpus luteum examined using an image analysis system. American Journal of Reproductive Immunology 28: 77–80.

Philippeaux M-M, Piguet P F 1993 Expression of tumor necrosis factor-α and its mRNA in the endometrial mucosa during the menstrual cycle. American Journal of Pathology 143: 480–486.

Phillips J, Everson M P, Moldoveanu Z, Lue C, Mestecky J 1990 Synergistic effect of 14–4 and IFNγ on expansion of polymeric Ig receptor (secretory component) and IgA binding by human epithelial cells. Journal of Immunology 145: 1740–1744.

Pisa P, Halapi E, Pisa E K et al 1992 Selective expression of interleukin 10, interferon γ and granulocyte-macrophage colony-stimulating factor in ovarian cancer biopsies. Proceedings of the National Academy of Sciences of the USA 89: 7708–7712.

Piver M S, Barlow J J, Bhattacharya M 1979 Treatment and immunodiagnosis of advanced ovarian adenocarcinoma: a preliminary report. Cancer Treatment Reports 63: 265–267.

Pomerantz R J, de la Monte S M, Donegan S P et al 1988 Human immune deficiency virus (HIV) infection of the uterine cervix. Annals of Internal Medicine 108: 321–327.

Porter C W, Highfill D, Minovich R 1970 Guinea pig ovary and testis: organization of common gonad specific antigens. International Journal of Fertility 15: 177–181.

Poulton T A, Crowther M E, Hay F C, Nineham L J 1978 Immune complexes in ovarian cancer. Lancet ii: 72–73.

Poulton T A, Crowther M E, Nineham L J, Mooney N A, Hay F C 1982 Sequential studies of circulating immune complexes in gynecological malignancies. American Journal of Reproductive Immunology 2: 265–269.

Priolo L, Minkoff H L 1992 HIV infection in women. Baillière's Clinical Obstetrics and Gynaecology 6: 617–628.

Prozorovskaya K N, Stefani D V, Antonova L V, Dub N V 1977 Immunoglobulins of the cervical mucus in healthy pregnancy. Voprosy Okhrany Materinstva i Detstva (Moscow) 22: 76–79.

Pulay T A, Benczur M, Vargu M 1982 Natural killer lymphocyte function in cervical cancer patients. Neoplasma 29: 237–240.

Rabinowe S L, Ravnikar V A, Dib S A, George K L, Dluhy R G 1989 Premature menopause: monoclonal antibody defined T lymphocyte abnormalities and antiovarian antibodies. Fertility and Sterility 51: 450–454.

Radhakrishna Pillai M, Balaram P, Hareendran N K, Binda S, Padmanabhan T K, Nair M K 1990 Clinical and prognostic significance of concanavalin-A-induced suppressor cell activity in malignant cervical neoplasia. British Journal of Obstetrics and Gynaecology 97: 357–361.

Ralston S H, Russell R G R, Gowen M 1990 Estrogen inhibits release of tumor necrosis factor from peripheral blood mononuclear cells in postmenopausal women. Journal of Bone and Mineral Research 5: 983–988.

Ramakrishnan S, Xu F J, Brandt S J, Niedel J E, Bast R C Jr, Brown E L 1989 Constitutive production of macrophage colony-stimulating factor by human ovarian and breast cancer cell lines. Journal of Clinical Investigation 83: 921–926.

Rand R J, Jenkins D M, Bulmer R 1977 T and B lymphocyte subpopulations in pre-invasive and invasive carcinoma of the cervix. Clinical and Experimental Immunology 30: 421–428.

Rebello R, Green F H Y, Fox H 1975 A study of the secretory immune system of the female genital tract. British Journal of Obstetrics and Gynaecology 82: 812–816.

Ritson A, Bulmer J N 1987 Endometrial granulocytes in human decidua react with a natural-killer (NK) cell marker, NKH1. Immunology 62: 329–331.

Rivera E S, Hersh E M, Bowen J M, Barnett J W 1979 Leucocyte migration inhibition assay of tumor immunity in patients with cervical squamous cell carcinoma. Cancer 43: 2297–2305.

Rizov B, Raychev R, Kozhumarova M 1973 Immunological reactions in cases of endocervicitis. In: Bratanov K, Edwards R G, Vulchanov V H (eds) Immunology of reproduction. Bulgarian Academy of Sciences Press, Sofia, pp 211–214.

Roche J K, Crum C P 1991 Local immunity in the uterine cervix: implications for cancer-associated viruses. Cancer Immunology and Immunotherapy 33: 203–209.

Rose E, Pillsbury D M 1944 Lupus erythematosus (erythematodes) and ovarian function: observations on a possible relationship, with report of six cases. Annals of Internal Medicine 21: 1022–1034.

Rubin S C, Lewis J L Jr 1986 Tumor antigens in ovarian malignancy. Clinical Obstetrics and Gynecology 29: 693–704.

Russo I, Metz C B 1974 Inhibition of fertilization in vitro by treatment of rabbit spermatozoa with univalent isoantibody. Journal of Reproduction and Fertility 38: 211–215.

Sacco A G, Moghissi K S 1979 Anti-zona pellucida activity in human sera. Fertility and Sterility 31: 503–506.

Sacco A G, Shivers C A 1973 Localization of tissue specific antigens in the rabbit ovary, oviduct and uterus by the fluorescent antibody technique. Journal of Reproduction and Fertility 32: 412–427.

Saha K, Bhatia G, Mukherjee S, Mitra A B, Luthra U K 1981 Fluctuations of immunoglobulin levels in cervical mucus during the various phases of female reproductive life and its alterations in uterine disorders. Indian Journal of Medical Research 74: 696–704.

Saifuddin A, Buckley C H, Fox H 1983 Immunoglobulin content of the endometrium in women with endometriosis. International Journal of Gynecological Pathology 2: 255–263.

Satam M N, Nadkarni J J, Nadkarni J S, Rajpal R M 1981 Immune status in untreated cervical cancer patients. Neoplasma 28: 111–116.

Satam M N, Suraiya J N, Nadkarni J J 1986 Natural killer and antibody-dependent cellular cytotoxicity in cervical carcinoma patients. Cancer Immunology and Immunotherapy 23: 56–59.

Sawonabar S, Ashman R B, Nahmias A J, Benigno B B, LaVia M F 1977 Rosette formation and inhibition in cervical dysplasia and carcinoma in situ. Cancer Research 37: 4332–4335.

Scambia G, Panici P B, Battaglia F et al 1991 Effect of recombinant human interferon alpha (2b) on receptors for steroid hormones and epidermal growth factor in patients with endometrial cancer. European Journal of Cancer 27: 51–53.

Schumacher G F B, Yang S L 1977 Cyclic changes of immunoglobulins and specific antibodies in human and Rhesus monkey cervical mucus. In: Insler V, Battendorf G (eds) The uterine cervix in reproduction. Georg Thieme, Stuttgart, pp 187–203.

Schwimmer W B, Ustay K A, Behrman S J 1967 Sperm-agglutinating antibodies and decreased fertility in prostitutes. Obstetrics and Gynecology 30: 192–195.

Sedmak D D, Hart W R, Tubbs R R 1986 Autoimmune oophoritis — a histopathological study of involved ovaries with immunologic characterization of the mononuclear cell infiltrate. International Journal of Gynecological Pathology 6: 73–81.

Sekiguchi M, Shibitsawa M, Asanuma K, Kaku R, Wagatsuma T, Kobayashi H 1982 Inhibition of leucocyte migration in agar by soluble extract from a human ovarian carcinoma cell line. Japanese Journal of Experimental Medicine 52: 119–124.

Seltzer V, Doyle A, Kadish A S 1983 Natural cytotoxicity in malignant and premalignant cervical neoplasia and enhancement of cytotoxicity with interferon. Gynecologic Oncology 15: 340–349.

Seth P, Balachandran N, Malaviya A N, Kumar S 1979 Circulating immune complexes in carcinoma of the uterine cervix. Clinical and Experimental Immunology 38: 77–82.

Shai S, Bar-Yoseph N, Peer E, Naot Y 1990 A reverse (antibody capture) enzyme-linked immunosorbent assay for detection of antisperm antibodies in sera and genital tract secretions. Fertility and Sterility 54: 894–901.

Sharp B M, Matta S G, Peterson P K, Newton R, Chao C, McCallan K 1989 Tumour necrosis factor-α is a potent ACTH secretagogue: comparison to interleukin-1β. Endocrinology 124: 3131–3133.

Shau H, Koren H S, Dawson J R 1983 Human natural killing against ovarian carcinoma. British Journal of Cancer 47: 687–695.

Sheid B, Boyce J 1984 Inhibition of lymphocyte mitogenesis by factor(s) released from macrophages isolated from ascitic fluid of advanced ovarian cancer patients. Cancer Immunology and Immunotherapy 17: 190–194.

Shemesh M, Meirom R, Zolti M, Ben-Rafael Z, Wollach D R 1990 Tumor necrosis factor (TNFα) and the endogenous prostaglandin inhibitor (PGIn) in bovine follicles. In: Mashiach S, Ben-Rafael Z, Laufer N, Schenker J (eds) Advances in in vitro fertilization and embryo transfer. Plenum Press, New York, pp 129–137.

Shivers C A, Dunbar B S 1977 Autoantibodies to zona pellucida: a possible cause for infertility in women. Science 197: 1082–1084.

Shulman S, Hu C-Y 1992 A study of sperm antibody in cervical mucus with a modified immunobead method. Fertility and Sterility 58: 387–391.

Sidhu G S, Koss K G, Barber H R K 1970 Relation of histologic factors to the response of Stage I epidermoid carcinoma of the cervix to surgical treatment. Obstetrics and Gynecology 35: 329–338.

Siklos P, Pete I, Ungar L, Hercz P, Bakacs T 1992 Enhanced K-cell activity in the peripheral blood of patients with gynaecological malignancies: the impact of radiotherapy. Journal of Experimental and Clinical Cancer Research 11: 253–258.

Silburn P A, Khoo S K, Daunter B, Hill R, Roberts T K, Mackay E V 1983 Types of immune complexes in the ascitic fluid of women with carcinoma of the ovary. International Archives of Allergy and Applied Immunology 71: 219–222.

Silburn P A, Neill J C, Khoo S K et al 1984 Immune complexes in ovarian cancer: association between IgM class complexes and antinuclear autoantibodies in ascitic fluid. International Archives of Allergy and Applied Immunology 74: 63–66.

Sinha D P, Andersen T D, Holborrow E J, Nandakumar V C 1977 Local immunological factors as possible cause of reduced sperm motility in the cervical mucus of infertile women. British Journal of Obstetrics and Gynaecology 84: 948–953.

Smith J R, Barton S E 1992 Gynaecological problems and infertility. Baillière's Clinical Obstetrics and Gynaecology 6: 187–197.

Smith J R, Kitchen V S, Botcherby M et al 1991 HPV and cervical neoplasia in HIV seropositive women. Abstracts of the MSSVD and GBGK Spring Meeting, Heidelberg, Germany, p 22.

Smith L H, Oi R H 1984 Detection of ovarian neoplasms: a review of the literature. III. Immunological detection and ovarian cancer-associated antigens. Obstetrical and Gynecological Survey 39: 346–360.

Snow K, Ball G D 1992 Characterization of human sperm antigens and antisperm antibodies in infertile patients. Fertility and Sterility 58: 1011–1019.

Snyder K A, Barber S R, Symbula M, Taylor P T, Crum C P, Roche J K 1991 Binding by immunoglobulin to the HPV-16-derived proteins L1 and E4 in cervical secretions of women with HPV-related cervical disease. Cancer Research 51: 4423–4429.

Soffer Y, Marcus Z H, Nebel L 1976 Reactions leucocytaires 'in vitro' aux spermatozoides humaines dans femmes infertiles. Journal de Gynécologie Obstétrique et Biologie de la Reproduction 5: 621–631.

Soffer Y, Caspi E, Weinstein Y 1983 Endometrial cell-mediated immunity and contraception: new perspectives. In: Dondero F (ed) Immunological factors in human contraception. Field Educational Italia Acta Medica, Rome, pp 161–167.

Sollid L M, Kvale D, Brandtzaeg P, Markussen G, Thorsby E 1987 Interferon-γ enhances expression of secretory component, the epithelial receptor for polymeric immunoglobulins. Journal of Immunology 138: 4303–4306.

Sotsiou F, Bottazzo G F, Doniach D 1980 Immunofluorescence studies of autoantibodies in steroid-producing cells, and to germ line cells in endocrine disease and infertility. Clinical and Experimental Immunology 39: 97–11.

Spriggs D R, Imamura K, Rodriguez C, Sariban E, Kufe D W 1988 Tumor necrosis factor expression in human epithelial tumor cell lines. Journal of Clinical Investigation 81: 455–460.

Spurrett B, Jones S D, Stewart G 1988 Cervical dysplasia and HIV infection. Lancet i: 237–238.

Stanislavov R, Nalbanski B, Protig M, Barov D 1983 The uterine cervix as a site of local immunity to spermal antigens. Akusherstvo i Ginekologiya (Sofia) 22: 144–147.

Starkey P M, Clover L M, Rees M C P 1991 Variation during the menstrual cycle of immune populations in human endometrium. European Journal of Obstetrics, Gynecology and Reproductive Biology 39: 203–207.

Steele R W, Dmowski W P, Marmer D J 1984 Immunologic aspects of human endometriosis. American Journal of Reproductive Immunology 6: 33–36.

Stern J E, Dixon P M, Manganiello P D, Brinck-Johnsen T 1992 Antisperm antibodies in women: variability in antibody levels in serum, mucus, and peritoneal fluid. Fertility and Sterility 58: 950–958.

Stevens V C, Powell J E, Lee A C, Griffin P D 1981 Anti-fertility effects from immunization of female baboons with C-terminal peptides of hCG beta subunit. Fertility and Sterility 36: 98–105.

Stewart C J R, Farquharson M A, Foulis A K 1992 The distribution and possible function of gamma interferon-immunoreactive cells in normal endometrium and myometrium. Virchows Archiv A Pathological Anatomy and Histology 420: 419–424.

Stratton J A, DiSaia P J 1982 Depressed mononuclear cell function in advanced neoplastic disease. American Journal of Reproductive Immunology 2: 111–116.

Sullivan D A, Underdown B J, Wira C R 1983 Steroid hormone

regulation of free secretory component in the rat uterus. Immunology 49: 379–386.

Sullivan D A, Richardson G S, MacLaughlin D T, Wira C R 1984 Variations in the level of secretory component in human uterine fluid during the menstrual cycle. Journal of Steroid Biochemistry 20: 509–513.

Sunderland C A, Davies J O, Stirrat G M 1984 Immunohistology of normal and ovarian cancer tissue with a monoclonal antibody to placental alkaline phosphatase. Cancer Research 44: 4496–4502.

Suri A, Talwar G P, Shaha C 1993 Oral immunization with sperm antigens. In: Griffin P D, Johnson P M (eds) Local immunity in reproductive tract tissues. Oxford University Press, Delhi, pp 427–440.

Suzuki M, Ogawa M, Tamada T, Nagura H, Watanabe K 1984 Immunohistochemical localization of secretory component and IgA in the human endometrium in relation to the menstrual cycle. Acta Histochemica et Cytochemica 17: 223–229.

Tabibzadeh S 1990 Evidence of T cell activation and potential cytokine action in human endometrium. Journal of Clinical Endocrinology and Metabolism 71: 645–649.

Tabibzadeh S 1991 Ubiquitous expression of TNF-α/cachectin immunoreactivity in human endometrium. American Journal of Reproductive Immunology 26: 1–4.

Tabibzadeh S S, Poubouridis D 1990 Expression of leukocyte adhesion molecules in human endometrium. American Journal of Clinical Pathology 93: 183–189.

Tabibzadeh S S, Gerber M A, Satyaswaroop P G 1986 Induction of HLA-DR antigen expression in human endometrial epithelial cells in vitro by recombinant gamma-interferon. American Journal of Pathology 125: 90–96.

Tabibzadeh S, Santhanam U, Seghal P B, May L T 1989 Cytokine induced production of IFN-β/IL6 by freshly explanted endometrial stromal cells: modulation by estradiol 17-β. Journal of Immunology 142: 3134–3139.

Takayama H, Wakamiya N, O'Hara C et al 1991 Tumour necrosis factor expression by human ovarian carcinoma in vivo. Cancer Research 51: 4476–4480.

Tartakovsky B, Ben-Yair E 1991 Cytokines modulate preimplantation development and pregnancy. Development Biology 146: 345–354.

Tay S K, Jenkins D, Maddox P, Campion M, Singer A 1987a Subpopulations of Langerhans' cells in cervical neoplasia. British Journal of Obstetrics and Gynaecology 94: 10–15.

Tay S K, Jenkins D, Maddox P, Singer A 1987b Lymphocyte phenotypes in cervical intraepithelial neoplasia and human papillomavirus infection. British Journal of Obstetrics and Gynaecology 94: 16–21.

Tay S K, Jenkins D, Maddox P, Hogg N, Singer A 1987c Tissue macrophage response in human papilloma virus infection and cervical intraepithelial neoplasia. British Journal of Obstetrics and Gynaecology 94: 1094–1097.

Taylor D D, Homesley H D, Doellgast G J 1983 'Membrane-associated' immunoglobulins in cysts and ascitic fluids of ovarian cancer patients. American Journal of Reproductive Immunology 3: 7–11.

Teland M, Reyniak J V, Shulman S 1978 Antibodies to spermatozoa. VIII. Correlation of sperm antibody activity with postcoital tests in infertile couples. International Journal of Fertility 23: 200–206.

Terho P, Meurman O 1981 Chlamydial serum IgG, IgA and local IgA antibodies in patients with genital tract infections measured by solid phase radioimmunoassay. Journal of Medical Microbiology 14: 77–87.

Teshima H, Wanebo H, Pinsky C, Day N K 1977 Circulating immune complexes detected by the 125 I-Clq deviation test in sera of cancer patients. Journal of Clinical Investigation 59: 1134–1142.

Thompson L A, Tomlinson M J, Barrett C L R, Bolton A E, Cooke I D 1991 Positive immunoselection — a method of isolating leukocytes from leukocytic reacted cervical mucus samples. American Journal of Reproductive Immunology 26: 58–61.

Thompson L A, Barrett C L R, Bolton A E, Cooke I D 1992 The leukocytic reaction in the human cervix. American Journal of Reproductive Immunology 28: 85–89.

Timonen T, Lehtovirta P, Saksela E 1987 Interleukin-2-stimulated natural killer cell activity against malignant and benign endometrium. International Journal of Cancer 40: 479–483.

Tomasi T B, McNabb P C 1980 The secretory immune system. In: Fudenberg H H, Stites D P, Caldwell J L, Wells J V (eds) Basic and clinical immunology. Lange Medical Publications, Los Altos, California, pp 240–250.

Tosner J, Fixa B 1979 Non-specific leucocyte migration inhibition of gynaecological carcinoma patients. Clinical and Experimental Immunology 38: 356–360.

Tötterman T H, Hayry P, Saksela E, Timonen T, Eklund B 1978 Cytological and functional analysis of inflammatory infiltrates in human malignant tumours: II. Functional investigations of the infiltrating inflammatory cells. European Journal of Immunology 8: 873–875.

Tourville D R, Ogra S S, Lippes J, Tomasi T B Jr 1970 The human female reproductive tract: immunohistological localization of γA, γG, γM, secretory 'piece' and lactoferin. American Journal of Obstetrics and Gynecology 108: 1102–1108.

Trnka V, Rejnek J, Dolezac A 1964 The protein spectrum of cervical secretions during the course of pregnancy. American Journal of Obstetrics and Gynecology 89: 215–217.

Tsuji Y, Fukuda H, Iuchi A, Ishizuka I, Isojima S 1992 Sperm immobilizing antibodies react to the 3-O-sulfated galactose residue of seminolipid on human sperm. Journal of Reproductive Immunology 22: 225–236.

Ueda K, Toyokawa M, Makamori H et al 1978 Immunosuppressive effect of serum in patients with ovarian carcinoma. Obstetrics and Gynecology 51: 225–228.

Ueda K, Toyokawa M, Makamori H et al 1979 The prognostic value of serum immunosuppressive effect in patients with ovarian cancer. Obstetrics and Gynecology 53: 480–483.

Urry R L, Laudle M R, Rote N S 1985 Autoimmune infertility and recurrent abortion. In: Scott J R, Rote N S (eds) Immunology in obstetrics and gynaecology. Century Crofts, Norwalk, p 77.

Vaccarello L, Wang Y L, Whiteside T L 1990 Sustained outgrowth of autotumor-reactive T lymphocytes from human ovarian carcinomas in the presence of tumor necrosis factor α and interleukin 2. Human Immunology 28: 216–227.

Vaccarello L, Kanbour A, Kanbour-Shakir A, Whiteside T L 1993 Tumor-infiltrating lymphocytes from ovarian tumors of low malignant potential. International Journal of Gynecological Pathology 12: 41–50.

Vaerman J P, Ferin J 1974 Local immunological response in the vagina, cervix and endometrium. In: Diczfalusy E (ed) Immunological approaches to fertility control. Karolinska Instutet, Stockholm, pp 281–301.

Vande Perre P, DeClercq A, Cogniaux-Lederc J, Nzaramba D, Butzler J P, Sprecher-Goldberger S 1988 Detection of HIV p17 antigen in lymphocytes but not epithelial cells from cervicovaginal secretions of women seropositive for HIV: implications for heterosexual transmission of the virus. Genitourinary Medicine 64: 30–37.

Van der Linde P W, Streefkerk M, teVelde E R, Schurman H J, Szabo B C, Kater L 1981 Tumor specific antibodies in sera from patients with squamous cell carcinoma of the uterine cervix: demonstration by a membrane immunofluorescence assay in cultured cervical carcinoma cells. Cancer Immunology and Immunotherapy 11: 201–206.

Van der Linde A W, Streefkerk M, Schurman H J, teVelde E R, Kater L 1983 Divergence between the occurrence of antibody and cellular immune reactivity to cervical carcinoma cell lines in preinvasive and microinvasive stages of cervical carcinoma. British Journal of Cancer 47: 147–153.

Van Niekerk C C, Boerman O C, Ramaekers F C S, Poels L G 1991 Marker profile of different phases in the transition of normal human ovarian epithelium to ovarian carcinomas. American Journal of Pathology 138: 455–463.

Van Niekerk C C, Ramaekers F C S, Hanselaar A G J M, Aldeweirelot J, Poels L G 1993 Changes in expression of differentiation markers between normal ovarian cells and derived markers. American Journal of Pathology 142: 157–177.

van Weissenbruch M M, Hoek A, van Vliet-Bleeker I, Schoemaker J, Drexage H A D 1991 Evidence for existence of immunoglobulins that block ovarian granulosa cell growth in vitro: a putative role in resistant ovary syndrome? Journal of Clinical Endocrinology and Metabolism 73: 360–367.

Vasquez A M, Kenny F M 1973 Ovarian failure and antiovarian autoantibodies in association with hypoparathyroidism, moniliasis and Addisons and Hashimoto's diseases. Obstetrics and Gynecology 41: 414–418.

Vasudevan D M, Balakrishnan K, Talwar G P 1971 Immunoglobulins in carcinomas of cervix. Indian Journal of Medical Research 59: 1653–1659.

Viac J, Guerin R I, Chardonnet Y, Bremond A 1990 Langerhans' cells and epithelial cell modifications in cervical intraepithelial neoplasia: correlation with human papilloma virus infection. Immunobiology 180: 328–338.

Vigano P, Vercellini P, Di Blasio A M, Colombo A, Candiani G B, Vignali M 1991 Deficient antiendometrium lymphocyte-mediated cytotoxicity in patients with endometriosis. Fertility and Sterility 56: 894–899.

Vigano P, Di Blasio A M, Busacca M, Sabbadini M G, Vignali M 1992 Danazol suppresses both spontaneous and activated human lymphocyte-mediated cytotoxicity. American Journal of Reproductive Immunology 28: 38–42.

Vijayakumar T, Ankathil R, Remani P, Sasidharan V K, Vijayan K K, Vasudevan D M 1986 Serum immunoglobulins in patients with carcinoma of the oral cavity, uterine cervix and breast. Cancer Immunology and Immunotherapy 22: 76–79.

Vos G H, Hammond M D, Vos D, Grobbelaar B G, Auslander M P, Marescotti G 1972 An evaluation of humoral antibody responses in patients with carcinoma of the cervix. Journal of Obstetrics and Gynaecology of the British Commonwealth 79: 1040–1046.

Wah R M, Anderson D J, Hill J A 1990 Asymptomatic cervicovaginal leukocytosis in infertile women. Fertility and Sterility 54: 445–450.

Waldman R H, Cruz J M, Rowe D S 1971 Immunoglobulin levels and antibody to Candida albicans in human cervicovaginal secretions. Clinical and Experimental Immunology 9: 427–434.

Waldman R H, Cruz J M, Rowe D S 1972 Intravaginal immunisation of humans with Candida albicans. Journal of Immunology 109: 662–664.

Wang Y F, Holstein A F 1983 Intraepithelial lymphocytes and macrophages in the human epididymis. Cell and Tissue Research 233: 517–521.

Watson J M, Sensintaffar J L, Berek J S, Martinez-Maza O 1990 Constitutive production of interleukin 6 by ovarian cancer cell lines and by primary ovarian tumor cultures. Cancer Research 50: 6959–6965.

Weed J C, Arquembourg P C 1980 Endometriosis: can it produce an autoimmune response resulting in infertility? Clinical Obstetrics and Gynecology 23: 885–895.

Weintraub I, Klisak I, Lagasse L D, Byfield J E 1973 Evidence for specific tumor cytotoxic antibodies in serum of cervical cancer patients. American Journal of Obstetrics and Gynecology 116: 986–992.

Weisz-Carrington P, Roux M E, McWilliams M, Phillips-Quaglata J M, Lamm M E 1978 Hormonal induction of the secretory immune system in the mammary gland. Proceedings of the National Academy of Sciences 75: 2928–2932.

Welch D B, Fabra A, Nakajima M 1990 Transforming growth factor β stimulates mammary adenocarcinoma cell invasion and metastatic potential. Proceedings of the National Academy of Sciences of the USA 87: 7678–7682.

Wild R A, Shivers C A 1985 Antiendometrial antibodies in patients with endometriosis. American Journal of Reproductive Immunology and Microbiology 8: 84–86.

Williamson H O, Phansey S A, Mathur S, Mathur R S, Baker E R, Fudenberg H H 1980 Myasthenia gravis, premature menopause and thyroid autoimmunity. American Journal of Obstetrics and Gynecology 137: 893–898.

Witkin S S, Toth A 1983 Relationship between genital tract infections, sperm antibodies in seminal fluid and infertility. Fertility and Sterility 40: 805–808.

Witkin S S, Bongiovanni A M, Armbruster T, Birnbaum S, Caputo T 1984 Analysis of sera from ovarian cancer patients for immune complexes. Journal of Clinical and Laboratory Immunology 14: 65–68.

Wolff H, Anderson D J 1988 Immunohistological characterization and quantification of leucocyte subpopulations in human semen. Fertility and Sterility 49: 497–504.

Wolff H, Politch J A, Martinez A, Haimovici F, Hill J A, Anderson D J 1990 Leukocytospermia is associated with poor semen quality. Fertility and Sterility 53: 528–536.

Wolff J P, De Oliveira C F 1975 Lymphocytes in patients with ovarian cancer. Obstetrics and Gynecology 45: 656–658.

Wong W F 1978 Sperm antibodies in the cervical mucus and sera and postcoital tests in infertile women. European Journal of Obstetrics, Gynecology and Reproductive Biology 8: 363–367.

Woodworth C D, Simpson S 1993 Comparative lymphokine secretion by cultured normal human cervical keratinocytes, papillomavirus-immortalized and carcinoma cell lines. American Journal of Pathology 142: 1544–1555.

Wu S, Rodabaugh K, Martinez-Mazu O et al 1992 Stimulation of ovarian tumor cell proliferation with monocyte products including interleukin-1, interleukin-6 and tumor necrosis factor-α. American Journal of Obstetrics and Gynecology 166: 997–1007.

Wu S, Boyer C M, Whitaker R S et al 1993 Tumor necrosis factor α as an autocrine and paracrine growth factor for ovarian cancer: monokine induction of tumor cell proliferation and tumor necrosis factor α expression. Cancer Research 53: 1939–1944.

Yaneva H 1974 Immunoglobulin secretion by normal human endometrium — an immunohistochemical study. Pathologie et Biologie 22: 607–610.

Yron I, Schickler M, Fisch B, Pinkas H, Ovadia J, Witz I P 1986 The immune system during the pre-cancer and the early cancer period: IL2 production by PBL from post-menopausal women with and without endometrial carcinoma. International Journal of Cancer 38: 331–338.

Yuan C C, Tsai L C, Hsu S C et al 1992 Production and characterization of a monoclonal antibody (Cx-99) against cervical carcinoma. British Journal of Cancer 65: 201–207.

Zbroja-Sontag W 1983 Cell mediated immunity in the blood of women with inflammatory and neoplastic lesions of the ovary. American Journal of Reproductive Immunology 4: 146–152.

Zbroja-Sontag W, Sikorski R, Kadel E 1982 Antibodies to ovarian antigens in different diseases of the ovary. American Journal of Reproductive Immunology 2: 58–63.

Zeller J M, Henig I, Radwanska E, Dmowski W P 1987 Enhancement of human monocyte and peritoneal macrophage chemiluminescence activities in women with endometriosis. American Journal of Reproductive Immunology and Microbiology 13: 78–82.

Zolti M, Meirom R, Shemesh M, Wollach D, Mashiach S, Shore L 1990 Granulosa cells as a source and target organ for tumor necrosis factor-α. FEBS Letters 261: 253–255.

42. Quantitative pathology of gynaecological tumours

J. P. A. Baak   G. J. Meijer   M. Brinkhuis   J. A. M. Beliën
J. Brugghe   M. Broeckaerts

INTRODUCTION

This chapter deals with quantitative pathological methods for assessing the diagnosis and prognosis of gynaecological cancer — the two essential steps in the selection of appropriate therapy. Although quantitative pathology as a tool in clinical oncology is fairly new, the application of quantitative microscopic techniques in cancer research is much older. As early as 1890, Hansemann hypothesized that all cancers are characterized by asymmetrical cell division which ultimately leads to cancer; this presupposed quantitative chromosomal changes in every cancer. The work of Caspersson and his colleagues in Stockholm in the 1930s marks the beginning of modern cytometry. In 1935, he showed a clear, high nucleic acid absorption band in a metaphase chromosome and a few years later it was shown that proteins and nucleic acids in epithelial tumours were different to those in normal cells (Caspersson & Santesson, 1942). With the advent of improved electronic equipment and digital computers in the 1950s and 1960s, rapid (static and flow) DNA cell analysis, cell sorting (Kamentsky et al, 1965; Atkin, 1971; Bohm & Sandritter, 1975) and quantitative chromatin pattern analysis could be applied on a much larger scale (Wied et al, 1968) than before the Second World War. Automation in cervical cytology was begun in 1954, but the use of completely automated cytological procedures for routine cervical screening has not yet been realized on a wide scale. Since the early 1960s several workers worldwide have measured cellular DNA content. It soon became clear that the total DNA content obtained did not usually discriminate benign, dysplastic and malignant lesions absolutely, although DNA histogram patterns could be categorized in different prognostically significant types. Wied and his colleagues started to develop quantitative descriptors of the morphological pattern. Programmes to reach this goal were expanded to a pattern recognition system, called TICAS (Wied et al, 1968, 1969).

The passage above refers to quantitative analysis of histo- and cytochemical components (*cytometry*) such as (total) DNA, RNA or chromatin pattern. The analysis of geometric non-chemical cell and tissue components (*morphometry and stereology*) has developed somewhat independently. For example, as early as 1925, such a morphometric analysis as counting of mitoses appeared to provide a strong prognostic factor in breast cancer (Greenhough, 1925), and already at that time measurement of the size of cancer cell nuclei was being performed. In 1925, Jacobj found that the volume of normal cells doubles before cell division. Some years later, Heiberg & Kemp (1929) substantiated the subjective impression that nuclei of cancer cells are larger than those of normal cells. Chalkley (1943) was the first to apply the stereological point-counting method to cancer tissues. In the late 1970s and early 1980s the application of morphometric and stereological analysis to pathologically changed tissues became increasingly popular and widely applied, particularly in cancer (Oberholzer, 1983; Baak, 1991). Morphometric and stereological techniques are fairly easy and inexpensive. DNA (flow) cytometry is more expensive, and both methods are useful. Today, many different techniques such as morphometry, stereology, image and flow cytometry are well established and routinely used in diagnostic quantitative pathology. Other techniques such as quantitative immunohistochemistry and cytochemistry, confocal laser scan microscopy, three-dimensional microscopy, neural nets, multimedia and artificial intelligence are still in their infancy (for an overview see Baak, 1991).

The causes of the sharp increase in interest in the application of quantitative pathology to cancer diagnosis and prognosis are:

a. The increased demand for quantitation and objectivity
b. The improvement in, and widespread availability of, adequate technology
c. The awareness that changes can be detected with quantitative analysis which would otherwise escape notice
d. The improved therapeutic possibilities for cancer patients

e. Most importantly, that the opinions of pathologists have not always proved consistent or reproducible. Quantitative pathological analyses are more reproducible and capable of preventing under- and overtreatment.

LACK OF REPRODUCIBILITY OF USUAL PATHOLOGY ASSESSMENTS

Pathologists usually agree with their own and with each other's diagnoses. However, there is a certain lack of diagnostic agreement between pathologists when classifying the same tumours. In 1979 the Multicentre Ovarian Tumour study was therefore undertaken to investigate consistency of grading criteria, inter- and intrapathologist reproducibility in grading and typing, and the value of prognostic assessments by four different pathologists. Histological sections from 198 ovarian tumours, predominantly of the common epithelial types, were randomly drawn from the archives of the different centres, histological typing was performed using the WHO recommendations, and the tumours were graded as benign, borderline or malignant (well, moderately or poorly differentiated). Intermediate grades were allowed. All slides were assessed twice by each pathologist (at about a 12-month interval) in a 'blind' fashion (without knowledge of stage, treatment or clinical outcome).

The results showed that pathologists use different criteria when grading ovarian tumours (Baak et al, 1986a) and that there is considerable intra- and interpathologist disagreement in typing and grading. Panel discussions are of little help with these differences (Baak et al, 1986b), which can cause differences in therapy. Moreover, there were considerable variations in the survival curves and in the five-year survival of patients of the same grade assessed by different pathologists (five-year survival 82–100% in borderline, 49–80% in well-differentiated, and 21–48% in moderately-differentiated tumours) (see Fig. 42.1). The intraobserver variation in assessments (also tested after a 6-month interval) was lower, but still present. It was concluded that histological grading has stronger prognostic value than typing. Unfortunately, there is considerable prognostic variability in grading (Baak et al, 1987a).

These are not isolated results; a large number of studies found serious discrepancies between pathologists in the diagnosis of gynaecological and other tumours (for an overview see Baak & Oort, 1983).

These data confirm the general impression that there is an obvious need for objective methods in certain areas of diagnostic pathology. Although grading is an improvement on the purely subjective approach, it still has a high degree of subjectivity. This explains why studies concerning grading between different pathologists in difficult areas of pathology give disagreement rates of up to 85%.

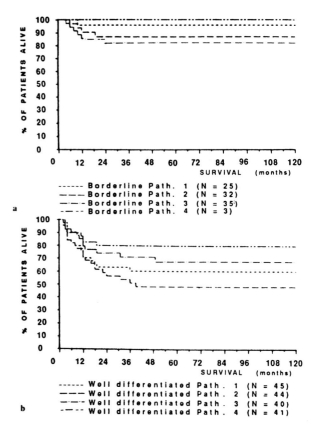

Fig. 42.1 Pathologist-dependent variability of survival of patients classified as suffering from **a** borderline and **b** well-differentiated ovarian tumours. (Reprinted with permission from Baak, 1991.)

Detailed analyses have shown that there are many potential sources of error in making a diagnosis and these are mainly related to lesions that form a continuous spectrum of change, from benign to malignant, where arbitrary criteria are needed to distinguish the different appearances (Fig. 42.2). Studies on the diagnosis of such lesions have identified a number of types of diagnostic shift, or error. Random shifts may be caused by poor perception; other factors may cause systematic shifts. Random shifts are due to a variety of reasons: day of the week, time, previous experience, fatigue.

In general, the diagnostic process is complex and only partially understood. A logical line cannot always be detected. In the ideal situation, several stages can be discerned (Fig. 42.3). The illustration portrays an idealized situation. In reality such emotionless analytical diagnosis rarely occurs for, in practice, many pathologists look down the microscope and immediately make a diagnosis. Subsequently, features are mentioned which they think led to the diagnosis. This is synthetic or inductive diagnosis making (template recognition), an important part of which is probably subconscious; most pathologists are aware of this. When a beginner asks a senior pathologist to explain a certain diagnosis, it may be difficult to give a clear answer. Clinical information may be useful and some-

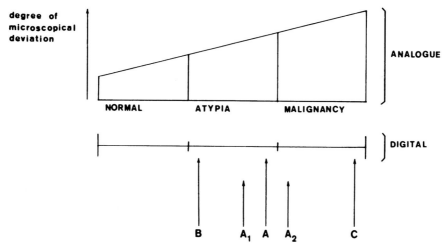

Fig. 42.2 The spectrum of deviations and examples of (mis)classification. (Reprinted with permission from Baak & Oort, 1983.)

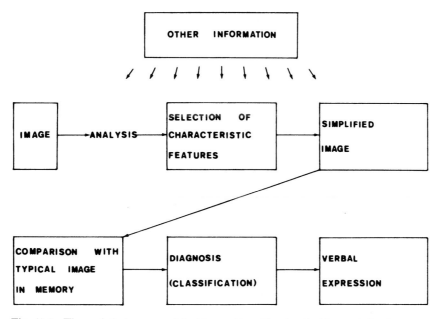

Fig. 42.3 The analytical process of decision-making. (Reprinted with permission from Baak & Oort, 1983.)

times essential to come to a certain diagnosis, but it may also obscure the pathologist's view. Psychological factors may also play a rôle. Such factors may result in a classification shift in continuous lesions, and hence to a diagnosis which is not strictly correct.

Another source of error in image analysis is optical illusion (Fig. 42.4).

A third type of error is related to the meaning of verbal expressions, and has only fairly recently been recognized in the literature. In histo- or cytopathological descriptions, the following words are often used — probable, likely, often, many, most, some — all expressing a certain numerical probability. However, different people assign a different value to the same words (Bryant & Norman, 1980; Toogood, 1980). For example, 'probably malignant' for one pathologist means: 'there is invasive growth or a metastasis somewhere, although I don't see it in the present section'. For another these words mean 'it is an atypical lesion, with some, but not all, the morphological features of malignancy'. The clinician interprets these statements and a variety of therapeutic measures may result. The factors which cause these errors can be largely overcome by quantitative analysis.

TECHNIQUES IN QUANTITATIVE PATHOLOGY

For the purpose of this chapter it is useful to distinguish the following techniques.

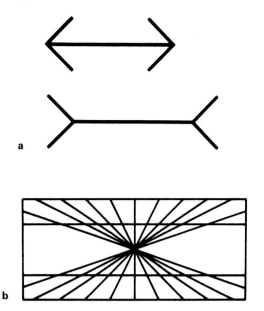

Fig. 42.4 Optical illusions: **a** the horizontal lines have the same length; **b** the horizontal lines in the centre are parallel.

Morphometry

This is generally used to denote measurement of geometric cell and tissue features. Measurements, though useful, are not always enough — calculations are necessary to obtain quantitative information about volume, surface, length and numerical density in the three-dimensional organ. For a given shape of the structures, the original three-dimensional diameter distribution of the structures in the organ can be calculated by stereological analysis of the two-dimensional distribution of profiles in the section.

Stereology

This is the body of mathematical methods that relate three-dimensional structural parameters to two-dimensional measurements obtainable from sections of the structure; 'morphometry' and 'stereology' are thus not synonymous (Weibel, 1979). Stereological methods have proved useful in diagnostic quantitative pathology. For in-depth accounts of stereological principles see Weibel (1979), Aherne & Dunnill (1982), Oberholzer (1983) and Baak (1991). A short summary of stereological techniques will follow here.

In a representative section of isotropic uniform random tissue, the volume percentage (volume per volume, or volume density V_v) of a structure, or structures, is equal to the area percentage (or area density) A_a. Density is here defined as 'quantity per unit volume, unit area or unit length' (Weibel, 1979). Thus, the terms volume density, surface density, length density and numerical density are often used in stereological papers.

The principle of volume density estimation by area density measurement was first published by Delesse (1847).

The area percentage can be assessed by paper weighing (tracing, cutting and weighing the structures or particles of interest, assuming paper of constant thickness). However, this method is time consuming, and the proportion points (P_p) of a point grid laid on the microscopic image can be an equally or even more precise estimation of the area percentage and thus of the volume percentage (Glagoleff, 1988). This method was first used in histopathology by Chalkley (1943):

$$V_v = A_a = P_p$$

Calculation of surfaces of structures in an organ (e.g. inner and outer surface of endometrial glands, or surface of the capillary wall in a tumour) can be expressed as surface per volume (S_v), or surface density (mm²/mm³):

$$S_v = 2\ I_L\ (mm^2/mm^3)$$

and by counting the number of transections Q in an area A, the length per volume (length density) can be calculated. Figures 42.5 and 42.6 illustrate these phenomena.

$$L_v = 2\ Q_A\ (mm/mm^3)$$

There are many more stereological formulas available, such as those used to calculate the mean curvature, shape factors and volume-weighted mean volume (Gundersen & Jensen, 1985; Sørensen et al, 1992). Recently, a very fast low resolution method, called syntactic structure analysis (SSA), has proved to be useful for assessing the prognosis of patients with stage 1c and 2 ovarian cancer (van Eerden et al, 1992). The principle is shown in Figure 42.7. One assessment takes only a few minutes per case, and SSA features probably are associated with differentiation and cell size (Kayser et al, 1987, 1990; van Diest et al, 1992).

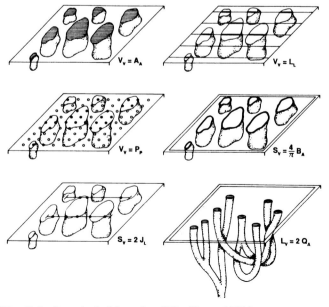

Fig. 42.5 Stereological formulas. (After Bouw, 1975.)

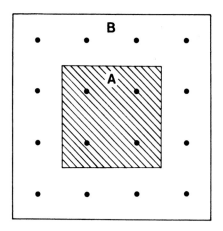

Fig. 42.6 The point-counting method. (Reprinted from Baak, 1991.)

Cytometry

This is the measurement of cytochemical, histochemical or molecular cell or tissue features. There are two types of cytometry: image (static) and flow. These will be dealt with in a later section of this chapter.

EQUIPMENT FOR QUANTITATIVE CELL AND TISSUE ANALYSIS

Despite wide recognition of the need for quantitative assessment of microscopical images, many pathologists have been put off these techniques because of the tedium involved in the acquisition of quantitative data. However, since the end of the 1970s, equipment for quantitative image analysis has appeared on the market which has not only enormously improved in performance, but also fallen in price.

Initially, instruments were mainly hardware designs, but they have become increasingly software-based. Prices vary considerably from US \$25 to \$350 000 and higher, depending on the complexity of possible analyses. It is possible to start with the basic elements and then slowly expand the system as needed.

The commercially available equipment for quantitation can be categorized as follows:

1. Point-counting
2. Digitizing graphic tablet systems
3. Mechanical scanners
4. Electron image sensors
5. Flow cytometers.

Table 42.1 summarizes their advantages and disadvantages.

The most important factor in the purchase of such a system is user-friendliness. Calibration should be easy. The user frequently wishes to perform a standard set of traces on a structure which is repeated throughout a tissue. A study of cells may entail tracing around different compartments (or phases) of the same cell (nucleolus, nucleus, cytoplasmic border), a digitizing interactive system should offer the possibility to perform nested operations (multiphase measurements) and store related results together. Four factors have fuelled the development of low cost digital image analysis by small microcomputers:

1. Wide availability of high power, relatively inexpensive desk-top computers with megabytes of memory (e.g. IBM PC or compatibles)

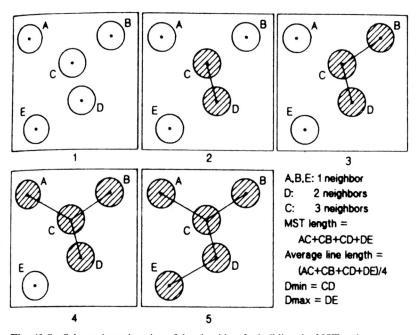

Fig. 42.7 Schematic explanation of the algorithm for building the MST and calculation of the spanning tree features. (Reprinted from van Diest et al, 1992.)

Table 42.1 Equipment for quantitative microscopy

Instruments	Method	Advantages	Disadvantages	Application
I. Non-automatic Projection microscope; eyepiece graticules	Stereology	Inexpensive	Slow	Mainly histology
II. Semi-automatic Interactive digitizing system	Morphometry; planimetry; stereology	Measurements of individual particles	Slow	Histology and cytology
Mechanical scanning	Scanning photometry	Accurate	Slow; tedious; expensive; artifacts	Histology and cytology
III. Automatic Electron image sensor scanners	Image cytometry	Fast; architecture kept; visual inspection	Artifacts; often insufficient image	Histology and cytology
Flow cytometer for analysis and sorting	Flow cytometry	Fast; sorting	Architecture lost; no visual inspection without sorting	Particles suspended in solution

2. Development of integrated circuits to perform high quality digital conversion of video signals at full frame rate
3. A fall in price and an improvement in the quality of stable, blemish-free, linear response solid state, charged-coupled device (CCD) cameras
4. Availability of inexpensive off-the-shelf add-on digital image processing PC boards and fairly powerful image processing software packages which run on PCs.

Between 1986 and 1988 there was an explosion in the number of systems based on microcomputers. In reality, digital image analysis may not always be the best way to start a quantitative pathology service, ease of use is frequently illusory, and the complexity of most histological images is not matched by sophistication of computer analysis (Marchevsky et al, 1987). For microscopic images contrast enhancement is a useful facility, but most important is the ability to perform full resolution shading correction to compensate for uneven illumination across the field. After detection of objects is achieved (usually after applying a binary threshold), image editing is essential to separate objects, remove artifacts and tidy up an image prior to measurement. An important error may be caused by interactive (non-automatic) segmentation. The threshold (black-level) is set by the user for optimal balance between the original and the binary image (to paraphrase recent sales literature). Interactive thresholding can introduce serious measurement bias and poor precision.

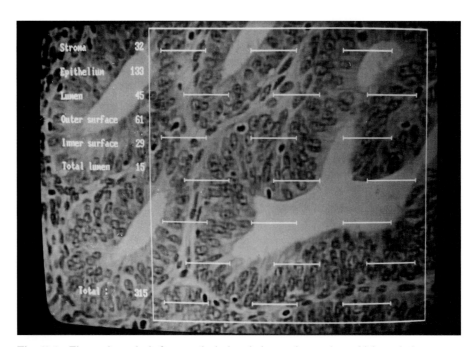

Fig. 42.8 Electronic graticule for stereological analysis superimposed on a high resolution, flicker-free monitor image of a software-based video overlay interactive morphometry/stereology system.

At present, most routine histological and cytological images are unsuitable for anything approaching fully automatic image analysis of morphometric features (such as area) and densitometric features (such as DNA); analysis by digital image processing systems requires considerable image editing before evaluation. For morphometric cell and tissue features, results identical in precision and accuracy may be obtained by an inexpensive interactive stereological method or digitizing graphic tablet video overlay system.

Currently, inexpensive video-overlay/frame grabber boards with software packages are available from US $5000 upwards that can run on a 286, 386 or 486 PC to perform point-counting, morphometric, stereological and DNA cytometric analyses. Such systems also can store and display multiple images per patient. The speed of some commercially available DNA image cytometers has increased tremendously and is as high as 1000 cells in three minutes, with a low coefficient of variation (comparable to flow cytometers) (see Figs 42.8–42.10).

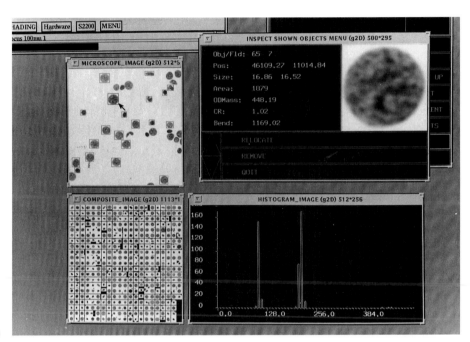

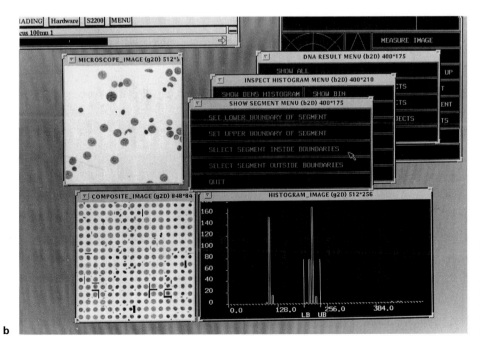

Fig. 42.9 Example of a very fast fully automated DNA image cytometer. Both the histogram and a composite image of all objects measured are displayed. Each image of each object can be magnified on the screen **a** and automatically relocated on the microscope to the nearest micrometre **b**.

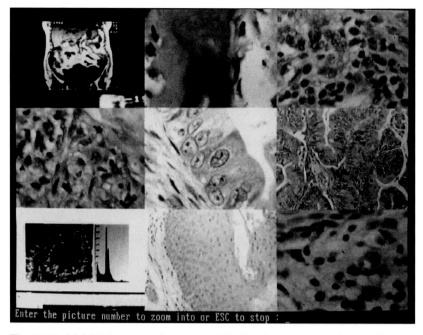

Fig. 42.10 Multiple images can be stored and displayed (top), one can browse through pages in an 'album', select one image and zoom in to display at full monitor size (bottom).

Table 42.2 (Additional) value and approximate price of different quantitative methods in diagnostic pathology

Method[1]	Value	Equipment/yr (kUS$)	Workforce[2]
MOR, STER	Strong	5	10
FCM	Varies	18 (9–45)	20
ICM, DIP	Varies	12 (8–30)	20
CLSM	Strong	50	50
AI	Varies	10 (1–30)	5
MMDB	Strong	6	10

[1] MOR = morphometry; STER = stereology; FCM = flow cytometry; ICM = image cytometry; DIP = digital image processing; CLSM = confocal laser scan microscopy; AI = artificial intelligence; MMDB = multimedia databases.
[2] Per 100 determinations. Including preparation, etc. Approximate prices.

Table 42.2 gives a summary of the price: performance ratio of the different methods. Clearly, a video overlay system, eventually with image processing possibilities for (DNA) cytometry, is by far the best buy.

RELIABILITY OF QUANTITATIVE PATHOLOGICAL ASSESSMENTS, STANDARDS, AND QUALITY CONTROL

Arguments for quantitative techniques are the reliability of assessments, i.e. their objectivity and reproducibility. However, quantitative assessments are subject to measurement errors which should and can be controlled as much as possible. Therefore, precautions should be taken to guarantee their reliability.

Terminology

Reproducibility denotes the degree of concordance in measurement results obtained from repeated assessments of a certain object or of samples from one population.

Precision expresses how closely the measurement results lie around the sample mean x.

Bias describes the degree of systematic over- or underestimation of the true value T by x.

The coefficient of variation (CV) expresses the absolute dispersion of a data distribution as a percentage of the mean statistic (mean).

Measurement error usually refers to precision.

The standard error (SE) is the standard deviation (SD) of a sampling distribution of a certain statistic obtained from different samples from one population. The SE of the mean (SEM) can be estimated as SD/Vn by a single sample. The more elements the sample contains, the smaller SEM becomes. Provided that the measurements are unbiased, the number of observations is large, and the feature is approximately normally distributed, a *confidence interval* of the sample mean M × ± 1.96 SEM indicates that the true mean lies within this interval with a probability of 95%. The borders of such an interval are called the *confidence limits*. The *coefficient of error* (CE) expresses SE as a percentage of the mean statistic (mean) as CE = (SE/mean) × 100%. It can be used to express the measurement precision.

Influencing factors

The following factors can influence quantitative assessments.

Preoperative factors

There is no way to control these and theoretically they form the practical limits. In view of the prognostic strength of quantitative assessments it is unlikely that these factors are an important source of error.

Specimen sampling

This should be standardized. We use the following standard rule for sampling from solid tumours (see Kempson, 1976): if possible, take at least ten sections from any tumour. For a very large specimen, take one section per cm diameter or per 100 g of tumour tissue, whichever is larger. For borderline tumours or well-differentiated carcinomas, careful searching for microinvasive and epithelium-rich areas is essential.

Variations in tissue and cell processing

These are also important. We have investigated the influence of fixatives (formaldehyde, Bouin's fluids, etc.) on the nuclear area and shape factors (Baak et al, 1989) and also on percentages of epithelium, stroma and lumen in endometrial tissue. The influence of delay in fixation, air-drying, acidity of 10% formalin (4% formaldehyde), Bouin and mercury-formalin fixatives, acetone and ethanol dehydration and under- and overstretching of the paraffin sections has been studied. Acidity had the strongest influence on the nuclear area: for pH < 3, the nuclear area is approximately 25% lower compared with a pH of 5–9. No significant differences in the nuclear area were detected in the range of pH 5 to pH 9. Once this factor was taken into account, the other factors studied had no influence. The pH also has a strong influence on the quality of DNA flow cytometry histograms. Figure 42.11 shows DNA flow histograms of the same tumour in different fixatives (Fleege et al, 1991). For quantitative pathology, therefore, at least one representative slice of each tumour must be fixed in buffered 4% formaldehyde with a controlled pH of 5–9. Beyer-Boon et al (1979) investigated the influence of routine fixation and staining procedures on quantitative *cytopathological* data. Air-drying gave increases of 58% and 33% in the nuclear and cellular areas, and a 9% increase in the nucleo-cytoplasmic ratio; other techniques resulted in a decrease in nuclear and cellular area and the nucleo-cytoplasmic ratio. Staining and mounting of cells appeared to have little effect, so the changes were mainly fixation-induced. Air-drying and the percent-

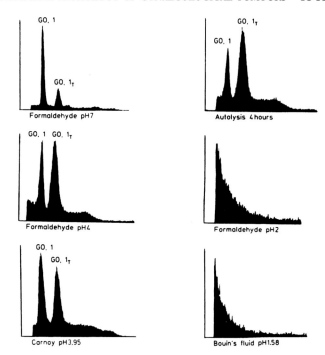

Fig. 42.11 DNA flow histograms of the same tumour with different fixatives. (Reprinted from Fleege et al, 1991.)

age of alcohol in the fixative are therefore important influencing factors.

Definition

At the microscopic level two crucial aspects are *definition* and ease of *segmentation* of particles and compartments. For example, immunostained antigens may lead to a very vague demarcation, as the intensity of the stain within one nucleus can range from very dark to very faint brown; different observers may use different thresholds of positivity when analysing such a slide (Baak et al, 1987b).

The experience of the operator

This is another potential source of inter- and intra-observer variation. Gamel et al (1985) studied the reproducibility of nucleolar measurements in ocular melanoma and demonstrated that measurements of an experienced operator were the more precise and less biased.

Measuring system parameters

For nuclear morphometrical analysis by means of an interactive digitizing system, there is a decrease of CV with increasing 'projected' diameter of the object measured at the digitizing tablet level that can be explained by the lower influence of manual tremor. From a minimal particle diameter of 15 mm onwards, the CV remains fairly stable below 1.0%. For measurements of cancer nuclei (average diameter range 6–12 micrometres) a total magnification at the digitizing tablet level of 2000× is usually sufficient. With an Intel 286 processor based digitizing system, maximum tracing speed should be 20 mm/s; higher speeds result in increased CVs. However, the influence of tracing speed may vary depending on the processor used in the computer. A video overlay system is preferable to a drawing tube system due to the visual control on the monitor of the match between the tracing and the object. Moreover a cursor (mouse) gives better results than a drawing pen (Fleege et al, 1988). DNA flow cytometric analyses of the same samples by different operators and on different machines can give enormous variations in the CVs of diploid peaks and especially also in the estimated percentage of S-phase cells.

Recently we found that quantitative immunochemistry by the CAS200 system by different observers is quite variable (Makkink-Nombrado & Baak, 1993 unpublished results).

Selection and sample size

The reliability of measurements also depends on the selection method and sample size. Selection is the cornerstone of diagnostic pathology. Likewise, in morphometry, careful choice of a particular *measurement field* or cells with certain qualitative attributes is often of the utmost importance. One has to cope with different biological phenomena within the selected measurement field. These are *object variation, object clustering* and *object gradients* (Fleege et al, 1991). The higher the degree of object variation, the more objects have to be measured to achieve a certain level of measurement precision. The more pronounced the object clustering, or presence of gradients, the more care should be taken that the selection method covers the measurement field uniformly. Regularly distributed points in the measurement field determine where to measure and which objects to select. Within one field the objects to be measured are selected systematically. Some commercially available morphometry systems provide the possibility for point-sampled selection, thus minimizing bias and improving reproducibility. Heterogeneity also plays an important rôle in flow cytometric analysis of DNA ploidy. Thus, adequate samples are required; sometimes it may be necessary to eliminate clearly diploid (benign) parts of a specimen. By doing this, aneuploid cell clones can be detected in 'diploid' tumours (Oud et al, 1987). Image cytometers have the advantage over flow cytometers that the cells and tissues studied can be visually inspected during or after the measurement, thus allowing the analysis and correction of irrelevant (benign) cells. In particular, when the aneuploid cells have a low frequency in relation to the normal diploid cells, the detection of eventual aneuploidy becomes unreliable with flow cytometry.

A measurement protocol

This should clearly describe where, what, how, and how much to measure. For example, different measurement protocols of mitosis counts can lead to results with completely different significance. The *criteria to classify an object as a mitosis* can be found in Fleege et al (1991).

Interpretation of results

Histogram interpretation of DNA flow and image cytometry and cell-cycle analysis data can also show variations (van Thiel et al, 1989; Bergers et al, 1995). Moreover, false-negative diploid histograms may be obtained when the aneuploid cells are overshadowed by large numbers of diploid tumour or non-malignant cells; therefore the smallest percentage of aneuploid cells detectable by flow cytometry is about 1–10%.

APPLICATIONS

The above makes clear that diagnostic quantitative gynaecological pathology is easy, inexpensive and useful. Secondly, it also makes clear that a diagnostic quantitative application is not a black box — it requires constant quality control and quality assurance. Thirdly, the number of applications is rapidly increasing, and the following can merely be an introduction to the expanding literature on the topic. Due to the amount of space available, the focus will be on (pre)malignancies. However, the reader should realize that studies of non-malignant physiological conditions are equally promising and useful. Furthermore, the cancer-related topics to be discussed are not exhaustive. For a detailed treatise, reference is made to an earlier publication (Baak, 1991).

Vulva

The prognosis of a *preinvasive vulvar lesion* is a matter of debate as cytological atypia does not reflect the same invasive potential as in cervical specimens. Studies on cellular size of *exfoliated cells* from normal, reactive and neoplastic vulvar skin were performed by Nauth et al (Nauth & Boon, 1983; Nauth et al, 1987). Cytoplasmic pleomorphism was associated with increasing malignancy, but there was a wide overlap between different conditions, and no clear distinction could be made. Furthermore, malignant cells are not always present in cytological specimens from cancers: Nauth & Boger (1982) detected malignant cells in only 51% of vulvar cancers.

Dalrymple et al (1989) investigated nuclear : cytoplasmic (N/C) ratios in *normal and perineoplastic vulvar* skin by point-counting, compared the findings with DNA content (static cytometry) and analysed them for changes occurring with age. There was no significant correlation between N/C ratio and age in 19 patients undergoing radical vulvectomy for squamous cell carcinoma, nor in 29 controls. However, controls showed N/C ratios lower than in the skin around the carcinomas. Distributions were significantly different; all controls showed diploid DNA patterns, but 15 of the carcinoma-associated cases (79%) were aneuploid. Stereological assessment of N/C ratio is easy, can be done on standard tissue sections and is a fast procedure — much faster than DNA cytometry. Thus, an N/C ratio > 0.27 should be regarded as a sign of malignancy (Table 42.3).

Depth of invasion is a known prognostic factor in *vulvar carcinoma*, despite the difficulty that, while the deepest point of invasion can be accurately located, the upper reference point is arbitrary. In 124 vulvar carcinoma cases, Kurzl et al (1988) compared three methods, all using the deepest point but with three upper reference points: the basement membrane of the most superficial dermal papilla, the tumour surface and the basement membrane of the deepest rete ridge. Measurement from the deepest point of invasion to the surface with a cut-point of 0.5 cm showed the best prognostic power. Prognosis of invasive vulvar cancer was further studied in 131 cases by Kearn et al (1992) by DNA flow cytometry measurements. Samples were prepared from paraffin-

Table 42.3 Nuclear:cytoplasmic (N/C) ratios and percentage of aneuploid cases in normal and perineoplastic vulvar skin (after Dalrymple et al, 1989)

	N/C ratio	% aneuploid
Normal	0.21–0.30	0
Perineoplastic	0.28–0.46	79

embedded tissue. Of these, 66 were found to be diploid, 52 aneuploid and 13 could not be evaluated. The five-year crude survival rate was 62% for the diploid and 23% for the aneuploid tumours (p < 0.001). The aneuploid tumours without lymph node metastases showed a five-year cancer-related survival rate of 44% as compared to 58% for the diploid tumours with nodal metastases. In a multivariate Cox regression analysis the most important independent prognostic parameters were (1) lymph node involvement (p < 0.0001), (2) tumour ploidy (p = 0.0001) and (3) tumour size (p = 0.0039).

Cervix

In the cervix, quantitative cell and tissue analysis is especially useful in *adenocarcinomas*; their incidence has increased from 5% in the 1950s to 15–20% in the 1980s, perhaps because adenocarcinoma in situ (AIS) has been underdiagnosed (Boon et al, 1981).

Although distinction between benign, atypical and adenocarcinomatous glands is usually easy, problems may arise in certain cases. Figure 42.12 shows that the mean shortest and longest axes of 50 randomly selected representative intact nuclei distinguish benign glands, histologically 'normal' glands (in the absence of inflammatory changes) adjacent to invasive adenocarcinoma, AIS and adenocarcinoma. The 'normal' glands adjacent to carcinoma have longer nuclear axes than truly benign glands. Measurements were performed in longitudinally sectioned glands in H&E-stained paraffin sections from 4% buffered formaldehyde-fixed tissue. One should measure in endocervical glands of biopsies, cones or hysterectomy specimens only; in cervical polyps, the isthmus or endometrium the rules may be different.

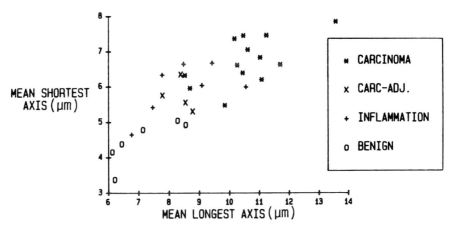

Fig. 42.12 Mean longest and shortest nuclear axes can help to distinguish endocervical glands in different conditions. (Reprinted from Baak, 1991.)

As to the prediction of outcome, subclassifications based on growth patterns and qualitative cellular features remain controversial. Fu et al (1987) studied nuclear DNA ploidy levels, standard deviations of nuclear area and percentage amounts of lumen and neoplastic tissue. Useful thresholds in discriminating recurrent disease, identified by logistic regression analysis, included a DNA ploidy level 3.0 c, percentage of lumen 34.6 and nuclear area mean and standard deviation 53.1 and 20.1 μm^2 (Table 42.4).

These parameters should provide useful guidelines in visual assessment of histological features with prognostic significance.

According to Richart (1987), *squamous carcinomas of the uterine cervix* are preceded by intraepithelial neoplasia (CIN). CIN is divided into three grades: CIN 1, CIN 2 and CIN 3. Lower grades often disappear spontaneously while higher grades carry a serious risk of becoming invasive. However, although a certain correlation exists between the degree of severity and progression to a higher grade or invasive carcinoma, conventional histopathology cannot predict the regressive or progressive nature of these lesions.

Using static and flow cytometric methods, DNA ploidy measurements of CIN and invasive carcinoma have been used to predict the clinical course more accurately. A large number of persistent and recurrent CIN lesions have an aneuploid DNA pattern, as do invasive carcinomas (Fu et al, 1981; Goppinger et al, 1986), but diploid DNA patterns of CIN and squamous cell carcinomas are often reported, especially in young women. This may be due to technical problems which can be overcome, at least partially (Oud et al, 1987), but it indicates that flow cytometrically assessed diploid DNA pattern is not always indicative of a good prognosis (Hanselaar et al, 1988). Other markers are needed for more accurate prediction of the clinical course in an individual patient. Developments in viral oncology have suggested that oncogenic human papillomaviruses (HPV) are implicated in the development of squamous and adenocarcinoma of the uterine cervix. HPV 16 and 18 have been detected in about 50% of cervical adenocarcinomas and their metastases (Walboomers et al, 1987). Morphometric features and DNA ploidy patterns of lesions associated with HPV have also been studied. In general, HPV 6 and 11 show a high correlation with polyploidization, presence of normal mitotic figures and a clinically benign course. In contrast, HPV 16 and 18 lesions are frequently aneuploid with abnormal mitotic figures. In fact, abnormal mitoses are a consistent marker of DNA aneuploidy (Crum et al, 1984). Fu et al (1988a) studied the correlation between HPV subtypes in 28 CIN lesions. Total mitotic index in HPV 6, 11 lesions, ranged from 0 to 6 (mean 2.5); abnormal mitoses were found in only one specimen. In HPV 16 and 18, 33 lesions, total mitotic index varied from 6 to 51 (mean 17.9) and abnormal mitotic figures were found in all specimens. Total mitotic index was the best individual discriminator. Fu et al (1989) also found that none of the regressive cases had a mitotic activity index above 7, and all persistent or progressive cases had a mitotic activity index of 7 or higher. Thus, simple quantitative analysis of H&E-stained sections can provide clues as to HPV type and malignant potential of cervical lesions.

In *invasive squamous cervical cancer*, a number of different factors are associated with prognosis. In a large recent study, stage, node status and grade maintained significance in multivariate analysis (Hopkins & Morley, 1991). Stendahl et al (1979) presented a system for reporting the malignancy grade score (MGS) based on the semi-quantitative evaluation of four parameters related to the tumour cell population and four variables associated with the tumour-host relationship. The authors reported a highly significant prognostic value of the malignancy grade score (Stendahl et al, 1979). Unfortunately, malignancy grading based on subjective interpretation of qualitative, and perhaps vaguely defined, criteria suffers from poor reproducibility. Nuclear DNA content by flow cytometry has shown excellent prognostic value (Jakobsen et al, 1985, 1988) Ji et al (1991) found that, despite an intimate association of HPV 16 and 18 in cervical carcinogenesis, the presence of their DNA in cancer biopsies does not seem to have any prognostic value. Willén et al (1987) found no correlation between FIGO stage and percentage of S-phase cells.

Morphometry has also been used in the prognostication of invasive cervical cancer (Atkin, 1964; Nødskov-Pedersen, 1971) and as a possible guide to the choice of treatment (Révész & Siracka, 1984). A combination of morphology and nuclear morphometry can identify high risk patients (van Nagell et al, 1988). Recently, it was found that unbiased estimates of the three-dimensional, volume-weighted mean nuclear volume (nuclear v_v) in pretreatment biopsies from 51 patients treated for cervical cancer in stages I–III were on average increased in euploid lesions (0.01), but the overall relationship between nuclear v_v and DI was poor (Sørensen et al, 1992). Single-factor analysis showed prognostic impact of clinical stage of disease ($2P = 0.0001$) and DI ($2P = 0.04$), whereas estimates of nuclear v_v were only of marginal prognostic significance ($2P = 0.07$). Cox multivariate regression

Table 42.4 Prognostic value of quantitative pathological features in stage I invasive cervical adenocarcinoma (after Fu et al, 1987)

Feature		8-year survival	P-value*
DNA ploidy	<3.0 c	74.4	0.0001
	>3.0 c	9.0	
% of lumen	>34.6	77.9	0.0006
	<34.6	24.4	
Mean nuclear	<53.1	74.5	0.0018
area (μm^2)	>53.1	19.7	

* Mantel-Cox statistic

analysis showed independent prognostic value of patient age and nuclear v_v along with clinical stage and DI. Although the number of cases was restricted and different stages were used, they concluded that estimates of mean nuclear volume are of prognostic value for objective malignancy grading in patients with squamous cell carcinoma of the uterine cervix (Sørensen et al, 1992). An advantage of nuclear volume estimates is the relative simplicity of the assessment.

The value of DNA cytometry and morphometric analysis in squamous cervical cancer is therefore promising and remains to be confirmed in larger studies.

Endometrium

Quantitative pathological analysis of endometrial samples can be used to distinguish between atypical hyperplasia and carcinoma to predict the progression risk of atypical hyperplasia and to grade cancers and predict their outcome.

Distinction and grading of atypical hyperplasias and carcinomas

According to Skaarland (1985a,b), discrimination between hyperplasia and carcinoma in cytological specimens is disappointing, but Fu et al (1988b) could correctly classify 88% of the specimens by a multivariate combination of morphometric (especially mean cell area) and densitometric parameters assessed by digital image techniques. Not only nuclear features in histological sections allow adequate classification, for it is possible to improve the accuracy by measurement and calculation of such architectural features as the volume percentage epithelium (VPE) and the inner (luminal) surface of the glands. DNA cytometry is of little value as aneuploidy occurs in both atypical hyperplasias and carcinomas, and in atypical hyperplasias flow cytometry-assessed aneuploidy is not a prognostic factor (Baak et al, 1994).

Other stereological gland parameters and, to a lesser degree, morphometric nuclear shape factors are also useful for distinction between mild and severe hyperplasias

Table 42.5 Descriptive statistics of morphometric features of mild and severe atypical hyperplasia

Feature	Hyperplasia		
	Mild	Severe	P (Wilcoxon two-sided)
VPE	22.3 ± 5.52	39.9 ± 8.64	0.00001
Outer surface density glands	10.5 ± 3.04	18.2 ± 5.23	0.00004
Volume % glands	33.7 ± 6.62	52.9 ± 12.27	0.00009
Length density lumina	32.3 ± 15.56	58.3 ± 23.38	0.0004
Inner surface density glands	6.6 ± 2.75	10.2 ± 3.46	0.004
Mean diameter lumen	72.1 ± 29.75	52.4 ± 14.4	0.03
Mean nuclear shape factor	0.69 ± 0.068	0.74 ± 0.054	0.04

and, in carcinomas, for more refined grading (Table 42.5 and 42.6).

Progression risk of endometrial atypical hyperplasia

Endometrial atypical hyperplasia is usually considered precancerous, but only 10–20% of cases develop into endometrial carcinoma (Gusberg & Kaplan, 1963; Kurman et al, 1985). Until recently, there were no adequate criteria to predict risk in an individual case and therefore hysterectomy is usually carried out for hyperplasia. This procedure is obviously thought to be the safer option, as there is often disagreement between pathologists on the differential diagnosis of atypical hyperplasia and well-differentiated carcinoma. Apparently, classification of hyperplasias is a historical problem and the difficulty in predicting the outcome probably contributes significantly to the frightening number of hysterectomies performed in the USA (500 000 per year at a cost of over $2 billion — Wall Street Journal, May 1993). Though the number of operations has declined by about 100 000 since the late seventies, the operation is still considered to be overused.

We have seen above how morphometric analysis can objectively support the distinction. Colgan et al (1983) described a morphometric classification rule to predict the risk of progression to cancer in atypical hyperplasia. Mean

Table 42.6 Descriptive statistics of morphometric features of well- and moderately to poorly differentiated carcinomas

Feature	Differentiation		
	Well	Moderate/poor	P (Wilcoxon two-sided)
Mean diameter glands	178.4 ± 71.50	316.8 ± 113.8	0.00029
Mean thickness epithelium	72.4 ± 35.80	134.8 ± 53.04	0.00033
Inner surface density glands	18.0 ± 5.52	10.7 ± 5.42	0.00031
Outer surface density glands	21.3 ± 7.84	12.4 ± 4.91	0.00039
VPE	67.0 ± 8.31	76.7 ± 5.53	0.00124
Volume % lumen	17.0 ± 8.57	9.2 ± 3.02	0.00196
Mean curvature glands	13.4 ± 5.40	24.5 ± 16.60	0.007
Mean nuclear axes ratio	1.77 ± 0.183	1.61 ± 0.171	0.01
Mean nuclear shape factor	0.728 ± 0.067	0.781 ± 0.072	0.03

and SD of the longest axis of the glandular nuclei were especially useful. Larger and more pleomorphic nuclei are correlated with a higher risk of progression and the following classification rule was used:

$$F = -7.13 + 1.24 \times \text{(mean maximal nuclear diameter)} - 3.00 \times \text{(SD/maximal nuclear diameter)}$$

where $F < 0$ means no progression; $F > 0$ means progression.

In their 24 cases, one of the 16 patients with no progression had $F > 0$ and three of the eight cases with progression to cancer had $F < 0$, i.e. 83% predicted correctly. To confirm this, morphometric analysis was applied to 42 cases of atypical hyperplasia with known outcome. The results were comparable with those described by Colgan's group (although the percentage correct was much lower — 32%) and also suggest that nuclear morphometry may help to avoid hysterectomy in approximately one-third of all cases of atypical hyperplasia (Ausems et al, 1985). Confirmation was especially important since it showed that the predictive value overcame the potentially blurring influence of variations in tissue processing and measuring procedure. A disadvantage was that many non-(pre)malignant conditions such as secretory endometrium had $F > 0$, with risk of serious overtreatment if Colgan's rule consisting of nuclear morphometric features only was 'blindly' applied. Therefore, we evaluated the usefulness of combining tissue architectural and nuclear features (Baak et al, 1988a) (Fig. 42.13).

The discrimination can be further improved by using a multivariate score:

$$D = +0.6229 + 0.0439 \times \text{(volume percentage stroma)} - 3.9934 \times \text{Ln (SD of short nuclear axis)} - 0.1592 \times \text{(outer surface density glands)}$$

Figure 42.14 shows discrimination by the D-score between atypical hyperplasias with and without progression to cancer, and Figure 42.15 shows an example of one case with complex atypical hyperplasia.

With these combined features hysterectomy may be avoided in up to two-thirds of cases of endometrial atypical hyperplasia. We found DNA flow cytometry to be of no value in predicting the outcome of atypical hyperplasia as the progression risk in diploid and aneuploid cases was the same (Baak et al, 1994).

Prognosis in endometrial cancer

The incidence of endometrial carcinoma has increased in recent years and in some countries it has become the second most frequent gynaecological tumour. Although

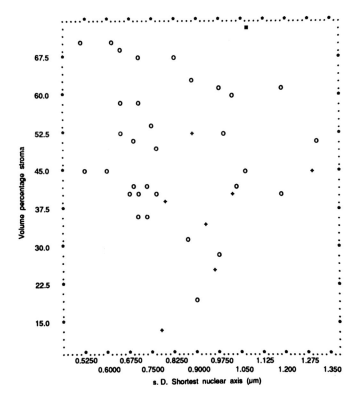

Fig. 42.13 Discrimination of endometrial atypical hyperplasias without (open circles) and with (stars) progression to cancer. (From Baak, 1988a.)

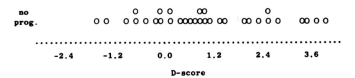

Fig. 42.14 The multivariate D-scores of atypical hyperplasias with and without progression to cancer. (From Baak, 1988a.)

a favourable outcome may be expected in about 75% of cases, a proportion of women with stage I endometrial carcinomas will die as a result of their neoplasm within a few years after initial treatment, and there are currently no accurate means of identifying those tumours that are likely to pursue a fatal course. Moreover, the death rate has not decreased and more precise predictors of outcome would be of considerable value to individualize therapy, which is essential to improve the prognosis for these patients. In general, stage, depth of myometrial invasion, nuclear and histological grade and histological type have some predictive value as to the aggressiveness of the disease, but none of these factors is very accurate. Moreover, histological

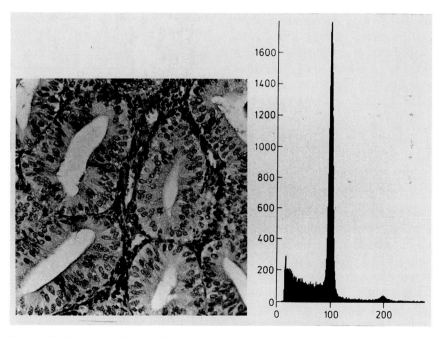

Fig. 42.15 Endometrial atypical hyperplasia. Stratification of nuclei, moderate nuclear atypicality, enlarged but otherwise simple glands, D = –0.59. Carcinoma detected 19 months after the curettage from which picture was taken. (From Baak, 1991.)

type and grade of endometrial carcinoma are not always perfectly reproducible.

It also has been reported that the incidence of steroid hormone receptors has prognostic value (Creasman et al, 1985; Lindahl et al, 1986), but not all authors could confirm this (Putten et al, 1989). Chromosomal instability leading to structural or numerical aberrations is recognized as an early feature of malignant transformation. Extensive cytogenetic studies have been carried out in a variety of tumours, but the procedure is laborious and not always available.

The results of DNA analysis studies are promising (Atkins, 1976; Moberger et al, 1985; Lindahl et al, 1987; Britton et al, 1990). Others found DNA ploidy in combination with other features to be important. For example, in the prospective study of Putten et al (1989) the morphometrical feature mean shortest nuclear axis proved to discriminate significantly between surviving and non-surviving stage I patients. It appeared that the mean shortest nuclear axis and the mean nuclear area were smaller in the group of survivors compared with the group of non-survivors (P < 0.008). The flow cytometrically assessed DNA ploidy was also highly discriminating (P < 0.01) (Fig. 42.16). Other single morphological features that discriminated significantly between surviving and dead patients were, in order of decreasing importance, depth of myometrial invasion of the tumour (significantly more often confined to the inner third in the surviving group than in the group of deceased patients, P < 0.01); mean nuclear shape factor, which was lower in the surviving

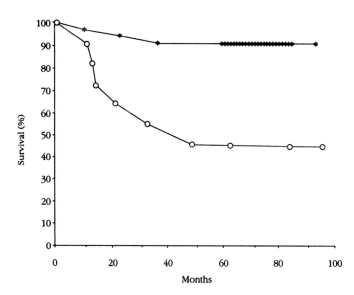

Fig. 42.16 Endometrial carcinoma stage I: Kaplan-Meier survival curve of patients with a diploid and non-diploid nuclear DNA content. Diploid tumours are associated with a favourable outcome. Three of the 39 patients with diploid tumours died (Mantel-Cox = 14.6, P = 0.0001). (Reproduced from Cancer 63: 1378–1387, 1989.)

group (P < 0.03); mean nuclear angle, which was larger in the surviving group (P < 0.03); and mean nuclear axes ratio (higher in the group of survivors, which thus had more ellipsoid nuclei). Using patient status at five-year follow-up as the decision threshold, the smallest and yet strongest set of independent parameters which discriminated best between survivors and non-survivors in stage I carcinomas was found with multivariate stepwise linear regression analysis. This combination consisted, in order of decreasing importance, of mean shortest axis of the nucleus, DNA ploidy, and depth of myometrial invasion ($R^2 = 0.78$, $P < 0.00001$). The combination of these three prognostic features resulted in an endometrial carcinoma stage I prognostic index (ECPI-1), formulated as follows:

$$ECPI\text{-}1 = 0.6494 \times \text{(mean shortest nuclear axis)}$$
$$+ 0.6939 \times \text{(code DNA)}$$
$$+ 0.2398 \times \text{(myometrial invasion)} - 5.7283;$$

in which (1) mean shortest nuclear axis is expressed in μm (with one decimal); (2) code DNA (1 = diploid, 2 = peri-tetraploid, 3 = aneuploid); and (3) myometrial invasion (1 = ≤ ⅓; 2 = > ⅓); using ECPI-1 < 0.87 = survivor and ECPI-1 ≥ 0.87 = non-survivor as a classification rule.

The prognostic rule consisting of these features overshadowed the value of all other features investigated. The overriding prognostic value of this highly reproducible rule was clear from the complete separation of 27 survivors and six non-survivors in the learning set of 33 patients. In an independent test set, all three non-survivors and 13 of the 14 survivors were correctly classified, thus confirming the accuracy and reliability of the developed rule to predict the outcome of future patients with stage I endometrial adenocarcinoma (Fig. 42.17).

Further evaluation of these results was carried out in a retrospective analysis of 77 patients with FIGO I endometrial cancer, diagnosed as such at our Institute between 1973 and 1979. Table 42.7 shows the prognostic value of the different features. Again, the ECPI-1 is by far the strongest factor (see Fig. 42.18). Technical difficulties

Table 42.7 Prognostic value of classical and quantitative pathological factors in Free University Hospital patients, 1973–1979, with 10–15 years follow-up (MC = Mantel-Cox statistic; P = probability of no difference)

Feature	MC	P
ECPI-1	51.1	< 0.0001
DNA ploidy	19.8	0.0001
Grade (revised)	19.7	0.0001
Invasion depth	12.2	0.0005
Mean shortest nuclear axis	4.6	0.03

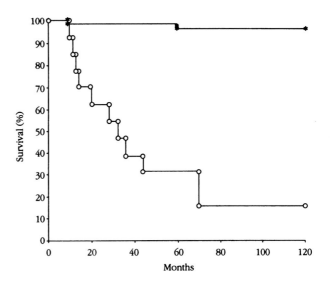

Fig. 42.18 Endometrial cancer stage I: Free University Hospital, 1973–1977, according to ECPI-1 score. Low, ★; high, ○.

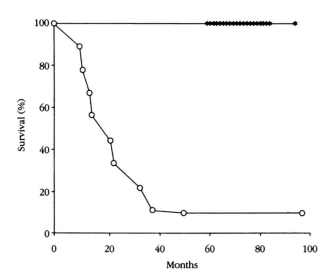

Fig. 42.17 Endometrial carcinoma stage I: Kaplan-Meier survival curve of patients according to the ECPI-1 score low (< 0.87, ★) and high (≥ 0.87, ○) values. The former have a favourable outcome (Mantel-Cox = 62.8, P < 0.00001). (Reproduced from Cancer 63: 1378–1387, 1989.)

as to the selection of nuclei to be measured (Fleege et al, 1990) and false negative (i.e. diploid) results with flow cytometry due to admixture of (diploid) stromal cells require special attention in the application of the method. These data are confirmed by a recent study of Ambros & Kurman (1992), who showed that in stage I cancers DNA ploidy and myometrial invasion are the strongest prognostic factors, next to vascular invasion (mean shortest nuclear axis was not evaluated). Sorbe et al (1994) also confirmed that the combination of DNA ploidy and mean shortest nuclear axis has strong prognostic value. It is of interest that mean shortest nuclear axis is correlated with mean nuclear volume (Nielsen & Nyholm, 1993), a feature with strong prognostic value in cancers of many other organs.

Due to these positive findings, the Gynaecologic Cancer Group of the Cancer Centre, Amsterdam, started a prospective study in late 1986. At present more than 600 patients have been enrolled, and again the (short-term follow-up) results are highly promising (Table 42.8). If this trend continues, one should consider treating high risk patients as advanced endometrial cancers with adjuvant chemotherapy in a prospective randomized trial.

Table 42.8 Interim results of prognostic short-term follow-up (18 months) evaluation of the IKA prospective endometrial carcinoma documentation project (stage I only, n = 220 patients). Many patients are censored

Feature	MC value	P*
Age (<65, >65)	8.1	0.001
Invasion	8.2	0.001
Grade	4.7	0.10
Mean shortest nuclear axis	8.1	0.01
Ploidy	8.6	0.01
ECPI-1 (<0.87, >0.87)	22.5	<0.0001

* Probability of no difference

As to the lack of prognostic value of steroid receptors in certain studies, this may be due to the use of cytosol techniques which may be polluted by non-malignant components. Immunohistochemical assays may be more reliable. Using this method, Sivridis et al (1993) found immunocytochemical technique oestrogen (EB) and progesterone binding sites (PB) in endometrial carcinoma. Tumours were considered as being 'binding-site' rich if more than 40% of the component epithelial cells were positive for hormone binding sites (HB). Over half of the adenocarcinomas studied were HB rich. Significantly higher five- and 10-year survival rates were found in women whose tumours were HB rich compared with those whose neoplasms were HB poor, and a similar trend was established for patients with a combined EB-rich/PB-rich status versus that of EB-poor/PB-poor. This beneficial effect of a rich type I and type II receptor site status on survival, however, was shown only to a limited extent for EB. These results were independent of adjuvant treatment and of all clinical and histopathological features of known prognostic importance, save tumour differentiation.

Epidermal growth factor receptors (EGF-R) have been correlated with different clinically relevant prognostic factors. The advanced tumours, stage III and IV, and tumours with a squamous cell component in the histological examination expressed EGF-R in a higher percentage. Specific EGF binding >7 fmol/mg^{-1} is associated with a reduced survival probability (Birmelin et al, 1992).

Stromal sarcomas

Neoplasms of the endometrial stroma are in general easily separated into three groups on the basis of morphology: stromal nodule, low-grade stromal sarcoma, and high-grade stromal sarcoma, but there may be confusion about their biological behaviour. August et al (1989) examined endometrial stromal tumours with clinical, morphological, and flow cytometric parameters. No patients with stromal nodules or low-grade stromal sarcomas displayed a mitotic rate $>10/10$ high power fields, nuclear pleomorphism, atypical mitotic figures, DNA aneuploidy, or an S-phase $>10\%$, and they all survived. Of the five cases with high-grade stromal sarcoma, four had mitotic rates $>10/$ 10 high power fields, nuclear pleomorphism, atypical mitotic figures, DNA aneuploidy, and an S-phase fraction $>10\%$. The fifth stromal sarcoma case had a high mitotic rate, but lacked other features associated with aggressive behaviour; this patient survived, but the other four patients died. Presence of the three features — nuclear pleomorphism, aneuploidy and S-phase $>10\%$ — seems to indicate a poor response to therapy and a gloomy prognosis. Mitotic activity seems a less useful prognostic indicator in stromal sarcomas.

Myometrium

Benign tumours of the myometrium are amongst the most common human tumours. In contrast, the incidence of uterine sarcoma is extremely low. The five-year survival is 3–75%; the variation may reflect the problem of diagnosis (Stegner, 1980). Although the degrees of hypercellularity, nuclear atypia and multinucleated tumour giant cells have some power to distinguish between leiomyomas and leiomyosarcomas, mitotic activity index is the most important feature for diagnosis and prognosis (Kempson & Bari, 1970; Christopherson et al, 1972; Saksela et al, 1974; Taylor & Norris, 1976; Eberl et al, 1980).

The usefulness of mitotic counting in histological diagnosis of uterine smooth muscle tumours has been both doubted (Silverberg, 1976) and recommended (Kempson, 1976; Norris, 1976). Agreement between different investigators that counting mitosis is of great predictive value cannot be ignored (Scully, 1976). In comparing different studies, lack of standardization of objectives used can be a problem. Eberl et al (1980) found that prognosis is mainly determined by the extent of tumour at diagnosis, but in stage I and II tumours mitotic activity correlates with prognosis. For $\times 400$, 1 mitotic figure per 2–10 high power fields (comparable with 1–5/10 high power fields) indicated good prognosis; if this figure is larger than 10, the prognosis is bad, in agreement with Novak & Woodruff (1974) and Hendrickson & Kempson (1980). The decision tree (see Fig. 42.19: Hendrickson & Kempson, 1980) can help in the diagnosis of particular case.

DNA cytometry was studied by Tsushima et al (1988) in 41 leiomyomas and 49 leiomyosarcomas. Among leiomyomas, 36 (88%) were diploid, 2 (5%) were tetraploid/polyploid and 3 (7%) were aneuploid; 9 leiomyosarcomas (18%) were diploid, 29 (59%) were tetraploid/polyploid and 11 (23%) were aneuploid. Aneuploidy seems to favour the diagnosis of leiomyosarcoma and may in future be incorporated into decision trees.

Gestational trophoblastic disease

It can be difficult to distinguish partial and complete moles. Their differentiation from hydropic abortions is a

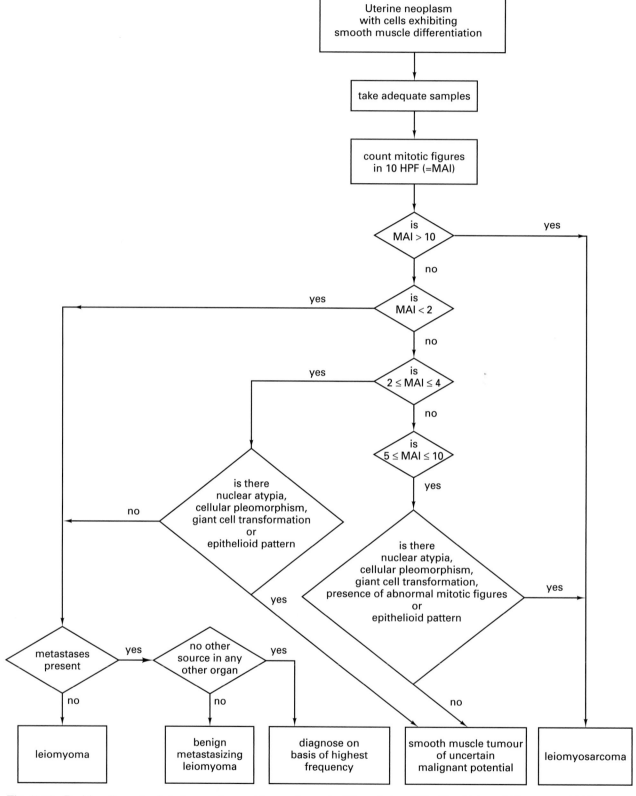

Fig. 42.19 Decision diagnosis of uterine neoplasms with smooth muscle differentiation. (After Hendrickson & Kempson, 1980.)

common problem for histopathologists. DNA cytometric analysis may help, as complete moles are diploid, whereas partial moles are usually considered triploid. Distinction of molar and hydropic gestations is clinically important as approximately 10% of patients with complete moles develop persistent trophoblastic disease (PTD) including invasive mole and choriocarcinoma. Hydatidiform mole is the preceding gestation in at least half of all cases of choriocarcinoma (Elston, 1981).

Of 88 cases originally diagnosed as molar pregnancies, 26 were triploid (2 complete, 20 partial moles, 4 hydropic abortions), 59 were diploid (46 complete moles, 10 partial moles, 3 hydropic abortions); 1 was tetraploid (partial mole); 2 were DNA aneuploid (1 partial, 1 complete mole). Most complete moles are diploid, in contrast to less than one-third of the partial moles (Hemming et al, 1987). Thus triploidy supports the diagnosis of partial mole. These figures were confirmed by Oven et al (1989) (3 of 4 partial moles triploid) and by Lage et al (1988) (5 of 7 partial moles triploid). Moreover, an increased hyperdiploid fraction was detected in cases of established persistent trophoblastic disease (Hemming et al, 1987). The high proliferation rate may explain the premalignant potential of complete hydatidiform moles. Nuclear morphometry also may help to predict progression to malignant trophoblastic disease after evacuation of a hydatidiform mole (Franke et al, 1985). In buffered formalin-fixed, H&E-stained 5 μm slides, mean nuclear area (MNA) in the three-or-more-layered trophoblastic lining of large villi in hydatidiform mole with progression is higher than non-progressive cases — 73.8 ($\pm$ 14.4) versus 49.2 ($\pm$ 11.7 μm^2). If MNA exceeds 90 μm^2, in the more-than-three-layered trophoblastic lining cells of large villi in hydatidiform moles, progression to malignant trophoblastic disease is probable.

Ovary

Borderline tumours

In borderline tumours of the common epithelial type (clear cell tumours not included), morphometric characteristics such as the mitotic activity index (MAI) and volume percentage epithelium (VPE) can be used to distinguish those with a favourable and those with an unfavourable disease course. MAI and VPE exceeded the prognostic value of histological type, nuclear and histological grade and even extent of disease (Baak et al, 1985). A combination of high MAI and VPE was associated with a very poor outcome (see Fig. 42.20). Nuclear area and shape factors also have prognostic value, but are less significant.

DNA aneuploidy does occur in borderline ovarian tumours and has been associated with a poor prognosis

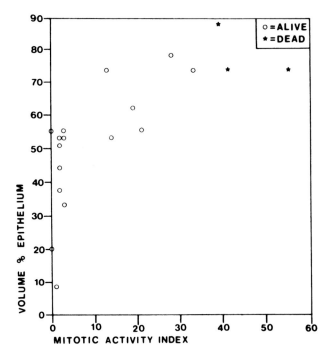

Fig. 42.20 Correlation of survival with mitotic activity index and volume percentage epithelium in borderline tumours. (From Baak et al, 1985.)

(Kearn et al, 1993). It has to be admitted that DNA flow cytometry fails to produce adequate histograms in 5–15% of all cases, especially in mucinous tumours. Klemi et al (1988) found that 7 of 43 borderline tumours were aneuploid (16%), but none of these patients died. Similar results were found in a Danish case-control study (Jakobsen et al, 1995). However, follow-up was short in the latter two studies, unlike the former two which found quantitative analysis to be of exceedingly strong prognostic value. *Thus, it can be concluded that a high MAI, VPE and mean nuclear area and aneuploidy are unfavourable signs in borderline tumours.*

Early cancers (FIGO I, II)

In FIGO I ovarian cancers quantitative pathological features such as nuclear size and nuclear DNA content have prognostic value (Erhardt et al, 1984; Baak et al, 1986c, 1987b). Approximately 20–40% of patients with a FIGO stage I ovarian carcinoma of the serous, mucinous or endometrioid types die within five years of diagnosis. In adequately staged FIGO stage I patients with at least five-year follow-up, the size of the tumour cell nuclei is of prognostic value. In addition, very significant prognostic information can be obtained by classifying the patients in three categories, based on the mitotic activity index (MAI) and the volume percentage epithelium (VPE), carefully excluding the rare histological types of common epithelial tumours (especially clear cell tumours). The five-year survival rates were 91% for 11 patients with MAI < 30 and VPE < 65 (category A), 67% for 9 patients with MAI < 30 and VPE ≥ 65 (category B) and 38% for 13 patients with MAI ≥ 30 (category C). DNA flow cytometry showed 25 of the tumours to be DNA diploid and 8 to be DNA aneuploid. The DNA content of the tumour cell nuclei also revealed prognostic information: the five-year survival figures for patients with DNA diploid and DNA aneuploid tumours were, respectively, 68% and 37%. Combination of morphometric and DNA flow cytometric features showed that in DNA diploid tumours, the morphometric features have additional prognostic value: survival rates of the diploid tumour cases within morphometric categories A, B and C were 91%, 63% and 50%, respectively. None of the eight patients with DNA aneuploid tumours was morphometrically favourable (category A) while seven were morphometrically unfavourable (in category C). The five-year survival rate of the latter patients with morphometrically unfavourable and DNA aneuploid tumour characteristics was only 29% (although they were FIGO stage I). Schueler et al (1993) found ploidy, as assessed by DNA flow cytometry, to be of prognostic value in FIGO stage I and II cancers as well. In a recent study we found the mean nuclear area to be the strongest prognostic factor in FIGO stage Ic and II cis-platin-treated patients. If MNA ≤ 50 μm², prognosis was excellent, above 50 μm² death rate was 50%. MNA exceeded state (Ic, II) as a prognostic factor (unpublished results). *Thus, in early ovarian cancer, ploidy, MAI, VPE and MNA are important prognostic variables, stronger than histological type and other classical features.*

Advanced ovarian cancers (FIGO stage III and IV)

For a full appreciation of new prognostic factors in advanced ovarian cancer (stage III and IV), tumours should be adequately debulked if possible and patients uniformly treated with cis-platin. Several studies which claim that quantitative pathological features are prognostically important in advanced ovarian cancers do not fulfil these criteria; their value is therefore questionable.

We found (Baak et al, 1988b) that in adequately debulked cis-platin-treated patients the following single features were associated with prognosis: SD of nuclear area, mean nuclear area (MNA), nuclear DNA content (diploid, peritetraploid, aneuploid), mitotic activity index (MAI) (< 30, ≥ 30) and volume percentage epithelium (VPE) (< 65%, ≥ 65%). In FIGO stage III and IV cancers, tumours with a mean nuclear area > 70 μm² (25–35% of cases) were nearly all aneuploid (only one diploid). Peritetraploidy was associated with a very poor prognosis, as was a MNA > 90. Roodenburg et al (1987) found DNA ploidy to be significant but later (Roodenburg et al, 1988) confirmed that MAI and VPE were stronger prognosticators than DNA ploidy. Weger et al (1989) also found MNA to be prognostically important and Högberg et al (1992) found a correlation between nuclear size and the amount of tumour at second-look operation. Haapasalo et al (1990) confirmed the prognostic value of mitotic counts. Multivariate analysis (Baak et al, 1988b) showed that statistically the most significant combination of features consisted of (in order of decreasing significance) mean nuclear area, presence or absence of bulky disease and FIGO stage (Mantel-Cox = 23.07, p < 0.00001, see Fig. 42.21). The multivariate advanced carcinoma of the ovary prognostic score (ACOPS) is calculated as follows:

ACOPS = 2.825
– [0.04070 × mean nuclear area (μm², to one decimal)]
– [0.67367 × FIGO (III, IV)]
– [0.60381 × bulky disease (1 = no, 2 = yes)]

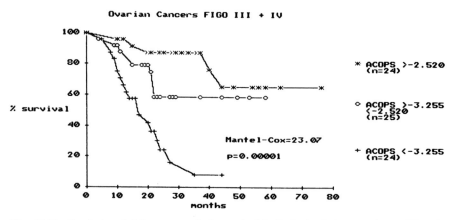

Fig. 42.21 Survival probability curves of adequately debulked, cis-platin-treated stage III and IV ovarian cancer patients by ACOPs. (From Baak et al, 1988b.)

ACOPS >-2.520 means favourable (60% five-year survival); <-3.255 means unfavourable (6% survival); in between, intermediate prognosis (45% survival). These data were recently confirmed in an independent study on a Dutch cis-platin trial with very long follow-up (more than 10 years) (van Diest et al, 1994). In this study the mean nuclear area and the above mentioned ACOP score proved to be the strongest factor in predicting survival. No other features studied (age, grade, etc.) provided additional prognostic value. *Thus, in borderline ovarian tumours and all stages of ovarian cancer, the MAI, MNA, VEPI and DNA ploidy should be determined routinely.*

FUTURE PERSPECTIVES

Digital image processing (DIP)

Developments in DIP technology are rapid and the price of such instruments is falling. In a feasibility study of breast cancer, mitoses could be detected with DIP by means of relatively simple thresholding and binary image manipulation (ten Kate et al, 1993). Furthermore, the epithelium percentage, which is an important prognostic factor, could be assessed fully automatically with DIP (Schipper et al, 1987). Within two or three years, it should be possible to have commercially available DIP computers which can detect nuclei in turnout sections automatically. Similar equipment for the measurement of DNA ploidy patterns of several thousand nuclei in a reasonable time (5–30 minutes) should be possible even sooner (preliminary laboratory versions are already available). Today certain commercially available DIP computers have the capability to quantitate immunoproducts, such as monoclonal antibodies directed against steroid receptors, and nuclear antigens associated with proliferation (Bacus et al, 1988; Cohen et al, 1988). However, the reproducibility may not always be as good as is sometimes believed (Fig. 42.22).

Laser scan microscopy

Laser scan microscopes (LSM) fill the gap between electron- and lightmicroscopes. They offer the possibility of detecting particles which are not quite visible with a lightmicroscope, and as such they can be of help in detecting minor changes in cells and their products. Furthermore, confocal LSMs offer better (x-, y-, z-) resolution than does the classical lightmicroscope and the reduced depth of field makes them very suitable for optical sectioning. Different forms of image processing are also possible, because laser scan microscopes are usually coupled with digital image processing computers. In this way, three-dimensional imaging of cancer sections may become possible (Tekola et al, 1995) (Figs 42.23 and 42.24).

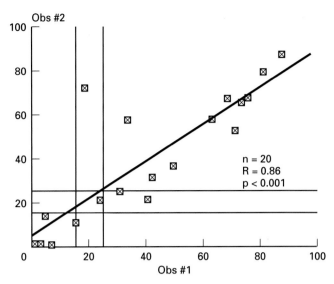

Fig. 42.22 Interobserver reproducibility of oestrogen receptor determination on a commercially available cytometer.

Therefore, laser scan microscopy is a promising new and potentially important imaging technique for quantitative pathological examination of (sub)cellular and tissue components (Baak et al, 1987c); it has also proved to be useful in the assessment of multidrug resistance (Schuurhuis et al, 1991; de Lange et al, 1992). Examples of quantitative molecular pathological applications will be described below.

Quantitative molecular pathology perspectives

In spite of the improved assessment of diagnosis and prognosis of (patients with) gynaecological tumours by morphometry, DNA flow cytometry and molecular biological methods, subgroups of patients remain for whom these methods at present fall short. For example, overtreatment of endometrial atypical hyperplastic lesions and CIN lesions can not be prevented by morphometry alone in all these patients. The prognostic accuracy of morphometry of high risk patients with cervical adenocarcinoma in situ is strong yet not absolute. On the other hand, neither do molecular biological methods, as assessed up till now, identify patients with progressive, recurrent or metastatic disease with 100% accuracy. For example, regression of HPV 16-associated lesions has been reported (Campion et al, 1986) and therefore HPV can not be used as a single predictor of CIN progression.

A combination of the methods described can be especially useful, as morphometric and DNA cytometric analysis in combination with molecular pathology provide much stronger prognostic information than each of the methods alone. For the cervix we have given an example of how combined molecular biological methods and

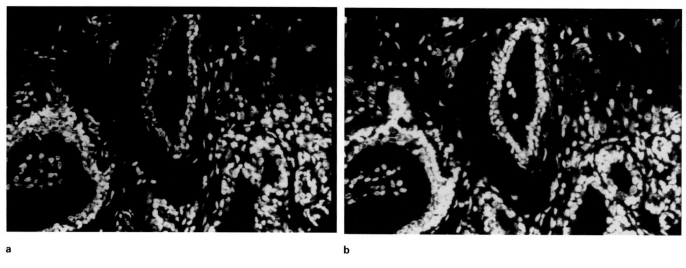

a

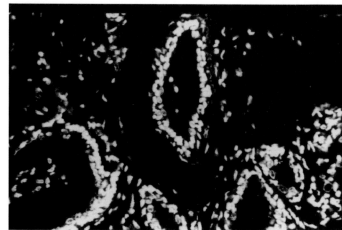

b

Fig. 42.23 Optical sections (taken at various focal depths in the specimen) used to reconstruct the 3-D global tissue structure. The confocal images were taken (clockwise from top left corner) at 2 μm, 10 μm, 15 μm, 18 μm depth respectively into the specimen. In the oval and circular glands of the confocal images, some nuclei start to appear and disappear depending on their orientation in space. (Reprinted from Tekola et al, 1995.)

c

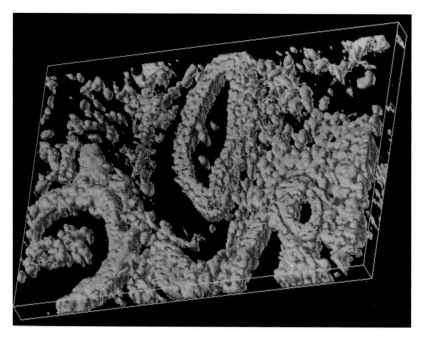

Fig. 42.24 3-D reconstruction of a breast cancer tissue section displayed in different orientations. The image on the left side is tilted away from the observer so that it will be seen from another perspective point. (Reprinted from Tekola et al, 1995.)

morphometry can be useful. Moreover, recently developed confocal laser scan microscopy seems extremely promising for combining quantitative and molecular pathological techniques. This combination can be very powerful, especially when assessed quantitatively, performed in situ on tissue sections, and done by non-autoradiographic yet sensitive means. For example, using biotinylated RNA probes followed by detection with gold/silver enhancement and visualization by confocal laser scan microscopy the detection of messenger RNA can be greatly improved (Baak et al, 1987c; Oudejans et al, 1988, 1989). Furthermore, using the polymerase chain reaction (PCR), it is theoretically possible to improve the detection of HPV nucleic acid to such an extent that, for example, one HPV molecule can be detected in a tissue section (by enzymatic amplification of the target nucleic acid) (Walboomers et al, 1988). Application of this method in tissue sections with preservation of morphology in combination with quantitative confocal laser scan microscopy is in progress. Such a highly sensitive quantitative technique is especially important as there is no clear relationship between the HPV DNA copy number per cell and the clinical stage of the disease studied by our group so far. In this context, it might be essential to be informed not only about the presence of HPV DNA but also about the specific activity of the DNA viral genome (RNA/proteins).

Indeed, little is known about the HPV expression at the single cell level and very sensitive methods are necessary to get insight into the correlation between HPV expression and the clinical outcome of the HPV-infected patients. Objective and accurate measurement of gene activity of certain genes such as (proto)-oncogenes, major histocompatibility complex class I (-related) genes (van den Brule et al, 1991) and viruses can be expected to contribute extensively to the proper assessment of diagnosis, prognosis and perhaps therapy of patients with gynaecological tumours.

CONCLUSIONS

Proof is very strong that in gynaecological tumours the prognostic value of morphometric and cytometric features, either alone or in combination, and as multivariate combinations with, for example, stage (ovary), depth of invasion (endometrium), lymph node status (vulva), exceeds that of classical pathological characteristics such as stage, type and grade. Moreover, the quantitative features are much more reproducible, can be applied on standard material, are relatively fast (5–20 minutes per determination per case) and are inexpensive (especially morphometric analysis). We strongly believe that these methods should lead to a refined patient-tailored therapy in women suffering from gynaecological tumours.

REFERENCES

Aherne W, Dunnill M S 1982 Morphometry. Edward Arnold, London.

Ambros R A, Kurman R J 1992 Identification of patients with stage I uterine endometrioid adenocarcinoma at high risk of recurrence by DNA ploidy, myometrial invasion, and vascular invasion. Gynecologic Oncology 45: 235–239.

Atkin N B 1964 Nuclear size in carcinoma of the cervix: its relation to DNA content and to prognosis. Cancer 17: 1391–1399.

Atkin N B 1971 Model DNA value and chromosome number in ovarian neoplasia: a clinical and histopathologic assessment. Cancer 27: 1064–1073.

Atkin N B 1976 Prognostic significance of ploidy level in human tumors: I. Carcinoma of the uterus. Journal of the National Cancer Institute 56: 909–910.

August C Z, Bauer K D, Lurain J, Murad T 1989 Neoplasms of endometrial stroma: histopathologic and flow cytometric analysis with clinical correlation. Human Pathology 20: 232–237.

Ausems E, van der Kamp J, Baak J P A 1985 Nuclear morphometry in the determination of the prognosis of marked atypical endometrial hyperplasia. International Journal of Gynecological Pathology 4: 180–185.

Baak J P A 1991 Manual of quantitative pathology in cancer diagnosis and prognosis. Springer-Verlag, Heidelberg.

Baak J P A, Oort J 1983 A manual of morphometry in diagnostic pathology. Springer-Verlag, Germany.

Baak J P A, Fox H, Langley F A, Buckley C H 1985 The prognostic value of morphometry in ovarian epithelial tumors of borderline malignancy. International Journal of Gynecological Pathology 4: 186–191.

Baak J P A, Delemarre J F M, Langley F A et al 1986a Grading ovarian tumors. Evaluation of decision making by different pathologists. Analytical Quantitative Cytology and Histology 8: 349–353.

Baak J P A, Langley F A, Talerman A et al 1986b Interpathologist and intrapathologist disagreement in ovarian tumor grading and typing. Analytical Quantitative Cytology and Histology 8: 354–357.

Baak J P A, Wisse-Brekelmans E C M, Langley F A et al 1986c Morphometric data to FIGO stage and histological type and grade for prognosis of ovarian tumours. Journal of Clinical Pathology 39: 1340–1346.

Baak J P A, Langley F A, Talerman A et al 1987a The prognostic variability of ovarian tumor grading by different pathologists. Gynecologic Oncology 27: 166–172.

Baak J P A, Wisse-Brekelmans E C M, Uyterlinde A M, Schipper N W 1987b Evaluation of the prognostic value of morphometric features and cellular DNA content in FIGO I ovarian cancer patients. Analytical Quantitative Cytology and Histology 9: 287–290.

Baak J P A, Thunnissen F B J M, Oudejans C B M, Schipper N W 1987c Potential clinical uses of laser scan microscopy. Applied Optics 26: 3413–3416.

Baak J P A, Nauta J J P, Wisse-Brekelmans E C M, Bezemer P D 1988a Architectural and nuclear morphometrical features together are more important prognosticators in endometrial hyperplasias than nuclear morphometrical features alone. Journal of Pathology 154: 335–341.

Baak J P A, Schipper N W, Wisse-Brekelmans E C M, Ceelen Th et al 1988b The prognostic value of morphometrical features and cellular DNA-content in cis-platin treated late ovarian cancer patients. British Journal of Cancer 57: 503–508.

Baak J P A, Noteboom E, Koevoets J J M 1989 The influence of fixatives and other variations in tissue processing on nuclear morphometric features. Analytical Quantitative Cytology and Histology 11: 219–224.

Baak J P A, Kuik D J, Bezemer P D 1994 The additional prognostic value of morphometric nuclear arrangement and DNA ploidy to other morphometrical and stereological features in endometrial hyperplasia. International Journal of Gynecological Cancer 4: 289–297.

Bacus S, Flowers J L, Press M F, Bacus J W, McCarty K S 1988 The evaluation of estrogen receptor in primary breast carcinoma by computer-assisted image analysis. American Journal of Clinical Pathology 90: 233–239.

Bergers E, van Diest P J, Baak J P A 1995 Reproducibility of semi-automated cell cycle analysis of flow cytometric DNA-histograms of fresh breast cancer material.

Beyer-Boon M E, van der Voorn-Den Hollander M J A, Arentz P W et al 1979 Effect of various routine cytopreparatory techniques on normal urothelial cells and their nuclei. Acta Pathologica Microbiologica Scandinavica (sect A) 87: 63–69.

Birmelin G, Zimmer V, Sauerbrei W, Pfleiderer A, Bauknecht T 1992 Relationship between epidermal growth factor receptor (EGF-R) and various prognostic factors in human endometrial carcinoma. International Journal of Gynecological Cancer 2: 66–74.

Bohm N, Sandritter W 1975 DNA in human tumors: a cytophotometric study. Current Topics in Pathology 60: 152–214.

Boon M E, Baak J P A, Kurver P H J et al 1981 Adenocarcinoma in situ of the cervix: an underdiagnosed lesion. Cancer 48: 768–773.

Bouw G M 1975 Growth and growth retardation of the human placenta. PhD thesis, Free University of Amsterdam.

Britton L C, Wilson T O, Gaffey T A, Cha S S, Wieland H S, Podratz K C 1990 DNA ploidy in endometrial carcinoma: major objective prognostic factor. Mayo Clinic Proceedings 65: 643–650.

Bryant G D, Norman G R 1980 Expressions of probability: words and numbers. New England Journal of Medicine 302: 411.

Campion M J van, Cuzick J, McCance D J, Singer A 1986 Progressive potential of mild cervical atypia: prospective, cytological, colposcopic and virological study. Lancet iii: 237–240.

Caspersson T O, Santesson L 1942 Studies on protein metabolism in the cells in epithelial tumors. Acta Radiologica (suppl) 46: 1–105.

Chalkley H W 1943 Methods for quantitative morphological analysis of tissue. Journal of the National Cancer Institute 4: 47–53.

Christopherson W M, Williamson E O, Gray L A 1972 Leiomyosarcomas of the uterus. Cancer 29: 1512–1517.

Cohen O, Brugal G, Seigneurin D, Demongeot J 1988 Image cytometry of estrogen receptors in breast carcinomas. Cytometry 9: 579–587.

Colgan T J, Norris H J, Foster W et al 1983 Predicting the outcome of endometrial hyperplasia by quantitative analysis of nuclear features using a linear discriminant function. International Journal of Gynecological Pathology 1: 347–352.

Creasman W T, Soper J T, McCarty K S Jr et al 1985 Influence of cytoplasmic steroid receptor content on prognosis of early stage endometrial carcinoma. American Journal of Obstetrics and Gynecology 151: 922–932.

Crum C P, Ikenberg H, Richard R M et al 1984 Human papillomavirus type 16 and early cervical neoplasia. New England Journal of Medicine 310: 880–883.

Dalrymple J C, Brough A K, Monaghan J M 1989 Morphometric analysis of nuclear/cytoplasmic ratios in normal and perineoplastic vulvar skin. Histopathology 14: 645–653.

de Lange J H M, Schipper N W, Schuurhuis G J et al 1992 Quantification by laser scan microscopy of intracellular doxorubicin distribution. Cytometry 13: 571–576.

Delesse M A 1847 Procédé méecanique pour déterminer la composition des roches. Comptes Rendue Hebdomadaires des Seances de l'Academie des Sciences 25: 544–545.

Eberl M, Pfeiderer A, Teufel G, Bachmasin F 1980 Sarcomas of the uterus: morphologic criteria and clinical course. Pathology Research and Practice 169: 165–172.

Elston C W 1981 Gestational tumours of trophoblast. In: Anthony P P, MacSween R M N (eds) Recent advances in histopathology. Edinburgh, Churchill Livingstone, pp 149–161.

Erhardt K, Auer G, Bjorkholm E et al 1984 Prognostic significance of nuclear DNA content in serous ovarian tumours. Cancer Research 44: 2198–2202.

Fleege J C, Baak J P A, Smeulders A W M 1988 Analysis of measuring system parameters that influence reproducibility of morphometric assessments with a graphic tablet. Human Pathology 19: 513–517.

Fleege J C, van Diest P J, Baak J P A 1990 Computer assisted efficiency testing of different sampling methods for selective nuclear graphic tablet morphometry. Laboratory Investigation 63: 270–275.

Fleege J C, van Diest P J, Baak J P A 1991 Reliability of quantitative pathological assessments, standards, and quality control. In: Baak J P A (Ed) Manual of quantitative pathology in cancer diagnosis and prognosis. Springer-Verlag, Heidelberg, pp 151–181.

Franke H R, Alons C L, Caron F J M et al 1985 Quantitative morphology: a study of the trophoblast. Virchows Archive A (Pathological Anatomy) 406: 323–331.

Fu Y S, Reagan J W, Richart R M 1981 Definition of precursor. Gynecologic Oncology 12: 220–231.

Fu Y S, Hall T L, Berek J S et al 1987 Prognostic significance of DNA ploidy and morphometric analyses of adenocarcinoma of the uterine cervix. Analytical Quantitative Cytology and Histopathology 9: 17–24.

Fu Y S, Huang S, Ionesco M et al 1988a Correlative study of human papillomavirus DNA, histopathology, and morphometry in cervical condyloma and intraepithelial neoplasia. International Journal of Gynecological Pathology 7: 298–307.

Fu Y S, Ferenczy A, Huang I, Gelfrand M M 1988b Digital imaging analysis of normal, hyperplastic and malignant endometrial cells in endometrial brushing samples. Analytical Quantitative Cytology and Histopathology 10: 139–149.

Fu Y S, Huang J, Halke R 1989 Comparative and quantitative analysis of regressive and persistent cervical intraepithelial neoplasia. Annual meeting United States-Canadian division, International Academy of Pathology, 5–10 March, 1989, San Francisco.

Gamel J W, Gleason J, Williams H et al 1985 Reproducibility of nucleolar measurements in human intraocular melanoma cells on standard histologic microslides. Analytical Quantitative Cytology and Histopathology 7: 74–177.

Glagoleff A A 1933 On the geometrical methods of quantitative mineralogic analysis of rocks. Transactions of the Institute of Economic Mineralogy, Moscow 59.

Goppinger A, Freudenberg N, Ross A et al 1986 The prognostic significance of the DNA distribution in squamous cell carcinomas of the uterine cervix. Analytical Quantitative Cytology and Histopathology 87: 662–678.

Greenhough R B 1925 Varying degrees of malignancy in cancer of the breast. Journal of Cancer Research 9: 452–463.

Gundersen H J G, Jensen E B 1985 Stereological estimation of the volume-weighted mean volume of arbitrary particles observed on random sections. Journal of Microscopy 138: 127–142.

Gusberg S B, Kaplan A L 1963 Precursors of corpus cancer. American Journal of Obstetrics and Gynecology 87: 662–678.

Haapasalo H, Collan Y, Seppa A, Gidlund A L, Atkin N B, Pesonen E 1990 Prognostic value of ovarian carcinoma grading methods — a method comparison study. Histopathology 16: 1–7.

Hanselaar A G J M, Vooijs G P, Oud P S et al 1988 DNA ploidy patterns in cervical intraepithelial neoplasia grade III with and without synchronous invasive squamous cell carcinoma. Cancer 62: 2537–2546.

Heiberg K H, Kemp T 1929 Über die Zahl der Chromosomen in Karzinomzellen beim Menschen. Virchows Archive A (Pathological Anatomy) 273: 693–700.

Hemming J D, Quirke P, Womack C et al 1987 Diagnosis of molar pregnancy and persistent trophoblastic disease by flow cytometry. Journal of Clinical Pathology 40: 615–620.

Hendrickson M R, Kempson R L 1980 Surgical pathology of the uterine corpus. Saunders, Philadelphia, pp 468–529.

Högberg T, Wang G, Risberg B et al 1992 Nuclear morphometry: a strong prognostic factor for survival after secondary surgery in advanced ovarian cancer. International Journal of Gynecological Cancer 2: 198–206.

Hopkins M P, Morley G W 1991 Squamous cell cancer of the cervix: prognostic factors related to survival. International Journal of Gynecological Cancer 1: 173–177.

Jacobj W 1925 Über das rhythmische Wachstum der Zellen durch Verdoppelung ihres Volumes. Archiv für Entwicklungsmechanik der Organismen 106: 630–631.

Jakobsen A, Bichel P, Vaeth M 1985 New prognostic factors in squamous cell carcinoma of cervix uteri. American Journal of Clinical Oncology 8: 39–43.

Jakobsen A, Bichel P, Kristensen G B, Nyland M 1988 Prognostic influence of ploidy level and histopathologic differentiation in cervical carcinoma stage Ib. European Journal of Cancer and Clinical Oncology 24: 969–972.

Jakobsen A, Bichel P, Nilsen R H 1995 Flow cytometry in borderline ovarian tumours. In Preparation.

Ji H X, Syrjänen S, Klemi P, Chang F, Tosi P, Syrjänen K 1991 Prognostic significance of human papillomavirus (HPV) type and nuclear DNA content in invasive cervical cancer. International Journal of Gynecological Cancer 1: 59–67.

Kamentsky L A, Melamed M R, Derman H 1965 Spectrophotometer: new instrument for rapid cell analysis. Science 150: 630–631.

Kayser K, Kiefer B, Toomes H et al 1987 Analysis of adenomatous structures in histopathology. Analytical Quantitative Cytology and Histopathology 9: 273–278.

Kayser K, Bubenzer J, Paul J 1990 Combined morphometrical and syntactic structure analysis as tools for histomorphological insight into human lung carcinoma growth. Annals of Cellular Pathology 2: 167–178.

Kearn J, Iversen T, Tropé C, Pettersen E O, Nesland J M 1992 Flow cytometric DNA measurements in squamous cell carcinoma of the vulva: an important prognostic method. International Journal of Gynecological Cancer 2: 169–174.

Kearn J, Tropé C, Kristensen G B, Abeler V M, Pettersen E O 1993 DNA ploidy; the most important prognostic factor in patients with borderline tumours of the ovary. International Journal of Gynecological Cancer 3: 349–358.

Kempson R L 1976 Mitosis counting (editorial). Human Pathology 7: 482–483.

Kempson R L, Bari N 1970 Uterine sarcomas. Classification, diagnosis and prognosis. Human Pathology 1: 331–349.

Klemi P J, Joensuu H, Kiilholma P et al 1988 Clinical significance of abnormal nuclear DNA content in serous ovarian tumours. Cancer 62: 2005–2010.

Kurman R J, Kaminski P F, Norris H J 1985 The behaviour of endometrial hyperplasia: a long-term study of "untreated" hyperplasia in 170 patients. Cancer 56: 403–412.

Kurzl R, Messerer D, Lohe K J et al 1988 Comparative morphometric study on the depth of invasion in vulvar carcinoma. Gynecologic Oncology 29: 12–25.

Lage J M, Driscoll S G, Yavner D L et al 1988 Hydatidiform moles: application of flow cytometry in diagnosis. American Journal of Clinical Pathology 89: 596–600.

Lindahl B, Alm P, Ferno M, Grundsell H, Norgren A, Tropé C 1986 Relapse of endometrial carcinoma related to steroid receptor concentration, staging, histologic grading and myometrial invasion. Anticancer Research 6: 1317–1321.

Lindahl B, Alm P, Fernö M, Killander D, Långström E, Norgren A, Tropé C 1987 Prognostic value of flow cytometrical DNA measurements in stage I–II endometrial carcinoma: correlations with steroid receptor concentration, tumor myometrial invasion, and degree of differentiation. Anticancer Research 7: 791–798.

Marchevsky A M, Gil J, Jeanty H 1987 Computerized interactive morphometry in pathology. Human Pathology 18: 320–331.

Moberger B, Auer G, Forsslund G et al 1985 The prognostic significance of DNA measurements in endometrial carcinoma. Cytometry 5: 430–436.

Nauth H F, Boger A 1982 New aspects of vulvar cytology. Acta Cytologica 26: 1–6.

Nauth H F, Boon M E 1983 Significance of the morphology of anucleated squames in the cytologic diagnosis of vulvar lesions. Acta Cytologica 27: 230–236.

Nauth H F, Neumann G K, Feilen K D 1987 Structural and morphometric analysis of parakeratotic and dyskeratotic cells exfoliated from various vulvar lesions. Correlation with data from cervical cytology. Analytical Quantitative Cytology and Histopathology 9: 243–252.

Nielsen A L, Nyholm H C J 1993 Stereological estimates of nuclear volume in endometrial adenocarcinoma of endometrioid type: reproducibility and intra-tumour variation. Histopathology 22: 17–24.

Nødskov-Pedersen S 1971 Degree of malignancy of cancer involving the cervix uteri, judged on the basis of clinical stage, histology, size of nuclei, and content of DNA. Acta Pathologica et Microbiologica Scandinavica (A) 79: 617–628.

Norris H J 1976 Mitosis counting (editorial). Human Pathology 7: 483–484.

Novak E R, Woodruff J D 1974 Sarcomas and allied lesions of the uterus. In: Novak's Gynecologic and obstetric pathology. Saunders, Philadelphia, pp 272–287.

Oberholzer M 1983 Morphometrie in der Klinischen Pathologie. Springer-Verlag, Heidelberg, pp 69–70.

Oud P S, Hanselaar A G J M, Pahlplatz M M M et al 1987 Image DNA index (ploidy) analysis in cancer diagnosis. Applied Optics 26: 3349–3355.

Oudejans C B M, ten Kate T, Meijer C J L M, Baak J P A 1996 Quantitative non-autoradiographic assessment of target mRNA copies in tissue sections. In preparation

Oudejans C B M, Krimpenfort P, Meijer C J L M, Ploegh H L 1989 Lack of expression of HLA-B27 gene in transgenic mouse trophoblast: conserved genetic pressures underlying extra-embryonic development. Journal of Experimental Medicine 169: 447–456.

Oven van M W, Schoots C J F, Oosterhuis J W et al 1989 The use of DNA flow cytometry in the diagnosis of triploidy in human abortions. Human Pathology 20: 238–242.

Putten H W H M, Baak J P A, Koenders T J M et al 1989 Prognostic value of quantitative pathologic features and DNA content in individual patients with stage I endometrial adenocarcinoma. Cancer 63: 1378–1387.

Révész L, Siracka E 1984 A morphometric study of vascularization in uterine cervix cancers. Cytometry 5: 442–444.

Richart R M 1987 Causes and management of cervical intraepithelial neoplasia. Cancer 60: 1951–1959.

Roodenburg C J, Ploem-Zaaijer J J, Cornelisse C J et al 1987 Use of DNA image cytometry in addition to flow cytometry for the study of patients with advanced ovarian cancer. Cancer Research 47: 3938–3941.

Roodenburg C J, Cornelisse C J, Hermans J, Fleuren G J 1988 DNA flow cytometry and morphometry as prognostic indicators in advanced ovarian cancer: a step forward in predicting the clinical outcome. Gynecologic Oncology 29: 176–187.

Saksela E, Lampinen V, Procope B 1974 Malignant mesenchymal tumours of the uterine corpus. American Journal of Obstetrics and Gynecology 120: 452–460.

Schipper N W, Smeulders A W M, Baak J P A 1987 Quantification of epithelial volume by image processing applied to ovarian tumors. Cytometry 8: 345–352.

Schueler J A, Cornelisse C J, Hermans J, Trimbos J B, van der Burg M E, Fleuren G J 1993 Prognostic factors in well-differentiated early stage epithelial ovarian cancer. Cancer 71: 787–795.

Schuurhuis G J, Broxterman H J, de Lange J H M et al 1991 Early multidrug resitance, defined by changes in intracellular doxorubicin distribution, independent of P-glycoprotein. British Journal of Cancer 64: 857–861.

Scully R E 1976 Mitosis counting (editorial). Human Pathology 7: 481–482.

Silverberg S G 1976 Reproducibility of the mitosis count in the histologic diagnosis of smooth muscle tumours of the uterus. Human Pathology 7: 451–454.

Sivridis E, Buckley C H, Fox H 1993 Type I and type II estrogen and progesterone binding sites in endometrial carcinomas: their value in predicting survival. International Journal of Gynecological Cancer 3: 80–88.

Skaarland E 1985a Morphometric analysis of nuclei in epithelial structures from normal and neoplastic endometrium: a study using the Isaacs cell sampler and Endoscann instruments. Journal of Clinical Pathology 38: 496–501.

Skaarland E 1985b Nuclear size and shape of epithelial cells from the endometrium: lack of value as a criterion for differentiation between normal, hyperplastic, and malignant conditions. Journal of Clinical Pathology 38: 502–506.

Sorbe B, Risberg B, Thornthwaite J 1994 Nuclear morphometry and DNA flow cytometry as prognostic methods for endometrial carcinoma. International Journal of Gynecological Cancer 4: 94–100.

Sørensen F B, Bichel P, Jakobsen A 1992 DNA level and stereologic estimates of nuclear volume in squamous cell carcinomas of the uterine cervix: a comparative study with analysis of prognostic impact. Cancer 69: 187–199.

Stegner H E 1980 Clinical aspects of uterine sarcoma. Pathology Research and Practice 169: 120–126.

Stendahl U, Willén H, Willén R 1979 Classification and grading of invasive squamous cell carcinoma of the uterine cervix. Acta Radiologica et Oncologica 18: 481–496.

Stendahl U, Willén H, Willén R 1980 Invasive squamous cell carcinoma of the uterine cervix. I. Definition of parameters in a histo-pathologic malignancy grading system. Acta Radiologica et Oncologica 19: 467–480.

Taylor H B, Norris H J 1976 Mesenchymal tumours of the uterus. IV. Diagnosis and prognosis of leiomyosarcomas. Archives of Pathology 82: 40–44.

Tekola P, Zhu Q, Baak J P A 1994 Confocal laser microscopy and image processing for 3-dimensional microscopy. Human Pathology 25: 12–21.

ten Kate T K, Beliën J A M, Smeulders A W M, Baak J P A 1993 Method for counting mitoses by image processing in feulgen stained breast cancer sections. Cytometry 14: 241–250.

Toogood J G 1980 What do we mean by "usually?" Lancet I: 1094.

Tsushima K, Stanhope C R, Gaffey T A et al 1988 Uterine leiomyosarcomas and benign smooth muscle tumors: usefulness of nuclear DNA patterns studied by flow cytometry. Mayo Clinic Proceedings 63: 248–255.

van den Brule A J C, Cromme F V, Snijders P J F et al 1991 Nonradioactive RNA in situ hybridization detection of human papillomavirus 16-E7 transcripts in squamous cell carcinomas of the uterine cervix using confocal laser scan microscopy. American Journal of Pathology 139: 1037–1045.

van Diest P J, Fleege J C, Baak J P A 1992 Syntactic structure analysis in invasive breast cancer: analysis of reproducibility, biologic background, and prognostic value. Human Pathology 23: 876–883.

van Diest P J, Baak J P A, Brugghe J, van den Burg M E L, van Oosterom A T, Neijt J P 1994 Quantitative pathologic features as predictors of long-term survival in patients with advanced ovarian cancer treated with cisplatin. International Journal of Gynecological Cancer 4: 174–179.

van Eerden J J, Meijer G A, van Diest P J, Baak J P A 1992 Syntactic structure analysis in FIGO stage Ic & II ovarian cancers. 7th International symposium on diagnostic quantitative pathology (morphometry in morphological diagnosis), Heraklion, Crete, October 5–9, 1992.

van Nagell J R, Powell D E, Gallion H H et al 1988 Small cell carcinoma of the uterine cervix. Cancer 62: 1586–1593.

van Thiel P H, van der Linden J C, Baak J P A et al 1989 Reproducibility of flow cytometric assessment of follicular tumours of the thyroid. Journal of Clinical Pathology 42: 260–263.

Walboomers J M M, Fokke H E, Polak M at al 1987 In situ localization of human papilloma virus type 16 DNA in a metastasis of an endocervical adenocarcinoma. Intervirology 27: 81–85.

Walboomers J M M, Melchers W J G, Mullink H et al 1988 Sensitivity of in situ detection with biotinylated probes of human papillomavirus type 16 DNA in frozen tissue sections of squamous cell carcinomas of the cervix. American Journal of Pathology 131: 587–594.

Weger A R, Ludescher Chr, Mikuz G, Kemmler G, Reitsamer R, Hausmaninger H, Lindholm J 1989 The value of morphometry to predict chemotherapy response in advanced ovarian cancer. Pathology Research and Practice 185: 676–679.

Weibel E R 1979 Stereological methods, vol I. Practical methods for biological morphometry. Academic Press, London.

Wied G L, Barrels P H, Bahr G F 1968 Taxonomic intra-cellular analytic system (TICAS) for cell identification. Acta Cytologica 12: 180–204.

Wied G L, Bartels P H, Bahr G F 1969 Computer-assisted identification of cells from uterine adenocarcinoma. II. measurements at 590 mm. Acta Cytologica 13: 21–26.

Willén R, Tropé C, Långstrom E, Ranstam J, Killander D, Clase L 1987 Prospective malignancy grading and flow cytometry DNA distribution in biopsy specimens from invasive squamous cell carcinoma of the uterine cervix. Anticancer Research 7: 235–252.

43. Molecular biology in gynaecological pathology

Michael Wells

INTRODUCTION

With the exception of human papillomavirus typing, molecular biology as applied to diagnostic gynaecological histopathology is still in its infancy. Despite the burgeoning number of reports there is little that can be reliably applied in day-to-day diagnostic practice. The current excitement lies largely in the area of molecular pathogenesis of cervical and ovarian epithelial neoplasia. At the time of writing, for example, the identification of the gene on chromosome 17q responsible for hereditary breast and ovarian cancer is imminent. The identification of genetic abnormalities is of enormous potential value in terms of screening, diagnosis and prognosis. Many of the molecular pathological studies have produced contradictory findings with regard to their clinical or prognostic significance. This is also true for many of the immunohistochemical studies of the protein products of oncogenes or tumour suppressor genes which, for the most part, are not considered here. The purpose of this chapter, however, is not to be nihilistic but to provide some insight into the potential application and significance of molecular pathological changes.

Certain fundamental facts such as the structure of chromosomes, the structure and function of DNA, the transcription into single-stranded messenger RNA (mRNA) and the synthesis of proteins will not be reiterated here. It should be remembered that the orientation of the two strands in double-stranded DNA is antiparallel, which means that, when bound together in a helix, one reads 5′ to 3′ and the other 3′ to 5′. Recombinant DNA technology depends upon two key steps: (a) cleavage of DNA sequences at specific sites by restriction endonucleases and (b) hybridization of complementary DNA sequences (Arends & Bird, 1992; Bennett & Moore, 1992; Herrington & McGee, 1992).

TECHNIQUES

Southern blotting

Once DNA has been fragmented by one or more restric-

tion enzymes the DNA may then be separated using agarose gel electrophoresis. Small molecules travel further along the gel than larger molecules. After staining with ethidium bromide the gel may be photographed under ultraviolet light. The bonds between the two strands of DNA are broken by treatment with sodium hydroxide. The gel is covered by a special nitrocellulose membrane to which the DNA is transferred and bound (the Southern blot). Northern blotting refers to the same procedure for mRNA.

Hybridization

Hybridization refers to the process by which a labelled complementary DNA sequence (probe) binds to the regions of DNA under study to produce a radioactive (or other) signal. The conditions (stringency) of the hybridization reaction may be varied to influence both specificity and sensitivity. For example, under high stringency conditions of high temperature and low salt concentration only perfectly matched sequences will hybridize.

DNA cloning

New DNA fragments can be cloned in appropriate vectors, commonly plasmids. The new gene or foreign DNA is usually cleaved with the same restriction enzyme as the plasmid vector, thus generating overhanging cohesive ends which hybridize and are ligated. The recombined DNA molecule is introduced into a small proportion of bacterial host cells, which may be selected by growth in the presence of the appropriate antibiotic.

Unrelated individuals may inherit restriction enzyme recognition sites at different places in the genome, so that cleavage produces DNA fragments of varying lengths, known as restriction fragment length polymorphisms (RFLPs). These are useful as markers at particular regions in the genome. Cloned DNA fragments can be characterized by base pair sequencing. They may also be labelled with radionucleotides or non-radioactive chromogens for use as probes.

In situ hybridization

In situ hybridization refers to the direct detection of nucleic acid (DNA or RNA) within cellular material so that the resulting signal can be viewed microscopically and the topographical relationships of the signal observed (Wilkinson, 1992). The DNA or RNA probes may be isotopically or non-isotopically labelled and the technique may be applied to chromosomes, cytological preparations or paraffin-embedded tissue sections. In gynaecological pathology in situ hybridization has been predominantly used for the diagnosis of human papillomavirus infection (Lewis & Wells, 1992).

In non-isotopic in situ hybridization (NISH) the most popular labelling molecules are biotin and digoxigenin. These have the advantages of being non-hazardous and easy to detect. A primary antibody directed against the label is added, and finally a secondary antibody. The primary or secondary antibody is labelled with a detection molecule which is visualized by a detection system, e.g. horseradish peroxidase or alkaline phosphatase.

Probes to DNA viruses are constructed with whole viral DNA or restriction enzyme fragments of specific viral sequences. More recently virus probes have been produced synthetically. These oligonucleotides, containing complementary sequences to DNA or RNA viruses, can be easily labelled and used as probes but their use in conjunction with non-isotopic detection systems is limited. This is due to a lack of sensitivity, resulting from the lower amount of label available on these short sequences.

Fluorescent in situ hybridization

Fluorescent in situ hybridization (FISH) combines the specificity of molecular genetics with traditional cyto-genetics; it is being widely incorporated into the clinical setting due to its speed, high resolution and reproducibility and the simple microscopy required for analysis.

FISH is a technique whereby a biotin- or digoxigenin-labelled nucleic acid probe, usually DNA, is hybridized using molecular methods to either metaphase chromosomes or to cells. Visualization of hybridized probes by fluorescence microscopy is achieved using fluorochromes such as fluorescein which are conjugated to avidin for detection of biotin or anti-digoxigenin (Speel et al, 1992; Van de Kaa et al, 1993; Van Lijnschoten et al, 1994).

Various types of probes are commercially available that address different applications of the technology. Types of FISH probes include: chromosome-specific repetitive probes, whole chromosome painting probes or locus-specific probes. Some applications of FISH include the following:

a. identification of marker chromosomes
b. characterization of chromosomal rearrangements

c. study of confined placental mosaicism
d. rapid assessment of ploidy and major trisomies.

Two colour probe combinations can also be used for the determination of numerical chromosomal abnormalities and gene amplification. Results can be analysed microscopically or flow cytometrically and areas showing focal chromosomal aberrations can be correlated with histological appearances (Persons et al, 1993).

Polymerase chain reaction

This technique, first described in 1985, has had a dramatic effect on the development of molecular biology and its applicability to the routine diagnostic laboratory (Wright & Wynford-Thomas, 1990; Templeton, 1992). The technique permits the analysis of DNA or RNA from any source. It can be used to amplify DNA fragments up to 10 kb in length. Because the polymerase chain reaction is so sensitive meticulous laboratory technique is essential to avoid contamination by previously amplified DNA.

A small proportion of DNA is placed in a tube. Two oligonucleotides (primer sequences) are added. These have base pair sequences matching two sequences of the DNA that flank the region of interest. A thermostable DNA polymerase is added and the mixture heated to just below 100°C; the DNA then dissociates into two strands. The solution is allowed to cool to 40–60°C and the single strands bind to the oligonucleotides, which are in excess. The oligonucleotide now acts as a primer for DNA polymerase and is extended to form a new double-stranded molecule. The cycle is repeated, with the amount of DNA doubling each time. Normally 20–40 cycles are performed in automated devices, producing a 10^5–10^6 amplification of target DNA within a few hours. Amplified products of known length can be rapidly identified by size fractionation in electrophoretic gels without the need for radioactive probes or blotting techniques.

When making double-stranded DNA, Taq polymerase attaches new residues to the 3′ end of the primers. Thus in the polymerase reaction DNA is essentially copied only between the two primers. After multiple copies of amplification, the predominant double-stranded DNA species in the sample is a fragment whose two ends are defined by the two primer oligonucleotides, i.e. not all the DNA in the original sample is amplified. RNA-dependent DNA polymerase (reverse transcripts) may be used to amplify single-stranded RNA molecules.

There are three major molecular pathological applications of the polymerase chain reaction:

1. Detecting very small amounts of DNA in limited clinical samples, including the analysis of individual cells. This is of particular importance with regard to infections such as HPV and HIV.

2. Identifying the specific new mutation in a particular gene that causes a given inherited disease in a patient.

3. Analysis to detect known mutations that always cause a particular disease or polymorphism.

Single-stranded conformational polymorphisms

Procedures for the detection of genetic mutations fall into two groups: the first detects known mutations whilst the second comprises methods to scan DNA sequences for unknown mutations. Most of these procedures depend on the amplification of sample DNA by PCR prior to analysis; the most widely used is single-stranded conformational polymorphism (SSCP) analysis (Grompe, 1993). This technique relies on the principle that amplified wild-type and mutant DNA assume different three-dimensional configurations when denatured into single strands. The single-stranded wild-type and mutant DNA will then show differential migration in a non-denaturing gel when electrophoresed side by side. PCR products with altered migration patterns can then be analysed by DNA sequencing to determine the exact nature of the alteration.

SCCP analysis is simple and relatively sensitive and multiple samples may be examined simultaneously. The technique detects 70–90% of mutations in PCR products of 200 base pairs or less but does not localize them within the fragment.

Genetic analysis of tissue after selective ultraviolet radiation microdissection and the polymerase chain reaction

Cells in histological sections can be selected for DNA amplification by painting the glass slide with black ink to cover the area of tissue of interest. The sections can then be irradiated with ultraviolet light which will result in degradation of all DNA except in the areas protected by black ink. Loss of heterozygosity studies can then be carried out by DNA extraction and amplification using appropriate primer sequences and the PCR (Shibata et al, 1992; Zheng et al, 1993).

In situ polymerase chain reaction

DNA extraction and PCR preclude histological correlation with molecular biological findings, and in situ hybridization is relatively insensitive with a detection threshold of approximately 20 copies per cell. In situ PCR (ISPCR) is a new molecular technique with potential to combine the high sensitivity of PCR with the precise topographical localization provided by in situ hybridization (Nuovo et al, 1991; Nuovo, 1992). The use of single primer pairs in ISPCR and the detection of in situ am-plificants by oligonucleotide probes should significantly increase the applicability of indirect ISPCR on dispersed cells and cytospins to studies other than viral infection. Diffusion artifact, however, is a significant problem with ISPCR applied to tissue sections, potentially leading to false positive results.

Comparative genomic hybridization for molecular cytogenetic analysis

Most molecular techniques are highly focused; they target one specific gene or chromosome region at a time and leave the majority of the genome unexamined. The recently described technique of comparative genomic hybridization allows comparison of DNA from malignant and normal cells so that entire genomes can be examined and regions of gain or loss of DNA identified (Kallioniemi et al, 1992). Biotinylated tumour DNA and digoxigenin-labelled normal genomic reference DNA are simultaneously hybridized to normal metaphase spreads. Hybridization of tumour DNA can be detected with green-fluorescing fluorescein isothiocyanate (FITC)-avidin, and the reference DNA with red-fluorescing rhodamine anti-digoxigenin. The fluorescence signals can then be quantitatively analysed by means of a digital image analysis system. Changes in the green : red ratio will reflect differences in the relative amounts of tumour and reference DNA bound at a given chromosomal locus.

DNA fingerprinting

The products of genes are generally similar between individuals but there is a greater variation in non-transcribed DNA. Distributed throughout the genome of any individual are many simple tandem repeat sequences, consisting of a variable number of repeats of a short sequence. These are referred to as 'mini-satellites' or, when composed of smaller sequences, 'micro-satellites'. Unique patterns due to different lengths of these sequences are present in each individual's genome. In DNA fingerprinting a probe is constructed which detects these mini-satellite regions by ligating together several copies of the core repeat sequence. The various restriction fragments are separated by electrophoresis and Southern blotted. The blot is then hybridized to a probe which detects the central core of the repeating unit. The resulting autoradiograph will show a large number of bands. Any individual will have inherited half of the bands from each parent, but the degree of polymorphism is so high that it appears that the banding pattern for each individual is unique. DNA fingerprinting can be performed on human blood and biological parentage established by comparison of test material with the maternal and paternal mini-satellite fragments (Jeffreys et al, 1985).

More recently, probes have been introduced which detect unique sequences which are very highly polymorphic. These are also based on variable numbers of tandem repeat sequences (VNTR) but may be specific for an individual chromosome. These probes are easier to read since each individual will usually have only two bands rather than the large number seen with the original probes (Bennett & Moore, 1992; Gruis et al, 1993).

DNA fingerprinting may be used to distinguish between a diploid complete hydatidiform mole (in which all of the chromosomes are inherited from the father) and a triploid partial mole (with two sets of paternal chromosomes and one set of maternal chromosomes) (Lane et al, 1992).

MOLECULAR PATHOLOGY

For thorough understanding of these issues a knowledge of oncogenes and their biological significance is essential (Curling & Watson, 1992).

Oncogenes

Oncogenes are genes governing the neoplastic behaviour of cells and were originally discovered in oncogenic RNA retroviruses. These viruses contain the enzyme, reverse transcriptase, which enables their RNA to be transcribed into complementary DNA which is then incorporated into the genome of the infected cell; these genes were called oncogenes.

It was subsequently discovered that DNA sequences identical to viral oncogenes are present in the genome of normal cells (cellular or proto-oncogenes). These cellular oncogenes produce proteins which are essential for normal cell and tissue growth and differentiation. It is when they are aberrant or inappropriately expressed that they result in the growth of a tumour.

Oncogenes can be classified into five groups according to the function of the gene product (oncoprotein):

1. Growth factors
2. Growth factor receptors (e.g. *erb*B, coding for epidermal growth factor receptor)
3. Intracellular transducers of growth factor signals (tyrosine kinase activity)
4. Nuclear-binding oncoproteins involved in the regulation of cellular proliferation (e.g. *myc*)
5. Cyclic nucleotide binding activity disrupting intracellular signalling (e.g. *ras*).

Oncogenes may be activated by:

A. Translocation — this is often evident from the karyotype; part of one chromosome which is known to bear an oncogene may be translocated to another chromosome where a gene known to be actively 'read' is situated.
B. Mutation.

C. Amplification — this can be recognized in chromosome preparations from tumour cells by the presence of homogeneously staining regions and double minute chromosomes.

Altered oncogene expression can result in either:

a. normal quantities of the oncoprotein molecule altered by mutation in such a way that it is abnormally active, or
b. normal oncoprotein produced in excessive quantities because of gene amplification or enhanced transcription.

Mutant oncoproteins may have less or greater biological activity than the normal molecule. This can have profound effects on receptor function and intracellular signalling.

Increased expression of oncogenes has been found in many tumours and may be detected by:

a. the presence of more of the oncogene product (oncoprotein) within the cells
b. increased production of mRNA transcripts of the oncogene
c. increased numbers of copies of the oncogene in the genome.

It is important to remember that no single oncogene is capable of promoting and inducing all of the biological properties required for tumour formation by itself. Oncogenes may co-operate with each other and multiple oncogene abnormalities are usually present within a single tumour. A distinction must be drawn between molecular analysis and the use of antibodies (monoclonal or polyclonal) to the oncogene protein product. The emphasis in this chapter will be on the findings of molecular analysis rather than immunohistochemistry.

Tumour suppressor genes (anti-oncogenes)

Anti-oncogenes or tumour suppressor genes are important in the negative control of cell growth (Tidy & Wrede, 1992). Mutations causing a loss, rather than gain, of function are associated with malignant development. The retinoblastoma (Rb-1) and p53 genes are members of this group of genes. There continues to be intense interest in the molecular pathology of p53.

p53 is a nuclear phosphoprotein, the gene for which has been cloned and localized to chromosome 17p13. The p53 gene was originally considered to be an oncogene, but is now believed to have the properties of a tumour suppressor gene (Levin et al, 1991). The current view regards the rôle of wild-type p53 as being that of the 'guardian of the genome', responsible for halting progression through the G1/S boundary of the cell cycle to allow time for DNA repair or, if cellular damage is too severe, inducing apoptosis. The association of p53 with human carcinogenesis is now well established with mutations in this tumour suppressor gene representing the most common genetic abnormality observed. Such mutations cause loss of suppressor function and induction of growth-promoting potential. Its rôle may also depend on the level of remaining wild-type p53 protein in the cell (Vogelstein & Kinzler, 1993).

Vulva, vagina and cervix

Human papillomaviruses

Certain 'high risk' types of human papillomaviruses (particularly HPV 16 and 18 but also HPV 31, 33, 35 and others) occur more frequently in high-grade cervical intraepithelial neoplasia (CIN) and invasive cervical squamous carcinoma. The most important potential application for HPV typing is in cervical cytology and, in particular, in the assessment of women with mildly abnormal (dyskaryotic) smears. Two things are becoming increasingly clear: firstly, women with a mildly dyskaryotic smear in the presence of HPV type 16 are at greater risk of harbouring a more severe histological lesion (Bavin et al, 1993); secondly, there is a greater risk of neoplastic progression from mild dyskaryosis in the presence of HPV type 16 (Gaarenstroom et al, 1994).

Integration of the viral genome into host DNA is usual in these lesions and the protein coding sequences of the viral early (E) or late (L) open reading frames appear to have a major rôle in oncogenesis (Scurry & Wells, 1992; Wells, 1992). Viral infection with integration usually occurs specifically, disrupting the genome between the E2 and L2 or L1 open reading frames, resulting in loss of the E2 regulatory protein and late regions associated with structural proteins, but increased expression of the transforming E6 and E7 regions (Thierry, 1993). The cell target appears to be basal squamous epithelial cells; in normal proliferating cells, transcription of the viral genes is regulated by host inhibitory factors which must be inactivated before transformation can occur.

The E6 protein of HPV 16 is capable of binding to cellular p53 protein to form a complex which neutralizes the normal function of p53. Binding capacity correlates with the in vivo transforming activity of different papillomavirus types. E6 protein from the 'benign' or 'low risk' HPV types 6 and 11 for example does not appear to form a complex with p53 (Werness et al, 1990). Co-operation of HPV E6 and cellular oncogenes c-*myc* and H-*ras*, which are inactivated in many cases of human cervical cancers, may be necessary to completely overcome the anti-oncogenic function of p53 in these tumours (Chen & Defendi, 1992). In vitro, complexed E6 promotes degradation of p53 via the ubiquitin-dependent protease system suggesting a possible route for deregulation of cell growth (Huibregtse et al, 1993). Replicative DNA repair after

damage requires wild-type p53; HPV 16 E6 has been shown to disrupt the normal response of cervical epithelial cells to DNA damage mediated by p53 and may thereby also allow the accumulation of genetic abnormalities associated with cervical oncogenesis (Kessis et al, 1993a).

Mutation of the p53 gene does not appear to be a common event in cervical carcinogenesis (Kessis et al, 1993b). Several studies have now reported an inverse relationship between the presence of HPV DNA and that of p53 gene mutation both in primary cervical carcinomas (Crook et al, 1992) and cell lines (Scheffner et al, 1991). The attractive hypothesis is therefore that p53 is inactivated in cervical carcinoma, either by complexing with HPV 16 protein (in HPV-positive tumours), or by p53 gene mutation in those that are HPV negative. This has not, however, been a consistent finding and other workers have shown that inactivation of the p53 gene by allelic loss or by point mutation is infrequent in cervical cancer, irrespective of the presence or absence of HPV infection (Fujita et al, 1992; Paquette et al, 1993; Busby-Earle et al, 1994). Such discrepancies raise the possibility of different pathogenetic factors being involved. Crook & Vousden have identified p53 point mutations in metastases arising from HPV-positive cervical carcinomas suggesting that acquisition of p53 mutation may play a rôle in the progression of some HPV-associated primary cancers (Crook & Vousden, 1992).

The results from immunohistochemistry have been somewhat confusing. Overexpression of p53 protein has generally been assumed to reflect p53 mutation, since wild-type protein is not usually demonstrable by immunohistochemistry. Recent reports suggest that p53 immunoreactivity does not correlate with mutation but may reflect the change of wild type from a suppressor to a promoter during the cell growth response, or a longer half-life of the protein due to binding by another protein (Cooper et al, 1993; Helland et al, 1993).

The prognostic significance of an established invasive cervical carcinoma being positive for human papillomaviruses is controversial. There is evidence in the literature that human papillomavirus detection in squamous cell carcinomas confers a better prognosis though a worsened prognosis for HPV type 18 positive tumours has been reported (Riou et al, 1990; Higgins et al, 1991; Girardi et al, 1992; Arends et al, 1993). Recently it has been suggested that there is a good prognosis group of tumours with HPV type 31,16 and 'unknown' and a poor prognosis group consisting of HPV type 33 and 18 and HPV-negative cases (Hagmar et al in press).

Human papillomaviruses are possibly also implicated in the aetiology of adenocarcinoma of the cervix though the relationship is less clear than is the case for squamous carcinoma since most studies show a lower incidence of infection than squamous neoplasia in both in situ and invasive adenocarcinoma. Types 16, 18 and 33 may be identified and type 18 seems to be predominant (Griffin et al, 1991; Duggan et al, 1993; Milde-Langosch et al, 1993; Duggan M A et al, 1994).

Smoking has been associated on epidemiological grounds with an increased risk of cervical neoplasia. Characteristic smoking-related DNA additional products have been demonstrated in cervical tissue and a significant difference in their levels detected between current and non-current smokers (Simons et al, 1993; Ali et al, 1994). Such findings suggest a causal relationship between smoking and cervical neoplasia. The carcinogenic constituents of cigarette smoke are likely to be important cofactors along with high risk human papillomavirus types in the aetiology of cervical neoplasia.

Oncogenes

The ras gene family has three main members: Harvey (Ha-ras), Kirsten (Ki-ras) and neuroblastoma (N-ras), which each code for a 21 000 protein product termed p21. p21 functions as a signal transducer relaying messages from the plasma membrane to intracytoplasmic effectors. The ras gene has been associated with a number of malignancies through various mechanisms including overexpression, mutation and amplification.

The oncogenes of the myc family code for products which localize to the nucleus, are elevated upon stimulation by mitogenic stimuli or growth factors, and probably affect transcription by binding to regulatory DNA regions or small ribonucleoproteins. The myc gene may be activated by rearrangement or amplification. It codes for a gene product known as p62 which may also be overexpressed.

Harvey ras is amplified as well as overexpressed in the majority of cervical carcinomas (Curling & Watson, 1992). It has been suggested that overexpression of c-myc is a significant independent indicator of the risk of overall relapse and distant metastases, even in early stage cervical carcinoma (Riou et al, 1992).

Endometrium

Endometrial hyperplasia and adenocarcinoma

Endometrial carcinomas have been shown to have mutations of Ki-ras, amplification of myc, c-erb-B2 and p53 mutation. Several reports have suggested that point mutations in codon 12 of Ki-ras are significant events in the aetiology of adenocarcinoma of the endometrium (Enomoto et al, 1991b; Ignar-Trowbridge et al, 1992; Imamura et al, 1992; Sasaki et al, 1993; Duggan B D et al, 1994). Other reports have failed to confirm this and have argued that the presence of Ki-ras does not contribute to the differential diagnosis of hyperplasia and carcinoma or predict the biological behaviour of established endometrial cancer (Sato et al, 1991). The fms oncogene encodes the receptor for macrophage colony-stimulating factor (CSF-1). fms mRNA has been identified in proliferative, but not secretory, endometrium as well as in endometrial adenocarcinoma. In general, much higher levels of mRNA were observed in malignant as compared to benign tissues and were associated with disease of high stage and grade (Kacinski et al, 1988).

A high degree of c-myc amplification has been reported in advanced stage disease, poorly-differentiated lesions and serous papillary adenocarcinoma (Borst et al, 1990). In a study of erb-B2 amplification in endometrial adenocarcinomas by Borst et al (1990), 11/16 had multiple copies of the gene and those patients with amplification had more advanced stage disease and poorly-differentiated lesions, a finding supported by others (Berchuk et al, 1991). Sasano et al (1990a) studied serous papillary carcinomas of the endometrium but observed no erb-B2 amplifications. At present such abnormalities are not established as prognostic indicators in endometrial cancer.

p53 mutations have also been demonstrated in human endometrial lesions (Okamoto et al, 1991a; Kohler et al, 1992; Honda et al, 1993). A recent report has shown p53 mutations in atypical endometrial hyperplasias identical to those seen in some endometrial cancers. Such mutations were not seen in endometrial hyperplasia without cytological atypia (Enomoto et al, 1993). These findings have not, however, been supported by others (Kohler et al, 1993c).

Ovary

Studies of families of ovarian cancer patients have shown that their sisters and mothers have approximately a five-fold increased risk of developing ovarian cancer (Easton & Peto, 1990). Of all the common cancers, this is the largest excess risk to relatives and argues for genetic susceptibility. Family studies also show that first degree relatives are at increased risk of breast cancer, leading to the suggestion of a common genetic mechanism. This suggestion has been partially confirmed by the recognition that a rare dominant gene termed BRCA-1, which has recently been mapped to chromosome 17q, increases the risk of cancer at both sites (Smith et al, 1992; Feunteun et al, 1993; Smith et al, 1993). An analysis of 214 families showed that for women carrying a mutation in this gene, the risk by the age of 60 for breast cancer was 0.54, for ovarian cancer was 0.30 and for either cancer was 0.68 (Easton et al, 1993).

Clinically, three distinct types of families with apparent predisposition to ovarian cancer are recognized:

1. Rare families in which the predisposition appears to be entirely to ovarian cancer
2. Families predisposed to both breast and ovarian cancers

3. Families with the Lynch type II syndrome with susceptibility to ovarian cancers and a variety of other cancers.

A number of other studies have investigated the genetic profile of ovarian neoplasia (Berek et al, 1993; Bast et al, 1994). They have shown a complicated loss of genetic material which changes between low- and high-grade tumours, stage of tumour and type of tumour. It is known that p53 is definitely implicated in ovarian neoplasia, with 36% of cases demonstrating point mutations (Marks et al, 1991; Mazars et al, 1991; Okamoto et al, 1991b; Eccles et al, 1992a; Jacobs et al, 1992; Kohler et al, 1993a,b; Milner et al, 1993; Berchuk et al, 1994). The rôle of the DCC (deleted in colon cancer) gene is more controversial with several authors reporting loss in the region of 18q but whether it is the DCC gene or a different region of 18q between D18S5 and D18S11 is controversial (Chenevix-Trench et al, 1992). Loss on 17q is frequent and may involve the breast/ovary cancer gene (Eccles et al, 1992b; Cliby et al, 1993; Foulkes et al, 1993a; Jacobs et al, 1993). Loss has been reported at sites close to known tumour suppressor genes on 5q, 13q and 8p (Gallion et al, 1992). Other frequently abnormal sites without known cancer tumour suppressor genes are on 11p, 6p and 6q, 9q and 14q (Foulkes et al, 1993a,b). Thus uncertainty still surrounds the actual tumour suppressor genes damaged.

The erbB-2 (HER-2/neu) oncogene encodes a protein kinase transmembrane receptor which binds a ligand similar to epidermal growth factor. The erbB-2 gene product is expressed by the ovarian surface epithelium of normal adult ovaries, although fetal expression has not been demonstrated (Press et al, 1990). Amplification of the erbB-2 gene is found in about 30% of ovarian cancers and it has been suggested that amplification and overexpression may be associated with a poor prognosis (Berchuk et al, 1990; Rubin et al, 1994).

Enomoto et al (1991a) have reported Ki-ras mutations in 27% of 37 ovarian tumours, particularly in mucinous cystadenocarcinomas, but overall their detection appears to be of no clinicopathological value in ovarian neoplasia. Amplification of the myc gene has been reported in up to 50% of ovarian malignancies (correlating with degree of nuclear atypia, increased mitotic activity and serous type tumours) but not in benign or borderline tumours (Sasano et al, 1990b; Schreiber & Dubeau, 1990). Over-expression of fms mRNA correlates with aggressive clinicopathological features (high stage and grade) in ovarian cancer (Kacinski et al, 1990).

Germ cell neoplasms

Germ cells undergo meiosis and by comparing heterozygous host markers to those markers seen in tumours, the stage of meiotic development that the tumour stem cell attained prior to neoplastic transformation can be de-termined (Mutter, 1992). The extent to which the tumour stem cell has progressed through meiotic development prior to neoplastic transformation correlates with histological subtype and natural history. When applied to mature ovarian teratomas, marker studies indicate various stages of neoplastic transformation (Dahl et al, 1990; Deka et al, 1990; Surti et al, 1990). The majority of ovarian mature cystic teratomas arise from an oocyte that has completed the first meiotic division, in a manner analogous to parthenogenesis. While essentially all post-meiosis 1 derived female germ cell tumours are benign, mature cystic teratomas or low-grade immature teratomas, pre-meiosis 1 lesions fall into several discrete subsets:

1. Pre-M1 immature teratomas tend to have worse prognostic features, such as aneuploidy compared to euploidy in post-M1 cases.
2. Multiple mature teratomas tend to be pre-M1.
3. Malignant tumours of embryonic histology (dysgerminoma, embryonal carcinoma, yolk sac tumour, mixed germ cell tumour) are always pre-M1. These, like their testicular counterparts, frequently have specific chromosomal abnormalities (Gibas & Talerman, 1993).

A non-random marker chromosome composed of two attached short arms of chromosome 12, an isochromosome of 12p or i(12p), has long been known to be present in 70–90% of testicular germ cell tumours and is very specific to these tumours. The number of comparable ovarian lesions that have been fully karyotyped is very small, but the accumulated sporadic reports indicate that this marker chromosome is frequently present in ovarian dysgerminomas (Atkin & Baker, 1987) and yolk sac tumours (Speleman et al, 1990; Vos et al, 1990).

Patients with dysgenetic gonads have a greatly increased risk of developing some types of germ cell tumours, especially gonadoblastoma. The risk for developing gonadoblastoma in a dysgenetic setting is highest when Y chromosome sequences can be documented directly, as by karyotype, or indirectly by detection of Y chromosome-derived proteins such as HY antigen. Molecular methods for identification of Y chromosome sequences in paraffin-embedded, fresh, or fixed tissues include PCR (Mutter & Pomponio, 1991) and fluorescent in situ hybridization (FISH). Fresh tissue may be suitable for karyotypic analysis. However, some patients who exhibit no cytological evidence of a Y chromosome have small portions of the Y chromosome if studied by more sensitive and specific molecular techniques (Shah et al, 1988).

The placenta

In situ hybridization has been applied to placentas for the detection of structural and numerical chromosomal abnormalities and for the detection of virus infections. In situ hybridization on chorionic villus biopsy has been successfully used in prenatal diagnosis for the confirmation of small structural abnormalities (Zahed et al, 1992). The validity of prenatal screening for numerical abnormalities for chromosomes 1,13,16,18,21, X and Y by means of fluorescence in situ hybridization (FISH) applied to interphase nuclei from fresh chorionic villus samples is still under debate (American College of Medical Genetics, 1993; Pandya et al, 1994).

Zahed et al (1992) carried out a preliminary study, wherein fresh interphase nuclei from 6 chorionic villus biopsies were obtained and probes for chromosome 13 and 21, 18, X and Y were used. They concluded that trisomy 18, X and Y can efficiently be detected but that the probe for chromosome 13 and 21 is inefficient. Pandya et al (1994) came to the same conclusion: ISH can be reliably applied to estimate fetal sex, trisomy 18, triploidy and monosomy X but not for detection of trisomy 21 and 13. The amount of information given by FISH never reaches that provided by traditional karyotyping. However, it can be very useful if rapid diagnosis is needed after ultrasonographic detection of congenital abnormalities or in pregnancies complicated by a high serum alphafetoprotein.

Interphase in situ hybridization has been applied to archival material of abortions and hydatidiform moles (Van de Kaa et al, 1991, 1993). In an attempt to discriminate hydropic abortions and partial moles from complete moles Van de Kaa et al (1991, 1993) estimated ploidy of, respectively, 7 and 23 abortions by in situ hybridization for chromosome 1, X and Y on whole tissue sections. In situ hybridization combined with image DNA cytometric analysis can contribute to the differential diagnosis between complete mole, partial mole and hydropic abortions.

FISH analysis of interphase nuclei of archival abortion material has also been compared to conventional karyotyping to see whether it could be used for retrospective analysis (chromosome 1,16,18,X,Y) (Van Lijnschoten et al, 1994). These chromosomes are involved in about 80% of all chromosomally abnormal spontaneous abortions. In 14 out of 18 cases the results matched completely. In three cases placental mosaicism and maternal contamination could account for the differences found. The remaining case could be explained by the assumption that the extra material was derived from chromosome 18. These studies only give information about numerical abnormalities of the chromosomes under investigation. In future comparative genomic hybridization might overcome this disadvantage.

Gestational trophoblastic disease

Complete moles

Most techniques confirm that complete moles are diploid and of paternal origin, having arisen by androgenesis with loss or inactivation of the oocyte nucleus. Fertilization may occur by a haploid sperm which duplicates or a diploid sperm which fails to undergo meiotic division resulting in a diploid homozygous complete mole (46,XX, with 46,YY apparently non-viable). A third method is synchronous fertilization by two haploid sperm resulting in diploid heterozygous complete mole (46,XX or 46,YY). Cases of triploidy or tetraploidy are also considered to lack the maternal contribution (Lane et al, 1992).

Partial moles

These arise with diploid fertilization of the oocyte but with retention of the female nucleus. They are XXX or XXY, rarely XYY, and are homozygous or heterozygous for the paternal contribution (Lane et al, 1992).

It seems likely that the excess paternal contribution therefore contributes to the development of molar disease, particularly if the maternal influence is completely lost as in complete mole. It would be expected that choriocarcinoma following complete mole would arise from paternally derived DNA. However, Azuma et al (1990) used restriction fragment length polymorphism analysis and showed that either maternal or paternal contributions were present.

The relative DNA content of molar disease has been investigated by cytogenetic analysis, flow cytometry, and AgNORs. Whilst giving valuable assessment of ploidy, only cytogenetics gives the relative maternal:paternal contribution but this may be problematic in routine diagnosis. There is a requirement for fresh tissue and specialist centres, interpretation of some chromosomal patterns may be difficult and there may be failure of growth in culture.

DNA fingerprinting has been used on fresh molar material to confirm the androgenetic origin of complete moles or to make the diagnosis in difficult cases (Fisher et al, 1989; Saji et al, 1989; Nobunaga et al, 1990; Takahashi et al, 1990). These assessments have confirmed the previous cytogenetic analyses of DNA parental contributions of complete and partial mole. The pieces of DNA required, however, are too large for extraction from archival material.

The smaller micro-satellites can be detected in material extracted from fresh or routinely processed specimens. These polymorphisms have alleles which may differ in length by only two base pairs and are not detectable by gel electrophoresis or Southern blotting. They can be amplified using the PCR technique so that they may be detected on a sequencing gel, using radioactive or fluorescent probes (Fisher & Newlands, 1993; Lane et al, 1993).

With both these techniques, if only paternal alleles are present, the gestation is confirmed as a complete mole. If unique maternal sequences are present, then complete mole is excluded. The latter situation may arise, however, with partial mole, hydropic abortion or in cases where the polymorphisms are not unique to either parent and further investigation is necessary. Peripheral blood may be used for comparison to confirm that maternal and paternal alleles are the same and not diagnostic. A panel of highly polymorphic sequences will give a higher probability of finding unique, diagnostic alleles.

Quantitative PCR using fluorescent probes and gene scanning equipment will determine the relative contribution of each allele and thus give the ploidy and parental contribution with the same test. This should be a rapid and useful method, not only of confirming the diploid androgenetic complete mole, but also of investigation into the nature of triploid partial moles, hydropic abortuses and cases of tetraploidy.

REFERENCES

Ali S, Astley S B, Sheldon T A, Peel K R, Wells M 1994 Detection and measurement of DNA adducts in the cervix of smokers and non-smokers. International Journal of Gynecological Cancer 4: 188–193.

American College of Medical Genetics 1993 Prenatal interphase fluorescence in situ hybridization (FISH): policy statement. American Journal of Medical Genetics 53: 526–527.

Arends M J, Bird C C 1992 Recombinant DNA technology and its diagnostic applications. Histopathology 21: 303–313.

Arends M J, Donaldson Y K, Duvall E et al 1993 Human papillomavirus type 18 associates with more advanced cervical neoplasia than human papillomavirus type 16. Human Pathology 24: 432–437.

Atkin N B, Baker M C 1987 Abnormal chromosomes including small metacentrics in 14 ovarian cancers. Cancer Genetics and Cytogenetics 26: 355–361.

Azuma C, Saji F, Nobunaga T et al 1990 Studies on the pathogenesis of choriocarcinoma by analysis of restriction fragment length polymorphisms. Cancer Research 50: 488–491.

Bast R C, Boyer C M, Xu F J et al 1994 Selected molecular targets for diagnosis and therapy and epithelial ovarian cancer. Cancer Molecular Biology 1: 87–93.

Bavin P J, Giles J A, Deery A et al 1993 Use of semi-quantitative PCR for human papillomavirus type 16 to identify women with high grade cervical disease in a population presenting with a mildly dyskaryotic smear report. British Journal of Cancer 67: 602–605.

Bennett P, Moore G 1992 Molecular biology for obstetricians and gynaecologists. Blackwell Scientific Publications, Oxford.

Berchuk A, Kamel A, Whitaker R et al 1990 Overexpression of HER-2/neu is associated with poor survival in advanced epithelial ovarian cancer. Cancer Research 50: 4087–4091.

Berchuk A, Rodriguez G, Kinney R B et al 1991 Overexpression of HER-2/neu in endometrial cancer is associated with advanced stage disease. American Journal of Obstetrics and Gynecology 164: 15–21.

Berchuk A, Kohler M F, Marks J R, Wiseman R, Boyd J, Bast R C 1994 The p53 tumour suppressor gene frequently is altered in gynecologic cancers. American Journal of Obstetrics and Gynecology 170: 246–252.

Berek J S, Martinez-Maza O, Hamilton T et al 1993 Molecular and biological factors in the pathogenesis of ovarian cancer. Annals of Oncology 4: 53–116.

Borst M P, Baker V V, Dixon D, Hatch K D, Shingleton H M, Miller D M 1990 Oncogene alterations in endometrial carcinoma. Gynecologic Oncology 38: 364–366.

Busby-Earle R M C, Steel C M, Williams A R W, Cohen B, Bird C C 1994 p53 mutations in cervical carcinogenesis: low frequency and lack of correlation with human papillomavirus status. British Journal of Cancer 69: 732–737.

Chen T M, Defendi V 1992 Functional interaction of p53 with HPV 8 E6, c-myc and H-ras in 3t3 cells. Oncogene 7: 1541–1547.

Chenevix-Trench G, Leary J, Kerr J et al 1992 Frequent loss of heterozygosity on chromosome 18 in ovarian adenocarcinoma which does not always include the DCC locus. Oncogene 7: 1059–1065.

Cliby W, Ritland S, Hartmann L et al 1993 Human epithelial ovarian cancer allelotype. Cancer Research 53: 2393–2398.

Cooper K, Herrington C S, Evans M F, Gatter K C, McGee J O'D 1993 p53 antigen in cervical condylomata, intraepithelial neoplasia and carcinoma: relationship to HPV infection and integration. Journal of Pathology 171: 27–34.

Crook T, Vousden K H 1992 Properties of p53 mutations detected in primary and secondary cervical cancers suggest mechanisms of metastasis and involvement of environment carcinogens. EMBO Journal 11: 3935–3940.

Crook T, Wrede D, Tidy J A, Mason W P, Evans D J, Vousden K H 1992 Clonal p53 mutation in primary cervical cancer: association with human papillomavirus-negative tumours. Lancet 239: 1070–1073.

Curling M, Watson J V 1992 Oncogenes in gynaecological cancer. In: Lowe D, Fox H (eds) Advances in gynaecological pathology. Churchill Livingstone, Edinburgh, pp 63–78.

Dahl N, Gustavson K H, Rune C, Gustavsson I, Pettersson U 1990 Benign ovarian teratomas: an analysis of their cellular origin. Cancer Genetics and Cytogenetics 46: 115–123.

Deka R, Chakravarti A, Surti U et al 1990 Genetics and biology of human ovarian teratomas. II. Molecular analysis of origin of nondisjunction and gene-centromere mapping of chromosome I markers. American Journal of Human Genetics 47: 644–655.

Duggan B D, Felix J C, Muderspach L I, Tsao J L, Shibata D K 1994 Early mutational activation of the c-ki-ras oncogene in endometrial carcinoma. Cancer Research 54: 1604–1607.

Duggan M A, Benoit J L, McGregor S E, Nation J G, Inoue M, Stuart G C E 1993 The human papillomavirus status of 114 endocervical adenocarcinoma cases by dot blot hybridization. Human Pathology 24: 121–125.

Duggan M A, Benoit J L, McGregor S E, Inoue M, Nation J G, Stuart G C E 1994 Adenocarcinoma in situ of the endocervix: human papillomavirus determination by dot blot hybridisation and polymerase chain reaction amplification. International Journal of Gynecological Pathology 13: 143–149.

Easton D F, Peto J 1990 The contribution of inherited predisposition to cancer incidence. Cancer Surveys 9: 395–416.

Easton D F, Bishop D T, Ford D, Crockford G P 1993 Genetic linkage analysis in familial breast and ovarian cancer: results from 214 families. American Journal of Human Genetics 52: 678–701.

Eccles D M, Brett L, Lessells A et al 1992a Overexpression of the p53 protein and allele loss at 17p13 in ovarian carcinoma. British Journal of Cancer 65: 40–44.

Eccles D M, Russell S E H, Haites N E et al 1992b Early loss of heterozygosity on 17q in ovarian cancer. Oncogene 7: 2069–2072.

Enomoto T, Weghorst C, Inoue M, Tanizawa O, Rice J 1991a K-ras activation occurs frequently in mucinous adenocarcinomas and rarely in other common epithelial tumors of the ovary. American Journal of Pathology 139: 777–785.

Enomoto T, Inoue M, Perantoni A et al 1991b K-ras activation in premalignant and malignant epithelial lesions of the human uterus. Cancer Research 51: 5304–5314.

Enomoto T, Fujita M, Inoue M et al 1993 Alterations of the p53 tumor suppressor gene and its association with activation of the c-K-ras-2 protooncogene in premalignant and malignant lesions of the human uterine endometrium. Cancer Research 53: 1883–1888.

Feunteun J, Narod S A, Lynch H T et al 1993 A breast-ovarian cancer susceptibility gene maps to chromosome 17q21. American Journal of Human Genetics 52: 736–742.

Fisher R A, Povey S, Jeffreys A J, Martin C A, Patel I, Lawler S D 1989 Frequency of heterozygous complete hydatidiform moles, estimated by locus-specific minisatellite and Y chromosome-specific probes. Human Genetics 82: 259–263.

Fisher R E, Newlands E S 1993 Rapid diagnosis and classification of hydatidiform moles with polymerase chain reaction. American Journal of Obstetrics and Gynecology 168: 563–569.

Foulkes W D, Black D M, Stamp G W H, Solomon E, Trowsdale J 1993a Very frequent loss of heterozygosity throughout chromosome 17 in sporadic ovarian carcinoma. International Journal of Cancer 54: 220–225.

Foulkes W D, Campbell T G, Stamp G W, Trowsdale J 1993b Loss of heterozygosity and amplification on chromosome 11q in human ovarian cancer. British Journal of Cancer 67: 268–273.

Foulkes W D, Ragoussis J, Stamp G W H, Alan G J, Trowsdale J W 1993c Frequent loss of heterozygosity on chromosome 6 in human ovarian carcinoma. British Journal of Cancer 67: 551–559.

Fujita M, Inoue M, Tanizawa O, Iwamoto S, Enomoto T 1992 Alterations of the p53 gene in human primary cervical carcinoma with and without human papillomavirus infection. Cancer Research 52: 5323–5328.

Gaarenstroom K N, Melkert P, Walboomers J M M et al 1994 Human papillomavirus DNA and genotypes: prognostic factors for progression of cervical intraepithelial neoplasia. International Journal of Gynecological Cancer 4: 73–78.

Gallion H H, Powell D E, Morrow J K et al 1992 Molecular genetic changes in human epithelial ovarian malignancies. Gynecologic Oncology 47: 137–142.

Gibas Z, Talerman A 1993 Analysis of chromosome aneuploidy in ovarian dysgerminoma by flow cytometry and fluorescence in situ hybridization. Diagnostic Molecular Pathology 2: 50–56.

Girardi F, Fuchs P, Haas J 1992 Prognostic importance of human papillomavirus type 16 DNA in cervical cancer. Cancer 69: 2502–2504.

Griffin N R, Dockley D, Lewis F A, Wells M 1991 Demonstration of low frequency of human papillomavirus DNA in cervical adenocarcinoma and adenocarcinoma in situ by the polymerase chain reaction and in situ hybridization. International Journal of Gynecological Pathology 10: 36–43.

Grompe M 1993 The rapid detection of unknown mutations in nucleic acids. Nature Genetics 5: 111–117.

Gruis N A, Abeln E C A, Bardoel A F J, Devileep, Franks R R, Cornelisse C J 1993 PCR-based microsatellite polymorphisms in the detection of loss of heterozygosity in fresh and archival tumour tissue. British Journal of Cancer 68: 308–313.

Hagmar B, Platz-Christensen J J, Johansson B et al 1995 HPV type in cervical squamous cell carcinoma; implications for survival. International Journal of Gynecological Cancer (in press).

Helland A, Hollm R, Kristensen G et al 1993 Genetic alterations of the TP53 gene, p53 protein expression and HPV infection in primary cervical carcinomas. Journal of Pathology 171: 105–107.

Herrington C S, McGee J O'D 1992 Diagnostic molecular pathology: a practical approach. IRL Press, Oxford.

Higgins G D, Davy M, Roder D, Uzelin D M, Philips G E, Burrell C H 1991 Increased age and mortality associated with cervical carcinomas negative for human papillomavirus RNA. Lancet 338: 910–913.

Honda T, Kato H, Imamura T et al 1993 Involvement of p53 gene mutations in human endometrial carcinomas. International Journal of Cancer 53: 963–967.

Huibregste J M, Scheffner M, Howley P M 1993 Cloning and expression of the cDNA for E6-AP, a protein that mediates the interaction of the human papillomavirus E6 oncoprotein with p53. Molecular and Cell Biology 13: 775–784.

Ignar-Trowbridge D, Risinger J I, Dent G A et al 1992 Mutations of the Ki-ras oncogene in endometrial carcinoma. American Journal of Obstetrics and Gynecology 167: 227–232.

Imamura T, Arima T, Karo H, Miyamoto S, Sasazuki T, Wake N 1992 Chromosomal deletions and K-ras gene mutations in human endometrial carcinomas. International Journal of Cancer 51: 47–52.

Jacobs I J, Kohler M F, Wiseman R W et al 1992 Clonal origin of epithelial ovarian carcinoma: analysis by loss of heterozygosity, p53 mutation and X-chromosome inactivation. Journal of the National Cancer Institute 84: 1793–1798.

Jacobs I J, Smith S A, Wiseman R W et al 1993 A deletion unit on chromosome 17q in epithelial ovarian tumors distal to the breast/ovarian cancer locus. Cancer Research 53: 1218–1221.

Jeffreys A J, Wilson V, Thein S L 1985 Individual-specific "fingerprints" of human DNA. Nature 316: 76–79.

Kacinski B M, Carter D, Mittal K et al 1989 High level of expression of fms proto-oncogene mRNA is observed in clinically aggressive human endometrial adenocarcinomas. International Journal of Radiation Oncology, Biology and Physics 15: 823–829.

Kacinski B M, Carter D, Mittal K et al 1990 Ovarian adenocarcinomas express fms-complementary transcripts and fms antigen, often with co-expression of CSF-1. American Journal of Pathology 137: 134–147.

Kallioniemi A, Kallioniemi O P, Sudar D et al 1992 Comparative genomic hybridization for molecular cytogenetic analysis of solid tumours. Science 258: 818–821.

Kessis T D, Slebos R J, Nelson W G et al 1993a Human papillomavirus 16 E6 expression disrupts the p53-mediated cellular response to DNA damage. Proceedings of the National Academy of Sciences USA 90: 3988–3992.

Kessis T D, Slebos R J, Han S M et al 1993b p53 gene mutations and MDMZ amplification are uncommon in primary carcinomas of the uterine cervix. American Journal of Pathology 143: 1398–1405.

Kohler M F, Berchuck A, Davidoff A M et al 1992 Overexpression and mutation of p53 in endometrial carcinoma. Cancer Research 52: 1622–1627.

Kohler M F, Marks J R, Wiseman R W et al 1993a Spectrum of mutation and frequency of allelic deletion of the p53 gene in ovarian cancer. Journal of the National Cancer Institute 85: 1513–1519.

Kohler M F, Kerns B J M, Humphrey P A, Marks J R, Bast R C, Berchuk A 1993b Mutation and overexpression of p53 in early-stage epithelial ovarian cancer. Obstetrics and Gynecology 81: 643–650.

Kohler M F, Nishii H, Humphrey P A et al 1993c Mutation of the p53 tumor-suppressor gene is not a feature of endometrial hyperplasia. American Journal of Obstetrics and Gynecology 169: 690–694.

Lane S A, Taylor G R, Quirke P 1992 The diagnosis of molar disease. In: Lowe D, Fox H (eds) Advances in gynaecological pathology. Churchill Livingstone, Edinburgh, pp 235–260.

Lane S, Taylor G R, Ozols B, Quirke P 1993 Diagnosis of complete molar pregnancy by microsatellites in archival material. Journal of Clinical Pathology 46: 346–348.

Levin A J, Momand J, Finlay C A 1991 The p53 tumor suppressor gene. Nature 351: 453–456.

Lewis F A, Wells M 1992 Detection of virus in infected human tissue by in situ hybridization. In: Wilkinson D G (ed) In situ hybridisation: a practical approach. Oxford University Press, Oxford, pp 121–136.

Marks J R, Davidoff A M; Kerns B J et al 1991 Overexpression and mutation of p53 in epithelial ovarian cancer. Cancer Research 51: 2979–2984.

Marshall C J 1991 Tumor suppressor genes. Cell 64: 313–326.

Mazars R, Pujol P, Maudelonde T, Jeanteur P, Theillet C 1991 p53 mutations in ovarian cancer: a late event. Oncogene 6: 1685–1690.

Milde-Langosch K, Schreiber C, Becker G 1993 Human papillomavirus detection in cervical adenocarcinoma by polymerase chain reaction. Human Pathology 24: 590–594.

Milner B J, Allen L A, Eccles D M et al 1993 p53 mutation is a common genetic event in ovarian carcinoma. Cancer Research 539: 2128–2132.

Mutter G L 1992 Germ cell neoplasia: molecular genetics. Course notes: The Molecular Biology of Women's Health: Breast and Reproductive Tract, Harvard Medical School.

Mutter G L, Pomponio R J 1991 Molecular diagnosis of sex chromosome aneuploidy using quantitative PCR. Nucleic Acids Research 19: 4203–4207.

Nobunaga T, Azuma C, Kimura T et al 1990 Differential diagnosis between complete mole and hydropic abortus by deoxyribonucleic acid fingerprints. American Journal of Obstetrics and Gynecology 163: 634–638.

Nuovo G 1992 PCR in situ hybridisation: protocols and applications. Raven Press, New York.

Nuovo G J, MacConnell P, Forde A, Delvenne P 1991 Detection of human papillomavirus DNA in formalin-fixed tissues by in situ hybridisation after amplification by polymerase chain reaction. American Journal of Pathology 139: 847–854.

Okamoto A, Sameshima Y, Yamada Y et al 1991a Allelic loss of chromosome 17p and p53 mutations in human endometrial carcinoma of the uterus. Cancer Research 51: 5632–5636.

Okamoto A, Sameshima Y, Yokoyama S et al 1991b Frequent allelic losses and mutations of the p53 gene in human ovarian cancer. Cancer Research 51: 5171–5176.

Pandya P P, Kuhn P, Brizot M, Cardy D L, Nicolaides K H 1994 Rapid detection of chromosomal aneuploidies in fetal blood and chorionic villi by fluorescence in situ hybridisation. British Journal of Obstetrics and Gynaecology 101: 493–497.

Paquette R L, Lee Y Y, Wilczynski S P et al 1993 Mutations of p53 and human papillomavirus infection in cervical carcinoma. Cancer 72: 1272–1280.

Persons D L, Hartmann L C, Herath J F et al 1993 Interphase molecular cytogenetic analysis of epithelial ovarian carcinomas. American Journal of Pathology 142: 733–741.

Press M F, Cordon-Cardo C, Alamon D J 1990 Expression of the HER-2/neu proto-oncogene in normal human adult and fetal tissues. Oncogene 5: 953–962.

Riou G, Farue M, Jeannel D, Bourhis J, Le Doussal V, Orth G 1990 Association between poor prognosis in early stage invasive cervical cancer and non-detection of HPV-DNA. Lancet 335: 1171–1174.

Riou G, Le M G, Favre M, Jeanell D, Bourhis J, Orth G 1992 Human papillomavirus — negative status and c-myc gene overexpression: independent prognostic indicators of distant metastasis for early stage invasive cervical cancers. Journal of the National Cancer Institute 84: 1525–1526.

Rubin S C, Finstad C L, Federici M G, Scheiner L, Lloyd K O, Hoskins W J 1994 Prevalence and significance of HER-2/neu expression in early epithelial ovarian cancer. Cancer 73: 1456–1459.

Saji F, Tokugawa Y, Kimura T et al 1989 A new approach using DNA fingerprinting for the determination of androgenesis as a cause of hydatidiform mole. Placenta 10: 399–405.

Sasaki H, Nishii H, Takahashi H et al 1993 Mutation of the Ki-ras protooncogene in human endometrial hyperplasia and carcinoma. Cancer Research 53: 1906–1910.

Sasano H, Comerford J, Wilkinson D S et al 1990a Serous papillary adenocarcinoma of the endometrium: proto-oncogene amplification, flow cytometry, estrogen and progesterone receptors and immunohistochemical analysis. Cancer 65: 1545–1551.

Sasano H, Garrett C T, Wilkinson D S, Silverberg S, Comerford J, Hyde J 1990b Proto-oncogene amplification and tumor ploidy in human ovarian neoplasms. Human Pathology 21: 382–391.

Sato S, Ito K, Ozawa N et al 1991 Analysis of point mutations at codon 12 of k-ras in human endometrial carcinoma and cervical adenocarcinoma by dot blot hybridization and polymerase chain reaction. Tohoku Journal of Experimental Medicine 165: 131–136.

Scheffner M, Munger K, Byrne J C, Howley P M 1991 The state of the p53 and retinoblastoma genes in human cervical carcinoma cell lines. Proceedings of the National Academy of Sciences USA 88: 5523–5527.

Schreiber G, Dubeau L 1990 C-myc proto-oncogene amplification detected by polymerase chain reaction in archival human ovarian carcinomas. American Journal of Pathology 137: 653–658.

Scurry J, Wells M 1992 Viruses in anogenital cancer. Epithelial Cell Biology 1: 138–145.

Shah K D, Kaffe S, Gilbert F, Dolgin S, Gertner M 1988 Unilateral microscopic gonadoblastoma in a prepubertal Turner mosaic with Y chromosome material identified by restriction fragment analysis. American Journal of Clinical Pathology 90: 622–627.

Shibata D, Hawes D, Li Z H, Hernandez A M, Spruck C H, Nichols P W 1992 Specific genetic analysis of microscopic tissue after selective ultraviolet radiation fractionation and the polymerase chain reaction. American Journal of Pathology 141: 539–543.

Simons A M, Phillips D H, Coleman D V 1993 Damage to DNA in cervical epithelium related to smoking tobacco. British Medical Journal 306: 1444–1448.

Smith S A, Easton D F, Evans D G, Ponder B A 1992 Allele losses in the region 17q12–21 in familial breast and ovarian cancer involve the wild-type chromosome. Nature Genetics 2: 128–131.

Smith S A, Easton D F, Ford D et al 1993 Genetic heterogeneity and localization of a familial breast-ovarian cancer gene on chromosome 17q12–q21. American Journal of Human Genetics 52: 767–776.

Speel A J M, Schutte B, Wiegant J, Ramaekers F C S, Hopman A H N 1992 A novel fluorescence detection method for in situ hybridization, based on the alkaline phosphatase-Fast Red reaction. Journal of Histochemistry and Cytochemistry 40: 1299–1308.

Speleman F, De Potter C, Dal Cin P et al 1990 i(12p) in a malignant ovarian tumor. Cancer Genetics and Cytogenetics 45: 49–53.

Surti U, Hoffner L, Chakravarti A, Ferrell R E 1990 Genetics and biology of human ovarian teratomas. I. Cytogenetic analysis and mechanism of origin. American Journal of Human Genetics 47: 635–643.

Takahashi H, Kanazawa K, Ikarashi T, Sudo N, Tanaka K 1990 Discrepancy in the diagnosis of hydatidiform mole by macroscopic and microscopic findings and the deoxyribonucleic acid fingerprint method. American Journal of Obstetrics and Gynecology 163: 112–113.

Templeton N S 1992 The polymerase chain reaction: history, methods and applications. Diagnostic Molecular Pathology 1: 58–72.

Thierry F 1993 Proteins involved in the control of HPV transcription. Papillomavirus Report 4: 27–32.

Tidy J A, Wrede D 1992 Tumor suppressor genes: new pathways in gynecological cancer. International Journal of Gynecological Cancer 2: 1–8.

Van de Kaa C A, Nelson K A M, Ramaekers F C S et al 1991 Interphase cytogenetics in paraffin sections of routinely processed. hydatidiform moles and hydropic abortions. Journal of Pathology 165: 281–287.

Van de Kaa C A, Hanselaar A G J M, Hopman A H N et al 1993 DNA cytometric and interphase cytogenetic analysis of paraffin-embedded hydatidiform moles and hydropic abortions. Journal of Pathology 170: 229–238.

Van Lijnschoten G, Albrechts J, Vallinga M et al 1994 Fluorescence in situ hybridization on paraffin-embedded material as a means for retrospective chromosome analysis. Human Genetics 94: 518–522.

Vogelstein B, Kinzler K W 1993 p53 function and dysfunction. Cell 70: 523–526.

Vos A, Oosterhuis J W, de Jong B et al 1990 Karyotyping and DNA flow cytometry of metastatic ovarian yolk sac tumor. Cancer Genetics and Cytogenetics 44: 223–228.

Wells M 1992 Human papillomavirus associated lesions of the lower female genital tract. In: Lowe D, Fox H (eds) Advances in gynaecological pathology. Churchill Livingstone, Edinburgh, pp 79–97.

Werness B A, Levine A J, Howley P M 1990 Association of human papillomavirus types 16 and 18 E6 proteins with p53. Science 248: 76–79.

Wilkinson D G 1992 In situ hybridisation: a practical approach. Oxford University Press, Oxford.

Wright P A, Wynford-Thomas D 1990 The polymerase chain reaction: miracle or mirage? A critical review of its uses and limitations in diagnosis and research. Journal of Pathology 162: 99–117.

Zahed L, Murere-Orlando M, Vekemans M 1992 In situ hybridization studies for the detection of common aneuploidies in CVS. Prenatal Diagnosis 12: 483–493.

Zheng J, Wan M, Zweizig S, Velicescu M, Yu M C, Dubeau L 1993 Histologically benign or low-grade malignant tumours adjacent to high-grade ovarian carcinomas contain molecular characteristics of high-grade carcinomas. Cancer Research 53: 4138–4142.

44. Immunohistochemical markers in gynaecological pathology

Elizabeth Benjamin

INTRODUCTION

The ability to detect antigens in tissue by immuno-cytochemistry has enabled pathologists to correlate morphology with functional and biochemical characteristics. Immunocytochemistry has therefore become a useful diagnostic tool and its potential range of application in gynaecological pathology continues to be widely investigated. It is in neoplastic disease, particularly ovarian neoplasms, that much of the work in this field has been concentrated. The interpretation of stains for immuno-cytochemical markers in gynaecological disease requires an understanding of the expression of these markers in normal tissues of the female genital tract and an awareness of the limitations of the techniques and markers used.

APPLICATIONS OF IMMUNOCYTOCHEMISTRY IN GYNAECOLOGICAL PATHOLOGY

Most immunocytochemical studies in gynaecological pathology have been directed towards the diagnosis and differential diagnosis of tumours. Immunohistochemistry can provide evidence of differentiation, give clues to histogenesis and, by identification of tumour products such as enzymes and hormones, give information about the functional activity of the neoplasm. Some of these tumour products may be measurable in the patient's serum and have formed the basis of the clinical monitoring of tumour markers. More recently, tumour antigens have been used as targets in antibody-directed irradiation for advanced ovarian cancer (Epenetos et al, 1986) and in imaging techniques such as radioimmunoscintigraphy (Jobling et al, 1990).

Antibodies have been commercially developed to demonstrate steroid hormone receptors, growth factors and oncogene products and may be useful in management and assessment of prognosis for patients with gynaecological cancer.

IMMUNOCYTOCHEMICAL METHODS

Immunocytochemical techniques are described in detail elsewhere (Polak & van Noorden, 1988).

Good fixation of tissue is essential for optimal preservation of antigen; both inadequate fixation and prolonged fixation may lead to loss of antigenicity. Paraffin wax-embedded fixed tissues are suitable for demonstration of many antigens and so permit the analysis of archival material. Some of the currently available monoclonal antibodies may unfortunately require the use of fresh tissue for optimal antigen detection.

Pre-treatment of paraffin wax-embedded tissue with proteolytic enzymes such as trypsin and pronase may be necessary to unmask antigenic sites. However this step is not required with all antibodies and indeed its indiscriminate use may be a source of error (Ordonez et al, 1988). More recently microwave irradiation has been employed in immunohistochemistry for antigen retrieval, as an alternative to proteolytic enzymes. Results suggest that this technique is successful in enhancing the range of antibodies that can be used to study formalin-fixed paraffin-embedded tissues. Certain antibodies that normally only react with frozen sections have been shown to work successfully in paraffin wax-embedded sections by this technique while the reactivity of other antibodies has been improved (Cattoretti et al, 1993). However, not all antibodies are suitable for use with this technique.

Immunohistochemistry is based upon antibody recognition of epitopes on target antigens, the antibody itself being labelled with a signal molecule. The signal molecule may be directly visualized, as with the use of fluorescein or rhodamine, which may be detected using ultraviolet light. In diagnostic histopathology, it is more common to use enzymes as signal molecules, the two most widely used being horseradish peroxidase and alkaline phosphatase. The signal molecule is allowed to react with a specific substrate in the presence of a chromogen to produce a coloured, insoluble reaction product. Many techniques have been introduced to increase the number of signal molecules attached to each antibody molecule, in order to enhance the sensitivity of the technique. The most commonly used techniques are:

a. Indirect immunoenzyme staining. In this technique, binding of a primary antibody to an antigen is detected by using a labelled antibody, against the primary antibody.

b. Enzyme-antienzyme technique (peroxidase, antiperoxidase, alkaline phosphatase, antialkaline phosphatase). In these techniques the primary antibodies are not labelled; instead antibodies raised against the signal enzyme molecule are used to make complexes with that molecule. These complexes can then be attached to the primary antibody through an intermediate antibody with binding sides directed both at the primary and the signal antibody. The advantage of this technique is that the enzyme labelled does not have to be chemically linked to the antibody, and the signal to antibody ratio is greatly increased by enhancing the sensitivity of the technique.

c. Avidin biotin method. This technique is based upon the binding affinity between avidin and biotin. Primary or secondary antibodies labelled with biotin are detected by using avidin, labelled with a signal molecule. Streptavidin, which has four biotin binding sites, is widely used.

In all these techniques, endogenous enzyme activity must either be recognized and discounted or blocked. Endogenous biotin may preclude the use of the avidin biotin technique in certain tissues such as the liver. All immunocytochemical procedures should incorporate appropriate controls to ensure that the results are valid.

LIMITATIONS OF IMMUNOCYTOCHEMISTRY

Discrepancies in reported immunocytochemical results occur for a variety of reasons. These include different conditions of fixation among laboratories and varying interlaboratory procedures. Tumour cell populations often exhibit considerable antigen heterogeneity (Breitenecker et al, 1989) so that tissue sampling is important. Another important cause is the different specificity of antibodies used. For example, different available antibodies to carcinoembryonic antigen (CEA) may not detect the same epitope and this may lead to discrepancies in reported detection rates of this marker in the same tumour type. Problems in the interpretation of immunocytochemical results may arise from non-specific staining as well as from cross-reactivity of antibodies. Immunohistochemistry must therefore be used as an adjunct to histopathological diagnosis on routine chromatic stains. To rely on a single antibody is dangerous and, wherever possible, a panel of antigen markers should be used. Immunocytochemical findings can be confirmed by other methods such as biochemical assays and radioimmunoassays.

OVARY

Common epithelial tumours

Tumour-associated antigens

Ovarian cancer associated or 'tumour-specific' antigens have been widely investigated. The necessity for screening markers for early detection of ovarian cancer is highlighted by the fact that more than 50% of patients are in advanced stage (stage 3 and 4) at the time of diagnosis. To date, the search for a true ovarian cancer specific antigen has proved frustrating but a number of antibodies raised against ovarian carcinoma tissue or cell lines have a rôle in diagnosis and management. Many of these antibodies have been investigated as diagnostic serum markers rather than for primary histopathological diagnosis. A wide range of antibodies that recognize tumour-associated antigens has been described (Bhattacharya et al, 1985; Smith & Teng, 1987; Daunter, 1990). Table 44.1 lists some of the tumour-associated antigens that have been investigated in ovarian carcinoma.

It has been shown that one or more serum markers may be elevated in patients with ovarian cancer and that the tumour may not always be the source of the raised serum concentration of the marker (Motoyama et al, 1990). It follows that the immunohistochemical identification of a marker in tumour tissue is a prerequisite to its use as a clinical marker to monitor disease progression. Most cancer-associated antigens are expressed by more than one type of tumour and sometimes by tumours of diverse histogenesis. Many are expressed in fetal tissues and can also be found in some normal adult tissues. Generally, the markers used for screening detect larger, advanced stage tumours (Saksela, 1993). What is required are markers sensitive to smaller, stage 1 tumours which would be more responsive to early intervention.

Cancer antigen 125. This tumour-associated antigen was derived from an ovarian serous carcinoma cell line (Bast et al, 1981). It is at present the most widely used tumour marker for ovarian carcinoma. It is expressed by over 80% of non-mucinous ovarian tumours (Kabawat et al, 1983) including serous, endometrioid, clear cell and undifferentiated carcinomas. Its clinical usefulness is, however, limited by the fact that it reacts with 22% of non-gynaecological cancers, including those of breast and gastrointestinal tract, as well as being found in benign gynaecological conditions (for a review, see Daunter, 1990). In situations where ovarian cancer is suspected, preoperative determination of CA125 has a high predictive value which increases with advancing age and advancing stage of tumour. A significant rise of CA125 after an initial fall or disappearance following treatment appears accurately to predict disease progression. Raised serum levels of CA125 may also occur in carcinoma of the Fallopian tube, cervix and endometrium. Unfortunately serum

Table 44.1 Some tumour-associated antigens to ovarian carcinoma

Monoclonal antibody	Antigen	Source of immunogen	Ovarian tumour reactivity	Reactivity with other gynaecological cancer	Reference
OC125	CA125 glycoprotein	Ovarian serous Ca	Serous*, endometrioid	Cervix, endometrium, Fallopian tube	Berkowitz et al (1983) Kabawat et al (1983)
OC133	80 kD glycoprotein	Ovarian serous Ca	Serous	Endocervix, endometrium	Bast et al (1981) Masuko et al (1984)
MOV2	High MW mucin/glycoprotein	Ovarian mucinous Ca	Mucinous*, serous, endometrioid	—	Tagliabue et al (1985)
OVTL3	—	Ovarian endometrioid Ca	Serous*, endometrioid, clear cell, mucinous	Endometrium	Poels et al (1986)
B72.3	Tumour-associated glycoprotein TAG-72.3	Breast carcinoma	Endometrioid, serous, mucinous	Cervix, endometrium	Thor et al (1986)
NB/70K	Glycoprotein subfraction OCA	Ovarian cancer	Serous, mucinous, endometrioid	Cervix, endometrium	Knauf & Urbach (1980)
1D3	High MW mucin	Ovarian cancer	Mucinous	—	Bhattacharya et al (1982)
4C7	—	Ovarian mucinous Ca	Mucinous, endometrioid, clear cell	—	Tsuji et al (1985)
3C2	—	Ovarian serous Ca	Serous, endometrioid	—	Tsuji et al (1985)
NS19-9	Ca19-9	Colonic carcinoma	Mucinous*, endometrioid, serous	—	Atkinson et al (1982)

* Main tumour reactivity

levels of 35 U/ml, the currently used cut-off value for positivity, are found in 1% of healthy controls. The antigen, probably a Müllerian differentiation antigen, is also present in normal endocervix, endometrium and Fallopian tube (Kabawat et al, 1983). Table 44.2 summarizes the reported frequency of the immunohistochemical demonstration of CA125 and other tumour markers in common epithelial tumours.

The antibody OC133 has similarities to CA125 but reacts with serous tumours only (Berkowitz et al, 1983; Masuko et al, 1984).

CA19-9. This antigen, carbohydrate-determinant 19-9, originally described in colonic carcinoma (Atkinson et al, 1982), is expressed by most mucinous ovarian carcinomas. It can also be expressed by a significant proportion of serous and other non-mucinous ovarian carcinomas (Table 44.2) and has been used in combination with CA125 for clinical monitoring.

Tumour-associated trypsin inhibitor (TATI). This peptide has been found in the urine of patients with ovarian cancer and elevated serum levels are encountered in association with different ovarian tumours and in the cyst fluids of mucinous tumours, for which it may be a useful marker. In mucinous ovarian tumours 40–75% of patients with local disease and 70–90% of patients with advanced disease are reported to be positive for TATI (Halila et al, 1988). Its use to complement CA125, commonly elevated in serous ovarian carcinomas, has been advocated.

Carcinoembryonic antigen (CEA). This has been extensively investigated in ovarian carcinoma with polyclonal and monoclonal antibodies. It is mainly expressed by mucinous carcinomas. Charpin et al (1982) showed an increasing incidence of expression from 15% in benign mucinous tumours to 100% in mucinous carcinoma. Other studies (Table 44.2) have confirmed a greater degree of expression in borderline and malignant mucinous tumours than in cystadenomas but CEA has also been demonstrated in some serous and other non-mucinous ovarian tumours.

There is wide variation in the reported detection rates of CEA in gynaecological cancer in the literature, a fact probably related to different specificities of CEA antibodies used (Wagener et al, 1984). CEA is a complex molecule with a number of epitopes and also cross-reactive antigens and it is probable that these factors contribute to the differences in detection rates of the antigen. The introduction of monoclonal antibodies to specific epitopes may improve the specificity of this tumour marker.

Table 44.2 Immunohistochemical markers in ovarian common epithelial tumours. (Data compiled from Nouwen et al, 1987; Hamilton-Dutoit et al, 1990; Motoyama et al, 1990.)

Tumour	CA125 % positive	CA19-9 % positive	CEA % positive	PLAP % positive
Serous				
Benign n=15	80	6	0	83
Borderline n=8	100	87	6	100
Malignant n=59	100	40	17	84
Mucinous				
Benign n=49	0	73	45	0
Borderline n=8	12.5	87	87	0
Malignant n=38	16	86	97	0
Endometrioid Ca n=27	66	64	25	66
Clear cell Ca n=20	75	70	15	0
Undifferentiated Ca n=17	82	52	23	57
Mixed Müllerian tumour n=5	80	80	40	33

Placental alkaline phosphatase (PLAP). PLAP levels are elevated in 6–64% of patients with ovarian cancer (Vergote et al, 1987). It is expressed by serous and endometrioid carcinomas (Nouwen et al, 1987; Hamilton-Dutoit et al, 1990) but not by mucinous tumours. There are two groups of tumour-associated PLAP — the Regan iso-enzyme, which is identical to term placental alkaline phosphatase, and a number of PLAP-like variants which include the Nagao iso-enzyme. These can be distinguished immunohistochemically (Hamilton-Dutoit et al, 1990) and both have been detected in serous carcinomas (Fig. 44.1).

Alpha amylase. This has been demonstrated in serous tumours of benign, borderline and malignant type (Bruns et al, 1982) and in endometrioid adenocarcinomas. The enzyme has also been demonstrated in some mucinous adenocarcinomas (Griffin & Wells, 1990). The antigen is normally detected in Müllerian-derived epithelia including Fallopian tube, endometrium and endocervix.

Intermediate filaments

Intermediate filaments are components of the cytoskeleton of cells and may be regarded as being tissue specific (Lazarides, 1980). Epithelial cells express cytokeratin; mesenchymal cells, vimentin; muscle cells, desmin; glial cells, glial fibrillary acidic protein and neuronal cells, neurofilament. There is more and more evidence that intermediate filaments are, however, not as tissue specific as originally thought: intermediate filament expression in different tissues may be similar and expression of one or more classes of intermediate filaments by the same cell may occur (Gould, 1985). The main intermediate filaments expressed by ovarian epithelial tumours are cytokeratin and vimentin (Dabbs & Geisinger, 1988).

Cytokeratins. About 30 cytokeratin polypeptides have been described to date. The low molecular weight cytokeratins 7, 8, 18 and 19 are universally expressed by ovarian carcinomas in concordance with the biochemical analysis of simple epithelial-type cytokeratin polypeptides (Moll et al, 1983). Stratification-related cytokeratin polypeptides allow foci of squamous differentiation, which may not be apparent in routine histological sections, to be identified. The stratification-associated cytokeratin peptides 4, 5 and 13 can identify such squamous foci in endometrioid, serous and anaplastic carcinomas (Van Niekerk et al, 1993). Stratification-related cytokeratins, however, are not detected in mucinous or clear cell tumours (Moll et al, 1991; Czernobilsky, 1992). Cytokeratins 10 and 11 are markers for keratinizing squamous epithelium and will identify differentiated squamous epithelium. Of the simple epithelial cytokeratin polypeptides, cytokeratins 8, 18 and 19 are present in all or the majority of cells of carcinomas. Cytokeratin 7 is of interest: it is present in nearly all ovarian tumours apart from mucinous tumours, in which its expression is markedly low (Moll et al, 1991; Van Niekerk et al, 1993). Cytokeratin 20 is a newly described cytokeratin polypeptide (Moll et al, 1992). It is expressed by mucinous ovarian tumours but not by non-mucinous, Müllerian-derived tumours, in which it is weak or absent. It is consistently expressed in colonic adenocarcinoma and may be of value in differential diagnosis.

Vimentin. Vimentin is expressed by ovarian carcinomas and has been consistently detected, though to a variable extent, in most carcinomas. Differences are apparent, however, in its expression by different types of ovarian

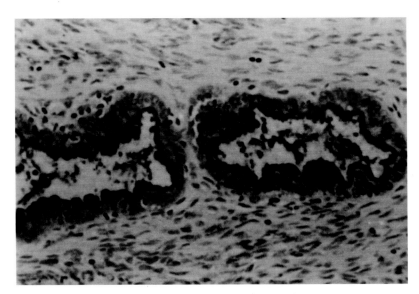

Fig. 44.1 Ovarian serous carcinoma stains with antibody to placental alkaline phosphatase. Immunoperoxidase × 350.

carcinoma. In one study vimentin was present in 71% of endometrioid carcinomas, 42% of serous carcinomas and 7% of clear cell carcinomas, but it was not detected in mucinous carcinomas (Dabbs & Geisinger, 1988). Viale et al (1988) also confirmed the co-expression of vimentin and cytokeratin in most ovarian serous and clear cell carcinomas and in some endometrioid carcinomas. Moll et al (1991) found strong positivity in serous tumours and the least expression in anaplastic tumours. They did not detect vimentin in mucinous and Brenner tumours. In a recent study Van Niekerk et al (1993), using four different antibodies to vimentin and frozen sections, claimed to have demonstrated focal vimentin positivity in the majority of mucinous tumours. Their results are at variance with all previous studies (Dabbs & Geisinger, 1988; Viale et al, 1988; Moll et al, 1991). It is of interest that the demonstration of vimentin in ovarian carcinoma parallels its expression in the Müllerian tract epithelia. Fallopian tube epithelium and endometrium express vimentin and endocervical mucinous epithelium does not. Ovarian surface epithelium, which is not of Müllerian derivation, but has a similar embryological origin from coelomic epithelium, also expresses vimentin. Desmin, indicative of smooth muscle differentiation, may be detected in the stroma of ovarian carcinomas: smooth muscle actin may also be expressed (Czernobilsky et al, 1989).

Glial fibrillary acidic protein. An interesting finding is the expression of glial fibrillary acidic protein by a subpopulation of tumour cells (5–15%) in some ovarian carcinomas (Moll et al, 1991). Glial fibrillary acidic protein was detected in 7 of 14 serous and endometrioid carcinomas but not in mucinous, anaplastic or clear cell carcinomas. No morphological differences were evident between cells staining for glial fibrillary acidic protein and those which did not. Positive staining cells were also noted in some endometrial carcinomas. Glial fibrillary acidic protein expression has also been reported in mixed Müllerian tumours and endometrial stromal cells but its biological significance in these settings is not known (Liao & Choi, 1986, 1987; Gershell et al, 1989; Erhmann et al, 1990).

Other markers

Epithelial markers such as epithelial membrane antigen (EMA), human milk fat globule (HMFG), and the epithelial cell surface antigen AuA1 are all expressed by ovarian carcinomas (Benjamin, 1987; Nouwen et al, 1987; Aguirre et al, 1989) in common with carcinomas elsewhere. They can be of value in the differential diagnosis of ovarian carcinomas and sex cord-stromal tumours as described later. Alpha-1-antitrypsin and alpha-1-antichymotrypsin may be expressed by most carcinomas whilst human chorionic gonadotrophin (hCG) and human placental lactogen

(hPL) are expressed in occasional cases (Ishikura & Scully, 1987; Khalifa & Sosterhenn, 1990).

The rare hepatoid carcinomas of the ovary may express alphafetoprotein (Ishikura & Scully, 1987): alphafetoprotein expression has also been described, rarely, in mucinous adenocarcinomas (Konishi et al, 1988). Neuroendocrine markers such as chromogranin A, neurone-specific enolase, serotonin and peptide hormones have been detected in neuroendocrine cells of ovarian carcinomas with the highest prevalence in mucinous tumours (Sasaki et al, 1989).

The small cell carcinoma of the ovary associated with hypercalcaemia (Dickersin et al, 1982) occurs in women in the second to fourth decades. Hypercalcaemia is found in two-thirds of cases in which preoperative measurements are done and serum calcium levels fall to normal where complete operative removal of the tumour is possible. The histogenesis of this tumour is unknown. Tumour cells universally express cytokeratin, one-third of cases express epithelial membrane antigen and approximately half are vimentin positive: neurone-specific enolase and chromogranin may also be detected. The presence of immunoreactive parathormone has been reported in some cases and may be causally related to the hypercalcaemia (Abeler et al, 1988; Scully, 1993).

Small cell carcinoma with hypercalcaemia needs to be differentiated from the primary pulmonary type of small cell carcinoma reported in the ovary (Eichorn et al, 1992). These tumours typically occur in menopausal and post-menopausal women and, in their histological and immunohistochemical features, are similar to pulmonary small cell carcinomas. Tumour cells express cytokeratin and, nearly always, epithelial membrane antigen, in contrast to the expression of the latter in only one-third of cases in the hypercalcaemic type of small cell carcinoma. Vimentin is usually absent and this may be of value in differential diagnosis as it is present in half the cases of the hypercalcaemic type of small cell carcinoma. Neurone-specific enolase and chromogranin may also be expressed. The presence of vimentin may help to separate the two subtypes of small cell carcinoma, which require different treatment regimes.

Brenner tumours

Immunohistochemical studies of the epithelial component of Brenner tumours have confirmed that this is antigenically similar to transitional epithelium (Shevchuck et al, 1980; Santini et al, 1989) which supports the concept of urothelial differentiation. Brenner tumour epithelium expresses low and high molecular weight cytokeratins. Nests of transitional epithelium contain cytokeratin 18 while those with squamoid features contain cytokeratins 10 and 11, which are markers of keratinizing squamous epithelium; mixed nests with both cytokeratin groups also occur (Lifschitz-Mercer et al, 1988). Vimentin is not demonstrable (Santini et al, 1989), a feature in common with mucinous ovarian neoplasms and urothelium. Vimentin is however demonstrable in the stromal cells of a Brenner tumour. Evidence of smooth muscle differentiation, characterized by desmin positivity, may also be found in the stroma (Seldenrijk et al, 1986). CEA has been detected in most benign, proliferating and malignant Brenner tumours (Shevchuck et al, 1980; Charpin et al, 1982). Positive staining for chromogranin, serotonin and neurone-specific enolase may be found in Brenner epithelium, consistent with the presence of argyrophilic cells (Aguirre et al, 1986; Santini et al, 1989).

Mixed Müllerian tumours

These tumours are more common in the uterus than in the ovary and are discussed with uterine tumours (see p. 1384).

Metastatic ovarian carcinomas

These are most commonly from the colon, stomach or breast. Of these, metastatic colonic carcinomas can be the most difficult to distinguish from a primary ovarian tumour (Lash & Hart, 1987). Immunostains for CA125 and placental alkaline phosphatase may be helpful as they are commonly expressed by many ovarian carcinomas. However both are also, occasionally, present in colonic carcinomas, while placental alkaline phosphatase is present in primary and metastatic gastric carcinomas.

Conventional antibodies to CEA stain most metastatic colonic carcinomas (Lash & Hart, 1987) and also mucinous and some non-mucinous ovarian carcinomas. Some of the monoclonal antibodies to specific epitopes of CEA may however prove to be more useful in this respect. Three such markers (CD-14, CEJ065 and SP-625) have been reported to show positive staining with virtually all primary and metastatic colonic carcinomas but to have little reactivity with ovarian carcinoma (Pavelic et al, 1991). They were less useful however in differentiating metastatic gastric and breast carcinoma.

Cytokeratin 7 is of interest in the differential diagnosis between primary and metastatic ovarian carcinoma. It has been reported to be consistently positive in primary ovarian epithelial tumours (Ramaekers et al, 1990; Moll et al, 1991; Ueda et al, 1993; Van Niekerk et al, 1993) but negative in colonic carcinomas and metastatic ovarian tumours of primary colonic origin. Although cytokeratin 7 has been reported to be usually absent in gastric carcinomas and their metastases by some workers (Ramaekers et al, 1990), others have found frequent, although weak, positivity (Ueda et al, 1993). Nevertheless, the presence of cytokeratin 7 expression in combination with vimentin positivity would help to separate primary ovarian carcino-

mas from most metastatic gastrointestinal carcinomas (Moll et al, 1991). Primary breast and pancreatic carcinomas were however found to express cytokeratin 7 (Ueda et al, 1993). Ueda et al (1993) also studied four cases of pseudomyxoma peritonei occurring in patients who had mucinous ovarian tumours, some of whom had co-existent appendicular pathology. They addressed the issue of whether pseudomyxoma in these patients was of ovarian or appendiceal origin. In three of their four cases cytokeratin 7 was negative and they attributed these cases to an appendiceal origin. The fourth case was cytokeratin positive and it was presumed to be of ovarian origin. These findings merit further investigation. Cytokeratin 20 has been reported to be of use in the differential diagnosis between metastatic colonic adenocarcinoma in the ovary and non-mucinous primary ovarian or Müllerian-derived tumours (Moll et al, 1992): it is, however, expressed by mucinous ovarian neoplasms.

Thus immunohistochemical profiles that might be useful in differential diagnosis are the expression of cytokeratin 7 and vimentin which mark most ovarian tumours, apart from mucinous tumours, but are generally absent in metastatic gastrointestinal tumours. Primary mucinous ovarian tumours are usually cytokeratin 7 negative and vimentin negative but do express cytokeratin 20. Cytokeratin 20 is expressed by most gastrointestinal carcinomas. Furthermore, the unusual expression of glial fibrillary acidic protein in an ovarian carcinoma would be more in favour of a tumour of Müllerian differentiation than one of gastrointestinal origin. Although glial fibrillary acidic protein has been found in ovarian and endometrial carcinomas the expression of this marker outside neural tissues is not unique to Müllerian-derived tumours as it has also been observed occasionally in renal carcinoma (Budka, 1986).

Sex cord-stromal tumours

Immunocytochemical studies on sex cord-stromal tumours are more limited than is the case for epithelial tumours. The main markers studied have been hormones and intermediate filaments.

Hormonal markers

Studies that correlate hormone production with morphology have demonstrated considerable overlap in hormonal content of sex cord-stromal tumours (Kurman & Nadji, 1985). Furthermore, immunocytochemical localization of a hormone cannot distinguish between its synthesis, storage or receptor binding at that site. Hormonal localization studies have several technical problems, including a high level of background staining and loss of antigenicity when using fixed tissues (Kurman & Nadji, 1985).

Granulosa-theca cell tumours have been shown to have

oestradiol and sometimes testosterone and progesterone within granulosa cells whilst theca cells contain oestradiol, progesterone and, occasionally, testosterone. In Sertoli–Leydig cell tumours, Sertoli cells contain testosterone, oestradiol and, less commonly, progesterone, or are devoid of hormones. The Leydig cells contain testosterone, oestradiol and sometimes progesterone (Kurman & Nadji, 1985). Confirmation of steroid hormone production by these tumours may be obtained by in vivo hormone measurements and in vitro incubation studies and steroid receptor assays.

A more recent immunohistochemical avenue of investigation of steroid hormone production has involved the demonstration of the steroidogenic enzymes, aromatase, 17α-hydroxylase and cholesterol side-chain cleavage cytochromes P-450, necessary for oestrogen, androgen and progesterone production respectively (Sasano et al, 1989). Immunostaining for 3β-hydroxysteroid dehydrogenase, which converts pregnenolone to progesterone, has also been investigated (Sasano et al, 1990). These studies have revealed little evidence of steroid synthesis in granulosa cells but the luteinized cells of thecomas show evidence of androgen and oestrogen production. In Sertoli–Leydig cell tumours there is evidence of progesterone, androgen and oestrogen production. Ovarian sclerosing stromal tumours produce androgens while steroid cell tumours are associated with progesterone, androgen and oestrogen production.

Intermediate filaments

Early studies of intermediate filaments in sex cord-stromal tumours reported immunostaining for vimentin but not for cytokeratins (Miettinen et al, 1985). Granulosa and theca cells of normal ovaries were also reported to show this pattern of expression. Subsequent studies, however, have shown that granulosa cells and Sertoli cells can express both cytokeratin and vimentin (Benjamin et al, 1987). In adult and fetal ovaries, granulosa cells express cytokeratin and vimentin whilst thecal cells and apparently undifferentiated stromal cells express vimentin only. This pattern of intermediate filament expression is also seen in fetal ovaries in the early stages of development.

Granulosa cell tumours

Adult and juvenile granulosa cell tumours may both express cytokeratin (Fig. 44.2a); immunoreactivity has been demonstrated in 20–68% of cases studied using antibodies to low molecular weight cytokeratins such as CAM 5.2, AE1/AE3 and MAK-6 (Benjamin et al, 1987; Aguirre et al, 1989; Costa et al, 1994). The extent of positive staining varies: it may be more prominent in tumours with insular, macrofollicular and microfollicular growth patterns and is usually absent in sarcomatoid tumours. Cytokeratin expression is perinuclear and varies from dot-like to more extensive perinuclear staining. Biochemical analysis has confirmed the presence of cytokeratin polypeptides 8 and 18 (Czernobilsky et al, 1987). Vimentin intermediate filaments are universally present (Fig. 44.2b) and are characteristically seen as globoid paranuclear staining. Desmoplakins have also been demonstrated immunohistochemically and correspond to the presence of desmosomal plaques of which they are the major constituent

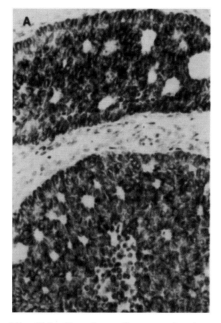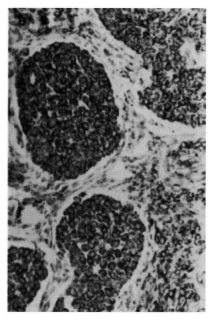

Fig. 44.2 Granulosa cell tumour showing: **a** cytoplasmic staining for cytokeratin antibody (CAM 5.2); **b** perinuclear staining with anti-vimentin, which also stains stromal cells. Immunoperoxidase × 300.

protein. It has been shown by immunoelectronmicroscopy that vimentin filaments attach to desmoplakin in desmosomes. The unusual combination of vimentin and desmoplakin may be a useful marker of granulosa cell tumours and an aid in distinguishing them from mesenchymal tumours (Czernobilsky et al, 1987).

Costa et al (1994) found no reactivity to desmin in 52 cases of adult and juvenile granulosa cell tumour but 92% of their cases showed focal immunoreactivity with antibodies to smooth muscle actin. Otis et al (1992) studied the expression of desmin in granulosa cells and found staining in minor thecomatous and fibromatous components but not in neoplastic granulosa cells. S100 expression with cytoplasmic and nuclear pattern of staining has been reported in granulosa cells and may be of value in the separation of granulosa from Sertoli cell tumours, in which S100 is only very rarely expressed (Costa et al, 1994).

The histogenesis of granulosa cell tumours is not settled; whether the origin of normal granulosa cells is from coelomic mesothelium or gonadal mesenchyme is still disputed. The presence of desmosomes and the immunocytochemical demonstration of cytokeratin and desmoplakins indicate that granulosa cells have epithelial differentiation but do not resolve the issue of histogenesis. A recently described marker of granulosa cell tumours is the peptide hormone inhibin which is produced by granulosa cells and Sertoli cells. In the cases studied so far, increased serum levels of inhibin correlated well with tumour burden (Lappohn et al, 1989; Nishida et al, 1991) and levels returned to normal after tumour resection; this appears to mark primary and recurrent disease.

Müllerian inhibiting substance, a glycoprotein hormone produced by fetal Sertoli cells which causes regression of the Müllerian duct in males during development, is another recently described serum marker for ovarian sex cord tumours (Gustafson et al, 1992). Raised serum levels of this hormone were found in a patient with a sex cord tumour with annular tubules and in three other patients with granulosa cell tumours.

Thecomas and fibromas

These uniformly express vimentin but not cytokeratin, a pattern similar to normal thecal and ovarian stromal cells (Miettinen et al, 1985; Benjamin et al, 1987). Cytokeratins were not detected in the previous studies but Van Niekerk et al (1993) detected cytokeratin polypeptides (7, 8, 18 and 19) in some tumours. Desmin immunoreactivity was reported in 39% of 23 fibromas and 13% of 23 thecomas (Costa et al, 1993).

Sertoli–Leydig cell tumours

The Sertoli cells in well-differentiated Sertoli–Leydig cell tumours express low molecular weight cytokeratins

(Benjamin et al, 1987). Poorly-differentiated tumours may show focal expression which sometimes corresponds to the presence of poorly-formed tubular structures. Vimentin may also be expressed but tends to be focal. Leydig cells have been reported to express only vimentin but cytokeratin has been demonstrated in testicular Leydig cell tumours (Duek et al, 1989). Sertoli–Leydig cell tumours with heterologous elements may additionally express intermediate filaments corresponding to their component tissues and neuroendocrine peptide hormones corresponding to the presence of argyrophilic cells. Alpha-fetoprotein has also been demonstrated in neoplastic Sertoli cells and Leydig cells and in tumour cells resembling liver cells (Young et al, 1984; Tetu et al, 1986; Chada et al, 1987).

Sex cord tumour with annular tubules

Both cytokeratin and vimentin positivity has been noted in the cells forming the annular tubules (Miettinen et al, 1985; Benjamin et al, 1987): stromal cells expressed vimentin. The origin of this tumour, whether of granulosa or Sertoli cell type, has been debated and the intermediate filament distribution is consistent with both cell types and does not distinguish between them.

Differential diagnosis of sex cord-stromal tumours

A number of neoplasms may mimic sex cord-stromal tumours. They include endometrioid carcinoma (which may resemble Sertoli–Leydig cell tumours and granulosa cell tumours), metastatic carcinoma (especially tubular Krukenberg tumours) and ovarian carcinoid tumours (Young & Scully, 1987). Conventional mucin stains are not always helpful in distinguishing these tumours: a periodic acid–Schiff-positive, diastase-resistant material resembling mucin may occur in granulosa cell and Sertoli–Leydig cell tumours. Similarly, expression of the intermediate filaments (cytokeratin and vimentin) also does not differentiate sufficiently between these tumour groups.

The epithelial markers — human milk fat globule antigen, epithelial membrane antigen and AuA1 — do, however, appear to be useful in distinguishing them (Fig. 44.3). Carcinomas consistently express these markers and sex cord-stromal tumours do not (Benjamin, 1987). Aguirre et al (1989) also failed to demonstrate staining with epithelial membrane antigen in 15 cases of adult granulosa cell tumours: all of their cases of endometrioid carcinoma expressed the antigen. They did, however, find positive staining for EMA in one of their 14 cases of Sertoli–Leydig cell tumour. Carcinoid tumours express human milk fat globule antigen and epithelial membrane antigen but not usually AuA1 (unpublished data) and they can be distinguished by reactivity with neuroendocrine markers, such as chromogranin.

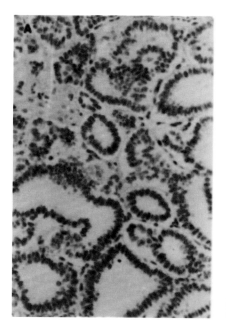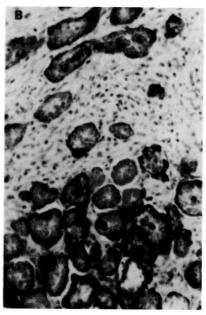

Fig. 44.3   Antibody to HMFG: **a** fails to stain an ovarian Sertoli–Leydig cell tumour; **b** shows strong reactivity in an ovarian carcinoma. Immunoperoxidase × 250.

Germ cell tumours

Germ cell tumours were among the earliest tumours to be studied immunohistochemically with the oncofetal markers beta-hCG and alphafetoprotein. The main application of these markers is in clinical monitoring as serum levels often closely reflect the histological composition of these tumours and tumour burden. The beta subunit of hCG can be detected at relatively low levels of concentration and withstands routine fixation. Detection of alphafetoprotein in fixed tissue is more likely to be hampered by denaturing of the antigen during processing (Kurman & Nadji, 1985). Serum concentrations of placental alkaline phosphatase (PLAP) and PLAP-like iso-enzymes are most consistently elevated in germ cell tumours (Hamilton-Dutoit et al, 1990). They are, however, sensitive rather than specific markers of germ cells. Reactivity of germ cell tumours has been shown to be mainly with the placental alkaline phosphatase-like (Nagao) iso-enzyme rather than the placental (Regan) iso-enzyme.

A separate locus coding for the Nagao (PLAP-like) iso-enzyme has been reported (Millan & Manes, 1988). The gene has been cloned and its product termed 'germ cell alkaline phosphatase'.

Dysgerminoma

Among available markers the most consistent immunocytochemical marker of dysgerminoma, and of testicular seminoma, is placental alkaline phosphatase and placental alkaline phosphatase-like enzymes. In a study of gonadal dysgerminomas and seminomas this enzyme was detected

in 86% of cases (Niehans et al, 1988). Placental alkaline phosphatase immunoreactivity in dysgerminomas is diffuse whereas it is patchy in other germ cell tumours. In the 3–5% of tumours that have syncytiotrophoblast giant cells, hCG is demonstrable and is localized within these cells; such cases may be associated with raised serum concentrations of hCG. Alphafetoprotein is not usually detectable in pure dysgerminomas.

Although cytokeratin expression was not found in early studies of dysgerminoma (Miettinen et al, 1985), it has been described in 14–80% of seminomas (Ramaekers et al, 1985; Denk et al, 1987) and has now also been detected in dysgerminomas (Van Niekerk et al, 1993) comprising polypeptides 7, 8 and 18. Vimentin reactivity is found in 30% of seminomas and dysgerminomas (Niehans et al, 1988). Epithelial membrane antigen is usually not expressed by dysgerminomas nor by most germ cell neoplasms other than choriocarcinomas, syncytiotrophoblast giant cells and teratomas. Immunostaining for placental alkaline phosphatase in the absence of epithelial membrane antigen expression is claimed to be unique to germ cell tumours (Niehans et al, 1988).

Lymphomas and malignant melanomas may rarely enter into the differential diagnosis of dysgerminomas. Absence of immunohistochemical markers such as leucocyte common antigen and S100 in neoplastic germ cells aids their immunohistochemical distinction.

Yolk sac tumours

These are the second commonest malignant ovarian germ cell tumour. Alphafetoprotein is the most important immunohistochemical marker and often correlates with raised serum levels; its localization may be diffuse or focal within the tumour. Hyaline globules seen in yolk sac tumours rarely show reactivity for alphafetoprotein (Eglen & Ulbright, 1987). Placental alkaline phosphatase is demonstrable in about half the cases (Niehans et al, 1988) whilst epithelial membrane antigen is rarely expressed. Cytokeratin is consistently present and CK 7, 8, 18 and 19 have been detected in tumour cells. Vimentin is rarely expressed and is focal, if present. CEA and alpha-1-antitrypsin may also be demonstrable in these tumours.

Embryonal carcinoma

Ovarian embryonal carcinomas usually form part of a mixed germ cell tumour. The cells of embryonal carcinoma may show focal expression of alphafetoprotein. Syncytiotrophoblast giant cells are often present and contain immunoreactive hCG (Kurman & Norris, 1976). A high proportion of embryonal carcinomas express placental alkaline phosphatase but not epithelial membrane antigen; most contain cytokeratin and occasionally vimentin (Niehans et al, 1988). The Ki-1 antigen (CD30), which was thought to be restricted to haemopoietic and lymphoid tissues, has now been shown to be expressed by embryonal carcinomas of testis and embryonal elements of mixed germ cell tumours but not by other germ cell tumours (Pallesen & Hamilton-Dutoit, 1988). The significance of this finding is uncertain but it may be of value as a marker of embryonal carcinoma. Alpha-1-antitrypsin, transferrin, ferritin and CEA have been demonstrated in embryonal carcinoma cells while human placental

lactogen and pregnancy-specific glycoprotein (SP1) have been found within syncytiotrophoblast giant cells (Krag-Jacobsen et al, 1981; Kurman & Nadji, 1985).

Choriocarcinoma

Non-gestational ovarian choriocarcinoma is usually part of a mixed germ cell tumour and rarely occurs as a pure tumour. As with gestational choriocarcinoma, beta-hCG is the main immunohistochemical marker for this tumour: it is found in syncytiotrophoblast cells. Human placental lactogen is also expressed and placental alkaline phosphatase is demonstrable in about half the cases (Niehans et al, 1988). Epithelial membrane antigen is also found in syncytiotrophoblastic cells and focal CEA expression can occur in cytotrophoblastic cells. Cytokeratins are expressed by both cell types; vimentin is usually negative, but may be present in mesenchymal stromal cells (Miettinen et al, 1985).

Teratomas

Ovarian teratomas contain elements derived from the three germ cell layers. Intermediate filament expression occurs in line with tissue differentiation and epithelial, mesenchymal and muscle components can be identified by immunostaining for cytokeratin, vimentin and desmin respectively. Mature glial tissue immunostains for glial fibrillary acidic protein and antibodies to neurofilament mark neuronal cells and fibres. Primitive neural epithelium of immature teratomas does not stain for glial fibrillary acidic protein (Fig. 44.4).

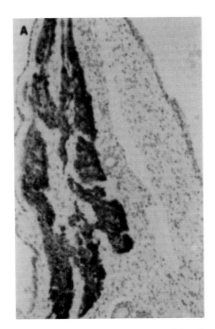 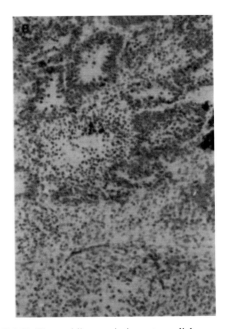

Fig. 44.4 Ovarian teratoma: **a** staining for glial fibrillary acidic protein in mature glial tissue; **b** primitive neuroepithelium with foci of melanin pigment fails to stain with GFAP. Immunoperoxidase × 250.

Endodermal-derived epithelium may focally stain for alphafetoprotein and occasionally be associated with a raised serum alphafetoprotein concentration (Ishiguro et al, 1981). Staining for hCG has been noted in syncytiotrophoblast giant cells in immature teratomas (Krag-Jacobsen et al, 1981; Calame & Shaberg, 1989). In a study of solid teratomas Calame & Shaberg (1989) found argyrophilic cells in all cases and immunoreactivity of these cells was reported to a range of peptides including glucagon, insulin, gastrin, secretin, somatostatin and pancreatic polypeptide. All solid teratomas also showed CEA reactivity.

The differential diagnosis between solid teratomas and malignant mixed Müllerian tumours is usually not difficult, in part because of the different age groups affected. Where this difficulty does arise, because of the range of tissues present in the ovarian tumour, the presence of markers such as glial fibrillary acidic protein, neurofilament, alphafetoprotein, hCG and neuroendocrine markers is more in favour of a teratoma than a mixed Müllerian tumour (Calame & Shaberg, 1989). There have, however, now been reports of the presence of glial tissue (and therefore glial fibrillary acidic protein) in uterine and ovarian mixed Müllerian tumours (Gershell et al, 1989; Ehrmann et al, 1990).

Struma ovarii and ovarian carcinoid tumours are monodermal or monophyletic teratomas. The presence of thyroglobulin and thyroid hormones can be demonstrated immunohistologically in struma ovarii (Hasleton & Whittaker, 1978). Primary ovarian carcinoid tumours have been shown to contain neuroendocrine markers such as chromogranin A (Wolpert et al, 1989) and a variety of endocrine peptides, including pancreatic polypeptides, glucagon, enkephalin and somatostatin. Immunoreactive

cells to such peptides have been found in 53% of trabecular carcinoids, 42% of strumal carcinoids and 7% of insular carcinoids (Sporrong et al, 1982). Strumal carcinoids may also contain thyroglobulin (Fig. 44.5) and calcitonin (Dayal et al, 1979).

Non-specific ovarian tumours

Mesenchymal tumours of the ovary are rare and most of the primary neoplasms comprise a few recorded cases. As with soft tissue tumours at other sites, immunohistochemistry can aid in their diagnosis. The most frequent among this group are smooth muscle tumours and problems may occasionally arise in the differential diagnosis between ovarian leiomyomas and fibrothecomas. Staining for desmin, although more extensive in leiomyomas, may also be present in fibrothecomas (Costa et al, 1993). Staining for smooth muscle actin has been reported to be useful in distinguishing these entities as it is negative in the fibrothecoma group but present in leiomyomas (Czernobilsky et al, 1989). However, Silva et al (1993) have reported smooth muscle actin expression in 90% of 23 thecomas and 11% of 23 fibromas. Whilst expression of desmin and smooth muscle actin aids in their diagnosis, immunohistochemical staining of smooth muscle tumours has to be interpreted in the context of morphological features as unexpected findings such as the expression of epithelial markers may be present. Recently, three cases of myxoid leiomyosarcoma of the ovary with unusual morphological appearances and inconclusive electronmicroscopy appearances were described (Nogales et al, 1993). The diagnosis was confirmed by positive staining of tumour cells for smooth muscle actin. Vimentin was also expressed but cytokeratins were negative in these tumours.

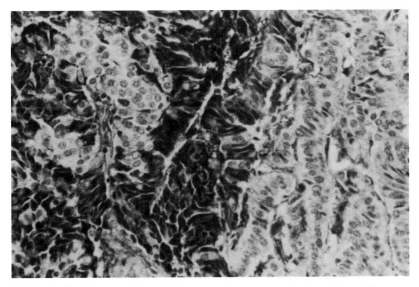

Fig. 44.5 Ovarian strumal carcinoid tumour showing cytoplasmic staining with antibody to thyroglobulin. Immunoperoxidase × 350.

Ovarian myxomas are rare neoplasms whose origin is disputed. They need to be distinguished from other lesions such as massive ovarian oedema, fibromas with myxoid change, myxoid smooth muscle tumours, sclerosing stromal tumours, myxoid neurofibromas, myxoid variants of several sarcomas and pseudomyxomatous pattern of mucinous carcinomas. Adequate sampling of these lesions is essential for diagnosis. Immunohistochemically, the tumour cells stain for smooth muscle actin and weakly for vimentin but not for desmin (Eichorn & Scully, 1991; Costa et al, 1993). Cytokeratins, epithelial membrane antigen, S100, Leu-7, neurone-specific enolase, neurofilament and factor VIII-related antigen are usually negative. Recently Costa et al (1993) have proposed that myxomas are a variant of the thecofibroma group of tumours, in which no remaining stromal tumour is detectable. Smooth muscle actin, which is expressed in myxomas, is an isoform of actin in smooth muscle cells and is also expressed by myoepithelial cells and myofibroblasts. They suggest that the immunohistochemical findings in myxomas are indicative of myofibroblastic differentiation. Immunohistochemistry is also of value in separating myxomas from other tumours in which myxoid change may occur. The expression of S100 can separate nerve sheath tumours and myxoid liposarcomas, whilst desmin immunostaining will identify smooth muscle tumours.

The ovaries may be the site of involvement by malignant lymphomas and leukaemias. The use of immunohistochemistry in the differential diagnosis of these neoplasms from other ovarian tumours is discussed in Chapter 31.

Adenomatoid tumours of the female genital tract

Adenomatoid tumours are now accepted to be a variant of benign mesotheliomas which occur exclusively in the genital tract of both males and females. In the female genital tract the Fallopian tube and myometrium are the most frequently involved sites and the ovaries rarely (Young et al, 1991). The tumour cells stain strongly for cytokeratin. The cystic spaces which they line, and which might be confused with haemangiomas or lymphangiomas, show no immunostaining to factor VIII-related antigen or *Ulex europaeus* lectin (Stephenson & Mills, 1986). The tumour cells may express vimentin but do not usually immunostain for carcinoembryonic antigen and epithelial membrane antigen.

UTERUS

Endometrium

Tumour-associated antigens

Many tumour-associated antigens have been studied to determine their value in distinguishing between normal endometrium, atypical hyperplasia and endometrial carci-

noma. CEA has been demonstrated in all cases of atypical hyperplasias and 60% of carcinomas (Hustin, 1978). CA1 antigen, a mucin-like glycoprotein, was found in some cases of atypical hyperplasia and endometrial carcinoma but reactivity was also present in secretory phase endometrium (Ferguson & Fox, 1984); a monoclonal antibody to the tumour-associated glycoprotein TAG-72 showed a similar pattern of reactivity (Thor et al, 1987). Binding of antibody to human milk fat globule membrane antigen showed a luminal pattern of distribution in normal endometrium and endometrial hyperplasia without atypia, while in atypical hyperplasia and endometrial carcinoma cytoplasmic expression was also present (Morris et al, 1989). None of these antibodies, however, has proved sufficiently discriminatory to be of value as a marker of neoplastic transformation. Some serum tumour markers elevated in ovarian carcinomas may also be elevated in endometrial carcinomas (see Table 44.1) and have been used for clinical monitoring.

Intermediate filaments

Endometrial carcinomas, in common with normal endometrial glands, express cytokeratin polypeptides 7, 8, 18 and 19 (Moll et al, 1983, 1991) which can be demonstrated by low molecular weight cytokeratin antibodies. In addition, stratification-related cytokeratin peptides 4, 5, 6, 13, 14 and 17 are found in endometrial carcinoma, within individual cells or groups of cells. Stratification-related cytokeratins are associated with squamous cell foci as well as in single cells, presumably indicative of an early stage of squamous differentiation (Moll et al, 1991). Vimentin positivity occurs in 70–80% of proliferative glands but drops to 20% or less in secretory glands (Dabbs et al, 1986). Endometrial stromal cells express vimentin only. Vimentin positivity occurs in 65–100% of cases of endometrial carcinoma (Dabbs et al, 1986; Moll et al, 1991) but is less in squamous foci than in glandular areas of tumour. This contrasts with lack of vimentin immunoreactivity in endocervical adenocarcinomas and normal endocervical glands (Dabbs et al, 1986). Demonstration of the presence of vimentin, therefore, may be a useful way of distinguishing between endometrial and endocervical adenocarcinomas (Fig. 44.6). It is likely, however, that in this context vimentin marks endometrioid differentiation rather than endometrial origin. Mucinous and clear cell carcinomas do not usually immunostain for vimentin, although focal positivity was noted in one clear cell carcinoma studied (Moll et al, 1991).

Other tumours

Small cell carcinomas, similar to those occurring in the cervix and ovary, rarely present in the endometrium. These are aggressive tumours associated with advanced stage at presentation. Most show cytokeratin positivity

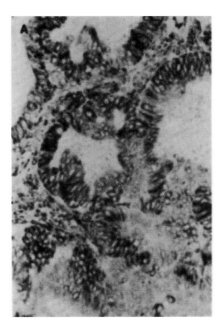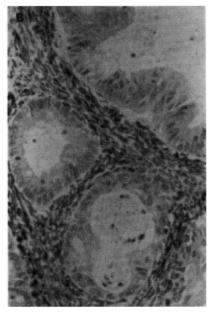

Fig. 44.6 Antibody to vimentin: **a** stains glands of endometrial adenocarcinoma; **b** fails to stain mucinous epithelium of endocervical adenocarcinoma. Immunoperoxidase × 250.

and approximately half express vimentin. Nearly all show NSE positivity but are CEA negative (Abeler et al, 1991; Huntsman et al, 1994). Markers for neuroendocrine differentiation such as chromogranin are only expressed infrequently and less consistently than reported in small cell cervical carcinomas (Gershell et al, 1988). These tumours need to be differentiated from rare lymphoid tumours of the uterus and uterine sarcomas. Whilst the former can usually be excluded by application of specific lymphoid markers, the distinction from uterine sarcomas may be more difficult, particularly in the presence of vimentin positivity. Cytokeratin positivity, however, is a helpful feature.

Smooth muscle tumours

Leiomyomas and leiomyosarcomas express vimentin and desmin. An unexpected immunocytochemical finding has been the demonstration of low molecular weight cytokeratin positivity in uterine and extrauterine leiomyomas and leiomyosarcomas (Brown D G et al, 1987; Norton et al, 1987). It is unclear whether positive staining indicates the presence of cytokeratin or cross-reactivity (Gusterson, 1987). Immunoreactivity to epithelial membrane antigen has also been described in extrauterine leiomyosarcomas (Miettinen, 1988) indicating that the presence of these epithelial markers cannot be taken, in isolation from their morphological features, as specific for carcinoma.

Endometrial stromal tumours

Vimentin is expressed by all stromal sarcomas but the

expression of cytokeratin is more controversial. Binder et al (1991) detected cytokeratin in three of five tumours in which no obvious epithelial differentiation was present, but other studies have not supported this finding (Lifschitz-Mercer et al, 1987; Puts et al, 1987). Tumour cells which immunostain for desmin may also be present (Del Poggetto et al, 1983). In stromal sarcoma cells, beta and gamma actin have been detected biochemically, and they are also present in normal endometrial stromal cells (Lifschitz-Mercer et al, 1987). The presence of smooth muscle differentiation within an endometrial stromal nodule may occur and be detectable by immunostains for smooth muscle (Lloreta & Prat, 1992). This should not be confused with myometrial invasion. Criteria such as circumscription and lack of invasion at the periphery of this lesion should be used to distinguish this from endometrial stromal sarcomas. Immunostaining with factor VIII antigen is helpful in delineating vascular space permeation by endometrial stromal sarcoma.

One example of stromomyoma was positive for desmin and vimentin but not cytokeratin, and two cases of uterine tumours that had sex cord-stromal features co-expressed cytokeratin and vimentin (Binder et al, 1991). Sex cordlike elements immunostain with desmin and musclespecific actin (Clement & Scully, 1992). Endometrial stromal sarcomas may also show extensive endometrioid glandular differentiation and such glands immunostain for cytokeratin and vimentin, as is the case with normal endometrial glands. It is likely that the diverse immunostaining patterns of stromal tumours reflect their postulated histogenesis from a primitive stem cell which differentiates along both epithelial and mesenchymal cell lines.

Mixed Müllerian tumours

These contain epithelial and mesenchymal elements and comprise adenofibroma, adenosarcoma, carcinofibroma and carcinosarcoma. Immunohistochemical studies have concentrated on carcinosarcomas. The epithelial component stains for cytokeratin and epithelial membrane antigen, and also focally for vimentin (Geisinger et al, 1987; Auerbach et al, 1988; Bitterman et al, 1990). The distribution of keratin, epithelial membrane antigen and vimentin in metastases (carcinoma) is reported to be similar to the epithelial component of the primary tumour (Bitterman et al, 1990). CEA has also been demonstrated (Calame & Shaberg, 1989). Epithelial differentiation may also be identified with these markers in spindle-shaped stromal cells and giant cells (Deligdisch et al, 1988). Homologous stromal sarcoma cells are vimentin positive and may focally express cytokeratin (Fig. 44.7). Desmin immunoreactivity has been found in 50% of cases (Auerbach et al, 1988) and a proportion of these also stain for myoglobin, indicative of striated muscle differentiation. Cross striations are usually identified only in differentiated rhabdomyoblasts whereas myoglobin staining may help to identify skeletal muscle differentiation at an earlier stage (Sahin & Benda, 1988). Other markers such as S100 may stain foci of chondrosarcoma, and alpha-1-antichymotrypsin stains stromal and giant cells (Auerbach et al, 1988).

Neuroectodermal differentiation has now been reported in uterine and ovarian mixed Müllerian tumours (Gershell et al, 1989; Ehrmann et al, 1990). Such tumours show immunostaining for glial fibrillary acidic protein in mature glial tissue. This is contrary to the previously held view that neural tissues never occur in mixed Müllerian tumours (Dehner et al, 1971). Clearly it is questionable whether such tumours do represent mixed Müllerian tumours or are in fact teratomas. Glial fibrillary acidic protein may be found in spindle cells of mixed Müllerian tumours in which no glial differentiation is present and can be produced by cultured cells of mixed Müllerian tumours and normal endometrial stromal cells (Liao & Choi, 1986, 1987). Recently GFAP has also been demonstrated in cells of some ovarian serous and endometrioid adenocarcinomas and endometrial carcinomas (Moll et al, 1991). This indicates that mixed Müllerian tumours are capable of a wider range of differentiation than was hitherto thought. The histogenesis of mixed Müllerian tumours, whether from primitive stem cells giving rise to epithelial and mesenchymal elements or from two independent stem cell lines developing in concert, is controversial. The immunocytochemical profile of these tumours almost certainly reflects their differentiation rather than their origin.

CERVIX

Immunocytochemical studies have been directed towards the demonstration of viral antigens and to tumour markers of cervical neoplasms. Markers that may be of use in predicting malignant transformation of squamous and glandular epithelium and in differentiating endocervical from endometrial adenocarcinoma have also been investigated.

Viral antigens

Human papillomavirus and the herpes simplex viral anti-

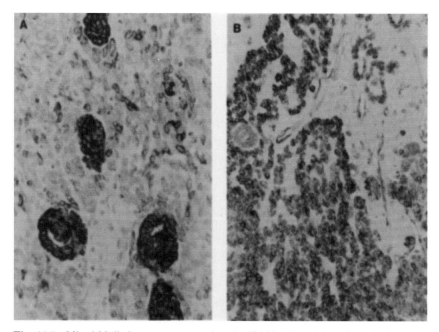

Fig. 44.7 Mixed Müllerian tumour: **a** cytokeratin (CAM 5.2) staining of poorly-formed epithelial structures and scattered stromal cells; **b** perinuclear staining of homologous stromal sarcoma cells with anti-vimentin. Immunoperoxidase × 250.

gens have been demonstrated in cervical lesions. It is now clear that immunohistochemical methods are not sufficiently specific or sensitive for detection of viral antigens: they have largely been superseded by DNA hybridization techniques and the polymerase chain reaction.

Tumour-associated markers

Squamous cell carcinoma antigen/TA-4 antigen. The squamous cell carcinoma antigen is a subfraction of the glycoprotein TA-4 derived from a cervical squamous cell carcinoma. Both have been used as markers in monitoring squamous and adenosquamous carcinomas of the cervix (Karo & Tongae, 1977; Duk et al, 1990). Raised serum levels may also occur with squamous cell carcinomas in other sites. The antigen has been demonstrated immunohistochemically in keratinizing and large cell non-keratinizing tumours. Undifferentiated and small cell carcinomas do not immunostain.

Carcinoembryonic antigen. Elevated serum CEA levels may be found in both squamous cell carcinoma and adenocarcinomas of the cervix and may be of value in predicting recurrence in patients who have tumours that contain CEA. It has been detected in 50–82% of squamous cell carcinomas and 75–100% of adenocarcinomas (Van Nagell et al, 1982; Bychkov et al, 1983).

Squamous lesions

Intermediate filaments

Cytokeratin expression in the uterine cervix is complex. Endocervical epithelium contains simple epithelial-type keratins 8, 18 and 19 while ectocervical epithelium contains stratification-type keratins 5 and 17 as well as several other cytokeratin polypeptides (Syrjanen et al, 1988). Low molecular weight (simple epithelial) cytokeratins have been investigated for use as markers of potential invasion in cervical intraepithelial neoplasia but the results are conflicting. Some studies have showed that cases of cervical intraepithelial neoplasia (CIN) 1 and 2 do not express these cytokeratins whereas some cases of CIN 3 and most invasive squamous carcinomas do express them (Bobrow et al, 1986; Angus et al, 1988). Others have disputed this, having found staining in only a small proportion of squamous cell carcinomas (Raju, 1988) and lack of staining in microinvasive squamous carcinoma (Wells et al, 1986). In HPV-infected cervical epithelium and CIN, disturbances in the pattern of cytokeratin expression have also been described (Morris et al, 1983; Syrjanen et al, 1988).

Involucrin

This is a differentiation antigen of squamous epithelium, unrelated to keratin. It is expressed in normal squamous epithelium, squamous metaplasias and viral condylomas.

Its expression is less in CIN (Warhol et al, 1982) but its value as a marker of CIN is reduced when there is significant inflammation, which itself results in decreased expression. It may however be of some value in distinguishing CIN 1 from immature squamous metaplasia and flat condylomas.

Glandular lesions

Carcinoembryonic antigen

As well as being a serum tumour marker in cervical adenocarcinoma, CEA has been reported to be of use in distinguishing benign glandular lesions from endocervical adenocarcinoma. Normal endocervix and 95% of cases of microglandular hyperplasias do not express CEA whereas 64% of adenocarcinomas do (Speers et al, 1983). Other studies have confirmed this (Michael et al, 1984; Steeper & Wick, 1986) and, furthermore, have shown that cases of minimal deviation adenocarcinoma consistently expressed CEA. Reports of CEA expression in adenocarcinoma in situ are more conflicting: Hurliman & Gloor (1984) detected CEA in 6 of 9 cases (67%) while Tobon & Dave (1988) detected it in only one of 11 cases. Alpha-amylase and human milk fat globule antigen have also been investigated as markers of endocervical glandular atypia; the pattern of human milk fat globule antigen staining is reported to be useful in distinguishing atypia from benign endocervical proliferations (Brown L J R et al, 1987). Results of staining for amylase are conflicting (Lee & Raju, 1988; Griffin et al, 1989).

The distinction between adenocarcinoma of endocervical and endometrial origin can sometimes be difficult in a cervical biopsy. The use of CEA to differentiate between these tumours was described by Wahlstrom et al (1979) who showed that 80% of endocervical tumours stained, in contrast to 8% of endometrial tumours. Other studies have shown no significant differences between the frequency and extent of expression of CEA in the two tumours irrespective of whether monoclonal or polyclonal antibodies are used (Maes et al, 1988).

Vimentin may be more useful than CEA in distinguishing endocervical from endometrial adenocarcinomas, as already described. Vimentin, however, can be expressed by the rare mesonephric carcinoma of the cervix and by mesonephric hyperplasia, in which vimentin positivity occurs in 10–30% of cells (Lang & Dallenbach-Hellweg, 1990). These entities do not however express CEA and the combination of vimentin positivity and absence of CEA may help to distinguish them from typical endocervical adenocarcinoma. Kudo et al (1990) have described a monoclonal antibody, IC5, that has a reactivity which they claim to be superior to that of CEA in invasive and in situ adenocarcinomas and adenosquamous carcinoma. Immunostains to the antibody were reported to be negative in intraepithelial and invasive squamous cell carcinomas and so could be used to distinguish between glandular and squamous neoplasms. The authors also claimed that it was useful in distinguishing endocervical from endometrial adenocarcinoma.

Small cell/neuroendocrine cervical carcinoma

Hormone production by cervical carcinomas is well recognized. Serotonin, somatostatin and ACTH may also occasionally be detected. Small cell undifferentiated carcinomas may express cytokeratin, epithelial membrane antigen and CEA. The most commonly demonstrated neuroendocrine markers include chromogranin A, Leu-7, neurone-specific enolase and synaptophysin (Gershell et al, 1988; Ueda et al, 1988).

Adenoid cystic carcinomas and adenoid basal carcinomas

These tumours have been studied immunohistochemically and express cytokeratin; CEA and EMA are present focally. Adenoid cystic carcinomas appear to differ from their salivary gland counterparts by failing to stain for S100 protein, which in salivary glands is expressed by the myoepithelial component. Ferry & Scully (1988) postulate that this tumour is a carcinoma resembling an adenoid cystic carcinoma rather than a true adenoid cystic carcinoma.

GESTATIONAL TROPHOBLASTIC LESIONS

The immunohistochemical profile of the three types of gestational trophoblastic cells — syncytiotrophoblast, cytotrophoblast and intermediate trophoblast — is well characterized. Human chorionic gonadotrophin is the most important diagnostic marker and is demonstrable in syncytiotrophoblastic cells and cells of the intermediate trophoblast but is absent in cytotrophoblast. Cytokeratin expression occurs in all types of trophoblastic cells in chorionic villi and in extravillous trophoblast. Its expression spans the early implantation site to term placentas (Young et al, 1988). Epithelial membrane antigen is expressed by intermediate trophoblast and syncytiotrophoblast but not usually by cytotrophoblast. However, a subpopulation of trophoblastic cells present in the chorion laeve and designated 'vacuolated cytotrophoblast' has been reported to immunostain for epithelial membrane antigen in addition to cytokeratin. These cells also immunostain for placental alkaline phosphatase but not for human chorionic gonadotrophin or placental lactogen (Yeh et al, 1989).

The timing of expression of human chorionic gonadotrophin, human placental lactogen and placental alkaline phosphatase in the developing placenta may be related to maturation of trophoblast (Young et al, 1988). Human placental lactogen is detectable at 12 days' gestation in syncytiotrophoblast and intermediate trophoblast. In intermediate trophoblast human placental lactogen expression

reaches a peak at 11–15 weeks' gestation and decreases thereafter. In syncytiotrophoblast, human placental lactogen expression increases till term and is demonstrable in virtually all syncytiotrophoblast cells in the term placenta. Human chorionic gonadotrophin is present focally in intermediate trophoblast, especially in the first trimester. In syncytiotrophoblast cells, human chorionic gonadotrophin is demonstrable from the 12th day of gestation, reaches a peak at six weeks and decreases thereafter; at term hCG is present only focally in these cells. The expression of placental alkaline phosphatase in the first trimester is more variable. However, by 15–16 weeks' gestation it becomes prominent in intermediate trophoblast and syncytiotrophoblast. It then increases till term when it shows a uniform distribution in syncytiotrophoblast and a focal distribution in intermediate trophoblast.

A number of other hormonal markers have been localized by immunoperoxidase in the developing placenta: these include pregnancy-specific beta-1 glycoprotein, placental protein 5, pregnancy-associated plasma protein A, oestradiol and progesterone. These have been mainly localized to syncytiotrophoblastic cells.

Partial and complete hydatidiform mole

The expression of the trophoblastic markers, hCG, hPL and placental alkaline phosphatase has been compared in complete hydatidiform moles and partial moles in order to identify immunohistochemical features that might be useful in distinguishing between them in cases of difficulty (Brescia et al, 1987). The distribution of these markers in syncytiotrophoblast revealed differences between the two conditions. The syncytiotrophoblast of classical hydatidiform moles showed marked staining for hCG and little staining for placental alkaline phosphatase, regardless of gestational age. Staining for hPL varied in distribution but its expression tended to rise with increasing gestational age. In contrast, in partial moles, there was moderate to widespread distribution of hPL and placental alkaline phosphatase but only a focal distribution of hCG.

Choriocarcinoma

In choriocarcinoma strong diffuse immunostaining for human chorionic gonadotrophin occurs in syncytiotrophoblastic cells whilst human placental lactogen is focally present. Placental alkaline phosphatase is also expressed. Both trophoblastic cells immunostain for cytokeratins whilst epithelial membrane antigen can be detected in syncytiotrophoblastic cells but not in cytotrophoblast.

Placental site trophoblastic tumour

This is a tumour of intermediate trophoblast. It needs to be distinguished from choriocarcinoma, from which it differs in biological behaviour and response to chemotherapy. Serum levels of human chorionic gonadotrophin are less elevated than in patients with choriocarcinomas and, in up to two-thirds of patients, levels are normal or only slightly elevated. Immunohistochemistry may aid in the differential diagnosis between these two entities. Tumour cells of placental site trophoblastic tumour show diffuse staining for cytokeratins and human placental lactogen whereas human chorionic gonadotrophin immunostaining is only focal. By contrast, in choriocarcinoma there is a diffuse pattern of staining for hCG and focal immunostaining for human placental lactogen, as already described. Some examples of malignant placental site trophoblastic tumour have shown a pattern of staining which is more atypical and resembles that of choriocarcinoma. It appears likely that a placental site trophoblastic tumour that synthesizes more human chorionic gonadotrophin than human placental lactogen is composed of less mature intermediate trophoblast than a typical placental site trophoblastic tumour (Young et al, 1988).

Placental site nodules

Characteristic immunohistochemical profiles have also been described in other lesions associated with intermediate trophoblast. Placental site nodules are nodules of acellular hyalinized tissue mixed with intermediate trophoblast, found in the endometrium or endocervix. Such nodules are thought to represent the persistence of a portion of the implantation site, and possibly represent implantation site vessels. These are detected as incidental findings in biopsies performed for menorrhagia or an abnormal cytological smear. Immunohistochemically, intermediate trophoblast in these lesions showed diffuse immunostaining for placental alkaline phosphatase, cytokeratin and EMA in 100%, 96% and 84% of cases studied, respectively. Weak or focal staining occurred with human placental lactogen in 78% of cases and human chorionic gonadotrophin in 42% of cases (Huettner & Gershell, 1994). Vimentin-positive cells present in the lesions were not typical intermediate trophoblast cells and were probably stromal cells.

Intermediate trophoblast in these lesions was similar to the intermediate trophoblast of the normal implantation site in the pattern of immunostaining to cytokeratin, EMA, human chorionic gonadotrophin and human placental lactogen. Placental alkaline phosphatase expression, however, was unusual in that whilst it is weak or absent in normal intermediate trophoblast, it was strongly positive in placental site nodules. In this respect the trophoblastic population of placental site nodules has similarities to the subpopulation of vacuolated cytotrophoblast described in the chorion laeve which also stains for placental alkaline phosphatase. The vacuolated intermediate trophoblastic cells present in placental site nodules morphologically resemble vacuolated cytotrophoblastic cells. Placental site nodules may need to be distinguished from hyalinized foci of decidual cells and this can be done by lack of immunostaining in decidual cells for cytokeratins, epithelial membrane antigen, placental alkaline phosphatase, human chorionic gonadotrophin and human placental lactogen (Young et al, 1988).

Multiple nodular proliferations of intermediate trophoblast cells have been described as an unusual complication following evacuation of hydatidiform moles (Silva et al, 1993). Such nodules occurred in the endometrium and myometrium and showed immunostaining for cytokeratin, epithelial membrane antigen, human placental lactogen and human chorionic gonadotrophin consistent with that of intermediate trophoblastic cells. It is likely that they are similar in nature to placental site nodules.

The facility to identify intermediate trophoblast by immunohistochemistry is also useful in identifying an early implantation site in uterine curettings. This would be important, for example, in a patient suspected to have an ectopic pregnancy (Young et al, 1988). Morphologically, the separation of intermediate trophoblast from decidual and smooth muscle cells may be difficult; however the presence of cytokeratin and human placental lactogen would separate intermediate trophoblast from decidual cells. Smooth muscle cells may rarely express cytokeratins but would be negative for human placental lactogen.

CONCLUSION

Immunocytochemical markers are useful for the clinical and pathological investigation of gynaecological disease. There are inherent limitations because of antigen heterogeneity in tumour cell populations and variation in specificity of currently available antibodies. As newer antibodies are introduced and more information on currently available ones grows, more selective immunotyping of tumours may be possible. This is already becoming the case with antibody markers to specific cytokeratin polypeptides and to specific CEA epitopes. Furthermore, techniques which enhance antigen retrieval in fixed tissues will extend the scope of immunohistochemical investigation in the future.

REFERENCES

Abeler V M, Kjorstad K E, Nesland J M 1988 Small cell carcinoma of the ovary: a report of six cases. International Journal of Gynecological Pathology 7: 315–329.
Abeler V M, Kjorstad K E, Nesland J M 1991 Undifferentiated carcinoma of the endometrium: a histopathologic and clinical study of 31 cases. Cancer 68: 98–105.

Aguirre P, Scully R E, Wolfe H J et al 1986 Argyrophil cells in Brenner tumors: histochemical and immunohistochemical analysis. International Journal of Gynecological Pathology 5: 223–234.
Aguirre P, Thor A D, Scully R E 1989 Ovarian endometrioid carcinomas resembling sex cord-stromal tumours: an immunohistochemical study. International Journal of Gynecological Pathology 8: 364–373.

Angus B, Kiberu S, Purvis J, Wilkinson L, Horne C H W 1988 Cytokeratins in cervical dysplasia and neoplasia: a comparative study of immunohistochemical staining using monoclonal antibodies NCL-5D3, CAM 5.2, and PKK1. Journal of Pathology 155: 71–75.

Atkinson B F, Ernst C S, Herlyn M, Steplewski Z, Sears H F, Koprowski H 1982 Gastrointestinal cancer associated antigen in immunoperoxidase assay. Cancer Research 42: 4820–4823.

Auerbach H E, Livolski V A, Merino M J 1988 Malignant mixed Müllerian tumors of uterus: an immunohistochemical study. International Journal of Gynecological Pathology 7: 123–130.

Bast R C, Fenney M, Lazarus H, Nadler L M, Colvin R B, Knapp R C 1981 Reactivity of a monoclonal antibody with human ovarian carcinoma. Journal of Clinical Investigation 68: 1331–1337.

Benjamin E 1987 Sex cord-stromal tumour or ovarian carcinoma? Use of epithelial surface markers in differential diagnosis. Journal of Pathology 152: 192A.

Benjamin E, Law S, Bobrow L G 1987 Intermediate filaments cytokeratin and vimentin in ovarian sex cord-stromal tumours with correlative studies in adult and fetal ovaries. Journal of Pathology 152: 253–266.

Berkowitz R, Kabawat S, Lazarus H, Colvin R B, Knapp R, Bast R C 1983 Comparison of a rabbit heteroantiserum and a murine monoclonal antibody raised against a human epithelial ovarian carcinoma cell line. American Journal of Obstetrics and Gynecology 146: 607–612.

Bhattacharya M, Chatterjee S K, Barlow J J, Fuji H 1982 Monoclonal antibodies recognising tumour associated antigen of human ovarian mucinous cystadenocarcinomas. Cancer Research 42: 1650–1654.

Bhattacharya M, Chatterjee S K, Barlow J J 1985 Ovarian tumour antigens and other markers. In: Hudson C N (ed) Ovarian carcinoma. Oxford University Press, Oxford, pp 169–189.

Binder S W, Nieberg R K, Cheg L, Al-Jitawi S 1991 Histological and immunohistochemical analysis of nine endothelial stromal tumors: an unexpected high frequency of keratin protein positivity. International Journal of Gynecological Pathology 10: 191–197.

Bitterman P, Chun B, Kurman R J 1990 The significance of epithelial differentiation in mixed mesodermal tumors of the uterus. American Journal of Surgical Pathology 14: 317–328.

Bobrow L G, Makin C A, Law S et al 1986 Expression of low molecular weight cytokeratin proteins in cervical neoplasia. Journal of Pathology 148: 135–140.

Breitenecker G, Neunteufel W, Bieglmayer C, Kolbl H, Schieder K 1989 Comparison between tissue and serum content of CA 125, CA 19-9 and carcinoembryonic antigen in ovarian tumors. International Journal of Gynecological Pathology 8: 97–102.

Brescia R J, Kuman R J, Main C S et al 1987 Immunocytochemical localisation of chorionic gonadotropin, placental lactogen and placental alkaline phosphatase in the diagnosis of complete and partial moles. International Journal of Gynecological Pathology 6: 213–229.

Brown D G, Theaker J M, Banks P M, Gatter K C, Mason D Y 1987 Cytokeratin expression in smooth muscle and smooth muscle tumours. Histopathology 11: 477–486.

Brown L J R, Griffin N R, Wells W 1987 Cytoplasmic reactivity with the monoclonal antibody HMFG1 as a marker of cervical glandular atypia. Journal of Pathology 15: 203–208.

Bruns D E, Mills S E, Savary J 1982 Amylase in fallopian tube and serous ovarian neoplasms: immunohistochemical localisation. Archives of Pathology and Laboratory Medicine 106: 17–20.

Budka H 1986 Non glial specificities of immunocytochemistry for the glial fibrillary acidic protein (GFAP). Acta Neuropathologica 72: 43–54.

Bychkov V, Rothman M, Bardawil W A 1983 Immunocytochemical localisation of carcino-embryonic antigen (CEA) alpha-fetoprotein (AFP) and human chorionic gonadotropin (HCG) in cervical neoplasia. American Journal of Clinical Pathology 79: 414–420.

Calame J J, Schaberg A 1989 Solid teratomas and mixed Müllerian tumors of the ovary: a clinical, histological and immunocytochemical comparative study. Gynecologic Oncology 33: 212–221.

Cattoretti G, Pileri S, Parravicini C et al 1993 Antigen unmasking on formalin-fixed paraffin-embedded tissue sections. Journal of Pathology 171: 83–98.

Chada S, Honnebier W J, Schaberg A 1987 Raised serum alpha

fetoprotein in Sertoli-Leydig cell tumor (androblastoma of ovary): report of two cases. International Journal of Gynecological Pathology 6: 82–88.

Charpin C, Bhan A K, Zurawski V R, Scully R E 1982 Carcinoembryonic antigens (CEA) and carbohydrate determinant 19-9 (CA 19-9) localisation in 121 primary and metastatic ovarian tumors: an immunohistochemical study with use of monoclonal antibodies. International Journal of Gynecological Pathology 1: 231–245.

Clement P B, Scully R E 1992 Endometrial stromal sarcoma of the uterus with extensive endometrioid glandular differentiation: a report of three cases that caused problems in differential diagnosis. International Journal of Gynecological Pathology 11: 163–173.

Costa M J, Morris R, De Rose P et al 1993 Histologic and immunohistochemical evidence for considering ovarian myxoma as a variant of the thecoma-fibroma group of ovarian stromal tumors. Archives of Pathology and Laboratory Medicine 117: 802–808.

Costa M J, De Rose P B, Roth L M, Brescia R J, Zaloudek C J, Cohen C 1994 Immunohistochemical phenotype of ovarian granulosa cell tumor: absence of epithelial membrane antigen has diagnostic value. Human Pathology 25: 60–66.

Czernobilsky B 1992 Intermediate filaments in ovarian tumors. International Journal of Gynecological Pathology 12: 166–169.

Czernobilsky B, Moll R, Leppien G, Schweikhart G, Franke W W 1987 Desmosomal plaque-associated vimentin filaments in human ovarian granulosa cell tumors of various histologic patterns. American Journal of Pathology 126: 476–486.

Czernobilsky B, Shezen E, Lifschitz-Mercer B et al 1989 Alpha smooth muscle actin in normal human ovaries, in ovarian stromal hyperplasia and in ovarian neoplasms. Virchow Archives B Cell Pathology 57: 55–61.

Dabbs D J, Geisinger K R 1988 Common epithelial ovarian tumors: immunohistochemical intermediate filament profiles. Cancer 62: 368–374.

Dabbs D J, Geisinger K R, Norris H T 1986 Intermediate filaments in endometrial and endocervical carcinomas. American Journal of Surgical Pathology 10: 568–576.

Daunter B 1990 Tumor markers in gynecologic oncology. Gynecologic Oncology 39: 1–15.

Dayal Y, Tashijan A H, Wolfe H J 1979 Immunocytochemical localisation of calcitonin producing cells in a strumal carcinoid with amyloid stroma. Cancer 43: 1331–1338.

Dehner L P, Norris H J, Taylor H B 1971 Carcinosarcomas and mixed Müllerian tumors of the ovary. Cancer 27: 207–216.

Deligdisch L, Plaxe S, Cohen C J 1988 Extra-uterine pelvic malignant mixed mesodermal tumors: a study of 10 cases with immunohistochemistry. International Journal of Gynecological Pathology 7: 361–372.

Del Poggetto C B, Virtanen I, Lehto V-P, Walstrom T, Saksela 1983 Expression of intermediate filaments in ovarian and uterine tumors. International Journal of Gynecological Pathology 1: 359–366.

Denk H, Moll R, Weybora W et al 1987 Intermediate filaments and desmosomal plaque proteins in testicular seminomas and non-seminomatous germ cell tumours as revealed by immunohistochemistry. Virchows Archives A Pathological-Anatomy 410: 295–307.

Dickersin R G, Kline I W, Scully R E 1982 Small cell carcinoma of the ovary with hypercalcemia: a report of eleven cases. Cancer 49: 188–197.

Duek W, Dieckmann K P, Loy V, Stein H 1989 Immunohistochemical determinations of oestrogen receptor, progesterone receptor and intermediate filaments in Leydig cell tumours, Leydig cell hyperplasia and normal Leydig cells of the human testis. Journal of Pathology 157: 225–234.

Duk J M, De Bruijn W A, Groenier H K H 1990 Cancer of the uterine cervix: sensitivity and specificity of serum squamous cell carcinoma antigen determinations. Gynecologic Oncology 29: 186–194.

Eglen D E, Ulbright T M 1987 The differential diagnosis of yolk sac tumor and seminomas. American Journal of Pathology 88: 328–332.

Ehrmann R L, Weidner N, Welch W R, Gleiberman I 1990 Malignant mixed Müllerian tumor of ovary with prominent neuroectodermal differentiation (teratoid carcinosarcoma). International Journal of Gynecological Pathology 9: 272–282.

Eichorn J H, Scully R E 1991 Ovarian myxoma: clinicopathologic and immunocytologic analysis of five cases and a review of the literature. International Journal of Gynecological Pathology 10: 156–169.

Eichorn J H, Young R H, Scully R E 1992 Primary ovarian small cell carcinoma of the pulmonary type: a clinicopathologic, immunohistologic and flow cytometric analysis of 13 cases. American Journal of Surgical Pathology 16: 926–938.

Epenetos A A, Hooker G E, Krauz T, Snook D, Bodmer W F, Taylor-Papadimitriou J 1986 Antibody-guided irradiation of malignant ascites in ovarian cancer: a new therapeutic method possessing specificity against cancer cells. Obstetrics and Gynecology 68: 71s–74s.

Ferguson A M, Fox H 1984 The expression of Ca antigen in normal, hyperplastic and neoplastic endometrium. British Journal of Obstetrics and Gynaecology 91: 1042–1045.

Ferry J A, Scully R E 1988 Adenoid cystic carcinoma and adenoid basal carcinoma of the uterine cervix: a study of 28 cases. American Journal of Surgical Pathology 12: 134–144.

Geisinger K R, Dabbs D J, Marshall R B 1987 Malignant mixed Müllerian tumors: an ultrastructural and immunohistochemical analysis with histogenetic considerations. Cancer 59: 1781–1790.

Gershell D J, Mazoujian G, Mutch D G, Rudloff M A 1988 Small cell undifferentiated carcinoma of the cervix: a clinicopathological, ultrastructural and immunocytochemical study of 15 cases. American Journal of Surgical Pathology 12: 684–698.

Gershell D J, Duncan D A, Fulling K 1989 Malignant mixed Mullerian tumor of the uterus with neuroectodermal differentiation. International Journal of Gynecological Pathology 8: 169–178.

Gould V E 1985 The co-expression of distinct classes of intermediate filaments in human neoplasms. Archives of Pathology and Laboratory Medicine 109: 984–985.

Griffin N R, Wells M 1990 Immunolocalisation of alpha amylase in ovarian mucinous tumors. International Journal of Gynecological Pathology 9: 41–46.

Griffin N R, Wells M, Fox H 1989 Modulation of the antigenicity of amylase in cervical glandular atypia, adenocarcinoma in situ and invasive adenocarcinoma. Histopathology 15: 267–279.

Gustafson M L, Lee M M, Scully R E et al 1992 Müllerian inhibiting substance as a marker for ovarian sex-cord tumor. New England Journal of Medicine 326: 466–471.

Gusterson B A 1987 Commentary: is cytokeratin present in smooth muscle? Histopathology 11: 549–551.

Halila H, Lentovirta P, Stenman U H 1988 Tumour-associated trypsin inhibitor in ovarian cancer. British Journal of Cancer 57: 304–307.

Hamilton-Dutoit S J, Lou H, Pallerson G 1990 The expression of placental alkaline phosphatase (PLAP) and PLAP-like enzymes in normal and neoplastic human tissues. Acta Pathologica, Microbiologica et Immunologica Scandinavica 98: 797–811.

Hasleton P S, Whittaker J L 1978 Benign and malignant struma ovarii. Archives of Pathology and Laboratory Medicine 102: 180–183.

Huettner P C, Gershell D J 1994 Placental site nodule: a clinicopathological study of 38 cases. International Journal of Gynecological Pathology 13: 191–198.

Huntsman D G, Clement P B, Gilks C B, Scully R E 1994 Small cell carcinoma of the endometrium. American Journal of Surgical Pathology 18: 364–375.

Hurliman J, Gloor E 1984 Adenocarcinoma in-situ and invasive adenocarcinoma of the uterine cervix: an immunohistological study with antibodies specific for several epithelial markers. Cancer 54: 103–109.

Hustin J 1978 Immunohistochemical demonstration of several tumor markers in neoplastic and preneoplastic states of the uterine mucosa. Gynecologic and Obstetric Investigation 9: 3.

Ishiguro T, Oshida Y, Tenzaki T, Oshima M, Susuki H 1981 AFP in yolk sac tumor and solid teratoma of ovary: significance of post operative serum AFP. Cancer 48: 2480–2482.

Ishikura H, Scully R E 1987 Hepatoid carcinoma of the ovary. Cancer 60: 2775–2784.

Jobling T W, Granowska K E, Britton K E et al 1990 Radioimmunoscintigraphy of ovarian tumors using a new monoclonal antibody SM-3. Gynecologic Oncology 38: 468–472.

Kabawat S E, Bast R C, Bhan A K, Welch W R, Knapp R C, Colvin R B 1983 Tissue distribution of a coelomic-epithelium related antigen recognised by the monoclonal antibody OC125. International Journal of Gynecological Pathology 2: 275–285.

Kato H, Tongae T 1977 Radioimmunoassay for tumor antigen of human cervical squamous cell carcinoma. Cancer 40: 1621–1628.

Khalifa M A, Sosterhenn I A 1990 Tumor markers of epithelial ovarian neoplasms. International Journal of Gynecological Pathology 9: 217–230.

Knauf S, Urbach G H 1980 Identification, purification and radioimmunoassay of NB/70K, a human tumour associated antigen. Cancer Research 41: 1351–1357.

Konishi I, Fujii S, Kataoka N et al 1988 Ovarian mucinous cystadenocarcinoma producing alpha-fetoprotein. International Journal of Gynecological Pathology 7: 182–189.

Krag-Jacobsen G K, Jacobsen M, Clausen P P 1981 Distribution of tumor associated antigens in the various histologic components of germ cell tumor of the testis. American Journal of Surgical Pathology 5: 257–266.

Kudo R, Sasano H, Kolzumi M, Orenstein J, Silverberg S G 1990 Immunohistochemical comparison of new monoclonal antibody ICS and carcino-embryonic antigen in the differential diagnosis of adenocarcinoma of the uterine cervix. International Journal of Gynecological Pathology 9: 325–336.

Kurman R J, Nadji M 1985 Immunocytochemistry of ovarian neoplasms. In: Roth L M, Czernobilsky B (eds) Tumors and tumor-like conditions of the ovary. Churchill Livingstone, New York, pp 207–232.

Kurman R J, Norris H J 1976 Embryonal carcinoma of the ovary: a clinicopathological entity distinct from endodermal sinus tumor resembling embryonal carcinoma of adult testis. Cancer 38: 2420–2433.

Lang G, Dallenbach-Hellweg G 1990 The histogenetic origin of cervical mesonephric hyperplasia and mesonephric adenocarcinoma of the uterine cervix studied with immunohistochemical methods. International Journal of Gynecological Pathology 9: 145–157.

Lappohn R E, Burger H G, Bouma J, Bangah M, Krans M, de Bruijn H W A 1989 Inhibin as a marker for granulosa-cell tumors. New England Journal of Medicine 321: 790–793.

Lash R H, Hart W R 1987 Intestinal adenocarcinomas metastatic to ovaries: a clinico-pathological evaluation of 22 cases. American Journal of Surgical Pathology 11: 114–121.

Lazarides E 1980 Intermediate filaments as mechanical integrators of cellular space. Nature 283: 249–250.

Lee Y, Raju G C 1988 The expression and localisation of amylase in normal and malignant glands of the endometrium and endocervix. Journal of Pathology 155: 201–205.

Liao S Y, Choi B H 1986 Expression of glial fibrillary acidic protein by neoplastic cells of Müllerian origin. Virchows Archives (Cell Pathology) 52: 185–193.

Liao S Y, Choi B H 1987 The cultured cells of malignant mixed Müllerian tumors and normal endometrium express glial fibrillary acidic protein: a light and EM immunocytochemical study. Laboratory Investigation 56: 43A.

Lifschitz-Mercer B, Czernobilsky B, Dgani R, Dallenbach-Hellweg G, Moll R, Franke W W 1987 Immunocytochemical study of an endometrial diffuse clear cell stromal sarcoma and other endometrial stromal sarcomas. Cancer 59: 1494–1499.

Lifschitz-Mercer B, Czernobilsky B, Shezen E, Dgoni R, Leitner O, Geiger B 1988 Selective expression of cytokeratin polypeptides in various epithelia of human Brenner tumor. Human Pathology 19: 640–650.

Lloreta J, Prat J 1992 Endometrial stromal nodule with smooth and skeletal muscle components simulating stromal sarcoma. International Journal of Gynecological Pathology 11: 293–298.

Maes G, Fleuren G J, Bara J, Nap M 1988 The distribution of mucins, carcino-embryonic antigen and mucus-associated antigens in endocervical and endometrial adenocarcinoma. International Journal of Gynecological Pathology 7: 112–122.

Masuko Y, Zalutsk M, Knapp R C, Bast R C 1984 Interaction of monoclonal antibodies with cell surface antigens of human ovarian carcinomas. Cancer Research 44: 2813–2819.

Michael H, Grawe L, Kraus F T 1984 Minimal deviation endocervical adenocarcinoma: clinical and histological features, immunohistochemical staining for carcino-embryonic antigen and differentiation from confusing benign lesions. International Journal of Gynecological Pathology 3: 261–276.

Miettinen M 1988 Immunoreactivity for cytokeratin and epithelial membrane antigen for leiomyosarcoma. Archives of Pathology and Laboratory Medicine 112: 637–640.

Miettinen M, Wahlstrom T, Virtanen I, Talerman A, Astengo-Osuna C 1985 Cellular differentiation in ovarian sex cord-stromal and germ cell tumors studied with antibodies to intermediate filament proteins. American Journal of Surgical Pathology 145: 127–148.

Millan J L, Manes T 1988 Seminoma derived Nagao isoenzyme is encoded by a germ cell alkaline phosphatase gene. Proceedings of the National Academy of Sciences, USA 85: 3024–3028.

Moll R, Levy R, Czernobilsky B, Hohlweg-Majert P, Dallenbach-Hellweg G, Franke W W 1983 Cytokeratins of normal epithelia and some neoplasms of the female genital tract. Laboratory Investigations 49: 599–610.

Moll R, Pitz S, Levy R, Weikel W, Franke W W, Czernobilsky B 1991 Complexity of expression of intermediate filament proteins including glial filament protein in endometrial and ovarian adenocarcinoma. Human Pathology 22: 989–1002.

Moll R, Lowe A, Laufer J, Franke W W 1992 Cytokeratin 20 in human carcinomas. American Journal of Pathology 140: 427–447.

Morris H B, Gatter K C, Pulford K et al 1983 Cervical wart virus infection, intraepithelial neoplasia and carcinoma: an immunohistochemical study using a panel of monoclonal antibodies. British Journal of Obstetrics and Gynaecology 90: 1069–1081.

Morris W P R, Griffin N R, Wells M 1989 Patterns of reactivity with the monoclonal antibodies HMFG 1, and HMFG 2 in normal endometrium, endometrial hyperplasia and adenocarcinoma. Histopathology 15: 179–186.

Motoyama T, Watanabe H, Takeuchi S, Watanabe T, Gotoh S, Okazaki E 1990 Cancer Antigen 125, carcinoembryonic antigen and carbohydrate determinant 19-9 in ovarian tumors. Cancer 66: 2628–2635.

Niehans G A, Manivel C, Copland G T, Scheithauer B W, Wick M R 1988 Immunohistochemistry of germ cell and trophoblastic neoplasms. Cancer 62: 1113–1123.

Nishida M, Jimi S, Haji M, Hayashi I, Kai T, Tasaka H 1991 Case report: juvenile granulosa cell tumor in association with a high serum inhibin level. Gynecologic Oncology 40: 90–94.

Nogales F C, Concha A, Plata C, Ruiz-Avila I 1993 Granulosa cell tumor of the ovary with diffuse true hepatic differentiation simulating stromal luteinization. American Journal of Surgical Pathology 17: 85–90.

Norton A J, Thomas J A, Isaacson P G 1987 Cytokeratin specific monoclonal antibodies are reactive with tumours of smooth muscle derivation: an immunohistochemical and biochemical study using antibodies to intermediate filament cytoskeletal proteins. Histopathology 11: 487–500.

Nouwen E J, Hendrix P G, Dauwe S, Eerdekens M W, de Broe M E 1987 Tumor markers in the human ovary. American Journal of Pathology 126: 230–241.

Ordonez N G, Manning J T, Brooks T E 1988 Effect of trypsinisation on the immunostaining of formalin fixed, paraffin-embedded tissues. American Journal of Surgical Pathology 12: 121–129.

Otis C N, Powell J L, Barbuto D 1992 Intermediate filamentous proteins in adult granulosa cell tumors: an immunohistochemical study of 25 cases. American Journal of Surgical Pathology 16: 962–968.

Pallesen G, Hamilton-Dutoit S J 1988 Ki-1(CD30) antigen is regularly expressed by tumor cells of embryonal carcinoma. American Journal of Pathology 133: 446–450.

Pavelic Z P, Pavelic L, Pavelic K, Peacock J S 1991 Utility of carcinoembryonic antigen monoclonal antibodies for differentiating ovarian adenocarcinoma from gastrointestinal metastasis to ovary. Gynecologic Oncology 40: 112–117.

Poels L G, Peters D, van Megen Y et al 1986 Monoclonal antibody against human ovarian tumor associated antigens. Journal of the National Cancer Institute 76: 781–791.

Polak J M, van Noorden S 1988 An introduction to immunocytochemistry: current techniques and problems. Revised edn. Microscopy Handbooks II, Oxford University Press, Oxford.

Puts J J G, Moesker O, Aldeweireldt H, Vooijs G P, Raemaekers F C S 1987 Application of antibodies to intermediate filaments in simple and complex tumors of the female genital tract. International Journal of Gynecological Pathology 6: 257–274.

Raju G C 1988 Expression of cytokeratin marker CAM 5.2 in cervical neoplasia. Histopathology 12: 437–443.

Ramaekers F, Feitz W, Moesker O et al 1985 Antibodies to cytokeratin and vimentin in testicular tumour diagnosis. Virchows Archives A Pathological Anatomy 405: 127–142.

Ramaekers F, van Niekerk C, Poels L et al 1990 Use of monoclonal antibodies to keratin in differential diagnosis of adenocarcinomas. American Journal of Pathology 136: 641–655.

Sahin A, Benda J A 1988 An immunohistochemical study of primary ovarian sarcoma. International Journal of Gynecological Pathology 7: 268–279.

Saksela E 1993 Prognostic markers in epithelial ovarian cancer. International Journal of Gynecological Pathology 12: 156–161.

Santini D, Gelli M C, Mazzoleni et al 1989 Brenner tumor of the ovary: a correlative, histologic, histochemical, immunohistological and ultrastructural investigation. Human Pathology 20: 787–795.

Sasaki E, Sasano N, Kimura N, Andoh N, Yajima A 1989 Demonstrations of neuroendocrine cells in ovarian mucinous tumors. International Journal of Gynecological Pathology 8: 189–200.

Sasano H, Oakamoto M, Mason J I et al 1989 Immunohistochemical studies of steroidogenic enzymes (aromatase, 17 alpha hydroxylase and cholesterol side-chain cleavage cytochromes P-450) in sex cord-stromal tumors of the ovary. Human Pathology 20: 452–457.

Sasano H, Mason J I, Sasaki E et al 1990 Immunohistochemical study of 3 beta hydroxy steroid dehydrogenase in sex cord-stromal tumors of the ovary. International Journal of Gynecological Pathology 9: 325–336.

Scully R E 1993 Small cell carcinoma of hypercalcemic type. International Journal of Gynecological Pathology 12: 148–152.

Seldenrijk C A, Willig A P, Baak J P A et al 1986 Malignant Brenner tumor. Cancer 58: 754–760.

Shevchuck M M, Fenoglio C M, Richart R M 1980 Histogenesis of Brenner tumors. II Histochemistry and CEA. Cancer 46: 2617–2622.

Silva E G, Tornos C, Lage J, Ordonez N G, Morris M, Kavanagh J 1993 Multiple nodules of intermediate trophoblast following hydatidiform moles. International Journal of Gynecological Pathology 12: 324–332.

Smith L H, Teng N H 1987 Clinical applications of monoclonal antibodies in gynecologic oncology. Cancer 60: 2068–2074.

Speers W C, Picaso L G, Silverberg S G 1983 Immunohistochemical localisation of carcino-embryonic antigen in microglandular hyperplasia and adenocarcinoma of the endocervix. American Journal of Clinical Pathology 79: 105–107.

Sporrong B, Falkmer S, Robboy S J 1982 Neurohormonal peptides in ovarian carcinoids. Cancer 49: 68–74.

Steeper T A, Wick M R 1986 Minimal deviation adenocarcinoma of the uterine cervix ("adenoma malignum"): an immunohistochemical comparison with microglandular endocervical hyperplasia and conventional adenocarcinoma. Cancer 58: 1131–1138.

Stephenson T J, Mills P M 1986 Adenomatoid tumours: an immunohistochemical and ultrastructural approach of their histogenesis. Journal of Pathology 148: 327–335.

Syrjanen S, Cintorino M, Armellini D et al 1988 Expression of cytokeratin polypeptides in human papilloma virus (HPV) lesions of the uterine cervix. 1. Relationship to grade of CIN and HPV type. International Journal of Gynecological Pathology 7: 23–38.

Taglialbue E, Menord S, Torre G D et al 1985 Generation of monoclonal antibodies reacting with human epithelial ovarian cancer. Cancer Research 45: 379–385.

Tetu B, Ordonez N G, Silva E G 1986 Sertoli-Leydig cell tumor of the ovary with alpha fetoprotein production. Archives of Pathology and Laboratory Medicine 110: 65–68.

Thor A, Ohuchi N, Szpak C A, Johnson W W, Schlom J 1986 Distribution of neofetal antigen associated glycoprotein-72 defined by monoclonal antibody B72.3. Cancer Research 46: 3118–3124.

Thor A, Viglione M J, Muraro R, Ohuchi N, Schlom J, Gorstein F 1987 Monoclonal antibody B72.3 reactivity with human endometrium: a study of normal and malignant tissues. International Journal of Gynecological Pathology 6: 235–247.

Tobon H, Dave H 1988 Adenocarcinoma in situ of the cervix: clinicopathologic observations of 11 cases. International Journal of Gynecological Pathology 7: 139–151.

Tsuji Y, Suzuki T, Nishiara H, Takemura T, Isojima S 1985 Identification of two different surface epitopes of human ovarian epithelial carcinomas by monoclonal antibodies. Cancer Research 45: 2358–2362.

Ueda G, Shimizu C, Shimizu H et al 1988 An immunohistochemical study of small-cell and poorly differentiated carcinomas of the cervix using neuroendocrine markers. Gynecologic Oncology 34: 164–169.

Ueda G, Sawada M, Ogawa H, Tanisawa O, Tsujimoto M 1993 Immunohistochemical study of cytokeratin 7 for the differential diagnosis of adenocarcinoma in the ovary. Gynecologic Oncology 51: 219–223.

Van Nagell J R, Hudson S, Gay E C et al 1982 Carcinoembryonic antigen in carcinoma of the uterine cervix. Cancer 49: 379–383.

Van Niekerk C C, Ramackers F C S, Hanselaar A G J M, Aldeweireldt J, Poels L G 1993 Changes in expression of differentiation markers between normal ovarian cells and derived tumors. American Journal of Pathology 142: 157–177.

Vergote I, Mathias O, Nustad K 1987 Placental alkaline phosphatase as a tumor marker in ovarian carcinoma. Obstetrics and Gynecology 69: 228–232.

Viale G, Gambacorta M, Dell'Orto P, Coggi G 1988 Coexpression of cytokeratins and vimentin in common epithelial tumours of the ovary: an immunocytochemical study of 83 cases. Virchows Archives of Pathology [A] 413: 91–101.

Wagener C, Petzold P, Kohler W, Totovic V 1984 Binding of five monoclonal anti-CEA antibodies with different epitope specificities to various carcinoma tissues. International Journal of Cancer 33: 469–475.

Wahlstrom T, Lindgren J, Korhonen M, Segala M 1979 Distinction between endocervical and endometrial adenocarcinoma with immunoperoxidase staining of carcinoembryonic antigen in routine histological tissue specimens. Lancet 2: 1159–1160.

Warhol M J, Antonioli D A, Pinkus G S, Burke L, Rice R H 1982 Immunoperoxidase staining for involucrin: a potential diagnostic aid in cervico-vaginal pathology. Human Pathology 13: 1095–1099.

Wells M, Brown L J R, Jackson P 1986 Low molecular weight cytokeratin proteins in cervical neoplasia (letter). Journal of Pathology 150: 69–70.

Wolpert H R, Fuller A F, Bell D A 1989 Primary mucinous carcinoid tumor of the ovary. International Journal of Gynecological Pathology 8: 156–162.

Yeh I T, O'Connor D M, Kurman R J 1989 Vacuolated cytotrophoblast in the chorion laeve. Placenta 10: 429–438.

Young R H, Scully R E 1987 Sex cord-stromal, steroid cell and other ovarian tumors with endocrine, paraendocrine and paraneoplastic manifestations. In: Kurman R J (ed) Blaustein's pathology of the female genital tract. Springer Verlag, New York, pp 607–658.

Young R H, Perez-Atayde A R, Scully R E 1984 Ovarian Sertoli-Leydig cell tumor with retiform and heterologous components: report of a case with hepatocytic differentiation and elevated serum alpha-fetoprotein. American Journal of Surgical Pathology 8: 709–718.

Young R H, Kurman R J, Scully R E 1988 Proliferations and tumors of intermediate trophoblast of the placental site. Seminars in Diagnostic Pathology 5: 223–237.

Young R H, Silva E G, Scully R E 1991 Ovarian and juxtaovarian adenomatoid tumors: a report of six cases. International Journal of Gynecological Pathology 10: 364–371.

45. Gynaecological cytopathology

D. V. Coleman

INTRODUCTION

One of the outstanding developments in modern gynaecological practice is the increasing reliance of gynaecologists on cytology as a method of investigating disease in the female genital tract. The ease with which these specimens can be collected and the non-invasive nature of the collection techniques make cytological methods particularly appropriate for the investigation of patients attending gynaecological outpatient clinics. Moreover, the high level of cytodiagnostic accuracy that can be achieved by the pathologist ensures that cytological techniques make a useful contribution to patient management.

The pathologist who provides a cytodiagnostic service to his or her gynaecological colleagues can expect to receive specimens from a variety of anatomical sites. The majority of specimens will be cervical smears but other types of specimens such as endometrial aspirates, vulvar scrapes, peritoneal washings, ascitic fluid and fine needle aspirates can be expected. Thus the pathologist needs to develop skills in the interpretation of a wide range of specimens and the aim of this chapter is to assist him or her with this task.

Cytological techniques lend themselves most readily to the detection of malignant disease in the female genital tract since tumour cells lack cohesiveness and exfoliate spontaneously or are readily dislodged (Coman, 1944). Several studies have shown that the earliest and smallest tumours can be detected by cytological methods even before the lesions are clinically apparent. Thus most specimens are taken to detect or exclude very early invasive cancers or preinvasive neoplastic disease. It is important to remember that other conditions such as viral or parasitic infections and hormonal imbalance can be diagnosed from cytological material and the pathologist should approach each case with an open mind to ensure that the maximum of clinically useful information is extracted from each sample.

The interpretation of a cytological specimen can be likened to detective work. As the cytologist advances across the microscope slide, field by field, he or she picks up clues to the nature of the epithelium from the appearance of the surface cells. Of course this approach has its limitations. It is not always possible to identify the tumour type accurately or to determine its grade or stage of development. Nor is it always possible to identify the precise location of the tumour from a cytological specimen. Despite these drawbacks cytology is an inexpensive and simple first line of investigation which is acceptable to clinician and patient alike. For a seriously ill patient who is unable to withstand open surgery, or for an obvious malignant tumour where tissue confirmation is needed, cytology provides a unique opportunity to make the definitive pathological diagnosis which is essential for sound clinical management.

GENERAL PRINCIPLES OF SPECIMEN COLLECTION AND PREPARATION

The accuracy of cytology as a diagnostic test depends on several factors. The most important of these are:

(i) the method used for the collection of the specimen
(ii) the laboratory techniques used to prepare the specimen for light microscopy
(iii) the skill and experience of the cytologist who is interpreting the specimen.

The following general principles apply to the collection and preparation of all cytology specimens.

Collection techniques

Specimen collection techniques should be adapted to ensure that the sample is collected directly from the suspect area or from an area very close to it. For example, an endometrial aspirate is more appropriate than a cervical smear for the detection of endometrial neoplasia. By the same token a cervical scrape is more likely to permit an accurate diagnosis of cervical neoplasia than an aspirate from the posterior fornix. The pathologist should be able to advise the clinician of the optimal collection techniques for a particular lesion. The advantages and disadvantages of the collection techniques available for the investigation of cervical, endometrial and ovarian lesions will be discussed under the appropriate heading.

Preparatory techniques

Preparatory techniques should be designed to ensure that the maximum number of cells are harvested from the specimen and as much cellular material as possible is processed for inspection in the light microscope. Thus fluid samples, e.g. cyst aspirates and peritoneal washings, should be concentrated by centrifugation or membrane filtration before smears are made and multiple smears prepared from the deposit. It is often advantageous to remove red blood cells from a heavily blood-stained specimen before processing using gradient separation techniques as the red blood cells may obscure the cells of interest in the sample. Moreover coverslip size should be selected to ensure that all the cells on the smear are available for inspection in the light microscope.

By convention, most cytological specimens are fixed in 95% alcohol and stained by the Papanicolaou method (Papanicolaou, 1942). This stain, when correctly applied, reveals details of nuclear structure and cytoplasm which are rarely seen in histological section but which are critical for the correct interpretation of cytological specimens. The Papanicolaou stain is particularly appropriate for those cases where an epithelial lesion is suspected as keratin-containing tumour cells appear strongly eosinophilic and mucin is translucent so that epithelial cells deep to the mucin layer are not obscured. Moreover the Papanicolaou stain ensures that individual cell nuclei within a cluster of epithelial cells can be visualized. The secret of successful Papanicolaou staining is rapid fixation of the specimen before the cells have time to dry. Of course, a range of other stains can be used on cytological material — haematoxylin and eosin, periodic acid–Schiff, Masson–Fontana — providing the specimens are appropriately fixed. The May–Grünwald–Giemsa stain is particularly useful in those cases where a non-epithelial lesion is suspected or the smears are so thin that air drying cannot be avoided. However, the Giemsa stain has a strong affinity for mucin so it should not be used routinely for gynaecological material. Immunocytochemical techniques and electron-microscopy have a place in the investigation of cytological specimens and these will be discussed under the appropriate headings.

For further details of preparatory techniques the reader is referred to Proctor (1989a,b) and Potter (1989).

Diagnostic accuracy

Assuming optimal collection and preparatory techniques

and a high level of interpretive skill on the part of the cytopathologist, the specificity of cytodiagnosis is very high, usually in the region of 99%. Unfortunately, false negative reporting is more difficult to control as this reflects sampling technique, but it should not be more than 10%. The sensitivity of most cytological investigatory techniques can be improved by repeated sampling and by review of the methods employed in specimen collection and preparation.

In most laboratories the preparation of cytology specimens is in the hands of the technologist, who may also be responsible for the processing of histological material. Many of the specimens submitted for cytological examination are presented in the form of alcohol-fixed smears which only require to be stained by the Papanicolaou method and mounted for analysis, and there is little scope for modification of preparatory techniques. In some cases, e.g. fine needle aspirates and peritoneal washings, diagnostic accuracy can be enhanced if special stains are applied and close communication between pathologist and technical staff is essential for good results.

CERVICAL CYTOPATHOLOGY

Cervical cytology is a safe, simple and non-invasive method of detecting neoplastic changes in the cervix. Because of these characteristics it is used worldwide as a method of screening healthy women for preinvasive and early invasive cancers of the cervix in an effort to reduce morbidity and mortality from this disease. Thus in the UK the majority of cervical smears submitted to the pathology laboratory are taken as part of the national screening programme for the prevention of cervical cancer. A small percentage of cervical smears are taken as part of the diagnostic work-up of women with symptoms and signs of malignant disease referable to the cervix.

It is important for both the pathologist and the clinician to be aware of the distinction between cervical smears that are taken for screening purposes and those that are taken as part of the diagnostic work-up of the patients, for although the principles underlying the collection, processing and interpretation of the specimens in the light-microscope are the same, the management of the patient is fundamentally different.

In the case of a cervical smear being taken for the purposes of screening, a negative cytology report is intended to reassure the clinician and the woman that she is free of cervical neoplasia. In the case of a cervical smear taken from a woman with symptoms suggestive of cervical cancer, a negative cytology report is an indication to the clinician that he may need to employ other diagnostic techniques to exclude cancer in his patient.

Cervical smears which are taken as part of a national cervical screening programme form a large component of the workload of most pathology laboratories. The work entailed in analysing them is considerable and is usually shared between the cytotechnologists and the pathologist. The cytotechnologist undertakes the primary screening and refers problem cases and abnormal smears to the pathologist for an expert medical opinion. In order for this relationship to be effective, the pathologist must be experienced in the interpretation of a wide range of smear patterns — both normal and abnormal. This experience can only be achieved by systematic screening of at least 5000 routine primary smears and by careful cytological/histological correlation of selected abnormalities illustrating the various patterns of cervical neoplasia. The pathologist must always attempt to provide a totally independent, unbiased, informed opinion on a problem smear and the practice of prior 'marking' of the equivocal cells by the cytotechnologist to facilitate their recognition by the pathologist is to be deplored.

In this section, the collection, preparation, method of analysis and reporting of cervical smears is discussed.

Specimen collection

The technique most widely used for the collection of cells from the cervix for cytological study is the cervical scrape. Other techniques which may be used to supplement the information obtained from the scrape include vaginal aspiration and cervical brush specimens.

Cervical scrape

Several studies have shown that this is the single most efficient method of detecting premalignant and early malignant lesions of the cervix (Wachtel, 1969). An excellent illustrated account of the technique has been prepared by the British Society for Clinical Cytology (1989). Copies of this booklet should be available in every pathology laboratory for distribution to nurses, clinicians and general practitioners who are concerned with smear taking.

The aim of the cervical scrape is to remove cells from the transformation zone, which is the most likely site of an early cancer. To achieve this the scrape should be obtained under direct vision with a vaginal speculum in position to expose the cervix. The scrape is taken with a wooden or plastic spatula which is inserted into the external os and rotated through 180° (Fig. 45.1).

The mucus and cells on the spatula are then transferred to a glass slide, the frosted end of which has been previously labelled in pencil with the patient's name. The transfer of material from spatula to slide should be made with a few deft strokes and the slide placed in fixative immediately by immersing it in a jar containing 95% ethanol (Fig. 45.2). The slide must remain in fixative for at least 30 minutes, after which it can be removed and stored at room temperature. Alternatively, a spray fixative or carbowax fixative can be used. Whichever method is

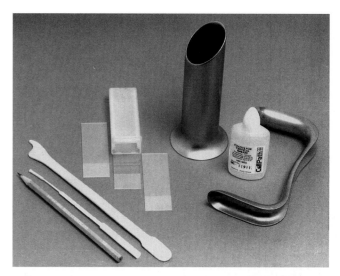

Fig. 45.1 Equipment required for taking a cervical smear showing speculum, glass slide with frosted end, spatula, endocervical brush, fixative and pencil.

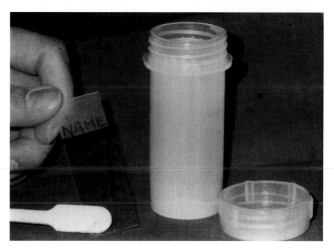

Fig. 45.2 Preparing a cervical smear: the cervical mucus and cells are transferred from the spatula on to the slide which must immediately be immersed in fixative.

employed, it is essential that the smear is not allowed to dry before fixation as this impairs the staining quality of the cells.

The effectiveness of cervical screening depends to a large extent on the quality of the smears and the skill with which they are taken. Up to 20% of preinvasive lesions may be missed due to poor smear taking. Many spatulae have been devised to assist the clinician with collection of specimens (Fig. 45.3) but the spatulae most frequently used in the UK are the Ayre spatula (Ayre, 1947) and the Aylesbury spatula (Wolfendale et al, 1987). The claims that a particular spatula is superior to another should be viewed with caution. Many of the so-called 'spatula trials' are poorly designed, lack objectivity and are rarely randomized. It seems unlikely that a single spatula design

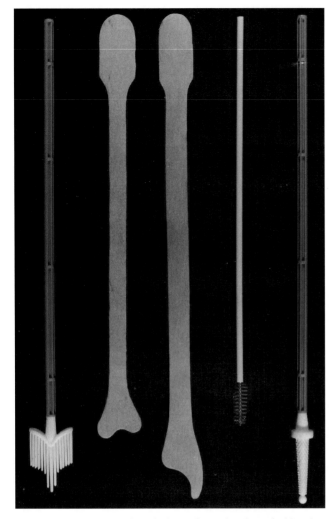

Fig. 45.3 Various types of cervical spatulae and endocervical brushes.

will be suitable for all cervices: 3% or 4% of smears may always be unsatisfactory even in skilled hands.

Vaginal aspirates

This method of obtaining exfoliated cells from the cervix was originally advocated by Papanicolaou for the diagnosis of uterine cancer (Papanicolaou & Traut, 1943). Specimens are obtained from the posterior vaginal fornix using a pipette and bulb. This method was soon shown to be much less sensitive than the cervical scrape for the detection of cervical neoplasia (Wachtel, 1969) and it is now rarely used. It may have a place in cases where the cervix cannot be visualized but these are rare.

Endocervical brush specimen

The presence of endocervical cells in a cervical smear is indicative that the smear has probably been taken from

the region of the transformation zone and is therefore an acceptable sample for analysis, The Cytobrush (Medscand AB, Malmo, Sweden) was developed to ensure sampling of the endocervical canal at the region of the squamocolumnar junction on the premise that the presence of these cells in a smear improved the detection rate of cervical cancer. Several studies have confirmed this hypothesis and endocervical sampling has proved to be particularly effective in detecting endocervical adenocarcinoma at an early stage in its development (Boon et al, 1986; Buntinx et al, 1991).

The instrument is shown in Figure 45.3. The brush is inserted into the external os and rotated through 360° and then withdrawn. The material on the brush is transferred to a glass slide by rolling it across the glass and the slide fixed immediately with a spray fixative. The information provided by the Cytobrush is limited as the smears do not contain cells from the ectocervix. Thus in every case a routine cervical scrape should accompany the Cytobrush specimen. A technique has been developed where both the Cytobrush and the cervical scrape can be spread on the same slide to reduce the time taken to screen the samples. When endocervical brush and ectocervical scrape were used in combination the number of adequate smears increased from 84% to 98% and the percentage of abnormal smears rose (Boon et al, 1986; Trimbos & Arentz, 1986; Taylor et al, 1987).

The addition of a Cytobrush sample to routine cervical screening adds significantly to the cost of the screening test and many clinicians prefer to use the Cytobrush on selected cases only. The indications for using the brush are fourfold.

(i) The brush should be used when the cervical os is too narrow to permit insertion of the pointed end of the spatula.

(ii) The brush should be used after cone biopsy or when the os is stenosed.

(iii) The brush should be used in postmenopausal women when the squamocolumnar junction may be high in the canal.

(iv) The brush should be used when the smear contains abnormal glandular cells of uncertain origin.

Interpretation and reporting of cervical smears

The concept of screening for preinvasive cancer of the cervix stems from observations made by Dr George Papanicolaou over 70 years ago (Papanicolaou, 1929). He was the first to describe the cell content of smears prepared from samples from women with diseased and healthy cervices and he developed a nomenclature to describe these cells which is in use today. The epithelial cells are classified on the basis of cell size and shape, the staining quality of the cytoplasm and the nuclear : cytoplasmic ratio. Thus careful attention has to be paid to these morphological features when interpreting the smear. It is important to remember that the epithelial cells in the smears are derived from the surface layers of the epithelium. The cytologist's skill lies in his or her ability to deduce from these surface cells the benign or malignant nature of the cervical epithelium.

The contents of a cervical smear from a normal cervix can be conveniently categorized as follows:

1. Squamous epithelial cells derived from the original (native) squamous epithelium of the cervix
2. Glandular epithelial cells from the endocervical canal
3. Metaplastic cells from the transformation zone
4. Cells from the endometrial lining and stroma
5. Leucocytes and erythrocytes
6. Commensal micro-organisms
7. Contaminants, e.g. spermatozoa
8. Cervical mucus.

Cells shed from the original (native) squamous epithelium

These cells are of three types and are designated superficial, intermediate and parabasal cells.

Superficial cells. These are large angular cells measuring 50 μm in diameter which are shed from the surface layers of a fully mature epithelium. They contain abundant cytoplasm, which usually stains a delicate pink colour with the Papanicolaou stain, and a nucleus which is pyknotic and measures less than 5 μm. The cells may be found singly or in sheets (Fig. 45.4).

Intermediate cells. These are slightly smaller than superficial cells and have a more rounded appearance (Fig. 45.5). They are shed from the surface layers of an epithelium which is showing a slightly diminished re-

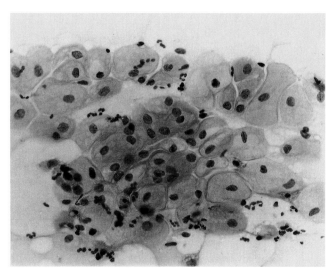

Fig. 45.5 Intermediate cells in a cervical smear. The intermediate cells have vesicular nuclei and a slightly more rounded appearance than the superficial cells and they are slightly smaller. ×475.

sponse to oestrogen or a progesterone effect. The cytoplasm is usually cyanophilic and the nuclei have a vesicular chromatin structure and range from 5–10 μm in diameter. The cells frequently appear in clumps.

In pregnancy, the intermediate cells assume a boat-like shape, with thickened borders and eccentric nucleus. When this pattern is seen the intermediate cells are sometimes referred to as 'navicular' cells (Fig. 45.6). Electron-microscopy has shown that under the influence of progesterone, the cytoplasm of the intermediate cells becomes packed with glycogen granules which accounts for the altered appearance of the cells.

Parabasal cells. These are usually shed spontaneously in smears from postmenopausal women when the

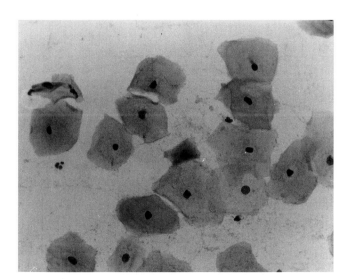

Fig. 45.4 Superficial cells in a cervical smear. Note the angular shapes of the cells, the abundant transparent cytoplasm and the pyknotic nuclei. The superficial cells are 50 μm in diameter. ×475.

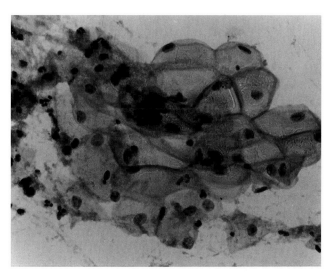

Fig. 45.6 Navicular cells: these are found in the smears of pregnant women. Note boat-shaped cells with thickened borders and eccentric nuclei. ×475.

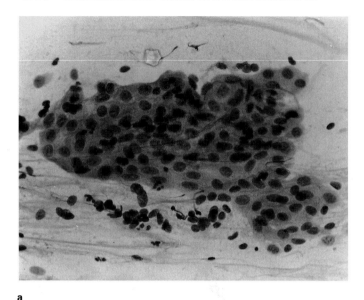

a

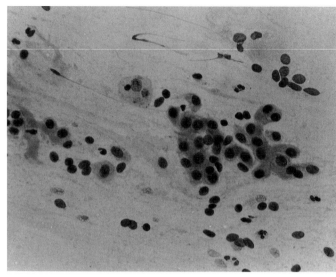

b

Fig. 45.7a,b a A sheet of parabasal cells in an atrophic smear. The smears are usually scanty and the cells may lie in dense sheets with occasional free nuclei in the background. b Discrete parabasal cells in an atrophic postmenopausal smear. Note uniform smear pattern composed of rounded cells about 30 μm in diameter and total absence of mature squames. ×500.

hormonal levels are diminished. Most frequently they appear as small rounded cells 15–30 μm in diameter with a round, centrally located nucleus which occupies about one-third of the volume of the cell (Fig. 45.7). These cells reflect the thin atrophic epithelium from which they are derived. The cytoplasm is often frayed and the nuclei often show degenerative changes such as vacuolation, pyknosis, and karyorrhexis. The smear may contain numerous free nuclei.

Occasionally, the parabasal cells have been forcibly detached from deeper layers of the epithelium by the spatula. This is manifest in the smear by the presence of parabasal cells with long cytoplasmic processes which reflect disruption of the intercellular bridges.

When undertaking the analysis of Papanicolaou-stained cervical smears it is important to remember that the colouration of the cytoplasm of the squamous epithelial cells is very variable. The Papanicolaou stain is notoriously susceptible to changes in pH so that the cytoplasm of superficial cells does not always take up the eosin and the cytoplasm of intermediate or parabasal cells is not always cyanophilic. Thus the classification of epithelial cells into superficial, intermediate and parabasal types should not be based on cytoplasmic colouration but rather on morphological features and on the nuclear : cytoplasmic ratio.

Glandular epithelial cells from the endocervical canal

These cells may appear singly or in sheets. When single they are readily recognized by their cylindrical shape, deli-

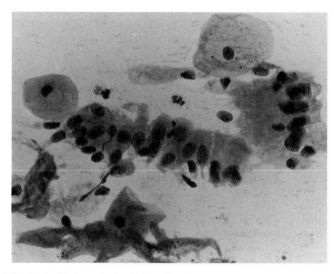

Fig. 45.8 Endocervical cells in palisade. ×475.

cate often vacuolated cytoplasm and basal nucleus. Cilia are rarely seen although a terminal bar may be recognized. When in sheets the cells appear in palisade formation or present a honeycomb appearance (Fig. 45.8). Single cells may present in smears en face (Fig. 45.9a). They appear as discrete rounded cells with scanty cytoplasm and are often indistinguishable from discrete parabasal cells (Fig. 45.9b). Endocervical cells that have been exfoliated from the endocervical canal and trapped in the cervical mucus exhibit degenerative changes. Nuclei lose their structure, the cytoplasm fragments and free nuclei abound.

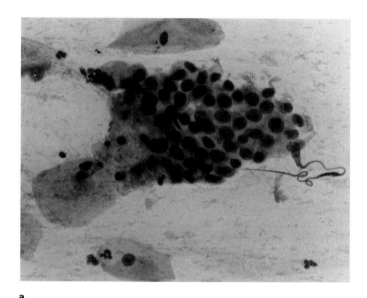

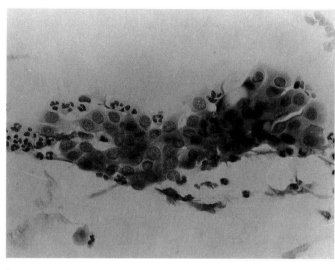

a

b

Fig. 45.9a,b   a Endocervical cells en face, forming a honeycomb pattern. ×500. **b** Endocervical cells in an atrophic smear. The atrophic endocervical cells are usually smaller and more cuboidal than the sheets of endocervical cells found in smears from premenopausal women. ×500.

Epithelial cells shed from immature and mature metaplastic epithelium

Although native squamous epithelium and metaplastic epithelium can be readily distinguished in histological section, this distinction is not so straightforward in cervical smears. Morphologically, the superficial and intermediate epithelial cells from native squamous epithelium are indistinguishable from surface cells shed from mature metaplastic epithelium. Similarly, epithelial cells derived from immature metaplastic epithelium or from areas of reserve cell hyperplasia resemble the parabasal cells found in atrophic smears (Fig. 45.10).

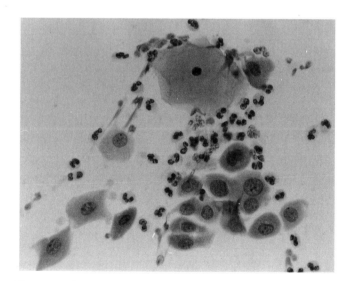

Fig. 45.10   Immature metaplastic cells. Note the similarity of some of the immature metaplastic cells to atrophic parabasal cells. However the presence of mature squames in the smear confirms the metaplastic origin of these cells. ×475.

Nevertheless, it is possible by careful analysis of the smear pattern to discriminate between immature metaplastic cells and atrophic parabasal cells in the smear. A cervical scrape taken from an atrophic cervix presents a uniform appearance as it will be composed almost entirely of parabasal cells. In contrast, a cervical scrape from an area of immature metaplastic change will contain both 'parabasal' type cells and more mature squamous cells (superficial or intermediate type) from the surrounding native epithelium.

Epithelial cells shed from other parts of the genital tract

Cells of endometrial origin may become trapped in the cervical mucus and may be present in the cervical smear. They have many of the characteristics of endocervical cells but are smaller (they rarely exceed 20 µm) and their nuclei contains both coarse and fine chromatin fragments. They are often described as having a 'pepper and salt' appearance. Endometrial cells are most likely to appear in smears taken at the onset of menstruation but they may also be found in the smears of women who have an intrauterine contraceptive device (IUCD) inserted into the uterus, reflecting the low-grade endometritis associated with the insertion of an IUCD.

Unlike endocervical cells, endometrial cells usually show marked degenerative changes. They may be shed singly, in which case they are difficult to distinguish from histiocytes, or in sheets when they appear as dense berry-like clusters (Fig. 45.11), or as large plaques comprising a central core of stromal cells and an outer rim of glandular cells (Fig. 45.12).

Occasionally, in smears taken near the end of menstruation, a large streak of endometrial cells intimately mixed

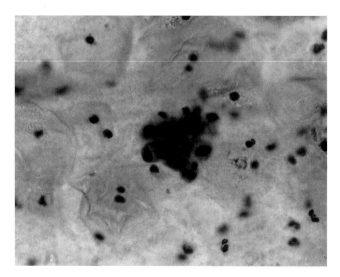

Fig. 45.11   Endometrial cells in a berry-like cluster. The nuclei are smaller and coarser than endocervical cells. ×475.

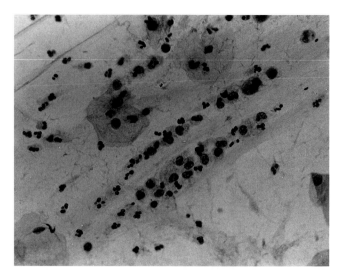

Fig. 45.13   A streak of histiocytes in a menstrual smear. Note the variation in shape and small size (12 μm diameter) of the histiocytes in comparison with the squamous cells (50 μm) in the smear. ×475.

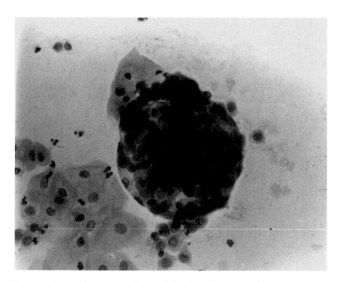

Fig. 45.12   A plaque of endometrial cells. Note central core of endometrial cells and surrounding rim of stromal cells. ×475.

with histiocytes may be seen in the smear (Fig. 45.13). This pattern has been designated 'the exodus' by some authors (Koss, 1992).

Commensal micro-organisms

Numerous organisms colonize the vagina in the absence of disease. They include lactobacilli (Döderlein), anaerobes, diphtheroids and coliforms, enterococci and coagulase-negative staphylococci, group B streptococci, *Gardnerella vaginalis*, *Candida albicans*, *Actinomyces israelii*, and *Staphylococcus aureus*. Of these, few are identifiable in cervical smears.

Döderlein bacilli in Papanicolaou-stained smears appear as blue-staining rod-shaped organisms 1–2 μm in

length. They are particularly abundant in smears taken in early pregnancy or in the late secretory phase of the menstrual cycle at which times, under the influence of progesterone, the cells lining the ectocervix and vagina are packed with glycogen granules. Döderlein bacilli metabolize the glycogen, destroying the cells in the process (see below, The cytolytic smear).

Candida, Gardnerella and Actinomyces will be discussed in the section on specific infections.

Other components of cervical smears

Leucocytes and histiocytes are invariably found in cervical smears. They may reflect a physiological response of the cervix tissue to external agents (e.g. smegma or semen) or they may reflect underlying cervicitis. The point at which the presence of neutrophils in a smear is deemed to reflect underlying pathological changes is ill defined. For practical purposes, if neutrophils are so abundant that they obscure most of the epithelial cells in the smear, acute cervicitis may be assumed. The presence of specific infectious organisms in addition to neutrophils is also generally indicative of an acute cervicitis.

The presence of histiocytes in the smear usually reflects chronic cervicitis although they may also be found in abundance in menstrual smears. Multinucleated histiocytes are commonly found in smears taken shortly after ablative therapy to the cervix or radiotherapy and in atrophic smears.

Red blood cells (RBCs) are common in the presence of true erosion or ectropion. In a menstrual smear, the large number of red blood cells present may render the smear unsuitable for analysis.

Postcoital smears may contain numerous spermatozoa which are readily recognized by their characteristic structure. However, seminiferous cells which usually accompany them are less readily classified as contaminants and may be misidentified as dyskaryotic cells.

A strange artifact, sometimes described as 'cornflake' artifact, may be found in smears. It usually only affects a few epithelial cells but if it is widespread the smear must be regarded as unsuitable for screening. The cause is unknown but it may be due to poor fixation.

Cervical mucus is present in many smears as elongated strands of amorphous basophilic material. As recorded elsewhere, the nature of cervical mucus changes during the menstrual cycle and the copious watery mucus in the second half of the cycle or in pregnancy can make smear preparation rather difficult as the cells do not readily adhere to the spatula. In the atrophic cervix, the mucus is thick and tenacious and may present as inspissated rounded droplets of intensely basophilic amorphous material in Papanicolaou-stained smears which may be mistaken for abnormal nuclei (Fig. 45.14).

Cytological patterns seen in normal cervical smears

Many pathologists regard the analysis of routine cervical smears as a tedious exercise devoid of the variety encountered in histological practice. Experienced cytologists would deny this, claiming that the variation in smear pattern is immense and the interpretation of cervical smears represents a continuous challenge. Analysis of cervical smear patterns shows that the content of an individual smear is determined by a number of factors, some of which are listed below:

1. Skill of the smear taker (Vooijs et al, 1986)
2. Hormonal status
3. Position of the squamocolumnar junction

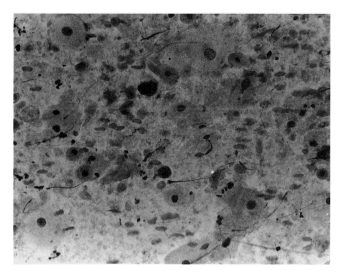

Fig. 45.14 Amorphous basophilic mucoid material frequently seen in atrophic smears. This material may be mistaken for tumour cell nuclei. ×475.

4. Shape and patency of the external os
5. Presence of disease in the cervix (local or general)
6. Recent ablative therapy, radiotherapy, chemotherapy or hormonal therapy
7. Instrument used to collect the sample.

Because of this it is essential for the cytologist to be aware of relevant clinical and therapeutic details such as age, date of last menstrual period, contraceptive use and clinical appearance of the cervix before he or she embarks on the microscopic analysis of the smear. Armed with this information the cytologist will be able to interpret the smear with a high degree of accuracy.

Some common smear patterns associated with hormonal changes are described in this section but it should be remembered that the patterns may be present in a variety of combinations and are too numerous to describe here.

Hormonal patterns

The squamous epithelium of the cervix and upper third of the vagina is derived from Müllerian epithelium and as such is responsive to endogenous oestrogen and progesterone. Thus the thickness of the epithelium alters throughout the menstrual cycle.

The squamous epithelium is at its most mature at mid-cycle when levels of unopposed oestrogen are at their highest. Smears taken at this time will be composed almost entirely of large superficial squames with eosinophilic cytoplasm and pyknotic nuclei. In contrast, in the secretory phase of the cycle, when oestrogen levels are diminished and progesterone levels increase, the epithelium is less mature and intermediate cells predominate in the smear. A similar pattern may be found in the early proliferative phase when oestrogen levels are diminished.

In the absence of steroid hormones, i.e. in postmenopausal women or in prepubertal girls, the epithelium is atrophic and the smears are composed almost entirely of parabasal cells. Because the epithelium is fragile and susceptible to infection, these atrophic smears may contain many free nuclei and numerous polymorphs. An atrophic pattern may sometimes be seen in the immediate postpartum period before the normal menstrual cycle is re-established.

Smears taken in the first trimester of pregnancy have a characteristic pattern. The high levels of progesterone are associated with a build-up of glycogen in the epithelial cells which will be manifest as navicular cells in the smears. There is a concomitant increase in the number of glycogenic bacteria in the cervix which cause intense cytolysis so that free nuclei, fragments of cytoplasm and Döderlein bacilli abound in the smear (Fig. 45.15).

A smear taken at the time of menstruation will usually be heavily blood-stained and may contain endometrial cells and histiocytes. The endometrial cells may be discrete or form plaques or berry-like clusters as previously

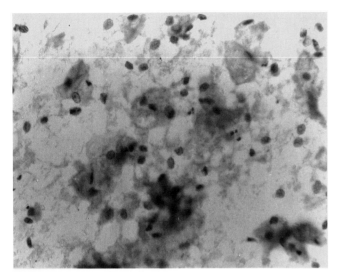

Fig. 45.15 A cytolytic smear: the Döderlein bacilli have destroyed the cytoplasm of the intermediate cells and free nuclei abound. Such a smear is not suitable for screening. ×475.

described. Smears taken at the end of menstruation may be composed of large streaks of histiocytes and endometrial cells intimately mixed. This pattern was described by Papanicolaou as the 'exodus'. Occasionally, the red blood cells in a cervical smear taken during menstruation may be so excessive that they obscure the squamous epithelial cells in the smear. However, this is not always the case and the squamous epithelial cells found in menstrual smears are usually of the intermediate type.

The patterns described above assume that there are no other factors influencing the maturation of the squamous epithelium. This, of course, is rarely the case and the patterns may be modified by infection, therapy and the administration of exogenous hormones, particularly oral contraceptives and hormone replacement therapy (HRT). It is important for the cytologist to take note of the hormonal pattern of the smear before preparing a cytology report and to ensure that it corresponds to the menstrual history of the patient. Any discrepancy may be of clinical significance; for example, a well-oestrogenized smear taken from a woman who is well past the menopause and who is not receiving exogenous oestrogens could be indicative of an oestrogen-producing tumour of the ovary.

The smear pattern in women who are taking oral contraceptives is usually of the intermediate type, reflecting the combined oestrogen/progesterone content of most contraceptive pills. Smears from women who are receiving hormone replacement therapy are well oestrogenized and contain numerous superficial cells instead of the atrophic parabasal cell pattern one might expect from a postmenopausal woman. Both tamoxifen and digitalis are known to be associated with an increase in the maturation of the cervical epithelium and with a predominance of superficial cells in the cervical smear. Unexpectedly, *Tricho-*

monas vaginalis infection is associated with maturation of the epithelium although the reason for this is unclear.

The smear in the presence of infection

The cervix in the sexually active female is a common site of inflammation which may occur as a result of trauma, parturition, abortion or sexually transmitted disease or may be due to prolonged irritation due to prolapse. Cervicitis is reflected in the cervical smear by the presence of leucocytes, red blood cells and numerous coccal forms of bacteria. The squamous and glandular epithelial cells invariably show degenerative or reactive changes. In some forms of infection, particularly those due to fungal infection or protozoa, the specific organisms can be identified in the smear. Several characteristic cytological patterns are described in this section.

Acute bacterial cervicitis

This form of cervicitis results from infection of the endocervical crypts with a range of bacteria which include *Neisseria gonorrhoeae*, *Gardnerella vaginalis* and *Chlamydia trachomatis*. Most forms of bacterial cervicitis are associated with a purulent exudate. In these cases the smear is characterized by the presence of polymorphonuclear leucocytes which may be so numerous that they obscure the epithelial cell elements in the smear. The smear may also be heavily blood-stained due to the friability of the cervix. In the presence of ulceration, streaks of necrotic cell debris may be present.

Numerous cocci or rod-shaped bacteria may be seen in the background but precise identification of the organism is rarely possible. The intracellular diplococci characteristic of *N. gonorrhoeae* have been recognized in smears but are an exceptional finding. Similarly, intracytoplasmic

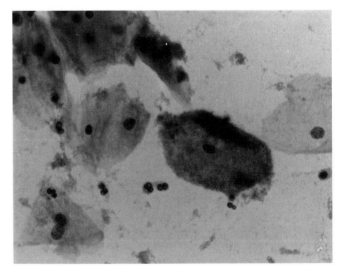

Fig. 45.16 Bacterial vaginosis: note presence of clue cells. ×475.

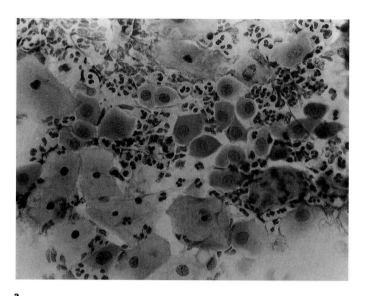
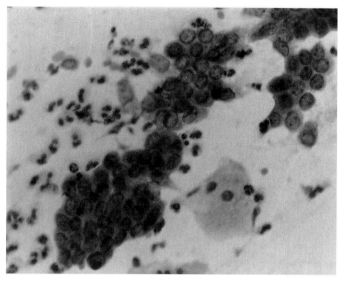

a
b

Fig. 45.17a,b a Degenerative changes in the presence of inflammation: note the slightly frayed cytoplasm of the superficial epithelial cells and swollen structureless nuclei of the immature metaplastic cells. Numerous polymorphs are also present, obscuring some cells. ×500. **b** Degenerative changes affecting the endocervical cells in the smear. These are characterized by loss of nuclear detail and frayed cytoplasm. ×500.

inclusions suggestive of chlamydial cervicitis can occasionally be recognized (Fig. 45.16). Bacterial vaginosis may be suspected by the presence of clue cells in the smear (Fig. 45.16).

In cases of acute cervicitis the epithelial cells show marked degenerative changes. (Fig. 45.17). These are particularly noticeable in endocervical cells, parabasal cells and immature metaplastic cells and therefore are most marked in smears from postmenopausal women or smears taken in the postnatal period. The degenerative changes are characterized by swelling and vacuolation of the nuclei, which lose their normal fine chromatin structure. Chromatin clumping, margination of the chromatin, pyknosis and karyorrhexis are also found. Fragmentation and loss of the cytoplasm is common in endocervical cells, parabasal cells and immature metaplastic epithelial cells resulting in the presence of numerous naked nuclei. These are not infrequently mistaken for trichomonads.

Mature or semimature squamous epithelial cells (superficial cells and intermediate cells) are much more resistant to the damaging effect of bacterial toxins and their nuclei usually only show slight swelling or shrinkage resulting in the formation of a perinuclear halo. The cytoplasm may be frayed and may contain engulfed polymorphs or cell debris. The remaining cytoplasm takes on a lilac hue and the power to discriminate between epithelial cell types on the basis of the colour of the cytoplasm is lost.

Chronic cervicitis

The cervical smear in chronic cervicitis is characterized by the presence of epithelial cells which reflect both the

damaging effect of the infection and attempts at repair. Thus the smear will contain degenerating epithelial cells with frayed vacuolated cytoplasm and pyknotic or fragmented nuclei in addition to sheets of regenerating epithelial cells. These are immature cells derived from the basal layers of the squamous epithelium or the reserve cell component of the endocervical epithelium which undergo metaplastic change to restore the epithelium to its original state. The regenerating cells have large active nuclei and a small rim of cytoplasm. The nuclei often appear hyperchromatic and may contain several small nucleoli and an occasional mitotic figure. The distinction between regenerating epithelial cells and cells shed from a neoplastic lesion can sometimes be difficult. The uniformity of appearance of the regenerating cells is a useful guide to their benign nature.

The composition of the inflammatory exudate in smears from patients with chronic cervicitis differs from acute cervicitis in that the exudate comprises many lymphocytes and macrophages. In the presence of chronic infection, the epithelium may show reactive changes such as parakeratosis and hyperkeratosis. The former is manifest in the smear as sheets of small orangeophilic keratinized squames with pyknotic nuclei. The latter is reflected in the smear as sheets of anucleate highly keratinized squames which often take on a yellow hue with the Papanicolaou stain.

Atrophic cervicitis

Postmenopausal women are particularly susceptible to chronic infection due to the atrophic nature of the epithe-

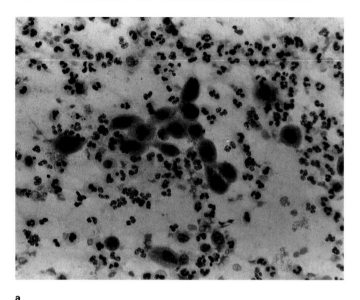

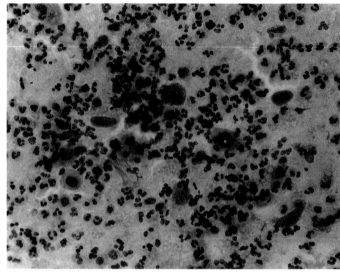

a

b

Fig. 45.18a,b Atrophic cervicitis: note degenerative changes in the parabasal cells which show pyknosis and karyorrhexis and altered cytoplasmic staining. There is a heavy inflammatory exudate in the background of the smear. ×500.

lium; the smears are composed of parabasal cells in varying stages of degeneration (Fig. 45.18). The nuclei are swollen and hypochromatic or shrunken and pyknotic. Karyorrhexis is very much in evidence and in some cells only a ghostly outline of the nucleus can be seen. In other cells the cytoplasm disintegrates resulting in the presence of numerous stripped nuclei in the smear. Where the cytoplasm is intact it may appear either eosinophilic, cyanophilic or amphophilic.

Although degenerative changes predominate in most smears from women with atrophic cervicitis, regenerative changes may also be seen. The presence of sheets of hyperchromatic nuclei in an otherwise atrophic smear can lead to problems of interpretation. The uniform morphology of the benign regenerating epithelial cells should enable the cytologist to make the correct diagnosis.

Multinucleated macrophages are sometimes a striking feature of the smear (Fig. 45.19).

Granulomatous cervicitis

The presence of granulomatous lesions in the cervix is most commonly due to infection with *Mycobacterium tuberculosis* but other possible causes for this pathological change include schistosomiasis, sarcoidosis, and lymphogranuloma venereum.

The smear may contain Langhans cells, epithelioid cells and numerous lymphocytes. The Langhans cells are characterized by their large size and multinucleation. They can be distinguished from multinucleated malignant cells by virtue of the uniformity of the nuclei within the giant cell, and from foreign body giant cells by virtue

of the peripheral location of the nuclei in the cells. The presence of amorphous caseating material in the smear is strongly suggestive of a tuberculous lesion. The demonstration of acid-fast bacteria in the smear will confirm this. In the absence of caseation, lymphogranuloma should be excluded.

Follicular cervicitis

This is a diagnosis that is sometimes made when large subepithelial deposits of lymphoid tissue are found in the cervix. The condition has been linked to the presence

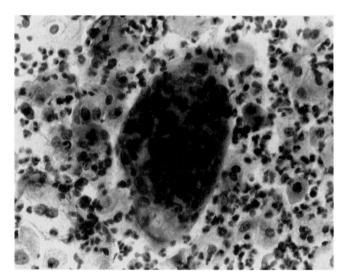

Fig. 45.19 Multinucleated giant cells in a cervical smear. These are commonly found in chronic cervicitis. ×475.

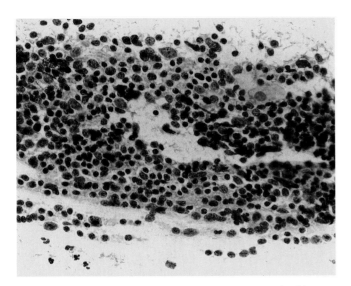

Fig. 45.20 Follicular cervicitis: this condition is characterized by sheets of mature and immature lymphoid cells and occasional tingible body macrophages. ×475.

of chlamydial infection by Hare et al (1981) but this association has not been confirmed. It can be recognized cytologically when the smear is found to contain streaks or swathes of small and large lymphocytes and tingible body macrophages derived from the ruptured follicles. The importance of this lesion for the cytologist stems from the fact that it may be misdiagnosed as infiltrating small cell carcinoma or lymphoma (Fig. 45.20).

Tuberculous cervicitis

The cells which typify tuberculous cervicitis histologically, viz Langhans giant cells and epithelioid cells, will only be seen in the cervical smear if there is extensive necrosis and caseation of the cervix and the cervical epithelium is breached (Coleman, 1969; Misch et al, 1976; Angrish & Verna, 1981). However these cells are not uncommonly found in smears in developing countries where patients present with advanced tuberculous disease. Langhans cells can be distinguished from other giant cells by the way the elongated nuclei are distributed at the periphery of the cytoplasm. The epithelioid cells contain elliptical or rounded nuclei with coarse chromatin and have scanty cytoplasm. Distinction between epithelioid cells and malignant cells is based on the small size of the granuloma-forming cells.

The presence of amorphous eosinophilic caseous material is consistent with a cytodiagnosis of tuberculosis provided the other cytological criteria of this infection are met. Other granulomatous lesions, e.g. lymphogranuloma inguinale, must be borne in mind and a definitive diagnosis of tuberculosis must be based on the demonstration of acid-fast bacilli in the smear.

Trichomoniasis

A definitive diagnosis of *Trichomonas vaginalis* can be made by examination of the cervical smear in over half the women presenting with this infection (Schnell et al, 1972). The diagnosis is based on the recognition in the smears of the organisms, which appear as slatey-grey pear-shaped objects 8–15 μm in diameter. They have an eccentrically placed fusiform nucleus which helps to distinguish them from fragments of cytoplasm or free endocervical cell nuclei. The axostyle which runs through the centre of the body and the four flagellae at the forward pole are rarely seen. Several highly refractile eosinophilic granules may be seen in the cytoplasm. The organisms are usually very numerous in the smear and frequently overlap the borders of the squamous epithelial cells (Fig. 45.21a,b).

Associated cytological features are the 'lilac' hue of the squamous epithelial cells in the smear due to the alkaline nature of the cervical discharge associated with the infection. The nuclei of the epithelial cells may be enlarged, pale or reduplicated and have enlarged chromocentres. They are often surrounded by a small but clear-cut perinuclear halo. Filamentous organisms of the genus leptothrix are occasionally found in the smears (Fig. 45.21c).

Most cases of *Trichomonas vaginalis* infection are associated with an inflammatory exudate. However, in 10% of cases no inflammatory response will be observed as the parasite appears to be in symbiosis with its host.

Candidiasis

Candida albicans is frequently present as a commensal in the lower female genital tract and only rarely gives rise to symptomatic disease. This is most likely to occur in pregnancy, diabetes mellitus, immunodeficiency states and after prolonged use of antibiotics. The delicate branching pseudohyphae and small rounded spores can be found intimately mixed with the epithelial cells in the smear. Candida spores and hyphae (Fig. 45.22) can be found in 20% of the cytolytic smears from pregnant women as the fungus flourishes in the acid pH of the vagina which is associated with prolonged oestrogen effect. The hyphae of *Candida albicans* cannot be distinguished morphologically from those of another fungus, *Torulopsis glabrata*, which is sometimes present in the female genital tract (Kearns & Gray, 1963; Marks et al, 1970).

Actinomyces

This group of bacteria is frequently found in cervical smears from women fitted with an intrauterine device (Gupta et al, 1976; Duguid et al, 1980). They appear as clumps of fine filaments with club-like tips arranged in a

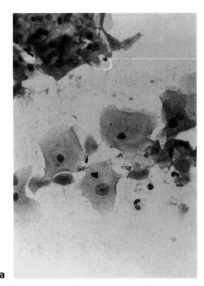

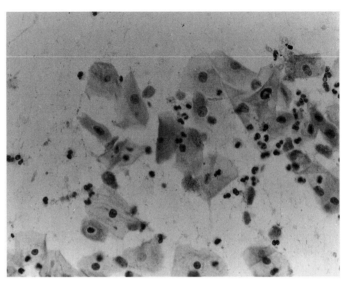

a

b

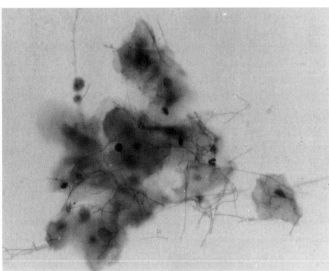

c

Fig. 45.21a–c   a *Trichomonas vaginalis*: these appear as pear-shaped grey-staining bodies about 8–10 μm in length. Note the small eccentric nucleus which is pathognomonic for these organisms and helps distinguish them from fragments of cytoplasm. They usually lie in close proximity to the squamous cells. ×500. **b** *Trichomonas vaginalis* infection: numerous trichomonads are present in this smear. Note the perinuclear halo and frayed cytoplasm. ×500. **c** Trichomonads and leptothrix in a cervical smear. Note the long filamentous organisms and the frayed cytoplasm of the epithelial cells. ×500.

sunburst pattern (Fig. 45.23). The inflammatory reaction associated with this infection is minimal. The bacteria grow as saprophytic clusters on the string of the intrauterine device. Their presence in the smear is rarely associated with disease and removal of the IUCD is only indicated if ascending infection is suspected. Actinomyces-like organisms have been described in cervical smears in association with non-pathogenic amoebae resembling *Entamoeba gingivalis* (Ruehsen et al, 1980).

Herpes simplex virus type 2

Combined clinical, cytological and virological studies have shown that the cytopathic effect of herpes simplex virus can be recognized in cervical smears (Morse et al, 1974; Coleman, 1979). The multinucleated giant cells (Fig. 45.24) are pathognomonic of this infection. These large cells may contain up to 100 nuclei which appear structureless and glassy or may contain a few angular chromatin fragments depending upon the stage of infection. A key feature of the giant cells is the margination of the nuclear chromatin and nuclear moulding. Large amphophilic intranuclear inclusions (Cowdray Type A inclusions) may be seen in the later stages of infection.

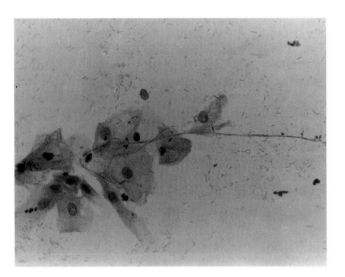

Fig. 45.22   Hyphae and spores of *Candida albicans* in a cervical smear. This is a common finding. ×475.

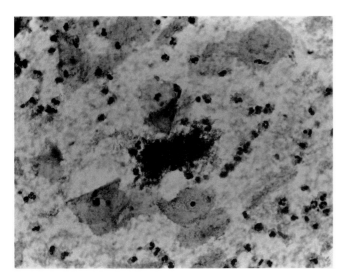

Fig. 45.23 Actinomyces-like organisms in a cervical smear. These are commonly found when an intrauterine contraceptive device is in situ. ×475.

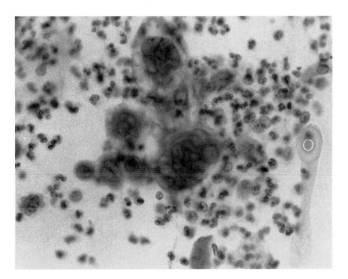

Fig. 45.24 Multinucleated giant cells found in herpes simplex infection of the cervix. Note ground-glass nuclei, margination of the chromatin and nuclear moulding. ×475.

A study, in which virus isolation and cervical cytology were performed consecutively on over 200 women, revealed that the multinucleated giant cells in the smear may be the only evidence of genital herpes (Morse et al, 1974).

Problems of differential diagnosis may be encountered in cervical smears. The multinucleated giant cells due to herpes simplex virus must be distinguished from multinucleated foreign body giant cells, malignant cells, Langhans cells and syncytiotrophoblast. They can be differentiated from foreign body giant cells and Langhans giant cells by the presence of nuclear moulding and ground-glass nuclei. Syncytiotrophoblast is rarely found in cervical smears except where smear taking coincides with miscarriage.

In cases of necrotizing cervicitis due to herpes simplex infection where the cervix appears ulcerated and haemorrhagic, the virus-infected cells in the cervical smear may be misdiagnosed as malignant cells. This mistake can be avoided if the morphology of the cells is carefully studied. Malignant cell nuclei are hyperchromatic and show a degree of anisonucleosis and pleomorphism not seen in herpes-infected cells. If there is doubt about the diagnosis, the slide can be reprocessed for electronmicroscopy and the viral agents demonstrated (Smith & Coleman, 1984).

Cytomegalovirus infection

The inclusion-bearing cells characteristic of this infection are rarely seen in cervical smears. A report of five cases and a review of the literature has been prepared by Huang & Naylor (1993). The virus-infected cells are large and contain a single eosinophilic intranuclear inclusion and multiple small cytoplasmic inclusions. These features will assist the differential diagnosis between cytomegalovirus infection (CMVI) and herpes simplex virus infection where the virus-infected cells are multinucleated and inclusion bodies are not found in the cytoplasm. Most patients in whom cytomegalovirus infection has been detected in cervical smears have a defect of cell-mediated immunity.

Human papillomavirus infection

Numerous epidemiological surveys of the prevalence of human papillomaviruses in the female genital tract have shown that the squamous epithelium of the uterine cervix is a common site of infection with these viruses (Munoz et al, 1988). A recent survey has shown that up to 30% of women aged 20–35 with otherwise clinically or cytologically normal cervices may harbour HPV 6, 11 or 16 (Prof. J. Peto, Institute of Cancer Research, Sutton, Surrey — personal communication). The prevalence of infection is somewhat less in older women and significantly higher in women with CIN or invasive cancer.

The surveys which report these very high prevalence rates of HPV DNA in the cervix have been carried out using the polymerase chain reaction to detect the viral DNA (Brule et al, 1989; Melchers et al, 1989). This is an extremely sensitive method of detecting the virus and can detect a single virus particle in 10^6 cells. Correlation of HPV DNA hybridization with clinical, colposcopic and histological studies has shown that the pattern of infection is very variable. Four common patterns are summarized below:

(i) HPV infection may result in the formation of clinically obvious condylomatous lesions on the ectocervix or at the external os.

(ii) Infection may result in the formation of flat lesions

which may occur in isolation or in association with an area of CIN.

(iii) HPV infection may occur within an area of CIN.

(iv) HPV DNA may be detected in a cervix in the absence of cytological or histological atypia or associated with minimal basal cell hyperplasia (latent infection).

Histologically, condylomas or flat lesions are characterized by the presence of koilocytotic atypia, parakeratosis, hyperkeratosis, individual cell keratinization and multinucleation. The cytological diagnosis of HPV infection depends to a large extent on the ability to recognize these changes in the cervical smear.

The presence of koilocytes in cervical smears is pathognomonic for HPV infection in the cervix (Fig. 45.25). Koilocytes are readily recognizable as superficial or intermediate squamous cells which have a large area of perinuclear clearing bounded by a rim of thickened cytoplasm. The nuclei of the koilocytes are often enlarged, hyperchromatic, multiple and irregular. If hyperkeratosis is present in the cervix this will be manifest in the smear by the presence of sheets of highly keratinized anucleate squames. Similarly, the presence of parakeratosis is manifest cytologically by the presence of small discrete highly keratinized squames with pyknotic nuclei which have been designated dyskeratocytes by Meisels (Meisels & Fortin, 1976; Meisels et al, 1977). The presence of these distinctive cells may reinforce the diagnosis of HPV infection. However a cytodiagnosis of HPV infection should *not* be made in the absence of koilocytes.

Although koilocytes can be readily recognized in a cervical smear the distinction between condylomatous change and a flat lesion cannot be made on cytological grounds. Moreover it is not possible cytologically to distinguish a discrete focus of HPV adjacent to an area of CIN and HPV involving an area of CIN. This is because the nuclear changes associated with HPV infection cannot be reliably distinguished from those found in neoplastic cells. Thus *management policies* for women whose smear contains koilocytes should not be based on the presence of HPV infection but on the degree of nuclear abnormality of the cells in the smear. This is further substantiated by the gap in our knowledge about the clinical significance of HPV infection in the cervix.

Meisels & Fortin (1976) and Purola & Savia (1977) were the first to describe the cytological changes associated with HPV infection of the cervix and the first to note the strong association with CIN and cervical cancer. Their observations were the stimulus for a programme of research which has greatly added to our understanding of cervical carcinogenesis and our knowledge of the epidemiology of HPV infection.

The association between the so-called high risk HPV types (HPV 16 and 18) and cervical cancer has led to the hypothesis that these viruses play a part in the oncogenic process (Zur Hausen, 1982). However, the tendency to regard all women with cytological evidence of HPV infection as high risk is misplaced. Firstly, cytology cannot discriminate between HPV types. Secondly, cytology is a relatively insensitive method of detecting HPV infection (Morse et al, 1988) and many women who harbour HPV 16 and 18 will not be detected by cervical cytology. Thirdly, prospective studies have shown that the lifetime risk of any woman acquiring HPV infection is very high,

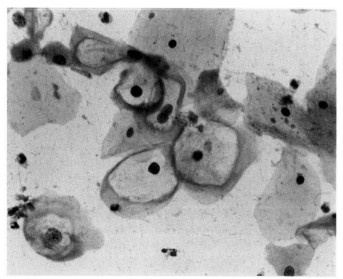

a

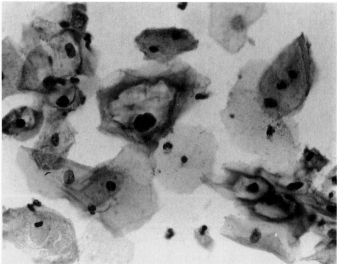

b

Fig. 45.25a,b   Koilocytes. **a** Note clearing of cytoplasm around the nucleus of the cell and condensation of cytoplasm at the periphery of the cell. The nucleus is only slightly enlarged in the cells shown here, suggesting that the cells are shed from a focus of HPV infection in the cervical epithelium. ×500. **b** Note cytoplasmic clearing and condensation at the periphery of the cell. On this occasion, the nucleus of the koilocyte is enlarged, hyperchromatic and irregular, indicating that the HPV infection may be superimposed on an area of CIN. ×500.

so that the individual risk of cervical cancer associated with these viruses is very small (Syrjanen et al, 1990).

Thus, until we have definitive evidence of a rôle for HPV in the genesis of cervical cancer, management of the patient with koilocytosis should be based on the degree of nuclear abnormality as described above.

Metaplastic, hyperplastic and other benign reactive changes in the cervix

Several different types of epithelium may be found in the cervix after puberty in addition to the native squamous and glandular epithelium present from birth. These include epithelium which reflects the changes of squamous metaplasia, tuboendometrioid metaplasia, intestinal metaplasia, hyperkeratosis, regeneration and repair. These epithelial patterns can be recognized in cervical smears and, unless they are recognized, may give rise to misdiagnosis.

Squamous metaplasia

It is important for the cytologist to be aware of the full range of histological changes associated with metaplastic change in the transformation zone. The normal physiological changes which occur at this site at puberty and pregnancy are described in Chapter 5. As stated earlier, mature squamous metaplastic epithelium cannot be distinguished from mature native squamous epithelium cytologically. However, the immature metaplastic cells and cells shed from an area of reserve cell hyperplasia can be recognized in the smear. They resemble the parabasal cells seen in atrophic smears but can be distinguished from them by the 'company they keep'. Immature metaplastic cells are always found in association with superficial and intermediate cells derived from adjacent mature squamous epithelium whereas smears from an atrophic cervix contain a single cell type.

Tuboendometrioid metaplasia

This pattern of metaplastic change occurs frequently, but not exclusively, in women who have had a cone biopsy or large loop excision of the transformation zone for CIN. It has been recorded in 69% of postconization hysterectomy specimens (Ismail, 1991, 1992). The epithelial cells characteristic of tuboendometrioid metaplasia are generally smaller than normal endocervical cells or immature squamous metaplastic cells and have a central or basally located round or oval nucleus. The nuclei may be hyperchromatic and have a small nucleolus but the distribution of the chromatin is even. The cells may appear in glandular clusters. Occasionally ciliated cells may be seen (Van et al, 1991; Ducatman et al, 1993).

Cells showing the changes of tuboendometrioid metaplasia in follow-up smears from women who have been

treated for CIN or GIN may be misinterpreted as evidence of recurrence of the neoplastic lesion (Hirschowitz et al, 1994). Differential diagnosis is based on the small sizes of the metaplastic cells, the absence of dyskaryosis and the uniform appearance of the hyperchromatic nuclei.

Examples of tubal metaplasia in the cervix have been described by Brown & Wells (1986), who found cervical glands lined with Fallopian tube-type columnar ciliated cells in 4% of cervices in which CIN 3 had been diagnosed. The presence of numerous ciliated columnar epithelial cells in the cervical smear should suggest this diagnosis.

Hyperkeratosis

Hyperplasia with hyperkeratosis of the ectocervix is frequently seen in prolapse. This is reflected in cervical smears by the presence of sheets of anucleate squames staining orange or yellow with the Papanicolaou stain (Fig. 45.26). Hyperkeratosis is also a feature of some squamous carcinomas and intraepithelial carcinomas, and the presence of anucleate squames in the cervical smear may mask underlying neoplastic change. It is also a feature of papillomavirus infection.

Regeneration and repair

Cervical smears taken from women with acute or chronic cervicitis may show evidence of regeneration and repair of the damaged endocervical or squamous epithelium. Thus it is not unusual for degenerative and regenerative changes to be seen in the same smear.

The regenerative changes are characterized by the presence of sheets of parabasal cells or endocervical cells

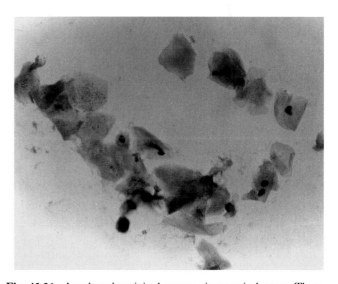

Fig. 45.26 Anucleate keratinized squames in a cervical smear. These reflect underlying hyperkeratosis which may be found in association with koilocytes. However, unlike the koilocyte, anucleate squames are not pathognomonic of HPV infection as hyperkeratosis may occur in association with chronic cervicitis and neoplasia. ×475.

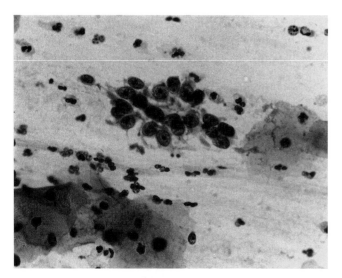

Fig. 45.27 Regenerating endocervical cells with enlarged nuclei and prominent nucleoli. Note uniform appearance of the cells which distinguished regenerative change from neoplastic change. ×475.

with large active nuclei, large nucleoli and little cytoplasm (Fig. 45.27). Mitotic figures may be seen. Regenerating epithelium may be misdiagnosed as neoplastic epithelium but recognition of the uniformity and the cohesiveness of the cells will enable the correct diagnosis to be made.

Iatrogenic changes

In this section the changes due to heat coagulation, cryosurgery, laser ablation, ionizing radiation, cytotoxic therapy and contraceptive use are considered and their effect on the cervical smear pattern discussed.

Changes due to electrodiathermy, cryotherapy and laser therapy

These modalities are commonly used for the treatment of CIN. Smears taken within a week of therapy have been found to contain degenerating and regenerating epithelial cells and necrotic cell debris. Holmquist et al (1976) described the cells in cervical smears immediately after laser treatment and observed elongation of the cells and their nuclei due to coagulation and distortion of the columnar cells. Secondary changes several weeks after therapy include florid squamous metaplasia indicating an active repair process. The regenerating cells may be misinterpreted as residual neoplastic cells leading to incorrect management of the patient. Clinicians should be advised that it is inappropriate to take a smear within three months of treatment as the cytological patterns are ambiguous.

Ionizing radiation

Unlike the effect of electrodiathermy or cryotherapy,

radiation changes may last for many years (Fig. 45.28). Smears taken immediately after irradiation of the cervix for malignant disease show evidence of radiation damage in both tumour cells and normal epithelial cells in the smear. Cytoplasmic vacuolation, multinucleation and phagocytosis are commonly seen. Large bizarre epithelial squames may be found many years after the administration of the X-ray treatment and the swollen nuclei and large nucleoli may give rise to diagnostic difficulty. As a rule, cells showing radiation changes have large pale-staining hypochromatic nuclei so that a diagnosis of recurrent or persistent malignant disease should be reserved for those cases where the potential for cell division (i.e. mitotic figures, prominent nucleoli or chromatin condensation) can be demonstrated in the abnormal cells.

Cytotoxic drugs and other drug therapy

The administration of cytotoxic drugs such as fluorouracil and cyclophosphamide for multifocal intraepithelial carcinoma has been associated with nuclear changes which are in themselves very similar to those found in intraepithelial neoplasia. The presence of epithelial cells with large hyperchromatic structureless nuclei should raise a suspicion that these cells are the result of treatment, but the pathologist is largely dependent on the clinical history to make this diagnosis.

It should also be borne in mind that patients receiving cytotoxic drugs may have impaired immunity resulting in opportunistic infection of the genital tract and an increased risk of cervical cancer (Penn & Starzl, 1972; Balachandran & Galagan, 1984). Changes consistent with herpes simplex virus and cytomegalovirus may be found in the cervical smears.

Tamoxifen therapy is associated with proliferation of the vaginal and cervical epithelium, and smears from postmenopausal women who are receiving this drug may have a high karyopyknotic index (Eells et al, 1990; Athanassiadou et al, 1992), as may patients who are receiving digoxin (Navab et al, 1965).

Intrauterine contraceptive device

The use of the intrauterine contraceptive device (IUCD) has been associated with chronic endometritis and smears from patients fitted with this device often contain endometrial cells regardless of the interval between cervical sampling and the onset of menstruation. The endometrial cells may be rather plump with prominent nuclei and nucleoli, leading to a misdiagnosis of endometrial hyperplasia (Fig. 45.29). Actinomyces-like organisms are commonly found in the smear. The presence of actinomyces in a smear from a patient with an IUCD is *not* per se an indication for treatment or removal of the device.

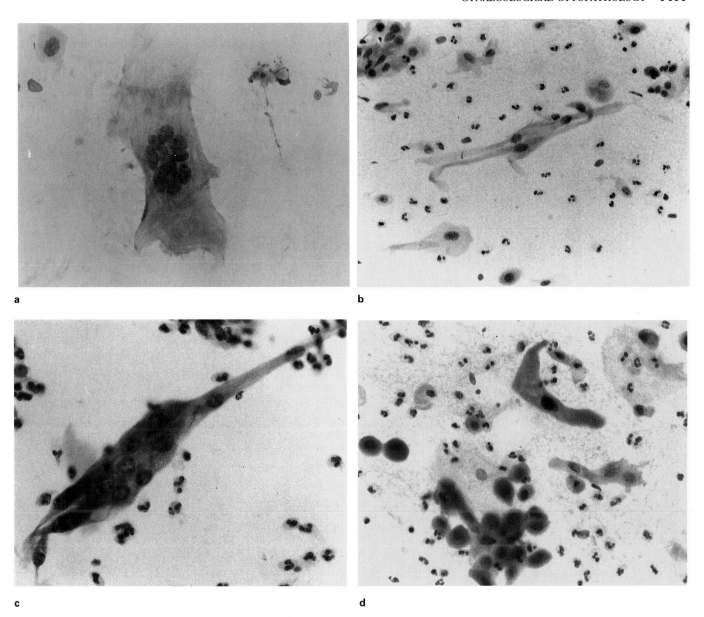

a

b

c

d

Fig. 45.28a–d Radiotherapy changes: these are very variable and are characterized by multinucleation — **a**, nuclear enlargement and hypochromasia — **b**, bizarre cellular shapes — **c**, increased volume and density of the cytoplasm associated with dense structureless nuclei — **d**, and by cytoplasmic and nuclear vacuolation. ×500.

Treatment may be indicated if the patient has symptoms of pelvic inflammatory disease. Psammoma bodies (Fig. 45.30) have been observed in smears from patients with an IUCD in the absence of malignant disease. They differ from the psammoma bodies associated with cancer in that they are usually small, the calcified rings are not so prominent, and they are not surrounded by tumour cells (Koss, 1992).

Squamous cell neoplasia

The spectrum of cervical disease encompassed by the term 'squamous cell neoplasia' is readily recognized in cervical smears. As a result, cervical screening programmes have been introduced in many countries throughout the world in an effort to prevent cervical neoplasia. Regrettably, those countries with the highest death rate from cervical cancer, such as India where over 100 000 women die each year from this disease, have the least developed screening programmes. On the other hand, in those countries where the cervical cancer prevention programme is well organized and cervical screening is offered on a systematic basis — e.g. British Columbia, Iceland, Sweden — deaths from cervical cancer have been significantly reduced (Holland & Stewart, 1990).

In this section, the cytological patterns characteristic of preinvasive and invasive squamous lesions of the cervix are described and screening strategy discussed.

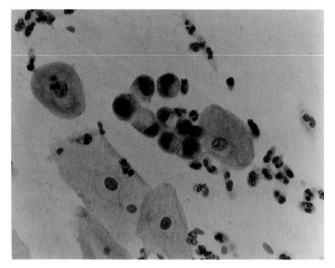

Fig. 45.29 Cytological changes in the presence of an IUCD. The cervical smears frequently contain atypical endometrial cells with prominent nuclei and abundant cytoplasm which may be mistaken for adenocarcinoma. ×500.

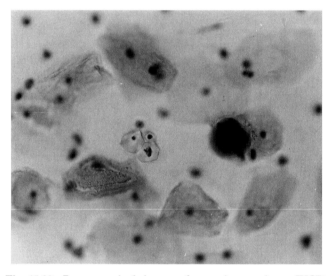

Fig. 45.30 Psammoma body in smear from patient wearing an IUCD. The concentric rings are not obvious and no tumour cells surround the structure. ×500.

Terminology

For many years the terminology used to describe cervical smears from patients with cervical neoplasia varied from one laboratory to another. This made comparative studies of cervical screening extremely difficult and prevented effective monitoring of the screening programme. Some centres used a numerical system for classifying cervical smears, e.g. the Papanicolaou classification or a modification of it. In other centres, the neoplastic cells were variously described as abnormal, atypical, dysplastic, abnormal or malignant, regardless of the severity of the underlying cervical lesion or whether it was precancerous or an invasive squamous carcinoma.

In 1986, the British Society for Cervical Cytology recommended a system of reporting abnormal cervical smears which was intended to standardize reporting throughout the UK (Evans et al, 1986). This system has been widely adopted and has provided a useful basis for establishing quality standards in the UK and monitoring laboratory performance. Within the terminology proposed by the British Society for Clinical Cytology the word 'dyskaryosis' (Gr: dys = abnormal; karyos = nucleus) is used to describe epithelial cells from preinvasive and invasive squamous lesions in cervical smears. The dyskaryotic cells can be further subdivided into those showing mild, moderate or severe dyskaryosis on the basis of previously defined nuclear and cytoplasmic changes to correspond with the epithelial abnormalities in the cervical epithelium from which they are shed, i.e. CIN 1, CIN 2 and CIN 3/ invasive cancer.

Dyskaryotic cells are characterized by the following features:

1. Nuclear enlargement, hyperchromasia and irregularity of the nuclear membrane.

2. Increased chromatin content and coarsely granular chromatin.

3. An altered nuclear:cytoplasmic ratio. The n:c ratio is usually greater than that normally seen in a parabasal cell (1:3).

4. The cytoplasm of dyskaryotic cells may also be abnormal. It may be highly keratinized.

In 1988 the National Cancer Institute (NCI) sponsored a workshop to address the standardization of cervical/ vaginal reports in the United States. A uniform system of reporting was proposed (the Bethesda System), which closely approximates to the UK system. The Bethesda System was further modified in 1993 and differs from the UK system with regard to the reporting of abnormal smears in two ways:

1. The term 'dyskaryosis' is not used. Instead the squamous cells in the smears are designated 'atypical' or 'abnormal'.

2. Only two categories of cervical intraepithelial neoplasia are recognized, namely low-grade squamous intraepithelial lesions and high-grade squamous intraepithelial lesions.

The category of low-grade squamous intraepithelial lesions incorporates lesions designated HPV, mild dysplasia or CIN 1 in the British system. The high-grade lesions incorporate lesions previously designated CIN 2, CIN 3, moderate and severe dysplasia and carcinoma in situ. The UK and the Bethesda systems are compatible for reporting and, as long as the laboratory is consistent in its approach to reporting and the clinicians are aware of the significance of the reports, either can be used.

The UK system is used in this chapter.

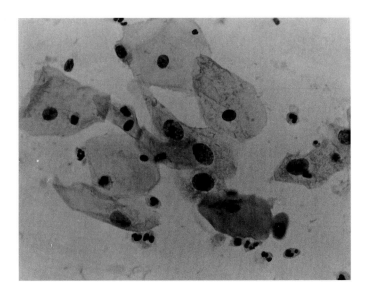

a

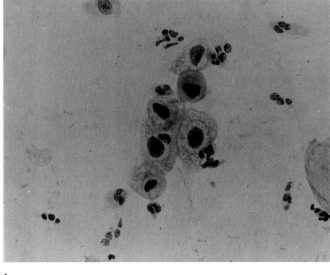

b

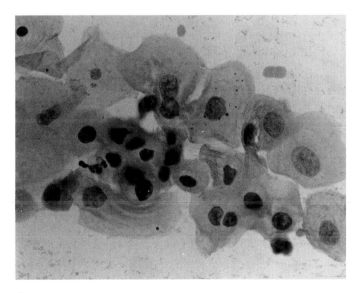

c

Fig. 45.31a–c Mild dyskaryosis reflecting CIN 1. The cells have abundant cytoplasm and the nuclei, which have an abnormal chromatin content and are irregular in shape, occupy less than half the area of the cytoplasm. ×500.

Cytology of CIN 1 and borderline changes

A cervical smear from an area of CIN 1 will contain squamous epithelial cells showing mild dyskaryosis. These cells are shed or scraped from the surface of the neoplastic lesion and are characterized by the presence of one (or more) irregular nucleus 3–4 μm in diameter which occupies less than one-half the area of the cytoplasm (Fig. 45.31). The nuclei have an increased chromatin content and appear hyperchromatic. If degenerative changes supervene the nuclei may appear pyknotic.

The cytoplasm is abundant and may be keratinized or show an unusual staining pattern. In the presence of co-existing papillomavirus infection of the neoplastic epithelium, koilocytosis may be observed. Overall, the cells in the cervical smear have the appearance of discrete superficial or intermediate cells with a slightly enlarged and irregular nucleus. In a small proportion of smears there may be doubt as to whether the nuclear morphology reflects neoplastic change or whether it is reflecting regenerative, degenerative or reactive changes in the cells. The smears are often described as showing 'nuclear changes bordering on dyskaryosis' (Fig. 45.32). Smears containing koilocytes with slightly enlarged hyperchromatic nuclei are sometimes assigned to this category.

Cytology of CIN 2

The cervical smear will contain cells showing a moderate degree of dyskaryosis. Thus the nucleus of the cell will be enlarged, hyperchromatic and irregular and occupy two-thirds of the cytoplasmic area (Fig. 45.33). The cells can be likened to superficial or intermediate cells with a greatly enlarged nucleus and are usually dispersed throughout the smear. Occasionally, koilocytosis is present reflecting co-existing HPV infection of the neoplastic epithelium.

Cytology of CIN 3

The severely dyskaryotic cells which characterize this lesion in cervical smears usually contain large irregular hyperchromatic nuclei with scanty cytoplasm. The nucleus measures 10–15 μm in diameter and occupies more than two-thirds of the cytoplasmic area (Figs 45.34 and 45.35). Hyperchromasia, irregular nuclear outline and coarse chromatin are readily detected even at low magnification. An enlarged nucleolus is rarely seen.

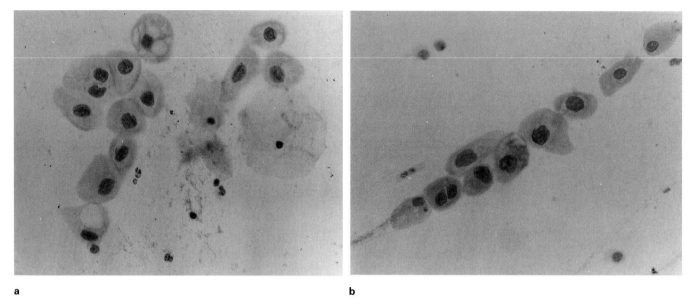

a   b

Fig. 45.32a,b Borderline changes in a cervical smear. **a** Note the enlarged nuclei and slight variation in nuclear size in cells with abundant cytoplasm. The cells resemble immature metaplastic cells. The nuclear chromatin is even and not increased. There is no evidence of infection or other obvious cause for these changes and neoplasia must be excluded. ×500. **b** Immature metaplastic cells with slight nuclear irregularity and enlargement may be found as a result of inflammatory change. In this case there is no evidence of acute cervicitis to explain these changes, hence a diagnosis of borderline change was made in this case. ×500.

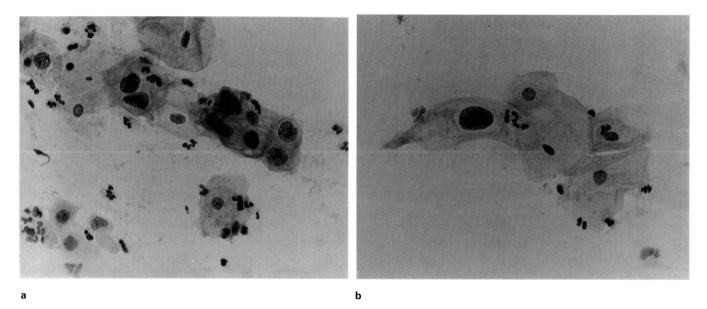

a   b

Fig. 45.33a,b Moderate dyskaryosis reflecting CIN 2. The nuclei are larger and more irregular than those shown in Fig. 45.31. ×500.

Cells showing a severe dyskaryosis are often found in streaks or loose aggregates in the smear, reflecting the loss of cell cohesion which is a feature of neoplasia. Abnormal nuclei totally devoid of cytoplasm may be seen due to loss of the rather fragile scanty cytoplasm (Fig. 45.36). These abnormal naked nuclei are frequently seen in atrophic smears. They can be distinguished from naked nuclei found in cytolytic smears by the pleomorphism and coarse chromatin of the stripped neoplastic nuclei.

Occasionally they are found in dense clusters which have been described as 'minibiopsies' of the neoplastic epithelium (Fig. 45.37) and are frequently overlooked (Robertson & Woodend, 1993). Examination of the clusters at high magnification will reveal abnormal cells with enlarged irregular nuclei which overlap each other reflecting the loss of polarity of the epithelium. They show marked anisonucleosis and very scanty cytoplasm. Mitotic figures may occasionally be seen.

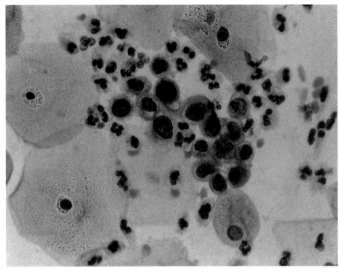

a

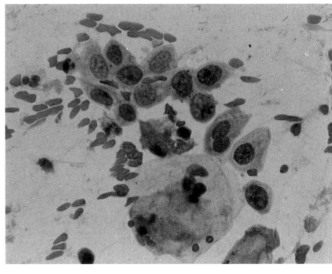

b

Fig. 45.34a,b Severe dyskaryosis reflecting CIN 3. The nuclei occupy more than two-thirds of the area of the cytoplasm and have a very abnormal chromatin content. There is marked anisonucleosis and irregularity of the nuclear membrane. The cells shown here have slightly more cytoplasm than those shown in Fig. 45.35, indicating that they have been shed from an area of CIN 3 where there is some surface differentiation.

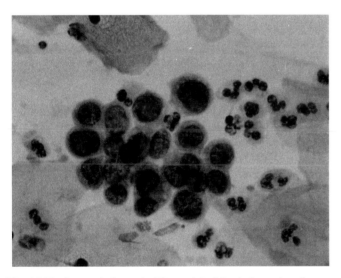

Fig. 45.35 Severe dyskaryosis. The nuclei of the dyskaryotic cells shown in this figure are surrounded by very little cytoplasm, indicating that they have been shed from an area of carcinoma in situ where there is no surface differentiation. ×475.

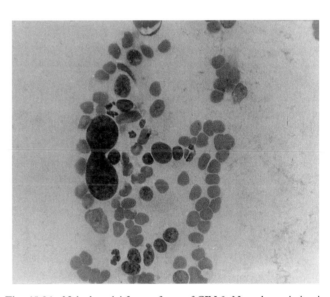

Fig. 45.36 Naked nuclei from a focus of CIN 3. Note the variation in size and shape. These may be particularly difficult to recognize in atrophic smears. ×500.

Smears taken from an area of CIN 3 where there is extensive surface differentiation may contain severely dyskaryotic cells with abundant cytoplasm. Similarly, the presence of a hyperkeratotic CIN lesion in the cervix will be reflected in the cervical smear by the presence of highly keratinized anucleate squames.

Koilocytosis is rarely seen in smears from an area of CIN 3. It should be remembered that more than one grade of CIN may be present in the cervix; hence more than one grade of dyskaryosis will be present in the cervical smear.

Microinvasive and clinically invasive squamous carcinoma

It must be made clear at the outset that it is not always possible to distinguish microinvasive and occult invasive squamous carcinoma from CIN in cervical smears. If there is any doubt about the differential diagnosis this should be made clear in the report to the clinician as patient management may be affected. Having made this point, however, the smear pattern in most cases of invasive squamous cancer of the cervix is usually quite distinctive.

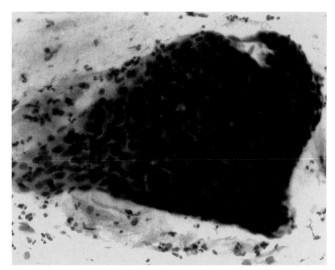

Fig. 45.37   A fragment of abnormal cervical epithelium from the smear which contains the cells shown in Fig. 45.36. This constitutes a minibiopsy and is not an unusual finding in abnormal smears as the dysplastic epithelium is very fragile and is readily detached when the smear is taken. ×475.

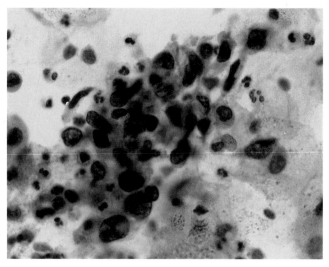

Fig. 45.39   Abnormal squames present in a smear from a case of invasive squamous carcinoma. Note the pleomorphism and malignant diathesis. ×475.

The smears from patients with *keratinizing squamous carcinoma* contain numerous abnormal cells which are shed from necrotic areas of the tumour. These cells often have highly keratinized orangeophilic cytoplasm and one or more hyperchromatic nuclei. The cancer cells have very bizarre shapes and exhibit far greater pleomorphism than the neoplastic cells seen in cervical smears from women with CIN (Figs 45.38 and 45.39). Nuclear sizes vary and the nuclei may be very large indeed (20–30 μm) or may be shrunken and pyknotic. Discrete spindle-shaped cells and tadpole-shaped cells are frequently seen. Epithelial whorls and phagocytosis of one tumour cell

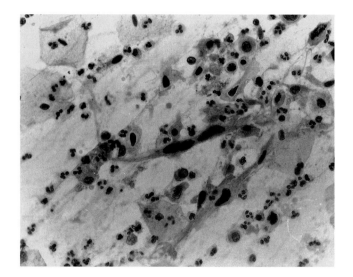

Fig. 45.38   Abnormal keratinized squemes illustrating the bizarre shapes of cells found in invasive squamous carcinoma. Spindle cells are rarely seen in cases of CIN. ×475.

by another are common. The presence of solid-looking plaques of keratin studded with irregular pyknotic nuclei and highly keratinized anucleate squames reflects the abnormal keratinization that is a feature of these tumours.

Occasionally undifferentiated tumour cells shed from less well differentiated parts of a keratinizing carcinoma may also be present in the smear (Fig. 45.40). These may appear as discrete cells with enlarged abnormal nuclei, one or more enlarged nucleoli and a small rim of cyanophilic cytoplasm. In addition, there may be dense clusters or sheets of poorly-differentiated tumour cells in the smears. The clusters are composed of overlapping nuclei with coarse chromatin and enlarged nucleoli. Nuclear moulding may be observed and anisonucleosis is always a prominent feature of these cell clusters. The cytoplasmic component of the cell clusters is usually scanty and cell borders are indistinct. Mitotic figures may be seen.

In cervical smears from patients with *non-keratinizing carcinoma (large cell type)*, these clusters of undifferentiated tumour cells described above predominate and bizarre keratinized cells are rarely seen.

As mentioned previously the distinction between intraepithelial, microinvasive and invasive carcinoma cannot always be made with confidence from the cervical smear. However, features additional to the cellular changes described above which support a diagnosis of an invasive lesion may be present. The presence of numerous red blood cells, polymorphs and necrotic debris in the smear are supportive evidence of an invasive lesion. This malignant diathesis reflects the ulceration associated with advanced cervical cancer and is rarely seen in the presence of a preinvasive lesion.

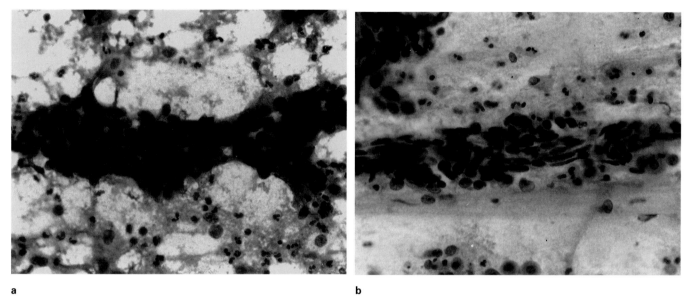

a   b

Fig. 45.40a,b Sheets of poorly-differentiated tumour cells from a non-keratinizing invasive squamous carcinoma. Note the densely packed hyperchromatic nuclei which vary in size and shape. Note the angulated shape of the cluster. Clusters of tumour cells from an adenocarcinoma are more likely to be rounded. ×500.

It is not unusual to detect highly keratinized abnormal squames in a cervical smear from a cancer that has been described in histological section as a non-keratinizing tumour. Most squamous carcinomas have a mixed cell population and the cervical smear reflects the necrotic cells at the tumour surface whereas the biopsy may be taken from a deeper area of rapid tumour growth.

Adenocarcinoma

A predominant feature in cervical scrapes taken from patients with *endocervical adenocarcinoma* is the large number of dyskaryotic endocervical cells in the smear. The neoplastic glandular cells exfoliate readily and may outnumber the cervical squames. They often appear as single cells but may present in papillary clusters or as a palisade of cells. Rosettes or balls of cells may also be seen (Figs 45.41 and 45.42).

The malignant glandular cells in a well-differentiated endocervical adenocarcinoma are characterized by their delicate, often vacuolated, cytoplasm, their columnar shape and their round eccentric enlarged hyperchromatic nuclei which may contain one or more prominent nucleoli (see Fig. 45.42b). Multinucleated endocervical cells may be seen and the morphology of individual cells ranges from within normal limits to the bizarre. The cytoplasm may be vacuolated, especially if the tumour is mucin secreting. Occasionally signet-ring cells are seen.

The differential diagnosis between poorly-differentiated adenocarcinoma of the cervix and a poorly-differentiated squamous carcinoma can be extremely difficult — both

lesions presenting as clusters of undifferentiated malignant cells in a heavily blood-stained smear. Equally difficult is the cytological detection of adenoma malignum (minimum deviation carcinoma). Szyfelbein et al (1984) described three such cases, two of which were found in patients with the Peutz–Jeghers syndrome. The smears contained numerous tall columnar cells with lacy cytoplasm arranged in palisade, sheets or acinar patterns with apparently normal nuclei. However, abnormal cells with prominent nucleoli were present in each smear reflecting the malignant nature of the lesion. Silverberg & Hurt (1975) reported five cases of adenoma malignum, four of which were reported as 'benign' in the cytological findings. Thus the pathologist needs to be alert to the possibility of this lesion when confronted with a smear containing numerous glandular epithelial cells.

The accuracy of a cytodiagnosis of glandular neoplasia has been questioned from time to time. It is generally agreed that the distinction between in situ and invasive endocervical adenocarcinoma cannot be made with confidence from the cytological appearances alone although the latter is more likely to be associated with a 'malignant diathesis'. Moreover distinction between endocervical adenocarcinoma and adenocarcinomas of endometrioid, clear cell and mixed adenosquamous type is not clear-cut in cervical smears although cases of an accurate cytodiagnosis of these rarer tumours have been recorded (Fig. 45.43). The distinction between primary endocervical adenocarcinoma of the cervix and metastatic endometrial carcinoma, ovarian carcinoma, breast carcinoma or even urothelial carcinoma metastatic in the cervix is

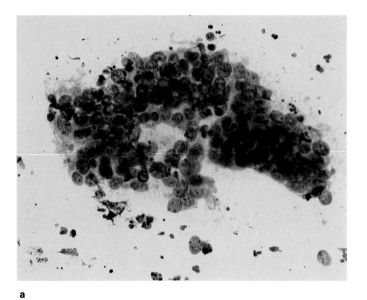

a

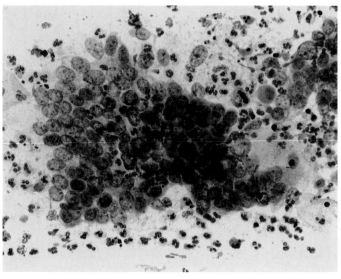

b

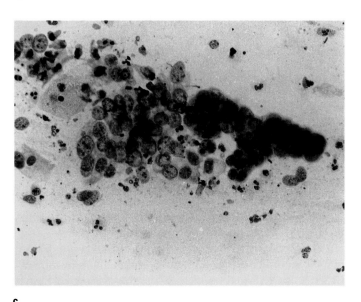

c

Fig. 45.41a,b Endocervical adenocarcinoma. **a** Note the large sheets of well-preserved endocervical cells which have a coarse chromatin structure and show a marked degree of anisonucleosis. Many cells are detached and there is loss of cohesion. ×500. **b** Endocervical adenocarcinoma showing tendency to rosette formation. ×500. **c** A cluster of malignant glandular cells where the palisade formation is preserved. ×500.

often difficult and relies heavily on accurate clinical information. Occasionally, psammoma bodies surrounded by tumour cells may be found in cervical smears. Their presence should promote a search for ovarian carcinoma.

Finally, the increasingly common use of the endocervical brush has revealed a wide range of glandular atypia which may be precursors of adenocarcinoma. Further research is needed to determine the significance of these lesions, but an awareness of them is essential to prevent diagnostic errors.

Other tumours

Ovarian carcinoma, sarcoma, malignant melanoma, mixed Müllerian tumour and choriocarcinoma have all been described in cervical smears. In some cases the tu-

mour cells were shed from the uterus, tubes and ovaries. In others the tumours had metastasized to the cervix.

Melanoma is characterized by the presence of discrete large epithelial cells with prominent nucleoli. In our experience of this rare entity the smear was covered with a brown deposit of melanin which obscured many of the tumour cells. In the absence of melanin, special stains such as the Masson–Fontana stain may assist the diagnosis.

Sarcomas may be recognized by the presence of pleomorphic tumour cells with reticulate irregular nuclei and delicate spidery cytoplasm. Many of the cells may be spindle-shaped cells so that the case may be misdiagnosed cytologically as a spindle cell variant of squamous carcinoma.

Carcinomas of the breast, bladder and endometrium not infrequently metastasize to the cervix. Diagnosis is assisted if a full clinical history is provided with the case.

Cells shed from a primary carcinoma of the endometrium, Fallopian tube and ovary may be detected in cervical smears. This distant site of the tumour can be suspected from the fact that the tumour cells are scanty and poorly preserved (see below).

The validity of a cervical smear report

The degree of confidence that can be placed in a cervical

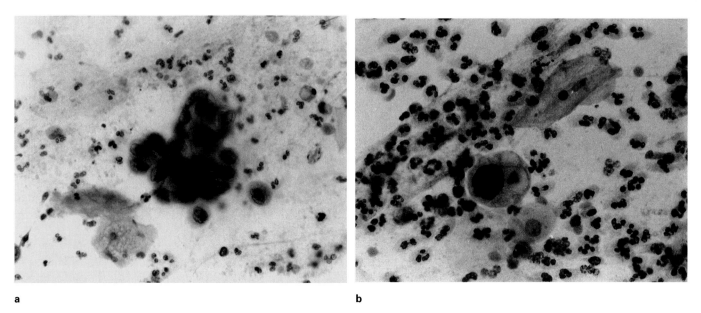

a   b

Fig. 45.42a,b Endocervical adenocarcinoma: in this smear the tumour cells appeared in balls or clusters — **a**, or as single cells — **b**. Note the rounded shape of the cluster of cells and the anisonucleosis. Note the large accentric nucleus and abundant vacuolated cytoplasm of the single tumour cell. ×500.

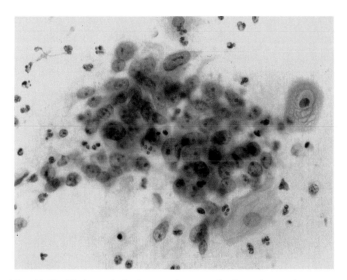

Fig. 45.43 Endocervical adenocarcinoma cells: hypochromatic tumour cells shed from a clear cell adenocarcinoma. ×475.

smear report has been a topic of concern for many years. Measurements of the sensitivity, specificity, and predictive value of the test indicate that this concern may well be justified.

Sensitivity of cervical screening

The sensitivity of the test, i.e. the ability of the test to detect all diseased people in the screened population, ranges from 50–80%, implying that the test fails to detect many women with precancerous and invasive cancer of the cervix.

In practice, the sensitivity of cervical cytology is difficult to estimate because the percentage of cases of preinvasive cancer that are missed on screening is not immediately apparent. They may only be recognized many years after the initial smear report when the patient presents with symptoms and signs of invasive cancer. Calculation of false negative rates based on rescreening of a defined population within a short interval (say one or two years) has been attempted (Yule, 1973) but even this approach is limited by the fact that not all women in the study will return for a repeat smear test and this may bias the result.

Three main causes for false negative reporting have been identified (Husain et al, 1974, Mitchell et al, 1990). They are:

(i) failure of the smear taker to obtain a smear that is truly representative of the transformation zone
(ii) failure of the laboratory to detect abnormal cells in the smear
(iii) failure of the tumour to exfoliate.

The cytologist is very reliant on the smear taker with regard to the adequacy of the smear. Criteria have been defined to assist with the identification of those cases where the transformation zone has not been sampled. The presence of endocervical cells, immature metaplastic cells and cervical mucus in a smear is acceptable (but not unequivocal) evidence that the transformation zone has been sampled. Similarly, the presence of numerous epithelial squames which are clearly displayed and covering two-thirds of the area of a microscope slide (44 × 24 mm^2) is considered evidence of satisfactory smear taking. Conversely scanty air-dried smears or smears where the epithelial cells of interest are obscured by debris or leucocytes or red blood cells are inadequate. Inadequate smears are common in patients with ulcerating invasive carcinoma of the cervix as polymorphs and red blood cells often obscure the tumour cell. Thus a clinical suspicion of malignancy must always override a negative smear report.

Both the British Society of Clinical Cytology and the Bethesda System for reporting cervical smears have set out guidelines for the recognition of satisfactory and unsatisfactory smears and the reader is referred to these guidelines for a detailed discussion of this topic.

A second reason for false negative reporting is screener error. That this occurs was clearly demonstrated by Yule (1973), who recalled 14 437 women taking part in a population screening programme for a second smear within three months of taking the first. Twenty nine additional positive cases were detected in the second smear giving a false negative rate of 16.9%. In 16 of the 29 cases review of the initial smear revealed tumour cells that had been missed on the first screening. Screener error has been attributed to fatigue or lack of training and quality control measures to combat these problems should be operating in every laboratory that undertakes cervical screening (Husain et al, 1974).

The remaining 13 cases may have been due to poor sampling technique or failure of the tumour to exfoliate. It may even have been due to tumour cells becoming trapped on the collecting instrument or becoming lost during processing of the slide (Rubio, 1977).

Specificity of a cervical smear report and positive predictive value

The specificity of the cervical smear test defines the ability of the test to correctly identify people who are free from CIN or invasive cancer and is generally based on the correlation between the cytological report and the biopsy findings. Although most studies where histology has been used as a gold standard report a specificity of 97% or more, this very pleasing result should be interpreted with caution. In the first place, the light microscope interpretation of cervical smears and cervical biopsies is a subjective exercise and diagnosis of CIN (particularly low-grade lesions) is subject to observer variation (Evans et al, 1974; Ismail et al, 1989; Robertson et al, 1989).

Secondly, correlation between the cytology and the histology may depend on the number of tissue sections examined: the greater the number of sections examined the more likely it becomes that an area of CIN will be found. Thirdly, the definition of a 'disease-free population' with regard to CIN is not clear-cut and a grey area exists both cytologically and histologically between low-grade neoplastic lesions in the cervix and atypia of the cervical epithelium due to inflammation or benign disease.

Thus, the 'cut-off' point in both cytology and histology will affect the specificity and the positive predictive value of the cervical smear test.

Reporting cervical smears

For many years, attempts to monitor the efficiency and the effectiveness of cervical screening have been hampered by the use of the variable criteria for the interpretation of smears and biopsies and by the wide range of terms used for reporting the specimens. Guidelines are now available for the reporting of cervical smears which it is anticipated will permit standardization and comparative studies of screening programmes.

A reporting format based on the terminology proposed by the British Society for Cervical Cytology is shown in Table 45.1. The guidelines proposed by the Bethesda System are shown in Table 45.2. The reader is referred to Evans et al (1986) and The Bethesda System (1993) for the original descriptions of these reporting modes.

Both the BSCC and the Bethesda system recommend that the cytology report should be written in narrative form and contain a description of the cells seen in the smears and the deductions that can be made from them.

Table 45.1 Preparation of cytology report based on BSCC guidelines

Cytological findings	Predicted histopathological changes	Recommendation for management
Smear unsuitable for cytological assessment (state reason)	—	—
Findings essentially normal, no evidence of neoplasia	Normal cervix: no evidence of neoplasia	Routine repeat smear (3 or 5 years)
Borderline changes (may include HPV changes)	Inflammation or neoplasia	Early repeat (6–12 months)
Mild dyskaryosis (may include HPV changes)	CIN 1	Early repeat (3–6 months)
Moderate dyskaryosis (may include HPV changes)	CIN 2	Repeat in 3 months or referral for colposcopy
Severe dyskaryosis	CIN 3	Refer for colposcopy
Severe dyskaryosis	Suggestive of invasive squamous carcinoma	Refer for colposcopy
Abnormal glandular cells present	Endocervical adenocarcinoma; endometrial hyperplasia or adenocarcinoma	
Abnormal cells suggestive of other tumour types	Other tumour types	

NB – Other findings of pathological significance, e.g. specific vaginal infection, endometrial cells in smears from postmenopausal women, or hormonal effects inconsistent with the clinical condition of the patient should also be described.

Table 45.2 The Bethesda System

ADEQUACY OF THE SPECIMEN
  Satisfactory for evaluation
  Satisfactory for evaluation but limited by . . . (specify reason)
  Unsatisfactory for evaluation . . . (specify reason)
GENERAL CATEGORIZATION (optional)
  Within normal limits
  Benign cellular changes: see Descriptive diagnosis
  Epithelial cell abnormality: see Descriptive diagnosis
DESCRIPTIVE DIAGNOSIS
  Benign cellular changes
    Infection
      Trichomonas vaginalis
      Fungal organisms morphologically consistent with *Candida* spp
      Predominance of coccobacilli consistent with shift in vaginal flora
      Bacteria morphologically consistent with *Actinomyces* spp
      Cellular changes associated with herpes simplex virus
      Other*
    Reactive changes
      Reactive cellular changes associated with:
      Inflammation (includes typical repair)
      Atrophy with inflammation ('atrophic vaginitis')
      Radiation
      Intrauterine contraceptive device (IUCD)
      Other
  Epithelial cell abnormalities
    Squamous cell
      Atypical squamous cells of undetermined significance: qualify[†]
      Low-grade squamous intraepithelial lesion (LSIL)
      encompassing: HPV* mild dysplasia/CIN 1
      High-grade squamous intraepithelial lesion (HSIL)
      encompassing: moderate and severe dysplasia, CIS/CIN 2 and CIN 3
      Squamous cell carcinoma
    Glandular cell
      Endometrial cells, cytologically benign in a postmenopausal woman
      Atypical glandular cells of undetermined significance: qualify
      Endocervical adenocarcinoma
      Endometrial adenocarcinoma
      Extrauterine adenocarcinoma
      Adenocarcinoma, NOS
  Other malignant neoplasms: specify
  Hormonal evaluation (applies to vaginal smears only)
  Hormonal pattern compatible with age and history
  Hormonal pattern incompatible with age and history: specify
  Hormonal evaluation not possible due to: specify

* Cellular changes of human papillomavirus (HPV) — previously termed *koilocytosis*, *koilocytotic atypia* and *condylomatous atypia* — are included in the category of LSIL.

[†] Atypical squamous or glandular cells of undetermined significance should be further qualified, if possible, as to whether a reactive or premalignant/malignant process is favoured.

Numerical classification systems such as those recommended by Papanicolaou should be avoided as they are open to misinterpretation. It is good clinical practice to include in the report a comment on the adequacy of the specimen and a sentence or two of advice on how the clinician should proceed. For example, in the event of a report indicating the presence of CIN, colposcopy may be advised. If an endometrial lesion is suspected, curettage should be requested. If samples are unsuitable for a reliable diagnosis, i.e. they contain too few cells or the cells of interest are obscured, this information should be included in the report.

The term 'borderline changes' in the BSCC guidelines roughly equates with 'atypical squamous cells of undetermined significance in the Bethesda system'. This category of report should be reserved for those cases where the cytologist is uncertain of the benign or neoplastic nature of the atypical cells.

History of cervical screening and screening strategy

The development of the cervical smear test for the prevention of cervical cancer stems from the pioneering work of Dr. George Papanicolaou which was carried out at Cornell University, New York, in the early part of the twentieth century (Carmichael, 1973). In 1928 Papanicolaou observed that vaginal aspirates from women with cervical cancer contain tumour cells. The clinical implications of his observation were not appreciated at the time and several years were to pass before the potential value of vaginal aspiration as a screening tool was appreciated. This followed publication of the seminal paper by Papanicolaou & Traut in 1943 in which the authors demonstrated that it was possible by a simple non-invasive cytological test to detect preinvasive and invasive cancer in healthy women. The first well woman cervical screening clinic was opened in Massachusetts in 1945; thereafter, clinicians world-wide recommended the regular screening of well women for precancerous lesions with the view to achieving the elimination of cervical cancer from the population.

The rapid introduction of cervical screening in many countries meant that no initial studies were carried out to evaluate the effectiveness of the test as a public health measure for reducing the burden of cancer in the population. This resulted in many years of uncertainty regarding the effectiveness of the programme. Much of the screening on offer was opportunistic, unmonitored and ineffective; in most countries where opportunistic screening was rife the mortality from cervical cancer was unchanged.

However, recent evaluation of screening in those countries or regions in which an organized screening programme has been in operation for at least twenty years, e.g. British Columbia, Finland, Sweden and the Grampian region of Scotland, has shown that cervical screening is an effective method of reducing mortality from cervical cancer although it is clear that the disease can never be totally eliminated by this method (IARC Working Group on Evaluation of Cervical Cancer Screening, 1984). Review of the screening activity in those countries where a reduction in mortality from cervical cancer has been achieved has shown that an important factor in determining the success of the programme has been total coverage of the population at risk.

Implementation of an effective screening programme depends on several factors. These have been identified by various groups (ICRF Coordinating Committee on Cervical Screening, 1984; Intercollegiate Working Party on Cervical Cytology Screening, 1987; Smith & Chamberlain, 1987) and guidelines for the implementation of a successful cervical screening programme have been prepared (Department of Health and Social Security Health Circular HSG (93)41, 1993; European guidelines for quality assurance in cervical cancer screening, Coleman et al, 1993).

The key to successful cervical screening is summarized below:

1. Identification of the population at risk. This requires an accurate computerized data base which must be continually updated to ensure that the appropriate target population is invited for screening and followed up.

2. Satisfactory arrangements for call and recall of the target population with clearly defined screening intervals.

3. Adequate resources for taking, examining and reporting on cervical smears and the management and follow-up of women with abnormal smears and the introduction of quality standards.

4. An informed client population who know and understand the significance of the test under offer.

5. Regular monitoring of the screening programme, both short term and long term.

6. Identification of a named individual who is responsible for the running and organization of the programme.

In 1986 an international collaborative study was set up to review the screening activity in eight countries in an attempt to estimate the risks of cervical cancer associated with different screening policies (IARC, 1986). The study found that screening every five years offered a high degree of protection against the development of invasive cervical cancer but appreciably less than that given by screening every three years (Table 45.3). The study demonstrated

Table 45.3 The effectiveness of different screening policies. Proportionate reduction in incidence of invasive squamous cell carcinoma of the cervix uteri assuming 100% compliance.

Policy	Age group	% Reduction in cumulative rate in age group	Numbers of smears per woman
Every 10 years	25–64	64	5
Every 5 years	35–64	70	6
Every 5 years	25–64	82	8
Every 5 years	20–64	84	9
Every 3 years	35–64	78	10
Every 3 years	25–64	90	13
Every 3 years	20–64	91	15
Every year	20–64	93	45

that, given limited resources, it is more effective to offer a single screening test to 80% of the target population than to offer regular five-yearly or three-yearly screening to fewer women. For the maximum benefit, screening should be aimed principally at women aged 35–60 years but should start some years before the age of 35 and the intervals between screening should be three years or less. A more recent study, taking protection from death from cervical cancer as the end point, has shown that a longer screening interval may be equally effective (Oortmarssen et al, 1992).

The introduction of quality standards in cervical cancer screening in the United States and the UK was a consequence of public concern about screening practice in those countries. This concern was the stimulus to the introduction of quality control guidelines which were concerned mainly with laboratory performance and relate to staff training, staff workload ratios, proficiency testing and laboratory accreditation. At the same time there has been a move towards the introduction of organized screening to achieve the maximum population coverage and ensure optimal use of national resources. The impact of these measures is currently being monitored and it is anticipated that in the long term (by the year 2000) they should lead to a significant reduction in mortality from cervical cancer.

CYTODIAGNOSIS OF PROLIFERATIVE DISORDERS AND CARCINOMA OF THE ENDOMETRIUM

Cytology is not widely used for the diagnosis of proliferative and neoplastic lesions of the uterine cavity in view of the difficulty in detecting endometrial lesions from cytological samples. However, smears prepared from routine cervical scrapes and aspirates from the vaginal pool may coincidentally contain abnormal cells from the endometrial cavity and it is important for the cytologist to be able to recognize these cells and to appreciate their clinical significance.

Instruments have been developed for direct cytological sampling of the endometrial cavity for the purposes of screening women who are at high risk of endometrial cancer and the value of this approach is also discussed in this section.

Normal endometrial cells in cervical scrapes and aspirates from the vaginal pool reflecting physiological change

The endometrial cells seen in cervical scrapes and posterior fornix aspirates have been spontaneously desquamated from the endometrial lining. They may occur singly or in small clusters or plaques and are poorly preserved.

They are likely to be found in routine smears in the absence of disease if the smear has been taken at the time of menstruation. According to Wachtel (1969), endometrial cells may be seen in smears taken two or three days before and after, as well as during, menstruation. Liu et al (1963) correlated the presence of endometrial cells in smears with onset of menstruation in over 2000 women and observed that endometrial cells could be found in 21% of smears taken during the first 10 days of the the cycle but in only 2% of smears taken after the eighteenth day of the cycle. Endometrial cells may also be found in smears from women fitted with a uterine contraceptive device or in smears from women on oral contraceptives who complain of breakthrough bleeding. In fact it is not uncommon to find normal endometrial cells in cervical smears and their significance must be related to the clinical status of the patient.

Normal and abnormal endometrial cells in vaginal pool smears and cervical scrapes reflecting pathological changes in the endometrium

Spontaneously exfoliated endometrial cells found in smears from postmenopausal women or women with unexplained intermenstrual bleeding must always be regarded as an indicator of disease of the uterine cavity even if the morphology of the cells appears to be within normal limits. They may reflect the presence of an endometrial polyp or endometrial hyperplasia.

Abnormal endometrial cells may occasionally be found in cervical smears and vaginal aspirates from women with advanced endometrial carcinoma. These cells may be distinguished from tumour cells shed from an endocervical carcinoma by their poorly preserved state. The cytoplasm frequently appears frayed and the nuclei small and hyperchromatic. The tumour cells may be found singly or in dense balls or clusters and are usually scanty (Fig. 45.44). The smear may have a high maturation index inappropriate for the age of the patient. Streaks of necrotic debris in the absence of red blood cells may be present in the smear.

Several studies have shown that it is inadvisable to rely on cervical smears or vaginal aspirates when endometrial carcinoma is suspected as careful evaluation of these techniques has shown that they are very inefficient for this purpose (Macgregor et al, 1966; Reagan & Ng, 1973; McGowan, 1974).

Cytological patterns found in direct endometrial aspirates

A large number of instruments have been devised for obtaining samples from the uterine cavity in an outpatient setting with a view to replacing endometrial biopsy by a simple non-invasive cytological technique.

Endometrial aspiration

One method of endometrial sampling relies on aspiration of cells from the uterine cavity. This was first attempted in 1943 by Cary, who aspirated material from the uterine cavity through a metal cannula inserted into the cervical

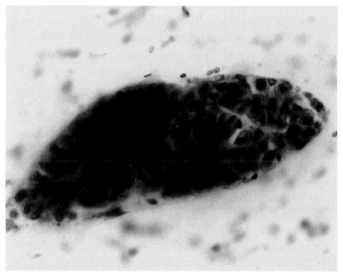 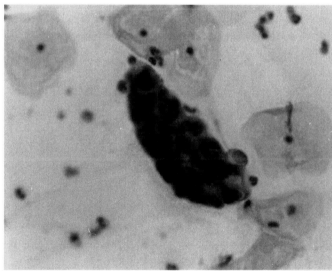

a   b

Fig. 45.44a,b Clusters of adenocarcinoma cells shed from the endometrium and trapped in the cervical mucus may be found in cervical smears. The presence of an occasional tumour cell or a few dense clusters which appear rounded up and poorly preserved such as the clusters shown here suggest an endometrial rather than an endocervical origin for the tumour. Note the superficial squames in the background of **b** indicating oestrogen production associated with the tumour. ×500.

os. The direct aspiration method was subsequently modified to include endometrial lavage under negative pressure (Dowling & Gravlee, 1964) but the technique was abandoned because diagnostic accuracy using this approach was poor. Experience has shown that lavage is unnecessary and direct aspiration can be very successful given a well-designed instrument; for many years the Isaacs endometrial sampler was in use at this hospital (Isaacs & Wilhoitte, 1974; Hutton et al, 1978; Ellice et al, 1981). This technique is safe, well tolerated by the patient and in skilled hands has proved to be a sensitive method of detecting endometrial lesions (An Foraker et al, 1979; Segadal & Iverson, 1980).

Endometrial brushing

An alternative approach to endometrial sampling involves dislodging cells from the uterine cavity by means of a small brush or other instrument. The cells or tissue fragments gathered in this way can be spread directly onto the slide, fixed in alcohol and stained by the Papanicolaou method or prepared as cell blocks. The first to use this approach was Ayre (1955), who inserted a small brush into the uterus via the endocervical canal. A modification of the original brush is currently in use (Uterobrush, Medscand AB, Malmo, Sweden). Other instruments which dislodge cells from the endometrial lining have been designed. Milan & Markley (1973) designed a plastic helix which could be rotated in the uterus (Mi Mark method). This approach was viewed critically by Crow et al (1980), who found that many of the specimens obtained by this method were unsatisfactory as they contained scanty material which was difficult to interpret. More recently the Endopap sampler — a T-shaped flexible plastic instrument that can be passed into the uterine cavity — has had favourable reports.

Cytological interpretation of endometrial aspirates and brushings

Endometrial cells in smears prepared from direct endometrial aspirates or brushings differ from the spontaneously exfoliated endometrial cells seen in cervical smears or vaginal aspirates in that the nuclear and cytoplasmic detail is well displayed so that it is possible to distinguish the subtle changes which occur in the endometrium throughout the menstrual cycle and in the postmenopausal woman. It is also possible to detect changes attributable to endometrial hyperplasia and carcinoma. However, a wide experience of the range of histological changes which can occur in the uterus is essential for accurate cytodiagnosis and endometrial cytology is wisely considered to be the preserve of the specialist.

Koss (1992) has identified certain features of endo-

metrial smears which must be assessed if a correct cyto-diagnosis is to be made. These include:

1. The number and cellularity of the endometrial clusters, especially in postmenopausal women where characteristically the smears are normally scanty.

2. The cohesiveness of the cell clusters. Loss of cohesion is a feature of advanced endometrial cancer although it may not be a feature of early cancers.

3. Nuclear abnormalities, particularly nuclear enlargement and the presence of enlarged irregular nucleoli.

4. Differentiation between endometrial cells and endocervical cells which may be contaminating the specimen.

Although these cytological guidelines are most valuable, it should be remembered that the identification of endometrial lesions, particularly the hyperplastic lesions, is based on architectural as well as cytological features of the tissue and the former are not readily appreciated in cytological smears.

Endometrial aspirates in the absence of disease

Endometrial cells shed from premenopausal women with a normal menstrual cycle are characterized by the presence of small clusters or sheets of endometrial cells. The clusters may be composed of 10–100 cells and the sheets appear as a flat monolayer. The nuclei are evenly spaced and not overlapping. The distinction between normal proliferative phase cells and secretory phase cells is subtle (Figs 45.45–45.47). The latter may exhibit slightly more foamy cytoplasm than the former. Tiny nucleoli seen only at high magnification and occasional mitoses have been described in proliferative stage smears. Stromal cells can be identified as discrete nuclei, smaller than the endometrial cells and with scanty cytoplasm.

Smears prepared from cells aspirated from the postmenopausal inactive endometrium contain scanty cells. The cells appear in small sheets (Fig. 45.48) and are rather pale staining. Stromal cells are generally sparse and much smaller than the glandular cells.

Cytological findings in endometrial adenocarcinoma

The cytological changes associated with adenocarcinoma and other malignant lesions of the endometrium have been well described by Reagan & Ng (1973) and by Koss (1992). In poorly-differentiated tumours (grade III) the neoplastic cells show a marked degree of anisonucleosis and nuclear pleomorphism. It is the well-differentiated carcinomas (grade I lesions) that are difficult to identify as the neoplastic cells are often no larger and only slightly more hyperchromatic than normal. The presence of abundant endometrial cells in an aspirate from a postmenopausal woman should raise the level of suspicion

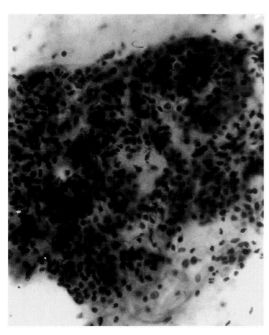

Fig. 45.45 Endometrial aspirate taken during the proliferative phase of the cycle. Note small evenly-spaced endometrial cells in large sheets and gland opening. ×300.

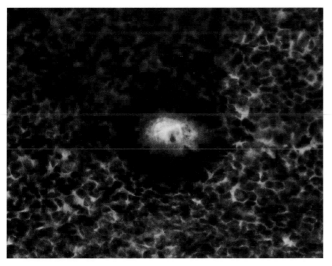

Fig. 45.46 Endometrial aspirate, proliferative phase shown above at higher magnification. Note gland opening. Mitotic figures were also seen (not shown). ×475.

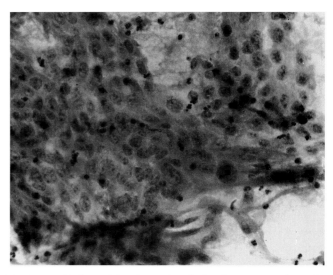

Fig. 45.47 Endometrial aspirate taken during the secretory phase of the cycle. Note pale-staining nuclei and more delicate and abundant cytoplasm. There is a leucocyte infiltrate. ×475.

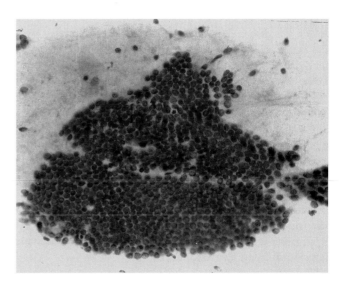

Fig. 45.48 Endometrial aspirate from a postmenopausal woman. Note scanty sheets of small even cells. No gland openings or mitoses were seen. ×285.

(Fig. 45.49). Occasionally, clear cell carcinoma may be recognized by its hobnail glands. Similarly, adenosquamous carcinoma and adenoacanthoma have been described in aspirated material. In the latter case contamination of the sample by cervical squames must be excluded.

Cytological findings in endometrial hyperplasia

Few cytologists admit to being able to diagnose endo-metrial hyperplasia with certainty. In those cases of hyperplasia without cytological atypia (e.g. simple hyperplasia) an exaggerated proliferative pattern involving both glands and stroma may be noted in the smear. Glandular cells appear in dense sheets of crowded cells with overlapped nuclei and scanty cytoplasm. The glandular nuclei are characteristically small and hyperchromatic. Stromal and glandular cells can rarely be distinguished although the former may appear slightly elongated (Morse, 1981).

In cases of hyperplasia with cytological atypia (atypical hyperplasia) nuclear pleomorphism is more marked and the distinction from endometrial carcinoma all but impossible (Morse, 1981).

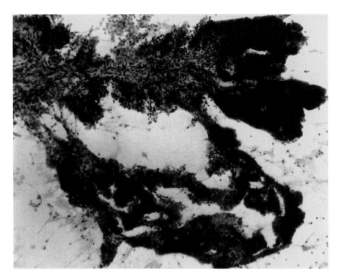

Fig. 45.49 Endometrial aspirate from a postmenopausal woman with a well-differentiated endometrial adenocarcinoma. The smears contained fronds of tumour cells. ×285.

Rôle of cytology in disorders of the endometrium

Given the problems of interpreting endometrial aspirates, their usefulness in clinical practice would seem to be rather limited. The efficacy of cytology depends very much on the skill and enthusiasm of the cytologist. Morse (1981) has had very satisfactory results with the Isaacs endometrial sampler. In a combined cytological/histological study of 212 women, a precise correlation was achieved in 149/157 cases where a satisfactory sample was obtained (95%). As expected, discrepancies occurred in the diagnosis of atypical hyperplasia. However, a case of endometrial carcinoma in a postmenopausal woman that was missed on conventional curettage was diagnosed on aspiration. An unsuspected ovarian carcinoma was also diagnosed on endometrial aspiration.

While it has to be accepted that aspiration may not be the preferred mode of investigation of the symptomatic patient, it also has to be acknowledged that lesions may be missed by curettage and a combined approach may be the most effective for the diagnosis of adenocarcinoma in the woman at risk.

It has been suggested that endometrial aspiration could have an important rôle in monitoring women on hormone replacement therapy — HRT (Morse, 1981). Routine aspiration at six-monthly intervals would be more acceptable to the patients receiving hormone replacement therapy than annual curettage. Early changes in the endometrial epithelium could be detected by studying sequential samples from these patients. However, not all operators are enthusiastic about this approach. Studd et al (1979) reported that two cases of adenocarcinoma were missed when 110 women on hormone replacement therapy were investigated by endometrial aspiration.

Endometrial aspiration was used by Koss et al (1981, 1982, 1984) to survey 2586 asymptomatic women for occult carcinoma of the endometrium and endometrial hyperplasia in an attempt to identify women over the age of 45 who may be at high risk for these diseases. Both smears and cell blocks were prepared from the aspirated material and both techniques provided adequate material for diagnosis. Sixteen occult carcinomas were diagnosed in the first round of screening and two cases were missed on screening and observed in women who subsequently developed symptoms. A prevalence rate for occult endometrial cancers of 7/1000 women was observed. The rate of endometrial hyperplasias was exceedingly low, casting doubt on the hypothesis proposed by Gusberg & Kaplan (1963) and revised by Welch & Scully (1977) and Fox & Buckley (1982) that endometrial hyperplasia may give rise to endometrial carcinoma.

CYTOLOGY OF VAGINAL LESIONS

Vaginal cytology

The indications for cytological investigation of the vagina are rather limited but nevertheless important.

Vaginal vault cytology is useful for monitoring the progress of women who have been treated for invasive carcinoma. It is also useful for identifying foci of vaginal intraepithelial neoplasia which may occur in women with CIN. It has a place in the investigation of diethylstilboestrol-exposed women who are at risk of vaginal adenosis and clear cell carcinoma. Smears from the upper third of the lateral vaginal wall may be used for hormonal evaluation.

The smears should be taken with the rounded end of the Ayre spatula and fixed immediately in 95% alcohol.

Follow-up after treatment of invasive cervical or endometrial cancer

Regular examination of smears from the vaginal vault from women who have been treated by hysterectomy for malignant disease will provide early evidence of a residual lesion or recurrence of the tumour even before it is visible to the naked eye. The tumour cells in the smear may show the features of the primary tumour or may be less well differentiated.

Caution is advised in the interpretation of these smears which may be complicated by the presence of granulation tissue or entrapment of Fallopian tube in the vaginal vault at the time of operation (Coleman & Evans, 1988).

Detection of vaginal intraepithelial neoplasia

Extension of CIN into the vaginal fornices has been observed in 1% of women. Vaginal extension of the cervical lesion may be suspected when a woman who appears to have been successfully treated for CIN continues to have abnormal smears in the absence of significant colposcopic findings. The grade of VAIN in these cases does not always correspond with the grade of CIN in the cervix.

Vaginal intraepithelial neoplasia may be detected in HIV-positive patients or renal allograft recipients, who are at risk of having multiple loci of intraepithelial carcinoma in the lower genital tract and anal region. These lesions, which appear to be associated with impaired immunological function, are rarely visible to the naked eye and vaginal cytology offers a reliable way of determining the extent of the epithelial abnormality. Preferred treatment of these cases is by local application of fluorouracil and cytology should be used to monitor response to treatment.

Vaginal adenosis and clear cell carcinoma

Foci of vaginal adenosis can be recognized in smears from women who have this condition. Vaginal adenosis can be suspected if the vaginal scrape contains glandular epithelial cells as well as squamous cells. Occasionally, metaplastic change will occur in a focus of adenosis and the vaginal smear will contain immature metaplastic squamous cells as well as mature squames. Routine cervical and vaginal smears are advised for DES-exposed women who are at risk of clear cell carcinoma.

Other uses of vaginal cytology

The vaginal epithelium is sensitive to oestrogen and progesterone. The changes induced are best seen in scrapes from the upper third of the vagina. Various indices have been devised to monitor the maturation of the vaginal epithelium over time. These include the karyopyknotic index, the eosinophilic index, the maturation index and the maturation value. For definition of these indices and critical review readers are referred to Wied et al (1983). The information concerning endocrine status to be derived from a single smear is unreliable and sequential smears are advised. Sequential smears have been used in the past to investigate infertility, amenorrhoea and threatened abortion but are of limited value and wherever possible should be superseded by precise biochemical steroid assay.

Vaginal cytology can be used to detect the rare primary and secondary tumours of the vagina and for the investigation of vaginal fistulas.

CYTOLOGY OF THE VULVA

Smears of the vulva in the absence of disease are composed of scanty squamous cells. Anucleate squames may also be found in smears taken from the labia majora. As the smears are mucus free and liable to air drying, Giemsa staining is preferred to Papanicolaou staining.

Cytology has a limited rôle to play in the investigation of some vesicular and ulcerating lesions of the vulva. Recognition of the characteristic cytological patterns described below can reduce the need for biopsy. However many lesions of the vulva are associated with marked hyperkeratosis of the surface epithelial layers and cytology has little to offer in these cases.

Herpes genitalis

Scrapes usually reveal the multinucleated giant cells seen in cervical smears.

Pemphigus vulgaris

Vulvar scrapes contain numerous discrete acantholytic cells consistent with the loss of cohesiveness which is a feature of this disease. The cells are rounded with large nuclei and scanty cytoplasm. The nuclei may contain a very prominent nucleolus and multinucleated cells are seen. Immunofluorescence of the smears will confirm the presence of immunoglobulin IgG on the surface of the cells.

Vulvar intraepithelial neoplasia (Bowen's disease, carcinoma in situ) and invasive squamous cell cancer of the vulva

These lesions are characterized by the presence of abnormal squames (Figs 45.50 and 45.51). The degree of dyskaryosis may be mild, moderate or severe. The abnormal squames are often scanty and large plaques of anucleate keratinized material may predominate in the smear.

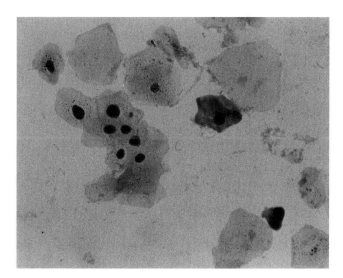

Fig. 45.50 Dyskaryotic cells in a vulvar scrape from a patient with vulvar intraepithelial cancer. The abnormal cells show a remarkable similarity to those seen in cervical smears from women with CIN. Note the presence of anucleate squames in the background. ×475.

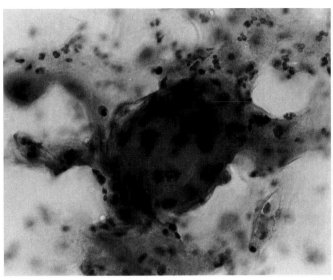

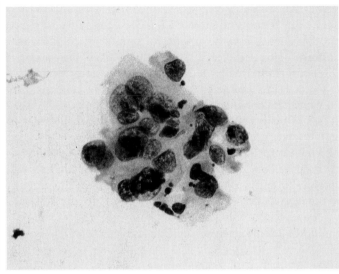

a
b

Fig. 45.51a,b Keratinized plaque studded with abnormal nuclei in a vulvar scrape from a woman with an ulcerating lesion which proved on biopsy to be a well-differentiated squamous carcinoma. ×500. **b** Malignant squamous cells in a vulvar scrape from an invasive squamous carcinoma of vulva. ×500.

Biopsy is indicated to differentiate between these various conditions.

Other lesions

Basal cell carcinoma, Paget's disease of the vulva and melanoma of the vulva have been described in vulvar scrapes.

CYTOLOGICAL DIAGNOSIS OF OVARIAN MASSES AND OTHER PELVIC LESIONS

Fine needle aspiration is a safe, simple and accurate method of cytodiagnosis which has an important rôle to play in the preoperative diagnosis of cancer. It can be used to investigate palpable lumps at almost any body site. Aspirates can also be obtained from internal organs under ultrasound or computer-guided tomography, thereby avoiding the need for open surgery in many cases.

Transrectal or transvaginal aspiration of the ovary has been advocated by several Scandinavian groups who have shown that the cytodiagnosis of a wide range of ovarian tumours is possible by this approach (Kjellgren et al, 1971; Kjellgren & Angstrom, 1979).

Despite the ease of access of the ovaries to fine needle aspiration the technique is rarely used outside Sweden for the investigation of ovarian masses because of the risk of tumour spread. There is always the possibility of rupturing a cyst that may be benign if removed intact, but which may result in peritoneal seeding if the contents are spilled.

Experience with fine needle aspiration of ovarian lesions at this hospital is limited to the examination of fluid obtained at laparoscopy from clinically benign ovarian cysts in young women in whom preservation of ovarian function was advisable.

Cytology of follicular cysts

The amount of fluid aspirated from these cysts does not usually exceed 20 ml as the cysts are normally small (about 8 cm in diameter). The fluid is usually clear and straw coloured and cells are scanty. Smears contain granulosa cells shed from the cyst lining which appear as small cells (about 30 μm in diameter) with a round hyperchromatic nucleus and scanty delicate cytoplasm. A few inflammatory cells may also be seen.

Cytology of corpus luteum cysts

The cyst fluid is usually blood-stained and quite cellular. Luteinized granulosa cells can be recognized in the smears by their small rounded hyperchromatic nuclei and abundant foamy cytoplasm. Occasionally, small cells with scanty cytoplasm may be seen which may be of thecal origin. The smears may also contain macrophages, inflammatory cells, red blood cells and fibrin strands.

Cytology of simple serous cysts

The fluid aspirated from these cysts is clear and contains few cells. The cells are columnar or cuboidal with basal nuclei and may appear in sheets or small papillary clusters. Occasionally terminal bars or ciliated cells or ciliated tufts of cytoplasm can be seen in the aspirate.

Cytology of mucinous cysts

The aspirates contain tall columnar cells with basal nuclei showing minimal anisonucleosis or pleomorphism. The cells may be embedded in a mucinous matrix. In such cases the lesion is usually malignant.

Mature cystic teratomas

These usually contain amorphous debris mixed with squamous cells and inflammatory cells including foreign body giant cells. Columnar epithelial cells of the type seen in the respiratory or intestinal tract may be recognized and ectodermal elements such as keratin whorls and hairs have been described.

Endometriotic cysts

Smears contain haemolysed blood in the background as well as histiocytes stuffed with haemosiderin. Dense clumps of degenerating endometrial cells with ill-defined nuclei and ragged cytoplasm may be seen.

Peritoneal washings and cul-de-sac aspiration (culdocentesis)

The technique of peritoneal washing at the time of laparotomy was pioneered by Keetel & Pixley (1958), who showed that this technique could detect spread of ovarian cancer in the absence of visible tumour, leading to more accurate staging of the disease and the adoption of a more aggressive treatment regime than might otherwise have been contemplated.

Initially, peritoneal lavage was used at the time of exploratory laparotomy to detect occult tumour in patients with clinically suspected ovarian cancer (Keetel & Pixley, 1958; Creasman & Rutledge, 1971). However the specimens were heavily mixed with blood and sheets of mesothelial cells as well as cells from the endometrial lining and Fallopian tubes, leading to 'false positive' reports; this approach is no longer recommended as good surgical practice (Spriggs, 1987). Subsequently the technique of peritoneal washing was carried out during second-look laparotomy in patients who had already received treatment for ovarian cancer in order to detect early recurrence of tumour (Quinn et al, 1980; Coffin et al, 1985).

Specimen collection

When the abdomen is first opened it should be inspected for the presence of seedlings on the serosal surfaces. Any free fluid is aspirated. If no seedlings are seen the peritoneal surfaces are washed with 50–100 ml of warm heparinized saline (10 units of heparin per ml saline) delivered through a disposable syringe (Ziselman et al, 1984) to which a blunt-ended cannula may be attached (McGowan, 1989). Specific areas lavaged are the likely sites for tumour metastases — the Pouch of Douglas, the right lower quadrant, the right paracolic gutter and the right subdiaphragmatic area. The fluid is then reaspirated and sent immediately for cytological examination. Delay impairs cell morphology. If delay is anticipated, the specimen should be stored at 4°C or a small quantity of 95% alcohol fixative (1 ml fixative per 10 ml fluid) added.

On receipt of the specimen by the laboratory, tissue fragments should be removed for histological examination. The suspension of cells is then processed by centrifugation and smears prepared from the cell pellet. Both air-dried and alcohol-fixed smears should be prepared routinely. Spare smears should be prepared for special stains if required. If the specimen is heavily blood-stained it is advisable to separate the red blood cells from the cells of interest in the fluid before centrifugation using a density gradient method (Proctor, 1989).

Cytology of peritoneal washings obtained at exploratory laparotomy in untreated patients

The principal benign components of the lavage fluid are mesothelial cells and macrophages and occasional inflammatory cells. Mesothelial cells appear in sheets and singly. Single mesothelial cells are rounded with a small rounded nucleus occupying a third of the cell and pale delicate cytoplasm. The sheets of mesothelial cells are remarkable for their large size. They may be composed of monolayers of many hundreds of cells reflecting the fact that the mesothelium has been forcibly detached by the irrigation procedure (Fig. 45.52). The nuclei may contain small chromocentres or a single nucleolus. The benign nature of the cells is obvious from the uniformity of their nucleus. Macrophages are recognizable by their foamy cytoplasm. Occasionally, ciliated columnar cells or ciliated tufts of cytoplasm thought to be derived from the Fallopian tubes are seen in the washing. Psammoma bodies have also been observed but do not have the same sinister significance that they have in cervical smears. In abdominal endometriosis, dense clusters of endometrial cells may be seen which may be misdiagnosed as malignant cells (Spriggs, 1987).

Malignant cells in peritoneal washings in patients with adenocarcinoma of the ovary

In washings obtained prior to radiotherapy or chemotherapy malignant glandular cells can usually be distin-

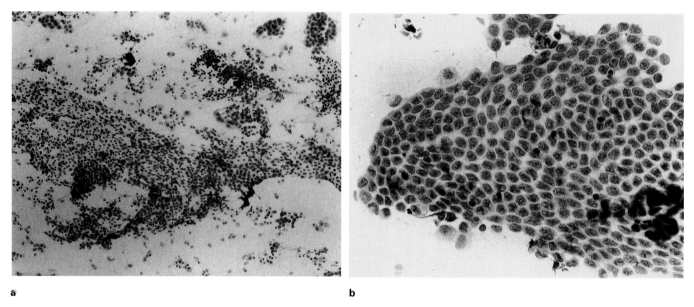

a   b

Fig. 45.52a,b   a Peritoneal washings showing sheets of benign mesothelial cells that were forcibly detached by the lavage procedure. ×300. **b** Same specimen at higher magnification. ×500.

guished from the mesothelial cells in the smears by their larger size and pleomorphism. Single adenocarcinoma cells have variable amounts of delicate cyanophilic vacuolated cytoplasm and may have one or more irregular hyperchromatic nuclei. Enlarged, irregular nucleoli may be present. The malignant cells most commonly observed in this way are from serous adenocarcinomas and show varying degrees of differentiation. Problems of differential diagnosis between malignant cells and mesothelial cells may arise in the case of borderline tumours of the ovary which may shed cells with atypical but not obviously malignant features. In cases of doubt a diagnosis of cancer should not be made.

Problems also exist in the recognition of tumour cells in lavage specimens taken at second-look laparotomy after chemotherapy or radiotherapy. Treatment may result in atypia of the mesothelial cells, affecting both nucleus and cytoplasm, leading to misdiagnosis. The changes induced in mesothelial cells by cytotoxic drugs include thickening of the cytoplasm, nuclear enlargement and irregularity. Coffin et al (1985) estimated that difficulties in differential diagnosis may occur in a third of second-look laparoscopies and with experience diagnostic accuracy could improve.

Immunocytochemical staining of peritoneal lavage specimens can be of value in discriminating between tumour cells and mesothelial cells. Coleman & Ormerod (1984) studied the value of immunocytochemical staining of lavage specimens using an antibody raised in rabbits against papillary cystadenocarcinoma of the ovary, designated CX-1. No staining of mesothelial cells was observed in 16 samples which were considered on cytological grounds

to be tumour free. However, distinct staining of tumour cells was noted in six of 10 lavage specimens containing malignant cells from an ovarian adenocarcinoma.

Peritoneal washing and the detection of other malignant lesions of the female genital tract

Peritoneal lavage has been used to detect peritoneal spread in patients with endometrial cancer. Several studies have shown that peritoneal spread of an endometrial cancer, even low-grade lesions, are associated with poor prognosis (Ide, 1984; Hirai et al, 1989; McLellan et al, 1989). Malignant lavage specimens have also been recorded in patients with carcinoma of the cervix (Ziselman et al, 1984; Roberts et al, 1986). It is possible that in some cases tumour cells from uterine neoplasms reach the peritoneal cavity via the Fallopian tubes.

Culdocentesis (cul-de-sac aspiration)

This involves aspiration of the Pouch of Douglas through the posterior vaginal wall. The benign mesothelial cells in cul-de-sac aspirates differ from those seen in peritoneal lavage specimens. They are larger and the nuclei appear to be more active with larger chromocentres and multiple small regular nucleoli. The cells appear in rounded three-dimensional clusters rather than flat sheets reflecting the fact that they are growing freely in the fluid (Fig. 45.53). Polymorphs and lymphocytes are frequently found in cul-de-sac specimens. The presence of psammoma bodies has been described in cul-de-sac specimens but in this situation they rarely indicate malignancy (Koss, 1992).

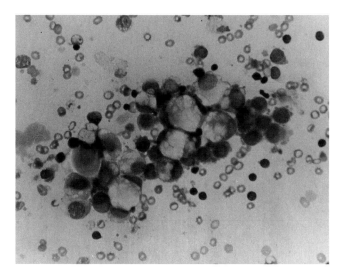

Fig. 45.53 Benign mesothelial cells in a peritoneal aspirate. Note how the cells are rounded up, indicating that they have been exfoliated rather than forcibly detached. There are numerous lymphocytes and red blood cells in the background of the smear. ×475.

Endometrial cell clusters may be found in aspirates from cases of pelvic endometriosis. Faecal contamination has also been described.

THE CYTOLOGY OF SEROUS EFFUSIONS

Accumulation of fluid in the peritoneal cavity is often secondary to inflammatory disease or malignant disease in the female genital tract. Free fluid may be found in association with acute salpingitis or tuberculous salpingitis. Serous and mucinous cystadenocarcinomas of the ovary frequently present as ascites. Ascites or hydrothorax may also be a feature of fibrothecoma of the ovary (Meigs' syndrome). For completeness, the cytology of ascitic fluid in these three conditions is described.

Peritonitis associated with acute salpingitis

Diagnosis usually presents little difficulty as the fluid appears purulent and the smears are composed almost entirely of polymorphs, fibrin strands and necrotic debris.

Tuberculous effusion

Large amounts of fluid may collect in the peritoneal cavity in cases of tuberculous peritonitis, leading to suspicion of malignancy. Even when aspirated to dryness, the fluid may collect again. Unfortunately the cytology of the cells harvested from the fluid shows a non-specific pattern. Lymphocytes may predominate but the mesothelial cells show marked reactive changes and may be quite numerous. Pure lymphocytic effusions associated with tuber-

culosis are described in textbooks but are rarely seen. The cells that are normally associated with tuberculosis, e.g. Langhans cells and endothelioid cells, are extremely rare and staining the cell deposit for acid-fast bacilli is rarely rewarding. Peritoneal biopsy and culture are required for definitive diagnosis in most cases.

Malignant effusions associated with metastatic ovarian cancer

Seventy per cent of ovarian cancers metastasize to the peritoneal cavity, hence malignant effusions due to ovarian carcinoma account for a large percentage of all malignant effusions. A feature of the smear is that it is often composed almost entirely of tumour cells, indicating that the tumour cells are proliferating freely in the fluid. The appearance of the tumour cells in cytological smears varies according to the degree of differentiation of the tumour.

In well-differentiated cystadenocarcinomas, the tumour cells may form round balls composed of many hundreds of cells. These may be so numerous that they are visible to the naked eye if a sample of fluid is held up to the light. In sections of cell blocks it can be seen that these balls of cells are usually hollow. In smears, however, they appear solid in three-dimensional balls or clusters of varying shapes and sizes (Fig. 45.54). The nuclei are usually pushed to the periphery of the sphere so that the sphere has a scalloped edge to it. Anisonucleosis is also a feature. Large vacuoles are present in the cytoplasm in serous cystadenocarcinoma. In mucin-secreting tumours, intracellular mucin can be demonstrated in the cells with special stains. In papillary serous cystadenocarcinomas, psammoma bodies may be present in large numbers.

In poorly-differentiated adenocarcinomas, the tumour cells appear singly or in small clusters. Diagnosis is facilitated by the presence of marked anisonucleosis and enlarged irregular nucleoli. Abnormal mitotic figures may be seen.

Electronmicroscopy of the adenocarcinoma cells in peritoneal fluid shows that their surface is covered with numerous microvilli. These sometimes form a tuft at one pole of the cell. This concentration of microvilli can sometimes be recognized at the light microscope level when the tumour cell appears to have acquired cilia. This pseudociliated appearance is almost exclusively found in effusions due to ovarian carcinomas and is seen most readily in Giemsa-stained smears.

It should be remembered that the cytological presentation of metastatic ovarian adenocarcinoma in smears of ascitic fluid is not specific. Tumour cells from a metastatic carcinoma of the colon, stomach or breast may have a similar appearance although their growth in the fluid is rarely so florid.

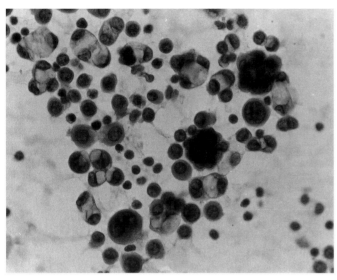
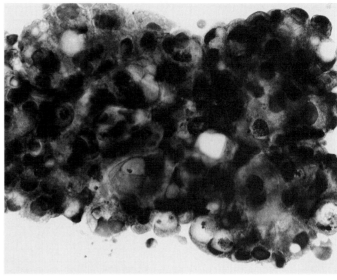

a   b

Fig. 45.54a,b **a** Malignant cells in a peritoneal aspirate. The tumour cells are lying singly and in small clusters. Note the abnormal eccentric nuclei and signet-ring appearance of the cells consistent with metastatic adenocarcinoma. ×500. **b** A large cluster of malignant cells in a peritoneal aspirate from the same case shown in **a**. ×500.

Peritoneal metastases from borderline ovarian tumours are difficult to distinguish from mesothelial cells. Two distinct cell populations should be identified before a diagnosis of malignancy is made.

Pseudomyxoma peritonei

This unusual condition is associated with the presence of mucin-producing tumours of the ovary which spread to the peritoneum. Mucin spills into the peritoneal cavity eliciting the formation of enormous volumes of free fluid. The fluid on aspiration is yellow and viscous and smears contain mucin strands but very few cells. Tumour cells, when they are present, appear remarkably bland and form sharply-defined small clusters of overlapping cells with nuclei and scanty cytoplasm. Occasionally, tumour cells are conspicuous by their absence.

Meigs' syndrome

Cytological smears prepared from the effusions associated with Meigs' syndrome contain numerous proliferating mesothelial cells. They may form balls which superficially ressemble the balls of cells seen in adenocarcinoma. However careful examination will reveal that the nuclei are small and do not protrude beyond the edge of the cluster and that the balls rarely contain more than 30 cells. A differential diagnosis of mesothelioma has also to be considered. Immunocytochemical stains may assist with the differential diagnosis.

For further details of the cytodiagnosis of effusions the reader is referred to Spriggs & Boddington's *Atlas of serous fluid cytopathology* (Kluwer Academic Publishers, Dordrecht, 1989).

REFERENCES

An Foraker S H, Kawada C Y, McKinney D 1979 Endometrial aspiration studies on Isaacs cell sampler with cytohistologic correlation. Acta Cytologica 23: 303–308.

Angrish K, Verna K 1981 Cytological detection of tuberculosis of the uterine cervix. Acta Cytologica 25: 160–162.

Athanassiadou P P, Kykou K A, Antoniades L G, Athanassiades P H 1992 Cytological evaluation of the effect of Tamoxifen in premenopausal and post menopausal women with primary breast cancer by analysis of the karyopyknotic indices of vaginal smears. Cytopathology 3: 203–208.

Ayre J E 1947 Selective cytology smear for diagnosis of cancer. American Journal of Obstetrics and Gynecology 53: 609–617.

Ayre J E 1955 Rotating endometrial brush: new technique for the diagnosis of fundal carcinoma. Obstetrics and Gynecology 5: 137–141.

Balachandran I, Galagan K S 1984 Cervical carcinoma in situ associated with azathioprine therapy; a case report and literature review. Acta Cytologica 28: 699–702.

Boon M E, Alons van Kordelaar J J M, Reitveld-Scheffers P E M 1986 Consequences of the introduction of combined spatula and cytobrush for sampling for cervical cytology. Acta Cytologica 30: 264–270.

British Society for Clinical Cytology 1989 Taking cervical smears (booklet and video). Aspen Corporate Communications. BSCC, The Quadrangle, Westmount Centre, Uxbridge Rd, Hayes UB4 0HB.

Brown L J, Wells M 1986 Cervical glandular atypia associated with squamous intraepithelial neoplasia: a premalignant condition? Journal of Clinical Pathology 39: 22–28.

Brule A, Claas E, DuMaine M et al 1989 Application of anticontamination primers in the polymerase chain reaction for the detection of human papillomavirus genotypes in cervical scrapes and biopsies. Journal of Medical Virology 29: 20–27.

Buntinx F, Boon M, Beck S, Knottnerus J, Essed G 1991 Comparison of cytobrush sampling, spatula sampling and combined Cytobrush and spatula sampling of the uterine cervix. Acta Cytologica 41: 64–68.

Carmichael D E 1973 Diagnosis by the vaginal smear. In: The Papanicolaou smear; life of George N Papanicolaou. Charles C Thomas, Springfield, Illinois, pp 54–61.

Cary W H 1943 A method of obtaining endometrial smears for study of their cellular content. Obstetrics and Gynecology 46: 422–423.

Coffin C M, Adcock L L, Dehner L P 1985 The second look operation of ovarian neoplasms: a study of 85 cases emphasising cytological and histologic problems. International Journal of Gynecological Pathology 4: 97–109.

Coleman D V 1969 A case of tuberculosis of the cervix. Acta Cytologica 13: 104–107.

Coleman D V 1979 Cytological diagnosis of virus infected cells in Papanicolaou smears and its application in clinical practice. Journal of Clinical Pathology 32: 1075–1089.

Coleman D V, Evans D M D 1988 Biopsy pathology and cytology of the cervix. Chapman & Hall, London.

Coleman D V, Ormerod M B 1984 Tumor markers in cytology. In: Koss L G, Coleman D V (eds) Advances in clinical cytology. Masson, New York, pp 33–47.

Coleman D, Day N, Douglas G et al 1993 European guidelines for quality assurance in cervical cancer screening: Europe Against Cancer Programme. European Journal of Cancer 29A (suppl 4): S1–S37.

Coman D R 1944 Decreased mutual adhesiveness; property of cells from squamous cell carcinomas. Cancer Research 4: 625–629.

Creasman W T, Rutledge F 1971 The prognostic value of peritoneal cytology in gynecologic malignant disease. American Journal of Obstetrics and Gynecology 110: 773–781.

Crow J, Gordon H, Hudson E 1980 An assessment of the Mi Mark endometrial sampling technique. Journal of Clinical Pathology 33: 72–80.

DHSS Health Service Guidelines 1993 National cervical screening programme HSG(93) Department of Health, London.

Dowling E A, Gravlee L C 1964 Endometrial cancer diagnosis: a new technique using a jet washer. Alabama Journal of Medical Sciences 1: 412–416.

Ducatman B S, Wang H H, Jonasson J G, Hogan C L, Antonioli D A 1993 Tubal metaplasia: a cytological study with comparison to other neoplastic and non-neoplastic conditions of the endocervix. Diagnostic Cytopathology 9: 98–103.

Duguid H L D, Parratt D, Traynor R 1980 Actinomyces-like organism in cervical smears from women using contraceptive devices. British Medical Journal 281: 534.

Eells T P, Alpern H D, Grzywacz C, MacMillan R W, Olson J E 1990 The effect of tamoxifen on cervical squamous maturation in Papanicolaou stained cervical smears of postmenopausal women. Cytopathology 1: 263–268.

Ellice R M, Morse A R, Anderson M C 1981 Aspiration cytology versus histology in the assessment of women attending a menopause clinic. British Journal of Obstetrics and Gynaecology 88: 421–425.

Evans D M D, Shelley G, Cleary B, Baldwin Y 1974 Observer variation and quality control of cytodiagnosis. Journal of Clinical Pathology 27: 945–950.

Evans D M D, Hudson E A, Brown C L et al 1986 Terminology in gynaecological cytopathology: report of the working party of the British Society for Clinical Cytology. Journal of Clinical Pathology 39: 933–944.

Fox H, Buckley C H 1982 The endometrial hyperplasias and their relationship to endometrial neoplasia. Histopathology 6: 493–510.

Gupta P K, Hollander D H, Frost J K 1976 Actinomyces in cervico-vaginal smears; an association with IUCD usage. Acta Cytologica 20: 295–297.

Gusberg S B, Kaplan A L 1963 Precursors of corpus cancer. IV Adenomatous hyperplasia as Stage 0 carcinoma of the endometrium. American Journal of Obstetrics and Gynecology 87: 662–678.

Hare M J, Toone E, Taylor Robinson D et al 1981 Follicular cervicitis — colposcopic appearances and association with Chlamydia trachomatis. British Journal of Obstetrics and Gynaecology 88: 174–180.

Hirai Y, Fujimoto I, Yamamuchi K, Hasumi K, Masabuchi K, Sano Y 1989 Peritoneal fluid cytology and prognosis in patients with endometrial carcinoma. Obstetrics and Gynecology 73: 335–338

Hirschowitz L, Eckford S, Phillpotts B, Midwinter A 1994 Cytological changes associated with tubo-endometrioid metaplasia of the uterine cervix. Cytopathology 5: 1–8.

Holland W, Stewart S 1990 Screening in adult women. In: Screening in health care. The Nuffield Provincial Hospitals Trust, London, pp 155–197.

Holmquist N D, Bellina J H, Danos M L 1976 Vaginal and cervical cytologic changes following laser treatment. Acta Cytologica 20: 290–294.

Huang J C, Naylor B 1993 Cytomegalovirus infection of the cervix detected by cytology and histology: a report of five cases. Cytopathology 4: 237–241.

Husain O A N, Butler E B, Evans D M D, McGregor J E, Yule R 1974 Quality control in cytology. Journal of Clinical Pathology 27: 935–944.

Hutton J E, Morse A R, Anderson M C, Beard R W 1978 Endometrial assessment with Isaacs cell sampler. British Medical Journal 1: 947–949

Ide P 1984 Prognostic value of peritoneal fluid cytology in patients with endometrial cancer stage I. European Journal of Obstetrics and Gynecology and Reproductive Biology 18: 343–349.

Imperial Cancer Research Fund (ICRF) Coordinating Committee on Cervical Screening 1984 Organisation of a programme for cervical cancer screening. British Medical Journal 289: 894–895.

Intercollegiate Working Party on Cervical Cancer Screening 1987 Report of the Intercollegiate Working Party on Cervical Cancer Screening. Royal College of Obstetricians and Gynaecologists, London.

International Agency for Research on Cancer (IARC) Working Group on Evaluation of Cervical Cancer Screening Programmes 1984 Screening for cervical cancer. British Medical Journal 289: 659–664.

International Agency for Research on Cancer (IARC) Working Group on Evaluation of Cervical Screening Programmes 1986 Screening for squamous cervical cancer: duration of low risk after negative results of cervical cytology and its implication for screening policies. British Medical Journal 293: 659–664.

Isaacs J H, Wilhoitte R W 1974 Aspiration cytology of the endometrium: office and hospital sampling procedures. Obstetrics and Gynecology 118: 679–684.

Ismail S M 1991 Cone biopsy causes cervical endometriosis and tuboendometrioid metaplasia. Histopathology 18: 107–114.

Ismail S M 1992 Cervical endometriosis and tuboendometrioid metaplasia. Histopathology 20: 279–280.

Ismail S M, Colclough A B, Dinnen J S et al 1989 Observer variation in histopathological diagnosis and grading of CIN. British Medical Journal 298: 707–710.

Kearns P R, Gray J E 1963 Mycotic vulvovaginitis. Obstetrics and Gynecology 22: 621–625.

Keetel W C, Pixley E 1958 Diagnostic value of peritoneal washings. Clinical Obstetrics and Gynecology 1: 592–606.

Kjellgren O, Angstrom T 1979 Transvaginal and transrectal aspiration biopsy in diagnosis and classification of ovarian tumours. In: Zajicek J (ed) Aspiration biopsy and cytology: part 2. Karger, Basel, pp 81–103.

Kjellgren O, Angstrom T, Bergman F, Wiklund D E 1971 Fine needle aspiration biopsy in diagnosis and classification of ovarian carcinoma. Cancer 28: 967–976.

Koss L G 1992 Diagnostic cytology and its histopathologic bases, 4th edn. Lippincott, Philadelphia.

Koss L G, Schreiber K, Oberlander S G, Moukhtar M, Levine H S, Moussouris H F 1981 Screening of asymptomatic women for endometrial cancer. Obstetrics and Gynecology 57: 681–691.

Koss L G, Schreiber K, Moussouris H, Oberlaender S G 1982 Endometrial carcinoma and its precursors: detection and screening. Clinical Obstetrics and Gynecology 25: 49–61.

Koss L G, Schreiber K, Oberlander S G, Moussouris H F, Lesser M 1984 Detection of endometrial carcinoma and hyperplasia in asymptomatic women. Obstetrics and Gynecology 64: 1–11.

Liu W, Barrow M J, Spitler M F, Kochis A F 1963 Normal exfoliation of endometrial cells in premenopausal women. Acta Cytologica 7: 211–214.

McGowan L 1974 Cytologic methods for the detection of endometrial cancer. Gynecologic Oncology 2: 272–278.

McGowan L 1989 Peritoneal fluid washings. Acta Cytologica 33: 414–415.

MacGregor J E, Fraser M E, Mann E M F 1966 The cytopipette in the diagnosis of early cervical carcinoma. Lancet i: 252–256.

McLellan R, Dillon M B, Currie J L, Rosenshein N B 1989 Peritoneal cytology in endometrial cancer: a review. Obstetrical and Gynecological Survey 44: 711–719.

Marks M, Langston C, Eickhoff T C 1970 Torulopsis glabrata: an opportunistic pathogen in man. New England Journal of Medicine 283: 1131–1136.

Meisels A, Fortin R 1976 Condylomatous lesions of the cervix and vagina: I Cytologic patterns. Acta Cytologica 20: 505–509.

Meisels A, Fortin R, Roy M 1977 Condylomatous lesions of the cervix: II Cytologic, colposcopic and histologic study. Acta Cytologica 21: 379–390.

Melchers W, Brule A, Walboomers J et al 1989 Increased detection rate of human papillomavirus in cervical scrapes by the polymerase chain reaction compared to modified FISH and Southern blotting analysis. Journal of Medical Virology 27: 329–335.

Milan A R, Markley R L 1973 Endometrial cytology by a new technique. Obstetrics and Gynecology 42: 469–475.

Misch K A, Smithies A, Twomey D, O'Sullivan J C, Onuigobo W 1976 Tuberculosis of the cervix: cytology as an aid to diagnosis. Journal of Clinical Pathology 29: 313–316.

Mitchell M, Medley G, Giles G 1990 Cervical cancers diagnosed after negative results on cervical cytology: perspective in the 1980s. British Medical Journal 300: 1622–1626.

Morse A R 1981 The value of endometrial aspiration in gynaecological practice. In: Koss L G, Coleman D V (eds) Advances in clinical cytology. Butterworths, London, pp 44–63.

Morse A R M, Coleman D V, Gardner S D 1974 An evaluation of cytology in the diagnosis of herpes simplex virus infection and cytomegalovirus infection of the cervix uteri. Journal of Obstetrics and Gynaecology of the British Commonwealth 81: 393–398.

Morse A, Wickenden C, Byrne M V et al 1988 HPV DNA hybridisation of cervical scrapes and comparison with cytological findings in Papanicolaou smears. Journal of Clinical Pathology 41: 296–299.

Munoz N, Bosch X, Kaldor J M 1988 Does human papillomavirus cause cervical cancer? The state of the epidemiological evidence. British Journal of Cancer 57: 1–5.

Navab A, Koss L G, La Due J S 1965 Estrogen-like activity of digitalis. Journal of the American Medical Association 194: 30–32.

Oortmarssen G J V, Habemma J D F, Ballegooijen M V 1992 Predicting mortality from cervical cancer after negative smear test results. British Medical Journal 305: 449–451.

Papanicolaou G N 1929 New cancer diagnosis. In: Proceedings of third race betterment conference. Race Betterment Foundation, Battle Creek.

Papanicolaou G 1942 A new procedure for staining vaginal smears. Science 95: 438.

Papanicolaou G, Traut H E 1943 Diagnosis of uterine cancer by vaginal smears. The Commonwealth Fund, New York.

Penn I, Starzl T E 1972 Malignant tumors arising de novo in immunosuppressed organ transplant recipients. Transplantation 14: 407–417.

Potter A R 1989 Immunocytochemical methods. In: Coleman D V, Chapman P A (eds) Clinical cytotechnology. Butterworth, London, pp 106–124.

Proctor D 1989a Preparatory techniques. In: Coleman D V, Chapman D A (eds) Clinical cytotechnology. Butterworth, London, pp 52–78.

Proctor D 1989b Staining techniques. In: Coleman D V, Chapman D A (eds) Clinical cytotechnology. Butterworth, London, pp 79–105.

Purola E, Savia E 1977 Cytology of gynaecologic condyloma acuminatum. Acta Cytologica 21: 26–31.

Quinn M A, Bishop G J, Cambell J J, Rodgerson J, Pepperell R J 1980 Laparoscopic follow up of patients with ovarian carcinoma. British Journal of Obstetrics and Gynaecology 87: 1132–1139.

Reagan J W, Ng A B P 1973 The cells of uterine adenocarcinoma, 2nd edn. Karger, Basel.

Roberts W S, Bryson S C, Cavenagh D, Roberts V C, Layman G H 1986 Peritoneal cytology and invasive carcinoma of the cervix. Gynecologic Oncology 24: 331–336.

Roberts J H, Woodend B 1993 Negative cytology preceding cervical cancer: causes and prevention. Journal of Clinical Pathology 46: 700–702.

Robertson A J, Anderson J M, Swanson Beck J et al 1989 Observer variability in histopathological reporting of cervical biopsy specimens. Journal of Clinical Pathology 42: 231–238.

Rubio C A 1977 The false negative smear. Obstetrics and Gynecology 49: 576–580.

Ruehsen M de M, McNeill R E, Frost J K, Gupta P K, Diamond L S, Honiberg B M 1980 Amoeba resembling Entamoeba gingivalis in the genital tract of IUD users. Acta Cytologica 24: 413–420.

Schnell J D, Andrews P, Plempel M 1972 Die Vaginale Kontamination der weiblechen Bevolkerung einer Grosstadt mit Trichomonadem und Hefen. Geburtshilfe und Frauenheilkunde 32: 1007–1014.

Segadal E, Iverson O E 1980 The Isaacs cell sampler: an alternative to curettage. British Medical Journal 2: 364–365.

Silverberg S C, Hurt W G 1975 Minimum deviation adenocarcinoma (adenoma malignum) of the cervix. American Journal of Obstetrics and Gynecology 123: 971–975.

Smith A, Chamberlain J P 1987 Managing cervical screening. In: Information technology in health care, Part B. Kluwer, London.

Smith J, Coleman D V 1984 Electron microscopy of cells showing viral cytopathic effects in Papanicolaou smears. Acta Cytologica 27: 605–613.

Spriggs A I 1987 Cytology of peritoneal washings. British Journal of Obstetrics and Gynaecology 94: 1–3.

Studd J W W, Thom M, Dische F, Driver M, Wade Evans T, Williams D 1979 Value of cytology for detecting endometrial abnormalities in climacteric women receiving hormone replacement therapy. British Medical Journal 1: 846–848.

Syrjanen K, Hakama M, Saarikoski S 1990 Prevalence, incidence and estimated life time risk of cervical human papillomavirus infections in non selected Finnish female population. Sexually Transmitted Diseases 17: 15–19.

Szyfelbein W M, Young R H, Scully R E 1984 Adenoma malignum of the cervix; cytologic findings. Acta Cytologica 25: 691–698.

Taylor P T, Anderson W A, Barber S R, Covell S L, Smith E B, Underwood P B 1987 The Papanicolaou smear: contribution of the endocervical brush. Obstetrics and Gynecology 70: 734–738.

The Bethesda System for Reporting Cervical/Vaginal Diagnoses 1993 Acta Cytologica 37: 115–124.

Trimbos B, Arentz N 1986 The efficiency of the cytobrush versus the cotton swab in the collection of endocervical cells in cervical smears. Acta Cytologica 30: 261–263.

Van L L, Novotny D, Dotters D J 1991 Distinguishing tubal metaplasia from endocervical metaplasia on cervical Papanicolaou smears. Obstetrics and Gynecology 78: 974–976.

Vooijs G P, Elias A, van der Graaf Y, Berg M P 1986 The influence of sample takers on the cellular composition of cervical smears. Acta Cytologica 30: 251–257.

Wachtel E G 1969 Exfoliative cytology in gynaecological practice, 2nd edn. Butterworth, London.

Welch W R, Scully R E 1977 Precancerous lesions of the endometrium. Human Pathology 8: 503–512.

Wied G, Bibbo M, Keebler C M 1983 Evaluation of endocrinologic conditions in exfoliative cytology. In: Wied G, Koss L G, Reagan J W (eds) Compendium on diagnostic cytology, 5th edn. International Academy of Cytology, Chicago, pp 28–39.

Wolfendale M R, Howe B, Guest R, Usherwood M McD, Draper G J 1987 Controlled trial of a new cervical spatula. British Medical Journal 294: 33–55.

Yule R et al 1973 The prevention of cancer of the cervix by cytological screening of the population. In: Easson E C (ed) Cancer of the uterine cervix. Saunders, London, pp 11–25.

Ziselman E M, Harkavy S E, Hogan M, Willa W, Atkinson B 1984 Peritoneal washing cytology; uses and diagnostic criteria in gynecologic neoplasms. Acta Cytologica 28: 105–110.

Zur Hausen H 1988 Human genital cancer: synergism between two virus infections or synergism between a virus infection and initiating events? Lancet ii: 1370–1372.

46. Development and anatomy of the placenta

Peter Kaufmann   Mario Castellucci

EARLY DEVELOPMENT OF THE HUMAN PLACENTA

Prelacunar stage

The development of the placenta begins as soon as the blastocyst implants. The implanting blastocyst, composed of 107–256 cells (Hertig, 1960), is a flattened vesicle. Most of the cells make up the outer wall (trophoblast), surrounding the blastocystic cavity (Fig. 46.1a). Apposed to its inner surface is a small group of cells that form the embryoblast.

The embryonic, or implantation, pole of the blastocyst is attached to the endometrium first (Fig. 46.1a, cf. also Fig. 46.10). The usual implantation site is the upper part of the posterior wall of the uterine body, near to the mid-sagittal plane (Fig. 46.12a); for additional details see Boyd & Hamilton (1970) and Denker & Aplin (1990).

During attachment, and following invasion of the endometrial epithelium, the trophoblastic cells of the implanting embryonic pole of the blastocyst proliferate to form a double-layered trophoblast (Heuser & Streeter, 1941). The outer of the two layers, directly facing the maternal tissue, is transformed into a syncytiotrophoblast by fusion of neighbouring trophoblast cells. The remaining cellular components of the blastocyst wall, which have not yet achieved contact with maternal tissues, remain discrete and are called cytotrophoblast (Fig. 46.1a and b). Throughout the following days, and with progressive invasion, additional parts of the blastocyst surface come into close contact with maternal tissues. This is followed by trophoblastic proliferation with subsequent fusion. The syncytiotrophoblastic mass increases by expanding over the surface of the implanting blastocyst as implantation progresses (Fig. 46.1b). At the implantation pole, it is not a smooth-surfaced mass but rather is covered with branching, finger-like extensions which deeply invade the endometrium. This first stage, lasting from day 7–8 post conception, has been defined as the pre-lacunar period by Wislocki & Streeter (1938).

The syncytiotrophoblast has lost its generative potency during fusion. The cytotrophoblast acts as stem cells which guarantee growth of the trophoblast by continuous proliferation, with subsequent fusion to form the syncytiotrophoblast. The latter is a continuous acellular system, not interrupted by intercellular spaces and not composed of individual syncytial units. Terms such as 'syncytial cells' or 'syncytiotrophoblasts' are inappropriate.

Lacunar stage

At day 8 post conception, small vacuoles appear in the enlarging syncytiotrophoblastic mass at the implantation pole. The vacuoles quickly enlarge and become confluent to form a system of so-called lacunae (Fig. 46.1b–d). The separating lamellae, or pillars, of syncytiotrophoblast are called the trabeculae. Their appearance marks the beginning of the lacunar or trabecular stage of placentation which lasts from day 8–13 post conception. Lacuna formation starts at the implantation pole. With advancing implantation and expansion of the syncytiotrophoblastic mass the process extends all over the blastocyst within a few days.

At day 12 post conception the blastocyst is so deeply implanted that the uterine epithelium closes over the implantation site (cf. Fig. 46.1c). At this time, the outer surface of the blastocyst is completely transformed into syncytiotrophoblast. At its inner surface, it is covered by a locally incomplete layer of cytotrophoblast. Since trophoblastic proliferation and syncytial fusion have started at the implantation pole, the trophoblastic wall is considerably thicker at this point, as compared to the anti-implantation pole (Figs 46.1c and 46.10, day 13 and 18). This difference in thickness is never made up by the thinner parts during the following developmental steps. The thicker trophoblast of the implantation pole is later transformed into the placenta, whereas the opposing thinner trophoblastic circumference only initially attempts to establish the same structure; later, it shows regressive transformation into the smooth chorion, the 'membranes' (Fig. 46.10, day 40). All data of placental development

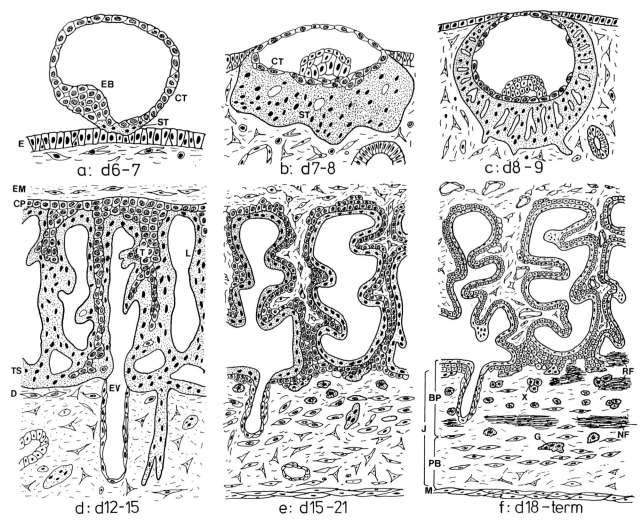

Fig. 46.1   Typical stages of early placental development: **a** and **b** prelacunar stages; **c** lacunar stage; **d** transition from lacunar to primary villous stage; **e** secondary villous stage; **f** tertiary villous stage. EB = embryoblast; CT = cytotrophoblast; ST = syncytiotrophoblast; E = endometrial epithelium; EM = extraembryonic mesoderm; CP = primary chorionic plate; T = trabeculae and primary villi; L = maternal blood lacunae; TS = trophoblastic shell; EV = endometrial vessel; D = decidua; J = junctional zone; BP = basal plate; PB = placental bed; M = myometrium; RF = Rohr fibrinoid; NF = Nitabuch fibrinoid; X = extravillous trophoblast (X cells); G = trophoblastic giant cell. (Modified with permission from Kaufmann & Scheffen, 1992.)

given in the following sections refers to the situation at the implantation pole.

Lacuna formation subdivides the trophoblastic covering of the blastocyst into three layers (Fig. 46.1d):

a. the primary chorionic plate, facing the blastocystic cavity
b. the lacunar system, together with the trabeculae
c. the trophoblastic shell, facing the endometrium.

The primary chorionic plate is composed of a more or less continuous stratum of cytotrophoblast. Towards the lacunae, the cytotrophoblast is covered by syncytiotrophoblast (Fig. 46.1d). At day 14 post conception, mesenchymal cells spread around the inner surface of the cytotrophoblast layer (Fig. 46.1d). There they transform into a loose network of branching cells, the extraembryo-

nic mesenchyme. Luckett (1978) found evidence that these primitive connective tissue cells were derived from the embryonic disc rather than being of trophoblastic origin.

Below the primary chorionic plate is the lacunar system. The lacunae are separated from each other by septa or pillars of syncytiotrophoblast, the trabeculae (Fig. 46.1c and d). Originally, these are solely syncytiotrophoblastic in nature. Around day 12 post conception, however, they are invaded by cytotrophoblast cells (Fig. 46.1d), which are derived from the primary chorionic plate. Within a few days, the cytotrophoblast spreads down the entire length of the trabeculae. Where the peripheral ends of the trabeculae join together, they form the outermost layer of the trophoblast, the trophoblastic shell (Hertig & Rock, 1941; Boyd & Hamilton, 1970). In the beginning, this is a purely syncytiotrophoblastic structure (Fig. 46.1d), but as soon as the cytotrophoblast reaches the shell via the trabeculae (about day 15 post conception), the former achieves a more heterogeneous structure (Fig. 46.1e).

In the early stages of implantation, the erosion of the maternal tissues occurs under the lytic influence of the syncytial trophoblast. The existence of cytotrophoblast at the base of the shell changes this situation. The proliferative activity of the cytotrophoblast and its rapid migration into the depth of the endometrium appear to be responsible for the further invasion and, thus, for the further expansion of the implantation area (Boyd & Hamilton, 1970; Pijnenborg et al, 1981). In the course of this process, numerous syncytial elements can be observed far removed from the trophoblastic shell (Fig. 46.1f), partly in the depth of the uterine wall. These so-called syncytiotrophoblastic or multinuclear giant cells are derived from invading cytotrophoblast which later fuse (Park, 1971; Robertson & Warner, 1974; Pijnenborg et al, 1981).

The endometrial stroma undergoes remarkable changes throughout this process. The presence of eroding trophoblast, by being a mechanical irritant and by hormonal activity, causes the endometrial stromal cells to proliferate and to enlarge, thus giving rise to the decidual cells (Welsh & Enders, 1985).

The invasive activities of the basal syncytiotrophoblast cause disintegration of the maternal endometrial vessel walls from day 12 post conception onwards, starting with the superficial capillary loops. Blood cells, leaving the altered capillaries, are found inside the lacunae (Boyd & Hamilton, 1970). At the same time, the disintegrating capillaries are surrounded by the basally expanding syncytiotrophoblast, which gradually replaces the capillary walls (Leiser & Beier, 1988). Further invasion of the trophoblast, with progressive destruction of the capillary limbs down to their arteriolar beginnings and their venular endings, provides the anatomical basis for the final formation of separate arterial inlets into the lacunar system as well as venous outlets.

Recent morphological (Hustin et al, 1988) and clinical studies in the human using Doppler, ultrasound and endoscopy (Schaaps & Hustin, 1988) suggest that true maternal blood flow in the normal human placenta is only established after the 12th week of pregnancy. In the earlier stages, it is postulated that only maternal plasma perfuses the intervillous space.

Early villous stages

Shortly after the first appearance of maternal erythrocytes in the lacunae, around day 13 post conception, blindly ending syncytial side branches form which protrude into the lacunae (Fig. 46.1d and e). With increasing length and diameter, these so-called primary villi are invaded by cytotrophoblast. Both processes mark the beginning of the villous stages of placentation. Further proliferative activities, with branching of the primary villi, initiate the development of villous trees, the stems of which are derived from the former trabeculae. Where the latter keep their contact with the trophoblastic shell, they are called anchoring villi (Fig. 46.1e and f). At the same time, the lacunar system is, by definition, transformed into the intervillous space.

Only two days later, mesenchymal cells derived from the extraembryonic mesenchyme of the primary chorionic plate begin to invade the villi, thus transforming them into secondary villi (Fig. 46.1e). Within a few days, the mesenchyme expands peripherally to the villous tips and to near the base of the anchoring villi (Wislocki & Streeter, 1938; Boyd & Hamilton, 1970). It does not, however, reach the trophoblastic shell which, during these early stages of placentation, remains free of fetal connective tissue.

Beginning between days 18 and 20 post conception, the first fetal capillaries can be observed in the mesenchyme (Fig. 46.1f). They are derived from haemangioblastic progenitor cells which locally differentiate from the mesenchyme (King, 1987; Demir et al, 1989). The same progenitor cells give rise to groups of haematopoietic stem cells which are always surrounded by the early endothelium and are thus positioned within the primitive capillaries. The appearance of capillary cross sections in the villous stroma marks the development of the first tertiary villi. Until term, all fetally vascularized villi can be subsumed under this name; and this is the vast majority of the villi. Henceforth, only transitory developmental stages of new villus formation (trophoblastic and villous sprouts) correspond to primary or secondary villi.

At about the same time as the fetal vascularization of the villi starts, the fetally vascularized allantois reaches the chorionic plate (Fig. 46.10) and fuses with the villous vessels. A complete feto-placental circulation is established around the beginning of the 5th week post conception, as soon as enough capillary segments are fused with each other to form a true capillary bed. Also during the following weeks, in confined areas of the placenta, intravascular haematopoiesis may be observed.

The expansion of the early villous trees takes place in the following way (Castellucci et al, 1990b): at the surfaces of the larger villi, local cytotrophoblast proliferation, with subsequent syncytial fusion, causes the production of syncytial sprouts. These are structurally comparable to the early primary villi, and are composed solely of trophoblast. Most of the syncytial sprouts degenerate, probably due to inappropriate local conditions, and only some are invaded by villous mesenchyme. Formation of fetal vessels within the stroma, with subsequent growth in length and width, is characteristic of the transformation into new mesenchymal villi. Along their surfaces new sprouts are produced.

Fetal and maternal circulations come into close proxim-

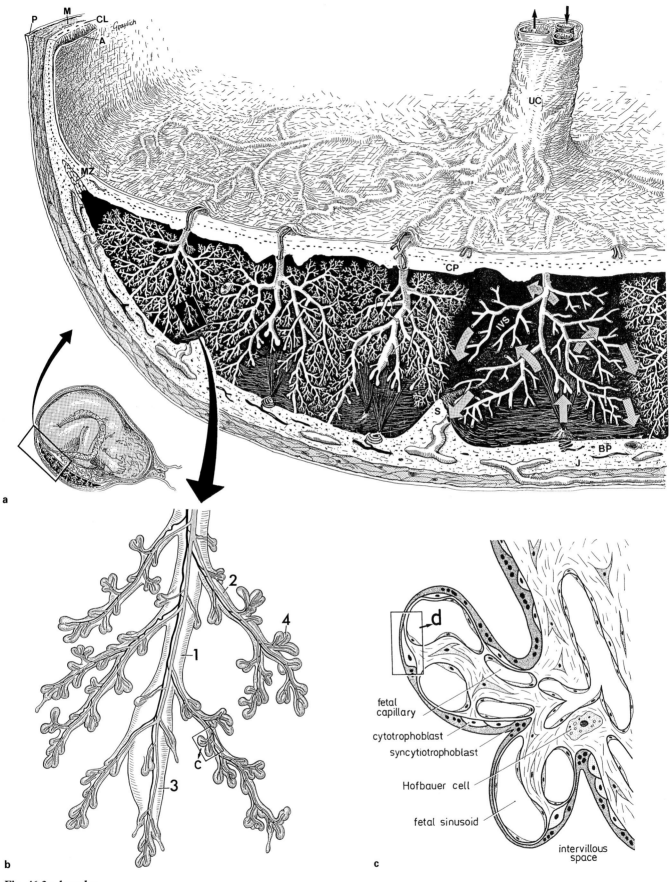

Fig. 46.2a, b and c

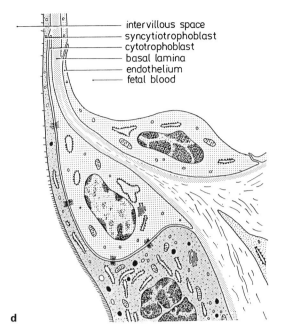

intervillous space
syncytiotrophoblast
cytotrophoblast
basal lamina
endothelium
fetal blood

d

Fig. 46.2 Basic structure of the mature human placenta.
a The maternal blood flow leaving the endometrial spiral arteries is directed into loose centres of the villous trees, so-called placentone centres. UC = umbilical cord; A = amnion; CL = chorion laeve; M = myometrium; P = perimetrium; MZ = marginal zone between placenta and fetal membranes, with obliterated intervillous space and ghost villi; CP = chorionic plate; IVS = intervillous space; S = placental septa; * = cell island, connected to a villous tree; BP = basal plate; J = junctional zone.
b Peripheral ramifications of a mature villous tree, consisting of a stem villus (1) which continues in a bulbous immature intermediate villus (3); the slender side branches are the mature intermediate villi (2); its surface is densely covered with grape-like terminal villi (4).
c Simplified lightmicroscopic diagram of two terminal villi, branching off a mature intermediate villus (right).
d Simplified electronmicroscopic diagram of the placental barrier, demonstrating its typical layers.
(**a** Reproduced with permission from Kaufmann & Scheffen, 1992; **b–d** modified with permission after Benirschke & Kaufmann, 1995.)

ity with each other as soon as an intravillous, i.e. fetal circulation, is established. Both bloodstreams are always separated by the placental barrier (Fig. 46.2c and d) which is made up of the following layers:

1. a continuous, uninterrupted layer of syncytiotrophoblast covering the villous surface and thus lining the intervillous space
2. an initially (first trimester) complete, but later (second and third trimesters) discontinuous layer of cytotrophoblast (Langhans cells)
3. a trophoblastic basal membrane
4. connective tissue
5. fetal endothelium, which is only surrounded by an ultrastructurally evident basal membrane in the last trimester.

Throughout the following periods of development, the tertiary villi undergo a complex process of differentiation, which results in various villous types which differ from

each other in terms of structure and function. This differentiation process is paralleled by qualitative and quantitative changes of the placental barrier (cf. Table 46.1, p. 1462): the syncytiotrophoblast is reduced in thickness from more than 20 μm to a mean of 3.5 μm. The cytotrophoblast diminishes and, at term, can be found in only 20% of the villous surface. The mean villous diameter decreases since the newly formed villous types are generally smaller than those preceding. Because of this latter process, the intravillous position of the fetal capillaries comes closer to the villous surface with advanced maturation. In many places, the capillary basal lamina may even fuse with that of the trophoblast, thus considerably reducing the barrier in terms of thickness and number of layers.

In summary, all these factors result in a reduction of the mean maternal–fetal diffusion distance from between 50 and 100 μm in the second month to between 4 and 5 μm at term (Table 46.1).

BASIC VILLOUS STRUCTURE AND VILLOUS COMPONENTS

The basic morphology of the placental villi can be seen from Figures 46.2 and 46.3. The maternal blood in the intervillous space is directly in contact with the syncytiotrophoblast which is the superficial layer of the placental villi. It must be pointed out that the syncytiotrophoblast is a continuous, uninterrupted syncytial layer (Fig. 46.3) that extends over the surfaces of all villous trees and is thus completely lining the intervillous space. The few reports that point to the existence of lateral cell membranes, subdividing the syncytium into 'syncytial units', appear to have an artifactual rather than a real basis. However, with advancing pregnancy, focal degeneration of the syncytiotrophoblast may occur, predominantly at the surfaces of the chorionic plate and the trophoblastic shell, but also at the villous surfaces. These local interruptions of the syncytiotrophoblast are closed within a few days by fibrinoid material. Below the syncytiotrophoblast varying numbers of cytotrophoblast cells (Langhans cells) can be found. The two components of the trophoblast layer are separated from the centrally located villous stroma by a basement membrane (Fig. 46.3). The villous stromal core consists of fixed connective tissue cells, connective tissue fibres, macrophages (Hofbauer cells), occasional mast cells and fetal vessels.

The trophoblastic mantle of the villi is the principal site for placental transfer and secretory functions. Most of these take place in the syncytiotrophoblast, whereas the underlying Langhans cells (Fig. 46.3b) act as proliferating stem cells that contribute to syncytiotrophoblastic growth by syncytial fusion (Fig. 46.4). Not only does syncytial growth depend on continuous incorporation of fusing cytotrophoblastic cells, but the regeneration of degenerating syncytial organelles and enzyme systems does so as well (Pierce & Midgley, 1963; Kaufmann et al, 1983). Thus, the villous cytotrophoblast (Langhans cells) act as stem cells, proliferating, differentiating, and subsequently fusing with the syncytium (Fig. 46.4). Proliferation of the cytotrophoblast is regulated by the oxygen supply (Fox, 1970), as in many other cell populations.

Corresponding to its functional pluripotency, the syncytiotrophoblast is structurally composed of mosaic-like patches (Fig. 46.3a) with varying ultrastructural and enzyme patterns:

1. The epithelial plates, or vasculo-syncytial membranes, offer a minimal maternofetal diffusion distance of 1–2 μm; these are the main sites of diffusional transfer of gases, water and the carrier transfer of glucose.

2. The thicker syncytial segments, with prevailing rough or smooth endoplasmic reticulum, are specialized areas for the secretion of proteo-hormones and placental proteins, metabolism of steroid hormones and materno-fetal protein transfer.

3. The so-called syncytial knots and sprouts are very heterogeneous structures, characterized by accumulations of nuclei more (sprouts) or less (knots) protruding into the intervillous space. Most of those found in histological sections are merely tangential sections of the villous surfaces (Fig. 46.9c) (Cantle et al, 1987). Only a few of the remaining true syncytial knots and sprouts are direct evidence of trophoblastic proliferation as first steps of villus formation (Fig. 46.5), others are local aggregations of old syncytial nuclei which have been accumulated within

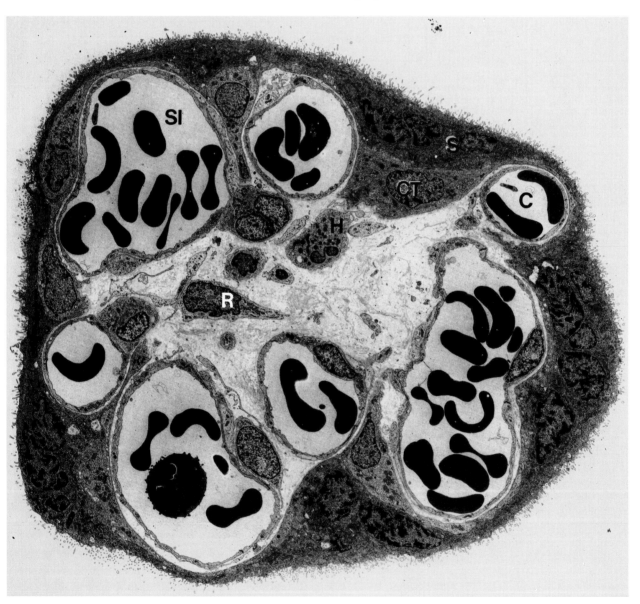

a

Fig. 46.3a

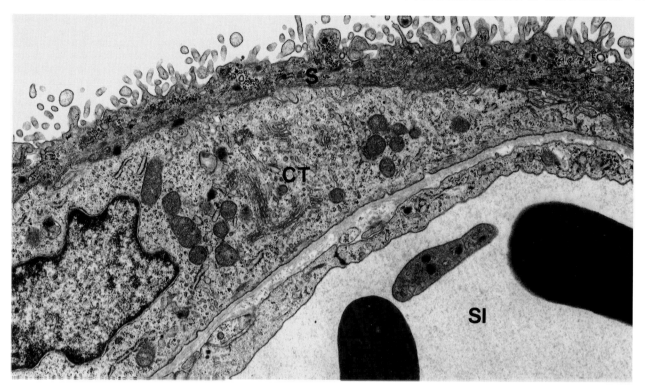

b

Fig. 46.3 **a** Ultrastructural features of a typical, well-fixed terminal villus. It illustrates the high degree of fetal capillarization with narrow capillaries (C) and dilated sinusoids (SI). The sparse connective tissue is composed of fixed connective tissue cells (R) and macrophages (H), enmeshed in loosely arranged connective tissue fibres. The stromal core is surrounded by the outer syncytiotrophoblast (S) which is composed of mosaic-like patches which vary in structure and thickness. Below the syncytiotrophoblast a few Langhans cells (villous cytotrophoblast) (CT) can be seen. × 2000. **b** Higher magnification of a Langhans cell (CT) of the villus shown in **a**. Most of the Langhans cells belong to this undifferentiated type of proliferating or resting stem cell. × 9800. (Reproduced with permission from Schiebler & Kaufmann, 1981.)

the syncytiotrophoblast by its continuous incorporation of cytotrophoblast (Fig. 46.4f).

The endothelium of the villous vessels (Fig. 46.3b) acts as a filter, limiting macromolecular transfer across the vessel wall to a certain molecular size (probably below 20 000 Dalton). The cells that surround the endothelium, i.e. the pericytes and smooth muscle cells, are thought to be active in vaso-regulation (Nikolov & Schiebler, 1973). Since nerves have never been observed in the placenta, vaso-regulation must be accomplished by humoral means, and/or by local mechanisms.

The connective tissue cells of the vessel adventitia shade into the components of the surrounding villous stroma, without any sharp demarcation line. We can differentiate between fixed stromal cells and Hofbauer cells. The former are responsible for the production of the extracellular matrix of the villous core. They show different morphological aspects related to the stromal architecture of the different villous types (see below).

The Hofbauer cells are fetal macrophages present throughout pregnancy in the human placenta (Figs 46.6c and 46.7). The surface morphology of these cells is characterized by lamellipodia, blebs, and microplicae. More-

over they have numerous, large intracytoplasmic vacuoles in the first half of pregnancy. As gestation progresses these vacuoles decrease in number and size, and intracytoplasmic granules, probably lysosomes, become more apparent (Enders & King, 1970; Castellucci et al, 1980; Castellucci & Kaufmann, 1990). The vacuoles and the large lamellipodia have been considered to be involved in the reduction of the quantity of fetal serum proteins in the stroma of the villus. This view is in agreement with the fact that the placenta lacks a lymphatic system to return proteins from the interstitial space to the blood vascular system (Enders & King, 1970; Castellucci et al, 1984).

Concerning the immunological aspects of these cells, it has been demonstrated that they possess Fc receptors for IgG (Moskalewski et al, 1975; Kameda et al, 1991; Sedmak et al, 1991), express CR3 (CD11) and are capable of immune and non-immune phagocytosis (Goldstein et al, 1988; Zaccheo et al, 1989). Hofbauer cells can express class I and II MHC determinants and, concerning the latter, first-trimester Hofbauer cells are rarely DR- and DP-positive; DQ antigens are not expressed (Bulmer & Johnson, 1984; Goldstein et al, 1988). Class II MHC antigens are acquired by increasing numbers of placental macrophages from the second trimester onwards

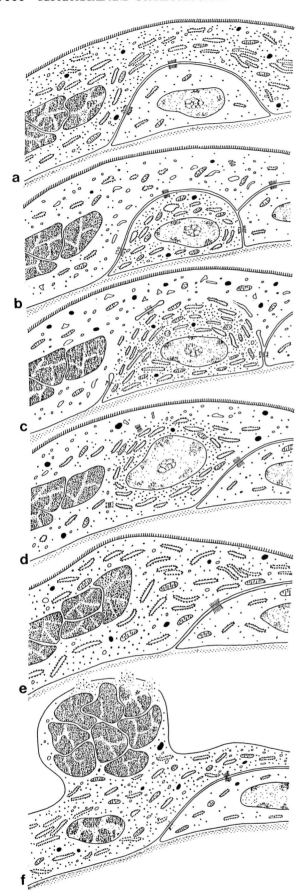

a

b

c

d

e

f

Fig. 46.4 Cytotrophoblastic contribution to growth and regeneration of syncytiotrophoblast. Below areas of syncytiotrophoblast which undergo loss of ribosomes (degranulation of the rough endoplasmic reticulum), Langhans cells start differentiation by developing a large number of organelles **a, b.** After disintegration of the separating cell membranes **c,** these organelles are transferred into the syncytiotrophoblast and thus regenerate the latter. As soon as these organelles age again, this process starts anew. In this way increasing numbers of trophoblastic nuclei are accumulated in the syncytiotrophoblast **e.** The oldest are clustered as syncytial knots, thereafter protruded as 'syncytial sprouts' and finally extruded into the intervillous space **f.** (Reproduced with permission from Kaufmann et al, 1983.)

(Castellucci et al, 1990a; Castellucci & Kaufmann, 1990). Several CD (cluster of differentiation) antigens are expressed by the Hofbauer cells as, for example, CD4 and CD14 (Goldstein et al, 1988; Zaccheo et al, 1989). Immunohistochemical application of antibodies against CD and similar antigens has indicated that more macrophages are present in the placental villi than is evident from histological and electronmicroscopical studies. Hofbauer cells produce IL1 (Flynn et al, 1982), which has diverse biological functions within and without the immune response (Platanias & Vogelzang, 1990; Dinarello, 1991). IL1 may regulate the remodelling of the core of the placental villi by influencing the behaviour of villous fibroblasts (Glover et al, 1987; Castellucci & Kaufmann, 1990; Thornton et al, 1990). Moreover, Hofbauer cells have been suggested to influence angiogenesis and vasculogenesis in the human placenta (Castellucci et al, 1980; King, 1987; Demir et al, 1989).

Several antibodies are available that may be used as easily applicable markers for the various villous components:

- trophoblast: anti-cytokeratin (Beham et al, 1988; Daya & Sabet, 1991)
- syncytiotrophoblast: anti-HPL (Beck et al, 1986; Gosseye & Fox, 1984); anti-βhCG (Kurman et al, 1984a,b); anti-transferrin receptor (Yeh et al, 1987; Bierings et al, 1988); the monoclonal NDOG1 (Sunderland et al, 1981)
- cytotrophoblast (Langhans cells): GB36 (at the end of pregnancy also expressed in syncytiotrophoblast) (Hsi et al, 1987a); anti-factor V (Hsi et al, 1987b)
- stromal cells: anti-vimentin (Khong et al, 1986; Beham et al, 1988)
- fibroblasts and smooth muscle cells, including myofibroblasts: anti-desmin (Beham et al, 1988; Nanaev et al, 1991a)
- macrophages (Hofbauer cells): anti-CD14/anti-leu-M3 (Zaccheo et al, 1989); alpha-1-antichymotrypsin (Braunhut et al, 1984);
- endothelium: anti-von Willebrand factor (Jaffe, 1987).

VILLOUS TREES

Structure of villous types

The ramifications of the villous trees can be subdivided into segments which differ mainly in their calibre, stromal structure, vessel structure, and position within the villous tree (Figs 46.5 and 46.6a). Five villous types have been described (Kaufmann et al, 1979; Sen et al, 1979; Castellucci & Kaufmann, 1982; Kaufmann, 1982; Castellucci et al, 1984, 1990b; Burton, 1987). Some can

be further subdivided. As will be discussed, all villous types derive from single precursors, the mesenchymal villi, which correspond to the so-called tertiary villi of the early stages of placentation.

The following villous types can be histologically identified:

1. Stem villi (Figs 46.5 and 46.6b) are characterized by a compact fibrous stroma, arteries and veins or arterioles, and by venules with a lightmicroscopically identifiable

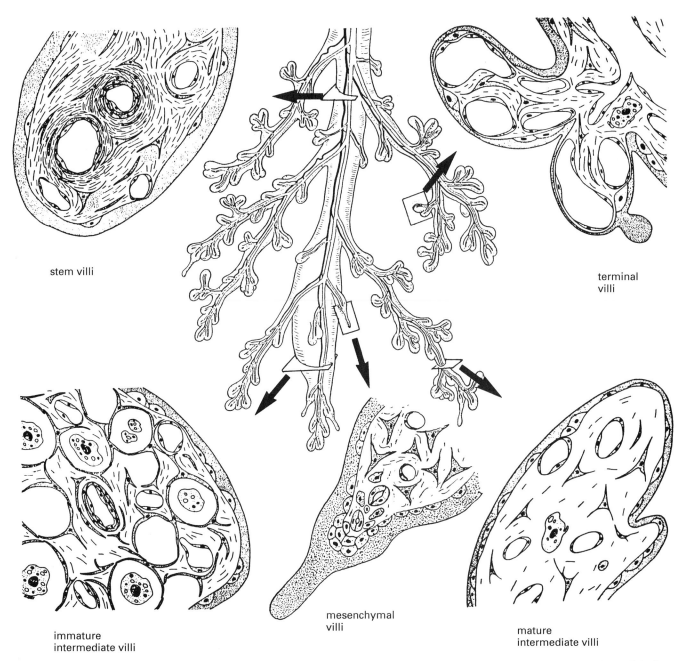

stem villi

terminal villi

immature intermediate villi

mesenchymal villi

mature intermediate villi

Fig. 46.5 Simplified representation of the peripheral branches of a mature placental villous tree, together with typical cross sections of the five villous types. For further details see text. (Modified with permission after Kaufmann & Scheffen, 1992.)

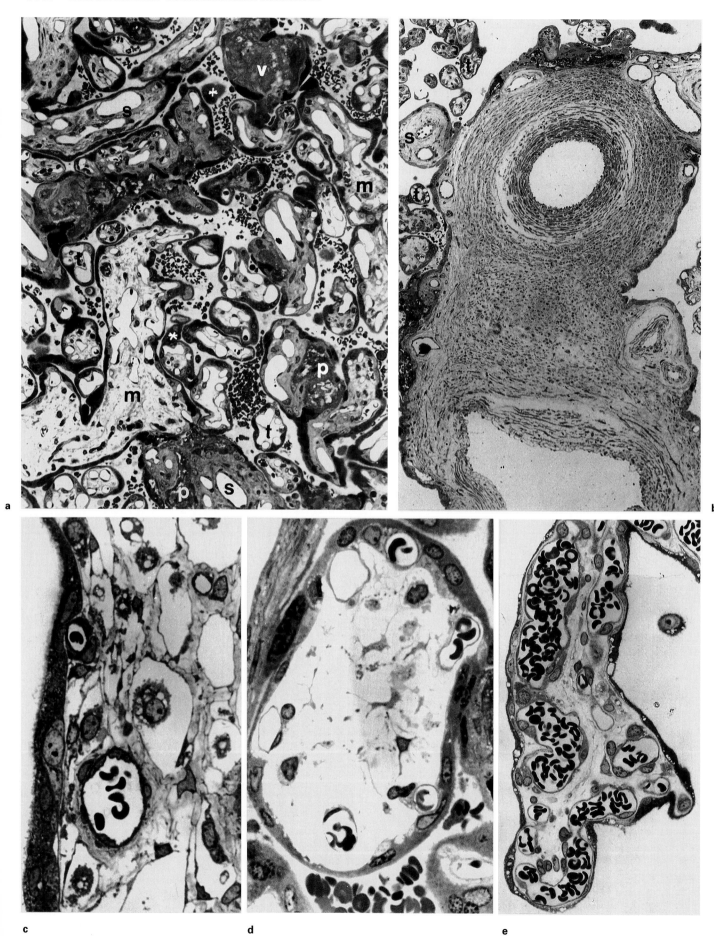

Fig. 46.6 Semithin plastic sections of human placental villi.
a This survey picture demonstrates the structural and staining variability of villous cross sections. s = stem villus; m = mature intermediate villus; t = terminal villus; * = tangential sections of villous trophoblastic surfaces; p = perivillous fibrin (fibrin-type fibrinoid); v = villous fibrinoid necrosis (mostly fibrin-type fibrinoid). × 165. (Reproduced with permission from Benirschke & Kaufmann, 1995.)
b Cross section of a large stem villus, surrounded by smaller stem villi (s) and terminal villi (t). Note that the adventitia of the artery (above) and of the vein (below) continue directly into the surrounding villous stroma. Superficially, numerous smaller cross sections of the paravascular capillary net of the stem villi are seen. × 115. (Reproduced with permission from Leiser et al, 1985.)
c Section of an immature intermediate villus from the 22nd week of pregnancy with its typical reticular stroma. The rounded, vacuolated macrophages (Hofbauer cells) are located in stromal channels which are devoid of collagen fibres and appear as empty holes (cf. Fig. 46.7). In faintly stained paraffin sections, such features can be misinterpreted as villous oedema. × 520. (Reproduced with permission from Kaufmann, 1981a.)
d Cross section of the typical poorly vascularized mature intermediate villus. Note the peripheral position of the narrow capillaries and the loose connective tissue. × 730. (Reproduced with permission from Benirschke & Kaufmann, 1995.)
e Longitudinal section of a richly vascularized terminal villus. The capillaries are locally dilated making the so-called sinusoids. The latter protrude the trophoblastic surface forming epithelial plates. × 430. (Reproduced with permission from Kaufmann et al, 1979.)

media and/or adventitia. Fetal capillaries are poorly developed and make up the so-called paravascular net (Arts, 1961; Leiser et al, 1985) which is underlying the trophoblast. The stem villi comprise the following structures:

a. the main stem (truncus chorii) (Fig. 46.11) of a villous tree which connects the latter with the chorionic plate (diameter 1000–3000 μm)

b. about four generations of short, thick branches (rami chorii) which are usually derived from the truncus already in the vicinity of the chorionic plate

c. up to 20 further generations of asymmetric dichotomous branchings (ramuli chorii) which are more slender branches (diameter ranging from 80–300 μm), extending into the periphery of the villous trees

d. a special group of stem villi is represented by the anchoring villi. These are ramuli chorii which connect to the basal plate by a cell column. The latter acts as the growth zone for this ramulus as well as for the basal plate.

The probable functional rôle of the stem villi is to support the mechanical stability of the villous tree and to provide the peripheral villi with fetal blood. About one-third of the total villous volume of the mature placenta is made up of this villous type.

2. Mature intermediate villi (Figs 46.5, 46.6d and 46.9b) are peripheral ramifications of villous stems, arranged in bundles of long, slender, multiply branching villi, their calibre at term ranging from 80 to about 120 μm. Most of their vessels are fetal capillaries, in between which are some small arterioles and venules. The vessels are embedded in a very loose connective tissue, with scanty fibres and cells, and occupy more than half of the villous volume. To their surfaces at least 95% of all terminal villi are connected (Fig. 46.9b and d). This demonstrates that these are the main sites of growth and differentiation of the terminal villi. As concluded from the increased degree of fetal vascularization, their share in maternofetal exchange cannot be ignored. Highly active enzyme patterns indicate their metabolic and endocrine activities. About 25% of the villous branches are of this type. The first typical mature intermediate villi are formed in the 25th week post menstruation.

3. Terminal villi (Figs 46.3a, 46.5, 46.6e and 46.9b) are the final, grape-like ramifications of the intermediate villi, characterized by their high degree of capillarization (> 50% of the stromal volume) and the presence of highly dilated sinusoids, showing mean capillary diameters of about 14 μm and maximum values of more than 40 μm (Kaufmann et al 1985). Moreover, they are characterized by the presence of epithelial plates (Amstutz, 1960) or vasculo-syncytial membranes. These are thinned anuclear syncytiotrophoblastic lamellae which are directly apposed to the sinusoidally dilated segments of the fetal capillaries (Fig. 46.3a).

One or a small group of terminal villi are connected to the intermediate villi by a narrow neck region (diameter about 40 μm), characterized by thin trophoblast surrounding a scant stromal core, most of which is occupied by two to four narrow capillaries. The extremely high degree of fetal vascularization in the terminal villi and neck region, and the minimal maternofetal diffusion distance of less than 4 μm, make this villous type the most appropriate for diffusional exchange. The terminal villous volume amounts to 30–40% of the villous tree. Terminal villi develop shortly after the first mature intermediate villi, roughly around the 27th week post menstruation (Table 46.2).

4. Immature intermediate villi (Figs 46.5, 46.6c and 46.7) are peripheral continuations of stem villi. They prevail in immature placentas and normally persist, in small groups, in the centres of the villous trees (placentones). They represent the immature forerunners of stem villi. By lightmicroscopy their typical structural feature is the presence of a voluminous reticularly structured connective tissue that is rich in Hofbauer cells and poor in fibres. As can be seen by electronmicroscopy, sail-like processes of the fixed stromal cells form a system of collagen-free intercommunicating channels parallel oriented to the major axis of the villi (Castellucci & Kaufmann, 1982). The Hofbauer cells lie mostly inside the channels. Functionally, the rôle of immature intermediate villi in the maternofetal exchange at maturity should be negligible. Their main functions probably are, firstly, to act as precursors of the stem villi, into which they are continuously transformed, and secondly to produce villous sprouts.

Immature intermediate villi may cause diagnostic problems, since their reticular stromal core has only a weak

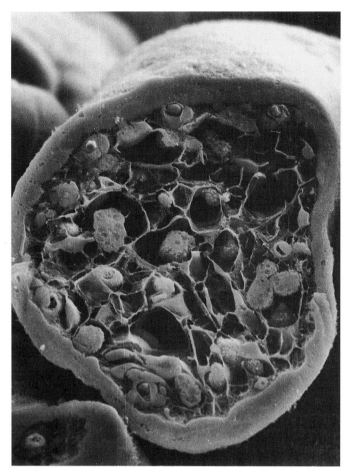

Fig. 46.7 Scanning electronmicrograph of a freeze-cracked immature intermediate villus demonstrating the three-dimensional view of reticular stroma with fixed connective tissue cells surrounding the stromal channels in which the macrophages can be found. × 550. (Reproduced with permission from Castellucci & Kaufmann, 1982.)

affinity for conventional stains due to the lack of collagen. The resulting histological picture is that of a seemingly oedematous villus which has accumulated much interstitial fluid (cf. Fig. 46.14c). We believe that many villi referred to as 'oedematous villi' in the literature are in fact normal, immature intermediate villi. They can be very numerous in several pathological conditions in which villous development and differentiation is impaired, as in, for example, most cases of maternofetal rhesus incompatibility (Pilz et al, 1980; Kaufmann et al, 1987).

5. Mesenchymal villi (Figs 46.5 and 46.14a and b). These are the first tertiary villi. They prevail in the early stages of pregnancy, where they are the forerunners of immature intermediate villi. In the mature placenta, the mesenchymal villi are inconspicuous. They are transient stages of villous development, derived from villous sprouts. They differentiate either via immature intermediate villi into stem villi (first to second trimester), or directly into mature intermediate villi (third trimester). Structurally, the mesenchymal villi can be identified by

their slender shape, by numerous Langhans cells, poorly developed fetal capillaries, and a connective tissue that consists mostly of large, poorly branched cells, surrounded by scanty bundles of connective tissue fibres. Immunohistochemically, they can be identified by the presence of tenascin which is diffusely present in the villous stroma whereas this morphogenetically important matrix molecule is only poorly expressed in other villous types (Castellucci et al, 1991a).

Development of the villous trees

The five villous types described above represent different stages of development and differentiation of the villous trees (Fig. 46.8) (Castellucci et al, 1990b). The process starts with trophoblastic sprouts which are produced by trophoblastic proliferation along the surfaces of mesenchymal and immature intermediate villi. Mesenchymal invasion into the trophoblastic sprouts leads to the formation of villous sprouts. As soon as capillaries are formed they are named mesenchymal villi. Until the 7th week post menstruation, mesenchymal villi may fibrose directly to primitive stem villi. However, from the 8th week post menstruation onwards, mesenchymal villi differentiate into immature intermediate villi, which produce ample new sprouts before they are transformed into stem villi (Fig. 46.8). From this date onwards, this is the only route for the formation of stem villi. As long as these processes are active, the placenta is rapidly growing though not differentiating.

This situation changes considerably during the third trimester, in which placental growth slows and villous differentiation starts. The mesenchymal villi no longer transform into immature intermediate villi but rather into mature intermediate ones which later produce terminal villi along their surfaces (Fig. 46.8). The remaining immature intermediate villi differentiate into stem villi. As a consequence, the number of immature intermediate villi steeply decreases towards term. Because of this fact, the base for the formation of new sprouts is also reduced, and the growth capacity of the villous trees gradually slows. Only in the centres of the villous trees (placentone centres) do some mesenchymal villi persist and continue to produce immature intermediate villi. It follows that at term these two villous types can only be found around the central cavity where they are responsible for the typical loose and apparently immature structure of the placentone centres (Fig. 46.2a) (cf. section on intervillous space and placentone architecture). There they serve as persistent growth zones of the villous trees (Schuhmann, 1981).

The above described events at the beginning of the last trimester are the most important steps for understanding villous development. At this time, the transformation of newly formed mesenchymal villi into immature intermediate villi switches to a transformation of the former into

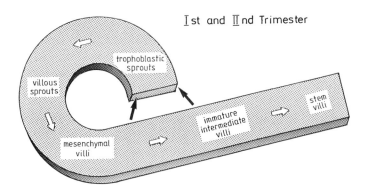

Ist and IInd Trimester

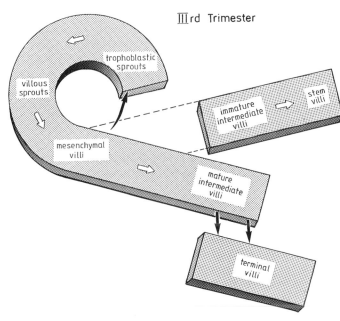

IIIrd Trimester

Fig. 46.8 Routes of villous development during early and late pregnancy. White arrows indicate the transformation of one villous type into another, whereas black arrows symbolize the formation of new villi along the surfaces of others. Throughout the first and second trimesters, trophoblastic sprouts are produced along the surfaces of mesenchymal and immature intermediate villi. They are transformed into mesenchymal villi and then differentiate into immature intermediate villi before they are transformed into stem villi. Throughout the third trimester, the mesenchymal villi become transformed into mature intermediate villi, which later produce terminal villi along their surfaces. The remaining immature intermediate villi continue to differentiate into stem villi. Thus their number steeply decreases towards term. Only in the centres of the villous trees may the villous developmental mode of the first and the second trimester persist until term. Because of this, the base for the formation of new sprouts is reduced and the growth capacity of the villous trees gradually slows. (Reproduced with permission from Castellucci et al, 1990b.)

mature intermediate villi (Fig. 46.8, Table 46.2). If this switch takes place early in gestation, the placenta differentiates prematurely but stops growing too soon, due to the deficit of immature intermediate and mesenchymal villi. By contrast, if the switch is delayed, the placenta is characterized by persisting immaturity and striking growth since immature, quickly growing villi prevail.

Angioarchitecture of the villous trees

Fetal arteries and veins are restricted to the stem villi (Fig. 46.6b), whereas arterioles and venules are mainly located in the smaller stem villi, as well as in mature and immature intermediate villi (Kaufmann et al, 1985; Leiser et al, 1985). All of the above larger fetal vessels are accompanied by a system of long, slender capillaries, the so-called paravascular net (Arts, 1961). In the mature, intermediate villi, the arterioles and venules turn into long coiled terminal capillary loops. In areas of maximum coiling, the capillaries stretch the surface of the mature intermediate villi, producing bulges, the terminal villi. This mechanism takes place in the course of the last trimester. As soon as the longitudinal growth of the capillaries exceeds that of the mature intermediate villi, the capillaries coil and cause the protrusion of the terminal villi. This process is accentuated under hypoxic conditions where capillary growth is stimulated (Bacon et al, 1984), resulting in a higher number of multiply branched terminal villi (cf. Fig. 46.9c and d) (Jackson et al, 1987; Kaufmann et al, 1987, 1988).

Particularly within the terminal villi, the capillaries may dilate considerably, thus forming sinusoids (Figs 46.3a and 46.6e). One capillary loop may supply several terminal villi 'in series', dilating and narrowing several times for each single terminal villus. The main function of the sinusoids is probably to reduce blood flow resistance and, thus, to guarantee an even blood supply to the long terminal capillary loops (mean 4000 μm) and the shorter paravascular capillaries (1000 μm) (Kaufmann et al, 1985). There is no convincing proof for the earlier view that the sinusoids are dilated, specialized venous parts of the capillary loops, which were thought to increase the maternofetal exchange rate by reducing the blood flow velocity.

Intervillous space and placentone architecture

The human placenta is of the haemochorial, villous type. After leaving the spiral arteries, the maternal blood circulates through the diffuse intervillous space and flows directly around the villi (Fig. 46.2a). Most anatomical investigations of the intervillous space have been made on delivered placentas which are no longer exposed to the in vivo effect of maternal blood pressure distending the intervillous space. Therefore, the usual appearance of the intervillous space of the delivered placenta is that of a system of extremely narrow clefts. Calculations based on intervillous blood volume and villous surface make it likely that the mean width ranges between 16 and 32 μm (Benirschke & Kaufmann, 1995).

Wigglesworth (1967) studied corrosion casts of fetal vessels and suggested that most villous trees are arranged as hollow-centred bud-like structures. When he injected the spiral arteries, he found that the injection mass collected in the loose centres of the villous trees. This is in agreement with Schuhmann's description of the 50–100 maternal arterial inlets as being located near the centres of the villous trees (Schuhmann & Wehler, 1971; Schuhmann, 1981). The 50–200 maternal venous outlets per placenta are thought to be arranged around the periphery of the villous trees. Thus, each fetomaternal circulatory unit is composed of one villous tree with a corresponding, centrifugally perfused, part of the intervillous space (Fig. 46.2a). This unit was called a 'placentone' by Schuhmann & Wehler (1971). Most placentologists agree that, under in vivo conditions, the majority of the 40–60 placentones are in contact with each other and that they overlap more or less broadly, since structural borderlines, such as placental septa, are absent (Becker & Jipp, 1963). It is our experience that the peripheral placentones are more clearly separated from each other and thus exhibit typical structural differences between their central and their peripheral zones. In the thicker, more central regions of the placenta, most villous trees overlap. This causes less distinct differences between maternal inflow and outflow areas of the placentone.

According to Schuhmann & Wehler (1971), the centres of typical placentones exhibit loosely arranged villi, mostly of the immature intermediate type, and provide a large intervillous space for the maternal arterial inflow. Schuhmann (1981) suggested that these central cavities are pressure-dependent in vivo structures which rapidly collapse after delivery. Sonographic findings support this view. According to Moll (1981) the central cavity guarantees fast and homogeneous distribution of blood into the surrounding mantle of smaller, more densely packed villi of mature intermediate and terminal type, without much loss of pressure (cf. Fig. 46.2a).

The perilobular zone of a placentone is that loosely arranged area of mature intermediate and terminal villi which separates neighbouring villous trees and which, subchorially, is connected to the subchorial lake. This is the venous outflow area.

The radioangiographic studies of Ramsey et al (1963) in the rhesus monkey, and of Borell et al (1958) in human placentas, are consistent with the placentone concept. Physiological studies concerning the intervillous circulation (Moll, 1981; Schmid-Schönbein, 1988) indicate that the actual filling velocities of the central cavities amount only to a few centimetres per second. After passage of the central cavity, a subsequent rather slow centrifugal spreading of the blood towards the subchorial and peripheral zone is observed. Wallenburg et al (1973) ligated single spiral arteries in rhesus monkeys and obtained obliteration of the intervillous space and degeneration of the corresponding villous tree. This experiment demonstrates that each villous tree depends on its own spiral artery. Even though the intervillous space is a widely open, freely communicating system, villous arrangement and pressure gradients are co-ordinated in such a way that blood

perfusion depends strictly on the original flow arrangement. Reversal of the direction seems to be impossible.

If one accepts these considerations, the zones of highest P_{O_2} in the intervillous space are in the placentone's centres where the immature intermediate villi, together with their sprouting mesenchymal side branches, are concentrated. 3H-thymidine incorporation is twice as high in the placentone centre as in the periphery (Geier et al, 1975). This is in seeming contrast to experimental and histological findings which suggested that low oxygen concentration serves as a stimulus for trophoblastic proliferation and villous sprouting (Alvarez, 1967; Alvarez et al, 1970; Fox, 1970). The most likely explanation for this discrepancy is that oxygen delivery to the centrally located, large villi in the central cavity and its vicinity is reduced, due to high blood flow velocity and long diffusion distances. The surrounding densely packed mantle of the placentone, although located nearer the venous pole, probably has the much higher oxygen delivery since blood flow velocity is reduced in the slender intervillous clefts and diffusion distances are short. This results in high mean P_{O_2} values at the villous surfaces and supports effective maternofetal oxygen transfer. At the same time, it inhibits villous proliferation and stimulates villous differentiation.

Whereas the centre of the placentone acts as a proliferative zone which guarantees placental growth until term, the periphery is the functionally fully active exchange and secretory area. This has also been demonstrated histochemically and biochemically by the higher activity of enzymes such as alkaline phosphatase (Schuhmann et al, 1976), and by the higher conversion rate of steroid hormones (Lehmann et al, 1973) in the placentones' periphery.

In most placentas, the immature placentone centres are present until term, at least in the more peripheral areas of the organ. Due to their size and distribution they are rarely present in routine histological sections. Only in cases of preterm maturation of the placenta (hypermaturity, maturitas praecox) do we regularly find mature placentone centres. Thus, such a placenta has lost its capacity to grow since only the immature intermediate villi and their immediate mesenchymal branches are able to sprout and act as growth zones.

For the histopathologist, the heterogeneity of the villous tree causes considerable problems. Since the average diameter of a placentone is two to four centimetres, histological sections will often not cover a representative part of the placentone and may not include both the immature growth zones and the highly differentiated mature tissue. Prevalence of one or the other tissue may influence the diagnosis. This danger is even greater when one considers that neighbouring villous trees may show varying degrees of maturation. This is of particular importance when performing morphometric evaluations of the placenta. Burton (1987) remarked: '... strict attention must be paid to the sampling regime if meaningful results are to be obtained. Sadly this has not always been taken into consideration in the past, and so many of the published claims must be qualified accordingly'. This problem is greater still when one uses small tissue samples — for example, those obtained from the placenta at caesarean section (Schweikhart & Kaufmann, 1977) or by chorion biopsy.

Three-dimensional interpretation of villous cross-sectional features

Placental histopathology is based on the lightmicroscopy of paraffin sections. Thus, the normal and pathological features of the placenta are usually described in terms of the two dimensions apparent in the lightmicroscope. The studies by Küstermann (1981), using reconstructions of serial paraffin sections, and by Burton (1986a, b; 1987), working with plastic serial sections, as well as those by Cantle et al (1987) and Kaufmann et al (1987), comparing lightmicroscopy of villous sections with scanning electronmicroscopy of comparable and identical material, revealed that the two-dimensional impression does not always reflect the real three-dimensional structure.

This is particularly true for the so-called syncytial knots (aggregations of syncytial nuclei with thickening of the syncytiotrophoblast), syncytial sprouts (mushroom-shaped syncytial protrusions with aggregated nuclei), and syncytial bridges (sprouts connected with a neighbouring villus), most of which prove to be only tangential sections of the villous surface. Their true interpretation is of importance for placental pathology since the histological appearance of syncytial sprouts, for example, is often accepted as a diagnostic indicator of placental ischaemia (Alvarez et al, 1964, 1969, 1970; Schuhmann & Geier, 1972). Küstermann's (1981) view that all syncytial sprouts, knots and bridges of the mature placenta have to be interpreted as sectional artifacts, has been largely corroborated by the studies of Burton (1986a) and Cantle et al (1987). The latter two investigations revealed that most of the above mentioned structures were flat sections but that also occasional true sprouts and bridges were present. At the same time, it became apparent (Kaufmann et al, 1987) that the diagnostic value of the so-called sprouts, even though mainly trophoblastic flat sections, was still useful. These are significant 'sectional artifacts' which point to a characteristic deformation of the terminal villi. It became evident from Cantle's material (1987) that branching, twisting, and coiling of villi (e.g. as a result of hypoxia) enhances the chance of tangential sectioning of trophoblastic surface (Fig. 46.9a–d). Since this deformation is usually caused by ischaemia the above conclusions drawn by Alvarez et al (1969, 1970) are generally correct. The diagnostic value of the two-dimensional finding of 'syncytial sprouts' still remains.

Küstermann (1981), Burton (1986a) and Cantle et al (1987) used various reconstruction methods to verify that most knots, sprouts, and bridges are only flat sections of bizarrely shaped villous surfaces, the incidence of this sectional artifact increasing with increasing thickness of the section. This is in agreement with the experience of all electronmicroscopists who have studied the placenta, that knots, sprouts, and bridges are common in paraffin sections (5–10 μm), but rare in semithin sections (0.5–1.0 μm), and mostly absent in the ultra-fine sections (0.05–0.1 μm) for electronmicroscopy. For placental histopathology this means that the thickness of paraffin sections greatly influences the incidence of trophoblastic flat sectioning resulting in 'knots', 'sprouts' and 'bridges'.

Although most knots, sprouts and bridges in the mature placenta must be considered sectional artifacts, there is a certain proportion of true syncytial protrusions. These trophoblastic specializations may serve as first steps of villous sprouting, i.e. formation of new villi (Fig. 46.5) (Boyd & Hamilton, 1970; Cantle et al, 1987; Castellucci et al, 1990b), as a mechanism of extrusion of old syncytial nuclei (Fig. 46.4f) (Martin & Spicer, 1973; Jones & Fox, 1977), or as simple mechanical aids to establish junctions between neighbouring villi (Cantle et al, 1987). Generally, in the young placenta, the majority of sprouts are true trophoblastic outgrowths. In paraffin sections of the mature placenta, the vast majority of these structures are artifacts due to thick sectioning and villous deformation (Fig. 46.9a–d).

The question of how to interpret 'knots', 'sprouts', and 'bridges' relates to the more relevant question of how to interpret villous shapes and branching patterns three-dimensionally. Burton (1986a) showed that three factors increase the chance of tangential sectioning of villi. These are branching, curving, and superficial notching. Long, slender, stretched villi (e.g. derived from a slightly immature placenta of about 32–36 weeks menstrual age) have an extremely low incidence of tangential sectioning. Thicker, bulbous villi, as in the early stages of pregnancy (Fig. 46.14a–d), gestational diabetes mellitus, persisting immaturity at term, and rhesus incompatibility, may show some more tangential sections due to the irregular surfaces of the bulbous immature intermediate villi. However, these cases also show an increased incidence of real trophoblastic sprouting as the first step of formation of new villi. The normal mature placenta, which has numerous short terminal villi branching from the surfaces of the mature intermediate villi (Fig. 46.9a,b), has a slightly higher incidence. The hypoxic, hypercapillarized placenta (e.g. pre-eclampsia) is characterized by multiply branched, fist-like terminal villi (Fig. 46.9d); it shows such a degree of flat sectioning that the two-dimensional picture may achieve a net-like appearance (Fig. 46.9c), in which most terminal villi are seemingly connected to each other by syncytial 'bridges'.

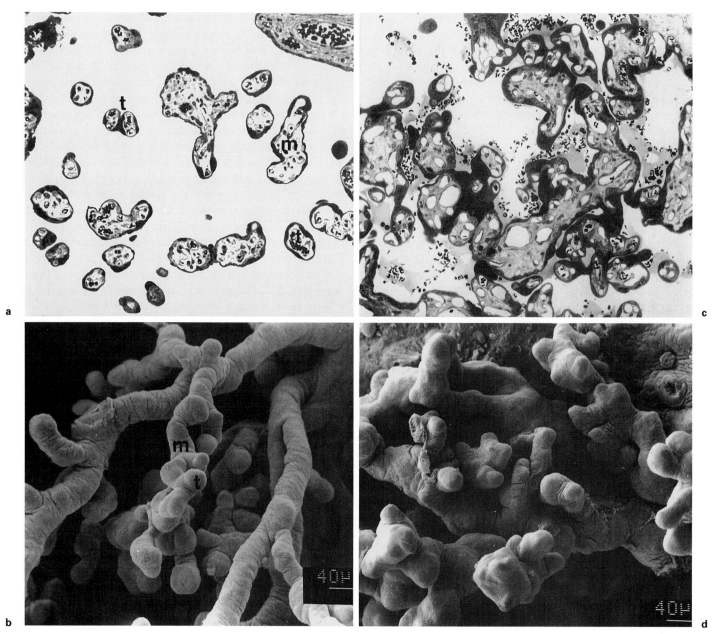

Fig. 46.9 Comparison of cross-sectional features with the three-dimensional shape of the villi. **a** and **b** Normal mature placenta. Sectioning of slender mature intermediate villi (m) covered with grape-like terminal villi (t) like those in the scanning electronmicrograph **b** results in numerous roundish to oval villous sections **a** and only a few trophoblastic flat sections, so-called sprouts and bridges. **c** and **d** Severe pre-eclampsia near term. Multiply indented, fist-like terminal villi branching off irregularly shaped mature intermediate villi like those in the scanning electronmicrograph **d** increase the chance of flat sectioning across trophoblastic surfaces. The resulting picture **c** is that of a seemingly net-like system with numerous trophoblastic 'sprouts' and 'bridges'. × 120. (Reproduced with permission from Kaufmann et al, 1987.)

NON-VILLOUS PARTS OF THE PLACENTA

Chorionic plate, umbilical cord, and membranes

The development of the chorionic plate, the umbilical cord and the membranes is closely related to that of the amnion. Throughout the last days of the 2nd week post conception, the blastocystic cavity is being filled by a loose meshwork of mesoderm cells, the so-called extra-embryonic mesoblast, which surrounds the embryoblast (Fig. 46.10, day 13). The embryoblast is composed of two vesicles, the amnionic vesicle and the primary yolk sac. Where both vesicles are in contact with each other, they form the double-layered embryonic disc. During the course of the following days, the extraembryonic meso-derm cells are rearranged in such a way that they only line the inner surface of the primary chorionic plate and the surfaces of the two embryonic vesicles (Fig. 46.10, day 18). Between both mesoderm layers the exocoelom cavity

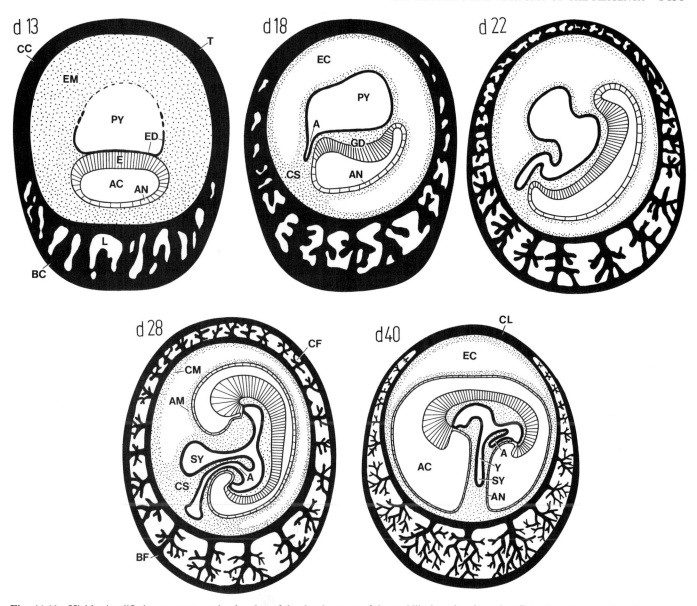

Fig. 46.10 Highly simplified, not true to scale, drawing of the development of the umbilical cord and amnion. Day 13 post conception: the embryonic disc consists of two epithelial layers — the ectoderm (E), which is contiguous with the amnionic epithelium (AN) and surrounds the amnionic cavity (AC), and the entoderm (ED), which partially surrounds the primary yolk sac cavity (PY). Both vesicles are surrounded by the extraembryonic mesoderm (EM) and by the trophoblast (black) which shows some lacunar spaces (L). BC = basal chorion; CC = capsular chorion; T = trophoblast. Day 18 post conception: at this stage at the presumptive caudal end of the germinal disk (GD), the allantoic invagination (A) has occurred. In the extraembryonic mesoderm, the exocoelom (EC) has cavitated. A mesenchymal bridge has developed that will ultimately form the umbilical cord, the 'connecting stalk' (CS). Day 22 and day 28 post conception: the embryo has begun to rotate and fold. The primary yolk sac is being subdivided into the intraembryonic intestinal tract and the secondary (extraembryonic) yolk sac (SY). Secondary yolk sac and allantois extrude from the future embryonic intestinal tract into the connecting stalk. The amnionic cavity partly filled with amnionic mesoderm (AM) and chorionic mesoderm (CM) largely surrounds the embryo because of its folding and rotation. Villous formation has occurred at the entire periphery of the chorionic vesicle, forming the so-called chorion frondosum (CF). BF = basal chorion frondosum. Day 40 post conception: the embryo has now fully rotated and folded. It is completely surrounded by the amnionic cavity. The umbilical cord has developed from the connecting stalk, as it has become covered by amnionic membrane. The exocoelom has become largely compressed by the expansion of the amnionic cavity. At the abembryonic pole of the chorionic vesicle, the recently formed placental villi gradually atrophy, thus forming the chorion laeve (CL). Only that portion which retains villous tissue, that which has the insertion of the umbilical cord, develops into the placental disc. Y = omphalo-mesenteric duct. (Modified with permission after Benirschke & Kaufmann, 1995.)

forms. It largely separates the embryo, together with its mesodermal cover, from the chorionic mesoderm. The exocoelom is only bridged by the mesoderm in one place, which lies basal to the amnionic vesicle. This mesenchy-

mal connection is referred to as the connecting stalk: this is the early forerunner of the umbilical cord and fixes the early embryo to the membranes.

During the same period (around day 18 post conception), a duct-like extension of the yolk sac, originating from the presumptive caudal region of the embryo, extends into the connecting stalk: this is the allantois, the primitive extraembryonic urinary bladder.

The three subsequent weeks are characterized by three developmental processes (Fig. 46.10):

a. The embryo rotates in such a way that the yolk sac vesicle, originally facing the region opposite the implantation site, is turned towards the implantation pole.

b. The amnionic vesicle enlarges considerably, extending around the embryo.

c. The originally flat embryonic disc is bent in the anterior-posterior direction, and rolled up in the lateral direction. It thus 'herniates' into the amnionic vesicle. The bending fetus subdivides the yolk sac into an intra-embryonic duct (the gut) and into an extraembryonic part (the omphalo-enteric or omphalo-mesenteric duct), which is peripherally dilated to form the extraembryonic yolk sac vesicle.

Both the allantois and the extraembryonic yolk sac extend into the mesenchyme of the connecting stalk (Fig. 46.10, day 28). Fluid accumulation within the amnionic cavity causes its expansion, so that it slowly compresses the exocoelom. Between days 28 and 40 post conception, the expanding amnionic cavity has surrounded the embryo to the extent that the connecting stalk, together with the allantois and the yolk sac, are compressed to a slender cord, which is surrounded by amnionic epithelium (Fig. 46.10, day 40): they thus form the umbilical cord. The cord lengthens as the embryo 'prolapses' backwards into the amnionic sac (Hertig, 1962).

By the 3rd week post conception, the extraembryonic yolk sac, the omphalo-mesenteric duct which connects with the embryonic gut, and the allantois become supplied with fetal vessels. All mammals use either allantoic or yolk sac vessels for the vascularization of the placenta. The human allantoic vessels — two allantoic arteries originating from the internal iliac arteries, and one allantoic vein which enters into the hepatic vein — invade the placenta and become connected to the villous vessels. The allantoic participation in placental vascularization gave rise to the name 'chorio-allantoic' placenta. The allantoic epithelium gradually disappears. Fusion of the allantoic vessels with the intravillous vessel system establishes a complete fetoplacental circulation in the course of the 5th week post conception.

During the same process of expansion that leads to the formation of the cord, the amnionic mesenchyme locally touches and finally fuses with the chorionic mesoderm, thus occluding the exocoelomic cavity. This process starts in the surroundings of the cord insertion at the chorionic plate and persists until the middle of pregnancy, when the amnionic cavity completely occupies the exocoelom, so that amnionic and chorionic mesenchyme fuse every-

where (Figs 46.10, day 40; 46.12a,b). Only cleft-like remnants of the exocoelom may be detectable in the later stages of pregnancy. As distinct from the cord, where the amnion firmly fuses with the underlying connective tissue,

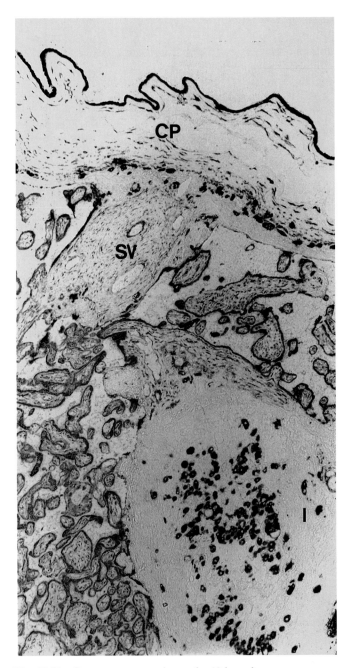

Fig. 46.11 Cryostat survey section at the 40th week post menstruation, showing the chorionic plate (CP) which is covered with the folded amnion, an off-branching stem villus (SV), numerous peripheral villous branches and a cell island (I). Because of the histochemical reaction for malate dehydrogenase, the amnionic epithelium and the large extravillous trophoblast cells within the chorionic plate and within the cell islands show intense staining, whereas villous trophoblast and connective tissue cells are weaker stained; the fibrinoid (matrix-type fibrinoid) of the cell island (I), embedding and surrounding the extravillous trophoblast cells, remains unstained. × 110. (Reproduced with permission from Schiebler & Kaufmann, 1981.)

fusion of the amnion with chorionic plate or membranes is never perfect, but rather amnion and chorion can always easily slide against each other. Histologically they seem to be separated by a system of slender, fluid-filled clefts, the intermediate, or spongy, layer of the chorionic plate and of the membranes (Figs 46.11 and 46.13a).

At day 14 post conception, the primary chorionic plate consists of three layers: extraembryonic mesenchyme, cyto-trophoblast, and syncytiotrophoblast (Fig. 46.1f). They separate the intervillous space from the blastocystic cavity. Trophoblastic proliferation with subsequent degeneration and fibrinoid transformation, together with fibrin deposition from the intervillous space (Langhans fibrinoid), cause continuous growth of the primary chorionic plate. Around the 4th and 5th week of pregnancy, allantoic blood vessels reach the primary chorionic plate via the connective stalk (Benirschke, 1965). Where stem villi branch off from the chorionic plate, branches of the allantoic vessels protrude into the stroma and fuse with the intravillous capillary system.

As soon as the amnionic sac has expanded to such a degree that the amnionic mesenchyme comes into close contact with the mesenchymal surface of the chorionic plate (8th–10th week post conception), the definitive cho-

rionic plate is formed (Fig. 46.10, day 40; Fig. 46.13a). For further details regarding the mature chorionic plate, see Weser & Kaufmann (1978) and Wiese (1975).

As already mentioned earlier, all villous developmental steps described above are valid only for the implantation pole, i.e. that part of the blastocystic circumference which was attached to the endometrium and which implanted first. The other parts of the blastocystic circumference, implanted a few days later, undergo a corresponding, although delayed development (Fig. 46.10, day 28). These areas are called the capsular chorion frondosum. Here, the first regressive changes can be observed, even during the process of villous vasculogenesis in the early part of the 4th week. The newly formed villi degenerate, and the surrounding intervillous space is obliterated. Finally, the chorionic plate, the obliterated intervillous space, villous remnants, and the basal plate fuse, forming a multilayered compact lamella, the smooth chorion or chorion laeve (Fig. 46.10, day 40). The first patches of the smooth chorion appear opposite to the implantation pole at the so-called anti-implantation pole. From there, they spread over about 70% of the surface of the chorionic sac until the 4th lunar month, when this process comes to a halt.

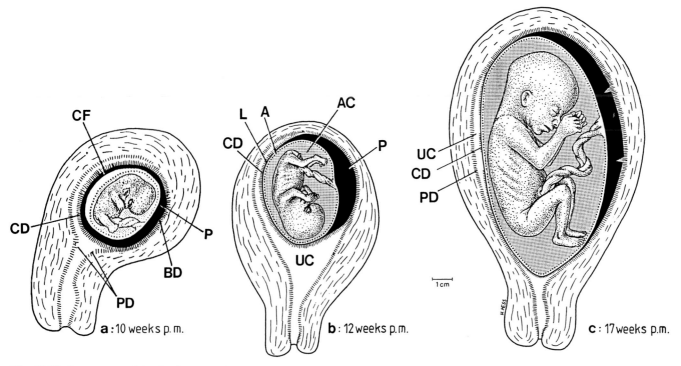

Fig. 46.12 Later stages of the development of the fetal membranes. **a** Up to 10 weeks post menstruation, the embryo is surrounded by the chorion frondosum (CF); its later specialization into chorion laeve and the placenta is indicated by a slight local increase in thickness (P) only. The chorion frondosum is covered by the capsular decidua (CD) which is continuous with basal decidua (BD) at the placental site, and with the parietal decidua (PD) which lines the uterine cavity. The amnion (dotted line) is not fused in most places with the chorion frondosum. **b** Two weeks later (12th week post menstruation), the original chorion frondosum has differentiated into the thick placenta (P) and the thinner fetal membranes that surround the amnionic cavity (AC). At this stage, the membranes are composed of inner amnion (A), intermediate chorion laeve (L), and outer capsular decidua (CD). Because of the embryo's small size, the uterine cavity (UC) is largely open. **c** From 17 weeks on, the membranes come into close contact with the uterine wall. The remainder of the capsular decidua (CD) fuse with the parietal decidua (PD) and largely close the uterine cavity (UC). From then on, the chorion laeve contacts the parietal decidua. (Modified with permission after Kaufmann, 1981a.)

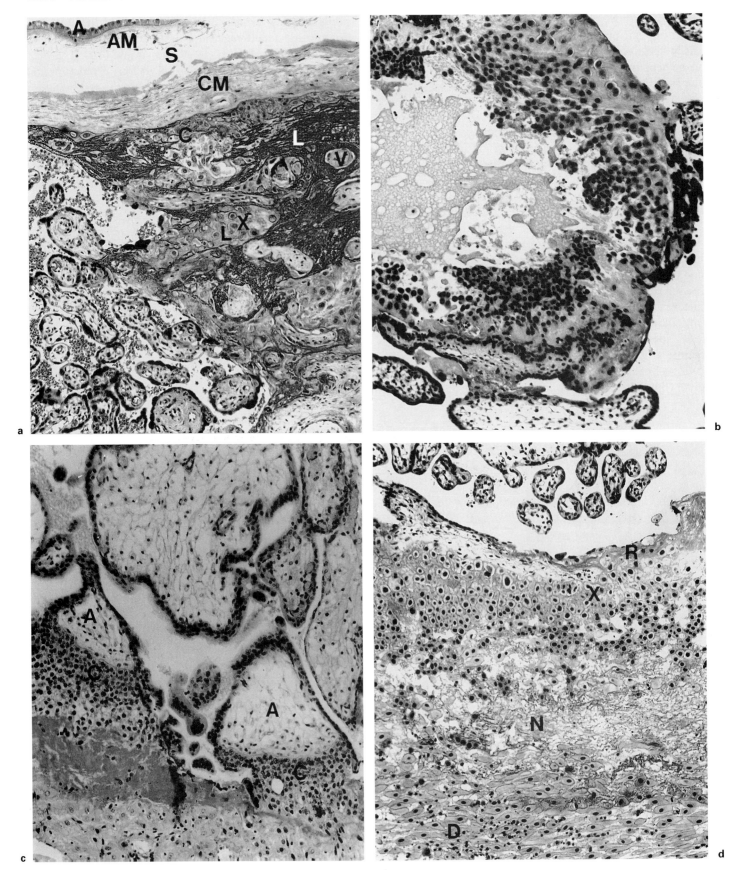

Fig. 46.13 Paraffin sections of non-villous parts of the placenta.
a The chorionic plate at the 40th week post menstruation; the typical layering of the mature chorionic plate with amnionic epithelium (A), amnionic mesenchyme (AM), spongy layer (S), chorionic mesenchyme (CM), chorionic cytotrophoblast (C), and Langhans fibrinoid (L) is evident. Clusters of trophoblast cells (X) and residues of buried villi (V) are typically incorporated in the Langhans fibrinoid. Note the histologically different appearance of the light, glossy fibrinoid (matrix-type fibrinoid) surrounding the trophoblast cells as compared to the darker, reticular fibrinoid (fibrin-type fibrinoid, derived from blood clot) in between. × 130. (Reproduced with permission from Benirschke & Kaufmann, 1995.)
b A cell island at the 19th week post menstruation. It is composed of matrix-type fibrinoid and clusters of extravillous trophoblast cells. In the centre a central cavity, a so-called cyst, can be observed. Such cavities have to be considered a result of degeneration with subsequent liquefaction. × 140. (Reproduced with permission from Kaufmann, 1981a.)
c Cell columns at the 15th week post menstruation. In early stages of pregnancy the anchoring villi (A) are connected to the basal plate (below) by broad or slender feet consisting of cytotrophoblast, the so-called cell columns (C). These are proliferative zones for the villous trophoblast as well as for the trophoblast of the basal plate. × 110. (Reproduced with permission from Benirschke & Kaufmann, 1995.)
d The basal plate at the 23rd week post menstruation. The typical layering of the basal plate is evident. Facing the intervillous space it is covered by an interrupted layer of Rohr's fibrinoid (R), followed by a nearly complete layer of cytotrophoblast (X). The latter is largely separated from the decidua cells (D) by a loose layer of Nitabuch's fibrinoid (N). The heterogeneous staining patterns of both fibrinoid layers point to their mixed composition of matrix-type and of fibrin-type fibrinoids. × 160. (Reproduced with permission from Benirschke & Kaufmann, 1995.)

With complete implantation, the decidua closes again over the blastocyst, bulging into the uterine lumen, and is called the capsular decidua (Fig. 46.12a). With increasing diameter of the chorionic sac, the capsular decidua locally comes into contact with the parietal decidua of the opposing uterine wall and between the 15th and 20th week post conception the two decidual layers fuse with each other, thus obstructing the uterine cavity (Fig. 46.12d). From this point onwards, the smooth chorion has contact over almost its entire surface with the decidual surface of the uterine wall, and may function as a paraplacental exchange organ. Due to the deficiency of a fetal vascularization of both the smooth chorion and the amnion, all paraplacental exchange between fetal membranes and fetus has to pass the amnionic fluid.

The structure of the fetal membranes at term was defined by Bourne (1962) and is described in Chapter 51. Apart from the amnion's involvement in the production and resorption of the amnionic fluid, there are findings which suggest that it is metabolically active; Mühlhauser et al (1992) found that the amnionic epithelium contains abundant carbonic anhydrase, an enzyme involved in removal of CO_2 and in pH regulation.

Basal plate and uteroplacental vessels

The trophoblastic shell is formed as the base of the lacunar system at day 8 post conception (Fig. 46.1c and

d). In the beginning, it is a purely syncytiotrophoblastic layer. From day 13 post conception onwards, cytotrophoblast reaches the shell, penetrates it (Fig. 46.1e), and intermingles with neighbouring cells of the endometrium; many of the latter have meanwhile transformed into decidual cells. As soon as invading trophoblast cells come into close contact with each other, they may fuse to form the syncytial giant cells of the junctional zone. Where they are separated from each other, they may undergo differentiation into so-called X cells (interstitial trophoblast or intermediate trophoblast) (Fig. 46.1f). The phagocytic activity of the trophoblast, as it invades more deeply, causes considerable tissue necrosis. Parts of the necrotic tissue are transformed into fibrinoid material. Where the latter is in close contact with the intervillous space, it is called Rohr's fibrinoid (Fig. 46.1f). The deeper layers of fibrinoid, which surround groups of trophoblastic and/or decidual cells, are called Nitabuch's fibrinoid. The entire maternofetal 'battlefield' stretches from the intervillous space down to the myometrium and is described as the junctional zone (Fig. 46.1f). The superficial part of this, which adheres to the placenta after placental separation, is the basal plate (Fig. 46.13d). It consists of the remainders of the original trophoblastic shell, together with the attached trophoblastic and endometrial cells, and much fibrinoid material (Hein, 1971; Kaufmann & Stark, 1971; Stark & Kaufmann, 1971). Those parts of the junctional zone that remain in the uterus after delivery are called the placental bed. This consists mainly of intact and necrotic endometrial tissue, with intermingled trophoblastic cells (Robertson & Warner, 1974).

Following erosion of the first endometrial capillaries at day 12 post conception, larger endometrial arteries (spiral arteries) and veins also become eroded and thus connected with the intervillous space. There is general agreement that the number of corresponding maternal vessels that supply the placenta, although originally high, is reduced considerably towards term by obliteration (Boyd & Hamilton, 1970). The final number of spiral arteries for the term placenta is about 100, that for venous openings 50–200.

As early as in the second month of pregnancy, the walls of the spiral arteries and veins show regressive changes. Endothelial necrosis is followed by focal and, later, general degeneration of the muscle cells of the media. In some places, all cellular elements may degenerate, thus transforming the vessels into flaccid tubes, constructed only of amorphous extracellular material (Brosens et al, 1967; de Wolf et al, 1973). This process is accompanied by dilatation of the lumina, in particular those near the intervillous space. Parallel to the above vessel changes, rounded trophoblast cells, so-called intra-arterial trophoblast, invade the arterial lumina from the intervillous space. In some places, these cells may completely obstruct the arterial lumina whilst in others they replace the degenerate endothelium to form a new vascular lining. Utero-placental veins undergo similar changes, though to a much lesser degree: they always remain free of intravascular trophoblast.

Even though they appear degenerative in nature, these pregnancy changes in the uteroplacental vessels are described as 'physiological processes' (Brosens, 1988), necessary for normal placentation. Complete absence of, or reduced, physiological vessel alterations are regularly combined with hypertensive pregnancy and complicated by fetal growth retardation (Brosens, 1988; Sheppard & Bonnar, 1988).

Placental septa

Placental septa are bizarre-shaped conglomerations of fibrinoid, intermingled with groups of trophoblastic and/or decidual cells, connected to the basal plate. They are not vascularized. They are columnar, or sail-like, structures rather than real septa (Becker & Jipp, 1963), dividing the intervillous space into separately maternally perfused chambers (Fig. 46.2a). They are interpreted as dislocations of basal plate tissue into the intervillous space, caused by lateral movement and folding of the uterine wall and basal plate over each other (Benirschke & Kaufmann, 1995).

Cell columns and cell islands

Cell columns are the trophoblastic connections of larger stem villi, the so-called anchoring villi, to the basal plate. These are segments of the villous tree that persist in the primary villus stage, since mesenchymal invasion during formation of secondary villi does not reach the most basal segments of the anchoring villi (Fig. 46.1f and 46.13c). Because of continuing cytotrophoblastic proliferation, the cell columns serve as segments of longitudinal growth of the anchoring villi. From their bases, cytotrophoblast may invade the basal plate (Fig. 46.13c), thus also contributing to the growth of the latter. Fibrinoid deposition at the surface of the cell columns slowly 'buries' them into the basal plate. As soon as they are completely incorporated into the latter, the cytotrophoblastic proliferation slows down. Following partial degeneration of the cells and complete disintegration of their structure, cell columns largely disappear in the course of the last trimester and can only rarely be observed in the term placenta.

Cell islands obviously are largely comparable structures. They, too, are formed from villous tips which have not been opened up by connective tissue and fetal vessels during the transition from primary, via secondary, to tertiary villi (Fig. 46.14a). The only difference is that these villous tips were not connected to the basal plate as anchoring villi. Also the cytotrophoblast of the cell islands proliferates and, afterwards, becomes largely embedded into fibrinoid which surrounds the clusters and strings of extravillous cytotrophoblast (Fig. 46.11). Sometimes central degeneration and liquefaction causes the development of fluid-filled cysts inside the cell islands.

Extravillous trophoblast

The vast majority of cellular and syncytial trophoblast from the implanted blastocyst is consumed in the development of the placental villi. The remaining trophoblast, which is not used for villus formation, the extravillous trophoblast, is the basic material for the development of all other parts of the placenta. These are the chorion laeve, the marginal zone, the chorionic plate, the basal plate including the cell columns, the septa and the cell islands.

The nomenclature of the extravillous trophoblast. Because some doubt originally existed regarding its derivation, the first name employed was 'X cells'. The trophoblastic nature of these cells was, however, finally proved by Y-specific fluorescence studies in placentas of male infants (Faller & Ferenci, 1973; Khudr et al, 1973). Since the cells are obviously heterogeneous in structure, many authors proposed new designations: extravillous trophoblast, extravillous cytotrophoblast, non-villous trophoblast, intermediate trophoblast, specialized trophoblast, interstitial trophoblast, intravascular trophoblast, intra-arterial trophoblast, trophoblastic giant cells, trophocytes, spongiotrophoblast-like cells, placental site giant cells, etc. Regrettably, each of these terms has a slightly different definition. We, therefore, use the term 'extravillous trophoblast' as the most general heading for all types of trophoblast occurring outside the villi. When syncytial elements can be excluded, the name 'extravillous cytotrophoblast' may be more appropriate.

One may speculate that all these forms of extravillous cytotrophoblast merely represent different stages of differentiation from a proliferating stem cell, via highly differentiated, metabolically active forms towards cellular degeneration (Kaufmann & Stark, 1971; Okudaira et al, 1971). There are, however, some immunohistochemical findings (Gosseye & Fox, 1984; Kurman et al, 1984a,b; Beck et al, 1986) which restrict this interpretation. They make it very likely that the extravillous cytotrophoblast is composed of several parallel lines of cell differentiation.

We propose the following nomenclature. The extravillous trophoblast is composed of:

a. extravillous syncytiotrophoblast (multinucleated giant cells — remainders of invading blastocystic syncytiotrophoblast, or newly fused syncytial elements)
b. extravillous cytotrophoblast (this term probably being largely identical with what has been called 'intermediate trophoblast' by Kurman et al, 1984a); this again is composed of two different entities:

i. the intra-arterial (intravascular) trophoblast, lining the spiral artery lumina and partly occluding these

ii. the interstitial trophoblast, comprising all those extravillous trophoblast cells that are not located inside vessel lumina, which show various degrees of differentiation from proliferation to degeneration, which are more or less in contact with fibrinoid; also this subgroup may not be homogeneous in nature.

In the pathological literature (cf. Benirschke & Kaufmann, 1995) a population of cells is referred to as 'placental site giant cells' or 'placental site cells', located at the maternofetal interface: these are, in fact, cells of the interstitial extravillous trophoblast. They have a basophilic cytoplasm and penetrate deeply into the decidua. Pathologists are often faced with the need to establish beyond doubt that an intrauterine pregnancy has been present and such cells allow them to distinguish clearly a placental site.

One of the crucial problems in histopathology is the discrimination between extravillous cytotrophoblast and decidua. Reliable markers for decidual cells, as opposed to trophoblastic cells, are anti-prolactin (Rosenberg et al, 1980) and anti-vimentin (Beham et al, 1988). Extravillous trophoblast can be identified by binding anti-cytokeratins (Beham et al, 1988; Daya & Sabet, 1991), anti-hPL (Kurman et al 1984a,b; Gosseye & Fox, 1984; Beck et al, 1986) and BC1 (Loke et al, 1992).

Fibrinoid

Fibrinoid material is present in both normal and pathological placentas at all stages of development. Fibrinoid deposition is a regular feature at all those locations where syncytiotrophoblast, as the usual lining of the intervillous space, has disappeared as a result of degenerative changes. Another important location is in the immediate maternofetal 'battlefield' of the junctional zone, the deeper part of the basal plate (Nitabuch's fibrinoid) (Fig. 46.13d).

Recent immunohistochemical studies (Frank et al, 1994; Lang et al, 1994) have shown that placental fibrinoid is heterogeneous in nature, two different types being distinguished. Fibrin-type fibrinoid shows intense reaction with anti-fibrin antibodies but does not contain extravillous trophoblast cells or extracellular matrix molecules. It is found particularly in perivillous fibrin and in the Rohr stria of the basal plate. Matrix-type fibrinoid is largely devoid of fibrin but contains numerous extracellular matrix molecules such as laminin, collagen IV and oncofetal fibronectin. These molecules embed clusters of extravillous trophoblast which are involved in the production of this material. Matrix-type fibrinoid is found within degenerating villi, cell islands, septa and the basal plate. Locally, both types may mix with each other.

Several functional rôles have been proposed for the two forms of placental fibrinoid, these including a contribution to the mechanical stability of the placenta, a substitute for the degenerating syncytiotrophoblast at the villous surface, shaping of the intervillous space, an immunological barrier and growth promotion for trophoblast.

CELL BIOLOGY OF THE PLACENTA

Some of the cell biological trends in modern placental research may become important in placental pathology in the near future.

Cell isolation and culture

Fundamental for the study of the human placenta has been the development of a technique to isolate the cytotrophoblast. This was established by Kliman et al (1986) and at present most laboratories use this technique, in some cases with certain modifications (Douglas & King, 1989; Bischof et al, 1991). Several methods have been used to isolate the Hofbauer cells using proteolytic enzymes (Flynn et al, 1982; Frauli & Ludwig, 1987), a combination of enzymatic digestion and density gradient centrifugation (Uren & Boyle, 1985), or using mechanical action and density gradient centrifugation without the use of enzymes (Zaccheo et al, 1989). Drake & Loke (1991) have recently established an easy technique to isolate endothelial cells from decidual vessels, whilst placental fibroblasts have been separated by Fant (1991). The ability to isolate and culture the various types of placental cells and to develop co-culture systems opens fascinating perspectives in obtaining better insights into cellular interactions during morphogenesis of the organ.

Growth factors, growth factor receptors and oncogenes

The human placenta undergoes dramatic structural reorganization and remodelling during its development, cellular differentiation and invasion of the endometrium. Growth factor genes and proto-oncogenes are generally linked to such processes. It has been established that the placenta produces a large number of polypeptide growth factors, possesses a complex array of their receptors and expresses several proto-oncogene protein products (for reviews see Adamson, 1987; Blay & Hollenberg, 1989; Ohlsson, 1989).

Epidermal growth factor receptor (EGF receptor) — a product of the proto-oncogene c-erbB-1 — is present in the syncytiotrophoblast as well as in the villous and extravillous cytotrophoblast (Bulmer et al, 1989; Ladines-Llave et al, 1991; Mühlhauser et al, 1993). EGF is detectable in amniotic fluid, umbilical vessels, and placental tissue (Scott et al, 1989). The question of placental production sites is still open. Morrish et al (1987) pointed out that this growth factor induces morphological differentiation together with increased production of hCG and hPL in vitro.

Structurally related to the protein product of c-erbB-1 is that of the proto-oncogene c-erbB-2 which encodes a receptor protein for an as yet unknown ligand, although some candidate ligands have recently been identified (Lupu et al, 1992; Peles et al, 1992). The latter proto-oncogene seems to play a rôle in human cancer. In some types of malignant tumours, c-erbB-2 protein product and EGF-R are both overexpressed, and this correlates with a reduction in patient relapse-free and overall survival (Slamon et al, 1987; Wright et al, 1989). These data suggest that the two receptors may contribute to the development and maintenance of the malignant phenotype. Interestingly, in the human placenta, which shares some aspects with invasive tumours, this co-expression is present in syncytiotrophoblast which, in contrast to invasive tumour cells, is non-proliferative; on the other hand, in the proliferating cells of the extravillous trophoblast, only EGF-R is expressed whereas c-erbB-2 characterizes the differentiating and hence non-proliferating cells (Mühlhauser et al, 1993).

Insulin-like growth factors IGF-1 and IGF-2 and their receptors are also expressed in the human placenta (Boehm et al, 1989; Ohlsson, 1989; Ohlsson et al, 1989). In particular, IGF-2 is expressed primarily in highly proliferative cytotrophoblastic structures, as for example in the cell islands and cell columns, while other cellular components such as villous cytotrophoblast or mesenchymal stromal cells harbour less active IGF-2 genes (Ohlsson et al, 1989). Because numerous IGF receptors are expressed in villous cytotrophoblast, it has been suggested that IGF mediates autocrine and/or short-range paracrine growth control of placental development (Ohlsson et al, 1989).

Platelet-derived growth factor (PDGF) and its receptors (PDGF-R) are expressed in the human placenta (Goustin et al, 1985; Marez et al, 1987; Taylor & Williams, 1988; Holmgren et al, 1991). PDGF is a potent mitogen for a variety of cells, particularly for mesenchymal ones, and there is evidence for its rôle in angiogenetic processes (Holmgren et al, 1991; Risau et al, 1992), as well as for stimulation of cell movement through chemotaxis (Westermark et al, 1990). PDGF consists of homo- and heterodimers of two subunits, PDGF-A and PDGF-B, the latter encoded by the cellular equivalent of the v-sis oncogene (Doolittle et al, 1983). It has been shown that PDGF is co-expressed with the myc proto-oncogene in proliferative cytotrophoblast, and it has been suggested that PDGF influences the 'pseudomalignant' phenotype of the early human placenta (Goustin et al, 1985). In addition, Holmgren et al (1991) have proposed an important rôle for PDGF-B and its receptors in placental angiogenic processes.

Another growth factor detected in the human placenta and related to, but different from, PDGF is the platelet-derived endothelial cell growth factor (PD-ECGF). By immunohistochemistry, it is mainly detected in the stromal cells of the chorionic villi and at the trophoblast level (Usuki et al, 1990). Ishikawa et al (1989) have established that PD-ECGF stimulates growth and chemotaxis of endothelial cells in vitro and angiogenesis in vivo.

Transforming growth factor β (TGFβ) and TGFβ messenger RNA have been isolated from human placenta (Frolik et al, 1983). This growth factor is a multifunctional peptide, involved in immunosuppressive activities and, depending on the cell type, in stimulation or inhibition of cell growth (Miller et al, 1990; Sporn & Roberts, 1990). Concerning the human placenta, it has been suggested that it may play an important rôle in the inhibition of trophoblastic invasion of the uterine wall during placental development (Dungy et al, 1991). It may regulate the local immune response and prevent rejection of the fetus (Kauma et al, 1990), Moreover, Morrish et al (1991) have shown that it acts as a major inhibitor of trophoblast differentiation and concomitant peptide secretion.

Proteases

The human placenta is an invasive tissue which shares some similarities with malignant tumours. It has been established that cell invasion and migration are processes related to the production of proteases and their inhibitors. In addition, the remodelling of the villous stroma during placental development could be also related to the secretion of matrix-degrading proteolytic enzymes by the various stroma cells. It has been shown that trophoblast expresses interstitial and type IV collagenolytic activities (Emonard et al, 1990; Moll & Lane, 1990; Librach et al, 1991) and the former has been also detected in villous fibroblasts (Moll & Lane, 1990). Inhibitors of such proteases as, for example, tissue inhibitor of metalloproteases (TIMP), are involved in the regulation of trophoblast invasion, the latter inhibitor being probably produced by trophoblast and decidual cells (Lala & Graham, 1990).

Plasminogen activators (uPA and tPA) and their inhibitors are present in amniotic fluid (Kjaeldgaard et al, 1989) and are produced by the trophoblast (Åstedt et al, 1986; Feinberg et al, 1989; Radtke et al, 1990; Librach et al, 1991; for reviews see Lala & Graham, 1990; Bischof & Martelli, 1992), Interestingly, plasminogen activator inhibitor type 1 (PAI-1) is mainly present in invading cytotrophoblast cells whereas PAI-2 is prominent in the villous syncytiotrophoblast (Feinberg et al, 1989). It is well known that the expression of proteases and their inhibitors is regulated by some growth factors as, for example, TGFβ (Lala & Graham, 1990). It seems therefore that trophoblast invasion is a very complex mechanism wherein proteases, their inhibitors, hormones, growth factors and different types of extracellular matrix interact (Lala & Graham, 1990; Bischof & Martelli, 1992).

Extracellular matrix

Recent research concerning extracellular matrix in the human placenta has strongly emphasized the rôle of its molecular constituents in morphogenetic and invasive processes. Tenascin (Castellucci et al, 1991a; Damsky et al, 1992) has been shown to be expressed in fetal stroma related both to proliferative trophoblast and to trophoblastic defects covered by fibrinoid.

Fibronectins are well known to be expressed in the villous stroma (Yamada et al, 1987; Virtanen et al, 1988; Earl et al, 1990). Moreover, they are also expressed in the cytotrophoblastic cell columns (Earl et al, 1990; Castellucci et al, 1991b; Damsky et al, 1992); in this area the oncofetal isoform — absent in the villous stroma — is specifically expressed, i.e. at the fetomaternal border of the basal plate (Feinberg et al, 1991). It has been speculated that this isoform could mediate implantation and placental-uterine attachment throughout gestation. Fibronectins are involved in attaching cells to extracellular matrix through integrins such as $\alpha5/\beta1$ (Damsky et al, 1992; for a review see Akiyama et al, 1990). In vitro studies have demonstrated that extracellular matrix-integrin interactions involve cytoskeletal structures transmitting extracellular signals that regulate various programmes of gene expression; these findings imply that cell shape may be a primary regulator of phenotypic expression (Ben-Ze'ev, 1986; Werb et al, 1986).

In the human placenta, unlike other organs, molecules such as, for example, laminin, collagen IV, and heparan sulphate — are not only detectable in the basement membrane but also weakly throughout the villous stroma (Yamada et al, 1987; Nanaev et al, 1991b; Rukosuev, 1992). The universal presence of these molecules in the extracellular matrix may facilitate remodelling of basement membranes and thus may increase the morphogenetic and functional flexibility of the various villous cell populations.

Furthermore, collagen types I, III, V and VI have been found by immunohistochemistry in the stroma of the chorionic villi (Amenta et al, 1986; Nanaev et al, 1991b; Rukosuev, 1992). Decorin, a small leucine-rich proteoglycan which seems to have a primary function in the organization of the extracellular matrix (Hardingham & Fosang, 1992), has also been detected in the villous stroma (Bianco et al, 1990). Interestingly, the core protein of decorin (whose synthesis is induced by TGFβ) binds and neutralizes TGFβ (Yamaguchi et al, 1990).

There is an increasing use of extracellular matrix molecules in in vitro studies of the trophoblast. It has been demonstrated that such molecules influence trophoblast differentiation (Kao et al, 1988; Nelson et al, 1990); they

can play a pivotal rôle in repair mechanisms (Nelson et al, 1990), may participate in modulating hormone and protein production (Castellucci et al, 1990c) and can influence the morphology and proteolytic activity of the trophoblast (Kliman & Feinberg, 1990; Bischof et al, 1991).

APPENDIX: BRIEF DESCRIPTION OF DEVELOPMENTAL STAGES

It is the intention of this synopsis to present only information on developmental stages that is directly applicable to the pathological and histological examination of human material. For this purpose, data from various sources has been pooled. Information concerning the embryo and fetus will only be given as far as it is of importance for the definition of the stage. Some of the quantitative data is summarized in Table 46.1. Qualitative data concerning villous development is outlined in Table 46.2. The data is based on the following publications (in parentheses): embryonic staging post conception (p.c.) (Carnegie staging — O'Rahilly, 1973); crown–rump length, embryonic and fetal weight, mean diameter of the chorionic sac, placental diameter and thickness, placental weight (Boyd & Hamilton, 1970; O'Rahilly, 1973; Kaufmann, 1981a); placental and uterine thickness in vivo (Johannigmann et al, 1972); length of umbilical cord (Winckel, 1893); structural and quantitative data concerning villous development (Benirschke & Kaufmann, 1995).

Day 1 post conception, Stage 1: one fertilized cell; diameter 0.1 mm.

Day 2 post conception, Stage 2a: from 2 to 4 cells; diameter 0.1–0.2 mm.

Day 3 post conception, Stage 2b: from 4 to ± 16 cells; diameter 0.1–0.2 mm.

Day 4 post conception, Stage 3: from 16 to ± 64 cells; diameter about 0.2 mm; free blastocyst.

Day 5 to early day 6 post conception, Stage 4: from about 128 to ± 256 cells; diameter 0.2–0.3 mm; blastocyst attached to the endometrium.

Late day 6 to early day 8 post conception, Stage 5a: implantation, prelacunar stage of the trophoblast; the flattened blastocyst measures about 0.3 × 0.3 × 0.15 mm. The blastocyst is partially implanted. The embryonic disc measures about 0.1 mm in diameter.

Late day 8 to day 9 post conception, Stage 5b, early lacunar or trabecular stage: diameter of chorionic sac 0.5 × 0.5 × 0.3 mm; embryonic disc about 0.1 mm. The syncytiotrophoblast at the implantation pole exhibits vacuoles as forerunners of the lacunar system.

Day 10 to day 12 post conception, Stage 5c, late lacunar or trabecular stage: diameter of chorionic sac 0.9 × 0.9 × 0.6 mm. Around day 11, implantation is complete; the defect in the endometrial epithelium becomes closed by a blood coagulum, and covered by epithelium on day 12. The syncytiotrophoblastic vacuoles fuse to

Table 46.1   Summary of mean data on placental development. All data refer to the end of the corresponding week or to the end of the corresponding month of pregnancy.

week post conception (p.c.)	week post menstruation (p.m.)	month post menstruation (p.m.)	crown–rump length (Kaufmann, 1981a)	embryonic/fetal weight (Kaufmann, 1981a)	placental weight (Kaufmann, 1981a)	placental weight per fetal weight (Kaufmann, 1981a)	mean length of umbilical cord (Winckel, 1893)	mean placental diameter (Boyd & Hamilton, 1970)	placental thickness postpartum (Boyd & Hamilton, 1970)	placental thickness, incl. uterine wall by ultrasound (Johannigmann et al, 1972)	villous volume per placenta (Knopp, 1960)	villous surface per placenta (Knopp, 1960)	mean trophoblastic thickness (Benirschke & Kaufmann, 1990)	volume of fetal vessel lumina per villous volume (Kaufmann, 1981a)	percentage of villous surface covered by Langhans cells (Kaufmann, 1972)	mean maternofetal diffusion distance (Kaufmann & Scheffen, 1992)
			mm	g	g	g/g	mm	mm	mm	mm	g (%)	cm	μm	%	%	μm
	1															
	2	1														
1	3															
2	4															
3	5		2.5													
4	6	2	5				5									
5	7		9										18.9	2.7		55.9
6	8		14	1.1	6	5.5					5 (83%)	830			85	
7	9		20	2									19.1	3.0		
8	10	3	26	5	14	2.8										
9	11		33	11									21.6	4.0		
10	12		40	17	26	1.5					18 (29%)	3020			80	
11	13		48	23			160	50								
12	14	4	56	30	42	1.4			10							
13	15		65	40			—	—								
14	16		75	60	65	1.1	180	75	12		28 (43%)	5440		6.0	80	40.2
15	17		88	90			220	75								
16	18	5	99	130	90	0.69							11.6	6.3		
17	19		112	180												
18	20		125	250	115	0.46	300	100	15	28	63 (55%)	14 800		6.6	60	22.4
19	21		137	320			330	100								
20	22	6	150	400	150	0.38										
21	23		163	480			—	—								
22	24		176	560	185	0.33	350	125	18	34	102 (55%)	28 100			55	21.6
23	25		188	650			370	125								
24	26	7	200	750	210	0.28										
25	27		213	870			—	—								
26	28		226	1000	250	0.25	400	150	20	33	135 (54%)	42 200	9.7	9.1	45	
27	29		236	1130			420	150								
28	30	8	250	1260	285	0.23										
29	31		263	1400			—	—								
30	32		276	1550	315	0.20	450	170	22	43	191 (61%)	72 200			35	20.6
31	33		289	1700			460	170								
32	34	9	302	1900	355	0.19										
33	35		315	2100			—	—								
34	36		328	2300	390	0.17	490	200	24	45	234 (50%)	101 000	5.2	21.3	25	11.7
35	37		341	2500		500	200									
36	38	10	354	2750	425	0.15										
37	39		367	3000			—	—								
38	40		380	3400	470	0.14	520	220	25	45	273 (58%)	125 000	4.1	28.4	23	4.8

form the lacunar system. First contact of lacunar system with eroded endometrial capillaries. At the implantation site, the endometrial thickness is 5 mm; first signs of decidualization.

Day 13 post conception, Stage 6, early primary villous stage (first free primary villi): the nearly round chorionic sac has a diameter of 1.2–1.5 mm; length of embryonic disc is 0.2 mm.

With expansion of the lacunar system, the syncytiotrophoblast becomes reduced to radially oriented trophoblastic trabeculae, the forerunners of the stem villi. After invasion of cytotrophoblast into the trabeculae, free trophoblastic outgrowths into the lacunae, so-called free primary villi, are formed. The trabeculae are now called 'villous stems'. By definition, from this date onwards, the lacunae are transformed into the intervillous space. Cytotrophoblast from the former trabeculae penetrates the trophoblastic shell and invades the endometrium.

Day 14 post conception, Stage 6, late primary villous stage: diameter of chorionic sac 1.6–2.1 mm; length of embryonic disc 0.2–0.4 mm. First appearance of primitive streak and of yolk sac. Placenta cf. day 13.

Day 15 to 16 post conception, Stage 7, early secondary villous stage: diameter of chorionic sac about 5 mm; length of embryonic disc < 0.9 mm. Appearance of notochordal process and primitive node (Hensen). Starting at the implantation pole and continuing to the anti-implantation pole, extraembryonic mesenchyme from the chorionic cavity invades the villi, transforming them into secondary villi. The bases of the villous stems, connecting the latter with the trophoblastic shell, remain free of mesenchyme and thus persist in the primary villous stage (forerunners of the cell columns).

Day 17 to 18 post conception, Stage 8, late secondary villous stage: diameter of chorionic sac < 8 mm; length of embryonic disc < 1.3 mm. On the embryonic disc, the notochordal and neurenteric canals, and the primitive pit can be discerned. For the structure of the placenta cf. days 15, 16.

Day 19 to 21 post conception, Stage 9, early tertiary villous stage: diameter of chorionic sac < 12 mm; length of embryonic disc = crown–rump length of the embryo 1.5–2.5 mm; 1–3 somites. Neural folds appear; first heart contractions.

In the villous mesenchyme fetal capillaries develop (tertiary villi). The villous diameters are largely homogeneous, presenting two differently sized groups of villi. The larger villi and their branches exhibit diameters of 120–250 μm. Histologically, the stroma of both is mesenchymal in nature. Along their surfaces, one finds numerous small (30–60 μm) sprouts.

Day 22 to 23 post conception, Stage 10: diameter of chorionic sac < 15 mm; crown–rump length 2–3.5 mm; 4–12 somites. Neural folds start to fuse, two visceral arches. Placenta cf. days 19 to 21.

Day 23 to 26 post conception, Stage 11: diameter of the chorionic sac < 18 mm; crown–rump length 2.5–4.5 mm; 13–20 somites. Closure of the rostral neuropore; optic vesicles identifiable.

The length of villi connecting chorionic plate with trophoblastic shell varies from 1 mm (anti-implantation pole) to 2 mm (implantation pole). The central two-thirds are supplied with mesenchyme and capillaries, the peripheral one-third remain in the primary villous stage (cell columns). Most villi contain loose mesenchyme, together with centrally positioned fetal capillaries (mesenchymal villi) (Fig. 46.14a). Peripherally, they continue into massive trophoblastic sprouts. The larger villi (> 200 μm) show moderate net-like fibrosis. The villous trophoblastic surface is composed of the outer syncytiotrophoblast and complete inner layer of cytotrophoblast. The chorionic plate, consisting of fetal mesenchyme, cytotrophoblast and syncytiotrophoblast, still lacks fibrinoid. The trophoblastic shell is transformed into the basal plate by intense mixing of decidual and trophoblastic cells. Tissue necrosis in the contact zone of both cell populations causes the appearance of the first loci of Nitabuch fibrinoid.

Day 26 to 29 post conception, Stage 12: diameter of chorionic sac < 21 mm; crown–rump length 3–5 mm; 21–29 somites. Closure of the caudal neuropore; three visceral arches; upper limb buds appear. Placenta cf. days 23 to 26.

Day 29 to 42 post conception, Stages 13 to 16: diameter of chorionic sac from 21–33 mm; crown–rump length 4–12 mm. Thirty and more somites; four limb buds and otic vesicle, first appearance of lens pit and optic cup, thereafter closure of lens vesicle; clear evidence of cerebral vesicles; hand plates; retinal pigment visible; foot plates.

Thickness of the chorion at the implantation pole about 6 mm at the anti-implantation pole about 3 mm. The uterine lumen is still open, parietal and capsular decidua are not yet in contact. The largest villi reach diameters < 400 μm. The overwhelming share of the villous stroma is still mesenchymal in nature (Fig. 46.14b). The villous cytotrophoblastic layer is incomplete. Near the end of this period, the majority of mesenchymal villi show increased numbers of macrophages, as well as appearance of the first stromal channels. These are the first signs of reticular transformation of their stroma towards immature intermediate villi. In the course of the 7th week post conception the newly formed medium-sized villi (150–250 μm) more or less completely show reticular stroma of immature intermediate villi. Peripheral portions of villous side branches, persisting in the primary villous stage, may increase in size by continuous cell proliferation with subsequent fibrinoid degeneration; they establish the first cell islands.

3rd month post menstruation 9th–12th week post menstruation, days 43–70 post conception; Stages 17 to 23: diameter of chorionic sac from 38–63 mm; crown–rump length

Table 46.2 Summary of the structural and developmental characteristics of the five villous types from the 4th to the 40th week post menstruation

Weeks post menstruation	Stem villi	Immature intermediate villi	Mesenchymal villi	Mature intermediate villi	Terminal villi
4			Only mesenchymal villi (120–250 μm) and trophoblastic sprouts (30–60 μm) are present. Large mesenchymal villi (>200 μm) may show diffuse and moderate stromal fibrosis.		
5					
6					
7			Within the mesenchymal villi, the first stromal channels appear.		
8			Numerous short mesenchymal villi (60–100 μm), partly continuous with slim trophoblastic sprouts, branching from the surfaces of immature intermediate villi.		
9		Numerous immature intermediate villi (100–200 μm) with reticular stroma; calibre of the largest vessels is 20–30 μm.			
10					
11		Increasing amount and size of immature intermediate villi (100–400 μm); calibre of stem vessels increased up to 100 μm; vessel walls with 2 to 3 concentric layers of cells.			
12					
13					
14					
15		Lightmicroscopically apparent bundles of collagen fibres arranged around vessel walls.			
16					
17	About 50% of all villi with calibres >150 μm show fusion of the fibrosed adventitial sheaths around the primitive arteries with those of the veins. This is the first step towards formation of the fibrosed stromal core of stem villi.		The amount of mesenchymal villi and of trophoblastic sprouts is slowly decreasing.		
18					
19					
20	First true stem villi appear. Smaller ones (150–300 μm) show centrally fibrosed core with arterial and venous adventitia being fused. Those >300 μm show a largely fibrosed core.	Immature intermediate villi are still the dominating villous type. Those with calibres from 100–150 μm show no stromal fibrosis. The larger ones show fibrosis of the walls of larger vessels.			
21					
22			The number of mesenchymal villi with poorly fibrosed and poorly vascularized stroma, rich in cells, considerably increases. They grow in length and in width (calibres 80–150 μm) and show a continuous transition into mature intermediate villi.		
23	Calibre >300 μm: completely fibrosed stroma; calibre <300 μm: superficial layer of reticular stroma below the trophoblast.	Number and size of immature intermediate villi is decreasing.			
24					
25					
26			Typical mesenchymal villi are rare and mostly located near to immature intermediate villi.	Mature intermediate villi with dense stroma, rich in stromal cells and poor in fibres, with calibres ranging from 100–150 μm are the dominating villous type.	Local spot-like groups of first typical terminal villi appear; they show calibres of about 60 μm, about half of their stromal volume being occupied by capillary lumina.
27					
28					
29	Calibre >200 μm: completely fibrosed stroma; calibre <200 μm: incomplete superficial rim of reticular stroma.				
30					
31		Still few evenly distributed immature intermediate villi can be found; the stroma is only partly reticular in nature.			
32					Increasing amount of evenly distributed terminal villi with sinusoidally dilated capillaries and few epithelial plates.
33					

Table 46.2 (*contd.*)

Weeks post menstruation	Stem villi	Immature intermediate villi	Mesenchymal villi	Mature intermediate villi	Terminal villi
34			Mesenchymal villi are histologically inconspicuous; the few identifiable ones are usually located around the central cavities.		Terminal villi are the dominating villous type; they amount to about 40% of total villous volume.
35	Usually, all stem villi are devoid of reticular stroma; however, below the trophoblast there still is a less densely fibrosed rim, rich in fibroblasts.	The few remaining immature intermediate villi are no longer evenly dispersed but rather concentrated as small groups in the centres of the villous trees lining the central cavities. The extremely loose reticular stroma shows only a few typical stromal channels.		The relative amount of mature intermediate villi is decreasing to about 25% of total villous volume. The calibre is reduced to 80–120 μm.	
36					
37					
38	All stem villi (except a few around the central cavity) are completely fibrosed. The trophoblast of the larger ones often is replaced by fibrinoid.				
39					
40					

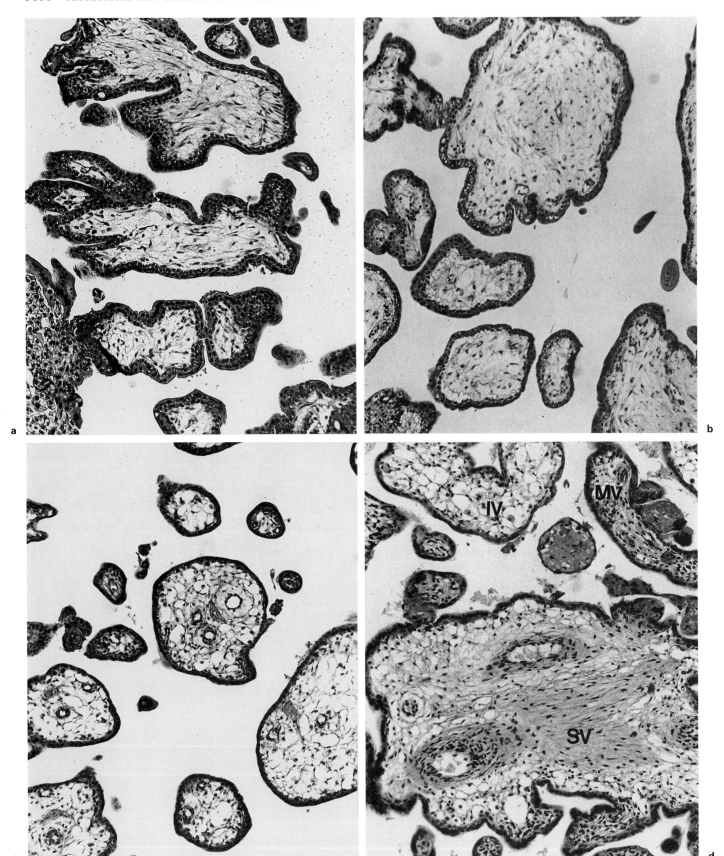

Fig. 46.14 **a** Paraffin section of placental villi of the 6th week post menstruation. Note the thick trophoblastic covering consisting of complete layers of cytotrophoblast and syncytiotrophoblast. Fetal capillaries are poorly developed or, in some places, still lacking. In the lower left corner, an early step in the formation of a cell island can be seen, attached to the villous surface. × 135.
b Paraffin section of placental villi of the 8th week post menstruation. All villi are vascularized. As one can see from the diffuse stromal structure, the villi still belong to the mesenchymal type. × 135.
c Paraffin section of placental villi of the 12th week post menstruation. The larger villi have achieved the reticular stroma of typical immature, intermediate villi. The smaller villi are mesenchymal in structure. The first small fetal arteries and veins can be seen. × 135.
d Paraffin section of placental villi of the 15th week post menstruation. The larger immature intermediate villi exhibit the first signs of central stromal fibrosis, originating from the larger fetal vessels, thus establishing the first stem villi (SV). Several typical immature intermediate villi (IV), as well as mesenchymal villi (MV) can be seen. As this is typical for mesenchymal villi of the second and third trimester, they are associated with degenerating villi being more or less transformed into fibrinoid. × 135.
(Reproduced with permission from Benirschke & Kaufmann, 1995.)

from 10–31 mm. Finger rays, toe rays, nipples and eyelids appear; upper limbs bent at the elbow region; first signs of finger separation. The embryonic weight increases throughout the 3rd month from 2 to 17 g.

The chorionic sac is covered by villi over its entire surface, and there is, as yet, no subdivision into smooth chorion and placenta. However, around the anti-implantation pole, increased degenerative changes in the villi and considerable fibrinoid deposition initiate formation of the chorion laeve. Parietal and capsular decidua may locally come into contact, but they remain still unfused. The early, moderately fibrosed mesenchymal villi (cf. days 23–26) near the chorionic plate meanwhile have achieved a diameter of up to 500 μm. The majority of villi measuring between 100 and 400 μm establish the typical reticular appearance of immature intermediate villi (Fig. 46.14 c,d). Small-sized villi with diameters below 100 μm show mesenchymal stroma. Trophoblastic and villous sprouts are numerous. In the 8th week post conception stem vessels are formed (luminal diameters 20–30 μm) with vessel walls consisting of two to three layers of cells. They do not show surrounding adventitial fibrosis. Until the 12th week post conception (Fig. 46.14c) some of these vessels show an increase in luminal width up to 100 μm; however, there is no change in their wall structure. Fibrinoid deposition at the intervillous surface of the chorionic plate is still an exception. The amnionic cavity has extended to such a degree that the amnionic mesoderm in many places comes into contact with the connective tissue layer of the chorionic plate.

4th month post menstruation, 13th–16th week post menstruation, 11th–14th week post conception: The maximum diameter of the chorionic sac increases throughout this period from 68 mm to 80–90 mm. The crown–rump length grows from 45 to 80 min.

The continuous degeneration of placental villi at the anti-implantation pole, which is free of villi from the middle of the 4th month onwards, as well as the villous proliferation at the implantation pole, initiate the differentiation of the chorionic sac into smooth chorion and placenta. The first real placental septa become visible. The cell columns become more deeply incorporated into the basal plate by fibrinoid deposition in their surroundings. The chorionic plate is in close contact with the amnion over its entire surface, giving it the definitive shape and layering.

Among the villi the immature intermediate ones with diameters of 100 to about 300 μm dominate (Fig. 46.14d). Their larger, centrally positioned fetal vessels show concentric adventitial fibrosis. Until the end of this month, this fibrosis increases to such an extent that in about half of the cases arterial and venous adventitia fuse, thus forming a fibrous central villous core (first real stem villi). The remaining parts of the stroma remain reticular in structure. In this stage, the first real stem villi can be easily distinguished from the much larger fibrosed original mesenchymal villi near the chorionic plate, which show only moderate fibrosis in a net-like pattern, extending all over the villous core. Mesenchymal villi (60–100 μm in diameter) and sprouts are numerous but, because of their size, they occupy only a minority of the total villous volume. Perivillous fibrinoid deposition becomes a usual finding on the villous surfaces.

5th month post menstruation, 17th–20th week post menstruation, 15th–18th week post conception: The crown–rump length increases from 80 to 130 mm. The placenta is clearly separated from the smooth chorion.

The structure of the stem villi is nearly the same as in the previous month; however, their number is considerably increased. In the 18th week post conception, the majority of the large-calibre villi, those exceeding 300 μm, are more or less completely fibrosed. Those ranging from 150–300 μm show central stromal fibrosis surrounding artery and vein, and a broad superficial layer of reticular stroma (Fig. 46.15a). Most villi have diameters between 100 and 150 μm and are still immature intermediate in character without, or with only sparse, adventitial fibrosis around the central vessels. Continuous development of fetal capillaries causes the reduction of mean maternal–fetal diffusion distance. Septa and cell islands, which originally consisted mainly of accumulations of cells, now grow considerably by apposition of fibrinoid. In their centres, cysts sometimes form.

6th month post menstruation, 21st–24th week post menstruation, 19th–22nd week post conception: The fetus grows from 130 to 180 mm crown–rump length.

The histological features change considerably: the ma-

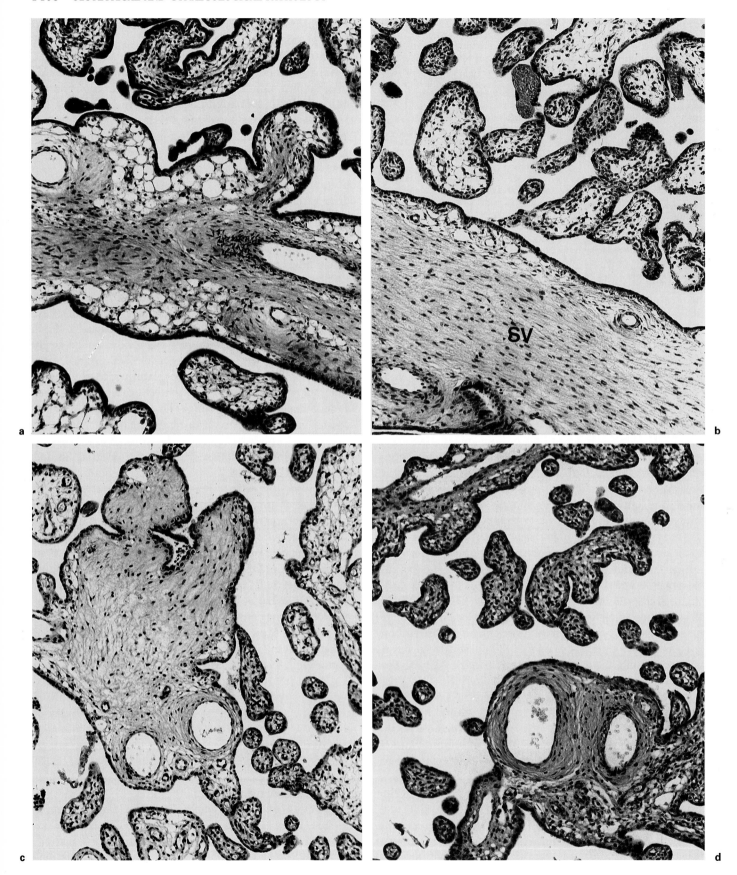

Fig. 46.15 **a** Paraffin section of placental villi of the 18th week post menstruation. The picture is comparable to that of the preceding stage. Formation of stem villi with stromal fibrosis is a little more expressed. × 135.
b Paraffin section of placental villi of the 21st week post menstruation. The stroma of the stem villi (SV) is largely fibrous. Only a thin superficial rim of reticular connective tissue hints at their derivation from immature intermediate villi. × 135.
c Paraffin section of placental villi of the 24th week post menstruation. As compared to the preceding stages, the variability in villous shapes and diameters is sharply increasing. The population of small slender villi, originally referred to as mesenchymal villi, has achieved structural characteristics of mature intermediate villi. × 135.
d Paraffin section of placental villi of the 29th week post menstruation. In this period, the mature intermediate villi and the stem villi are the prevailing villous types. × 135. (Reproduced with permission from Benirschke & Kaufmann, 1995.)

jority of immature intermediate villi become transformed into stem villi. Those exceeding 300 μm in calibre are more or less completely fibrosed, those ranging from 100–300 μm still have a discontinuous thin superficial layer of reticular stroma (Fig. 46.15b) The majority of stem villi measure around 200 μm in thickness, some achieve diameters of more than 1000 μm. Size and number of immature intermediate villi is slowly decreasing. Unlike all earlier stages, the originally stub-like mesenchymal villi expand in diameter (80–150 μm) and in length, achieving nearly filiform shapes. Their stroma is characterized by an increasing number of cells. These events mark their initial transformation into mature intermediate villi rather than immature intermediate villi. In this stage, in routine paraffin sections it is impossible to distinguish between mesenchymal and newly formed mature intermediate villi (Fig. 46.15c).

7th month post menstruation, 26th–28th week post menstruation, 23rd–26th week post conception: As compared to the 6th month, there are only quantitative changes. The crown–rump length increases from 180 to 230 mm.

The distribution of structure and calibre of the villi is similar to what was seen during the 6th month. The number of immature intermediate villi with reticular stroma decreases in favour of stem villi and mature intermediate villi. The latter represent the dominating villous type, being identifiable by their calibre (100–150 μm), their mostly elongated sectional shape and their highly numerical density of stromal cells. In locally restricted areas, obviously in the periphery of the villous trees, the first small groups of grape-like, highly capillarized terminal villi (calibre 60–80 μm) appear. Cell columns are surrounded by increasing amounts of fibrinoid and become deeply invaginated into the basal plate. The syncytiotrophoblastic covering of the chorionic plate becomes replaced by an initially thin layer of fibrinoid which, throughout the following weeks, grows in thickness and forms the Langhans stria.

8th month post menstruation, 29th–32nd week post menstruation, 27th–30th week post conception: crown–rump length 230 to 280 mm.

Steeply increasing numbers of mature intermediate villi and of terminal villi, which both exhibit calibres from 40–150 μm, are the reason for considerably increased numbers of villi per section (Fig. 46.15d). Besides a majority of villi of small calibre there are mainly stem villi of large calibre. Stem villi exceeding 20 μm in diameter are more or less completely fibrosed. Smaller ones still exhibit a discontinuous superficial reticular rim. The few still existing immature intermediate villi are rather evenly dispersed. As a result of beginning sinusoidal dilatation of the fetal capillaries in the newly formed terminal villi, the amount of vasculo-syncytial membranes (epithelial plates) is increased, and the mean trophoblastic thickness as well as the mean maternofetal diffusion distance are considerably reduced.

9th month post menstruation, 33rd–36th week post menstruation, 31–34th week post conception: crown–rump length 280 to 330 mm.

Histologically, the developmental processes described for the preceding month become even more prominent: the mean maternal–fetal diffusion distance and the mean trophoblastic thickness are further reduced. Cytotrophoblast is present only at 25% of the villous surfaces and difficult to identify in paraffin sections, due to the slender form and light staining of the cells. The largest stem villi reach 500–1500 μm in diameter. The originally reticular superficial zone of the stroma shows an increased number of fibroblasts for a few weeks, as compared to the more central highly fibrous parts of the stem villi (Fig. 46.16a). This difference usually is no longer observed at term. Larger parts of the syncytiotrophoblast of the stem villi are replaced by fibrinoid. The vast majority of villi are mature intermediate and terminal villi (Fig. 46.16b). The mature intermediate ones still have large diameters of 100–150 mm. A few evenly distributed immature intermediate villi, with calibres of 100–200 μm, can regularly be found in nearly all villous trees, indicating still active placental growth.

10th month post menstruation, 37th–40th week post menstruation, 35th–38th week post conception: the mean crown–rump length is raised from 330 mm to its final value of 380 mm. The mean placental weight increases from 400 to 470 g. There are considerable individual variations. Early clamping of the cord following delivery of the baby may even increase placental weight by as much as 100 g.

The permutation of villous types differs from the foregoing stage in several aspects. There are considerably increased numbers of terminal villi (about 40% of the total villous volume of the placenta) (Fig. 46.16c,d) and a higher degree of capillarization of the latter. This is mainly

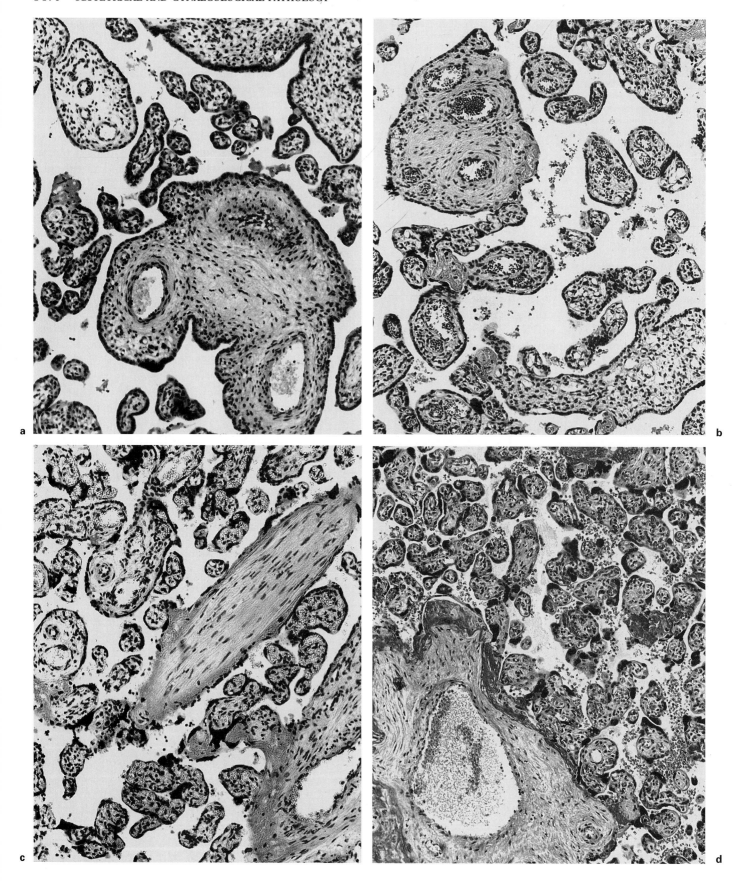

Fig. 46.16 a Paraffin section of placental villi of the 33rd week post menstruation. The number of immature intermediate villi is decreasing. The majority of villi are stem villi and mature intermediate villi; the latter are intermingled with the first few terminal villi which, because of their similar diameters, are difficult to differentiate from mature intermediate villi in paraffin sections. The stem villi are still not fully fibrosed but rather show a thin superficial stromal layer which has few fibres and is rich in connective tissue cells. × 135.
b Paraffin section of placental villi of the 35th week post menstruation. The distribution of villous types is largely comparable to that demonstrated for the preceding stage. × 135.
c Paraffin section of placental villi of the 38th week post menstruation. Dominating villous types are mature intermediate villi and terminal villi, both of small calibre. In between, several stem villi of varying calibre can be seen. As is typical for near term placentas, the trophoblastic cover of the stem villi is partly replaced by fibrinoid. The stromal core is completely fibrosed. Reticular stroma or cellular connective tissue (which, as a typical sign of immaturity, was visible below the trophoblast in earlier stages throughout the last few weeks) is absent. × 135.
d Paraffin section of placental villi of the 40th week post menstruation. The calibre distribution is not very different from that of the 38th week. Despite this, some remarkable changes exist: the fibrinoid deposits around the larger stem villi (mostly fibrin-type fibrinoid) are considerably increased; also, because of the irregular shapes of terminal villi at term, numerous flat sections of villous surfaces can be seen. In this figure, these appear as dark spots of seemingly accumulated nuclei. × 135. (Reproduced with permission from Benirschke & Kaufmann, 1995.)

due to the fact that many of the capillary cross sections are dilated sinusoidally to maximum values of 40 μm. In well-preserved, early-fixed placentas, which did not suffer from fetal vessel collapse, the terminal fetal villous capillary lumina amount to 40% or more of the villous volume. About 20% of the villi are stem villi. In the fully mature placenta, the fibrous stroma reaches the trophoblastic or fibrinoid surface of the stem villi everywhere; a superficial reticular rim, or a superficial accumulation of fibroblasts, as in the 9th month, should be absent at term (Fig. 46.16c,d). This has to be interpreted as a sign of persisting immaturity. The syncytiotrophoblastic mantle of the larger stem villi is degenerate in most places, and very often it is replaced by fibrinoid (Fig. 46.16d). About 30–40% of the villous volume is made up of intermediate villi which, histologically, can be differentiated from the terminal villi by their slender, elongated and usually winding and branching shape, by the reduced degree of fetal capillarization, by the absence of larger fetal vessels with lightmicroscopically identifiable media and adventitia, and by the high proportion of connective tissue cells. Their diameter has reached its definitive value of 80–120 μm. In normal mature placentas, the few persisting immature intermediate villi should be concentrated in the centre of the villous trees rather than being evenly distributed. The latter situation always indicates persisting immaturity of the placenta. If the central cavities of the placentones are not collapsed the immature intermediate villi delineate the remains of the latter. The cell bodies of the still existing villous cytotrophoblast are so thin at

times that they may be difficult to identify; thus many investigators tend to underestimate their quantity, or even deny their existence. The amount of perivillous fibrinoid is extremely variable. In normal placentas we have never observed complete absence.

Additional quantitative results concerning placental development and composition of the term placenta are given in Tables 46.1 and 46.2. When examining these tables and comparing the results from different authors, it is important to note that placental morphometry is heavily influenced by the mode of sampling and by the preparation of the material. Because of the high degree of maternal and fetal vascularization, the placenta reacts immediately to changes in intravascular pressure. Thus, the mode of birth, the time elapsing from cessation of maternal and fetal blood flows to tissue fixation and the nature of cord clamping directly influence the volumetric relations of villi and intervillous space. Normally, immersion fixation of the entire placenta or of small pieces should be sufficient. The more advanced methods, such as perfusion fixation (Burton et al, 1987) or puncture biopsy of the still maternally perfused placenta during caesarean section (Voigt et al, 1978; Sen et al, 1979), are very time-consuming. When studying immersion-fixed material, however, one should keep in mind that this material differs quantitatively and qualitatively from the in vivo conditions.

For further details we refer to the following publications: placental growth development in relation to birth weight (Bouw et al, 1978); relationship of placental weight to body size at 7 years of age, and to abnormalities in children (Naeye, 1987); fetal and placental weights in relation to maternal weight (Auinger & Bauer, 1974); ultrasonographic measurements of volumetric growth of the placenta (Bleker et al, 1977); weight development of placenta and membranes in early pregnancy (Abramovich, 1969); ratio of gestational sac volume to crown–rump length in early pregnancy (Goldstein et al, 1986); villous surface area and villous volume densities in various placental regions and along different levels of the chorial basal axis (Teasdale, 1978; Boyd et al, 1980; Cabezon et al, 1985; Bacon et al, 1986); local variations of villous surface, fetal vascularization, and amount of vasculo-syncytial membranes in the placentone (maternal-fetal circulatory unit) (Schuhmann et al, 1986); total villous surface in relation to fetal weight, in normal and various pathological cases (Clavero-Nunez & Botella-Llusia, 1963); morphometric data affecting placental oxygen diffusion (Mayhew et al, 1984, 1986); computer measurement of the mass of syncytiotrophoblast (Boyd et al, 1983); ultrastructural morphometric analysis of the villous syncytiotrophoblast (Sala et al, 1983); microvillous surface enlargement of the villous surface (Teasdale & Jean-Jacques, 1985); comparison of villous structure following immersion and perfusion fixation (Burton et al, 1987).

REFERENCES

Abramovich D R 1969 The weight of placenta and membranes in early pregnancy. Journal of Obstetrics and Gynaecology of the British Commonwealth 76: 523–526.

Adamson E D 1987 Review article: expression of proto-oncogenes in the placenta. Placenta 8: 449–466.

Akiyama S K, Nagata K, Yamada K M 1990 Cell surface receptors for extracellular matrix components. Biochimica Biophysica Acta 1031: 91–110.

Alvarez H 1967 Syncytial proliferation in normal and toxemic pregnancies. Obstetrics and Gynecology 29: 637–643.

Alvarez H, De Bejar R, Aladjem S 1964 La placenta human: aspectos morfologicos y fisio-patologicos. 4th Uruguayan Congress for Obstetrics and Gynecology I: 190–261.

Alvarez H, Morel R L, Benedetti W L, Scavarelli M 1969 Trophoblast hyperplasia and maternal arterial pressure at term. American Journal of Obstetrics and Gynecology 105: 1015–1021.

Alvarez H, Benedetti W L, Morel R L, Scavarelli M 1970 Trophoblast development gradient and its relationship to placental hemodynamics. American Journal of Obstetrics and Gynecology 106: 416–420.

Amenta P S, Gay S, Vaheri A, Martinez-Hernandez A 1986 The extracellular matrix is an integrated unit: Ultrastructural localization of collagen types I, III, IV, V, VI, fibronectin, and laminin in human term placenta. Collagen Related Research 6: 125–152.

Amstutz E 1960 Beobachtungen über die Reifung der Chorionzotten in der menschlichen Placenta mit besonderer Berücksichtigung der Epithelplatten. Acta Anatomica 42: 122–130.

Arts N F T 1961 Investigations on the vascular system of the placenta. Part I. General introduction and the fetal vascular system. American Journal of Obstetrics and Gynecology 82: 147–158.

Åstedt B, Hägerstrand I, Lecander I 1986 Cellular localisation in placenta of placental type plasminogen activator inhibitor. Thrombosis and Haemostasis 56: 63–65.

Auinger W, Bauer P 1974 Zum Zusammenhang zwischen Kindsgewicht, Placentagewicht, Muttergewicht und Muttergröße. Archiv für Gynäkologie 217: 69–83.

Bacon B J, Gilbert R D, Kaufmann P et al 1984 Placental anatomy and diffusing capacity in guinea pigs following long-term maternal hypoxia. Placenta 5: 475–488.

Bacon B J, Gilbert R D, Longo L D 1986 Regional anatomy of the term human placenta. Placenta 7: 233–241.

Beck T, Schweikhart G, Stolz E 1986 Immunohistochemical location of HPL, SP1 and β-HCG in normal placentas of varying gestational age. Archives of Gynecology 239: 63–74.

Becker V, Jipp P 1963 Über die Trophoblastschale der menschlichen Plazenta. Geburtshilfe und Frauenheilkunde 23: 466–474.

Beham A, Denk H, Desoye G 1988 The distribution of intermediate filament proteins, actin and desmoplakins in human placental tissue as revealed by polyclonal and monoclonal antibodies. Placenta 9: 479–492.

Benirschke K 1965 In: Wynn R M (ed) Fetal homeostasis. Academic Press, New York, p 328.

Benirschke K, Kaufmann P 1995 Pathology of the human placenta, 3rd edn. Springer, New York.

Ben-Ze'ev A 1986 The relationship between cytoplasmic organization, gene expression and morphogenesis. Trends in Biochemical Sciences 11: 478–481.

Bianco P, Fisher L W, Young M F, Termine J D, Robey P G 1990 Expression and localization of the two small proteoglycans biglycan and decorin in developing human skeletal and non-skeletal tissues. Journal of Histochemistry and Cytochemistry 38: 1549–1563.

Bierings M B, Adriaansen H J, Van Dijk J P 1988 The appearance of transferrin receptors on cultured human cytotrophoblast and in vitro-formed syncytiotrophoblast. Placenta 9: 387–396.

Bischof P, Martelli M 1992 Proteolysis in the penetration phase of the implantation process. Placenta 13: 17–24.

Bischof P, Friedli E, Martelli M, Campana A 1991 Expression of extracellular matrix degrading metalloproteinases by cultured human cytotrophoblast cells. Effects of cell adhesion and immunopurification. American Journal of Obstetrics and Gynecology 165: 1791–1801.

Blay J, Hollenberg M D 1989 The nature and function of polypeptide growth factor receptors in the human placenta. Journal of Developmental Physiology 12: 237–248.

Bleker O P, Kloosterman G J, Breur W, Mieras D J 1977 The volumetric growth of the human placenta: a longitudinal ultrasonic study. American Journal of Obstetrics and Gynecology 127: 657–661.

Boehm K D, Kelley M F, Ilan J 1989 Expression of insulin-like growth factors by the human placenta. In: Leroith D, Raizada M K (eds) Molecular and cellular biology of insulin-like growth factors and their receptors. Plenum, New York, pp 179–193.

Borell U, Fernström I, Westman A 1958 Eine arteriographische Studie des Plazentarkreislaufs. Geburtshilfe und Frauenheilkunde 18: 1–9.

Bourne G L 1962 The human amnion and chorion. Lloyd-Luke, London.

Bouw G M, Stolte L A M, Baak J P A, Oort J 1978 Quantitative morphology of the placenta. 3. The growth of the placenta and its relationship to birth weight. European Journal of Obstetrics, Gynecology and Reproductive Biology 8: 73–76.

Boyd J D, Hamilton W J 1970 The human placenta. Heffer & Sons, Cambridge.

Boyd P A, Brown R A, Stewart W J 1980 Quantitative structural differences within the normal term human placenta: a pilot study. Placenta 1: 337–344.

Boyd P A, Brown R A, Coghill G R, Slidders W, Stewart W J 1983 Measurement of the mass of syncytiotrophoblast in a range of human placentae using an image analysing computer. Placenta 4: 255–262.

Braunhut S J, Blanc W A, Ramanarayanan M, Marboe C, Mesa-Tejada R 1984 Immunocytochemical localization of lysozyme and alpha-1-antichymotrypsin in the term human placenta: an attempt to characterize the Hofbauer cell. Journal of Histochemistry and Cytochemistry 32: 1204–1210.

Brosens I 1988 The utero-placental vessels at term — the distribution and extent of physiological changes. In: Placental vascularization and blood flow. Trophoblast Research 3: 61–68.

Brosens I, Robertson W B, Dixon H G 1967 The physiological response of the vessels of the placental bed to normal pregnancy. Journal of Pathology and Bacteriology 93: 569–579.

Bulmer J N, Johnson P M 1984 Macrophage populations in the human placenta and amniochorion. Clinical and Experimental Immunology 57: 393–403.

Bulmer J N, Thrower S, Wells M 1989 Expression of epidermal growth factor receptor and transferrin receptor by human trophoblast populations. American Journal of Reproductive Immunology 21: 87–93.

Burton G J 1987 The fine structure of the human placental villus as revealed by scanning electron microscopy. Scanning Microscopy 1: 1811–1828.

Burton G J 1986b Scanning electron microscopy of intervillous connections in the mature human placenta. Journal of Anatomy 147: 245–254.

Burton G J 1986a Intervillous connections in the mature human placenta: instances of syncytial fusion or section artifacts? Journal of Anatomy 145: 13–23.

Burton G J, Ingram S C, Palmer M E 1987 The influence of mode of fixation on morphometrical data derived from terminal villi in the human placenta at term: a comparison of immersion and perfusion fixation. Placenta 8: 37–51.

Cabezon C, De La Fuente F, Jurado M, Lopez G 1985 Histometry of the placental structures involved in the respiratory interchange. Acta Obstetrica et Gynecologica Scandinavica 64: 411–416.

Cantle S J, Kaufmann P, Luckhardt M, Schweikhart G 1987 Interpretation of syncytial sprouts and bridges in the human placenta. Placenta 8: 221–234.

Castellucci M, Kaufmann P 1982 A three-dimensional study of the normal human placental villous core: II. Stromal architecture. Placenta 3: 269–285.

Castellucci M, Kaufmann P 1990 Hofbauer cells. In: Benirschke K, Kaufmann P (eds) Pathology of the human placenta, 2nd edn. Springer, New York, pp 71–80.

Castellucci M, Zaccheo D, Pescetto G 1980 A three-dimensional study of the normal human placental villous core. I. The Hofbauer cells. Cell and Tissue Research 210: 235–247.

Castellucci M, Schweikhart G, Kaufmann P, Zaccheo D 1984 The stromal architecture of immature intermediate villus of the human placenta: functional and clinical implications. Gynecological and Obstetrical Investigation 18: 95–99.

Castellucci M, Mühlhauser J, Zaccheo D 1990a The Hofbauer cell: the macrophage of the human placenta. In: Andreani D, Bompiani G, Di Mario U, Faulk W P, Galluzzo A (eds) Immunobiology of normal and diabetic pregnancy. John Wiley & Sons, Chichester, pp 135–144.

Castellucci M, Scheper M, Scheffen I, Celona A, Kaufmann P 1990b The development of the human placental villous tree. Anatomy and Embryology 181: 117–128.

Castellucci M, Kaufmann P, Bischof P 1990c Extracellular matrix influences hormone and protein production by human chorionic villi. Cell and Tissue Research 262: 135–142.

Castellucci M, Classen-Linke I, Mühlhauser J, Kaufmann P, Zardi L, Chiquet-Ehrismann R 1991a The human placenta: a model for tenascin expression. Histochemistry 95: 449–458.

Castellucci M, Crescimanno C O, Arezio P, Mühlhauser J, Cinti S, Kaufmann P 1991b Extracellular matrix molecules in the morphogenesis of the human placenta. Placenta 12: 376.

Clavero-Nunez J A, Botella-Llusia J 1963 Ergebnisse von Messungen der Gesamtoberfläche normaler und krankhafter Placenten. Archiv für Gynäkologie 198: 56–60.

Damsky C H, Fitzgerald M L, Fisher S J 1992 Distribution patterns of extracellular matrix components and adhesion receptors are intricately modulated during first trimester cytotrophoblast differentiation along the invasive pathway, in vivo. Journal of Clinical Investigation 89: 210–222.

Daya D, Sabet L 1991 The use of cytokeratin as a sensitive and reliable marker for trophoblastic tissue. American Journal of Clinical Pathology 95: 137–141.

Demir R, Kaufmann P, Castellucci M, Erbengi T, Kotowski A 1989 Fetal vasculogenesis and angiogenesis in human placental villi. Acta Anatomica 136: 190–203.

Denker H-W, Aplin J D (eds) 1990 Trophoblast invasion and endometrial receptivity: novel aspects of the cell biology of embryo implantation. Trophoblast Research IV.

de Wolf F, de Wolf-Peeters C, Brosens I 1973 Ultrastructure of the spiral arteries in the human placental bed at the end of normal pregnancy. American Journal of Obstetrics and Gynecology 117: 833–848.

Dinarello C A 1991 Interleukin-1 and interleukin-1 antagonism. Blood 77: 1627–1652.

Doolittle R F, Hunkapiller M W, Hood L E et al 1983 Simian sarcoma virus oncogene, v-sis, is derived from the gene (or genes) encoding a platelet derived growth factor. Science 221: 275–277.

Douglas G C, King B F 1989 Isolation of pure villous cytotrophoblast from term human placenta using immunomagnetic microspheres. Journal of Immunological Methods 119: 259–268.

Drake B L, Loke Y W 1991 Isolation of endothelial cells from human first trimester decidua using immunomagnetic beads. Human Reproduction 6: 1156–1159.

Dungy L R, Siddiqi T A, Khan S 1991 Transforming growth factor-β1 expression during placental development. American Journal of Obstetrics and Gynecology 165: 853–857.

Earl U, Estlin C, Bulmer J N 1990 Fibronectin and laminin in the early human placenta. Placenta 11: 223–231.

Emonard H, Christiane Y, Smet M, Grimaud J A, Foidart J M 1990 Type IV and interstitial collagenolytic activities in normal and malignant trophoblast cells are specifically regulated by the extracellular matrix. Invasion and Metastasis 10: 170–177.

Enders A C, King B F 1970 The cytology of Hofbauer cells. Anatomical Record 167: 231–252.

Faller T H, Ferenci P 1973 Der Aufbau der Placenta-Septen. Untersuchungen mir Hilfe der Quinacrinfluorescenzfärbung des Y-Chromatins. Zeitschrift für Anatomie und Entwicklung Geschichte 142: 207–217.

Fant M E 1991 In vitro growth rate of placental fibroblasts is developmentally regulated. Journal of Clinical Investigation 88: 1697–1702.

Feinberg R F, Kao L-C, Haimowitz J E et al 1989 Plasminogen activator inhibitor types 1 and 2 in human trophoblasts. PAI-1 is an immunocytochemical marker of invading trophoblasts. Laboratory Investigation 61: 20–26.

Feinberg R F, Kliman H J, Lockwood C J 1991 Is oncofetal fibronectin a trophoblast glue for human implantation? American Journal of Pathology 138: 537–543.

Flynn A, Finke J H, Hilfiker M L 1982 Placental mononuclear phagocytes as a source of interleukin-1. Science 218: 475–477.

Fox H 1970 Effect of hypoxia on trophoblast in organ culture. American Journal of Obstetrics and Gynecology 107: 1058–1064.

Frank H G, Malekzadeh F, Kertschanska S et al 1994 Immunohistochemistry of two different types of placental fibrinoid. Acta Anatomica 150: 55–68.

Frauli M, Ludwig H 1987 Immunocytochemical identification of mitotic Hofbauer cells in cultures of first trimester human placental villi. Archives of Gynecology and Obstetrics 241: 47–51.

Frolik C A, Dart L L, Meyers C A, Smith D M, Sporn M B 1983 Purification and initial characterization of a type β transforming growth factor from human placenta. Proceedings of the National Academy of Sciences USA 80: 3676–3680.

Geier G, Schuhmann R, Kraus H 1975 Regional unterschiedliche Zellproliferation innerhalb der Plazentone reifer menschlicher Plazenten: autoradiographische Untersuchungen. Archiv für Gynakologie 21: 31–37.

Glover D M, Brownstein D, Burchette S, Larsen A, Wilson C B 1987 Expression of HLA class II antigens and secretion of interleukin-1 by monocytes and macrophages from adults and neonates. Immunology 61: 195–201.

Goldstein J, Braverman M, Salafia C, Buckley P 1988 The phenotype of human placental macrophages and its variation with gestational age. American Journal of Pathology 133: 648–659.

Goldstein S R, Subramanyam B R, Snyder J R 1986 Ratio of gestational sac volume to crown–rump length in early pregnancy. Human Pathology 31: 320–321.

Gosseye S, Fox H 1984 An immunohistological comparison of the secretory capacity of villous and extravillous trophoblast in the human placenta. Placenta 5: 329–348.

Goustin A S, Betsholtz C, Pfeifer-Ohlsson S et al 1985 Coexpression of the sis and myc proto-oncogenes in developing human placenta suggests autocrine control of trophoblast growth. Cell 41: 301–312.

Hardingham T E, Fosang J D 1992 Proteoglycans: many forms and many functions. FASEB Journal 6: 861–870.

Hein K 1971 Licht- und elektronenmikroskopische Untersuchungen an der Basalplatte der reifen menschlichen Plazenta. Zeitschrift für Zellforschung 122: 323–349.

Hertig A T 1960 La nidation des oeufs humains fecondes normaux et anormaux. In: Ferin J, Gaudefroy M (eds) Les fonctions de nidation uterine et leurs troubles. Masson, Paris, pp 169–213.

Hertig A T 1962 The placenta: some new knowledge about an old organ. Obstetrics and Gynecology 20: 859–866.

Hertig A T, Rock J 1941 Two human ova of the previllous stage having an ovulation age of about eleven and twelve days respectively. Contributions to Embryology, Carnegie Institution of Washington 29: 127–156.

Heuser C H, Streeter G L 1941 Development of the macaque embryo. Contributions to Embryology, Carnegie Institution of Washington 29: 15–55.

Holmgren L, Glaser A, Pfeifer-Ohlsson S, Ohlsson R 1991 Angiogenesis during human extraembryonic development involves the spatiotemporal control of PDGF ligand and receptor gene expression. Development 113: 749–754.

Hsi B L, Yeh C-J G, Samson N, Fehlmann M 1987a Monoclonal antibody GB 36 raised against human trophoblast recognizes a novel epithelial antigen. Placenta 8: 209–217.

Hsi B L, Faulk W P, Yeh C-J G, McIntyre J A 1987b Immunohistology of clotting factor V in human extraembryonic membranes. Placenta 8: 529–535.

Hustin J, Schaaps J P, Lambotte R 1988 Anatomical studies of the utero-placental vascularization in the first trimester of pregnancy. Trophoblast Research 3: 49–60.

Ishikawa F, Miyazono K, Hellman U et al 1989 Identification of angiogenic activity and the cloning and expression of platelet-derived endothelial cell growth factor. Nature 338: 557–562.

Jackson M R, Mayhew T M, Haas J D 1987 Morphometric studies on villi in human term placentae and the effects of altitude, ethnic grouping and sex of newborn. Placenta 8: 487–495.

Jaffe E A 1987 Cell biology of endothelial cells. Human Pathology 18: 234–239.

Johannigmann J, Zahn V, Thieme V 1972 Einführung in die Ultraschalluntersuchung mit dem Vidoson. Elektromedica 2: 1–11.

Jones C J P, Fox H 1977 Syncytial knots and intervillous bridges in the human placenta: an ultrastructural study. Journal of Anatomy 124: 275–286.

Kameda T, Koyama M, Matzuzaki N, Taniguchi T, Saji F, Tanizawa O 1991 Localization of three subtypes of Fcꝑ receptors in human placenta by immunohistochemical analysis. Placenta 12: 15–26.

Kao L-C, Caltabiano S, Wu S, Strauss J F III, Kliman H J 1988 The human villous cytotrophoblast: interaction with extracellular matrix proteins, endocrine function, and cytoplasmic differentiation in the absence of syncytium formation. Developmental Biology 130: 693–702.

Kaufmann P 1972 Untersuchungen über die Langhanszellen in der menschlichen Placenta. Zeitschrift fur Zellforschung 128: 283–302.

Kaufmann P 1981a Entwicklung der Plazenta. In: Becker V, Schiebler Th H, Kubli F (eds) Die Plazenta des Menschen. Thieme, Stuttgart.

Kaufmann P 1981b Fibrinoid. In: Becker V, Schiebler Th H, Kubli F (eds) Die Plazenta des Menschen. Thieme, Stuttgart.

Kaufmann P 1982 Development and differentiation of the human placental villous tree. Bibliotheca Anatomica 22: 29–39.

Kaufmann P, Scheffen I 1992 Placental development. In: Polin R, Fox W (eds) Neonatal and fetal medicine — physiology and pathophysiology. Saunders, Orlando.

Kaufmann P, Stark J 1971 Die Basalplatte der reifen menschlichen Placenta. I. Semidünnschnitt-Histologie. Zeitschrift für Anatomie und Entwicklung Geschichte 135: 1–19.

Kaufmann P, Sen D K, Schweikhart G 1979 Classification of human placental villi. I. Histology and scanning electron microscopy. Cell and Tissue Research 200: 409–423.

Kaufmann P, Nagl W, Fuhrmann B 1983 Die funktionelle Bedeutung der Langhanszellen der menschlichen Plazenta. Verhandlungen der Anatomischen Gesellschaft 77: 435–436.

Kaufmann P, Bruns U, Leiser R, Luckhardt M, Winterhager E 1985 The fetal vascularization of term human placental villi. II. Intermediate and terminal villi. Anatomy and Embryology 173: 203–214.

Kaufmann P, Luckhardt M, Schweikhart G, Cantle S J 1987 Cross-sectional features and three-dimensional structure of human placental villi. Placenta 8: 235–247.

Kaufmann P, Luckhardt M, Leiser R 1988 Three-dimensional representation of the fetal vessel system in the human placenta. Trophoblast Research 3: 113–137.

Kauma S, Matt D, Strom S, Eierman D, Turner T 1990 Interleukin-1β, human leukocyte antigen HLA-DRα, and transforming growth factor-β expression in endometrium, placenta, and placental membranes. American Journal of Obstetrics and Gynecology 163: 1430–1437.

Khong T Y, Lane E B, Robertson W B 1986 An immunocytochemical study of fetal cells at the maternal-placental interface using monoclonal antibodies to keratins, vimentin and desmin. Cell and Tissue Research 246: 189–195.

Khudr G, Soma H, Benirschke K 1973 Trophoblastic origin of the X-cell and the placental giant cell. American Journal of Obstetrics and Gynecology 115: 530–533.

King B F 1987 Ultrastructural differentiation of stromal and vascular components in early macaque placental villi. American Journal of Anatomy 178: 30–44.

Kjaeldgaard A, Pschera H, Larsson B, Gaffney P, Åstedt B 1989 Plasminogen activators and inhibitors in amniotic fluid. Fibrinolysis 3: 203–206.

Kliman H J, Feinberg R F 1990 Human trophoblast-extracellular matrix (ECM) interactions in vitro: ECM thickness modulates morphology and proteolytic activity. Proceedings of the National Academy of Sciences 87: 3057–3061.

Kliman H J, Nestler J E, Sermasi E, Sanger J M, Strauss J F III 1986 Purification, characterization and in vitro differentiation of cytotrophoblasts from human term placenta. Endocrinology 118: 1567–1582.

Knopp J 1960 Das Wachstum der Chorionzotten vom 2. bis 10. Monat. Zeitschrift für Anatomie und Entwicklung Geschichte 122: 42–59.

Kurman R J, Main C S, Chen H-C 1984a Intermediate trophoblast: a distinctive form of trophoblast with specific morphological, biochemical and functional features. Placenta 5: 349–370a.

Kurman R J, Young R H, Norris H J, Main C S, Lawrence W D, Scully R E 1984b Immunocytochemical localization of placental lactogen and chorionic gonadotropin in the normal placenta and trophoblastic tumors, with emphasis on intermediate trophoblast and the placental site trophoblastic tumor. International Journal of Gynecological Pathology 3: 101–121.

Küstermann W 1981 Über "Proliferationsknoten" und "Syncytialknoten" der menschlichen Placenta. Anatomischer Anzeiger 150: 144–157.

Ladines-Llave C A, Maruo T, Manalo A S, Mochizuki M 1991 Cytologic localization of epidermal growth factor and its receptor in developing human placenta varies over the course of pregnancy. American Journal of Obstetrics and Gynecology 165: 1377–1382.

Lala P K, Graham C H 1990 Mechanisms of trophoblast invasiveness and their control: the role of proteases and protease inhibitors. Cancer Metastasis Reviews 9: 369–379.

Lang I, Hartmann M, Blaschitz A et al 1994 Differential lectin binding to the fibrinoid of human full term placenta: correlation with a fibrin antibody and the PAF-Halmi method. Acta Anatomica 150: 170–177.

Lehmann W D, Schuhmann R, Kraus H 1973 Regionally different steroid biosynthesis within materno-fetal circulation units (placentones) of mature human placentas. Journal of Perinatal Medicine 1: 198–204.

Leiser R, Beier H M 1988 Morphological studies of lacunar formation in the early rabbit placenta. Trophoblast Research 3: 97–110.

Leiser R, Luckhardt M, Kaufmann P, Winterhager E, Bruns U 1985 The fetal vascularisation of term human placental villi. I. Peripheral stem villi. Anatomy and Embryology 173: 71–80.

Librach C L, Werb Z, Fitzgerald M L et al 1991 92-kD type IV collagenase mediates invasion of human cytotrophoblasts. Journal of Cell Biology 113: 437–449.

Loke Y W, Hsi B L, Bulmer J N et al 1992 Evaluation of a monoclonal antibody, BC-1, which identifies an antigen expressed on the surface membrane of human extravillous trophoblast. American Journal of Reproductive Immunology 27: 77–81.

Luckett W P 1978 Origin and differentiation of the yolk sac and extraembryonic mesoderm in presomite human and rhesus monkey embryos. American Journal of Anatomy 152: 59–97.

Lupu R, Colomer R, Kannan B, Lippman M E 1992 Characterization of a growth factor that binds exclusively to the erbB-2 receptor and induces cellular responses. Proceedings of the National Academy of Sciences USA 89: 2287–2291.

Marez A, Nguyen T, Chevallier B, Clement G, Dauchel M C, Barritault D 1987 Platelet derived growth factor is present in human placenta: purification from an industrially processed fraction. Biochimie 69: 125–129.

Martin B J, Spicer S S 1973 Ultrastructural features of cellular maturation and aging in human trophoblast. Journal of Ultrastructure Research 43: 133–149.

Mayhew T M, Joy C F, Haas J D 1984 Structure-function correlation in the human placenta: the morphometric diffusing capacity for oxygen at full term. Journal of Anatomy 139: 691–708.

Mayhew T M, Jackson M R, Haas J D 1986 Microscopical morphology of the human placenta and its effects on oxygen diffusion: a morphometric model. Placenta 7: 121–131.

Miller D, Pelton R, Deryick R, Moses H 1990 Transforming growth factor-β. A family of growth regulatory peptides. Annals of the New York Academy of Sciences 593: 208–217.

Moll W 1981 Physiologie der maternen plazentaren Durchblutung. In: Becker V, Schiebler Th H, Kubli F (eds) Die Plazenta des Menschen. Thieme, Stuttgart, pp 172–194.

Moll U M, Lane B L 1990 Proteolytic activity of first trimester human placenta: localization of interstitial collagenase in villous and extravillous trophoblast. Histochemistry 94: 555–560.

Morrish D W, Bhardwaj D, Dabbagh L K, Marusyk H, Siy O 1987 Epidermal growth factor induces differentiation and secretion of human chorionic gonadotropin and placental lactogen in normal human placenta. Journal of Clinical Endocrinology and Metabolism 65: 1282–1290.

Morrish D W, Bhardwaj D, Paras M T 1991 Transforming growth factor β1 inhibits placental differentiation and human chorionic gonadotropin and placental lactogen secretion. Endocrinology 129: 22–26.

Moskalewski S, Ptak W, Czarnik Z 1975 Demonstration of cells with IgG receptor in human placenta. Biology of the Neonate 26: 268–273.

Mühlhauser J, Crescimanno C, Rajaniemi H, Castellucci M, Kaufmann P 1992 Localization of carbonic anhydrase isoenzymes in amnion and human placenta by immunofluorescence techniques. Anatomischer Anzeiger 174 (suppl): 128.

Mühlhauser J, Crescimanno C, Kaufmann P, Höfler H, Zaccheo D, Castellucci M 1993 Differentiation and proliferation patterns in human trophoblast revealed by c-erbB-2 oncogene product and EGF-R. Journal of Histochemistry and Cytochemistry 41: 165–173.

Naeye R L 1987 Do placental weights have clinical significance? Human Pathology 18: 387–391.

Nanaev A K, Shirinsky V P, Birukov G 1991a Immunofluorescent study of heterogeneity in smooth muscle cells of human fetal vessels using antibodies to myosin, desmin, and vimentin. Cell and Tissue Research 266: 535–540.

Nanaev A K, Rukosuev V S, Shirinsky V P et al 1991b Confocal and conventional immunofluorescent and immunogold electron microscopic localization of collagen types III and IV in human placenta. Placenta 12: 573–595.

Nelson D M, Crouch E C, Curran E M, Farmer D R 1990 Trophoblast interaction with fibrin matrix: epithelialization of perivillous fibrin deposits as a mechanism for villous repair in the human placenta. American Journal of Pathology 136: 855–861.

Nikolov S D, Schiebler T H 1973 Über das fetale Gefäßsystem der reifen menschlichen Placenta. Zeitschrift for Zellforschung 139: 333–350.

Ohlsson R 1989 Growth factors, protooncogenes and human placental development. Cell Differentiation and Development 28: 1–16.

Ohlsson R, Holmgren L, Glaser A, Szpecht A, Pfeifer-Ohlsson S 1989 Insulin-like growth factor 2 and short-range stimulatory loops in control of human placental growth. EMBO Journal 8: 1993–1999.

Okudaira Y, Hashimoto T, Hamanaka N, Yoshinare S 1971 Electron microscopic study on the trophoblastic cell column of human placenta. Journal of Electron Microscopy 20: 93–106.

O'Rahilly R 1973 Developmental stages in human embryos. Part A, Publication 631. Carnegie Institute of Washington, Washington.

Park W W 1971 Choriocarcinoma: a study of its pathology. Heinemann, London, pp 13–27.

Peles E, Bacus S S, Koski R A et al 1992 Isolation of the neu/HER-2 stimulatory ligand: a 44 kd glycoprotein that induces differentiation of mammary tumor cells. Cell 69: 205–216.

Pierce G B, Midgley A R 1963 The origin and function of human syncytiotrophoblastic giant cells. American Journal of Pathology 43: 153–173.

Pijnenborg R, Robertson W B, Brosens I, Dixon G 1981 Trophoblast invasion and the establishment of haemochorial placentation in man and laboratory animals. Placenta 2: 71–92.

Pilz I, Schweikhart G, Kaufmann P 1980 Zur Abgrenzung normaler, artefizieller und pathologischer Strukturen in reifen menschlichen Plazentazotten. III. Morphometrische Untersuchungen bei Rh-Inkompatibilität. Archives of Gynecology and Obstetrics 229: 137–154.

Platanias L C, Vogelzang N J 1990 Interleukin-1: biology, pathophysiology, and clinical prospects. American Journal of Medicine 89: 621–629.

Radtke K-P, Wenz K-H, Heimburger N 1990 Isolation of plasminogen activator inhibitor-2 (PAI-2) from human placenta: evidence for vitronectin/PAI-2 complexes in human placenta extract. Biological Chemistry Hoppe-Seyler 371: 1119–1127.

Ramsey E M, Corner G W Jr, Donner M W 1963 Serial and cineradioangiographic visualization of maternal circulation in the primate (hemochorial) placenta. American Journal of Obstetrics and Gynecology 86: 213–225.

Risau W, Drexler H, Mironov V et al 1992 Platelet-derived growth factor is angiogenic in vivo. Growth Factors 7: 261–266.

Robertson W B, Warner B 1974 The ultrastructure of the human placental bed. Journal of Pathology 112: 203–211.

Rosenberg S M, Maslar I A, Riddick D H 1980 Decidual production of prolactin in late gestation: further evidence for a decidual source of amniotic fluid prolactin. American Journal of Obstetrics and Gynecology 138: 681–685.

Rukosuev V S 1992 Immunofluorescent localization of collagen types I, III, IV, V, fibronectin, laminin, entactin, and heparan sulphate proteoglycan in human immature placenta. Experientia 48: 285–287.

Sala A M, Valeri V, Matheus M 1983 Stereological analysis of syncytiotrophoblast from human mature placenta. Archives of Anatomy and Microscopy 72: 99–106.

Schaaps J P, Hustin J 1988 In vivo aspect of the maternal-trophoblastic border during the first trimester of gestation. Trophoblast Research 3: 3–48.

Schiebler T H, Kaufmann P 1981 Reife Plazenta. In: Becker V, Schiebler T H, Kubli F (eds) Die Plazenta des Menschen. Georg Thieme, Stuttgart, pp 51–100.

Schmid-Schönbein H 1988 Conceptional proposition for a specific microcirculatory problem: Maternal blood flow in hemochorial multivillous placentae as percolation of a "porous medium". Trophoblast Research 3: 17–38.

Schuhmann R 1981 Plazenton: Begriff, Entstehung, funktionelle Anatomie. In: Becker V, Schiebler T H, Kubli H (eds) Die Plazenta des Menschen. Thieme Verlag, Stuttgart, pp 199–207.

Schuhmann R, Geier G 1972 Histomorphologische Placentabefunde bei EPG-Gestose. Archiv für Gynäkologie 213: 31–47.

Schuhmann R, Wehler V 1971 Histologische Unterschiede an Plazentazotten innerhalb der materno-fetalen Strömungseinheit. Ein Beitrag zur funktionellen Morphologie der Plazenta. Archiv für Gynäkologie 210: 425–439.

Schuhmann R, Kraus H, Borst R, Geier G 1976 Regional unterschiedliche Enzymaktivität innerhalb der Placentone reifer menschlicher Placenten. Histochemische und biochemische Untersuchungen. Archiv für Gynäkologie 220: 209–226.

Schuhmann R, Stoz F, Maier M 1986 Histometrische Untersuchungen an Plazentonen menschlicher Plazenten. Zeitschrift für Geburtshilfe und Perinatologie 190: 196–203.

Schweikhart G, Kaufmann P 1977 Zur Abgrenzung normaler, artefizieller und pathologischer Strukturen in reifen menschlichen Plazentazotten. I. Ultrastruktur des Syncytiotrophoblasten. Archiv für Gynäkologie 222: 213–230.

Scott S M, Buenaflor G G, Orth D N 1989 Immunoreactive human epidermal growth factor concentrations in amniotic fluid, umbilical artery and vein serum, and placenta in full-term and preterm infants. Biology of the Neonate 56: 246–251.

Sedmak D D, Davis D H, Singh U, van de Winkel J G J, Anderson C L 1991 Expression of IgG Fc receptor antigens in placenta and on endothelial cells in humans: an immunohistochemical study. American Journal of Pathology 138: 175–181.

Sen D K, Kaufmann P, Schweikhart G 1979 Classification of human placental villi. II. Morphometry. Cell and Tissue Research 200: 425–434.

Sheppard B L, Bonnar J 1988 The maternal blood supply to the placenta in pregnancy complicated by intrauterine fetal growth retardation. Trophoblast Research 3: 69–82.

Slamon D J, Clark G M, Wong S G et al 1987 Human breast cancer: correlation of relapse and survival with amplification of the HER-2/Neu oncogene. Science 235: 177–182.

Sporn M, Roberts A 1990 The transforming growth factor-betas: past, present and future. Annals of the New York Academy of Sciences 593: 1–6.

Stark J, Kaufmann P 1971 Die Basalplatte der reifen menschlichen Placenta. II. Gefrierschnitthistochemie. Zeitschrift für Anatomie und Entwicklung Geschichte 135: 185–201.

Sunderland C A, Redman C W G, Stirrat G M 1981 Monoclonal antibodies to human syncytiotrophoblast. Immunology 43: 541–546.

Taylor R N, Williams L T 1988 Developmental expression of platelet-derived growth factor and its receptor in the human placenta. Molecular Endocrinology 2: 627–632.

Teasdale F 1978 Functional significance of the zonal morphologic differences in the normal human placenta. American Journal of Obstetrics and Gynecology 130: 773–778.

Teasdale F, Jean-Jacques G 1985 Morphometric evaluation of the microvillous surface enlargement factor in the human placenta from mid-gestation to term. Placenta 6: 375–381.

Thornton S C, Por S B, Walsh B J, Penny R, Breit S N 1990 Interaction of immune and connective tissue cells: I. The effect of lymphokines and monokines on fibroblast growth. Journal of Leukocyte Biology 47: 312–320.

Uren S, Boyle W 1985 Isolation of macrophages from human placenta. Journal of Immunological Methods 78: 25–34.

Usuki K, Norberg L, Larsson E et al 1990 Localization of platelet-derived endothelial cell growth factor in human placenta and purification of an alternatively processed form. Cell Regulation 1: 577–596.

Virtanen I, Laitinen L, Vartio T 1988 Differential expression of the extra domain-containing form of cellular fibronectin in human placentas at different stages of maturation. Histochemie 90: 25–30.

Voigt S, Kaufmann P, Schweikhart G 1978 Zur Abgrenzung normaler, artefizieller und pathologischer Strukturen in reifen menschlichen Plazentazotten. II. Morphometrische Untersuchungen zum Einfluss des Fixationsmodus. Archiv für Gynäkologie 226: 347–362.

Wallenburg H C S, Hutchinson D L, Schuler H M, Stolte L A M, Janssens J 1973 The pathogenesis of placental infarction. II. An experimental study in the rhesus monkey placenta. American Journal of Obstetrics and Gynecology 116: 841–846.

Welsh A O, Enders A E 1985 Light and electron microscopic examination of the mature decidual cells of the rat with emphasis on the antimesometrial decidua and its degeneration. American Journal of Anatomy 172: 1–29.

Werb Z, Hembry R M, Murphy G, Aggeler J 1986 Commitment to expression of the metalloendopeptidases, collagenase and stromelysin: relationship of inducing events to changes in cytoskeletal architecture. Journal of Cell Biology 102: 697–702.

Weser H, Kaufmann P 1978 Lichtmikroskopische und histochemische Untersuchungen an der Chorionplatte der reifen menschlichen Placenta. Archiv für Gynäkologie 225: 15–30.

Westermark B, Siegbahn A, Heldin C-H, Claesson W L 1990 B-type receptor for platelet-derived growth factor mediates a chemotactic response by means of ligand-induced activation of the receptor protein-tyrosine kinase. Proceedings of the National Academy of Sciences USA 87: 128–132.

Wiese K-H 1975 Licht- und elektronenmikroskopische Untersuchungen an der Chorionplatte der reifen menschlichen Placenta. Archiv für Gynäkologie 218: 243–259.

Wigglesworth J S 1967 Vascular organization of the human placenta. Nature 216: 1120–1121.

Winckel F K L W 1893 Lehrbuch der Geburtshilfe, 2. Aufl. Veit, Leipzig.

Wislocki G B, Streeter G L 1938 On the placentation of the macaque (Macaca mulatta) from the time of implantation until the formation of the definitive placenta. Contributions to Embryology of the Carnegie Institute 27: 1–66.

Wright C, Angus B, Nicholson S et al 1989 Expression of c-erbB-2 oncoprotein: a prognostic indicator in human breast cancer. Cancer Research 49: 2087–2090.

Yamada T, Isemura M, Yamaguchi Y et al 1987 Immunohistochemical localization of fibronectin in the human placentas at their different stages of maturation. Histochemistry 86: 579–584.

Yamaguchi Y, Mann D M, Ruoslahti E 1990 Negative regulation of transforming growth factor-β by the proteoglycan decorin. Nature 346: 281–284.

Yeh C-J G, Hsi B L, Samson M et al 1987 Monoclonal antibodies (GB 16, GB 18, GB 19, GB 22) raised against human placental microvilli recognize the transferrin receptor. Placenta 8: 627–638.

Zaccheo D, Pistoia V, Castellucci M, Martinoli C 1989 Isolation and characterization of Hofbauer cells from human placental villi. Archives of Gynecology and Obstetrics 246: 189–200.

47. General pathology of the placenta

H. Fox

Until relatively recently the literature on placental pathology was disfigured by an undue emphasis on functionally unimportant macroscopic lesions, by a lack of precise histopathological detail and by the use of archaic terminology. In this chapter a contemporary approach to placental pathology will be presented in which it is hoped to avoid these blemishes: the central theme of this approach is that placental changes must be assessed in functional terms and that no lesion, however pathologically impressive it may appear, can be considered as significant if it cannot be shown to impair fetal oxygenation, development or growth. It is readily accepted, however, that the pathologist committed to this attitude is faced with a grave disadvantage when examining the delivered placenta for it is becoming increasingly clear that many, probably most, of the complications of pregnancy traditionally attributed to 'placental insufficiency' are a result, not of intrinsic changes within the placenta, but of abnormalities in maternal uteroplacental blood flow. These in turn appear to be largely due to inadequate conversion, by extravillous trophoblast, of the spiral arteries into uteroplacental vessels (see Ch. 48). The pathologist must therefore examine the placenta in the light of the frustrating knowledge that the most important pathological processes affecting the organ are present in vessels which are not usually available for study. It should be noted that this chapter is largely concerned with the pathology of the third-trimester placenta: changes encountered in placentas from pregnancies terminating during the early stages are discussed in Chapter 53. Certain specialized aspects of placental pathology are considered in Chapters 49, 55 and 61.

MACROSCOPIC ABNORMALITIES OF THE PLACENTA

These can be usefully, though obviously arbitrarily and somewhat artificially, grouped into four categories:

1. Developmental abnormalities
2. Lesions which reduce the mass of functioning villi
3. Haematomas and thrombi
4. Miscellaneous abnormalities which are devoid of functional significance.

Developmental abnormalities

Placenta extrachorialis

This is the commonest developmental anomaly of the placenta, being found in about 25% of all placentas (Fox, 1978). In this abnormality the chorionic plate, from which the villi arise, is smaller than the basal plate and hence the transition from villous to membranous chorion takes place not at the edge of the placenta but at some distance within the circumference of the fetal surface of the placenta, thus leaving a ridge of villous tissue projecting beyond the limits of the chorionic plate (Fig. 47.1). If the transition from villous to membranous chorion is marked by a flat ring of membranes the placenta is classed as 'circummarginate' (Fig. 47.2) whilst if this ring is plicated with a raised, often rolled, edge the placenta is of the 'circumvallate' type (Figs 47.3 and 47.4). Either of these two anomalies may be either complete or partial (Fig. 47.5) whilst a placenta may be circummarginate in one area and circumvallate in another.

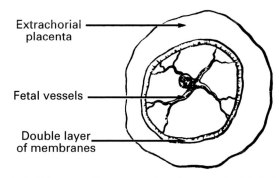

Fig. 47.1 Diagrammatic representation of an extrachorial placenta as viewed from the fetal aspect. (From Fox, 1978. Reproduced by permission of W. B. Saunders.)

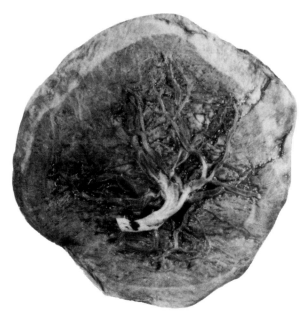

Fig. 47.2 A circummarginate placenta viewed from the fetal aspect. (From Fox, 1978. Reproduced by permission of W. B. Saunders.)

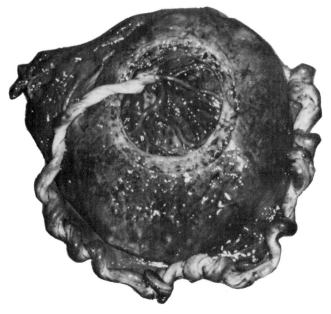

Fig. 47.4 An extreme degree of circumvallate placentation: viewed from the fetal aspect.

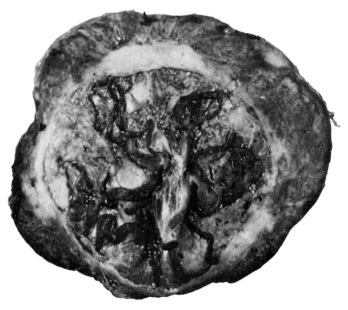

Fig. 47.3 A circumvallate placenta viewed from the fetal aspect. (From Fox, 1978. Reproduced by permission of W. B. Saunders.)

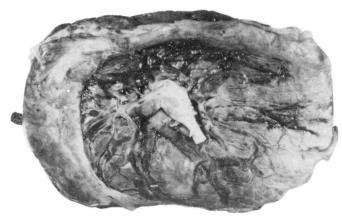

Fig. 47.5 A partially circumvallate placenta viewed from the fetal aspect. On the left side the placenta is vallate but on the right side it is normal. (From Fox, 1978. Reproduced by permission of W. B. Saunders.)

The pathogenesis of placenta extrachorialis is unknown but suggested theories include poor development of the chorion frondosum, low intra-amniotic pressure, unduly shallow implantation of the ovum, marginal haemorrhage during early pregnancy and genetic factors: none of these hypotheses carries much conviction and a more persuasive view is that extrachorial placentation is a consequence of excessively deep implantation of the blastocyst (Torpin, 1966).

Opinion has been sharply divided about the clinical significance of extrachorial placentation, some maintaining that it is simply an anatomical variant of no clinical importance (Wentworth, 1968) and others claiming that it is causally related to a high incidence of abortion, antepartum bleeding, premature labour and perinatal death (Wilson & Paalman, 1967; Lal, 1976). Some of this confusion has been due to the inclusion of both circummarginate and circumvallate placentas under the single heading of placenta extrachorialis for it is now clear that the circummarginate form is totally devoid of clinical significance (Benson & Fujikura, 1969; Fox & Sen, 1972). By contrast the circumvallate placenta, whether partial or complete, is associated with an increased incidence of low birth weight (Fox & Sen, 1972; Rolschau, 1978; Sandstedt, 1979; Liu, 1990) though it should be noted that the affected infants are, to use a paradoxical phase, 'heavy' small babies, a point emphasized by the fact that circumvallate placentation is not associated with any excess perinatal mortality. It is not currently known whether the increased incidence of low birth weight associated with circumvallate placentas is because this is, possibly because of distortion or constriction of the intervillous space, an inadequate form of placentation or whether both the abnormal placental form and the fetal growth defect are mutually dependent upon a common causal factor.

It has been claimed, in a relatively small and still unconfirmed study, that circumvallate placentas are associated with an increased incidence of congenital malformations, these ranging from minor deviations to those incompatible with life and showing no bias towards any organ or system (Lademacher et al, 1981). Kaplan (1993) has claimed that circumvallate placentation is associated with prematurity but data to support this contention has not been provided.

Placenta membranacea

In this anomaly all, or most, of the membranes are covered on their outer aspect by placental villi. Exceptionally there may be focal thickening to form a placental disc (Hurley & Beischer, 1987; Wilkins et al, 1991) but more commonly the gestational sac is diffusely covered by villous tissue. This condition, which is extremely rare occurring in between 1 in 20 000 and 1 in 40 000 pregnancies (Greenberg et al, 1991), has been variously attributed to pre-existing endometritis, poor development of the decidual blood supply, endometrial hyperplasia, unduly deep blastocyst implantation and a faulty trophoblastic anlage (Fox, 1978). Irrespective of pathogenesis, this anomaly is of grave import for the fetus: a placenta membranacea must of necessity also be a placenta praevia and in virtually every case recurrent antepartum bleeding, often from quite an early stage of pregnancy, is associated with either abortion or premature onset of labour. The outlook for fetal survival is particularly poor for not only is the fetus at risk from early delivery but it is also usually markedly underweight for the length of the gestational period (Janovski & Granowitz, 1961), this suggesting that this is an inefficient mode of placentation. In about one-third of cases a placenta membranacea is also a placenta increta (Greenberg et al, 1991).

Accessory lobe

Adjacent to the main placenta may be found one or more accessory lobes of variable size (Fig. 47.6). The accessory lobe may be linked to the main placental mass by a narrow

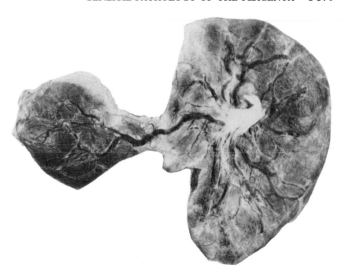

Fig. 47.6 A placenta with an accessory lobe which is joined to the main placental mass by a bridge of membranes. The cord is inserted into the main placenta and a vessel is running intramembranously to the lobe.

isthmus of chorionic tissue but it is not infrequently entirely separate and connected only by the membranes. The vascular supply to the lobe is usually from a vessel which runs an intramembranous course as a branch from an artery on the fetal surface of the placenta. Accessory lobes are found in about 30% of pregnancies and are usually devoid of clinical significance: occasionally, however, the lobe is retained in utero after delivery of the main placenta, this leading to subinvolution and postpartum bleeding, whilst very rarely trauma to the vessels running intramembranously to the lobe results in serious fetal haemorrhage (Hata et al, 1988).

An accessory lobe has been attributed to unduly superficial implantation of the blastocyst with subsequent development on both anterior and posterior walls of the uterus, to implantation into the lateral or apical sulcus or to partial failure of the normal process of villous atrophy in the chorion laeve.

Bilobate placenta

This consists of two approximately equal lobes which may be connected by a bridge of chorionic tissue or which may be quite discrete from each other (Fig. 47.7). The umbilical cord is usually inserted between the two lobes, sometimes into a connecting bridge but often velamentously. This anomaly occurs in approximately one in 350 pregnancies (Earn, 1951) and its only clinical association is with an unusually high incidence of first-trimester bleeding (Fujikura et al, 1970). The pathogenesis of this anomaly is believed to be superficial implantation of the fertilized ovum with subsequent attachment of the placenta to both anterior and posterior uterine walls (Torpin & Barfield, 1968).

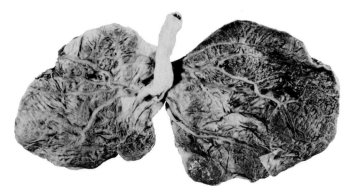

Fig. 47.7 A bilobate placenta with the cord inserted between the two placental lobes.

Fenestrate placenta

This is an exceptionally rare abnormality of unknown pathogenesis in which the central portion of a discoidal placenta is missing (Fig. 47.8): sometimes there is an actual hole in the centre of the placenta but more commonly the deficit is of villous tissue only. The only clinical significance of this abnormality is that it may be mistakenly thought that the missing portion is still retained in the uterus and the mother thus subjected to an unnecessary uterine exploration.

Ring-shaped placenta

In this extremely uncommon anomaly, also known as a 'girdle' or 'annular' placenta, the placenta is annular in shape and resembles a segment of a hollow cylinder:

sometimes a complete ring of placental tissue is seen but more commonly a portion of the ring atrophies, resulting in a placenta which is horeshoe-shaped. This condition, which is probably due to a distortion of the normal process of orderly villous atrophy in early gestation, is associated with a high incidence of both ante- and postpartum bleeding whilst the fetus is often of low birth weight for the length of the gestational period.

Lesions reducing mass of functional villi

Perivillous fibrin deposition

Some degree of fibrin deposition around villi occurs in almost all placentas but in a proportion is sufficiently extensive to be macroscopically visible either as a firm white plaque, often but not invariably in the marginal angle (Fig. 47.9), or as an area of irregular, whitish mottling (Fig. 47.10). Histologically these lesions are seen to consist of widely separated villi entrapped in fibrin which fills in and obliterates the intervillous space (Fig. 47.11). The syncytiotrophoblast of the entrapped villi degenerates and disappears but the villous cytotrophoblast persists and may proliferate not only to form a cellular mantle around individual villi (Fig. 47.12) but also to spread out into the surrounding fibrin (Fig. 47.13). The stroma of the included villi becomes markedly fibrotic whilst their fetal vessels undergo sclerosis and eventual obliteration. Lesions of this type occur in about 25% of placentas from uncomplicated term pregnancies and this incidence is not increased in prolonged pregnancy or in pre-eclampsia, indeed it is often unusually low in placentas from the latter group.

The entrapped villi are not, in any sense of the word, infarcted but are nevertheless of no functional value to the fetus in so far as they are clearly excluded from playing any rôle in maternofetal transfer mechanisms. However,

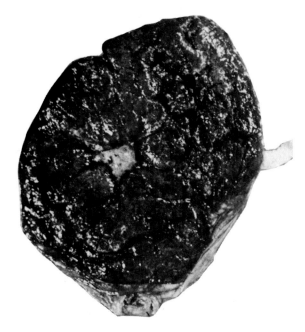

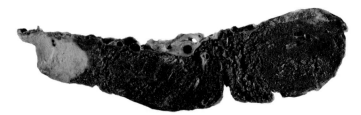

Fig. 47.9 A peripherally situated plaque of perivillous fibrin which fills in the lateral angle of the placenta.

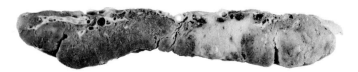

Fig. 47.8 A fenestrate placenta viewed from the maternal aspect. There is a focal deficiency of villous tissue in the centre of the placenta but the chorionic plate is complete.

Fig. 47.10 A centrally situated focus of perivillous fibrin which is irregular in outline and rather poorly delineated.

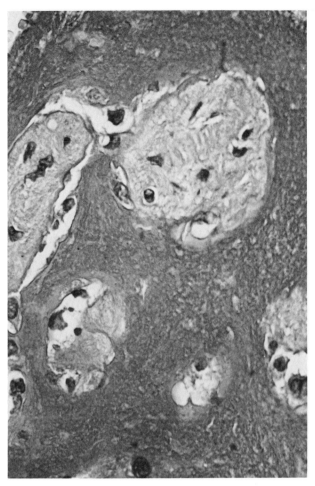

Fig. 47.11 Villi entrapped in a plaque of perivillous fibrin. The villi are fibrotic, avascular and have lost their trophoblastic covering. H & E × 350.

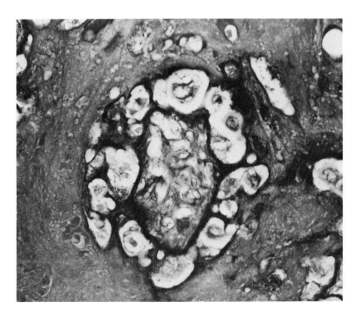

Fig. 47.12 Proliferation of cytotrophoblastic cells to form a mantle around a villus embedded in a plaque of fibrin. PAS × 450.

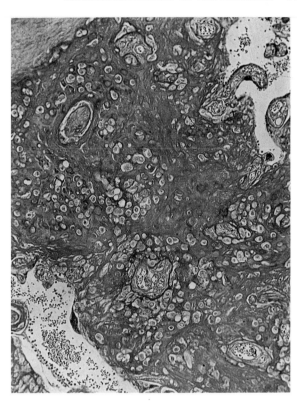

Fig. 47.13 A plaque of perivillous fibrin in which there has been marked proliferation of the villous cytotrophoblastic cells, many of which have become detached from their parent villi and have spread out into the enveloping fibrin. PAS × 65. (From Fox, 1978. Reproduced by permission of W. B. Saunders.)

macroscopically visible perivillous fibrin plaques, despite clearly reducing the mass of functional villous tissue, are devoid of any clinical significance, this applying not only to small lesions but also to those in which as many as 25–30% of the villi are entrapped in fibrin (Fox, 1967a, 1978). The clinical banality of this lesion is explicable in terms of its pathogenesis. The fibrin surrounding the villi is formed from maternal blood in the intervillous space. As the villous syncytiotrophoblast is in direct contact with the maternal blood, and can thus be regarded as playing an endothelial-like rôle, it was in the past thought that thrombosis occurred as a result of syncytial 'degeneration': electronmicroscopy has, however, clearly shown that the initial stage in the development of this lesion is an adherence of platelets to healthy villous syncytiotrophoblast (Moe & Jorgensen, 1968) and there can be little doubt that fibrin deposition occurs as a result of turbulence, eddy currents and stasis of maternal blood within the intervillous space. The greater, however, the maternal blood flow through the closed irregular intervillous space the greater is the possibility of turbulence, stasis and fibrin deposition and it therefore follows that perivillous fibrin plaques tend to form particularly in placentas with an excellent maternal blood supply, this accounting for the low incidence of these plaques in placentas from pre-eclamptic women and the very low incidence of fetal hypoxic complications associated with the presence of this placental lesion (Fox, 1967a).

The outstanding significance of perivillous fibrin plaques is that they bear eloquent witness to the fact that the placenta can withstand the loss of 30% of its functioning villous population without any evidence of physiological embarrassment. Very occasionally however there is a truly massive perivillous deposition of fibrin, with 80–90% of the villous parenchyma being incorporated into fibrinous masses (Fig. 47.14): the placenta can clearly not withstand a loss of villous tissue of this magnitude and, very exceptionally, fetal death can ensue from perivillous fibrin deposition of this degree.

Infarction

A fresh placental infarct is well demarcated, dark red and moderately firm (Fig. 47.15). As the infarct ages it becomes progressively harder and its colour changes successively to brown, yellow and white, an old infarct thus appearing as a hard white plaque with a smooth, or slightly granular, amorphous cut surface (Fig. 47.16). Histologically the early infarct is characterized by aggregation of the villi in the affected area with marked narrowing, often obliteration, of the intervillous space (Fig. 47.17):

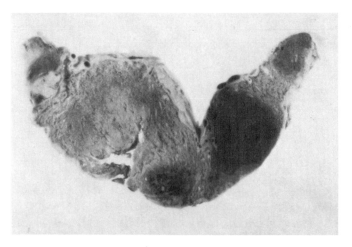

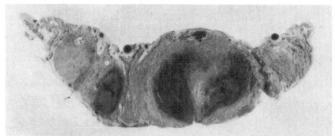

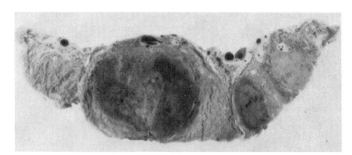

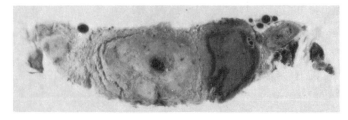

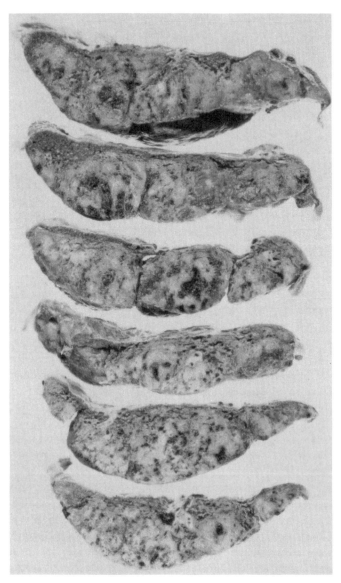

Fig. 47.14 An extreme example of perivillous fibrin deposition: approximately 90% of the villous parenchyma is incorporated into fibrinous plaques.

Fig. 47.15 Multiple fresh infarcts in a placenta. The infarcted areas are dark red, firm and well delineated.

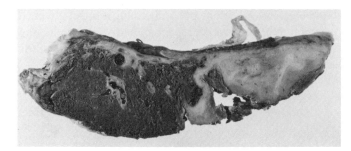

Fig. 47.16 An old placental infarct. This is seen as a white, amorphous plaque. (From Fox, 1978. Reproduced by permission of W. B. Saunders.)

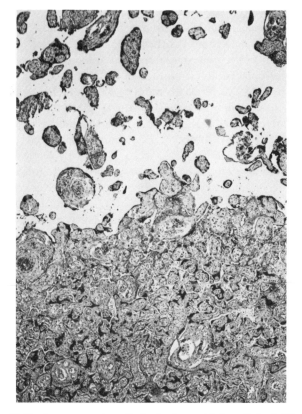

Fig. 47.17 Low power view of a fresh placental infarct (below). The villi are aggregated and the intervillous space obliterated. H & E × 50. (From Fox, 1978. Reproduced by permission of W. B. Saunders.)

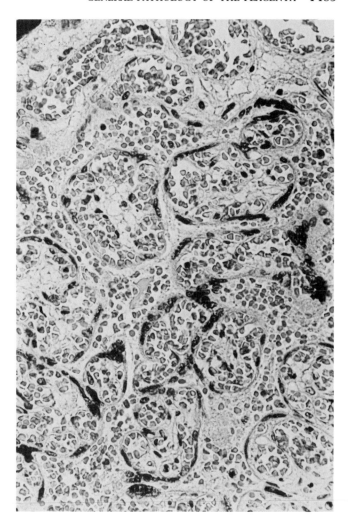

Fig. 47.18 Higher power view of a fresh placental infarct. The villous vessels are congested and the intervillous space is markedly narrowed. H & E × 360.

the villous fetal vessels are dilated and congested whilst the syncytial nuclei show early necrotic changes, such as pyknosis or karyorrhexis (Fig. 47.18). As the infarct ages the syncytial nuclei eventually disappear and there is a progressive coagulative necrosis of the villi: the fetal erythrocytes trapped in the vessels of the infarcted villi undergo haemolysis and the endothelium of these vessels degenerates (Fig. 47.19). The old infarct simply consists therefore of crowded 'ghost villi' showing, it should be noted, no fibrosis or cytotrophoblastic proliferation (Fig. 47.20). There is no evidence of circulation of maternal blood through the narrowed intervillous space within the infarct

though what little is left of this space often contains fibrin which is probably derived from plasma which has leaked out from the necrotic fetal villous vessels: there is commonly deposition of fibrin, derived from maternal blood, around the periphery of the infarct and non-infarcted villi are frequently entrapped within this peripheral fibrinous shell. There may be a polymorphonuclear leucocytic infiltration of the infarcted area but such a cellular infiltrate is often either scanty or entirely absent.

Small areas of infarction, involving less than 5% of the villous parenchyma, are common, occurring in 25% of placentas from uncomplicated pregnancies, and are of no clinical importance (Fox, 1967b, 1978). It is widely agreed, however, that extensive placental infarction, involving more than 10% of the villous parenchyma, is associated with a high incidence of fetal hypoxia, growth retardation and intrauterine death (Kloosterman & Huidekoper, 1954; Little, 1960; Fox, 1967b; Naeye, 1977). At first sight it appears obvious that these fetal complications are a direct result of loss of viable villous

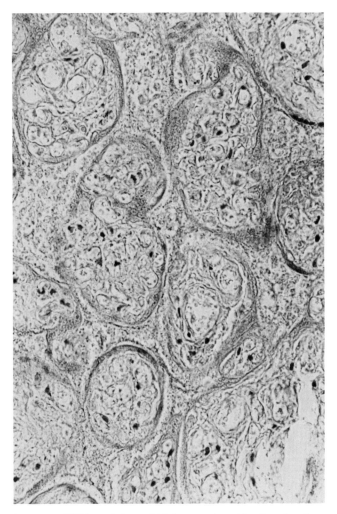

Fig. 47.19 Villi in an infarct which is somewhat older than that shown in Fig. 47.18. Villous congestion is less obvious and many of the erythrocytes in the fetal vessels have undergone haemolysis. The villous syncytiotrophoblast is almost entirely necrotic. H & E × 360.

tissue and, indeed, it has been these apparent ill-effects of placental infarction which have led many to the belief that the placenta is normally at the full stretch of its physiological capacity and has little or no functional reserve. This is an apparently logical corollary of the observation that the placenta can not withstand the loss of 10% of its functioning tissue without dire consequences for the continuing growth and viability of the fetus but is too simplistic a view for, as already discussed, a similar, or even greater, loss of villi due to their entrapment in fibrin is of no importance. This is an apparent paradox unless it is borne in mind that the villi are oxygenated from the maternal blood and that although many maternal vessels open into the intervillous space there is little or no mixing of arterial streams, the individual vessels being, in functional terms, end arteries; an infarct is therefore due to a localized obstruction to the maternal uteroplacental circulation either by a retroplacental haematoma or by a thrombus (Brosens & Renaer, 1972; Wallenburg et al 1973). If the comparatively uncommon infarcts due to retroplacental haematomas are excluded it is clear that extensive infarction is due to widespread thrombotic occlusion of maternal uteroplacental vessels: this is not an event which would be expected to occur in a healthy vascular tree and it is therefore no coincidence that extensive placental infarction is usually only seen in placentas from pre-eclamptic women for it is in these that a vascular abnormality, in the form of an acute atherosis (Robertson, 1976, 1981; Khong, 1991), is found which predisposes to thrombosis. Far more importantly, however, there is in this condition, whether thrombosis is superadded or not, a severely restricted maternal blood flow to the placenta as a result of inadequate transformation of the spiral arteries into

Fig. 47.20 Villi in an old infarct. The villi have a 'ghost-like' appearance whilst the villous trophoblast is almost entirely lost. H & E × 360.

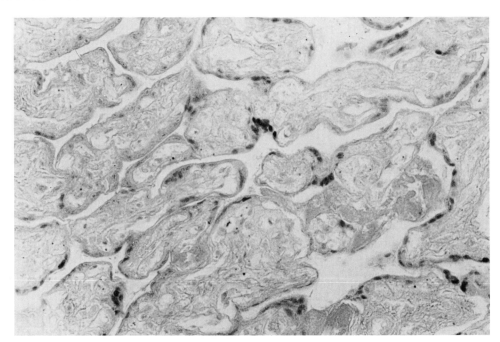

uteroplacental vessels (Robertson et al, 1975; Robertson, 1976, 1981). Thus extensive infarction occurs only against a background of a markedly abnormal maternal vasculature and a restricted maternal blood flow to the placenta and it is these factors, rather than the loss of villi due to infarction, which are the real cause of the fetal complications. The true significance of extensive placental infarction is therefore that it is the visible hallmark of a severely compromised circulation to the placenta. It is true that the situation is further worsened in such cases by infarction being superimposed on a placenta, the functional reserve of which may have been already dissipated by uteroplacental ischaemia, but the infarction per se is not the cause of the fetal complications and would be of no consequence if it occurred in a placenta with an adequate maternal blood supply.

Fetal artery thrombosis

This lesion is seen macroscopically as a roughly triangular area of pallor within the placental substance, the base of the triangle abutting onto the basal plate (Fig. 47.21): there is no alteration in parenchymal texture or consistence. Histological examination reveals a sharply localized area of avascular villi (Fig. 47.22) which contrast starkly with their immediately adjacent fully vascularized neighbours (Fig. 47.23): the stroma of these villi becomes fibrotic and the fetal vessels undergo an obliterative sclerosis though their trophoblast remains intact and viable. An organizing, or organized, thrombosis is seen occluding a fetal stem artery at the apex of the lesion.

The cause of fetal artery thrombosis is usually unknown but Kraus (1993) and Rayne & Kraus (1993) have suggested that they are indicative of a hypercoagulable state in the fetus and may be associated with a maternal coagulopathy, such as that found in association with anticardiolipin antibodies or protein S deficiency. Fetal artery thrombosis is a relatively common condition, found in about 4% of placentas from live births, and is usually clinically unimportant. The banal nature of this abnor-

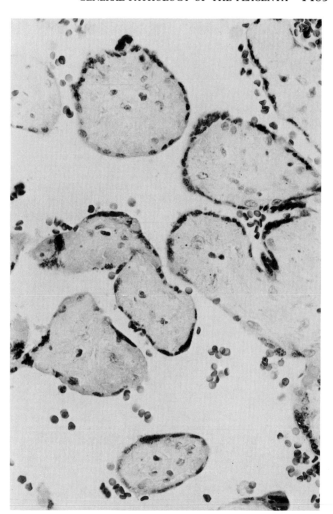

Fig. 47.22 Avascular villi resulting from a fetal artery thrombosis. H & E × 360. (From Fox, 1978. Reproduced by permission of W. B. Saunders.)

mality is still further evidence of the functional reserve capacity of the placenta, for even lesions in which 20–30% of the villi are rendered avascular are not associated with any effect on fetal well-being, despite the obvious fact that the avascular villi are effectively excluded from playing any rôle in maternofetal transfer activity. Very occasionally, it is true, placentas are encountered in which multiple occlusions of fetal vessels, again occurring for no discernible cause, result in 50%, or more, of the villi being rendered avascular (Fox, 1966): under such circumstances fetal death can, and does, occur, for the placenta can not withstand a deletion of villous tissue of this magnitude.

Primary defect in placental growth

It is widely assumed that a below normal villous mass may result in inadequate growth of the placenta, that the physiological capacity of the placenta is related to its weight and that the functional deficiencies of a small placenta will restrict fetal growth: in other words, a small

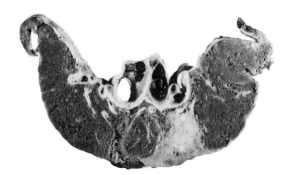

Fig. 47.21 A localized area of pallor in a placenta, due to a fetal artery thrombosis. (From Fox, 1978. Reproduced by permission of W. B. Saunders.)

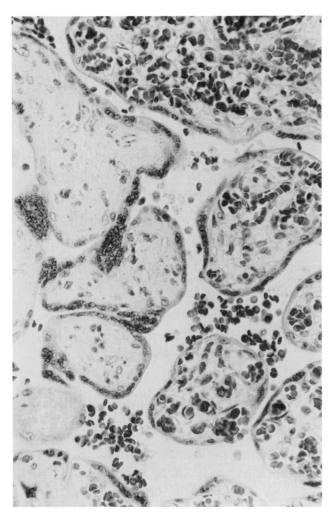

Fig. 47.23 Avascular villi consequent on thrombosis of a fetal stem artery (left) contrast with their immediately adjacent fully vascularized neighbours (right). H & E × 360. (From Fox, 1978. Reproduced by permission of W. B. Saunders.)

placenta will result in an abnormally small fetus. However, a knowledge of placental weight is, in itself, of little or no value, especially when taking into account the extreme difficulty of obtaining an accurate assessment of placental mass and the grossly inaccurate and misleading nature of the values obtained by weighing the placenta in the delivery room or in the laboratory (Fox, 1978). Placental : fetal weight ratios are clearly more meaningful but, although there have been a number of reviews of the significance of this ratio (Little, 1961; Thomson et al, 1969; Lemtis & Hadrich, 1974; Molteni et al, 1978), it would not, despite claims to the contrary (Teasdale, 1982), be an undue oversimplification to draw the conclusion that these studies suggest only that small babies have small placentas and large babies have large placentas. It then becomes almost a matter of faith whether one believes that the baby is small because the placenta is small or that the placenta is small because the baby is small.

Certain facts suggest, however, that placental mass is unlikely to be a limiting factor for fetal growth. Thus if fetal weight were narrowly limited by placental mass this would imply that the term placenta does not have any functional reserve capacity. Simple pathological studies of such trivial lesions as perivillous fibrin deposition and fetal artery thrombosis indicate that this is most unlikely to be true whilst experimental studies, involving either surgical reduction of placental mass (Cefalo et al, 1977; Robinson et al, 1979) or artificially increased fetal oxygen consumption (Lorijn & Longo, 1980), have confirmed the striking functional reserve of the placenta. Furthermore, the placenta has a normally unrealized potential for further incremental growth, a fact indicated by the unduly large placentas found in conditions such as pregnancy at high altitude, severe maternal anaemia and maternal heart failure (Clavero-Nunez, 1963; Beischer et al, 1970; Kruger & Arias-Stella, 1970; Agboola, 1975; Godfrey et al, 1991).

The combination of a considerable reserve capacity and of a potential for further growth makes it unlikely that placental mass limits fetal weight, the placenta, in fact, usually being small because the baby is small. Under these circumstances the placenta, although small, has probably reached a size sufficient either to meet the nutritional and gaseous needs of the small fetus or one which is fully capable of transferring to the fetus the limited supply of maternal oxygen and nutrients. A knowledge of placental weight is therefore of very little value.

Haematomas and thrombi (Fig. 47.24)

Retroplacental haematoma

This is a haematoma which lies between, and separates, the basal plate of the placenta and the uterine wall: it is apparent on the maternal aspect of the placenta and bulges up towards the fetal surface with compression and often, though not invariably, infarction of the overlying villous tissue. An old haematoma is firmly adherent to the placenta and although a fresh one may become detached during delivery it leaves a characteristic crateriform depression in the maternal surface: it should be noted that adherent clot is always easily separated from the placenta and does not indent the surface.

Retroplacental haematomas have been variously attributed to rupture of a maternal uteroplacental artery or obstruction of the placental venous outflow; placental bed biopsies have suggested that, in some cases, the bleeding may originate from vascular malformations in the placental bed (Dommisse & Tiltman, 1992). They are found in approximately 5% of all placentas, though their incidence is increased threefold in those from pre-eclamptic women (Fox, 1978); there is no consistent relationship between the presence of a retroplacental haematoma and a clinical history of abruptio placentae.

The haematoma separates the overlying villi from the maternal blood vessels, but many haematomas are small,

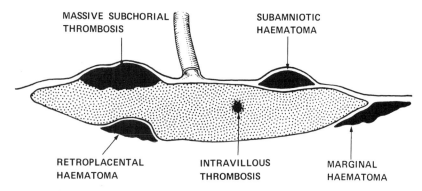

MASSIVE SUBCHORIAL
THROMBOSIS

SUBAMNIOTIC
HAEMATOMA

RETROPLACENTAL
HAEMATOMA

INTRAVILLOUS
THROMBOSIS

MARGINAL
HAEMATOMA

Fig. 47.24   Diagram of the sites of the various haematomas and thrombi that can occur in and around the placenta. (From Fox, 1978. Reproduced by permission of W. B. Saunders.)

detected only on pathological examination and of no clinical significance. It is, however, not surprising that large lesions, in which 40% or more of the villous population is acutely deprived of its blood supply, are associated with a high incidence of fetal hypoxia and death.

Subamniotic haematoma

This occurs on the fetal surface of the placenta as a plum-coloured tumefaction which lifts the amnion off from the chorion. Most are fresh and result from tearing of surface chorionic veins by excessive cord traction during delivery. Old haematomas, which are often accompanied by thrombosis of chorionic veins, tend to be associated with a low birth weight (DeSa, 1971), though the nature of this relationship is far from clear.

Marginal haematoma

This is seen as a crescentic lesion at one edge of the placenta: the haematoma is usually also adherent to the maternal surface of the immediately adjacent membranes. There is good evidence that haematomas of this type occur in cases where the placenta is partially implanted in the lower uterine segment but with its lateral margin being some distance from the internal os, i.e. a lateral placenta praevia (Wilkin, 1965). Marginal bleeding is thought to result from rupture of venous channels at the lower placental margin during the process of obliteration of the lower uterine segment. The lesion is of no clinical importance.

Massive subchorial thrombosis

This lesion, also known as a Breus' mole, is a thrombus, measuring more than 1 cm in thickness, which separates the chorionic plate from the underlying villous tissue (Fig. 47.25). The thrombus is often lobulated or bulbous and may distort the fetal surface of the placenta by forming bulging protuberances into the amniotic cavity.

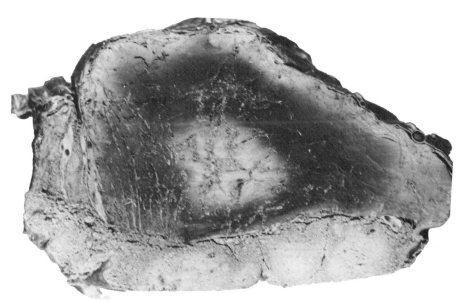

Fig. 47.25   A massive subchorial haematoma. The chorionic plate (above) has been completely stripped off from the villous tissue (below) by a massive accumulation of thrombus.

The thrombus probably originates from maternal blood and it has been speculated that it results from extensive obliteration of the venous channels draining the intervillous space. Massive subchorial thrombi are usually found in placentas from abortuses but Shanklin & Scott (1975) have described seven examples associated with the delivery, usually prematurely, of a liveborn child: their clinical significance is not known.

Not all subchorial thrombi are massive and although small lesions of this type have attracted little attention it is probable that they are more common than is usually realized: such lesions are, however, probably of no clinical significance (Pearlstone & Baxi, 1993).

Intervillous thrombosis

This is a villus-free nodular thrombus within the intervillous space (Fig. 47.26). The thrombi usually lie approximately midway between the maternal and fetal surfaces of the placenta, measure between 1 cm and 2 cm in diameter and are soft and dark red when fresh, such early lesions also being known as Kline's haemorrhages: as the thrombi age they become gradually converted into hard, white, laminated plaques.

Thrombi of this type are found in up to 40% of all placentas (Fox, 1978), contain an admixture of fetal and maternal blood (Kaplan et al, 1982) and mark a site of fetal bleeding into the intervillous space. Fetal haemorrhage is almost certainly a consequence of rupture of a villus at a site of syncytial attenuation and it is probable that thrombosis occurs because of release of a thromboplastic substance from the site of villous syncytial damage (Batcup et al, 1983). Large intervillous thrombi may be associated with elevated maternal serum alphafetoprotein levels (Salafia et al, 1988; Jauniaux et al, 1990).

Miscellaneous macroscopic abnormalities

These include subchorionic fibrin plaques, septal cysts and grossly visible calcification, all of which are devoid of functional significance. It is probably worth stressing that placental calcification, often regarded as evidence of either

placental senescence or 'degeneration', is of no pathological or clinical importance. Calcification is not more common, or extreme, in placentas from prolonged or abnormal pregnancies than it is in placentas from uncomplicated term pregnancies and is not associated with any fetal complications (Fox, 1978). The cause of the calcification is unknown but it occurs most commonly in first pregnancies and its incidence is related directly to low maternal age, high maternal socio-economic status and delivery during the summer months (Tindall & Scott, 1969; Russell & Fielden, 1969; Brandt, 1973). Placental calcification appears to occur earlier in pregnancy in cigarette smokers (Brown et al, 1988).

HISTOLOGICAL ABNORMALITIES OF THE PLACENTA

Villous abnormalities

It is preferable to classify villous abnormalities on a functional, rather than a purely morphological, basis. These may be grouped into:

1. Abnormalities of villous maturation and differentiation
2. Changes secondary to a reduced maternal uteroplacental blood flow
3. Changes secondary to a reduced fetal villous blood flow
4. Abnormalities of unknown pathogenesis.

Abnormalities of villous maturation and differentiation

During the nine months of a normal gestation there is a progressive change in the predominant type of villus seen on histological examination of the placenta, this being a morphological expression of the continuing growth and evolution of the villous tree (Kaufmann, 1982). Most of the villi present in the first trimester are stem villi whilst intermediate-type villi dominate during the second trimester: from about the 30th week of gestation terminal villi (Fig. 47.27) begin to bud off from the intermediate villi and these form the bulk of the villous population in the term placenta (Kaufmann et al, 1979; Kaufmann, 1981; Schiebler & Kaufmann, 1981). Histologically this changing pattern is reflected in a progressive change from large villi with small, centrally placed, fetal vessels to small villi with sinusoidally dilated fetal capillaries which lie in an immediately subtrophoblastic position. These histological changes are often regarded as being manifestations of an ageing process but are, in reality, indicative of the maturation, not so much of the villi themselves, but of the villous tree. The net result of these villous changes is a marked increase in the surface area of the trophoblast which is in contact with the maternal blood in the intervillous space, an approximation to each other of the maternal and fetal circulatory systems, an increased concentration gradient between maternal and fetal blood and

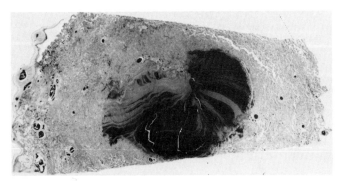

Fig. 47.26 A fresh, red laminated intervillous thrombus.

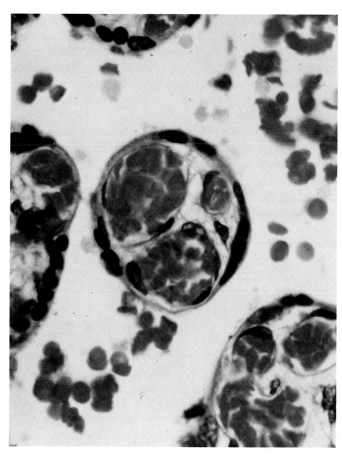

Fig. 47.27 A typical terminal villus. It is small and sinusoidally dilated vessels occupy most of its cross sectional area. H & E × 780. (From Fox, 1978. Reproduced by permission of W. B. Saunders.)

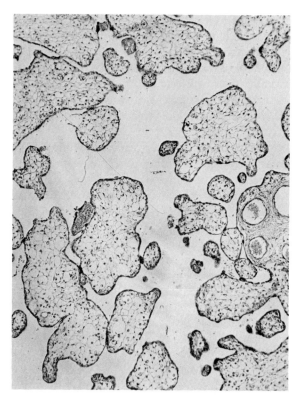

Fig. 47.28 Villi in a placenta from an uncomplicated pregnancy terminating spontaneously at the 36th week of gestation. There is, for this stage of pregnancy, a marked deficiency of terminal villi, most of the villi being of the intermediate type. H & E × 54. (From Fox, 1978. Reproduced by permission of W. B. Saunders.)

a crowding of flow lines, the small terminal villi being the form of villous structure which is optimally adapted for maternofetal transfer; it has been estimated that this process of maturation of the villous tree increases the transfer capacity of the placenta sixfold between the 20th and 40th weeks of gestation (Aherne, 1975). It is thus clear that villous tree maturation is essential for fully effective functioning of the placenta and the corollary of this is that a failure of the villous tree to undergo full maturation, with a resulting paucity of terminal villi at term, will result in a decreased functional efficiency of the placenta. It is therefore not surprising that a deficiency of the terminal villi (Fig. 47.28) towards the end of gestation (a phenomenon usually simply classed as 'villous immaturity') is associated with a high incidence of fetal growth retardation (Becker, 1975, 1981). The relatively simple concept of villous immaturity has, however, been expanded in recent years into an elaborate subclassification based on the use of such terms as 'arrested ramification', 'discordant retardation', 'intercalary defective ramification', 'centroperipheral discontinuity of vascularization' and 'concordant retardation', it being suggested that each of these particular patterns, which are not easily recognizable to

many students of placental pathology, represents a particular form of maturational arrest resulting from an insult offered to the placenta at a specific stage of gestation (Kloos & Vogel, 1974; Hopker & Ohlendorf, 1979). It remains to be proven however that this complex classification is founded on any firm basis of fact.

If it is simply accepted that inadequate maturation of the villous tree is usually easily recognizable in the term placenta by the preponderance of large villi with abundant loose stroma and relatively small vessels which have not moved out fully to a peripheral position then a good association does exist between the presence of this abnormality and poor fetal nutrition, though it would be remarked that most small for gestational age infants have fully mature placentas. It should also be noted that this association only holds if there is a generalized immaturity of the villi for in all term placentas a few highly immature villi are always to be found scattered amongst an otherwise fully mature villous population, usually in the centre of a lobule (Bleyl & Stefek, 1965; Fox, 1968). These are an indication of continuing placental growth with the formation of fresh villi.

It is not always fully appreciated that villous maturation

is accompanied by progressive topographical differentiation of the villous trophoblast, the two processes being intertwined though independent of each other. The villous trophoblast has both a transfer and a synthetic function and it would be reasonable to expect that there must be some spatial segregation of these disparate activities within a single tissue, different areas of the syncytiotrophoblast becoming specifically adapted for the optimal fulfilment of one particular activity. During the first trimester the villous trophoblast appears remarkably homogeneous at the lightmicroscopic level but electron-microscopy shows that even at this early stage there is ultrastructural evidence of regional functional differentiation (Dempsey & Luse, 1971). In the term placenta the morphological evidence of functional segregation becomes more overt and is indicated most prominently by the development of vasculosyncytial membranes (Fig. 47.29), these being attenuated, anuclear areas of syncytiotrophoblast which overlie, and appear almost to fuse with, the

wall of an adjacent dilated fetal villous capillary (Getzowa & Sadowsky, 1950). The suggestion that the vasculosyncytial membranes represent the principal site of, and are specialized areas for, maternofetal oxygen transfer was originally based on the thinning of the trophoblast but it is now recognized that gas transfer across the placenta is flow limited rather than membrane limited (Longo, 1981): the evidence for the membranous areas being specialized zones rests, however, on more than just the localized thinning for these areas differ both histochemically and ultrastructurally from the non-membranous areas of the trophoblast (Amstutz, 1960; Burgos & Rodriguez, 1966; Fox & Agrafojo-Blanco, 1974), whilst there is a good correlation between a paucity of vasculosyncytial membranes and a high risk of fetal hypoxia (Fox, 1967c; 1968). A lack of vasculosyncytial membranes indicates a failure of trophoblastic differentiation but it should be stressed that such a phenomenon is not simply a manifestation of failure of villous maturation for placentas are sometimes encountered in which the villi are in all other respects fully mature but lack vasculosyncytial membranes, a finding indicative of an isolated failure of trophoblastic differentiation. On the other hand, it is common for placentas in which there has been a failure of maturation of the villous tree to also have inadequate membrane formation, there appearing to be in this instance a combined failure of the two closely associated processes of maturation and differentiation.

It should be noted here that, as already remarked, the histological features which characterize both maturation and differentiation within the villi have been widely misinterpreted as ageing changes, thus leading to the tenaciously held belief that the placenta progressively ages during the course of a normal pregnancy and is, at term, in, or on the verge of, a decline into morphological and functional senescence (Rosso, 1976). A critical review of the evidence for placental ageing reveals, however, little or no indication that the placenta undergoes a true ageing process and indicates that the mature placenta is far from being senescent in either morphological or functional terms (Fox, 1979a, 1982; Fox & Faulk, 1981).

Changes secondary to a reduced maternal uteroplacental blood flow

Villi in placentas subjected to a reduced maternal uteroplacental blood flow, e.g. in severe maternal preeclampsia, show a consistent and characteristic pattern of abnormalities which is identical to that noted in villous tissue grown in vitro under conditions of low oxygen tension (Fox, 1970; MacLennon et al, 1972). There is an undue prominence and number of villous cytotrophoblastic cells (Fig. 47.30), together with irregular thickening of the trophoblastic basement membrane: although the syncytiotrophoblast usually appears remarkably nor-

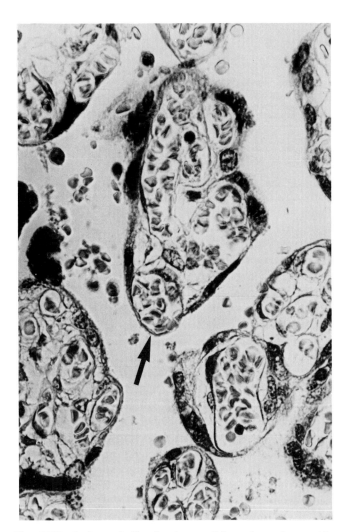

Fig. 47.29 A placental villus showing a well-formed vasculosyncytial membrane (arrowed). H & E × 464.

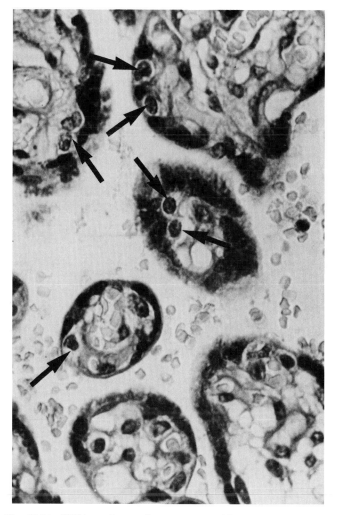

Fig. 47.30 Villi in a placenta from a woman with severe pre-eclampsia. Many prominent cytotrophoblastic cells (arrowed) are seen. PAS × 520.

mal on lightmicroscopy, small focal areas of syncytial necrosis are seen on ultrastructural examination (Jones & Fox, 1980).

The cytotrophoblastic cells are the trophoblastic stem cells for, even during rapid periods of trophoblastic growth, it is only in these cells that DNA synthesis and mitotic activity occurs, the syncytiotrophoblast appearing to be formed by a breaking down of the limiting membrane of the cytotrophoblastic cells (Carter, 1964). The electronmicroscope has also allowed for the recognition of the 'intermediate' type of cytotrophoblastic cell which has a cytoplasmic complexity lying somewhere between that of the simple, rather primitive, resting cytotrophoblastic cell, with its paucity of cytoplasmic organelles, and that of the organelle-rich syncytiotrophoblast (Tighe et al, 1967): such cells are regarded as being in the process of conversion into syncytiotrophoblast. The cytotrophoblastic stem cells can therefore be considered as forming a germinative zone though one which is, in the later stages of pregnancy, largely quiescent, the cytotrophoblastic cells becoming

progressively less numerous and prominent as gestation proceeds; their inactivity at term indicates that there is little need for the formation of fresh trophoblast at this time.

If, however, the necessity of forming new syncytiotrophoblast arises, as is the case when this tissue suffers ischaemic damage as a result of a reduced maternal blood flow, the germinative zone will be reactivated and the cytotrophoblastic cells proliferate in an attempt to repair and replace injured syncytial tissue: thus the cytotrophoblastic cells become more numerous and unusually prominent whilst mitotic figures are seen with modest frequency, all features suggesting a resurgence of activity. That there is a true proliferation of these cells has been confirmed by Arnholdt et al (1991) using a monoclonal antibody to Ki67. At the electronoptical level many of the proliferating cells are seen to be of the intermediate type, this indicating rapid and continuing conversion into syncytiotrophoblast, and freshly formed syncytial tissue can sometimes be recognized. This repair process is a highly successful one for it often requires prolonged search to detect residual focal areas of syncytial damage at the ultrastructural level (Jones & Fox, 1980).

The trophoblastic basement membrane thickening which is seen in the villi of placentas subjected to ischaemia is probably an incidental by-product of the cytotrophoblastic cell hyperplasia for basement membrane protein is almost certainly secreted, in part at least, by these cells and an unusual degree of proliferative activity on their part would therefore be accompanied by an excessive production of basement membrane material: this is a situation akin to that found in diabetic microangiopathy, in which thickening of the capillary basement membrane is secondary to an increased turnover of endothelial cells (Vracko & Benditt, 1970).

The essential response of the placenta to ischaemia is therefore a reparative one, with gross trophoblastic damage being efficiently repaired.

Changes secondary to a reduced fetal blood flow

These are seen in their purest form in the localized group of villi which, whilst fully oxygenated from the maternal blood, have been deprived of their fetal circulation by thrombosis of a fetal stem artery: such villi invariably show stromal fibrosis and an excess formation of syncytial knots and it is of interest to note that identical changes occur in the monkey placenta after ligation of a fetal stem artery (Myers & Fujikura, 1968). These changes, stromal fibrosis and excess syncytial knot formation, are seen in generalized form whenever there is an overall reduction of fetal perfusion of the placenta as occurs, for example, in some cases of prolonged pregnancy, and are invariably found as a post mortem change (Fig. 47.31) in placentas from fetuses which have been dead in utero for several days

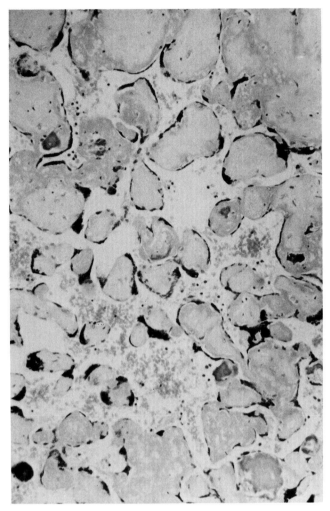

Fig. 47.31 Villi in placenta from a case of longstanding fetal intrauterine death. The villi show stromal fibrosis and a marked excess of syncytial knots. H & E × 200. (From Fox, 1978. Reproduced by permission of W. B. Saunders.)

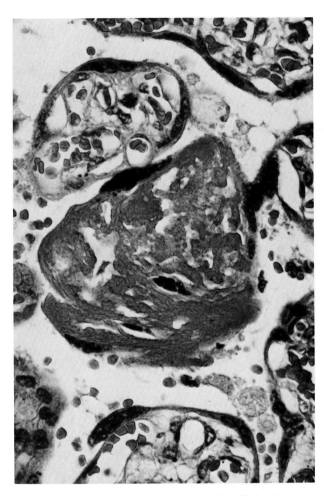

Fig. 47.32 A villus which has undergone complete fibrinoid necrosis. PAS × 600.

or weeks before delivery (Fox, 1978; Genest, 1992). Why these particular changes should result from an impairment of fetal blood flow through the placenta is unknown but the placental villi do not in any way depend upon the fetal blood supply for either their oxygenation or supply of nutrients and hence there is no good reason why a reduced fetal perfusion should affect the functional activity of the placenta: it is therefore not surprising that neither stromal fibrosis nor excess syncytial knot formation can be correlated with any evidence of adverse effects, during life, on the fetus (Fox, 1978).

It should, perhaps, be noted that syncytial knots, which are focal clumps of syncytial nuclei that protrude into the intervillous space from the villous surface, are not, as is often thought to be the case, a manifestation of any degenerative change in the trophoblast or a reaction to uteroplacental ischaemia (Jones & Fox, 1977; Fox, 1978):

their appearance in the placenta as gestation progresses is a time-related phenomenon but is not a true ageing change.

Abnormalities of unknown pathogenesis

Prominent amongst these is fibrinoid necrosis of placental villi. The first stage in the evolution of this lesion is the appearance of a small nodule of homogeneous, acidophilic, PAS-positive material at one point in the villous trophoblast. This nodule progressively enlarges as fresh fibrinoid material is laid down on its deep aspect so as to form a mass which gradually bulges into, and compresses, the villous stroma, this process continuing until the whole villus is converted into a fibrinoid nodule (Fig. 47.32). The syncytiotrophoblast of the affected villus is normal in the early stages of evolution of this lesion but eventually atrophies and is largely lost, though even at a late stage a few remnants of this tissue remain around the periphery of the fibrinoid material. This particular villous abnormality remains as something of an enigma: there is clear evidence that the fibrinoid material appears first in a cytotrophoblastic cell and is not due to deposition within the villus of fibrin derived from the maternal blood in the intervillous space (Wilkin, 1965; Liebhart, 1971) but how and why it develops is far from clear. The lesion has been variously attributed to an immunological reaction within villous tissue (McCormick et al, 1971) and to amyloid deposition as an ageing change (Burstein et al, 1973): it is now certain that the fibrinoid material is not amyloid whilst the possibility that the fibrinoid material is deposited as a result of an antigen-antibody reaction within villous tissue currently receives little support but has not yet been totally excluded. A pathologist noting an excess of villi showing this change in a placenta is not currently in a position to draw any conclusions from this observation.

Villous oedema (Fig. 47.33) is of unknown origin: most accounts of placental pathology indicate that this abnormality is easy to recognize but, in practice, its distinction from villous immaturity is difficult and there is no doubt

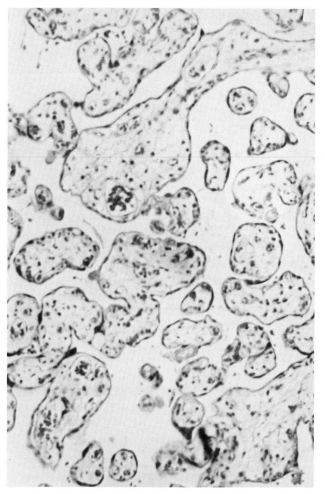

Fig. 47.33 Oedematous villi in a full-term placenta from a diabetic woman. H & E × 120. (From Fox, 1978. Reproduced by permission of W. B. Saunders.)

that normal intermediate villi are often wrongly classed as oedematous (Kaufmann et al, 1987; Benirschke & Kaufmann, 1995). Nevertheless villous oedema does occur, though it can probably only be recognized when of quite marked degree; under such circumstances the presence of villous oedema correlates well with an increased placental water content (Barker et al, 1994).

It is clearly tempting to attribute villous oedema to a functional inadequacy of the villous fetal circulation but no firm evidence exists to support this view. It is usually considered that villous oedema is of no functional importance but it has been suggested that the increased size of the placental villi decreases the capacity of the intervillous space and hence restricts maternal blood flow to the placenta (Alvarez et al, 1972; Kovalovszki et al, 1990): haemodynamic studies to support this assertion are currently lacking. Naeye et al (1983) also considered villous oedema to be indicative of fetal hypoxia but Sen-Schwarz et al (1989) could not confirm this.

In some placentas there is an obvious excess of fetal vessels within the terminal villi, a condition described as chorangiosis by Altshuler (1984). For recognition of this entity Altshuler suggested that there should be at least 10 different lightmicroscopic fields in 10 different placental areas with 10 villi that have 10 capillary lumens in each villus. He correlated this villous abnormality with a poor neonatal outcome and suggested that it represented a response to decreased maternal uteroplacental blood flow. There has, however, been little further study of this abnormality and its significance remains uncertain.

Abnormalities of the fetal stem arteries

Fibromuscular sclerosis

This is characterized by a marked hyperplasia of the fibrous and muscular tissue of the media with a proliferation of intimal fibrous tissue which grows into, and eventually obliterates, the vascular lumen (Fig. 47.34). Fibromuscular sclerosis is seen in localized form in stem arteries supplying areas of villous infarction and in stem arteries distal to an occluding thrombus whilst a generalized fibromuscular sclerosis of the fetal stem arteries is found only in placentas from stillbirths, being absent from placentas of fresh stillbirths but becoming increasingly more prominent as the time interval between fetal demise and delivery increases (Fox, 1978; Genest, 1992). These observations point inescapably to the conclusion that fibromuscular sclerosis is a reactive change consequent upon a cessation of fetal blood flow through the affected vessels.

Obliterative endarteritis

This term is applied to an abnormality of the fetal stem

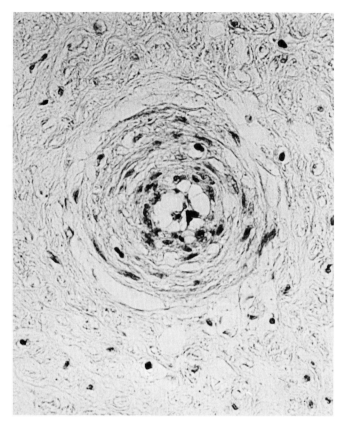

Fig. 47.34 Fibromuscular sclerosis of a fetal stem artery in a placenta from a case of intrauterine fetal death. H & E × 650.

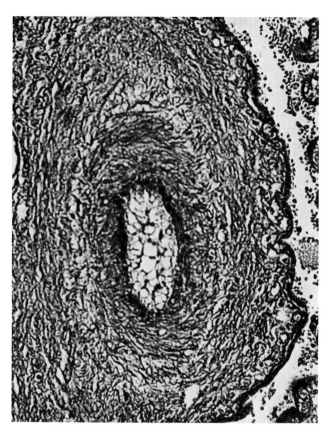

Fig. 47.35 Obliterative endarteritis in a fetal stem artery. PAS × 150. (From Fox, 1978. Reproduced by permission of W. B. Saunders.)

arteries of the placenta which is characterized by apparent swelling and proliferation of clear endothelial cells with narrowing, sometimes to an extreme degree, of the vascular lumen (Fig. 47.35). Ultrastructural studies of stem arteries showing this change have revealed, however, that the apparent swelling and proliferation of the endothelial cells is due to their partial displacement into the vascular lumen by herniations of medial smooth muscle cell cytoplasm into the intima: the clarity of the apparently swollen endothelial cells is a fixation artifact (van der Veen et al, 1982). An obliterative endarteritis appears therefore not to be a pathological lesion in the true sense of the word for the smooth muscle herniation is almost certainly a reflection of, and due to, vasoconstriction. If vasoconstriction is prolonged it can lead to widespread sclerosis of small vessels in the distal part of the villous tree (Giles et al, 1985; McCowan et al, 1988; Fok et al, 1990), a change associated with an increased resistance in the placental vascular bed (Trudinger et al, 1985b; Bracero et al, 1989; Zacutti et al, 1992; Hitschold et al, 1993).

Constriction of the fetal stem arteries is an indirect response to diminished maternal uteroplacental blood flow (Stock et al, 1980) and is part of an attempt by the deprived fetus to divert blood to the cerebral and coronary circulations.

PLACENTAL CHANGES IN SPECIFIC COMPLICATIONS OF PREGNANCY

The literature on this topic is vast: it is also contradictory, confusing, chaotic and, all too often, totally unscientific. This has been largely due to the study of too few placentas in many series, the widespread lack of any control groups, the consideration of placentas from pregnancies of varying duration as a homogeneous group and a failure to examine a particular complication in isolation: this last defect has been a particular source of unwarranted conclusions and is seen, for example, in studies of placentas from diabetic women in which those from otherwise uncomplicated pregnancies were grouped together with those in whom there was also superimposed pre-eclampsia. This literature has been reviewed in detail elsewhere (Fox, 1978; Fox & Jones, 1983) and does not merit reconsideration here, the findings described below being largely based upon the personal observations of the author and his colleagues.

Maternal disorders

Pre-eclampsia

Placentas from pre-eclamptic women tend, on average,

to be smaller than those from uncomplicated pregnancies but the decrease is only slight and a proportion of such placentas are unusually large: the placental : fetal weight ratio is generally increased (Nummi, 1972; Holzl et al, 1974; Soma et al, 1982). There is no excess of extrachorial placentation and the incidence of placental infarction ranges from about 33% in cases of mild pre-eclampsia to approximately 60% in patients with the severe form of the disease: extensive infarction (involving more than 10% of the parenchyma) is found in about 30% of placentas from cases of severe pre-eclampsia but is not a feature of the milder forms of this disease. It will be appreciated that most placentas from pre-eclamptic women therefore either show no infarction or are only infarcted to an extent too limited to be of functional significance. Retroplacental haematomas are found unduly frequently, occurring in about 12–15% of cases, but there is no excess of any other gross lesion.

Histologically (Fig. 47.36) the villi are usually of normal maturity for the length of the gestational period and the only consistent abnormalities are hyperplasia of the villous cytotrophoblastic cells and thickening of the villous trophoblastic basement membrane. In some cases there is also a degree of fetal underperfusion, probably because of vasoconstriction of the fetal stem arteries (manifest as an 'obliterative endarteritis'), and this adds an element of stromal fibrosis and excess syncytial knot formation to the histological picture.

At the ultrastructural level the cytotrophoblastic hyperplasia and the basement membrane thickening are confirmed whilst the villous syncytiotrophoblast shows patchy focal necrosis (Fig. 47.37), loss and distortion of microvilli on the free surface, diminished pinocytotic activity, a reduced number of secretory droplets and dilatation of the rough endoplasmic reticulum (Jones & Fox, 1980; Soma et al, 1982).

The changes seen in the placenta of the pre-eclamptic woman therefore exemplify those, previously described, which are associated with a reduced maternal uteroplacental blood flow: all the abnormalities in the trophoblast are explicable on this basis whilst the reduced fetal villous perfusion, resulting from fetal artery vasoconstriction, is also probably a response to uteroplacental ischaemia for it has been shown experimentally that a decreased maternal blood flow to the placenta results in a marked reduction in fetal placental blood flow (Stock et al, 1980).

That maternal uteroplacental blood flow is decreased in pre-eclampsia is well established (Browne & Veall, 1953; Dixon et al, 1963; Lippert et al, 1980; Lunell et al, 1982; Campbell et al, 1986; McParland & Pearce, 1988; Steel et al, 1988; Bewley et al, 1991) and the pathological

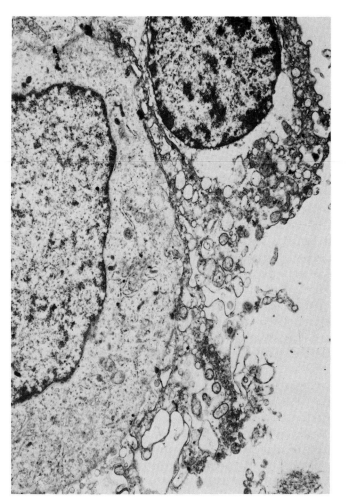

Fig. 47.37 Electronmicrograph of villous trophoblast in a woman with pre-eclampsia. The syncytiotrophoblast is necrotic but an underlying cytotrophoblastic cell appears normal. × 9000. (From Fox, 1978. Reproduced by permission of W. B. Saunders.)

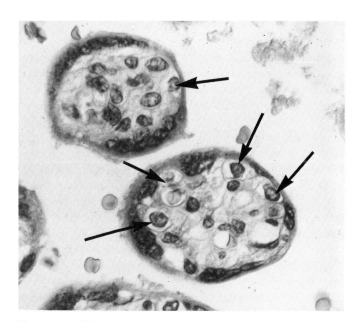

Fig. 47.36 Villi in a term placenta from a woman with severe pre-eclampsia. The villi are of normal maturity but are underperfused and show an excess of cytotrophoblastic cells (arrowed). H & E × 840. (From Fox, 1978. Reproduced by permission of W. B. Saunders.)

basis for this, which is an inadequate transformation by extravillous intravascular trophoblast of the spiral arteries into uteroplacental vessels, has been clearly defined in recent years (see Ch. 48). All the changes seen in placentas from pre-eclamptic patients can reasonably be attributed to this reduction in maternal blood flow and no other pathogenetic factor need be invoked: the functional consequences of the ischaemic damage to the placenta are, however, hard to assess. The reduced syncytial pinocytotic activity is indicative of a decreased transfer capacity whilst the paucity of secretory droplets attests to impaired synthetic activity. Whether, however, these functional changes reflect true syncytial damage or are simply a consequence of a diminished oxygen supply is debatable. It is nevertheless clear that any damaging effects of pre-eclampsia on the placenta are limited by the extremely efficient repair process which the trophoblast mounts against ischaemic attack and it is highly probable that the ill effects of pre-eclampsia on fetal growth, oxygenation and viability are due, not to placental damage, but to an inadequate maternal supply of oxygen and nutrients (Fox, 1988).

The maternal ill effects are thought, by contrast, to be due to the release into the circulation of some substance from the ischaemic placenta which has a damaging effect on maternal endothelial cells (Roberts et al, 1989; Redman, 1991).

Essential hypertension

In most studies of placental abnormalities in hypertensive disease during pregnancy placentas from women with essential hypertension have been grouped together with those from patients with pre-eclampsia and this has led to the effective submergence of any possible differences between the two groups of placentas. In fact the changes seen in the placentas of women suffering from essential hypertension are qualitatively, but not quantitatively, identical to those noted in pre-eclampsia. Thus at the lightmicroscopical level villous cytotrophoblastic hyperplasia and trophoblastic basement membrane thickening are seen whilst on electronmicroscopy abnormalities identical in nature to those observed in pre-eclampsia are noted: it is of particular interest, however, that these changes are much less marked in placentas from women with essential hypertension than is the case in placentas from pre-eclamptic patients (Jones & Fox, 1981).

The placental abnormalities in essential hypertension can, in their entirety, be attributed to uteroplacental ischaemia (Fox, 1988). A reduced uteroplacental blood flow has been noted in essential hypertension (Browne & Veall, 1953) and it must be assumed that this results from the increased vascular resistance offered by the uterine vasculature, in which a hyperplastic arteriosclerosis has been described (Robertson, 1976; Sheppard & Bonnar,

1980a). This hyperplastic change is not seen in the intradecidual portion of the spiral arteries of the placental bed, which undergo physiological change in the normal manner, and is either absent or minimal in the intramyometrial segments of these vessels; it is reasonable to assume, however, that this vascular abnormality is present in the radial arteries and, although the effects of the increased vascular resistance may be at least partially offset by the increased pulse pressure, there is probably some limitation of blood flow. The ischaemic damage suffered by the placenta in essential hypertension is, however, relatively slight and most unlikely to influence adversely placental function: it is not surprising that uncomplicated essential hypertension in pregnancy is not associated with any excess incidence of fetal growth retardation or of perinatal mortality (Chamberlain et al, 1978; MacGillivray & Campbell, 1980).

Diabetes mellitus

The placenta of the diabetic woman tends, on average, to be heavier than that of the non-diabetic (Thomson et al, 1969; Nummi, 1972) whilst a small proportion accord with the traditional belief that such placentas are unduly heavy, bulky and oedematous; nevertheless many placentas from diabetic patients are similar both in weight and in general macroscopic appearances to those from non-diabetics. Fetal artery thrombosis, usually involving only one vessel, occurs unduly frequently in these placentas but otherwise there is no excess of gross lesions.

About 40% of placentas from diabetic patients have a villous pattern which is normal for the length of the gestational period: in the remaining 60% the maturity of the villous tree is at odds with the length of the pregnancy, some appearing unduly immature and others showing an apparently accelerated maturation, there being no consistent trend which can be discerned in this discordance. Villous oedema is common but villous vascularity is very variable: in many placentas the villi are normally vascularized, in some they are hypovascular and poorly perfused whilst in others the villous vessels are numerous and prominent. Asmussen (1982a,b) attributes this latter finding to capillary proliferation and regards it as a manifestation of fetal diabetic microangiopathy, a view not fully plausible. Villous cytotrophoblast cells are often numerous and prominent whilst the trophoblastic basement membrane commonly shows a moderate degree of focal or diffuse thickening. In those villi which are poorly perfused some degree of stromal fibrosis and excess syncytial knot formation are seen.

At the ultrastructural level small, scattered foci of syncytial necrosis (Fig. 47.38) are noted (Jones & Fox, 1976a) but most of the syncytium appears fully viable and the microvilli on its free border are normal in number, size and shape. The syncytial rough endoplasmic reticulum

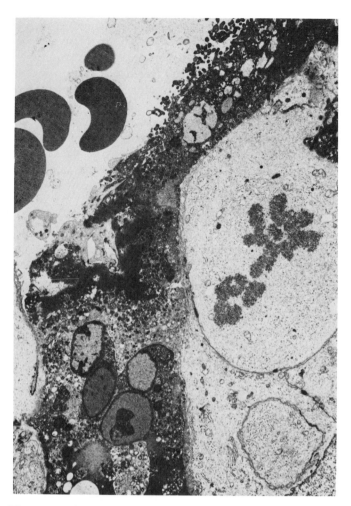

Fig. 47.38 Electronmicrograph of villous trophoblast in a placenta from a diabetic woman. A focal area of syncytial necrosis is seen and below this a cytotrophoblastic cell is undergoing mitotic division. × 4500. (From Fox, 1978. Reproduced by permission of W. B. Saunders.)

tends to be a little dilated but pinocytotic activity is either normal or augmented whilst the number of secretory droplets is often increased. The excess of villous cytotrophoblastic cells is also apparent at the electronmicroscopic level and most of these cells are of the intermediate type.

The pathological findings apply to placentas from women with well-established diabetes mellitus but it is of particular interest to note that qualitatively identical abnormalities are seen in placentas from women suffering from gestational (Class A) diabetes (Jones & Fox, 1976b; Fox 1979b); although the changes seen in the placenta of the frankly diabetic woman tend to be more marked and to occur with greater consistency than do those in the gestational diabetic's placenta there is nevertheless a degree of overlap and the morphological abnormalities in the placenta of a woman with mild, excellently controlled, transitory gestational diabetes may be as marked as those in a placenta of a woman suffering from longstanding, moderately controlled, overt diabetes.

It is clear that in diabetes mellitus the trophoblast is damaged, the syncytial necrosis and the subsequent cytotrophoblastic hyperplasia-repair reaction being eloquent witness of this. The pathogenesis of the syncytial injury is, however, thoroughly obscure. The absence of microvillous damage and the lack of impairment of secretory and transfer activity suggest that the syncytial damage is not due to ischaemia and indeed there is no evidence that there is any significant reduction in maternal uteroplacental blood flow in diabetic women whose pregnancies are not complicated by pre-eclampsia: placental bed biopsies in such patients show no evidence of any maternal vascular lesion (Emmrich et al, 1975), the spiral arteries appear usually to undergo a normal conversion to uteroplacental vessels (Robertson, 1979) and haemodynamic studies have not detected any decrease in maternal blood flow (Lunell & Sarby, 1979). A possible immunological basis for the placental lesions has been canvassed (Galbraith & Faulk, 1979; Hoet et al, 1992) but in our present state of knowledge it has to be assumed that the trophoblastic damage is in some way related to the abnormal metabolic milieu to which this tissue is exposed in the diabetic patient. Jones & Fox (1976a,b) were not, however, able to show that there was any correlation between the severity of extent of the placental abnormalities and either the severity of the diabetic state or the degree of control achieved: more recently Bjork & Persson (1982) have suggested that the placental changes can be better correlated with the degree of metabolic control attained in early pregnancy.

Irrespective of how the placenta is damaged it would not appear that its functional capacity is in any way impaired. Trophoblastic damage is rapidly repaired, secretory and transfer activity appears to be enhanced and there is, quite possibly, increased villous growth (Teasdale, 1981), all features indicating a retention, or even an augmentation, of normal physiological activity.

Intrahepatic cholestasis of pregnancy

Lightmicroscopic examination of placentas from women with intrahepatic cholestasis of pregnancy (IHC) has yielded little of note (Liebhart & Wojcicka, 1970; Fisk & Storey, 1988) but electronmicroscopy has shown a marked increase in syncytial osmiophilic bodies, dilatation of syncytial rough endoplasmic reticulum and an apparent maturational arrest of the cytotrophoblastic cells, the trophoblastic basement membrane appearing normal (Costoya et al, 1980). These findings have been attributed to toxic damage which arrests cytotrophoblastic maturation, inhibits the release of syncytial secretory products and arrests release of protein from the syncytial endoplasmic reticulum (Fox & Jones, 1983). It should be emphasized, however, that the presence of a toxic substance in IHC, though often mooted, has never been proved whilst the further suggestion that the syncytial osmiophilic bodies represent trophoblastic deposition of the abnormal lipoprotein found in maternal serum in IHC (Costoya et al, 1980) is purely speculative.

The significance of the trophoblastic lesions and their contribution to the increased perinatal mortality which characterizes this disorder are currently unknown.

Systemic lupus erythematosus

It has been suggested that the high perinatal mortality rate associated with this disease may be due to placental damage resulting either from immune complex deposition (Grennan et al, 1978) or from ischaemia as a result of a necrotizing vasculitis of the vessels of the placental bed (Abramowsky et al, 1980).

In the light of current knowledge, however, it appears likely that the placental changes described by Abramowsky et al (1980) were due to the presence of circulating antiphospholipid antibodies which, whilst occurring in some otherwise fully normal women, are found unduly frequently in patients with systemic lupus erythematosus. Antiphospholipid antibodies are associated with a high incidence of abortion and preterm fetal death (Triplett, 1992) and studies of placentas from women with these antibodies have demonstrated a high incidence of thrombosis of the maternal uteroplacental vessels, decidual necrosis and extensive infarction (De Wolf et al, 1982; Out et al, 1991; Silver et al, 1992; Rayne & Kraus, 1993; Benirschke & Kaufmann, 1995).

Maternal exposure to toxins

Remarkably little is known about the effects on the placenta of maternal exposure to drugs, toxic chemicals, environmental pollutants or food additives; the only example of possible toxic damage to the placenta which has, so far, received extensive attention has been that due to maternal cigarette smoking.

Cigarette smoking. Cigarette smoking is associated with a decrease in fetal weight but has no significant effect on placental weight, this resulting in a decreased fetoplacental weight ratio (Wingerd et al, 1976; Christianson, 1979; Salafia et al, 1992a). Placentas from smoking mothers do not show any excess of gross lesions and the only reasonably consistent findings on lightmicroscopy are an excess of villous cytotrophoblastic cells and irregular thickening of the trophoblastic basement membrane (Naeye, 1978, 1979; van der Veen & Fox, 1982; van der Velde et al, 1983). Electronmicroscopy confirms the presence of a villous cytotrophoblastic hyperplasia, most of these cells being of the intermediate type and sometimes showing mitotic activity, and of trophoblastic basement membrane thickening (Asmussen, 1978, 1980; van der Veen & Fox, 1982); occasional cytotrophoblastic cells

show, however, marked degenerative changes. Much of the villous syncytiotrophoblast has a normal fine structure but small areas of syncytial necrosis are often present whilst focal areas are seen in which there is a markedly complicated infolding of the surface plasma membrane (Fig. 47.39) with local loss of syncytial cytoplasm and reduction in the number of, and assumption of bizarre forms by, the microvilli. Syncytial pinocytotic activity tends to be reduced and the number of syncytial secretory droplets is decreased. Degenerative changes are sometimes noted in the endothelial cells of the fetal villous vessels.

Many of the abnormalities seen in the placenta of smokers are typical of ischaemic damage and it does appear highly probable that maternal uteroplacental blood flow is reduced in smokers: it has been shown experimentally that infusion of nicotine into pregnant animals results in a sharp decrease in uterine blood flow (Resnik et al, 1979; Suzuki et al, 1980) whilst in the pregnant human the smoking of a single cigarette causes an acute decrease in intervillous blood flow (Lehtovirta & Forss, 1978). These effects of nicotine are presumably mediated by its

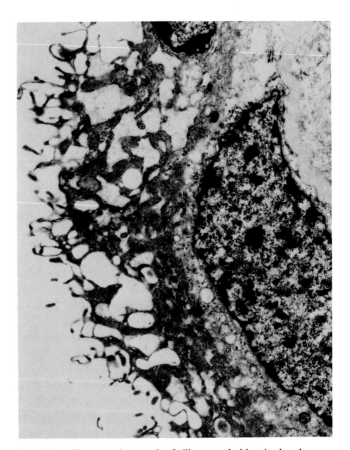

Fig. 47.39 Electronmicrograph of villous trophoblast in the placenta of a cigarette-smoking woman. This shows a focal area of infolding of the free plasma membrane and dilatation of the rough endoplasmic reticulum. The underlying cytotrophoblastic cell is of the intermediate type. × 15 120. (Reproduced by kind permission of the editors and publishers of *Placenta*.)

ability to induce vasoconstriction of the uterine vasculature but not all the placental abnormalities are explicable solely on the basis of ischaemia, this applying particularly to the degenerative changes in cytotrophoblastic cells and to the curious focal infoldings of the syncytial plasma membrane. Damage of this type could be due to any of the two thousand chemical compounds found in tobacco smoke but a good case can be made out for the toxic rôle of cadmiun: cadmium is a known constituent of tobacco smoke, has been shown experimentally to have a particular propensity for causing placental necrosis in pregnant animals (Levin et al, 1981; Di Sant' Agnese et al, 1983) and is present in much higher concentration in placentas from smokers than from non-smokers (Peereboom et al, 1979). It is also possible that exposure of the placenta to the polycyclic hydrocarbons present in tobacco smoke may lead to inhibition of trophoblastic oxidative enzyme systems (Longo, 1980).

Irrespective of the exact manner by which the placenta suffers injury in smokers it seems highly unlikely that the damage inflicted could be held responsible for the increased incidence of low birth weight babies amongst the infants of smoking women. Any ischaemic damage suffered by the villous trophoblast appears to be readily and efficiently repaired, most of the trophoblast appears fully normal and any presumed loss of placental transfer activity could well be compensated for by the increased placental growth which occurs in cigarette smokers. Reduced fetal growth is therefore probably due partly to an inadequate maternal supply of oxygen and nutrients and partly to the direct effects of nicotine and carbon dioxide on the fetus.

Dioxin poisoning. The placental changes occurring after maternal exposure to dioxin have been studied in cases therapeutically aborted after the Seveso disaster in Italy (Remotti et al, 1981). At the lightmicroscopic level no abnormality was seen but electronmicroscopy revealed the presence of numerous osmiophilic microprecipitates in, and deep to, the trophoblastic basement membrane. These bodies contain calcium, iron, potassium and sulphur and it has been suggested that they are evidence of a toxic impairment of the metabolic pathways for transtrophoblastic transfer of mineral elements. The truth or otherwise of this contention and the possible functional significance, if any, of this morphological finding, are currently unknown.

Alcohol. There has, to date, been only one detailed study of placental morphology in cases of maternal alcohol abuse (Baldwin et al, 1982). The only positive findings which were clearly independent of low socioeconomic status were an excess of infarcts and of plaques of perivillous fibrin (neither of extensive degree) and features, such as villous stromal fibrosis and excess syncytial knot formation, suggestive of reduced fetal villous perfusion. This study suffered from a lack of any statement of

associated smoking habits or drug usage but nevertheless points the way to further pathological examination of placentas from maternal abusers of alcohol, particularly those whose infants are growth-retarded or show evidence of the fetal alcohol syndrome.

Cocaine. A detailed study of 13 placentas from pregnancies during which the mother had used cocaine failed to reveal any characteristic morphological changes (Gilbert et al, 1990).

Pregnancies of abnormal duration

Prolongation of pregnancy

Prolongation of pregnancy to, or beyond, 42 weeks of gestation is associated with an increased perinatal mortality, a high incidence of fetal hypoxia and frequent evidence of intrauterine malnutrition, ill effects traditionally attributed to placental senescence (Vorherr, 1975).

Placentas from prolonged pregnancies usually appear macroscopically normal though a proportion are unduly heavy: there is no excess of either gross calcification or infarction. On lightmicroscopy between 25% and 35% of placentas from prolonged pregnancies show no histological abnormality whilst in between 15% and 20% the villi are underperfused from the fetal side with a corresponding excess of syncytial knots and increased stromal fibrosis (Fig. 47.40). The villi in a small (10–15%) proportion of these placentas show evidence of mild ischaemia, i.e. cytotrophoblastic proliferation and trophoblastic basement membrane thickening, whilst in 40% there is a combination of inadequate fetal perfusion and mild ischaemic changes.

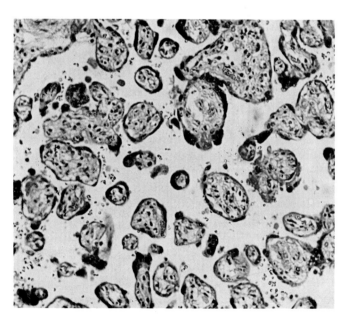

Fig. 47.40 Villi in a placenta of a woman delivered at the 42nd week of gestation. The villi are poorly perfused and show excessive syncytial knot formation. H & E × 110.

At the ultrastructural level the villous trophoblast shows changes which are qualitatively, but not quantitatively, similar to those seen in pre-eclampsia, e.g. focal syncytial necrosis, cytotrophoblastic hyperplasia, a reduction in the number of syncytial microvilli, reduced syncytial pino-cytotic activity, a paucity of syncytial secretory droplets and irregular thickening of the trophoblastic basement membrane (Jones & Fox, 1978a).

That uteroplacental ischaemia, albeit of relatively mild degree, does occur in a significant proportion of prolonged pregnancies seems very probable for it has been recognized for some time that a decrease in maternal blood flow is not infrequently noted in prolonged human gestations (Robertson & Dixon, 1969) whilst experimental studies in rats have also demonstrated a markedly diminished maternal placental blood flow in artificially prolonged pregnancies (Yamagushi et al, 1975). It remains far from clear why there should be a partial failure of the maternal vascular blood flow to the placenta in prolonged pregnancies whilst the reduction, in many cases, of fetal villous blood flow is of equally obscure origin. Neither change could, however, be reasonably considered as an ageing phenomenon and, as already remarked, there is little or no convincing evidence that the placenta undergoes a true ageing process during the limited time span of a human pregnancy (Fox, 1979a). It is of interest in this respect that a claim to have detected lipofuscin pigment in the placenta (Parmley et al, 1981) has now been refuted (Haigh et al, 1984). It is probable, therefore, that the combination of relatively mild ischaemia and diminished fetal perfusion in a high proportion of cases would serve adequately to explain the ill effects of prolonged pregnancy without there being any necessity to resort to a purely hypothetical condition of placental senescence.

Unduly short pregnancy

In many cases premature onset of labour is a consequence of, and secondary to, premature rupture of the membranes whilst in many other instances labour occurs early in relation to a particular complication of pregnancy, e.g. severe pre-eclampsia. Idiopathic primary premature onset of labour is therefore a relatively rare event; placentas from such cases are macroscopically unremarkable and there is no excess of placental infarcts (Salafia et al, 1992b). Histologically the villi are usually both morphologically normal and of normal maturity for the length of the gestational period but a small proportion, about 10%, depart from this pattern and have a villous morphology typical of the fully mature term organ (Aladjem, 1968; Becker, 1975; Fox, 1978), this phenomenon representing an asynchrony between placental and fetal maturation. These placentas are of considerable theoretical interest for it is at least hypothetically possible that, in this small proportion

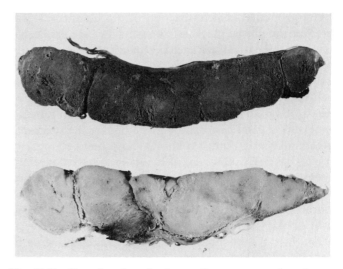

Fig. 47.41 Above is a slice of a placenta from an uncomplicated delivery whilst below is a similar slice of a placenta from a case of severe maternofetal rhesus isoimmunization. Note that the latter placenta is markedly pale but not unduly bulky. (From Fox, 1978. Reproduced by permission of W. B. Saunders.)

of cases, premature onset of labour has been predisposed to by the accelerated maturation of the placenta.

Fetal disorders

Maternofetal rhesus isoimmunization

Many placentas from cases of maternofetal rhesus incompatibility appear normal to the naked eye though some are unusually pale (Fig. 47.41). In a proportion of cases, however, the placenta is unduly heavy and bulky, sometimes being overtly oedematous or hydropic. In a minority of these placentas lightmicroscopy shows no histological abnormality but in most there is some degree of failure of full maturation of the villous tree together with a variable amount of villous stromal oedema (Fig. 47.42). Cytotrophoblastic cells are present in excess numbers and there is often some thickening of the trophoblastic basement membrane (Fox, 1978; Pilz et al, 1980). A number of observers have also commented on the presence of focal necrosis of the villous syncytiotrophoblast (Hellman & Hertig, 1938; Kline, 1948; Thomsen & Berle, 1960; Holzl et al, 1975).

Electronoptical examination confirms the presence of patchy syncytial necrosis (Jones & Fox, 1978b): the areas of necrosis are usually small but sometimes are quite extensive. Most of the villous syncytiotrophoblast is, however, fully viable and contains non-vacuolated endoplasmic reticulum together with a normal complement of pinocytotic vesicles and secretory droplets: microvilli are present in normal numbers. The excess of villous cytotrophoblastic cells is also confirmed by electronmicroscopy and most of these cells are of the intermediate type,

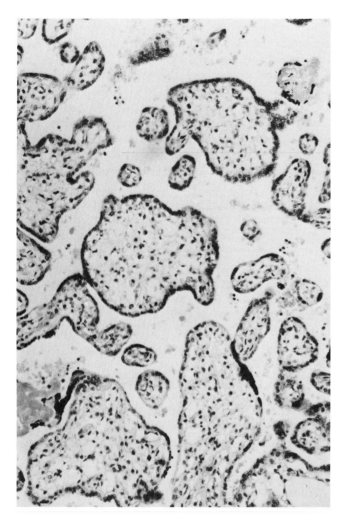

Fig. 47.42 Villi in a placenta from a case of severe maternofetal rhesus isoimmunization. There is a failure to achieve full maturation of the villous tree and the villi are moderately oedematous. H & E × 192. (From Fox, 1978. Reproduced by permission of W. B. Saunders.)

some showing mitotic activity (Kaufmann et al, 1977; Jones & Fox, 1978b).

The pathogenesis of the trophoblastic lesions in maternofetal rhesus incompatibility is far from clear. There is no evidence that maternal uteroplacental blood flow is reduced in this condition and the observed morphological changes do not suggest ischaemic damage: fetal anaemia plays no rôle in evoking syncytial injury for the trophoblast does not depend, in any way, on the fetal circulation for its supply of oxygen or nutrients. Rhesus haemolytic disease is clearly an immunologically mediated disease and it is therefore tempting to suggest that the trophoblastic injury is similarly of an immunological nature. It is certainly possible to envisage the placenta as containing D antigen and thus serving as a target for antibody-mediated immune attack: it is, however, now generally accepted that rhesus factors are tissue-specific alloantigens found only on erythrocytes (Bagshawe & Lawler, 1975) and it is

therefore extremely unlikely that the syncytial necrosis encountered in this disease is immunologically mediated: it should also be noted that no evidence has been found of immune complex deposition in the placental tissues.

Currently, therefore, the cause of the placental damage in maternofetal rhesus isoimmunization is unknown. The injury inflicted on the placenta is unlikely to be of any great importance for the damage suffered is clearly too limited in extent to have any significant effect on placental functional activity whilst the repair capacity of the placenta, as evidenced by the cytotrophoblastic proliferation, is unimpaired and syncytial pinocytotic and secretory activity appear unaffected. However, because of the common failure of the villous tree to undergo full maturation it is nevertheless probable that the placenta is, in this disorder, functioning at less than optimal capacity; yet it is almost certain that any defect in trophoblastic transfer capacity resulting from the arrested or retarded villous tree maturation is offset, and compensated for, by the increased growth of the placenta which is commonly found in rhesus disease.

Congenital nephrotic syndrome

In this condition the placental villous tree is often immature and the villi oedematous (Kouvalainen et al, 1962). Inferrera et al (1980) have made a detailed study of a placenta from a child with this form of renal disease: the villous trophoblast appeared immature but otherwise normal on lightmicroscopy. At the ultrastructural level the villous syncytiotrophoblast showed no abnormality of note whilst the cytotrophoblastic cells were of the resting stem cell type. The trophoblastic basement membrane showed an irregular nodular thickening. Inferrera and his colleagues suggested that the congenital nephrotic syndrome is characterized by the secretion of an abnormal basement membrane protein, both in the placenta and in the renal glomeruli.

Metabolic disorders

Vacuolation of the villous syncytiotrophoblast has been described in the placentas of fetuses with Gm_1-gangliosidosis and has been attributed to storage of ganglioside within the trophoblastic tissue (Lowden et al, 1973; Roberts et al, 1991) whilst foamy change has been noted in the cytoplasm of the syncytiotrophoblast, extravillous cytotrophoblast and villous Hofbauer cells in the placenta of a fetus with mucolipidosis type II (Powell et al, 1976). Nelson et al (1993) have described foamy Hofbauer cells in cases of fetal beta-glucuronidase deficiency and similar changes have also been seen in sialidosis (Mahmood & Haleem, 1989) and aspartylglucosaminuria (Aula et al, 1984).

The ultrastructural appearances of the placenta in a wide range of fetal metabolic disorders have been described and reviewed by Jones et al (1990).

Intrauterine growth retardation

There are many well-established causes of intrauterine fetal growth retardation, such as pre-eclampsia, fetal infection, congenital fetal malformation, maternal cigarette smoking, etc., but after elimination of these there remains a residue of cases for which there is no obvious maternal or fetal cause: it is the placenta of such infants which is considered here, whilst recognizing, of course, that even these instances of 'idiopathic' intrauterine growth retardation are almost certainly a heterogeneous group in aetiological terms.

Placentas from cases of idiopathic intrauterine growth retardation usually show no excess of macroscopic abnormalities (Fox, 1978; Garcia, 1982) though an increased incidence of infarcts, albeit usually small ones, has been noted in some studies (Bjoro, 1981; Salafia et al, 1992c). The placentas are small but placento-fetal weight ratios are usually normal. On histological examination many placentas from growth-retarded infants are fully normal but a majority show evidence of ischaemic insult with villous cytotrophoblastic hyperplasia and trophoblastic basement membrane thickening (Fox, 1978, 1981, 1994). The villous tree is usually normally mature but there is a high incidence of villitis (see Ch. 49).

At the ultrastructural level many, but not all, placentas from growth-retarded infants show lesions, such as focal syncytial necrosis together with loss and distortion of the microvilli, which are similar to those seen in placentas from women suffering from pre-eclampsia, though the abnormalities are usually less well marked (Sandstedt, 1979; Sheppard & Bonnar, 1980b; van der Veen & Fox, 1983).

The pathological findings suggest, therefore, that there is a restriction of maternal uteroplacental blood flow in many instances of normotensive fetal growth retardation and this concept is in accord with experimental studies in which artificially produced reduction in maternal blood flow to the placenta resulted in a deficit in fetal growth (Wigglesworth, 1964; O'Shaughnessy, 1981). That there is in fact a diminished maternal blood flow to the placenta in many cases of idiopathic intrauterine growth retardation is now well established, both by the use of older haemodynamic techniques (Chatfield et al, 1975; Lunell et al, 1979) and by Doppler studies (Campbell et al, 1983; Trudinger et al, 1985a; McCowan et al, 1988; Jacobson et al, 1990; Bewley et al, 1991; Schulman, 1993). The pathological basis for this limitation of maternal blood supply has also been clarified in so far as abnormalities have been observed in the maternal utero-placental vasculature. In many, though not all, cases of intrauterine growth retardation the normal physiological changes in these vessels occur incompletely with inadequate transformation of the spiral arteries into utero-placental vessels (Khong et al, 1986; Khong & Robertson, 1992), a subject considered more fully in Chapter 48. An acute atherosis also occurs in the maternal uterine vasculature in some cases of normotensive intrauterine growth retardation (Sheppard & Bonnar, 1976, 1981; Althabe et al, 1985; Khong, 1991) and in two studies birth weight has been most markedly reduced in those cases in which atherosis complicated inadequate physiological change (McFadyen et al, 1986; Frusca et al, 1989).

As a response to the uteroplacental ischaemia there is, as already discussed, vasoconstriction of the fetal stem arteries in the placenta, manifest histologically by an 'endarteritis obliterans', with secondary changes in the distal villous tree such as sclerosis of vessels and an increased number of syncytial knots.

It is clear that a reduction in maternal uteroplacental blood supply is a major, and indeed causal, factor in many cases of inadequate fetal growth and in such cases there is no evidence that placental damage or malfunction plays any rôle in the production of a growth-retarded fetus. This is, however, not the whole story for it has emerged in recent years that there is a clear relationship between confined placental mosaicism and fetal growth retardation (Kalousek et al, 1991; Kalousek, 1994; Kalousek & Langlois, 1994). The histopathological findings related to confined placental mosaicism have not yet been defined but it has been suggested that this cytogenetic abnormality may be associated with inadequate placentation and hence with uteroplacental ischaemia (Fox, 1994).

CONCLUSIONS

It will be apparent from this chapter that our knowledge of placental pathology is still largely at a descriptive stage: it is justifiable to attempt to draw functional inferences from altered morphological patterns but many of the possible physiological consequences of trophoblastic damage that have been commented on in this chapter are matters of opinion rather than of fact. It is nevertheless clear that the placenta has a very considerable functional reserve capacity, can repair any damage it suffers with commendable ease and often shows compensatory mechanisms which tend to limit the ill effects of both tissue injury and of an unfavourable maternal milieu. It therefore appears unlikely that the placenta is ever functionally inadequate to a degree that it fails in its principal function of transferring oxygen and nutrients from maternal to fetal circulations and no attempt has been made in this chapter to describe the placental changes in, and hence perpetuate the myth of, placental insufficiency.

REFERENCES

Abramowsky C R, Vegas M E, Swinehart G, Gyves M T 1980 Decidual vasculopathy of the placenta in lupus erythematosus. New England Journal of Medicine 303: 668–672.

Agboola A 1975 Placental changes in patients with a low haematocrit. British Journal of Obstetrics and Gynaecology 82: 225–227.

Aherne W 1975 Morphometry. In: Gruenwald P (ed) The placenta and its maternal supply line. MTP Press, Lancaster, pp 80–97.

Aladjem S 1968 Placenta of the premature infant. American Journal of Obstetrics and Gynecology 102: 111–112.

Althabe D, Labarrere C, Telenta M 1985 Maternal vascular lesions in placentae of small-for-gestational age infants. Placenta 6: 369–373.

Altshuler G 1984 Chorangiosis: an important placental sign of neonatal morbidity and mortality. Archives of Pathology and Laboratory Medicine 108: 71–74.

Alvarez H, Sala M A, Benedetti W L 1972 Intervillous space reduction in the edematous placenta. American Journal of Obstetrics and Gynecology 112: 819–820.

Amstutz E 1960 Beobachtungen uber die Reifung der Chorionzotten in menschlichen Placenta mit besonderer Berucksichtigung der Epithelplatten. Acta Anatomica 42: 12–30.

Arnholdt H, Meisel F, Fandrey K, Lohrs U 1991 Proliferation of villous trophoblast of the human placenta in normal and abnormal pregnancies. Virchows Archives B Cellular Pathology 60: 365–372.

Asmussen I 1978 Ultrastructure of the human placenta at term: observations on placentas from newborn children of smoking and non-smoking mothers. Acta Obstetricia et Gynecologica Scandinavica 56: 119–126.

Asmussen I 1980 Ultrastructure of the villi and fetal capillaries in placentas delivered by smoking and non-smoking mothers. British Journal of Obstetrics and Gynaecology 87: 239–245.

Asmussen I 1982a Ultrastructure of the villi and fetal capillaries of the placentas delivered by non-smoking diabetic women (White Group D). Acta Pathologica, Microbiologica et Immunologica Scandinavica Section A 90: 95–101.

Asmussen I 1982b Vascular morphology in diabetic placentas. Contributions to Gynecology and Obstetrics 9: 76–85.

Aula P, Rapola J, von Koskull H, Ammala P 1984 Prenatal diagnosis and fetal pathology of aspartylglucosaminuria. American Journal of Medical Genetics 19: 359–367.

Bagshawe K, Lawler S 1975 The immunogenicity of the placenta and trophoblast. In: Edwards R G, Howe C V S, Johnson H H (eds) Immunobiology of trophoblast. Cambridge University Press, London, pp 171–182.

Baldwin V J, MacLeod P M, Benirschke K 1982 Placental findings in alcohol abuse in pregnancy. Birth Defects: Original Article Series 18: 89–94.

Barker G, Boyd R D H, D'Souza S W et al 1994 Placental water content and distribution. Placenta 15: 47–56.

Batcup G, Tovey L A D, Longster G 1983 Feto-maternal blood group incompatibility studies in placental intervillous thrombosis. Placenta 4: 449–453.

Becker V 1975 Abnormal maturation of villi. In: Gruenwald P (ed) The placenta and its maternal supply line. MTP Press, Lancaster, pp 232–243.

Becker V 1981 Pathologie der Ausreifung der Plazenta. In: Becker V, Schiebler T H, Kubi F (eds) Die Plazenta des Menschen. Thieme, Stuttgart, pp 266–281.

Beischer N A, Sivasamboo R, Vohra S, Silpisornkosal S, Reid S 1970 Placental hypertrophy in severe pregnancy anaemia. Journal of Obstetrics and Gynaecology of the British Commonwealth 77: 398–409.

Benirschke K, Kaufmann P 1995 Pathology of the human placenta, 3rd edn. Springer Verlag, New York.

Benson R C, Fujikura T 1969 Circumvallate and circummarginate placenta: unimportant clinical entities. Obstetrics and Gynecology 34: 799–804.

Bewley S, Cooper D, Campbell S 1991 Doppler investigation of uteroplacental blood flow resistance in the second trimester: a screening study for pre-eclampsia and intrauterine growth retardation. British Journal of Obstetrics and Gynaecology 98: 871–879.

Bjork O, Persson B 1982 Placental changes in relation to the degree of metabolic control in diabetes mellitus. Placenta 3: 367–378.

Bjoro K 1981 Gross pathology of the placenta in intrauterine growth retardation. Annales Chirurgiae et Gynecologiae Fennae 70: 316–322.

Bleyl U, Stefek E 1965 Zur Morphologie und diagnostischen Bewertung der lockeren jugendlichen Zotten in reifen meschlichen Plazenten. Beitrage zur pathologischen Anatomie und zur allgemeinen Pathologie 131: 168–182.

Bracero L A, Beneck D, Kirshenbaum N et al 1989 Doppler velocimetry and placental disease. American Journal of Obstetrics and Gynecology 161: 388–393.

Brandt G 1973 Atiologie und Pathogenese der Kalkablagerung in der Plazenta. Geburtshilfe und Frauenheilkunde 33: 119–124.

Brosens I, Renaer R M 1972 On the pathogenesis of placental infarcts in pre-eclampsia. Journal of Obstetrics and Gynaecology of the British Commonwealth 79: 794–799.

Brown H L, Miller J M, Khawli D, Gabert H A 1988 Premature placental calcification in maternal cigarette smokers. Obstetrics and Gynecology 71: 914–917.

Browne J C Mc C, Veall N 1953 The maternal placental blood flow in normotensive and hypertensive women. Journal of Obstetrics and Gynaecology of the British Empire 60: 141–147.

Burgos M H, Rodriguez E M 1966 Specialized zones in the trophoblast of the human term placenta. American Journal of Obstetrics and Gynecology 96: 342–356.

Burstein R, Frankel S, Soule S D, Blumenthal H T 1973 Ageing of the placenta: autoimmune theory of senescence. American Journal of Obstetrics and Gynecology 116: 271–274.

Campbell S, Griffin D R, Pearce J M et al 1983 New Doppler technique for assessing uteroplacental blood flow. Lancet 1: 675–677.

Campbell S, Pearce J M, Hackett G et al 1986 Qualitative assessment of uteroplacental blood flow: early screening test for high-risk pregnancies. Obstetrics and Gynecology 68: 649–653.

Carter J E 1964 Morphologic evidence of syncytial formation from the cytotrophoblastic cells. Obstetrics and Gynecology 23: 647–656.

Cefalo R C, Simkovich K W, Abel F, Hellegers A E, Chez R A 1977 Effect of potential surface area reduction in fetal growth. American Journal of Obstetrics and Gynecology 129: 434–439.

Chamberlain G, Philipp E, Howlett B, Masters K 1978 British births 1970. Vol 2 Obstetric care. Heinemann, London.

Chatfield W R, Rogers T G H, Brownlee B E W, Rippon P E 1975 Placental scanning with computer-linked gamma camera to detect impaired placental blood flow and intrauterine growth retardation. British Medical Journal 2: 120–122.

Christianson R E 1979 Gross differences observed in the placentas of smokers and non-smokers. American Journal of Epidemiology 110: 178–187.

Clavero-Nunez J A 1963 La placenta de las cardiacas. Revista Espanola de Obstetricia y Ginecologia 22: 129–134.

Costoya A L, Leontic E A, Rosenberg H G, Delgada M A 1980 Morphological study of placental terminal villi in intrahepatic cholestasis. Placenta 1: 361–368.

Dempsey E W, Luse S A 1971 Regional specialization in the syncytial trophoblast of early human placentae. Journal of Anatomy 108: 545–556.

De Sa O J 1971 Rupture of foetal vessels on placental surface. Archives of Disease in Childhood 46: 495–501.

De Wolf F, Carreras L O, Moerman P et al 1982 Decidual vasculopathy and extensive placental infarction in a patient with repeated thromboembolic accidents, recurrent fetal loss, and a lupus anticoagulant. American Journal of Obstetrics and Gynecology 142: 834–929.

Di Sant' Agnese P A, Jenson K D, Levin A, Miller R K 1983 Placental toxicity of cadmium in the rat: an ultrastructural study. Placenta 4: 149–164.

Dixon H G, Browne J C Mc C, Davey D A 1963 Choriodecidual and myometrial blood flow. Lancer ii: 369–373.

Dommisse J, Tiltman A J 1992 Placental bed biopsies in placental abruption. British Journal of Obstetrics and Gynaecology 99: 651–654.

Earn A A 1951 Placental anomalies. Canadian Medical Association Journal 64: 118–120.

Emmrich P, Birke R, Godel E 1975 Beitrag zur Morphologie der myometrialen und dezidualen Arterien bei normalen schwangerschaften, EPH-Gestogen und mutterlichen Diabetes mellitus. Pathologia et Microbiologica 43: 38–61.

Fisk N M, Storey G N B 1988 Fetal outcome in obstetric cholestasis. British Journal of Obstetrics and Gynaecology 95: 1137–1143.

Fok R Y, Pavlova Z, Benirschke K et al 1990 The correlation of arterial lesions with umbilical artery Doppler velocimetry in the placentae of small-for-dates pregnancies. Obstetrics and Gynecology 75: 578–583.

Fox H 1966 Thrombosis of foetal arteries in the human placenta. Journal of Obstetrics and Gynaecology of the British Commonwealth 75: 961–965.

Fox H 1967a Perivillous fibrin deposition in the human placenta. American Journal of Obstetrics and Gynecology 98: 245–251.

Fox H 1967b The significance of placental infarction in perinatal morbidity and mortality. Biologica Neonatorum 11: 87–105.

Fox H 1967c The incidence and significance of vascule-synctial membranes in the human placenta. Journal of Obstetrics and Gynaecology of the British Commonwealth 74: 28–33.

Fox H 1968 Villous immaturity in the term placenta. Obstetrics and Gynecology 31: 9–12.

Fox H 1970 Effect of hypoxia on trophoblast in organ culture: a morphologic and autoradiographic study. American Journal of Obstetrics and Gynecology 107: 1058–1064.

Fox H 1978 Pathology of the placenta. Saunders, Philadelphia.

Fox H 1979a The placenta as a model for organ aging. In: Beaconsfield P, Villee C (eds) Placenta — a neglected experimental animal. Pergamon, Oxford, pp 351–378.

Fox H 1979b Placental changes in gestational diabetes. In: Sutherland H W, Stowers J M (eds) Carbohydrate metabolism in pregnancy and the newborn 1978. Springer, Berlin, pp 102–113.

Fox H 1981 Placental malfunction as a factor in intrauterine growth retardation. In: van Assche F A, Robertson W B (eds) Fetal growth retardation. Churchill Livingstone, Edinburgh, pp 117–125.

Fox H 1982 The role of the placenta in perinatal mortality. In: Milunsky A, Friedman E A, Gluck L (eds) Advances in perinatal medicine, volume 2. Plenum, New York, pp 193–244.

Fox H 1988 The placenta in pregnancy hypertension. In: Rubin P C (ed) Handbook of hypertension. Vol 10 Hypertension in pregnancy. Elsevier, Amsterdam, pp 16–37.

Fox H 1994 The placenta in intrauterine growth retardation. In: Ward R H T, Smith S K, Donnai D (eds) Early fetal growth and development. RCOG Press, London, pp 223–235.

Fox H, Agrofojo-Blanco A 1974 Scanning electron microscopy of the human placenta in normal and abnormal pregnancies. European Journal of Obstetrics, Gynecology and Reproductive Biology 4: 45–50.

Fox H, Faulk W P 1981 The placenta as an experimental model. Clinics in Endocrinology and Metabolism 10: 57–72.

Fox H, Jones C J P 1983 Pathology of trophoblast. In: Loke Y W, Whyte A (eds) Biology of trophoblast. Elsevier, Amsterdam, pp 137–185.

Fox H, Sen D K 1972 Placenta extrachorialis: a clinico-pathological study. Journal of Obstetrics and Gynaecology of the British Commonwealth 79: 32–35.

Frusca T, Morassi L, Pecorelli S et al 1989 Histological features of uteroplacental vessels in normal and hypertensive patients in relation to birthweight. British Journal of Obstetrics and Gynaecology 96: 835–839.

Fujikura T, Benson R C, Driscoll S G 1970 The bipartite placenta and its clinical features. American Journal of Obstetrics and Gynecology 107: 1013–1017.

Galbraith R M, Faulk W P 1979 Immunological considerations of the materno-fetal relationship in diabetic pregnancy. In: Markatz A R, Adams P A J (eds) The diabetic pregnancy: a perinatal perspective. Grune & Stratton, London, pp 111–121.

Garcia A G P 1982 Placental morphology of low-birth-weight infants born at term: gross and microscopic study of 50 cases. Contributions to Gynecology and Obstetrics 9: 100–112.

Genest D R 1992 Estimating the time of death in stillborn fetuses. II. Histologic evaluation of the placenta: a study of 71 stillborns. Obstetrics and Gynecology 80: 585–592.

Getzowa S, Sadowsky A 1950 On the structure of the human placenta with full term and immature foetus, living or dead. Journal of Obstetrics and Gynaecology of the British Empire 37: 388–396.

Gilbert W M, Lafferty C M, Benirschke K, Resnik R 1990 Lack of specific placental abnormality associated with cocaine use. American Journal of Obstetrics and Gynecology 163: 998–999.

Giles W B, Trudinger B J, Baird P J 1985 Fetal umbilical flow velocity wavelengths and placental resistance: pathologic correlation. British Journal of Obstetrics and Gynaecology 92: 31–38.

Godfrey K M, Redman C W, Barker D J, Osmond C 1991 The effect of maternal anaemia and iron deficiency on the ratio of fetal weight to placental weight. British Journal of Obstetrics and Gynaecology 98: 886–891.

Greenberg J A, Sorem K A, Shifren J L, Riley L E 1991 Placenta membranacea with placenta increta: a case report and literature review. Obstetrics and Gynecology 78: 512–514.

Grennan D M, McCormick J N, Wejtacha D, Carty M, Behan W 1978 Immunological studies of the placenta in systemic lupus erythematosus. Annals of the Rheumatic Diseases 37: 129–134.

Haigh M, Chawner L E, Fox H 1984 The human placenta does not contain lipofuscin pigment. Placenta 5: 459–464.

Hata K, Hata T, Aoki T et al 1988 Succenturiate placenta diagnosed by ultrasound. Gynecological and Obstetrical Investigation 25: 273–276.

Hellman L M, Hertig A T 1938 Pathological changes in the placenta associated with erythroblastosis of the fetus. American Journal of Pathology 14: 111–120.

Hitschold T, Weiss E, Beck T et al 1993 Low target birth weight or growth retardation? Umbilical Doppler flow velocity waveforms and histometric analysis of fetoplacental vascular tree. American Journal of Obstetrics and Gynecology 168: 1260–1264.

Hoet J J, Reusens-Billen B, Catalano P M 1992 Immunological aspects of diabetic pregnancies. In: Coulam C B, Faulk W P, McIntyre J A (eds) Immunological obstetrics. Norton, New York, pp 517–528.

Holzl M, Lüthje D, Seck-Ebersbach R 1974 Placentaverlandungen bei EPH-Gestose: morphologischer Befund und Schweregrad der Erkrankung. Archiv Fur Gynakologie 217: 315–334.

Holzl M, Lüthje D, Dietrich H 1975 Placentaveranderungen bei Rh Inkompatibilitat unter besonderer Berucksichtigung von Zottenreifungsstorungen. Zentralblatt fur Gynakologie 97: 859–870.

Hopker W W, Ohlendorf B 1979 Placental insufficiency: histomorphologic diagnosis and classification. Current Topics in Pathology 66: 57–81.

Hurley V A, Beischer N A 1987 Placenta membranacea: case report. British Journal of Obstetrics and Gynaecology 94: 798–802.

Inferrera C, Barresi G, Chimicata S, de Luca F, Baviera G, Gulli V, Gemelli M 1980 Morphologic considerations on the placenta in congenital nephrotic syndrome of Finnish type. Virchows Archives A Pathological Anatomy and Histology 389: 13–26.

Jacobson S L, Imhof R, Manning M et al 1990 The value of Doppler assessment of the uteroplacental circulation in predicting pre-eclampsia or intrauterine growth retardation. American Journal of Obstetrics and Gynecology 162: 110–114.

Janovski N A, Granowitz E T 1961 Placenta membranacea: report of a case. Obstetrics and Gynecology 18: 206–212.

Jauniaux E, Gidd D, Moscoso G, Campbell S 1990 Ultrasonographic diagnosis of a large placental intervillous thrombosis associated with elevated maternal serum alpha-fetoprotein level. American Journal of Obstetrics and Gynecology 163: 1558–1560.

Jones C J P, Fox H 1976a An ultrastructural and ultrahistochemical study of the placenta of the diabetic woman. Journal of Pathology 119: 91–99.

Jones C J P, Fox H 1976b Placental changes in gestational diabetes: an ultrastructural study. Obstetrics and Gynecology 48: 274–280.

Jones C J P, Fox H 1977 Syncytial knots and intervillous bridges in the human placenta: an ultrastructural study. Journal of Anatomy 124: 275–286.

Jones C J P, Fox H 1978a Ultrastructure of the placenta in prolonged pregnancy. Journal of Pathology 126: 173–179.

Jones C J P, Fox H 1978b An ultrastructural study of the placenta in maternofetal rhesus incompatibility. Virchows Archives A Pathological Anatomy and Histology 279: 229–241.

Jones C J P, Fox H 1980 An ultrastructural and ultrahistochemical study of the human placenta in maternal pre-eclampsia. Placenta 1: 61–76.

Jones C J P, Fox H 1981 An ultrastructural and ultrahistochemical study of the human placenta in maternal essential hypertension. Placenta 2: 195–204.

Jones C J P, Lendon M, Chawner L E, Jauniaux E 1990 Ultrastructure of the human placenta in metabolic storage disease. Placenta 11: 395–411.

Kalousek D K 1994 Current topic: confined placental mosaicism and intrauterine fetal development. Placenta 15: 219–230.

Kalousek D K, Langlois S 1994 The effects of placental and somatic chromosomal mosaicism on fetal growth. In: Ward R H T, Smith S K, Donnai D (eds) Early fetal growth and development. RCOG Press, London, pp 245–256.

Kalousek D K, Howard-Peebles P N, Olson P B et al 1991 Confirmation of CVS mosaicism in term placentae and high frequency of intrauterine growth retardation association with confined placental mosaicism. Pre-natal Diagnosis 11: 743–750.

Kaplan C 1993 Placental pathology for the nineties. Pathology Annual 28: 15–72.

Kaplan C, Blanc W A, Elias J 1982 Identification of erythrocytes in intervillous thrombi: a study using inmunoperoxidase identification of hemoglobins. Human Pathology 13: 554–557.

Kaufmann P 1981 Entwicklung der Plazenta. In: Becker V, Schiebler Tk H, Kubli F (eds) Die Plazenta des Menschen. Thieme, Stuttgart, pp 13–50.

Kaufmann P 1982 Development and differentiation of the human placental villous tree. Bibliotheca Anatomica 22: 29–39.

Kaufmann P, Gentzen D M, Davidoff M 1977 Die Ultrastruktur von Langhanszellen in pathologischen menschlichen Plazenten. Archiv fur Gynakologie 222: 319–322.

Kaufmann P, Sen D K, Schweikhart G 1979 Classification of human placental villi. I Histology. Cell and Tissue Research 200: 409–423.

Kaufmann P, Luckhardt M, Schweikhart G, Cantle S J 1987 Cross sectional features and three dimensional structure of the human placental villi. Placenta 8: 235–247.

Khong T Y 1991 Acute atherosis in pregnancies complicated by hypertension, small-for-gestational-age infants, and diabetes mellitus. Archives of Pathology and Laboratory Medicine 115: 722–725.

Khong T Y, Robertson W B 1992 Spiral artery disease. In: Coulam C B, Faulk W P, McIntyre J A (eds) Immunological obstetrics. Norton, New York, pp 492–501.

Khong T Y, De Wolf F, Robertson W B et al 1986 Inadequate maternal vascular response to placentation in pregnancies complicated by pre-eclampsia and by small-for-gestational-age infants. British Journal of Obstetrics and Gynaecology 93: 1049–1059.

Kline B S 1948 Microscopic observations of the placental barrier in transplacental erythrocytotoxic anaemia (erythroblastosis fetalis) and in normal pregnancy. American Journal of Obstetrics and Gynecology 56: 226–237.

Kloos K, Vogel M 1974 Pathologie der Perinatalperiode. Thieme, Stuttgart.

Kloosterman G J, Huidekoper B L 1954 The significance of the placenta in obstetrical mortality. Gynaecologica 138: 529–550.

Kouvalainen K, Hjelt I, Hallman N 1962 Placenta in congenital nephrotic syndrome. Annales Paediatrici Fenniae 8: 181–188.

Kovalovszki L, Villanyi E, Banko G 1990 Placental villous edema: a possible cause of antenatal hypoxia. Acta Paediatrica Hungarica 30: 209–215.

Kraus F T 1993 Placental thrombi and related problems. Seminars in Diagnostic Pathology 10: 275–283.

Kruger H, Arias-Stella J 1970 The placenta and the newborn infant at high altitudes. American Journal of Obstetrics and Gynecology 106: 586–591.

Lademacher D S, Vermeulen R C W, Harten J J, Arts N F T 1981 Circumvallate placenta and congenital malformation. Lancet i: 732.

Lal K 1976 Placenta extrachorialis: a clinico-pathological study. Journal of Obstetrics and Gynaecology of India 25: 181–185.

Lehtorvirta P, Forss M 1978 The acute effect of smoking on intervillous blood flow of the placenta. British Journal of Obstetrics and Gynaecology 85: 720–731.

Lemtis H, Hadrich G 1974 Uber die Gewichtsabnaume des Mutterkuchens nach der Geburt und die Bedeutung fur die Quotienten aus Plazenta und Kindsgewicht. Geburtshilfe und Frauenheilkunde 34: 618–622.

Levin A A, Plautz J R, di Sant' Agnese P A, Miller R K 1981 Cadmium: placental mechanisms of fetal toxicity. Placenta (suppl 3): 303–318.

Liebhart M 1971 Some observations on so-called fibrinoid necrosis of placental villi: an electron-microscopic study. Pathologia Europaea 6: 217–220.

Liebhart M, Wojcicka J 1970 Microscopic patterns of placenta in cases of pregnancy complicated by intrahepatic cholestasis (idiopathic jaundice). Polish Medical Journal 9: 1589–1600.

Lippert T H, Cloeren S F, Kidess E, Fridrich R 1980 Assessment of uteroplacental haemodynamics in pre-eclampsia. In: Bonnar J, MacGillivray I, Symonds E M (eds) Pregnancy hypertension. MTP Press, Lancaster, pp 267–270.

Little W A 1960 Placental infarction. Obstetrics and Gynecology 15: 109–130.

Little W A 1961 The significance of placental/fetal weight ratios. American Journal of Obstetrics and Gynecology 79: 154–157.

Liu Q X 1990 Pathology of the placenta from small for gestational age infants. Chinese Journal of Obstetrics and Gynecology 25: 331–334.

Longo L D 1980 Environmental pollution and pregnancy: risks and uncertainties for the fetus and infant. American Journal of Obstetrics and Gynecology 137: 162–175.

Longo L D 1981 The interrelations of maternal-fetal transfer and placental blood flow. Placenta (suppl 2): 45–64.

Lorijn R H W, Longo L D 1980 Clinical and physiologic implications of increased fetal oxygen consumption. American Journal of Obstetrics and Gynecology 136: 451–457.

Lowden J A, Cruz R, Conen P E, Rudd N, Doran T A 1973 Prenatal diagnosis of Gm$_1$-gangliosidosis. New England Journal of Medicine 288: 225–228.

Lunell N O, Sarby B 1979 Utero-placental blood flow: methods of determination, clinical application and the effect of beta-mimetic agonists. In: Sutherland H W, Stowers J M (eds) Carbohydrate metabolism in pregnancy and the newborn 1978. Springer, Berlin, pp 86–101.

Lunell N O, Sarby B, Lewander R, Nylund L 1979 Comparison of uteroplacental blood flow in normal and in intrauterine growth-retarded pregnancy. Gynecologic and Obstetric Investigation 10: 106–118.

Lunell N O, Nylund L, Lewander R, Sarby B 1982 Uteroplacental blood flow in pre-eclampsia: measurement with indium-113m and a computer linked gamma camera. Clinical and Experimental Hypertension B1: 105–117.

McCormick J N, Faulk W P, Fox H, Fudenberg H H 1971 Immunohistological and elution studies of the human placenta. Journal of Experimental Medicine 91: 1–13.

McCowan L M, Ritchie K, Mo Ly et al 1988 Uterine artery flow velocity waveforms in normal and growth-retarded pregnancies. American Journal of Obstetrics and Gynecology 158: 499–504.

McFadyen I R, Price A B, Geirsson R T 1986 The relation of birth weight to histological appearances in vessels of the placental bed. British Journal of Obstetrics and Gynecology 93: 47–51.

MacGillivray I, Campbell D M 1980 The effect of hypertension and oedema on birth weight. In: Bonnar J, MacGillivray I, Symonds E M (eds) Pregnancy hypertension. MTP Press, Lancaster, pp 307–311.

MacLennon A H, Sharpe F, Shaw-Dunn J 1972 The ultrastructure of human trophoblast in spontaneous and induced hypoxia using a system of organ culture: a comparison with ultrastructural changes in pre-eclampsia and placental insufficiency. Journal of Obstetrics and Gynaecology of the British Commonwealth 79: 113–121.

McParland P, Pearce J M 1988 Doppler blood flow in pregnancy. Placenta 9: 427–450.

Mahmood K, Haleem A 1989 Placental morphology in sialidosis: report of a case. Annals of Saudi Medicine 9: 302–304.

Moe N, Jorgensen I 1968 Fibrin deposits on the syncytium of the normal human placenta: evidence of their thrombogenic origin. Acta Pathologica et Microbiologica Scandinavica 72: 519–541.

Molteni R A, Stanley J S S, Battaglia F C 1978 Relations of fetal and placental weight in human beings: fetal/placental weight ratios at various gestational ages and birthweight distributions. Journal of Reproductive Medicine 21: 327–332.

Myers R A, Fujikura T 1968 Placental changes after experimental abruptio placentae and fetal vessel ligation of rhesus monkey placenta. American Journal of Obstetrics and Gynecology 100: 846–851.

Naeye R L 1977 Placental infarction leading to fetal or neonatal death: a prospective study. Obstetrics and Gynecology 50: 583–588.

Naeye R L 1978 Effects of materal cigarette smoking on the fetus and placenta. British Journal of Obstetrics and Gynaecology 85: 732–737.

Naeye R L 1979 The duration of maternal cigarette smoking, fetal and placental disorders. Early Human Development 3: 229–237.

Naeye R L, Maisels J, Lorenz R P, Botti J J 1983 The clinical significance of placental villous edema. Pediatrics 71: 588–594.

Nelson J, Kenny B, O'Hara D et al 1993 Foamy changes of placental cells in probable beta-glucuronidase deficiency associated with fetal hydrops. Journal of Clinical Pathology 46: 370–371.

Nummi S 1972 Relative weight of the placenta and perinatal mortality: a retrospective clinical and statistical analysis. Acta Obstetricia et Gynecologica Scandinavica (suppl 17): 1–69.

O'Shaughnessy R W 1981 Uterine blood flow and fetal growth. In: van Assche F A, Robertson W B (eds) Fetal growth retardation. Churchill Livingstone, Edinburgh, pp 101–116.

Out H J, Kooijman C D, Bruinse H W, Derksen R H 1991 Histopathological findings in placentae from patients with intrauterine fetal death and anti-phospholipid antibodies. European Journal of Obstetrics and Gynecology and Reproductive Biology 41: 179–186.

Parmley T H, Gupta P K, Walker M A 1981 'Aging' pigments in term human placenta. American Journal of Obstetrics and Gynecology 139: 760–763.

Pearlstone M, Baxi L 1993 Subchorionic hematoma: a review. Obstetrical and Gynecological Survey 48: 65–68.

Peereboom J W C, de Voogt P, de Hatten B, van der Welde W, Peereboom-Stegenan J H J C 1979 The use of the human placenta as a biological indicator for cadmium exposure. In: Proceedings of the Second Conference on the Management of Control of Heavy Metals in the Environment. CEP Consultants, Edinburgh, pp 7–10.

Pilz I, Schweikhart G, Kaufmann P 1980 Zur Abgrenzung normaler, artefizieller und pathologischer Strukturen in reifen menschlichen Plazentazotten. III Morphometrische Untersuchungen bei Rhesus-Inkompatabilitat. Archives of Gynecology 229: 137–154.

Powell H C, Benirschke K, Favara B E, Pfluoger O H 1976 Foamy changes of placental cells in fetal storage disorders. Virchows Archives A Pathological Anatomy and Histology 369: 191–196.

Rayne S C, Kraus F T 1993 Placental thrombi and other vascular lesions: classification, morphology, and clinical correlations. Pathology Research and Practice 189: 2–17.

Redman C W G 1991 Pre-eclampsia and the placenta. Placenta 12: 301–308.

Remotti G, de Virgilis G, Bioanco V, Candiani R 1981 The morphology of early trophoblast after dioxin poisoning in the Seveso area. Placenta 2: 55–62.

Resnik R, Brisk G W, Wilkes M 1979 Catecholamine-mediated reduction in uterine blood flow after nicotine infusion in the pregnant ewe. Journal of Clinical Investigation 63: 1133–1136.

Roberts D J, Ampola M G, Lage J H 1991 Diagnosis of unsuspected fetal metabolic storage disease by routine placental examination. Pediatric Pathology 11: 647–656.

Roberts J M, Taylor R N, Musci T J et al 1989 Pre-eclampsia: an endothelial cell disorder. American Journal of Obstetrics and Gynecology 161: 1200–1204.

Robertson W B 1976 Utero-placental vasculature. Journal of Clinical Pathology 20: Supplement, Royal College of Pathologists 10: 9–17.

Robertson W B 1979 Uteroplacental blood flow in maternal diabetes. In: Sutherland H W, Stowers J M (eds) Carbohydrate metabolism in pregnancy and the newborn 1978. Springer, Berlin, pp 63–75.

Robertson W B 1981 Maternal blood supply in fetal growth retardation. In: van Assche F A, Robertson W B (eds) Fetal growth retardation. Churchill-Livingstone, Edinburgh, pp 126–138.

Robertson W B, Dixon H G 1969 Uteroplacental pathology. In: Klopper A, Diczfalusy E (eds) Fetus and placenta. Blackwell, Oxford.

Robertson W B, Brosens I, Dixon H G 1975 Uteroplacental vascular pathology. European Journal of Obstetrics, Gynecology and Reproductive Biology 5: 47–65.

Robinson J S, Kingston E J, Jones C T, Thornburn G D 1979 Studies on experimental growth retardation in sheep: the effect of removal of endometrial caruncles on fetal size and metabolism. Journal of Developmental Physiology 1: 379–398.

Rolschau J 1978 Circumvallate placenta and intrauterine growth retardation. Acta Obstetrica et Gynecologica Scandinavica (suppl) 72: 11–14.

Rosso P 1976 Placenta as an aging organ. Current Concepts in Nutrition 4: 23–41.

Russell J G B, Fielden P 1969 The antenatal diagnosis of placental calcification. Journal of Obstetrics and Gynaecology of the British Commonwealth 76: 813–816.

Salafia C M, Silberman L, Herrera N E, Mahoney M J 1988 Placental pathology at term associated with elevated midtrimester maternal serum alpha-fetoprotein cocentration. American Journal of Obstetrics and Gynecology 158: 1064–1066.

Salafia C M, Vintzileos A M, Lerer T, Silberman L 1992a Relationships between maternal smoking, placental pathology, and fetal growth. Journal of Maternal-Fetal Medicine 1: 90–95.

Salafia C M, Vogel C A, Bantham K F et al 1992b Preterm delivery: correlations of fetal growth and placental pathology. American Journal of Perinatology 9: 190–193.

Salafia C M, Vintzileos A M, Silberman L et al 1992c Placental pathology of idiopathic intrauterine growth retardation at term. American Journal of Perinatology 9: 179–184.

Sandstedt B 1979 The placenta and low birth weight. Current Topics in Pathology 66: 1–55.

Schiebler T H, Kaufmann P 1981 Reife Placenta. In: Becker V, Schiebler T H, Kubli F (eds) Die Plazenta des Menschen. Thieme, Stuttgart, pp 51–100.

Schulman H 1993 Uteroplacental flow velocity. In: Chervenak F A, Isaacson G C, Campbell S (eds) Ultrasound in obstetrics and gynecology. Little, Brown, Boston, pp 569–577.

Sen-Schwarz S, Ruchelli E, Brown D 1989 Villous oedema of the placenta: a clinicopathological study. Placenta 10: 297–307.

Shanklin D R, Scott J S 1975 Massive subchorial thrombohaematoma (Breus' mole). British Journal of Obstetrics and Gynaecology 82: 476–487.

Sheppard B L, Bonnar J 1976 The ultrastructure of the arterial supply of the human placenta in pregnancy complicated by fetal growth retardation. British Journal of Obstetrics and Gynaecology 83: 948–959.

Sheppard B L, Bonnar J 1980a Uteroplacental arteries and hypertensive pregnancy. In: Bonnar J, MacGillivray I, Symonds E M (eds) Pregnancy hypertension. MTP Press, Lancaster, pp 213–219.

Sheppard B L, Bonnar J 1980b Ultrastructural abnormalities of placental villi in placentae from pregnancies complicated by fetal growth retardation: their relationship to decidual spiral arterial lesions. Placenta 1: 145–156.

Sheppard B L, Bonnar J 1981 An ultrastructural study of uteroplacental spiral arteries in hypertensive and normotensive pregnancy and fetal growth retardation. British Journal of Obstetrics and Gynaecology 88: 695–705.

Silver M M, Laxer R M, Laskin C A et al 1992 Association of fetal heart block and massive placental infarction due to maternal antibodies. Pediatric Pathology 12: 131–139.

Soma H, Yoshida K, Mulkaida T, Tabuchi Y 1982 Morphologic changes in the hypertensive placenta. Contributions to Gynecology and Obstetrics 9: 58–75.

Steel S A, Pearce J M, Chamberlain G V P 1988 Doppler ultrasound of the uteroplacental circulation as a screening test for severe pre-eclampsia with intrauterine growth retardation. European Journal of Obstetrics and Gynecology and Reproductive Biology 28: 279–287.

Stock M A, Anderson D F, Phernetton T M et al 1980 Vascular response of the fetal placenta to local occlusion of the maternal placental vasculature. Journal of Developmental Physiology 2: 339–346.

Suzuki K, Minei I J, Johnson E E 1980 Effect of nicotine on uterine blood flow in the pregnant rhesus monkey. American Journal of Obstetrics and Gynecology 136: 1009–1013.

Teasdale F 1981 Histomorphometry of the placenta of the diabetic woman: class A diabetes mellitus. Placenta 2: 241–252.

Teasdale F 1982 Morphometric evaluation. Contributions to Gynecology and Obstetrics 9: 17–28.

Thomsen K, Berle P 1960 Placentabefund bei Rh-Inkompatibilitat. Archiv fur Gynakologie 192: 628–643.

Thomson A M, Billewicz W Z, Hytten F E 1969 The weight of the placenta in relation to birthweight. Journal of Obstetrics and Gynaecology of the British Commonwealth 76: 865–872.

Tighe J R, Garrod P R, Curran R C 1967 The trophoblast of the human chorionic villus. Journal of Pathology and Bacteriology 93: 559–567.

Tindall V R, Scott J S 1965 Placental calcification: a study of 3025 singleton and multiple pregnancies. Journal of Obstetrics and Gynaecology of the British Commonwealth 72: 356–373.

Torpin R 1966 Evolution of a placenta circumvallata. Obstetrics and Gynecology 27: 99–101.

Torpin R, Barfield W E 1968 Placenta duplex: report of a case studied by reconstruction of the fetal sac. Journal of the Medical Association of Georgia 37: 78–80.

Triplett D A 1992 Obstetrical complications associated with antiphospholipid antibodies. In: Coulam C B, Faulk W P, McIntyre J A (eds) Immunological obstetrics. Norton, New York, pp 377–403.

Trudinger B J, Giles W B, Cook C M 1985a Uteroplacental blood flow velocity time waveforms in normal and complicated pregnancy. British Journal of Obstetrics and Gynaecology 92: 39–45.

Trudinger B J, Giles W B, Cook C M et al 1985b Fetal umbilical flow velocity waveforms and placental resistance: clinical significance. British Journal of Obstetrics and Gynaecology 92: 23–30.

van der Veen F, Fox H 1982 The effects of cigarette smoking on the human placenta: a light and electron microscopic study. Placenta 3: 243–256.

van der Veen F, Fox H 1983 The human placenta in idiopathic intrauterine growth retardation: a light and electron microscopic study. Placenta 4: 65–78.

van der Veen F, Walker S, Fox H 1982 Endarteritis obliterans of the fetal stem arteries of the human placenta: an electron microscopic study. Placenta 3: 181–190.

van der Welde W J, Copius Peereboom-Stegeman J H J, Treffers P E, James J 1983 Structural changes in the placenta of smoking mothers: a quantitative study. Placenta 4: 231–240.

Vorherr H 1975 Placental insufficiency in relation to post-term pregnant and fetal postmaturity: evaluation of fetoplacental function: management of the postterm gravida. American Journal of Obstetrics and Gynecology 123: 67–103.

Vracko R, Benditt E 1970 Capillary basal lamina thickening: its relationship to endothelial cell death and replacement. Journal of Cell Biology 47: 281–285.

Wallenburg H C S, Stolte I A M, Jansenns J 1973 The pathogenesis of placental infarction. I. A morphological study on the human placenta. American Journal of Obstetrics and Gynecology 116: 835–840.

Wentworth P 1968 Circumvallate and circummarginate placentas. American Journal of Obstetrics and Gynecology 102: 44–47.

Wigglesworth J S 1964 Experimental growth retardation in the foetal rat. Journal of Pathology and Bacteriology 88: 1–13.

Wilkin P 1965 Pathologie du placenta. Masson, Paris.

Wilkins B S, Batcup G, Vinall P S 1991 Partial placenta membranacea. British Journal of Obstetrics and Gynaecology 98: 675–679.

Wilson D, Paalman R J 1967 Clinical significance of circumvallate placenta. Obstetrics and Gynecology 29: 774–778.

Wingerd J, Christianson R E, Levitt W V, Schoen E J 1976 Placental ratio in white and black women: relation to smoking and anemia. American Journal of Obstetrics and Gynecology 124: 671–675.

Yamagushi R, Ushioda E, Nishakawa Y, Shintani M 1975 Uteroplacental blood flow in normal and prolonged pregnancies pursued with tracer microspheres. Acta Obstetrica Gynaecologica Japonica 22: 175–181.

Zacutti A, Borruto F, Bottacci G et al 1992 Umbilical blood flow and placental pathology. Clinical and Experimental Obstetrics and Gynecology 19: 63–69.

48. Pathology of the pregnant uterus

Michael Wells   Omar Mohamdee

INTRODUCTION

To fulfil its function of reproduction the female genital tract undergoes extensive physiological and structural adaptations to pregnancy. Because it has to contain and nurture the growing fetus, the uterus manifests such adaptations to a degree more obvious than other parts of the genital tract but there is still much ignorance of the mechanisms involved. Even less is known about defects in the adaptation of the uterus to the pregnant state that may have a bearing on the aetiology and pathogenesis of many pregnancy disorders. In the great majority of abnormal pregnancies, for obvious reasons, the uterus is not available for study by the morphologist who has to make what deductions he/she can about the disorder in question from the delivered fetal placenta and, in cases of perinatal death, from autopsy studies of the neonate. The uterus involutes postpartum and any pregnancy-associated defect on the maternal side of the placenta disappears in the process and may not reappear in subsequent pregnancies. The additional information gleaned so far has been derived from occasional pregnancy hysterectomy specimens, from the technique of placental bed biopsy (Dixon & Robertson, 1958; Robertson et al, 1986) and from autopsies in cases of maternal death (Rushton & Dawson, 1982), the last fortunately now an uncommon occurrence. Regrettably, in that circumstance the case is usually the subject of a coroner's enquiry where the emphasis is more upon the cause of death and less upon the elucidation of the pathology of the condition leading to the fatality (Ch. 63).

It is reasonable to assume that any serious anatomical or physiological abnormality, congenital or acquired, of the uterine tissues will be inimical to a pregnancy. It follows that aberrations in the normal interaction between fetal and maternal tissues necessary to achieve the required symbiosis are likely to be crucial determinants of many pregnancy disorders. Pre-eclampsia, intrauterine fetal growth retardation, spontaneous abortion, antepartum and postpartum haemorrhage are but a few examples of probably defective feto-maternal interactions. This chapter will therefore be devoted to a review of what is currently known and, perhaps more importantly, to what remains to be discovered about human placentation and its imperfections.

NORMAL UTERINE ADAPTATIONS TO PREGNANCY

Endometrium

Conception occurs probably in most instances soon after release of the oocyte from the follicle at mid-cycle, that is about day 15 or 16 of a normal 28-day cycle. The zygote then develops through the morula stage in the Fallopian tube and, if it survives the journey, reaches the cavity of the uterus a few days later to mature into a blastocyst prior to nidation in the prepared endometrium about day 21 of the cycle. By this time the endometrium, having been primed by oestrogen in the first half of the cycle, is at full glandular secretory activity but the stroma at this stage shows no evidence of predecidualization. The maturation of the conceptus to a blastocyst and the secretory activity of the endometrium would appear to require fairly precise synchronization if nidation is to be successful. There is evidence (Noyes, 1972) that a predecidualized stroma is inhibitory to implantation and this may be a factor, amongst others, that could help to explain the high loss of early pregnancies, in the first two post-conception weeks (Edmonds et al, 1982).

It is remarkable that histopathologists are still unable to differentiate the features of a luteal phase endometrium where conception, but not nidation, has occurred from those of the more usual secretory endometrium of a non-conception cycle (Arronet et al, 1973). In the latter circumstance the glands begin to undergo involutionary changes about day 23 whereas the stroma flourishes to produce a pronounced predecidual reaction by the time of menstruation. In the former circumstance two factors operate to produce subtle changes in the endometrium. If the conceptus is viable and has begun to produce hCG the corpus luteum is sustained instead of involuting, ensuring a rising level of plasma progesterone, while the hCG itself has a direct effect on the endometrium (Arias-Stella, 1973). Most observers (Hertig, 1964; Buxton & Olson, 1969; Karow et al, 1971) agree that the glands, instead of collapsing into the typical 'saw-tooth' appearance associated with secretory exhaustion (Fig. 48.1), continue to secrete with the epithelium becoming increasingly vacuolated and thrown into pseudopapillary folds, giving a hypersecretory impression (Fig. 48.2). The stroma retains the oedematous, congested appearance character-

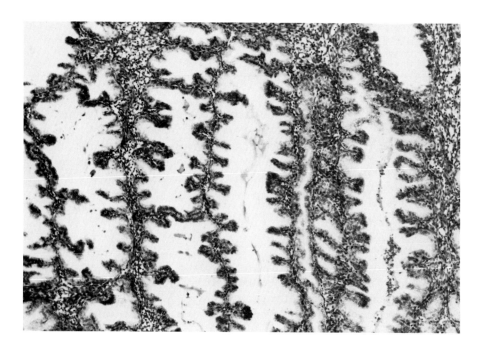

Fig. 48.1 Mid to late luteal phase endometrium with collapse of the glands due to cessation of secretory activity producing the characteristic 'saw-tooth' appearance. H & E × 80.

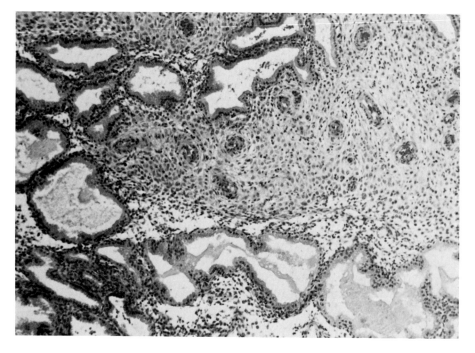

Fig. 48.2 Endometrium from a woman who had missed her period for a few days with no other evidence of pregnancy. Hyperplastic glands actively secreting and spiral arteries cuffed with predecidua combine to produce the picture of gestational hyperplasia. H & E × 80.

istic of the mid-secretory endometrium until the formation of the true decidua of a well-established pregnancy (Fig. 48.3). The more easily recognizable Arias-Stella phenomenon, with its nuclear pleomorphism and hyperchromicity added to the hyperplastic glandular changes (Fig. 48.4), does not develop fully until about four or five weeks after conception; it is now regarded as being due to a direct influence of progesterone upon endometrial glands.

One cell type, prominent in late secretory endometrium and in the decidua of early pregnancy, the endometrial granulocyte or K cell (Kornchenzellen), is now recognized

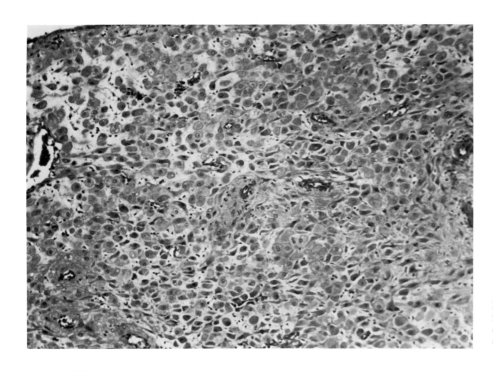

Fig. 48.3 Decidua vera in curettings from a first-trimester abortion. The stroma has been converted to a sheet of plump glycogen-rich cells. H & E × 80.

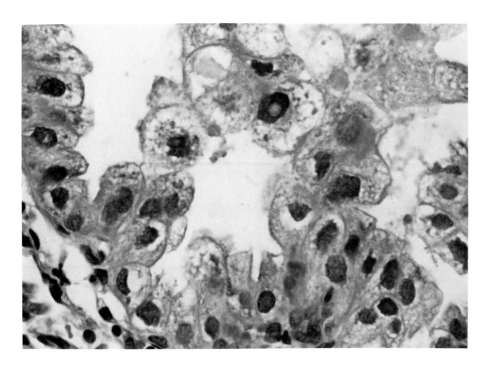

Fig. 48.4 Cytological detail of the Arias-Stella phenomenon: the glandular epithelial nuclei vary in size and are hyperchromatic with crenated nuclear membranes while the cytoplasm is vacuolated to a greater or lesser degree. H & E × 560.

to be a large granular lymphocyte. They contain large phloxinophilic granules (Fig. 48.5) and are seen best in the decidua vera clustered around vessels and the slit-like glands in early pregnancy (Fig. 48.6). When degranulated they are difficult to distinguish from the other round cells seen at the site of placentation.

Myometrium

It is self-evident that the uterus must enlarge *pari passu* with the growing conceptus but whether it does so by hypertrophy of existing smooth muscle or by hyperplasia is still debated. The answer is almost certainly that both

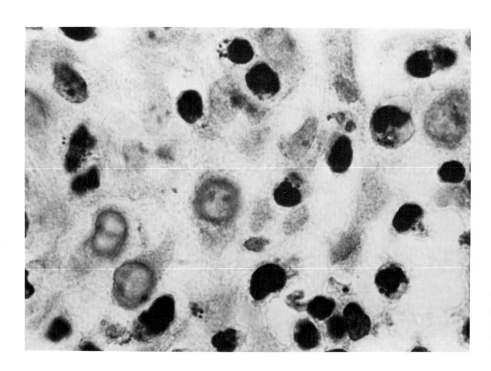

Fig. 48.5 The large, pale decidual cells contrast with the smaller, darkly staining endometrial granulocytes which contain spherical phloxinophilic granules. Phloxine tartrazine × 1400.

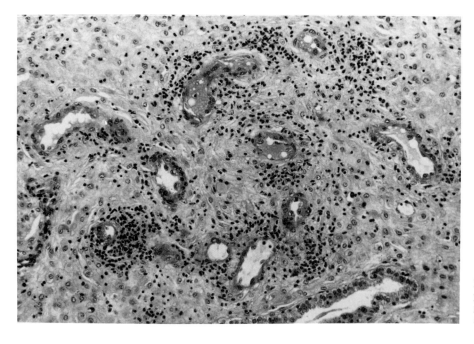

Fig. 48.6 Decidua vera (parietalis) of early pregnancy with concentration of endometrial granulocytes in the region of glands and spiral arteries. H & E × 130.

processes are at work as mitoses are not difficult to find in the myometrium of the early pregnant uterus (Fig. 48.7). The relative contributions of the two mechanisms to increasing uterine bulk remain to be determined. A significant addition to the weight and size of the uterus is made by increased collagen synthesis, the production of more of the complex ground substance and, no doubt, from increased fluid storage (Hytten & Leitch, 1971).

Blood vessels

The major vessels of the uterus are involved also in the

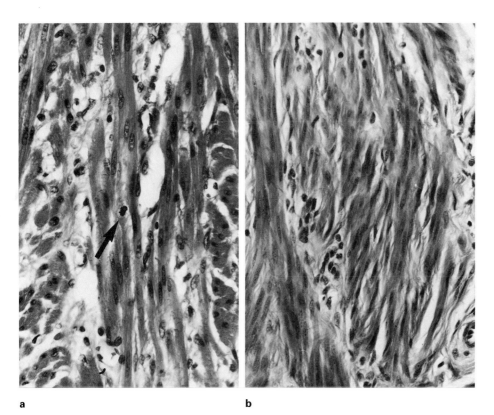

a   b

Fig. 48.7 Myometrium in the first trimester of pregnancy **a** showing hypertrophied smooth muscle, mitosis (arrow) and increase in intercellular constituents. Non-pregnant uterus **b** at same magnification for contrast. H & E × 250.

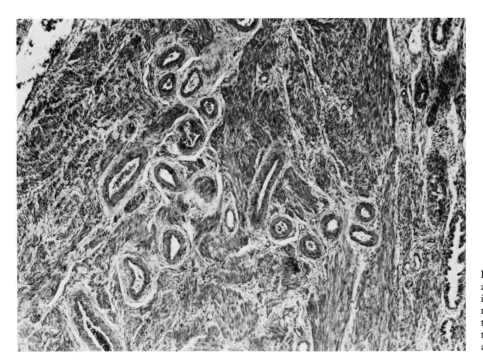

Fig. 48.8 Complex of larger radial arteries and their smaller branches, the spiral arteries, in the inner myometrium (endometrium, right). The latter are colonized by migratory trophoblast (see Fig. 48.18) during the second trimester in their conversion to uteroplacental arteries. H & E × 40.

processes of hypertrophy and hyperplasia (Burchell et al, 1978; Ramsey & Donner, 1980). The uterine and ovarian arteries and their accompanying veins increase in length and calibre dramatically as the pregnant uterus enlarges which is only to be expected as there is a tenfold increase in blood supply to the pregnant uterus during the third trimester (Browne & Veall, 1953). Similar accommodating changes have to take place in the arcuate system of blood vessels and its radial branches in the substance of the uterus. The latter arteries are the parent vessels of the spiral arteries supplying the endometrium of the non-pregnant uterus, some of which are destined to become the uteroplacental arteries of the pregnant uterus (Fig. 48.8).

Figure 48.9 gives a diagrammatic representation of the blood supply to the non-pregnant uterus as an aid to the understanding of human placentation and its disorders.

EARLY PLACENTATION

The development of the fetal placenta has been dealt with in Chapter 46 but, because human placentation is haemochorial and, as such, requires a more intimate and complex reaction of fetal with maternal tissues, it is necessary to return to the subject to deal with the maternal aspect.

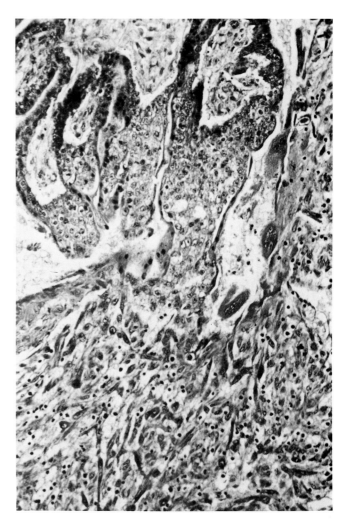

Fig. 48.10   Eight-week (six weeks post-conception) gestation: anchoring villi with streamers of non-villous trophoblast infiltrating the basal decidua. H & E × 625.

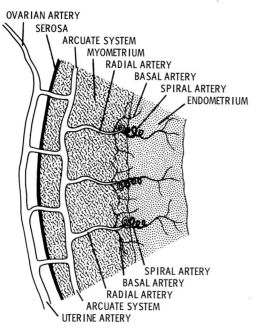

Fig. 48.9   Diagram of the blood supply to the non-pregnant uterus. During pregnancy the spiral arteries of the placental site or bed are converted to uteroplacental arteries by the action of migratory trophoblast. The small basal arteries are not involved and remain as nutritive vessels to the inner myometrium and basal decidua.

Migratory trophoblast

A phenomenon common to all species with haemochorial placentation is the elaboration of migratory trophoblast, the pattern of which varies in different species (Pijnenborg et al, 1981a; Ramsey, 1982). Invasion of uterine tissues occurs to a greater or lesser degree, depending on the species, but an essential feature is the opening up of maternal vessels by non-villous trophoblast. In the human the migratory trophoblast in the early stages of placentation derives from the cytotrophoblastic shell elaborated around the conceptus in the first two or three weeks of gestation (Boyd & Hamilton, 1970). In the ensuing weeks, when placental villi are forming and developing, streamers of such cells can be seen emanating from anchoring villi in the basal decidua (Fig. 48.10) that is on the abembryonic side of the conceptus. By about six weeks post-conception, or eight weeks gestation by dating from the last menstrual period, the basal decidua is extensively overrun by migratory cytotrophoblast (Fig. 48.11), some of which,

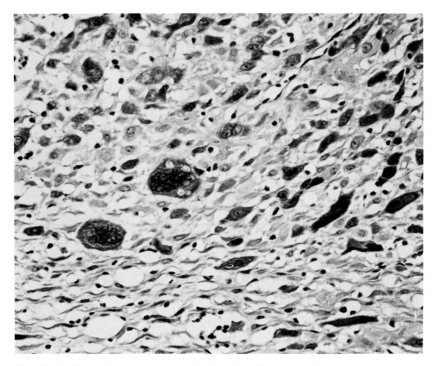

Fig. 48.11   First-trimester pregnancy: the basal decidua is extensively overrun by migratory interstitial cytotrophoblast, some of which has converted to syncytial placental bed giant cells. This picture often is inappropriately named 'syncytial endometritis'; placental site reaction is a better term. H & E × 200.

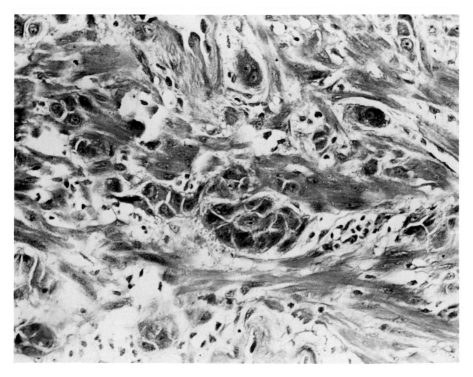

Fig. 48.12   Ten week gestation: migratory cytotrophoblast has infiltrated into the myometrium and clumps of cells are in the process of forming syncytial giant cells. H & E × 250.

usually that nearer to the myometrium, is in the early stage of symplasmic fusion to form syncytiotrophoblast (Pijnenborg et al, 1980), the characteristic placental bed (or site) giant cells.

By about 10 weeks gestation the inner few millimetres of the myometrium of the placental bed are heavily colonized by this interstitial migratory cytotrophoblast (Fig. 48.12) but here the scene is altogether different with cytotrophoblast and smooth muscle co-existing in apparent harmony (Pijnenborg et al, 1981b). The function of non-villous interstitial migratory trophoblast is not at all clear. There is evidence (Boyd & Hamilton, 1970; Pijnenborg et al, 1981b) that it is an important source of the hormones elaborated by trophoblast but even if this proves to be so it still does not reveal the functions of these cells. A good case has been made that one function is the 'priming' of the myometrial segments of the spiral arteries of the placental bed preparatory to their conversion to uteroplacental arteries (Pijnenborg et al, 1983). There is a tendency for the interstitial migratory cytotrophoblast to concentrate around the myometrial blood vessels and this proximity is associated with the development of oedema and disruption of the normal architecture of the vessel wall (Fig. 48.13). The ultimate fate of migratory cytotrophoblast that reaches the myometrium is unknown although much of it by symplasmic fusion is converted to placental bed giant cells (Robertson & Warner, 1974; Pijnenborg et al, 1981b). These latter cells

are almost certainly static end cells; only the uninuclear cytotrophoblast apparently has the property of mobility. It seems likely that an undetermined proportion of the original invasive trophoblast perishes in the myometrium or is simply dispersed by the expansion of the placental site. The placental bed giant cells can be regarded as the survivors until term (Fig. 48.14) and it is doubtful that they have a rôle to play in the second half of pregnancy. Be that as it may, they usually disappear within about a week after parturition (Boyd & Hamilton, 1970). In pregnancies in which physiological changes fail to occur in spiral arteries at the decidual-myometrial junction, there is normal migration of interstitial trophoblast into the uterine wall, but the prevalence of multinucleated giant cells at this junction is much increased before 36 weeks gestation. This may be an expression of disturbed migration of trophoblastic cells into the arterial wall (Gerretsen et al, 1983).

Development of the uteroplacental vasculature

One subset of non-villous trophoblast, if indeed it is a distinctive variety, does have an observable function, the attack upon and opening up of the maternal vessels. In the early weeks of gestation sheets of cytotrophoblast proliferating from the original cytotrophoblastic shell (Harris & Ramsey, 1966), and later from the tips of villi (Pijnenborg et al, 1980), can be seen penetrating the walls of decidual

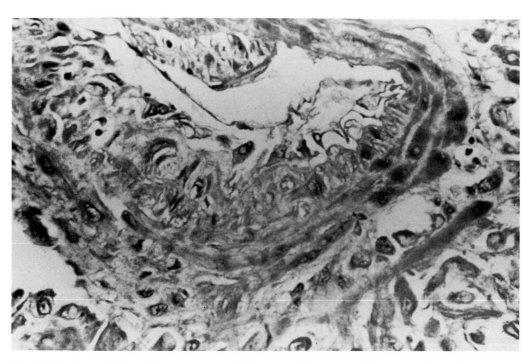

Fig. 48.13 Concentration of migratory cytotrophoblast around the myometrial segment of a spiral artery associated with oedema and disruption of the architecture of the vessel wall. H & E × 400.

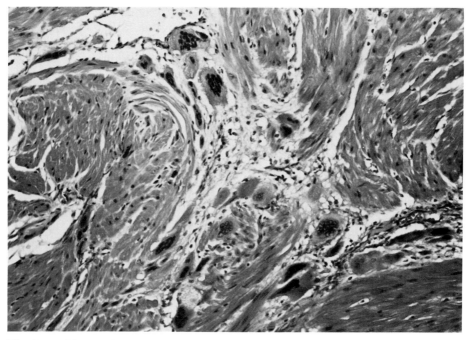

Fig. 48.14 Placental bed at term: residual, partially effete, syncytial giant cells in the myometrium. H & E × 130.

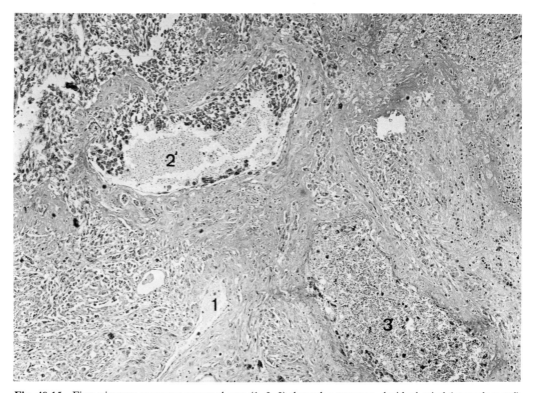

Fig. 48.15 First-trimester pregnancy: several cuts (1, 2, 3) through a tortuous, decidual spiral (uteroplacental) artery. In 1 the lumen is empty while in 2, the opening into the intervillous space, endovascular cytotrophoblast is entering the vessel from an anchoring villus. Segment 3 shows degenerative change in its walls as it is colonized by trophoblast. H & E × 250.

spiral arteries and forming plugs of such cells in the lumens (Fig. 48.15). These cells have the remarkable capacity to migrate in a retrograde fashion down the intima of the colonized vessel, gradually being incorporated into the vessel wall to become truly endovascular. The interaction between the mural trophoblast and the tissues native to the vessel wall is accompanied by extensive fibrinoid deposition (Fig. 48.16), a mixture of insuded maternal fibrin and microfibrillary material elaborated by the trophoblast (De Wolf et al, 1973). The net effect is the ultimate conversion of the decidual segments of the spiral arteries of the placental bed to distended sinusoidal

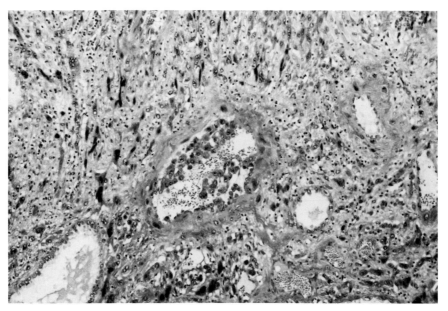

Fig. 48.16   Decidual spiral artery with cytotrophoblast in the lumen and within its wall, the latter phenomenon accompanied by fibrinoid deposition. Plentiful cyto and syncytial interstitial non-villous trophoblast and endometrial granulocytes can be seen in the surrounding decidua. H & E × 150.

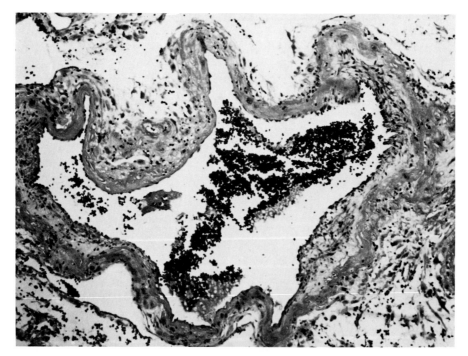

Fig. 48.17   Third-trimester pregnancy: at this stage the decidual segment of the uteroplacental artery has evolved into a distended, sinusoidal vessel, the wall of which is composed largely of fibrinoid and fibrous tissue with little musculo-elastic tissue remaining. H & E × 80.

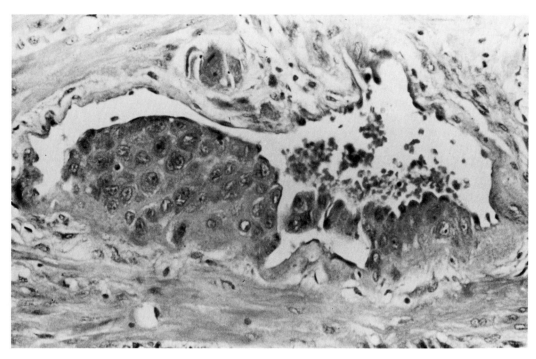

Fig. 48.18 Sixteen weeks gestation: myometrial spiral artery, already altered in morphology (see Fig. 48.13) to resemble a vein, containing an intimal collection of cytotrophoblast from the second endovascular migration. H & E × 520.

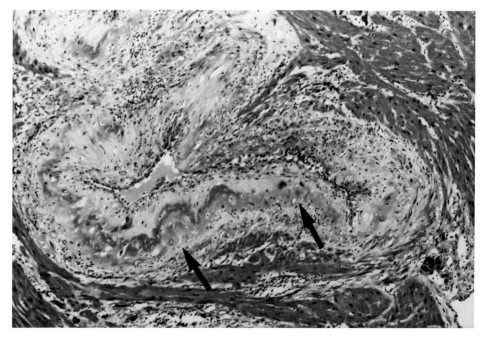

Fig. 48.19 Third-trimester pregnancy: myometrial spiral artery with fully developed physiological changes. The uteroplacental artery, which is artifactually collapsed, has a wall composed largely of fibrinoid with incorporated trophoblast (arrows) and fibrous tissue, there being little residual musculo-elastic tissue. H & E × 130.

vessels lacking musculoelastic tissue so that they become virtually passive fibrinoid tubes (Fig. 48.17). It was to this mode of conversion of the small spiral arteries to large capacity uteroplacental arteries that Brosens et al (1967) gave the name 'physiological changes'.

In many species there are separate waves of endovascular trophoblast migration (Pijnenborg et al, 1981a) and this feature has been found also in human pregnancy (Robertson et al, 1975; Pijnenborg et al, 1983). The physiological vascular changes of the decidual segments of the spiral arteries are completed in essentials by about the tenth week of gestation as is the definitive form of the fetal placenta. Subsequent growth of the placental site would then appear to be simply by expansion commensurate with growth of the feto-placental unit (Gruenwald, 1972). However, all is not yet completed because it is doubtful if the uteroplacental vasculature elaborated for the first trimester could satisfy the increasing demands made upon it in the second and third trimesters. At about 14–16 weeks gestation the second wave of endovascular trophoblast migration descends upon the myometrial segments of the spiral arteries (Fig. 48.18) which, it will be recalled, had already been altered in their morphology (Fig. 48.13), presumably because of their close association with migratory interstitial cytotrophoblast. An interaction identical to that which took place in the decidual arteries between the endovascular trophoblast and the vessel wall then ensues in the myometrial segments (De Wolf et al, 1980a) with progressive distension of the vessel, probably going on well into the third trimester (Fig. 48.19). Although no detailed studies of the decidual or myometrial veins have been undertaken, a similar transformation of the decidual veins has been noted (Brosens et al, 1967) but for some unknown reason the myometrial veins are left relatively undisturbed in their morphology although they increase enormously in calibre. A system has thus been elaborated of a low resistance, high conductance (Moll et al, 1975) arterial supply to the intervillous space of the fetal placenta capable of delivering something in excess of half a litre of blood per minute during the third trimester. Figure 48.20 gives a diagrammatic representation of the fully developed blood supply to the placenta.

PLACENTAL BED PATHOLOGY

Hypertensive disorders of pregnancy

During a normal pregnancy there is a tendency for the blood pressure to fall slightly until mid-gestation then to rise gradually to the pre-pregnancy level or somewhat higher in the last few weeks and during labour (Hytten & Leitch, 1971). Particularly in primipara (Chesley, 1980), the disorder now known as pre-eclampsia (the terms 'toxaemia of pregnancy' and 'pre-eclamptic toxaemia' should

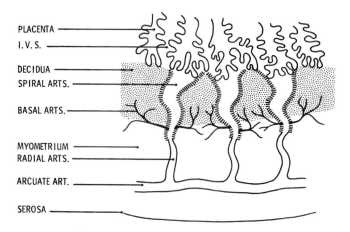

Fig. 48.20 Diagram of the uteroplacental blood supply during the third trimester. The venous drainage, which in general parallels the arterial supply, is not shown. Note that the basal arteries (black) are not involved with physiological vascular changes.

be abandoned as there is no evidence of a toxin in the disorder) may appear in the third trimester and is characterized by a rapidly rising blood pressure, proteinuria and, in severe cases, generalized oedema. Diagnosis and definitions present difficulties when the clinical manifestations are mild or variable, but the classification of Davey & MacGillivray (1988), which groups patients with hypertension and/or proteinuria in pregnancy into clearly defined categories, should be useful. Failing intervention by the clinician the disorder may be complicated by epileptiform fits, overt eclampsia, before, during or after labour, and death may result from cerebral haemorrhage, renal or liver failure and other complications. Women who have essential hypertension or renal disease have a greater than average risk of developing superimposed pre-eclampsia.

The aetiology of the disorder is still unknown, but evidence is accumulating that a defective interaction between trophoblast and uterine tissues, possibly of an immunological nature, is at the root of the problem (MacGillivray, 1983). The pathology of pre-eclampsia is now better defined, at least in its morphological aspects, providing a more logical approach to the determination of aetiological factors. In the first place it seems likely that the stage is set during the second trimester for the clinical manifestations of the disorder in the third trimester. Consistently in cases of pre-eclampsia, whether arising *de novo* or superimposed upon essential hypertension or renal disease, the second wave of endovascular trophoblast migration into the myometrial segments of the spiral (uteroplacental) arteries does not occur (Brosens et al, 1972) so that these arterial segments remain unaffected by the adaptive physiological vascular changes (Fig. 48.21, cf. Fig. 48.19) throughout the whole course of pregnancy. In addition, complete absence of physiological changes throughout the entire length of both decidual and myometrial segments of some

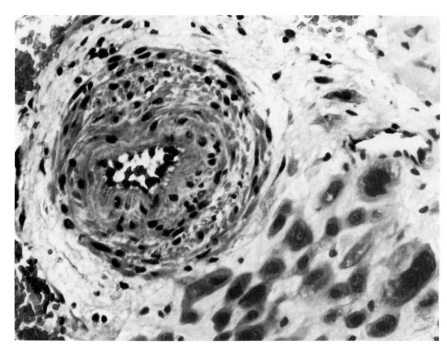

Fig. 48.21 Pregnancy complicated by pre-eclampsia: the myometrial segment of the spiral artery, having *not* been colonized by the second wave of endovascular trophoblast migration, shows no physiological changes (cf. Fig. 48.19) despite the presence of abundant interstitial trophoblast, including giant cells, near the vessel. H & E × 360.

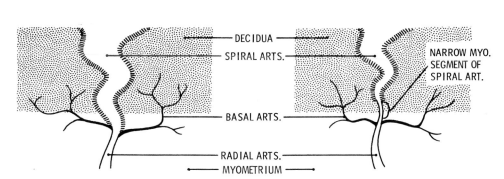

Fig. 48.22 Extent of physiological changes in the uteroplacental arteries in normal and pre-eclamptic pregnancies. In the latter the failure of the second wave of endovascular trophoblast migration leaves the myometrial segments of the spiral arteries as constricted high resistance vessels from the second trimester until term.

spiral arteries has been demonstrated in a study of basal plates of placentas (Khong et al, 1986). More recently, partial and incomplete physiological changes restricted to less than 50% of the circumference of vessels have been noted in a study of placental bed spiral arteries in hypertensive pregnancies (Pijnenborg et al, 1991), suggesting that the inhibition of trophoblastic invasion is by no means a uniform process or an 'all or none' phenomenon. These findings all point to a defect in the normal interaction between migratory trophoblast and maternal uterine tissues, which could be due to increased resistance on the part of maternal tissue or to decreased aggressiveness of

the trophoblast or a combination of both. Whatever the mechanism may be, the consequence during the late second trimester and for the whole of the third is a compromised blood supply to the intervillous space (Fig. 48.22). It was initially thought to be puzzling why the rise in blood pressure and the onset of proteinuria should be delayed by up to 10 weeks or more, since the second wave of endovascular trophoblast migration normally gets under way by the sixteenth week of gestation at the latest. However, the timing and extent of the trophoblastic invasion may be more variable than is usually assumed. In normal pregnancy, about 32% of spiral arteries have undergone physiological changes by 16–18 weeks (Pijnenborg et al, 1983), but almost all of the 100–150 arteries show physiological changes by term. This suggests that trophoblastic invasion of the myometrial segments, and the development of physiological changes in the spiral arteries, continues throughout pregnancy and is not restricted to the first two trimesters (Pijnenborg et al, 1991).

Nevertheless, Khong et al (1986) consider that there have been sufficient investigations of the placental bed at or near term in normal pregnancies and enough of normal pre-term pregnancies to confirm that intraluminal/endovascular trophoblast must be a rare finding in the third trimester of normal pregnancy (Brosens et al, 1967). Therefore the presence of luminal endovascular trophoblast in uteroplacental arteries in the third trimester in abnormal pregnancies complicated by pre-eclampsia and/or babies with a birth weight less than the tenth centile for gestational age, is taken as evidence of defective interaction between fetal and maternal tissues (Khong et al, 1986).

When the clinical manifestations of pre-eclampsia do appear, pathological lesions are inflicted upon the uteroplacental arteries and their branches and upon small arteries in the decidua vera remote from the placental bed. The archetypal lesion, acute atherosis (Fig. 48.23), was first described by Hertig (1945), elaborated upon by Zeek & Assali (1950), and has been the subject of many studies since (Dixon & Robertson, 1958; Brosens, 1964; Maqueo et al, 1964; Robertson et al, 1967, 1975, 1976; Sheppard & Bonnar, 1976, 1980; Gerretsen et al, 1981) with more recent reviews by Labarrere (1988) and Khong (1991). The arteriopathy is characterized by a fibrinoid-type necrosis of the whole vessel wall in small decidual arteries with the distinctive feature of an accumulation of lipophages in the damaged wall and an inconstant infiltrate of round cells in the vicinity. Ultrastructural studies (De Wolf et al, 1975; Sheppard & Bonnar, 1976) have shown that the lipid-bearing cells are of two types, damaged myointimal cells and macrophages phagocytosing cell debris, so that there is some analogy with the development of atheroma to justify the name given to this idiosyncratic vasculopathy of pre-eclampsia. The pathogenesis of the lesion is unresolved with altered haemodynamic influences and inappropriate immunological feto-maternal reactions or a combination of both as the current chief contenders (Robertson et al, 1967; Kitzmiller & Benirschke, 1973). Immunohistochemical studies often reveal extensive deposition of IgM and C3 in decidual arteries with acute atherosis in pre-eclampsia and these deposits have also been found in similar vessels in pregnant patients with autoimmune diseases (Laberrere et al, 1986) and in atherosis-like lesions from rejected renal and cardiac homograft transplants (Porter, 1974; Palmer et al, 1985) and after hepatic transplantation (Demetris et al, 1985). Acute atherosis is restricted to the pregnant uterus, however, and its topography is of interest in that it is seen best and in its pure form in the small arteries in the decidua vera or parietalis remote from any trophoblast, the nearest

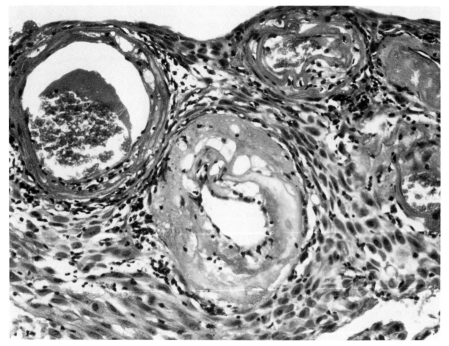

Fig. 48.23 Acute atherosis in the decidua vera of a pregnancy complicated by pre-eclampsia. The spiral arteries show extensive fibrinoid necrosis with intramural lipophages and a mild perivascular mononuclear infiltrate. H & E × 250.

being the thin rim of chorion of the membranes. Similarly, in the placental bed, it affects small basal arteries which do not communicate with the intervillous space and also the decidual and myometrial segments of the uteroplacental spiral arteries that have *not* undergone physiological changes (Fig. 48.24) and therefore contain

no trophoblast in their walls. It is therefore difficult to accept that some form of immunological reaction between trophoblast and the maternal vessel wall is involved. If such a reaction were humoral, with the formation of immune complexes, it could be anticipated that acute atherosis would be found in pre-eclamptic women at sites

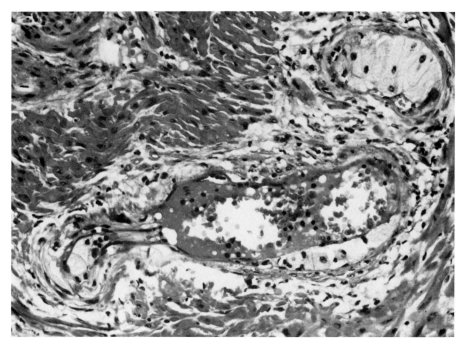

Fig. 48.24 Pre-eclampsia: myometrial spiral artery, unaffected by physiological changes, showing advanced acute atherosis. H & E × 250.

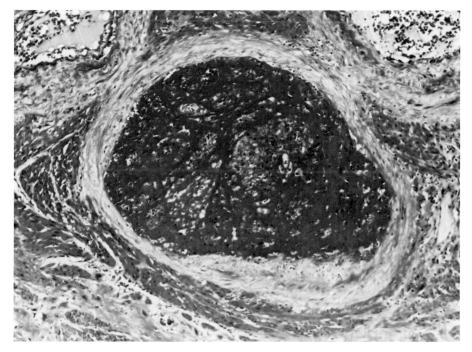

Fig. 48.25 Placental bed biopsy from a case of severe pre-eclampsia showing occlusive thrombosis of a uteroplacental artery. H & E × 100.

other than the uterus and such has never been reported although necrotizing arterial lesions occur in the liver, brain and other organs in fatal cases of eclampsia (Govan, 1976). The higher incidence and severity of chronic villitis of unknown aetiology in placentas from pre-eclamptic cases has led to the suggestion that this may represent a feto-maternal immunological reaction (Labarrere & Althabe, 1985, 1986). Whatever the pathogenesis of the vasculopathies of pre-eclampsia may be, there can be little doubt that they offer the best explanation for occlusive thrombosis (Fig. 48.25) with resultant placental infarction (Brosens & Renaer, 1972), decidual necrosis, placental abruption and antepartum haemorrhage (Fig. 48.26), all of which are relatively common complications of the hypertensive disorders of pregnancy.

When pre-eclampsia is superimposed upon pre-existing essential hypertension or renal disease the resultant pathology is more complex. Women with essential hypertension who complete their pregnancies without developing pre-eclampsia usually deliver babies of normal or even above normal weight (MacGillivray, 1975). In these circumstances it will be found that the maternal vascular response to placentation is perfectly adequate with the development of physiological changes in the uteroplacental arteries right down to the terminations of the parent radial arteries. In other cases of chronic hypertension and where pre-eclampsia does complicate the pregnancy the physiological changes will be found to be restricted to the decidual segments of the uteroplacental arteries but, pre-

sumably because of the effect of the hypertension on the high resistance myometrial segments, unchanged by the action of endovascular trophoblast, these segments show remarkable hyperplastic changes with apparent luminal stenosis (Fig. 48.27). Since such vascular pathology is not usually seen outside the uterus in hypertensive women of this age group, this exaggerated response to hypertension in the uteroplacental vasculature is probably related to the special haemodynamic requirements of the pregnant uterus. However, there is a suggestion that, in arteries with partial physiological changes in hypertensive pregnancies, sub-intimal proliferation may represent an over-reaction to physiological trophoblastic invasion (Pijnenborg et al, 1991). Endothelial vacuolation in uteroplacental arteries is also common in cases of chronic hypertension (Pijnenborg et al, 1991).

The deleterious effects of pre-eclampsia upon the hyperplastic vessels make bad matters worse as acute atherosis is now superimposed upon arteriosclerosis (Fig. 48.28). It is scarcely surprising that a pregnant woman with essential hypertension who subsequently develops pre-eclampsia carries a much higher than average risk of perinatal morbidity and mortality for her baby. A similar sequence of events may occur in women with overt or latent renal disease during pregnancy and, in fact, a woman who has recurrent pre-eclampsia in sequential pregnancies should be investigated for the possibility of latent renal disease or other predisposing disorders (Chesley, 1980).

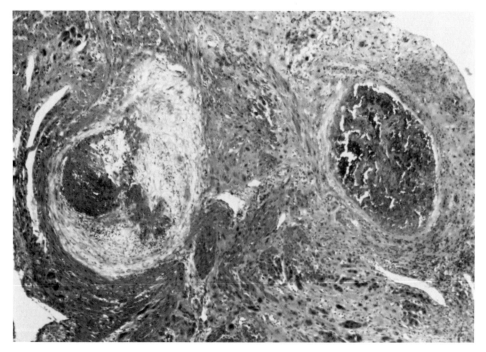

Fig. 48.26 Placental bed biopsy from a severe case of pre-eclampsia with placental abruption: recent upon organizing thrombosis of a uteroplacental artery with decidual necrosis (right). H & E × 80.

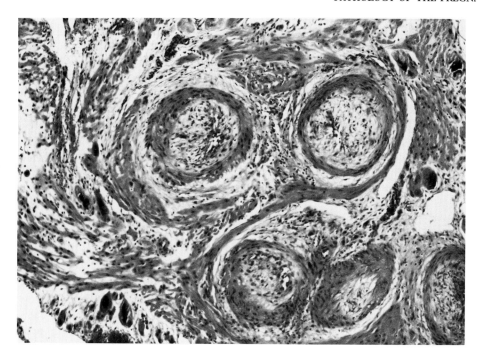

Fig. 48.27   Severe essential hypertension subsequently complicated by pre-eclampsia: the myometrial segments of the spiral (uteroplacental) arteries show marked hyperplastic arteriosclerosis but no trophoblast-induced physiological changes. The myometrium contains placental bed giant cells. H & E × 130.

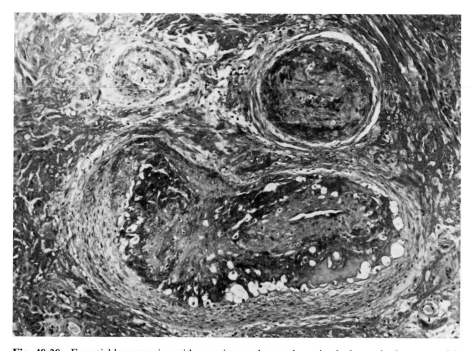

Fig. 48.28   Essential hypertension with superimposed pre-eclampsia: the hyperplastic myometrial spiral arteries are further damaged by acute atherosis with numerous foam cells in the fibrinoid necrosis. H & E × 130.

Intrauterine fetal growth retardation

In most, but not in all, cases of pregnancy hypertension with proteinuria the neonate is in the lower centiles for birth weight, even allowing for the higher incidence of premature delivery. The inadequate uteroplacental blood supply and associated vascular and placental lesions provide an acceptable explanation for this outcome but what about those cases of intrauterine growth retardation (IUGR) where there is no hypertension or other cause, such as maternal cigarette smoking, to incriminate? It has been claimed (Sheppard & Bonnar, 1976, 1980) that severe intrauterine growth retardation is always associated with atherotic lesions of the uteroplacental arteries and resultant placental damage irrespective of the level of the blood pressure and that an inadequate physiological vascular response to placentation is inconstant in intrauterine growth retardation and in pre-eclampsia. Others disagree (Brosens et al, 1977; Gerretsen et al, 1981), maintaining that acute atherosis, defined as a necrotizing arteriopathy affecting vessels *not* showing trophoblast-induced physiological changes, is virtually pathognomonic of pre-eclampsia and that restriction of the physiological changes to the decidual vessels is consistent in pre-eclampsia but inconstant and variable in idiopathic intrauterine growth retardation.

In two studies (McFadyen et al, 1986; Frosca et al, 1989), mean adjusted birth weight was markedly reduced in those cases with atherosis compared to those with only inadequate physiological changes. Absence of trophoblastic invasion and acute atherosis have been described in spiral arteries of the decidual portion of the placental bed in cases of intrauterine growth retardation without maternal hypertension (De Wolf et al, 1980b) and in spiral arteries of the basal plate, intermingled with vessels showing normal physiological changes (Althabe et al, 1985) (Fig. 48.29). Lesions described as being similar to those found in chronic vasculitis with necrosis and lymphocytic infiltration of the arterial wall have been observed in

parietal decidua concomitantly with atherotic-like lesions, suggesting that these vasculopathies represent different stages of the same lesion (Althabe et al, 1985). However, they may also be an expression of maternal 'aggression' towards fetal tissues leading to a defective vascular response to placentation, the consequence of which is low fetal birth weight. An interesting observation was that when acute atherosis occurred during pregnancies with intrauterine growth retardation unassociated with maternal hypertension, it was *not* observed in maternal arteries underlying the amnio-chorion (Khong, 1991).

A small fetus is usually attached to a small placenta and it could be argued that the placenta is small commensurate with the fetus (Gruenwald, 1975; Fox, 1976) rather than that the fetus is small because of a damaged and inadequate placenta. In a majority of cases of intrauterine growth retardation the small fetus cannot be explained by so-called 'placental insufficiency' for which there is little morphological or other evidence (Fox, 1976, 1981). Intrauterine growth retardation probably starts early in gestation although it is usually only detected clinically in the third trimester and it is false to argue that the small feto-placental unit is the result of acute lesions occurring late in the third trimester (Robertson et al, 1981). Furthermore, acute atherosis also occurs in the placental bed and in the decidua vera in cases of pre-eclampsia, admittedly a minority, where there is no intrauterine growth retardation. It would require detailed studies of the intact pregnant uterus with the placenta in situ, for obvious rea-

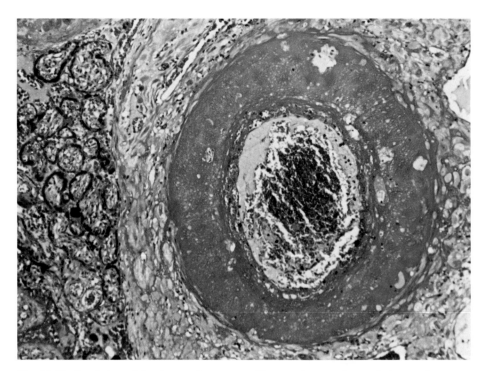

Fig. 48.29 Basal plate of the placenta from a case of intrauterine growth retardation *not* due to hypertensive disorders. The artery shows complete fibrinoid change with a few lipid-containing cells in the damaged wall, a vasculopathy indistinguishable from acute atherosis. H & E × 80.

sons almost impossible to achieve, to assess the anatomy and pathology of the uteroplacental vasculature in cases of idiopathic intrauterine growth retardation as was done in cases of pre-eclampsia (Robertson et al, 1967).

Other systemic disorders

Diabetes mellitus

Diabetes mellitus complicating pregnancy brings its own special problems. Despite better control of glucose metabolism there is still a higher than average incidence of complications during pregnancy, of perinatal morbidity and mortality and of congenital malformations in babies born to diabetic mothers. Not unnaturally, because of the well-known deleterious effect of diabetes on large and small blood vessels, attention has been focused on the placenta (Fox, 1978, 1979) and, in particular, upon the uteroplacental vasculature (Driscoll, 1965). The results of many studies, however, have been equivocal because of the failure by the authors to distinguish vasculopathies attributable to other complications of diabetic pregnancies, such as hypertensive disorders, from those due to the diabetes per se (Robertson, 1979). A study (Kitzmiller et al, 1981), carefully avoiding these pitfalls, recorded acute vasculopathies (extensive atherosis and fibrinoid deposits) in the decidua of 30% of pregnant diabetic women who did not have established hypertension or pre-eclampsia and similar vasculopathies in 50% of diabetic women with hypertension. Deposits of IgM and C3 were detected in arteries with atherosis.

Although poorly controlled diabetic pregnancies are characteristically associated with larger than average fetuses, it is interesting that when the diabetes is strictly controlled intrauterine growth retardation is an occasional outcome. It may be that despite the control of carbohydrate metabolism the complex basic metabolic defects of the diabetic state exert an unfavourable influence on the uteroplacental vasculature to the extent of promoting atheromatous lesions in the senescent uteroplacental arteries (Fig. 48.30) in the later stages of pregnancy.

Systemic lupus erythematosus

A woman with systemic lupus erythematosus (SLE) on becoming pregnant may experience a worsening of her condition and have an abortion, stillbirth or deliver a baby with intrauterine growth retardation (Jungers et al, 1982). Hypertension with proteinuria due to lupus nephritis produces a syndrome akin to pre-eclampsia and acute atherosis may be found in the decidua (Abramowsky et al, 1980). Labarrere et al (1986) have also found this lesion in the basal and parietal decidua of patients with SLE, associated with absence of physiological changes in the basal plate. Massive deposits of IgM and a smaller amount of C3 and C1q were also present in these acute atherotic lesions. Similar findings were also noted in cases of scleroderma and idiopathic thrombocytopenic purpura. In some women with SLE and in others without the stigmata of SLE a plasma factor, somewhat paradoxically called lupus anticoagulant, may be present (Carreras et al, 1981; Vermulen et al, 1981; Branch et al, 1985). This factor, an immunoglobulin, inhibits the production of vascular prostacyclin thereby promoting the aggregation of platelets, presumably by unopposed adenosine diphos-

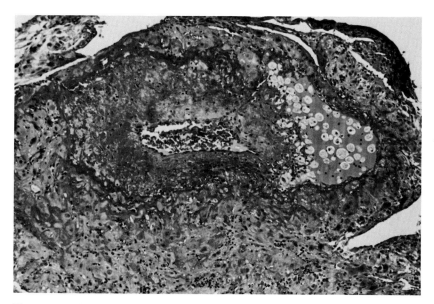

Fig. 48.30 Placental bed biopsy at 38 weeks gestation from a woman with insulin-dependent diabetes and a 'light-for-dates' fetus: the decidual uteroplacental artery shows advanced degenerative 'atheromatous' change with numerous lipophages in the damaged vessel wall. H & E × 80.

phate (ADP) and thromboxane activity, leading to venous and arterial thromboses during pregnancy with consequent recurrent abortions, stillbirths and, when less severe, intrauterine growth retardation.

OTHER DEFECTS OF PLACENTATION

It is self-evident that the complex interactions between fetal and maternal tissues essential for the establishment and maintenance of haemochorial placentation will misfire on occasions but we known remarkably little, as is obvious from the situation in pre-eclampsia, about the mechanisms and even of the morphological background of many such mishaps. Perhaps the most compelling aspect of human placentation requiring elucidation relates to the promotional and controlling factors regulating trophoblast migration, presumably resident in or mediated by the fetus. Accepting that trophoblast migration is a *sine qua non* of haemochorial placentation, what calls a halt to the interstitial trophoblast once it penetrates for a few millimetres into the myometrium of the human placental bed? Similarly, why does endovascular trophoblast move down the decidual spiral arteries and stop in these vessels at the deciduomyometrial junction at about 10 weeks gestation, there to await a further signal about a month later to proceed to the myometrial segments but to go no further than their origins from the radial arteries? What effects the disappearance of non-villous migratory trophoblast normally within about a week of an abortion or term pregnancy? The answers to these questions could explain much that is unknown about many pregnancy disorders.

Spontaneous abortion

Although the pathology of abortion is dealt with fully in Chapter 53, a few observations are probably relevant to the subject of defective placentation. Accepting that a high proportion of reproductive failures in the first trimester are attributable to chromosomal aberrations, the question must arise as to the nature of the built-in mechanism for rejecting these deviations from the norm and why, on occasions, it fails to operate and allows the continued survival of fetuses with severe congenital anomalies. The abortion of abnormal conceptuses is one enigma but the abortion of apparently normal conceptuses is another. It is reasonable to suggest that in cases of the latter category there is a failure in the symbiotic adjustment between fetal and maternal tissue and, in particular, failure to establish an efficient uteroplacental circulation.

Earlier observations included that of Burchell et al (1978) that when the ascending branches of the uterine arteries are bifid instead of single there is a higher incidence of abortion and intrauterine growth retardation during pregnancy. It was also felt that, on occasions, the damage inflicted on the maternal vessels by endovascular trophoblast may prove to be too great, leading to thromboses with placental bed necrosis, haemorrhage and abruption (Fig. 48.31) as is the case in ectopic pregnan-

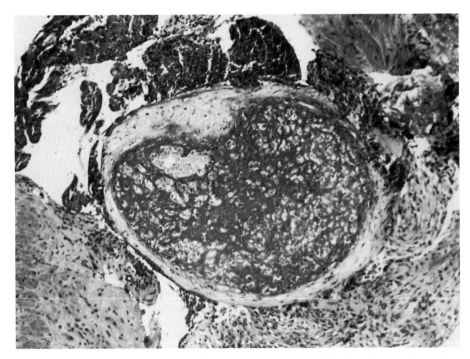

Fig. 48.31 Curettage specimen from a first-trimester spontaneous abortion: the uteroplacental artery at the deciduomyometrial junction is occluded by recent thrombosis: cause or effect? H & E × 80.

cies. The problem with making such a deduction on histological examination of an abortus and curettage specimen is that fetal death predates the abortion by some time and apparent vascular catastrophes may be the result and not the cause of the abortion. The absence of thrombosis in the course of the transformation of the spiral to the uteroplacental arteries is surprising enough in itself (Pijnenborg et al, 1980) although there is evidence (Hutton et al, 1980) that the placenta, and presumably trophoblast, elaborates a substance, probably an ADPase, inhibitory to platelet aggregation. It has been suggested also that prostaglandin production by the placenta and uterus has an important rôle in regulating the uteroplacental vasculature (Wallenburg, 1981).

In the presumed first reported study of the placental bed in recurrent and idiopathic sporadic miscarriages, spiral arteries in the placental bed showed preservation of musculo-elastic tissue with no evidence of involvement with migratory extravillous trophoblast in the decidual segments in the first-trimester miscarriages and in both the decidual and myometrial segments in the second-trimester miscarriages (Khong et al, 1987). It would appear that an abnormal uteroplacental vasculature is no more likely to be associated with chromosomally defective fetuses than with chromosomally normal fetuses. These findings were confirmed by Hustin et al (1990) in a study of a larger series of complete, intact, first-trimester spontaneous abortion products. They postulated that the defective physiological changes in spiral arteries were associated with a reduction in trophoblast invasion, which followed defective trophoblast growth. This allowed free flow of blood in the intervillous space at a time when it was harmful for the growing conceptus, leading to tearing apart of the trophoblastic shell with consequential separation at a cleavage line similar to that found in term placentas.

Trophoblastic disease

Once again, although this subject is dealt with at length in Chapter 52 it may well have a bearing on placentation and its regulatory mechanisms. In the great majority of examples of molar pregnancy there is failure to form an embryo but placental development, albeit abnormal, continues and excessive villous trophoblast proliferation is a common feature. If the control of trophoblast proliferation and migration is mediated by the fetus it is perhaps not surprising that growth of the placenta continues in molar pregnancy in an aberrant fashion as no fetus is present. It is interesting that although whole villi may infiltrate into, and very occasionally through, the uterus, excessive infiltration of the myometrium by migratory non-villous trophoblast is not a noticeable feature of molar pregnancy. We are not aware of any study that has been made of the uteroplacental vasculature in molar pregnancy, a difficult

undertaking these days when hysterectomy is rarely performed for the disorder. Persistent trophoblastic disease with, as the term implies, survival and continued growth of trophoblast beyond its normal life span following an abortion or term pregnancy, is yet another example of failure of control of this inherently aggressive fetal tissue. At the worst extreme is the fortunately rare development of the highly malignant choriocarcinoma. Wells & Bulmer (1988) have summarized the results of immunohistological studies which, overall, are similar to those described in normal pregnancy.

Placenta creta

This condition is subdivided into placenta accreta where there is undue adhesion to the placental bed, increta where anchoring villi penetrate deeply into the myometrium (Fig. 48.32) and percreta where villi infiltrate right through the wall of the uterus. This undue adhesiveness or invasiveness may be total, more commonly partial or focal, and the depth of penetration may vary in different areas of the placental bed. The aetiology and pathogenesis of the condition are still debated but analysis of series of cases (Benirschke & Driscoll, 1967; Fox, 1972, 1978) provides information about its incidence, associations and natural history.

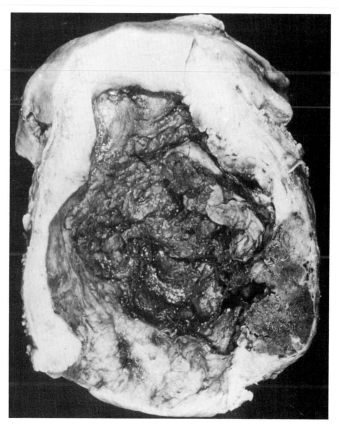

Fig. 48.32 Hysterectomy specimen from a case of placenta increta: penetration by placental villi deep into the lower segment myometrium has almost reached the serosa.

The disorder tends to increase with the age and parity of the pregnant woman, being rare in primipara, and there is an inconstant association with previous uterine infection, manual removal of the placenta in the preceding pregnancy, surgical operations (particularly caesarean section) on the uterus, other uterine disorders such as leiomyomas and adenomyosis (Khong & Robertson, 1987) and with myotonic dystrophy (Freeman, 1991). Not surprisingly, perhaps, there is an association with placenta praevia in over 30% of cases.

The popular explanation for the development of placenta creta is a focal or diffuse deficiency of decidua permitting the anchoring villi and the fibrinoid basal plate to attach directly to the underlying myometrium and, in more severe cases, to penetrate deeply into the myometrium. Examination of sections (Fig. 48.33) through the adherent areas reveals an absence or paucity of decidua but with an excess of the cytotrophoblast that is a normal feature of the basal plate in late pregnancy (Fig. 48.34). Decidua has been regarded as a barrier

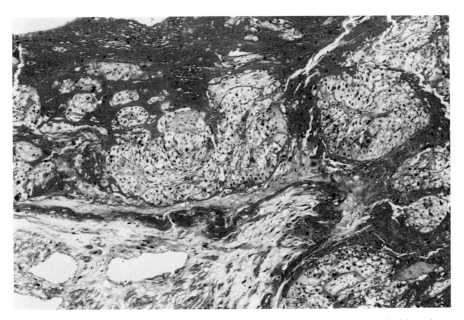

Fig. 48.33 Placenta accreta: the fibrinoid of the basal plate, without intervening decidua, abuts directly on the myometrium. The cytotrophoblast, a normal feature of the basal plate, is unusually prominent and hypertrophic. H & E × 130.

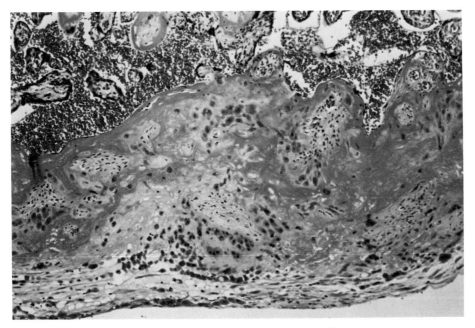

Fig. 48.34 Basal plate of a normal placenta showing fibrinoid, non-villous cytotrophoblast and adherent basal decidua. H & E × 80.

to prevent undue invasiveness of trophoblast (Kirby & Cowell, 1968; Finn & Porter, 1975) on evidence largely derived from experimental work in rodents. A further refinement was the claim that a pericellular coating of glycoproteinous fibrinoid protected trophoblastic cells from immune attack (Kirby et al, 1964; Currie & Bagshawe, 1967). Both postulates have been questioned on morphological and other grounds (Wynn, 1972; Robertson & Warner, 1974; Pijnenborg et al, 1981a) and any barrier effect must at best be temporary as cytotrophoblast manifestly sweeps through the decidua early in pregnancy to reach the myometrium. It does not follow that an absence of decidua in the placental bed at or near term means that the decidua was not there originally. Haemochorial placentation requires the formation of a decidualized uterine mucosa but, during placentation, there is much necrosis and destruction of decidual cells and there seems to be a proper balance between that decidua and the invasive trophoblast; in effect the decidua appears to constitute a temporary restraining, rather than an obstructive, tissue. A more likely explanation, therefore, of the pathogenesis of placenta accreta is that nidation is achieved and the early stage of placentation is effected in a normal part of the endometrium but, as the placental site extends and enlarges, in areas of the placental bed such as those near scars or in the lower segment, isthmus or upper cervical canal of the uterus where decidualization is less than adequate, the invasive non-villous trophoblast overwhelms the poorly decidualized mucosa to achieve deep penetration (Robertson et al, 1985). This would account for the fact that placenta creta is usually only partial and, in cases

of placenta praevia, restricted to that part of the placenta embedded in the lower segment, isthmus and cervical canal (Fig. 48.35).

The fact that placenta creta is rare in primipara and increases in incidence with age and parity suggests that the balance between invasive trophoblast and the constraining action of decidua shifts progressively in favour of the former. This idea would be in keeping also with the not infrequent history in cases of placenta creta of the necessity for manual removal of the placenta in the previous pregnancy. The deep penetration of anchoring villi in placenta creta is accompanied by an extension of endovascular trophoblast migration with physiological vascular changes in larger calibre arteries such as the radials (Fig. 48.36) accounting for the torrential haemorrhage that may accompany attempted removal of the placenta in cases of placenta praevia with creta.

Khong & Robertson (1987) have confirmed the presence of an unusual uteroplacental vasculature in which physiological changes were present much more deeply than normally, in large arteries of the radial/arcuate system deep in the myometrium while there were some superficial spiral arteries and some arteries deeper in the placental bed in closer proximity to abundant trophoblast without physiological changes. They also found that there was no apparent diminution of decidua parietalis or, in cases of focal accreta, of adjacent basalis. The extravillous trophoblast was mainly uninuclear or binuclear, with a paucity of placental bed syncytial giant cells, in contrast to the findings in late normal placentation. There was an apparent proliferation of interstitial trophoblast at the

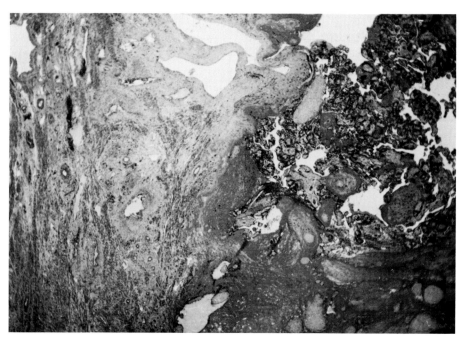

Fig. 48.35 Placenta praevia creta: the placenta (right) is deeply embedded in the lower uterine segment (left) in close proximity to large distended blood vessels. H & E × 18.

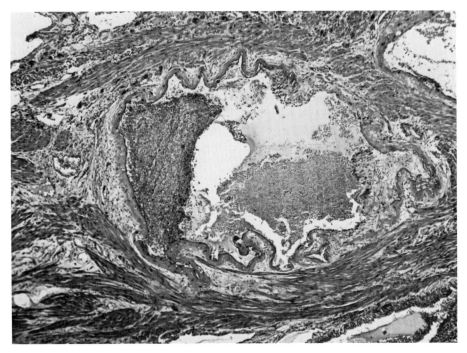

Fig. 48.36 Placenta accreta: physiological vascular changes in a radial artery deep in the myometrium. H & E × 35.

junction of placenta with myometrium, but the density of interstitial trophoblast deeper in the myometrium was lower than in normal placentation. These findings suggest that there is defective interaction between maternal tissues, particularly decidua, and migratory trophoblast in the early stages of placentation, resulting in undue adherence of the placenta or penetration into the uterus coupled with the development of an abnormal utero-placental circulation.

This hypothesis is supported by the albeit rare presentation of placenta creta before 20 weeks gestation, only about 10 cases of which have been reported (Harden et al, 1990) and the incidental finding of direct attachment of villi to the uterine musculature at the implantation site of an unsuspected 2.5 cm embryo in a uterus from a 'grand multip' removed during the course of a prolapse repair (Begneaud et al, 1965).

Immunohistologically, the phenotype of extravillous trophoblast populations is identical to that seen in normal placental tissue (Earl et al, 1987).

Antepartum haemorrhage

The pathology of uterine bleeding during the second half of pregnancy, apart from that associated with late abortion, premature labour, placenta praevia and blood dyscrasias, is something of a mystery. Clinically, antepartum haemorrhage (APH) presents as revealed or concealed 'accidental haemorrhage' of varying degrees of severity from the trivial to the potentially life-threatening

for the fetus and mother. Pathologically it is associated with placental abruption, retroplacental bleeding and haematoma formation. That the condition is relatively common in minor degree is evidenced by the not infrequent finding of small retroplacental haematomas (Fig. 48.37) of various ages on the maternal surface of delivered placentas where the pregnancies and deliveries had been perfectly normal. Manifestly the bleeding is maternal and comes from the uteroplacental circulation but the precise cause of the bleeding is unknown (Fox, 1978) although it is presumed by most to be triggered off by decidual necrosis with involvement of uteroplacental arteries; a minority consider the bleeding to come from ruptured veins.

Ignorance of the pathogenesis of the various lesions of the basal decidua and basal plate is due to the fact that all pathological studies and deductions so far have had to be made on the delivered fetal placenta. An extensive review of the placentas from 21 784 deliveries by Gruenwald et al (1968) produced valuable clinicopathological correlations of what they termed clinical 'abruption' and pathological 'separation', the former obviously detected by the obstetricians and the latter only by the pathologists. They could shed no light on the actual pathogenesis of the retro-placental pathology. A similar state of affairs emerges from a more recent review (Gorodeski et al, 1982). It is remarkable that serious vascular complications occur but rarely in the uteroplacental circulation during its establishment and evolution considering that Virchow's classical triad for thrombogenesis — damage to the vessel wall, changes in haemodynamics and alteration in the constitu-

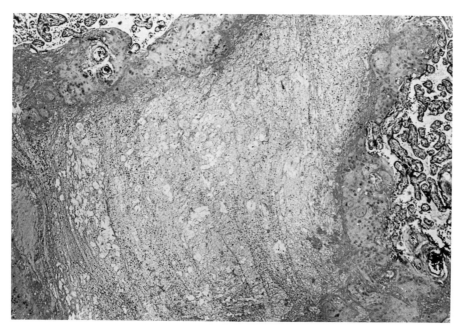

Fig. 48.37 Placenta from a normal pregnancy with a small retroplacental haematoma of some age in the basal decidua. H & E × 35.

ents of the blood — all occur during placentation. No doubt adjustments to systemic haemostatic mechanisms afford some protection against vascular complications but, as previously suggested, trophoblast must be equipped to protect itself against the deleterious effects of thrombosis in the vessels it colonizes. It can safely be assumed however that, as in all biological processes, there are occasional failures. This is certainly the case in the hypertensive disorders of pregnancy where decidual necrosis, placental abruption and haemorrhage are common, as already illustrated, but here the vascular lesions are a consequence, *inter alia*, of the raised blood pressure and, in general, they occur in vessels that have not been altered by trophoblast action. Furthermore, antepartum haemorrhage generally co-exists with placental infarction only when a large retroplacental haematoma is formed, the latter most likely the immediate cause of the former. It would therefore seem likely that mechanisms other than thromboses in the uteroplacental vasculature will have to be found to explain antepartum haemorrhage in otherwise normal pregnancies, which constitute the largest proportion of this category of pregnancy complications.

In the very occasional hysterectomy specimen available from normotensive pregnancies complicated by severe antepartum haemorrhage, abnormal vascular configurations akin to arteriovenous malformations have been detected (Fig. 48.38). This finding, however, can be taken only as a hint that not every uteroplacental artery of the 120 or so transformed spiral arteries in normal pregnancy (Brosens & Dixon, 1966) results in an architecturally perfect, or even adequate, vessel following the complicated

interactions between trophoblast and the vessel wall in the first and second trimesters of pregnancy.

In a recent study of placental bed biopsies in placenta abruption, however, Dommisse & Tiltman (1992) found vascular malformations in four out of 12 biopsies, three of which were from normotensive pregnancies. These lesions appeared to be somewhat different in structure from those previously detected. Although varying in size, each was a markedly dilated, complex vessel which, for the most part, resembled a vein with recent, non-occlusive thrombus in the lumen and a thin wall which contained no elastic lamina, trophoblast or fibrin. Elsewhere, however, the wall was thickened and showed sub-intimal fibrosis with fibrin and trophoblast deep to the thickening, and numerous smaller channels at the periphery. Near two of these malformations there was marked intramyometrial haemorrhage and, in one, this appeared to arise from the abnormal vessel. These lesions may represent arteriovenous communications and the sub-intimal fibrosis may indicate attempts at 'arterialization' of veins subjected to arterial pressures; haemorrhages from such vessels may well be under sufficient pressure to track between muscle fibres. In seven of the 12 biopsies, there was absence of physiological transformation of uteroplacental arteries, but four of these were from hypertensive patients.

Postpartum haemorrhage

After delivery of the newborn and its placenta there is a rapid contraction of the parturient uterus accompanied by an equally rapid adjustment of haemostatic mechanisms

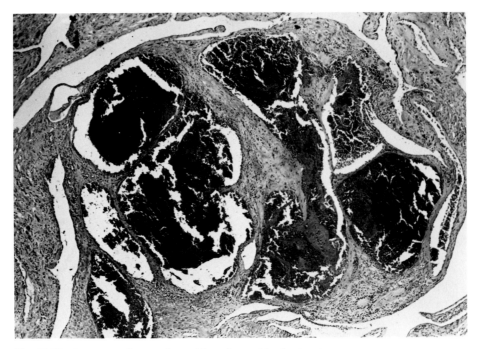

Fig. 48.38   Antepartum haemorrhage ultimately requiring hysterectomy.

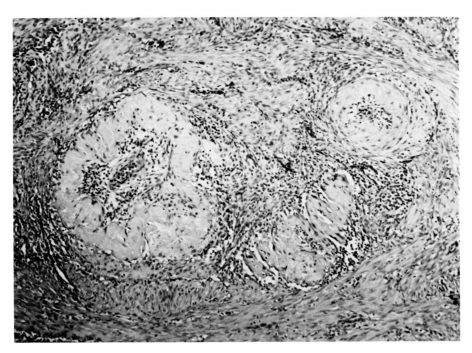

Fig. 48.39   Placental bed about a week postpartum with early involution of uteroplacental arteries including canalization of thrombosed lumens. H & E × 80.

(Bonnar et al, 1969) to promote closure and thrombosis in the sheared decidual segments of the uteroplacental arteries and veins (Fig. 48.39). Failure of either or both processes may lead to serious primary postpartum bleeding. A commoner mishap occurring at various intervals after labour is secondary postpartum haemorrhage (PPH). It is often assumed that this form of haemorrhage is due to 'retained products of conception', implying retention of portions of the fetal placenta, but only in a minority of cases is a so-called placental polyp revealed on curettage (Fig. 48.40). In some, postpartum infection undoubtedly plays a rôle but in the majority curetted material yields neither placental villi nor evidence that infection is a major factor. The usual finding is of organizing hyaline

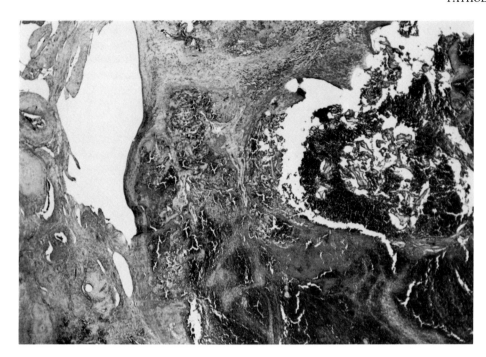

Fig. 48.40 Curettage specimen from a case of postpartum haemorrhage (PPH): a 'placental polyp' including retained villi admixed with haemorrhagic fibrinoid and partial involution of uteroplacental vessels (left). H & E × 18.

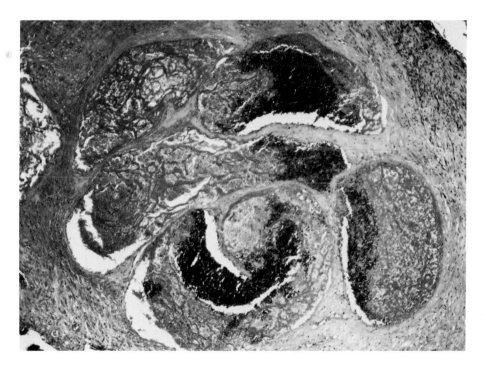

Fig. 48.41 Secondary postpartum haemorrhage: subinvolution of a leash of uteroplacental vessels which contain recent thrombi of various ages. H & E × 80.

and decidualized tissue, perhaps containing effete non-villous trophoblast, but the most significant feature is the presence of distended and partially hyalinized portions of the uteroplacental vessels containing organizing thrombi of various ages, much of it very recent (Fig. 48.41), indicating partial failure or delay in the involution of the placental bed (Ober & Grady, 1961; Robertson, 1976).

Involution of the pregnant uterus to the non-pregnant state is an ill-understood subject. It is remarkable that by the time of the first menstrual period following parturition the myometrial and endometrial segments of the spiral arteries that had been altered almost beyond recognition to become uteroplacental arteries have reverted to the original morphology of small arteries in the uterus, or elsewhere in the body for that matter.

No systemic study has documented the disappearance of extravillous trophoblast from the placental bed following normal delivery, but it is generally considered that trophoblast persists for only 7–10 days postpartum. In a study of 22 cases of subinvolution, Andrew et al (1989) demonstrated the presence of extravillous trophoblast in a perivascular location and this was seen in larger amounts and more frequently around subinvoluted vessels than around involuted vessels in the same specimen. Trophoblast was not seen in control tissues which contained no subinvoluted vessels. Normally involuted vessels showed intimal proliferation with regeneration of the internal elastic lamina and hyalinization of the medial tissue. Normal uteroplacental arteries showed replacement of endothelium by endovascular trophoblast in the first two trimesters, but they had generally re-endothelialized in the third trimester. The subinvoluted vessels possessed *no* endothelial lining and this may account for the presence of thrombi within these vessels. Persistence of endovascular trophoblast was seen in two of the cases of subinvolution. These findings suggest yet another abnormal maternofetal relationship in vessels of the placental bed, this time in the postpartum period, manifesting itself as subinvolution.

It would appear that it is interference with this process of vascular involution and reconstitution which is the commonest cause of secondary postpartum haemorrhage. The larger blood vessels of the uterus, that is the radials and arcuates, hardly ever involute completely so that it is usually easy to distinguish the histology of the parous from the nulliparous myometrium by the legacies of pregnancies left in the blood vessels. When the residua of pregnancies are excessive, the characteristic vascular features of intimal hyperplasia and medial lamination of hyalinized material (Fig. 38.42) form part of the bulky uterus of so-called subinvolution. Whether or not these features account for the symptomatologies, such as menorrhagia, associated with a clinical diagnosis of subinvolution of the uterus in the older parous woman has not been established.

Acknowledgements

We are most grateful to Professor W. B. Robertson for allowing us to update his chapter which originally appeared in the third edition. We are indebted to the following publishers and editors for their permission to reproduce Professor W. B. Robertson's illustrations already in print: Butterworths, London (Figs 48.1, 48.6, 48.33, 48.36 and 48.39), John Wiley and Sons, NY (Figs 48.8, 48.20 and 48.22), Appleton-Century-Crofts, NY (Fig. 48.28), Churchill Livingstone, Edinburgh (Fig. 48.30), the Royal College of Pathologists and the *Journal of Clinical Pathology* (Figs 48.9, 48.27, 48.41 and 48.42), *Placenta* (Figs 48.10, 48.12, 48.13, 48.15 and 48.18), the *European Journal of Obstetrics, Gynecology and Reproductive Biology* (Fig. 48.19) and the *Journal of Pathology* (Figs 48.21, 48.25 and 48.26).

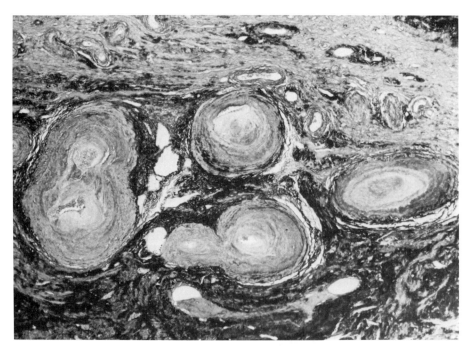

Fig. 48.42 Non-pregnant uterus from a 'grand multipara': the arcuate and radial arteries show laminated medial and intimal thickenings and there is much elastica-like material around the vessels. Orcein–van Gieson × 35.

REFERENCES

Abramowsky C R, Vegas M E, Swinehart G, Gyves M T 1980 Decidual vasculopathy of the placenta in lupus erythematosus. New England Journal of Medicine 303: 668–672.

Althabe D, Labarrere C, Telenta M 1985 Maternal vascular lesions in placentae of small-for-gestational-age infants. Placenta 6: 265–276.

Andrew A C, Bulmer J N, Wells M, Morrison L, Buckley C H 1989 Subinvolution of the uteroplacental arteries in the human placental bed. Histopathology 15: 395–405.

Arias-Stella J 1973 Gestational endometrium. In: Norris H J, Hertig A T, Abell M R (eds) The uterus. Williams & Wilkins, Baltimore, pp 185–212.

Arronet G H, Berquist C A, Parekh M C, Latour J P A, Marshall K G 1973 Evaluation of endometrial biopsy in the cycle of conception. International Journal of Fertility 18: 220–225.

Begneaud W, Dougherty C M, Mickal A 1965 Placenta accreta in early gestation; report of 2 cases. American Journal of Obstetrics and Gynecology 92: 267–268.

Benirschke K, Driscoll S G 1967 The pathology of the human placenta. Springer Verlag, Berlin.

Bonnar J, McNicol C P, Douglas A S 1969 Fibrinolytic enzyme system and pregnancy. British Medical Journal 3: 387–389.

Boyd J D, Hamilton W J 1970 The human placenta. Heffer, Cambridge.

Branch D W, Scott J R, Kochenour N K, Hershgold E 1985 Obstetric complications associated with the lupus anticoagulant. New England Journal of Medicine 313: 1322–1326.

Brosens I 1964 A study of the spiral arteries of the decidua basalis in normotensive and hypertensive pregnancies. Journal of Obstetrics and Gynaecology of the British Commonwealth 71: 222–230.

Brosens I, Dixon H G 1966 The anatomy of the maternal side of the placenta. Journal of Obstetrics and Gynaecology of the British Commonwealth 73: 357–363.

Brosens I, Renaer M 1972 On the pathogenesis of placental infarcts in preeclampsia. Journal of Obstetrics and Gynaecology of the British Commonwealth 79: 794–799.

Brosens I, Robertson W B, Dixon H G 1967 The physiological response of the vessels of the placental bed to normal pregnancy. Journal of Pathology and Bacteriology 93: 569–579.

Brosens I, Robertson W B, Dixon H G 1972 The role of the spiral arteries in the pathogenesis of preeclampsia. In: Wynn R M (ed) Obstetrics and gynecology annual 1. Appleton-Century-Crofts, NY, pp 177–191.

Brosens I, Dixon H G, Robertson W B 1977 Fetal growth retardation and the arteries of the placental bed. British Journal of Obstetrics and Gynaecology 84: 656–664.

Browne J C M, Veal L N 1953 The maternal placental blood flow in normotensive and hypertensive women. Journal of Obstetrics and Gynaecology of the British Empire 60: 141–147.

Burchell R C, Creed F, Rasoulpour M, Whitcomb M 1978 Vascular anatomy of the human uterus and pregnancy wastage. British Journal of Obstetrics and Gynaecology 85: 698–706.

Buxton C L, Olson L E 1969 Endometrial biopsy inadvertently taken during conception cycle. American Journal of Obstetrics and Gynecology 105: 702–706.

Carreras L O, Machin S J, Denman R et al 1981 Arterial thrombosis, intrauterine death and lupus anticoagulant: detection of immunoglobulin interfering with prostacyclin formation. Lancet 1: 244–246.

Chesley L C 1980 Evolution of concepts of eclampsia. In: Bonnar J, MacGillivray I, Symonds E M (eds) Pregnancy hypertension. MTP Press, Lancaster, pp 1–11.

Currie G A, Bagshawe K D 1967 The masking of antigens on trophoblast and cancer cells. Lancet 1: 708–710.

Davey D A, MacGillivray I 1988 The classification and definition of the hypertensive disorders of pregnancy. American Journal of Obstetrics and Gynecology 158: 892–898.

Demetris A J, Lasky S, Van Thiel D H et al 1985 Pathology of hepatic transplantation: a review of 62 adult allograft recipients immunosuppressed with a cyclosporin/steroid regimen. American Journal of Pathology 118: 151–161.

De Wolf F, De Wolf-Peeters C, Brosens I 1973 Ultrastructure of the spiral arteries in the human placental bed at the end of normal pregnancy. American Journal of Obstetrics and Gynecology 117: 833–848.

De Wolf F, Robertson W B, Brosens I 1975 The ultrastructure of acute atherosis in hypertensive pregnancy. American Journal of Obstetrics and Gynecology 123: 164–174.

De Wolf F, De Wolf-Peeters C, Brosens I, Robertson W B 1980a The human placental bed: electron microscopic study of trophoblastic invasion of spiral arteries. American Journal of Obstetrics and Gynecology 137: 58–70.

De Wolf F, Brosens I, Renaer M 1980b Fetal growth retardation and the maternal arterial supply of the human placenta in the absence of sustained hypertension. British Journal of Obstetrics and Gynaecology 87: 678–685.

Dixon H G, Robertson W B 1958 A study of the vessels of the placental bed in normotensive and hypertensive women. Journal of Obstetrics and Gynaecology of the British Empire 65: 803–809.

Dommisse J, Tiltman A J 1992 Placental bed biopsies in placental abruption. British Journal of Obstetrics and Gynaecology 99: 651–654.

Driscoll S G 1965 The pathology of pregnancy complicated by diabetes mellitus. Medical Clinics of North America 49: 1053–1067.

Earl U, Bulmer J N, Briones A 1987 Placenta accreta: an immunohistological study of trophoblast populations. Placenta 8: 273–282.

Edmonds D K, Lindsay K S, Miller J F et al 1982 Early embryonic mortality in women. Fertility and Sterility 38: 447–453.

Finn C A, Porter D G 1975 The uterus. Elek Science, London, pp 74–85.

Fox H 1972 Placenta accreta, 1945–1969. Obstetrical and Gynecological Survey 27: 475–490.

Fox H 1976 The histopathology of placental insufficiency. Journal of Clinical Pathology 29 suppl (Royal College of Pathologists) 10: 1–8.

Fox H 1978 Pathology of the placenta. Saunders, London.

Fox H 1979 Placental changes in gestational diabetes. In: Sutherland H W, Stowers J M (eds) Carbohydrate metabolism in pregnancy and the newborn 1978. Springer Verlag, Berlin, pp 102–113.

Fox H 1981 Placental malfunction as a factor in intrauterine growth retardation. In: Van Assche A, Robertson W B (eds) Fetal growth retardation. Churchill Livingstone, Edinburgh, pp 117–125.

Freeman R M 1991 Placenta accreta and myotonic dystrophy: two case reports. British Journal of Obstetrics and Gynaecology 98: 594–595.

Frosca T, Morassi L, Pecorelli S, Grigolato P, Gastaldi A 1989 Histological features of uteroplacental vessels in normal and hypertensive patients in relation to birthweight. British Journal of Obstetrics and Gynaecology 96: 835–839.

Gerretsen G, Huisjes H J, Elema J D 1981 Morphological changes of the spiral arteries in the placental bed in relation to preeclampsia and fetal growth retardation. British Journal of Obstetrics and Gynaecology 88: 876–881.

Gerretsen G, Huisjes H J, Hardouk M J, Elema J D 1983 Trophoblast alterations in the placental bed in relation to physiological changes in spiral arteries. British Journal of Obstetrics and Gynaecology 90: 34–39.

Gorodeski I G, Bahari C M, Schachter A, Neri A 1982 Abruption and premature separation of placenta previa. European Journal of Obstetrics, Gynecology and Reproductive Biology 13: 75–85.

Govan A D T 1976 The histology of eclamptic lesions. Journal of Clinical Pathology 29 suppl (Royal College of Pathologists) 10: 63–69.

Gruenwald P 1972 Expansion of placental site and maternal blood supply of primate placentas. Anatomical Record 173: 189–204.

Gruenwald P 1975 The supply line of the fetus: definitions relating to fetal growth. In: Gruenwald P (ed) The placenta and its maternal supply line. MTP Press, Lancaster, pp 1–17.

Gruenwald P, Levin H, Yousen H 1968 Abruption and premature separation of the placenta. American Journal of Obstetrics and Gynecology 102: 604–614.

Harden M A, Walters M, Valente P T 1990 Postabortal hemorrhage due to placental increta: a case report. Obstetrics and Gynecology 75 (2): 523–526.

Harris J W S, Ramsey E M 1966 The morphology of human uteroplacental vasculature. Contributions to embryology, no 260. Carnegie Institution of Washington Publication 625, 38: 43–58.

Hertig A T 1945 Vascular pathology in the hypertensive albuminuric toxemias of pregnancy. Clinics 4: 602–613.

Hertig A T 1964 Gestational hyperplasia of endometrium. Laboratory Investigation 13: 1153–1157.

Hustin J, Jauniaux E, Schaaps J P 1990 Histological study of the materno-embryonic interface in spontaneous abortion. Placenta 11: 477–486.

Hutton R A, Chow F P R, Craft I L, Dandona P 1980 Inhibitors of platelet aggregation in the fetoplacental unit and myometrium with particular reference to the ADP-degrading property of placenta. Placenta 1: 125–130.

Hytten F E, Leitch I 1971 The physiology of human pregnancy, 2nd edn. Blackwell, Oxford.

Jungers P, Dougados M, Pelissier C et al 1982 Lupus nephropathy and pregnancy: report of 104 cases in 36 patients. Archives of Internal Medicine 142: 771–776.

Karow W G, Gentry W C, Skeels R F, Payne S A 1971 Endometrial biopsy in the luteal phase of the cycle of conception. Fertility and Sterility 22: 482–495.

Khong T Y 1991 Acute atherosis in pregnancies complicated by hypertension, small-for-gestational-age infants and diabetes mellitus. Archives of Pathology and Laboratory Medicine 115: 722–725.

Khong T Y, Robertson W B 1987 Placenta creta and placenta praevia creta. Placenta 8: 399–409.

Khong T Y, De Wolf F, Robertson W B, Brosens I 1986 Inadequate maternal vascular response to placentation in pregnancies complicated by pre-eclampsia and by small-for gestational age infants. British Journal of Obstetrics and Gynaecology 93: 1049–1059.

Khong T Y, Liddell H S, Robertson W B 1987 Defective haemochorial placentation as a cause of miscarriage: a preliminary study. British Journal of Obstetrics and Gynaecology 94: 649–655.

Kirby D R S, Cowell T P 1968 Trophoblast-host interactions. In: Fleischmajer P, Billingham R E (eds) Epithelial-mesenchymal interactions. Williams & Wilkins, Baltimore, pp 64–77.

Kirby D R S, Billington W D, Bradbury S, Goldstein D J 1964 Antigen barrier of the mouse placenta. Nature London 204: 548–549.

Kitzmiller J L, Benirschke K 1973 Immunofluorescent study of placental bed vessels in preeclampsia of pregnancy. American Journal of Obstetrics and Gynecology 115: 248–251.

Kitzmiller J L, Watt N, Driscoll S G 1981 Decidual arteriopathy in hypertension and diabetes in pregnancy: immunofluorescent studies. American Journal of Obstetrics and Gynecology 141: 773–779.

Labarrere C, Althabe O 1985 Chronic villitis of unknown etiology and maternal arterial lesions in pre-eclamptic pregnancies. European Journal of Obstetrics, Gynecology and Reproductive Biology 20: 1–11.

Labarrere C, Althabe O 1986 Chronic villitis of unknown etiology and decidual maternal vasculopathies in sustained chronic hypertension. European Journal of Obstetrics, Gynecology and Reproductive Biology 21: 27–32.

Labarrere C A, Catoggio L J, Mullen E G, Althabe O H 1986 Placenta lesions in maternal auto-immune diseases. American Journal of Reproductive Immunology and Microbiology 12: 78–86.

Labarrere C 1988 Review article: acute atherosis: a histopathological hallmark of immune aggression? Placenta 9: 95–108.

McFadyen I R, Price A B, Geirsson R T 1986 The relation of birthweight to histological appearances in vessels of the placental bed. British Journal of Obstetrics and Gynaecology 93: 476–481.

MacGillivray I 1975 Clinical aspects of uteroplacental insufficiency. European Journal of Obstetrics, Gynecology and Reproductive Biology 5: 101–108.

MacGillivray I 1983 Preeclampsia: the hypertensive disease of pregnancy. Saunders, London.

Maqueo M, Azuela J C, De la Vega M D 1964 Placental pathology in eclampsia and preeclampsia. Obstetrics and Gynecology 24: 350–356.

Moll W, Kunzel W, Herberger J 1975 Hemodynamic implications of hemochorial placentation. European Journal of Obstetrics, Gynecology and Reproductive Biology 5: 67–74.

Noyes R W 1972 Disorders of gamete transport and implantation. In: Assali N S (ed) Pathophysiology of gestation, vol 1. Academic Press, NY, pp 64–143.

Ober W B, Grady H G 1961 Subinvolution of the placental site. Bulletin of the New York Academy of Medicine 37: 713–730.

Palmer D C, Tsar C C, Roodman S T et al 1985 Heart graft arteriosclerosis: an ominous finding on endomyocardial biopsy. Transplantation 39: 385–388.

Pijnenborg R, Dixon G, Robertson W B, Brosens I 1980 Trophoblastic invasion of human decidua from 8 to 18 weeks of pregnancy. Placenta 1: 3–19.

Pijnenborg R, Robertson W B, Brosens I, Dixon H G 1981a Trophoblast invasion and the establishment of haemochorial placentation in man and laboratory animals. Placenta 2: 71–92.

Pijnenborg R, Bland J M, Robertson W B, Dixon H G, Brosens I 1981b The pattern of interstitial trophoblastic invasion of the myometrium in early human pregnancy. Placenta 2: 303–316.

Pijnenborg R, Bland J M, Robertson W B, Brosens I 1983 Uteroplacental arterial changes related to interstitial trophoblast migration in early human pregnancy. Placenta 4: 397–414.

Pijnenborg R, Anthony J, Davey D A et al 1991 Placental bed spiral arteries in the hypertensive disorders of pregnancy. British Journal of Obstetrics and Gynaecology 98: 648–655.

Porter K A 1974 Renal transplantation. In: Heptinstall R M (ed) Pathology of the kidney. Little Brown, London, pp 977–1042.

Ramsey E M 1982 The placenta: human and animal. Praeger, NY.

Ramsey E M, Donner M W 1980 Placental vasculature and circulation. Thieme, Stuttgart.

Robertson W B 1976 Uteroplacental vasculature. Journal of Clinical Pathology 29 suppl (Royal College of Pathologists) 10: 9–17.

Robertson W B 1979 Utero-placental blood supply in maternal diabetes. In: Sutherland H W, Stowers J M (eds) Carbohydrate metabolism in pregnancy and the newborn 1978. Springer Verlag, Berlin, pp 63–75.

Robertson W B, Warner B 1974 The ultrastructure of the human placental bed. Journal of Pathology 112: 203–211.

Robertson W B, Brosens I, Dixon H G 1967 The pathological response of the vessels of the placental bed to hypertensive pregnancy. Journal of Pathology and Bacteriology 93: 581–592.

Robertson W B, Brosens I, Dixon H G 1975 Uteroplacental vascular pathology. European Journal of Obstetrics, Gynecology and Reproductive Biology 5: 47–65.

Robertson W B, Brosens I, Dixon H G 1976 Maternal uterine vascular lesions in the hypertensive complications of pregnancy. In: Lindheimer M D (ed) Hypertension in pregnancy. Wiley, NY, pp 115–127.

Robertson W B, Brosens I, Dixon H G 1981 Maternal blood supply in fetal growth retardation. In: Van Assche A, Robertson W B (eds) Fetal growth retardation. Churchill Livingstone, Edinburgh, pp 126–138.

Robertson W B, Brosens I, Landells W N 1985 Abnormal placentation. Obstetrics and Gynecology Annual 14: 411–426.

Robertson W B, Khong T Y, Brosens I, De Wolf F, Sheppard B L, Bonner J 1986 The placental bed biopsy: review from three European centres. American Journal of Obstetrics and Gynecology 155: 401–412.

Rushton D I, Dawson I M P 1982 The maternal autopsy. Journal of Clinical Pathology 35: 909–921.

Sheppard B L, Bonnar J 1976 The ultrastructure of the arterial supply of the human placenta in pregnancy complicated by fetal growth retardation. British Journal of Obstetrics and Gynaecology 83: 948–959.

Sheppard B L, Bonnar J 1980 Uteroplacental arteries and hypertensive pregnancy. In: Bonnar J, MacGillivray I, Symonds E M (eds) Pregnancy hypertension. MTP Press, Lancaster, pp 213–219.

Vermulen J, Carreras L O, Van Assche A 1981 Repeated abortion and intrauterine death in women with a lupus anticoagulant. In: Van Assche A, Robertson W B (eds) Fetal growth retardation. Churchill Livingstone, Edinburgh, pp 156–160.

Wallenburg H C S 1981 Prostaglandins and the maternal placental circulation: review and perspectives. Biological Research in Pregnancy 2: 15–22.

Wells M, Bulmer J N 1988 The human placental bed: histology, immunohistochemistry and pathology. Histopathology 13: 493–498.

Wynn R M 1972 Cytotrophoblastic specialisations: an ultrastructural study of the human placenta. American Journal of Obstetrics and Gynecology 114: 339–355.

Zeek P M, Assali N S 1950 Vascular changes in the decidua associated with eclamptogenic toxemia of pregnancy. American Journal of Clinical Pathology 20: 1099–1109.

49. Infections of the placental villi (villitis)

Peter Russell

INTRODUCTION

Recognition of pathological changes in the placenta presupposes a knowledge of its normal anatomy and histology. Diffidence in their ability to recognize these normal features may cause many pathologists to avoid examining placentas and thus under-utilize a valuable source of a tissue diagnosis in cases of suspected intra-uterine fetal infection. The often subtle changes of chronic placental inflammation are frequently either dismissed or misinterpreted as being of an ischaemic or degenerative nature. As all chorionic tissue is fetal, focal or diffuse inflammation of placental villi (villitis) should be regarded as evidence of potential infection in the associated fetus or newborn, irrespective of whether or not cultural studies lead to isolation of an organism. Chronic villitis with plasma cell infiltration has been suggested as being of immunological origin (Homberger et al, 1971; Labarrere et al, 1982); however these lesions are more likely to be a consequence of infection, even if immunological aberrations are also present.

There are two main routes of feto-placental infection, ascending and haematogenous: variations on these two main themes are shown in Figure 49.1. These two routes result in quite different patterns of inflammatory reaction, and whilst there is clearly some degree of overlap between these and their consequent patterns of inflammatory reaction to various organisms, in general villitis is a manifestation of chronic haematogenous infection whilst acute chorioamnionitis or 'amniotic infection syndrome' (discussed in Ch. 51) is due to infection via an ascending route.

Villitis is an 'intrinsic inflammatory response occurring within one or more villi, the proliferating or infiltrating cells being fetal in origin. This inflammatory response is initiated by the fetus against an external antigenic stimulus' (Altshuler & Russell, 1975). Villitis should be distinguished from maternal sinusoidal inflammatory cells chemotactically attracted to the periphery of infarcted villi. The lesions of villitis tend to be focal and extensive

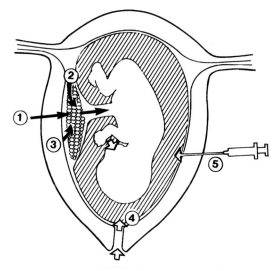

Fig. 49.1 Pathways of feto-placental infection; haematogenous via (1) maternal bloodstream, (2) direct spread from residual endometrial infection, (3) via ascending decidual infection; ascending via (4) amniotic fluid infection or (5) iatrogenic amniotic fluid infection (amniocentesis).

sampling may be required to demonstrate their presence in mild cases (Fig. 49.2). At the other extreme much of the placental parenchyma is involved (Fig. 49.3). Focal lesions are usually randomly distributed in the placenta although some cases show a propensity to involve the basal or 'anchoring' villi adjacent to the maternal decidua (Fig. 49.4).

The placenta has a limited ability to respond specifically to different infective organisms and much histological overlap in inflammatory patterns is observed with the variety of micro-organisms known to infect the feto-placental unit (Table 49.1). Various patterns of villitis are observed, describing evolution and repair stages and secondary changes in the placenta consequent upon inflammatory processes (Altshuler & Russell, 1975; Russell, 1980). Subtle variations in these, however, can be noted and may allow the pathologist to direct clinicians to a particular avenue of cultural or serological confirmation;

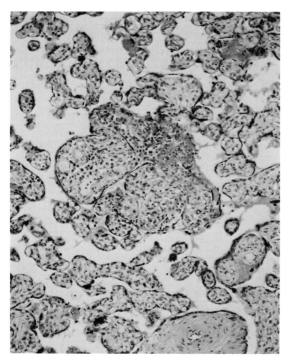

Fig. 49.2 Mild focal villitis showing a small group of disrupted villi with an intrinsic inflammatory infiltrate, stromal fibroplasia and peripheral fibrin deposition. H & E × 150.

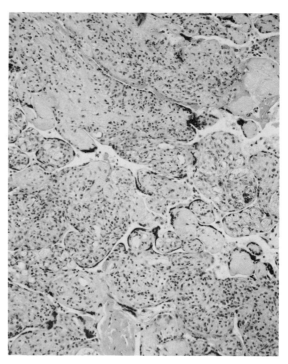

Fig. 49.3 Severe villitis. Much of the placental parenchyma is involved in the chronic proliferative inflammation with scarred acellular villi in areas where inflammation has subsided. H & E × 150.

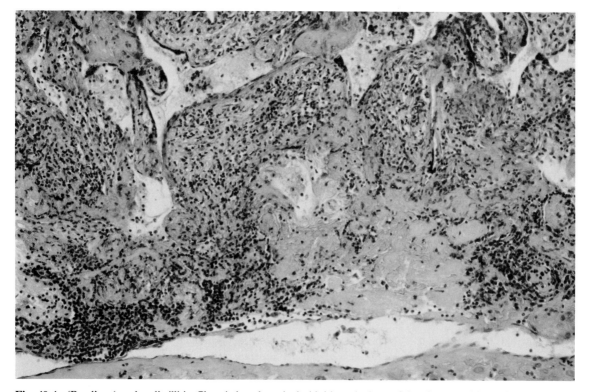

Fig. 49.4 'Basal' or 'parabasal' villitis. Chronic lymphocytic deciduitis at the base of the placenta with contiguous spread to the adjacent placental villi. H & E × 210.

Table 49.1   Organisms associated with haematogenous infection

BACTERIA
  Staphylococcus
  Streptococcus
  Pneumococcus
  Listeria monocytogenes
  Mycobacterium tuberculosis
  Mycobacterium leprae
  Enteric bacteria
  Salmonella
  Brucella
  Campylobacter fetus
  Vibrio cholerae
  Francisella tularensis
  Treponema pallidum
  Borrelia
  Leptospira

MYCOPLASMAS

CHLAMYDIA

RICKETTSIAE
  Rickettsia bacilliformis
    (Bartonella)

FUNGI
  Coccidioides immitis
  Cryptococcus

PARASITES AND PROTOZOA
  Toxoplasma gondii
  Plasmodia
  Schistosoma
  Trypanosoma cruzi

VIRUSES
  Herpesvirus
    Cytomegalovirus
    Herpes simplex virus
    Varicella zoster
    Epstein–Barr virus
  Rubella
  Poxvirus
    Variola alastrim
    Vaccinia
  Hepatitis B
  Picornavirus
    Poliomyelitis
    ECHO
    Coxsackie A and B
    Hepatitis A
  Paramyxovirus
    Mumps
    Measles
    Influenza
  Arbovirus
    Western equine encephalitis
  Human immunodeficiency virus

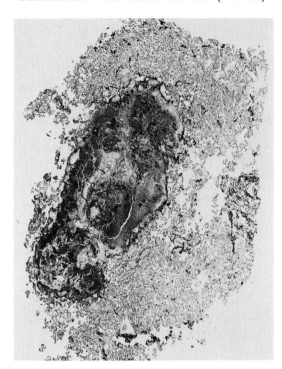

Fig. 49.5   Congenital listeriosis. Macroscopically visible septic focus sharply demarcated and with a central abscess cavity. H & E × 12.

occasionally the causative organism can be identified by light- or electronmicroscopy. Although the following descriptions are of placental changes only, the reader is directed, for further clinicopathological correlation, to the landmark publications by Blanc (1961, 1981).

BACTERIAL INFECTIONS

Listeria monocytogenes

These short Gram-positive rods are facultative anaerobes and may be confused with diphtheroids: they do, however, have specific cultural requirements. *Listeria monocytogenes* is a well-known cause of abortion and fetal wastage in animals and, although it is an uncommon human pathogen, a significant majority of reported isolates have been in neonates and pregnant women (Rappaport et al, 1960; Seeliger, 1961). Listeriosis is least rare in Scandinavia and Australia, and has only occasionally been reported as a cause of reproductive failure elsewhere.

Affected placentas typically show parenchymal abscesses (Fig. 49.5) together with chorioamnionitis and funisitis. Therefore, it is far from clear whether infection is principally by the ascending or haematogenous route or if both types of infection occur simultaneously (Sarrut & Alison, 1967; Blanc, 1981). Microabscesses and septic infarcts are widely distributed in the placenta of second- and third-trimester pregnancies and the larger of these are visible grossly. Histologically, early lesions are composed of groups of necrotic villi and fibrin heavily infiltrated with neutrophils. Central abscess cavities later develop and slightly older lesions have a rim of palisaded histiocytes (Fig. 49.6), this feature appearing to be specific for listeriosis. More granulomatous lesions may be seen nearby (Fig. 49.7) and smaller satellite foci showing acute villous vasculitis or subtrophoblastic collections of neutrophils in single villi are also noted. These latter two patterns are less specific, both being present in the absence of listeriosis (see villitis of unknown aetiology — Fig. 49.25). Sarrut & Alison (1967) have made the important point that organisms are not always demonstrable in the lesions.

Mycobacterium tuberculosis

The reduced fertility of patients with pelvic tuberculosis and the rarity of miliary tuberculosis complicating pregnancy make placental and congenital tuberculosis singularly uncommon (Ramos et al, 1974; Kaplan et al, 1980). Illustrated descriptions of the placental pathology of tuberculosis have dated therefore from the turn of the century (Schmorl & Kockel, 1894; Schmorl & Geipl, 1904) and these have included details of fetuses in whom transplacental passage of acid-fast bacilli had occurred. This, however, in rare even in the presence of widespread placental tuberculosis (Rich, 1950).

Tuberculous placental lesions are essentially the same as those in other organs, varying from characteristic miliary tubercles to large zones of caseation. Such foci are

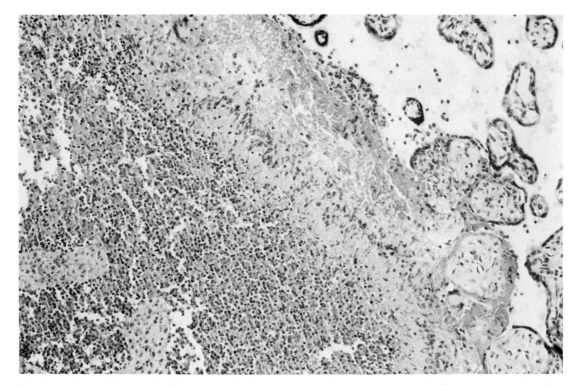

Fig. 49.6 Congenital listeriosis. The margin of a microabscess showing central neutrophil infiltration and peripherally palisaded histiocytes. H & E × 210.

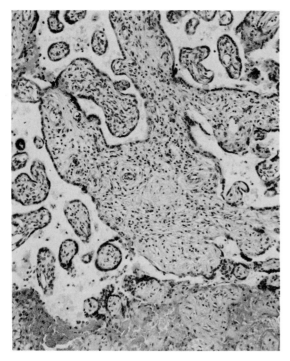

Fig. 49.7 Chronic granulomatous villitis adjacent to a microabscess of placental listeriosis. H & E × 150.

centred in villi or in intervillous spaces. A non-specific deciduitis may be noted but membranitis occurs only in isolated cases (Benirschke & Driscoll, 1967). Blanc (1981) makes the point that, because of the rarity of placental tuberculosis, the presence of giant cells in a case of villitis should prompt a careful exclusion of varicella and vaccinia.

Mycobacterium leprae

Placentas from women with leprosy (particularly lepromatous leprosy) tend to be small (Duncan, 1980) but no other abnormality has been documented. Lepra bacilli have been found in placentas of leprous patients within both villous tissues and the maternal intervillous space (Sugai & Monobe, 1912) but in neither this study nor that of others (King & Marks, 1958; Duncan et al, 1984) have any histologically definable lesions been demonstrated.

Enteric and other Gram-negative organisms

Coliforms may, at various times, be common pathogens in perinatal disease. Chorioamnionitis is the typical lesion associated with such bacteria, indicating an ascending pathway of placental infection as described by Blanc (1961). In those rare cases in which villitis occurs in association with coliform infections (e.g. criminal abortions or maternal septicaemia), membranitis is also often present, supporting this concept. Scott & Henderson (1972) reported a case of intrauterine fetal transfusion in which the transfused blood was contaminated with the Gram-negative *Acinetobacter calcoaceticus*, this organism being isolated from the blood of mother and fetus after delivery: the placenta was free of membranitis but showed a villitis. Maternal septicaemia was probably consequent upon fetal, and therefore villous, bacteraemia originating from contaminated blood in the fetal abdomen.

The histology of villitis due to Gram-negative organisms is characteristic. Lesions are marked by maternal intervillous fibrin and leucostasis around villi showing various stages of evolution of microabscesses (Fig. 49.8). Organisms are sufficiently abundant that a Gram stain is often not necessary for their recognition.

Brucella

Documentation of inflammatory lesions in the human placenta due to the Brucella group of bacteria is poor. Thus, although brucellosis is a significant cause of pregnancy loss and placentitis in animals, only rare isolates of *Brucella melitensis* (Sarram et al, 1974) and *Brucella abortus* (Trifonova, 1959; Poole et al, 1972) have been made from human placental and/or aborted material. In these cases, descriptions of placental lesions were limited to terms such as 'necrosis' and 'necrobiosis'.

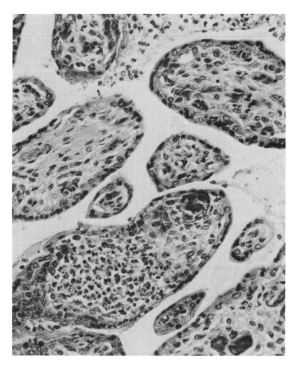

Fig. 49.8 Acute suppurative villitis due to *E. coli* from a septic abortion. Neutrophil infiltrates within villi and in intervillous spaces are noted. Bacterial colonies are centred on villous vessels. H & E × 300.

Campylobacter fetus

The organism is a curved, Gram-negative coccobacillus, with fastidious anaerobic cultural requirements. It is well known as a venereally transmitted cause of abortion in sheep and cattle but has only rarely been implicated in human reproductive failure (Eden, 1966). Some authors have pointed to epidemiological similarities between listeriosis and *Campylobacter fetus* infection (Willis & Austin, 1966) and have suggested the rarity of diagnosis of the latter to be at least partly due to lack of awareness as well as difficulty in its microbiological identification.

Human infection was first described by Vinzent et al in 1947; since then, investigators have reported infrequent isolates of *Campylobacter fetus* from aborted fetal material (Hood & Todd, 1966) and from neonates (Willis & Austin, 1966).

Rare documentation of placental pathology has been provided by Vinzent (Vinzent, 1949; Vinzent et al, 1950) and somewhat more recently by Gilbert et al (1981), who described widespread foci of placental necrosis with an associated intense neutrophil response. Organisms were present in these lesions.

Francisella tularensis

Tularaemia is acquired by contact with infected rabbits, ticks or flies. The organism is a Gram-negative coccobacillus, an uncommon pathogen in the mainland United States and Russia and rare elsewhere.

Lide (1947) has described the only case to date of placental villitis due to *Francisella tularensis*. The placenta, associated with a 2400 g macerated stillborn fetus, exhibited many confluent intervillous granulomatous lesions, several of which were centrally necrotic. Cellular infiltrates were a mixture of neutrophils, lymphocytes and histiocytes. Similar lesions were present in fetal tissues and abundant organisms were demonstrated in inflammatory foci and elsewhere.

Treponema pallidum

Almost all countries of the world are experiencing a resurgence of syphilis and with it the risk of intrauterine infection of this ancient disease. To place the pathologist's rôle in perspective it is appropriate that we be disabused of some popular misconceptions relating to intrauterine syphilis. Firstly, evidence indicates that spirochaetes can cross the placenta and invade the fetus regardless of the stage of gestation (Hager, 1978), and indeed have been reported in first-trimester placentas (Harter & Benirschke, 1976). Absence of a host inflammatory response may indicate either an immunologically immature host or a very early (inductive) phase of the infection (Walter et al,

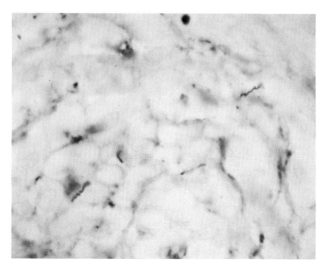

Fig. 49.9 Placenta in congenital syphilis. Spirochaetes are readily demonstrated in untreated cases. Warthin–Starry × 1500.

1982b). Secondly, the spirochaetes are so sensitive to penicillin that even a single maternal dose will preclude their histological identification within the placenta. In untreated cases, the presence of spirochaetes — best stained for by the Warthin–Starry method — is pathognomonic (Fig. 49.9). Thirdly, if the mother commences therapy more than a few weeks before delivery or if the infant, though infected, appears normal, then the associated pla-

centa will be essentially normal (Blanc, 1981). The place of placental examination is thus in the diagnosis or documentation of suspected but untreated cases, be they liveborn, stillborn or aborted, and particularly if serological confirmation is not readily available.

The placenta tends to be large and pale (Malan et al, 1990) but not oedematous and presents a triad of histological features, none of which is specific, but which together are highly suggestive of congenital syphilis (Hormann, 1954; Russell & Altshuler, 1974; Walter et al, 1982b). The first of these is relative immaturity — the villi being larger than normal and showing peripheral budding, immature trophoblast and marked hypercellularity due partly to more obvious Hofbauer cells. Nucleated red blood cells are present in the fetal circulation (Fig. 49.10). These changes relate to infective haemolytic anaemia in the infant; their severity depends on the degree of anaemia, and they are similar to those found with other intrauterine fetal anaemias. The second feature is an endovascular proliferation leading to obstruction of stem villous vessels (Fig. 49.11). This feature is seen in other congenital infections (cytomegalovirus, rubella, villitis of unknown aetiology) but is much more prominent in intrauterine syphilis. Distal villi become acellular and atrophic as a consequence. Perivascular proliferation also may be noted, but this is similar to the change in stem villous vessels after prolonged intrauterine death and its

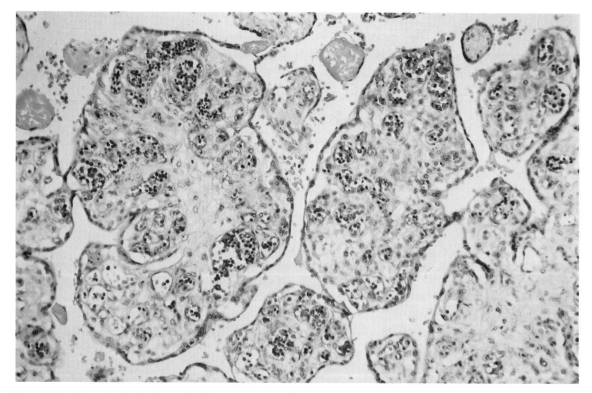

Fig. 49.10 Placental relative immaturity from a term case of congenital syphilis. The changes illustrated here are indistinguishable from those of intrauterine toxoplasmosis or of immunohaemolytic anaemia. H & E × 210.

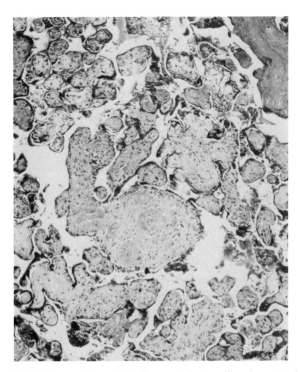

Fig. 49.11 Congenital syphilis. The central stem villus shows marked endovascular proliferation to the point of vessel obstruction. H & E × 120.

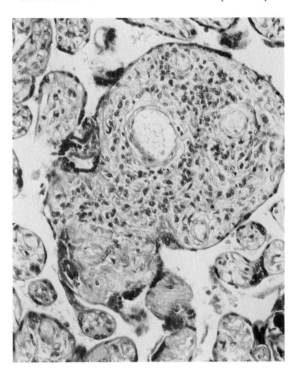

Fig. 49.12 Congenital syphilis. Focal villitis showing an almost pure plasma cell infiltrate with only occasional lymphocytes. H & E × 360.

significance is therefore less clear. The third feature is a focal proliferative villitis which varies from lymphocytic to granulomatous (Russell & Altshuler, 1974) but which characteristically is marked by numerous plasma cells (Fig. 49.12). The only other placental disorder showing as prominent a plasma cell infiltrate is cytomegalovirus infection (q.v.) and the background histological changes of this differ significantly from those of congenital syphilis.

MYCOPLASMAS

A relationship between genital mycoplasmas and chorioamnionitis has been demonstrated (Shurin et al, 1974; Embree et al, 1980) but too few investigations have been performed to assess any possible association between mycoplasma infection and villitis.

CHLAMYDIAE

Chlamydia trachomatis

To date, no placental lesion has been attributed to this organism in humans, but it is a common inhabitant of the female genital tract, is known to be a cause of salpingitis and postpartum endometritis, and may have abortifacient potential. The relationship of Chlamydia trachomatis to villitis of unknown aetiology has been the subject of some investigation (Russell, 1980). Initial suggestions of a link

between villitis of unknown aetiology, non-bacterial ophthalmia neonatorum and low birth weight, however, have not led to a clear relationship between this placental lesion and positive chlamydial cultures.

FUNGAL INFECTIONS

Coccidioidomycosis, a highly communicable disease caused by Coccidioides immitis and most prevalent in the south west of the United States, has been reported to produce various placental lesions of necrotic, caseous and purulent types (Figs 49.13 and 49.14). Tubercle-like granulomas have also been noted. It would appear, however, that even in the presence of severe placental infection, passage of the organism to the fetus does not occur (Vaughan & Ramirez, 1951; Baker, 1955; Spark, 1981). Cryptococcus neoformans has recently been demonstrated to infect the placenta in a woman with acquired immunodeficiency syndrome (Kida et al, 1989). Multiple colonies of encapsulated budding yeasts were present in the intervillous (maternal) spaces, but there was no significant inflammatory response, and transmission of the fungus to the fetus did not occur. Histoplasmosis is a common fungus infection capable of causing serious disease, but there has not been a reported case of placental infection with this organism. Similarly, although Candida albicans and Torulopsis glabrata (Quirke et al, 1980) may be associated with chorioamnionitis, they do not produce a villitis.

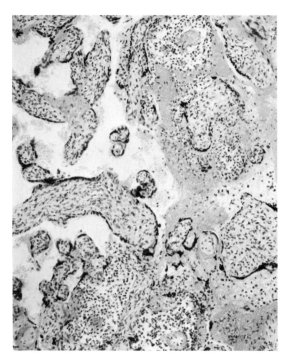

Fig. 49.13 Placental coccidioidomycosis. An acute suppurative villitis in which sporangia are seen (top and bottom). H & E × 150. (Material courtesy of Dr. Geoffrey Altshuler, Oklahoma City.)

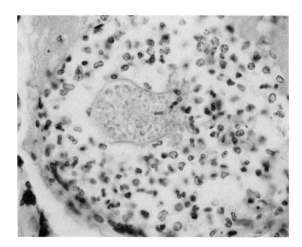

Fig. 49.14 Placental coccidioidomycosis. A ruptured sporangium with release of endospores. H & E × 600. (Material courtesy of Dr. Geoffrey Altshuler, Oklahoma City.)

PARASITIC AND PROTOZOAN INFECTIONS

Toxoplasma gondii

The organism *Toxoplasma gondii* is an obligate intracellular parasite, the life cycle of which has now been delineated (Frenkel et al, 1970). 'The great majority of babies born to women who acquire toxoplasmosis during pregnancy are unaffected or minimally so' (Desmonts & Couvreur, 1974). The occasional severe cases of congenital toxoplasmosis seem to derive principally from second-trimester maternal infections.

Placentas associated with *Toxoplasma gondii* infection may show no macroscopic abnormality but are more often large and pale, and thus resemble those of erythroblastosis fetalis or congenital syphilis. This similarity is also apparent at the microscopic level with patchy villous hyperplasia and immaturity and nucleated red blood cells within fetal vessels (Altshuler, 1973; Altshuler & Russell, 1975), these being a result of the associated fetal anaemia. A chronic focal proliferative villitis is also typically present with lymphocytes and histiocytes predominating (Elliott, 1970; Susani, 1981; Garcia et al, 1983; Abdel-Salam et al, 1990; Popek, 1992), plasma cells being rarely seen. Older lesions show fibrosis of villi: the inflammatory process characteristically involves single or small groups of villi. A chronic lymphocytic deciduitis is noted in the fetal membranes and maternal floor of the placenta (Benirschke & Driscoll, 1967), and rarely a funisitis (Garcia, 1968).

The parasite is usually encysted and most readily found in the amnion and chorion, less often in the decidua. An inflammatory response is characteristically absent (Fig. 49.15), indeed placentas have been documented in which encysted *Toxoplasma gondii* were present without any of the other stigmata of placental toxoplasmosis (Glasser & Delta, 1965).

Plasmodia

Malaria is still endemic in many countries and transmission to the human fetus has been known to occur for half

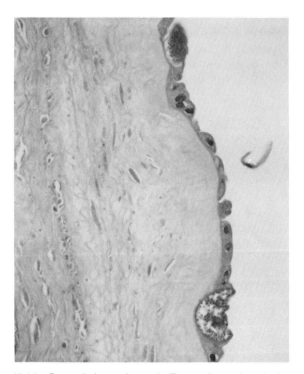

Fig. 49.15 Congenital toxoplasmosis. Encysted organisms in the amnion. Note complete absence of an inflammatory response. H & E × 600.

a century (Wickramasuriya, 1935), parasites having been demonstrated in tissues of both liveborn and stillborn infants.

Placental changes (Galbraith et al, 1980a,b; Walter et al, 1982a; Bulmer et al 1993a,b) include parasitized erythrocytes in the maternal sinusoids, if the placenta is delivered during a malarial bout, and pigment deposition. Less specifically, heavy monocytic infiltrates (some cells containing ingested malarial pigment) are noted in intervillous spaces, excess intervillous fibrin is deposited and a very mild focal lymphocytic and histiocytic villitis may also occur (Wickramasuriya, 1935, Benirschke & Driscoll, 1967). Trophoblastic basement membrane thickening, cytotrophoblastic prominence and villous fibrinoid necrosis have also been noted (Bulmer et al, 1993b).

Ultrastructurally, there is focal damage to syncytiotrophoblast and trophoblastic basal lamina thickening (Walter et al, 1982a).

Schistosoma

Schistosomiasis is probably the most common parasitic disease of man, affecting approximately 150 million individuals in the geographically endemic areas — namely Africa, South and Central America and the Far East. Placental bilharziasis was first described by Sutherland et al in 1965 and is characterized by a lack of inflammatory response to schistosomal ova, although two cases have demonstrated focal granulomas (Bittencourt et al, 1980). Placental involvement appears to occur particularly in women with urinary or genital tract schistosomiasis (Renaud et al, 1972) and without affecting the outcome of the pregnancy or fetus. Extensive time-consuming examination of the placenta for ova may be obviated by the method of digestion of placental segments in sodium hydroxide followed by lightmicroscopic examination of the sediment (Sutherland et al, 1965).

Trypanosoma cruzi

Chagas' disease is almost entirely confined to South and Central America and has infection of the sarcoplasm of heart muscle with leishmanial forms of the organism as its hallmark (Olivier et al, 1972). It differs from the closely related African trypanosomiasis ('sleeping sickness') which is characterized by lymph node and cerebral infestation. Chronically affected chagasic mothers transmit the disease transplacentally to about 10% of their offspring and fetal infection may recur with successive pregnancies.

The most complete documentation of placental Chagas' disease has been by Bittencourt (Bittencourt, 1960, 1963; Bittencourt et al, 1972). Widespread and severe granulomatous villitis is noted with a mixed histiocytic and giant cell infiltrate. Older lesions show villous scarring. Hofbauer cells contain leishmanial forms of the parasite (Fig. 49.16), these being occasionally difficult to find.

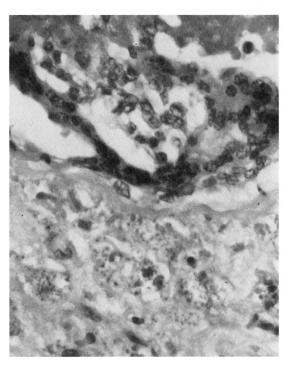

Fig. 49.16 Placental Chagas' disease. Leishmanial forms of the organism are present in stromal Hofbauer cells. H & E × 600.

VIRUSES

Cytomegalovirus

Cytomegalovirus (CMV) infection is common in pregnancy with about 5% of pregnant women actively excreting the virus in their urine and an even greater percentage via the cervix uteri. A significant proportion of recently delivered women also excrete CMV in their breast milk. However, current evidence suggests that infection acquired during or just after delivery is not specially harmful and that intrauterine infection is responsible for most of the havoc caused by this virus. It has been further shown that congenital viraemia associated with primary maternal infection is much more likely to lead to a symptomatically affected infant than that associated with recurrent maternal disease (Stagno et al, 1982).

Grossly, the placenta may be normal but with severely affected infants is more likely to be bulky and pale. The range of changes detailed histologically (Monif & Dische, 1972; Benirschke et al, 1974; Altshuler & Russell, 1975; Blanc, 1978; Garcia et al, 1989) is influenced by fetal age and the chronicity of the infection, but reasonably constant features are:

a. An acute necrotizing villitis, particularly in early cases, with nuclear debris and stromal hyalinization (Fig. 49.17). Trophoblast is relatively spared compared to other villitides but the fetal vessels often show an acute vasculitis with luminal obliteration or thrombosis. Older lesions show villous scarring.

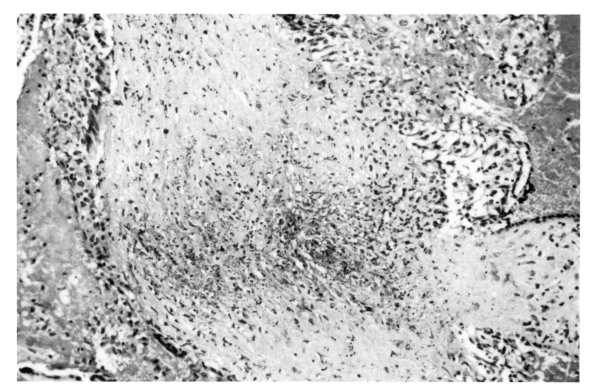

Fig. 49.17 Acute necrotizing villitis of CMV infection. Stromal hyalinization and 'dusting' with nuclear debris are prominent. H & E × 210.

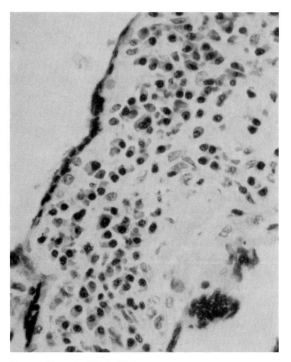

Fig. 49.18 Chronic CMV villitis with a prominent plasmacytic infiltrate. H & E × 600.

b. A lymphoplasmacytic infiltrate in which plasmacytes may be very prominent indeed (Fig. 49.18).

c. Focal or generalized villous oedema (Fig. 49.19) with prominence of the Hofbauer cells, these latter often assuming unusual configurations (Blanc, 1981). This change is distinct from the relative immaturity and erythroblastosis-like changes occasioned by the fetal anaemia often also present (see Fig. 49.10 of congenital syphilis).

d. Deposition of haemosiderin can be seen in villous stroma and is probably a marker of the vascular damage so prominent in CMV villitis. Calcific deposits may also be present in old lesions.

e. Cytomegalic cells (Fig. 49.20) are often difficult to find, particularly in chronic cases, but are specific for this disease. Immunocytochemical studies have demonstrated viral antigens in the villous Hofbauer cells (Schwartz et al, 1992) and in the endothelial cells of the villous fetal vessels (Muhlemann et al, 1992). Blanc (1978) has observed a reasonable correlation between the severity of these various placental changes and the outcome for the fetus/infant.

A further interesting lesion is focal necrotizing deciduitis subjacent to the placenta or fetal membranes. Typical inclusions are not seen in or near these lesions yet they may prove to be relevant in view of the suggestion that an additional mode of pathogenesis of congenital CMV

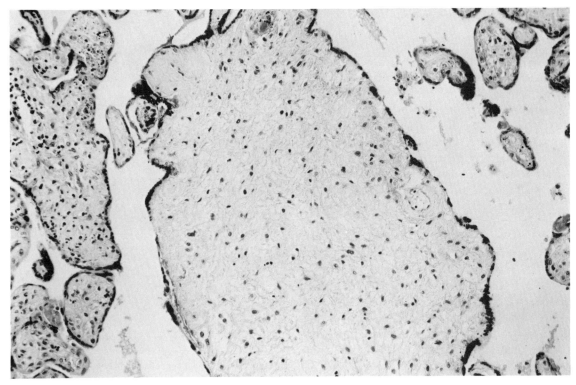

Fig. 49.19 Chronic CMV villitis with focal villous oedema. An active proliferative inflammation is seen in the villi to the left. H & E × 210.

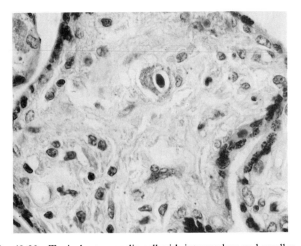

Fig. 49.20 Typical cytomegalic cell with intranuclear and smaller cytoplasmic granular inclusions. H & E × 600.

is transmission of reactivated latent virus to the fetus from the endometrium (Alford et al, 1980). Perhaps also related to CMV infection is the so-called 'haemorrhagic endovasculitis and haemorrhagic villitis' of Sander (1980) which accentuates the vasculotropic properties of this virus (described in the section on Villitis of unknown aetiology).

Herpes simplex virus

Haematogenous and ascending routes of feto-placental infection have both been documented for this virus. Clinically, the ascending route is the more important with haematogenous and mixed patterns occurring only infrequently (Hanshaw, 1973). Descriptions of placental pathology are limited to a few cases. Some demonstrate acute or subacute necrotizing membranitis (Altshuler, 1974; Blanc, 1978) with oedema, and a chorioamnionic mononuclear infiltrate with nearby cells containing typical intranuclear inclusions. Similar changes may be noted in the umbilical cord.

Acute transplacental herpes infection has been correlated with multiple foci of bland placental necrosis (Witzleben & Driscoll, 1965; Blanc, 1978). Intranuclear inclusions suggestive of herpesvirus infection have been observed but the lesions are further typified by a relative lack of inflammatory cell infiltration. It is interesting to note, therefore, that Blanc (1981) also describes a lymphocytic villitis in 'chronic' herpes infection of the placenta.

Varicella

Most cases of congenital chickenpox have occurred following maternal infection late in pregnancy (Keutel, 1968) and are mild. Occasional reports of early gestational infection with this herpesvirus note the possibility of teratogenic effects on the fetus (Srabstein et al, 1974).

The reports of chickenpox placentitis by Garcia (1963) and Blanc (1978, 1981) indicate a spectrum of lesions varying from acute necrotizing focal villitis in early and severe cases, with progressive or subacute disease manifesting itself as a granulomatous villitis in which histiocytic giant cells are noted. These latter may exhibit eosinophilic intranuclear inclusions (also present in the decidual cells). Affected villi are bound by maternal fibrin and produce macroscopically visible foci, so-called 'rice seeds' (Garcia, 1963). Plasma cells are not observed in acute or subacute stages but are sometimes present in chronic cases (Blanc, 1981).

Epstein–Barr virus

Ornoy et al (1982) have reported placental lesions in association with maternal infectious mononucleosis. Their five cases were derived from therapeutic terminations for maternal disease and two of three fetuses examined had viral myocarditis. The placentas variously showed a perivasculitis and necrotizing deciduitis in the maternal floor, an acute chorionitis and a villitis notable for vascular obliteration and for mononuclear and plasma cell infiltration. Trophoblastic necrosis and villous oedema were also found.

Rubella

Most instances of congenital rubella syndrome are associated with acute maternal viraemia during an epidemic. However, it is well to note that as well as these and sporadic primary infections, re-infection of pregnant women can lead to fetal involvement (Northrop et al, 1972; Eilard & Strannegard, 1974) and that women can excrete the virus from the uterine cervix for prolonged periods of time (Seppala & Vaheri, 1974), thus raising the possibility of an ascending viral infection of the conceptus.

Placentas tend to be smaller than normal but macroscopically otherwise unremarkable (Garcia et al, 1985). The reported series of placental rubella (Tondury & Smith, 1966; Driscoll, 1969; Ornoy et al, 1973; Garcia et al, 1985) indicate that focal lesions progress through similar stages to those described for CMV infection. Early lesions are characterized by a necrotizing villitis in which acute endovasculitis is particularly prominent (Fig. 49.21). Endothelial necrosis may be accompanied by erythrocyte fragmentation but not haemorrhage. Clusters of affected villi are bound together by intervillous fibrin consequent upon trophoblast damage. While some continuation of the inflammatory process manifests itself as neutrophilic or lymphocytic infiltrates (but rarely plasma cells), much of the acute villitis subsides leaving atrophic scarred avascular villi (Fig. 49.22). Blanc (1981) has stressed the

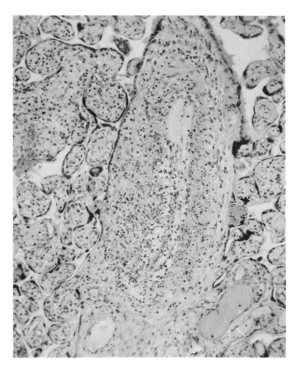

Fig. 49.21 Rubella villitis showing an acute endovasculitis in the central stem villus. H & E × 150.

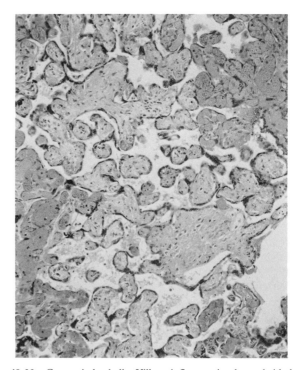

Fig. 49.22 Congenital rubella. Villous inflammation has subsided leaving scarred avascular villi. H & E × 150.

various vascular changes in the inflammatory process including endothelial cushions and old calcified thrombi. Eosinophilic inclusions may be found in the endothelial cells as well as in the trophoblast.

Villous immaturity and oedema are not features of this viral placentitis and, with the absence of haemosiderin deposition and erythroblastosis, readily distinguish it from CMV villitis. A chronic lymphocytic deciduitis is sometimes present (Benirschke & Driscoll, 1967) but occasionally the placentas are histologically normal (Fox, 1978).

Vaccinia and variola

Sporadic reports have appeared in the literature of prenatal poxvirus infection occurring as a complication of vaccination in pregnancy (Wielenga et al, 1961; Entwistle et al, 1962; Hood & McKinnon, 1963) and of congenital variola minor (Garcia, 1963). These have documented focal necrotizing villitis with eosinophilic inclusions. It is to be hoped that these lesions remain of historical interest only and the preterist is referred to the above reports for histological detail.

Hepatitis B

Hepatitis B virus can infect the fetus transplacentally as well as intrapartum, particularly if clinical infection of the mother occurs in the third trimester. In most instances the infection manifests itself only as a transient antigenaemia but clinical hepatitis may result with long-term sequelae (Gillespie et al, 1970).

Placentas of infants with biopsy-proven congenital hepatitis have shown a diffuse relative immaturity but no inflammatory infiltrate (Altshuler & Russell, 1975). Similar changes have been observed in placentas from infants with hepatitic mothers. These changes could be a direct effect of the virus but more likely represent a non-specific marker of the associated jaundice and/or anaemia.

Picornavirus

Polio, ECHO, coxsackie A and B and hepatitis A viruses have been shown to infect the fetus transplacentally, and these viruses have, on occasion, been isolated from placentas (Mehrotra, 1986; Prabhu & Pendharkar, 1986). ECHO viruses are briefly described as producing a non-specific proliferating, necrotizing and reparative villitis and an acute intervillositis (Garcia et al, 1990). In the single report of intrauterine coxsackie A infection (Batcup et al, 1985), a severe necrotizing villitis with diffuse perivillous fibrin deposition has been described. Coxsackie-virus A9 was cultured. Investigations have suggested a link between early intrauterine coxsackie B infection and the hypoplastic left heart syndrome (Trevenen et al, 1982). From other cases of picornavirus infection histologically examined, however, morphological placental abnormalities have not been identified (Baskin et al, 1950; Kilbrick & Benirschke, 1958).

Paramyxovirus

Mumps, measles and influenza viruses (Yawn et al, 1971; Moroi et al, 1991) have all been documented as crossing the placenta but significant placental lesions have been observed in only the first of these infections. Garcia et al (1980) have described widespread necrotizing villitis with nuclear dust and necrotic material in the intervillous space. Granulomas containing giant cells and epithelioid cells were noted in some villi. Eosinophilic cytoplasmic inclusions were described in villous fibroblasts as well as in decidual cells.

While haematogenous infection is assumed for each of these infections, Blanc (1981) raises the possibility of ascending amniotic infection in two reported cases of congenital giant cell pneumonia, possibly measles, as an alternative. Abnormalities in the placentas were absent in these cases.

C virus

C-type particles have been identified electronmicroscopically in normal human placentas (Kalter et al, 1973; Vernon et al, 1974) and in placentas from patients with systemic lupus erythematosus (Imamura et al, 1976), but the significance of this finding is as yet unknown.

Human immunodeficiency virus

Histopathological features specific for HIV infection have not been identified, although HIV antigen may be identified immunohistochemically in the trophoblast of placentas which show other evidence of placental infection such as chorioamnionitis (Chandwani et al, 1991).

VILLITIS OF UNKNOWN AETIOLOGY

Microbiological, serological or electronmicroscopic techniques may be used to confirm or exclude specific causes of the agglomerate of histological features referred to as 'villitis' in the preceding sections. Even in the absence of such confirmation, some cases of villitis are sufficiently typical to permit a firm diagnosis on histological grounds alone. There will be, despite our best efforts, however, a very significant residuum of cases in which these techniques fail to identify a causative agent and the villitis remains non-specific or of unknown aetiology.

Villitis of unknown aetiology has been estimated as occurring in 6–10% of *all* placentas in Australia and North America (Altshuler & Russell, 1975; Russell, 1979; Blanc, 1981; Kaplan et al, 1985) and about 13% of placentas within the United Kingdom (Knox & Fox, 1984) and is thus by far the commonest type of villitis. Clinical consequences for the infant are usually insignificant, for which reason attention is not drawn to the placenta and knowledge of the existence of this lesion amongst pathologists and obstetricians alike is very sporadic. It has recently been linked with preterm delivery where its incidence is inversely proportional to the presence of chorionic or umbilical vasculitis (Salafia et al, 1991). In severe cases it is undoubtedly an important cause of retarded intrauterine growth (Altshuler et al, 1975; Labarrere et al, 1982; Bjoro & Myhre, 1984; Althabe & Labarrere, 1985; Kaplan et al, 1985) and may be associated with otherwise unexplained stillbirth. The mechanism by which it causes intrauterine growth retardation is not known — possibly by destruction of placental tissue (although this appears rarely of sufficient severity to account for significant fetal malnutrition), possibly by the inhibitory effect on the fetal growth of the associated infective organism (although no organism/s has been identified and the infants do not show other signs of intrauterine infection). Villitis of unknown aetiology also recurs in successive pregnancies in a proportion of cases (Russell, 1979, 1980; Redline & Abramowsky, 1985). The assumption that this inflammatory process is infective in origin is based on the similarity of the histological lesions to those occurring in association with villitides of known infections. Other possibilities include a type of host-versus-graft reaction (Labarrere et al 1989, 1990). Until such time as it is known whether the inflammatory cells are of fetal or maternal origin, and whether the inciting antigen is intrinsic or extrinsic (Fox, 1991), this dilemma will remain unsolved.

The range of severity of placental lesions is seen in Figures 49.2 and 49.3 and, as noted earlier, most lesions are randomly distributed in the placenta with a basal component (Fig. 49.4) in about one-fifth of cases. Recurrent cases show the same range of severity, although reports in the literature are biased towards the clinically spectacular (Dollmann & Schmitz-Moormann, 1972; Russell et al, 1980; Blanc, 1981). In my experience and that of others (Redline & Abramowsky, 1985), although there is marked variation in severity of the villitis between patients, recurrent cases show remarkable consistency in severity of the inflammatory process between placentas of successive pregnancies.

The cellularity of the lesions varies from lymphocytic (Fig. 49.23) and resembling active rubella villitis to quite granulomatous (Fig. 49.24) and showing features common to placental chickenpox. Less commonly an acute necrotizing villitis is present (Fig. 49.25) with features indistinguishable from the early placental lesions of listeriosis (acute chorioamnionitis, however, is absent, the infants are unaffected and listeria organisms are not found). Residual scarring follows subsidence of the inflammation. Vascular involvement of the stem villi may produce acellular hyaline atrophy of the terminal villi.

'Haemorrhagic endovasculitis' is a variant described by Sander (Sander, 1980; Sander & Stevens, 1984; Sander et al, 1986) which, to date, is poorly reported from regions outside the Michigan-Great Lakes area of the United

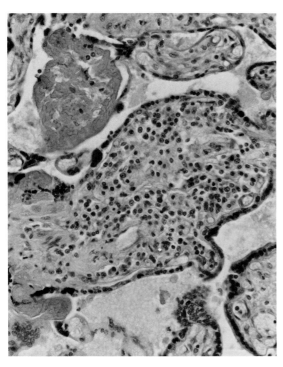

Fig. 49.23 Villitis of unknown aetiology. A lymphocytic infiltrate with relative sparing of villous architecture. H & E × 300.

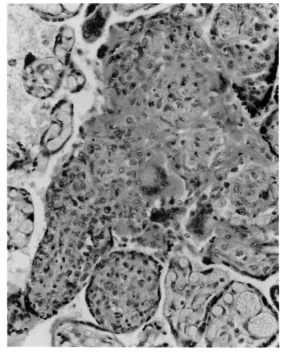

Fig. 49.24 Granulomatous villitis of unknown aetiology featuring histiocytic giant cells and resembling that associated with intrauterine chickenpox. H & E × 300.

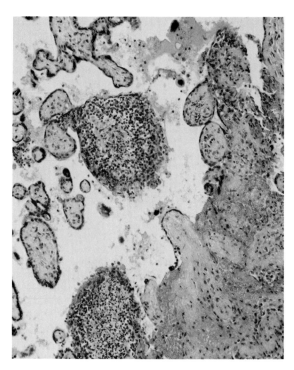

Fig. 49.25 Acute necrotizing villitis of unknown aetiology from a case of recurrent reproductive failure (Russell et al, 1980). Indistinguishable lesions are also seen in congenital listeriosis. H & E × 150.

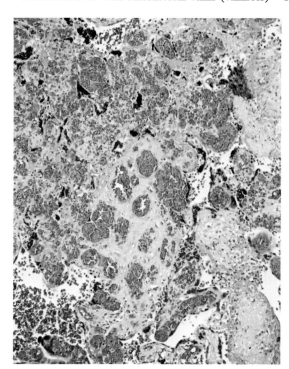

Fig. 49.26 Haemorrhagic endovasculitis and villitis. Note villous engorgement and diffuse villous haemorrhage (top left) and villous scarring (bottom right). H & E × 150. (Material courtesy of Dr. Charles H. Sander, East Lansing.)

States (Shen-Schwarz & Macpherson, 1988; Altshuler, 1991). There is a 50% mortality in the associated infants, a significant recurrence rate and two-thirds of cases exhibit villitis of unknown aetiology elsewhere in the placenta. A recent series of cases has been reported in association with non-immune fetal hydrops (Novak et al, 1991). Vascular changes — microthrombi (recent and organizing), intimal proliferation and focal necrosis in larger stem villous vessels, red cell fragmentation, and villous stromal haemorrhages with haemosiderin — include features which may add up to a type of microangiopathic

haemolytic anaemia which Sander (1980) suggests is possibly post-infectious in nature. Similar lesions, however, have been induced in short-term placental organ cultures (Silver et al, 1988) and I have observed identical lesions in otherwise normal term placental tissue retained in utero for short periods of time, when no such lesions were demonstrable in the placenta delivered with the infant. Such observations suggest that the pathogenesis of haemorrhagic endovasculitis relates to the haemodynamics within the placenta prior to its delivery or prior to the in utero death of the fetus.

REFERENCES

Abdel-Salam A M, Eissa M H, Mangoud A M, Eissa T M, Morsy T A 1990 Pathologic examination of the placenta in human cases of toxoplasmosis. Journal of Egyptian Society of Parasitology 20: 549–554.

Alford C A, Stagno S, Pass R F 1980 Natural history of perinatal cytomegaloviral infection. In: Ciba Foundation Symposium 77. Excerpta Medica, Amsterdam, pp 125–147.

Althabe O, Labarrere C 1985 Chronic villitis of unknown aetiology and intrauterine growth-retarded infants of normal and low ponderal index. Placenta 6: 369–373.

Altshuler G 1973 Toxoplasmosis as a cause of hydranencephaly. American Journal of Diseases of Children 125: 251–252.

Altshuler G 1974 Pathogenesis of congenital herpesvirus infection. American Journal of Diseases of Children 127: 427–429.

Altshuler G 1991 The placenta. In: Sternberg S S, Mills S E (eds) Surgical pathology of the female reproductive system. Raven Press, New York, pp 17–36.

Altshuler G, Russell P 1975 The human placental villitides: a review of chronic intrauterine infection. Current Topics in Pathology 60: 63–112.

Altshuler G, Russell P, Ermocilla R 1975 The placental pathology of small for gestational age infants. American Journal of Obstetrics and Gynecology 121: 351–359.

Baker R L 1955 Pregnancy complicated by coccidioidomycosis: report of two cases. American Journal of Obstetrics and Gynecology 70: 1033–1038.

Baskin J L, Soule E M, Mill D S 1950 Poliomyelitis of the newborn: pathologic changes in two cases. American Journal of Diseases of Children 80: 10–21.

Batcup G, Holt P, Hambling M H, Gerlis L M, Glass M R 1985 Placental and fetal pathology in coxsackie virus A9 infection: a case report. Histopathology 9: 1227–1235.

Benirschke K, Driscoll S G 1967 The pathology of the human placenta. Springer-Verlag, Berlin.

Benirschke K, Mendoza G R, Bazeley P L 1974 Placental and fetal manifestations of cytomegalovirus infection. Virchows Archiv Abteilung B Zell Pathologie 16: 121–139.

Bittencourt A C 1960 Sobre a forma congenita da doenca de Chagas. Revista do Instituto de Medicina Tropical de Sao Paulo 2: 319–334.

Bittencourt A C 1963 Placentite chagasica e transmissao congenita da doenca de Chagas. Revista do Instituto de Medicina Tropical de Sao Paulo 5: 62–67.

Bittencourt A C, Barbosa H S, Rocha T, Sodre I, Sodre A 1972 Incidencia da transmissao congenita da doenca de Chagas em partos prematuros na maternidade tsylla balbino (Salvador, Bahia). Revista do Instituto de Medicina Tropical de Sao Paulo 14: 131–134.

Bittencourt A L, Cardoso de Almeida M A, Iunes M A, Casulari da Motta L D 1980 Placental involvement in Schistosomiasis mansoni: report of four cases. American Journal of Tropical Medicine and Hygiene 29: 571–575.

Bjoro K Jr, Myhre E 1984 The role of chronic non-specific inflammatory lesions of the placenta in intra-uterine growth retardation. Acta Pathologica Microbiologica et Immunologica Scandinavica 92: 133–137.

Blanc W A 1961 Pathways of fetal and early neonatal infection: viral placentitis, bacterial and fungal choriamnionitis. Journal of Pediatrics 59: 473–496.

Blanc W A 1978 Pathology of the placenta and cord in some viral infections. In: Viral diseases of the fetus and newborn. W B Saunders, Philadelphia, pp 237–258.

Blanc W A 1981 Pathology of the placenta, membranes and umbilical cord in bacterial, fungal and viral infections in man. In: Naeye R L, Kissane J M (eds) Perinatal diseases (IAP Monograph Series, no. 22). Williams & Wilkins, Baltimore, pp 67–132.

Bulmer J, Rasheed F N, Francis N et al 1993a Placental malaria. I. Pathological classification. Histopathology 22: 211–218.

Bulmer J, Rasheed F N, Morrison L et al 1993b Placental malaria. II. A semi-quantitative investigation of the pathological features. Histopathology 22: 219–225.

Chandwani S, Greco A, Mittal K, Antoine C, Krasinski K, Borkowsky W 1991 Pathology and human immunodeficiency virus expression in placentas of seropositive women. Journal of Infectious Diseases 163: 1134–1138.

Desmonts G, Couvreur J 1974 Congenital toxoplasmosis: a prospective study of 378 pregnancies. New England Journal of Medicine 290: 1110–1116.

Dollmann A, Schmitz-Moormann P 1972 Rekurrierende Plazentalinsuffizienz durch villose Plazentitis mit extremer fetaler Hypotrophie. Geburtshilfe und Frauenheilkinde 32: 795–801.

Driscoll S G 1969 Histopathology of gestational rubella. American Journal of Diseases of Children 118: 49–53.

Duncan M E 1980 Babies of mothers with leprosy have small placentae, low birth weights and grow slowly. British Journal of Obstetrics and Gynaecology 87: 471–479.

Duncan M E, Fox H, Harkness R A, Rees R J W 1984 The placenta in leprosy. Placenta 5: 189–198.

Eden A N 1966 Perinatal mortality caused by Vibrio fetus. Journal of Pediatrics 68: 297–304.

Eilard T, Strannegard O 1974 Rubella reinfection in pregnancy followed by transmission to the fetus. Journal of Infectious Diseases 129: 594–596.

Elliott W G 1970 Placental toxoplasmosis. American Journal of Clinical Pathology 53: 413–417.

Embree J E, Krause V W, Embil J A, MacDonald S 1980 Placental infection with Mycoplasma hominis and Ureaplasma urealyticum: clinical correlation. Obstetrics and Gynecology 56: 475–481.

Entwistle D M, Bray P T, Laurence K M 1962 Prenatal infection with vaccinia virus: report of a case. British Medical Journal 1: 238–239.

Fox H 1978 Pathology of the placenta. W B Saunders, London, pp 286–325.

Fox H 1991 Current topic: trophoblastic pathology. Placenta 12: 479–486.

Frenkel J K, Dubey J P, Miller N L 1970 Toxoplasma gondii in cats: fecal stages identified as coccidian oocysts. Science 167: 893–896.

Galbraith R M, Faulk W P, Galbraith G M P, Holbrook T W, Bray R S 1980a The human materno-fetal relationship in malaria: I. Identification of pigment and parasites in the placenta. Transactions of the Royal Society of Tropical Medicine and Hygiene 74: 52–60.

Galbraith R M, Fox H, Hsi B, Galbraith G M P, Bray R S, Faulk W P 1980b The human materno-fetal relationship in malaria: II. Histological, ultrastructural and immunopathological studies of the placenta. Transactions of the Royal Society of Tropical Medicine and Hygiene 74: 61–72.

Garcia A G P 1963 Fetal infection in chickenpox and alastrim with histopathologic study of the placenta. Pediatrics 32: 895–901.

Garcia A G P 1968 Congenital toxoplasmosis in two successive sibs. Archives of Disease in Childhood 43: 705–709.

Garcia A G P, Pereira J M S, Vidigal N, Lobato Y Y, Pegado C S, Castelo Branco J P 1980 Intrauterine infection with mumps virus. Obstetrics and Gynecology 56: 756–759.

Garcia A G P, Coutinho S G, Amendoeira M R, Assumpcao M R, Albano N 1983 Placental morphology of newborns at risk for congenital toxoplasmosis. Journal of Tropical Pediatrics 29: 95–103.

Garcia A G P, Marques L C S, Lobato Y Y, Fonseca M E F, Wigg M D 1985 Placental pathology in congenital rubella. Placenta 6: 281–295.

Garcia A G P, Fonseca E F, Marques R L, Lobato Y Y 1989 Placental morphology in cytomegalovirus infection. Placenta 10: 1–18.

Garcia A G P, Basso N G S, Fonseca M E F, Outani H N 1990 Congenital ECHO virus infection — morphological and virological study of fetal and placental tissue. Journal of Pathology 160: 123–127.

Gilbert G L, Davoren R A, Cole M E, Radford N J 1981 Midtrimester abortion associated with septicaemia caused by Campylobacter jejuni. Medical Journal of Australia 1: 585–586.

Gillespie A, Dorman D, Walker-Smith J A, Yu J S 1970 Neonatal hepatitis and Australia antigen. Lancet 2: 1081.

Glasser L, Delta B G 1965 Congenital toxoplasmosis with placental infection in monozygous twins. Pediatrics 35: 276–283.

Hager W D 1978 The transplacental transmission of spirochaetes in congenital syphilis: a new perspective. Sexually Transmitted Diseases 5: 122–123.

Hanshaw J B 1973 Herpesvirus hominis infections in the fetus and the newborn. American Journal of Diseases of Children 126: 546–555.

Harter C H, Benirschke K 1976 Fetal syphilis in the first trimester. American Journal of Obstetrics and Gynecology 124: 705–711.

Homberger C, Chaughan P, Blanc W A 1971 Lymphoplasmacytic placentitis, fetal infection and placental immunoglobulin synthesis. Abstract, Pediatric Pathology Meeting, International Academy of Pathology, Montreal, March 1971.

Hood C K, McKinnon G E 1963 Prenatal vaccinia. American Journal of Obstetrics and Gynecology 85: 238–240.

Hood M, Todd J M 1960 Vibrio fetus — a cause of human abortion. American Journal of Obstetrics and Gynecology 80: 506–511.

Hormann G 1954 Placenta und Lues: ein Beitrag zur Diagnose und Prognose konnataler Syphilis. Archiv fur Gynakologie 184: 481–521.

Imamura M, Phillips P E, Mellors R C 1976 The occurrence and frequency of type C virus-like particles in placentas from patients with systemic lupus erythematosus and from normal subjects. American Journal of Pathology 83: 383–394.

Kalter S S, Helmke R J, Heberling R L, Panigel M, Fowler A K, Strickland J E, Hellman A 1973 C-type particles in normal human placentas. Journal of the National Cancer Institute 50: 1081–1084.

Kaplan C, Benirschke K, Tarzy B 1980 Placental tuberculosis in early and late pregnancy. American Journal of Obstetrics and Gynecology 137: 858–860.

Kaplan C G, Bienstock J, Baker D A 1985 Villitis of unknown etiology: incidence and implications in an unselected population (abstract). Laboratory Investigation 52: 33A.

Keutel J 1968 Angeborene Varicellen. Bericht uber einen Fall: Literaturubersicht — immunologische Gesichtspunkte. Archiv fur Kinderheilkunde 102: 266–274.

Kida M, Abramowsky C R, Santoscov C 1989 Cryptococcosis of the placenta in a woman with acquired immunodeficiency syndrome. Human Pathology 20: 920–921.

Kilbrick S, Benirschke K 1958 Severe generalised disease (encephalohepatomyocarditis) occurring in the newborn period and due to infection with Coxsackie virus group B: evidence of intrauterine infection with this organism. Pediatrics 22: 857–875.

King J A, Marks R A 1958 Pregnancy and leprosy: a review of 52 pregnancies in 26 patients with leprosy. American Journal of Obstetrics and Gynecology 59: 190–194.

Knox W F, Fox H 1984 Villitis of unknown aetiology: its incidence and significance in placentae from a British population. Placenta 5: 395–402.

Labarrere C, Althabe O, Telenta M 1982 Chronic villitis of unknown aetiology in placentae of idiopathic small for gestational age infants. Placenta 3: 309–317.

Labarrere C, Faulk W P, McIntyre J A 1989 Villitis in normal term human placentae: frequency of the lesion determined by monoclonal antibody to HLA-DR antigen. Journal of Reproductive Immunology 16: 127–135.

Labarrere C A, McIntyre J A, Faulk W P 1990 Immunohistologic evidence that villitis in human normal term placentas is an immunologic lesion. American Journal of Obstetrics and Gynecology 162: 515–522.

Lide T N 1947 Congenital tularemia. Archives of Pathology 43: 165–169.

Malan A F, Woods D L, van der Elst C W, Meyer M P 1990 Relative placental weight in congenital syphilis. Placenta 11: 3–6.

Mehrotra R 1986 Histopathological and immunohistochemical changes in placenta due to acute viral hepatitis during pregnancy. Indian Journal of Medical Research 83: 282–292.

Monif G R G, Dische R M 1972 Viral placentitis in congenital cytomegalovirus infection. American Journal of Clinical Pathology 58: 445–449.

Moroi K, Saito S, Kurata T, Sato T, Yanagida M 1991 Fetal death associated with measles virus infection of the placenta. American Journal of Obstetrics and Gynecology 164: 1107–1108.

Muhlemann K, Miller R K, Metlay L et al 1992 Cytomegalovirus infection of the human placenta: an immunocytochemical study. Human Pathology 23: 1234–1237.

Northrop R L, Gardner W M, Geittmann W F 1972 Rubella reinfection during early pregnancy. Obstetrics and Gynecology 39: 524–526.

Novak P M, Sander C M, Yang S S, von Oeyen P T 1991 Report of fourteen cases of nonimmune hydrops fetalis in association with hemorrhagic endovasculitis of the placenta. American Journal of Obstetrics and Gynecology 165: 945–950.

Olivier, Olivier, Segal 1972 A bibliography on Chagas disease 1909–1969. Washington, U.S.D.A. and University of Maryland.

Ornoy A, Segal S, Nishmi M, Simcha A, Polishuk W Z 1973 Fetal and placental pathology in gestational rubella. American Journal of Obstetrics and Gynecology 116: 949–956.

Ornoy A, Dudai M, Sadovsky E 1982 Placental and fetal pathology in infectious mononucleosis: a possible indicator for Epstein-Barr virus teratogenicity. Diagnostic Gynecology and Obstetrics 4: 11–16.

Popek E J 1992 Granulomatous villitis due to Toxoplasma gondii. Pediatric Pathology 12: 281–288.

Poole P M, Whitehouse D B, Gilchrist M M 1972 A cause of abortion consequent upon infection with Brucella abortus biotype 2. Journal of Clinical Pathology 25: 882–884.

Prabhu S R, Pendharkar C A 1986 Histopathological study of placenta in viral hepatitis. Indian Journal of Pathology and Microbiology 29: 137–144.

Quirke P, Hwang W, Validin C 1980 Congenital Torulopsis glabrata infection in man. American Journal of Clinical Pathology 78: 137–140.

Ramos A D, Hibbard L T, Craig J R 1974 Congenital tuberculosis. Obstetrics and Gynecology 43: 61–64.

Rappaport F, Rabinovitz M, Toaff R, Krochik N 1960 Genital listeriosis as a cause of repeated abortion. Lancet 1: 1273–1275.

Redline R W, Abramowsky C R 1985 Clinical and pathologic aspects of recurrent placental villitis. Human Pathology 16: 727–731.

Renaud R, Brettes P, Castanier C, Loubiere R 1972 Placental bilharziasis. International Journal of Gynaecology and Obstetrics 10: 24–30.

Rich A R 1950 The pathogenesis of tuberculosis, 2nd edn. C C Thomas, Springfield.

Russell P 1979 Inflammatory lesions of the human placenta. II: Villitis of unknown aetiology in perspective. American Journal of Diagnostic Gynecology and Obstetrics 1: 339–346.

Russell P 1980 Inflammatory lesions of the human placenta. III: The histopathology of villitis of unknown aetiology. Placenta 1: 227–244.

Russell P, Altshuler G 1974 The placental abnormalities of congenital syphilis. American Journal of Diseases of Children 128: 160–163.

Russell P, Atkinson K, Krishnan L 1980 Recurrent reproductive failure due to severe placental villitis of unknown etiology. Journal of Reproductive Medicine 24: 93–98.

Salafia C M, Vogel C A, Vintzileos A M, Bantham K F, Pezzullo J, Silberman L 1991 Placental pathologic findings in preterm birth. American Journal of Obstetrics and Gynecology 165: 934–938.

Sander C 1980 Hemorrhagic endovasculitis and haemorrhagic villitis of the placenta. Archives of Pathology and Laboratory Medicine 104: 371–373.

Sander C H, Stevens N G 1984 Hemorrhagic endovasculitis of the placenta: an in depth morphologic appraisal with initial clinical and epidemiologic observations. Pathology Annual 19 (Part 1): 37–79.

Sander C H, Kinnane L, Stevens N G, Echt R 1986 Haemorrhagic endovasculitis of the placenta: a review with clinical correlation. Placenta 7: 551–574.

Sarram M, Feiz J, Foruzandeh M, Gazanfarpour P 1974 Intrauterine fetal infection with Brucella melitensis as a possible cause of second trimester abortion. American Journal of Obstetrics and Gynecology 119: 657–661.

Sarrut S, Alison F 1967 Etude du placenta dans 21 cas de listeriose congenitale. Archives Francais de Pediatrie 24: 285–302.

Schmorl G, Geipl L 1904 Uber die Tuberkulose der menschlichen Plazenta. Munchener Medizinische Wochenschrift 51: 1676–1679.

Schmorl G, Kockel K V 1894 Die Tuberkulose der menschlichen Placenta und ihre Beziehung zur kongenitalen Infection mit Tuberkulose. Beitrag zur pathologischen Anatomie und zur allgemeine Pathologie 16: 313–339.

Schwartz D A, Khan R, Stoll B 1992 Characterization of the fetal inflammatory response to cytomegalovirus placentitis: an immunohistochemical study. Archives of Pathology and Laboratory Medicine 116: 21–27.

Scott J M, Henderson A 1972 Acute villous inflammation in the placenta following intrauterine transfusion. Journal of Clinical Pathology 25: 872–875.

Seeliger H P R 1961 Listeriosis. Hafner Publishing, New York.

Seppala M, Vaheri A 1974 Natural rubella infection of the female genital tract. Lancet 1: 46–47.

Shen-Schwarz S, Macpherson T A 1988 The clinical significance of hemorrhagic endovasculitis of the placenta. American Journal of Obstetrics and Gynecology 159: 48–51.

Shurin P A, Alpert S, Rosner B, Driscoll S G, Kass E H 1974 Genital mycoplasmas — association with chorioamnionitis. Pediatric Research 8: 428.

Silver M M, Yeger L, Lines L D 1988 Hemorrhagic endovasculitis-like lesion induced in placental organ culture. Human Pathology 19: 251–256.

Spark R P 1981 Does transplacental spread of coccidioidomycosis occur? Report of a neonatal fatality and review of the literature. Archives of Pathology and Laboratory Medicine 105: 347–350.

Srabstein J C, Morris N, Larke R P B, de Sa D J, Castelini B B, Sum E 1974 Is there a congenital varicella syndrome? Journal of Pediatrics 84: 239–243.

Stagno S, Pass R F, Dworsky M E, Henderson R E, Moore E G, Walton P D, Alford C A 1982 Congenital cytomegalovirus infection: the relative importance of primary and recurrent maternal infection. New England Journal of Medicine 306: 945–949.

Sugai T, Monobe J 1912 Uber histologische Befunde in der Placenta Tuberculose — und Leprakranker. Zentralblatt fur Bakteriologie, Parasitenkunde, Infektionkrankheiten und Hygeine 13: 232.

Susani M 1981 Granulomatous placentitis in toxoplasmosis. Wiener Klinische Wochenschrift 93: 24–28.

Sutherland J C, Berry A, Hynd M, Proctor N S F 1965 Placental bilharziasis — report of a case. South African Journal of Obstetrics and Gynaecology 3: 76–80.

Tondury G T, Smith D W 1966 Fetal rubella pathology. Journal of Pediatrics 68: 867–879.

Trevenen C L, Hwang W-S, Williams T 1982 Hypoplastic left heart syndrome: possible etiologic role of Coxsackie B virus. Laboratory Investigation 46: 16P.

Trifonova S F 1959 Pathomorphology of the placenta in brucellosis. Akusherstvo i Ginekologiya 2: 41–44.

Vaughan J E, Ramirez H 1951 Coccidioidomycosis as a complication of pregnancy. California Medicine 74: 121–125.

Vernon M L, McMahon J M, Hackett J J 1974 Additional evidence of type-C particles in human placentas. Journal of the National Cancer Institute 52: 987–989.

Vinzent R 1949 Une affection mecomme de la grossesse: l'infection placentaire a vibrio fetus. Presse Medical 57: 1230–1232.

Vinzent R, Dumas J, Picard N 1947 Septicemie grave au cours de la grossesse due a un vibrion: avortement consecutif. Bulletin de l'Academie Nationale de Medicine 131: 90–92.

Vinzent R, Delarue J, Hebert H 1950 L'infection placentaire a vibrio fetus. Annales de Medicine 51: 23–68.

Walter P R, Garin Y, Blot P 1982a Placental pathologic changes in malaria. A histologic and ultrastructural study. American Journal of Pathology 109: 330–342.

Walter P R, Blot P, Ivanoff B 1982b The placental lesions in congenital syphilis: a study of six cases. Virchows Archiv [A] 397: 313–326.

Wickramasuriya G A W 1935 Some observations on malaria occurring in association with pregnancy. Journal of Obstetrics and Gynaecology of the British Empire 42: 816–834.

Wielenga G, van Tongeren H A E, Ferguson A H, van Rijssel T G 1961 Prenatal infection with vaccinia virus. Lancet 1: 258–260.

Willis M D, Austin W J 1966 Human Vibrio fetus infection. American Journal of Diseases of Children 112: 459–462.

Witzleben C L, Driscoll S G 1965 Possible transplacental transmission of herpes simplex infection. Pediatrics 36: 192–199.

Yawn D H, Pyeatte J C, Joseph J M, Eichler S L, Garcia-Bunnel R 1971 Transplacental transfer of influenza virus. Journal of the American Medical Association 216: 1022–1023.

50. Pathology of the umbilical cord

Hans G. Kohler   Gillian Batcup

INTRODUCTION

Traditionally the umbilical cord symbolizes the close bond between mother and unborn child. In anatomical terms, the cord links the fetal circulation with that of the placenta.

The obvious function of the cord, conveying oxygenated blood with nutrients to the fetus and returning spent blood with waste products to the placenta, has probably caused other funicular functions to be overlooked — or at any rate to receive too little attention. We are thinking here of the cord's part in the feto-placental turnover of water (Plentl, 1961) or in the paraplacental supply to the fetus (Schmidt, 1965). These functions are still awaiting further elucidation.

In this contribution the collective term 'umbilical cord failure' refers to lesions interfering with the blood flow in the cord. In addition to functional breakdown prejudicing the life and well-being of the fetus, the pathologist must also pay attention to lesions that by themselves are not necessarily of serious consequence but which are frequently associated with more sinister conditions; thus a single umbilical artery points to other malformations (and to intrauterine growth retardation) whilst leucocytic infiltration of the cord should lead to a search for infection in both placenta and infant. Oedema of the umbilical cord, if not explained by prematurity alone, can be a warning sign of impending cardiorespiratory insufficiency, in particular of respiratory distress syndrome, whilst a thin cord accords well with intrauterine growth retardation.

A third group of lesions are of unpredictable clinical significance, e.g. tumours of the cord, but are of some theoretical interest. In this group one might also include malformations of the cord (other than single umbilical artery and velamentous cord insertion). Lastly there is a residual group of lesions (or morphological features) to be discussed, as well as some pertinent problems, that cannot be accommodated under any other heading.

ANATOMY AND HISTOLOGY OF THE CORD

The umbilical cord consists in essence of two arteries and one vein surrounded by Wharton's jelly which, in turn, is coated by one or more layers of amniotic epithelium: the cells in this are generally of flat squamous type but are occasionally cuboidal. In addition to these essential constituents, the umbilical cord often contains vestigial structures, such as remnants of vitelline duct, allantois and primitive vessels dating back to its formation by fusion of the body stalk (with the allantois) and yolk stalk in the sixth week of the embryo. From a later period in fetal life (seventh to tenth week post ovulation) when much of the early or primitive intestine is extruded into the cord ('physiological umbilical hernia') intestinal elements may be left behind and these can occasionally give rise to unexpected and puzzling histological pictures (Fig. 50.1) (Harris & Wenzl, 1963). Very rarely, when structures arising from these remnants differentiate in the direction of gastric mucosa, 'peptic' ulceration may cause serious damage to umbilical blood vessels (Blanc & Allan, 1961). Jauniaux et al (1989) examined 1000 cords and found no fewer than 231 with one type of embryonic remnant or another.

Wharton's jelly is, according to Maximov (1927), 'the classical object for the study of mucous or myxoid tissue', which is not found in adult mammals. It is composed of scanty, large stellate cells which appear flat in profile and are arranged concentrically around the blood vessels. These cells, which have many of the features of myofibroblasts (Takechi et al, 1993), give rise to collagenous fibres, which increase in number with gestational age: they also show a tendency to concentric arrangement. Cells and fibres are embedded in a homogeneous ground substance which in the fresh state reacts chemically as mucin. In the fixed specimen granular filamentous deposits appear which stain metachromatically with thionin, Unna's methylene blue or cresyl echt violet. Zawisch (1955) em-

1559

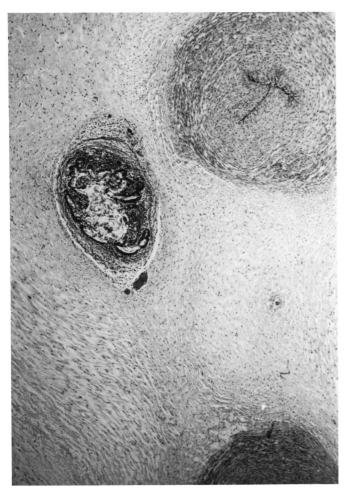

Fig. 50.1 Vestigial structures in the umbilical cord. A remnant of the omphalo-enteric duct is present (left) and this is showing differentiation into intestinal-type epithelium. H & E × 40.

phasizes that Wharton's jelly is not only a cushioning medium against external trauma, but also enables blood inside more or less closely adjacent vessels to flow in opposite directions. This author also draws attention to the jelly's metabolic activity, in particular to perpetual polymerization and depolymerization of mucopolysaccharides. The regular presence of mast cells in the umbilical cord is emphasized by Moore (1956). The umbilical cord arteries — the intra-abdominal umbilical arteries are not necessarily included — differ from other arteries by the virtual absence of an internal elastic lamina. The external elastic lamina is also indistinct, but elastic fibres are interspersed with the plain muscle fibres of the media. The adventitia merges imperceptibly with the surrounding Wharton's jelly, which Zawisch (1955) has called the 'adventitia of the umbilical vessels'. Vasa vasorum are not seen, save in exceptional cases, nor are perivascular lymphatics (Angiolillo & Picinelli, 1965), but Clarke (1965) claims to have demonstrated vasa vasorum by X-ray microscopic study.

The 'valves' of Hoboken are a peculiar feature of the umbilical cord arteries (Boyd & Hamilton, 1970). They are not real valves, but constrictions of the lumen, occurring at varying intervals (Spivack, 1936); the claim that their absence prejudices fetal life (Kovacs, 1951), has not been confirmed. Scharl (1986) sees Hoboken's 'valves' as a transient phenomenon which may have some significance in controlling potential blood loss of the neonate.

The question whether nerves are present in the umbilical cord has been hotly debated for at least 200 years but is still not fully decided. Recent publications include those of Bettzieche (1978), presenting evidence for the presence of nerve fibres in the cord, and Reilly & Russell (1977) and Fox & Khong (1990) against.

LENGTH OF CORD

The length of the umbilical cord has been the subject of both investigation and speculation. Various authors have established normal ranges and mean values by measuring the cord in normal babies in larger or smaller numbers. Fox (1978) has summarized several publications, concluding that the average length is between 54 and 61 cm. The minimal length of the cord allowing normal vertex delivery at term has been calculated to be 32 cm, a figure which no doubt is on the safe side. An arbitrary figure of 100 cm is often used as the maximum normal length and this appears justifiable, as according to Purola (1968) only 0.5% of all cords exceed this length.

A too-short cord may lead to obstetric problems, especially with breech presentation, and makes external version difficult or impossible. Shortness of the cord may conceivably be a factor in some cases of abruptio placentae, intrafunicular haemorrhage and even inversion of the uterus. Too long a cord, on the other hand, is likely to facilitate entanglement, prolapse of the cord and even thrombosis (Benirschke & Driscoll, 1967; Benirschke, 1994).

Most of the discussions on the obstetric implications of abnormally long or short cords are, however, based on small groups of cases or even on single case reports, and large-scale statistical enquiries into the relative frequency of various obstetrical complications in relation to abnormal cord length do not appear to have been undertaken.

In the past, interest in this field has been directed mainly towards potential adverse effects of the extremes of cord length and little attention was paid to factors influencing cord growth. Miller et al (1981) have, however, thrown some light on the aetiology of variation in cord length. In an admittedly small series, they found an interesting positive correlation between very short cords and various conditions restricting the mobility of the fetus, such as oligohydramnios, narrow uterine cavity due to submucous leiomyomas and also amniotic strands that have a tethering effect on the fetus. These clinical observations,

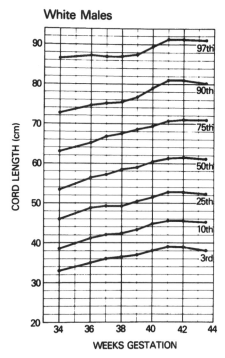

Fig. 50.2 Umbilical cord length by gestational age in white males in the United States. (From Mills et al, 1983. Courtesy of the Editor of Placenta.)

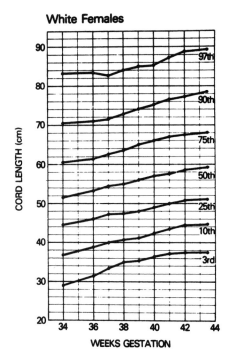

Fig. 50.3 Umbilical cord length by gestational age in white females in the United States. (From Mills et al, 1983. Courtesy of the Editor of Placenta.)

suggesting a stimulating influence of fetal activity on the longitudinal growth of the cord, are in harmony with the experimental results of Moessinger et al (1982) and are also compatible with the findings of Mills et al (1983) in so far as these last-named authors report longitudinal growth of the cord continuing up to term. The association of a short umbilical cord with various fetal anomalies of the 'amniotic band spectrum' has been confirmed by Grange et al (1987).

The standard tables (Figs 50.2 and 50.3) compiled by Mills et al, within the framework of the 'Collaborative Perinatal Project — NINDB', are based on strictly standardized measurements of the cords of 9620 male and 9068 female white American neonates, ranging in gestational age from 34–43½ weeks. In each weekly group there is great scatter, but mean values increase consistently from week to week until there is a plateau, or even a slight drop after 42 weeks in the case of males, whilst in females growth continues, albeit at a flatter gradient.

The thickness of the umbilical cord will be discussed in conjunction with umbilical cord oedema and 'thin cord syndrome'. Umbilical cord circumference at birth was measured and discussed by Patel et al (1989).

PLACENTAL INSERTION OF THE UMBILICAL CORD

The attachment of the umbilical cord to the placenta is a link in the umbilical circulation and, at times, a vulnerable one. The histology of this attachment — both normal and abnormal — has been investigated by Scheuner (1964, 1965).

The umbilical cord can insert anywhere on the fetal surface (Fig. 50.4) of the placental disc and occasionally outside it. McLennan (1968) has pointed out that there are no natural categories of central, moderately eccentric, markedly eccentric, and marginal insertions, but a continuous series. The frequency of insertion at various points within this series is, therefore, determined by the laws of probability.

If we try to extend this concept 'beyond the margin', i.e. to include velamentous insertion, the continuous series of quantitative changes comes to an abrupt end because velamentous insertion is, in a sense, a negation of the concept of placental attachment. The distal end of the cord is not attached to the placenta at all, but to the extra-placental membranes, the chorion laeve, either at an obtuse angle or completely flush. The cord 'gets lost' in the membranes, Wharton's jelly peters out and the divested umbilical vessels have to find their way to the placental margin unprotected and exposed to mechanical injury (Fig. 50.5). The concept that velamentous insertion is not a variant of the norm, but a definite anomaly, is hard to refute.

Both the pathogenesis of placenta velamentosa and its relation to associated developmental defects have been subjects of disagreement. Basically, two opposite views have been championed. Franqué (1900) postulated an

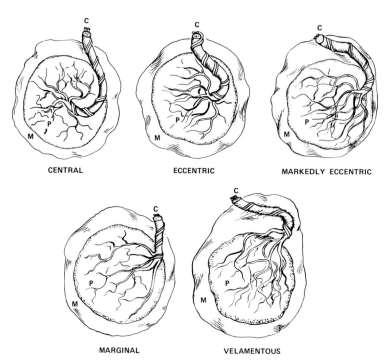

CENTRAL   ECCENTRIC   MARKEDLY ECCENTRIC

MARGINAL   VELAMENTOUS

Fig. 50.4   Diagrammatic representation of various insertion sites of the umbilical cord. (From Fox, 1978. Courtesy of W. B. Saunders.)

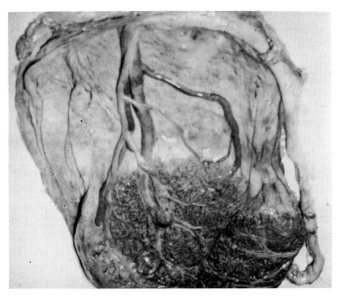

Fig. 50.5   Velamentous insertion of the cord.

abnormal implantation by which the body stalk comes to be attached to the chorion in apposition to the decidua capsularis; i.e. to that part of the chorion which later becomes the chorion laeve. Placenta velamentosa is therefore a primary abnormality and this hypothesis accords well with the fact that a velamentous cord insertion is not infrequently associated with a low-lying placenta.

Strassmann (1902), on the other hand, had a more dynamic attitude to the problem. He considered that an originally satisfactory implantation, firmly based on decidua basalis, could, as a result of growth and expansion, later become inadequate; the growth of the placenta would then of necessity be directed towards a better perfused decidua. In consequence an originally central insertion would become eccentric, even marginal. If then the chorion frondosum in the area around the insertion regresses to become chorion laeve, the result is a placenta velamentosa, albeit a secondary one. This theory, implying a gradual transition from central insertion, to eccentric, marginal and velamentous is admirably suited to support a gradual increase of fetal abnormalities, as the cord insertion moves in a centrifugal direction. Such a 'differential' in the frequency of associated abnormalities was indeed observed and reported by Krone (1961, 1966). His results were, however, not confirmed by Uyanwah-Akpom & Fox (1977), who found an increased number of light-for-date babies but not of malformations associated with velamentous cord insertion.

A third party, as it were, has emerged more recently. Robinson et al (1983) have found a positive correlation of velamentous (but not marginal!) cord insertion with structural defects and have gone one step further: analysing the type of defect, they found that an undue proportion consisted of deformations (as distinct from malformations), i.e. those abnormal body forms that can be accounted for by intrauterine space restriction or other limitation of the fetus's mobility. These authors, who are more inclined to accept Strassmann's 'tropotrophism' rather than Franqué's 'atypical implantation', believe that restricted intra-amniotic space and similar factors account for the abnormal morphology of both fetus and placenta.

At present, none of these hypotheses is proven. The series of observations proffered in evidence is too small to settle the argument on a statistical basis, though as yet no other approach is available. Moreover, the logical link between the nature of the evidence and the theory it is meant to support is not so close as to exclude other explanations and we agree with Fox (1978) that more than one theory could be valid.

The frequency of velamentous cord insertion, observed in a number of published investigations surveyed by Fox (1978), varies considerably, between 0.24% (Rucker & Tureman, 1945) and 13.6% (Raaflaub, 1959). No doubt, the enquiries that have yielded these grossly discrepant results are not fully comparable in respect of the methods of ascertainment. In the more 'sober' investigations the frequency is around 1%. In the material examined at Leeds Maternity Hospital 35 velamentous insertions were found in 2000 umbilical cords, an incidence of 1.75%. (This search of placental records was prompted by the wish to have a 'standard of comparison' for the finding of eight velamentous insertions in 116 single umbilical artery cords, i.e. approximately 7%.)

From a clinician's point of view velamentous insertion is important not so much because of the frequency or otherwise of associated fetal anomalies but because of its vulnerability to injury in the form of external pressure on the blood vessels and/or laceration of these. The risk for the life and health of the fetus is enhanced if the velamentous portion is overlying the internal os, a condition known as vasa praevia. Here the presenting part of the fetus, as it descends, is bound to press on the unprotected umbilical blood vessels and, if labour is allowed to proceed, rupture of these vessels would be inevitable. Even where the umbilical vessels are not directly in the way of the presenting part, i.e. away from the internal os, the risk of haemorrhage still exists with either spontaneous or artificial rupture of the membranes (Vestermark et al, 1990). Occasionally, massive bleeding may occur even before rupture of the membranes (Bilek et al, 1962). In order to prevent a disaster caused by medical interference, Barham (1968) has proposed to examine first the internal os by amnioscope whenever either artificial rupture or 'sweep' of the membranes is contemplated, though amnioscopy itself is not without risk.

In principle, similar complications as with velamentous insertion can occur whenever unprotected blood vessels are exposed to trauma, e.g. the vessels between the lobes of a bipartite placenta or between the main lobe and an accessory lobe in placenta succenturiata. In practice this seems to happen less often. Vasa praevia in a bilobed placenta can apparently be compatible with labour and delivery uncomplicated by either massive haemorrhage or fetal distress, as in case 2 of Kouyoumdjian (1980). This

author calls vasa praevia 'a unique obstetric complication in which the fetus is at maximum risk, while the mother is at no risk at all (except for the occasional association with placenta praevia): the fetal mortality has remained virtually unchanged since the condition was first recognised more than 200 years ago'; this is at present too despondent a view. An increased incidence of vasa praevia has been reported in pregnancies achieved by in vitro fertilization (Burton & Saunders, 1988).

Vasa praevia is not infrequently associated with twin pregnancy (Whitehouse & Kohler, 1960; Benirschke & Driscoll, 1967). Where there are sufficiently large anastomosing vessels between the two placental portions (usually only in monochorionic twinning and by no means in all instances), the second twin may also exsanguinate 'by proxy' (Knapp, 1896; Whitehouse & Kohler, 1960, case 2). Vasa praevia affecting both twins concordantly is hardly feasible, but the case described by Gaulis (1953) comes very close to such a situation. Concordant velamentous insertion, however, is not very rare and has been observed more than once by the present reviewers. In some instances one twin had the more usual velamentous insertion at the margin of the disc, whilst the other's umbilical vessels reached the placenta via the membranous septum.

Polar insertion of the umbilical cord is an extreme form of velamentous insertion: the attachment to the membranes is at the pole opposite to the placenta (Herberz, 1938) whilst, in the ultravelamentous insertion, the vessels do not follow the shortest but the longest course to the placental margin. The potential risk of injury in these variants of placenta velamentosa is likely to be increased.

The two essential elements of velamentous insertion are well illustrated by two rare variants: interpositio velamentosa, in which the cord attaches to the membranes but the vessels retain their protective coat of Wharton's jelly, and insertio furcata, in which the site of insertion is on the fetal surface but loss of Wharton's jelly occurs before the fetal surface is reached. Both conditions were first described by Ottow (1922, 1923).

LESIONS PREJUDICING BLOOD SUPPLY TO THE FETUS (UMBILICAL CORD FAILURE)

Thrombosis of umbilical cord vessels

Obstruction of feto-placental blood flow by a thrombosed funicular blood vessel (Fig. 50.6) is an infrequent occurrence, but probably not as infrequent as used to be believed. The uncertainty about the incidence is surpassed, however, by dubiousness concerning the significance of this lesion.

Edith Potter, whose experience and expertise in perinatal pathology is second to none, admitted — in a personal communication to S. K. Nayak (Nayak, 1967) — that she

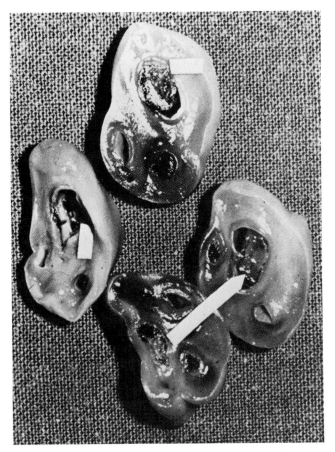

Fig. 50.6 Umbilical vein thrombosis. (From Nayak, 1967. Courtesy of the Editor of the Australian and New Zealand Journal of Obstetrics and Gynaecology.)

had never seen a case. In contrast, six cases of umbilical vein thrombosis were found in an unselected prospective examination of 7738 cords by Heifetz (1988), an incidence of 1:1290 and therefore not a rarity. Ten years earlier, a review of the (scanty) literature prompted Fox (1978) to conclude 'that an infant can survive an umbilical cord thrombosis and this lesion in itself is unlikely to cause fetal death' and earlier 'in most cases it appears probable that fetal demise had been due principally to the condition of which the thrombotic episode is a complication rather than to the thrombosis itself'.

This conclusion has been vindicated by the results of Heifetz's research. His six infants were all liveborn and had normal Apgar scores, even though one of them had suffered fetal distress. All but one had an additional umbilical cord lesion: haematoma or funisitis or both. The fact that not a single instance of umbilical artery thrombosis was found in Heifetz's prospective series is remarkable but should not be considered to have absolute validity. For the sake of a wider and perhaps more balanced view of the problem, Heifetz also presents the results of two retrospective investigations — one comprising 14 thrombosed cords from some 3500 high risk pregnancies, selection being within the discretion of the clinicians con-

cerned. The other retrospective inquiry was based on records of some 30 000 perinatal autopsies: 32 instances of umbilical vessel thrombosis were recorded. Furthermore this author reviewed 68 published cases — a bibliographical achievement in addition to this study's other merits. The overall impression gained from this 'multiple tier' investigation is that venous thrombosis occurs more frequently than arterial, but the latter is more often associated with perinatal morbidity and mortality. One infant, however, whose umbilical cord had a 'triple thrombosis' (i.e. both arteries as well as the vein) did quite well. Neither Fox nor Heifetz attempt to explain how so severe a disturbance of the feto-placental circulation as umbilical thrombosis can occur without any apparent serious effect on fetal life and health. Hopefully the new non-invasive techniques of monitoring umbilical blood flow may shed some light on this puzzling problem.

Haematoma, haemorrhage, rupture, aneurysms and varicosities

Reports of umbilical cord haematomas in the earlier literature almost invariably begin with a quasi-apologetic insistence on the rarity of this lesion. Interest in umbilical cord vessels — mainly aimed at establishing the number of arteries in the cord — may have revealed that funicular haematoma is not quite so rare and need not always have serious consequences: nonetheless, many of the recorded cases were associated with fetal or neonatal deaths (Clare et al, 1979). In recent years antepartum diagnosis of cord haematoma, especially by the techniques of ultrasound and cardiotocography, has aroused some interest (Dillon & O'Leary, 1981; Ruvinsky et al, 1981; Virot et al, 1981; Ronero et al, 1982).

Haematoma, haemorrhage and rupture may profitably be discussed together because of their pathogenetic relationship. Extravasation from one of the umbilical cord vessels or from a vascular tumour (Dohmen & Bubenzer, 1978) or, indeed, any lesion affecting the vessels, will give rise to a haematoma if the bleeding is confined to Wharton's substance. If the epithelial sheath of the cord is broken, blood will enter the amniotic cavity and will become apparent when the membranes are ruptured. Bleeding from an intrafunicular haematoma, by 'overflow' or by secondary rupture, is another possibility.

Partial rupture of the cord, involving severe laceration of a blood vessel, will usually cause flank haemorrhage, but haematoma formation may also occur. Complete rupture is bound to cause haemorrhage and may result in exsanguination of the fetus, though cases of complete rupture with a surviving, if shocked, infant have been reported (Leinzinger, 1972).

Haematoma formation (Fig. 50.7) in the absence of haemorrhage into the amniotic sac can also lead to substantial fetal blood loss; this is usually less severe, but

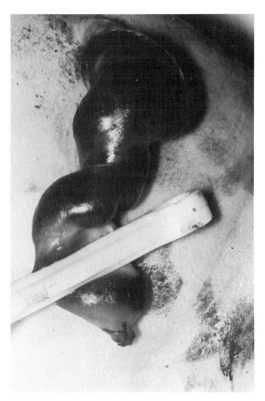

Fig. 50.7 A haematoma of the umbilical cord.

exceptionally can amount to four-fifths of the estimated total blood volume of the fetus (Ruvinsky et al, 1979). However, a sizeable haematoma can press on the blood vessels, particularly the umbilical vein, and in this way reduce or even stop the supply of oxygenated blood to the fetus. This consideration is perhaps not completely invalidated by Bret & Bardiaux (1960) who in fatal cases found the vessels enveloped by haematoma to be not compressed but widely patent and congested. Freisfeld (1936), on the other hand, described the umbilical vein in his case as compressed by cord haematoma.

The causation of a haematoma can be obvious if due to medical intervention (Ronero et al, 1982; Keckstein et al, 1990; Benirschke, 1994) but in non-iatrogenic cases, even where a break in the continuity of a vessel wall can be demonstrated, the underlying condition responsible for this break may still be obscure. Clare et al (1979) reported a disrupted wall of the umbilical vein in a 44-week gestation; whether this split in the media was cause or effect of haemorrhage is difficult to say. A dissecting aneurysm of the umbilical vein at the site of the haematoma was found by Lupovitch & McInerney (1968); their case was additionally complicated by prolapse of the cord. Schreier & Brown (1962), who described a fusiform haematoma of 6 cm diameter some 15 cm from the umbilicus, found thinning and necrosis of the wall of the umbilical vein and interpreted this as a congenital defect predisposing to haemorrhage; the infant survived.

Mechanical 'insults', such as prolapse, entanglement, as well as torsion or thrombosis, are potential or actual causes of vascular engorgement and distension; for a variety of reasons the vein is more often affected than the arteries. This distension is bound to have a thinning effect on the wall, possibly aggravated by hypoxaemia. This makes the concept of bleeding by diapedesis, postulated by Bret & Bardiaux (1960), a probability in at least some cases.

Very few reports on cord haematoma have been published in Great Britain since the classical review of Browne (1925). Evason (1952) records a haematoma close to the umbilicus which was cast off when the dried-up umbilical stump separated, leaving behind a clean navel and a healthy infant. Irani (1964) reported three cases, two fatal. In a personal observation (HGK), a liveborn male infant with signs of respiratory distress had a haematoma of nearly 5 cm diameter which was so close to the umbilicus that a diagnosis of exomphalos was being considered. The infant died on his fifth day and, at autopsy, extensive cerebral hypoxic damage was revealed as well as anoxic lesions in liver, kidneys and peritoneum. From Germany, Honer (1976) reported a haematoma-associated neonatal death at the age of 17 hours.

Notwithstanding this and other case histories, there can be little doubt that many haematomas, probably a majority, go unnoticed if they are of moderate size; they certainly go unpublished. The inexperienced worker should, however, be warned that certain artifacts may easily be mistaken for haematomas by the unsuspecting, in particular where cord blood had been sampled during the third stage of labour.

Torsion, stricture

Torsion of the umbilical cord means an excessive degree of twisting around a longitudinal axis with the result that the blood vessels are compressed and eventually occluded. The subject is highly controversial and opinions are divided not only among clinicians, but also among pathologists. Probably a majority of those interested in this field consider torsion of the cord a genuine, if not very common, cause of intrauterine death, but a vocal minority maintain that torsion is a postmortem effect, brought about by passive movements of the fetus resulting from uterine contractions, and therefore irrelevant to the cause of fetal death.

The problem of torsion is bedeviled by two peculiarities. One is that there is a strong resemblance to physiological twisting or spiralling of the cord. It is difficult to decide where spiralling ends and torsion begins; torsion short of obstructing the umbilical blood flow is a 'non-event'. A recent contribution to this subject is by Herman et al (1992).

The other source of misgivings is the fact that most

stillbirths with torsion are macerated, and this is clearly the origin of the belief that it is a postmortem effect. Moreover, maceration can mask some lesions and simulate others; this tends to reduce the pathologist's confidence. Torsion in fresh stillbirths is extremely rare, probably because it does not trigger off or enhance uterine activity and fetal death in utero may go unnoticed for some time. It is certainly not as overtly dramatic an event as the term 'umbilical cord catastrophe' might suggest. Only occasionally is fetal death from umbilical cord complications preceded by increased, even violent, movements (McClintock, 1943).

The cardinal feature of torsion, which distinguishes it from marked physiological twisting, is the focal character of the lesion and the associated thinness of the cord. It is 'reduced to a thickness and consistency of thin whipcord' (Corkill, 1961), i.e. 2 or 3 mm at most. Characteristically, this focal lesion is situated near the umbilicus (Fig. 50.8), though Weber (1963) has shown that it can also occur nearer the placental end of the cord. This author has demonstrated that localized thinning of the cord and local reduction or absence of Wharton's jelly are not necessarily and exclusively the effect of torsion, but may pre-exist and predispose to torsion, though occasionally seen as isolated lesions. Such strictures have been seen in non-macerated cords and in the absence of torsion. In most instances, the lumen of the umbilical vessels is severely constricted or even fully obliterated. The tenor of Weber's contribution is that the 'strictures' are the primary and essential lesion, torsion being merely its complication: this view is certainly plausible but needs clarification and confirmation. (In Weber's publication the term 'constriction' is being used, which, in this context, we avoid because it suggests the presence of an external constricting agent.) The nature of strictures or coarctations is poorly understood, no doubt because they are seen but infrequently. A localized deficiency of Wharton's jelly seems to be their essence, but whether this is due to a primary fault in development or a result of focal degeneration is uncertain.

Mucoid degeneration of Wharton's jelly

This somewhat hypothetical degeneration was proposed by Bergman et al (1961) as an explanation of more or less severe deficiency of Wharton's jelly. As a result, the blood vessels of the cord are less well protected against compression and other mechanical interference. One of the two cases of these authors was a stillbirth. In all three instances of the same lesion reported by Labarrere et al (1985) fetal death occurred.

No information is available about any possible connection between mucoid degeneration and insertio furcata, stricture, the 'thin cord' syndrome or Malpas' 'constrictive sclerosis'.

Strangulation

Strangulation of the umbilical cord by membranous strands is discussed in Chapter 51 with other lesions of the 'amniotic band spectrum'.

Entanglement of the umbilical cord

In its stricter sense this term denotes intertwining of the umbilical cords of two fetuses (Fig. 50.9). This is possible only in monoamniotic twin pregnancies (or similar situations in 'higher' multiple pregnancy). It has also been observed in a case of 'pseudo-monoamniotic' twin pregnancy, where the (dichorionic) septum had been destroyed by a diagnostic procedure (Megory et al, 1991). In its wider sense — in which it will be used here — cord entanglement additionally comprises true knots and circumvolution of the cord around the infant's neck ('nuchal cord') or body. One might define entanglement as an anomalous position of the cord, brought about by a coiling or looping process and potentially interfering with blood flow in the umbilical cord. Strangulation of the cord by amniotic strands is not included under this heading, because it is essentially the strand that is wound around the cord rather than the cord around the strand, even though occasionally this latter process is also involved (James et al, 1969).

Three questions are bound to be asked with regard to the several forms of cord entanglement:

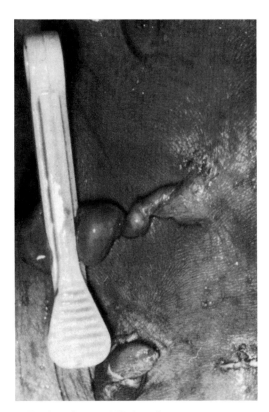

Fig. 50.8   Torsion of the umbilical cord.

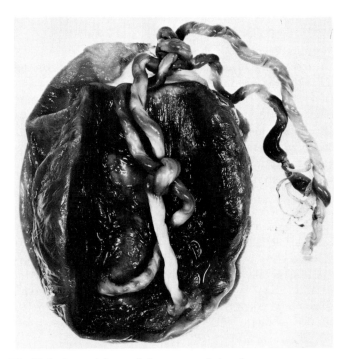

Fig. 50.9 Intertwining cords in monoamniotic twins.

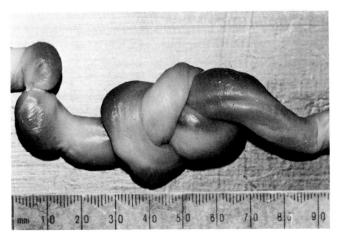

Fig. 50.10 A true knot of the umbilical cord.

1. How frequently do they occur?
2. How do they arise?
3. How serious a threat to fetal life and well-being do they present?

The frequency of each of the three types of entanglement is of a different order of magnitude. Entwining is at the 'bottom of the league table' owing to the relative rarity of monoamniotic twinning, but within this small population intertwining is relatively frequent, though its overall incidence is likely to be less than 1 in 10 000 deliveries.

True knots (Fig. 50.10) are more common: the reported frequencies vary from 0.04% (Corkill, 1961) to 1.05% (Spellacy et al, 1966). The subject has been thoroughly reviewed by Hartge (1979). True knots must be distinguished from 'false knots' (Fig. 50.11) which are either varicose umbilical vessels or focal accumulations of Wharton's jelly. We agree with Benirschke & Kaufmann (1990) that false knots should not be discussed at all under the heading of umbilical cord knots, because they are not knots (though they might legitimately be labelled 'nodes'). We believe that finding an appropriate niche for this morphological irregularity will only be possible after the undertaking of a more thorough anatomical exploration than has hitherto been available. Until then we regretfully follow the old custom but accept the view that false knots are not causally associated with any clinical complications.

Circumvolutions around the neck or around another part of the body occur fairly frequently: 24.6% and 2.09% respectively in the series of Spellacy et al (1966), based on a total number of 17 190 deliveries, whilst Scheffel &

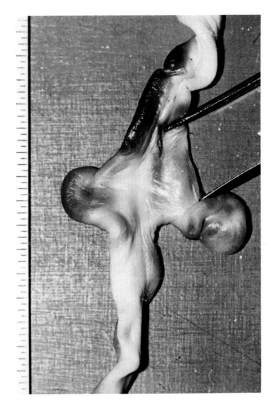

Fig. 50.11 A false knot of the umbilical cord.

Langanke (1970) report a combined incidence of 16.25% (of a total of 61 810) of encirclements of neck or any other organ. Dippel (1964) reports an incidence of 32.5% (in 1021 deliveries) of 'all entanglements', in which this author includes also prolapse (and occult prolapse) of the umbilical cord.

The question of the cause or causes of entanglements is more difficult to answer. Certainly, a sufficiently long cord is a *sine qua non* for any of the three forms of entanglement (Benirschke, 1994). Whether the cord length measured after delivery is always an accurate reflection of cord length prior to entanglement may be debatable; extrapolating from the work of Miller et al (1981) on causes of short umbilical cord one could conceive of entanglement as having a lengthening effect on the cord. It is likely, but by no means proven, that active movements by a living fetus are necessary for entwining, knot formation and circumvolution. Any of these incidents requires a sufficiently spacious amniotic cavity, so is more likely to occur before mid-pregnancy, or not long after, when the space available is relatively greater than in later gestation. Hydramnios, however, may facilitate entanglement even in the last trimester. Crawford (1962, 1964) presents some evidence that the incidence of circumvolution rises sharply after the 39th week, but there have been no confirmatory reports of this observation.

The effects of entanglement depend on the tightness of the knots etc. and, related to this, the tautness of the cord involved. Complete obstruction and cessation of umbilical blood flow is the exception rather than the rule. Scheffel & Langanke (1970), report a less than 2% fetal mortality with nuchal cords and 8.7% with true knots; but by no means in all fatal cases of these two groups was the cord entanglement necessarily the cause of death. Moreover, a niggling suspicion exists that the total incidence of true knots (0.19%) may have been under-recorded; these would almost certainly be recorded when the fetus was stillborn, but not necessarily when the infant lived. 'Over-recording' of true knots may also occur; novice pathologists examining placentas may fall into the trap set by some midwives by tying the loose end of the cord into a knot.

Many investigators, including Schafer & Mikulicz-Radecki (1961), Dippel (1964) and Fisher (1964), have come to the conclusion that entanglement, though rarely the cause of fetal death, may not so rarely cause fetal distress and neonatal depression.

The physiological effects of cord entanglement, in particular the level of blood gases in infants born with nuchal cords, were measured immediately after delivery by Stembera & Horska (1972). Their conclusions accord well with clinical experience: coiling of the cord around the neck, in the absence of other complications and with a healthy placenta, does not cause acidosis. If, however, placental reserve is diminished, the situation can become critical.

In assessing the effects of circumvolution of the neck, one should not only consider the effects on the umbilical, but also on the fetal cervical blood vessels, especially the jugular veins. The pressure exerted by the cord is not likely to impede the carotid blood flow, but may well suppress jugular venous drainage. Congestion of cerebral and meningeal vessels and intracranial haemorrhage can be found in some such infants.

Entanglement and, in particular, circumvolution reduce the effective length of the umbilical cord. When the extremities are involved in the process of entanglement,

as in the case reported by Corridan et al (1980), fetal movements can cause traction and thus trigger off abruptio placentae.

Intertwining of cords of monoamniotic twins, though not common, even in busy maternity units, has generated a considerable literature. No figures are available about its incidence within the group of monoamniotic twins, but it is certainly more 'newsworthy' than uncomplicated monoamniotic twinning, so the literature may present a misleading picture. Most of the cases reported before the middle of this century were fatal, but more recently the picture has radically changed. Even the closely 'braided' cords in the case reported by Golan et al (1982) did not prove fatal to either twin, and the twins recorded by Lumsden et al (1981) and by Annan & Hutson (1990) have also survived. This brighter outlook is presumably due to generally improved obstetric management, but no technique has yet been devised for in utero disentangling of entwined cords. So, presumably, much of the fetal loss was not exclusively due to the umbilical cord anomaly but also to associated factors.

Intertwining is not the only umbilical cord complication of monoamniotic twinning. The cord of one twin may be coiled around the neck of the other. Several examples of this anomaly are referred to later in the paragraph on iatrogenic and forensic considerations.

A pathologist dealing with a stillbirth in which the only lesion found is a cord around the neck, or a true knot, faces a dilemma. The pitfall of blindly accepting the cord anomaly as the cause of fetal demise should of course be avoided. On the other hand, he or she should not dismiss the suggestion without assessing the state of the umbilical cord and without a thorough search for complicating factors, such as oedema or thrombosis. If all the circumstances are taken into account, a true 'cord catastrophe' may occasionally emerge as the most likely cause of death.

Prolapse

Umbilical cord prolapse has much in common with cord entanglement, but does not qualify for inclusion under that heading because looping of the cord is not an essential part of the process. However, the umbilical blood flow is jeopardized, at least potentially, by pressure from outside, because the presenting part of the fetus is pressing the cord against the pelvic brim. Kinking of the cord can also be involved. Sinnathuray (1967) has emphasized the part played by umbilical vascular spasm in perinatally fatal cases of prolapsed cord. Manifest prolapse, as distinct from its preliminary stages (viz cord presentation and occult prolapse), is defined by Kaser & Pallaske (1967) as a situation in which a coil of umbilical cord can be felt in the vagina or can be seen at the vulva. At least one case, however, is on record in which the cord did not prolapse into the vagina but through an incompletely healed caesarean incision into the abdominal cavity (Lenke & Osterkamp, 1980).

The frequency of umbilical cord prolapse appears to have diminished in recent decades. Possibly there are also some environmental variations. Thus a fair comparison is not possible between two of the largest published series: Savage et al (1970) from Brooklyn, NY, USA report an incidence of six per 1000 (516 in 83 624 deliveries) during the years 1951–1965 inclusive; Kouam & Miller (1980) from Berlin report 38 cases in 20 698 deliveries, an incidence of 1.8 per 1000. (Their mortality figures are even less suited for comparison. Savage et al record a 'crude' mortality of 38%, and Kouam & Miller a 'corrected' mortality of 10.5%.) We may conclude that the incidence of prolapse, at least in the recent past and in countries with good obstetric services, is of a similar order of magnitude as that of true knots.

In contrast to true knots, however, several factors predisposing to prolapse are clinically detectable and can serve as a warning: these include premature labour, premature rupture of membranes, hydramnios and abnormal presentation of the fetus; so, to some extent, a prophylactic policy is possible.

'TELL-TALE' LESIONS OF THE UMBILICAL CORD

The single umbilical artery

The single umbilical artery is not only by far the most frequent developmental abnormality of the umbilical cord, but probably also the most common malformation in general.

The presence of only one artery instead of the usual two had occasionally been observed and recorded for over 400 years. The first published observation we owe to Gabriele Fallopio (1523–1562). The leading anatomist of that time, Andreas Vesalius (1514–1564) considered this finding important enough to refer to it in his *Fabrica corporis humani*.

Over the next three centuries many sporadic instances were recorded, usually in the context of other fetal abnormalities. It was Josef Hyrtl (1810–1894) who dealt in some detail with the phenomenon of the single umbilical artery in his monograph on *The blood vessels of the human afterbirth* (Hyrtl, 1870) and who emphasized the relatively frequent occurrence of single umbilical artery as an isolated abnormality.

A statistical and epidemiological approach was introduced by Benirschke, who first established the frequency of single umbilical artery in a series of perinatal autopsy records (Benirschke & Brown, 1955) and later in an unselected prospective series of 1500 consecutive deliveries (Benirschke & Bourne, 1960). A flood of similar investigations in the 1960s and 1970s followed and well over

300 000 (this figure, of course, refers to published investigations only) umbilical cords were examined in this respect in unselected series. In addition, several postmortem series were published as well as individual cases or small groups. In Table 50.1 only series of 5000 umbilical cords or more are included.

All these major investigations aimed to establish: (a) the incidence of single umbilical artery in a particular population and (b) the frequency of other congenital anomalies associated with it (Table 50.1). The results show a considerable variation both in the general incidence of single umbilical artery (0.27–1.0%) and in the frequency of associated malformations (8.7–46%).

It is most probable that differences in single umbilical artery frequency are at least in part due to differences in technique of umbilical cord examination and other factors, e.g. hidden selectivity. There can be no doubt, however, that genuine differences exist between various populations. Froehlich & Fujikura (1966) have reported an incidence of single umbilical artery among their white infants more than double that among blacks, but whether this difference — clearly significant because of the large numbers involved and because of their uniform protocol — is due solely to racial differences or possibly also to socio-economic or other factors is not known.

Differences in the frequency of associated malformations in single umbilical artery infants are also not fully explained. To some extent, they may be due to dissimilar standards in examination and documentation and also in the interpretation of the term 'malformation'.

Table 50.1 Reported incidence of single umbilical artery and of associated fetal malformation in prospective investigations

Author	Number examined	SUA* (%)	Incidence of malformation in fetuses with SUA* (%)
Thomas (1961)	6970	27 (0.39)	5 (18.5)
Feingold et al (1964)	6080	32 (0.52)	15 (46)
Fujikura (1964)	5972	38 (0.6)	7 (18.4)
Papadatos & Paschos (1965)	7886	32 (0.41)	10 (31.2)
Peckham & Yerushalmy (1965)	5848	51 (0.87)	12 (23.5)
Froehlich & Fujikura (1966)	26 539	203 (0.76)	58 (28.6)
Lewenthal et al (1967)	5135	50 (0.97)	12 (24)
Segovia (1967)	10 000	60 (0.6)	8 (13.3)
Ainsworth & Davies (1969)	12 078	113 (0.94)	38 (33.6)
Jean et al (1969)	11 115	112 (1)	17 (15.1)
Kristoffersen (1969)	8751	41 (0.47)	11 (23.4)
Cederqvist (1970)	9422	53 (0.27)	17 (32)
Broussard et al (1972)	9697	45 (0.46)	4 (8.8)
Le Marec et al (1972)	5619	31 (0.53)	10 (33)
Froehlich & Fujikura (1973)	39 773	344 (0.9)	30 (8.7)
Bryan & Kohler (1974)	20 000	144 (0.72)	26 (18.2)**
Eberst et al (1979)	22 293	137 (0.6)	24 (17.5)
Grall et al (1983)	42 815	194 (0.46)	44 (23)

* In parentheses — incidence expressed as a percentage
** These figures differ slightly from those originally published, because one already published case (of Lobdell–DiGeorge's syndrome) with single umbilical artery had been omitted (Kohler, 1968)

One of the motives for routinely checking the number of cord vessels was the prospect of earlier detection of malformations that were not apparent on clinical examination of the newborn. To assess the practical value of this policy the authors of two of the largest series, Froehlich & Fujikura (1973) and Bryan & Kohler (1975), carried out follow-up examinations of single umbilical artery infants who had appeared normal at birth. Froehlich & Fujikura reported no abnormality of significance among their infants apart from a curious frequency of inguinal hernia, possibly predisposed to by some minor and concealed abnormality. Bryan & Kohler, on the other hand, detected relevant abnormalities in 10 out of 96 single umbilical artery children who had been discharged from the newborn nursery as normal and could be traced for follow-up.

Malformations are not the only clinically relevant concomitant of single umbilical artery. Low birth weight is found relatively more frequently in single umbilical artery infants than in those with two umbilical arteries. In some cases this is fully accounted for by preterm birth, but in a very considerable number intrauterine growth retardation is responsible. Of course, many of the severely malformed infants are also light for dates, but we are concerned here with those who are free of additional malformation. In the series of Bryan & Kohler, these amounted to 25 or 17.5% of the total single umbilical artery population or 22% of the 'normal' single umbilical artery infants. By the time they were followed up, all of them had 'caught up' in weight with the exception of those few who had previously undetected congenital anomalies.

Surviving single umbilical artery children may in later life still show some effects of their vascular abnormality, i.e. when the umbilical artery has lost all functional relevance. Meyer & Lind (1974) found differences in size and histology of the two common iliac arteries. On the side of the single umbilical artery the iliac artery is larger and of elastic type, but on the 'missing' side smaller and of muscular type. Complementary investigations were carried out by Berry et al (1976) on living and otherwise normal single umbilical artery children at the Leeds Maternity Hospital. Using a non-invasive Doppler ultrasonic technique, these workers found excessive compliance of iliac arteries (but not of the arteries of the lower extremity) on the side of the single umbilical artery. This is explained as a consequence of the greater blood flow through one iliac artery when only one umbilical artery is available. Essentially similar results were obtained by Johnsonbaugh (1973) who used trans-umbilical aortography in newly-born single umbilical artery infants. In the same publication the negative result is reported of an investigation into suggested differences in length of the lower extremities in single umbilical artery infants.

It is generally acknowledged that, with very few exceptions, the absence of one artery from the umbilical cord reflects a similar intra-abdominal deficiency, but this intra-abdominal situation is by no means uniform. Broadly, two vascular patterns have been described: the more common pattern is that in which one artery is missing but the other one is found in a more or less normal contralateral position; the less common pattern is that in which neither left nor right umbilical artery is found. In this latter variant, the single artery in the cord is the continuation of an abdominal midline artery which branches off the abdominal aorta anywhere below the origin of the superior mesenteric artery even as low as the bifurcation of the aorta. This has been interpreted as a persistent omphaloenteric or vitelline artery (Ballantyne, 1897). It seems that some intermediate forms also occur and Dawson (1922) was not at all convinced of the vitelline origin of the midline umbilical artery and considered it as a displaced umbilical artery. We cannot, however, agree with Dawson that this 'midline single umbilical artery is found exclusively in sireniform fetuses. Bryan & Kohler (1974) report one case in which this variant was found as part of a malformation complex of which exomphalos was the most striking feature. So far only one recorded instance of 'midline single umbilical artery has come to our knowledge in which no major malformation was associated (Gisel, 1938). The association with other malformations is by no means a prerogative of the 'midline single umbilical artery.

The suggestion that single umbilical artery is especially, if not exclusively, associated with a particular malformation or group of malformations is sometimes implied in discussions of the subject. From the considerable amount of data that has accumulated, it is clear that single umbilical artery is not specifically associated with *any particular malformation*. It is true, however, that certain types of malformation are found more often than others in the company of single umbilical artery. These include: sirenomelia, acardiac twins, exomphalos and the so-called VATER complex (Kohler, unpublished observation).

Aetiology

The net results of the numerous prospective investigations in the last 30 years are somewhat meagre in so far as elucidation of the aetiology of single umbilical artery is concerned. This may in part be due to incomplete documentation of epidemiologically relevant factors. One aetiological factor that seems to be well established, thanks to the investigations by Lilja and her colleagues (1991), is maternal cigarette smoking. Maternal smoking might also be an aetiological factor in the branching and proliferation of umbilical blood vessels (see later).

From the findings of Froehlich & Fujikura (1966, 1973) and of others who have commented on the marked difference in frequency between black and white (northern) Americans, one might suspect a strong genetic element in the aetiology. However, this is not borne out by observations in uni-ovular ('identical') twins. Countless instances are found in the prospective series and many more in retrospective or sporadic case reports of single umbilical artery detected in one of monozygous (and also dizygous) twins, but only three examples of *concordant* single umbilical artery in uni-ovular twins are known to the present authors (Fasolis & Okely, 1966; Jaluvka & Pfeifer, 1967; Mortimer & Kohler, 1982, unpublished).

Quite recently we found reference to another three cases of single umbilical artery concordance of twins in a publication from Sweden (Lilja, 1991). A case of single umbilical artery concordance in dizgous twins is included in the series of Fujikura (1964). Recurrence in the same family is also rare — three times in one of the present authors' experience of some 45 000 umbilical cords, in the same maternity unit. The significance of multiple pregnancy as an aetiological factor is also still obscure; Benirschke & Driscoll (1967) emphasize a greater frequency of single umbilical artery in one partner of twins than in singletons. This might perhaps not be surprising, as many other malformations, including sirenomelia (Kohler, 1972), are more frequent in twins than in singletons. However, Bryan & Kohler (1974) found single umbilical artery marginally less frequently in twins than in singletons, and other investigators are divided on this point.

The association of single umbilical artery with karyotypic anomalies is frequently mentioned and in almost every series a few sporadic cases are included; these were infants with obvious malformations. Only one series, albeit small, is known to us in which all phenotypically 'normal' single umbilical artery infants were karyotyped: not a single case of chromosomal aberration came to light (Johnsonbaugh, 1973). Franzolin et al (1983), however, claim to have demonstrated less obvious karyotypic anomalies in some single umbilical artery infants in the *absence* of gross malformations. We have, however, the impression from recent publications that karyotypic anomalies are more frequently found in single umbilical artery infants, than is likely to be due to chance association (Byrne & Blanc, 1985; Salter et al, 1990).

The significance of maternal diabetes in this context is still a matter of dispute. Froehlich & Fujikura (1966) found a history of maternal diabetes in some 5% of their single umbilical artery cases, i.e. considerably more than in their control population. Bryan & Kohler (1974), on the other hand, failed to find any increase whatsoever in their single umbilical artery series.

Morphogenesis of single umbilical artery

Very little work has been done in the second half of this century to extend our knowledge of normal and abnormal development of umbilical arteries. The only interesting idea has come from Monie (1970), who demonstrated that the body stalk contains at first a vascular plexus which 'streamlines' itself into a single primitive umbilical artery; subsequently it is supplemented and eventually replaced by the two 'definitive' umbilical arteries. Single umbilical artery could therefore be the result of arrested development at the stage of the primitive single umbilical artery. Monie's views are compatible with those of Dawson (1922) who considers the midline variety of single umbilical artery as a displaced umbilical vessel, not a persistent arteria omphalo-mesoraica.

Altshuler et al (1975) claim to be able to distinguish, by simple histological examination, umbilical arteries that have all but disappeared by regression from those that have never been formed. We do not know of any further publications along these lines.

The question of the relationship between single umbilical artery and any malformations associated with it still remains unanswered: is the single umbilical artery, by reducing placental circulation and/or generally upsetting the balance of the fetal vascular system, the direct cause of those other morphological changes, or is the causal relationship a less direct one? A third possibility, i.e. that the associated anomalies are to blame in some way for the atrophy or aplasia of one umbilical artery, has not been seriously discussed in recent years. If the deficiency of one umbilical artery is to be regarded as the cause of any associated anomalies, one would expect the latter to arise at a later time than the establishment in normal embryos of the 'definitive' umbilical circulation. This seems not to be the case, for example, in sirenomelia, the classical example of an single umbilical artery-associated anomaly; the teratogenetic process is initiated before the umbilical arteries are normally formed. (This conclusion is based, admittedly, on an extrapolation of the experimental data of Wolff (1936), who produced symmelia in chick embryos by irradiation of the primitive streak.)

In the absence of direct evidence, we feel unable to reject completely the immediate causal rôle of single umbilical artery, which for 100 years or more has been championed by investigators of great credibility, experience and skill (Weigert, 1886; Ballantyne, 1904; Chaurasia, 1974). For the time being the verdict must remain 'unproven'.

Supernumerary umbilical vessels

Heightened interest in the blood vessels of the umbilical cord, and especially the numerous prospective investigations concerning a missing umbilical artery, resulted in the occasional — or more than occasional — finding of cords with more than three vessels on cross section. Such a finding calls for additional cuts across the cord in order to eliminate 'looping' as a cause of excessive vessel lumina. Looping is a common experience, related to uneven length of blood vessels within individual cords.

Other possible explanations for an additional vessel lumen are branching and anastomosis (Kelber, 1976). These are deviations from the norm as yet of unknown frequency and significance.

The possibility that accessory vessels found in the umbilical cord may be partial remnants of an incompletely regressed (right) umbilical vein has been considered by Meyer et al (1969). They found no fewer than 16 cases with 4 vessels in 310 cords of heterogeneous origin, mainly from normal deliveries.

What one might regard as a 'genuine and complete' supernumerary cord vessel, viz a persistent right umbilical vein in both its proximal (i.e. intra-abdominal) and distal (i.e. funicular) portions. Bell et al (1986) have reported a case and reviewed five other instances; all six had associated anomalies and each had only one umbilical artery (!). Obviously, it is not always sufficient to count the vessel lumina. The infant reported by Bell et al had been exposed in utero to anticonvulsant drugs. Experimentally, Monie et al (1957) had produced persistence of the right umbilical vein in rats by deficiency of folic acid.

An interesting new approach has been opened by Gupta et al (1993). In 644 umbilical cords — all from high risk pregnancies — they found no fewer than 40 instances (6.2%) in which more than the usual three 'vascular profiles' were seen. Correlating various clinical and pathological features with the 'multivascular' umbilical cord, Gupta and colleagues found a highly significant association with maternal smoking (10 or more cigarettes/day). There was also a positive correlation with inflammatory cell infiltration of the cord. The authors suggest that branching and/or proliferation of umbilical blood vessels may be a response to stress-producing insults.

Inflammation

Inflammation of the umbilical cord (funisitis or funiculitis) almost always implies an infection and an infiltration by acute inflammatory cells. Polymorphs are initially evident within the walls of the umbilical vessels, from where they may migrate into Wharton's jelly. This sequence of events denotes a fetal origin of the migrating inflammatory cells and indicates that infection of the cord has occurred during fetal life. Funiculitis is difficult to diagnose macroscopically, and the umbilical cord may appear normal to the naked eye, even in the presence of histologically evident inflammation. However, certain pathogenic organisms, notably *Listeria monocytogenes* and *Candida albicans*, may be manifest as minute white or cream-coloured abscesses visible on the surface of the cord and chorionic plate. Candida infections are often associated with a mixed macrophage and polymorph infiltration, denoting a more chronic infection, and the fungal elements may be demonstrated by special stains.

Funiculitis has a strong association with chorio-amnionitis of both the peripheral fetal membranes and chorionic plate, and has a similar association with prolonged rupture of the membranes and prematurity. However, the incidence of inflammation in the cord is lower than in the membranes, chorionic plate and subchorionic fibrin layer. Chellam & Rushton (1985), in a study of placentas from live and stillborn infants weighing less than 2.5 kg, recorded a frequency of 48.5% for chorioamnionitis but of only 9.5% for umbilical cord inflammation.

Necrotizing funisitis is, according to Craver & Baldwin (1992), characterized by perivascular bands of necrotic Wharton's jelly containing more or less degenerate inflammatory cells. These bands — reminiscent of an Ouchterlony diffusion plate — suggest a diffusible toxin in the amniotic fluid. Perinatal morbidity and mortality are increased. The aetiology is likely to be of infectious nature, but so far no specific pathogen can be incriminated, though a few cases have been attributed to maternal syphilis (Fojaco et al, 1989).

Inflammatory cell infiltration of the umbilical cord is included under the heading 'tell-tale lesions' because its detection may draw attention to infection in the placenta or in the fetus, or may strengthen suspicion formed on clinical grounds. For this reason it may be helpful to speed up the diagnosis by using a frozen section technique, for which the umbilical cord is highly suitable (Benirschke & Clifford, 1959; Kerisit et al, 1981).

Oedema

Oedema of the umbilical cord (Fig. 50.12) is fairly common, but in the past was often disregarded except perhaps when it was one aspect of generalized hydrops. Only cases of extreme oedema (e.g. Walz, 1947) found their way into the literature as curiosities. In recent years, thanks to the work of Scott and her colleagues (Scott & Jordan, 1972; Coulter et al, 1975; Scott & Wilkinson, 1978), the relative frequency of cord oedema, and its association with various cardiorespiratory afflictions of the newborn, have attracted some attention. Standards for diagnosis and documentation had to be introduced and Scott chose a simple method of recording two umbilical cord diameters at right angles in the same plane. The site of cross section should be as near as practicable to the fetal end, avoiding any focal swelling of the cord or engorgement of umbilical blood vessels. Multiplication of the two diameters gives the 'diameter product'. Oedema is considered to be present when the diameter product is 1.3 (corresponding to a cross section area of approximately 1.0 cm^2) or more. A cord with a diameter product of 0.6 or less is regarded as abnormally thin.

This method may be open to criticism, as cord thickness is often irregular and therefore unreliable as a parameter; furthermore, thickness is related also to factors other than water content. However, it has proved useful in prac-

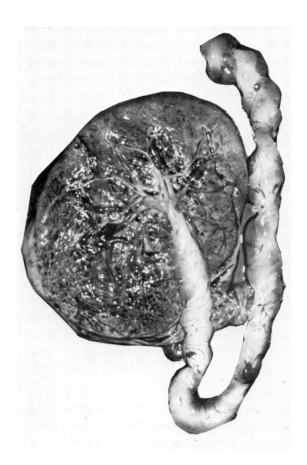

Fig. 50.12 Oedema of the umbilical cord. (From Fox, 1978. Courtesy of W. B. Saunders.)

tice. Water content determinations (Scott & Wilkinson, 1978) have shown a good correlation with diameter product: cords with a diameter product of 1.3 or more had a water content of 92% or more (average 93.5%), whilst 'thin, wrinkled cords', with a diameter product of 0.6 cm or less, had an average water content of 89.2%. The normal range gave results around 90%. However, an additional group of 'thin, wet cords' had to be recognized: these were cords with a diameter product in the low normal or abnormally low ranges, but a definitely high water content. In practice, thin wet cords are readily picked out; they usually belong to preterm babies, often with additional complications.

The clinical conditions found in infants with oedema of the umbilical cord are those in which the infant's circulatory efficiency may be below par, in particular respiratory distress syndrome and transient respiratory distress. Rolschau's (1978) conclusion that oedema of the umbilical cord is 'of no significance to the infant' is not in accord with our experience. It may be advisable to include the measurement of cord diameters in the routine examination of the placenta.

The water content of the umbilical cord has also been investigated by Sloper et al (1979), who found mean val-

ues of 88.9% (±2.73) for infants born at term, and 91.9% (±1.99) for preterm babies. These workers emphasize the higher water content of the fetal against the placental end of the cord and conclude that their findings 'suggest a metabolically active role for the umbilical cord', confirming, in this respect, the findings of Plentl (1961).

It may be as well to remember that abnormal thickness at the infant's end of the umbilical cord ('giant umbilical cord') can be associated with a patent urachus (Chantler et al, 1969; Ente et al, 1970).

Thin cord

The term 'thin cord syndrome' has been introduced by Hall (1961) and used (untranslated) by German authors (Kloos & Vogel, 1974; Becker et al, 1981). It was coined to characterize two infants, of whom one was stillborn, the other liveborn with a history of fetal distress. Hall suggests that the thin cord is due to a deficiency of Wharton's jelly and therefore more sensitive to various mechanical insults such as prolapse, entanglement and especially torsion; he does not raise the question whether the deficiency is primary or secondary. Criteria for diagnosis are not specified. However, Scott & Wilkinson (1978) (see preceding section) found a diameter product of 0.6 or less in 'thin wrinkled cords' of infants who frequently were dismature or postmature. (The term dismature refers to discordance or disparity or discrepancy between gestational age (by dates) and maturity assessed by weight and other physical criteria. The frequently seen spelling 'dysmature' is linguistically wrong, as the syllable 'dys' means painful or ugly or bad; none of these connotations is intended.) The question whether the thin cord is a cause or effect of intrauterine growth retardation remains unanswered, at least for the time being.

An interesting case with both quantitative and qualitative deficiency of Wharton's jelly was reported by Malpas (1968). The diameter product was less than 0.2, the texture unusually firm and there was some ill-defined cellular infiltration in the absence of any other evidence of infection. The author speaks of 'constrictive sclerosis'. Malpas also speculates about the effect of this abnormal cord on the balance of intervillous and intravillous pressure in relation to abruptio placentae, which complicated his case. He concludes that premature placental detachment may have fetal as well as maternal causes.

Meconium staining of the cord

Meconium staining of the umbilical cord has the same significance as similar discolouration of the fetal surface of the placenta, though it has recently been claimed that meconium can induce necrosis of umbilical vessels and necrosis of the cord (Altschuler et al, 1992; Benirschke, 1994). In our experience, listeriosis is associated with heavy meconium staining more frequently, perhaps also more intensely, than other infections.

Jaundice

Jaundice can be more conspicuous in the umbilical cord than in any other superficial tissue. It used to be seen frequently in severe haemolytic disease of the newborn when this condition was more common than it is now. It prompts us to suspect that not only water, but bile pigments too, can cross the vessel wall and Wharton's jelly.

TUMOURS AND MALFORMATIONS

Tumours of the umbilical cord

The only umbilical cord tumour generally accepted as a true neoplasm is the teratoma. Few examples have been reported, the latest by Smith & Majmudar (1985). Other cases of teratoma are reviewed by Fox (1978).

None of the reported teratomas were claimed to be malignant in the customary histological sense, but some were associated with fetal death (e.g. Kreyberg, 1958) either causally or coincidentally. (An example of causal association is mechanical interference with the umbilical circulation by a cord tumour, no matter what its histogenesis or degree of differentiation.)

Whilst clinical interest in umbilical cord teratoma is limited by its rarity, students of oncogenesis have debated its origin. There is fairly general agreement that all teratomas arise from germ cells. These are first detectable in the yolk sac, then migrate via the midgut to arrive eventually at the genital ridge where they form the primordium of the gonad. Teratomas are believed to take their origin from cells that have 'dropped out' on the long march or have actively strayed away. The point at issue is whether cord teratomas are derived from cells left behind in the yolk sac or from cells that have got as far as the gut, but which from the seventh to the tenth week of fetal life are displaced into the umbilical cord; from there the germ cells could migrate into the cord mesenchyme.

A tumour in the wider sense of the word, but not a true neoplasm, the haemangioma of the umbilical cord is in most respects closely similar to the chorionic haemangioma (or chorangioma) of the placenta. Both these tumours are derived from fetal blood vessels and are regarded as hamartomatous in nature, i.e. dysplastic rather tha neoplastic.

Haemangiomas of the cord, like those of the placenta, can act as arteriovenous shunts. Many instances are reported of circulatory impairment (e.g. Benson & Joseph, 1961) and even hydrops (e.g. Jones et al, 1972) complicating placental chorangioma, but only one case of non-immune fetal hydrops associated with a haemangioma of the cord has been reported (Seifer et al, 1985). This is perhaps explained by differences in vascular architecture of cord and placenta. A haemangioma of the cord is likely to interfere with umbilical blood supply to the fetus, before reaching great size, whilst a chorangioma can expand, mainly at the expense of the intervillous space.

Some haemangiomas have been found in association with stillborn fetuses (Zeman & Rauchenberg, 1970): Dohmen & Bubenzer (1978) observed a fatal haematoma within a cavernous haemangioma, whilst a pedunculated cord haemangioma was reported by Nieder & Link (1970). Bleeding is the most frequent complication of these tumours.

From these and other published reports (Heifetz & Rueda-Pedraza, 1983) as well as our own observations it would appear that umbilical cord haemangiomas are only likely to be noted if they are visible — and conspicuous — to the naked eye; among these, only those cases associated with fetal death (or with clinically manifest damage to the newborn) stand a chance of being reported. Cord haemangiomas are, however, now diagnosable prenatally by ultrasound (Ghidini et al, 1990) and this may well lead to an increased awareness of their presence and a more accurate estimate of their incidence.

Barson et al (1980) and Resta et al (1988) have reported raised alphafetoprotein levels in maternal serum in association with haemangiomas of the umbilical cord.

Several angiomyxomas of the cord have been reported in recent years, including one by Fortune & Ostor (1980) who define this type of tumour as a combination of haemangioma with myxomatous degeneration of Wharton's jelly. In their case the fetus was macerated and immature: autopsy did not reveal any alternative cause of death, nor was any significant abnormality found in the placenta, so the authors concluded that death was due to the haemodynamic effects of the angiomyxoma. Yavner & Redline (1989) described a huge angiomyxoma at the fetal end of the cord whilst Jauniaux et al (1990) reported an angiomyxoma which involved the entire length of the cord.

As a curiosity we mention a case from the older literature: Kaufmann (1890) described a 'myxosarcoma teleangiectodes', which in all probability was a benign angiomyxoma. The infant was liveborn and in the first few days the swelling, at the fetal end of the cord, increased in size; this was apparently the reason for giving it the label of malignancy, but bleeding into the tumour is a more likely explanation.

A case of umbilical cord metastasis of a fetal neuroblastoma has been reported by Andersen & Hariri (1983).

Malformations

Mention has already been made of lesions consisting of vestiges of gut and its appendages that have been left behind when the 'physiological umbilical hernia' was reduced (at the end of the tenth week post conception). If a substantial portion of gut fails to be reduced we are faced with the pathological condition of neonatal umbilical hernia.

Some confusion has arisen from inexact terminology, implicitly equating umbilical hernia with omphalocele or exomphalos. Potter (1961) points out that the more severe forms of exomphalos are due to a failure in the formation of the embryo's body stalk much earlier in prenatal life than the 'physiological umbilical hernia'. This is, of course, a more profound disturbance of development, frequently associated with other severe abnormalities including complete or near complete aplasia ('achordia') of the umbilical cord (Bohm, 1982).

The umbilical cord changes seen in conjunction with a patent urachus ('giant umbilical cord') have been referred to in the discussion on thickness of the umbilical cord.

Abnormal connections between cord and fetal body (Fig. 50.13) have been reported in at least two cases of anencephaly with placenta attached to the meninges (Askanazy, 1939; Donnai et al, 1982).

Partial fusion of umbilical cords may occur in monochorionic (but not necessarily monoamniotic) twins, the fusion being located at the distal (i.e. placental) end of the cord. This sets the scene for a peculiar variant of feto-fetal transfusion. Kloosterman (1958) reported such a case, in which both infants were afflicted with Rh haemolytic disease, but only one infant was hydropic. Zennegg (1966) reported fusion of the cords (though vascular anastomoses of cord vessels are not obvious from the illustration), with one twin hydropic. Howorka & Kapczynski (1972) reported diamniotic, monochorionic twin fetuses with their fused cords apparently running in part between the two amniotic membranes.

MISCELLANEOUS CONDITIONS

Surface ulceration of the umbilical cord

This is apparently a rare and puzzling anomaly, but Bendon et al (1991) have been able to report three cases. The lesions show no obvious signs of infective aetiology; they appear to be related to funicular blood vessels, especially the arteries and may erode these. This results in haemorrhage, chiefly into the liquor amnii. All three infants observed by Bendon et al had some form of small intestinal atresia. The nature of this association is obscure but the clinical significance is clear. Blood loss from umbilical cord ulcers can be serious. Moreover, the ulceration may be a warning sign in respect of small gut atresia. As noted previously, the possibility has been raised that meconium may induce cord necrosis and ulceration.

Umbilical cord pseudocyst

This term denotes a localized oedematoid change in the texture of Wharton's jelly, possibly the effect of mucoid degeneration. As far as we know, there is no clinical significance attached to it.

Umbilical cord calcification

In contrast to the placenta the umbilical cord is only very rarely the seat of calcification. Even in cases of unusually massive calcium deposits in the placenta the umbilical cord can be free of calcification. Moreover, in two still-

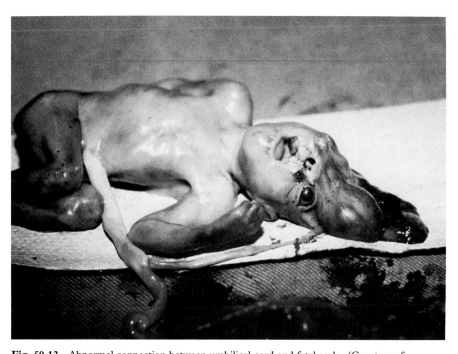

Fig. 50.13 Abnormal connection between umbilical cord and fetal scalp. (Courtesy of Dr. D. Donnai, Manchester.)

born infants with generalized arterial calcification (Ivemark et al, 1962) the umbilical arteries were free. A fairly recent publication by Khong & Dilly (1989) emphasizes the heterogeneity of this disorder and suggests there may be two distinct lesions, one arising in the vessel wall, the other in the (thrombosed) lumen.

Iatrogenic and forensic aspects of the umbilical cord

One of the effects of the expansion of sophisticated diagnostic and therapeutic techniques in obstetrics and perinatology is an increase in lesions caused by medical intervention. Prior to the introduction of intrauterine transfusion (Liley, 1963) and the ever extending use of diagnostic amniocentesis, iatrogenic lesions were uncommon. Almost the only common obstetric practices that were likely to injure the umbilical cord and/or fetal membranes were artificial rupture and 'sweep' of membranes. These were especially hazardous in the absence of any means to exclude the presence of vasa praevia.

Complications of amniocentesis are of great variety but here we wish to draw attention only to those involving the umbilical cord and membranes.

In both amniocentesis and intrauterine transfusion, injury to an umbilical cord vessel can lead to bleeding into the amniotic cavity or to haematoma formation or both. Damage to fetal membranes in the course of amniocentesis can manifest itself as 'spontaneous' rupture of membranes (Teramo & Sipinen, 1978), as extramembranous pregnancy (Vago & Chavkin, 1980), as intrauterine amputation caused by amniotic strands (Rehder & Weitzel, 1978; Moessinger et al, 1981) and as strangulation of the umbilical cord (Robertson et al, 1981).

Inadvertently severing the cord of an undelivered second twin must be every obstetrician's nightmare. Yet no fewer than six instances (and possibly more) of mono-amniotic twin pregnancy with this complication are on record (Podzahradsky, 1912; Hagood & Stokes, 1953; Tagawa, 1974; Ong et al, 1976; Kassam & Tompkins, 1980; McLeod & McCoy, 1981). In each case the first twin, presenting by the head, had around his/her neck an umbilical cord which was divided in order to facilitate delivery of the trunk. When this was achieved, the first twin's cord was seen to be intact and the real situation was recognized. Accelerated delivery of the second twin resulted in double live birth in each of the six quoted reports, but in at least one instance (Kassam & Tompkins, 1980) the second twin suffered irreversible hypoxic damage.

Only one report of an untoward effect of amnioscopy is known to us; a focal infiltration of leucocytes was found in the cervical membranes, presumably an effect of pressure by the amnioscope (Horky & Aman, 1967).

Criminal intrusion into the amnion is virtually synonymous with attempted abortion. Relatively few such cases have been examined by forensic pathologists in recent years and no detailed study of the fetal membranes in this context is available.

The umbilical cord is a favourite instrument of infanticide. From a personal communication by Dr M. A. Green in 1983, we understand that strangulation of the newly-born infant's neck by umbilical cord is not uncommon in the experience of forensic pathologists. 'Damage to the cord is obvious to the naked eye, a thin stretched segment in the part which had been put around the neck; also areas of haemorrhage into Wharton's jelly . . .'. In such cases, and in many others of concealed confinement, the cord would be 'torn rather than cut . . . The technique recommended is to immerse the ends in water and examine them with a hand lens, so that the frayed edges of the torn end can be identified.'

REFERENCES

Ainsworth P, Davies P A 1969 Single umbilical artery: a five year study. Developmental Medicine and Child Neurology 11: 297–302.

Altshuler G, Tsang R C, Ermocilla R 1975 Single umbilical artery: correlation of clinical status and umbilical cord histology. American Journal of Diseases of Children 129: 697–700.

Altshuler G, Arizawa M, Molnar-Nadasdy G 1992 Meconium-induced umbilical cord vascular necrosis and ulceration: a potential link between the placenta and poor pregnancy outcome. Obstetrics and Gynecology 79: 760–766.

Andersen H J, Hariri J 1983 Congenital neuroblastoma in a fetus with multiple malformations: metastasis in the umbilical cord as a cause of intrauterine death. Virchows Archiv A Pathological Anatomy and Histology 400: 219–222.

Angiolillo M, Picinelli M L 1965 Il problema dei vasi nutrizi del funicolo ombilicale a termine. Monitore Zoologica Italiano 73: 66–73.

Annan B, Hutson R C 1990 Double survival despite cord entanglement in monoamniotic twins: case report. British Journal of Obstetrics and Gynaecology 97: 950–951.

Askanazy M 1939 Quand les vaisseaux ombilicaux (placentaires) entrent-ils dans la tete du foetus? Schweizer Zeitschrift fur Allgemeine Pathologie 2: 1–16.

Ballantyne J W 1897 The occurrence of a non-allantoic or vitelline placenta in the human subject. Transactions of the Edinburgh Obstetric Society 23: 58–81.

Ballantyne J W 1904 Manual of antenatal pathology and hygiene, vol 2. The embryo. William Green, Edinburgh.

Barham K A 1968 The use of amnioscopy in the detection of meconium. Australian and New Zealand Journal of Obstetrics and Gynaecology 8: 9–16.

Barson A J, Donnai D, Read A P 1980 Haemangioma of the cord: further cause of raised alphafetoprotein. British Medical Journal 281: 1252.

Becker V, Schiebler T H, Kubli F (eds) 1981 Die Plazenta des Menschen. Georg Thieme, Stuttgart.

Bell A D, Gerlis L M, Variend S 1986 Persistent right umbilical vein — case report and review of literature. International Journal of Cardiology 10: 167–176.

Bendon R W, Tyson R W, Baldwin V J, Cashner K A, Mimouni F, Miodovnik M 1991 Umbilical cord ulceration and intestinal atresia:

a new association? American Journal of Obstetrics and Gynecology 164: 582–586.

Benirschke K 1994 Obstetrically important lesions of the umbilical cord. Journal of Reproductive Medicine 39: 262–272.

Benirschke K, Bourne G L 1960 The incidence and prognostic implication of congenital absence of one umbilical artery. American Journal of Obstetrics and Gynecology 79: 251–254.

Benirschke K, Brown W H 1955 On aplasia of an umbilical artery. Obstetrics and Gynecology 6: 399–404.

Benirschke K, Clifford S M 1959 Intrauterine bacterial infection of the newborn infant: frozen sections of the cord as an aid to early detection. Journal of Pediatrics 54: 11–18.

Benirschke K, Driscoll S G 1967 The pathology of the human placenta. Springer Verlag, Berlin.

Benirschke K, Kaufmann P 1990 The pathology of the human placenta. Springer, Berlin.

Benson P F, Joseph M C 1961 Cardiomegaly in a newborn due to a placental chorioangioma. British Medical Journal 1: 102–105.

Bergman P, Lundin P, Malmstrom T 1961 Mucoid degeneration of the Wharton's jelly: an umbilical cord anomaly threatening foetal life. Acta Obstetricia et Gynecologica Scandinavica 40: 372–378.

Berry C L, Gosling R G, Laogvn A A, Bryan E M 1976 Anomalous iliac compliance in children with a single umbilical artery. British Heart Journal 38: 510–515.

Bettzieche H 1978 Studien zur Frage der Innervation der Nabelschnur. Zentralblatt fur Gynakologie 100: 799–804.

Bilek K, Rothe K, Piskaczek K 1962 Insertio velamentosa Blutung vor dem Blasensprung. Zentralblatt fur Gynakologie 84: 1536–1541.

Blanc W A, Allen G W 1961 Intrafunicular ulceration of persistent omphalo-mesenteric duct with intra-amniotic hemorrhage and fetal death. American Journal of Obstetrics and Gynecology 82: 1392–1396.

Bohm N 1982 Das fehlende Nabelschnur-Syndrom. Tagung der deutschen Gesselschaft fur Pathologie. Abstract in Zentralblatt fur Allgemeine Pathologie 128: 267.

Boyd J D, Hamilton W J 1970 The human placenta. Heffer, Cambridge.

Bret A J, Bardiaux M 1960 Hematome du cordon. Revue Francaise de Gynecologie et d'Obstetrique 55: 81–142.

Broussard P, Raudrant D, Picaud J J, Boughlet C, Dumont M 1972 Artere ombilicale unique: etude de 45 cas: valeur de l'examen systematique du placenta. Journal de Gynecologie d'Obstetrique et de Biologie de la Reproduction 1: 551–558.

Browne F J 1925 Abnormalities of the umbilical cord. Journal of Obstetrics and Gynaecology of the British Empire 32: 17–48.

Bryan E M, Kohler H G 1974 The missing umbilical artery. I. Prospective study based on a maternity hospital. Archives of Disease in Childhood 49: 844–852.

Bryan E M, Kohler H G 1975 The missing umbilical artery. II. Paediatric follow-up. Archives of Disease in Childhood 50: 714–718.

Burton G, Saunders D M 1988 Vasa-praevia: another cause for concern in in-vitro-fertilization pregnancies. Australian and New Zealand Journal of Obstetrics and Gynaecology 28: 180–181.

Byrne J, Blanc W A 1985 Malformation and chromosome anomalies in spontaneously aborted fetuses with single umbilical artery. American Journal of Obstetrics and Gynecology 151: 340–342.

Cederqvist L 1970 Die Bedeutung des Fehlens einer Arterie in der Nabelschnur. Acta Obstetricia et Gynecologica Scandinavica 49: 113–117.

Chantler C, Baum J D, Wigglesworth J S, Scopes J W 1969 Giant umbilical cord associated with a patent urachus and fused umbilical artery. Journal of Obstetrics and Gynaecology of the British Commonwealth 76: 273–274.

Chaurasia B D 1974 Single umbilical artery with caudal defects in human fetuses. Teratology 9: 287–298.

Chellam V G, Rushton D I 1985 Chorioamnionitis and funiculitis in the placentas of 200 births weighing less than 2.5 kg. British Journal of Obstetrics and Gynaecology 92: 808–814.

Clare N M, Hagashi R, Khodr G 1979 Intrauterine death from umbilical cord hematoma. Archives of Pathology and Laboratory Medicine 103: 46–47.

Clarke J A 1965 An X-ray microscopic study of the vasa vasorum of the human umbilical arteries. Zeitschrift fur Zellforschung 66: 243–249.

Corkill T F 1961 The infant's vulnerable life line. Australian and New Zealand Journal of Obstetrics and Gynaecology 1: 154–160.

Corridan M, Kendall E D, Begg J D 1980 Cord entanglement causing premature placental separation and amniotic fluid embolism. British Journal of Obstetrics and Gynaecology 87: 935–940.

Coulter J B S, Scott J M, Jordan M M 1975 Oedema of the cord and respiratory distress in the newborn. British Journal of Obstetrics and Gynaecology 82: 453–459.

Craver R D, Baldwin V J 1992 Necrotising funisitis. Obstetrics and Gynecology 79: 64–70.

Crawford J S 1962 Cord around the neck: incidence and sequelae. Acta Paediatrica Scandinavica 51: 594–603.

Crawford J S 1964 Cord around the neck: further analysis of incidence. Acta Paediatrica Scandinavica 53: 553–557.

Dawson A B 1922 The origin and occurrence of the single umbilical artery in normal and abnormal human fetuses. Anatomical Record 24: 321–343.

Dillon W P, O'Leary J 1981 Detection of fetal cord compromise secondary to umbilical cord hematoma with the non-stress test. American Journal of Obstetrics and Gynecology 141: 102–105.

Dippel A L 1964 Malignant umbilical cord entanglements. American Journal of Obstetrics and Gynecology 88: 1012–1019.

Dohmen W, Bubenzer J 1978 Hamatom als Komplikation eines kavernosen Hamangioms der Nabelschnur. Zeitschrift fur Geburtshilfe und Perinatologie 182: 312–315.

Donnai D, Read A P, Brandreth C L, Donnai P 1982 Prenatal detection of aberrant tissue bands and cord abnormalities. Journal of Obstetrics and Gynaecology 2: 203–205.

Eberst B, Borg G, Harzolf G, Ritter J, Gander R 1979 L'artere ombilicale unique. Revue Francaise de Gynecologie et d'Obstetrique 74: 37–40.

Ente H, Penzer P H, Kenigsberg K 1970 Giant umbilical cord associated with patent urachus: an external clue to internal anomaly. American Journal of Disease of Children 120: 82–83.

Evason F H 1952 Haematoma of the umbilical cord. British Medical Journal 2: 1081 (letter to editor).

Fasolis S, Okely C 1961 Agenesia dell 'arteria ombelicale destra in entrambi gli individui di copia gemallare. Folia Heredito Pathologica 10: 115.

Feingold M, Fine R N, Ingall D 1964 Intravenous pyelography in infants with single umbilical artery. New England Journal of Medicine 270: 1178–1180.

Fisher E L 1964 Cord entanglement and fetal prognosis. Obstetrics and Gynecology 23: 608–610.

Fojaco R M, Hensley G T, Moskowitz L 1989 Congenital syphilis and necrotizing funisitis. Journal of the American Medical Association 261: 1788–1790.

Fortune D W, Ostor A G 1980 Angiomyxomas of the umbilical cord. Obstetrics and Gynecology 55: 375–378.

Fox H 1978 Pathology of the placenta. Saunders, London.

Fox S B, Khong T Y 1990 Lack of innervation of human umbilical cord: an immunohistological and histochemical study. Placenta 11: 59–62.

Franqué O V 1900 Zur Pathologie der Nachgeburtsheile. Zeitschrift fur Geburtshilfe und Gynakologie 43: 463–498.

Franzolin A, Mathers A, Ferrari N 1983 Cytogenetic and dermatoglyphic studies of newborns with a single umbilical artery. Zeitschrift fur Geburtshilfe und Perinatologie 187: 44–47.

Freisfeld R 1936 Uber einen Fall von Nabelschnurhamatom. Zentralblatt fur Gynakologie 60: 1699–1701.

Froehlich L A, Fujikura T 1966 Significance of single umbilical artery: report from the collaborative study of cerebral palsy. American Journal of Obstetrics and Gynecology 94: 274–279.

Froehlich L A, Fujikura T 1973 Follow-up of infants with single umbilical artery. Pediatrics 52: 22–29.

Fujikura T 1964 Single umbilical artery and congenital malformations. American Journal of Obstetrics and Gynecology 88: 829–830.

Gaulis G L 1953 Double insertion velamenteuse praevia: grossesse gemelolaire univitelline. Bulletin de Federation des Societes de Gynecologie de d'Obstetrique de la langue Francaise 5: 162–163.

Ghidini A, Romero R, Eisen R N, Smith G J, Hobbins J C 1990 Umbilical cord hemangioma: prenatal identification and review of the literature. Journal of Ultrasound Medicine 9: 297–300.

Gisel A 1938 Persistenz der Arteria omphalo-mesoraica und Fehlen der Nabelarterien bei einer Neugeborenen. Zeitschrift fur Anatomie und Entwicklungsgeschichte 108: 686–694.

Golan A, Amit A, Baram A, David M P 1982 Unusual cord intertwining in monoamniotic twins. Australian and New Zealand Journal of Obstetrics and Gynaecology 22: 165–167.

Grall J Y, Coudrais C, Jovan H, Priov G, Aras P L, Kerisit J 1983 L'artere ombilicale unique: a propos de 194 observations. Annals d'Anatomie et Cytologie Pathologiques 31: 111–114.

Grange D K, Arya S, Opitz J M, Laxova R, Herrmann J, Gilbert E F 1987 The short umbilical cord. Birth Defects Original Article Series 23: 191–214.

Gupta I, Hillier V F, Edwards J M 1993 Vascular branching in the umbilical cord: an indication of maternal smoking habits and intrauterine distress. Placenta 14: 117–123.

Hagood M, Stokes R H 1953 Double survival of monoamniotic twins. American Journal of Obstetrics and Gynecology 65: 1152–1154.

Hall S P 1961 The thin cord syndrome: a review with a report of two cases. Obstetrics and Gynecology 18: 507–509.

Harris L E, Wenzl J E 1963 Heterotopic pancreatic tissue and intestinal mucosa in the umbilical cord. New England Journal of Medicine 268: 721–722.

Hartge R 1979 Uber das Vorkommen yon Nabelschnurknoten. Geburtshilfe und Frauenheilkunde 39: 976–980.

Heifetz S A 1988 Thrombosis of the umbilical cord: analysis of 52 cases and literature review. Pediatric Pathology 8: 37–54.

Heifetz S A, Rueda-Pedraza E 1983 Hemangiomas of the umbilical cord. Pediatric Pathology 1: 385–398.

Herberz O 1938 Polar insertion, rare variant of velamentous insertion. Duodecim 54: 698–703.

Herman A, Zabow P, Segal M et al 1992 Extremely large number of twists of the umbilical cord causing torsion and intrauterine fetal death. International Journal of Gynaecology and Obstetrics 35: 165–167.

Honer M 1976 Komplikationen am Schangerschaftsende und unter der Geburt durch ein Nabelschnurhamatom. Zentralblatt fur Gynakologie 98: 848–859.

Horky Z, Amon K 1967 Rundcellulare Infiltration der Eihaute nach Amnioskopie. Geburtshilfe und Frauenheilkunde 27: 1065–1076.

Howorka E, Kapczynski W 1972 Unvollstandige Nabelschnurteilung zwischen zwei Zwillingsfruchten und zwischenhautiger Verlauf eines gemeinsamen paraplazentaren Nabelschnurabschnittes. Zentralblatt fur Gynakologie 94: 422–423.

Hyrtl J 1870 Die Blutgefasse der menschlichen Nachgeburt in normalen und anormen Verhaltnissen. Braumuller, Wien.

Irani P K 1964 Haematoma of the umbilical cord. British Medical Journal 2: 1436–1437.

Iremark B I, Lagergren C Z, Ljungquist A 1962 Generalised arterial calcification associated with hydramnios in two stillborn infants. Acta Paediatrica 51 (suppl 135): 103–110.

Jaluvka V, Pfeifer K 1967 Uber das Fehlen einer Arteria umbilicalis bei beiden eineiigen Zwillingen. Zentralblatt fur Allgemeine Pathologie 110: 320–328.

James P D, Beilly J O W, Steele S J 1969 An unusual cause of intrauterine death. Journal of Obstetrics and Gynaecology of the British Commonwealth 76: 752–754.

Jauniaux E, de Munter C, Vanesse M, Wilkin P, Hustin J 1989 Embryonic remnants of the umbilical cord; morphological and clinical aspects. Human Pathology 20: 458–462.

Jauniaux E, Mosconso G, Chitty L et al 1990 An angiomyxoma involving the whole length of the umbilical cord: prenatal diagnosis by ultrasonography. Journal of Ultrasound Medicine 9: 419–422.

Jean C, Dupre A, Carrier C 1969 L'artere umbilicale unique: etude de 112 observations. Canadian Medical Association Journal 100: 1088–1091.

Johnsonbaugh R E 1973 Unilateral short lower extremity and single umbilical artery. American Journal of Diseases in Children 126: 186–187.

Jones C E M, Rivers R P A, Taghizadeh A 1972 Disseminated intravascular coagulation and fetal hydrops in a newborn infant in association with a chorangioma. Pediatrics 50: 901–907.

Kaser O, Pallaske H J 1967 Geburt. In: Kaser O, Friedling V, Ober K G, Thomsen K, Zander J (eds) Gynakologie und Geburtshilfe, vol II. Georg Thieme, Stuttgart, pp 754–759.

Kassam S H, Tompkins M G 1980 Monoamniotic twin pregnancy and modern obstetrics: report of a case with a peculiar cord complication. Diagnostic Gynecology and Obstetrics 2: 213–220.

Kaufmann E 1890 Uber eine Geschwulstbildung des Nabelstranges. Virchows Archiv 121: 513–522.

Keckstein G, Tschurtz S, Schneider V et al 1990 Umbilical cord haematoma as a complication of intrauterine intravascular blood transfusion. Prenatal Diagnosis 10: 59–65.

Kelber R 1976 Gespaltene 'solitare' Nabelschnurarterie. Archiv fur Gynakologie 220: 319–323.

Kerisit J, Senecal J, Fisselier M P, Cosmier M, DePawe G, de Queiroz F 1981 L'examen histologique extemporare du cordon ombilical. Journal de Gynecologie, d'Obstetrique et de Biologie de la Reproduction 10: 45–49.

Khong T Y, Dilly S A 1989 Calcification of umbilical artery: two distinct lesions. Journal of Clinical Pathology 42: 931–934.

Kloos K, Vogel M 1974 Pathologie der Perinatalperiode. Grundlage, Methodik und erste Ergebnisse einer Kyematopathologie. Georg Thieme, Stuttgart.

Kloosterman G J 1958 Intrauterine exsanguinatie? Nederlands Tijdschrift voor Verloskunde en Gynaecologie 58: 391–401.

Knapp L 1896 Eineiige Zwillingsplazenta, velamentose Insertion Verblutung beider Fruchte unter der Geburt. Archiv fur Gynakologie 51: 586–594.

Kohler H G 1972 An unusual case of sirenomalia. Teratology 6: 295–301.

Kouam L, Miller E C 1980 Einige Aspekte zum Nabelschnurvofall. Zentralblatt fur Gynakologie 102: 724–733.

Kouyoumdjian A 1980 Velamentous insertion. Obstetrics and Gynecology 56: 737–742.

Kovacs F 1951 Mangel der plazentaren und Nabelschnurgefassklappen als Ursache manches intrapartalen Fruchttodes. Archiv fur Gynakologie 179: 615–634.

Kreyberg L 1958 A teratoma-like swelling in the umbilical cord, possibly of acardius nature. Journal of Pathology and Bacteriology 75: 109–112.

Kristofferson K 1969 The significance of absence of one umbilical artery. Acta Obstetricia et Gynecologica Scandinavica 48: 195–214.

Krone H A 1961 Die Bedeutung des Eibettstorungen fur die Entstehung menschilicher Missbildungen. Fischer, Stuttgart.

Krone H A 1966 Ursache und Bedeutung der pathologischen Nabelschnurinsertion. Geburtshilfe und Frauenheilkunde 26: 509–512.

Labarrere C, Sebastiani M, Siminovick M, Torassa E, Althabe O 1985 Absence of Wharton's jelly around umbilical arteries: an unusual cause of perinatal mortality. Placenta 6: 555–559.

Leinzinger E 1972 Totaler Nabelschnurabriss intra partum bei Hydramnion. Zentralblatt fur Gynakologie 94: 1233–1238.

LeMarec R, Kerisit J, de Villartay A, Ferraud B, Toulouse R, Senecal J 1972 L'artere ombilicale unique: etude de 31 cas. Journal de Gynecologie, d'Obstetrique et de Biologie de la Reproduction 1: 825–841.

Lenke R, Osterkamp T 1980 A prolapsed umbilical cord into the abdominal cavity in a woman with a previous Caesarian section. American Journal of Obstetrics and Gynecology 138: 1224–1225.

Leventhal H, Alexander D J, Ben-Adereth N 1967 Single umbilical artery: a report of 50 cases. Israel Journal of Medical Sciences 3: 899–902.

Liley A W 1963 Intrauterine transfusion of foetus in haemolytic disease. British Medical Journal 11: 1107–1109.

Lilja M 1991 Infants with single umbilical artery studied in a national registry: general epidemiological characteristics. Paediatric and Perinatal Epidemiology 5: 27–36.

Lumsden M A, Choong K-H, Gillmer H D 1981 Monoamniotic twin pregnancy: cord entanglement associated with periods of extreme fetal tachycardia. Journal of Obstetrics and Gynaecology 1: 220–222.

Lupovitch A, McInerney T S 1968 Hematoma of the umbilical cord: a dissecting aneurysm of the umbilical vein. American Journal of Obstetrics and Gynecology 102: 902–904.

McClintock K 1943 Intrauterine rupture of the umbilical cord. British Medical Journal 1: 446.

McLennan J E 1968 Implications of the eccentricity of the umbilical cord. American Journal of Obstetrics and Gynecology 101: 1124–1130.

McLeod F N, McCoy D R 1981 Monoamniotic twins with an unusual cord complication: case report. British Journal of Obstetrics and Gynaecology 88: 774–775.

Malpas 1968 A case of constrictive sclerosis of Wharton's jelly associated with detachment of the placenta. Journal of Obstetrics and Gynaecology of the British Commonwealth 75: 678–679.

Maximov A 1927 Bindegewebe mit besonderen Eigenschaften: (a) Gallert Oder Schleimgeweve. In: Mollendorff W V (ed) Handbuch der mikroskopischen Anatomie des Menschen II. Springer-Verlag, Berlin, pp 323–324.

Megory E, Weiner E, Shalev E, Ohel G 1991 Pseudomonoamniotic twins with cord entanglement following genetic funipuncture. Obstetrics and Gynecology 78: 915–917.

Meyer W W, Lind J 1974 Iliac arteries in children with a single umbilical artery: structure calcifications and early atherosclerotic lesions. Archives of Disease in Childhood 49: 671–679.

Meyer W W, Lind J, Moinian M 1969 An accessory fourth vessel of the umbilical cord. American Journal of Obstetrics and Gynecology 105: 1063–1068.

Miller M E, Higginbottom M, Smith D W 1981 Short umbilical cord: its origin and relevance. Pediatrics 67: 618–621.

Mills J L, Harley E E, Moessinger A C 1983 Standards for measuring umbilical cord length. Placenta 4: 423–426.

Moessinger A C, Blanc W A, Byrne J, Andrews D, Warburton D 1981 Amniotic band syndrome associated with amniocentesis. American Journal of Obstetrics and Gynecology 141: 588–591.

Moessinger A C, Blanc W A, Maronez P A, Polsen D C 1982 Umbilical cord length as an index of fetal activity: experimental study and clinical implication. Pediatric Research 16: 109–112.

Monie I W 1970 Genesis of single umbilical artery. American Journal of Obstetrics and Gynaecology 108: 400–405.

Monie I W, Nelson M M, Evans H M 1957 Persistent right umbilical vein as a result of vitamin deficiency during gestation. Circulation Research 5: 187–190.

Moore R D 1956 Mast cells of human umbilical cord. American Journal of Pathology 32: 1179–1183.

Nayak S A 1967 Thrombosis of the umbilical cord vessels. Australian and New Zealand Journal of Obstetrics and Gynaecology 7: 148–154.

Nieder J, Link M 1970 Ein Beitrag zur Pathologie der Nabelschnurgeschwulste. Zentralblatt fur Gynakologie 92: 420–428.

Ong H C, Puvan I S, Chan W F 1976 An unusual complication in a twin pregnancy: umbilical cord of twin 2 around the neck of twin 1. Australian and New Zealand Journal of Obstetrics and Gynaecology 16: 57–58.

Ottow B 1922 Interpositio velamentosa funiculi umbilicalis. Archiv fur Gynakologie 116: 176–199.

Ottow B 1923 Uber die insertio furcata der Nabelschnur. Archiv fur Gynakologie 118: 378–382.

Papadatos C, Paschos S 1965 Single umbilical artery and congenital malformations. Obstetrics and Gynecology 26: 367–370.

Patel D, Dawson M, Kalyanam P 1989 Umbilical cord circumference at birth. American Journal of Disease in Children 143: 638–639 (letter to editor).

Peckham C H, Yerushalmy J 1965 Aplasia of one umbilical artery: incidence by race and certain obstetric factors. Obstetrics and Gynecology 26: 359–366.

Plentl A A 1961 Transfer of water across the perfused umbilical cord. Proceedings of the Society of Experimental Biology and Medicine 107: 622–626.

Podzahradsky O 1912 Ein Fall von monoamniotischen Zwillingen. Wiener Klinische Wochenschrift 25: 413–416.

Potter E L 1961 Pathology of the fetus and infant, 2nd edn. Year Book Publishers, Chicago.

Purola E 1968 The length and insertion of the umbilical cord. Annales Chirurgiae et Gynecologiae Fenniae 57: 621–622.

Raaflaub W 1959 Zur Kausalitat der Nabelschnurkomplikationen. Gynaecologia 148: 145–148.

Rehder H, Weitzel H 1978 Intrauterine amputations after amniocentesis. Lancet 1: 382.

Reilly F D, Russell P T 1977 Neurohistochemical evidence supporting an absence of adrenergic and cholinergic innervation in the human placenta and umbilical cord. Anatomical Record 188: 277–285.

Resta R G, Lauthy D A, Mahony B S 1988 Umbilical cord hemangioma associated with extremely high alpha-fetoprotein levels. Obstetrics and Gynecology 72: 488–491.

Robertson R D, Rubinstein L M, Wolfson W L, Lebherz T B, Blanchard J B, Crandall B F 1981 Constriction of the umbilical cord as a cause of fetal demise following midtrimester amniocentesis. Journal of Reproductive Medicine 26: 325–327.

Robinson L K, Jones K L, Benirschke K 1983 The nature of structural defects associated with velamentous and marginal insertion of the umbilical cord. American Journal of Obstetrics and Gynecology 146: 191–193.

Rolschau J 1978 The relationship between some disorders of the umbilical cord and intrauterine growth retardation. Acta Obstetricia et Gynecologica Scandinavica (suppl) 72: 15–21.

Ronero R, Chervenak F A, Cousta D, Berkowitz R I, Hobbin J C 1982 Antenatal sonographic diagnosis of umbilical cord hematoma. American Journal of Obstetrics and Gynecology 143: 719–720.

Rucker M P, Tureman G R 1945 Vasa previa. Virginia Medical Monthly 72: 202–207.

Ruvinsky E D, Wiley Th L, Morrison J C, Blake P G 1981 In-utero diagnosis of umbilical cord hematoma by ultrasonography. American Journal of Obstetrics and Gynecology 140: 833–834.

Salter D N Jr, Keene C L, Sun C C J, Schwartz S 1990 The association of single umbilical artery with cytogenetically abnormal pregnancies. American Journal of Obstetrics and Gynecology 163: 922–925.

Savage E W, Kohl S G, Wynn R M 1970 Prolapse of the umbilical cord. Obstetrics and Gynecology 36: 502–509.

Schafer G, Mikulicz-Radecki F R 1961 Uber die Gefahrung des Intrauterinen Wohlergeheus des Kindes durch Nabelschnurumschlingung nebst Bemerkungen zu deren Entstehung. Munchener Medizinische Wochenshchrift 103: 2261–2265.

Scharl A 1986 Neue Erkenntnisse uber die "Hobokenschen Klappen" der Nabelschnurarterie. Zeitschrift fur Geburtshilfe und Perinatologie 190: 266–274.

Scheffel T H, Langanke D 1970 Die Nabelschurkomplikationen an der Universitats Frauenklinik Leipzig 1955 Bis 67. Zentralblatt fur Gynakologie 92: 429–434.

Scheuner G 1964 Uber die Verankerung der Nabelschnur an der Placenta. Gegenbaurs Morphologisches Jahrbuch 106: 73–89.

Scheuner G 1965 Uber die Mikroskopische Struktur der Insertio velamentosa. Zentralblatt fur Gynakologie 87: 38–49.

Schmidt W 1965 Uber den paraplazentaren, fruchtwassergebundenen Stofftransport beim Menschen. Histochemische Untersuchung der in den Eihauten angereicherten Stoffe. Zeitschrift Fur Anatomie und Entwicklungsgeschichte 124: 321–334.

Schreier R, Brown S 1962 Hematoma of the umbilical cord: report of a case. Obstetrics and Gynecology 20: 798–800.

Scott J M, Jordan M M 1972 Placental insufficiency and the small for dates baby. American Journal of Obstetrics and Gynecology 113: 823–832.

Scott J M, Wilkinson R 1978 Further studies on the umbilical cord and its water contents. Journal of Clinical Pathology 31: 944–948.

Segovia J P 1967 Anomalias vasculares del cordon umbilical (conespecial considerocion a la arterio umbilical unica). Revista de Obstetricia y Ginecologia de Venezuela 27: 421–427.

Seifer D B, Ferguson I J E, Behrens C M 1985 Non-immune hydrops fetalis in association with hemangioma of the umbilical cord. Obstetrics and Gynecology 66: 283–286.

Sinnathuray T A 1967 Prolapse of the umbilical cord. MD Thesis, University of Singapore.

Sloper K S, Brown R S, Baum J D 1979 Water content of umbilical cord. Early Human Development 3: 205–210.

Smith D, Majmudar B 1985 Teratoma of the umbilical cord. Human Pathology 16: 190–193.

Spellacy W M, Graven H, Fisch R O 1966 The umbilical cord: complications of true knots, nuchal coils and cord around body. American Journal of Obstetrics and Gynecology 94: 1136–1142.

Spivack M 1936 On the anatomy of the so called 'valves' of umbilical vessels with especial reference to the 'valvulae Hobokenii'. Anatomical Record 66: 127–148.

Stembera Z K, Horska S 1972 The influence of coiling of the umbilical cord around the neck of the fetus on its gas metabolism and acidbase balance. Biology of the Neonate 20: 214–225.

Strassmann P 1902 Placenta praevia. Archiv fur Gynakologie 67: 112–275.

Tagawa T 1974 Monoamniotic twin pregnancy and double survival with a peculiar cord complication. Winsconsin Medical Journal 73: 131–133.

Takechi K, Kuwubara Y, Mizuno M 1993 Ultrastructural and immunohistochemical studies of Wharton's jelly umbilical cord cells. Placenta 14: 238–245.

Teramo K, Sipinen S 1978 Spontaneous rupture of membranes after amniocentesis. Obstetrics and Gynecology 52: 272–275.

Thomas J 1961 Untersuchungsergebnisse uber die Aplasie eine Nabelarterie unter besonderer Berucksichtigung der Zwillingsschwangerschaft. Geburtshilfe und Frauenheilkunde 21: 984–992.

Uyanwah-Akpom P O, Fox H 1977 The clinical significance of marginal and velamentous insertion of the umbilical cord. British Journal of Obstetrics and Gynaecology 84: 941–943.

Vago T, Chavkin J 1980 Extramembranous pregnancy: an unusual complication of amniocentesis. American Journal of Obstetrics and Gynecology 137: 511–512.

Vestermark V, Christensen I, Kay L, Windfeldt M 1990 Spontaneous intra-uterine total rupture of a velamentous umbilical cord: a case report. European Journal of Obstetrics, Gynecology and Reproductive Biology 35: 279–281.

Virot S, Mace J, Virot J G, Blanc J M 1981 L'hematome du cordon rapport de l'echographie. Revue Francaise de Gynecologie et d'Obstetrique 77: 131–135.

Walz W 1947 Uber das Odem der Nabelschnur. Zentralblatt fur Gynakologie 69: 144–145.

Weber J 1963 Constriction of the umbilical cord as a cause of fetal death. Acta Obstetricia et Gynecologica Scandinavica 42: 259–267.

Weigert C 1886 Zwei Falle von Missbildung eines Ureter and einer Samenblase mit Bemerkungen uber einfache Nabelarterien. Virchows Archiv 104: 10–20.

Whitehouse D B B, Kohler H G 1960 Vasa praevia in twin pregnancy. Journal of Obstetrics and Gynecology of the British Empire 67: 281–285.

Wolff E 1936 Les cases de la teratogenese experimentale des vertebres amniotes d'apres resultats de methods directes. Archive d'Anatomie, d'Histologie et d'Embryologie 22: 1–375.

Yavner D L, Redline R W 1989 Angiomyxoma of the umbilical cord with massive cystic degeneration of Wharton's jelly. Archives of Pathology and Laboratory Medicine 113: 935–937.

Zawisch C 1955 Die Wharton'sche Sulze und die Gefasse des Nabelstranges. Zeitschrift fur Zellforschung 42: 94–133.

Zeman V, Rauchenberg M 1970 Kavernozni a kapilarni hemangiomy pupecniku. (Cavernous and capillary haemangiomata of the umbilical cord.) Ceskoslovenska Pediatrie 25: 663–665.

Zennegg M 1966 Obrzek vogolniony jednego z blizniakow wprzpadku wady rozwojowej pepowiny. (Generalised oedema in twins related to congenital malformation of the umbilical cord.) Ginekologia Polska 37: 787–789.

51. Pathology of the fetal membranes

Gillian Batcup   Hans G. Kohler

INTRODUCTION

The term 'fetal membranes' is sometimes used synonymously with the now obsolescent 'secundinae' or the colloquial 'afterbirth', i.e. comprising all the extrafetal components of the conceptus. More often, however, its meaning is restricted to the amniotic and chorionic membranes and it is used in this sense in this chapter. In conformity with most other accounts of the subject, the chorionic plate of the placenta, or 'chorion frondosum', an integral part of the placenta proper, will be referred to only where a need arises from the context. So, unless stated otherwise, 'chorion' or 'chorionic membrane' means chorion laeve or parietal chorion or chorion reflexum (this last term is semantically incorrect: the parietal chorion is not reflected, but the decidua is).

The obvious function of the 'bag of waters' is to contain the amniotic fluid, which in addition to its cushioning effect provides a physically, chemically and physiologically suitable environment for the fetus. There can be no doubt that the amnion contributes to the pool of liquor amnii, but how much and when is not yet fully known.

The studies of Schmidt (1965, 1967), Schmidt et al (1971) and of other investigators have shown that the fetal membranes also supply nutrients to the fetus. The swallowing of liquor by the fetus serves not only the purpose of controlling the quantity of fluid, but also that of fetal nutrition (Pitkin & Reynolds, 1975).

THE MICROSCOPIC ANATOMY OF AMNION AND CHORION

This has been studied sporadically by a number of investigators in the nineteenth and early twentieth centuries. A chapter on fetal membranes in the standard work on human histology (Schroeder, 1930) is disappointing. A gap existed throughout the decades and was eventually filled by Bourne's scholarly monograph (1962). This was based mainly on the author's lightmicroscopic studies, but took also into account results of investigations using the electronmicroscope. Since then little additional information has been unearthed in the field of lightmicroscopy (Schmidt et al, 1982a, b; Jirasek, 1983), but ultrastructural research, both by transmission electronmicroscopy and by scanning electronmicroscopy (van Herendael et al, 1978; Minh et al, 1981; Wang & Schneider, 1982, 1983), has yielded interesting results.

Bourne's (1962) semidiagrammatic representation of the various layers of amnion and chorion has been copied in several subsequent publications and we have no hesitation in following suit (Fig. 51.1). In paying tribute to Bourne's descriptive skill and attention to detail, the present authors have to admit that in routine sections for diagnostic histology they have, more often than not, been unable to identify all of Bourne's layers. This has probably also been the experience of other diagnostic histopathologists; even morphologists with a special interest in this field, e.g. Schmidt (1956), have reduced the number of layers of the amniochorion by combining Bourne's compact and fibroblast layers as the 'amniotic connective tissue', whilst cellular and reticular layers jointly form the 'chorionic connective tissue'.

It has been known for some time that fetal membranes have neither innervation nor blood supply, but blood vessels are present in the reticular layer of the chorionic plate of the placenta; these, however, enjoy 'extra-territorial status' and do not supply the surrounding tissue. In the chorion laeve a similar situation exists with regard to aberrant or velamentous chorionic vessels. This does not necessarily preclude any form of interchange between these blood vessels and the surrounding chorion. Traumatic damage to the vessels may cause a subchorial or intrachorial haematoma.

Of the layers shown in Figure 51.1, two are of special interest: the amniotic epithelium, because it immediately faces the liquor amnii and is therefore in the 'front line', and the spongy layer ('intermediate stratum' of continental authors) because of its rôle in the formation of amniotic strands. Bourne classifies it as a part of the amnion, because in monochorionic, diamniotic twins, where by

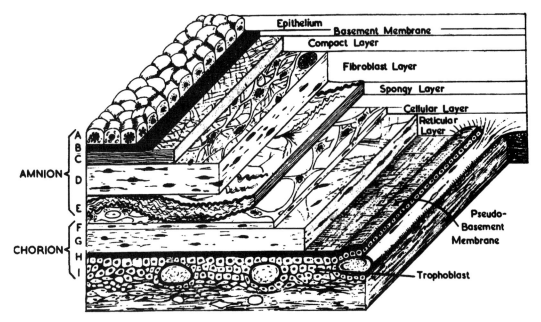

Fig. 51.1 Diagrammatic representation of the constituent layers of the amniochorion. (From Bourne, 1960. Courtesy of the Editor of the American Journal of Obstetrics and Gynecology.)

definition the septum between the two amniotic sacs consists of two layers of amnion only (in mirror image apposition), a spongy layer can be demonstrated.

Macrophages comparable to the Hofbauer cells of the chorionic villus are normally quite inconspicuous; they can, however, become very prominent when stuffed with meconium. Plain muscle fibres or their predecessors were seen by Remak (1854) and by Wang & Schneider (1982).

It is customary to describe the normal amniotic epithelium as cuboidal; more precisely, most of the cells are of cuboidal type, but both columnar and flat epithelial cells are part of the normal pictures. They occur in varying numbers at various sites, but it appears that columnar cells are more frequently found on the placental amnion, flat cells being more common on the extraplacental amnion and also on the umbilical cord. A common feature of amniotic epithelial cells is the presence of:

1. Intercellular bridges or bars near the free margin, believed to increase the mechanical coherence of the layer
2. Intercellular canaliculi serving the liquid exchange with the amniotic fluid
3. Microvilli on the apical surface believed to mediate absorption of fluid
4. 'Bleb' formation and extrusion.

Bourne (1962) distinguishes abnormal columnar cells from normal ones on morphological grounds. The abnormal cells are recognized by their nuclei being nearer the apex, in contrast to the basal nuclei of most normal cells, and also by a greater number of vacuoles and by an increased diameter of intercellular canals. The varieties distinguished are:

1. 'Palisade deformity' with cells of approximately equal height and intact intercellular bars and markedly distended intercellular canals
2. 'Club-shaped deformity' with marked differences in cellular height causing an entirely uneven 'cobblestone surface', whilst the nuclei are in an apical position, about to be extruded.

Another cellular abnormality in the amniotic epithelium concerns the position of the nuclei: if these are situated at varying distances from the basement membrane a spurious impression of multiple layers of epithelial cells may be created; this is known as pseudostratification.

A combination, or perhaps a medley, of the aforementioned lesions (with the addition of focal cell death and exfoliation), is named 'epithelial disorganization' or 'bristling amnion'. Marked anisocytosis and poikilocytosis of epithelial cells with conspicuous vacuoles, cellular fragmentation and occasional denudation of the basement membrane, suggest serious damage to the amniotic lining. The question of what causes this damage presents itself. In many cases the answer is obvious: there may have been marked meconium staining on naked-eye examination and/or meconium particles are seen in Hofbauer cells, but meconium in the liquor cannot always be demonstrated, nor is the bristling amnion invariably found when meconium is present. A time factor may be involved. Even where meconium irritation is established as a cause, other influences may have an aggravating or modifying effect, such as pH, oxygen tension, lecithin : sphingomyelin (L:S) ratio, surface tension, etc. Regrettably, the basic findings of Bourne have not been followed up by correlation studies.

Squamous metaplasia of amniotic epithelium

Squamous plaques are a morphological variant (one hesitates to call it a lesion), frequently seen in otherwise normal specimens (Fig. 51.2), sometimes also in the neighbourhood of lesions such as necrosis, exfoliation or disorganization. The area around the placental insertion of the umbilical cord is more likely to be affected than others (Benirschke & Driscoll, 1967).

Foci of squamous metaplasia are usually inconspicuous to the naked eye, but can be readily found if looked for. In most instances they are of pinhead to nailhead size, but may be a good deal larger and only slightly raised above the amniotic surface. Normally the plaques can be felt by a sensitive index finger, can resist attempts at scraping off and are obviously opaque if the amniotic membrane is stripped off and viewed against transmitted light, in contrast to the translucent appearance of the normal amnion. Microscopically, a focus consists of multiple layers of very flat, stratified epithelium, more or less clearly demarcated from the surrounding normal tissue; some keratin is often visible, but no lanugo hair or vernix is seen.

Squamous metaplasia has no known aetiology, nor any regular clinical or pathological association, but has sometimes been confused with amnion nodosum (see below). We agree with Bourne (1962) and with Benirschke & Driscoll (1967) that 'metaplasia' is a misnomer in view of the close histogenetic relationship of the epithelia of amnion and of fetal epidermis (Lister, 1968).

The amniotic epithelium in polyhydramnios and oligohydramnios

No lightmicroscopic studies of the effects of polyhydramnios on the amniotic epithelium appear to have been published. Leonardi & Rigano (1966), using transmission electronmicroscopy, saw both swollen and shrunken cells; these were interpreted as different phases in the process of liquor absorption. Pollard et al (1976, 1979), using scanning electronmicroscopy, could not find any significant distinctive features in the amnion of pregnancies complicated by polyhydramnios, but Wang et al (1979) emphasize an increase in the number of microvilli on both apical and lateral surfaces of amniotic epithelial cells in association with polyhydramnios.

In pregnancies with oligohydramnios, Pollard et al found a change in emphasis rather than any entirely different features. The findings in this group suggested: (a) increased cell shrinkage, probably related to more concentrated liquor, and (b) reduction of intracellular canaliculi.

However, in most cases of oligohydramnios the morphological picture of the amniotic surface is likely to be overshadowed by amnion nodosum.

Amnion nodosum

This term is readily understood and also literally correct, if not very revealing; it denotes the presence on the amniotic surface of multiple, often numerous, greyish or yellowish-grey nodules of pinpoint to nailhead size (Fig. 51.3), rarely forming confluent plaques. They can be wiped off the amnion surface by gentle pressure.

Microscopically, the nodules consist of dead squamous cells, lanugo hair (Fig. 51.4), lipid droplets (vernix) and amorphous matter. Some of the older nodules may be overgrown by amniotic epithelium. Whilst there is nothing indicative of an inflammatory or granulomatous nature, there can be, in the older lesions at least, some evidence of organization in which the amniotic connective tissue is involved. For a description and discussion of ultrastructural features the reader is referred to Salazar & Kanbour (1974).

For more than 100 years these nodules had been seen by various observers, reported, forgotten and 'rediscovered'. It was not until 1950 that their association with urinary tract anomalies was pointed out by Landing (1950). The rôle of oligohydramnios as the crucial factor was further emphasized by Scott & Bain (1958) and their interpretation is now widely accepted. The composition of the nodules clearly suggests their origin from particles that are normally suspended in the amniotic fluid. Most, if not all, of these particles come from the fetal skin and other fetal sources, e.g. meconium, but some contribution by the amnion itself cannot be excluded. When a normal quantity of liquor is available, these particles are kept in a

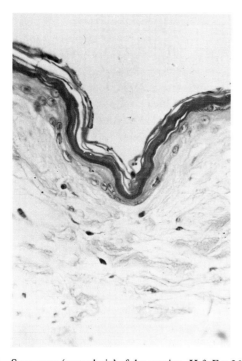

Fig. 51.2 Squamous 'metaplasia' of the amnion. H & E × 360. (From Fox, 1978. Courtesy of W. B. Saunders.)

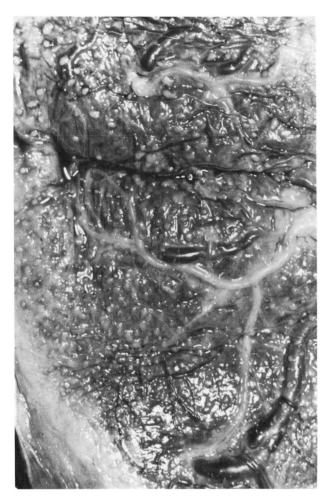

Fig. 51.3 Macroscopic appearances of amnion nodosum in the amnion covering the fetal surface of the placenta. The tiny nodules are seen most clearly above and to the left.

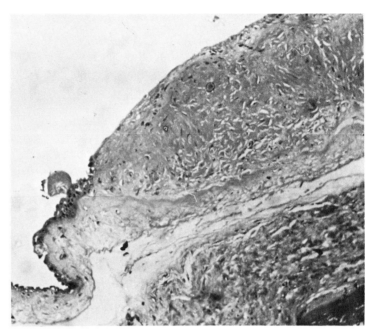

Fig. 51.4 Histological appearances of amnion nodosum. Cellular fragments are embedded in amorphous eosinophilic material. H & E × 250. (From Fox, 1978. Courtesy of W. B. Saunders.)

dynamic, more or less constant, state of suspension. A serious reduction in the quantity of suspending medium might well favour aggregation of particulate matter and deposition on the amniotic surface, especially as the 'fluid cushion' between fetal skin and amnion is much reduced or eliminated.

It is not surprising that amnion nodosum is not demonstrable in all instances of oligohydramnios but occasionally can be detected in its absence. There is also clearly some difference between diminished production of liquor amnii, as in urinary tract malformations or in intrauterine growth retardation on the one hand, and excessive loss due to leakage on the other. Bain et al (1964) have not found any instance of amnion nodosum in 12 infants born after prolonged leakage of liquor whilst other fetal stigmata of oligohydramnios were clearly present. In our own experience of several cases of extramembranous pregnancy (see below) and of infants born after moderately prolonged drainage of liquor, amnion nodosum may be difficult or impossible to demonstrate by naked eye, but a microscopic search is sometimes rewarding.

The detection of amnion nodosum in the membranes of a living infant can occasionally be of clinical importance, especially when oligohydramnios has not been diagnosed earlier. It may warn the neonatal paediatrician of the probability of 'hypoplastic' lungs. Rarely it may lead to the diagnosis of an operable abnormality of the urinary tract such as an urethral valve.

CHORIOAMNIONITIS

The chorioamniotic layer of the peripheral membranes is continuous with that which comprises the fetal surface of the placenta, and shares with it an ability to react to inflammatory stimuli. Macroscopic diagnosis of membrane inflammation is unreliable, and the chorioamnion may appear normal to the naked eye in the presence of microscopic inflammatory changes; conversely, an opacity of the fetal surface of the placenta may be caused by noninflammatory conditions, the most common of which is a thickening of the subchorionic fibrin layer. Chorioamnionitis is thus best diagnosed by microscopy (Fig. 51.5). The term almost always implies an acute inflammation of the amnion and chorion due to infection, although evidence of a more chronic process is occasionally apparent. Inflammatory changes in the decidua are not confined solely to infections. In otherwise normal deliveries, the decidua capsularis adjacent to the chorioamnion of the peripheral membranes commonly shows scattered acute inflammatory foci, and while these may be due to infection, they are more frequently associated with small areas of decidual necrosis occurring around the time of birth.

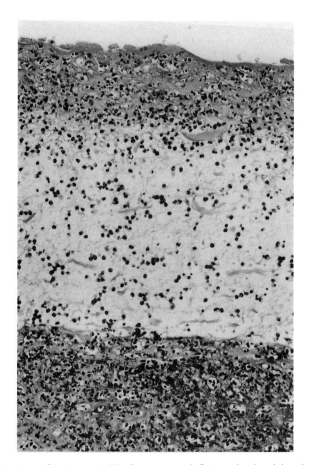

Fig. 51.5 Chorioamnionitis. Severe acute inflammation involving the full thickness of the chorionic plate with degeneration of the amniotic epithelium on the fetal surface of the placenta. H & E × 178.

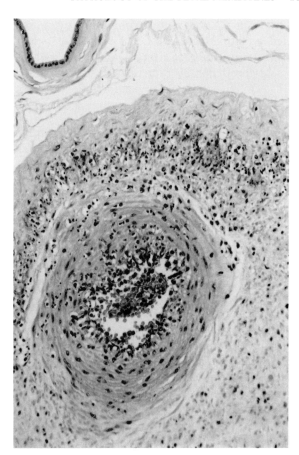

Fig. 51.6 Chorioamnionitis. Fetal polymorphonuclear leucocytes migrating through the wall of a vessel in the chorionic plate. H & E × 178.

The acute inflammatory infiltrate of the chorioamnion is of dual origin (Naeye, 1988). Polymorphs from the maternal circulation first accumulate in the subchorionic fibrin layer of the placenta and in the decidua capsularis of the peripheral membranes. From there they migrate inwards across the chorion and amnion to reach the amniotic cavity and fetus. In an established infection, polymorphs of fetal origin contribute to the inflammatory infiltration by migrating through the walls of vessels in the placental chorionic plate and umbilical cord (Fig. 51.6).

Chorioamnionitis of longer duration is characterized by an infiltration of macrophages in addition to polymorphs, and a concentration of the infiltrate immediately below the amnion. The amniotic epithelial cells may become columnar, or alternatively may show degenerative changes, with focal epithelial loss and exposure of the basement membrane. The causative organisms are rarely visible in routine sections, but occasionally it is possible to demonstrate bacterial clusters or aggregates of fungal elements.

Clinically evident amniotic infection, recognized by the presence of maternal pyrexia, tachycardia and leucocytosis, fetal tachycardia, uterine tenderness and purulent vaginal loss, occurs far less frequently than histological

chorioamnionitis, and reliance on such manifestations will always underestimate the true incidence. Naeye (1988) has estimated that clinical findings of infection in the mother or neonate are present in only about 10% of cases showing histological evidence of chorioamnionitis.

Attempts to identify organisms by culture are not always successful, partly due to the relatively fastidious growth requirements of the mycoplasmas and certain anaerobic bacteria. Pankuch et al (1984) were able to recover bacteria from 18 of 25 (72%) placentas with histologically proven chorioamnionitis. More elaborate techniques in the culture of fetal membranes and amniotic fluid have yielded a variety of aerobic and anaerobic bacteria (in either a pure or a mixed growth), *Candida* species, *Mycoplasma hominis* and *Ureaplasma urealyticum* (Hurley, 1988; Romero et al, 1989). Viruses are not considered to be causative agents for chorioamnionitis.

More rapid methods of identification or diagnosis have been assessed. Romero et al (1989) have found a Gram stain of the amniotic fluid to have a 79.1% sensitivity and a 99.6% specificity in the prediction of a positive amniotic fluid culture. Mycoplasma and ureaplasma species gave false negative results, since these organisms are not visible on a Gram stain. Other amniotic fluid investigations have included endotoxin assay, leucocyte esterase assay and gas-liquid chromatography for the measurement of organic acids produced by bacterial metabolism (Gibbs & Duff, 1991). Taken alone, the maternal blood neutrophil count does not correlate well with chorioamnionitis, but estimation of the non-specific acute phase C-reactive protein in maternal serum can be useful in predicting histological chorioamnionitis, especially if the upper limit of normal values is set at a relatively high level (Fisk et al, 1987). More specific methods of diagnosis utilizing the polymerase chain reaction are likely to become available in the near future.

Chorioamnionitis usually originates in the membranes adjacent to the cervical os, as an ascending infection caused by vaginal organisms, although occasionally transabdominal diagnostic or therapeutic procedures, such as amniocentesis, fetoscopy or intrauterine transfusion, are responsible (Kaplan, 1993). Organisms resulting in an ascending infection may arise from the indigenous vaginal population; infectious agents isolated from vaginal swabs in pregnancy are largely similar to those isolated from infected fetal membranes and amniotic fluid (McDonald et al, 1991). Organisms may also be introduced by the male partner. The association between coitus and chorioamnionitis is most evident in communities characterized by a low socio-economic status. Naeye & Ross (1982), in a study of urban black mothers in South Africa, found the peak frequency of chorioamnionitis limited to the extraplacental membranes to be present when labour and delivery took place within two days of the last coitus. Spread of the infection, as evident by a peak frequency of inflammation in the placental chorionic plate, was present when delivery occurred within four days. Toth et al (1988) studied a population of 193 pregnant women in New York, three-quarters of whom were of black or Hispanic origin, and found a correlation between premature rupture of the membranes (a condition often attributed to chorioamnionitis) and a history of multiple sexual partners.

Chorioamnionitis has several important associations, and is known to be both a cause and a result of membrane rupture. Prolonged rupture of the membranes was one of the first associations to be recognized, and Fox & Langley (1971) in a study of 1000 consecutive livebirth deliveries of all gestational ages found histological chorioamnionitis to have occurred in 54.5% of cases where the membranes had been ruptured for more than 24 hours. This is the most frequent association at term gestation. It is now well established, however, that chorioamnionitis has a strong temporal relationship with preterm labour and preterm premature rupture of the membranes, the latter being defined as spontaneous rupture of the fetal membranes prior to the onset of preterm labour and occurring in more than

one-third of all preterm births (Zaaijman et al, 1982). There is now good evidence that chorioamnionitis may act as a precipitating agent, both for preterm labour and for membrane rupture (Naeye, 1988; Romero & Mazor, 1988; Drife, 1989). Hillier et al (1988) were able to isolate organisms from the area between the amnion and chorion in 61% of placentas from women who delivered before 37 weeks' gestation, but in only 21% of placentas from women without preterm labour who delivered at term. The recovery of any organism from the chorioamnion was strongly associated with histological chorioamnionitis, and the most frequent isolates from the placentas of infants delivered prematurely were *Ureaplasma urealyticum* and *Gardnerella vaginalis*.

McDonald et al (1991) studied the vaginal flora of women in preterm labour and found two distinct bacterial groupings, the first of which was represented by *Gardnerella vaginalis* and *Bacteroides* species, and the second by enteropharyngeal organisms, such as *Escherichia coli* and *Klebsiella* species. Both types of bacteria were isolated with even greater frequency when labour occurred before 34 weeks' gestation. Chorioamnionitis is also particularly prevalent in very premature deliveries. Russell (1979) found chorioamnionitis to be present in 54.5% of placentas delivered between 20 and 28 weeks' gestation; Naeye (1988) has estimated that chorioamnionitis is responsible for almost 70% of spontaneous preterm deliveries between 24 and 26 weeks' gestation, but for only about 30% of preterm deliveries at 34–36 weeks.

The evidence for chorioamnionitis occurring before membrane rupture was initially indirect, and was inferred, for example, by the higher incidence of histological chorioamnionitis in cases where the fetal membranes ruptured just before the onset of preterm labour, as compared with the incidence where rupture occurred just after this event (Naeye & Peters, 1980). The culture of amniotic fluid obtained by amniocentesis from patients with preterm labour and intact membranes has now demonstrated such infection unequivocally. Romero et al (1989) found the incidence of positive amniotic fluid culture in these patients to be 21.6% where the delivery occurred before 37 weeks' gestation. The most frequently isolated organisms were *Ureaplasma urealyticum*, *Fusobacterium* species and *Mycoplasma hominis*.

Other conditions associated with chorioamnionitis include polyhydramnios, cervical incompetence (Naeye & Peters, 1978) and multiple pregnancy, all of which tend to augment the area of fetal membrane exposed at the cervical os, thus increasing the likelihood of an ascending infection. Paradoxically, cervical cerclage, designed to prevent preterm labour and infection, may actually increase their incidence, either by suture line infections (McDonald, 1980) or by the release of cervical prostaglandins (Charles & Hurry, 1983). Partial placenta membranacea, a condition characterized by the abnormal preservation of chorionic villi over the fetal membranes, is also associated with chorioamnionitis (Wilkins et al, 1991).

Some of the consequences of placental infection have already been described, and include maternal septicaemia and preterm premature rupture of the membranes. The major hazard to the fetus is that of premature delivery (Zaaijman et al 1982), but occasionally a serious neonatal infection can supervene. In addition, Naeye (1988) has described an association between chorioamnionitis and fetal hypoxia. Low Apgar scores in premature infants were found to be correlated with placental villous oedema and compression or constriction of villous vessels. Vascular constriction may be due to an imbalance in circulating prostaglandins, a condition known to occur in other pathological conditions such as pre-eclampsia (Boura & Walters, 1991).

The higher incidence of histological chorioamnionitis in very premature deliveries is partly related to the changes in bactericidal and bacteriostatic activity of the amniotic fluid as pregnancy progresses. Bratlid & Lindback (1978) found the bacteriolytic activity to increase threefold from the 25th gestational week to term. The antibacterial activity has been variously ascribed to lysozyme, immunoglobulins, β-lysin and a zinc-peptide complex (Hurley, 1988), and is dependent on the mother's nutritional state. Tafari et al (1977), in a study of amniotic fluid samples obtained from Ethiopian patients, found that loss of antimicrobial activity and lower zinc concentrations were related to maternal undernourishment.

The mechanism whereby placental infection initiates labour is not fully understood but there is strong evidence that local formation of prostaglandins is of major importance. The regulation of placental eicosanoid biosynthesis in normal and complicated pregnancies has recently been reviewed by Mitchell (1991). (Eicosanoids are substances formed from carbon-20 polyunsaturated fatty acids.) Prostaglandins are derived from the carbon-20 polyunsaturated arachidonic acid, which in turn is a breakdown product of glycerophospholipids. Non-esterified arachidonic acid is increased in the amniotic fluid in normal labour, while the arachidonic acid content of the amnion decreases. Amnion contains phospholipases A_2 and C, both of which are involved in the liberation of arachidonic acid from glycerophospholipids. Phospholipase activity is calcium-dependent, and regulation may be provided by platelet activating factor. A number of other cytokines and hormones are also capable of modifying prostaglandin biosynthesis.

The influence of bacteria and the inflammatory process on prostaglandin production has been investigated by a variety of cultural and biochemical techniques. Lamont et al (1985) found that when amnion cells in tissue culture were exposed to bacterial products from *Escherichia coli*

and *Streptococcus faecalis*, their prostaglandin E output rose considerably. Prostaglandins E_2 and $F_{2\alpha}$ levels in amniotic fluid were found by Romero et al (1986) to be higher in those patients with positive amniotic fluid cultures than in a control group whose amniotic fluid was sterile. An evaluation of prostaglandin production by fetal membranes was undertaken by López Bernal et al (1989), who found that inflamed amnion and choriodecidua from spontaneous preterm deliveries generated large amounts of prostaglandin E over a two-hour incubation period. It is probable that chorioamnionitis exerts its effect in a number of ways. Some pathogenic bacteria are known to possess phospholipase A_2 activity, and may thus stimulate the production of prostaglandins and initiate labour (Lamont et al, 1985). In addition, the inflammatory cytokines interleukin 1 and tumour necrosis factor can stimulate amnion cells to produce prostaglandin E_2, possibly by induction of cyclo-oxygenase which forms part of the pathway in the conversion of arachidonic acid to prostaglandins (Mitchell, 1991). The further elucidation of these complex biochemical interreactions is a necessary preliminary step towards the rational management of preterm labour associated with infection.

THE AMNIOCHORION AND FETAL DYSMORPHOLOGY

Premature rupture of membranes has so far been considered mainly with regard to its relationship to premature labour and its implications for fetal and maternal infections. In certain, largely obscure, circumstances, however, rupture of the membranes may occur so early and/or in such an abnormal fashion, that it has a profound effect on the fate of the pregnancy and on the gross morphological features of the fetus.

That early rupture of the membranes can lead to abortion is well known and will not be further discussed. Persistent or intermittent discharge ('draining') of amniotic fluid following early rupture is termed 'hydrorrhoea amnialis' or 'amniorrhoea' and can lead to secondary oligohydramnios.

Oligohydramnios (and anhydramnios) from whatever cause is apt to produce a class of abnormalities that are collectively termed postural deformities or deformations (Dunn, 1976). These include Potter's facies (Potter, 1946; Thomas & Smith, 1974), talipes, congenital dislocation of the hip, large, shovel-like hands (Bain & Scott, 1960) and features of arthrogryposis. Breech presentation is a common association of oligohydramnios. Loose skin is occasionally seen (Potter, 1961) whilst shortness of the umbilical cord, presumably an effect of diminished fetal mobility, has been discussed in Chapter 50. The reduced size and weight of the lungs in oligohydramnios (Potter, 1965) may be due either to mechanical compression of the fetal thorax (Potter, 1961) or to liquor not being inhaled (Kohler, 1972; Kohler & Rymer, 1973) or to a combination of both.

Extramembranous pregnancy

In addition to producing the fetal stigmata of oligo-hydramnios, long-standing rupture of membranes causes arrested growth of the parietal membranes and retraction of the free margin. As a result the body of the fetus is to a greater or lesser extent outside the amniotic cavity and surrounded by neither amnion nor chorion. This condition is termed extramembranous pregnancy and is almost invariably associated with placenta extrachorialis. The latter, however, is a very common condition (Scott, 1960); its reported frequency varies and, depending on the criteria applied, can be as high as 32% (Wentworth, 1968). So only a very small fraction of the total number of placentae extrachoriales are associated with extramembranous pregnancy. The causal relationship between placenta extrachorialis and extramembranous pregnancy is not clear.

The free margin of the ruptured membranes, commonly thickened in hem-stitch fashion, may leave superficial impression marks on the infant's skin (Kohler et al, 1970) (Figs 51.7 and 51.8).

According to Fox (1978) the gestational ages of infants from extramembranous pregnancy range from 27–35 weeks. This conclusion was based on published reports, most of them originating in the days when relatively little attention was paid to fetal loss before 28 weeks of gestation. From our experience in recent years we would estimate the peak of incidence as being between 25 and 28 weeks or even earlier.

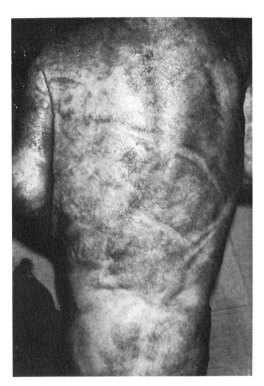

Fig. 51.8 Extramembranous pregnancy. Impressions produced in infant's skin by the margins of the membranous sac. (From Kohler et al, 1970. Courtesy of the Editor of the Journal of Obstetrics and Gynaecology of the British Commonwealth.)

Perinatal mortality in extramembranous pregnancy is still high though a fairly recent report (van Drooge & Okken, 1982) relates to two infants who both survived the neonatal period: in the past as often as not the diagnosis used to be made at autopsy. A pathologist should think of extramembranous pregnancy as a possibility whenever a history of amniorrhoea, or an unrecorded time of rupture of membranes, is associated with fetal signs of oligo-hydramnios and/or with a placenta extrachorialis. The diagnosis can be clinched by showing that fetal volume substantially exceeded the capacity of the membranous sac. Provided the placenta and membranes had not been damaged at delivery, it is usually possible to estimate the capacity of the sac fairly accurately, thanks to the seam-like free margin, by filling it with measured amounts of water. The volume of the fetus can be determined by its water displacement. In the pathogenesis of extramembranous pregnancy, mechanical trauma, no doubt, plays a part, but other aetiological factors may also be relevant, if elusive. One of the earliest reports of extramembranous pregnancy (Tarnier, 1895) blames a 12 cm long hairpin, pushed accidentally through the abdominal wall and into the pregnant uterus, without causing abortion. A more recent report, on the other hand, links extramembranous pregnancy with amniocentesis at 19 weeks' gestation (Vago & Chavkin, 1980).

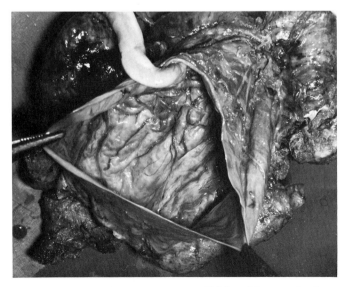

Fig. 51.7 Extramembranous pregnancy. Thickened free margin of small membranous sac. (From Kohler et al, 1970. Courtesy of the Editor of the Journal of Obstetrics and Gynaecology of the British Commonwealth.)

Extra-amniotic pregnancy

Occasionally the amnion may rupture in early or mid-pregnancy, whilst the chorion stays intact, giving rise to extra-amniotic (intrachorionic) pregnancy. This dissociation is possible thanks to the loose texture of the intermediate stratum (spongy layer of Bourne) which both separates and holds together amnion and chorion. Like the extraembryonic coelom, from which it originates, the spongy layer consists of reticular connective tissue with lubricating mucus in its mesh.

In the examination of the term placenta the amniotic membrane can readily be detached from the chorion which is, according to Meudt (1966), a sign of maturity; indeed, sometimes there seems to be no cohesion at all. It is reasonable to assume that this change in the spongy layer is the effect of some proteolytic enzyme. Whether a similar proteolytic effect could occasionally be brought about in early gestation and thus predispose to selective rupture is at present entirely a matter of speculation. Whatever its pathogenesis, the consequences of isolated amnion rupture show much variation.

Three different types of outcome have been recognized:

1. The collapsed amniotic membrane may fuse more firmly with the chorion and form a thickened patch on its inner surface (Torpin, 1968). This would have no appreciable effect on the fetus and, in most instances, would go unnoticed.

2. Just as rarely recorded are cases in which the retracting amnion forms a 'cuff' or a 'collar' around the root of the umbilical cord (Fig. 51.9). Here, too, there is no proven clinical significance. The case reported by Kohler & Jenkins (1976) was complicated by premature labour, but the association could have been coincidental.

3. Of much greater interest is the third possible consequence of early amnion rupture, i.e. the splitting up of the membrane into a multitude of shreds and strands, either at the time of rupture or subsequently (Torpin, 1968). These strands or strings float freely in the liquor amnii but can attach themselves to the chorion or to the fetal skin. ('Strands' and 'strings' are in this section being used synonymously. The term 'amniotic bands' that has usually been applied to these structures is avoided, because some authors have used it to denote circular skin lesions, i.e. 'ring constrictions' that can be *caused* by the strands.) Thus a digit or a forearm or a leg may be encircled, rarely an upper arm or a thigh. Encirclement of the trunk (Clair, 1936) is rarer still (presumably because a strand would have to be rather long to be effective). Fingers and toes are at greater risk of circumvolution by relatively short strands not only because of their lesser circumference, but also because they are likely, by active movement, to 'stray' into the vicinity of what has remained of the amnion.

Torpin (1968) believes that the length of the strands

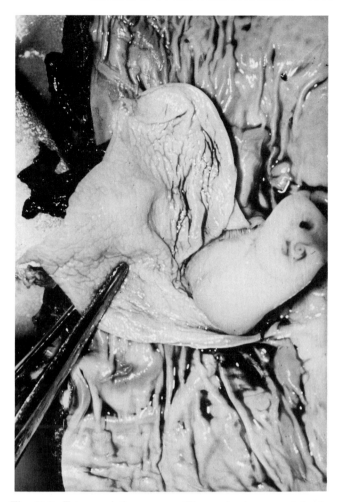

Fig. 51.9 Extra-amniotic pregnancy. The amnion is represented only by a small, shrunken, but grossly thickened remnant which forms a 'collar' around the insertion of the cord. (From Kohler & Jenkins, 1976. Courtesy of the Editor of the British Journal of Obstetrics and Gynaecology.)

is related to the gestational age at which amnion rupture has occurred. He also finds that strings consist not only of amnion, but also of fibrous tissue derived from the chorion. Possibly the process of detachment as such may lead to the formation of strands consisting of spongy layer; this process could be likened to the pulling apart of two surfaces that had been covered by glue which had not completely set: strings of semi-solid glue will form and solidify.

Amniotic extremital defects are not exclusively caused by strands. The late Sir Denis Browne (personal communication), suggested that holes in the membranes could be caused by a thrust-out extremity, in very much the same way as an old-fashioned and poor quality rubber glove could be pierced by a finger. In such an event the membrane would retract in a proximal direction on the thrust-out extremity and constrict it. The result is illustrated in Figure 51.10. Yet another variety of amniogenic damage was described (and illustrated) by Turner (1960): an

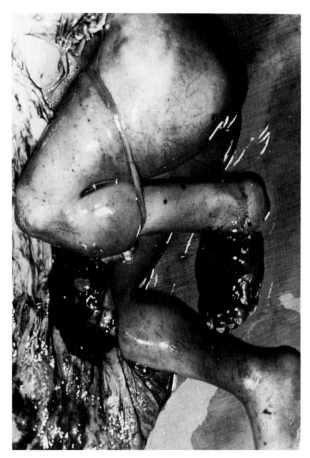

Fig. 51.10 Gangrene of fetal foot secondary to retraction of pierced membranes.

amnion pouch in which a foot of the fetus was caught, the neck of the pouch cutting into the soft tissue of the heel.

Extremital defects that might have been caused by amniotic strands (so-called intrauterine amputations) were first recorded in the seventeenth century by Jan Baptista van Helmont (1652) and Thomas Bartholinus (1673) (Kohler, 1962), but only in 1832 were constricting strands recognized by Montgomery as causal agents (Montgomery, 1832, 1833). He believed the strands consisted of solidified lymph, but the veterinary anatomist Gurlt (1833) suggested that the strands were actually rolled up or twisted fragments of ruptured membrane. This explanation was widely accepted, but in 1930 the embryologist Streeter *ex cathedra* rejected any part played by amniotic strands in the pathogenesis of extremital lesions (Streeter, 1930). His views were largely based on the examination of museum specimens without regard to clinical histories, and the proposed alternative explanation was, as he admitted, rather hazy. Nevertheless, Streeter's opinion found wide support, especially in the Anglo-Saxon world, and rather few authors dared disagree with him (Lennon, 1947; Potter, 1952; Browne, 1957;

MacGregor, 1960). By the time Kohler's (1962) review of the subject appeared the climate of opinion had begun to change and a return to a less biased approach was signalled by the publication of Torpin's monograph (1968) *Fetal malformations caused by amnion rupture*. In the last 20 years or so amniotic strands and related lesions have been restored to their rightful position as pathological agents in limb and skin defects. Beyond that, they are being held responsible for an increasing number of more severe malformations involving the central nervous system and viscera (see below).

Fetal injuries attributable to amniotic strands (and similar structures)

Extremital lesions (Fig. 51.11) are the most common ones in the field. They include the following, more or less in this sequential order: circular grooves ('ring constrictions') of varying depth; localized peripheral oedema, which may deepen the circular grooves and, occasionally, be so severe as to merit the term 'elephantiasis' (Senkel et al, 1979); ischaemic changes ranging from gangrene (Chaussier, 1812; Glessner, 1963; Glaun et al, 1971) to mummification and shrivelling (Schaeffer, 1775; Zagorski, 1834; Chemke et al, 1973) and finally separation of the distal part, which only in a few instances was found at delivery (Chaussier, 1812; Watkinson, 1825; Torpin & Faulkner, 1966).

In addition to reduction anomalies, *syndactyly* has been a feature in no fewer than 106 case records out of some 400 reviewed by Torpin and accepted as relevant to his theme. Syndactyly in this context is due to strands bind-

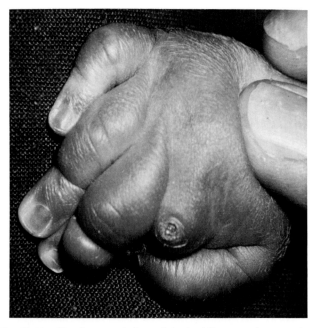

Fig. 51.11 Circular constrictions of the fetal fingers and amputation of one finger by amniotic strands.

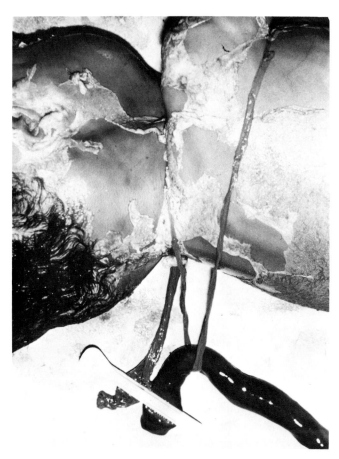

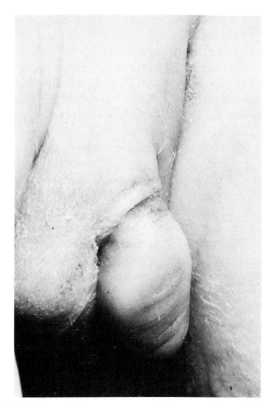

Fig. 51.13   Constriction groove around the root of the penis in an extramembranous pregnancy.

Fig. 51.12   Constriction of fetal neck by amniotic strand. (Courtesy of Drs W. Jones and G. Batcup.)

ing together the fingers (or occasionally the toes) like a bunch of flowers. Characteristically, the fusion is found in the distal phalanges.

Whilst lesions of amniogenic origin are rarely found on the trunk (Clair, 1936; Imber et al, 1974) cases of superficial amniotic lesions on the neck are even rarer (Fig. 51.12), but several reports of *acephaly* have appeared over the centuries. Not all of these cases are acceptable, but three reports (Ehrhardt, 1956; Benesova & Viznerova, 1962; Swinburne, 1967) are sufficiently precise to regard a diagnosis of 'intrauterine decapitation' as justified.

Encirclement of the penis has so far not been reported. At the autopsy of an immature neonate one of us (HGK) saw an almost complete circumferential groove of the shaft of the penis (Fig. 51.13). The infant had Potter's facies and other signs of oligohydramnios. The placenta, of circum-marginate type and with a deficiency of parietal membranes, suggested extramembranous pregnancy. Some strands were seen on the fetal surface of the membranes, but none actually on the penis.

Constriction of the umbilical cord by strands of amnion (Fig. 51.14) is invariably fatal. This conclusion could be drawn from the 34 case reports that were published in the 100 years from the first description (Braun, 1865)

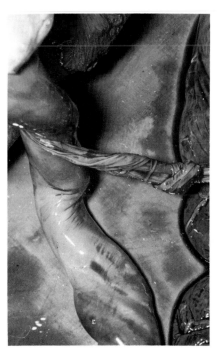

Fig. 51.14   Strangulation of the umbilical cord by a membranous strand. (From Kohler & Collins, 1972. Courtesy of the Editor of the Journal of Obstetrics and Gynaecology of the British Commonwealth.)

and reviewed by Torpin (1968). Indeed, a non-fatal case would be rather elusive. The exceedingly high mortality rate contrasts with notably lower figures for various forms of cord entanglement. The reason apparently is that amniotic strands can cut through Wharton's jelly quite effectively, in contrast to the blunt impact of the entangled cord or other external agents. Since Torpin's review the number of published reports has increased considerably. This is largely due to enhanced interest in both perinatal mortality in general and in amniotic lesions in particular. Even so, this cause of fetal loss is probably still under-diagnosed and under-reported. A real, if small, increase in incidence is likely to have occurred as a result of the wider use of diagnostic amniocentesis. Historically, it may be of interest that in the long dispute over the validity of the 'amniogenic theory', the opponents of this theory never attempted to account for strangulation of the umbilical cord by any other explanation.

Co-existent encirclement of umbilical cord and of extremities has been reported several times, in recent years by Senkel et al (1979).

Amnion strands swallowed by the fetus have been demonstrated by Zelenka et al (1959), Torpin et al (1964) and Jahoda & Schaller (1972). As long as they remain fixed at one end to the sac of membranes, they can effectively immobilize the fetus (or aggravate the immobilization caused by oligohydramnios).

Skin defects due to amnion strands, other than those caused by circumferential pressure (ring constrictions) have occasionally been described. Ahlfeld (1894) had tried to explain such lesions by assuming that an amniotic strand had been firmly attached to fetal skin and then forcefully pulled off, leaving a focal defect, but very few recorded observations support this hypothetical pathogenesis.

An alternative explanation is applicable only where there is an actual 'amputation'. Here the protruding bone of the 'amputation stump' is in a vantage position to cause skin defects on the medial aspect of the other leg by scratching and rubbing (Fig. 51.15). Where localized skin defects are found in the absence of any other amniogenic lesion, it may be wise first to exclude an alternative aetiology.

Oblique facial clefts are peculiarly complex malformations (Fig. 51.16). In addition to the lesion implied by the name, the fetus also has other anomalies, including severe cranial defects, e.g. exencephaly. Extremital reductions of more or less obvious amniogenic type are usually also present. Membranous strands or sheets, sometimes quite conspicuous, may be seen in relation to a facial cleft or extremital lesion or both. The clefts can run in any direction from near vertical to near horizontal; they do not mark or exaggerate natural anatomical boundaries and defy explanation in terms of retarded or arrested organogenesis (Politzer, 1936; Custer, 1943). The subject has been reviewed by Jones et al (1974) who conclude that

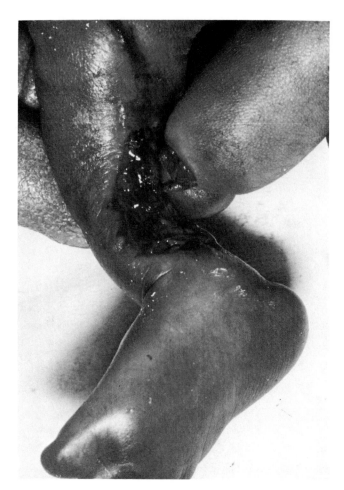

Fig. 51.15 Fetal skin damage due to pressure from protruding bone of an amputation stump caused by an amniotic strand. (Courtesy of Drs G. Batcup and W. Jones.)

'the problem of brain development in this disorder is not a primary one, but is secondary to the effect of tissue bands on the organisation of the calvarium . . . this might allow for better function and performance than would usually be anticipated in cases having this degree of microcephaly and encephalocele as a result of a primary defect of brain development'. The authors also emphasize their fruitless attempt to find in their seven cases any evidence of exogenous teratogens such as drugs or viruses, etc., nor were they able to detect any relevant family history that might incriminate either hereditary or long-lasting environmental factors.

These conclusions are deepened and extended in a subsequent publication (Higginbottom et al, 1979), in which the concept of *amniotic band disruption complex* is introduced. The implication of the term is that amnion tissue, not necessarily in the form of strands or strings and not just by encirclement, can interfere with embryonal development, e.g. by adhesion to the vault of the skull or to the anterior abdominal wall and can have a disruptive effect on organs already formed. 'Whereas late rupture of the amnion creates disruption and deformation principally of

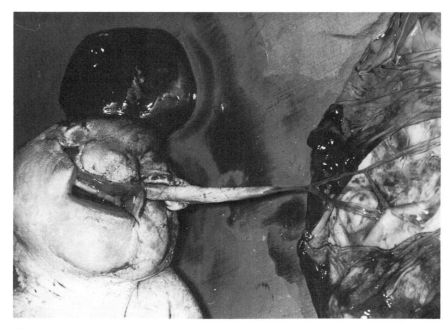

Fig. 51.16   Amniotic band disruption complex with an oblique facial cleft.

the limbs, early rupture appears to result in multiple malformations, disruptions, deformations and frequently prenatal wastage. Infants from the early group present with anencephaly, encephalocele, abdominal or thoracic eventration and severe limb abnormalities . . .' (Higginbottom et al, 1979). This concept resolves the dilemma in interpretation which arises when typical amputation or constriction lesions are found in a fetus alongside more fundamental defects. The distinction between early and late rupture is a useful suggestion, provided it is interpreted as a spectrum rather than a rigid boundary. It might even be compatible with Grosser's concept (1939) of the origin of amnion anomalies from incomplete expansion of the amniotic sac and persistence of magma reticulare.

The ideas on which the 'amniotic band disruption complex' are based are hardly new; they were developed and much discussed in the nineteenth century and extensively reviewed by Ballantyne (1904). They were eclipsed in the wake of Streeter (1930) but not quite extinct (e.g. Benesova & Viznerova, 1962).

The reader may feel sceptical, if not cynical, about this remarkable resurrection. In fairness, however, one has to acknowledge that the proposers have themselves indicated the criteria by which their theory is susceptible to proof or disproof:

1. A multiplicity and variety of abnormalities with 'no rhyme nor reason' in their composition.
2. The individual lesions can not readily be explained by 'traditional' disordered development
3. No known teratogen or adverse environmental influence
4. No relevant family history or other evidence of genetic disorders
5. Demonstrable abnormalities of the fetal membranes, in particular of the amnion
6. Good outlook for future pregnancies: no more than random risk of recurrence
7. Relatively good therapeutic prospects in some of the surviving infants.

REFERENCES

Ahlfeld F 1894 Eine neue typische Form durch amniotische Faden hervorgebrachter Verbildung. In: Festschrift sur Feier des 50 Jubileums der Gesellschaft fur Geburtshilfe und Gynakologie in Berlin. Alfred Holder, Wien, pp 1–8.

Bain A D, Scott J S 1960 Renal agenesis and severe urinary tract dysplasia: a review of 50 cases with particular reference to associated anomalies. British Medical Journal 1: 841–846.

Bain A D, Smith I I, Gould I K 1964 Newborn after prolonged leakage of liquor amnii. British Medical Journal 2: 598–599.

Ballantyne J W 1904 Manual of antenatal pathology and hygiene, vol 2. The embryo. William Green, Edinburgh.

Benesova D, Viznerova A 1962 Prispevek k vrozenym vchylkam

vyvolanym amnialnimi srosty. Ceskoslovenska Pediatrie 17: 490–501.

Benirschke K, Driscoll S G 1967 The pathology of the human placenta. Springer Verlag, Berlin.

Boura A L A, Walters W A W 1991 Autacoids and the control of vascular tone in the human umbilical-placental circulation. Placenta 12: 453–477.

Bourne G L 1960 The microscopic anatomy of the amnion and chorion. American Journal of Obstetrics and Gynecology 79: 1071.

Bourne G L 1962 The human amnion and chorion. Lloyd Luke, London.

Bratlid D, Lindback T 1978 Bacteriolytic activity of amniotic fluid. Obstetrics and Gynecology 51: 63–66.

Braun G 1865 Die strangformige Aufwickelung des Amnion um der Nabelstrang des reifen Kindes: eine seltene Ursache des intrauterinen Foetaltodes. Oesterreichische Zeitschrift fur Praktische Heilkunde 11: 165–166, 182–183.

Browne D 1957 The pathology of congenital rings. Archives of Disease in Childhood 32: 517–519.

Charles D, Hurry D J 1983 Chorioamnionitis. Clinics in Obstetrics and Gynaecology 10: 123–148.

Chaussier N 1812 Discours prononce a l'hospice de la maternite, vol 1 (no 2). Quoted after Torpin, 1968.

Chemke J, Graft G, Hurwitz N, Liban E 1973 Amniotic band syndrome. Obstetrics and Gynecology 41: 332–336.

Clair 1936 Grossesse extra-amniotique avec bride amniotique ayant provoque vue lesion cutanee chez l'enfant. Bulletin de la Societe d'Obstetrique et Gynecologie 25: 278–280.

Custer E M 1943 Uber das Wesen der schragen Gesichtsspalte. Ein Beitrag zur Morphologie, Systematik und Genese der Gesichtsspalten. Inaugural dissertation, Zurich.

Drife J 1989 Infection and preterm birth. British Journal of Obstetrics and Gynaecology 96: 1128–1130.

Dunn P M 1976 Congenital postural deformities. British Medical Bulletin 32: 71–76.

Ehrhardt L 1956 Seltene Spontanamputation durch Amniostrang: Akephalos. Zentralblatt fur Gynakologie 78: 1509–1513.

Fisk N M, Fysh J, Child A G, Gatenby P A, Jeffery H, Bradfield A H 1987 Is C-reactive protein really useful in preterm premature rupture of the membranes? British Journal of Obstetrics and Gynaecology 94: 1159–1164.

Fox H 1978 Pathology of the placenta. Saunders, London.

Fox H, Langley F A 1971 Leukocytic infiltration of the placenta and umbilical cord: a clinico-pathological study. Obstetrics and Gynecology 37: 451–458.

Gibbs R S, Duff P 1991 Progress in pathogenesis and management of clinical intraamniotic infection. American Journal of Obstetrics and Gynecology 164: 1317–1326.

Glaun B P, Weinberg E G, Malan A F 1971 Peripheral gangrene in a newborn. Archives of Disease in Childhood 46: 105–107.

Glessner J R 1963 Spontaneous intrauterine amputation. Journal of Bone and Joint Surgery 45A: 351–355.

Grosser O 1939 Entwicklungsgeschichtliche Grundlagen amniotischer Missbildungen. Verhandlungen der Deutschen Pathologischen Gesellschaft 31: 213–277.

Gurlt E 1933 Uber die von selbst erfolgte Abtrennung der Glieder des Fotus im Uterus. Medizinische Zeitung von dem Verein fur Heilkunde in Preussen 2: 13.

Higginbottom M C, Jones K L, Hall B D, Smith D W 1979 The amniotic band disruption complex: timing of amnionic rupture and variable spectra of consequent defects. Journal of Pediatrics 95: 544–549.

Hillier S L, Martius J, Krohn M, Kiviat N, Holmes K K, Eschenbach D A 1988 A case-control study of chorioamniotic infection and histologic chorioamnionitis in prematurity. New England Journal of Medicine 319: 972–978.

Hurley R 1988 Chorioamnionitis. Journal of Obstetrics and Gynaecology 8: 368–370.

Imber G, Guthrie Jr R H, Goul Jr D 1974 Congenital band of the abdomen and the amniotic etiology of bands. American Journal of Surgery 127: 753–754.

Jahoda E, Schaller A 1972 Uber einen vom Fetus verschslluckten Amnionstrang. Zentralblatt fur Gynakologie 94: 1229–1232.

Jirasek J E 1983 Anatomie Choria. Cesko-Slovenska Gynekologie 48.

Jones K L, Smith D W, Hall B D et al 1974 A pattern of cranio-facial and limb defects secondary to aberrant tissue bands. Journal of Pediatrics 84: 90–95.

Kaplan C 1993 Placental pathology for the nineties. Pathology Annual 28: 15–72.

Kohler H G 1962 Congenital transverse defects of limbs and digits: 'intrauterine amputation'. Archives of Disease in Childhood 37: 263–276.

Kohler H G 1972 An unusual case of sirenomelia. Teratology 6: 295–301.

Kohler H G, Collins M L 1972 Ligation of the umbilical cord by torn amniotic membrane. Journal of Obstetrics and Gynaecology of the British Commonwealth 79: 183–184.

Kohler H G, Jenkins D M 1976 Extra-amniotic pregnancy. British Journal of Obstetrics and Gynaecology 83: 251–253.

Kohler H G, Rymer B A 1973 Congenital cystic malformation of the lung and its relation to hydramnios. Journal of Obstetrics and Gynaecology of the British Commonwealth 80: 130–134.

Kohler H G, Peel K R, Hoar F 1970 Extramembranous pregnancy and amniorrhoea. Journal of Obstetrics and Gynaecology of the British Commonwealth 77: 809–812.

Lamont R F, Rose M, Elder M G 1985 Effect of bacterial products on prostaglandin E production by amnion cells. Lancet ii: 1331–1333.

Landing B H 1950 Amnion nodosum, a lesion of the placenta apparently associated with deficient secretion of fetal urine. American Journal of Obstetrics and Gynaecology 60: 1339–1342.

Lennon G G 1947 Fetal pathology (with special reference to the role of amniotic bands). Journal of Obstetrics and Gynaecology of the British Empire 54: 830.

Leonardi R, Rigano A 1966 Sull'ultrastrutture e sulla funzione dell'epitelio amniotico umano. Rivista di Ostetricia e Ginecologia 21: 33–56.

Lister U M 1968 Ultrastructure of the human amnion, chorion and fetal skin. Journal of Obstetrics and Gynaecology of the British Commonwealth 75: 327–341.

López Bernal A, Hansell D J, Khong T Y, Keeling J W, Turnbull A C 1989 Prostaglandin E production by the fetal membrane, in unexplained preterm labour and preterm labour associated with chorioamnionitis. British Journal of Obstetrics and Gynaecology 96: 1133–1139.

McDonald H M, O'Laughlin J A, Jolley P, Vigneswaran R, McDonald P J 1991 Vaginal infection and preterm labour. British Journal of Obstetrics and Gynaecology 98: 427–435.

McDonald I A 1980 Cervical cerclage. Clinics in Obstetrics and Gynaecology 7: 461–479.

MacGregor A R 1960 Pathology of infancy and childhood. Livingstone, Edinburgh.

Meudt R 1966 Beitrag zur Frage der Festigkeit der menschlichen Eihaut. Gynaecologia 162: 430–434.

Minh H-N, Smadja A, St Mair P P, Orcel K 1981 Electron microscopic study of intercellular canalicular systems in the parietal fetal membranes. British Journal of Obstetrics and Gynaecology 88: 1104–1109.

Mitchell M D 1991 Current topic: the regulation of placental eicosanoid biosynthesis. Placenta 12: 557–572.

Montgomery W F 1832 Observations on the spontaneous amputation of the foetus in utero, with an attempt to explain the occasional cause of its production. Dublin Journal of Medical and Chemical Science 1: 140–144.

Montgomery W F 1833 Further observations on spontaneous amputation of the limbs of the foetus in utero. Dublin Journal of Medical and Chemical Science 2: 49–51.

Naeye R L 1988 Acute bacterial chorioamnionitis. Progress in Clinical and Biological Research 281: 73–86.

Naeye R L, Peters E C 1978 Amniotic fluid infections with intact membranes leading to perinatal death: a prospective study. Pediatrics 61: 171–177.

Naeye R L, Peters E C 1980 Causes and consequences of premature rupture of fetal membranes. Lancet i: 192–194.

Naeye R, Ross S 1982 Coitus and chorioamnionitis: a prospective study. Early Human Development 6: 91–97.

Pankuch G A, Appelbaum P C, Lorenz R P, Botti J J, Schachter J, Naeye R L 1984 Placental microbiology and histology and the pathogenesis of chorioamnionitis. Obstetrics and Gynecology 4: 802–806.

Pitkin R M, Reynolds W A 1975 Fetal ingestion and metabolism of amniotic fluid protein. American Journal of Obstetrics and Gynecology 123: 356–357.

Politzer C 1936 Die Projektion der embryonalen Gesichtsfurchen auf des Gesicht des Erwachsenen und die Entstehung der schragen Gesichtsspalte. Beitrage zur Pathologischen Anatomie 97: 557–567.

Pollard S M, Aye N N, Symonds E M 1976 Scanning electron microscopic appearances of normal human amnion and umbilical cord after term. British Journal of Obstetrics and Gynaecology 83: 470–477.

Pollard S M, Symonds E M, Aye N N 1979 Scanning electron microscopic appearances in the amnion in polyhydramnios and oligohydramnios. British Journal of Obstetrics and Gynaecology 86: 228–232.

Potter E L 1946 Facial characteristics of infants with bilateral renal agenesis. American Journal of Obstetrics and Gynecology 51: 885–888.

Potter E L 1952 Pathology of the fetus and the newborn, 1st edn. Year Book Publishers, Chicago.

Potter E L 1961 Pathology of the fetus and infant, 2nd edn. Year Book Publishers, Chicago.

Potter E L 1965 Bilateral absence of ureters and kidneys: a report of 50 cases. Obstetrics and Gynecology 25: 3–12.

Potter E L, Craig J M 1976 Pathology of the fetus and the infant. Lloyd Luke (Medical Books), London.

Remak R 1854 Uber die Zusammenziehung des Amnios. Archiv fur Anatomie, Physiologie und Wissenschaftliche Medizin 21: 369–373.

Romero R, Mazor M 1988 Infection and preterm labor. Clinical Obstetrics and Gynecology 31: 553–584.

Romero R, Emamian M, Quintero R, Wan M, Hobbins J C, Mitchell M D 1986 Amniotic fluid prostaglandin levels and intra-amniotic infections. Lancet i: 1380.

Romero R, Sirtori M, Oyarzun E et al 1989 Infection and labor. V. Prevalence, microbiology and clinical significance of intraamniotic infection in women with preterm labor and intact membranes. American Journal of Obstetrics and Gynecology 161: 817–824.

Russell P 1979 Inflammatory lesions of the human placenta. 1. Clinical significance of acute chorioamnionitis. American Journal of Diagnostic Gynecology and Obstetrics 1: 127–137.

Salazar H, Kanbour A I 1974 Amnion nodosum: ultrastructure and pathogenesis. Archives of Pathology 98: 39–46.

Schaeffer J V T 1775 Foetus cum matre per nervos commercium. Thesis, Erlangae.

Schmidt W 1956 Der Feinbau der reifen menschlichen Eihaute. Zeitschrift fur Anatomie 119: 203–222.

Schmidt W 1965 Uber den paraplazentaren, fruchtwassergebundenen Stofftransport beim Menschen. Histochemische Untersuchung der in den Eihouten angereicherten Stoffe. Zietschrift Fur Anatomie und Entwicklungsgeschichte 124: 321–334.

Schmidt W 1967 Uber den paraplacentaren, fruchtuassergebundenen Stofftransport beim Menschen Nacheis der vom Amnion abgegebenen Lipide im Fruchtwasser und um Dunndarm des Keimes. Zeitschrift fur Anatomie und Entwicklungsgeschichte 126: 276–288.

Schmidt W, Eberhagen D, Svejcar J, Kurth E M 1971 Uber den paraplacentaren, fruchtwassergebundenen Stofftransport beim Menschen. 3. Quantitative und qualitative Analyse der im Fruchtwasser enthaltenen Stoffe. Zeitschrift fur Anatomie und Entwicklungsgeschichte 135: 210–221.

Schmidt W, Pfaller K, Schwarzfurtner H 1982a Licht und elektronenmikroskopische Untersuchungen an den Eihauten des Menschen. 1. Amnion und Zwischenschicht. Zentralblatt fur Gynakologie 104: 385–396.

Schmidt W, Pfaller K, Klima G 1982b Licht und elektronenmikroskopische Untersuchungen an den Eihauten des Menschen. 2. Chorion und Decidua. Zentralblatt fur Gynakologie 104: 1137–1148.

Schroeder R 1930 Die Eihaute vor und rach der Losung. In: Von Mollendorf W (ed) Handbuch der mikroskopischen Anatomie des Menschen. Springer, Berlin, vol VII, pp 493–495.

Scott J S 1960 Placenta extrachorialis (placenta marginata and placenta circumvallata): a factor in antepartum haemorrhage. Journal of Obstetrics and Gynaecology of the British Empire 67: 904–918.

Scott J S, Bain A D 1958 Amnion nodosum. Proceedings of the Royal Society of Medicine 51: 512–513.

Senkel V, Behling H, Hinske G 1979 Intrauterine fetale Komplikationen durch Amnionstrange. Zentralblatt fur Gynakologie 101: 809–812.

Streeter G L 1930 Focal deficiencies in fetal tissues and their relation to intrauterine amputation. Contributions to Embryology, Carnegie Institution of Washington 22: 1–44.

Swinburne L M 1967 Spontaneous intrauterine decapitation. Archives of Disease in Childhood 42: 636–641.

Tafari N, Ross S M, Naeye R L, Galask R P, Zaar B 1977 Failure of bacterial growth inhibition by amniotic fluid. American Journal of Obstetrics and Gynecology 128: 187–189.

Tarnier S 1895 Sejour prolonge d'un foetus vivant entre les membranes de l'oeuf rompu traumatiquement. France Medicale 42: 588.

Thomas I T, Smith D W 1974 Oligohydramnios: cause of non-renal features of Potter's syndrome, including pulmonary hypoplasia. Journal of Pediatrics 84: 811.

Torpin R 1968 Fetal malformations caused by amnion rupture during gestation. Thomas, Springfield.

Torpin R, Faulkner A 1966 Intrauterine amputation with the missing member found in the fetal membranes. Journal of the American Medical Association 198: 185.

Torpin R, Miller G T, Culpepper B W 1964 Amnion strand swallowed by the fetus. American Journal of Obstetrics and Gynecology 910: 829–831.

Toth M, Witkin S S, Ledger W, Thaler H 1988 The role of infection in the etiology of preterm birth. Obstetrics and Gynecology 71: 723–726.

Turner E J 1960 Intrauterine constriction band. Journal of Pediatrics 57: 890–891.

Vago T, Chavkin J 1980 Extramembranous pregnancy: an unusual complication of amniocentesis. American Journal of Obstetrics and Gynecology 137: 511–512.

van Drooge P H, Okken A 1982 Extramembraneuze zwangerchap. Nederlands Tijdschrift voor Geneeskunde 126: 1819–1823.

van Herendael B J, Oberti C, Brosens I 1978 Microanatomy of the human amniotic membrane: a light microscopic, transmission and scanning electron microscopic study. American Journal of Obstetrics and Gynecology 131: 872–880.

Wang T, Schneider J 1982 Myofibroblasten im bindegewebe des menschlichen Amnions. Zeitschrift fur Geburtshilfe und Perinatologie 186: 164–168.

Wang T, Schneider J 1983 Amniotic epithelium in toxemia of pregnancy. Chinese Medical Journal 95: 751–756.

Wang T, Reale E, Schneider J 1979 Das Amnionepithel bei Hydramnion. Fortschritte der Medizin 97: 1009–1012.

Watkinson 1825 Case of a foetus in which the left foot was separated from the leg during gestation. London Medical and Physical Journal 54: 38–39.

Wentworth P 1968 Circumvallate and circummarginate placentas: their incidence and clinical significance. American Journal of Obstetrics and Gynecology 102: 44–47.

Wilkins B S, Batcup G, Vinall P S 1991 Partial placenta membranacea. British Journal of Obstetrics and Gynaecology 98: 675–679.

Zaaijman J du T, Wilkinson A R, Keeling J W, Mitchell R G, Turnbull A C 1982 Spontaneous premature rupture of the membranes: bacteriology, histology and neonatal outcome. Journal of Obstetrics and Gynaecology 2: 155–160.

Zagorski P 1834 Monstrostatis singularis specimen. Memoirs de l'Academie Imperiale des Sciences de St Petersbourg (series 6) 3: 3–7.

Zelenka J, Syrova E, Trckova-Miksova E 1959 Objemna cast amnioe blany spontanne vysla se stolici ctyrdenniho novorozence. (A substantial portion of the amniotic membrane excreted in the stools of a four days old neonate.) Plzensky Lekarsky Sbornik 10: 61.

52. Gestational trophoblastic disease

C. W. Elston

INTRODUCTION

The lesions grouped together under this broad title represent a wide range of disease processes, from a specific type of abortion, hydatidiform mole, to the malignant neoplasm, choriocarcinoma. This apparent paradox is explained by the close histogenetic and clinical links between them and the importance of applying the correct therapy in an individual case. Because of its secretion of an ideal tumour marker substance, human chorionic gonadotrophin (hCG), the treatment of choriocarcinoma can be accurately monitored, and this has proved invaluable in reducing the previously high mortality. Choriocarcinoma evokes further interest because of its unique status as a naturally occurring neoplastic allograft and the implications this carries for the mechanism of nidation and intrauterine fetal survival.

CLASSIFICATION

In common with many tumours the histogenesis of trophoblastic neoplasia was first established correctly in Germany towards the end of the nineteenth century. The first description of choriocarcinoma was probably by Chiari in 1877. Although he stressed the origin from the placental bed, and the relationship with a previous gestation, he failed to recognize that it arose from the trophoblast. Sänger (1889) produced a comprehensive classification of primary uterine neoplasms, but in separating off the trophoblastic tumours he incorrectly presumed that they were sarcomatous and therefore arose from the decidua.

The correct origin from the trophoblast was finally deduced by Marchand (1894) after a classical clinicopathological study. He later established the fetal origin of the trophoblast, and introduced the term 'chorionepithelioma' (Marchand, 1898). This interpretation was quickly accepted in continental Europe and the United States, but not in England due to the obstinacy of the Obstetrical Society of London (Ober & Fass, 1961). It finally took a

Scotsman to convince the learned members of the Society (Teacher, 1903a,b) and the trophoblastic origin of choriocarcinoma has not been challenged seriously since then.

The next important step was the recognition by Ewing (1910) that the histological appearances in trophoblastic lesions were more important in relation to the degree of malignancy than had previously been claimed. He devised a morphological classification under the broad term 'chorioma' with the following subdivisions:

1. Hydatid mole
2. Chorioadenoma destruens
3. Choriocarcinoma
4a. Syncytial endometritis
4b. Syncytioma.

This formed the basis of the modern classification of trophoblastic neoplasia, and has only required modification in recent years. The inclusion of a non-neoplastic condition such as hydatidiform mole may at first appear illogical, since it is a distinctive type of abortion rather than a tumour (Fox, 1989) and in the great majority of cases there are no neoplastic sequelae. A hydatidiform mole is the preceding gestation in at least 50% of cases of choriocarcinoma and this, and the fact that patients with postmolar trophoblastic disease may be treated with cytotoxic agents on the basis of elevated gonadotrophin excretion alone, is sufficient justification for classifying the two lesions together.

Ewing devised the term chorioadenoma destruens to denote the type of hydatidiform mole which retained its villous structure and penetrated into the myometrium, occasionally extending into pelvic structures but rarely metastasizing. It behaved as a locally malignant process and Ewing considered the lesion to be intermediate between a classical hydatidiform mole and choriocarcinoma. The more straightforward descriptive term 'invasive mole' is now preferred (Park, 1971; Elston, 1978; Hertz, 1978), although the pathogenesis is still uncertain. Park (1967) proposed that abnormal trophoblast which forms villi has only a locally malignant potential, whilst that which does

1597

not form villi has a 'metastasizing' malignant potential, but this is not supported by cases of trophoblastic disease in which metastatic nodules have been shown to contain villi (e.g. Delfs, 1957; Ring, 1972; Kohorn et al, 1978). Tow (1966), based on his experience in treating trophoblastic disease in Singapore, suggested that invasive mole be renamed 'villous choriocarcinoma' and that classical choriocarcinoma be called 'avillous choriocarcinoma'. He argued that the villous form was merely an early stage of avillous choriocarcinoma and that, in his practice at least, both lesions received the same treatment. These ideas received some support on theoretical grounds from Brewer (1967) and use of the classification has been continued in Singapore (Ratnam & Chew, 1976). The available evidence, however, indicates that invasive mole rarely, if ever, progresses to true choriocarcinoma (Chun & Braga, 1967; Park, 1971) but rather that the presence of molar villi is a marker of an inherently less aggressive trophoblastic proliferation. Tow's proposal was not incorporated into the classification recommended by the International Union Against Cancer (1967), nor has it been supported elsewhere (Bagshawe, 1969; Park, 1971; Elston, 1978; WHO Scientific Group, 1983; Silverberg & Kurman, 1992)). Since the prognosis of invasive mole is very different from that of choriocarcinoma, and the presence of molar villi is a clear distinguishing feature, there are excellent practical reasons for keeping the two lesions separate.

A disadvantage of the Ewing classification is the fact that it was devised at a time when histological material was available in nearly all cases and no provision is made for cases of trophoblastic disease lacking a definite tissue diagnosis. Today, most patients with persistence of trophoblastic proliferation following a hydatidiform mole are monitored by gonadotrophin assay and may receive prophylactic chemotherapy without a firm tissue diagnosis of invasive mole or choriocarcinoma being established. The International Union Against Cancer (1967) used the unsatisfactory category 'uncertain' to denote such cases, but the more precise terminology 'persistent trophoblastic disease' is preferred (Elston, 1976, 1978; Hertz, 1978).

When Marchand (1895) correctly established the histogenesis of choriocarcinoma from the villous trophoblast he recognized an uncommon variant which he termed atypical choriocarcinoma. Ewing (1910) subsequently divided the latter entity into two forms, syncytial endometritis and syncytioma. The lesion which Ewing termed syncytial endometritis is characterized by an infiltration of intermediate trophoblastic cells through the decidua and adjacent myometrium at the placental bed. This terminology is inappropriate, for the appearances are not those of a pathological process, but rather a florid form of the normal physiological permeation of the gestational implantation site by extravillous trophoblast. The preferred terminology is 'exaggerated placental site reaction' (Elston, 1991; Silverberg & Kurman, 1992) and the lesion is worth

including in a classification of trophoblastic disease for two reasons: it defines the normal end of the spectrum, and its presence in a curettage for postpartum or postabortal bleeding may lead the unwary into a mistaken histological diagnosis of malignancy.

The lesion which Ewing termed syncytioma proved much more difficult to characterize because of its relative rarity. The striking resemblance to the placental site trophoblast and the benign course without metastatic spread led a number of authorities to conclude that the process was not neoplastic (Ober et at, 1971; Kurman et al, 1976; Elston, 1981). However, subsequent reports of fatal cases associated with metastasis clearly indicated a neoplastic process (Scully & Young, 1981; Eckstein et al, 1982; Young & Scully, 1984). It is now accepted that these lesions are tumours derived from the intermediate trophoblast of the placental bed, and the terminology proposed by Young et al (1988), 'placental site trophoblastic tumour (PSTT)', has been adopted by the International Society of Gynecological Pathologists (Silverberg & Kurman, 1992). It is therefore suggested that a modern histopathological classification of trophoblastic disease should include the categories indicated below:

Hydatidiform mole
- Complete
- Partial

Invasive hydatidiform mole
Persistent trophoblastic disease
Placental site trophoblastic tumour
Trophoblastic lesions, miscellaneous
- Exaggerated placental site
- Trophoblastic lesions, unclassified.

This classification is based on that proposed by the International Society of Gynecological Pathologists (Silverberg & Kurman, 1992), but includes the clinicopathological designation of persistent trophoblastic disease as suggested by Elston (1978) and Hertz (1978) to account for those cases in which there is evidence of trophoblastic proliferation, but a specific morphological diagnosis cannot be made.

AETIOLOGICAL FACTORS

No single aetiological factor has been implicated as the cause of trophoblastic neoplasia but, as is the case with many tumours, numerous risk factors have been identified.

Much of the investigative interest has centred on epidemiological factors, which have been reviewed by Elston (1981), Grimes (1984) and Bracken (1987). It was long suspected that trophoblastic disease occurs more frequently in the Far East and developing countries than in the Western Hemisphere and this was confirmed by a geographical study based on small samples from the United

States and several Asian countries (Joint Project, 1959). Initial estimates suggested that the difference in frequency amounted to some 10–20 times. This was based on comparison of such frequencies for hydatidiform mole as 1:125 for Taiwan (Wei & Ouyang, 1963) and 1:200 for the Philippines (Acosta-Sison, 1967) with 1:2000 for the United States (Hertig & Sheldon, 1947). Unfortunately, as pointed out by Hertz (1978), the WHO Scientific Group (1983) and Bracken (1987), much of the epidemiological data is of dubious value due to differences in methods of recording data and problems of diagnostic accuracy. Some studies have included both complete and partial hydatidiform moles whilst others, particularly those published more than two decades ago, recorded only complete moles. Very few series have collected sufficient data to estimate the frequency of choriocarcinoma accurately. Many studies show marked selection bias because they are based on hospital populations only, without correction for uncomplicated births in the community. This is reflected in the wide range of frequencies reported throughout the world (Table 52.1); Bracken (1987) estimated that for hydatidiform mole this varied from 0.5 to 2.5:1000 pregnancies. For the reasons stated above it is still difficult to obtain accurate comparisons between 'high' and 'low' risk areas. Womack & Elston (1985), using the frequency of hydatidiform mole per live births only, compared figures from Nottingham U.K. with those from Aichi, Japan (Ishizuka, 1976), and found a fourfold increase in the latter. Closely similar results were obtained by Graham et al (1990) who used the Nottingham data as a comparison for the frequency in Abu Dhabi, Middle East. It can be concluded that trophoblastic disease, and hydatidiform mole in particular, occurs approximately four times more frequently in the 'high risk' areas of Asia, Africa, Latin

Table 52.1 Estimated frequency of trophoblastic disease in relation to the number of gestations

Author	Year	Country	Frequency Hydatidiform mole	Choriocarcinoma
Asia				
King	1956	Hong Kong	1:530 pregnancies	1:496 deliveries
Reddy & Rao	1969	India	1:463 pregnancies	
Poen & Djojopranoto	1965	Indonesia	1:85 pregnancies[a]	1:570 pregnancies[a]
			1:373 pregnancies[b]	1:1800 pregnancies[b]
Ishizuka	1976	Japan	1:522 pregnancies	
Llewellyn-Jones	1965	Malaysia	1:760 pregnancies	1:8000 pregnancies
Acosta-Sison	1967	Philippines	1:200 pregnancies	1:1382 pregnancies
Tan et al	1982	Singapore	1:868 deliveries	
Wei & Ouyang	1963	Taiwan	1:125 deliveries	1:8000 pregnancies
Africa				
Agboola	1979	Nigeria	1:379 deliveries	
Leighton	1973	Uganda	1:971 deliveries	
Australasia				
Duff	1989	New Zealand	1:1497 pregnancies	
Olesnicky et al	1985	Australia	1:1357 deliveries	
Europe				
Bagshawe et al	1986	U.K.	1: 650 pregnancies	
Franke et al	1983	Netherlands	1:1580 pregnancies	
Kolstad & Hognestad	1965	Norway	1:1300 deliveries	1:20 000 deliveries
Ringertz	1970	Sweden	1:1560 pregnancies	1:41 000 deliveries
Vejerslev et al	1984	Denmark	1:3158 pregnancies	
Womack & Elston	1985	U.K.	1:1400 deliveries	
Middle East				
Ghali	1969	Iraq	1:276 deliveries	
Graham et al	1990	United Arab Emirates	1:491 deliveries	
Matalon & Modan	1972	Israel	1:1300 pregnancies	
Latin America				
Aguero et al	1973	Venezuela	1:1088 pregnancies	
Marquez-Monter et al	1963	Mexico	1:220 pregnancies	
North America				
Hayashi et al	1982	U.S.A.	1:923 pregnancies	
Hertig & Sheldon	1947	U.S.A.	1:2000 deliveries	
Martin	1978	U.S.A. (Alaska)[c]	1:257 deliveries	
Yen & MacMahon	1968	U.S.A.	1:1450 deliveries	
Yuen & Cannon	1981	Canada	1:1205 pregnancies	

[a]Incidence in hospital serving 'low' socioeconomic population
[b]Incidence in hospital serving 'high' socioeconomic population
[c]Population of relatively recent East Asian descent

America and the Middle East than in the 'low risk' areas of Australasia, Europe and North America. This is a much lower difference than had been suggested previously. However, the relative risk for persistent trophoblastic disease in the United Kingdom (Womack & Elston, 1985) and Japan (Ishizuka, 1976) is closely similar, 8% and 9.6% respectively.

The reasons for the geographical variation in frequency of trophoblastic disease are unclear. Complete hydatidiform mole is commonest at the extremes of the reproductive period (Yen & MacMahon, 1968; Hayashi et al, 1982; Atrash et al, 1986; Bagshawe et al, 1986, Graham et al, 1990) and it has been suggested that the tendency for child bearing to continue late into reproductive life in higher incidence areas may account for some of the excess cases (British Medical Journal, 1975). Overall parity does not appear to be a risk factor after correction for maternal age (Yen & MacMahon, 1968; La Vecchia et al, 1985). Although a number of studies have shown an increased frequency of hydatidiform mole in women with repeated abortion (Yen & MacMahon, 1968; La Vecchia et al, 1985; Messerli et al, 1985; Acaia et al, 1988) this is not supported by Atrash et al (1986). There appears to be a considerably increased risk of a subsequent mole in women following a first hydatidiform mole (Franke et al, 1983; Sand et al, 1984; La Vecchia et al, 1985; Bagshawe et al, 1986). Reports on ethnic differences have been conflicting, partly because of the difficulty in carrying out truly multiracial studies. No association with ethnic group was found by the Joint Project (1959) but in Hawaii McCorriston (1968) found a higher incidence of trophoblastic disease in Orientals compared with Europeans of the same socio-economic class and native Hawaiians of a lower status. Jacobs et al (1982a) estimated that the incidence of complete moles in Hawaiians of Filipino origin was five times that of caucasians. In Malaysia no ethnic difference was found for Kuala Lumpur (Llewellyn-Jones, 1965) and although Teoh et al (1971) claimed that hydatidiform mole occurred more frequently among Indians and Eurasians in Singapore this was not confirmed by Lee et al (1981). In the United States, Yen & MacMahon (1968) found a higher incidence of molar disease in blacks than whites, but this was not confirmed by Hayashi et al (1982). Martin (1978), however, showed that the risk is increased in Alaskan natives compared with caucasian Americans. In the Middle East, Graham et al (1990) found that the increased risk of complete mole was greater in Gulf arabs than in other ethnic groups.

Although the Joint Project (1959) suggested that socio-economic factors, and in particular nutritional status, were of aetiological importance this has not been generally substantiated (Bracken, 1987; Buckley, 1987). Information on environmental factors is limited. Cigarette smoking has only been investigated in a small number of studies and the data is conflicting and inconclusive (Berkowitz et al, 1985; La Vecchia et al, 1985). Bracken (1987) has reviewed studies on exposure to herbicides, especially in South East Asia, and concluded that case selection bias renders the data unreliable. Use of oral contraceptives has been found to be unrelated to risk of hydatidiform mole (Berkowitz et al, 1985; La Vecchia et al, 1985; Messerli et al, 1985).

The possibility of a link with an oncogenic virus must remain unresolved. De Ruyck (1951) claimed to have isolated a virus from both hydatidiform mole and choriocarcinoma, but this has never been confirmed by other workers, nor has any other infective agent been incriminated. In a study from Romania, Nastac et al (1980) extracted DNA from human cervical carcinomas and inoculated young hamsters and rabbits. Material from one human tumour apparently produced tumours in four out of ten hamsters, including a choriocarcinoma. The authors implied that incorporation of oncogenic herpesvirus into the cervical carcinoma cell genome had occurred, although they could not identify viral antigens in the DNA extracts. Such results must be interpreted with caution, and clearly further studies are required before a viral aetiology can be confirmed or refuted.

Perhaps the most significant advance in the understanding of the pathogenesis of trophoblastic disease has come from the field of cytogenetics. The early studies used the relatively crude technique of estimating genetic sex by the distribution of Barr bodies in the trophoblastic and stromal cells of hydatidiform mole. Although the reported prevalence varied widely there was general agreement that hydatidiform moles were predominantly of female genetic sex (Park, 1957; Atkin, 1965; Tominaga & Page, 1966; Elston, 1970). It has since been shown convincingly that the great majority of classical (complete) hydatidiform moles are of 46,XX constitution (Kajii & Ohama, 1977; Vassilakos et al, 1977; Szulman & Surti, 1978a,b; Jacobs et al, 1980; Lawler et al, 1982b).

The application of chromosome marker studies, based on the technique of quinacrine staining (Q banding) described by Caspersson (1971) which allows precise identification of each chromosome in the human karyotype, produced a more significant advance. Data derived from Q and C (Giemsa staining of centromeric regions) banding suggested that complete moles are of androgenetic origin (Kajii & Ohama, 1977; Wake et al, 1978; Lawler et al, 1979; Jacobs et al, 1980; Lawler et al, 1982b). Analysis of the results of karyotyping in over 400 complete moles indicated that between 92 and 96% have a 46,XX karyotype, due to fertilization of an egg with no effective genome by a haploid (23,X) sperm which then duplicates without cytokinesis (Kajii & Ohama, 1977; Jacobs et al, 1980; Wake et al, 1984: Lawler & Fisher, 1987a; Surti, 1987), that is, they are homozygous in origin. These conclusions have been supported by HLA studies (Yamashita et al, 1979) and gene probing using restriction fragment length polymorphisms (RFLP) (Wallace et al, 1982; Surti et al, 1983; Ko et al, 1991). Between 4 and 8% of complete moles are heterozygous with a 46,XY karyotype. These cases arise from dispermy — fertilization of the 'empty' ovum by two separate haploid sperms carrying 23,X and 23,Y chromosomes respectively (Wake et al, 1978; Surti et al, 1979; Ohama et al, 1981; Patillo et al, 1981; Kajii et al, 1984; Lawler & Fisher, 1987a; Surti, 1987). Rare cases of heterozygous 46,XX complete mole have also been described (Lawler & Fisher, 1987a).

Many of the early cytogenetic studies of partially hydropic abortuses were difficult to interpret because of a lack of consistency in the morphological findings, but several showed an association between hydropia and triploidy (Makino et al, 1964; Schlegel et al, 1966; Carr, 1969). Vassilakos et al (1977) included in their category of partial hydatidiform mole some cases with atrophic trophoblast and found a variety of chromosomal abnormalities, predominantly triploidy but also including trisomies. Szulman & Surti (1978a,b) defined the syndrome of partial mole more precisely and included only those cases which exhibit definite trophoblastic hyperplasia. In their studies the great majority of partial moles have had a triploid karyotype (Surti, 1987) and this has been substantially confirmed by other groups (Jacobs et al, 1982b; Lawler et al, 1982a; Lawler & Fisher, 1991). Triploidy occurs in approximately 1% of conceptions that lead to clinically apparent pregnancies, and about 80% of triploid abortuses are partial moles (Szulman et al, 1981a). Jacobs et al (1982b) have shown that if the additional haploid component is paternal (diandry) then a molar gestation ensues, and if it is maternal (digyny) the result is a non-molar gestation. The diandric origin of triploid partial moles has been confirmed by cytogenetic studies, chromosomal heteromorphisms, RFLP and HLA typing in the same way as in complete mole (Couillon et al, 1978; Szulman et al, 1981a; Lawler et al, 1982b; Vejerslev et al, 1987; Lawler & Fisher, 1991).

Although the great majority of hydatidiform moles reported to date have fallen into the groups described above, the total number of cases analysed is still relatively small and a number of unusual reports have appeared, including hypodiploid, triploid and tetraploid complete moles and diploid and tetraploid partial moles (Vejerslev et al, 1987; Elston, 1991; Lawler & Fisher, 1991). In the majority of these cases the karyotype showed an excess of paternal over maternal chromosomes, supporting the view that it is the ratio of maternal to paternal chromosomes and not ploidy which is important in the evolution of molar gestations (Vejerslev et al, 1987).

Anecdotal cases such as those referred to above highlight a particular problem associated with the analysis of chromosomal abnormalities in molar gestations: the fact that fresh tissue is required for tissue culture cytogenetics. Furthermore, selection bias may occur since cytogenetic analysis can only be carried out on cells that can be induced to grow; cells that do not grow, and those with a long cell cycle, will be missed. Flow cytometry permits the evaluation of the DNA content of cells in all stages of the cycle including interphase. A considerable further advantage has been conferred by the development of techniques for extracting DNA from formalin-fixed tissues (Hedley et al, 1983) thus obviating the need for fresh specimens. Flow cytometry has confirmed that the majority of complete moles are diploid, with a high cell proliferation, and that most partial moles are triploid with a low cell proliferation (Fisher et al, 1987; Hemming et al, 1987; Lage et al, 1988, 1991; Koenig et al, 1993). A small number of cases of complete mole showing triploidy (Hemming et al, 1987), complete and partial mole showing tetraploidy (Hemming et al, 1987, 1988; Lage et al, 1989) and complete and partial mole with DNA aneuploidy (Hemming et al, 1987) have also been recorded.

All these genetic studies have done much to clarify the defects behind hydatidiform mole (Bagshawe & Lawler, 1982; Lawler & Fisher 1987a) and some progress is being made to elucidate the link with choriocarcinoma. In fact the majority of patients with complete mole have no further sequelae and it has been established that the risk of persistent trophoblastic disease is no greater that 10% (Ishizuka, 1976; Womack & Elston, 1985; Bagshawe et al, 1986). It has been suggested that complete moles which are heterozygous have a greater disposition to persistent trophoblastic disease than those which are homozygous (Sasaki et al, 1982; Wake et al 1984, 1987). Heterozygosity has been demonstrated in four cases of invasive mole (Wake et al, 1984) and three cases of postmolar choriocarcinoma (Wake et al, 1981; Sasaki et al, 1982; Fisher & Lawler, 1984). However, in a relatively large series Lawler & Fisher (1991) found no difference in the requirement for chemotherapy between patients with homozygous and heterozygous complete moles, and Mutter et al (1993), using PCR on paraffin-embedded tissue, have shown that there is no increase in risk of metastasis for Y-chromosome positive compared with Y-chromosome negative moles. Furthermore, two recent studies have shown a much higher prevalence of heterozygosity than had been reported previously (Fisher et al, 1989; Kovacs et al, 1991). Indeed, in Kovac's study genetic 'fingerprinting' of 22 complete moles showed heterozygosity in 40%. More interestingly half of these heterozygous moles contained *maternal* contributions. These findings, if substantiated by other groups, suggest that the pathogenesis of complete mole is more heterogeneous than previously suspected and that molar disease can arise from biparental fertilization events. The potential for persistent trophoblastic disease following partial hydatidiform mole has been much less clear cut. Several studies have shown no sequelae at all (Szulman & Surti, 1982; Lawler et al, 1982a; Lawler & Fisher, 1991) but numerous anecdotal cases have been published in which definite persistent trophoblastic disease has developed after partial mole (Elston, 1976; Stone & Bagshawe, 1976; Szulman et al, 1978, 1981b; Looi & Sivanesaratnam, 1981; Berkowitz et al, 1983; Gaber et al 1986; Bagshawe et al, 1990). There is no doubt, therefore, that partial mole does carry a risk but it is much less than that for complete mole (Bagshawe et al, 1990; Lage et al, 1991).

The comparative rarity of choriocarcinoma has limited the opportunities for detailed cytogenetic analysis, and no consistent pattern of abnormality has emerged. Aneuploidy was found in two cases by Makino et al (1963) and in choriocarcinoma transplanted to the hamster cheek pouch (Galton et al, 1963). Other studies have shown grossly abnormal karyotypes with a wide range of ploidies and a number of chromosomal re-arrangements (Wake et al, 1981; Sasaki et al, 1982; Sheppard et al, 1985; Lawler & Fisher, 1986). In a study by Davis & Foster (1984), using quinacrine staining on histological sections, 14 of 19 choriocarcinomas were found to be Y-body positive. Genetic examination has been carried out in very few cases of placental site trophoblastic tumour. Two tumours have been shown to be diploid (Eckstein et al, 1985; Lathrop et al, 1988) in contrast with the findings detailed above for choriocarcinoma.

One factor which has limited research into the aetiology of trophoblastic disease is the relative lack of a suitable experimental model. The spontaneous development of choriocarcinoma in animals is exceedingly rare, the first convincing account being in a rhesus monkey (Lindsey et al, 1969). The experimental induction of choriocarcinoma has also proved difficult. For example, the uterine tumour induced in pregnant rats by dimethylbenzanthracene (Stein-Werblowksy, 1960) and originally classified as choriocarcinoma has since been designated as sarcomatous (Bagshawe, 1969). Other experiments have met with limited success; for example, one animal out of a batch of pregnant armadillos given oral thalidomide developed metastatic choriocarcinoma (Marin-Padilla & Benirschke, 1963), and a tumour resembling choriocarcinoma was produced in two out of 15 pregnant rabbits after electro-coagulative destruction of the lateral thalamic nucleus (Kushima et al, 1967). However, in Japan several groups have been able to produce histologically confirmed malignant trophoblast by reverting to the use of dimethylbenzathracene in pregnant rats, with evidence of hormonal activity in some cases (Shintani et al, 1966; Miyamoto et al, 1972; Komuro, 1976; Tanaka, 1976). Because of the difficulties referred to above, other workers have preferred to develop techniques involving the heterologous transplantation of human choriocarcinoma cell lines (Hertz, 1967; Pattillo & Gey 1968; Lewis et al, 1969) and basic insights into the endocrinology, ultrastructure and immunology of trophoblastic neoplasia have been obtained (Hertz, 1978). Interestingly, expression of four onco-proteins — c-fms, c-fos, c-myc and c-ras — has been identified by in situ hybridization in BeWo and JaR cell lines (Muller et al, 1983; Bartocci et al, 1986; Rettenmier et al, 1986; Sarkar et al, 1986; Pollard et al, 1987). The c-fms proto-oncogene product is related to the receptor for colony stimulating factor 1 (CSF-1) (Sheer et al, 1985) and c-fms expression has been identified in the syncytiotrophoblast of hydatidiform moles (Yokoyama et al, 1988; Cheung et al, 1993). Cheung et al demonstrated a difference in the intensity of c-fms expression between normal placentas and hydatidiform mole and have suggested that c-fms may therefore have a rôle in the genesis of molar disease. This is an intriguing proposal which clearly requires further study and confirmation.

Since gestational choriocarcinoma is derived from the trophoblast, a fetal tissue, and proliferates in the maternal host, it occupies a unique status as a neoplastic allograft. The remarkable success of cytotoxic therapy in gestational trophoblastic disease, particularly in comparison with the far less favourable results in trophoblastic tumours of teratomatous origin, points strongly to a genetic disparity between the patient and the tumour. This is supported by morphological studies which show that a lymphoplasmacytoid cell infiltrate, similar to that seen in cellular allograft rejection, is present in approximately 90% of choriocarcinomas (Elston, 1969). The intensity of the infiltrate is related to prognosis, and survival is better in patients with a marked reaction (Elston, 1969; Elston & Bagshawe, 1973; Elston, 1976). Similar findings have been reported by Park (1971), Mogensen & Olsen (1973) and also by Ito et al (1981), who advocate a system which includes both intensity of cellular reaction and vascular permeation by tumour cells. Junaid et al (1976) found a cellular reaction in less than half their cases in Nigeria, with no correlation with prognosis. This may be due to the late presentation of many of their patients, since prognosis deteriorates markedly the longer the interval between the antecedent gestation and the start of treatment (Bagshawe, 1976).

Confirmation that the lymphoplasmacytoid infiltrates are the morphological expression of tumour rejection is as yet incomplete, and much of the evidence is conflicting. Although Bagshawe (1969) has demonstrated that patients with gestational choriocarcinoma may develop tolerance to skin grafts from their husbands, results of immunotherapy have been inconclusive (Hertz, 1978; Goldstein & Berkowitz, 1982).

Most current research has been concentrated on the immunogenicity of trophoblastic tissue, and in particular on antigenic differences between patients and their partners, using both the HLA and ABO systems (Berkowitz et al, 1986a,b; Lawler & Fisher, 1987a). Circulating immune complexes including paternal HLA antigens have been identified in the serum of women following evacuation of complete moles (Lahey et al, 1984; Lawler &

Fisher, 1987b). The majority of patients who require chemotherapy for postmolar trophoblastic disease have antibodies to paternal HLA antigens and it appears that hydatidiform mole may be more immunogenic than a normal conceptus. This may be related to the androgenetic origin of most complete moles which expose the maternal immune system to a double dose of paternal antigen. Class I HLA antigens are expressed in the stroma of chorionic villi (Faulk & Temple, 1976; Sunderland et al, 1981; Fisher & Lawler, 1984a) but not on trophoblastic cells, although class I determinants have been identified on non-villous trophoblast and proliferating trophoblast of complete moles (Sunderland et al, 1985; Bulmer et al, 1988). Several studies indicate that HLA class I antigens are also expressed in gestational choriocarcinoma (Tursz et al, 1981; Berkowitz et al, 1986a,b). Circulating immune complexes containing paternal antigens have been detected in the sera of patients with choriocarcinoma (Shaw et al, 1979; Lahey et al, 1984), and immunohistological studies have identified HLA class I antigen in malignant trophoblastic cells, including the BeWo cell line (Trowsdale et al, 1980; Anderson & Berkowitz, 1985; Berkowitz et al, 1986a,b; Bulmer et al, 1988).

Theoretically HLA compatibility may influence the progression of gestational trophoblastic neoplasia. If the patient and her partner are histocompatible the trophoblastic tumour that bears paternal antigens might not be immunogenic in the maternal host. Some groups have claimed that histocompatibility is more common with metastatic trophoblastic disease (Mogensen & Kissmeyer-Nielsen, 1968, 1971; Tomoda et al, 1976) but this has not been confirmed by others (Rudoph & Thomas, 1970; Lawler et al, 1971; Lewis & Terasaki, 1971; Mittal et al, 1975; Berkowitz et al, 1981; Yamashita et al, 1981); Lawler (1978) concluded that the HLA system does not exert a strong influence on the chances of a woman developing a trophoblastic tumour.

In contrast there is substantial evidence that the ABO blood group system is of great importance in trophoblastic disease, and affects both risk and prognosis (Bagshawe et al, 1971; Smith et al, 1993). An increased frequency of blood group A has been found in women with choriocarcinoma (Llewellyn-Jones, 1965; Dawood et al, 1971) and the risk for women of blood group A is increased if the spouse is group O rather than group A (Bagshawe, 1973). In a study of complete moles Lawler & Fisher (1987b) found that no patients who were ABO compatible with their partner required treatment while 30% of those with partners of unlike mating type progressed to trophoblastic disease. The risk of a group O woman developing choriocarcinoma is also increased if her spouse is group A, whilst patients of group B and AB have the worst prognosis (Bagshawe, 1976). This data is incorporated into a prognostic index used at Charing Cross Hospital, London (Newlands et al, 1992), which has been shown to be more accurate than anatomical staging alone (Smith et al, 1993).

A number of human trophoblast-associated membrane antigens have been characterized in recent years, including the trophoblast-leucocyte common antigen system (termed TLX antigens) and placental-type alkaline phosphatase (PLAP) (Johnson et al, 1981; McLaughlin et al, 1982; Faulk & McIntyre 1983; Bulmer & Johnson, 1985). Both have been identified in molar trophoblast (Berkowitz et al, 1986b; Bulmer et al, 1988) but PLAP was not found in choriocarcinoma by Bulmer et al (1988), although only seven cases were studied. The TLX antigen system appears to have a central rôle in regulating maternal-fetal immunological interactions within placental and uterine tissues (Faulk & McIntyre, 1983) and it is likely that the expression of both TLX and PLAP on molar trophoblast may be important in the immunobiology of gestational trophoblastic disease (Berkowitz et al, 1986b). Although our understanding of these immunobiological aspects is still limited, further investigation may help to characterize those aggressive molar pregnancies and gestational tumours which require intensive hormonal follow-up and chemotherapy.

HYDATIDIFORM MOLE

Hydatidiform mole may be regarded as an abnormal product of conception which is usually associated with a 'blighted' ovum (Elston, 1978; Fox, 1989). Although the great majority of patients who abort a hydatidiform mole have no further sequelae, the lesion is included in the spectrum of trophoblastic disease because of its close aetiological link with choriocarcinoma. Persistent trophoblastic disease occurs in no more than 10% of patients with a hydatidiform mole (Womack & Elston, 1985), but a mole is the preceding gestation in at least 50% of cases of choriocarcinoma (Elston, 1978). Unfortunately it is not possible at the time of molar abortion to predict which patients are at risk for the development of persistent trophoblastic disease (Elston & Bagshawe, 1972a) and there is no alternative to clinical follow-up using urinary or serum gonadotrophin assay in order to identify at an early stage those patients likely to require cytotoxic therapy (Bagshawe et al, 1986). Since follow-up is recommended for a minimum of 6 months and often 12 months, during which time contraception should be practised (Bagshawe et al, 1986; Gal & Friedman, 1987; Newlands et al, 1992), it is not a procedure to be undertaken lightly and accurate patient selection is vital. For patients with the classical type of hydatidiform mole this poses few problems either clinically or pathologically. Genuine diagnostic difficulty does occur in the assessment of products of conception in which focal hydropic change is present (Rushton, 1981) and it has been shown that pathologists are poor at recognizing correlations between villous morphology and karyotypic abnormalities (Van Lijnschoten et al, 1993). It is also clear that consistency and reproducibility of diagnosis are poor when histological criteria alone are used to distinguish between hydropic abortion and partial hydatidiform mole and partial mole and complete mole (Javey et al, 1979; Messerli et al, 1987; Conran et al, 1993; Howat et al, 1993). Howat et al (1993) concluded that the histological criteria were either not being applied correctly or they are lacking in practical use. Similar findings were obtained by Conran et al (1993) who, however, achieved good agreement when data concerning DNA content (determined by flow cytometry) was included in their analysis.

In this situation it is the histopathologist who assumes considerable responsibility in the management of the patient. The choice lies between oversupervision of patients who have no risk of developing choriocarcinoma and the danger of inadequate follow-up of patients who are at increased risk of developing postmolar trophoblastic disease. Park (1971) and Elston (1978, 1991) have proposed that, at a practical level, the distinction between a simple hydropic abortion and a molar gestation should be made on the characteristics of the trophoblast. This has been confirmed by Howat et al (1993), who found that the most useful histological feature in partial mole is the presence of an atypical circumferential growth pattern of trophoblast rather than the polar accentuation seen in normal first-trimester pregnancies.

The clinicopathological features of complete and partial hydatidiform mole are discussed below.

Clinical features

A molar gestation may occur at any time during the childbearing period, but there is an increased risk for women over the age of 40 and at the lower end of the reproductive range (Smalbraak, 1957; Yen and MacMahon, 1968; Elston, 1978; Bagshawe et al, 1986). It appears that the risk for women under the age of 20 is greater with a complete mole than a partial mole (Jacobs et al, 1982a; Szulman & Surti, 1982). The proportion of partial moles in retrospective series varies enormously, from 3% up to 35% (Berkowitz et al, 1979; Czernobilsky et al, 1982; Womack & Elston, 1985; Bagshawe et al, 1986, 1990), whilst Lawler & Fisher (1991) found that just under 25% of moles in a prospective study were of partial type. It is probable that many partial moles are overlooked, either because products of conception are not routinely sent for histological examination, or due to underdiagnosis by histopathologists.

The main presenting symptom in complete molar gestations is vaginal bleeding towards the end of the first trimester (Newlands et al, 1992). Abdominal distension and uterine enlargement of a size greater than expected for dates are present in about 50% of patients and the pre-

eclampsia syndrome in about 25% (Lurain, 1987). Ovarian enlargement is an uncommon finding, usually caused by theca-lutein cysts. Fetal heart sounds are absent, with the very rare exception of co-existing twin pregnancy. A clinical diagnosis of complete mole should always be confirmed by ultrasonography before evacuation (Reid et al, 1983; Lurain, 1987); in combination with an elevated serum hCG level a diagnostic accuracy of nearly 90% is achieved (Romero et al, 1985).

In contrast a pre-evacuation diagnosis of partial mole is made in less than 10% of cases (Czernobilsky et al, 1982; Szulman & Surti, 1982) and the majority are not diagnosed until products are examined histologically. Similar clinical features to complete mole may be present but to a lesser degree. Fetal heart sounds may or may not be heard. If the diagnosis is suspected clinically, ultrasonography should be performed, but convincing evidence of villous hydropia will be found in only a minority of cases (Naumoff et al, 1981).

Urinary and serum levels of hCG are always elevated in a molar gestation. The level varies markedly from case to case, and may even be within the range for a normal pregnancy, but serum values in excess of 1×10^6 IU/l are not uncommon in a patient with a complete mole. Rather lower levels are usually found in partial mole. It is clearly of considerable practical value to obtain hCG measurements in patients suspected of having a molar gestation to serve as a baseline for subsequent follow-up.

Initial clinical management is evacuation of the uterus, preferably by suction rather than curettage (Bagshawe et al, 1986). A second evacuation is only recommended if indicated by clinical symptoms such as bleeding, or if there is ultrasonographic evidence of residual molar tissue (Newlands et al, 1992).

Morphology

Complete hydatidiform mole

Macroscopic appearances. The gross appearances of a complete hydatidiform mole are very characteristic. The 'bunch of grapes' appearance from which the name is derived (Figs 52.1 and 52.2) is due to the conversion of chorionic villi into strings and clusters of vesicles which vary in diameter from approximately 1–30 mm. The molar placenta is increased in weight, often in excess of 2000 g. It is rare for a gestational sac to be identified but occasionally the remains of a chorionic cavity or even fetal tissue may be identified and there are a number of case reports in the literature of complete mole and co-existing twin pregnancy (Jones & Lauersen, 1975; Suzuki et al, 1980; Fisher et al, 1982; Vejerslev et al, 1986; Deaton et al, 1989; Miller et al, 1993) and triplet pregnancy (Azuma et al, 1992). The author has anecdotal evidence that due to greater clinical awareness and use of ultrasonography,

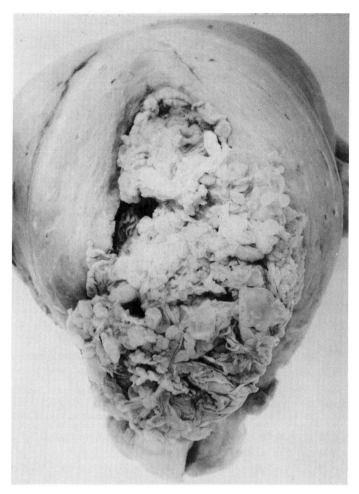

Fig. 52.1 An opened uterus containing a complete hydatidiform mole within the endometrial cavity. (From Fox H 1978 *Pathology of the placenta*, Saunders, Philadelphia. Reproduced by permission of Prof. Fox and W.B. Saunders Co.)

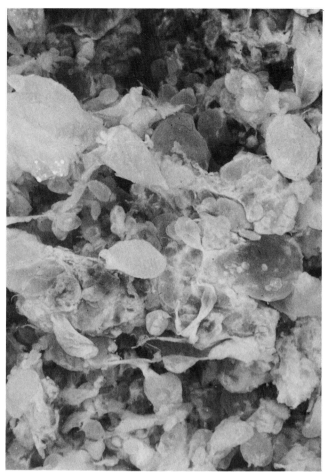

Fig. 52.2 Close-up view of another complete mole to show the variation in size of vesicles.

an increasing number of patients with complete mole are presenting at an earlier stage than previously. In these cases the classical gross appearances may not be fully developed, leading to an erroneous assumption that the changes represent a partial rather than a complete mole (Paradinas, 1994).

Microscopical appearances. The microscopical appearances are distinctive. The chorionic villi become distended by the accumulation of stromal fluid, resulting in a variable degeneration of the connective tissue, from mild oedema to central liquefaction (Fig. 52.3). The enlarged villi are generally rounded but collapsed villi may have an irregular shape (Figs 52.3 and 52.4). There is usually a complete absence of fetal stromal blood vessels; Elston (1970) found residual vessels in only 12% of cases. The appearance of the trophoblast is variable. In some hydropic villi it may appear flattened and atrophic (Fig. 52.4), but proliferation of cytotrophoblast is always seen. This may be focal and of a slight degree (Fig. 52.3) or more extensive and marked (Fig. 52.5), and is accompanied by

a lacy network of syncytiotrophoblast. Before the introduction of accurate methods for the measurement of hCG it was advocated that the morphological appearances of the trophoblast of complete moles could be used to predict which patients were likely to progress to develop choriocarcinoma (Hertig and Sheldon, 1947; Hertig & Mansell, 1956). Hertig and colleagues proposed a grading system, initially with six categories and subsequently with three, and claimed that there is an increasing risk of malignancy with increasing trophoblastic 'hyperplasia' and atypia. Although some studies have supported these findings (Schiffer et al, 1960; Douglas, 1962; Deligdisch et al, 1978; Sugimori et al, 1980) most have not (Hunt et al, 1953; Smalbraak, 1957, 1959; Logan & Motyloff, 1958; Tow & Yung, 1967; Elston & Bagshawe, 1972a; Genest et al, 1991). Elston & Bagshawe examined a series of hydatidiform moles, which, because of the referral nature of their unit, had a higher than average rate of subsequent choriocarcinoma (21% compared with 2%). They found no comparable excess of grade 3 moles, nor was

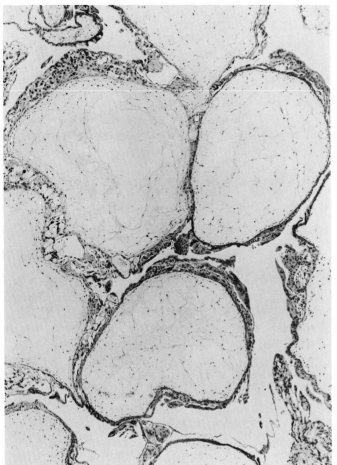

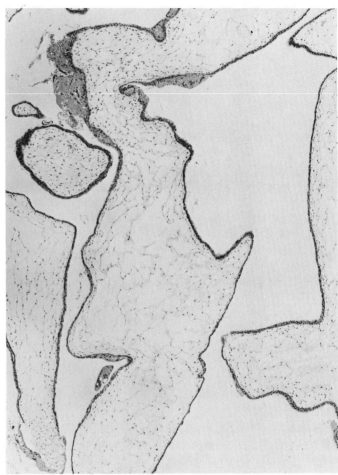

Fig. 52.3 Complete hydatidiform mole exhibiting villous hydropia with central liquefaction and absent stromal blood vessels. There is a slight degree of trophoblastic hyperplasia. H & E × 40.

Fig. 52.4 Part of another complete hydatidiform mole in which much of the trophoblast is atrophic. Very slight focal trophoblastic proliferation is present, at the top left. H & E × 40.

there any increase in the number of choriocarcinomas derived from the grade 3 moles which did occur. They concluded that there is no value in attempting to predict potential malignant behaviour from the histological appearances of a hydatidiform mole and this view became generally accepted although Hertig's teaching still had its adherents, mainly in the United States (Driscoll, 1977; Deligdisch et al, 1978). Genest et al (1991), from the New England Trophoblastic Disease Center, have now confirmed Elston & Bagshawe's work, and it is to be hoped that histological grading of hydatidiform mole will finally be abandoned as utterly inappropriate.

In summary, the histological diagnosis of a complete hydatidiform mole is relatively straightforward if the pathologist receives the total amount of tissue evacuated. This is usually the case when modern disposal vacuum suction systems are used, but if a small sample only is sent to the laboratory it is important to obtain clear details of the original gross appearances.

Ultrastructure. A number of ultrastructural studies have been carried out on hydatidiform moles but the results have been rather inconclusive and conflicting, probably due to problems in the selection of material and the small numbers of cases studied. Wynn & Davies (1964b) examined a single mole and concluded that in general the trophoblast resembled that of the normal placenta. An intermediate trophoblastic cell was prominent, with a spectrum of transition from typical cytotrophoblast to mature secretory syncytiotrophoblast. They considered that the hydropic change in hydatidiform mole was dependent on the functional activity of the overlying trophoblast, ceasing if the trophoblast became atrophic or degenerate. Most other studies have confirmed the similarity of molar cytotrophoblastic cells to the normal (Gonzalez-Angulo et at, 1966; Okudaira & Strauss, 1967; Fox & Kharkongor, 1971; Sen et al, 1973). The appearances of molar syncytiotrophoblast appear to be more variable and abnormal (Ockleford & Clode, 1983). Prominent and irregular surface microvilli are frequently seen and lipid droplets are increased (Fig. 52.6) with an expanded dilated endo-

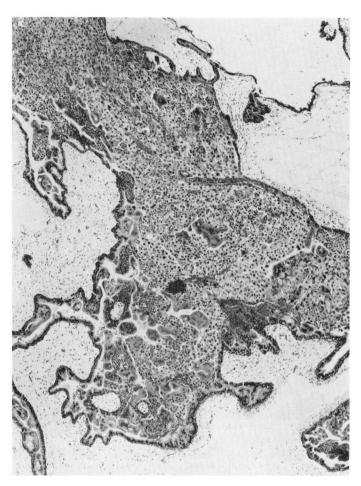

Fig. 52.5 Complete hydatidiform mole showing marked proliferation of cytotrophoblast, accompanied by syncytiotrophoblast. H & E × 40.

plasmic reticulum (Gonzalez-Angulo et al, 1966; Fox & Kharkongor, 1971; Sen et al, 1973). Ockleford & Clode (1983), using scanning electronmicroscopy, have found abnormal microvillous structures which they refer to as 'microgibbosities'. Mitochondrial appearances have been remarkably variable: small with irregular cristae (Larsen, 1973), normal (Sen et al, 1973), and enlarged (Fox & Kharkongor, 1971). The presence of intermediate trophoblastic cells was noted by Gonzalez-Angulo et al, and by Sen et al, but not by Fox & Kharkongor.

There has been little speculation on the significance of these ultrastructural findings; Fox & Kharkongor (1971) concluded that the appearances seen by them were related to trophoblastic hyperplasia rather than neoplasia, whilst Ockleford & Clode (1983) suggested that the microgibbous elongated microvilli were consistent with a dysplastic epithelium.

Partial hydatidiform mole

Macroscopic appearances. The gross appearances

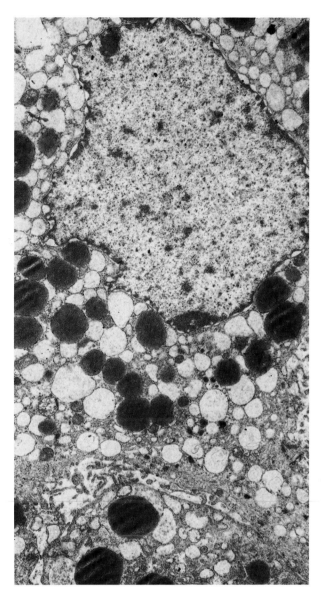

Fig. 52.6 Electronmicrograph of syncytiotrophoblast from a complete mole. There is abundant dilated endoplasmic reticulum with numerous lipid droplets. × 12 750.

are variable. The placental tissue is never as bulky as with a complete mole, and usually has the same volume as any other spontaneous abortion. In some cases the placental tissue appears normal save for occasional small vesicles (Fig. 52.7) whilst in others, although scanty tissue only is obtained, it all appears vesicular. A recognizable fetus, or fetal parts, is frequently present.

Microscopical appearances. Microscopically there is a variable degree of hydropic change which mirrors the gross appearances, and areas with a relatively normal immature structure are often found. Blood vessels containing fetal cells may be preserved. In the hydropic villi central cisternal formation is a characteristic feature and

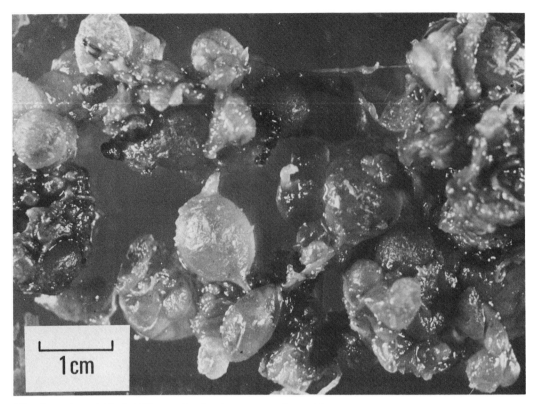

Fig. 52.7 A partial hydatidiform mole, showing scanty molar vesicles.

the outline is frequently indented or scalloped, producing a 'geographical' outline with infoldings resembling 'fjords' (Figs 52.8 and 52.9). So-called trophoblastic 'inclusions' may be evident in the villous mesenchyme; these are probably due to tangential cutting of infolded fjords (Figs 52.10 and 52.11). The component which particularly distinguishes a partial mole from a simple hydropic abortion is the presence of trophoblastic hyperplasia and its distinctive circumferential pattern (compare Fig. 52.13 with Fig. 52.14). This is a subtle change and it has been confirmed by proliferating cell nuclear antigen (PCNA) studies that the degree of trophoblastic proliferation in partial moles is at a low level (Suresh et al, 1993). Many villi show little or no hyperplasia or at most a focal proliferation (Fig. 52.12) whilst in other villi the change may be more extensive (Fig. 52.13). Cytotrophoblastic cells may be difficult to identify and the most characteristic change is the presence of multiple circumferential collections of syncytiotrophoblastic cells (Fig. 52.13). Care must be taken not to mistake the active trophoblast seen at the poles of the villi, mainly in first-trimester abortions, and due to tangential cutting, for molar proliferation (Fig. 52.15).

In summary, no single morphological feature can be considered entirely pathognomonic for the diagnosis of partial hydatidiform mole. The presence of irregular, scalloped outlines to hydropic villi and cisternal formations are suggestive of the diagnosis. If these are seen a careful assessment of the appearances of the trophoblast should be made, and there is general agreement that a diagnosis of partial mole should only be entertained if a definite circumferential pattern is seen (Szulman, 1987; Lage, 1990; Elston, 1991; Conran et al, 1993; Howat et al, 1993). If there is any doubt all available material must be sectioned, and Lage (1990) has suggested that up to 10 blocks may be required before a diagnosis of partial mole can be excluded.

Differential diagnosis of hydropic products of conception

In ideal circumstances the diagnosis of hydatidiform mole would be made on the basis of clinical features combined with histological and genetic data, but this is not a practical proposition for the vast majority of cases, especially as fresh tissue is required for cytogenetic analysis. For this reason a number of other techniques have been investigated to evaluate their usefulness in aiding the diagnosis of hydropic products of conception.

Flow cytometry, using the technique described by Hedley et al (1983), can be carried out on DNA extracted from paraffin blocks to determine ploidy status. Routine histological material is therefore available for analysis and several studies have confirmed the diploid status of the

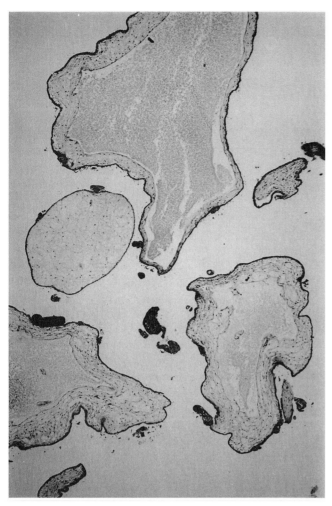

Fig. 52.8 Partial hydatidiform mole. Note the irregular 'scalloped' outline, cisternal formation and scanty circumferential collections of trophoblast. H & E × 36.

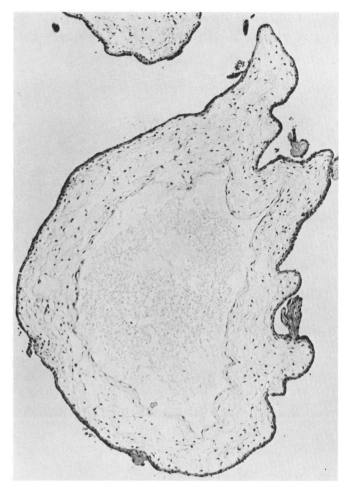

Fig. 52.9 Villus from a partial mole showing central cisternal formation and an indented outline. H & E × 80. (Reprinted with permission from Elston, 1989.)

great majority of complete moles and the presence of triploidy in most partial moles (Fisher et al, 1987; Hemming et al, 1987; Lage et al, 1988, 1991; Koenig et al, 1993). This technique is therefore a useful alternative to cytogenetics, particularly in the distinction of partial mole from complete mole (Bagshawe et al, 1990). For example, as pointed out earlier, a complete mole, evacuated at a relatively early gestational age, may lack the classical gross vesicular appearances and be mistaken microscopically for a partial mole; diploidy, established by flow cytometry, would provide strong evidence in support of the diagnosis of complete rather than partial mole.

Chromosomal aberrations at the cellular level can be demonstrated by in situ hybridization (ISH) using chromosome specific probes, so-called 'interphase cytogenetics'. Van de Kaa and colleagues (1991) used this technique to study paraffin sections from a small number of hydatidiform moles. By using probes for the centromeric region of chromosomes I and X and the Q arm of

Y they demonstrated that it is a useful technique which enables chromosome ploidy analysis to be established, with preservation of histological appearances. They have now applied the technique to a larger series of cases of hydatidiform mole, complete and partial, and compared the results with cases of hydropic abortion (Van de Kaa et al, 1993). In combination with DNA cytometry they have found DNA polyploidy in complete moles with a high GO/ G1 exceeding rate, significantly different from hydropic abortions, and concluded that these techniques are useful in distinguishing those two entities. However, no significant differences were found between triploid partial moles and hydropic abortions. The finding that a high proportion of complete moles in this series exhibited polyploidy rather than diploidy, as reported in all previous studies, clearly requires further confirmation. The polymerase chain reaction (PCR) has been used to detect variable number tandem repeat sequences in DNA (Jeffreys et al, 1988) and by using the appropriate primers PCR can also

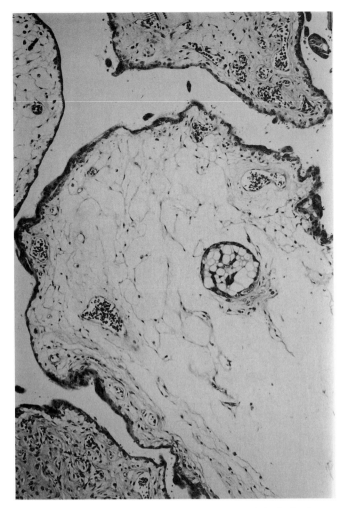

Fig. 52.10 Villus from a partial mole. A trophoblastic inclusion is present and blood vessels containing red cells are also seen. H & E × 90. (Reprinted with permission from Elston, 1989.)

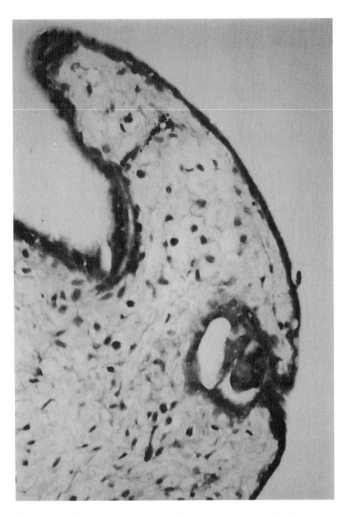

Fig. 52.11 Villus from a partial mole, showing a trophoblastic 'inclusion' produced by tangential cutting of an infolded fjord. H & E × 225. (Reprinted with permission from Elston 1989.)

be used to detect Y chromosome specific sequences and thus identify the sex of an individual (Witt & Erickson, 1989). Fukuyama et al (1991) and Azuma et al (1991) have demonstrated the androgenetic nature of a small number of complete hydatidiform moles using this technique and two further studies have confirmed the utility of PCR in this respect, using DNA extracted from formalin-fixed paraffin-embedded material (Fisher & Newlands, 1993; Lane et al, 1993) in both complete and partial mole. It appears that by identifying paternal contributions to the molar genome PCR has considerable potential in the diagnosis and classification of problem cases of hydatidiform mole.

Facilities for such specialized techniques as flow cytometry, ISH and PCR are, of course, not available in most routine laboratories, but in cases of diagnostic difficulty arrangements should be made for paraffin blocks to be sent to expert centres for analysis.

Since the morphological appearances of typical hyda-

tidiform moles, especially those of complete type, indicate that a degree of trophoblastic proliferation occurs, it is theoretically possible that markers of cell proliferation might be of diagnostic value. It has been shown that silver-stained nucleolar organizer region-associated proteins (AgNORs) tend to be more numerous in the nuclei of malignant tumours than benign tumours or hyperplastic conditions (Crocker & Skilbeck, 1987; Smith & Crocker, 1988; Suarez et al, 1989), but there has been debate as to whether AgNOR counts represent cellular ploidy or proliferation. Suresh et al (1990) have investigated the possible use of AgNOR counts in distinguishing hydropic abortions from hydatidiform moles. They found that AgNOR counts could not be correlated with proliferative activity and concluded that they were more likely to be a reflection of ploidy status. Although this study has not yet been confirmed by others it appears that AgNOR counts do not provide useful information in the diagnosis of molar trophoblastic disease. Proliferating cell nuclear

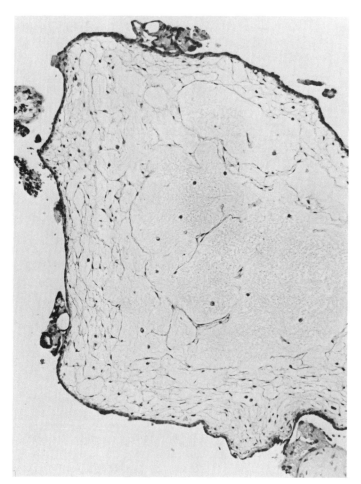

Fig. 52.12 Another villus from the same case as Fig. 52.9. Note the scanty but circumferential collections of syncytiotrophoblast. H & E × 100.

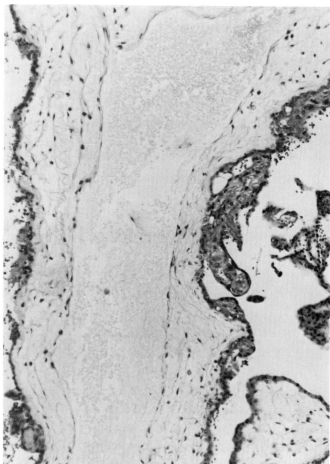

Fig. 52.13 Villus from another partial mole in which the circumferential trophoblastic collections are more prominent. H & E × 108.

antigen (PCNA) is a highly conserved 36 kd nuclear protein which is an auxiliary protein of DNA polymerase delta and is present in proliferating cells (Mathews et al, 1984; Bravo et al, 1987). The monoclonal antibody PC10 recognizes nuclear PCNA in routinely fixed paraffin-embedded tissues and has been used to study cell proliferation in a variety of tissues (Hall et al, 1990; Hall & Woods, 1990). Cheung et al (1993) have examined the expression of PC10 in choriocarcinoma, complete and partial mole and spontaneous abortions. They found much higher counts in choriocarcinoma than in the other three entities, but no difference between the moles and the abortions. Similarly Suresh et al (1993) have shown that there is no difference in PC10 expression between spontaneous abortion and partial mole; indeed their results indicated that trophoblastic *proliferation* is not a feature of partial mole. It must be concluded that PCNA expression is of no value in the distinction between spontaneous abortion and molar disease.

In conclusion, the great majority of cases of hydatidi-form mole will continue to be diagnosed on morphological grounds alone, but, increasingly, newer molecular biological techniques will be necessary to evaluate difficult or borderline cases. Those techniques which can be applied to formalin-fixed paraffin-embedded material clearly have the greater potential in routine practice, and in this respect flow cytometry, interphase cytogenetics using in situ hybridization and the polymerase chain reaction show the most promise.

Prognosis

Although hydatidiform mole is properly classified as a specific type of abortion, and is not a neoplastic condition, it is regarded as a premalignant condition because of its close association with choriocarcinoma. The careful follow-up of patients with hydatidiform mole has undoubtedly contributed to the dramatic reduction in mortality from choriocarcinoma, but paradoxically there is an unnecessary anxiety concerning the overall prognosis of

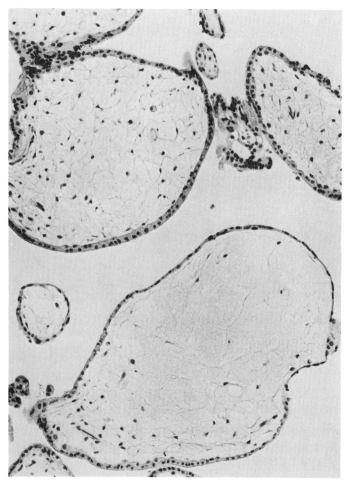

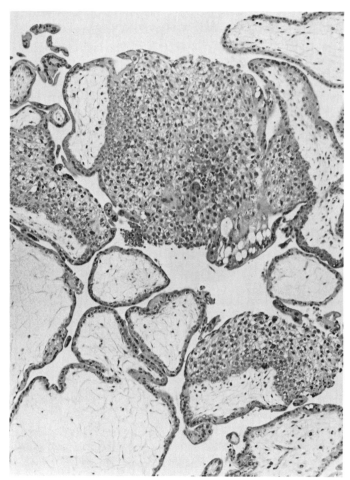

Fig. 52.14 Hydropic abortion. The villus at the top left shows slight stromal hydropia but the trophoblast is relatively normal. The enlarged villus below exhibits moderate hydropic change with early central liquefaction and attenuated trophoblast. H & E × 160.

Fig. 52.15 First-trimester spontaneous abortion, with apparent proliferation of cytotrophoblast at poles of villi due to tangential cutting. H & E × 100.

molar gestations. It must be stressed that the majority of patients with hydatidiform mole have no sequelae, and in modern clinical practice persistent trophoblastic disease ensues in no more than 10% of patients (Curry et al, 1975; Womack & Elston, 1985; Bagshawe et al, 1986; Lurain & Sciarra, 1991). There would be a significant benefit in reduction of unnecessary follow-up if the small group of patients who will develop persistent trophoblastic disease could be identified at the time of the original diagnosis. It has already been pointed out (p. 1606) that this cannot be achieved from assessment of morphological appearances of the molar trophoblast (Elston & Bagshawe, 1972a; Genest et al, 1991). Hemming et al (1988) investigated the value of flow cytometry in this respect. Although they found that cases which developed persistent trophoblastic disease all had high hyperdiploid fractions, the values fell within the range for all diploid hydatidiform moles. The authors concluded that flow cytometry cannot be used to predict the possible behaviour of hydatidiform mole in an individual patient. Methods which provide an

estimate of cellular proliferation such as AgNOR counts (Suresh et al, 1990) and PCNA (Cheung et al, 1993) have also proved unhelpful, and it must be concluded that there is no alternative to careful follow-up for all patients with complete hydatidiform mole. In the United Kingdom this is facilitated by the registration of patients with hydatidiform mole with the Royal College of Obstetricians and Gynaecologists, which ensures access to accurate radioimmunoassay in specialized laboratories (Bagshawe et al, 1986; Newlands et al, 1992). Patients are monitored by regular assay of hCG levels (urinary or serum) so that treatment can be instituted promptly when indicated. When the hCG level returns to normal patients are advised not to start another pregnancy until the hCG level has been normal for at least six months. Bagshawe et al (1986) found that when the hCG level fell to normal within eight weeks of evacuation follow-up could safely be limited to six months. In those patients where the hCG level is still elevated beyond eight weeks from the date of evacuation follow-up is continued for two years. This caution is highlighted by a recent report from Elmer et al (1993). They cited the case of a patient who required chemotherapy for persistent trophoblastic disease after hCG levels had returned to normal within 25 weeks of the evacuation of a complete hydatidiform mole and remained normal for over a year before rising again. The main criteria for treatment are a raised serum hCG (> 20 000 IU/l) more than 4 weeks after evacuation, rising hCG values, prolonged uterine haemorrhage and radiological evidence of metastatic lesions (Newlands et al, 1992). Following a complete mole, between 7 and 8% of patients require chemotherapy (Bagshawe et al, 1986; Newlands et al, 1992), and the mortality is extremely low at 0.2% Bagshawe et al, 1986).

The case for adequate follow-up for patients with complete hydatidiform mole is clearly established, but until comparatively recently much less has been known about the behaviour of partial moles. Some groups suggested that follow-up is not required (Vassilakos & Kajii, 1976; Lawler et al, 1982a) and data from two series of patients appeared to support this view (Szulman & Surti, 1982; Lawler & Fisher, 1987a). The total number of cases reported in this way was much too small to reach a definite conclusion, however, and a number of anecdotal case reports have demonstrated that persistent trophoblastic disease does develop after partial hydatidiform mole. Cases with histopathological confirmation include metastatic molar disease (Elston, 1976), invasive mole (Szulman et al, 1981b; Gaber et al, 1986) and, probably, choriocarcinoma (Looi & Sivanesaratnam, 1981; Gardner & Lage, 1992). Several series of patients who required chemotherapy for persistent trophoblastic disease after the evacuation of partial moles have now been reported, from New England, U.S.A. (Berkowitz et al, 1983; Berkowitz & Goldstein, 1988; Berkowitz et al, 1988; Rice et al, 1990), Charing Cross Hospital, U.K. (Bagshawe et al, 1990) and Aichi Prefecture, Japan (Goto et al, 1993), although they provide greatly differing estimates of the risk — 6.6% (New England), 2.8% (Aichi) and 0.5% (Charing Cross). This probably reflects differences in referral pattern and criteria for post-evacuation chemotherapy. There is, however, no doubt that patients with partial mole do require to be followed up in the same way as those with complete mole. In some centres the protocol is less rigid than that for complete mole and surveillance may cease as soon as hCG levels return to normal (Szulman, 1987).

INVASIVE HYDATIDIFORM MOLE

An invasive mole can be defined as a molar gestation in which hydropic villous trophoblast penetrates the myometrium or its blood vessels (Hertig & Mansell, 1956). By implication, this also includes cases of hydatidiform mole in which molar 'metastasis' occurs.

Ewing (1910) separated invasive mole (he used the term 'chorioadenoma destruens') from choriocarcinoma on clinicopathological grounds, since the presence of formed molar villi was a distinguishing histological feature which was matched by the more hopeful prognosis. This distinction has been accepted by most authorities (Hertig & Mansell, 1956; Ober et al, 1971; Park, 1971; Elston, 1991; Silverberg & Kurman, 1992). Dehner (1980) has commented that invasive mole has ceased to be an important clinicopathological entity, because hysterectomy is rarely performed now in trophoblastic disease and invasion is difficult to assess in curettings. Whilst these points have some validity they do not provide a serious argument for abandoning the concept of invasive mole. Patients with proven invasive mole rarely require follow-up cytotoxic therapy, whilst patients with choriocarcinoma invariably do. Although the diagnosis will be made less frequently than in the past there are strong practical reasons for retaining invasive mole as a diagnostic category separate from choriocarcinoma.

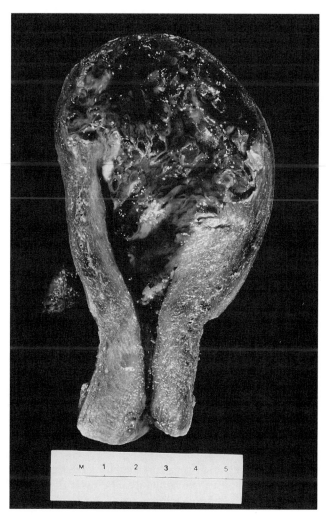

Fig. 52.16 Invasive mole of the increta type. Molar villi penetrate into the myometrium at the fundus. (Reproduced by kind permission of Professor D. Hourihan.)

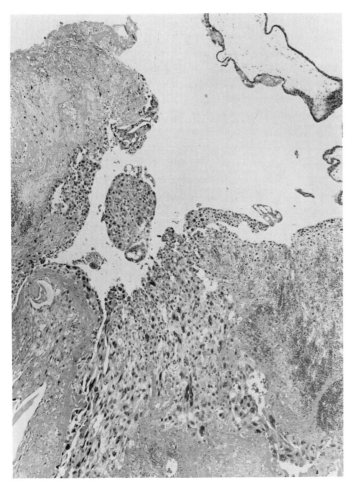

Fig. 52.17   Invasive mole of the accreta type. This field shows the molar implantation site with a villus above and trophoblast attached to decidua below. H & E × 40.

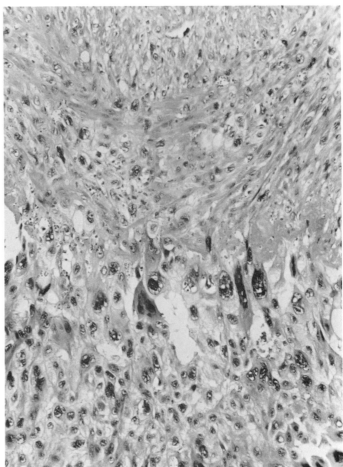

Fig. 52.18   Same case as Fig. 52.17. Proliferating trophoblast above is attached to myometrium below. H & E × 100.

The great majority of invasive moles occur in association with complete hydatidiform mole, but anecdotal cases occurring after a partial mole have been reported (Szulman et al, 1981b; Gaber et al, 1986).

Morphology

Macroscopic appearances.   The gross appearances are variable and dependent on the extent of invasion. There may be little abnormality in the uterine cavity except for the presence of haemorrhage and vesicles at the implantation site. A haemorrhagic cavity of variable size may be present, with obvious penetration into the myometrium (Fig. 52.16). Less commonly the molar tissue extends so deeply that the uterus is perforated, or there is extension into adjacent structures such as the broad ligament. In some cases the original hydatidiform mole is still present within the uterine cavity.

Microscopical appearances.   Microscopically the main diagnostic feature is the presence within the myometrium of molar villi showing trophoblastic proliferation.

The villi may vary considerably in size and occasionally are inconspicuous. It is therefore important that in any uterus containing a proliferative trophoblastic lesion a careful search should be made for molar villi in order to avoid an erroneous diagnosis of choriocarcinoma. The amount of trophoblastic proliferation is also variable, and although there is usually at least a moderate degree of hyperplasia, in some cases little trophoblastic overgrowth is seen. In the majority of cases a florid placental site reaction will persist, and this should not be mistaken for choriocarcinomatous invasion.

Hertig (1950) drew an analogy between the degree of invasion of an invasive mole and placenta accreta, increta and percreta. It is probable that in all hydatidiform moles there is at least a technical breach of the decidua and therefore minimal invasion, and the sooner a hysterectomy is performed after evacuation of a mole the more likely it is that evidence of local invasion will be found (Gore & Hertig, 1967).

In the accreta type of invasive mole, seen most frequently when the original hydatidiform mole is still con-

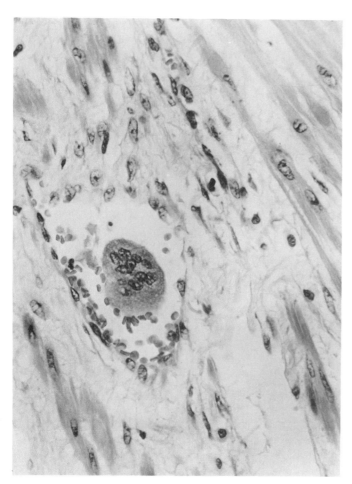

Fig. 52.19 A blood vessel deep in the myometrium contains a small trophoblastic embolus. Same case as Figs 52.17 and 52.18. H & E × 390.

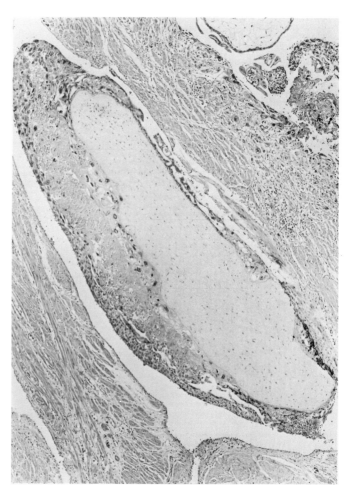

Fig. 52.20 Invasive mole of the increta type. A molar villus lies within a dilated venous sinus deep within the myometrium. H & E × 40.

tained in the uterus at hysterectomy, or where the mole was aborted shortly before hysterectomy, molar villi are attached directly to superficial myometrium without intervening decidua (Figs 52.17 and 52.18). There is no deep invasion of the myometrium, although small trophoblastic emboli may be found (Fig. 52.19).

The majority of cases fall into the increta category. Hydropic villi extend deeply into the myometrium, but the serosa remains intact. Most of the invasion takes place through dilated venous channels (Fig. 52.20) and direct myometrial muscle invasion is limited. Foci of haemorrhage may occur but are usually confined to the molar tissue rather than myometrium.

In a minority of cases molar villi penetrate through the full thickness of the uterine wall (percreta type). This results in uterine perforation or extension into the adjacent parametrium.

Ultrastructure. The ultrastructure of invasive mole has been studied by Wynn & Harris (1967) and Okudaira & Strauss (1967). Apart from evidence of more active trophoblast the appearances are similar to those seen in a complete hydatidiform mole.

Metastatic lesions

For most tumours the development of metastases is one of the main criteria for the diagnosis of malignancy. Because trophoblastic disease covers a wide spectrum of processes which includes both neoplastic and non-neoplastic conditions, such a simplistic view is inappropriate. Trophoblastic cells have been detected in the peripheral blood of pregnant women (Couone et al, 1984; Mueller et al, 1990) and deportation of benign trophoblastic fragments has also been described in normal pregnancy (Attwood & Park, 1961) and in eclampsia (Schmorl, 1893; Veit, 1901; Bardawil & Toy, 1959). Metastatic lesions are also well recognized in molar pregnancies, but it is extremely important to appreciate that their development does not necessarily mean that choriocarcinoma has supervened; indeed they more usually indicate simply that the mole is invasive.

The reported frequency of metastases in hydatidiform mole varies widely, with a range from 24% (Greene, 1959) to 40% (Wilson et al, 1961). In a selected series of patients in the United Kingdom, Elston (1970) found a

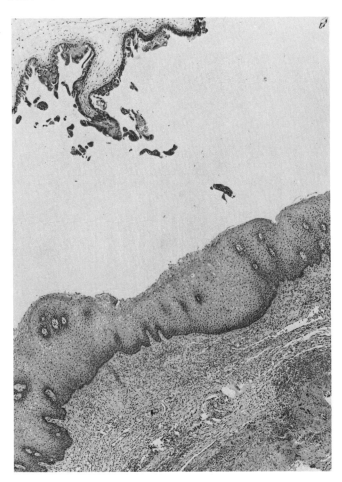

Fig. 52.21 Molar 'metastasis' to the vagina. The molar villus was obtained at biopsy of a haemorrhagic vaginal nodule, part of which is visible at the bottom right. H & E × 40.

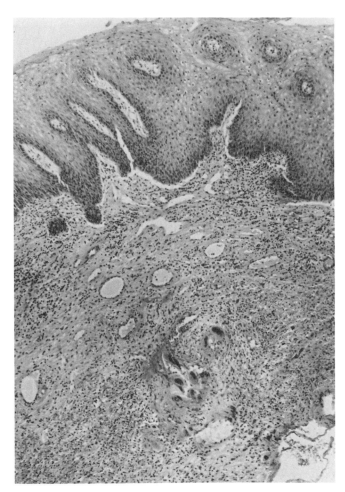

Fig. 52.22 Benign trophoblastic deportation in a patient with a hydatidiform mole. This is a vaginal nodule showing part of a haemorrhagic cavity in which syncytial giant cells are seen. H & E × 40.

frequency of 36% which agrees closely with the figure of 35% obtained by Tow (1966) from a review of the literature. Such figures are clearly an overestimate of the true frequency, due to selection of patients who have developed complications, and it must be re-emphasized that persistent trophoblastic disease, which includes patients with metastatic lesions, only occurs in approximately 10% of patients with hydatidiform mole (Womack & Elston, 1985; Bagshawe et al, 1986).

In the majority of cases of molar disease metastatic lesions occur in the lungs. Their detection is usually based on clinical assessment and radiological evidence, without histological confirmation. There are, however, a number of reports in which lung lesions have been excised or biopsied and shown to be composed of either hydropic molar villi or benign deported trophoblastic fragments (Delfs, 1957; Reed et al, 1959; Jacobson & Enzer, 1959; Wilson et al, 1961; Ring, 1972; Johnson et al, 1979). Vaginal metastases which contain molar villi or benign trophoblast have also been recorded (Haines, 1955; Bardawil et al, 1957; Dinh-De & Minh, 1961; Hsu et al, 1962; Thiele & de Alvarez, 1962; Elston, 1976) (Figs

52.21–52.23), and rarer metastatic sites include brain (Ishizuka, 1967), spinal cord (Hsu et al, 1962) and paraspinal connective tissue (Delfs, 1957). Such metastatic lesions are almost always benign in nature, and death attributed to histologically proven metastases has only rarely been reported (Hsu et al, 1962; Ishizuka, 1967). Malignancy can only be assumed to have developed in such patients when metastases have been confirmed histologically to have the appearances of choriocarcinoma. It is indefensible to institute potentially dangerous therapy for a simple hydatidiform mole when conservative management of metastases is sufficient; the pathologist bears a considerable responsibility in his or her assessment of such lesions.

Prognosis

Most published figures concerning the mortality of invasive mole have been from the era before chemotherapy became available. The highest recorded mortality is 20% in the Far East (Prawirohardjo et al, 1957), whilst a figure of 14% was obtained by Greene (1959) in a selected series

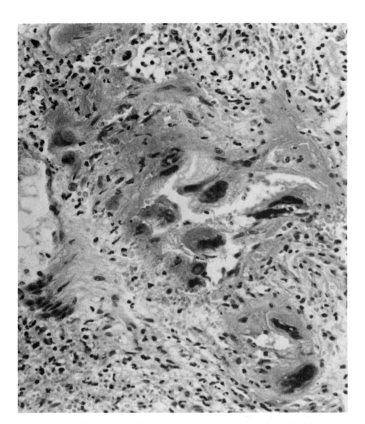

Fig. 52.23 Higher magnification of nodule shown in Fig. 52.22. There are scanty syncytiotrophoblastic cells but no chorionic villi. H & E × 220. (Reprinted with permission from Elston, 1989.)

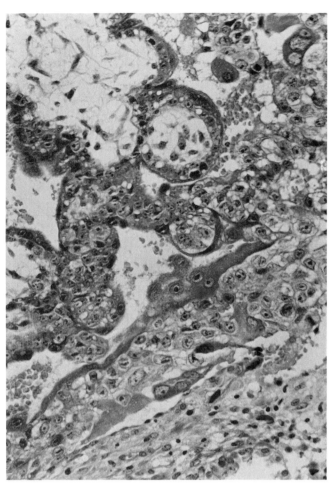

Fig. 52.24 Implanting 15-day blastocyst. The villous stroma is above and the decidua below. In the centre cores of mononuclear cytotrophoblast are surrounded by multinucleated syncytiotrophoblast which forms the margins of the intervillous space containing maternal red cells. H & E × 220.

in the United States. Ober (1965) reviewed the world literature and found nine deaths in 145 cases (6%), which is closely similar to Ishizuka's (1967) figures for Japan of an 8% mortality. Since the introduction of chemotherapy a diagnosis of invasive mole is made less frequently than before, with a decline in the use of hysterectomy, and most cases will be included within the broad classification of persistent trophoblastic disease. Accurate statistics are not readily available, but no deaths from histologically confirmed invasive mole occurred in the Charing Cross series (Elston, 1978), and this now seems to be the general experience (Du Beshter et al, 1987). Most deaths in the past were attributable to local catastrophic events such as haemorrhage or uterine perforation rather than to the development of malignant trophoblastic disease. It is clear that the mortality from invasive mole is now very low, emphasizing the limited aggressiveness of the lesion.

CHORIOCARCINOMA AND PLACENTAL SITE TROPHOBLASTIC TUMOUR

Choriocarcinoma and placental site trophoblastic tumour form two distinct clinicopathological entities; to have a proper understanding of their histogenesis it is important to outline the morphological and physiological features of normal trophoblast. During placentation the outer cell

layer of the blastocyst proliferates to form the trophoblastic cell mass. After about seven days the trophoblast differentiates into two layers: the inner layer is composed of large mononuclear cells with clear cytoplasm, the cytotrophoblast, and the outer layer is made up of a multinucleated syncytium, the syncytiotrophoblast. It is well established that the syncytiotrophoblast is derived from the cytotrophoblast by cell fusion, and is incapable of cell division. A third type of trophoblastic cell, which is also derived from the cytotrophoblast, has now been recognized. These cells are mononuclear but exhibit similar amphophilic cytoplasm to syncytiotrophoblast. Since they share morphological characteristics with both other types of trophoblast they have been designated intermediate trophoblast (Kurman et al, 1984). During implantation intermediate trophoblast migrates from the cytotrophoblastic cell columns at the anchoring tips of villi to infiltrate widely in the placental bed (Pijnenborg et al, 1981). It is these cells which also invade and partially replace the endothelium of the decidual portion of spiral arteries

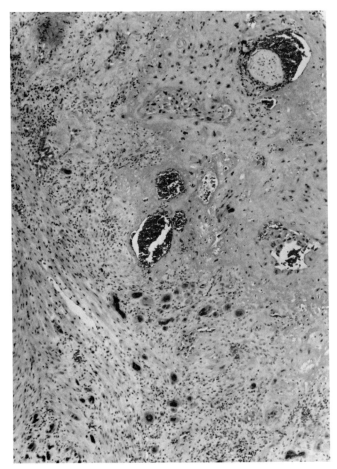

Fig. 52.25 Placental site reaction. Products of conception from a spontaneous abortion. A villus at the top right is embedded in decidua. Extravillous trophoblastic cells are seen at the bottom left. H & E × 64.

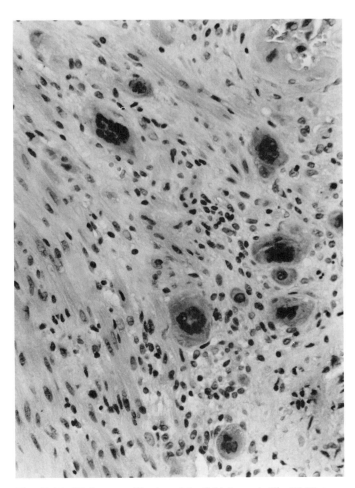

Fig. 52.26 Higher magnification of the field shown in Fig. 52.25, to show intermediate trophoblastic cells infiltrating between muscle bundles. H & E × 220.

(Kurman et al, 1984), a facet of implantation essential for subsequent fetal development. Thus the villous trophoblast comes to be composed predominantly of cyto-trophoblast and syncytiotrophoblast (Fig. 52.24) with a small component of intermediate trophoblast, and the extravillous trophoblast is composed mainly of intermediate trophoblast with a minor amount of syncytiotrophoblast (Figs 52.25 and 52.26). A range of protein hormones, steroid hormones and enzymes is secreted by the placenta. The majority are confined to the syncytiotrophoblast but the localization of two, hCG and human placental lactogen (hPL), has led to a more complete characterization of the various types of trophoblast (Kurman et al, 1984). Normally cytotrophoblast is devoid of both hCG and hPL. Syncytiotrophoblast contains hCG in large amounts in the first trimester, decreasing as pregnancy proceeds, and only small amounts of hPL at any stage. Intermediate trophoblast, in contrast, contains moderate amounts of hPL throughout with only focal amounts of hCG (Fig. 52.27). It is now firmly established that choriocarcinoma arises from the villous trophoblast and placental site trophoblastic tumour from the intermediate cells of extravillous trophoblast.

Choriocarcinoma

Clinical features

It is generally held that gestational choriocarcinoma occurs in approximately 1:20 000–1:40 000 pregnancies in the Western Hemisphere; rather higher figures are quoted for Third World countries but the accuracy of some studies is dubious (Table 52.1, p. 1599). It may present at any age during the reproductive period. Elston (1970) found a range from 17–56 years with an average age of 27 years; there was a mean gravidity of 2 with a range of 1–9. The most accurate estimates of the nature of the preceding gestation are derived from the era before cytotoxic therapy for gestational trophoblastic disease became fully established; from published data choriocarcinoma is preceded by hydatidiform mole in approximately 50% of cases in the Western Hemisphere, but in the Far East this association appears to be stronger (Table 52.2). Nowadays, in those countries or districts with registration and follow-up schemes for hydatidiform mole a definite diagnosis of choriocarcinoma is only rarely established, as treatment for persistent trophoblastic disease is usually initiated on the basis of raised hCG levels alone. In the

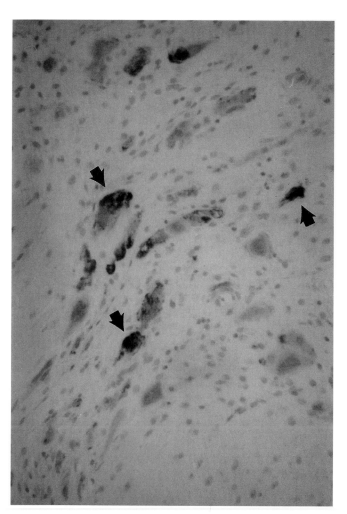

Fig. 52.27 Localization of hPL in intermediate trophoblast of placental site (arrowheads). Same case as Figs 52.25 and 52.26. Immunoperoxidase–hPL × 235.

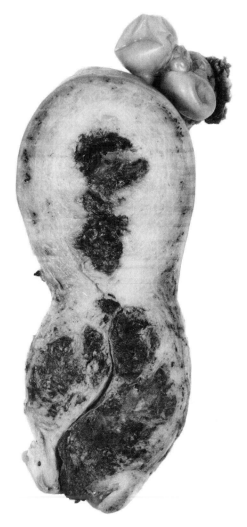

Fig. 52.28 Sagittal section of uterus to show dark haemorrhagic nodules of choriocarcinoma in the body, and similar deposits in the cervix. (From Fox H 1978 *Pathology of the placenta*, Saunders, Philadelphia. Reproduced by permission of Prof. H. Fox and W.B. Saunders Co.)

absence of this close clinical surveillance vaginal haemorrhage, often severe and prolonged, is the main presenting symptom, and this usually occurs within a few weeks of the related preceding gestation. Less frequently, patients will present with a distant metastasis. Rarely this may be as multiple pulmonary emboli or pulmonary hypertension due to intravascular tumour growth in the pulmonary arteries (Bagshawe & Brooks, 1959; Seckl et al, 1991); the correct diagnosis is easily established from the raised serum hCG levels. In those cases in which choriocarcinoma follows an apparently normal pregnancy it is assumed that

the tumour arose in the 'normal' placenta; direct evidence for this occurrence is available in anecdotal case reports of intraplacental choriocarcinoma which have been reviewed by Christopherson et al (1992) and Lage & Roberts (1993). The literature on the rare occurrence of gestational choriocarcinoma in the Fallopian tube was reviewed comprehensively by Ober & Maier (1982).

Table 52.2 Percentage of each type of antecedent gestation in choriocarcinoma

Author	Antecedent gestation				
	Hydatidiform mole		Abortion	Term delivery	Tubal pregnancy
Novak & Seah (1954)	U.S.A.	39	38	23	0
Hertig & Mansell (1956)	U.S.A.	50	25	22.5	2.5
Elston (1970)	U.K.	49	28	20.5	2.5
Acosta-Sison (1967)[a]	Philippines	60	23	11	0
Ratnam & Chew (1976)	Singapore	78.3	7.5	11.3	2.9

[a]Six cases ab initio.

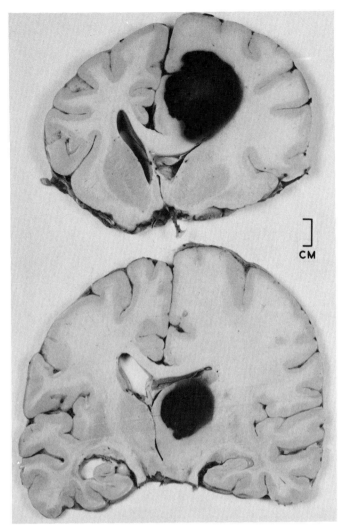

Fig. 52.29   Metastatic choriocarcinoma in brain. The coronal slices show two separate haemorrhagie nodules.

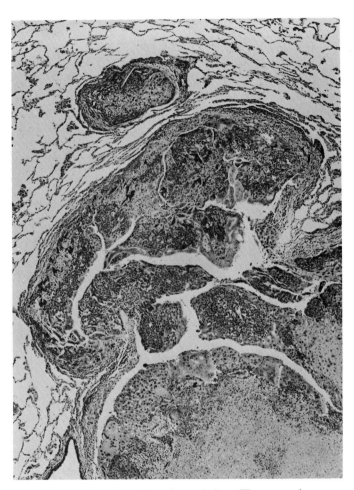

Fig. 52.30   Metastatic choriocarcinoma in lung. The tumour is located entirely within branches of the pulmonary artery. The patient presented with pulmonary hypertension. H & E × 40.

Morphology

Macroscopic appearances.   The gross appearances of choriocarcinoma are remarkably similar from case to case. Typically there is a well-circumscribed nodular lesion, 0.5 cm up to 5 cm in diameter, with a dominantly haemorrhagic structure. The colouration depends largely on the age of the nodule; in recent lesions there is a consistent red colour throughout, but in older lesions the central part gradually takes on a more yellow-brown appearance due to organization of the haemorrhagic and necrotic tumour tissue. In the uterus the primary nodules may be single or multiple, and may project into the endometrial cavity or extend deeply into the myometrium (Fig. 52.28). Local metastatic nodules may be present in the cervix or vagina. At distant metastatic sites the same haemorrhagic nodular pattern is usually seen (Fig. 52.29), but in the lungs in rare cases, as noted previously, the malignant trophoblast may be entirely intravascular, causing occlusion of pulmonary arteries by thromboembolus (Fig. 52.30).

Microscopical appearances.   In the typical primary nodule the malignant trophoblast is located at the periphery and little is found in the centre. This occurs to a much greater extent in choriocarcinoma than in other solid tumours, because, uniquely, it lacks an intrinsic tumour vasculature. The malignant trophoblast relies for cell nutrition on its permeation of the host blood vessels and such vessels are only present at the peripheral tumour-host interface. In this respect the malignant trophoblast of choriocarcinoma behaves in exactly the same physiological way as the normal trophoblast of the human placenta. The analogy can be taken further in considering the detailed microscopical structure. Choriocarcinoma has a very characteristic bilaminar pattern which recapitulates the appearances of the trophoblast of the early implanting blastocyst (Fig. 52.24). Central cores of mononuclear cytotrophoblastic cells are surrounded by rims of multinucleated syncytiotrophoblastic cells (Figs 52.31–52.33). The syncytiotrophoblast is usually arranged around maternal blood spaces which resemble the intervillous space of normal placentation (Fig. 52.32), but occasionally cyto-

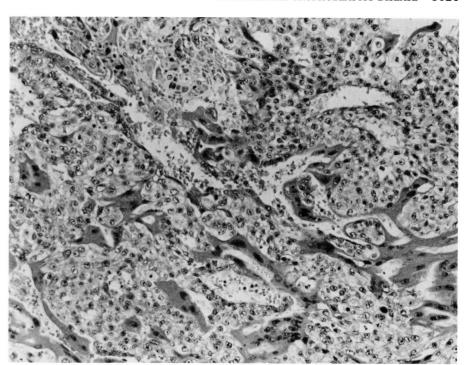

Fig. 52.31 Choriocarcinoma, composed of sheets of cytotrophoblast and syncytiotrophoblast. H & E × 100.

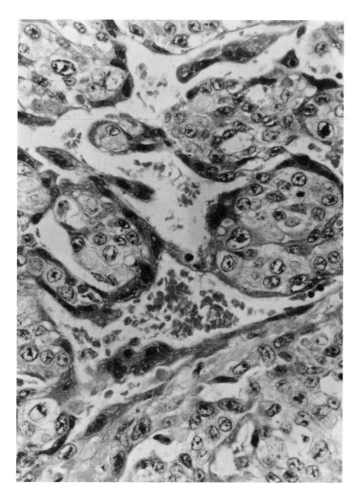

Fig. 52.32 High power view of a choriocarcinoma to show the typical bilaminar structure. Note the maternal red cells in pseudointervillous spaces. H & E × 320.

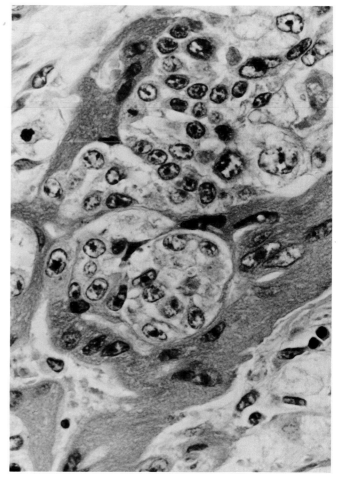

Fig. 52.33 Another choriocarcinoma, showing central cores of cytotrophoblast surrounded by syncytiotrophoblast. Note the prominent nucleoli, particularly in the cytotrophoblast. H & E × 580.

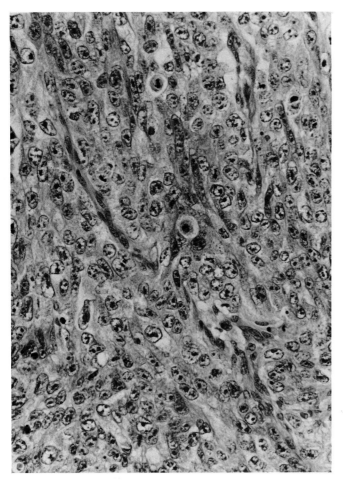

Fig. 52.34 Choriocarcinoma in which there is a predominance of cytotrophoblast. H & E × 220.

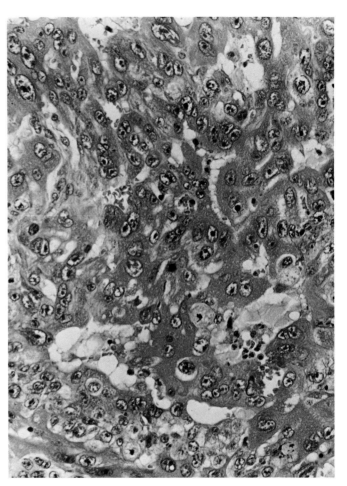

Fig. 52.35 Part of another choriocarcinoma exhibiting a predominantly syncytiotrophoblastic structure. H & E × 220.

trophoblast and syncytiotrophoblast are present as separate sheets of tumour tissue (Figs 52.34 and 52.35). It is extremely rare for a tumour to be composed entirely of one cell type but one element may sometimes be greatly in excess of the other. The nuclei of the cytotrophoblastic cells are large and vesicular with prominent nucleoli which are often multiple. The cytoplasm is generally clear but occasionally focally granular. The syncytial nuclei may also appear vesicular with prominent nucleoli, but are smaller than cytotrophoblastic nuclei. The syncytial cytoplasm is deeply eosinophilic and frequently appears as a lacy network. Mitoses are confined to the cytotrophoblast and are rarely excessive. There is no correlation between the degree of mitotic activity and prognosis.

Although extensive myometrial invasion is a prominent feature of typical choriocarcinoma, it is unusual to find muscle destruction or necrosis, and where malignant trophoblast is in contact with myometrium preservation of the latter is excellent. This is mainly because invasion rarely takes place directly into muscle but rather via the venous sinuses, which become markedly dilated in choriocarcinoma.

As noted previously, choriocarcinoma lacks an intrinsic

stromal vasculature and there is, therefore, always some permeation of the venous sinuses at the periphery of the tumour (Fig. 52.36). This is the first step in the progression of myometrial invasion towards the uterine venous plexus (Fig. 52.37). Tumour can also proliferate within the vessels and embolize along the venous sinuses until they impact and occlude the lumen (Fig. 52.38). The tumour nodule thus formed erodes the endothelium of the vessels and expands into the adjacent myometrium (Fig. 52.39). In this way it is possible for uterine perforation to occur, although the great bulk of the tumour in the myometrium is intravascular.

A variable infiltrate of lymphoplasmacytoid cells may be present, in close association with malignant trophoblast. This may be intense, and the severity correlates with prognosis (Elston & Bagshawe, 1973).

Although it is accepted that gestational choriocarcinoma arises from the villous trophoblast of the placenta, choriocarcinoma, by definition, is distinguished from invasive mole by the absence of true chorionic villi. Occasional non-molar cases have been described in which residual chorionic villi have been identified within the tumour or in adjacent myometrium (Novak & Seah, 1954;

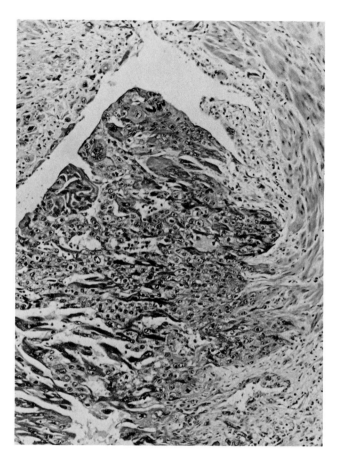

Fig. 52.36 Periphery of a choriocarcinoma. Malignant trophoblast is seen invading into a dilated venous sinus. H & E × 100.

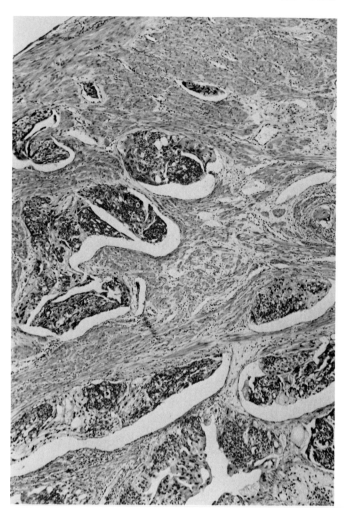

Fig. 52.37 Choriocarcinoma with extensive vascular invasion. The main tumour mass is at the bottom right and embolic tumour is present in dilated venous sinuses out to the serosa at the top left; intervening myometrium is intact. H & E × 40. (From Fox H 1978 *Pathology of the placenta*, Saunders, Philadelphia. Reproduced by permission of Prof. H. Fox and W.B. Saunders Co.).

Elston, 1978). In such cases the villi do not exhibit molar change and are either degenerate or appear normal microscopically (Fig. 52.40). There is no reason why the vestiges of the placental tissue from which the tumour has arisen should not persist, and, indeed, it is surprising that it does not happen more often, but the occurrence is exceedingly rare. Of even greater rarity is the finding of very early choriocarcinomatous change within an otherwise normal placenta (MacRae, 1951; Driscoll, 1963; Brewer & Mazur, 1981; Tsukamoto et al, 1981; Fox & Laurini, 1988; Hallam et al, 1990; Christopherson et al, 1992; Lage & Roberts, 1993); to date less than 20 cases have been reported in the literature. The placental primary is often very small and may only be found after a careful and extensive search. Microscopically intraplacental choriocarcinoma arises from the cytotrophoblast of apparently normal chorionic villi which do not show hydropic change. The characteristic bilaminar structure is seen as a mantle investing the villi, but true invasion is not seen (Fox & Laurini, 1988; Lage & Roberts, 1993). Metastases, when they occur, also have the typical bilaminar stucture, without the presence of formed villi. Such findings suggest that in the majority of cases of choriocarcinoma which follow a normal pregnancy the tumour arises in situ from villous trophoblast rather than in re-

tained or persistent trophoblast following the gestation. An unusual case has recently been reported in which an intraplacental chorangioma was associated with a proliferation of trophoblast resembling choriocarcinoma (Jauniaux et al, 1988). The authors used the term chorangiocarcinoma and could find no evidence of a similar example in the literature. In describing their cases of intraplacental choriocarcinoma Fox & Laurini (1988) speculated on the existence of intramolar choriocarcinoma which at that time had not been described. Choriocarcinoma in situ has now been reported in a single case of partial hydatidiform mole (Heifetz & Czaja, 1992), but the findings should be interpreted with caution. The patient did not require chemotherapy and Elston & Bagshawe (1972a) noted very similar florid proliferating trophoblast to that described by Heifetz & Czaja in a series of complete moles in which there was no correlation with subsequent persistent trophoblastic disease.

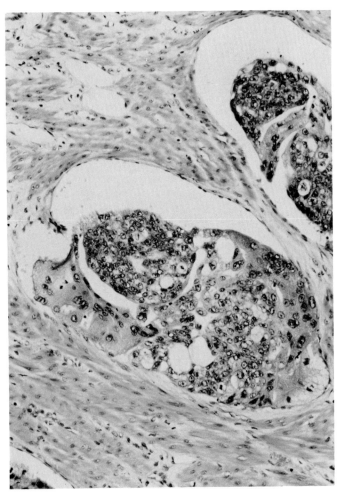

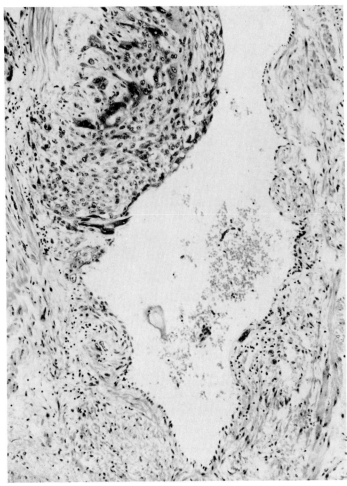

Fig. 52.38 Higher magnification of the tumour shown in Fig. 52.37. A tumour embolism has impacted in a venous sinus and is attached to the vessel wall, replacing the endothelium. H & E × 140 (From Fox H 1978 *Pathology of the placenta*, Saunders, Philadelphia. Reproduced by permission of Prof. H. Fox and W.B. Saunders Co.).

Fig. 52.39 Choriocarcinoma within a venous sinus. Part of the vessel wall is replaced by tumour which is invading into the adjacent myometrium. H & E × 100 (From Fox H 1978 *Pathology of the placenta*, Saunders, Philadelphia. Reproduced by permission of Prof. H. Fox and W.B. Saunders Co.).

Little variation in microscopical pattern is seen between tumours at primary and metastatic sites. The same basic structure is preserved in the metastases, with central necrosis and peripheral malignant trophoblast. In long-standing metastases, or in patients treated with cytotoxic therapy, the tumour nodule may be almost completely necrotic with little surviving tumour tissue.

Ultrastructure

In the small number of studies reported, the general appearances have resembled those of normal early placental trophoblast, although nuclei are slightly larger with infolded nuclear membranes. The cytotrophoblastic mitochondria tend to be enlarged and prominent, and the endoplasmic reticulum of the syncytiotrophoblast is slightly increased (Wakitani, 1962; Knoth et al, 1969;

Larsen, 1973). Phagocytic activity, not normally present in trophoblast, has been observed in the syncytiotrophoblast of choriocarcinoma (Knoth et al, 1969; Larsen, 1973). Infererra (1967) found both intermediate and undifferentiated trophoblastic cells in addition to relatively normal cytotrophoblast and syncytiotrophoblast. Because of the scarcity of suitable material from patients with choriocarcinoma, studies have also been carried out on cell lines of transplanted human choriocarcinoma in experimental animals (Wynn & Davies, 1964a; Larsen et al, 1967; Knoth et al, 1969). Essentially similar appearances to those described above were found. In addition Larsen et al (1967), studying choriocarcinoma transplanted to the hamster liver, noted desmosomes connecting tumour cells to liver cells and compared the invasiveness of choriocarcinoma with that of the normal fertilized ovum.

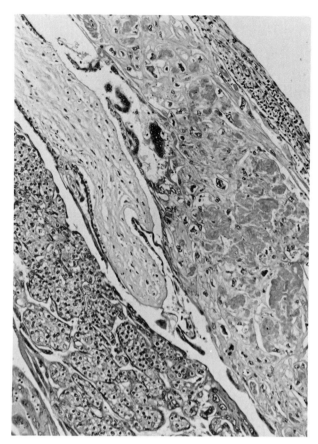

Fig. 52.40 Chorionic villus lying within a choriocarcinoma. The neoplastic trophoblast does not arise from the villus, nor is the latter invasive. H & E × 100.

Metastatic spread

It is difficult to obtain an accurate estimate for the frequency of metastases in choriocarcinoma due to the wide variation in published figures (Table 52.3). Some studies are based entirely on autopsy records, whilst others include clinical data without histological confirmation. The series reported by Hou & Pang (1956), Elston (1970), Ober et al (1971), Junaid et al (1974) and Mazur et al (1982) are all composed of personal or collective autopsy cases. Those reported by Elston and Mazur et al are probably the most representative of the modern chemotherapy era, and confirm that the lungs, brain and liver are the

most frequent metastatic sites. They are in keeping with clinical estimates obtained by Hunter et al (1990).

Prognosis

Prior to the establishment of the Mathieu Memorial Chorioepithelioma Registry in the United States in 1946 (Brewer, 1959) anecdotal evidence suggested that choriocarcinoma was highly malignant and always fatal. This over-gloomy view was dispelled by the first statistical report from the Registry, as Novak & Seah (1954) found a minimum two-year survival of 15% in the 74 patients on whom data was available. Treatment in all cases was hysterectomy, with pelvic irradiation in one. In a later report from the Registry based on 147 cases, a similar figure for five-year survival was obtained (Brewer et al, 1961).

The dramatic improvement in survival due to the use of cytotoxic therapy began as a result of observations made by Hertz and co-workers that folic acid was essential for the growth of the female genital tract and embryonic development (Hertz, 1978). Thiersch (1952) also found that it was possible to induce abortion in women treated with small doses of the folic acid antagonist 4-aminopteroyl-glutamic acid. These facts led to the treatment of the first patient with choriocarcinoma by methotrexate, and in 1956 Li et al reported complete remission in two patients with choriocarcinoma and one with invasive mole. By 1961 Hertz et al were able to present the results of 5 years experience with chemotherapy in 63 patients, 44 of whom had choriocarcinoma. They estimated that in comparison with previous results from the literature prolonged survival had been raised from 6% to 48%. As more experience was gained results improved and it was possible to obtain sustained remission in over 80% of patients if treatment was initiated early in the course of the disease.

Sustained remission rates of nearly 90% for metastatic trophoblastic disease and virtually 100% for localized disease have now been achieved, and it is clear that the best results are obtained in patients in whom treatment is monitored in an expert centre (Berkowitz & Goldstein, 1988; Jones, 1990; Lurain & Sciarra, 1991; Newlands et al, 1992). At Charing Cross Hospital, London, a prognostic scoring system is used to stratify patients so that they

Table 52.3 Distribution of distant metastases in choriocarcinoma

Study		Lung	Brain	Liver	Kidney	Intestines	Lymph node	No of cases
					Percentage involvement			
Park & Lees	(1950)	60	17	16	13	9	6	263
Hou & Pang	(1956)	96	90	50	43	21	0	25
Elston	(1970)	80	40	20	20	15	0	27
Ober et al	(1971)	100	61	60	47	40	15	44
Junaid et al	(1974)	94	33	39	26	17	5	100
Mazur et al	(1982)	97	50	50	33	23	23	30

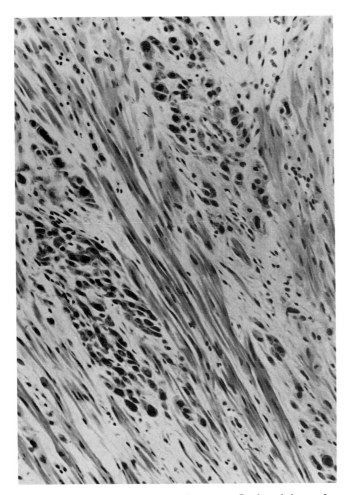

Fig. 52.41 Placental site trophoblastic tumour. Cords and sheets of intermediate trophoblastic cells infiltrate between muscle bundles. H & E × 160.

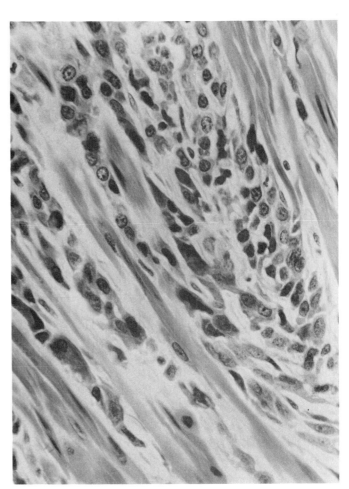

Fig. 52.42 Higher magnification of Fig. 52.41 showing mononuclear and multinucleated intermediate trophoblastic cells, with preservation of muscle bundles. H & E × 392.

receive appropriate therapy (Newlands et al, 1992). This is based on a number of factors, including the type of antecedent gestation, interval from pregnancy to diagnosis, hCG level at diagnosis, ABO blood groups (patient and partner) and number of metastases. Patients are divided into low, medium and high risk categories. Even in the high risk category overall survival is 85%. The poorest prognosis occurs in those patients, fortunately exceedingly rare, with intraplacental choriocarcinoma. Most of these patients present with widespread maternal metatases (and occasionally fetal) (Christopherson et al, 1992; Lage & Roberts, 1993) and there is a high mortality; in only two fully documented cases were there no sequelae (Driscoll, 1963; Fox & Laurini, 1988).

Placental site trophoblastic tumour

Clinical features

Placental site trophoblastic tumour is uncommon, but the overall frequency is difficult to assess because of the paucity of recorded cases. McLellan et al found 52 cases

in the literature in 1991 and only a small number of cases have been recorded since then. The age range and parity of the patients appear similar to those of patients with choriocarcinoma. One case of placental site trophoblastic tumour in a postmenopausal woman has been recorded (McLellan et al, 1991). The clinical presentation is variable, and in contrast with choriocarcinoma, in which haemorrhage is the commonest symptom, approximately half the patients report a period of amenorrhoea, which may last up to two years. A further distinction from choriocarcinoma is the rarity of a preceding molar gestation, approximately 5% compared with at least 50%. In about 75% of cases the antecedent gestation is a normal full-term pregnancy. The genetic origin of two cases, one from a normal conceptus and one from a hydatidiform mole, was established by Fisher et al (1992) using RFLPs and a Y-chromosome specific probe. A rare but distinctive complication is the occurrence of an associated nephrotic syndrome (Park, 1975; Eckstein et al 1982; Young & Scully, 1984; Young et al, 1985). In most of the cases reported the nephrotic syndrome resolved after hyster-

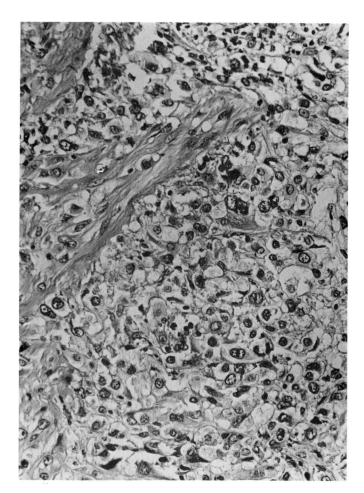

Fig. 52.43 Another placental site trophoblastic tumour in which the cells are predominantly mononuclear. H & E × 200.

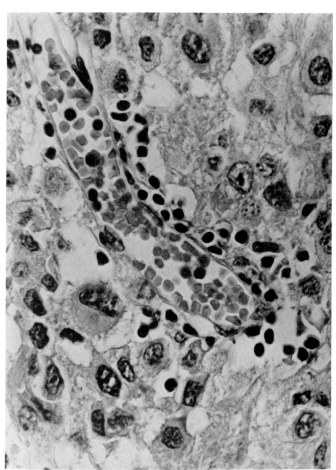

Fig. 52.44 Some case as Fig. 52.43 showing the trophoblastic cells infiltrating around a preserved myometrial capillary. H & E × 584.

ectomy (Eckstein et al, 1982; Young & Scully, 1984), and the mechanism of the renal lesion is thought to be immune complex production and chronic intravascular coagulation associated with tumour products (Young & Scully, 1984; Young et al, 1985).

Morphology

Macroscopic appearances. The gross appearances are much more variable than in choriocarcinoma. There may be a localized nodule, which in some cases projects into the endometrial cavity, but more often there is an ill-defined mass in the myometrium. The lesion is usually tan to yellow in colour, without striking haemorrhage, and foci of necrosis may be present. The degree of invasion is variable; in some cases only superficial involvement of the myometrium occurs whilst in others there may be penetration through to the serosa.

Microscopical appearances. The pattern of infiltration by the trophoblastic cells recapitulates the appearances seen at the normal placental bed (Figs 52.25 and 52.26). There is a diffuse infiltrate of mononuclear and multinucleated trophoblastic cells arranged in cords, islands and sheets between myometrial bundles (Figs 52.41 and 52.42). In contrast with the bilaminar pattern of choriocarcinoma the infiltrate is rather monotonous and resembles the intermediate trophoblast. The majority of cells are mononuclear with clear cytoplasm but multinucleated forms having amphophilic cytoplasm are also present (Figs 52.42 and 52.43). Where cords of cells infiltrate amongst myometrial bundles they may have a spindle cell appearance. A major point of distinction from choriocarcinoma is the preservation of intact venous sinuses or capillaries within the tumour mass (Fig. 52.44). Infiltration of vessel walls may be seen but intravascular proliferation is less obvious. Islands of tumour necrosis may be present, usually in areas of poor vascularity. Mitoses can usually be identified, but counts are variable and rarely high.

Immunostaining reveals an entirely different pattern to that seen in choriocarcinoma. Abundant amounts of hPL are seen in a diffuse pattern (Fig. 52.45) whilst hCG is present only focally (Fig. 52.46).

In the uncommon cases in which metastases occur

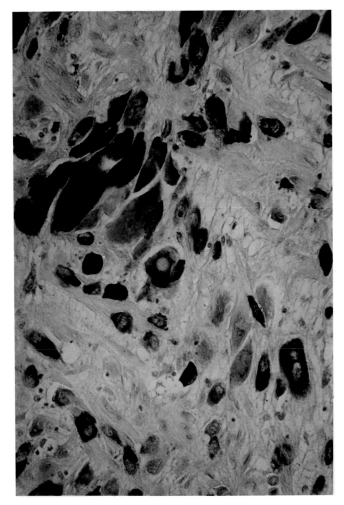

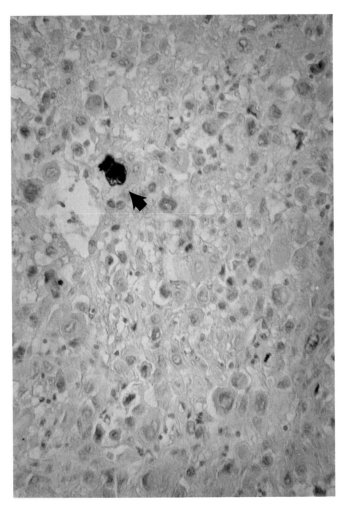

Fig. 52.45 Placental site trophoblastic tumour. The majority of cells show diffuse staining for hPL. Immunoperoxidase – hPL × 235.

Fig. 52.46 Same case as Fig. 52.45. Immunostaining reveals hCG in only one cell in this field (arrowhead). Immunoperoxidase – hCG × 235.

the morphological appearances are similar to those at the primary site.

Prognosis

Until comparatively recently it appeared that placental site trophoblastic tumour was a relatively benign and frequently self-limiting process; in 1981 Elston found only one death in 19 cases from the literature, and that was due to postoperative complications. Subsequently several fatal cases have been reported (Scully & Young, 1981; Twiggs et al, 1981; Eckstein et al, 1982; Gloor et al, 1983) and Young et al (1988) in a further review found seven deaths out of 38 fully documented cases in whom follow-up data of over one year's duration or to death was available. They were aware of a further 48 cases seen in consultation, four of whom were considered to have malignant tumours. Young et al (1988) therefore estimated that between 10 and 15% of patients with placental site trophoblastic tumour have a malignant outcome, with an overall mortality

of up to 10%. More accurate figures will only become available when a larger database is established.

The morphological features of placental site trophoblastic tumour cannot be used with confidence to predict prognosis and malignant cases have been described in which the original appearances suggested exaggerated placental site reaction (Collins et al, 1990; Orrell & Sanders, 1991). It has been proposed that estimation of the number of mitoses may be a helpful prognostic factor (Scully & Young, 1981; Mazur & Kurman, 1987; Lathrop et al, 1988; Young et al, 1988), since most fatal cases which have been reported have had counts of 5 or more per high power field. Leaving aside the inherent inaccuracy of expressing counts per 'high power field' without stating the field area (Ellis & Whitehead, 1981), fatal cases with low mitotic counts have occurred (Gloor et al, 1983; Young et al, 1985) and Eckstein et al (1982) found no correlation between mitotic activity and prognosis. It is therefore necessary to conduct full follow-up in all patients (Finkler et al, 1988; Dessau et al, 1990). It should also be noted that a curettage specimen from a placental site trophoblastic tumour may not be representative of the whole tumour and counts may appear falsely high or low.

In marked contrast with choriocarcinoma the treatment of choice is surgical rather than cytotoxic therapy (Newlands et al, 1992). In some cases curettage alone seems to have been curative (Ober et al, 1971; Kurman et al, 1976) and this indicates that the tumour may regress even if excision is incomplete. For the majority of patients, however, hysterectomy is indicated (Finkler et al, 1988; Lathrop et al, 1988; Dessau et al, 1990; Newlands et al, 1992) and this has the added advantage that the extent of local involvement can be assessed properly from full histopathological examination of the specimen. Hoffman et al (1993) have also advocated pelvic node dissection for staging purposes. Cytotoxic therapy has been used in some cases (Twiggs et al, 1981; Finkler et al, 1988; Lathrop et al, 1988; Dessau et al, 1990) but the results have been disappointing and only occasionally has long-term remission been achieved (Dessau et al, 1990; Hoffman et al, 1993).

BIOPSY AND DIFFERENTIAL DIAGNOSIS OF TROPHOBLASTIC LESIONS

In the general field of tumour pathology it has become increasingly important that a tissue diagnosis of malignancy is established before potentially dangerous treatment, such as radiotherapy or cytotoxic therapy, is embarked upon. Paradoxically, this maxim is no longer true for the one solid tumour in which it is possible to obtain a high level of lasting cures, choriocarcinoma. This is largely due to the secretion by trophoblastic cells of hCG, which has proved to be an ideal tumour marker. The development of the radioimmunoassay method for the measurement of gonadotrophin excretion in the urine (Bagshawe, 1969) and the beta subunit of hCG in the serum (Kardana & Bagshawe, 1976) means that initial tumour load and response to therapy can now be assessed with great accuracy (Newlands et al, 1992). The pathological distinction between benign and malignant trophoblastic lesions has become blurred, and many patients with postmolar trophoblastic disease are treated prophylactically without a definite diagnosis ever being established. This has had the inevitable effect of diminishing the use made of histological methods in both the initial diagnosis and management of trophoblastic disease. However, although most patients with trophoblastic disease are eventually treated in special centres, the initial diagnosis is usually made in the referring hospital. Patients most frequently present with menstrual irregularity or frank uterine haemorrhage, and histological examination of endometrial curettings is still the most widely used diagnostic procedure in this situation. Indeed, curettings containing chorionic villi or fragments of trophoblast are one of the commonest diagnostic problems in routine gynaecological histopathology. Whilst most specimens are straightforward retained products of conception, in a minority the trophoblast may appear abnormal and the possibility of trophoblastic disease has to be considered. Such biopsies may prove difficult to interpret, and there is unfortunately a tendency amongst pathologists to overdiagnose malignancy.

Elston & Bagshawe (1972b) carried out a detailed investigation into the reliability of the histological diagnosis of trophoblastic disease from uterine curettings. They stressed the importance of the clinical, and in particular, obstetric history, and defined three histological groups: trophoblast associated with villous structures, simple or suspicious trophoblast and trophoblast diagnostic of choriocarcinoma. In a subsequent review Elston (1981) suggested that for practical purposes the interpretation of trophoblastic curettings could be considered in two broad groups, depending on the presence or absence of chorionic villi. Since the establishment of placental site trophoblastic tumour as a neoplastic process it has also become necessary to include lesions derived from the extravillous trophoblast in the differential diagnosis of non-villous trophoblastic curettings.

The majority of specimens containing chorionic villi are derived from spontaneous or induced abortions and should pose few diagnostic problems. The villi are of normal size, the stroma, which is loose but not oedematous, contains fetal blood vessels, and the trophoblast is two-layered. The presence of small irregular villi may suggest a chromosomal abnormality such as triploidy, although correlation between morphological features and karyotypic abnormalities is poor (Van Lijneshoten et al, 1993; Fox, 1993). Nevertheless, if hydropic change is also present the possibility of partial hydatidiform mole must be considered, as described previously. Curettings taken in the investigation of postpartum haemorrhage may also reveal villous placental tissue which is often degenerate and inflamed. The introduction of hCG assay in the management and follow-up of patients with hydatidiform mole has reduced the need for uterine curettage (Newlands et al, 1992). For example, if curettage is performed within 48 hours of molar evacuation hydropic molar villi are almost always present but this finding has no particular diagnostic or prognostic significance. During follow-up it may be appropriate to carry out uterine curettage for the investigation of abnormal bleeding. It is of great importance that these specimens are interpreted with caution by the histopathologist. If they contain obvious molar villi a diagnosis of choriocarcinoma cannot, by definition, be made. The correct terminology is persistent postmolar trophoblastic disease, and therapeutic decisions will be based more on hCG levels and radiographic findings than the histological appearances. Nevertheless, the presence of molar villi is an indication that the patient is more likely to have an invasive mole than choriocarcinoma and only a small proportion of these patients will require cytotoxic therapy. It follows that with any trophoblastic proliferation a careful search must be made for formed villi; all available material should be blocked and multiple sections examined if necessary. The majority of postmolar curettages will be carried out within the first three months of follow-up, but molar villi may persist in the uterus for many months (Elston & Bagshawe, 1972b).

A range of appearances is seen in curettings containing trophoblast in the absence of chorionic villi. In many curettages performed for 'missed' abortion or 'retained products' the only finding is haemorrhagic and necrotic decidua in which residual placental site reaction may be visible (Figs 52.25 and 52.26). Even though chorionic villi are not present it may be helpful to the clinicians to report the presence of the placental site reaction, thus indicating that a gestation has taken place. In doubtful cases the presence of extravillous trophoblast can be confirmed very easily using immunostaining for low molecular weight cytokeratin, which distinguishes trophoblast from decidua

(Sasagawa et al, 1986). Similar appearances may also be found in postpartum curettings. In some cases the placental site trophoblast may be particularly florid, placing the appearances in the category of exaggerated placental site reaction. The differential diagnosis of placental site trophoblastic tumour should be considered in these circumstances and the distinction between the two may on occasion be difficult, especially if the tissue sample is small (Young et al, 1988; Orrell & Sanders, 1991). Proximity to the preceding gestation, a limited degree of decidual and myometrial infiltration and scanty mitoses favour a diagnosis of placental site reaction but in a small number of cases it is impossible to make a definite diagnosis and careful follow-up is advisable. The possibility of a placental site nodule should also be considered (Young et al, 1990). These can usually be distinguished from placental site trophoblastic tumour by their small size and circumscription, extensive hyalinization, degenerative appearance and lack of mitoses.

Trophoblastic fragments may also be encountered in the absence of any placental site reaction. There may

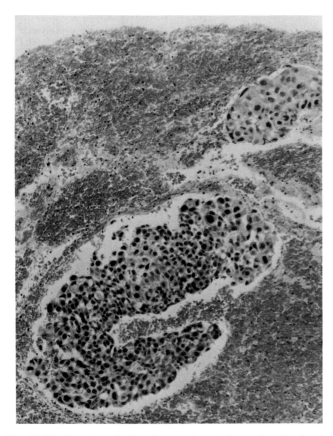

Fig. 52.47 Simple trophoblast in an endometrial curetting. Small fragments of trophoblast with pyknotic nuclei are seen; no clear distinction into cyto- or syncytiotrophoblast is evident. H & E × 100.

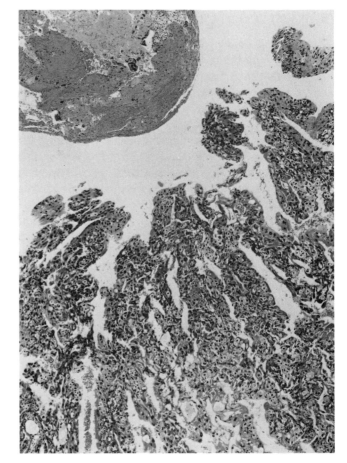

Fig. 52.48 Suspicious trophoblast. The large sheet of trophoblastic tissue on the right has a recognizable bilaminar structure, but no invasion was present. H & E × 40.

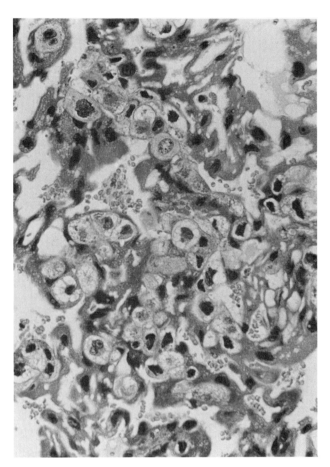

Fig. 52.49 Higher magnification of Fig. 52.48, showing clearly separate cytotrophoblast and syncytiotrophoblast. H & E × 220.

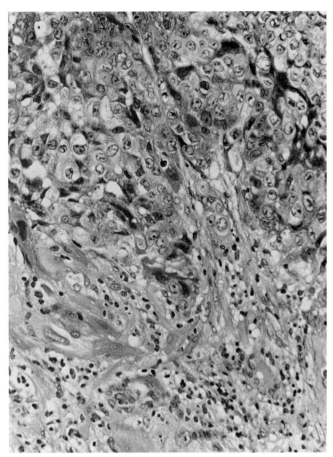

Fig. 52.50 Biopsy diagnostic of choriocarcinoma. Typical bilaminar trophoblast invades myometrium. H & E × 220.

be small collections of monomorphous, usually syncytial, trophoblastic cells set within necrotic debris (Fig. 52.47). Considerable nuclear abnormality may be present and care must be taken not to ascribe these atypical features to neoplastic change; they probably indicate hypoxia due to the growth pattern of trophoblast lacking an intrinsic vasculature. If larger sheets of trophoblast are seen with a bilaminar arrangement of cyto- and syncytiotrophoblast reminiscent of choriocarcinoma (Figs 52.48 and 52.49) but without evidence of invasion, the appearances are labelled as suspicious trophoblast. Only when bilaminar trophoblast exhibits unequivocal invasion can the appearances be considered diagnostic (Fig. 52.50). Differentiation of choriocarcinoma from placental site trophoblastic tumour should not be difficult on morphological grounds because of the contrast between the bilaminar structure of the former and the largely monomorphous appearance of the latter. Immunostaining for hCG and hPL should be used to resolve doubtful cases. This may also be helpful in distinguishing placental site trophoblastic tumour from uterine sarcomas and poorly differentiated carcinoma, although it must be recognized that trophoblastic differen-

tiation with hCG production has been observed rarely in endometrial carcinomas (Civantos & Rywlin, 1972; Pesce et al, 1991). Interpretation of curettings containing trophoblast without chorionic villi depends to a large extent on the nature of the preceding gestation. If this was a hydatidiform mole then the same cautious approach as that employed with villous curettings is indicated. A diagnosis of persistent trophoblastic disease is applied and careful follow-up continued. A minority of patients will subsequently require cytotoxic therapy. If the preceding gestation was a normal pregnancy or a spontaneous abortion then the presence of non-villous trophoblast is an almost certain indication that the patient has developed choriocarcinoma or placental site trophoblastic tumour. Immediate full investigation should be implemented, and virtually every patient in this group will require further therapy. It is important to make the distinction between the two lesions if at all possible. As pointed out previously, if the features point towards choriocarcinoma cytotoxic therapy is indicated, but if placental site trophoblastic tumour is suspected the treatment of choice is surgery.

REFERENCES

Acaia B, Parazzini F, La Vecchia C et al 1988 Increased frequency of complete hydatidiform mole in women with repeated abortion. Gynecologic Oncology 31: 310–314.

Acosta-Sison H 1967 Trophoblastic or chorionic tumors as observed in the Philippines. In: Holland J F, Hreshchyshyn M M eds Choriocarcinoma: transactions of a conference of the International Union against Cancer. Springer-Verlag, Berlin, pp 35–36.

Agboola A 1979 Trophoblastic neoplasia in an African urban population. Journal of the National Medical Association 71: 935–937.

Aguero O, Kizer S, Pinedo G 1973 Hydatidiform mole in Concepcion Palacios Maternity Hospital. American Journal of Obstetrics and Gynecology 116: 1117–1120.

Anderson D J, Berkowitz R S 1985 Gamma-interferon enhances expression of Class I MHC antigens in the weakly HLA-positive human choriocarcinoma cell line Be Wo but does not induce MHC expression in the HLA-negative choriocarcinoma cell line Jar. Journal of Immunology 135: 2498–2501.

Atkin N B 1965 In: Park W W ed The early conceptus, normal and abnormal. Livingstone, London, pp 130–134.

Atrash H K, Hogue C J R, Grimes D A 1986 Epidemiology of hydatidiform mole during early gestation. American Journal of Obstetrics and Gynecology 154: 906–909.

Attwood H D, Park W W 1961 Embolism to the lungs by trophoblast. Journal of Obstetrics and Gynaecology of the British Commonwealth 68: 611–617.

Azuma C, Saji F, Tokugawa Y et al 1991 Application of gene amplification by polymerase chain reaction to genetic analysis of molar mitochondrial DNA: the detection of anuclear empty ovum as the cause of complete mole. Gynecologic Oncology 40: 29–33.

Azuma C, Saji F, Takemura M et al 1992 Triplet pregnancy involving complete hydatidiform mole and two fetuses: genetic analysis by deoxyribonucleic acid fingerprint. American Journal of Obstetrics and Gynecology 166: 664–667.

Bagshawe K D 1969 The clinical biology of the trophoblast and its tumours. Arnold, London.

Bagshawe K D 1973 Recent observations related to chemotherapy and immunology of gestational choriocarcinoma. Advances in Cancer Research 18: 231–263.

Bagshawe K D 1976 Risk and prognostic factors in trophoblastic neoplasia. Cancer 38: 1373–1385.

Bagshawe K D, Brooks W D W 1959 Subacute pulmonary hypertension due to chorionepithelioma. Lancet 1: 653–658.

Bagshawe K D, Lawler S D 1982 Unmasking moles. British Journal of Obstetrics and Gynaecology 89: 255–257.

Bagshawe K D, Rawlings G, Pike M, Lawler S D 1971 ABO blood groups in trophoblastic neoplasia. Lancet i: 553–557.

Bagshawe K D, Dent J, Webb J 1986 Hydatidiform mole in England and Wales 1973–83. Lancet 2: 673–677.

Bagshawe K D, Lawler S D, Paradinas F et al 1990 Gestational trophoblastic tumours following initial diagnosis of partial hydatidiform mole. Lancet 335: 1074–1076.

Bardawil W A, Toy B L 1959 The natural history of choriocarcinoma; problems of immunity and spontaneous regression. Annals of the New York Academy of Sciences 60: 197–251.

Bardawil W A, Hertig A T, Velardo J T 1957 Regression of trophoblast. 1 Hydatidiform mole: a case of unusual features; possible metastasis and regression; review of literature. Obstetrics and Gynecology 10: 614–625.

Bartocci A, Pollard J W, Stanley E R 1986 Regulation of colony-stimulating factor-1 during pregnancy. Journal of Experimental Medicine 164: 956–961.

Berkowitz R S, Goldstein D P 1988 Diagnosis and management of the primary hydatidiform mole. Obstetrics and Gynecology Clinics of North America 15: 491–502.

Berkowitz R S, Goldstein D P, Bernstein M 1979 Natural history of partial hydatidiform moles. Lancet i: 719.

Berkowitz R S, Hornig-Rohan J, Martin-Alosco S et al 1981 HL-A antigen frequency distribution in patients with gestational choriocarcinoma, their husbands. Placenta (suppl 3): 263–267.

Berkowitz R S, Goldstein D P, Bernstein M R 1983 Natural history of partial molar pregnancy. Obstetrics and Gynecology 66: 677–681.

Berkowitz R S, Cramer D W, Bernstein M R et al 1985 Risk factors for complete molar pregnancy from a case-control study. American Journal of Obstetrics and Gynecology 152: 1016–1020.

Berkowitz R S, Umpierre S A, Taylor-Emery S, Goldstein D P, Anderson D J 1986a Immunobiology of complete molar pregnancy and gestational trophoblastic tumor. Cancer and Metastasis Reviews 5: 109–123.

Berkowitz R S, Umpierre S A, Johnson P M, McIntyre J A, Anderson D J 1986b Expression of trophoblast-leukocyte common antigens and placental-type alkaline phosphatase in complete molar pregnancy. American Journal of Obstetrics and Gynecology 155: 443–446.

Berkowitz R S, Goldstein D P, Bernstein M R 1988 Partial molar pregnancy: a separate entity. Contemporary Obstetrics and Gynecology 31: 99–102.

Bracken M B 1987 Incidence and aetiology of hydatidiform mole: an epidemiological review. British Journal of Obstetrics and Gynaecology 94: 1123–1135.

Bravo R, Frank R, Blundell P A, MacDonald-Bravo H 1987 Cyclin/PCNA is the auxiliary protein of DNA delta. Nature 326: 515–517.

Brewer J I 1959 The Albert F Mathieu Chorionepithelioma Registry. Annals of the New York Academy of Sciences 80: 140–142.

Brewer J I 1967 Light microscopy of gestational trophoblastic disease. In: Lund C W, Choate J W eds Transcript of 4th Rochester Trophoblast Conference Rochester, New York, pp 6–24.

Brewer J I, Mazur M T 1981 Gestational choriocarcinoma: its origin in the placenta during seemingly normal pregnancy. American Journal of Surgical Pathology 5: 267–277.

Brewer J I, Rhinehart J J, Dunbar R W 1961 Choriocarcinoma: a report of the 5 or more years survival from the Albert Mathieu Chorionepithelioma Registry. American Journal of Obstetrics and Gynecology 81: 574–583.

British Medical Journal 1975 Epidemiological aspects of choriocarcinoma. Leading article. British Medical Journal ii: 606–607.

Buckley J 1987 Epidemiology of gestational trophoblastic diseases. In: Szulman A E, Buchsbaum H J eds Gestational trophoblastic disease. Springer-Verlag, New York, pp 8–26.

Bulmer J N, Johnson P M 1985 Antigen expression by trophoblast populations in the human placenta and their possible immunobiological relevance. Placenta 6: 127–140.

Bulmer J N, Johnson P M, Sasagawa M, Takeuchi S 1988 Immunohistochemical studies of fetal trophoblast and maternal decidua in hydatidiform mole and choriocarcinoma. Placenta 9: 183–200.

Carr D H 1969 Cytogenetics and the pathology of hydatidiform degeneration. Obstetrics and Gynecology 33: 333–342.

Caspersson T, Lomakka G, Lech L 1971 The 24 fluorescence patterns of human metaphase chromosomes distinguishing characters and variability. Hereditas 67: 89–102.

Cheung A N Y, Srivastava G, Pittaluga S, Man T K, Collins R J 1993 Expression of C-myc and C-fms oncogenes in trophoblastic cells in hydatidiform mole and normal human placenta. Journal of Clinical Pathology 46: 204–207.

Chiari H 1877 Über drei Fälle von primären Carcinom im Fundus und Corpus des Uterus. Medizinische Jährbücher 7: 364–368.

Christopherson W A, Kanbour A, Szulman A E 1992 Choriocarcinoma in a term placenta with maternal metastases. Gynecologic Oncology 46: 239–245.

Chun D, Braga C A 1967 Choriocarcinoma in Hong Kong. In: Wood C, Walters W A W eds Proceedings of the 5th World Congress of Gynaecology and Obstetrics. Butterworth, New South Wales, pp 398–405.

Civantos F, Rywlin A M 1972 Carcinomas with trophoblastic differentiation and secretion of chorionic gonadotrophins. Cancer 29: 789–798.

Collins R J, Ngan H Y S, Wong L C 1990 Placental site trophoblastic tumor: with features between an exaggerated placental site reaction and a placental site trophoblastic tumor. International Journal of Gynecological Pathology 9: 170–177.

Conran R M, Hitchcock C L, Popek E J et al 1993 Diagnostic considerations in molar gestations. Human Pathology 24: 41–48.

Couillon P, Hors J, Boué J, Boué A 1978 Identification of the origin of triploidy by HLA markers. Human Genetics 41: 35–44.

Couone A W, Multon D, Johnson P M, Adolfini M 1984 Trophoblast cells in peripheral blood from pregnant women. Lancet ii: 841–843.

Crocker J, Skilbeck N 1987 Nucleolar organiser region associated proteins in cutaneous melanocytic lesions: a quantitative study. Journal of Clinical Pathology 40: 885–889.

Curry S L, Hammond C B, Tyrey L, Creasman W T, Parker R T 1975 Hydatidiform mole: diagnosis, management and long term follow-up of 347 patients. Obstetrics and Gynecology 45: 1–3.

Czernobilsky B, Barash A, Lancet M 1982 Partial moles: a clinicopathological study of 25 cases. Obstetrics and Gynecology 59: 75–77.

Davis J P, Foster K J 1984 Sex assignment in gestational trophoblastic neoplasia. American Journal of Obstetrics and Gynecology 148: 722–725.

Dawood M Y, Teoh E S, Ratnam S S 1971 ABO blood group in trophoblastic neoplasia. American Journal of Obstetrics and Gynecology 78: 918–923.

Deaton J L, Hoffman J S, Saal H, Allred C, Koulos J P 1989 Molar pregnancy coexisting with a normal fetus: a case report. Gynecologic Oncology 32: 394–397.

Dehner L P 1980 Gestational and nongestational trophoblastic neoplasia: a historic and pathobiologic survey. American Journal of Surgical Pathology 4: 43–58.

Delfs E 1957 Quantitative chorionic gonadotrophin: prognostic value in hydatidiform mole and chorionepithelioma. Obstetrics and Gynecology 9: 1–24.

Deligdisch L, Driscoll S G, Goldstein D P 1978 Gestational trophoblastic neoplasms: morphologic correlations of therapeutic response. American Journal of Obstetrics and Gynecology 130: 801–806.

De Ruyck R 1951 Mise en évidence du virus choriotrope dans quatre case de môle hydatidiforme, et dans un cas de métastase pulmonaire de chorio-épithéliome. Bulletin de L'Assocation Francaise pour l'Etude du Cancer 38: 252–268.

Dessau R, Rustin G J S, Dent J, Paradinas F J, Bagshawe K D 1990 Surgery and chemotherapy in the management of placental site tumor. Gynecologic Oncology 39: 56–59.

Dinh-De T, Minh H N 1961 Hydatidiform mole with recurrent vaginal metastases. American Journal of Obstetrics and Gynecology 82: 660–663.

Douglas G W 1962 Malignant change in trophoblastic tumors. American Journal of Obstetrics and Gynecology 84: 884–894.

Driscoll S G 1963 Choriocarcinoma: an 'incidental finding' within a term placenta. Obstetrics and Gynecology 21: 96–101.

Driscoll S G 1977 Gestational trophoblastic neoplasms: morphologic considerations. Human Pathology 8: 529–539.

Du Beshter B, Berkowitz R S, Goldstein D P, Cramer D W, Bernstein M R 1987 Metastatic gestational trophoblastic disease: experience at the New England Trophoblastic Disease Centre, 1965–1985. Obstetrics and Gynecology 69: 390–395.

Duff G B 1989 Gestational trophoblastic disease in New Zealand, 1980–1986. Australian and New Zealand Journal of Obstetrics and Gynaecology 29: 139–142.

Eckstein R P, Paradinas F J, Bagshawe K D 1982 Placental site trophoblastic tumour (trophoblastic pseudo tumour): a study of four cases requiring hysterectomy including one fatal case. Histopathology 6: 221–226.

Eckstein R P, Russell P, Friedlander M M, Tattersall M H N, Bradfield A 1985 Metastasizing placental site tumor: a case study. Human Pathology 16: 632–636.

Ellis P S J, Whitehead R 1981 Mitosis counting — a need for reappraisal. Human Pathology 12: 3–4.

Elmer D B, Granai C O, Ball H G, Curry S L 1993 Persistence of gestational trophoblastic disease for longer than 1 year following evacuation of hydatidiform mole. Obstetrics and Gynecology 81: 888–890.

Elston C W 1969 Cellular reaction to choriocarcinoma. Journal of Pathology 97: 261–268.

Elston C W 1970 A histopathological study of trophoblastic tumours: with special reference to the cellular reaction to choriocarcinoma. MD Thesis, University of London.

Elston C W 1976 The histopathology of trophoblastic tumours. Journal of Clinical Pathology 29 (suppl 10): 111–131.

Elston C W 1978 Trophoblastic tumours of the placenta. In: Fox H (ed) Pathology of the placenta. Saunders, London, pp 368–425.

Elston C W 1981 Gestational tumours of trophoblast. In: Anthony P P, MacSween R N M (eds) Recent advances in histopathology. Churchill Livingstone, Edinburgh, pp 149–161.

Elston C W 1991 Trophoblastic disease: a review with emphasis on recent advances and problems in differential diagnosis. In: Damjanov I, Cohen A H, Mills S E, Young R H (eds) Progress in reproductive and urinary tract pathology. Field & Wood, New York, pp 31–72.

Elston C W, Bagshawe K D 1972a The value of histological grading in the management of hydatidiform mole. Journal of Obstetrics and Gynaecology of the British Commonwealth 79: 717–724.

Elston C W, Bagshawe K D 1972b The diagnosis of trophoblastic tumours from uterine curettings. Journal of Clinical Pathology 25: 111–118.

Elston C W, Bagshawe K D 1973 Cellular reaction in trophoblastic tumours. British Journal of Cancer 28: 245–256.

Ewing J 1910 Chorioma: a clinical and pathological study. Surgery Gynecology and Obstetrics 10: 366–392.

Faulk W P, McIntyre J A 1983 Immunological studies of human trophoblast: markers, subsets and function. Immunological Reviews 75: 139–175.

Faulk W P, Temple A 1976 Distribution of B2 microglobulin and HLA in chorionic villi of human placentae. Nature 262: 799–802.

Finkler N J, Berkowitz R S, Driscoll S G, Goldstein D P, Bernstein M R 1988 Clinical experience with placental site trophoblastic tumors at the New England Trophoblastic Disease Centre. Obstetrics and Gynecology 71: 854–857.

Fisher R A, Lawler S D 1984a Heterozygous complete hydatidiform moles: do they have a worse prognosis than homozygous complete moles. Lancet ii: 51.

Fisher R A, Lawler S D 1984b The expression of major histocompatability antigens in the chorionic villi of molar placentae. Placenta 5: 237–242.

Fisher R A, Newlands E S 1993 Rapid diagnosis and classification of hydatidiform moles with polymerase chain reaction. American Journal of Obstetrics and Gynecology 168: 563–569.

Fisher R A, Sheppard D M, Lawler S D 1982 Twin pregnancy with complete hydatidiform mole (46,XX) and fetus (46,XY): genetic origin proved by analysis of chromosome polymorphisms. British Medical Journal 284: 1218–1220.

Fisher R A, Lawler S D, Ormerod M G, Imrie P R, Povey S 1987 Flow cytometry used to distinguish between complete and partial hydatidiform moles. Placenta 8: 249–256.

Fisher R A, Povey S, Jeffreys A J et al 1989 Frequency of heterozygous complete hydatidiform moles, estimated by locus-specific minisatellite and Y chromosome-specific probes. Human Genetics 82: 259–263.

Fisher R A, Paradinas F J, Newlands E S, Boxer G M 1992 Genetic evidence that placental site trophoblastic tumours can originate from a hydatidiform mole or a normal conceptus. British Journal of Cancer 65: 355–358.

Fox H 1989 Editorial: hydatidiform moles. Virchows Archives A Pathological Anatomy 415: 387–389.

Fox H 1993 Commentary: histological classification of tissue from spontaneous abortions: a valueless exercise? Histopathology 22: 599–600.

Fox H, Kharkongor N F 1971 Ultrastructure of molar trophoblast. Journal of Obstetrics and Gynaecology of the British Commonwealth 78: 652–659.

Fox H, Laurini R N 1988 Intraplacental choriocarcinoma: a report of two cases. Journal of Clinical Pathology 41: 1085–1088.

Franke H R, Risse E K J, Kenemans P, Vooijs G P, Stolke J G 1983 Epidemiologic features of hydatidiform mole in the Netherlands. Obstetrics and Gynecology 62: 613–616.

Fukuyama R, Takata M, Kudoh J et al 1991 DNA diagnosis of hydatidiform mole using the polymerase chain reaction. Human Genetics 87: 216–218.

Gaber L W, Redline R W, Mostoufi-Zadeh M, Driscoll S G 1986 Invasive partial mole. American Journal of Clinical Pathology 85: 722–724.

Gal D, Friedman M 1987 Follow up and contraception. In: Szulman A E, Buchsbaum H J (eds) Gestational trophoblastic disease. Springer-Verlag, New York, pp 179–185.

Galton M, Goldman P B, Holt S F 1963 Karyotypic and morphologic characterisation of a serially transplanted human choriocarcinoma. Journal of the National Cancer Institute 31: 1019–1035.

Gardner H A R, Lage J L 1992 Choriocarcinoma following a partial mole: a case report. Human Pathology 23: 468–471.

Genest D R, Laborde O, Berkowitz R S, Goldstein D P, Bernstein M R, Lage J 1991 A clinicopathologic study of 153 cases of complete hydatidiform mole (1980–1990): histologic grade lacks prognostic significance. Obstetrics and Gynecology 78: 402–409.

Ghali F H 1969 Incidence of trophoblastic neoplasia in Iraq. American Journal of Obstetrics and Gynecology 105: 992–993.

Gloor E, Ribolzi J, Dialdas J, Barrelet L, Hurlimann J 1983 Placental site trophoblastic tumors (trophoblastic pseudotumor) of the uterus with metastases and fatal outcome. American Journal of Surgical Pathology 7: 483–486.

Goldstein D P, Berkowitz R S 1982 Gestational trophoblastic neoplasms: clinical principles of diagnosis and management. WB Saunders, Philadelphia.

Gonzalez-Angulo A, Marquez-Monter H, Zavala B J, Yabur E, Salazar H 1966 Electron microscopic observations in hydatidiform mole. Obstetrics and Gynecology 27: 455–467.

Gore H, Hertig A T 1967 Problems in the histologic interpretation of the trophoblast. Clinical Obstetrics and Gynecology 10: 269–289.

Goto S, Yamada A, Ishizuka T, Tomoda Y 1993 Development of post molar trophoblastic disease after partial molar pregnancy. Gynecologic Oncology 48: 165–170.

Graham I H, Fajardo A M, Richards R L 1990 Epidemiological study of complete and partial hydatidiform mole in Abu Dhabi: influence of maternal age and ethnic group. Journal of Clinical Pathology 43: 661–664.

Greene R R 1959 Chorioadenoma destruens. Annals of the New York Academy of Sciences 80: 143–151.

Grimes D A 1984 Epidemiology of gestational trophoblastic disease. American Journal of Obstetrics and Gynecology 150: 309–318.

Haines M 1955 Hydatidiform mole and vaginal nodules. Journal of Obstetrics and Gynaecology of the British Empire 62: 6–11.

Hall P A, Woods A L 1990 Immunohistochemical markers of cell proliferation: achievements, problems and prospects. Cell and Tissue Kinetics 23: 531–549.

Hall P A, Levison D A, Woods A L et al 1990 Proliferating cell nuclear antigen (PCNA) immunolocalisation in paraffin sections: an index of cell proliferation with evidence of deregulated expression in some neoplasms. Journal of Pathology 162: 285–294.

Hallam L A, MacLaren K M, El-Jabbour J N, Helm C W, Smart G E 1990 Intraplacental choriocarcinoma: a case report. Placenta 11: 247–251.

Hayashi K, Bracken M B, Freeman D H, Hellenbrand K 1982 Hydatidiform mole in the United States (1970–1977): a statistical and theoretical analysis. American Journal of Epidemiology 115: 67–77.

Hedley D W, Friedlander M L, Taylor I W, Rugg C A, Musgrove E A 1983 Method for analysis of cellular DNA content of paraffin embedded pathological material using flow cytometry. Journal of Histochemistry and Cytochemistry 31: 1333–1335.

Heifetz S A, Czaja J 1992 In situ choriocarcinoma arising in partial hydatidiform mole: implications for the risk of persistent trophoblastic disease. Pediatric Pathology 12: 601–611.

Hemming J D, Quirke P, Womack C et al 1987 Diagnosis of molar pregnancy and persistent trophoblastic disease by flow cytometry. Journal of Clinical Pathology 40: 615–620.

Hemming J D, Quirke P, Womack C et al 1988 Flow cytometry in persistent trophoblastic disease. Placenta 9: 615–621.

Hertig A T 1950 Hydatidiform mole and chorionepithelioma. In: Meigs J B, Sturgis S H eds Progress in gynecology, vol 2. Grune & Stratton, New York, pp 372–394.

Hertig A T, Mansell H 1956 Tumors of the female sex organs. Part 1. Hydatidiform mole and choriocarcinoma. In: Atlas of tumour pathology, section 9, fascicle 33. Armed Forces Institute of Pathology, Washington, D C.

Hertig A T, Sheldon W H 1947 Hydatidiform mole: a pathologico-clinical correlation of 200 cases. American Journal of Obstetrics and Gynecology 53: 1–36.

Hertz R 1967 Serial passage of choriocarcinoma of women in the hamster cheek pouch. In: Holland J F, Hreshchyshyn M M eds Choriocarcinoma: transactions of a conference of the International Union against Cancer. Springer Verlag, Berlin, pp 26–28.

Hertz R 1978 Choriocarcinoma and related gestational trophoblastic tumors in women. Raven Press, New York.

Hertz R, Lewis J L Jr, Lipsett M B 1961 Five years experience with the chemotherapy of metastatic choriocarcinoma and related trophoblastic tumors in women. American Journal of Obstetrics and Gynecology 82: 631–640.

Hoffman J S, Silverman A D, Gelber J, Cartun R 1993 Placental site trophoblastic tumor: a report of radiologic, surgical and pathologic methods of evaluating the extent of disease. Gynecologic Oncology 50: 110–114.

Hou P-C, Pang S-C 1956 Chorionepithelioma: an analytical study of 28 necropsied cases with special reference to the possibility of spontaneous regression. Journal of Pathology and Bacteriology 72: 95–104.

Howat A J, Beck S, Fox H et al 1993 Can histopathologists reliably diagnose molar pregnancy? Journal of Clinical Pathology 46: 599–602.

Hsu C T, Huang I C, Chen T Y 1962 Metastases in benign hydatidiform mole and chorioadenoma destruens. American Journal of Obstetrics and Gynecology 84: 1414–1424.

Hunt W, Dockerty M B, Randall L M 1953 Hydatidiform mole: clinico-pathological study involving 'grading' as a measure of possible malignant change. Obstetrics and Gynecology 1: 593–609.

Hunter V, Raymond E, Christensen C et al 1990 Efficacy of the metastatic survey in the staging of gestational trophoblastic disease. Cancer 65: 1647–1650.

Inferrerra C, Pullé C, Rigano A, Palmara D 1967 Aspetti ultrastrutturali e citochimici del coriocarcinoma uterino. Archivo di Osetricia e Ginecologia 72: 707–744.

International Union Against Cancer 1967 In: Holland J F, Hreshchyshyn M M (eds) Choriocarcinoma: transactions of a conference of the International Union Against Cancer. Appendix 1. Springer Verlag, Berlin, Heidelberg, pp 116–118.

Ishizuka N 1967 Chemotherapy of chorionic tumors. In: Holland J F, Hreshchyshyn M M (eds) Choriocarcinoma: transactions of a conference of the International Union against Cancer. Springer Verlag, Berlin, pp 116–118.

Ishizuka N 1976 Studies of trophoblastic neoplasia. Gann 18: 203–216.

Ito H, Sekine T, Komuro N et al 1981 Histologic stromal reaction of the host with gestational choriocarcinoma and its relation to clinical stage, classification and prognosis. American Journal of Obstetrics and Gynecology 140: 781–786.

Jacobs P A, Wilson C M, Sprenkle J A, Rosenshein N B, Migeon B R 1980 Mechanism of origin of complete hydatidiform moles. Nature 286: 714–716.

Jacobs P A, Hunt P A, Matsuura J S, Wilson C C, Szulman A E 1982a Complete and partial hydatidiform mole in Hawaii: cytogenetics, morphology and epidemiology. British Journal of Obstetrics and Gynaecology 89: 258–266.

Jacobs P A, Szulman A E, Funkhouser J, Matsuura J S, Wilson C C 1982b Human triploidy: relationship between parental origin of the additional haploid complement and development of partial hydatidiform mole. Annals of Human Genetics 46: 223–231.

Jacobson F J, Enzer N 1959 Hydatidiform mole with 'benign' metastasis to lung. American Journal of Obstetrics and Gynecology 78: 868–875.

Jauniaux E, Zucker M, Meuris S et al 1988 Chorangiocarcinoma: an unusual tumour of the placenta: the missing link? Placenta 9: 607–613.

Javey H, Borazjani G, Behmard S, Langley F A 1979 Discrepancies in the histological diagnosis of hydatidiform mole. British Journal of Obstetrics and Gynaecology 86: 480–483.

Jeffreys A J, Wilson V, Neumann R, Keyte J 1988 Amplification of human minisatellites by the polymerase chain reaction: towards DNA fingerprinting of single cells. Nucleic Acids Research 16: 10953–10971.

Johnson P M, Cheng H M, Molloy C M, Stern C M M, Slade M B 1981 Human trophoblast-specific surface antigens identified using monoclonal antibodies. American Journal of Reproductive Immunology 1: 246–254.

Johnson T R, Comstock C H, Anderson D G 1979 Benign gestational trophoblastic disease metastatic to pleura: unusual cause of hemothorax. Obstetrics and Gynecology 53: 509–511.

Joint Project for Study of Choriocarcinoma and Hydatidiform Mole in Asia 1959 Geographic variation in the occurrence of hydatidiform mole and choriocarcinoma. Annals of the New York Academy of Sciences 80: 178–195.

Jones W B 1990 Gestational trophoblastic disease: what have we learned in the past decade? American Journal of Obstetrics and Gynecology 162: 1286–1295.

Jones W B, Lauersen N H 1975 Hydatidiform mole with coexistent fetus. American Journal of Obstetrics and Gynecology 122: 267–272.

Junaid T A, Hendrickse J P de V, Oladiran B, Edington G M, Williams A O 1974 Choriocarcinoma in Ibadan, Nigeria. Journal of the National Cancer Institute 53: 1597–1599.

Junaid T A, Hendrickse H P de V, Oladiran B, Edington G M, Williams A O 1976 Choriocarcinoma in Ibadan: clinicopathological studies. Human Pathology 7: 215–222.

Kajii T, Ohama K 1977 Androgenic origin of hydatidiform mole. Nature 268: 633–634.

Kajii T, Kurashigo H, Ohama K, Uchino F L 1984 XY and XX complete moles: clinical and morphological correlations. American Journal of Obstetrics and Gynecology 150: 57–64.

Kardana A, Bagshawe K D 1976 A rapid, sensitive and specific radioimmunoassay for human chorionic gonadotrophin. Journal of Immunological Methods 9: 297–305.

King G 1956 Hydatidiform mole and chorion epithelioma. The problem of the borderline case. Proceedings of the Royal Society of Medicine 49: 381–390.

Knoth M, Hesseldahl H, Larsen J F 1969 Ultrastructure of human choriocarcinoma. Acta Obstetrica et Gynecologica Scandinavica 48: 100–118.

Ko T-M, Hsieh C-Y, Ho H-N, Hsieh F-J, Lee T-Y 1991 Restriction fragment length polymorphism analysis to study the genetic origin of complete hydatidiform mole. American Journal of Obstetrics and Gynecology 164: 901–906.

Koenig C, Demopoulos R I, Vamvakos E C et al 1993 Flow cytometric DNA ploidy and quantitative histopathology in partial moles. International Journal of Gynecological Pathology 12: 235–240.

Kohorn E I, McGinn R C, Gee B L, Goldstein D P, Osathanondh R 1978 Pulmonary embolisation of trophoblastic tissue in molar pregnancy. Obstetrics and Gynecology 51: 155–205.

Kolstad P, Hognestad J 1965 Trophoblastic tumours in Norway. Acta Obstetrica et Gynecologica Scandinavica 44: 80–88.

Komuro N 1976 Experimental induction of chorionepithelioma in pregnant rats. Acta Obstetrica et Gynaecologica Japonica 23: 32–42.

Kovacs B W, Shahbahrami B, Tast D E, Curtin J P 1991 Molecular genetic analysis of complete hydatidiform moles. Cancer Genetics Cytogenetics 54: 143–152.

Kurman R J, Scully R E, Norris H J 1976 Trophoblastic pseudotumor of the uterus: an exaggerated form of 'syncytial endometritis' simulating a malignant tumor. Cancer 38: 1214–1226.

Kurman R J, Young R H, Norris H J, Lawrence W D, Scully R E 1984 Immunocytochemical localisation of placental lactogen and chorionic gonadotrophin in the normal placenta and trophoblastic tumors with emphasis on intermediate trophoblast and the placental site trophoblastic tumor. International Journal of Gynecological Pathology 3: 101–121.

Kushima K, Noda K, Makita M 1967 Experimental production of chorionic tumour in rabbits. Tohuku Journal of Experimental Medicine 91: 209–214.

Lage J M 1990 Diagnostic dilemmas in gynecologic and obstetric pathology. Seminars in Diagnostic Pathology 7: 146–155.

Lage J M, Roberts D J 1993 Choriocarcinoma in a term placenta: pathologic diagnosis of tumor in an asymptomatic patient with metastatic disease. International Journal of Gynecological Pathology 12: 80–85.

Lage J M, Driscoll S G, Yavner D L et al 1988 Hydatidiform moles: application of flow cytometry in diagnosis. American Journal of Clinical Pathology 89: 596–600.

Lage J M, Weinberg D S, Yavner D L, Bieber F R 1989 The biology of tetraploid hydatidiform moles: histopathology, cytogenetics and flow cytometry. Human Pathology 20: 419–425.

Lage J M, Berkowitz R S, Rice L W, Goldstein D P, Bernstein M R, Weinberg D S 1991 Flow cytometric analysis of DNA content in partial hydatidiform moles with persistent gestational trophoblastic tumor. Obstetrics and Gynecology 77: 111–115.

Lahey S J, Steele G, Rodrick M L et al 1984 Characterisation of antigenic components from circulating immune complexes in patients with gestational trophoblastic neoplasia. Cancer 53: 1316–1321.

Lane S A, Taylor G R, Ozols B, Quirke P 1993 Diagnosis of complete molar pregnancy by microsatellites in archival material. Journal of Clinical Pathology 46: 346–348.

Larsen J F 1973 Ultrastructure of the abnormal human trophoblast. Acta Anatomica Supplement 1: 47–74.

Larsen J F, Ehrmann R L, Bierring F 1967 Electron microscopy of human choriocarcinoma transplanted into hamster liver. American Journal of Obstetrics and Gynecology 99: 1109–1124.

Lathrop J C, Lauchlan S, Nayak R, Ambler M 1988 Clinical characteristics of placental site trophoblastic tumor (PSTT). Gynecologic Oncology 31: 32–42.

La Vecchia C, Franceschi S, Parazzini F et al 1985 Risk factors for gestational trophoblastic disease in Italy. American Journal of Epidemiology 121: 457–464.

Lawler S D 1978 HLA and trophoblastic tumours. British Medical Bulletin 34: 305–308.

Lawler S D, Fisher R A 1986 Genetic aspects of gestational trophoblastic tumors. In: Ichinoe K (ed) Trophoblastic diseases. Ikagu-Shoin, Tokyo, pp 23–33.

Lawler S D, Fisher R A 1987a Genetic studies in hydatidiform mole with clinical correlations. Placenta 8: 77–88.

Lawler S D, Fisher R A 1987b Immunological aspects. In: Szulman A E, Buchsbaum H J eds Gestational trophoblastic disease. Springer-Verlag, New York, pp 77–87.

Lawler S D, Fisher R A 1991 A prospective genetic study of complete and partial hydatidiform moles. American Journal of Obstetrics and Gynecology 164: 1270–1277.

Lawler S D, Klouda P T, Bagshawe K D 1971 The HL-A system in trophoblastic neoplasia. Lancet ii: 834–837.

Lawler S D, Pickthall V J, Fisher R A et al 1979 Genetic studies of complete and partial hydatidiform moles. Lancet ii: 580.

Lawler S D, Fisher R A, Pickthall V J, Povey S, Evans M W 1982a Genetic studies on hydatidiform moles. I. The origin of partial moles. Cancer Genetics and Cytogenetics 5: 309–320.

Lawler S D, Povey S, Fisher S, Pickthall V J 1982b Genetic studies on hydatidiform moles. II. The origin of complete moles. Annals of Human Genetics 46: 209–222.

Lee Y S, Cheah E, Szulman A E 1981 The pattern of hydatidiform moles in Singapore. Australian and New Zealand Journal of Obstetrics and Gynaecology 21: 230–233.

Leighton P C 1973 Trophoblastic disease in Uganda. American Journal of Obstetrics and Gynecology 117: 341–344.

Lewis J L Jr, Terasaki P T 1971 HL-A leukocyte antigen studies in women with gestational trophoblastic neoplasms. American Journal of Obstetrics and Gynecology 111: 547–554.

Lewis J L Jr, Davis C R, Ross G T 1969 Hormonal, immunologic and chemotherapeutic studies of transplantable human choriocarcinoma. American Journal of Obstetrics and Gynecology 104: 472–478.

Li M C, Hertz R, Spencer D B 1956 Effect of methotrexate therapy upon choriocarcinoma and chorioadenoma. Proceedings of the Society of Experimental Biology and Medicine 93: 361–366.

Lindsey J R, Wharton C R, Woodruff J D, Baker J H 1969 Intrauterine choriocarcinoma in a rhesus monkey. Pathologica Veterinaria 6: 378–384.

Llewellyn-Jones D 1965 Trophoblastic tumours: geographical variations in incidence and possible aetiological factors. Journal of Obstetrics and Gynaecology of the British Commonwealth 72: 242–248.

Logan B J, Motyloff L 1958 Hydatidiform mole: a clinical and pathological study of 72 cases, with reference to their malignant tendencies. American Journal of Obstetrics and Gynecology 75: 1134–1148.

Looi L M, Sivanesaratnam V 1981 Malignant evolution with fatal outcome in a patient with partial hydatidiform mole. Australian and New Zealand Journal of Obstetrics and Gynaecology 21: 51–52.

Lurain J R 1987 Natural history. In: Szulman A E, Buchsbaum H J eds Gestational trophoblastic disease. Springer-Verlag, New York, pp 69–76.

Lurain J R, Sciarra J J 1991 Study and treatment of gestational trophoblastic disease at the John I Brewer Trophoblastic Disease Center, 1962–1990. European Journal of Gynaecological Oncology 12: 425–428.

MacRae D J 1951 Chorionepithelioma occurring during pregnancy. Journal of Obstetrics and Gynaecology of the British Empire 58: 373–380.

McCorriston C C 1968 Racial incidence of hydatidiform mole: a study in a contained polyracial community. American Journal of Obstetrics and Gynecology 101: 377–381.

McLaughlin P J, Cheng H M, Slade M B et al 1982 Expression on cultured human tumour cells of placental trophoblast membrane antigens and placental alkaline phosphatase defined by monoclonal antibodies. International Journal of Cancer 30: 21–26.

McLellan R, Buscema J, Currie J L, Woodruff J D 1991 Placental site trophoblastic tumor in a postmenopausal woman. American Journal of Clinical Pathology 95: 670–675.

Makino S, Sasaki M S, Fukuschima T 1963 Preliminary notes on the chromosomes of human chorionic lesions. Proceedings of the Japanese Academy 39: 54–58.

Makino S, Sasaki M S, Fukuschima T 1964 Triploid chromosome constitution in human chorionic lesions. Lancet ii: 1273–1275.

Marchand F 1894 Verhandlung ärztlicher Verein zu Marburg. Klinische Wochenschrift Berlin 31: 813–814.

Marchand F 1895 Über die sogenannten 'decidualen, Geschwülste Anschluss an normale Geburt, Abort, Blasenmole, und Extrauterinschwangerschaft. Monatsschrift für Geburtshilfe und Gynäkologie 1: 419–428 and 513–562.

Marchand F 1898 Über das maligne Chorion-Epitheliom, nebst Mittheilung von 2 neuen Fallen. Zeitschrift für Geburtshilfe und Gynakologie 39: 173–258.

Marin-Padilla M, Benirschke K 1963 Thalidomide-induced alterations in the blastocyst and placenta of the armadillo, dasypus novemcintus mexicanus, including a choriocarcinoma. American Journal of Pathology 43: 999–1016.

Marquez-Monter H, de la Vega G A, Robles M, Bolio-Cicero A 1963 Epidemiology and pathology of hydatidiform mole in the General Hospital of Mexico: study of 104 cases. American Journal of Obstetrics and Gynecology 85: 856–864.

Martin P M 1978 High frequency of hydatidiform mole in native Alaskans. International Journal of Gynaecology and Obstetrics 15: 395–396.

Matalon M, Modan B 1972 Epidemiologic aspects of hydatidiform mole in Israel. American Journal of Obstetrics and Gynecology 112: 107–112.

Mathews M B, Berstein R M, Franza B R Jr, Garrels J I 1984 Identity of the proliferating cell nuclear antigen and cyclin. Nature 303: 374–376.

Mazur M T, Kurman R J 1987 Choriocarcinoma and placental site trophoblastic tumor. In: Szulman A E, Buchsbaum J H eds Gestational trophoblastic disease. Springer-Verlag, New York, pp 45–68.

Mazur M T, Lurain J R, Brewer J J 1982 Fatal gestational choriocarcinoma: clinicopathological study of patients treated at a trophoblastic disease center. Cancer 50: 1833–1846.

Messerli M L, Lilienfeld A M, Parmley T, Woodruff J D, Rosenshein N B 1985 Risk factors for gestational trophoblastic neoplasia. American Journal of Obstetrics and Gynecology 153: 294–300.

Messerli M L, Parmley T, Woodruff J D et al 1987 Inter- and intra-pathologist variability in the diagnosis of gestational trophoblastic neoplasia. Obstetrics and Gynecology 69: 622–626.

Miller D, Jackson R, Ehlen T, McMurtrie E 1993 Complete hydatidiform mole coexistent with a twin live fetus: clinical course of four cases with complete cytogenetic analysis. Gynecologic Oncology 50: 119–123.

Mittal K K, Kachru R B, Brewer J I 1975 The HL-A and ABO antigens in trophoblastic disease. Tissue Antigens 6: 57–69.

Miyamoto M, Nilsuwarn N, Angsubhakorn S 1972 The morphology of experimental chorionic tumours in rats. Acta Pathologica Japonica 22: 343–352.

Mogensen B, Kissmeyer-Nielsen F 1968 Histocompatibility antigens of the HL-A locus in generalised gestational choriocarcinoma. Lancet i: 721–725.

Mogensen B, Kissmeyer-Nielsen F 1971 Current data on HL-A and ABO typing in gestational choriocarcinoma and invasive mole. Transplantation Proceedings 3: 1267–1269.

Mogensen B, Olsen S 1973 Cellular reaction to gestational choriocarcinoma and invasive mole. Acta Pathologica et Microbiologica Scandinavica Section A 81: 453–456.

Mueller U W, Hawes C S, Wright A E et al 1990 Isolation of fetal trophoblast cells from peripheral blood of pregnant women. Lancet 336: 197–200.

Muller R, Tremblay J M, Adamson E D, Verman I M 1983 Tissue and cell type-specific expression of two human c-onc genes. Nature 304: 454–456.

Mutter G L, Pomponio R J, Berkowitz R S, Genest D R 1993 Sex chromosome composition of complete hydatidiform moles: relationship to metastasis. American Journal of Obstetrics and Gynecology 168: 1547–1551.

Nastac E, Athanasiu P, Predescu E et al 1980 Experimental investigations in hamsters and rabbits with DNA extracted from human uterine tumors. Virologie 31: 37–39.

Naumoff P, Szulman A E, Weinstein B, Mazer J, Surti U 1981 Ultrasonography of partial hydatidiform mole. Radiology 140: 467–470.

Newlands E S, Fisher R A, Searle F 1992 The immune system in disease: gestational trophoblastic tumours. Balliere's Clinical Obstetrics and Gynaecology 6: 519–538.

Novak E, Seah C S 1954 Choriocarcinoma of the uterus: study of 74 cases from the Mathieu Memorial Chorionepithelioma Registry. American Journal of Obstetrics and Gynecology 67: 933–957.

Ober W B 1965 Clinical and pathological aspects of abnormal trophoblast: discussion. In: Park W W ed The early conceptus, normal and abnormal. Livingstone, London, pp 141–144.

Ober W B, Fass R O 1961 The early history of choriocarcinoma. Journal of the History of Medicine and Allied Sciences 16: 49–73.

Ober W B, Maier R C 1982 Gestational choriocarcinoma of the Fallopian tube. Diagnostic Gynecology and Obstetrics 3: 213–231.

Ober W B, Edgcomb J R, Price E B Jr 1971 The pathology of choriocarcinoma. Annals of the New York Academy of Sciences 172: 299–426.

Ockleford C D, Clode A 1983 Microgibbosities in hydatidiform mole. Journal of Pathology 141: 181–189.

Ohama K, Kajii T, Okamoto E et al 1981 Dispermic origin of XY hydatidiform moles. Nature 292: 551–552.

Okudaira Y, Strauss L 1967 Ultrastructure of molar trophoblast: observations on hydatidiform mole and chorioadenoma destruens. Obstetrics and Gynecology 30: 172–187.

Olesnicky G, Long A R, Quinn M A et al 1985 Hydatidiform mole in Victoria: aetiology and natural history. Australian and New Zealand Journal of Obstetrics and Gynaecology 21: 1–6.

Orrell J M, Sanders D S A 1991 A particularly aggressive placental site trophoblastic tumour. Histopathology 18: 559–561.

Paradinas F J 1994 The histological diagnosis of hydatidiform mole. Current Diagnostic Pathology 1: 24–31.

Park W W 1957 The occurrence of sex chromatin in chorionepitheliomas and hydatidiform moles. Journal of Pathology and Bacteriology 74: 197–206.

Park W W 1967 The pathology of trophoblastic tumors. In: Holland J F, Hreshchyshyn M M (eds) Choriocarcinoma: transactions of a conference of the International Union against Cancer. Springer-Verlag, Berlin, pp 3–8.

Park W W 1971 Choriocarcinoma: a study of its pathology Heinemann, London.

Park W W 1975 Possible functions of nonvillous trophoblast. European Journal of Obstetrics, Gynecology and Reproductive Biology 5: 35–46.

Park W W, Lees J C 1950 Choriocarcinoma. A general review, with analysis of 516 cases. Archives of Pathology 49: 73–104 and 205–241.

Pattillo R A, Gey G O 1968 The establishment of a cell line of human hormone synthesising trophoblastic cells in vitro. Cancer Research 28: 1231–1236.

Pattillo R A, Sasaki S, Katayama K P, Roesler M, Mattingly R F 1981 Genesis of 46 XY hydatidiform mole. American Journal of Obstetrics and Gynecology 141: 104–105.

Pesce C, Merino M J, Chambers J T, Nogales F 1991 Endometrial carcinoma with trophoblastic differentiation: an aggressive form of uterine cancer. Cancer 68: 1799–1802.

Pijnenborg R, Bland J M, Robertson W B, Dixon G, Brosens I 1981 The pattern of interstitial trophoblastic invasion of the myometrium in early human pregnancy. Placenta 2: 303–316.

Poen H T, Djojopranoto M 1965 The possible etiologic factors of hydatidiform mole and choriocarcinoma: preliminary report. American Journal of Obstetrics and Gynecology 92: 510–513.

Pollard J W, Bartocci A, Arceci R, Orlofsky A, Ladner M B, Stanley E R 1987 Apparent role of the macrophage growth factor CSF-1, in placental development. Nature 330: 484–486.

Prawirohardjo S, Martiono K S, Sutomo T 1957 Hydatidiform mole and choriocarcinoma in Indonesia. First Asiatic Congress of Obstetrics and Gynecology, Tokyo, pp 112–129.

Ratnam S S, Chew S C 1976 The natural history of gestational trophoblastic disease. In: First Inter-Congress of the Asian Federation of Obstetrics and Gynaecology, pp 1–7.

Reddy D, Rao N 1969 Trophoblastic tumours. I. Hydatidiform mole. Indian Journal of Medical Science 23: 527–537.

Reed S, Coe J I, Bergquist K 1959 Invasive hydatidiform mole metastatic to the lungs: report of a case. Obstetrics and Gynecology 13: 749–753.

Reid M H, McGahan J P, Oi R 1983 Sonographic evaluation of hydatidiform mole and its look-alikes. American Journal of Roentgenology 140: 307–311.

Rettenmier G W, Sacca R, Furman W L et al 1986 Expression of the human c-fms proto-oncogene product (colony-stimulating factor-1 receptor) on peripheral blood mononuclear cells and choriocarcinoma cell lines. Journal of Clinical Investigation 77: 1740–1743.

Rice L W, Berkowitz R S, Lage J M, Goldstein D P, Bernstein M R 1990 Persistent gestational trophoblastic tumor after partial hydatidiform mole. Gynecologic Oncology 36: 358–362.

Ring A M 1972 The concept of benign metastasizing hydatidiform moles. American Journal of Clinical Pathology 58: 111–117.

Ringertz N 1970 Hydatidiform mole, invasive mole and choriocarcinoma in Sweden, 1958–1965. Acta Obstetricia et Gynecologica Scandinavica 49: 195–203.

Romero R, Horgan G, Kohorn E I et al 1985 New criteria for the diagnosis of gestational trophoblastic disease. Obstetrics and Gynecology 66: 553–558.

Rudolph R H, Thomas E D 1970 Histocompatibility studies in patients with trophoblastic tumors. American Journal of Obstetrics and Gynecology 108: 1126–1129.

Rushton D I 1981 Examination of products of conception from previable human pregnancies. Journal of Clinical Pathology 34: 819–835.

Sand P K, Lurain J R, Brewer J I 1984 Repeat gestational trophoblastic disease. Obstetrics and Gynecology 63: 140–144.

Sänger M 1889 Zwei aussergewöhnliche Falle von Abortus. Zentralblatt für Gynäkologie 13: 132–134.

Sarkar S, Kacinski B M, Kohorn E I et al 1986 Demonstration of myc and ras oncogene expression by hybridisation in situ in hydatidiform mole and in the BeWo choriocarcinoma cell line. American Journal of Obstetrics and Gynecology 154: 390–393.

Sasagawa M, Watanabe S, Ohmomo Y et al 1986 Reactivity of two monoclonal antibodies (Troma I and CAM 5.2) on human tissue sections: analysis of their usefulness as a histological trophoblast marker in normal pregnancy and trophoblastic disease. International Journal of Gynecological Pathology 5: 345–356.

Sasaki M, Katayama P K, Roesler M et al 1982 Cytogenetic analysis of choriocarcinoma cell lines. Acta Obstetrica et Gynecologica Japonica 36: 2253–2256.

Schiffer M A, Pomerance W, Mackles A 1960 Hydatidiform mole in relation to malignant disease of the trophoblast. American Journal of Obstetrics and Gynecology 90: 516–531.

Schlegel R J, Nen R, Leao J C et al 1966 Arborising amniotic polyps in triploid conceptuses: a diagnostic anatomic lesion? American Journal of Obstetrics and Gynecology 96: 357–361.

Schmorl G 1893 Pathologisch-anatomische Untersuchungen über Puerperal-eklampsie. Vogel, Leipsig.

Scully R E, Young R H 1981 Trophoblastic pseudotumor: a reappraisal. American Journal of Surgical Pathology 5: 75–76.

Seckl M J, Rustin G J S, Newlands E S, Gwyther S J, Bomanji J 1991 Pulmonary embolism, pulmonary hypertension and choriocarcinoma. Lancet 338: 1313–1315.

Sen D K, Sinnatharay T A, Lau K A 1973 The ultrastructure of molar trophoblast. Australian and New Zealand Journal of Obstetrics and Gynaecology 13: 35–39.

Shaw A R E, Dasgupta M K, Kovithavongs T et al 1979 Humoral and cellular immunity to paternal antigen in trophoblastic neoplasia. International Journal of Cancer 24: 586–593.

Sheer C J, Rettenmier C W, Sacca R, Roussel M F, Look A T, Stanley E R 1985 The c-fms proto-oncogene product is related to the receptor for the mononuclear phagocyte growth factor, CSF-1. Cell 41: 665–676.

Sheppard D M, Fisher R A, Lawler S D 1985 Karyotypic analysis and chromosomal polymorphisms in four choriocarcinoma cell lines. Cancer Genetics and Cytogenetics 16: 251–258.

Shintani S, Glass L E, Page E W 1966 Studies of induced malignant tumors to placental and uterine origin in the rat. 1. Survival of placental tissue following fetectomy. 2. Induced tumors and their pathogenesis with special reference to choriocarcinoma. 3. Identification of experimentally induced choriocarcinoma by detection of placental hormone. American Journal of Obstetrics and Gynecology 95: 542–563.

Silverberg S G, Kurman R J 1992 Tumors of the uterine corpus and gestational trophoblastic disease. Atlas of tumor pathology, third series, fascicle 3. Armed Forces Institute of Pathology, Washington, DC.

Smalbraak J 1957 Trophoblastic growths: a clinical, hormonal and histopathologic study of hydatidiform mole and choriocarcinoma. Elsevier, Amsterdam.

Smalbraak J 1959 Problems in the classification of hydatidiform moles. Annals of the New York Academy of Sciences 80: 105–120.

Smith D B, Newlands E S, Bagshawe K D 1993 Correlation between clinical staging (FIGO) and prognostic groups with gestational trophoblastic disease. British Journal of Obstetrics and Gynaecology 100: 157–160.

Smith R, Crocker J 1988 Evaluation of nucleolar organiser region-associated proteins in breast malignancy. Histopathology 12: 113–125.

Stein-Werblowsky R 1960 Induction of chorionepitheliomatous tumour in the rat. Nature 186: 980.

Stone M, Bagshawe K D 1976 Hydatidiform mole: two entities. Lancet i: 535–536.

Suarez V, Newman J, Hiley C, Crocker J, Collins M 1989 The value of AgNOR numbers in neoplasms and non-neoplastic epithelium of the stomach. Histopathology 14: 61–66.

Sugimori H, Kashiuara Y, Tsukamoto N, Taki I 1980 Histological grading of hydatidiform mole. Acta Obstetrica et Gynecologica Japonica 32: 1951–1956.

Sunderland C A, Redman C W, Stirrat G M 1981 HLA A, B, C antigens are expressed on nonvillous trophoblast of the early human placenta. Journal of Immunology 127: 2614–2615.

Sunderland C A, Redman C W G, Stirrat G M 1985 Characterisation and localisation of HLA antigens on hydatidiform mole. American Journal of Obstetrics and Gynecology 151: 130–135.

Suresh U R, Chawner L, Buckley C H, Fox H 1990 Do AgNOR counts reflect cellular ploidy or cellular proliferation? A study of trophoblastic tissue. Journal of Pathology 160: 213–215.

Suresh U R, Hale R J, Fox H, Buckley C H 1993 Use of proliferation cell nuclear antigen immunoreactivity for distinguishing hydropic abortions from partial hydatidiform moles. Journal of Clinical Pathology 46: 48–50.

Surti U 1987 Genetic concepts and techniques. In: Szulman A E,

Buchsbaum H J (eds) Gestational trophoblastic disease. Springer-Verlag, New York, pp 111–121.

Surti U, Szulman A E, O'Brien S 1979 Complete (classic) hydatidiform mole with 46 XY karyotype of paternal origin. Human Genetics 51: 153–155.

Surti U, Leppert K, White R 1983 Analysis of hydatidiform moles by RFLPs and chromosome heteromorphisms. American Journal of Human Genetics 35: 72A.

Suzuki M, Matsunobu A, Wakita K, Nishijima M, Osanai K 1980 Hydatidiform mole with a surviving coexisting fetus. Obstetrics and Gynecology 56: 384–388.

Szulman A E 1987 Partial hydatidiform mole. In: Szulman A E, Buchsbaum H J (eds) Gestational trophoblastic disease. Springer-Verlag, New York, pp 37–44.

Szulman A E, Surti U 1978a The syndromes of hydatidiform mole. I. Cytogenetic and morphologic correlations. American Journal of Obstetrics and Gynecology 131: 665–671.

Szulman A E, Surti U 1978b The syndromes of hydatidiform mole. II. Morphologic evolution of the complete and partial mole. American Journal of Obstetrics and Gynecology 132: 20–27.

Szulman A E, Surti U 1982 The clinicopathologic profile of the partial hydatidiform mole. Obstetrics and Gynecology 59: 597–602.

Szulman A E, Surti U, Berman M 1978 Patient with partial mole requiring chemotherapy. Lancet ii: 1099.

Szulman A E, Philippe E, Boué J G, Boué A 1981a Human triploidy: association with partial hydatidiform moles and nonmolar conceptuses. Human Pathology 12: 1016–1021.

Szulman A E, Ma H K, Wong E, Hsu C 1981b Residual trophoblastic disease in association with partial hydatidiform mole (retrospective study in Hong Kong). Obstetrics and Gynecology 57: 392–394.

Tan K C, Karim S M, Ratnam S S 1982 Hydatidiform mole in Singapore. Annals of Academic Medicine of Singapore 11: 545–548.

Tanaka T 1976 Studies on histogenesis of experimentally induced chorioepithelioma in rats. Acta Obstetrica et Gynecologica Japonica 23: 43–54.

Teacher J H 1903a On chorionepithelioma (the so-called deciduoma malignum) and the occurrence of chorionepitheliomatous and hydatidiform mole-like structures in tumours of the testis. Transactions of the Obstetrical Society of London 45: 256–302.

Teacher J H 1903b On chorionepithelioma and the occurrences of chorionepitheliomatous and hydatidiform mole-like structures in teratoma. Journal of Obstetrics and Gynaecology of the British Empire 4: 1–64 and 145–199.

Teoh E S, Dawood M Y, Ratnam S S 1971 Epidemiology of hydatidiform mole in Singapore. American Journal of Obstetrics and Gynecology 110: 415–420.

Thiele R A, de Alvarez R R 1962 Metastasizing benign trophoblastic tumors. American Journal of Obstetrics and Gynecology 84: 1395–1406.

Thiersch J B 1952 Therapeutic abortions with a folic acid antagonist, 4-aminopteroylglutamic acid (4 amino PGA) administered by the oral route. American Journal of Obstetrics and Gynecology 63: 1298–1304.

Tominaga T, Page E W 1966 Sex chromatin of trophoblastic tumors. American Journal of Obstetrics and Gynecology 96: 305–309.

Tomoda Y, Fuma M, Saiki N, Ishizuka N, Akaza T 1976 Immunologic studies in patients with trophoblastic neoplasia. American Journal of Obstetrics and Gynecology 126: 661–667.

Tow W S H 1966 The classification of malignant growths of the chorion. Journal of Obstetrics and Gynaecology of the British Commonwealth 73: 1000–1001.

Tow W S H, Yung R H 1967 The value of histological grading in prognostication of hydatidiform mole. Journal of Obstetrics and Gynaecology of the British Commonwealth 74: 292–293.

Trowsdale J, Travers P, Bodmer W F, Patillo R 1980 Expression of HL-A, -B, and -C and B2-microglobulin antigens in choriocarcinoma cell lines. Journal of Experimental Medicine 152: 11S–17S.

Tsukamoto N, Kashimura Y, Sano M, Saito T, Kanda S, Taki I 1981 Choriocarcinoma occurring within the normal placenta with breast metastasis. Gynecologic Oncology 11: 348–363.

Tursz T, Lipinski M, Guillard M et al 1981 Characterisation of antibodies reacting with husband's lymphocytes in sera from patients with trophoblastic malignancies. Tissue Antigens 17: 376–385.

Twiggs L B, Okagaki T, Phillips G L, Stroemer J R, Adcock L L 1981 Trophoblastic pseudotumor — evidence of malignant disease potential. Gynecologic Oncology 12: 238–248.

Van de Kaa C A, Nelson K A M, Ramaekers F C S, Vooijs P G, Hopman A H N 1991 Interphase cytogenetics in paraffin sections of routinely processed hydatidiform moles and hydropic abortions. Journal of Pathology 165: 281–287.

Van de Kaa C A, Hanselaar A G J, Hopman A H N et al 1993 DNA cytometric and interphase cytogenetic analyses of paraffin-embedded hydatidiform moles and hydropic abortions. Journal of Pathology 170: 229–238.

Van Lijnschoten G, Arends J W, Leffers P et al 1993 The value of histomorphological features of chorionic villi in early spontaneous abortion for the prediction of karyotype. Histopathology 22: 557–563.

Vassilakos P, Kajii T 1976 Hydatidiform mole; two entities. Lancet i: 259.

Vassilakos P, Riotton G, Kajii T 1977 Hydatidiform mole: two entities: a morphologic and cytogenetic study with some clinical considerations. American Journal of Obstetrics and Gynecology 127: 167–170.

Veit J 1901 Über deportation von Chorionzotten. Zeitschrift für Geburtshilfe und Gynäkologie 44: 466–504.

Vejerslev L O, Mogensen B, Olsen S 1984 Hydatidiform mole: preliminary results from the current Danish investigation. Second World Congress on Trophoblastic Neoplasms, Singapore, p 1 (abstract).

Vejerslev L O, Dueholm M, Nielsen F H 1986 Hydatidiform mole: cytogenetic marker analysis in twin gestation: report of two cases. American Journal of Obstetrics and Gynecology 155: 614–617.

Vejerslev L O, Fisher R A, Surti U, Wake N 1987 Hydatidiform mole: cytogenetically unusual cases and their implications for the present classification. American Journal of Obstetrics and Gynecology 157: 180–184.

Wake N, Takagi N, Sasaki M 1978 Androgenesis as a cause of hydatidiform mole. Journal of the National Cancer Institute 60: 51–53.

Wake N, Chapman V, Matski S, Sandberg A A 1981 Chromosomes and cellular origin of choriocarcinoma. Cancer Research 41: 3137–3143.

Wake N, Seki T, Fujita H et al 1984 Malignant potential of homozygous and heterozygous complete moles. Cancer Research 44: 1226–1230.

Wake N, Fujino T, Hoshi S 1987 The propensity to malignancy of dispermic heterozygous moles. Placenta 8: 319–326.

Wakitani T 1962 Electron microscopic observations on the chorionic villi of the normal human placenta and chorioepithelioma malignum. Mie Medical Journal 12: 43–64.

Wallace D C, Surti U, Adams C W, Szulman A E 1982 Complete moles have paternal chromosomes but maternal mitochondrial DNA. Human Genetics 61: 145–147.

Wei P Y, Ouyang P C 1963 Trophoblastic diseases in Taiwan: a review of 157 cases in a 10 year period. American Journal of Obstetrics and Gynecology 85: 844–849.

WHO Scientific Group 1983 Gestational trophoblastic disease. WHO Technical Report Series 692. WHO, Geneva.

Wilson R B, Hunter J S, Dockerty M B 1961 Chorioadenoma destruens. American Journal of Obstetrics and Gynecology 81: 546–559.

Witt M, Erickson R P 1989 A rapid method for detection of Y-chromosomal DNA from dried blood specimens by the polymerase chain reaction. Human Genetics 82: 271–274.

Womack C, Elston C W 1985 Hydatidiform mole in Nottingham: a 12-year retrospective epidemiological and morphological study. Placenta 6: 95–105.

Wynn R M, Davies J 1964a Ultrastructure of transplanted choriocarcinoma and its endocrine implications. American Journal of Obstetrics and Gynecology 88: 618–634.

Wynn R M, Davies J 1964b Ultrastructure of hydatidiform mole: correlative electron microscopic and functional aspects. American Journal of Obstetrics and Gynecology 90: 293–307.

Wynn R M, Harris J A 1967 Ultrastructure of trophoblast and endometrium in invasive mole (chorioadenoma destruens). American Journal of Obstetrics and Gynecology 99: 1125–1135.

Yamashita K, Wake N, Araki T, Ichinoe K, Makoto K 1979 Human lymphocyte antigen expression in hydatidiform mole: androgenesis following fertilization by a haploid sperm. American Journal of Obstetrics and Gynecology 135: 597–600.

Yamashita K, Ishikawa M, Shimizu T, Kuroda M 1981 HLA antigens in husband–wife pairs with trophoblastic tumor. Gynecologic Oncology 12: 68–74.

Yen S, MacMahon B 1968 Epidemiologic features of trophoblastic disease. American Journal of Obstetrics and Gynecology 101: 126–132.

Yokoyama S, Niimi S, Tsuroaka M 1988 The expression of c-myc, c-fms, c-sis oncogenes in the trophoblast of normal pregnancy and trophoblastic disease. Acta Obstetrica et Gynaecologica Japonica 40: 1867–1874.

Young R H, Scully R E 1984 Placental site trophoblastic tumor: current status. Clinical Obstetrics and Gynecology 27: 248–258.

Young R H, Scully R E, McCluskey R T 1985 A distinctive glomerular lesion complicating placental site trophoblastic tumor: report of two cases. Human Pathology 16: 35–42.

Young R H, Kurman R J, Scully R E 1988 Proliferations and tumors of the placental site. Seminars in Diagnostic Pathology 5: 223–237.

Young R H, Kurman R J, Scully R E 1990 Placental site nodules and plaques: a clinicopathological analysis of 20 cases. American Journal of Surgical Pathology 14: 1001–1009.

Yuen B H, Cannon W 1981 Molar pregnancy in British Columbia: estimated incidence and post evacuation regression patterns of the beta subunit of human chronic gonadotrophin. American Journal of Obstetrics and Gynecology 139: 316–319.

53. Pathology of abortion

D. Ian Rushton

INTRODUCTION

Abortion is today an emotive word most commonly used by the lay public and the media in the context of social or therapeutic terminations. Miscarriage is more generally applied to the spontaneous expulsion of an early pregnancy. The legalistic and litigious implications of the former have tended to overshadow the latter, the most common single complication of pregnancy, spontaneous abortion. One of the major rôles of natural selection is to ensure those members of a species best fitted for reproduction reach the age of puberty. It should be self-evident that spontaneous abortion is the greatest single contributor to the elimination of maldeveloped organisms, from the moment of fertilization to the onset of reproductive maturity in man.

Since the majority of patients suffering a clinically apparent abortion will subsequently have a normal pregnancy it is generally considered by both clinician and pathologist that little is to be gained from the examination of products of conception. The pregnancy is over, and with appropriate, usually empirical, guidance and reassurance the patient may be safely encouraged to attempt a further pregnancy. From the purely practical view products of conception will form a major part of the work load of any histopathologist serving an obstetrical and gynaecological unit. The lack of clinical interest may result in the pathologist giving such material scant attention, indeed such specimens may never reach the laboratory. The lack of pathological interest is emphasized by the scant attention spontaneous abortion is given in many text books of gynaecological pathology.

Interest in the pathology of early pregnancy has been revived by the introduction of antenatal diagnostic techniques such as serum alphafetoprotein screening (Clarke & Chard, 1981), ultrasound scanning of the conceptus in utero (Duenhoelter & Satos-Ramos, 1981), diagnostic amniocentesis (Willner & Hirschorn, 1981), fetoscopy (Benzie, 1981) and, more recently, trophoblastic biopsy (Williamson et al, 1981). These techniques have resulted in a new and growing source of pathological specimens which require examination, if for no other reason than to confirm the original antenatal diagnosis. The examination of these specimens has revealed a general ignorance of the pathology of early human development among both general and paediatric histopathologists. Indeed, many would consider these embryos and fetuses the province of the embryologist rather than the pathologist. It is, however, worth remembering that the embryologist without adequate pathological knowledge may fail to recognize significant disease processes, particularly those which do not result in disturbances or morphogenesis.

Since the majority of therapeutically terminated pregnancies are performed because of malformations which may also be found among spontaneous abortions, the genetic counselling services provided for the former group must of necessity be applicable to those patients who abort embryos or fetuses with similar malformations spontaneously. It therefore follows that there is a need for the proper examination of spontaneously expelled products of conception. Indeed, many more chromosomally abnormal and anatomically deformed conceptuses are lost spontaneously than are terminated following early antenatal diagnosis.

The pathology of early pregnancy and our knowledge of the natural history of disease in the embryo, fetus and placenta, has in many respects advanced little since the days of Ballantyne (1902), his *Manual of antenatal pathology and hygiene* remaining a major reference source to this day. The correlation of morphological, endocrinological and clinical data has only just begun. Few reports on the environmental factors purportedly responsible for spontaneous abortion even consider the nature of the aborted products (Elias & Simpson, 1980). Such an approach to aetiological factors would be unacceptable in most other fields of medicine. The search for aetiological factors responsible for malignant disease relies initially on an accurate morphological and histological description of the disease under investigation. Until such detailed studies are made of early human pregnancy wastage it will not be surprising to find both clinicians and pathologists who feel that spontaneous abortion is worthy of only minimal interest. It is to be hoped this chapter will encourage a more constructive approach to early pregnancy wastage in man by pathologists.

INCIDENCE OF SPONTANEOUS ABORTION

Clinical spontaneous abortion is but the tip of an iceberg of pregnancy wastage, the greater part of which occurs unbeknown to the mothers concerned. Data from many animal species has demonstrated early losses as high as 50% (Hafez, 1967; Hendrickx & Binkerd, 1980). Early morphological data from human pregnancies collected from surgically removed uteri and tubes suggested that at least one-third of fertilized ova were abnormal (Hertig et al, 1956). More recently the combination of highly sensitive endocrinological investigations and ultrasound examination of the uterus indicates that over 40% of pregnancies fail to develop beyond the first few weeks after fertilization (Robinson, 1975; Miller et al, 1980). Yet data based on clinical admissions to hospital would seem to indicate a spontaneous abortion rate of only 10–20% (Petterson, 1968). This discrepancy is of course the result of the very early wastage occurring prior to the first missed menstrual period, in many instances prior to implantation. A significant number of delayed heavy periods may be the result of early abortions and are not considered as evidence of pregnancy by many women since they only accept that they are pregnant when they have missed at least two menstrual periods. Patients having recurrent very early abortions may therefore present as having problems of infertility (Block, 1978).

CLASSIFICATION OF PRODUCTS OF CONCEPTION

Prior to consideration of the aetiology and pathology of spontaneous abortion it is necessary to consider the classifications of products of conception since comparison of data within the literature is impossible without knowledge of the individual author's approach to the grouping of the multiplicity of specimens which may arise from failed human pregnancies (Table 53.1).

The first systematic classification of spontaneous abortions was that of Mall & Meyer (1921). These authors divided the products of conception into seven categories: those consisting only of placental villi; those of chorion without amnion or cyema (embryo); those of amnion and chorion; those with a chorionic vesicle (gestation sac) or vesicles containing nodular embryonic remnants; those with cylindrical cyemata or stunted cyemata; and those with a fetus compressus. Hertig (1968) used a similar classification. Fujikura et al (1966) produced a simplified anatomical classification of abortions which was subsequently adopted more or less intact by the Geneva Conference on the standardization of procedures for chromosome studies in abortion (1966). The need for standardization was clear since many early reports on the cytogenetic abnormalities in spontaneous abortions failed to include any description of the products of conception. The latter two classifications are based, like earlier versions, on the macroscopic appearance of the products of conception and take no account of the placenta other than identifying it as being present when appropriate. Since the eventual failure of many pregnancies is dependent on failure of placental function and the placenta has a direct interface with maternal tissues it was concluded that a classification based on the morphology of the pla-

Table 53.1 Classifications of spontaneous abortions by different authors

Mall & Meyer, 1921	Fujikura et al, 1966	Geneva Conference, 1966	Hertig, 1968	Rushton, 1978
1. Villi only	1. Incomplete specimens	Incomplete specimen	1. Villi only	1. Blighted ova
2. Chorion without amnion or cyema	2. Ruptured empty sac a. with cord stump b. without cord stump	Ruptured sac a. with cord stump b. without cord stump	2. Chorion only (empty)	a. majority of villi with microscopic hydatidiform change
3. Chorion with amnion	3. Intact empty sac	Intact empty sac	3. Chorion and amnion only	b. mixed between (a) and (c)
4. Chorionic vesicles with nodular cyemata	4. Embryo or fetus with or without a chorionic sac	Embryo or fetus with or without a chorionic sac	4. Chorion, amnion and nodular embryo	c. majority of villi with stromal fibrosis and vascular obliteration
5. Cylindrical cyemata	a. normal embryo or fetus	a. normal embryo	5. Chorion, amnion and cylindrical embryo	2. Macerated embryos and fetuses
6. Stunted cyemata	b. deformed embryo	b. macerated normal embryo	6. Chorion, amnion and stunted embryo	a. with an embryo or fetus
7. Fetus compressus	c. abnormal embryo or fetus	c. focal embryonic abnormality	7. Chorion, amnion and macerated fetus	b. without an embryo or fetus
	d. indeterminate abnormality	d. focal embryonic abnormality (macerated)		3. Fresh embryo and fetus
		e. severely disorganized embryo		a. with an embryo or fetus
		f. severely disorganized embryo (macerated)		b. without an embryo or fetus

centa might be more closely related to the mechanism of abortion than the appearance of the embryo or fetus. The wide range of abnormalities associated with specific chromosomal abnormalities typifies the problem of using the gross features for classification. Thus trisomy 21 may result in a spectrum of abnormalities from a blighted ovum to a mentally retarded adult. Whether or not the pregnancy survives is dependent on as yet unknown factors but, as will become apparent, the timing of the effect leading to failure of the pregnancy influences the histological appearance of the placenta. It also provides some insight into the rôle of the conceptus as a determining factor in its own survival.

Details of the classification are given elsewhere (Rushton, 1978). There are three basic categories:

Group I: Blighted ova

a. In which the majority of villi show microscopic hydatidiform (hydropic) change.
b. In which there is a mixed pattern of villi from (a) and (c) with approximately equal proportions of both types.
c. In which the majority of villi show secondary changes associated with embryonic death and cessation of the intravillous circulation.

Group II: Macerated embryos or fetuses

a. With an embryo or fetus present.
b. Without an embryo or fetus, intrauterine death being diagnosed by the histological appearances of the placenta. Where a fetus is present it may show anatomical abnormalities.

Group III: Fresh embryos or fetuses

a. With an embryo or fetus present.
b. Without an embryo or fetus present, the viability of the fetus being determined from the histopathology of the placenta.
As in group II, embryos and fetuses may be anatomically abnormal.

If all pregnancies between 0 and 28 weeks' gestation are grouped in this manner then the mean ovulation age (menstrual age less two weeks) for Group I is 9.4 weeks, Group II 14.1 weeks and Group III 18.6 weeks, the latter group forming the bulk of the mid-trimester abortions in which environmental factors are of major importance. Groups II and III may of course be classified on macroscopic examination of the conceptus if an embryo or fetus is present and a certain proportion of those in Group II on examination of the placenta prior to histological study. The characteristic appearances of each of these groups will now be discussed more fully.

Group I: Blighted ova

The majority of these conceptuses are lost prior to, or about the time of, the third missed period. In many instances only curetted fragments may be received but the classical finding is an intact sac (Fig. 53.1) containing only clear fluid. Some may contain either an amorphous embryo (Fig. 53.2) or a stunted macerated embryo (Fig. 53.3). Frequently the largest single component of

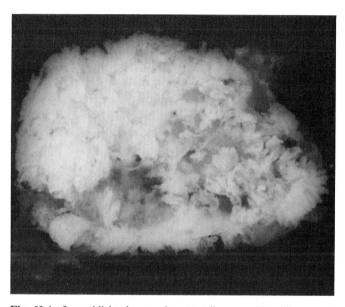

Fig. 53.1 Intact blighted ovum almost totally covered by villi, some of which show early hydatidiform change. × 4.

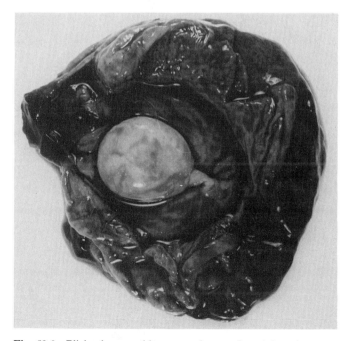

Fig. 53.2 Blighted ovum with an amorphous embryo 1.7 cm in diameter aborted at 14 weeks' gestation. (Courtesy of the Editor of the Journal of Medical Genetics.)

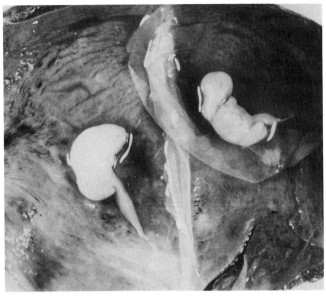

Fig. 53.3 Twin stunted and abnormal embryos between 1 and 1.5 cm crown–rump length aborted at 13 weeks' gestation.

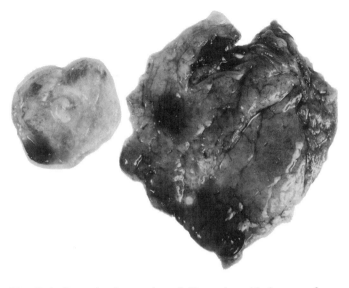

Fig. 53.4 Stunted embryo and sac (left) together with the mass of decidua indicating the relative proportions of the component parts of a blighted ovum at 12 weeks' gestation.

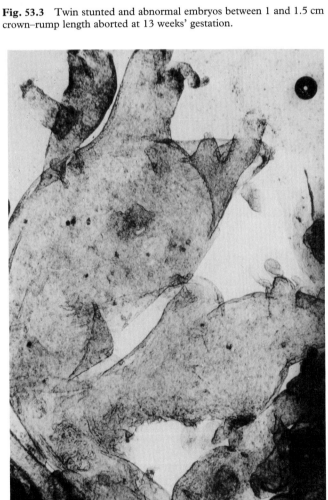

Fig. 53.5 Avascular swollen villi from a blighted ovum showing microscopic hydatidiform change. × 46.

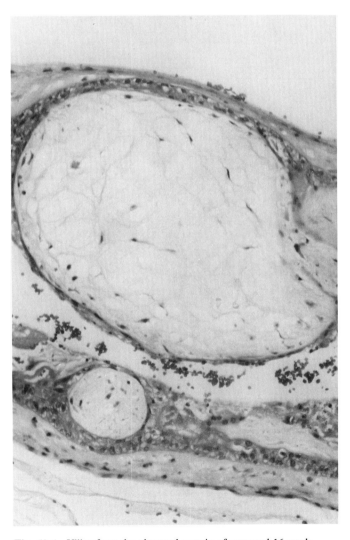

Fig. 53.6 Villus from the placental margin of a normal 16-week pregnancy showing microscopic hydatidiform change. H & E × 175.

the products which are aborted is the decidua, which may form a uterine cast (Fig. 53.4). This may or may not contain a gestation sac, in many instances the sac having been aborted prior to the shedding of the decidua. The external surface of the sac may be partially or completely covered by villi, which under the dissecting microscope may closely resemble villi of hydatidiform moles (Fig. 53.5). Some sacs are devoid of a villous covering, the villi often remaining embedded in the attached decidua. When compared with a conceptus of a similar gestational age which is developing normally there is usually a true reduction in the number of villi.

There is a spectrum of histological changes in the villi which has a counterpart in the normal early human conceptus. In a normal pregnancy the blastocyst initially has a complete covering of trophoblast and primary villous structures develop over its entire surface. Following implantation the villi on the surface nearest to the uterine cavity and on the lateral surfaces of the sac stop developing and regress while those at the site of the future pla-

centa (the chorion frondosum) continue to develop. The histological appearances of the villi that fail to develop are of two types:

(i) villi in which the trophoblast becomes attenuated and the stroma swollen and cystic (hydropic or microscopic hydatidiform change) (Fig. 53.6)
(ii) villi in which the trophoblast initially appears normal and the stroma becomes fibrotic and relatively acellular (Fig. 53.7).

The former type of villus occurs more peripherally, the latter being sited on the margin of the normal placenta. It is suspected that these two types of villi depend for their ultimate structure on the extent to which they are vascularized, the first type never being vascularized and the second being partially vascularized (Rushton, 1985). The first type of villus is typical of the blighted ovum in which there is no evidence of any embryonic development. The vast majority of villi may show this form (Fig. 53.8) and may be referred to as being hydropic though the author

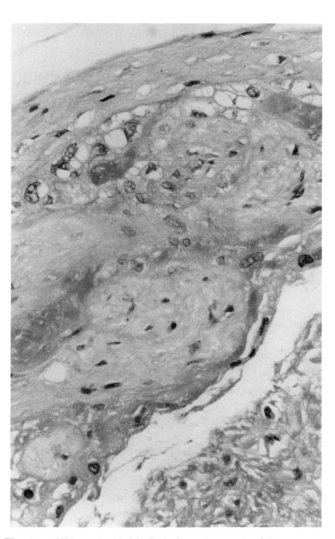

Fig. 53.7 Villus embedded in fibrin from the margin of the same placenta showing stromal fibrosis. H & E × 350.

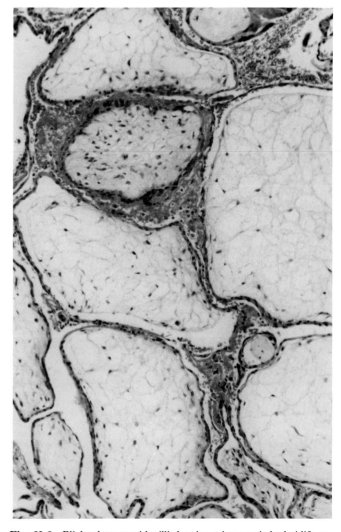

Fig. 53.8 Blighted ovum with villi showing microscopic hydatidiform change predominating. H & E × 140.

prefers the term microscopic hydatidiform change since in all respects other than the presence of trophoblastic hyperplasia they are similar to true molar villi. The trophoblast is typically attenuated though the growing tips of the villi may be capped by active trophoblast (see Fig. 53.11). This may occasionally cause concern to the pathologist but the presence of a chorionic plate from which the villi arise and the absence of active trophoblast on the larger villi exclude the diagnosis of true hydatidiform mole.

The second pattern of villous development is characteristically found in the blighted ova in which there is some evidence of embryonic development, i.e. a cord root, yolk sac remnant, amorphous, stunted or cylindrical embryo (Fig. 53.9).

The villi initially retain a bilaminar trophoblast and frequently contain vascular remnants, these being typified by collapsed capillaries containing effete red cells (Fig. 53.10).

It has been suggested that the assessment of red cell maturation in embryonic or placental vessels is of value in determining the gestational age of the conceptus (Ruchelli et al, 1990). The longer the conceptus is retained in utero the less apparent the vascular remnants become, the stroma is densely collagenized and the trophoblast degenerates and is eventually largely replaced by fibrin deposited on the surface of the villus. The obliteration of the villous vascular tree extends to the chorionic plate.

Between the two characteristic patterns there are a group of conceptuses in which both types of villi may be evident. In these cases it is assumed that partial vascularization has occurred. A macroscopic variant of this group is the Breus' or carneous mole in which the specimen appears externally to consist almost entirely of blood clot (Fig. 53.11), but on slicing frequently contains an intact gestation sac in which there is no embryo and which is

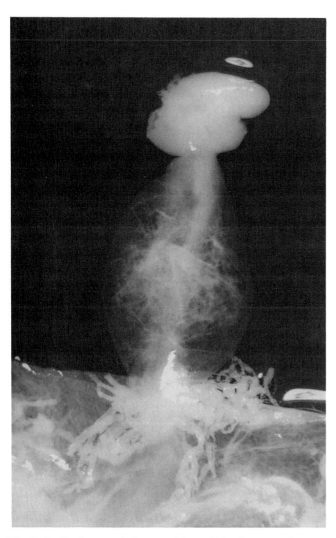

Fig. 53.9 Cord root and placenta with a nubbin of macerated embryonic tissue 3–4 mm in diameter attached to the tip. × 10. (From Barson A J (ed) *Fetal and neonatal pathology*. Praeger, New York.)

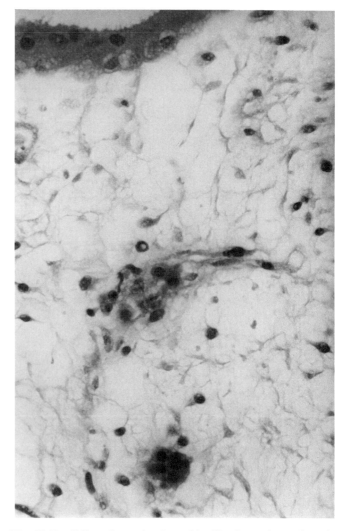

Fig. 53.10 Collapsed vascular channel in villus from a late embryonic death containing effete nucleated red cells. H & E × 560.

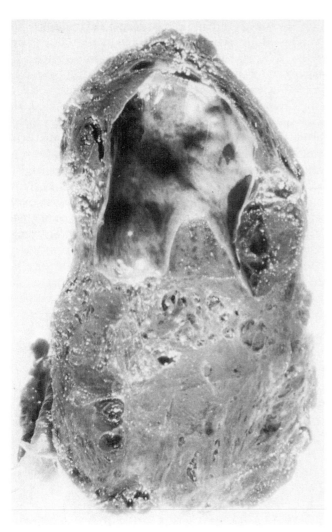

Fig. 53.11 Breus' mole consisting mainly of blood clot surrounding an empty but intact sac. × 1.5.

surrounded by blood clot and haemorrhagic necrotic decidua. The mechanisms involved in the pathogenesis of Breus' mole are unknown but Hustin et al (1990) have proposed that inadequate trophoblastic plugging of the spiral arteries during implantation may result in 'bleeding' into the intervillous space leading to abortion. In certain cases this mechanism might lead to a Breus' mole.

Group II: Macerated fetuses

The severely macerated, often compressed and distorted, fetus is readily identifiable (Fig. 53.12). If the gestation sac is complete the amniotic fluid is frequently brown and turbid and the longer the conceptus is retained after fetal death, the smaller the quantity of fluid. The reduction in volume leads to compression and distortion of the fetus. Confusion may arise if the amniotic fluid is infected since the fetal skin may appear to be macerated but appropriate histological studies of the skin, umbilical cord and membranes allow distinction of these changes. In the absence of amniotic fluid and embryo or fetus the membranes and cord are red-brown to brown in colour. It is however possible to assess the condition of the embryo or fetus by histological examination of the placenta. Macroscopically the placentas are firm with pale cut surfaces, often with widespread intervillous fibrin deposition which is frequently most marked on the maternal surface of the placenta, the so-called maternal floor infarction (Benirschke & Driscoll, 1967): this lesion will be discussed below. The histological changes which occur in the placentas of intrauterine deaths are sequential and characteristic (Wilkin, 1965; Rushton, 1981a) and it is not the death of the fetus itself which is critical but the cessation of

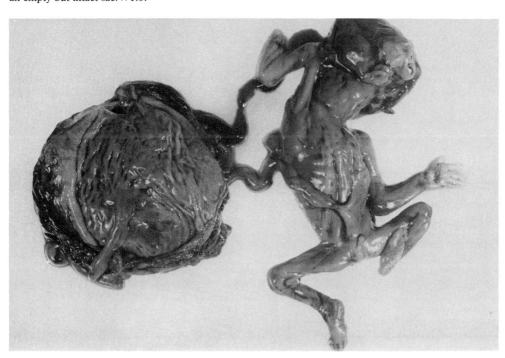

Fig. 53.12 Severely moulded macerated fetus and placenta aborted at 16 weeks' gestation.

the circulation through the villous vessels; thus similar changes may be found in retained placental products after an otherwise normal delivery, in areas of otherwise normal placentas where the fetal vasculature has become occluded, in the placenta of the dead fetus in which one or more fetuses survive in multiple pregnancies and in the experimental occlusion of part of the placental circulation (Millen, 1956; Myers & Fujikura, 1968; Fox, 1978).

Indeed, though there are some modifications in the placental response to cessation of the fetal circulation with gestation the basic changes described below may be seen in Group Ic blighted ova, mid-trimester abortions and stillbirths. Some of the lesions may also be found in placentas in which there is good clinical evidence of a failing fetal circulation prior to delivery of a live birth (Rushton, unpublished data).

The characteristic microscopic lesions may be summarized as follows:

1. The vessels within the villi collapse and trap nucleated red cells within their lumens. Initially these cells are well preserved but eventually they become impregnated with calcium and iron-containing salts. This process of mineralization extends to involve the vessel walls (Fig. 53.13).

2. The collapsed vessels are gradually obliterated, the stem vessels often being apparent as cords of concentric fibrous tissue within the centre of villi. This is often erroneously termed obliterative endarteritis though there is no evidence of any inflammatory component. In parallel with these vascular changes the stroma of the villi becomes fibrous and less cellular. Contraction of the fibrous tissue distorts the shape of the villi and as a result trophoblast surrounded by basement membrane (Fig. 53.14) may appear to be included within the substance of the villi.

3. The process of mineralization extends to involve the villous stroma, where it usually manifests as fine granular deposits of material which stain with both von Kossa and

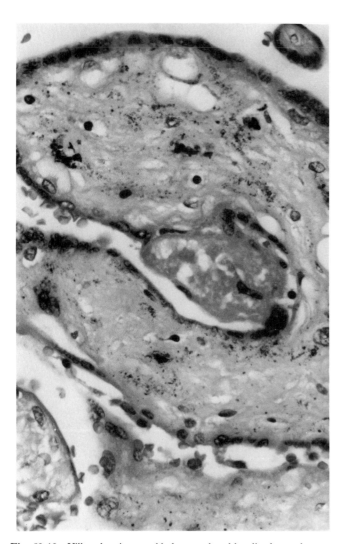

Fig. 53.13 Villus showing speckled stromal and localized vascular mineralization associated with fetal death at 18 weeks' gestation. H & E × 350.

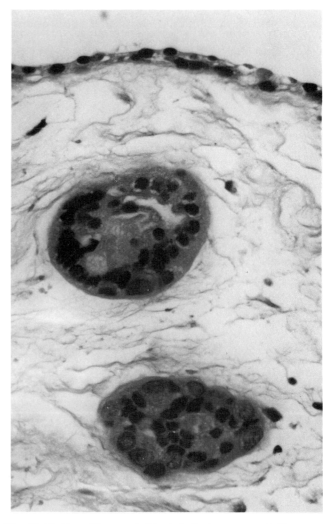

Fig. 53.14 Intravillous trophoblastic inclusions surrounded by basement membrane. H & E × 560.

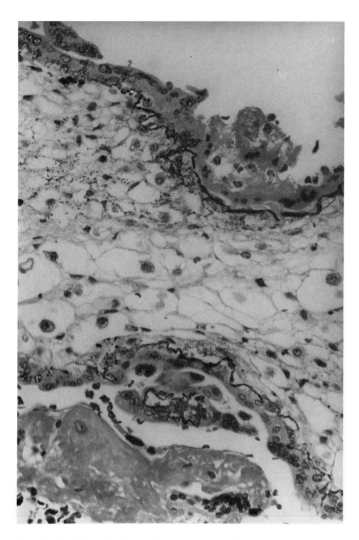

Fig. 53.15 Mineralization of the trophoblastic basement membrane and villous stroma. H & E × 350.

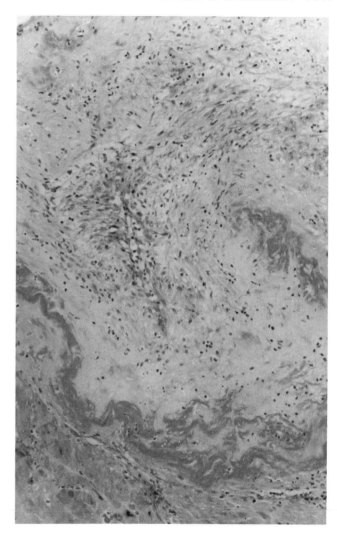

Fig. 53.16 Almost totally obliterated spiral artery within the decidua of a missed abortion. H & E × 140.

Perls techniques. Similar material is deposited on the trophoblastic basement membrane (Fig. 53.15). The deposition of iron and calcium is related to gestational age and the normal transfer activity of the placenta which varies with fetal needs.

4. Initially the trophoblast is well preserved and bilaminar but the syncytium gradually loses its regular appearance and deposits of fibrin form on the surface which progressively extend to cover the surface of the villus. In this respect it is of note that human chorioepithelial brush border membrane vesicles inhibit platelet aggregation (Iioka et al, 1993), a function that may be compromised following fetal death. Surviving cytotrophoblast may persist even in totally enveloped villi. The syncytium may also form knots in some areas. Eventually only small islands of trophoblast may persist. Fibrin deposition commences at the base of the placenta, and the striae of Rohr and Nitabuch become fused. If the pregnancy is retained in utero for several weeks the greater part of the inter-

villous space becomes obliterated. The reduced maternal circulation in the placenta is reflected in obliterative lesions in the spiral arteries of the placental bed (Fig. 53.16). It should be emphasized that these changes are not primarily ischaemic and as such the process cannot be described as infarctive in nature, though it has been termed maternal floor infarction (Fig. 53.17).

Group III: Fresh fetuses

Minor degrees of maceration or infection may occasionally present difficulties in interpretation but the archetypal conceptus of this group is derived from a pregnancy that has been progressing normally. Fetal and placental growth may appear appropriate for the estimated length of gestation though in threatened abortions ultrasound studies indicated that a significant number of fetuses are growth retarded (Mantoni & Pederson, 1982). However, morphological studies of the fetus and placenta also show that

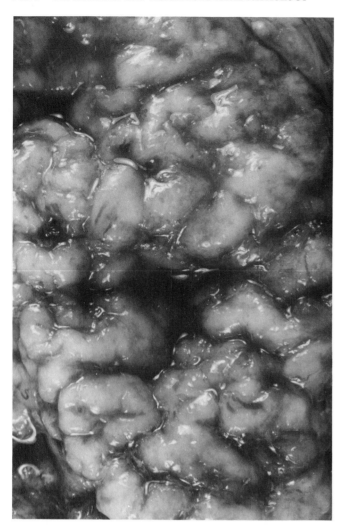

Fig. 53.17   Maternal surface of the placenta showing the typical gyriform pattern of maternal floor infarction. H & E × 5.

a proportion of mothers underestimate the gestation of their pregnancies if the duration of the pregnancy is determined from the last menstrual period compared with that estimated from fetal size (Rushton, 1984). This discrepancy can be explained, if it is assumed that vaginal bleeding occurs at or about the time of the first, or second, missed menstrual period. Bleeding at these times would also be consistent with the conceptus either implanting in an adverse site or not implanting normally due to uterine pathology. This interpretation adds weight to the hypothesis that disturbances in the environment of the conceptus may be a major factor leading to mid-trimester abortion. It should also be emphasized that the placentas of these abortions may show an apparent acceleration of maturation due to the underestimation of their true gestation. Disturbed placental maturation may result, however, from uteroplacental ischaemia (Rushton, 1988) and defective haemochorial placentation (Khong et al, 1987).

This simple classification, based largely on the morphology of the placenta, does not take into account the many aetiological factors associated with spontaneous abortion though it does allow a possible explanation of the process of expulsion of abnormal conceptions. Furthermore it is only a generalized description of relatively simple histological changes in placental structure.

AETIOLOGY OF SPONTANEOUS ABORTIONS

It has unfortunately become common practice to equate aetiology with the mechanisms of abortion when discussing early pregnancy wastage. This is particularly true of embryonic and fetal malformations. Thus, while many abnormalities are known to be present within a population of spontaneous abortions, it is by no means clear how they are related to the failure of the pregnancy and the subsequent expulsion from the uterus. Since, with the possible exception of certain chromosomal abnormalities, it is known that a proportion of cases with any individual lesion will survive to term, the prenatal selection process is not 100% effective. Indeed, if it were, the need for prenatal diagnosis would be obviated. Thus we may consider certain abnormalities of the conceptus to be associated with spontaneous abortion but it does not follow that they are, per se, the cause of abortion. This may appear to be pedantic but the acceptance of a cause and effect hypothesis has resulted in complacency about the mechanisms concerned in the elimination of the abnormal conceptus.

Since spontaneous abortion may, in a strict biological sense, be considered as a physiological response to numerous and varied abnormalities of the conceptus it is not unreasonable to anticipate that a final common pathway, dependent on the failure of specific biological processes, will have evolved which leads to expulsion from the uterus. The identification of such a pathway and the reasons for its failure might eventually result in a more accurate method of distinguishing between those patients threatening to abort who are destined to lose their pregnancies and those whose pregnancies will continue to produce viable infants.

In considering aetiological factors associated with abortion it is helpful to divide them into two major categories: those in which there is an inherent defect within the conceptus, often consistent with survival (a fault in the seed), and those in which the fault lies in the environment of the conceptus (the soil). This has a limited clinical value since, in our present state of knowledge, those in the former category are beyond therapeutic help while a proportion of those in the latter group may be amenable to treatment either in the index pregnancy or in subsequent pregnancies.

Faults in the conceptus

It is probable that the vast majority of spontaneous abortions follow inherent defects within the conceptus. It has been known for many years that a high proportion of early abortions were morphologically abnormal though it was disputed whether these were the result of maternal factors or inherent defects of the conceptus (Mall & Meyer, 1921). The advent of cytogenetic studies confirmed theoretical expectations that many early losses were chromosomally abnormal.

Chromosomal abnormalities

Chromosomal abnormalities of the conceptus are theoretically likely to arise at one of four major stages in the reproductive process.

1. Abnormalities of gametogenesis in the female resulting in a chromosomally abnormal ovum
2. Abnormalities of gametogenesis in the male resulting in a chromosomally abnormal sperm
3. An error occurring during fertilization
4. An error occurring during the early cell division within the fertilized ovum.

While it is not known with certainty at what stage the majority of the anomalies arise, preliminary data on trisomy, polyploidy and structural abnormalities (but not monosomic conceptuses, which make up about 10% of detected abnormalities) indicates that about one-quarter are due to abnormalities in female gametogenesis and approximately 4–5% occur in each of the other groups (Jacobs & Hassold, 1980). The relatively low proportion of cases arising as a result of abnormal male gametogenesis may be a reflection of the influence of the abnormal karyotype on the capabilities of the sperm to reach and to fertilize the egg. At the time of fertilization a major hazard is delay after ovulation, such delay making the ovum more sensitive to other teratogenic agents such as temperature (Witschi, 1970). The age of the egg may also be important in determining both the decline in fertility with age (Navot et al, 1991) and the increased abortion rate, which has consequences in assessing the risks associated with prenatal diagnosis (Cohen Overbeek et al, 1990). A small proportion of abnormal karyotypes result from parental chromosomal abnormalities, most commonly balanced translocations, which give rise to an unbalanced embryonic karyotype. Such couples may have recurrent abortions (Stenchever et al, 1977; Heritage et al, 1978; Kajii & Ferrier, 1978; Simpson, 1981). However, the majority of chromosomal abnormalities arise *de novo* and though they may be associated with a slightly increased risk of a subsequent pregnancy being affected they are usually isolated events in a couple's reproductive history. This is fortunate from the practical viewpoint since it eliminates the need for routine cytogenetic examination of all products of conception.

Many large series of spontaneous abortions have been studied by standard cytogenetic techniques and using the more recently developed methods of chromosomal banding (Warburton et al, 1980). In general it is believed that the earlier the abortion the more likely there is to be a chromosomally abnormal conceptus, though data relating to abortuses of less than four weeks gestation is rare (Mikamo, 1970). In six series, including their own, Warburton et al (1980) demonstrated a karyotypic abnormality in conceptuses up to 28 weeks gestation ranging from approximately 30–50%, while in those conceptuses between eight and 11 weeks the range was 40–60%. The chromosomal abnormalities found in spontaneous abortions do not reflect the incidence of the same abnormalities found in the newborn viable fetus since there is considerable variability in the prenatal mortality among differing karyotypes. Thus, in newborn babies, balanced structural chromosomal abnormalities occur in about one in 500 pregnancies and autosomal trisomies and sex chromosome abnormalities each in one in 800 pregnancies (Hamerton et al, 1975). In one series of spontaneous abortions (Boué & Boué, 1978) 61.5% of almost 1500 abortions were chromosomally abnormal, approximately half having an autosomal trisomy, one-fifth being triploid and one-sixth being monosomic for a sex chromosome. The variability of prenatal wastage among differing karyotypes is illustrated in Table 53.2. While the vast majority of chromosomal abnormalities are eliminated in early pregnancy and a few survive as live births a significant number of stillbirths and neonatal deaths have chromosomal abnormalities, reported incidences being between 5.6% and 7.2% (Machin & Crolla, 1974; Bauld et al, 1974). Thus chromosomal abnormalities, like other forms of reproductive wastage, show a continuum which extends from conception to adult life, 'the continuum of reproductive wastage' (Lilienfeld & Pasamanick, 1955). The majority of chromosomal abnormalities of the early conceptus do not produce characteristic morphological syndromes but in a few instances a relatively specific pattern of fetal and or placental pathology may allow the morbid anatomist to diagnose the underlying chromosomal abnormality with a high degree of accuracy. These will be discussed below.

Table 53.2 Embryonic survival rates associated with differing chromosomal abnormalities in the conceptus (Edwards et al, 1967)

Karyotype	Embryonic survival (%)
XO	2
XXY	80%
XXX	
Trisomy	
13–15	4
16	<1
17–18	30
21–22	30
Other	<1
Triploidy	<1
Tetraploidy	<1

Metabolic disease

The rôle of metabolic disorders in spontaneous abortion is controversial. The major reason for implicating these disorders is an extension of the argument which predicted that the low incidence of chromosomal abnormalities in the liveborn babies almost certainly indicated a higher incidence in early pregnancy, a conclusion which has been fully substantiated. Serious metabolic disorders are likely to result in embryonic or fetal death, and since abortion may not follow immediately such conceptuses are likely to be macerated and unsuitable for tissue culture studies which might demonstrate a metabolic defect. Unless these metabolic disorders are reflected in placental cells which may still be viable at the time of expulsion, detection will be impossible unless tissue is obtained prior to fetal death in those mothers having recurrent but otherwise unexplained abortions. Appleman et al (1991) have proposed that chorionic villus sampling be used for karyotyping missed abortions and clearly this approach is valid to obtain cultures to identify inherited metabolic disorders. The advent of trophoblastic biopsy may eventually provide evidence for or against this hypothesis. The metabolic disorders likely to be implicated are failures of the sequential initiation of essential biochemical processes and may well not affect the fetus until primary organogenesis is complete. Thus they may explain some of the macerated anatomically normal fetuses aborted in the late first trimester and early second trimester. Such disorders remain hypothetical at present but rarely they may be suspected by the demonstration of pathological lesions in the fetus (Rushton, 1981b) or placenta.

Congenital anatomical malformations

Many of the chromosomal abnormalities are associated with gross disturbances in embryogenesis; indeed, in many, no embryo may form. Thus in the earliest abortuses it is difficult to consider anatomical malformations in the same way as is done after organogenesis is complete. Care in interpretation of anatomical abnormalities in early pregnancy is needed and in particular cognizance of the developmental stages of the embryo at any specific gestation is essential. A similar pattern of variable prenatal selection and survival applies to anatomical abnormalities as to chromosomal anomalies. Some minor malformations of the limbs show a strikingly high prenatal mortality and do much to emphasize the dichotomy between the presence of a malformation and the mechanism of abortion. The same is true of cleft lip and palate, which has an incidence in spontaneous abortions of up to eight per 1000 while it occurs in between one and three per 1000 liveborn infants. Such data should be interpreted with caution, however, if it is based on anatomical studies in the absence of cytogenetic investigations since cleft lip and palate are not uncommon among certain chromosomal abnormalities, such as trisomy 13 and 18. Yet the same selective process operates with major malformations not generally associated with an abnormal karyotype. Thus the incidence of neural tube defects is between nine and 40 times that in the newborn and six times that in therapeutic terminations (Fantel et al, 1980).

Infections

Infections lie somewhere between the soil and the seed. There are three major ways in which infections may affect the conceptus.

1. They may produce a severe, sometimes fatal, systemic infection in the mother which results in the loss of the pregnancy without the organism necessarily involving the conceptus.
2. They may kill the embryo or fetus by direct infection via the maternal bloodstream and placenta or via the membranes and amniotic fluid.
3. They may be teratogenic, as in the case of rubella.

It should be noted that some drugs used to treat severe infections may be teratogenic and that a combination of a teratogen and pyrexia may enhance the effect of that teratogen.

When infection reaches the conceptus via the maternal bloodstream and leads to death or malformation of the embryo or fetus it is reasonable to argue that the infection was associated with abortion. However, when the route is via the female genital tract, membranes and amniotic fluid, caution must be used in interpreting their interrelationship since premature rupture of the membranes may precede the infection which acts as an additional irritant that may precipitate premature labour. In many instances ascending infections must be considered secondary and opportunistic.

It is now known that the non-pregnant uterine cavity is not always sterile and that bacteria can be isolated from asymptomatic women (Hensell et al, 1989). The significance of such colonization in infected abortions is unknown. Specific infections have been related to spontaneous abortion in man, and infection is a well-recognized cause of pregnancy wastage in animals (Hoerlein, 1967). In man numerous organisms have been implicated though in many instances their true significance is controversial. They probably only contribute to a small proportion of the total wastage in most populations but are of importance since they may be amenable to treatment. As has been suggested it may be impossible to separate the effects of infection on the mother's metabolic and physical state from those due to direct infection of the fetus. Thus influenza epidemics may be associated with an increased abortion and stillbirth rate (Klein et al, 1976) but since viraemia is very uncommon fetal infection may not occur even in fatal maternal disease (Ramphal et al, 1980), and it is likely that much of the increased fetal wastage is a non-specific effect of severe maternal disease. In the absence of demonstrable lesions in the uterus, placenta, membranes, embryo or fetus, claims that a particular organism is the cause of, or results in, abortion must be viewed with some scepticism even if the organism is grown from the products of conception. The birth canal is a highly infected environment which can contaminate the products of conception with many organisms which may be totally unrelated to the aetiology of the abortion. Even in those cases where the organism is known to be harmful to the conceptus, as in the case of rubella where epidemics are associated with an increased abortion rate (Robbins & Heggie, 1970), the sequence of events from infection to abortion remains as enigmatic as in those associated with chromosomal or anatomical abnormalities of the conceptus.

Since almost any infection of the mother may result in severe systemic manifestations almost all the major human pathogens may be suspect but those in Table 53.3 have either been shown to infect the conceptus or are strongly suspected of doing so on either microbiological or statistical and epidemiological data. They may therefore be implicated in some spontaneous abortions.

Faults in the soil

Structural abnormalities of the female genital tract, be they acquired or congenital, and hormonal dysfunction

Table 53.3 Infections which may be associated with spontaneous abortion (Blanc, 1981; Rosenberg et al, 1981)

Organisms	Haematogenous spread	Ascending infection
Viruses	Cytomegalovirus Rubella Rubeola Hepatitis Mumps Herpes simplex Poliomyelitis Varicella zoster Variola alastrim Vaccinia Coxsackie Influenza	Herpes simplex Cytomegalovirus
Bacteria	Enteric bacteria Gram-positive Listeria Campylobacter	Vaginal and perineal commensals Listeria Camplyobacter Brucella
Other	*Treponema pallidum* *Vibrio fetus* Leptospira Mycoplasmas Rickettsiae Toxoplasma Plasmodia Trypanosoma Schistosoma Chlamydia	*Candida albicans* Aspergillus Actinomyces Mycoplasmas Trichomonas *Vibrio fetus* Chlamydia

are frequently implicated as causes of spontaneous abortion. With few exceptions these are unlikely to become the concern of the morbid anatomist and histopathologist and therefore only warrant a brief comment. They do, however, provide the clinician with some grounds for optimism in that some may be treatable.

Hormonal dysfunction

There is a vast literature on hormonal dysfunction and its possible rôle in early pregnancy wastage (Schweditsch et al, 1979; Duff et al, 1980). It is confusing, controversial and frequently irrelevant. More often than not the endocrinological status of a patient with an abnormal conceptus is reflected in the results rather than a failing pregnancy due to some unspecified deficiency in the maternal endocrine system. The clinical application of this endocrinological data has been twofold:

1. To use it to attempt to predict the outcome of pregnancies of those threatening to abort or those who have aborted recurrently prior to the monitored pregnancy. Such investigations, like studies of cervical mucus and vaginal cytology, have been largely superseded by ultrasound scanning of the uterine contents in early pregnancy (Robinson, 1975).

2. To attempt to formulate therapeutic regimes to replace hormones believed to be deficient in early pregnancy, particularly in those who have suffered recurrent abortions. The use of such regimens presupposes that hormonal deficiency is a cause rather than an effect of early pregnancy wastage. It is this supposition that remains controversial. Progesterone, which plays a major rôle in preparation and maintenance of the endometrium before and during the early weeks of pregnancy, is considered the most likely culprit. Progesterone production is dependent on either pituitary of trophoblastic stimulation of the corpus luteum. Deficient production by the corpus luteum is associated with what is frequently termed the luteal phase defect.

Luteal phase deficiency is associated with high FSH and reduced oestradiol levels in the follicular phase consistent with abnormal follicular metabolism (Hamilton et al, 1990). This may affect oocyte release and/or compromise the oocyte directly as well as influence endometrial development (Li et al, 1990), though whether the latter is due to glandular or vascular disturbances remains uncertain (Buckley, 1991). Thus the effects of luteal phase deficiency may be both on the seed and the soil. However, it may be argued that it is the abnormal conceptus that is at fault and not the corpus luteum (Quagliarello et al, 1981). It is notable that in those studies where abortion has occurred in spite of replacement therapy it is unusual to find evidence of proper examination of the conceptus, either morphologically or cytogenetically. Whether hCG deficiency, be it primary (pituitary) or secondary (trophoblastic), is a cause of abortion is unsettled but clinical evidence is that supplements of progesterone in early pregnancy are probably ineffective (Shearman & Garrett, 1963) in the majority of cases.

Fortunately the vogue for giving oestrogen, particularly diethylstilboestrol (DES), has been abandoned but its use three to four decades ago has resulted in catastrophic results in the female offspring of some mothers given DES in early pregnancy (Herbst et al, 1971). Thyroid disorders have been associated with increased abortion rates (Man et al, 1971) and both hypo- and hyperthyroidism must be excluded or treated in patients with recurrent abortions, though their rôle is disputed (Strobino et al, 1980).

Anatomical abnormalities of female genital tract

Congenital anatomical abnormalities of the female genital tract, characterized by incomplete fusion of the Müllerian ducts, occur in between 2 and 3% of uteri examined clinically in the immediate postpartum period (Hay, 1958; Greiss & Mauzy, 1961). Details of these abnormalities are described elsewhere (Ch. 2). Such abnormalities of the female genital tract are not usually associated with an increase in first-trimester abortions but second-trimester losses may reach 25–50% (Elias & Simpson, 1980). Much of this wastage follows the inability of the abnormal uterus to expand to contain the enlarging conceptus.

Acquired structural abnormalities are typified by the uterine leiomyomas. These may occur at diverse sites within the uterus and appendages, those most commonly associated with spontaneous abortion being submucosal. In this site they may be associated with an attenuated endometrium and poor decidualization, they may encroach on the uterine cavity interfering with the growth of uterine contents or they may enlarge and degenerate rapidly (red degeneration) under the influence of the hormonal stimulus of pregnancy. Uterine leiomyomas may be associated with sterility and recurrent abortion (Elias & Simpson, 1980) and an increased malformation rate (Matsunaga & Shiota, 1980).

Functional disturbances of uterine activity may also be associated with spontaneous and recurrent abortion, incompetent cervix being the most common clinical diagnosis. This may occur in as many as one in 125 pregnancies (Jennings, 1972). The incompetence is usually the result of prior trauma to the cervix, as may occur after the termination of pregnancy, in premature instrumental deliveries or surgery to the cervix.

Immunological disorders (see also Ch. 62)

Since the conceptus consists of cells foreign to its host it is not unreasonable to anticipate that immunological rejection might be a significant factor in spontaneous abortion. The effects of pregnancy on the maternal immunological system and the immunology of pregnancy are as yet incompletely understood (Gudson, 1976; Mendenhall, 1976). In spite of much research, however, there is no incontrovertible evidence that immunological mechanisms play a significant rôle in human abortion, though abortion can be induced in animals by immunological techniques (Diczfalusy, 1974). Both ABO blood group antigens and HLA antigens have been studied. Evidence concerning the former is conflicting: thus Takano & Miller (1972) demonstrated an increased incidence of feto-maternal ABO incompatibility in mothers who abort while Pearce & Lau (1963) had been unable to show such a relationship. Lauritsen (1975) suggested a significant number of spontaneous abortions were due to ABO incompatibility. Equally confusing is the evidence for and against HLA tissue antigens which differ in the parents. The present situation may still be summarized as follows (Jenkins, 1976).

1. Repeated abortions may sensitize the mother to paternal antigens since the number of lymphocytes transformed by paternal antigens is highest in those mothers with the most abortions whereas repeated normal pregnancies lead to a fall in the maternal lymphocyte responsiveness to paternal antigens.
2. Habitual aborters may reject paternal skin grafts more rapidly than non-aborters. A change of husband may result in a successful pregnancy in these mothers.
3. The development of HLA antibodies to paternal antigens by the mother is associated with an increase in male infants, suggesting the male infant may evoke a greater maternal response.
4. Immunological selection does not appear to act in inbred populations but may do so in outbred animals.
5. Anti-HLA antibodies may occur in mothers aborting spontaneously but there is no convincing evidence that they are the cause of abortion. They may well be an effect of pregnancy failure.
6. No evidence has been forthcoming that indicates immunological mechanisms are concerned in the elimination of chromosomally abnormal conceptuses.
7. No morphological evidence of an immune response has been demonstrated in the uterus, placenta or fetus from human spontaneous abortions.

However, until the maternal acceptance of a foreign graft within the uterus is better understood it is not possible to discount immunological disorders as a cause of abortion.

The apparently successful treatment of mothers suffering recurrent abortions with leucocyte infusions from ABO compatible donors (Taylor & Page-Faulk, 1981) suggests that immunological factors may play a rôle in some habitual aborters. It has also been shown that some abortion-prone women do not have a blocking antibody in their blood which prevents maternal lymphocytes from detecting antigens on the surface of trophoblast (Stimson et al, 1979) whereas this blocking factor was found in normal primigravidae. The significance of this finding is considered at greater length in Chapter 62.

Morphological studies of the placental bed in miscarriages (Michel et al, 1990) have shown abnormalities in missed abortions and in some but not all cases where immunotherapy has been used, in particular a reduction in immunosuppressor cells. These results however do not allow distinction between cause and effect and it is possible that the changes follow embryonic death rather than play a causative rôle in abortion.

The behaviour of mothers with immunological disorders may also provide clues to the maternal response to the conceptus. These have been reviewed (Denman, 1982): the effect of pregnancy on such diseases is unpredictable and only mothers with systemic lupus erythematosus for at least six months prior to conception appear to have an increased risk of abortion (Zulman et al, 1980). Immunological factors have been incriminated in recurrent abortions associated with systemic lupus erythematosus (Bresnihan et al, 1977; Bulmash, 1978; Hartikainen-Sori & Kaila, 1980). It is also perhaps worth noting that acute atherosis typical of that described in the uterine vessels in pre-eclamptic toxaemia is occasionally present in decidual vessels curetted after spontaneous abortion (Khong et al, 1987; Rushton, 1988) and that these lesions have been likened to those found in the vessels of rejected transplants (Scott & Jenkins, 1976).

Since the majority of spontaneous abortions are not followed by a further abortion it would seem unlikely that immunological mechanisms are concerned in most cases unless successful pregnancy induces maternal tolerance to paternal antigens. They may however be concerned in a few women having recurrent abortions.

Miscellaneous factors

Maternal factors such as age and parity as well as systemic disease may result in varying risks of early pregnancy wastage. Haemoglobinopathies, diabetes mellitus, renal failure, hypertension, dietary deficiencies, cardiac, pulmonary and alimentary disorders may all compromise maternal reproductive capability though the rôle of some of these disorders, e.g. diabetes mellitus (Crane & Wahl, 1981), is controversial. Smoking and alcohol (Harlap & Shiono, 1980), hormonal therapy during conception and early pregnancy (Schardein, 1980), anaesthetic agents (Knill-Jones et al, 1975), sterilizing agents used by hospital staff (Hemminki et al, 1982) and many other environmental toxins and pollutants as well as drugs have been incriminated. The link between these factors and spontaneous abortion is based on epidemiological and statistical data, little or no account being taken of the products of conception of those pregnancies that fail. Furthermore many of these studies are retrospective and rely on maternal recall which may be modified by the psychological effects of pregnancy failure. Since some of these factors are clearly either avoidable or preventable they warrant careful consideration and further study. None appears to produce a specific pattern of abortion though some may produce characteristic lesions in the liveborn, e.g. fetal alcohol syndrome.

This list of diseases, environmental agents and maternal factors which are related to spontaneous abortion is by no means complete but it does emphasize the complexity of the problem and hopefully the need to correlate the pathology of the products of abortion with any suspect factor or agent.

CORRELATION OF CHROMOSOMAL ABNORMALITIES AND MORPHOLOGICAL ANOMALIES

The correlation of embryonic and fetal phenotypes with chromosomal abnormalities has been reviewed by Fantel et al (1980) and Warburton et al (1980). While it is impossible to match their classifications directly with the classification described above, certain facts can be established and these are summarized in Table 53.4. The overall distribution of abortuses, based on their morphological characteristics from the author's series (Rushton, 1978) and from Fantel et al (1980), is comparable in that for Group I (blighted ova) cases the percentage distributions are 43.0 and 53.3 and for Groups II (macerated fetuses) and III (fresh fetuses) 56 and 46.7 respectively. Unclassified specimens, including those with decidua and blood clot only, make up 28.9% and 24.2% respectively, though over half of the latter cases may have been classifiable using placental histological criteria. The data of Warburton et al (1980) would suggest that approximately 50% of Group I cases, over 25% of Group II cases, and over 5% of Group III cases will have chromosomal abnormalities, it being impossible to classify the latter two groups accurately since abnormal fetuses (24% of which were chromosomally abnormal) and incomplete fetuses (35.4% chromosomally abnormal) were not broken down by their degree of maceration by Fantel et al (1980). The same proviso applies to placental fragments, of which 43.3% showed chromosomal abnormalities. It might be anticipated that many of the incomplete fetuses were macerated. Thus a broad spectrum of chromosomal abnormalities appears to be associated with a more limited pattern of morphological changes in the conceptus. The current data from large series of karyotyped abortions indicates that the highest incidence of anomalies is between eight and 11 weeks' gestation. This would seem to contradict the evidence of Mikamo (1970) who demonstrated

Table 53.4 Comparative distribution of three series of spontaneous abortions emphasizing different biological parameters: placental morphology (Rushton, 1978), morphology of the entire conceptus (Fantel et al, 1980) and chromosomal abnormalities (Warburton et al, 1980)

Rushton		Fantel et al			Warburton et al	
Group	Distribution (%)	Group	Distribution (%)		Group	Chromosomal abnormalities (%)
I	43*	IIa	13.4		IIa	51.2
		IIb	11.9	44.9	IIb	
		III	6.8	(53.3)§	III	
		IVb	13.8		IVb	
II	29*	IVa	28.6		Normal macerated fetuses	26.8
		IVc	7.5	39.3	Normal fresh fetuses	4.6
		IVd	3.2	(46.7)§		
III	28*					
Unclassified	28.9	I	24.2†		Abnormal fetuses	24.0
					Incomplete fetuses	35.4
					Placental fragments	43.3

*These figures exclude unclassified cases
†Includes blood clot and decidua
§Corrected for unclassified cases

that the earlier the abortion, the more likely there was to be a chromosomal abnormality. Since the majority of chromosomal defects occur as the result of events occurring prior to, or during, fertilization with a few arising during the initial divisions of the fertilized ovum, such a distribution might be predicted. However, since in the early stages of development the survival of the conceptus depends on the combined functions of the corpus luteum and the trophoblastic component of the zygote, the abnormal conceptus may remain in situ for several weeks, even in the absence of embryonic development. Thus the mean age of blighted ova (Group I) is between nine and ten weeks (ovulation age) while the mean age at which hydatidiform moles are aborted is approximately 18 weeks (Beischer et al, 1970). In the latter there is a chromosomal abnormality, though of a different nature to those discussed above (see Ch. 52). No embryo forms but trophoblastic function (or certain aspects of it) is such that the conceptus survives into the mid-trimester though the chromosomal defect is known to arise at the time of fertilization. Some chromosomal abnormalities will result in failure of trophoblastic function and such pregnancies will be lost before or during implantation and thus be omitted from both clinical and cytogenetic series. These data provide an overall picture of the effects of chromosomal abnormalities on the conceptus but do not allow the correlation of specific morphological features with specific chromosomal abnormalities. Indeed the morphological disturbances in the vast majority of instances are entirely non-specific and in those conceptuses where the morphological appearances are indicative of a specific chromosomal abnormality, the embryo or fetus has developed to a stage where specific anatomical malformations can be identified. The three commonest chromosomal abnormalities in spontaneous abortions — autosomal trisomy, triploidy and monosomy for a sex chromosome —

constitute between 80% and 90% of all chromosomal abnormalities (Boué & Boué, 1978). Almost all these abnormalities may be associated with morphological lesions, ranging from a blighted ovum to a newborn with a definable clinical syndrome, this being particularly true of trisomies 13, 18 and 21 and of the 45,XO karyotypes: Patau's, Edwards', Down's and Turner's syndromes respectively.

It would be erroneous, and naive, to assume that spontaneous abortions will necessarily show the same abnormalities as the newborn since the latter represent a highly selected population. As yet the mechanisms which determine the survival of individual fetuses with specific chromosomal abnormalities are unknown though in simplistic terms it may be assumed that the anatomical and metabolic disturbances in those that are aborted are likely to be more fundamental than those in the survivors. The majority that fail to survive are, as has been emphasized, lost before the end of the first trimester. Since therapeutic termination is normally performed several weeks later, when conceptuses are identified with chromosomal abnormalities following diagnostic amniocentesis, they might be expected to have anatomical abnormalities more closely allied to those seen in the newborn infant. Indeed selective termination of abnormal pregnancies between 16 and 22 weeks of gestation is likely to include all those fetuses that would have survived to term as well as a few late abortions and stillbirths. It is as yet not possible to predict the fate that would have befallen any individual fetus with an identified chromosomal abnormality, but where the chromosomal defect has been diagnosed prenatally and termination has not been performed, 24% of trisomy 21, 33% of trisomy 13 and 75% of trisomy 18 fetuses died spontaneously in utero (Hook, 1978) while only 3.3% of sex chromosome aneuploidys, translocations, variants and mosaics were lost. A further more fundamental difference appears to exist between therapeutically terminated fetuses, newborn infants and spontaneous abortions with the same chromosomal abnormality. Thus Boué et al (1976) demonstrated that the cell doubling time in spontaneously aborted conceptuses with trisomy 21 was significantly longer than in either of the former groups and that in general life span of cell cultures from aneuploid tissues was shorter than normal cells. Both these factors may partially explain the selective mortality of individual conceptuses. The significance of these findings may be clarified in the future by trophoblastic biopsy which can be performed before natural abortion occurs.

The anatomical malformations associated with specific chromosomal defects are described in detail in texts on congenital malformations (Warkany, 1971) or clinical genetics (Hamerton, 1971) and do not warrant repetition. Many are found in the terminated fetus but unequivocal confirmation of the prenatal diagnosis may only be obtained by cytogenetic studies. It is not clear whether the distribution of these anomalies is different in the terminated group from that in newborn infants.

The abnormalities found in certain chromosomally abnormal spontaneous abortions will now be described.

Trisomic conceptuses

Trisomy of virtually all the autosomal chromosomes has been described in spontaneous abortions: thus Kajii et al (1980) found all but trisomy 1, 5, 17 and 19 in a series of 639 cases of which just over half were successfully karyotyped. The most common trisomy among spontaneous abortions is trisomy 16 (King et al, 1982), this being rarely observed in the viable fetus. A comprehensive review of the phenotypic expressions of lethal chromosomal abnormalities by Boué and colleagues (1976) revealed that there were frequently discrepancies between the developmental ages of the embryos and the malformations present. The placental villi were reduced in number and hypoplastic. Between 30% and 70% contained isolated trophoblastic cells in their stroma (Fig. 53.18), a feature emphasized by Honoré and colleagues (1976). The majority of trisomies were blighted ova without evidence of embryonic development. Trisomies 7, 8, 12 and 22 were associated with disorganized embryos. Three-quarters of trisomy 16 conceptuses were blighted ova. No gross abnormalities were observed in association with trisomy 21 whereas facial abnormalities, including cyclopia, were present in some examples of trisomy 13, 14 and 15. While cyclopia is probably most frequently associated with trisomy 13 (Fugimato et al, 1973) it has also been described in triploidy (Deligdisch et al, 1978) and trisomy 18 (Lang et al, 1976). Growth retardation is a feature of trisomy 18 but is equivocal in trisomy 13 and may be absent in trisomy 21 (Golbus, 1978). However, Stephens & Shepard (1980) described 13 fetuses between 127 and 180 mm crown–rump length with trisomy 21 and found evidence

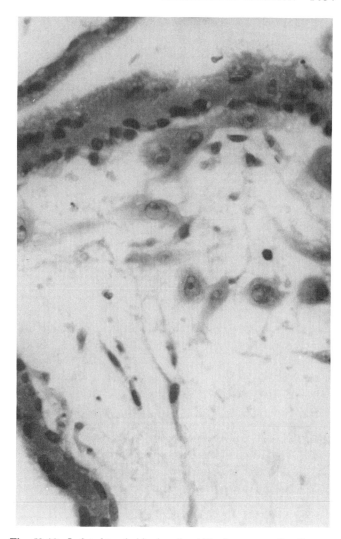

Fig. 53.18 Isolated trophoblastic cells within the stroma of a villus. Trisomy 18. H & E × 560.

of growth retardation. This, together with three other features — a simian crease, clinodactyly of the fifth finger and cardiac septal defects — were the commonest abnormalities and the presence of any two was considered suggestive of Down's syndrome in the fetus (Fig. 53.19).

Triploid conceptuses

These frequently show a discrepancy between the size of the gestation sac and the embryo, the latter appearing too small.

The embryo or fetus may be malformed, the most common abnormality being a neural tube defect. The most characteristic lesion however is the presence of partial molar degeneration of the placenta (Fig. 53.20), in the presence of an amniotic sac with or without a fetus (see Ch. 52).

The pattern of placental development in triploid conceptuses is influenced by the parental origin of the additional haploid set of chromosomes (genomic imprinting — see below) with a diandric triploid characteristically having a well-grown fetus and a large cystic placenta and the digynic triploid having a growth-retarded fetus and small non-cystic placenta (McFadden & Kalousek, 1991).

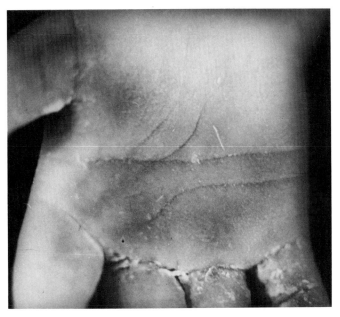

Fig. 53.19 Simian crease on the hand of a terminated fetus with trisomy 21. × 2. (From Barson A J (ed) *Fetal and neonatal pathology.* Praeger, New York.)

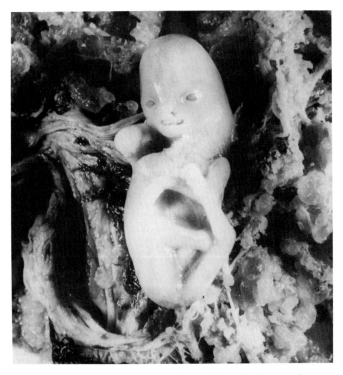

Fig. 53.20 Fetus and placenta showing partial molar degeneration aborted at 17 weeks' gestation. Triploidy. × 1.5.

Harris et al (1981) examined 40 examples: 26 were embryos of between five and seven weeks' gestation, six were intact sacs containing only clear fluid, four showed early embryonic growth disorganization and four were fetuses. The four most characteristic abnormalities were retarded limb development, facial dysplasia, subectodermal haemorrhages and cystic chorionic villi. Ornoy et al (1978) observed cells within the villous stroma similar to those described in trisomic placentas. Limb abnormalities were emphasized by Gosden et al (1976).

Tetraploid conceptuses are usually blighted ova and may include villi showing microscopic or macroscopic molar change in addition to abnormal stromal cells within the villi.

Monosomy X conceptuses

Boué et al (1976) found that two-thirds consisted of an intact sac with a cord root with attached embryonic remnants. A further group appeared to be anatomically normal while the late mid-trimester abortions, occurring

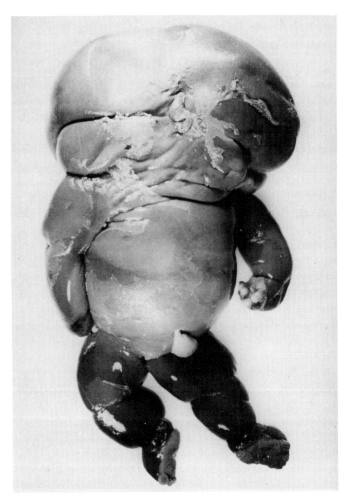

Fig. 53.21 45,XO fetus with hydrops and massive nuchal cystic hygromata. (Courtesy of the Editor of the Journal of Clinical Pathology.)

typically between 16 and 24 weeks' gestation, showed cystic hygromata of the neck (Fig. 53.21). The fetuses are externally female, frequently hydropic and many showed anatomical abnormalities of the cardiovascular and renal tracts. The ovaries may appear normal (Singh & Carr, 1966; Rushton et al, 1969). Many of these fetuses are macerated but even when known to be alive in utero may be associated with an elevated amniotic fluid alphafeto-protein level (Rushton, 1977; Seller, 1977). Fetuses with cysts of the head and neck are not uncommon and care should be taken to ensure that such cysts do not com-municate with the central nervous system, as occurs in Meckel's syndrome (Fig. 53.22). They may also consist of masses of oedematous mesenchyme with no central lu-men, particularly in association with trisomy 18 and 21 (Fig. 53.23).

The placenta of the 45,XO fetus frequently shows secondary features associated with fetal death including maternal floor infarction. In some fetuses which are alive until just prior to delivery there may be evidence of a fail-ing fetal circulation with extensive trophoblastic basement membrane mineralization (Fig. 53.24).

PATTERN OF MORPHOLOGICAL ABNORMALITIES

The above data provide information pertinent to the dis-tribution and identification of chromosomal abnormalities in spontaneous abortions and may aid the identification of specific karyotypic abnormalities from the morphology of the conceptus but they do not give a comprehensive account of the overall pattern of malformations in the aborted conceptus. The most extensive and detailed analysis of the pattern of morphological abnormalities in spontaneous abortions is that of Poland et al (1981). These authors studied 1961 women and 2020 products of conception. These were divided into embryos (less than 30 mm crown–rump length or eight weeks' gestation) and fetuses (more than 30 mm and less than 165 mm crown–rump length or 18 weeks' gestation). Of the 2020 speci-mens 1126 (56%) were embryos, 813 (40%) fetuses, 31

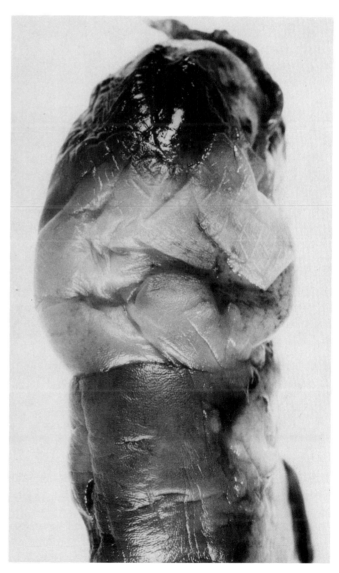

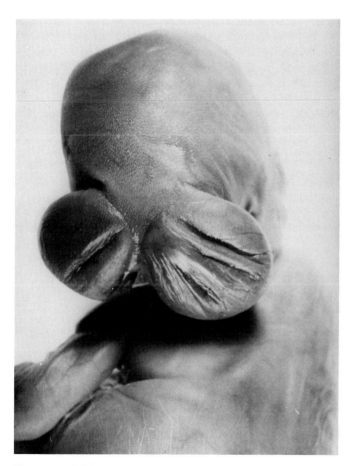

Fig. 53.22 Bifid occipital encephalocele in fetus with Meckel's syndrome.

Fig. 53.23 Nuchal swelling consisting of loose oedematous mesenchyme in fetus with trisomy 18.

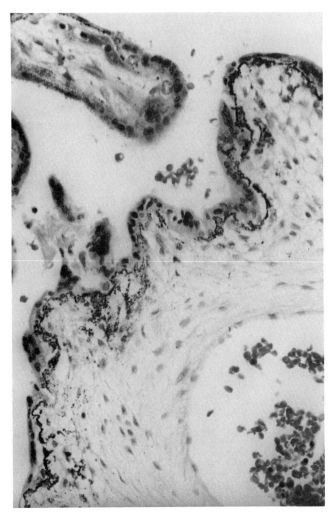

Fig. 53.24 Trophoblastic basement membrane mineralization in a 45,XO conceptus. Note the widely patent vessel within the villus. H & E × 350. (From Barson A J (ed) *Fetal and neonatal pathology*. Praeger, New York.)

moles (2%) and 50 were unclassifiable. 84% of the embryos and 26% of the fetuses were abnormal. The conceptuses with growth disorganization (GD) were subclassified into four groups:

GD₁ — intact chorionic sac with no embryo or
body stalk   337
GD₂ — amorphous embryonic tissue or body stalk   179
GD₃ — grossly disorganized embryo up to 10 mm
in length with some identifiable anatomical
features   133
GD₄ — major distortion of body shape   31

The vast majority of these would clearly fall into the Group I category of this author's classification (Table 53.5).

A further 78 embryos showed developmental inconsistences in which one or more developmental markers appeared out of phase. These data allow comparison of the prevalence of anatomical abnormalities in abortions, stillbirths and live births (Table 53.6).

Table 53.5 Macroscopic appearances of products of conception and classification according to the present grouping

	Proposed grouping
1. Gestation sac	
A. Intact containing	
(i) Fluid	1
(ii) Stunted, amorphous or cylindrical embryo	1
(iii) Macerated embryo or fetus	2
(iv) Fresh embryo or fetus	3
B. Ruptured	
(i) Absent cord root	1
(ii) Identifiable cord root	
a. Macerated	1 or 2*
b. Fresh	3
c. Equivocal	1, 2 or 3*
2. Embryo or fetus	
(i) Stunted, amorphous or cylindrical	1
(ii) Macerated	2
(iii) Fresh	3
(iv) Equivocal	2 or 3*
3. Placenta	
(i) Absent cord root	1
(ii) Identifiable cord root	
a. Macerated	2
b. Fresh	3
c. Equivocal	1, 2 or 3*
4. Curettings	
(i) Placental tissue	U*
(ii) Decidua	U
(iii) Blood clot	U
(iv) Other	U

*These specimens may be classifiable following examination of placenta histology
U = unclassifiable.
Identifiable pathological abnormalities other than those listed may be recorded but do not influence the grouping.

Table 53.6 Prevalence of abnormalities in spontaneous abortions, stillbirths and live births per 1000 cases (Poland et al, 1981)

Abnormality	Embryos	Fetuses	Stillbirths	Live births
General defects				
Growth disorganization	699	—	—	—
Developmental inconsistency	68	—	—	—
Systemic defects				
Central nervous system	23	12	49	1
Cyclopia	8	7	—	—
Eye, ear, neck	16	46	4	3
Cardiovascular system	15	96	15	7
Respiratory system	1	33	1	0.5
Alimentary system, body wall	12	76	10	5
Genitourinary system	1	54	11	5
Musculoskeletal	18	53	13	5
Other	3	28	—	—

In 79% of cases the placenta was examined. Two-thirds were considered to be normal while 21% showed cystic change, a figure comparable with other reported series (Fox, 1978). Cystic change was present in 39% of placentas from embryos with growth disorganization, 11% of cases with an abnormal embryo or fetus and in 6% where they were normal. This series included 53 pairs of twins

(Livingstone & Poland, 1980), an incidence of one in 35 pregnancies: 25 pairs were both embryos, 26 both fetuses and two consisted of one embryo and one fetus; 88% of the embryos and 21% of the fetuses were abnormal. Mono-zygotic twins were 17.5 times as frequent as dizygotic pairs, indicating a high prenatal mortality in the former.

The incidence of chromosomal abnormalities in 228 karyotyped embryos was 58% of those with growth dis-organization, 67% of those with other abnormalities and 25% of those considered to be anatomically normal. The comparative data for karyotyped fetuses was 22% in those which were abnormal and 2% in those with no abnormality.

The most recent data from Vancouver published by Kalousek (1987, 1991) expands this series, is classified by the same method (Table 53.7) and cannot be easily com-pared with the author's classification. This data shows that 62% of the specimens were either growth disorgan-ized or ruptured/fragmented sacs; these include almost 80% of the specimens with chromosomal abnormalities. The highest incidence of chromosomal abnormalities was found in those embryos with localized defects though these made up only 8% of the total specimens in her series. It is also of note that successful karyotyping was completed in approximately 64% of embryos with local-ized defects as against 17–30% in other specimens (with the exception of 15 GD_4 specimens where eight were karyotyped). It is therefore impossible to determine the true incidence of karyotypic abnormalities in these differ-ent morphological categories.

In summary it is clear that it is as yet impossible to match completely the findings in different series of abor-tions since the approaches to their study have varying emphasis depending on the author's major interests. The majority of chromosomally abnormal conceptuses fail to reach the end of the period of embryogenesis. The few that do may or may not show specific anatomical abnor-malities which are comparable to those found in the new-born with the same karyotypic abnormality. However, morphological diagnosis of a chromosomal abnormality is undoubtedly less reliable than in the newborn and

Table 53.7 Morphological classification, karyotyping and incidence of chromosomal abnormalities, percent (modified from Kalousek, 1991)

Specimens	Incidence	Karyotyped	Chromosomal abnormality
Complete			
Embryos with growth disorganization	24	20.5	56
Normal embryos	10	24.1	20
Embryos with local defect(s)	8	64.3	93
Fragmented/degenerate embryos	8	23.9	75
Incomplete			
Ruptured/fragmented sacs	38	29.7	63
Decidua only	12	0	N/A

any suspected chromosomal defect requires cytogenetic confirmation.

Recently several attempts have been made to correlate placental morphology with karyotype without success (Rehder et al, 1989; van Lijnschoten et al, 1993). This is perhaps not surprising in that villi are, in morphological terms, relatively simple structures and have only a limited capacity to vary from the norm. In an attempt to improve the sensitivity of histological methods to identify chromo-somally abnormal abortuses from examination of the placenta, Jauniaux & Hustin (1992) have added features found at the maternofetal interface. These included ab-sence of interstitial trophoblast, intravascular trophoblas-tic plugs and vascular changes in the spiral arteries. These lesions may all reflect the greater disturbance in tropho-blastic function that may be associated with chromosomal abnormalities. Certainly trophoblastic function does ap-pear to be abnormal in some forms of miscarriage as assessed by determination of circulating maternal levels of certain placental proteins (Johnson et al, 1993) though these findings are also open to the criticism that they are an effect of the deterioration of the fetus before it dies.

It must not be assumed that anatomical malformations found in therapeutically terminated pregnancies will be identical to those occurring in spontaneous abortions with the same karyotype of the same gestation.

MOSAICISM, UNIPARENTAL DISOMY AND GENOMIC IMPRINTING

The advent of chorionic villus sampling has greatly expanded our knowledge of the cytogenetics of early pregnancy and its influence on development. Early results revealed discrepancies between the karyotypes of the sampled villi and the fetus which were initially thought to be due to technical errors. As larger series were published, however, it became apparent that this was a true discrep-ancy and that differences between the fetal and placental karyotype might be of clinical significance.

Cell division may be disturbed at any time between conception and death as an adult. An aneuploid cell line arising *de novo* in an adult will be numerically insignificant and will probably die out or be eliminated, though some cell lines may have the potential for abnormal growth and malignancy. In the early stages of development, however, when the conceptus consists of only a small number of cells the appearance of an abnormal cell line may be of major significance. The proportion of abnormal cells will be very much larger (as high as 50% if it arises during the division of the fertilized ovum, with a possibility of rising if the growth of the abnormal cell line outstrips that of the diploid cells) and the mechanisms for the elimination of such cells will not be in place. Furthermore the abnormal cell line may become compartmentalized as the conceptus becomes increasingly organized, initially into the embryonic and placental components and later into organs and tissues.

The concurrent presence of two or more cell lines with different karyotypes arising from a common cell line in one individual results in mosaicism (the presence of two or more cell lines arising from different individuals results in chimaerism). Depending on the timing and site of origin of the abnormal cell line mosaicism may be generalized, affecting all components of the conceptus, or it may be confined, affecting a particular compartment either of the embryo or the placenta. If the conceptus has an aneuploid karyotype from fertilization abnormal cell division may then result in the appearance of a normal cell line.

Confined placental mosaicism (CPM) was first described by Kalousek & Dill (1983) and three forms are recognized (Kalousek 1990, 1991), the origin of which can be explained on embryological principles. Cells in the fertilized ovum destined to form the trophoblast must of necessity differentiate very early if implantation is to be successful. These trophoblastic cells form the major part of the blastocyst, indeed in mice it is known that the embryo is derived from only three cells of the blastocyst (Markert & Petters, 1978). The trophoblastic cells form the trophoblastic shell and primary villi. The latter subsequently obtain a central core of connective tissue from the extraembryonic mesoderm to form secondary villi (days 9–18) and blood vessels from cells of embryonic origin from day 18 to become tertiary villi. These tertiary villi therefore contain three cellular components — those of the trophoblast, those of the villous core and those of embryonic origin. Thus there are three types of CPM possible with a diploid fetus.

Type 1

Cytotrophoblast	Mosaic or non-mosaic aneuploidy
Villous stroma	Normal
Fetal tissues	Normal

Type 2

Cytotrophoblast	Normal
Villous stroma	Mosaic or non-mosaic aneuploidy
Fetal tissues	Normal

Type 3

Cytotrophoblast	Mosaic or non-mosaic aneuploidy
Villous stroma	Mosaic or non-mosaic aneuploidy
Fetal tissues	Normal

Apart from the mechanism described above, mosaicism may also arise in the placenta by loss of a twin (the so-called vanishing twin which may be a blighted ovum) with survival of some of that twin's placental tissue (Callen et al, 1991; Reddy et al, 1991).

The incidence of CPM is in the order of 2%, i.e. about ten times the incidence of complete mosaicism (Kalousek et al, 1991; Wang et al, 1993). The latter authors found 51 cases among 2612 consecutive chorionic villus sam-

ples, of which 20 were type 1, 24 type 2 and 7 type 3. They found that mosaicism was statistically associated with spontaneous abortion. There is some dispute as to the relationship between CPM and intrauterine fetal growth retardation and the effects on pregnancy outcome (Johnson et al, 1990; Kalousek, 1990; Kennerknecht & Terinde, 1990; Breed et al, 1991; Kalousek et al, 1991; Leschot & Wolf, 1991; Fryburg et al, 1992; Kennerknecht et al, 1992; Wapner et al, 1992) though the majority of authors support the view that intrauterine growth retardation and other perinatal problems can be associated with CPM. The survival of the fetus to late pregnancy or term in those pregnancies with an aneuploid fetus is benefited by the presence of a karyotypically normal placenta (Kalousek et al, 1989). Much is yet to be learnt about the interrelationship between the chromosomal constitution of the component parts of a pregnancy and their effects on reproductive failure, intrauterine fetal growth and pregnancy outcome. Once again it would appear that factors inherent in the conceptus rather than maternal factors are the major determinants of pregnancy outcome.

The mechanism leading to a pregnancy with a diploid fetus and mosaic trisomic placenta or a trisomic placenta is most likely to be loss of one of the trisomic chromosomes in the postzygotic period. Such a loss may result in the two remaining chromosomes of the trisomic triplet being derived either from each parent or from one parent, in the latter case resulting in uniparental disomy which should affect 1 in 3 such conceptuses (Hall, 1990; Engel & Delozier-Blanchet, 1991; Kalousek et al, 1993). Since it is known that normal development is dependent on the presence of both maternal and paternal copies of some chromosomes (Surani et al, 1988; Norris et al, 1990) uniparental disomy may be expected to have an adverse effect on reproductive outcome, this being mediated by the process of genomic imprinting. In man probably the most clear-cut example of genomic imprinting involves chromosome 15, maternal uniparental disomy resulting in Prader–Willi syndrome and paternal uniparental disomy in Angelmann's syndrome (Cassidy et al, 1992; Purvis-Smith et al, 1992; Smeets et al, 1992).

Only a few chromosomes have so far been identified in placentas with trisomic cell lines, i.e. 2, 7, 9, 15 and 16. Kalousek et al (1993) have recently described the effects of uniparental disomy for chromosome 16 in man. They investigated 9 cases of antenatally diagnosed trisomy 16 confined to the placenta. Fetal death, intrauterine growth retardation or low birth weight occurred in 6, with 4 of 5 cases of intrauterine growth retardation showing fetal uniparental disomy for chromosome 16. There was a correlation between the level of trisomic cells in the placenta and intrauterine growth retardation — the fewer the abnormal cells the better the growth. This study does not allow separation of the effects of uniparental disomy from those related to the proportions of trisomic cells in the placentas of growth-retarded conceptuses. The rôle of uniparental disomy and genomic imprinting in human pregnancy wastage is yet to be fully explored but may provide insight into some of the many unexplained anatomically normal losses with, and possibly without, growth retardation in the late first and mid trimesters.

Much may be learnt from the recent advances in the cytogenetics of reproductive wastage; in particular the rôles of placental mosaicism, genomic imprinting and uniparental disomy have hardly been explored.

EXAMINATION OF PRODUCTS OF CONCEPTION

Detailed information on the techniques for the examination of the embryo, fetus and placenta has been given elsewhere (Berry, 1980; Rushton, 1981a, 1982) but a brief outline is supplied below.

Embryos and fetuses

Larger fetuses and placentas may be examined separately. They may be of sufficient size to undergo a routine perinatal autopsy (Langley, 1971; Barson, 1981; Pryce-Davies, 1981). Smaller fetuses and embryos may be examined by the techniques described by Berry (1980). All specimens may be examined in the fresh or fixed state, though it is obvious that if bacteriological, virological, biochemical or cytogenetic studies are indicated fresh tissue will be required. It is therefore best for all products of conception to be sent to the laboratory unfixed. Dissection of small fetuses after fixation can be performed in the same manner as with zoological specimens, using a cork board to pin the conceptus out. The embryonic and fetal measurements should, under ideal circumstances, be those determined by ultrasonography, thus allowing comparison of the prenatal and postnatal parameters. These data will therefore include crown–rump and crown–heel length, biparietal diameter, abdominal and head circumference, foot length and weight. Foot length is particularly valuable since a severely macerated embryo or fetus may have disintegrated prior to or during delivery and the foot may be the only identifiable measurable part. Since head circumference is not a reliable indicator of hydrocephaly in early pregnancy, the head should be either examined by ultrasound after delivery to determine ventricular size or the thickness of the cerebral ventricles measured after opening the skull (Fig. 53.25). Gross ventricular dilatation may be evident in the presence of a normal size cranial vault.

External examination of the fetus (or embryo)

Gross abnormalities such as anencephaly, spina bifida or omphalocele will be obvious even to cursory examination but some abnormalities readily identifiable in the full-term infant are not identifiable in the second trimester,

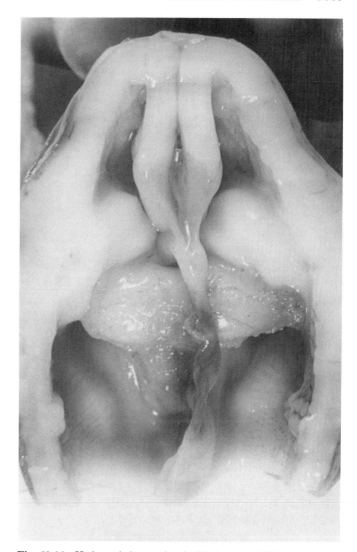

Fig. 53.25 Hydrocephaly associated with the Arnold–Chiari malformation and spinal bifida. The head was of normal size for the gestation of 22 weeks.

e.g. mongoloid facies (Fig. 53.26). Care should be taken to examine the hands, feet and genitalia. If the fetus is from a pregnancy terminated following prenatal diagnosis of a chromosomal abnormality, the latter must be confirmed cytogenetically. However, routine cytogenetic examination of all spontaneous abortions is not usually within the capability of most cytogenetic laboratories. There are however certain clues which may suggest a chromosomal abnormality and may indicate cytogenetic studies of the conceptus, these having been enumerated above. It is advantageous to record all embryonic or fetal abnormalities photographically if possible since such records are much more easily compared than written descriptions.

Macerated fetuses present particular problems and examination is frequently considered valueless. Abnormalities may be erroneously diagnosed if it is not appreciated that after fetal death the resorption of amniotic fluid re-

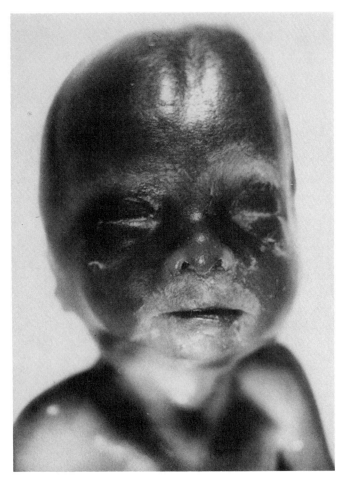

Fig. 53.26 Facies of a 22-week fetus with trisomy 21. None of the normal facial features of Down's syndrome is evident. (Courtesy of the Editor of the Journal of Clinical Pathology.)

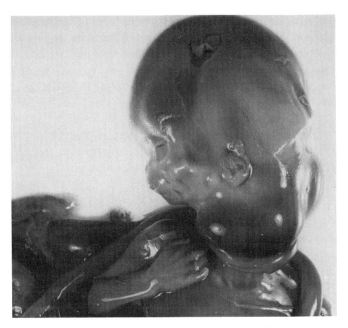

Fig. 53.27 Cord round the neck of a macerated fetus. Note the oedema above the cord entanglement.

sults in compression and distortion of the head and limbs. These distortions do not preclude further examination and gross external malformations should be readily identified. Radiological examination of all embryos and fetuses is recommended as an aid to the determination of gestational age and may be of particular value in macerated fetuses where vertebral ossification centres may be identified (Berry, 1980). In a few macerated fetuses the cause of intrauterine death may be apparent: thus entanglement of the umbilical cords may occur in monoamniotic twins while cord entanglement may be a cause of death in singleton pregnancies (Fig. 53.27).

Embryos and fetuses aborting spontaneously after diagnostic amniocentesis warrant particularly careful examination to exclude iatrogenic causes. It should be emphasized that there is no time limit between amniocentesis and abortion since fetal death due to injury may not result in expulsion of the conceptus for several weeks.

Internal examination

Under ideal circumstances full dissections should be per-

formed on all fetuses. They are essential on terminated fetuses with suspected abnormalities. Epidemiological data on the incidence of malformations within an aborted population relies on such dissections. Only a small proportion of the abnormalities demonstrated will be of clinical importance but in an individual case the finding of a malformation with a known pattern of inheritance will clearly be of great significance to the parents concerned. As yet, many of the more common genetic disorders cannot be diagnosed in the embryo or fetus with absolute certainty, this being particularly true of metabolic disorders where tissue culture and biochemical assays are required. Other diseases such as cystic fibrosis and muscular dystrophies still defy histopathological diagnosis. In general terms if the fetus is externally normal then a genetically significant abnormality is likely to be missed in about 2% of fetuses if a full examination is not completed. The exclusion of congenital heart disease, polycystic disease of the kidneys and hepatic lesions requires histological confirmation.

Examination of the placenta, cord and membranes

There are four indications for the examination of the placenta.

1. To exclude lesions likely to affect the management of the mother after delivery, e.g. trophoblastic disease (see Ch. 52).

2. To discover lesions related to or responsible for the expulsion of the conceptus, e.g. retroplacental haemorrhage, infection, criminal abortion, therapeutic abortion.

3. To discover lesions which may have resulted in fetal (or embryonic) death, e.g. uteroplacental ischaemia.

4. To distinguish between primary lesions related to the cause of abortion and secondary lesions usually related to cessation of the intravillous circulation. These are detailed elsewhere (Rushton, 1981a, 1982).

Examination of the placenta should be considered to be as important as examination of the embryo or fetus. In many cases only placental and decidual tissue will be available. Bacteriological, virological, biochemical and cytogenetic studies may be performed on fresh placental tissue.

The following data may be recorded: weight, shape, size, thickness, cord length and number of vessels within the cord, colour, translucency and smoothness of the membranes, evidence of trauma, the site and distribution of haemorrhage and its origin (maternal or fetal). The cut surface may reveal excavating retroplacental haemorrhage, infarction, subchorionic thrombosis (haematoma), pallor and molar change. Microscopic examination of the cord, membranes and placenta will aid in the confirmation of these lesions and also in the identification of more specific lesions, e.g. identification of organisms causing infection.

OTHER PATHOLOGY ASSOCIATED WITH SPONTANEOUS ABORTION (see Table 53.8)

Infections

The manifestations of infection in the placenta and fetus cannot be discussed in detail and the reader is referred to reviews and texts on infections in pregnancy (Ciba Foundation Symposium, 1973; Remington & Klein, 1976; Blanc, 1981; Rosenberg et al, 1981).

The most common manifestation of infection in spontaneous abortions is chorioamnionitis with or without involvement of the umbilical cord, embryo or fetus (see also

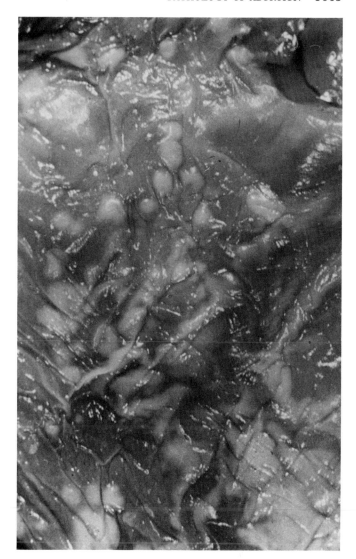

Fig. 53.28 Nodular amnionitis due to candidiasis. × 3. (Courtesy of the Editor of the Journal of Clinical Pathology.)

Table 53.8 Percentage distribution of additional pathology in fresh and macerated abortions

	Fresh	Macerated
Chorioamnionitis	25.5	10.3
Maternal floor infarction	N/A	22.1
Retroplacental haemorrhage	12.6	5.6
Malformations	5.3	11.2
Uteroplacental ischaemia	5.8	10.0
Hydrops	1.4	8.5
Multiple pregnancies	3.4	3.0
Cord complications	0	3.0
Amniotic bands	0	1.5
IUCD	1.2	0
Placenta praevia	1.2	0
Villitis	0.9	1.1
Molar change	0	1.1
Two vessels in cord	0.6	0
Placenta accreta	0.5	0
Placenta membranacea	0.5	0
No specific pathology	37.1	23.8

Chs 50 and 51). Chorioamnionitis was found in 10.3% of placentas from macerated conceptuses and 25.5% of fresh fetuses (Rushton, 1988). In the majority of cases it is bacterial in origin. In certain circumstances the lesions may be nodular (Fig. 53.28), this being characteristic of *Candida albicans* infection. There may also be white spots on the fetal skin. Appropriate staining techniques reveal the nature of the organism. The focal nature of the lesion may be apparent microscopically in the absence of any macroscopic lesion. Candida infection is an ascending infection and the organism can usually be isolated from the vagina.

Villitis, inflammation of the villous stroma (see also Ch. 49), with varying degrees of trophoblastic necrosis may be non-specific or due to known pathogens such as vaccinia virus (Rushton, 1981a) or listeriosis. Rarely the fetus may be infected in the absence of placental lesions as in herpes simplex infection (Fig. 53.29), the fetus having

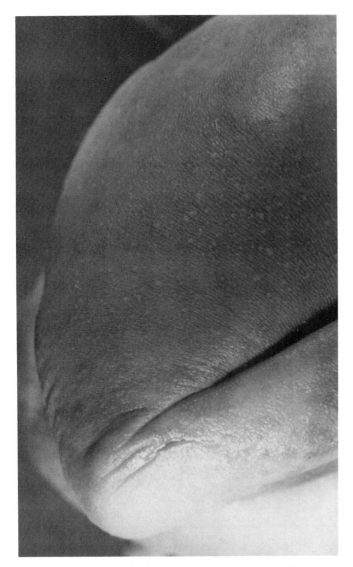

Fig. 53.29 Herpes simplex infection of fetal skin at 23 weeks' gestation. × 1.5.

multiple minute spots on the skin but no evidence of generalized infection. Occasionally infection may be suspected from endometrial curettings; thus, cytomegalovirus infection of the endometrium has been reported in association with spontaneous abortion (Dehner & Askin, 1975). However, since virtually all decidual and endometrial curettings obtained from the patient who aborts spontaneously show varying degrees of inflammatory response there must be specific changes present for an individual infection to be identified. Bacterial culture usually results in a mixed growth of organisms and routine virological studies are not feasible. The introduction of immunoperoxidase techniques may allow identification of specific organisms but it is unlikely that they will be generally available and they will in most instances not be cost effective. Occasionally, infective abortion may be associated with intrauterine contraceptive devices and it is of course a well-recognized hazard of criminal abortion.

Retroplacental and subchorionic haemorrhage

Retroplacental haemorrhage occurs in approximately 5% of Group II cases and 10% of Group III abortions (Rushton, 1988). While some of these haemorrhages may be central and excavating, the majority are marginal. They are usually of recent origin though a few may show stratification indicative of sequential bleeds (Fig. 53.30), a feature that may be reflected by a clinical history of threatened abortion.

The causes of these haemorrhages are unknown and while some may be related to trauma or to the site of implantation the majority remain unexplained. Such haemorrhages form a continuum with placental abruption and retroplacental haemorrhage in later pregnancy and they may be responsible for embryonic or fetal death. When associated with expulsion of a fresh fetus it is not always apparent whether they are the result of abortion or play a causal rôle in the loss of the pregnancy.

Subchorionic haemorrhage (see Ch. 47) may occur at any stage of gestation, though it is more common in early pregnancy. It is often considered to be a consequence of embryonic or fetal death but this is not invariably true (Shanklin & Scott, 1975). It is also considered to be the underlying factor in Breus' mole (Breus, 1892). As the name implies it typically consists of a large mass of clot sited immediately beneath the chorionic sac. The villous tissue between the thrombus and the decidua may appear normal or be separated from the chorionic plate. The lesion described by Breus, on the other hand, extends to the decidua and the conceptus appears as a solid mass of blood clot often with an empty intact gestation sac in its centre (Fig. 53.11). Villi are usually sparse and poorly vascularized. Thus in the author's opinion the two lesions are not identical and may have different aetiologies. Massive disruptive haemorrhage of the decidua is also a common finding in spontaneous abortions and since many retroplacental haemorrhages are in fact dissecting haemorrhages of the decidua, the true carneous mole may be more closely allied to these haemorrhages than to subchorionic haemorrhages seen in later pregnancy.

Uteroplacental ischaemia

Uteroplacental ischaemia is now a well-recognized and pathologically defined entity of major clinical importance in later pregnancy where it may be associated with placental infarction, fetal growth retardation, fetal death and maternal hypertensive disease, particularly pre-eclampsia.

The normal physiological response of the placental bed vessels to pregnancy (Brosens et al, 1967) and the response of the same vessels in hypertensive pregnancy (Robertson et al, 1967) clearly indicates that vascular adaption is disturbed in the latter instance in the first trimester of pregnancy, though there is no evidence of maternal disease. It therefore follows that a proportion of spontaneous abortions are likely to show evidence of vascular lesions in the placental bed, this being borne out by the ultrasound finding that some cases of threatened abortion are growth retarded (Mantoni & Pederson, 1982), though of course there may be other causes for fetal growth retardation.

The classic placental lesion associated with uterine vascular disease is the placental infarct and a significant degree of infarction is found in approximately 5% of macerated abortions (Group II) and 3% of fresh abortions (Group III). The extent of the infarction is consistent with it being responsible for fetal death in a few cases (Fig. 53.31). Since these patients are usually admitted

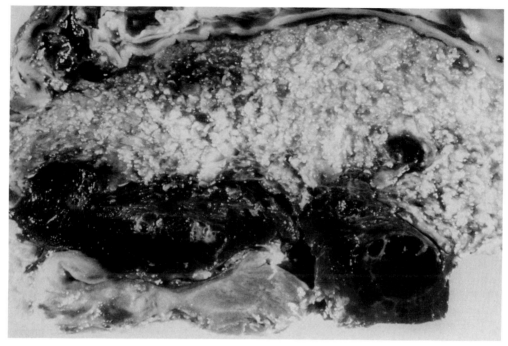

Fig. 53.30 Marginal retroplacental haemorrhages of varying age. × 2.

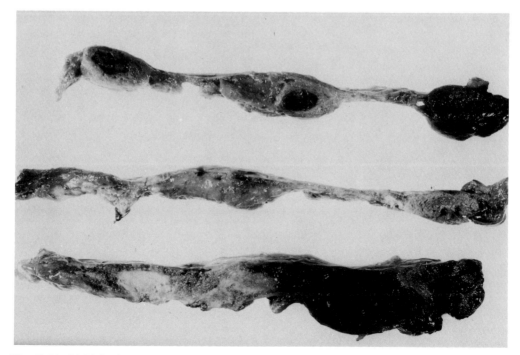

Fig. 53.31 Multiple placental infarcts, areas of thinning and local thrombosis. × 1.

after abortion has occurred, or occasionally while it is in progress, little is known of their clinical status.

While it is still not completely clear whether 'acute atherosis' is pathognomonic of pre-eclampsia (Robertson, 1976) or is also a feature of pregnancies with growth-retarded fetuses in the absence of maternal pre-eclampsia (Sheppard & Bonnar, 1976) it may be possible to reconcile these opposing views if the latter represents preclinical (forme fruste) pre-eclampsia. The importance of identifying these cases in a population of spontaneous abortions is twofold: firstly, the aetiology of these abortions is clearly different from the majority of early pregnancy losses; secondly, preliminary data suggests such lesions may recur in subsequent pregnancies (Rushton, 1988). The detailed pathology of the uterine vasculature in pregnancy is discussed elsewhere (Ch. 48).

Maternal floor infarction of the placenta

Maternal floor infarction of the placenta is a term coined by Benirschke & Driscoll (1967) for a placental lesion which was described approximately a century ago by Garrigues (1884), though the latter author likened the consistency of these placentas to lard (lardaceous placenta). The term is misleading in that it does not appear to be a primary ischaemic lesion, nor do the histological changes correspond to those seen in true placental infarction. Benirschke & Driscoll (1967) believed the lesion to be very rare and were uncertain of its significance though it was associated with intrauterine fetal death.

Macroscopically (Figs 53.17 and 53.32) there is a ridged, almost gyriform, pattern to the maternal aspect of the placenta, the gyri being pale yellow in colour. Slicing

shows a layer of slightly opalescent material of variable thickness from 1–2 mm to almost the entire thickness of the placenta. Within this material are irregular vascular channels. The material has the staining properties of fibrin.

Microscopic examination reveals progressive fibrin deposition beginning by fusion of the striae of Rohr and Nitabuch and extending to involve increasing volumes of the intervillous space from the basal aspect towards the chorionic plate.

The villi embedded within the fibrin are not infarcted. They are fibrotic and occasional cytotrophoblastic cells can be identified. The vascular channels contain small collections of syncytial cells attached to their walls (Fig. 53.33). As the fibrin encroaches on the intervillous space there is a fibroblastic obliteration of the lumen of the decidual vessels in the placental bed due to intimal thickening (Fig. 53.16). These vascular lesions closely resemble those in the postpartum uterus. Thus, while the character-

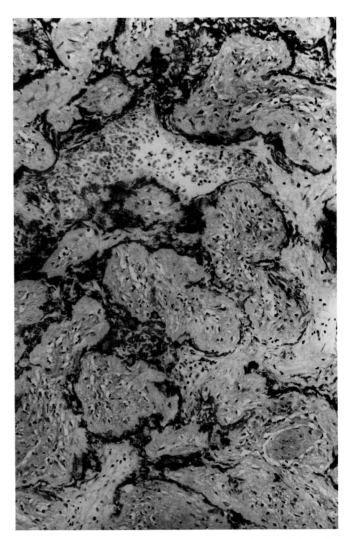

Fig. 53.33 Maternal floor infarction. The fibrotic but non-infarcted villi are embedded in fibrin with occasional intervillous vascular channels. Martius Scarlet Blue × 140.

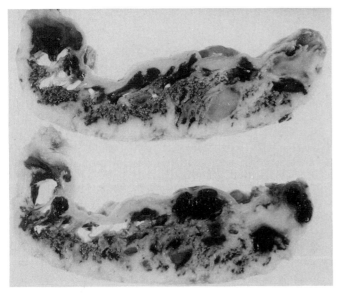

Fig. 53.32 Advanced maternal floor infarction with a thick basal layer of fibrinoid material, large dilated thrombosed vascular channels and septal cyst formation. × 1.2.

istic lesion described by Benirschke & Driscoll (1967) may be uncommon, if all the stages of evolution of the lesion are considered then some 28.7% of Group II abortions show this change (Rushton, 1988). It is not seen in association with live births though it may be present in twin placentas where one twin dies some weeks prior to delivery. The relative rarity of the classic lesion is almost certainly a reflection of the time required for the characteristic features to develop, most mothers aborting before they do so. The significance of this lesion will be discussed when the mechanisms of abortion are considered.

Abnormalities of placentation

Abnormal sites of implantation are responsible for a number of spontaneous abortions though it is difficult to assess how many. Ultrasound studies of early pregnancies may eventually clarify this problem. It would not be surprising if cervical pregnancies did abort. However it is difficult to assess the importance of low implantation when placental growth is incomplete. Morbidly adherent placentas were found in 1 in 200 spontaneous abortions in the author's series, the diagnosis being made on the histological criterion of direct apposition of villi and myometrium. Placenta membranacea was found in 1 in 200 specimens. It is difficult to see how these lesions might result in spontaneous abortion; while the incidence is high compared with term pregnancies, other factors may be responsible for their early expulsion from the uterus. Extrachorial placentation (circummarginate and circumvallate placenta) is difficult to diagnose in early pregnancy (Fox, 1978) but in Group III abortions the incidence appears comparable with that in full-term placentas.

Pathology of the umbilical cord (see also Ch. 50)

The high incidence and mortality of monoamniotic twins in spontaneous abortions would suggest that cord complications may be a significant factor in the death of some of these conceptuses. Cord complications, usually entanglement, were found in 2.9% of Group II cases and their absence in Group III abortuses may be an indication that cord entanglement is a significant cause of death in early pregnancy, though it is possible that the entanglement occurred after death.

The number of examples of single umbilical artery in the author's series is very small but all have been related to fetal malformations and as such they probably occur with the same relative frequency as in later pregnancy since a single umbilical artery per se is unlikely to cause fetal death or be responsible for abortion.

Javert (1957) stressed the importance of cord lesions as a cause of death, in particular emphasizing variations in length, torsion and knots. Fox (1978) argues that only about 3% of abortions in Javert's series could be attributed to cord complications, a figure almost identical to that of 2.9% in my own series (Rushton, 1988).

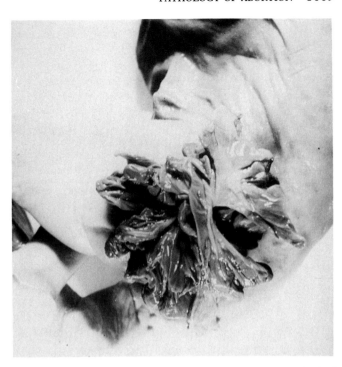

Fig. 53.34 Small intestine and mesentery protruding from the flank of a procured abortion.

PROCURED OR CRIMINAL ABORTION

Criminal abortion is, or appears to be, relatively uncommon in those societies where liberal abortion laws obtain. It is not possible to obtain a reliable estimate of the proportions of abortions which are criminally induced though figures from one per thousand (Hertig, 1968) to 40% are quoted (Gradwohl, 1968). In a hospital population the lower figure is appropriate but if criminal abortion is assessed on the basis of maternal mortality then obviously the incidence will appear much greater. Indeed such cases may first come to the pathologist's attention when he or she is presented with a maternal death at autopsy. The techniques for examination of products of conception (Rushton, 1981a, 1982) and performance of a maternal autopsy (Rushton & Dawson, 1982) are described elsewhere (see also Ch. 63).

The methods used to procure abortion and the complications associated with criminal intervention in pregnancy may be found in texts on forensic pathology, the major maternal problems being infection, trauma and air embolism.

The products of conception may reveal evidence of injury (Fig. 53.34), infection and inappropriate placental lesions, i.e. lesions which do not coincide with the anatomical structure of the placenta (Fig. 53.35).

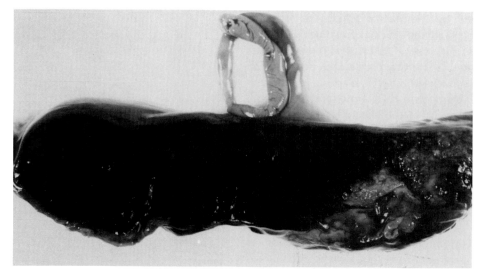

Fig. 53.35 Placenta of a procured abortion showing massive intervillous thrombosis not related to the normal anatomical units of the placenta.

THERAPEUTIC ABORTION FOR FETAL OR MATERNAL DISEASE

There are two major indications for the examination of products of conception from terminated pregnancies. In those cases where an antenatal diagnosis has been made this must be confirmed by the appropriate techniques, be it by morphological, cytogenetic or biochemical methods. It is also essential that those terminated fetuses, where the prenatal diagnostic results are abnormal and the fetus is macroscopically normal, are fully examined. An unexplained elevation of the maternal serum or amniotic fluid alphafetoprotein may necessitate detailed examination of the kidneys including both light- and electronmicroscopy since the congenital nephrotic syndrome will be missed in the absence of such studies. Even in the absence of facilities for electronmicroscopy the demonstration of dilated renal tubules containing deeply eosinophilic proteinaceous casts and numerous droplets within the proximal tubular epithelium are highly suggestive of this diagnosis (Fig. 53.36).

The second indication for examination is to exclude placental or fetal damage resulting from the investigative procedure: the author has seen examples of retroplacental haemorrhage, rupture of the membranes with amniotic fluid leakage, transfixion of the umbilical cord and lethal internal injuries of the fetus following diagnostic amniocentesis. It is estimated that there is only a 1% fetal mortality associated with diagnostic amniocentesis (Medical Research Council Working Party, 1978), but in the case of fetoscopy the fetal death rate may be significantly greater (Ward et al, 1981).

It is also essential to monitor the outcome of all pregnancies where borderline results are obtained using prenatal diagnosis. A marginally elevated alphafetoprotein level

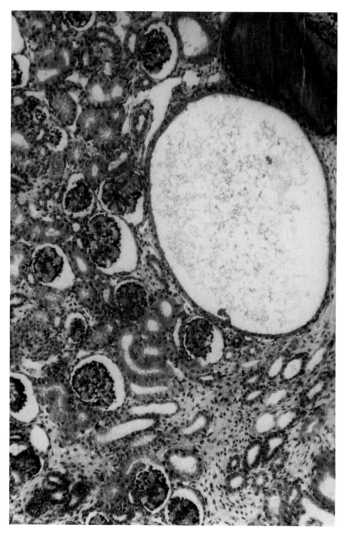

Fig. 53.36 Kidney of an 18-week fetus with congenital nephrotic syndrome. Note the isolated cysts, some with proteinaceous casts and the deeply staining granular proximal tubular epithelium. H & E × 140.

in the amniotic fluid may be an early indication of impending fetal death. In the newborn, abnormalities which might be the result of trauma or chronic loss of amniotic fluid, e.g. positional talipes, pulmonary hypoplasia and amnion nodosum should be sought.

When pregnancy is terminated for maternal disease, be it organic or psychiatric, it is not safe to assume that the conceptus will be normal. About 2% of these terminations have a chromosomal abnormality (Geneva Conference, 1966) and a similar proportion may have anatomical abnormalities. In early suction terminations placental abnormalities of the type described in Group I spontaneous abortions occur in about 5% of cases (Rushton, unpublished data). Since in many countries these terminations are not examined, pathologically accurate data is difficult to obtain. However, the demonstration of abnormalities in these conceptuses may not only provide important epidemiological data but it will also be of considerable psychological benefit to the mother concerned. The method of termination employed is reflected to some degree in the appearances of the placenta in the later pregnancies, the morphological and histological features having been reviewed by Fox (1978). These may be summarized as follows:

1. Intra-amniotic hypertonic saline: the placenta is pale with focal or continuous subchorionic haemorrhage (Fig. 53.37). The membranes may be oedematous with necrosis of the amniotic epithelium. Vessels in the chorionic plate and umbilical cord may be thrombosed. There is focal decidual necrosis.

2. Extra-amniotic hypertonic saline: the appearances may be similar to those seen with intra-amniotic injection but no specific lesions may be evident in a proportion of cases.

3. Intra-amniotic hypertonic urea may result in the lesions seen with hypertonic saline. Hypertonic glucose does not produce any lesions.

4. Prostaglandins may be given intra- or extra-amniotically, the former being the most common method in current use. No specific lesions have been identified using either method.

It is worthy of note that since 1970 the Confidential Enquiries into Maternal Deaths show that deaths due to legal termination exceed those due to spontaneous abortion and since 1973 exceed those due to illegal abortion (Report on the Confidential Enquiries, 1982).

MECHANISMS OF SPONTANEOUS ABORTION

The mechanisms concerned in the expulsion of abnormal conceptuses are still ill understood. As has been indicated, a proportion are due to local environmental problems within the uterus, a small number are criminally induced and some are therapeutically terminated. However, in the

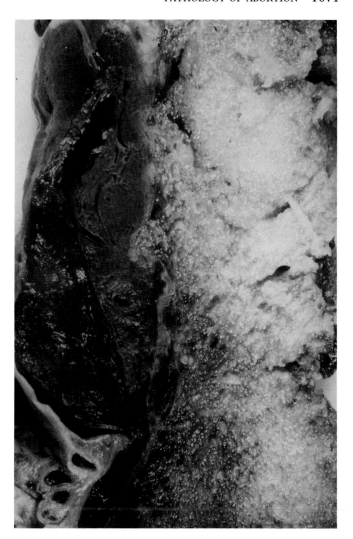

Fig. 53.37 Subchorionic thrombosis associated with a termination of pregnancy using hypertonic saline.

vast majority the mechanisms are obscure and certainly cannot be directly related to embryonic or fetal abnormalities. In Groups I and II of the current classification, which account for about 70% of our hospital population of spontaneous abortions, there is one common factor: absence of an embryonic or fetal circulation within the placental villi, either because the villi failed to develop a vascular network or because the circulation ceased as a result of fetal death. It is evident (Rushton, 1984, 1985) that the absence of a circulation within the villous tree has profound effects on the metabolic function of the trophoblast which result in failure of normal hormonal synthesis.

Morphologic changes in the syncytium may predispose to platelet and fibrin deposition on the villous surface and, under idealized circumstances, progressive obliteration of the intervillous space, a reduced maternal blood supply to the placenta and regressive changes in the uteroplacental vasculature. The eventual decline in placental function results in increased uterine irritability and eventually expulsion of the conceptus. This hypothesis obviates the need to implicate immunological factors as a cause of abortion and proposes that the developmental status of the embryo or fetus play an essential rôle in determining the outcome of pregnancy. Whether immunological factors are responsible for some fetal deaths remains enigmatic. In summary it is the conceptus which, in the majority of spontaneous abortions, determines its own fate by its ability to develop normally and survive. The loss of the conceptus is a result of placental and not embryonic or fetal abnormalities. Much remains to be explained but a better understanding of the natural mechanisms of spontaneous abortion and the reason why the elimination of all abnormal conceptuses does not occur may eventually lead to a more rational approach to the management of the complications of early pregnancy and the therapeutic termination of unwanted pregnancies.

CONCLUSIONS

Much can be learnt from the examination of both spontaneously aborting and terminated early pregnancies. It is hoped that in future pathological examination of spontaneous abortions will become routine and that initial indications that the nature of the aborted products of conception is of value in the counselling of patients will be confirmed (Poland et al, 1977). Routine cytogenetic studies on spontaneous abortions are not feasible and not warranted. In those who abort recurrently the obstetrician or gynaecologist should be advised that parental chromosomal studies are more appropriate.

Finally it is worth emphasizing that under ideal circumstances the study of the epidemiology of spontaneous abortions and the abnormalities found in geographically defined populations may be a more sensitive indicator of a new environmental teratogen than the finding of abnormalities in viable fetuses.

REFERENCES

Appleman Z, Rosensaft J, Chemke B, Caspi B, Ashkenazi M, Mogilner M B 1991 Trisomy 9 confined to the placenta: prenatal diagnosis and neonatal follow up. American Journal of Medical Genetics 40: 464–466.

Ballantyne J W 1902 Manual of antenatal pathology and hygiene. William Green & Sons, Edinburgh.

Barson A J 1981 The perinatal postmortem. In: Barson A J (ed) Laboratory investigation of fetal disease. Wright, Bristol, ch 21, pp 476–497.

Bauld R, Sutherland G R, Bain D 1974 Chromosome studies in investigation of stillbirths and neonatal deaths. Archives of Disease in Childhood 49: 782–788.

Beischer N A, Bettinger H F, Fortune D W, Pepperell R 1970 Hydatidiform mole and its complications in the State of Victoria. Journal of Obstetrics and Gynaecology of the British Commonwealth 77: 263–276.

Benirschke K, Driscoll S G 1967 The pathology of the human placenta. Springer-Verlag, New York, pp 232.

Benzie R J 1981 Fetoscopy and fetal blood sampling. In: Barson A J (ed) Laboratory investigation of fetal disease. Wright, Bristol, ch. 14, pp 320–336.

Berry C L 1980 The examination of embryonic and fetal material in diagnostic histopathology laboratories. Journal of Clinical Pathology 33: 317–326.

Blanc W A 1981 Pathology of the placenta, membranes and umbilical cord in bacterial fungal and viral infections in man. In: Naeye R L, Kissane J M, Kaufman N (eds) Perinatal diseases. International Academy of Pathology Monograph, Williams & Wilkins, Baltimore, pp 67–132.

Block S K 1978 Occult pregnancy as a factor in unexplained infertility. Journal of Reproductive Medicine 21: 251–253.

Boué A, Boué J 1978 Consequences of chromosome aberrations on the development of human conceptuses. In: Van Juhsingha E N, Tesh J M, Fara G M (eds) Advances in the detection of congenital malformations. European Teratology Society 99: 33–49.

Boué J, Phillipe E, Giroud A, Boué A 1976 Phenotypic expression of lethal chromosomal abnormalities in human abortuses. Teratology 14: 3–13.

Breed A S P M, Mantingh A, Vosters R et al 1991 Follow up and pregnancy outcome after a diagnosis of mosaicism on CVS. Prenatal Diagnosis 11: 577–580.

Bresnihan B, Griger R R, Oliver M et al 1977 Immunological mechanism for spontaneous abortion in systemic lupus erythematosus. Lancet ii: 1205–1207.

Breus C 1892 Das Tuberose Subchoriale-Hamatom der Decidua. Deuticke, Leipzig.

Brosens I, Robertson W B, Dixon H G 1967 The physiological response of the vessels of the placental bed to normal pregnancy. Journal of Pathology and Bacteriology 93: 569–579.

Buckley C H 1991 LPD. A glandular or vascular problem. Journal of Pathology 165: 95–96.

Bulmash J M 1978 Systemic lupus erythematosus and pregnancy. In: Wynn R M (ed) Obstetrics and gynecology annual, vol 7. Appleton-Century-Crofts, Norwalk, CT, pp 153–194.

Callen D F, Fernandez H, Hull Y J, Svigos J M, Chambers H M, Sutherland G R 1991 A normal 46XX infant with a 46XX/69XXX placenta: a major contribution to the placenta is from a resorbed twin. Prenatal Diagnosis 11: 437–442.

Cassidy S B, Lai L-W, Erickson R P et al 1992 Trisomy 15 with loss of the paternal 15 as a cause of Prader-Willi Syndrome due to maternal disomy. American Journal of Human Genetics 51: 701–708.

Ciba Foundation Symposium 10 (New Series) 1973 Intrauterine infection. Elsevier Excerpta Medica, North-Holland, Amsterdam.

Clarke P C, Chard T 1981 Alphafetoprotein assay. In: Barson A J (ed) Laboratory investigation of fetal disease. Wright, Bristol, ch 8, pp 173–189.

Cohen Overbeek T E, Hop W C J, den Ouden M, Pijpers L, Jahoda M G J, Wladimiroff J W 1990 Spontaneous abortion rate and advanced maternal age; consequences of prenatal diagnosis. Lancet 336: 27–29.

Crane J P, Wahl N 1981 The role of maternal diabetes in repetitive spontaneous abortion. Fertility and Sterility 36: 477–479.

Dehner L P, Askin F B 1975 Cytomegalovirus endometritis: report of a case associated with spontaneous abortion. Obstetrics and Gynecology 45: 211–214.

Deligdisch L, Legum C, Peyser M R, Toaff R 1978 Cyclopia associated with triploidy and hydatidiform mole: a case report. Teratology 18: 257–262.

Denman A M 1982 Pregnancy and immunological disorders. British Medical Journal i: 999–1000.

Diczfalusy E 1974 Steps in the human reproductive process susceptible to immunological interference. In: Diczfalusy E (ed) Karolinska Symposia on Research Methods in Reproductive Endocrinology, 7th Symposium. Immunological approaches to fertility control. Karolinska Institutet, Stockholm, pp 13–37.

Duenhoelter J H, Santos-Ramos R 1981 Intrauterine diagnosis by ultrasound. In: Barson A J (ed) Laboratory investigation of fetal disease. Wright, Bristol, ch 10, pp 218–236.

Duff G B, Evans J J, Legge M 1980 A study of investigations used to predict outcome of pregnancy after threatened abortion. British Journal of Obstetrics and Gynaecology 87: 194–198.

Edwards J H, Yuncken C, Rushton D I, Richards S, Mittwoch U 1967 Three cases of triploidy in man. Cytogenetics 6: 81–104.

Elias S, Simpson J L 1980 Evaluation and clinical management of patients at apparent increased risk of spontaneous abortions. In: Porter I H, Hook E B (eds) Human embryonic and fetal death. Academic Press, New York, pp 331–353.

Engel E, Delozier-Blanchet C D 1991 Uniparental disomy, isodisomy, and imprinting: probable effects in man and strategies for their detection. American Journal of Medical Genetics 40: 432–439.

Fantel A G, Shepard T H, Vadheim-Roth C, Stephens T D, Coleman C 1980 Embryonic and fetal phenotypes: prevalence and other associated factors in a large study of spontaneous abortion. In: Porter I H, Hook E B (eds) Human embryonic and fetal death. Academic Press, New York, pp 71–87.

Fox H 1978 Pathology of the placenta, vol 7. Major problems in pathology. Saunders, London.

Fryburg J S, Dimalo M S, Mahoney M J 1992 Postnatal placental confirmation of trisomy 2 and trisomy 16 detected at chorionic villus sampling: a possible association with intra uterine growth retardation and elevated maternal serum alpha fetoprotein. Prenatal Diagnosis 12: 157–162.

Fugimato A, Ebbin A J, Towner J W, Wilson M G 1973 Trisomy 13 in two infants with cyclopia. Journal of Medical Genetics 10: 294–304.

Fujikura T, Froehlich L A, Driscoll S G 1966 A simplified anatomic classification of abortions. American Journal of Obstetrics and Gynecology 95: 902–905.

Garrigues H J 1884 Missed abortion: sclerosis of the placenta. American Journal of Obstetrics 17: 963–964.

Geneva Conference 1966 Standardisation of procedures for chromosome studies in abortion. Cytogenetics 5: 361–393.

Golbus M S 1978 Development in the first half of gestation of genetically abnormal human fetuses. Teratology 18: 333–336.

Gosden C M, Wright M O, Paterson W G, Grant K A 1976 Clinical details, cytogenetic studies and cellular physiology of a 69 XXX fetus with comments on the biological effect of triploidy in man. Journal of Medical Genetics 13: 371–380.

Gradwohl's Legal Medicine 1968 Camps F E (ed). Wright, Bristol, ch 23.

Greiss F C, Mauzy C H 1961 Genital anomalies in women: an evaluation of diagnosis, incidence and obstetrics performance. American Journal of Obstetrics and Gynecology 82: 330–339.

Gudson J P 1976 Maternal immune responses in pregnancy. In: Scott J S, Jones W R (eds) Immunology of human reproduction. Academic Press, London, ch 5, pp 103–126.

Hafez E S E 1967 Reproductive failure in domestic mammals. In: Bernirschke K (ed) Comparative aspects of reproductive failure. Springer-Verlag, New York, pp 42–95.

Hall J G 1990 Genomic imprinting: review and relevance to human diseases. American Journal of Human Genetics 46: 857–873.

Hamerton J L 1971 Human cytogenetics. Clinical cytogenetics, vol II. Academic Press, New York.

Hamerton J L, Canning N, Ray M, Smith S 1975 A cytogenetic survey of 14 069 newborn infants (1) Incidence of chromosome abnormalities. Clinical Genetics 8: 223–243.

Hamilton M P R, Fleming R, Coutts J R T, MacNaughton M C, Whitfield C R 1990 Luteal phase deficiency: ultrasonic and biochemical insights into pathogenesis. British Journal of Obstetrics and Gynaecology 97: 569–575.

Harlap S, Shiono P H 1980 Alcohol, smoking and incidence of spontaneous abortions in the first and second trimester. Lancet ii: 173–176.

Harris M J, Poland B J, Dill F J 1981 Triploidy in 40 human spontaneous abortuses: assessment of phenotype in embryos. Obstetrics and Gynecology 57: 600–606.

Hartikainen-Sori A L, Kaila J 1980 Systemic lupus erythematosus and habitual abortion: case report. British Journal of Obstetrics and Gynaecology 87: 729–731.

Hay D 1958 The diagnosis and significance of minor degrees of uterine abnormality in relation to pregnancy. Journal of Obstetrics and Gynaecology of the British Empire 65: 557–582.

Hemminki K, Mutanen P, Saloniemi I, Niemi M L, Vaino H 1982 Spontaneous abortions in hospital staff engaged in sterilizing instruments with chemical agents. British Medical Journal ii: 1461–1463.

Hendrickx A G, Binkerd P E 1980 Fetal deaths in non human primates: In: Porter I H, Hook E B (eds) Human embryonic and fetal death. Academic Press, New York, pp 45–69.

Hensell D L, Obregon V L, Heard M C, Nobles B J 1989 Endometrial bacteria in asymptomatic non pregnant women. Journal of Reproductive Medicine 34: 872–874.

Herbst A L, Ulfelder H, Poskanzer D C 1971 Adenocarcinoma of the vagina: association of maternal stilbestrol therapy with tumor appearance in young women. New England Journal of Medicine 284: 878–881.

Heritage D W, English S C, Young R B, Chen A T L 1978 Cytogenetics of recurrent abortions. Fertility and Sterility 29: 414–417.

Hertig A T 1968 Human trophoblast. Thomas, Springfield, Illinois, p 167.

Hertig A T, Rock J, Adams E C 1956 A description of 34 human ova within the first 17 days of development. American Journal of Anatomy 98: 435–459.

Hoerlein A B 1967 Bacterial infertility in domestic animals. In: Benirschke K (ed) Comparative aspects of reproductive failure. Springer-Verlag, Berlin, pp 268–279.

Honoré L H, Dill F J, Poland B J 1976 Placental morphology in spontaneous human abortuses with normal and abnormal karyotypes. Teratology 14: 151–166.

Hook E B 1978 Spontaneous deaths of fetus with chromosomal abnormalities diagnosed prenatally. New England Journal of Medicine 299: 1036–1038.

Hustin J, Jauniaux E, Schapps J P 1990 Histological study of the materno-embryonic interface in spontaneous abortion. Placenta 11: 477–486.

Iioka H, Akada S, Shimamoto T et al 1993 Platelet aggregation inhibiting activity of human placental chorioepithelial brush border membrane vesicles. Placenta 14: 75–83.

Jacobs P A, Hassold T J 1980 The origins of chromosome abnormalities in spontaneous abortion. In: Porter I H, Hook E B (eds) Human embryonic and fetal death. Academic Press, New York, pp 289–298.

Jauniaux E, Hustin J 1992 Histological examination of first trimester spontaneous abortions: the impact of materno-embryonic interface features. Histopathology 21: 409–414.

Javert C T 1957 Spontaneous and habitual abortion. McGraw-Hill, New York.

Jenkins D M 1976 Pre-eclampsia/eclampsia (gestosis) and other pregnancy complications with a possible immunologic basis. In: Scott J S, Jones W R (eds) Immunology of human reproduction. Academic Press, London, ch 10, pp 317–320.

Jennings C L 1972 Temporary submucosal cerclage for cervical incompetence. Reports of forty eight cases. American Journal of Obstetrics and Gynecology 113: 1097–1102.

Johnson A, Wapner R J, Davis G H, Jackson L G 1990 Mosaicism in chorionic villus sampling: an association with poor perinatal outcome. Obstetrics and Gynecology 74: 573–577.

Johnson M R, Riddle A F, Grudzinskas J G, Sharma V, Collins W P, Nicholiades K H 1993 The role of trophoblast dysfunction in the aetiology of miscarriage. British Journal of Obstetrics and Gynaecology 100: 353–359.

Kajii T, Ferrier A 1978 Cytogenetics of abortion and abortuses. American Journal of Obstetrics and Gynecology 131: 33–38.

Kajii T, Ferrier A, Nikawa N, Takahara H, Ohama K, Avirachan S 1980 Anatomic and chromosomal anomalies in 639 spontaneous abortions. Human Genetics 55: 87–98.

Kalousek D K 1987 Anatomic and chromosome anomalies in specimens of early spontaneous abortion: seven year experience. In: Gilbert E F, Opitz J M (eds) Genetic aspects of developmental pathology. National Foundation — March of Dimes, Birth Defect: Original Article Series XXIII (1). AR Liss, New York, pp 153–168.

Kalousek D K 1990 Confined placental mosaicism and intrauterine development. Pediatric Pathology 10: 69–77.

Kalousek D K 1991 Pathology of abortion: chromosomal and genetic correlations. In: Kraus F T, Damjanov I, Kaufman N (eds) Pathology of reproductive failure. Williams & Wilkins, Baltimore, pp 228–256.

Kalousek D K, Dill F J 1983 Chromosomal mosaicism confined to the placenta in human conceptions. Science 221: 665–667.

Kalousek D K, McGillivray B C, Barret I J 1989 Placental mosaicism and intrauterine survival of trisomies 13 and 18. American Journal of Human Genetics 44: 338–343.

Kalousek D K, Howard-Peebles P N, Olson S B et al 1991 Confirmation of CVS mosaicism in term placentae and high frequency of intrauterine growth retardation associated with confined placental mosaicism. Prenatal Diagnosis 11: 743–750.

Kalousek D K, Langlois S, Barrett I et al 1993 Uniparental disomy for chromosome 16 in humans. American Journal of Human Genetics 52: 8–16.

Kennerknecht I, Teringe R 1990 Intrauterine growth retardation associated with chromosomal aneuploidy confined to the placenta: three observations: triple trisomy 6, 21, 22: trisomy 16; and trisomy 18. Prenatal Diagnosis 10: 539–544.

Kennerknecht I, Kramer S, Grab D, Terinde R, Vogel W 1992 No association of intrauterine growth retardation and confined placental mosaicism: a prospective study. Prenatal Diagnosis (suppl 12): S104.

Khong T Y, Liddell H S, Robertson W B 1987 Defective haemochorial placentation as a cause of miscarriage: a preliminary study. British Journal of Obstetrics and Gynaecology 94: 649–655.

King C R, Pernoll M L, Prescott G 1982 Reproductive wastage. In: Wynn R M (ed) Obstetrics and gynecology annual, vol 11. Appleton-Century-Crofts, Norwalk, Connecticut, pp 59–110.

Klein J O, Remington J S, Marcy S M 1976 An introduction to infections of the fetus and newborn infant. In: Remington J S, Klein O J (eds) Infectious diseases of the fetus and newborn infant. Saunders Philadelphia, ch 1, p 7.

Knill-Jones R P, Newman B, Spence A A 1975 Anaesthetic practice and pregnancy. Lancet ii: 807–809.

Lang A P, Schlager M, Gardner H A 1976 Trisomy 18 and cyclopia. Teratology 14: 195–204.

Langley F A 1971 The perinatal post mortem examination. Journal of Clinical Pathology 24: 159–169.

Lauritsen J G, Grunnet N, Jonson E M 1975 Maternal-fetal ABO incompatibility as a cause of spontaneous abortion. Clinical Genetics 7: 308–316.

Leschot N J, Wolf H 1991 Is placental mosaicism associated with poor perinatal outcome? Prenatal Diagnosis 11: 403–404.

Li T C, Dockery P, Rogers A W, Cooke I D 1990 A quantitative study of endometrial development in the luteal phase: comparison between women with unexplained infertility and normal fertility. British Journal of Obstetrics and Gynaecology 97: 576–582.

Lilienfeld A M, Pasamanick B 1955 The association of maternal fetal factors with the development of cerebral palsy and epilepsy. American Journal of Obstetrics and Gynaecology 70: 93–101.

Livingstone J E, Poland B J 1980 A study of spontaneously aborted twins. Teratology 21: 139–148.

McFadden D E, Kalousek D K 1991 Two different phenotypes of fetuses with chromosomal triploidy: correlation with parental origin of the extra haploid set. American Journal of Medical Genetics 38: 535–538.

Machin G A, Crolla J 1974 Chromosome constitution of 500 infants dying during the perinatal period. Humangenetik 23: 182–198.

Mall F P, Meyer A W 1921 Studies on abortuses: a survey of pathologic ova in the Carnegie embryological collection. In: Contributions to Embryology (Publications of the Carnegie Institution) 12: 1–364.

Man E B, Holden R H, Jones W S 1971 Thyroid function in human pregnancy VII Development and retardation of 4 year old progeny of euthyroid and hypothyroxemic women. American Journal of Obstetrics and Gynaecology 109: 12–19.

Mantoni M, Pederson J F 1982 Fetal growth delay in threatened abortion: an ultrasound study. British Journal of Obstetrics and Gynaecology 89: 525–527.

Markert C L, Petters R M 1978 Manufactured hexaparental mice show that adults are derived from three embryonic cells. Science 202: 56–58.

Matsunaga E, Shiota A 1980 Ectopic pregnancy and myoma uteri: teratogenic effects and maternal characteristics. Teratology 21: 61–69.

Medical Research Council Working Party on Amniocentesis 1978 An assessment of the hazards of amniocentesis. British Journal of Obstetrics and Gynaecology 85 (suppl 2): 1–41.

Mendenhall H W 1976 The immunology of the fetal maternal relationship. In: Scott J S, Jones W R (eds) Immunology of human reproduction. Academic Press, London, ch 3, pp 61–80.

Michel M Z, Khong T Y, Clark D A, Beard R W 1990 A morphological and immunological study of human placental bed biopsies in miscarriage. British Journal of Obstetrics and Gynaecology 97: 984–988.

Mikamo K 1970 Anatomic and chromosomal anomalies in spontaneous abortions. American Journal of Obstetrics and Gynecology 106: 243–254.

Millen R S 1956 The fate of the placenta left in situ following the delivery of a fetus in abdominal pregnancy. American Journal of Obstetrics and Gynecology 71: 1348–1350.

Miller J F, Williamson E, Glue J, Gordon Y B, Grudzinkas J D, Sykes A 1980 Fetal loss after implantation. Lancet ii: 554–556.

Myers R A, Fujikura T 1968 Placental changes after experimental abruptio placentae and fetal vessels ligation of rhesus monkey placenta. American Journal of Obstetrics and Gynecology 100: 846–851.

Navot D, Bergh P A, Williams M A et al 1991 Poor oocyte quality rather than implantation failure as a cause of age related decline in female fertility. Lancet 337: 1375–1377.

Norris M L, Barton S C, Surani M A H 1990 The differential roles of parental genomes in mammalian development. Oxford Reviews of Reproductive Biology 12: 225–244.

Ornoy A, Kohn G, Benzur Z, Weinstein D, Cohen M H 1978 Triploidy in human abortions. Teratology 18: 315–320.

Pearce W, Lau G F 1963 ABO incompatible pregnancies and reproductive performance. International Journal of Fertility 8: 495–502.

Petterson F 1968 Epidemiology of early pregnancy wastage. Stockholm Svenska Bokforlaget, Norstedts, Bonniers, p 25.

Poland B J, Miller J R, Jones D C, Trimble B K 1977 Reproductive counselling in patients who have had a spontaneous abortion. American Journal of Obstetrics and Gynaecology 127: 685–691.

Poland B J, Miller J R, Harris M, Livingston J 1981 Spontaneous abortion: a study of 1961 women and their conceptuses. Acta Obstetrica et Gynecologica Scandinavica suppl 102.

Pryce-Davies J 1981 The perinatal autopsy. In: Anthony P P, MacSween R N M (eds) Recent advances in histopathology. Churchill Livingstone, Edinburgh, pp 65–82.

Purvis-Smith S G, Saville T, Manass S et al 1992 Uniparental disomy 15 resulting from correction of an initial trisomy 15. American Journal of Human Genetics 50: 1348–1350.

Quagliarello J, Szlachter N, Nisselbaum J S, Schwartz M K, Steinetz B, Weiss G 1981 Serum relaxin and HGG concentrations in spontaneous abortions. Fertility and Sterility 36: 399–401.

Ramphal R, Donnelly W H, Small P A 1980 Fatal influenzal pneumonia in pregnancy: failure to demonstrate transplacental transmission of influenza virus. American Journal of Obstetrics and Gynecology 138: 347–348.

Reddy K S, Petersen M B, Antonarakis S E, Blakemore K J 1991 The vanishing twin: an explanation for discordance between chorionic villus karyotype and fetal phenotype. Prenatal Diagnosis 11: 679–684.

Rehder H, Coerdt W, Eggers R, Klink F, Schwinger E 1989 Is there a correlation between morphological and cytogenetic findings in placental tissue from early missed abortions? Human Genetics 82: 377–385.

Remington J S, Klein J O (eds) 1976 Infectious diseases of the fetus and newborn infant. Saunders, Philadelphia.

Report on the Confidential Enquiries into Maternal Deaths in England and Wales 1976–1978 1982 Department of Health and Social Security, Report on Health and Social Subjects 26. Her Majesty's Stationery Office, London.

Robbins F C, Heggie A D 1970 The rubella problem. In: Fraser F C, McKusick V A (eds) Congenital malformations. Proceedings of the

Third International Conference. Excerpta Medica, New York, pp 340–348.

Robertson W B 1976 Uteroplacental vasculature. Journal of Clinical Pathology 29, supplement (Royal College of Pathologists) 10: 9–17.

Robertson W B, Brosens I, Dixon H G 1967 The pathological response of the vessels of the placental bed to hypertensive pregnancy. Journal of Pathology and Bacteriology 93: 581–592.

Robinson H P 1975 Diagnosis of early pregnancy failure by sonar. British Journal of Obstetrics and Gynaecology 82: 849–857.

Rosenberg H S, Kohl S, Vogler C 1981 Viral infections of the fetus and neonate. In: Naeye R L, Kissane J H, Kaufman N (eds) Perinatal diseases. International Academy of Pathology Monograph. Williams & Wilkins, Baltimore, pp 133–200.

Ruchelli E D, Shen-Schwartz S, Martin J, Surti U 1990 Correlation between pathologic and ultrasound findings in first trimester abortions. Pediatric Pathology 10: 743–756.

Rushton D I 1977 Amniotic fluid alphafetoprotein levels in Turners syndrome. Lancet i: 1158.

Rushton D I 1978 Simplified classification of spontaneous abortions. Journal of Medical Genetics 15: 1–9.

Rushton D I 1981a Examination of products of conception from previable human pregnancies. Journal of Clinical Pathology 34: 819–835.

Rushton D I 1981b Fetal and neonatal liver disease. Diagnostic Histopathology 4: 17–48.

Rushton D I 1982 Examination of abortions. In: Barson A J (ed) Fetal and neonatal pathology. Praeger Scientific, Eastbourne, pp 27–64.

Rushton D I 1984 Classification and mechanisms of spontaneous abortion. Perspectives in Pediatric Pathology 8: 269–287.

Rushton D I 1985 The nature and causes of spontaneous abortion with normal karyotypes. In: Kalter H (ed) Issues and reviews in teratology, vol 3. Plenum Press, New York, pp 21–63.

Rushton D I 1988 Placental pathology in spontaneous miscarriage. In: Beard R W, Sharp F (eds) Early pregnancy failure. Proceedings of the 18th Royal College of Obstetrics and Gynaecologists Study Group. RCOG, London, pp 149–157.

Rushton D I, Dawson I M P 1982 The maternal autopsy. Journal of Clinical Pathology 35: 909–921.

Rushton D I, Faed M J W, Richards S E M, Bain A D 1969 The fetal manifestations of the 45XO karyotype. Journal of Obstetrics and Gynaecology of the British Commonwealth 76: 266–272.

Schardein J L 1980 Congenital abnormalities and hormones during pregnancy: a clinical review. Teratology 22: 251–270.

Schweditsch M O, Dubin N H, Jones G S, Wentz A C 1979 Hormonal consideration in early normal pregnancy and blighted ovum syndrome. Fertility and Sterility 31: 252–257.

Scott J S, Jenkins D M 1976 Immunogenetic factors in aetiology of pre-eclampsia (gestosis). Journal of Medical Genetics 13: 200–207.

Seller M J 1977 Amniotic fluid alphafetoprotein and Turners syndrome. Lancet i: 955.

Shanklin D R, Scott J S 1975 Massive subchorial thrombohaematoma (Breus' mole). British Journal of Obstetrics and Gynaecology 82: 476–487.

Shearman R P, Garrett W J 1963 Double blind study of the effect of 17-hydroxyprogesterone caproate on abortion rate. British Medical Journal 1: 292–295.

Sheppard B L, Bonnar J 1976 The ultrastructure of the arterial supply of the human placenta in pregnancy complicated by fetal growth retardation. British Journal of Obstetrics and Gynaecology 83: 948–959.

Simpson J L 1981 Pregnancies in women with chromosomal abnormalities. In: Schulman J D, Simpson J L (eds) Genetic disease in pregnancy: maternal effects and fetal outcome. Academic Press, New York, ch 13, pp 440–471.

Singh R P, Carr D H 1966 The anatomy and histology of XO human embryos and fetuses. Anatomical Record 155: 369–384.

Smeets D F C M, Mamel B C S, Nelen M R et al 1992 Prader-Willi syndrome and Angelmann syndrome in cousins from a family with a translocation between chromosomes 6 and 15. New England Journal of Medicine 326: 807–811.

Stenchever M A, Parks K J, Daines T L, Allen M A, Stenchever H R 1977 Cytogenetics of habitual abortion and other reproductive wastage. American Journal of Obstetrics and Gynecology 127: 143–151.

Stephens T D, Shepard T H 1980 The Down syndrome in the fetus. Teratology 22: 37–41.

Stimson W H, Strachan A F, Shepherd A 1979 Studies of the maternal immune response to placental antigens absence of a blocking factor from the blood of abortion prone women. British Journal of Obstetrics and Gynaecology 86: 41–45.

Strobino B R, Kline J, Shrout P, Stein Z, Susser M, Warburton D 1980 Recurrent spontaneous abortion: definition of a syndrome. In: Porter I H, Hook E B (eds) Human embryonic and fetal death. Academic Press, New York, pp 315–329.

Surani M A, Reid W, Allen N D 1988 Transgenes as molecular probes for genomic imprinting. Trends in Genetics 4: 59–62.

Takano K, Miller J R 1972 ABO incompatibility as a cause of spontaneous abortion: evidence from abortuses. Journal of Medical Genetics 9: 144–150.

Taylor C, Page-Faulk W 1981 Prevention of recurrent abortion with leucocyte transfusions. Lancet ii: 68–69.

van Lijnschoten, Arends J W, Leffers P et al 1993 The value of histomorphological features of chorionic villi in early spontaneous abortion for the prediction of karyotype. Histopathology 22: 555–563.

Wang B B T, Rubin C H, Williams J 1993 Mosaicism in chorionic villus sampling: an analysis of incidence and chromosomes involved in 2612 consecutive cases. Prenatal Diagnosis 13: 179–190.

Wapner R J, Simpson J L, Golbus M S et al 1992 Chorionic mosaicism: association with fetal loss but not with adverse perinatal outcome. Prenatal Diagnosis 12: 347–355.

Warburton D, Stein Z, Kline J, Susser M 1980 Chromosome abnormalities in spontaneous abortion: data from the New York study. In: Porter I H, Hook E B (eds) Human embryonic and fetal death. Academic Press, New York, pp 261–288.

Ward R H T, Modell B, Fairweather D V I, Shirley I M, Richards B A, Hetherington C P 1981 Obstetrics outcome and problems of mid-trimester fetal blood sampling for antenatal diagnosis. British Journal of Obstetrics and Gynaecology 88: 1073–1080.

Warkany J 1971 Congenital malformations: notes and comments. Year Book Medical Publishers, Chicago.

Wilkin P 1965 Pathologie du placenta: etude clinique et anatomo-clinique. Masson, Paris, pp 213–235.

Williamson R, Eskdale J, Coleman D V, Niazi N, Loeffler F E, Modell B 1981 Direct gene analysis of chorionic villi: a possible technique for first trimester antenatal diagnosis of haemoglobinopathies. Lancet II: 1125–1127.

Willner J P, Hirschorn K 1981 Prenatal cytogenetic diagnosis. In: Barson A J (ed) Laboratory investigation of fetal disease. Wright, Bristol, ch 7, pp 151–172.

Witschi E 1970 Teratogenic effects from over ripeness of the egg. In: Fraser F C, McKusick V A (eds) Congenital malformations: Proceedings of the Third International Conference. Excerpta Medica, New York, pp 157–169.

Zulman J I, Talal N, Hoffman G S, Epstein W V 1980 Problems associated with the management of pregnancies in patients with systemic lupus erythematosus. Journal of Rheumatology 7: 37–49.

54. Pathology of the human secondary yolk sac

Francisco F. Nogales

INTRODUCTION

The human yolk sac is an ephemeral endodermal organ which is active only during a few weeks of the first trimester of intrauterine life. However, its evolutionary importance as one of the most primitive organs of vertebrates is attested to by its various specialized rôles, be these nutritional or mediatory in the exchanges between the embryo and its environment.

The yolk sac serves distinct purposes in different species. In the human, although many of its functions still remain speculative, it must play a very important part in the welfare of the embryo, since development does not permit a waste of space, time or energy which could be devoted to something else (Diamond, 1991). Moreover, its large volume, complex cellular architecture and secretion of various substances would not be warranted if it were merely a vestigial structure. We now know that, apart from its early relationship with germ cell production, it is the initial source of haematopoiesis and also very possibly a transfer organ between the embryo and environment. Furthermore, its specialized protein secretion profile and close circulatory relationship with the embryo point towards a prehepatic rôle, before the definitive liver is functioning.

The relatively little available knowledge of the human yolk sac stems from the difficulty of obtaining adequate material for its study. This is due partly to an ethical problem but also to a general lack of awareness of its morphology and rôle during embryogenesis. However, recent studies using in vivo imaging techniques have demonstrated many of the different aspects of its developmental dynamics and clinical relevance (Mantoni & Pederson, 1979; Crooij et al, 1982; Reece et al, 1987; Ferrazzi et al, 1988; Green & Hobbins, 1988; Nyberg et al, 1988; Reece et al, 1988; Bree & Marn, 1990; Jauniaux et al, 1991a).

DEVELOPMENT, HISTOLOGY AND IMMUNOHISTOCHEMISTRY

The secondary human yolk sac undergoes rapid developmental changes during a period starting from the 4th week after the last menstrual period until the 11th–12th week. These changes have been summarized by Branca (1913) into three stages or periods: formation, function and regression. There is still some controversy surrounding the sequence of events leading to the formation of the secondary human yolk sac and the chronology of histological changes in the function and regression periods (Enders & King, 1993).

Formation period

At the time of implantation, a primary yolk sac cavity lined by endoderm and surrounded by extraembryonic mesoderm is already present in the embryo. At this time the primary yolk sac of the previllous stage is also called Heuser's or exocoelomic membrane. Its endoderm originates as a thin layer present under the trophoblast which eventually delaminates to form the primary yolk sac. When the earliest chorionic villi appear at day 12–15 post conception, the primary yolk sac starts to give rise to a secondary vesicle, or secondary yolk sac. The mechanism of this is still not clear, but involves collapse, re-expansion and fragmentation of the primary yolk sac (Enders & King, 1993); the surrounding extraembryonic mesodermal cells, possibly derived initially from the endoderm (Luckett, 1978; Enders et al, 1986; Enders & King, 1988), liquefy and the peripheral area then delineates the extraembryonic coelom and contributes to the formation of the outer 'mesothelial' lining of the secondary yolk sac vesicle and also the mesenchymal cells of the secondary yolk sac. At 16 days post conception (Fig. 54.1), corresponding to a stage 7 embryo (O'Rahilly, 1973), the secondary yolk sac is trilaminar with a prominent endodermal layer formed by cuboidal cells that already secrete alphafetoprotein (AFP) and fetal antigen 1 (FA1) an embryonal antigen produced by endoderm (Fay et al, 1988; Tornehave et al, 1989; Palomino et al, unpublished data). These proteins are localized diffusely in the cytoplasm and in canalicular structures (Fig. 54.2) which may

1677

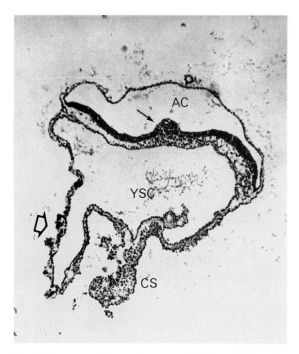

Fig. 54.1 Trilaminar 16 day embryo, stage 7. The amniotic cavity (AC), yolk sac cavity (YSC) and the connecting stalk (CS) are evident. The notochord (arrow) is prominent. The secondary yolk sac (large arrow) appears partially collapsed. H & E × 18.

correspond to the inter- or intracellular canaliculi that have been described at electronmicroscopic level (Hesseldahl & Falck-Larsen, 1969; Takashina, 1989; Jauniaux & Moscoso, 1992). At the same time, epidermal growth factor (EGF) is also secreted and endodermal cells show strong positivity for low molecular weight cytokeratins and vimentin. However, neither ferritin nor A_1AT has as yet been detected.

At this stage, the mesothelial layer (Figs 54.2 and 54.3) is prominent and composed of dome-shaped cuboidal cells with a smooth membrane contour. It has isolated secretory canaliculi and shows inconspicuous mesenchymal cells and isolated haematopoietic cells.

Function period

The occurrence of haematopoiesis signals the commencement of this period, at about the beginning of the 5th week. The yolk sac maintains haematopoiesis and secretory activity until approximately the 9th week (Gitlin & Perricelli, 1970; Gitlin et al, 1972; Gitlin & Biasucci, 1979; Jauniaux & Moscoso, 1992).

As from the 5th week, the secondary human yolk sac grows to attain a size larger than the amniotic cavity (Hamilton et al, 1972). The yolk sac cavity now communicates with the ventral part of the trilaminar embryo and the endodermal lining of the yolk sac is continuous with the visceral endoderm. At the 6th week the ample implantation area of the yolk sac begins to constrict and elongate, ultimately forming the yolk stalk which attaches the free-

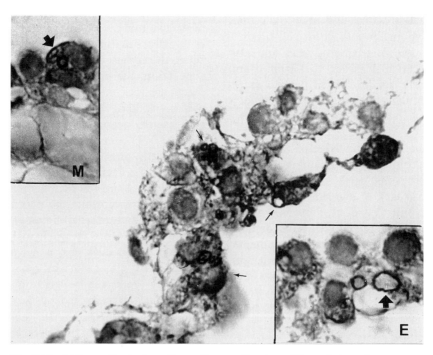

Fig. 54.2 AFP secretion in the yolk sac of a stage 7 embryo. The endoderm shows marked staining for AFP (small arrows). Ring-like secretory structures (insets, arrows) are present in both endoderm (E) and mesothelium (M). H & E × 1200.

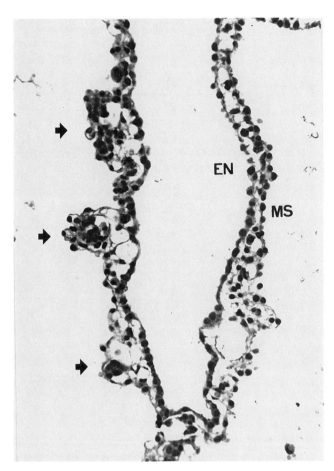

Fig. 54.3 Close up view of preceding embryo. Endoderm (EN) lines the yolk sac cavity, the outer surface is lined by mesothelial cells derived from the extraembryonic mesenchyme. In the intervening mesenchyme, haemopoiesis (arrows) is initiated. H & E × 240.

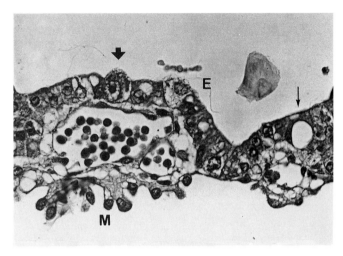

Fig. 54.4 Yolk sac from the 5th week. The endoderm (E) is composed of large cells with abundant cytoplasm. Some of its cells exhibit large nuclei with prominent nucleoli (large arrow) and intercellular canaliculi (small arrow). Mesothelial cells (M) and blood islands are prominent. H & E × 450.

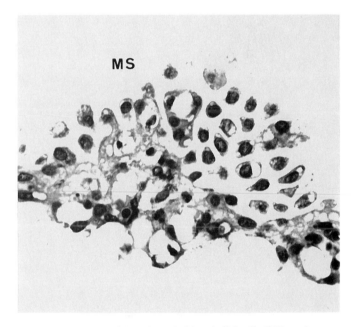

Fig. 54.5 Yolk sac of the 5th week. Mesothelial cells (MS) project into the exocoelomic cavity. H & E × 450.

floating, globular sphere of the secondary sac to the ventral part of the embryo. Eventually the stalk is reduced to form the vitelline duct which contains the vitelline vessels connecting the yolk sac to the embryo, forming a preportal circulation.

Macroscopically, during this period the yolk sac is a transparent spheroid, the walls of which are reticulated due to the presence of vessels and blood islands. Transvaginal ultrasonography demonstrates a growth from 3 mm to 4.5 mm (Bree & Marn, 1990; Jauniaux et al, 1991a), often with daily variations in size.

Histologically, the yolk sac wall becomes progressively thicker, due to simultaneous growth of endoderm, haematopoietic foci and mesenchyme (Figs 54.4 and 54.5). During all this time, the mesothelium remains as a single outer layer of cells. From the 5th to the 7th or 8th week the *endoderm* shows active mitotic growth forming downward projections of cell columns (Fig. 54.6) which eventually become branching tubules (Fig. 54.7). Infoldings of the growing endoderm are present by the beginning of the 5th week. The cells have large nuclei with prominent

nucleoli (Fig. 54.4). By the 7th week, the cell cytoplasm becomes large and polygonal (Fig. 54.8) and appears clear with fine eosinophilic granulations. At this stage, the vitelline tissue has a solid appearance with tubular areas (Fig. 54.8). Electronmicroscopically, endodermal cells are joined by desmosomes and tight junctions. The free cell surface facing the cavity or tubules shows numerous microvilli and occasional cilia (Takashina, 1993). A slender, discontinuous, subendodermal basement membrane is present temporarily at the 6th–7th week (Nogales et al, 1977; Takashina, 1989). Intercellular canaliculi between

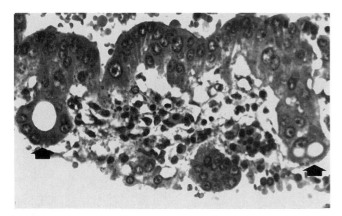

Fig. 54.6 Yolk sac of the 4th–5th week. There is a downward growth of columns of endoderm, which begins to form tubules (arrows). The cells show large nucleoli and the cytoplasm is dark. Haemalum & Saffron × 450.

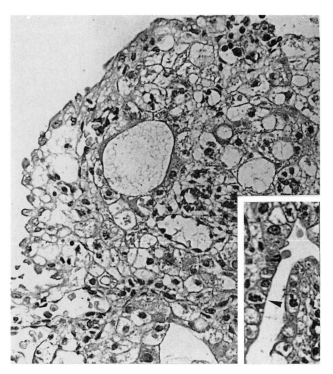

Fig. 54.8 Yolk sac of the 7th week. The wall is thick, endodermal cells are now large and clear with abundant tubules. Mitoses are still present in the tubular lining (inset, arrow). H & E × 240.

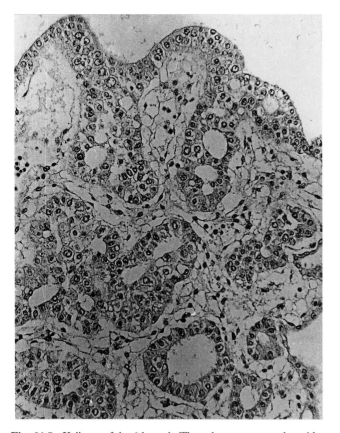

Fig. 54.7 Yolk sac of the 6th week. The columns are complex with abundant tubules, and mesenchyme is evident. H & E × 240.

endodermal cells are lined by regular microvilli (Hesseldahl & Falck-Larsen, 1969; Jauniaux & Moscoso, 1992). The cytoplasm contains well developed Golgi complexes, abundant profiles of rough endoplasmic reticulum, glycogen and pinocytotic and coated vesicles. Amorphous material is also present. Immunohistochemically, numerous proteins are present, either diffusely in

the cytoplasm or concentrated in the surface of the tubular system (Figs 54.2 and 54.9). AFP, FA1, A_1AT, transferrin, ferritin, apolipoproteins, fetal haemoglobin and growth factors such as fibroblast, epidermal and insulin-like are found, as well as many other substances which are produced at this time (Gitlin & Biasucci, 1979; Shi et al, 1985). Co-expression of vimentin and keratin is evident in the endodermal cells. The immunohistochemical profile, together with similarities in morphology, suggests a hepatic rôle for the secondary yolk sac at a time when the embryonal liver is not active or fully developed.

The *mesenchyme* is the seat of haematopoiesis during this period. At the end of the 4th week, haematopoietic stem cells (burst and colony forming units and erythroid progenitors) are present in the mesenchyme (Migliaccio & Migliaccio, 1993) and possibly by the 5th week have colonized the developing liver. The stem cell from which the definitive blood cells are derived appears to originate in the yolk sac, perhaps in the endoderm (Hoyes, 1969) as this has an intimate relationship with blood cells in various stages of maturation. Macrophages are also found in both extra- and intravascular locations and are thought to be the precursor cell from which the Kupffer cells of the liver originate (Enzan, 1993). A single layer of *mesothelium* covers the external surface of the yolk sac during the function period and its cells are prominent with developing cytoplasmic projections. Ultrastructurally, mesothelial cells show a marked surface specialization with microvilli that are longer and thicker than those of the endodermal layer (Jauniaux & Moscoso, 1992; Takashina, 1993) and have complex interdigitations. Their cytoplasm is poorer in organelles but richer in vacuoles and pinocytotic vesicles than in the endodermal cells, implying an active absorptive function. A slender basement membrane is present. Immunohistochemically, secretory canaliculi are not observed in the mesothelial cells except at the end of the formation period; there is a weak positivity, however, for HbF, A_1AT and caeruloplasmin which is probably due to proteins absorbed from the exocoelomic fluid. Only fetal antigen 2 (FA2), a protein present in mesenchyme and its derivatives and basement membranes (Fay et al, 1988; Tornehave et al, 1989), is strongly positive here as well as in the mesenchyme. Mesothelial cells also show co-expression of vimentin and low molecular weight keratins.

The most characteristic morphological feature of the secondary yolk sac during this period is the *complex system of tubules and canaliculi* which undergo progressive development. Inter- or intracellular canaliculi are visible first and resemble bile canaliculi (Fig. 54.2). Progressively, large tubular lumina form among the columns of endodermal cells which become dilated. Most of these tubules are connected both with the intercellular canaliculi (Fig. 54.9) and the yolk sac cavity by narrow openings although some do not seem to comunicate with the cavity. The function of the tubular system is as yet unknown; it has been proposed that it may be involved in the transport of blood cells to the cavity (Takashina, 1989); however, its likely rôle would seem to be the secretion and transport of different proteins. As early as the beginning of the 4th week, the intercellular canaliculi are the seat of intense secretion of AFP and FA1. From the 5th week until the 8th week, canaliculi and the tubular surface concentrate secretion of AFP, FA1, A_1AT, ferritin, apolipoproteins, fetal haemoglobin, fibroblast and epidermal growth factors. There is a high level of AFP in the exocoelomic fluid during the functional period of the yolk sac (Jauniaux et al, 1991b). The secondary yolk sac probably behaves as an active transport membrane between the maternal environment and the embryo; yolk sac mesothelium is involved in the transfer of maternal proteins filtered into the extraembryonic coelom (Jauniaux et al, 1991b). Certainly, in the Rhesus monkey, mesothelial cells are capable of absorbing exogenous proteins (King & Wilson, 1983) and it is possible that this occurs in the human (Gonzalez-Crussi, 1979). Perhaps, then, the tubulo-canalicular system carries the proteins absorbed from the exocoelom as well as its own embryonal proteins secreted by the endoderm, resulting finally in the incorporation of both maternal and embryonal proteins into the primitive embryonal circulation in the yolk sac. In this way the proteins would reach the embryo via the yolk sac cavity, i.e. the vitelline duct and preportal circulation.

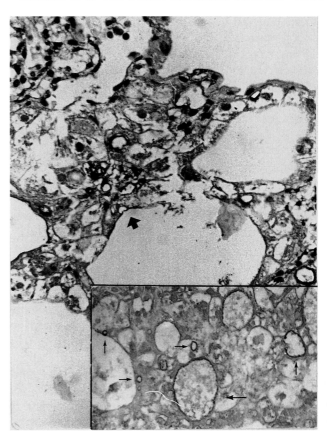

Fig. 54.9 Immunohistochemical findings in the yolk sac of the function period at the 7th week. FA1 is diffusely present in the endodermal cells, tubular surface and intercellular canaliculi (arrow). Inset corresponds to AFP deposited diffusely in cytoplasmic surface of tubuli and intercellular canaliculi, which seem to connect with the tubular system (arrows). H & E × 240.

Regression period

By the beginning of the 8th week, the secondary yolk sac undergoes gradual and organized regression which is complete by the 11th week. Regression probably occurs as a result of programmed cell death and may be assisted by the ischaemia resulting from the pressure caused by expansion of the growing amniotic cavity. Macroscopically, the yolk sac wall becomes opaque and loses its reticular appearance, becoming adherent to the membranes and resulting, on completion of regression, in a flattened disc which can be seen in the term placenta. Ultrasonographically, by the 9th to 10th week (Jauniaux et al, 1991a; Ferrazzi & Garbo, 1993) the yolk sac is seen to reach its largest size of 6 mm after which it collapses. The vitelline duct is obliterated and remains only in the proximal end of the umbilical cord as a duct lined with mucinous epithelium (Jauniaux et al, 1989). Its only remainder in adults is the ileal Meckel's diverticulum.

Endoderm

From the 8th week regression phenomena occur in the

endodermal cells: at first, the free membranes of cells lining tubules lose their microvilli, intercellular canaliculi and other organelles (Jauniaux & Moscoso, 1992). Progressively, some cells fragment and become detached and shed into the vitelline cavity. The cytoplasm becomes laden with large intracytoplasmic globules which may coalesce to form AFP-positive hyaline globules (Nogales et al, 1988) which correspond to the vacuoles with heterogeneous contents seen ultrastructurally. The overall architecture becomes distorted, first distended at the 9th week and then collapsed. Dystrophic calcification of necrotic endodermal cells is frequent although it does not always occur and in some cases the yolk sac appears as a cyst with a slender wall and clear contents.

Mesenchyme

Regression is characterized by the progressive growth and expansion of the mesenchyme which actively proliferates (Figs 54.10 and 54.11) to replace the wall as a physiological scar. At the end of the 8th week (Fig. 54.10) active mesenchymal growth dissects the endodermal sheets of cells undergoing necrobiosis and collagen-producing fibroblasts occupy the interstitium, leaving vessels and haematopoietic foci entrapped. The latter have disappeared by the 10th–11th week at which time the wall is fibrous (Fig. 54.12). Immunohistochemically, fibroblasts are pos-

itive for keratin, vimentin and FA2 but negative for actin and AFP.

Mesothelium

During the regression period, this undergoes similar ultrastructural changes to those seen in the the endoderm with loss of microvilli. At lightmicroscopic level the cells initially appear swollen and vacuolated but eventually become flattened.

YOLK SAC LESIONS OCCURRING IN ABORTED CONCEPTUSES

During spontaneous abortion the yolk sac shows a series

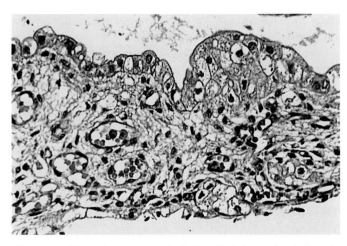

Fig. 54.11 Regression at 9th week. Only a single layer of endoderm is present. The wall thickness is composed of fibrous tissue, some vessels have nucleated blood cells. H & E × 230.

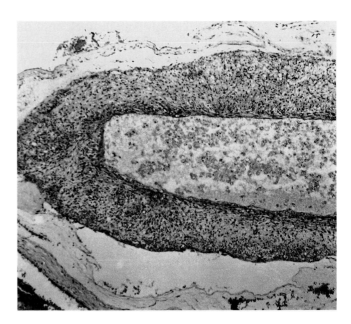

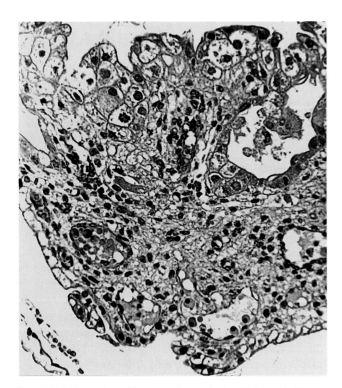

Fig. 54.10 Beginning of the regression period at 8th+4week. The mesenchyme is expanded. Haemopoiesis is focal and scarce. Endodermal cells are still large, and have a clear cytoplasm. H & E × 240.

Fig. 54.12 Yolk sac at 11th week. Endodermal cells are desquamated in the cavity. The wall is entirely fibrous. Adherence of membranes is seen. H & E × 46.

of deviations from its normal morphology. These differences are seen as (a) actual histological changes, (b) an altered chronology of developmental events and (c) topographical alterations of the yolk sac. Since the causes of abortion vary, involving both various environmental and genetic factors, the changes and their significance may be difficult to assess. The morphological lesions are neither clear-cut nor specific and different types of lesion may overlap in the same specimen. Some pathological processes precede others in the natural series of events, although, at any given time, there may be various lesions at different stages of the same process. It is also difficult in some cases to differentiate the changes from normal regression phenomena. Experimentally (Pinter et al, 1986; Brent et al, 1990; Reece et al, 1993) and clinically (Kaplan et al, 1985) yolk sac damage can lead to malformation or abortion; however, histopathological examination has not as yet revealed with certainty any primary lesions.

The present classification of lesions (Nogales et al, 1992a, 1993) is a descriptive one which correlates well with ultrasonographic findings. Correlation between ultrasonography and pathology greatly helps to ascertain the dynamics of the yolk sac during spontaneous abortion. Normal yolk sacs and two main categories of lesions can be differentiated morphologically in spontaneous abortion (Table 54.1):

1. Cases with preservation of the normal architecture concurrent with marked alterations in size and expansion when correlated with its expected morphology at a given gestational age
2. Retrogressive changes with marked distortion of the structure by phenomena such as necrosis, fibrosis, calcification or oedema.

When correlated with parameters such as gestational age, situation, embryonic status and placental vascularity, both groups show an evident difference in their onset: altered expansion changes occur an average of three weeks earlier than the average gestational age for retrogressive changes, indicating that they possibly represent an earlier form of injury. Retrogressive lesions are likely to be secondary to retention of a dead conceptus. Embryonal alterations, as expressed by Poland's classes (Poland et al,

1981), are frequently associated with both expansion changes and retrogressive lesions, thus indicating that an early embryonal death is followed by an earlier than normal involution of the yolk sac.

Analysis of placental vascularity reveals an association between early placentas with poorly vascularized villi and sacs with expansion changes, implying that insufficient placental vascularity may possibly determine an altered development of the yolk sac by interfering with its normal growth, or accelerating regression.

The situation of the yolk sac is also altered during spontaneous abortion; in general, pathologically retrogressive sacs adhere to the amniotic membranes at a much earlier age than normal, even as soon as the 6th week of gestation, whereas this phenomenon is not observed in normal sacs until the 10th to the 11th week.

Immunohistochemically, the pattern of secretion of different proteins varies greatly in yolk sac lesions when compared to the usual secretory pattern: yolk sacs with altered expansion changes have poor and patchy secretory features and yolk sacs with retrogressive changes, with the exception of oedematous sacs, show a practically total absence of secretion.

Macroscopical features

In abortions, the secondary yolk sac appears as a free floating vesicle in over half the cases, with transparent or opaline walls depending on the degree of maceration. There is a wide variation in size, ranging from over-dilated cystic sacs which can reach up to 1 cm in size to very small ones of under 1 mm. Overall, there is a poor correlation with the expected size for gestational age, reflecting an extended time of retention. In general, sizes are smaller than those found by ultrasonography (Nogales et al, 1992a) which frequently shows diameters close to normal sacs (Ferrazzi & Garbo, 1993). This could be explained partly by artifact occurring after extraction and manipulation. Adherent sacs are found in 40% of cases as small cysts or white, pearly elevations on the surface of membranes. Calcified sacs are intensely white dots embedded in the membranes.

Microscopical features

Normal yolk sacs

These were found in a fifth of our cases. Their architecture, with minor alterations, is analogous with that expected for the gestational age. The endoderm in sacs corresponding to the functional period is well preserved, with a characteristic immunohistochemical profile. Changes observed included a marked cytoplasmic vacuolation in both endoderm (Fig. 54.13) and mesenchyme co-existing with mitotic cells, possibly indicating an in vivo ischaemic lesion. Moderate nuclear irregularity was also noted.

Table 54.1 Classification and percentage of morphological patterns of the secondary human yolk sac in spontaneous abortion

Normal	18.5 %
Altered expansion changes	
Hypoplastic	6.7%
Cystic	6.7%
Retrogressive changes	
Necrosis	22.7%
Fibrosis	15.1%
Calcification	24.4%
Oedema	5.9%

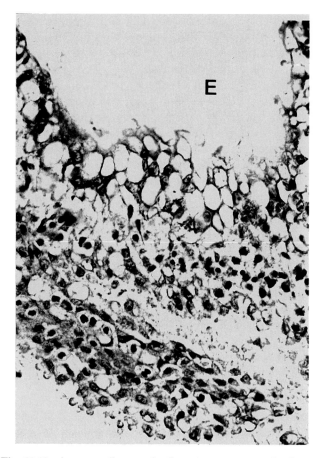

Fig. 54.13 A structurally normal yolk sac in spontaneous abortion. The endodermal cells (E), however, show extensive vacuolation. H & E × 240.

When the embryo is present in these cases, it is of normal external appearance and without any obvious microscopical changes. Placental villi in this group show normal vascularity and structure. Large haemorrhagic areas were noted in the placental bed.

Altered expansion changes

(i) Hypoplastic yolk sacs account for a tenth of all cases and show a preserved architecture with all three layers, but with a marked decrease in size and cellularity. They are found at an average age of 8 weeks. In these, the endoderm is reduced to a single cuboidal layer without formation of tubuli or columns (Fig. 54.14). Canaliculi are hardly seen; haematopoiesis is patchy or absent. The secretion of AFP and other antigens is weak and reduced to groups of cells. EGF and HbF staining is also weaker than in normal sacs. Hypoplastic yolk sacs possibly occur when there is a developmental failure causing early growth arrest of yolk sac and embryo. Even haematopoiesis is poorly developed but nucleated red blood cells can be seen in the placental vessels indicating that there has been haematopoietic colonization before growth arrest. Trisomies may show this injury pattern.

(ii) Cystic yolk sacs occur in the same proportion as hypoplastic sacs but are found at a higher average gestational age. Their cavity is extended and distended with a very thin delicate wall in which the endoderm is reduced to a flattened endothelioid layer (Figs 54.15 and 54.16); demonstration in these cells of different yolk sac antigens is patchy and poor. In some cases, mitoses occur in both

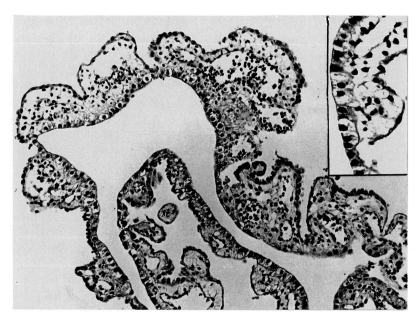

Fig. 54.14 Hypoplastic yolk sac in spontaneous abortion. Although the structure is preserved and there is some haematopoiesis, endodermal cells (inset) fail to develop or undergo formation of tubules. Intercellular channels are not seen by AFP or FA1 immunohistochemistry. H & E × 120; × 240.

endoderm and mesothelium (Nogales et al, 1992a). No canaliculi or tubuli are found. Haematopoiesis in these sacs is barely discernible and reduced to isolated red blood cells. Some cystic sacs have an immature appear-

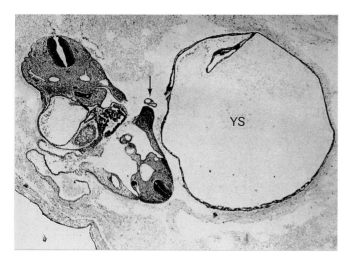

Fig. 54.15 Cystic yolk sac (YS) co-existing with a vital embryo. An arrow points to the sectioned vitelline stalk. H & E × 46.

ance, similar to that found at the 5th week, even when the gestational age is 9 weeks or more. The ultrasonographic appearances of cystic sacs (Ferrazzi et al, 1988; Rempen, 1988) correlate well with the histological changes. Serial ultrasonograms demonstrate that a large proportion of cystic sacs evolve within a week into retrogressive sacs (Nogales et al, 1993).

Some cystic sacs may represent a primary developmental failure, since they have very immature features and mitotic activity and are associated with highly disorganized embryos. In other cases, however, they might occur secondary to embryonal demise; there is an accumulation of exocoelomic fluid due to an unchecked inflow together with a dead embryo incapable of fluid uptake. This is seen experimentally (Dunton et al, 1986) in rodents, where cystic sacs occur after embryonal death.

Ectopic somatic endoderm is found in the walls of cystic or hypoplastic sacs; it consists of gland-like spaces present in the mesenchyme of the yolk sac wall lined by an epithelium resembling that of organ-forming endoderm (Nogales et al, 1992b), the vesicles of certain yolk sac tumours (Fig. 54.17) and the epithelium of the vitelline duct or allantoic rests. These ectopic foci are usually multiple and may represent a developmental failure, perhaps

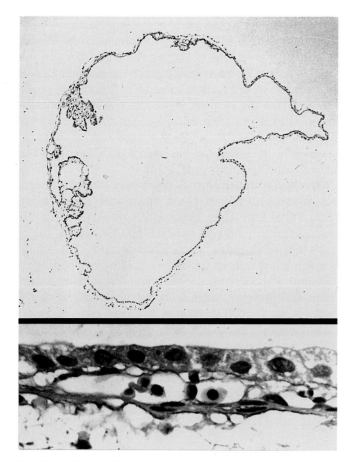

Fig. 54.16 Cystic yolk sac at the 7th week (top). The endoderm is only represented by a single line of cells, neither the mesenchyme nor the mesothelium is evident (bottom). H & E × 46; × 230.

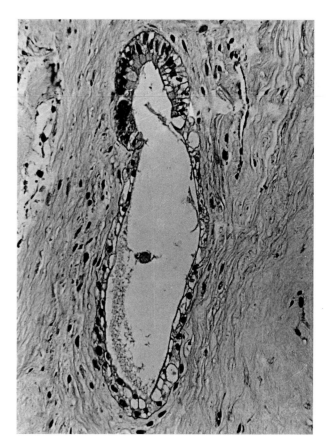

Fig. 54.17 Endodermal (somatic) differentiation in an abnormal yolk sac. The structure resembles allantoic, omphalomesenteric structures as well as early gut. Polyvesicular vitelline tumours show similar structures. H & E × 240.

a true malformation of the yolk sac or an expression of the somatic visceral potential of the extraembryonal endodermal cells (Nogales et al, 1992b).

Retrogressive changes

These occur in over 60% of cases of examined abortion material with a later average gestational age than the sacs in the previous group. Here, two well-defined lesions are found: sacs with an overlapping sequence of necrosis, fibrosis and calcification and those with an oedematous aspect.

(i) Necrosis, fibrosis and calcification (Figs 54.18 and 54.19). These phenomena occur physiologically during yolk sac regression and evolution and should only be considered of pathological significance if they occur before the 11th week of gestation. Coagulative type necrosis may involve the entire thickness of the wall or just the pericavitary endodermal layer. In both circumstances, the endodermal layer is shed into the cavity and cells disaggregate. Immunohistochemically, only traces of secretion of remaining proteins can be found. Fibrosis of the mesenchymal layer is an active phenomenon with evident mitosis (Nogales et al, 1992a). It seems to begin in the subendodermal areas and progresses to replace the entire wall and entrap endodermal cells and tubules. Occasionally, AFP-positive globules are found in the scars (Nogales et al, 1988). Fibrosis finally becomes acellular and the yolk sac is transformed into a solid round scar. Calcification is a dystrophic phenomenon that involves necrotic endodermal cells and fibrous scars, forming a calcified

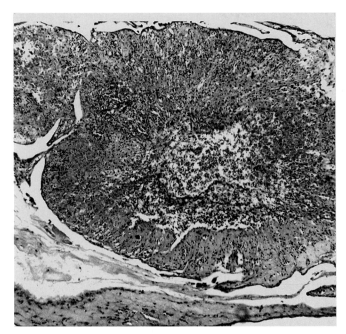

Fig. 54.19 Fibrous yolk sac with central necrosis at the 8th week. H & E × 23.

nodule adherent to the membranes. Calcified sacs, if found ultrasonographically before the 11th week, are considered highly suggestive of embryonal death (Ferrazzi et al, 1988; Harris et al, 1988). Massive necrosis may be the result of complete ischaemia. Possibly, fibrosis and subendodermal necrosis may reflect ischaemia which is only partial and still permits a degree of fibroblastic proliferation. Since the yolk sac is an organ with end circulation, it is likely that hypoxia plays an important rôle in the pathogenesis of these involutionary lesions. Most of the cases in this group are associated with retention and maceration of the conceptus.

(ii) Oedematous change represents 10% of all retrogressive changes and is found at an average age of 10 weeks. The three-layer structure is preserved, but the mesenchyme is markedly widened and basophilic due to deposition of abundant extracellular matrix (Fig. 54.20) in which a few cells of fibroblastic and macrophagic type are found. Parietal acellular blebs and dilations are found. There are, however, large blood islands and well-developed vessels. The endoderm is flattened but still shows immunohistochemical evidence of all proteins secreted during the function period. Endodermal canaliculi are also detected but are irregularly distributed. The mesothelium appears vacuolated. These sacs coincide invariably with hydropic and poorly vascularized villi. The embryo, when present, always shows severe growth disorganization (Nogales et al, 1993).

MISCELLANEOUS

Other aspects of yolk sac pathology include infection

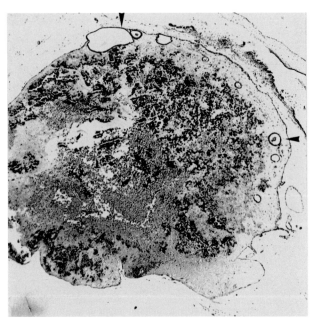

Fig. 54.18 Necrotic and calcified yolk sac at the 7th week; tubules (arrows) are still present. H & E × 24.

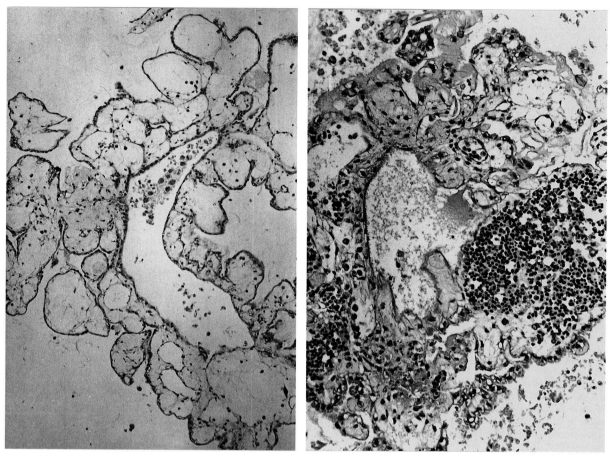

Fig. 54.20 Two oedematous yolk sacs coincident with severe growth disorganization and mostly avascular placental villi. Both the endoderm and mesothelium appear poorly developed. The mesenchyme is expanded by extensive deposits of extracellular matrix. Haematopoiesis (right) is preserved, but appears in unusually large islands. H & E × 48; ×120.

(Nogales et al, 1992a), double, shared yolk sacs in twins (Arey, 1923) and vitelline duct cysts (Barzilai et al, 1989).

CONCLUSIONS

In conclusion, little is known of the pathogenesis of yolk sac lesions and their relevance in the mechanism of spontaneous abortion. Even the physiological rôle of the yolk sac and parts of its development are still poorly understood. It would seem that normal yolk sacs associated with normal embryos and placentas may be associated with pregnancy wastage of environmental origin rather than because of embryonal malformation. Among the histopathological lesions, an altered expansion with hypoplasia would result from early embryonal death followed by growth arrest. Cystic sacs could have two possibly independent origins: one associated with immature features, which could represent a developmental incapacity for full differentiation, and the other a passive phenomenon secondary to failure of selective permeability of the wall and lack of fluid uptake by the dead embryo. Retrogressive lesions represent a stereotyped involution phenomenon parallel to the usual regression but occurring at a much earlier date as a result of embryonal death. Oedematous sacs, however, together with the presence of ectopic somatic endoderm, are possibly of malformative type.

REFERENCES

Arey L B 1923 Two embryologically important specimens of tubal twins. Surgery Gynecology and Obstetrics 36: 407–415.

Barzilai M, Lyons E A, Levi C S, Lindsay D J 1989 Vitelline duct cyst or double yolk sac. Journal of Ultrasound Medicine 8: 523–526.

Branca A 1913 Recherches sur la structure, l'evolution et le rôle de la vesicule ombilicale de l'homme. Journal d'Anatomie et Physiologie 49: 171–211.

Bree R L, Marn C S 1990 Transvaginal sonography in the first trimester: embryology, anatomy and hCG correlation. Seminars of Ultrasound, Computerized Tomography and Magnetic Resonance 11: 12–21.

Brent R L, Beckman B M, Koszalka T R 1990 Experimental yolk sac dysfunction as a model for studying nutritional disturbances in the embryo during early organogenesis. Teratology 41: 405–413.

Crooij M J, Westhuis M, Schoemaker J, Exalto N 1982 Ultrasonographic measurement of the yolk sac. British Journal of Obstetrics and Gynaecology 89: 931–934.

Diamond J 1991 The rise and fall of the third chimpanzee. Vintage, London, p 52.

Dunton A, Al-Alousi L A, Pratten M K, Beck F 1986 The giant yolk sac: a model for studying early placental transport. Journal of Anatomy 145: 189–206.

Enders A C, King B F 1988 Formation and differentiation of extraembryonic mesoderm in the rhesus monkey. American Journal of Anatomy 181: 327–340.

Enders A C, King B F 1993 Development of human yolk sac. In: Nogales F F (ed) The human yolk sac and yolk sac tumors. Springer-Verlag, Heidelberg, pp 1–48.

Enders A C, Schlafke S, Hendrickx A G 1986 Differentiation of the embryonic disc, amnion and yolk sac in the rhesus monkey. American Journal of Anatomy 177: 161–185.

Enzan H 1993 Macrophages in the human yolk sac. In: Nogales F F (ed) The human yolk sac and yolk sac tumors. Springer-Verlag, Heidelberg, pp 84–109.

Fay T N, Jacobs I, Teisner B et al 1988 Two fetal antigens (FA1 and FA2) and endometrial proteins (PP12, PP14), isolated from amniotic fluid: preliminary observations in fetal and maternal tissues. European Journal of Obstetrics and Gynecology and Reproductive Biology 29: 73–85.

Ferrazzi E, Garbo S 1993 Ultrasonography of the human yolk sac. In: Nogales F F (ed) The human yolk sac and yolk sac tumors. Springer-Verlag, Heidelberg, pp 161–179.

Ferrazzi E, Brambati B, Lanzani A et al 1988 The yolk sac in early pregnancy failure. American Journal of Obstetrics and Gynecology 158: 137–142.

Gitlin D, Biasucci A 1979 Development of γG, γA, γM, β1c/β1a, C1 esterase inhibitor, ceruloplasmin, transferrin, hemopexin, haptoglobin, fibrinogen, plasminogen, α1-antitrypsin, orosomucoid, β-lipoprotein, α2 macroglobulin and prealbumin in the human conceptus. Journal of Clinical Investigation. 48: 1433–1446.

Gitlin D, Perricelli A 1970 Synthesis of serum albumin, prealbumin and α-foetoprotein, α1-antitrypsin and transferrin by the human yolk sac. Nature 228: 995–997.

Gitlin D, Perricelli A, Gitlin G M 1972 Synthesis of α-fetoprotein by liver, yolk sac and gastrointestinal tract of the human conceptus. Cancer Research 32: 979–982.

Gonzalez-Crussi F 1979 The human yolk sac and yolk sac (endodermal sinus) tumors: a review. Perspectives in Pediatric Pathology 5: 179–215.

Green J J, Hobbins J C 1988 Abdominal ultrasound examination of the first trimester fetus. American Journal of Obstetrics and Gynecology 159: 165–175.

Hamilton W J, Boyd J D, Mossman H W 1972 Human embryology. Heffers, Cambridge.

Harris R D, Vincent L M, Askin F B 1988 Yolk sac calcification: a sonographic finding associated with intrauterine embryonic demise in the first trimester. Radiology 166: 109–110.

Hesseldahl H, Falck-Larsen J 1969 Ultrastructure of human yolk sac: endoderm, mesenchyme, tubules and mesothelium. American Journal of Anatomy 126: 315–336.

Hoyes A D 1969 The human foetal yolk sac: an ultrastructural study of four specimens. Zeitschrift für Zellforschung 99: 469–490.

Jauniaux E, Moscoso J G 1992 Morphology and significance of the human yolk sac. In: Barnea E R, Hustin J, Jauniaux E (eds) The first twelve weeks of gestation. Springer-Verlag, Heidelberg, pp 192–213.

Jauniaux E, DeMunter C, Vanesse M, Wilkin P, Hustin J 1989 Embryonic remnants of the umbilical cord: morphologic and clinical aspects. Human Pathology 20: 458–462.

Jauniaux E, Jurkovic D, Heuriet Y, Rodesch F, Hustin J 1991a Development of the secondary human yolk sac: correlation of sonographic and anatomical features. Human Reproduction 6: 1160–1166.

Jauniaux E, Jurkovic D, Gulbis B, Gervy C H, Ooms H A, Campbell S 1991b Biochemical composition of exocoelomic fluid in early human pregnancy. Obstetrics and Gynecology 78: 1124–1128.

Kaplan L C, Matsuoka R, Gilbert E F, Opitz J M, Kurnit D M 1985 Ectopia cordis and cleft sternum: evidence for mechanical teratogenesis following rupture of the chorion or yolk sac. American Journal of Medical Genetics 21: 187–202.

King B F, Wilson J M 1983 A fine structural and cytochemical study of the rhesus monkey yolk sac: endoderm and mesothelium. Anatomical Record 205: 143–158.

Luckett W P 1978 Origin and differentiation of the yolk sac and extraembryonic mesoderm in presomite human and rhesus monkey embryos. American Journal of Anatomy 152: 59–98.

Mantoni F, Pederson J F 1979 Ultrasound visualization of the human yolk sac. Journal of Clinical Ultrasound 7: 459–461.

Migliaccio G, Migliaccio A R 1993 The kinetics of hematopoiesis in the human yolk sac. In: Nogales F F (ed) The human yolk sac and yolk sac tumors. Springer-Verlag, Heidelberg, pp 70–84.

Nogales F F, Silverberg S G, Bloustein P A, Martinez-Hernandez A, Pierce G B 1977 Yolk sac carcinoma (endodermal sinus tumor): ultrastructure and histogenesis of gonadal and extragonadal tumors in comparison with normal human yolk sac. Cancer 39: 1462–1474.

Nogales F F, Fernandez P L, Alvaro T 1988 Alpha-fetoprotein-positive globules in involuting human yolk sac (letter). Human Pathology 19: 995.

Nogales F F, Beltran E, Fernandez P L 1992a The pathology of secondary human yolk sac in spontaneous abortion: findings in 103 cases. In: Fenoglio C, Woolf M, Rilke F (eds) Progress in surgical pathology, vol 12. Field and Wood, New York, pp 291–303.

Nogales F F, Beltran E, Pavcovitch M, Bustos M 1992b Ectopic somatic endoderm in secondary human yolk sac. Human Pathology 23: 921–924.

Nogales F F, Beltran E, Gonzalez F 1993 Morphological changes of the secondary human yolk sac in early pregnancy wastage. In: Nogales F F (ed) The human yolk sac and yolk sac tumors. Springer-Verlag, Heidelberg, pp 174–195.

Nyberg D A, Mack L A, Harvey D, Wang K 1988 Value of the yolk sac in evaluating early pregnancies. Journal of Ultrasound Medicine 7: 129–135.

O'Rahilly R 1973 Developmental stages in human embryos. Carnegie Institute, Washington, DC, pp 65–68.

Pinter E, Reece A, Leranth C Z et al 1986 Arachidonic acid prevents hyperglycemia-associated yolk sac damage and embryopathy. American Journal of Obstetrics and Gynecology 155: 691–702.

Poland B J, Miller J R, Harris M, Livingston J 1981 Spontaneous abortion: a study of 1961 women and their conceptuses. Acta Obstetricia et Gynecologica Scandinavica 102 (suppl): 1–32.

Reece E A, Pinter E, Green J C, Mahoney M J, Naftolin F, Hobbins J C 1987 Significance of isolated yolk sac visualized by ultrasonography. Lancet i: 269.

Reece E A, Scioscia A L, Pinter E, Hobbins J C, Green J, Mahoney M S, Naftolin F 1988 Prognostic significance of the human yolk sac assessed by ultrasonography. American Journal of Obstetrics and Gynecology 159: 1191–1194.

Reece E A, Pinter E, Naftolin F 1993 Experimental models of injury in the mamalian yolk sac. In: Nogales F F (ed) The human yolk sac and yolk sac tumors. Springer-Verlag, Heidelberg, pp 135–171.

Rempen A 1988 Der Embryonale Dottersack bei gestörten Frühschwangerschaft. Geburtshilfe und Frauenheilkunde 48: 804–808.

Shi W K, Hopkins B, Thompson S, Heath J K, Luke B M, Graham C F 1985 Synthesis of apolipoproteins, alphafoetoprotein, albumin and transferrin by the human foetal yolk sac and other foetal organs. Journal of Embryology and Experimental Morphology 85: 191–206.

Takashina T 1989 Hematopoiesis in the human yolk sac. American Journal of Anatomy 184: 237–244.

Takashina T 1993 Histology of the secondary human yolk sac with special reference to hematopoiesis. In: Nogales F F (ed) The human yolk sac and yolk sac tumors. Springer-Verlag, Heidelberg, pp 48–70.

Tornehave D, Fay T N, Teisner B, Cheminitz J, Westergaard J, Grudzinskas J G 1989 Two fetal antigens (FA1 and FA2) and endometrial proteins (PP12, PP14), isolated from amniotic fluid: localization in the fetus and adult female genital tract. European Journal of Obstetrics and Gynecology and Reproductive Biology 30: 221–232.

55. Non-trophoblastic tumours of the placenta

H. Fox

INTRODUCTION

Non-trophoblastic tumours of the placenta fall into three groups:

1. Tumours arising within the placenta
2. Metastatic deposits from a maternal neoplasm
3. Metastases from a fetal neoplasm.

PRIMARY NON-TROPHOBLASTIC TUMOURS OF THE PLACENTA

The only primary non-trophoblastic tumours of the placenta which have been convincingly described are the relatively common haemangioma, the extremely rare teratoma and the even rarer hepatocellular adenoma. Even these arouse some doubt as to their nosological status for the haemangioma is probably a hamartomatous malformation rather than a true neoplasm, whilst many believe that all apparent teratomas of the placenta are, in reality, examples of fetus acardius amorphus.

Haemangioma

Haemangiomas, also known as 'chorangiomas' or 'chorioangiomas', are relatively common and occur in approximately 1% of all placentas (Table 55.1). Placental haemangiomas are usually single but occasionally multiple, the apparent record being the 25 discrete tumours, each with its own pedicle, in the placenta described by Fisher (1940). There have been rare instances of placentas which were diffusely infiltrated by haemangiomatous tissue (Szarthmary, 1934; Burger et al, 1952; Bret et al, 1953; Karnauchow, 1957; Gruenwald, 1963; Berge, 1966; Muller & Rieckert, 1967; Battaglia & Woolever, 1968; Du et al, 1968; Blom & Gevers, 1974; Jaffe et al, 1985; Angelone et al, 1989), a condition known as chorangiomatosis.

Most placental haemangiomas are not visible on the external surface of the placenta: they are small and within the placental substance and hence are unlikely to be noticed unless the placenta is systematically sliced. These small intraplacental tumours are usually round and well demarcated from the surrounding normal villous tissue by an easily visible capsule: their cut surface is smooth and firm and may be yellow, brown, tan, red or white. They often bear a superficial resemblance to an intervillous thrombus from which, however, they can be distinguished by their lack of lamination. Large haemangiomas, i.e. measuring more than 5 cm in diameter (Fig. 55.1), are rare and usually readily apparent on naked-eye examination of the intact placenta; they are seen most commonly as bulging protuberances on the fetal surface but a minority occur on the maternal aspect where they may appear to replace the whole, or part, of a lobe. Occasionally a haemangioma is situated entirely within the membranes and is attached to the placenta only by a vascular pedicle. These large haemangiomas usually have a purplish-red, glistening, encapsulated, smooth or bosselated outer surface which is sometimes deeply grooved by bands of fibrous tissue; they may be round, ovoid or reniform and on section appear highly vascular.

Histologically, most placental haemangiomas have a microscopic appearance similar to that seen in haemangiomas elsewhere in the body, with numerous blood

Table 55.1 Incidence of haemangiomas in systematically studied placentas

Author	Number of placentas examined	Number of haemangiomas
Siddall (1926)	600	6
Zeek & Assali (1952)	562	4
Shaw-Dunn (1959)	500	7
Thomsen (1961)	660	7
van Assche et al (1963)	100	4
Wentworth (1965)	620	8
Wilkin (1965)	376	3
Fox (1966)	500	5
Phillipe et al (1969)	1000	7
Wallenburg (1971)	700	7
Nessmann-Emmanuelli et al (1978)	1200	4

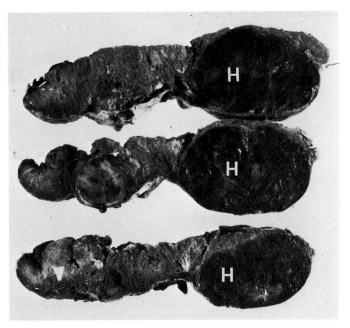

Fig. 55.1 A large haemangioma (H) in a placenta. (From *Pathology of the placenta* by courtesy of the Editor, Dr. E. V. D. K. Perrin.)

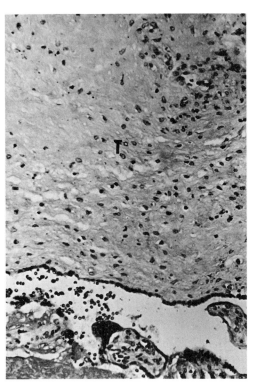

Fig. 55.3 A placental haemangioma (above) which shows a 'cellular' pattern and is formed largely of loose, mesenchymal tissue. Elsewhere there was a transition to a more typical 'angiomatous' pattern (see Fig. 55.4). H & E × 150. (From H. Fox *Pathology of the placenta* by courtesy of W. B. Saunders.)

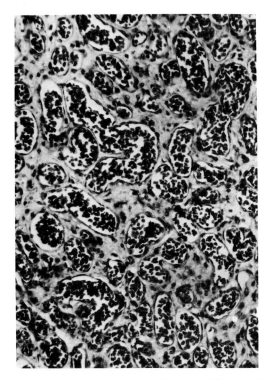

Fig. 55.2 Histological appearances of a placental haemangioma which is showing a typical 'angiomatous' pattern. H & E × 150. (From H. Fox *Pathology of the placenta* by courtesy of W. B. Saunders.)

vessels set in a loose, scanty, fibrous stroma (Fig. 55.2); the vessels are usually small and of capillary size but may be markedly dilated to give a cavernous appearance. Sometimes, however, there is a predominance of the stromal component (Fig. 55.3) with only a few ill-formed vessels

set in abundant loose, immature, cellular mesenchymal tissue. Degenerative changes, such as necrosis, calcification, myxoid change, hyalinization or even fat accumulation (Reddy et al, 1969), may complicate and confuse the histological picture. This variation in histological pattern is often used as a basis for classifying placental haemangiomas into 'angiomatous', 'cellular' and 'degenerate' types (Marchetti, 1939). This histological classification is useful for descriptive purposes but is basically a false subdivision for the cellular type is simply a less mature and less differentiated form of the angiomatous variety. Furthermore many haemangiomas show a variable picture, being cellular in some areas and angiomatous in others, often with a gradual transition between the two histological patterns (Fig. 55.4). Most haemangiomas do, however, show a predominantly angiomatous appearance and thus present little in the way of diagnostic difficulty, though those rare tumours which have a cellular pattern throughout have occasionally been misdiagnosed as fibromas, myxomas or leiomyomas (Tapia et al, 1985).

In most instances a haemangioma has a distinct capsule of either fibrous tissue or attenuated syncytiotrophoblast (Fig. 55.5) but occasionally there is only a pseudocapsule of compressed villous tissue. Mitotic figures are occasionally seen in placental haemangiomas and very rarely these are fairly numerous and associated with some degree of

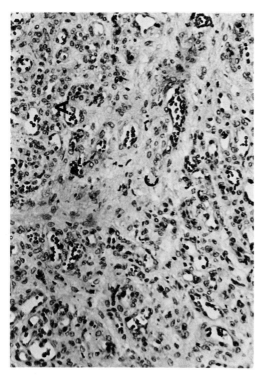

Fig. 55.4 Another area of the placental haemangioma shown in Fig. 55.3: here there is a transition from a 'cellular' to an 'angiomatous' pattern. H & E × 150. (From H. Fox *Pathology of the placenta* by courtesy of W. B. Saunders.)

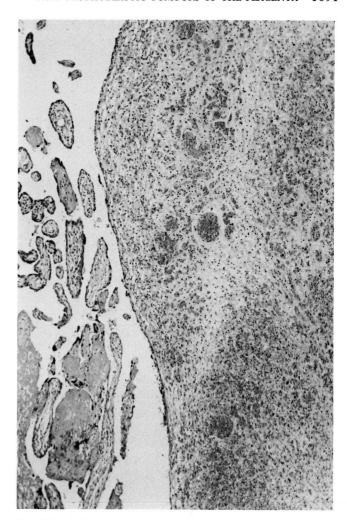

Fig. 55.5 A placental haemangioma (on the right) is limited by a distinct capsule of attenuated syncytiotrophoblast. H & E × 90. (From *Pathology of the placenta* by courtesy of the Editor, Dr. E. V. D. K. Perrin.)

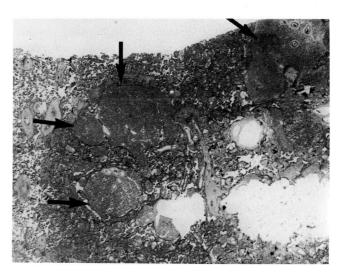

Fig. 55.6 Multiple nodules of haemangiomatous tissue (arrowed) in the substance of a placenta. H & E × 2. (From H. Fox *Pathology of the placenta* by courtesy of W. B. Saunders.)

endothelial or stromal cell atypia. Such findings have sometimes led to a diagnosis of sarcoma (Cary, 1914; Ahrens, 1953) but no placental haemangioma has ever behaved in a malignant fashion: it has nevertheless been suggested that such tumours be regarded as 'atypical haemangiomas' (Majlessi et al, 1983) and this is probably a prudent form of terminology. A very unusual, and conceptually challenging, placental tumour has been described by Jauniaux et al (1988) and Trask et al (1994). This is a typical haemangioma with a surrounding mantle of atypical proliferating trophoblast which closely resembles choriocarcinomatous tissue. Both the status and the significance of this neoplasm, classed as a 'chorangiocarcinoma', are thoroughly obscure.

Chorangiomatosis, in which multiple nodules of angiomatous tissue are scattered throughout the placental substance (Fig. 55.6), should be distinguished from 'chorangiosis', a condition in which a significant proportion of the villi contain an excess of fetal vessels (Altshuler, 1984). In a number of reports in the literature chorangiosis has been incorrectly used as a synonym for chorangiomatosis whilst it has often been mooted that chorangiosis forms a link between normal villi and a haemangioma. The concept of chorangiosis, which is defined as 10 or more villi in 10 fields, viewed under a × 10 objective, containing 10 or more fetal vessels has been subjected to criticism but nevertheless appears to be valid: there is, however, no evidence that chorangiosis is a transitional phase in the development, or a forme fruste, of chorangiomatosis.

Associated changes

Placentas containing a haemangioma are usually otherwise normal but a small proportion are unduly heavy, sometimes weighing, after removal of the tumour, over 1000 g (Sen, 1970; Potashnik et al, 1973). The cause of this placentomegaly is obscure: the suggestion that it is due to vascular stasis consequent upon tumoral compression of the umbilical veins (Pensa, 1932) is unconvincing, though it is true that a few heavy placentas associated with a haemangioma have been notably oedematous (Earn & Penner, 1950; Lantejoul & Heraux, 1951).

There is little evidence to support the contention that a circumvallate form of placentation may result from the presence of a haemangioma (Eton, 1956) and the claim that there is an association between placental haemangiomas and a single umbilical artery (Froehlich et al, 1971) remains to be substantiated. A unique example of a coexistent haemangioma and a hydatidiform mole has been reported (Vermelin et al, 1957), a combination which is rather curious in view of the avascularity of a mole. One placental haemangioma has been associated with bilateral ovarian theca-lutein cysts (King et al, 1991), a somewhat surprising finding because there is no evidence that placental haemangiomas secrete hCG.

Nature and origin

The angiomatous nature of these tumours has been fully confirmed by electronmicroscopic and immunohistochemical studies (Kim et al, 1971; Cash & Powell, 1980) but it is still a matter of dispute as to whether they are true neoplasms or hamartomas. The occasional presence of mitotic figures and the frequent evidence of disproportionate growth between the haemangioma and the rest of the placenta have persuaded some that they are true neoplasms (Scott, 1924; Mugnai, 1938; Crainz, 1942; Davies, 1948; McInroy & Kelsey, 1954; Shaw-Dunn, 1959) but it is probably a majority opinion that haemangiomas are hamartomas which arise as a malformation of the primitive angioblastic tissue of the placenta, i.e. the chorionic mesenchyme. The appearances of the cellular type of placental haemangioma mimic closely those seen in a primary villous stem during the stage of angiogenesis and it is indeed probable that haemangiomas arise as a result of distorted angiogenesis within a single primary villous stem, a view fully supported by an immunohistochemical study of their cytoskeletal profile (Lifschitz-Mercer et al, 1989). This hypothesis implies that haemangiomas arise during the early stages of placental development (Snoek & Wilkin, 1952) and it has therefore to be admitted that

haemangiomas have never been observed in placentas from first-trimester abortions, being apparently confined to second- and third-trimester placentas.

Clinical effects

Most placental haemangiomas are of no clinical importance but those measuring more than 5 cm in diameter may be associated with a variety of complications which can affect the mother, the developing fetus or the neonate. Recently it has been claimed that some haemangiomas of smaller size may be clinically important (Mucitelli et al, 1990) but this remains to be confirmed by further studies.

Complications during pregnancy. A high proportion of large haemangiomas are accompanied by polyhydramnios, the reported incidence of this association ranging from 16–33% (Fox, 1967). The development of polyhydramnios is clearly related to the size of the haemangioma, for Siddall (1926) found that if the tumour was 'larger than a hen's egg' the incidence of polyhydramnios was 48.7% whilst with smaller rumours the incidence of complication was only 11%: there are no convincing reports of polyhydramnios complicating haemangiomas measuring less than 5 cm in diameter. It has been maintained that the diagnosis of polyhydramnios is, in many cases of placental haemangioma, unfounded, being based only on the excessive size of the uterus, a sign that could be due solely to an unusually large placental mass: nevertheless, the volume of the amniotic fluid has been measured on several occasions and figures such as 5, 6 or 10 litres (Merlino, 1939; Bury, 1954; de Costa et al, 1956; Bonneau et al, 1968) leave little doubt as to the authenticity of the polyhydramnios. The excess of fluid is independent of associated fetal abnormalities (Fox, 1967; Wallenburg, 1971) and is of obscure cause. It has been suggested that liquor accumulates because of compression of the umbilical veins by the tumour (Klaften, 1929) but there is no evidence that those haemangiomas situated in close proximity to the cord are complicated unduly frequently by polyhydramnios (Wallenburg, 1971) and an excess of liquor has been noted in association with tumours situated entirely within the membranes (Fox, 1966). Kotz & Kaufman (1939) thought that the increased fluid was due to transudation from vessels on the fetal surface of the haemangioma but this mechanism would not account for those cases in which polyhydramnios has complicated tumours situated entirely on the maternal surface of the placenta. McInroy & Kelsey (1954) put forward the ingenious view that the polyhydramnios was a result of an increased excretion of fetal urine, the stimulus for this being the return to the fetus of waste products in blood which had bypassed the placenta by circulating through the functionally inactive haemangioma. Wallenburg (1971) has raised the possibility that the excess of amniotic fluid is due to a fluid imbalance consequent upon fetal congestive cardiac failure, this in turn being secondary to the haemangioma acting as a peripheral arteriovenous shunt. Which, if any, of these theories is correct is a matter for conjecture but it is worth pointing out that a few haemangiomas have been accompanied by oligohydramnios (Resnick, 1953; Engel et al, 1981; Wunsch & Furch, 1983), the cause of this being even more cryptic.

Antepartum bleeding may occasionally complicate a placental haemangioma, either as a result of retroplacental haemorrhage from a tumour on the maternal aspect of the placenta (Sulman & Sulman, 1949) or as a consequence of rupture of the vascular pedicle of a pedunculated tumour, a catastrophe that may lead to fetal exsanguination (Bukovinszky et al, 1960). It has been suggested that there may be an association between placental haemangioma and abruptio placentae which is independent of bleeding from the tumour and is due to increased stress being brought to bear on the uteroplacental vasculature by altered haemodynamics in the intervillous space (Kohler et al, 1976), but this remains to be proven. There have also been recurrent claims for an association between placental haemangioma and an increased incidence of pre-eclampsia (Heggtveit et al, 1965; Wentworth, 1965; Phillipe et al, 1969; Froehlich et al, 1971; Sieracki et al, 1975) but the evidence for this is unconvincing.

It is often thought that placental haemangiomas predispose to premature onset of labour and, indeed, in many series almost a third of pregnancies have terminated prematurely; nearly always, however, this is due to labour being precipitated by polyhydramnios, and pregnancies not complicated by an excess of liquor usually proceed to term (Fox, 1967; Wallenburg, 1971).

It should be noted that placental haemangiomas, especially those large enough to be of possible clinical significance, can now be readily diagnosed by ultrasound (Spirt et al, 1980; O'Malley et al, 1981; Liang et al, 1982; Wunsch & Furch, 1983; Scharl & Shlensker, 1987), even as early as the 19th week of gestation (Nahmanovici et al, 1982); furthermore, a placental haemangioma may be associated with elevated levels of alphafetoprotein either only in the maternal blood (Mann et al, 1983; Kapoor et al, 1989; Franca-Martins et al, 1990; Thomas & Blakemore, 1990) or in both maternal blood and amniotic fluid (Schnitger et al, 1980).

Complications during labour. There have been exceptional instances in which a very large placental haemangioma has obstructed vaginal delivery (Emge, 1927) whilst on rare occasions the tumour has become detached from the placenta during labour and either passed separately per vaginam (Shaw-Dunn, 1959; Bonneau et al, 1968) or retained in utero after expulsion of the placenta with subsequent subinvolution and postpartum bleeding.

Complications affecting the fetus and neonate. The overall mortality in cases of placental haemangioma

is only minimally increased (Fox, 1967) and this slight excess of deaths is confined to those rare cases in which there is either a very large tumour or multiple tumours in the placenta. Intrauterine fetal distress and death can occur in such cases and have been generally ascribed to hypoxia consequent upon fetal blood passing through the physiological dead space of the tumour and thus being returned to the fetus in an oxygen-depleted state (Shaw-Dunn, 1959; Yule & O'Connor, 1964; Kandom-Moyo et al, 1972). The view that fetal distress can be due to pressure of a large haemangioma on the normal placental tissue (Cardwell, 1988) has little to recommend it. Fetal death can be due, however, to cardiac failure as a consequence of the haemangioma acting as a peripheral arteriovenous shunt (Knoth et al, 1976) or to compression of the cord by an unusually bulky tumour (Rodan & Bean, 1983).

The liveborn infant whose placenta contains a haemangioma is usually normal though a few, again those with large or multiple tumours, are small for gestational age (Gruenwald, 1963; Vesanto et al, 1963; Muller & Rieckert, 1967; King & Lourien, 1978), this growth deficit being also attributed to bypassing of the functional placental tissue by fetal blood which is shunted through the tumour and returned to the fetus in a nutrient-poor state.

There is some dispute as to whether placental haemangiomas are associated with an excess of fetal malformations (Glaser et al, 1988). There does certainly appear to be a rather high incidence of skin angiomas in infants whose placenta contained a haemangioma (Ciulla, 1939; Bret & Duperrat, 1944; de Costa et al, 1956; Froehlich et al, 1971; Leblanc & Carrier, 1979) but whilst in some studies there has not been an increased incidence of any other form of malformation (Fox, 1967) in others there was a remarkably high incidence of congenital abnormalities (15%), albeit all of a rather trivial nature (Froehlich et al, 1971). Examples have been reported of placental haemangiomas occurring, probably coincidentally, in association with the Beckwith–Wiedemann (Drut et al, 1992) and the Wolf–Hirschhorn (Verloes et al, 1991) syndromes.

The newborn infant whose placenta contains a large mass of haemangiomatous tissue is subject to a number of complications, usually of a transitory nature, which are thought to be a direct consequence of the placental tumour (Table 55.2). Prominent amongst these is cardiomegaly which is probably due to the increased cardiac output required for shunting blood through the haemangioma which can, in haemodynamic terms, be considered as a peripheral arteriovenous shunt (Reiner & Fries, 1965). Neonatal oedema is uncommon and in some cases is a manifestation of cardiac failure (Eldar-Geva et al, 1988; Imakita et al, 1988; Nuttinen et al, 1988): in others, however, it is a consequence of neonatal hypoalbuminaemia, a deficiency which may be due either to transuda-

Table 55.2 Reported instances of transitory neonatal disorders ascribed to placental haemangiomas

Cardiomegaly
Begg (1961)
Benson & Joseph (1961)
Reinke & Fries (1965)
Du et al (1968)
Rauchenberg & Zeman (1971)
Wallenburg (1971)
Jones et al (1972)
Leonidas et al (1975)
Leblanc & Carrier (1979)
Tonkin et al (1980)
Green & Iams (1984)
Eldar-Geva et al (1988)
Nuttinen et al (1988)

Oedema
Phillip (1931)
Horn (1948)
Lantejoul & Heraux (1951)
Resnick (1953)
Battaglia & Woolever (1968)
Monteforte (1968)
Mandelbaum et al (1969)
Jones et al (1972)
Sweet & Robertson (1973)
Blom & Gevers (1974)
Sims et al (1976)
Burnard et al (1979)
Tonkin et al (1980)
Green & Iams (1984)
Stockhausen et al (1984)
Imakita et al (1988)

Anaemia
Battaglia & Woolever (1968)
Du et al (1968)
Mandelbaum et al (1969)
Wurster et al (1969)
Jones et al (1972)
Sumathy et al (1973)
Blom & Gevers (1974)
Sims et al (1976)
Bauer et al (1978)
Wunsch & Furch (1983)
Stockhausen et al (1984)
Chazotte et al (1990)

Thrombocytopenia
Froehlich et al (1971)
Jones et al (1972)
Sims et al (1976)
Bauer et al (1978)
Lopez-Herce Cid et al (1983)
Jaffe et al (1985)

Table 55.3 Reported cases of placental teratoma

Morville (1925)
Kuster (1928)
Perez et al (1939)
Fox & Butler-Manuel (1964)
Fujikura & Wellings (1964)
Joseph & Vogt (1973)
Kobos & Sporny (1982)
Smith & Pounder (1982)
Nickell & Stocker (1987)
Svanholm & Thordsen (1987)
Reus & Geppert (1988)
Unger (1989)
Fernandez-Figueras et al (1989)
Block et al (1991)

uted to platelet injury within the rumour vessels (Du et al, 1968) but can also be a manifestation of disseminated intravascular coagulation triggered off by a thromboplastic substance released from the haemangioma (Jones et al, 1972; Jaffe et al, 1985): neonatal thrombocytopenia due to a placental haemangioma has led to fatal intracranial haemorrhage (Lopez-Herce Cid et al, 1983).

Recurrence. Very little is known about the possibility of recurrence of placental haemangiomas in successive pregnancies but Ludighausen & Sahiri (1983) have described a case in which multiple large haemangiomas were present in the placenta of a woman's first and third pregnancies, both of which resulted in intrauterine fetal death; her second pregnancy was uncomplicated by placental haemangiomas and resulted in a live child. Chan & Leung (1988) have reported a not dissimilar patient who, in successive pregnancies, had a placenta containing multiple haemangiomas, these being associated in both gestations with intrauterine fetal death.

Teratoma

Placental teratomas are extremely rare, only a few cases having been reported (Table 55.3). These tumours always lie between the amnion and chorion, usually on the fetal surface of the placenta but sometimes within the membranes at the placental margin (Fig. 55.7): they are smooth, round or oval and their diameter ranges from 2.5–7.5 cm. The tumour has no umbilical cord and receives its blood supply from a branch of a fetal artery on the surface of the placenta. All reported placental teratomas have been solid throughout and have contained a melange of squamous epithelium, skin appendages, gastrointestinal epithelium, fat, muscle, thyroid tissue, neural tissue and mesenchyme: these tissues have always been mature and no example of an immature teratoma of the placenta has been described.

Not everyone agrees, however, that placental teratomas exist and some argue that all such apparent tumours are examples of fetus acardius amorphus (Benirschke &

tion of protein from the vessels of the tumour or to chronic fetomaternal bleeding. Du et al (1968) suggested that fetal anaemia was a result of sequestration of blood within the haemangioma but this can also be due to a massive fetomaternal haemorrhage (Blom & Gevers, 1974; Sims et al, 1976; Stiller & Skafish, 1986; Santamaria et al, 1987) or to a microangiopathic haemolytic anaemia following injury inflicted on fetal red cells as they traverse the labyrinthine vascular channels of the tumour (Wallenburg, 1971; Bauer et al, 1978). The infrequently encountered neonatal thrombocytopenia has been attrib-

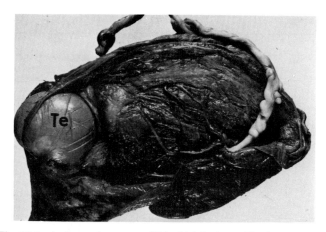

Fig. 55.7 A placental teratoma (Te) which is situated in the membranes adjacent to the main placental mass. The teratoma did not have an umbilical cord, showed no evidence of axial organization and contained skin, neural tissue, fat, cartilage and bone. (From H. Fox *Pathology of the placenta* by courtesy of W. B. Saunders.)

Driscoll, 1967; Smith & Pounder, 1982). It has been suggested that a distinction can be drawn between these two conditions (Fox & Butler-Manuel, 1964) on the following grounds:

1. A fetus acardius amorphus has a separate umbilical cord which is attached either to the placenta of its twin or to a separate placenta: such a cord may be poorly developed or rudimentary. By contrast a teratoma does not have a cord and is vascularized by a branch of a fetal artery on the placental surface.

2. It is usual to regard a fetus acardius amorphus as being totally disorganized but in fact a complete failure of organization is very unusual and in most cases central skeletal development is apparent with partial or complete formation of a vertebral column. This degree of organization is not seen in a teratoma, in which any bone present is usually totally disorganized.

These distinguishing criteria have, however, recently been criticized by Stephens et al (1989), who claimed, in particular, that lack of an umbilical cord does not help in the distinction between a teratoma and a fetus amorphus. These authors do allow that the extent of skeletal development is a more valid criterion but nevertheless come to the conceptually nihilistic conclusion that distinction of a placental teratoma from a fetus amorphus is meaningless.

At first sight it seems difficult to explain the histogenesis of placental teratomas but it is possible that they are derived from germ cells which migrate out from the evagination of primitive gut which is always present in the umbilical cord during the early stages of embryogenesis. Such germ cells could be arrested in the connective tissue of the cord and could give rise to a teratoma of the cord. If, however, they continue their migration they will pass into the loose connective tissue between the amnion and the fetal surface of the placenta and could then continue into the extraplacental membranes between amnion and chorion. All the placental teratomas which have been described have developed along the line of this proposed route of aberrant migration of germ cells.

Hepatocellular adenoma

A placental tumour of this type has been described by Chen et al (1986). This measured 7 cm in diameter and histologically resembled fetal liver. It is probable that this arose from heterotopic liver tissue which can occur in the placenta, presumably from displaced yolk sac elements.

PLACENTAL METASTASES FROM MATERNAL NEOPLASMS

Malignant disease in a pregnant woman, although uncommon, is by no means rare: nevertheless, there have been fewer than 50 reports of metastasis of a solid, non-lymphomatous maternal neoplasm to the placenta (Table 55.4), this possibly bearing greater witness to the infrequency of pathological examination of the placenta than to the rarity of placental involvement in disseminated maternal malignant disease. By far the commonest maternal neoplasm to involve the placenta is malignant melanoma which accounts for approximately half of the reported cases of placental metastatic disease. This predominance of malignant melanoma is not, however, surprising for tumour spread to the placenta occurs only by the bloodstream and only in patients with widely disseminated neoplastic disease: these criteria are exactly met by many cases of malignant melanoma, a neoplasm which, further, is not uncommon in relatively young women of reproductive age. Next in frequency to malignant melanoma are carcinomas of the breast and bronchus, this being probably a reflection not only of the high incidence of these neoplasms but also of their tendency to spread by the bloodstream at an early stage of their evolution. There have been remarkably few instances of gastrointestinal neoplasms which have metastasized to the placenta whilst reports of cervical carcinoma involving the placenta are notable by their extreme rarity; this latter deficiency is particularly striking in view of the fact that cervical neoplasms are amongst the commonest tumours to complicate pregnancy but one which is probably explicable by the tendency of cervical carcinomas to spread principally by the lymphatic, rather than the vascular, route. The only well-documented maternal sarcomas which have involved the placenta have been a vaginal angiosarcoma, a Ewing's sarcoma of bone, an orbital rhabdomyosarcoma and an angiosarcoma of the breast.

Placentas involved by a malignant melanoma are often, though not invariably, macroscopically abnormal: tumour deposits may be visible as black or brown nodules of varying size within the placental substance though the deposits

Table 55.4 Placental metastases from solid non-lymphomatous maternal neoplasms

Author	Maternal disease	Placenta			
		Gross deposits	Tumour cells in intervillous space	Villous invasion	Spread to fetus
Walz (1906)	Myxosarcoma thigh	+	+	+	0
Markus (1910)	Malignant melanoma	+	+	+	0
Senge (1912)	Carcinoma stomach	+	+	+	0
Gray et al (1939)	Carcinoma adrenal	0	+	+	0
Holland (1949)	Malignant melanoma	+	+	+	+
Bender (1950)	Carcinoma ethmoid	0	+	0	0
Bender (1950)	Carcinoma stomach	0	+	0	0
Cross et al (1951)	Carcinoma breast	+	+	0	0
Barr (1953)	Carcinoma bronchus	0	+	0	0
Byrd & McGanity (1954)	Malignant melanoma	+	+	0	0
Reynolds (1955)	Malignant melanoma	0	+	0	0
Freedman & McMahon (1960)	Malignant melanoma	+	+	0	0
Horner (1960)	Carcinoma ovary	0	+	0	0
Moschella (1961)	Malignant melanoma	+	+	0	0
Hesketh (1962)	Carcinoma bronchus	0	+	0	0
Pisarki & Mrozewski (1964)	Carcinoma breast	+	+	+	0
Rosemond (1964)	Carcinoma breast	0	+	0	0
Brodsky et al (1965)	Malignant melanoma	+	+	+	+
Rewell & Whitehouse (1966)	Carcinoma breast	0	+	0	0
Jones (1969)	Carcinoma bronchus	0	+	0	0
Metler et al (1970)	Carcinoma breast	0	+	0	0
Stephenson et al (1971)	Malignant melanoma	+	+	+	0
Rothman et al (1973)	Carcinoma rectum	+	+	0	0
Angate et al (1975)	Carcinoma breast	0	+	0	0
Gillis et al (1976)	Malignant melanoma	+	+	0	0
Smythe et al (1976)	Carcinomatosis — primary site unknonwn	0	+	0	0
Smythe et al (1976)	Carcinoma pancreas	0	+	0	0
Smythe et al (1976)	Malignant melanoma	0	+	0	0
Sokol et al (1976)	Malignant melanoma	+	+	+	0
Frick et al (1977)	Vaginal angiosarcoma	+	+	0	0
Russell & Laverty (1977)	Malignant melanoma	+	+	+	0
Looi & Wang (1979)	Malignant melanoma	0	+	+	0
Cailliez et al (1981)	Squamous cell carcinoma of cervix	+	+	+	0
Read & Platzer (1981)	Carcinoma bronchus	+	+	0	0
Greenberg et al (1982)	Ewing's sarcoma of bone	+	+	+	0
Orr et al (1982)	Squamous cell carcinoma of neck	+	+	+	0
Sedgley et al (1985)	Angiosarcoma of breast				
Suda et al (1986)	Adenocarcinoma of lung	0	+	0	0
Moller et al (1986)	Malignant melanoma	+	+	+	0
Anderson et al (1989)	Malignant melanoma	0	+	+	0
Delerive et al (1989)	Bronchial carcinoma	0	+	0	0
Patsner et al (1989)	Carcinoma ovary	0	+	0	0
Schmitt et al (1989)	Adenoid cystic carcinoma of trachea	0	+	0	0
Dildy et al (1989)	Bronchial carcinoma	0	+	0	0
Pfuhl & Panitz (1991)	Carcinoma breast	0	+	+	0
Pollack et al (1993b)	Medulloblastoma	0	+	0	0
Brossard et al (1994)	Malignant melanoma	0	+	0	0
Brossard et al (1994)	Medulloblastoma	0	+	0	0
O'Day et al (1994)	Orbital rhabdomyosarcoma	+	+	0	0

may appear white, and can be mistaken for infarcts, if the melanoma is of the amelanotic variety. Not uncommonly the placenta is generally rather firm and has a brown or grey tinge. Histologically, malignant melanoma cells are seen as clumps or sheets within the intervillous space (Fig. 55.8): central necrosis is not uncommon in large masses of tumour cells and it should be noted that, to the unwary eye, the neoplastic cells may be mistaken for pro-liferating cytotrophoblast (Fig. 55.9). Invasion of the villi

by melanoma cells is an inconstant finding, the villi often being enveloped by tumour cells without any obvious tissue invasion (Fig. 55.10): nevertheless, infiltration of the villous stroma, and sometimes the fetal villous vessels, has been noted in approximately half of the reported cases. The villous Hofbauer cells often contain abundant melanin pigment, this occurring independently of the villous invasion by malignant cells and being responsible for the generalized discolouration of the placenta.

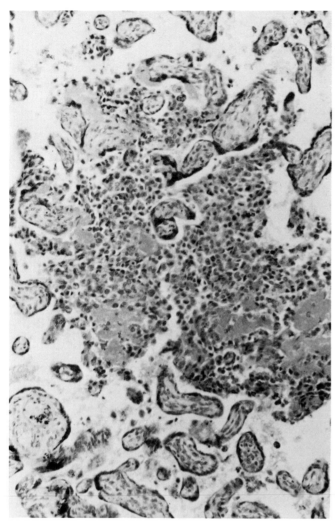

Fig. 55.8   Sheet-like masses of metastatic malignant melanoma cells in the intervillous space. H & E × 95. (From *Pathology of the placenta* by courtesy of the Editor, Dr. E. V. D. K. Perrin. Sections kindly supplied by Dr. P. Russell, Sydney.)

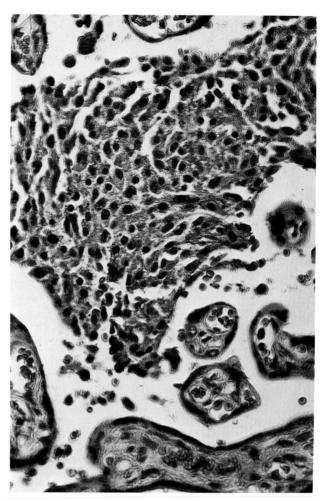

Fig. 55.9   A higher power view of a placental metastasis from a cutaneous malignant melanoma. The malignant cells are forming sheets within the intervillous space. H & E × 120. (From H. Fox *Pathology of the placenta* by courtesy of W. B. Saunders.)

Placentas containing metastatic deposits of non-melanotic neoplasms often appear normal to the naked eye, visible tumour deposits being present in only about a third of cases; the tumour nodules may be of pin-head size only but can attain a diameter of 2 cm. Histologically, sheets of neoplastic cells are seen in the intervillous space (Fig. 55.11); villous or fetal vascular invasion is uncommon.

There have been two well-documented reports of placental involvement by maternal malignant lymphoma (Kurtin et al, 1992; Pollack et al, 1993a) and there have been a few descriptions of placental leukaemic deposits in cases in which the mother has been suffering from the acute form of this disease (Bierman et al, 1956; Rigby et al, 1964; Nummi et al, 1973; Honoré & Brown, 1990), the leukaemic cells being confined to the intervillous space (Fig. 55.12) where they appeared as sheets or clumps.

The presence of malignant cells within the intervillous space is usually classed as a placental 'metastasis' but it should be noted that the tumour cells are still within the maternal vascular system and are often not obviously invading placental tissue: this has led some to decry the use of the term 'metastasis' in this context and to regard the presence of intervillous tumour cells as simply a se-questration effect (Demaille & Cappelaere, 1979). Never-theless, the large sheets of malignant cells found in the intervillous space in many instances do suggest that tu-mour growth is occurring in this intravascular site and that the cells must have a point of contact with placental structures. The reasons for the common failure of neo-plastic cells in the intervillous space to invade villous tis-sue are, however, far from clear. Possibly the trophoblast simply acts as a physical or mechanical barrier though it has often been suggested that the fetal tissue of the

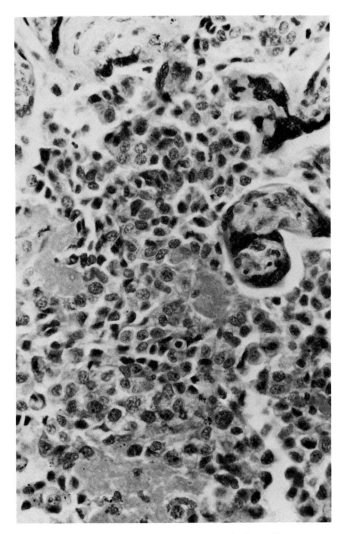

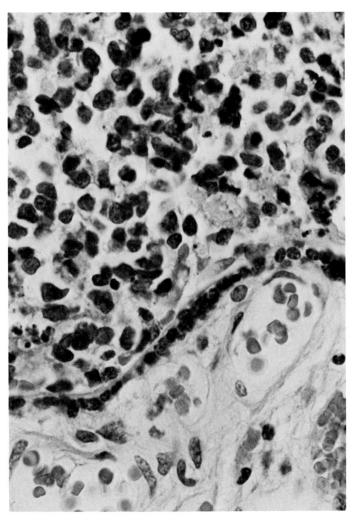

Fig. 55.10 Metastatic malignant melanoma in the intervillous space. The neoplastic cells surround, but do not invade, a villus. H & E × 220. (Courtesy of Dr. P. Russell, Sydney.)

Fig. 55.11 A metastatic deposit of Ewing's sarcoma in the intervillous space adjacent to an intact villus. H & E × 800. (From Greenberg et al, 1982. Courtesy of Dr. P. Greenberg and W. B. Saunders.)

placenta rejects the antigenically alien maternal tumour cells by an immunological reaction; proponents of this latter view have, however, not usually remarked on the lack of immunocompetent cells in the villi which are resisting attack. Some light has possibly been shed on this problem by a study of a placenta from a woman with acute lymphoblastic leukaemia in which phagocytosis and destruction of tumour cells within the villous trophoblast was clearly demonstrable on electronmicroscopic examination (Wang et al, 1983). Whether this remarkable phenomenon is confined to leukaemic cells or is typical of a more generalized trophoblastic response to neoplastic cells awaits further elucidation.

Whatever the true nature of the placental 'barrier' may be, it is clearly not always inviolate for, as already noted, it is breached in a proportion of cases with resulting malignant infiltration of the villous stroma and, occasionally,

of the fetal villous vessels. Indeed malignant cells can pass over into the fetus though, despite some claims to the contrary, there have been only two fully documented and definite cases of transplacental spread of a maternal neoplasm to the fetus, both being malignant melanomas. The child described both by Weber et al (1930) and by Holland (1949) died at 8 months of age whilst the infant reported by Brodsky et al (1963) died after 48 days of life; widespread deposits of malignant melanoma were present in both children and it is of particular interest that in both cases malignant cells had been seen in the fetal vessels of the placenta. It can not be assumed, however, that the mere presence of tumour cells within fetal vessels is absolute proof of spread to the fetus for in a number of cases in which this phenomenon has been noted there has been no subsequent evidence of neoplastic disease in the infant.

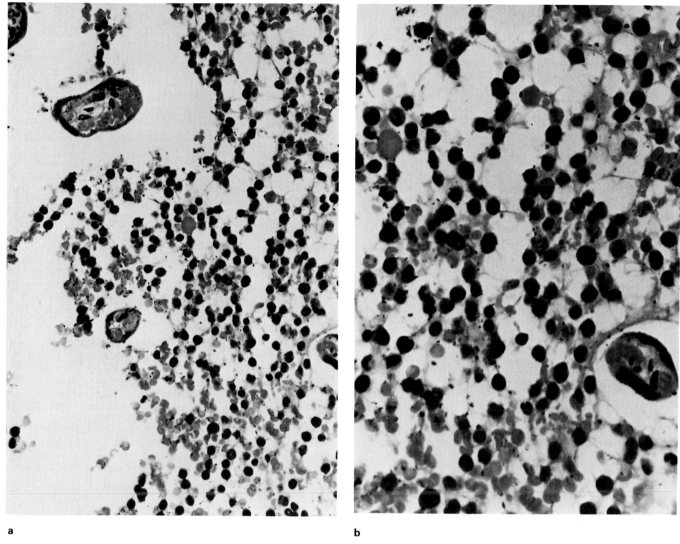

a   b

Fig. 55.12 **a** Leukaemic cells in the intervillous space of a placenta from a woman suffering from acute leukaemia. H & E × 50. **b** Higher power view of part of the field shown in **a**. H & E × 420. (Courtesy of Professor D. Jenkins, Cork.)

PLACENTAL METASTASES FROM FETAL NEOPLASMS

Dissemination of a malignant fetal neoplasm to the placenta is extremely uncommon though it is probable that the apparent rarity of this phenomenon has been accentuated by the fact that most congenital tumours are not clinically apparent at birth and by the infrequency with which placentas are submitted to routine histological examination.

The fetal neoplasm which has attracted most attention has been the neuroblastoma and there have been approximately a dozen well-documented reports of placental involvement by such a tumour (Strauss & Driscoll, 1964; Anders et al, 1970; Hustin & Chef, 1972; Jurkovic et al, 1973; Johnson & Halbert, 1974; Perkins et al, 1980;

Stovring, 1980; van der Slikke & Balk, 1980; Smith et al, 1981; Mutz & Sterling, 1991). The descriptions given of the gross and microscopic features of the placentas in these cases have been strikingly uniform for all were bulky, pale, oedematous and heavy (commonly weighing over 1000 mg) and all bore a close resemblance to the hydropic placenta of severe erythroblastosis fetalis. Tumour deposits were not macroscopically visible in any case and the detection of neoplastic involvement was dependent upon histological examination. Microscopy revealed plugging of the fetal stem and villous vessels (Figs 55.13 and 55.14) by clumps and nests of neuroblastomatous cells, the extent of fetal vascular invasion being, however, very variable. In some placentas the tumour cells were widely disseminated throughout the fetal vasculature and were, in one case, seen in every villus (Strauss & Driscoll, 1964);

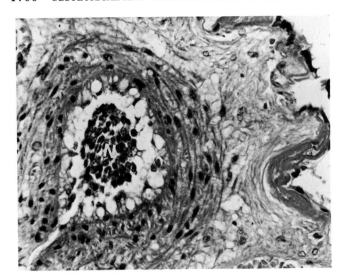

Fig. 55.13 A fetal stem artery in a placenta from a fetus with a widely metastasizing thoracic neuroblastoma. The arterial lumen is plugged by a clump of neuroblastomatous cells. H & E × 120. (Photograph kindly supplied by Dr. I. Jurkovic, Czechoslovakia, and reprinted from H. Fox *Pathology of the placenta* by courtesy of W. B. Saunders.)

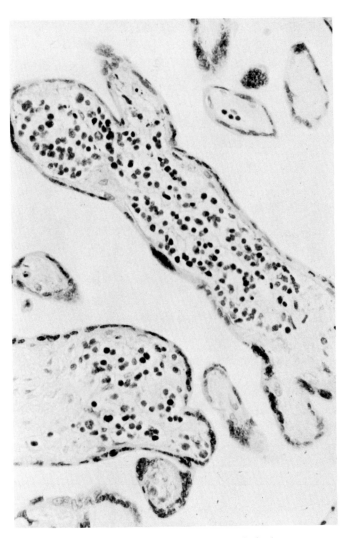

Fig. 55.15 Villi in a placenta containing metastatic fetal neuroblastoma. The neoplastic cells have broken out from the fetal vessels and are infiltrating the villous stroma. H & E × 90. (Section kindly supplied by Dr. D. Haust, London, Ontario, and reprinted from *Pathology of the placenta* by courtesy of the Editor, Dr. E. V. D. K. Perrin.)

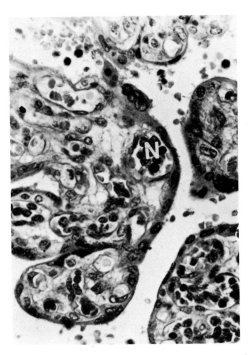

Fig. 55.14 Villi from the placenta illustrated in Fig. 55.13. Many of the fetal villous vessels contain groups of neuroblastoma cells. H & E × 120. (Photograph kindly supplied by Dr. I. Jurkovic, Czechoslovakia, and reprinted from H. Fox *Pathology of the placenta* by courtesy of W. B. Saunders.)

more commonly, neoplastic cells were seen within the fetal vessels in at least one villus per low power field. In only one case (Fig. 55.15) have neuroblastomatous cells extended out from the fetal vessels to invade the villous stroma (Perkins et al, 1980).

The villi in the involved placentas are usually large, immature and oedematous with, sometimes, a proliferation of villous stromal mesenchymal cells; these villous abnormalities are present both in villi vascularized by tumour-containing vessels and in villi free of neoplastic cells.

It is not clear whether the failure, in most cases, of the neuroblastomatous cells to penetrate into the villous stroma is due to mechanical or immunological factors. Strauss & Driscoll (1964) thought that an immunological defence mechanism of some type was involved, basing this view on the resemblance of these placentas to those seen in severe materno-fetal rhesus incompatibility and on their finding, in one case, of nuclear debris in the perivascular villous stroma. The validity or otherwise of this concept is currently an imponderable but the placental abnormalities are certainly not due solely to the presence of neoplastic cells, for identical villous abnormalities have been observed in a placenta from a baby with congenital neuroblastoma which had not spread to involve the

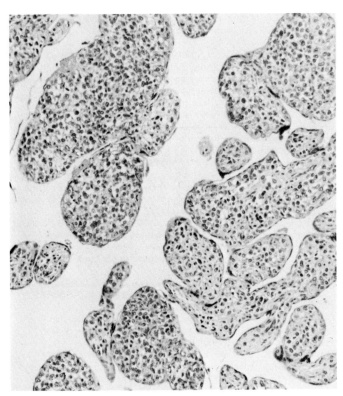

Fig. 55.16 Placental villi from a case of fetal leukaemia. Villous vessels and stroma contain numerous leukaemic cells. H & E × 70. (From *Pathology of the placenta* by courtesy of the Editor, Dr. E. V. D. K. Perrin.)

placenta (Birner, 1961). This observation lends credence to the view that placental oedema and bulkiness is due simply to mechanical obstruction of placental venous return by a large fetal intra-abdominal mass.

There has been one instance of a fetal hepatoblastoma metastasizing to the placenta (Robinson & Rolande, 1985) and a fetal malignant melanoma, arising in a giant melanocytic naevus, has also metastasized to the placenta (Schneiderman et al, 1987): the placenta in the latter case was extremely bulky and malignant melanoma cells were present both within the fetal villous vessels and within the stroma of the villi. Nests, or aggregates, of intravillous naevus cells have also been described in placentas from fetuses with benign giant skin naevi (Holaday & Castrow, 1968; Werner, 1972; Demian et al, 1974; Sotelo-Avila et al, 1988) and have usually been described as 'metastases': it is, however, more probable that the naevus cell

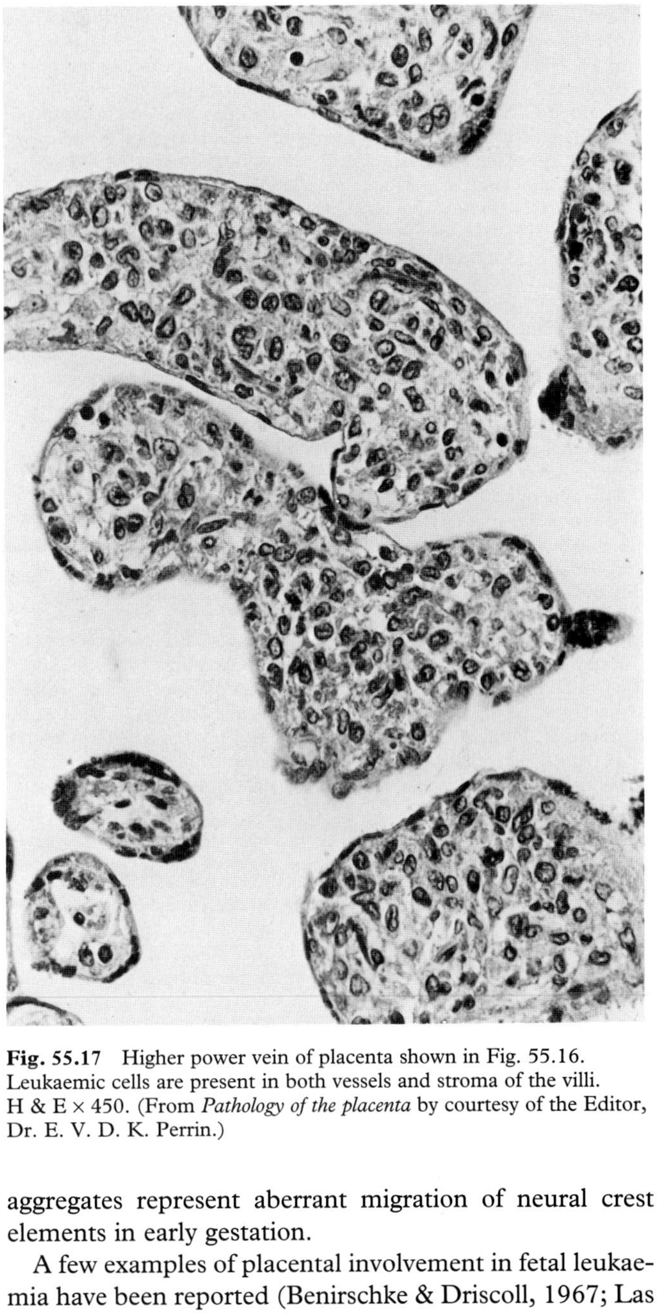

Fig. 55.17 Higher power vein of placenta shown in Fig. 55.16. Leukaemic cells are present in both vessels and stroma of the villi. H & E × 450. (From *Pathology of the placenta* by courtesy of the Editor, Dr. E. V. D. K. Perrin.)

aggregates represent aberrant migration of neural crest elements in early gestation.

A few examples of placental involvement in fetal leukaemia have been reported (Benirschke & Driscoll, 1967; Las Heras et al, 1980; Gray et al, 1986). In these cases leukaemic cells have been present in the fetal villous vessels and usually, though not invariably, in the villous stroma (Figs 55.16 and 55.17). Placentas involved in fetal leukaemia are usually unduly bulky and oedematous.

REFERENCES

Ahrens C A 1953 Vier Falle von Plazentatumoren. Zeitschrift fur allgemeinen Pathologie und pathologische Anatomie 90: 144.
Altshuler G 1984 Chorangiosis: an important placental sign of neonatal morbidity and mortality. Archives of Pathology and Laboratory Medicine 108: 71–74.
Anders D, Frick R, Kindermann G 1970 Metastasierendes Neuroblastom des Feten mit Aussaat in die Plazenta. Geburtshilfe und Frauenheilkunde 30: 969–975.

Anderson J F, Kent S, Machin G A 1989 Maternal malignant melanoma with placental metastasis: a case report with literature review. Pediatric Pathology 9: 35–42.
Angate A Y, Loubiere R, Battesti F, Coulibaly A O, Fretillere N 1975 Metastase placentaire secondaire a un cancer du sein avec survie de trente et un mois de l'enfant. Chirurgie (Paris) 101: 121–128.
Angelone A, Caruso A, Berghella A, Sindici G, Bianchi O 1989 Sur un

caso di emangioma diffuso della placenta. Minerva Ginecologica 41: 625–628.

Barr J S 1953 Placental metastases from a bronchial carcinoma. Journal of Obstetrics and Gynaecology of the British Empire 60: 895–897.

Battaglia F C, Woolever C A 1968 Fetal and neonatal complications associated with recurrent chorioangiomas. Pediatrics 41: 62–66.

Bauer C R, Fojaco R M, Bancalari E, Fernandez-Rocha L 1978 Microangiopathic hemolytic anemia and thrombocytopenia in a neonate associated with a large placental chorioangioma. Pediatrics 62: 574–577.

Begg J D A 1961 A further case of chorangioma. Journal of Obstetrics and Gynaecology of the British Empire 68: 229–231.

Bender S 1950 Placental metastases in malignant disease complicated by pregnancy with a report of two cases. British Medical Journal 1: 980–991.

Benirschke K, Driscoll S G 1967 The pathology of the human placenta. Springer Verlag, Berlin.

Benson P F, Joseph M C 1961 Cardiomegaly in a newborn due to a placental chorioangioma. British Medical Journal 1: 102–105.

Berge T 1966 Placental chorioangiomatosis. Acta Pathologica et Microbiologica Scandinavica 66: 465–470.

Bierman H R, Aggeler P M, Thelander H, Kely K H, Cordes L 1956 Leukemia and pregnancy: a problem in transmission in man. Journal of the American Medical Association 161: 220–223.

Birner W F 1961 Neuroblastoma as a cause of antenatal death. American Journal of Obstetrics and Gynecology 82: 1388–1391.

Block D, Cruikshank S, Kelly K, Stanley M 1991 Placental teratoma. International Journal of Gynaecology and Obstetrics 34: 377–380.

Blom A H, Gevers R H 1974 Een patiente met diffuse choriangiomatosis placentae. Nederlands Tijdschrift voor Geneeskunde 118: 7–10.

Bonneau H, Fouque J P, Varette I, Blanc B, Danjoux R 1968 A propos de deux cas de chorio-angiomes placentaires. Bulletin de la Federation des Societes de Gynecologie et d'Obstetrique de Langue Francaise 20: 56–59.

Bret J, Duperrat B 1944 Angiome du placenta. Gynecologie et Obstetrique (Paris) 44: 334.

Bret A J, Loewe-Lyon M Me, Duperrat B, Gauthier R 1953 L'Hemangiome racemeux du placenta. Presse Medicale 61: 1193–1196.

Brodsky I, Baron M, Kahn S B, Lewis G Jr, Teillem M 1965 Metastatic malignant melanoma from mother to fetus. Cancer 18: 1048–1050.

Brossard J, Abish S, Bernstein M L et al 1994 Maternal malignancy involving the products of conception: a report of malignant melanoma and medulloblastoma. American Journal of Pediatric Medicine and Oncology 16: 380–383.

Bukovinszky L, Jakobovitz A, Barna J 1960 Plazentatumor mit Gefaseruptur. Zentralblatt fur Gynakologie 82: 502–506.

Burger P, Fruhling L, Wurch T 1952 Reticulohemangio-endotheliome diffus du placenta avec hydramnios et monstre coelosome porteur de malformations multiples. Revue Francaise de Gynecologie et Obstetrique 47: 45–54.

Burnard N J, Merino W T, LiVolsi V A 1979 Chorangiosis of the placenta and hydrops fetalis. American Journal of Diagnostic Gynecology and Obstetrics 1: 257–260.

Bury R D 1954 A case of placental haemangioma. Proceedings of the Royal Society of Medicine 47: 911.

Byrd B F, McGanity W J 1954 The effect of pregnancy on the clinical course of malignant melanoma. Southern Medical Journal 47: 196–199.

Cailliez D, Moirot M H, Fessaro C, Hemet J, Philippe E 1980 Localization placentaire d'un carcinome du col uterin. Journal de Gynecologie, Obstetrique et Biologie de la Reproduction 9: 461–463.

Cardwell M S 1988 Antenatal management of a large placental chorangioma: a case report. Journal of Reproductive Medicine 33: 68–70.

Cary W H 1914 Report of a well-authenticated case of sarcoma of the placenta. American Journal of Obstetrics 69: 658–664.

Cash J, Powell D 1980 Placental chorangioma. American Journal of Surgical Pathology 4: 87–92.

Chan K W, Leung C Y 1988 Recurrent multiple chorioangiomas and intrauterine death. Pathology 20: 77–78.

Chazotte C, Girz B, Koenigsberg M, Cohen M R 1990 Spontaneous infarction of placental chorioangioma and associated regression of hydrops fetalis. American Journal of Obstetrics and Gynecology 163: 1180–1181.

Chen K T, Ma C K, Kassel S H 1986 Hepatocellular adenoma of the placenta. American Journal of Surgical Pathology 10: 436–440.

Ciulla U 1939 Angioma fetale associato angioma placentare. Atti della Society do Ostetricia e Ginecologia 35: 48–53.

Crainz F 1942 L'angioma della placenta. Monitore Ostetrico-Ginecologico di Endocrinologia e Metabolismo 14: 827–895.

Cross R G, O'Connor M H, Holland P D J 1951 Placental metastasis of a breast carcinoma. Journal of Obstetrics and Gynaecology of the British Empire 58: 810–811.

Davies D V 1948 A benign tumour of the placenta. Journal of Obstetrics and Gynaecology of the British Empire 55: 44–46.

de Costa E J, Gerbie A B, Andresen R H, Allanis I C 1956 Placenta tumors: hemangiomas with special reference to an associated clinical syndrome. Obstetrics and Gynecology 7: 249–259.

Delerive C, Locquet F, Mallat A, Jamim A, Gosselin B 1989 Placental metastasis from maternal bronchial oat cell carcinoma. Archives of Pathology and Laboratory Medicine 113: 556–558.

Demaille A, Cappelaere P 1979 Les metastases placentaires. Bulletin du Cancer 66: 139–145.

Demian S D E, Donnelly W H, Frias J L, Monif C R G 1974 Placental lesions in congenital giant pigmented nevi. American Journal of Clinical Pathology 61: 438–442.

Dildy G A, Moise K J, Carpenter R J, Klima T 1989 Maternal malignancy metastatic to the products of conception: a review. Obstetrical and Gynecological Survey 44: 535–540.

Drut R, Drut R M, Toulouse J C 1992 Hepatic hemangio-endotheliomas, placental chorioangiomas and dysmorphic kidneys in Beckwith-Wiedemann syndrome. Pediatric Pathology 12: 197–203.

Du J, Ko C, Lauchlan S C 1968 Multiple chorangiomata of the placenta associated with fetal anemia. Canadian Medical Association Journal 99: 862–864.

Earn A A, Penner D W 1950 Five cases of chorangioma. Journal of Obstetrics and Gynaecology of the British Empire 57: 442–444.

Eldar-Geva T, Hochner-Ceinikier D, Ariel I, Ron M, Yagel S 1988 Fetal high-output cardiac failure and acute hydramnios caused by large placental chorioangioma: a case report. British Journal of Obstetrics and Gynaecology 95: 1200–1203.

Emge L A 1927 Dystocia caused by a hemangioma of the placenta. American Journal of Obstetrics and Gynecology 14: 35–40.

Engel K, Hahn T, Kayschnia R 1981 Sonographische Diagnose eines Plazentatumors mir hochgradiger Mangelentwicklung, Aysbiloug einer Anhydramnie und nachfollen dem Fruchtion. Geburtshilfe und Frauenheilkunde 41: 570–573.

Eton B 1956 A case of chorioangioma. Journal of Obstetrics and Gynaecology of the British Empire 63: 290–294.

Fernandez-Figueras M T, Vaz-Romero M, Sancho-Poch F J, Diaz-de-Losada J P 1989 Teratoma of the placenta: a case report. European Journal of Obstetrics, Gynecology and Reproductive Biology 32: 160–172.

Fisher J F 1940 Chorioangioma of the placenta. American Journal of Obstetrics and Gynecology 40: 493–498.

Fox H 1966 Haemangiomata of the placenta. Journal of Clinical Pathology 19: 133–137.

Fox H 1967 Vascular tumors of the placenta. Obstetrical and Gynecological Survey 22: 697–711.

Fox H, Butler-Manuel R 1964 A teratoma of the placenta. Journal of Pathology and Bacteriology 88: 137–140.

Franca-Martins A M, Graubard Z, Holloway G A, Van der Merwe F J 1990 Placental haemangioma associated with acute fetal anaemia in labour. Acta Medica Portugesa 3: 187–189.

Freedman W L, McMahon F J 1960 Placental metastasis: review of literature and report of a case of metastatic melanoma. Obstetrics and Gynecology 16: 550–560.

Frick R, Rummell H H, Heberling D, Schmidt W D 1977 Placenta-Metastasen mutterlicher Neoplasien: Angioblastische Sarkom der Vagina mit Placentarer Aussatt. Geburtshilfe und Frauenheilkunde 37: 216–220.

Froehlich L, Fujikura T, Fisher P 1971 Chorioangiomas and their clinical implications. Obstetrics and Gynecology 37: 51–59.

Fujikura T, Wellings S R 1964 A teratoma-like mass on the placenta of a malformed infant. American Journal of Obstetrics and Gynecology 89: 824–825.

Gillis H II, Mortel R, McGavran M H 1976 Maternal malignant melanoma metastatic to the products of conception. Gynecologic Oncology 4: 30–42.

Glaser G, Junemann A, Tunte W et al 1988 Plazentares Chorangiom und kindliche Fehlbildungen. Geburtshilfe und Frauenheilkunde 48: 450–452.

Gray E S, Balch N J, Kohler H, Thompson W D, Simpson J G 1986 Congenital leukaemia: an unusual cause of stillbirth. Archives of Disease in Childhood 61: 1001–1006.

Gray J, Kenny M, Sharpey-Schafer E P 1939 Metastasis of maternal tumour to products of gestation. Journal of Obstetrics and Gynaecology of the British Empire 46: 8–14.

Greenberg P, Collins J D, Voet R L, Jariwala L 1982 Ewing's sarcoma metastatic to placenta. Placenta 3: 191–197.

Green E E, Iams J D 1984 Chorioangioma: a case presentation. American Journal of Obstetrics and Gynecology 148: 1146–1148.

Gruenwald P 1963 Chronic fetal distress and placental insufficiency. Biologica Neonatorium 5: 215–265.

Heggtveit H A, Arvaho R de Nuyens A H 1965 Chorioangioma and toxemia of pregnancy. American Journal of Obstetrics and Gynecology 91: 291–292.

Hesketh P 1962 A case of carcinoma of the lung with secondary deposits in the placenta. Journal of Obstetrics and Gynaecology of the British Empire 69: 514.

Holaday W J, Castrow F F 1968 Placental metastasis from fetal giant pigmented nevus. Archives of Dermatology 98: 486–488.

Holland E 1949 A case of transplacental metastasis of malignant melanoma of mother to foetus. Journal of Obstetrics and Gynaecology of the British Empire 56: 529–536.

Honoré L H, Brown L B 1990 Intervillous placental metastasis with maternal myeloid leukemia. Archives of Pathology and Laboratory Medicine 114: 450.

Horn A W 1948 Chorioangiofibroma. Medical Journal of Australia 2: 183–184.

Horner E N 1960 Placental metastases. Case report: maternal death from ovarian cancer. Obstetrics and Gynecology 15: 566–572.

Hustin J, Chef R 1972 Nphroblastome diffuse bilaterale: reflexions sur un nouveau cas. Journal de Gynecologie, Obstetrique et Biologie de la Reproduction 1: 373–384.

Imakita M, Yutani C, Ishibashi-Ueda H, Murakami M, Chiba Y 1988 A case of hydrops fetalis due to placental chorangioma. Acta Pathologica Japonica 38: 941–945.

Jaffe R, Seigal A, Rat J et al 1985 Placental chorioangiomatosis: a high risk pregnancy. Postgraduate Medical Journal 64: 453–455.

Jauniaux E, Zucker M, Meuris S et al 1988 Chorangiocarcinoma: an unusual tumour of the placenta: the missing link? Placenta 9: 607–613.

Johnson A T, Halbert D 1974 Congenital neuroblastoma presenting as hydrops fetalis. North Carolina Medical Journal 35: 289–291.

Jones C E M, Rivers R P A, Taghizadeh A 1972 Disseminated intravascular coagulation and fetal hydrops in a newborn infant in association with a chorangioma of placenta. Pediatrics 50: 901–907.

Jones E M 1969 Placental metastases from bronchial carcinoma. British Medical Journal 2: 491–492.

Joseph T J, Vogt P J 1973 Placental teratomas. Obstetrics and Gynecology 41: 574–578.

Jurkovic I, Fric I, Boor A 1973 Placenta pri neuroblastome. Ceskoslovenska Pediatrie 28: 443–445.

Kandom-Moyo J, Jajeri H, Winisdoerffer C, Philippe E, Beauvais P, Dreyfus J 1972 Souffrance foetal et chorio-angiome: etude du rhythme cardiaque foetal: a propos de 2 cas. Journal de Gynecologie, Obstetrique et Biologie de la Reproduction 1: 575–579.

Kapoor R, Gupta A K, Sing S, Sood A, Saha M M 1989 Antenatal sonographic diagnosis of chorioangioma of the placenta. Australasian Radiology 33: 288–289.

Karnauchow P N 1957 Chorioangiomatosis of the placenta. Obstetrics and Gynecology 9: 317–321.

Kim C G, Benirschke K, Connolly K S 1971 Chorangioma of the placenta: chromosomal and electron microscopic studies. Obstetrics and Gynecology 37: 372–376.

King C R, Lourien E 1978 Chorioangioma of the placenta and intrauterine growth failure. Journal of Pediatrics 93: 1027–1028.

King P A, Lopes A, Tang M H, Lam S K, Ma H K 1991 Theca-lutein ovarian cysts associated with placental chorioangioma: case report. British Journal of Obstetrics and Gynaecology 98: 322–323.

Klaften E 1929 Choriohaemangioma placentae. Zeitschrift fur Geburtshilfe und Gynakologie 95: 426–437.

Knoth M, Rygaard J, Hesseldahl H 1976 Choriangioma with hydramnios and intrauterine fetal death. Acta Obstetricia et Gynecologica Scandinavica 55: 279–281.

Kobos J, Sporny S 1982 Ein teratom der Plazenta. Zentralblatt fur allgemeine Pathologie und pathologischen Anatomie 126: 317–320.

Kohler H G, Iqbal N, Jenkins D M 1976 Chorionic haemangiomata and abruptio placentae. British Journal of Obstetrics and Gynaecology 83: 667–670.

Kotz J, Kaufman M S 1939 Chorioangioma of the placenta. Medical Annals of the District of Columbia 8: 106–110.

Kurtin P J, Gaffrey T A, Habermann T M 1992 Peripheral T-cell lymphoma involving the placenta. Cancer 70: 2963–2968.

Kuster 1928 Adultes Teratom ('Dermoid') der Placenta. Archiv fur Gynakologie 133: 93–99.

Lantejoul P, Heraux A 1951 Un cas de tumeur benigne du placenta. Presse Medical 5: 1409.

Las Heras J, Leal G, Haust M D 1986 Congenital leukemia with placental involvement: report of a case with ultrastructural study. Cancer 58: 2278–2281.

Leblanc A, Carrier C 1979 Chorio-angiome placentaire, angiomes cutanes et cholestase neonatale. Archives Francaises de Pediatrie 36: 484–486.

Leonidas J C, Beatty E C, Hall R T 1975 Chorangioma of the placenta: a cause of cardiomegaly and heart failure in the newborn. American Journal of Roentgenology, Radium Therapy and Nuclear Medicine 123: 703–707.

Liang S T, Wood J S K, Wong V C W 1982 Chorioangioma of the placenta: an ultrasonic study. British Journal of Obstetrics and Gynaecology 89: 480–482.

Lifschitz-Mercer B, Fogel M, Kushnir I, Czernobilsky B 1989 Chorangioma: a cytoskeletal profile. International Journal of Gynecological Pathology 8: 349–356.

Looi L M, Wang F 1979 Malignant melanoma metastases in chorionic villi: a case report. Malaysian Journal of Pathology 2: 73–75.

Lopez-Herce Cid J, Escriba Polo R, Escudero Loy R 1983 Corioangioma placentario y hemorraghia intracraneal neonatal. Anales Espanoles de Pediatria 19: 405–406.

Ludighausen M V, Sahiri I 1983 Chorangiome der Plazenten als Ursache wiederhalter Totgeburten. Geburtshilfe und Frauenheilkunde 43: 233–235.

McInroy R A, Kelsey H A 1954 Chorio-angioma (haemangioma of placenta) associated with acute hydramnios. Journal of Pathology and Bacteriology 68: 519–523.

Majlessi H F, Wagner K M, Brooks J 1983 Atypical cellular chorangioma of the placenta. International Journal of Gynecological Pathology 1: 403–408.

Mandelbaum B, Ross M, Riddle C B 1969 Hemangioma of the placenta associated with fetal anemia and edema: report of a case. Obstetrics and Gynecology 34: 335–338.

Mann L, Alroomf L, McNay M, Ferguson-Smith M A 1983 Placental haemangioma: case report. British Journal of Obstetrics and Gynaecology 90: 983–984.

Marchetti A A 1939 Consideration of certain types of benign tumors of the placenta. Surgery, Gynecology and Obstetrics 68: 733–743.

Markus N 1910 Gleichzeitige Entwicklung eines Melanosarcoma ovarii und Carcinoma hepatis in der Schwangerschaft. Eklampsie. Placentametastase. Archiv fur Gynakologie 92: 659–678.

Merlino A 1939 Contributo allo studio del corion-angioma. Archivo di Ostetricia e Ginecologia 3: 422–439.

Metler S, Werner B, Meyer J 1970 Przeruty raka sutka do lozyska (Mammary cancer metastases to the placenta). Ginekologia Polska 41: 301–307.

Moller D, Ipsen L, Asschenfeldt P 1986 Fatal course of malignant melanoma during pregnancy with dissemination to the products of conception. Acta Obstetricia et Gynecologica Scandinavica 65: 501–505.

Monteforte C 1968 Osservagioni su due casi di corionangioma. Archivo di Ostetricia e Ginecologia 73: 329–344.

Morville P 1925 Une teratome placentaire. Gynecologie et Obstetrique (Paris) 2: 29–32.

Moschella S L 1961 A report of malignant melanoma of the skin in sisters. Archives of Dermatology 84: 1024–1025.

Mucitelli D R, Charles E Z, Kraus F T 1990 Chorioangiomas of intermediate size and intrauterine growth retardation. Pathology Research and Practice 186: 455–458.

Mugnai 1938 Alcune considerazioni su un casi di 'angioma coriale'. Monitore Ostetrico-Ginecologico e Endocrinologia e Metabolismo 10: 261–290.

Muller G, Rieckert H 1967 Beitrag zur Frage Placentar-insuffizienz an Hand eines diffusen Chorangiomes. Archiv fur Gynakologie 204: 79–88.

Mutz I D, Sterling R 1991 Konnatales Neuroblastom und Plazentametastasen. Monatsschrift fur Kinderheilkunde 139: 154–156.

Nahmanovici C, Pancrazi J, Philippe E 1982 Chorioangiome placentaire: diagnostie echographique a la 19° semaine. Journal de Gynecologie, Obstetrique et Biologie de la Reproduction 11: 593–597.

Nessmann-Emmanuelli C, Breart G, Kone-Pale B et al 1978 Correlations entre la pathologie placentaire et les pathologies maternelles et neonatales. Journal de Gynecologie Obstetrique et Biologie de la Reproduction 7: 933–944.

Nickell K A, Stocker J T 1987 Placental teratoma: a case report. Pediatric Pathology 7: 645–650.

Nummi S, Koivisto M, Hakosalo J 1973 Acute leukaemia in pregnancy with placental involvement. Annales Chirurgiae et Gynaecologiae Fenniae 62: 394–398.

Nuttinen E M, Puistola A, Herva R, Joivisto M 1988 Two cases of large placental chorioangioma with fetal and neonatal complications. European Journal of Obstetrics, Gynaecology and Reproductive Biology 29: 315–320.

O'Day M P, Nielsen P, Al-Bolomi I, Wilkins I A 1994 Orbital rhabdomyosarcoma metastatic to the placenta. American Journal of Obstetrics and Gynecology 171: 1382–1383.

O'Malley B P, Toi A, deSa D J, Williams G L 1981 Ultrasound appearances of placental chorioangioma. Radiology 138: 159–160.

Orr J W, Grizzle W E, Huddleston J F 1982 Squamous cell carcinoma metastatic to placenta and ovary. Obstetrics and Gynecology 59 (suppl): 81s–83s.

Patsner B, Mann W J Jr, Chumas J 1989 Primary invasive ovarian adenocarcinoma with brain and placental metastases: a case report. Gynecologic Oncology 33: 112–115.

Pensa A 1932 Contributo allo studio dei corioangiomi. Monitore Ostetrico-Ginecologico di Endocrinologia e Metabolismo 4: 519–651.

Perez M L, Brachetto-Brian D, Ferrari G A 1939 Sobre una observacion de teratoma de la placenta. Archives de la Societa Argentina de Anatomia Normal y Patologica 1: 771–780.

Perkins D G, Kopp C M, Haust M D 1980 Placental infiltration in congenital neuroblastoma: a case study with ultrastructure. Histopathology 4: 383–389.

Pfuhl J P, Panitz H G 1991 Plazentametastasen maternaler maligner Tumoren. Gynakologe 24: 174–175.

Phillip E 1931 Choriohamangiom. Zeitschrift fur Geburtshilfe und Gynakologie 99: 599–604.

Phillipe E, Muller G, Dehalleux J M, Mot E, de Afakis P, Gandar R 1969 Le chorio-angiome et ses complications foeto-maternelles. Revue Francaise de Gynecologie et d'Obstetrique 64: 335–341.

Pisarki T, Mrozewski A 1964 Przerzut raka sutka do lozyska. (The mammary gland cancer metastases to the placenta). Ginekologia Polska 35: 277–286.

Pollack R N, Sklarin N T, Rao S, Divon M Y 1993a Metastatic placental lymphoma associated with maternal human immunodeficiency virus infection. Obstetrics and Gynecology 81: 856–857.

Pollack R N, Pollack M, Rochon L 1993b Pregnancy complicated by medulloblastoma with metastases in the placenta. Obstetrics and Gynecology 81: 858–859.

Potashnik.G, Ben Adereth N, Leventhal H 1973 Chorioangioma of the placenta: clinical and pathological implications. Israel Journal of Medical Sciences 9: 904–908.

Rauchenberg M, Zeman V 1971 Chorioangian placenty. Casopis Lekaru Ceskych 110: 727–733.

Read E J, Platzer P B 1981 Placental metastases from maternal carcinoma of the lung. Obstetrics and Gynecology 58: 387–391.

Reddy C R R, Rao A V N, Sulochana G 1969 Haemangiolipoma of placenta. Journal of Obstetrics and Gynaecology of India 19: 653–655.

Reiner L, Fries E 1965 Chorangioma associated with arteriovenous aneurysm. American Journal of Obstetrics and Gynecology 93: 58–64.

Resnick L 1953 Chorangioma, with report of a case associated with oligohydramnios. South African Medical Journal 27: 57–60.

Reus W A, Geppert M 1988 Teratom der Plazenta. Geburtshilfe und Frauenheilkunde 48: 459–461.

Rewell R E, Whitehouse W L 1966 Malignant metastasis to the placenta from carcinoma of the breast. Journal of Pathology and Bacteriology 91: 255–256.

Reynolds A G 1955 Placental metastasis from a malignant melanoma. Obstetrics and Gynecology 6: 205–209.

Rigby P G, Hanson T A, Smith R S 1964 Passage of leukemic cells across the placenta. New England Journal of Medicine 271: 124–127.

Robinson H B Jr, Rolande R P 1985 Fetal hepatoblastoma with placental metastases. Pediatric Pathology 4: 163–167.

Rodan B A, Bean W J 1983 Chorioangioma of the placenta causing intrauterine fetal demise. Journal of Ultrasound Medicine 2: 95–97.

Rosemond G P 1964 Management of patients with carcinoma of the breast in pregnancy. Annals of the New York Academy of Sciences 114: 851–856.

Rothman L A, Cohen C J, Astarloa J 1973 Placental and fetal involvement by maternal malignancy: a report of rectal carcinoma and review of the literature. American Journal of Obstetrics and Gynecology 115: 1023–1034.

Russell P, Laverty C R 1977 Malignant melanoma metastases in the placenta: a case report. Pathology 9: 251–255.

Santamaria M, Benirschke K, Carpenter P M, Baldwin V J, Pritchard J A 1987 Transplacental hemorrhage associated with placental neoplasms. Pediatric Pathology 7: 601–615.

Scharl A, Schlensker K H 1987 Chorioangiome — sonographische Diagnose und klinische Bedeutung. Zeitschrift fur Perinatologie 191: 250–253.

Schmitt F C, Zelhandi-Felho C, Bacchi M, Castilho E D, Bacchi C E 1989 Adenoid cystic carcinoma of trachea metastatic to the placenta. Human Pathology 20: 193–195.

Schneiderman H, Wu A Y, Campbell W A et al 1987 Congenital melanoma with multiple prenatal metastases. Cancer 60: 1371–1377.

Schnitger A, Lieogren S, Radberg C, Johansson S G O, Kjessler B 1980 Raised maternal serum and amniotic fluid alpha-fetoprotein levels associated with a placental haemangioma. British Journal of Obstetrics and Gynaecology 87: 824–826.

Scott R A 1924 Benign tumors of the placenta: a review of the literature and report of a chorio-angioma. Surgery, Gynecology and Obstetrics 39: 216–221.

Sedgely M G, Ostor A G, Fortune D W 1985 Angiosarcoma of the breast metastatic to breast and ovary. Australian and New Zealand Journal of Obstetrics and Gynaecology 25: 299–302.

Sen D K 1970 Placental hypertrophy associated with chorioangioma. American Journal of Obstetrics and Gynecology 107: 652–654.

Senge J 1912 Sekundare Carcinosis der Placenta bei primarem Magenkarzinom. Beitrage zur pathologischen Anatomie und zur allgemeinen Pathologie 53: 532–549.

Shaw-Dunn R A 1959 Haemangioma of placenta (chorio-angioma). Journal of Obstetrics and Gynaecology of the British Empire 66: 51–61.

Siddall R S 1926 The occurrence of chorangiofibroma (chorioangioma). Bulletin of the Johns Hopkins Hospital 38: 355–364.

Sieracki J G, Panke T W, Horvat B L, Perrin E V, Nanda B 1975 Chorioangiomas. Obstetrics and Gynecology 46: 155–159.

Sims D G, Barron S L, Wadhera V, Ellis H A 1976 Massive chronic feto-maternal bleeding associated with placental chorio-angiomas. Acta Paediatricia Scandinavica 65: 271–273.

Smith C R, Chan H S L, de Sa D J 1981 Placental involvement in congenital neuroblastoma. Journal of Clinical Pathology 34: 785–789.

Smith L A, Pounder D J 1982 A teratoma-like lesion of the placenta: a case report. Pathology 14: 85–87.

Smythe A R, Underwood P B, Kreutner A Jr 1976 Metastatic placental tumors: report of three cases. American Journal of Obstetrics and Gynecology 125: 1149–1151.

Snoek J, Wilkin P 1952 Le chorio-angiome: tumour benign du placenta. Bulletin de la Federation des Societes Gynecologie et d'Obstetrique de Langue Francaise 4: 644–651.

Sokol R J, Hutchison P, Cowan D, Reed G B 1976 Amelanotic melanoma metastatic to the placenta. American Journal of Obstetrics and Gynecology 124: 431–432.

Sotelo-Avila C, Graham M, Hanby D E, Rudolph A J 1988 Nevus cell aggregates in the placenta: a histochemical and electron microscopic study. American Journal of Clinical Pathology 89: 395–400.

Spirt B, Gordon L, Cohen W, Yambao T 1980 Antenatal diagnosis of chorioangioma of the placenta. American Journal of Roentgenology 13: 1273–1275.

Stephens T D, Spall R, Urter A G, Martin R 1989 Fetus amorphus or placental teratoma? Teratology 40: 1–10.

Stephenson H E Jr, Terry C W, Lukens J N et al 1971 Immunologic factors in human melanoma 'metastatic' to products of gestation (with exchange transfusion of infant to mother). Surgery 69: 515–522.

Stiller A C, Skafish P R 1986 Placental chorioangioma: a rare cause of feto-maternal transfusion with maternal hemorrhage and fetal distress. Obstetrics and Gynecology 67: 296–298.

Stockhausen H B, Hansen H G, Monkemeier D, Muhrer A 1984 Riesenhamangiom der Plazenta als Ursache einer lebensbedrohlichen Neugeborenenamie mit Hydrops congenitum. Monatsschrift fur Kinderheilkunde 132: 182–185.

Stovring S 1980 Kongenit neuroblastom med metastaser til placenta. Ugeskrift fur Laeger 142: 2977–2978.

Strauss L, Driscoll S G 1964 Congenital neuroblastoma involving the placenta: reports of two cases. Pediatrics 34: 23–31.

Suda R, Repke J T, Steer R, Niebyl J R 1986 Metastatic adenocarcinoma of the lung complicating pregnancy: a case report. Journal of Reproductive Medicine 31: 1113–1116.

Sulman F G, Sulman E 1949 Increased gonadotrophin production in a case of detachment of placenta due to placental haemangioma. Journal of Obstetrics and Gynaecology of the British Empire 56: 1033–1034.

Sumathy V, Grimes E M, Miller G L 1973 Chorioangioma of placenta. Missouri Medicine 70: 647–649.

Svanholm H, Thordsen C 1987 Placental teratoma. Acta Obstetricia et Gynecologica Scandinavica 66: 179–180.

Sweet L, Robertson N R C 1973 Hydrops fetalis with chorioangioma of the placenta. Journal of Pediatrics 82: 91–94.

Szarthmary Z 1934 Ueber Geschwulste der Placenta. Archiv fur Gynakologie 155: 453–468.

Tapia R H, White V A, Ruffolo E H 1985 Leiomyoma of the placenta. Southern Medical Journal 78: 863–864.

Thomas R L, Blakemore K J 1990 Chorioangioma: a new inclusion in the prospective and retrospective evaluation of elevated maternal serum alpha-fetoprotein. Prenatal Diagnosis 10: 691–696.

Thomsen K 1961 Hamangiome in der menschlichen Plazenta. Zentralblatt fur Gynakologie 83: 289–290.

Tonkin I L, Setzer E S, Ermocilla R 1980 Placental chorangioma: a rare cause of congestive heart failure and hydrops fetalis in the newborn. American Journal of Roentgenology 134: 181–183.

Trask C, Lage J M, Roberts D J 1994 A second case of "chorangiocarcinoma" presenting in a term pregnancy: choriocarcinoma in situ with associated villous vascular proliferation. International Journal of Gynecological Pathology 13: 87–91.

Unger J L 1989 Placental teratoma. American Journal of Clinical Pathology 92: 371–373.

van Assche A, Brosens I, Lauwerijns J 1963 Het chorangioma van de placenta: voorstelling van vier gevallen. Bulletin de la Societe Royale Belge de Gynecologie et d'Obstetrique 33: 483–488.

van der Slikke J W, Balk A G 1980 Hydramnios with hydrops fetalis and disseminated fetal neuroblastoma. Obstetrics and Gynecology 55: 250–253.

Verloes A, Schaaps J P, Herens C et al 1991 Prenatal diagnosis of cystic hygroma and chorioangioma in the Wolf-Hirschhorn syndrome. Prenatal Diagnosis 11: 129–132.

Vermelin H, Braye M, Collette C I 1957 Association de chorioangiome placentaire et de degenerescence molaire. Bulletin de la Federation des Societes de Gynecologie et d'Obstetrique de Langue Francaise 9: 225.

Vesanto T, Jarvinen P A, von Numers C 1963 Placentan hemangioomasta. Duodecim 79: 808–811.

Vettenranta K, Heikinheimo M, Sipponen P, Rapola J, Ruth V 1987 Placental hemangioma: a cause of neonatal hypovolemia. Duodecima 103: 1095–1097.

Wallenburg H C S 1971 Chorioangioma of the placenta: thirteen new cases and a review of the literature from 1939 to 1970 with special reference to clinical complications. Obstetrical and Gynecological Survey 26: 411–425.

Walz K 1906 Ueber Placentartumoren. Verhandlungen der Deutschen Gesellschaft fur Pathologie 10: 279–281.

Wang T, Harman W, Hartge R 1983 Structural aspects of a placenta from a case of maternal acute lymphatic leukaemia. Placenta 4: 185–196.

Weber F P, Schwartz K, Hellenschied R 1930 Spontaneous inoculation of melanotic sarcoma from mother to foetus. British Medical Journal 1: 537–539.

Wentworth P 1965 The incidence and significance of haemangiomata of the placenta. Journal of Obstetrics and Gynaecology of the British Commonwealth 72: 81–88.

Werner C 1972 Melaninablagerungen in der Plazenta bei neurokutaner Melanophakomatose des Feten. Geburtshilfe und Frauenheilkunde 32: 891–894.

Wilkin P 1965 Pathologie du placenta. Masson, Paris.

Wunsch M, Furch W 1983 Sonographische Diagnose eines Grossen Plazentatumors in der Spatschwangerschaft: Falldarstellung und Uberlegungen zur Geburstleitung. Geburtshilfe und Frauenheilkunde 43: 236–239.

Wurster D H, Hoefnagel D, Benirshke K, Allen F H 1969 Placental chorangioma and mental deficiency in a child with 2/15 translocation: 46 XX, (2q;ms;15q+). Cytogenetics 8: 389–399.

Yule R, O'Connor D 1964 Haemangioma of the placenta. Medical Journal of Australia 1: 157–158.

Zeek P M, Assali N S 1952 The formation regression and differential diagnosis of true infarcts of the placenta. American Journal of Obstetrics and Gynecology 64: 1191–1200.

56. Pathology of the kidney in pregnancy

David R. Turner

INTRODUCTION

Before considering renal disease in pregnancy it is important to appreciate that even in normal pregnancy there are major alterations in the results of tests of renal function which complicate the assessment of renal disease. Thus the glomerular filtration rate normally increases by up to 50% (Sims & Krantz, 1958) and the effective renal plasma flow increases correspondingly, particularly during the second trimester, returning to normal values at the time of delivery. In consequence, serum creatinine and urea levels fall during the second trimester and return to normal at term. Therefore tests of renal function in pregnancy must be viewed against this background since a 'normal' value obtained in a pregnant woman may in fact represent impaired renal function.

When a patient is found to have evidence of renal disease in pregnancy it may prove to be a chronic process which preceded the pregnancy or a recent development which has either been precipitated by some aspect of the pregnancy itself or has occurred coincidentally. In any of these cases it is necessary to consider the effect of the disease on the pregnancy as well as the effect of pregnancy on the progression of the disease. The problems which need to be covered can be conveniently included under the following headings: infections, causes of acute renal failure in pregnancy and the puerperium, pre-eclampsia, hypertension and renal diseases co-existing with pregnancy.

INFECTION

Acute pyelonephritis

Acute pyelonephritis is an important and serious complication of pregnancy which usually develops in women with asymptomatic bacteriuria (Eschenbach, 1976). Clinically these patients develop loin pain and fever, and are obviously ill with symptoms of co-existing lower urinary tract infection. Most patients are treated with antibiotics and recover, so histological examination is not relevant, but where material has become available the classical

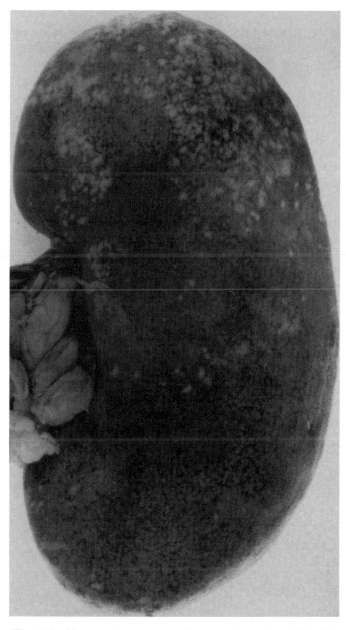

Fig. 56.1 Macroscopic appearance of severe acute pyelonephritis with almost confluent yellow 'spots' on the capsular surface of the kidney.

1707

pathology of acute pyelonephritis is observed. The kidney is enlarged and acutely inflamed. The surface may show areas containing yellowish 'spots' (Fig. 56.1) which on cut surfaces are seen to overlie yellowish streaks extending out from the medulla into the cortex. The renal pelvis is also acutely inflamed as are the ureters and bladder. Histological examination of the renal parenchyma confirms the patchy involvement of the organ with groups of renal tubules filled with neutrophil polymorphs spilling over into the surrounding renal interstitium which is correspondingly distended by the cellular infiltrate and oedema (Fig. 56.2). It should be noted that in addition to the neutrophil polymorphs the cellular infiltrate contains numerous macrophages, lymphocytes and plasma cells, the proportions varying according to the time scale of the infection.

If the acute inflammation progresses unchecked then destruction of the renal parenchyma can occur causing extensive loss of tubular epithelial cells, invasion of

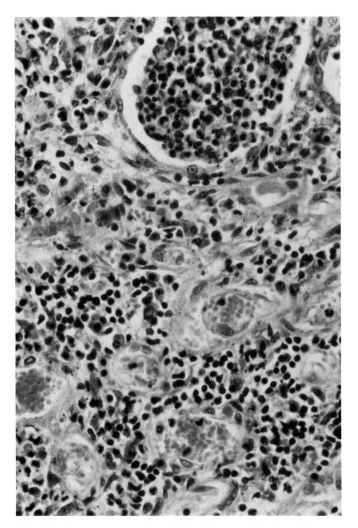

Fig. 56.2 Severe acute pyelonephritis with neutrophils distending a tubule top right and inflammatory cells within the interstitial tissues.

glomeruli, abscess formation, septicaemia and even necrosis of renal papillae. However, the most usual result is resolution of infection assisted by antibiotic therapy.

As mentioned above, the majority of patients who are likely to develop acute pyelonephritis during pregnancy can be identified at their first antenatal visit as having 'asymptomatic bacteriuria'. This has been defined by Whalley (1967) as 'a condition consisting of an absence of symptoms at a time when the patient has true bacteriuria (as opposed to simple contamination)'.

Normal urine is sterile and with symptomatic infection of the urinary tract one would expect to find a pathogenic organism such as *Esch. coli* present with a bacterial colony count in excess of 10^5 of organisms/ml in the vast majority of cases. Accidental contamination of the urine by non-pathogenic organisms during collection of the specimen usually gives a colony count of less than 10^4 organisms/ml.

Assuming a clean specimen of urine has been collected, a colony count of 10^5 organisms/ml in a patient without symptoms is highly likely to represent bacteriuria. Colony counts of between 10^4 and 10^5 are equivocal and should be confirmed in a repeat test. Obviously the precision of the urine collection is important in these assessments and needs to be performed in a uniform manner so that comparisons between groups of patients can be meaningful. The clean catch method with cleansing of the hands and periurethral area with antiseptic soap followed by spreading of the labia prior to voiding urine is probably the most practical technique. There is an 80% reliability with one test and a 95% reliability when repeated.

The prevalence of bacteriuria in pregnancy is quoted at between 2% and 10% in different studies with the figures being consistently higher in the lower social classes. Whether this relates to the greater use of antibiotics by the upper social classes or lack of hygiene in the lower social classes is not established.

What is clearly established is that antibiotics given to those pregnant women with bacteriuria will largely prevent them from developing acute pyelonephritis (Lindheimer & Katz, 1977a). Only about one-third of cases of bacteriuria will proceed to clinical infection if left untreated which suggests that the bacteriuric patients are not a homogeneous group. Indeed, it seems that those with upper urinary tract involvement are more likely to proceed to clinical infection than those with lower tract involvement. A number of methods have been examined for their suitability in distinguishing between these two categories. Fairley (1970) described the use of ureteral catheterization to identify asymptomatic infection involving the upper urinary tract. The maximal urinary concentrating ability is impaired in some 14–40% of pregnancy bacteriurics and this impairment is restored by eradicating the bacteria (Norden & Tuttle, 1965). Similar circumstantial evidence can be cited in relation to serum antibody levels which tend to be elevated in about a third of bacteriurics (Reeves & Brumfitt, 1968). The fluorescent antibody test (Thomas et al, 1974) is capable of demonstrating the presence of a coating of immunoglobulin on the surface coat of bacteria when infection of the upper urinary tract is present. However, there is dispute about the interpretation of this test. So far there is no perfect system for identifying with certainty all cases with infection of the upper urinary tract and it is therefore prudent to treat all bacteriurias. Indeed even the test system for bacteriuria is not perfect and a small percentage of patients with subclinical urinary tract infection will not be identified and treated. This probably explains why some cases of acute pyelonephritis in pregnancy have no preceding history of bacteriuria.

The bacteriuria which is seen in early pregnancy is almost certainly an extension of the asymptomatic bacteriuria seen in schoolgirls (1.2% of population) with some enhancement following the onset of regular sexual intercourse, rather than representing something special to pregnancy.

When a patient has had one or more attacks of acute pyelonephritis in pregnancy it is recommended that the urinary tract should be examined postpartum for abnormalities. This is best delayed for several weeks (12 or so) to give time for the changes of pregnancy to regress. Only occasionally do such examinations demonstrate scarring of the kidneys. In those cases the scarring is generally taken to represent damage due to reflux nephropathy acquired in childhood and not the result of recent infection. Other structural abnormalities such as aberrant collecting systems, calculi and neurogenic bladders are also relatively uncommon findings in women who have had acute pyelonephritis in pregnancy. The predisposition of the urinary tract to infection during pregnancy was originally blamed solely on obstruction of the ureters by pressure on the pelvic brim by the enlarging uterus. However, it is now appreciated that inhibition of peristalsis of the smooth muscle in the wall of the ureter by progesterone is also an important factor in causing dilatation of the ureters and urinary stasis, which thereby predisposes to bacterial infection. Although *Esch. coli* account for 80% of urinary tract infections in pregnancy, other organisms such as Klebsiella, enterobacter, proteus species and enterococci may be responsible.

It is clearly established that patients with symptomatic pyelonephritis in pregnancy have twice the expected rate of premature deliveries (Lancet leading article, 1985). Conflicting results have been obtained for the relationship between bacteriuria in pregnancy and prematurity, presumably because the bacteriurias represent a non-homogeneous group. As mentioned above this non-homogeneity is increased by treatment with antibiotics and subsequent relapse of a proportion of cases.

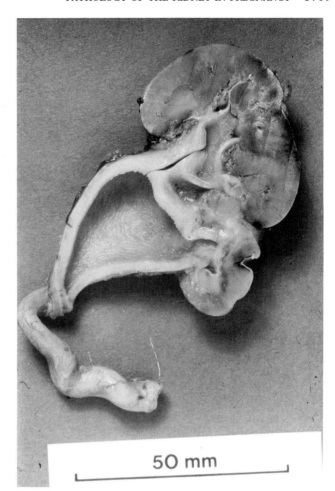

Fig. 56.3 Macroscopic appearance of segmental scarring in a kidney from a young child with reflux and secondary infection.

Chronic pyelonephritis

Chronic pyelonephritis represents a chronic inflammatory destruction of renal parenchyma which may be related to a variety of causes including obstruction in the renal tract and vesico-ureteric reflux. The pattern of scarring is often of a segmental nature with a predilection for the upper and lower poles of the kidney. The calyces of the renal pelvis may be dilated and pulled outwards in relation to the scarred areas (Fig. 56.3). The evidence of chronic inflammation is usually seen best in the renal parenchyma adjacent to the renal pelves where aggregates of lymphocytes and plasma cells are found. Even germinal centres may develop in this site. Elsewhere in the renal parenchyma chronic inflammatory cells may also be present in a patchy distribution. In the early stages destruction of renal tubules is evident in scarred areas with a tendency to crowding of residual glomeruli. The residual atrophic tubules contain protein casts which stain intensely with eosin giving an appearance similar to that seen in thyroid follicles (Fig. 56.4). As the scarring progresses the

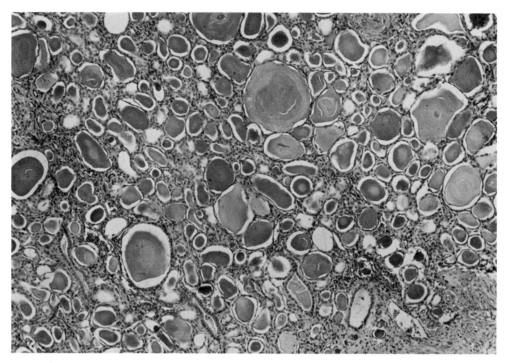

Fig. 56.4   End-stage picture of atrophic tubules in chronic pyelonephritis with intensely staining eosinophilic casts within the renal tubules.

glomeruli develop sclerotic changes, which may be either segmental or involve whole glomeruli, followed by their disappearance. Thus gradually both tubules and glomeruli disappear from the scarred areas leaving the blood vessels as a dominant feature, the latter having become more prominent as a result of thickening of their walls and crowding due to loss of intervening parenchyma.

Where obstruction is a major factor in the genesis of chronic pyelonephritis the effect of pressure atrophy contributes to the loss of renal parenchyma, which may become generally thinned as a consequence in addition to segmental scarring.

In non-obstructive pyelonephritis the causative factors include vesico-ureteric reflux in infancy together with abnormal structure of some renal papillae (Ransley & Risdon, 1978) which permit the ingress of urine into the corresponding collecting ducts (so-called intrarenal reflux). However the situation is complicated by the fact that vesico-ureteric reflux and obstruction may co-exist and furthermore vesico-ureteric reflux tends to disappear with time so the basic cause of renal scarring may well not be demonstrable by the time a woman in the reproductive phase of life is found to have scarred kidneys.

For the woman who begins pregnancy with chronic pyelonephritis, however acquired, there is a higher chance of both asymptomatic and symptomatic bacteriuria as compared with control groups. The overall prognosis for pregnancy is determined more by the presence or absence of hypertension and by the adequacy of residual renal function. The prognosis is usually favourable in the ab-

sence of hypertension, assuming that renal function is adequate, while the presence of hypertension and renal insufficiency are associated with a poor prognosis (Lindheimer & Katz, 1977b). Indeed Kincaid-Smith (1983) quotes rapid deterioration of renal function in four patients with reflux nephropathy who started pregnancy with impaired renal function.

Interstitial nephritis

A variety of different disease processes have been included with chronic pyelonephritis under the general term interstitial nephritis. These include analgesic nephropathy, Balkan nephropathy, drug-induced interstitial nephritis and metabolic disturbances such as hyperuricaemia, oxalosis and nephrocalcinosis. No detailed studies of the interrelationship of these disorders with pregnancy seem to be available. The general impression, however, is gained that provided renal function is not seriously impaired at the start of pregnancy the prognosis is good.

Renal tuberculosis

The diagnosis of renal tuberculosis is usually heralded by the finding of symptoms of dysuria, frequency and haematuria accompanied by sterile pyuria. Acid-fast bacilli may be identified in a smear of centrifuged urine or a positive culture may be required to establish the diagnosis. It is considered safe for pyelography to be carried out after the twentieth week of pregnancy to establish the extent of the disease.

Renal involvement in tuberculosis is never primary and always results from blood-borne spread (although the primary site of infection may have healed). Furthermore it cannot be assumed to be limited to one site; the whole of the renal tract must be regarded as being potentially involved.

The disease begins with the development of tuberculoid granulomas within the renal interstitium. The granulomas are composed of Langerhans type giant cells and epithelioid macrophages. The acid-fast bacilli may be very difficult to identify both in terms of their size and relative scarcity in histological sections. As the granulomas enlarge they undergo necrosis centrally and coalesce to form a larger necrotic mass surrounded by a palisade of macrophages and giant cells (Fig. 56.5). Ultimately this mass may encroach upon one of the calyces and can then discharge its cheese-like contents into the urinary system leaving a cavity within the renal parenchyma. Such cavities remain as a permanent marker of renal destruction and indeed have a predisposition to dystrophic calcification which fortuitously makes them more readily visible by X-rays. Involvement of the urinary tract may lead to progressive chronic inflammation of the ureters and bladder. However, modern anti-tuberculous chemotherapy usually cuts short the disease process before it has become extensive.

There is general agreement that pregnancy does not significantly affect the course and prognosis of patients with tuberculosis apart, perhaps, from the possibility of more frequent relapses in the puerperium (Sulavick, 1975), In-deed, provided the patient has adequate renal function and a normal blood pressure at the start, renal tuberculosis is not a contraindication to a successful pregnancy (Felding, 1968).

ACUTE RENAL FAILURE IN PREGNANCY

This can be defined as the sudden development of renal insufficiency from any cause in a pregnant patient previously thought to have normal kidneys. A marked rise in blood urea nitrogen and serum creatinine levels are found together with a decrease in urine output to less than 400 ml/d in the majority of cases, although a non-oliguric form of acute renal failure with impaired function but normal urine volume is also recognized. Causative factors include events which may occur at any time and are not therefore specific to pregnancy (1a below) and others which are particular complications of pregnancy (1b below).

1a. Causative factors not limited to pregnancy which may lead to acute renal failure
Septicaemic shock
Hypovolaemic shock due to haemorrhage or dehydration
Intravascular haemolysis
Administration of nephrotoxic agents
Urinary tract obstruction
Fulminant glomerulonephritis
Myoglobinuria

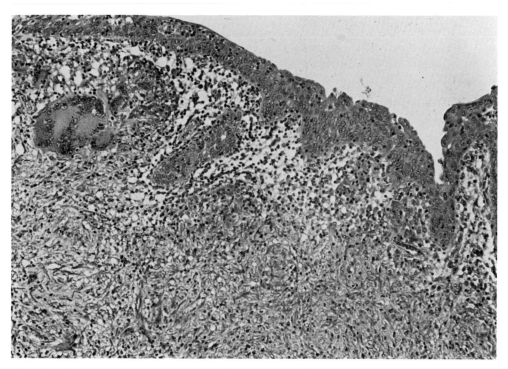

Fig. 56.5 Numerous granulomas and giant cells beneath the calyceal epithelium in a case of renal tuberculosis.

1b. Special complications of pregnancy which may lead to acute renal failure

Septic abortion
Acute pyelonephritis
Eclampsia
Hyperemesis gravidarum
Acute fatty liver in pregnancy
Abruptio placentae
Prolonged intrauterine death
Amniotic fluid embolism
Uterine haemorrhage
Postpartum idiopathic acute renal failure

} Particularly prone to progress to bilateral renal cortical necrosis

Studies using angiography and isotope methods indicate that there is usually a demonstrable vasoconstriction and/or reduction of vascular supply to the renal cortex in cases of acute renal failure (Hollenberg et al, 1970). The corollary of this is a reduction in renal blood flow to less than half its normal value and almost total cessation of glomerular filtration. If this condition is of short duration, due either to a relatively transient problem or due to rapid and effective therapeutic measures, the functional disturbance is entirely reversible. This readily reversible type of acute renal failure is described as prerenal failure, and one would not expect to find any significant morphological abnormality within the renal tissue.

Acute tubular necrosis

The longer the period in which renal cortical blood flow is severely restricted, the greater the chance that tissue necrosis will occur. The most vulnerable cells in terms of metabolic activity are the proximal tubular epithelial cells, closely followed by the distal tubular epithelial cells. The first morphological evidence of cell damage occurs in the thick ascending loop of Henle (Brezis et al, 1984). Cytoplasmic swelling and vacuolation may be seen first in a focal distribution, subsequently becoming confluent, as the ischaemic period increases (Fig. 56.6). Nuclear degeneration and loss are the markers of cell death (Fig. 56.7). Fortunately the regenerative capacity of the tubular epithelial cells is considerable, such that, provided the devastation is not complete, a sufficient number of cells will survive with the capacity to reconstitute the tubular epithelium. If a renal biopsy is performed in the regenerative stage, the tubular epithelial cells may be seen to be much flatter than normal and lack many of their normal features of differentiation (Fig. 56.8). Occasional mitotic figures are an encouraging sign that regeneration is progressing. In many cases necrosis is not identified at any stage but by electronmicroscopy a loss of differentiation can be identified; microvilli and basolateral infoldings disappear.

The patient will require to be supported during the period of functional failure of her kidneys by peritoneal

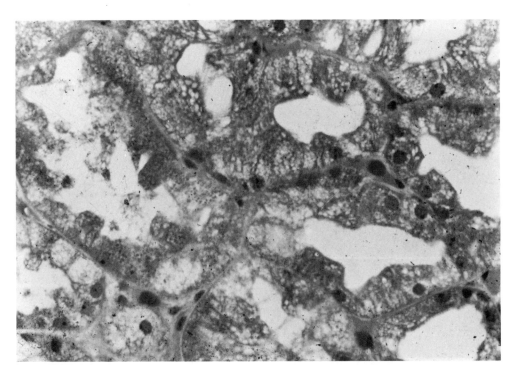

Fig. 56.6 Tubular necrosis with cytoplasmic swelling and vacuolation.

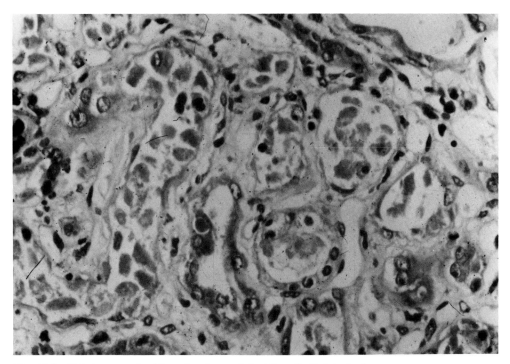

Fig. 56.7   Tubular necrosis with nuclear loss and shedding of cells into the lumen.

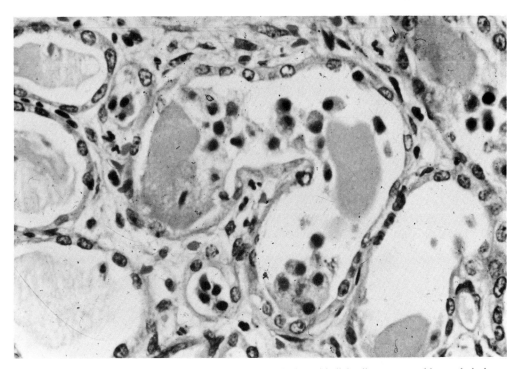

Fig. 56.8   The reparative stage of the tubular necrosis with the epithelial cells represented by a relatively undifferentiated flattened layer of cells.

dialysis or haemodialysis according to what local facilities are available. Mortality is less than for acute renal failure in non-obstetric patients (Grünfeld et al, 1980; Turney et al, 1990).

Bilateral renal cortical necrosis

When renal ischaemia is particularly severe and prolonged the degree of necrosis is correspondingly severe, and affects all the constituent structures of the renal cortex where vascular spasm exerts its maximal effect (Fig. 56.9). Much weight has been placed on the finding of intravascular thrombi involving glomeruli and arterial vessels. However, the relative infrequency of these lesions in many cases suggests that they could not solely account for the extent or distribution of the necrosis which occurs. Although cortical necrosis is seen in both pregnant and non-pregnant states there is a marked predisposition for it to be associated with obstetric complications (Kleinknecht et al, 1973). This suggests that there are some facets of pregnancy which aggravate renal cortical ischaemia when it occurs. In normal pregnancy the levels of fibrinogen, factor VII, factor VIII and factor X are all increased and fibrinolysis is reduced (Bonnar, 1976) so that it is tempting to assume that intravascular thrombi could develop more readily than in the non-pregnant state. However, therapeutic attempts to prevent or reverse the assumed intravascular coagulation with heparin and fibrinolytic agents have proved remarkably ineffective in preventing cortical necrosis. Although it is often possible to demonstrate evidence of defibrination in patients with obstetric complications this does not seem to be consistently greater in those cases which proceed to cortical necrosis. Furthermore, when intravascular thrombi are identified in renal cortical necrosis they tend to be identified in the terminal stages rather than in early biopsies, suggesting that they are more likely to represent an additional feature rather than the primary event.

It would seem therefore that Sheehan's original hypothesis (Sheehan & Moore, 1952) that the usual primary event in renal cortical necrosis is severe and prolonged vascular spasm is still supported by the available evidence. He regarded the intravascular thrombi as evidence of a terminal relaxation of vascular spasm leading to blood flow through necrotic vessels and glomeruli and consequent thrombosis of these vessels. It would perhaps be naive to assume that all examples of cortical necrosis were explicable by a single pathogenetic mechanism. The prognosis for renal cortical necrosis is obviously poor and often leads to death, haemodialysis or renal transplantation (Grünfeld et al, 1980). It should be noted that some cases of patchy involvement of the renal cortex have been known to recover a useful degree of renal function (Heptinstall, 1992). There is therefore a danger that a renal biopsy may provide a falsely gloomy picture if only a small piece of totally necrotic material is obtained.

Acute renal failure in pregnancy septicaemia

Following the change in social attitudes which permitted

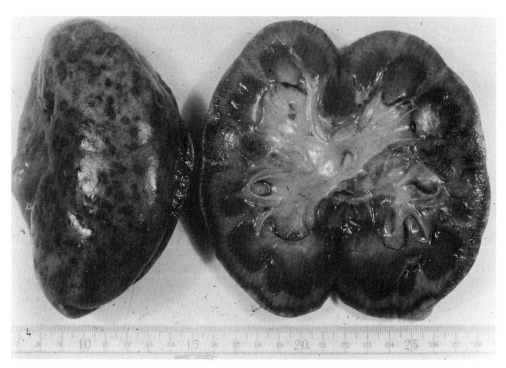

Fig. 56.9 Bilateral renal cortical necrosis with pallor of the cortical tissue due to infarction of all its tissue components. (Provided by Prof. R. Risdon.)

the legalization of abortion the incidence of septic abortion has fallen considerably. It remains, however, an important cause of acute renal failure in early pregnancy with a peak incidence around 16 weeks gestation. Septicaemia may also occur in pregnancy as a complication of acute pyelonephritis and puerperal sepsis. The marked hypotensive effect of overwhelming infection causes renal ischaemia, and intravascular coagulation may be superimposed. This latter process may be triggered by endotoxins in the circulation or by intravascular haemolysis due to clostridial infection (Emmanuel & Lindheimer, 1976).

Parallels are inevitably drawn between the occasional development of renal cortical necrosis as a consequence of pregnancy septicaemia and the generalized Shwartzman reaction, which can be triggered by giving a single dose of endotoxin in pregnant animals. Certainly endotoxin has the capacity to induce intravascular coagulation. In practice, however, pregnancy septicaemia does not usually progress to renal cortical necrosis.

Pre-eclampsia

Acute renal failure may develop within the setting of severe pre-eclampsia. Here it is postulated that renal cortical ischaemia is caused by the severe swelling of the glomerular capillary endothelium to the extent that the capillary lumens are obliterated causing post-glomerular ischaemia. A minority of such cases progress to cortical necrosis. There is some evidence that the older multiparous patients are more liable to have such a fatal outcome, possibly due to undetected hypertension or renal vascular disease (Grünfeld et al, 1980). Intravascular haemolysis has also been postulated as being responsible in part for the renal cortical ischaemia in eclampsia but the mechanism for this is uncertain.

Abruptio placentae

There is a particularly high incidence of renal cortical necrosis developing in patients with acute renal failure due to abruptio placentae. The estimated blood loss is usually less than would be expected from the degree of renal ischaemia produced, suggesting that hypovolaemia is only part of the problem. The defibrination syndrome is usually also present (Kleiner & Greston, 1976).

Prolonged intrauterine death and amniotic fluid embolism

The defibrination syndrome is often encountered in association with prolonged intrauterine death and amniotic fluid embolism. These complications of pregnancy are then particularly prone to lead to acute renal failure and renal cortical necrosis.

Acute fatty liver of pregnancy

This rare complication of pregnancy, which is primarily a problem from the hepatological aspects, has been linked with tetracycline usage by some authors (Kunelis et al, 1965). Acute renal failure is a frequent complication but the morphological changes seen in the kidneys are usually unimpressive apart from fatty vacuolation of the tubular epithelial cells. The liver failure is the main clinical problem. In some cases where renal failure has developed, thrombi have been seen in the microvasculature of the renal cortex (Morrin et al, 1967) but this development has not been shown convincingly to be a prime cause of the renal failure. Slater & Hague (1984) have described sub-endothelial electron-dense deposits and mesangial cell interposition in four cases of acute fatty liver of pregnancy with renal involvement. The precise mechanism responsible for these effects was unclear.

Idiopathic postpartum acute renal failure

This syndrome was first described by Scheer & Jones (1967), Wagoner et al (1968) and Robson et al (1968) and is relatively rare yet often fatal when it does occur. Microangiopathic haemolytic anaemia is often present and accelerated hypertension frequently develops. The pregnancy has usually been uneventful until shortly after parturition when a typical case will present with a flu-like illness reminiscent of the prodromal phase of the haemolytic uraemic syndrome. The histological changes seen in the kidney are very similar to those seen in scleroderma with renal involvement. There is marked cellular proliferation and accumulation of mucopolysaccharide ground substance in the subintimal zone of arterial vessels (Fig. 56.10). Fibrinoid necrosis is seen particularly in the walls of arterioles (Fig. 56.11). The glomeruli may show ischaemic changes as a consequence of the vascular occlusion or segmental necrosis with crescent formation may occur. Fibrin is usually demonstrable, using immunochemical techniques, in the walls of arterioles and small arteries and in parts of some glomeruli. In glomeruli which are showing neither ischaemic collapse nor necrosis the capillary walls are initially thickened by a pale material in the subendothelial zone which may contain fibrin tactoids. Subsequently, mesangial cell interposition may occur and cause a reduplication of the glomerular capillary basement membranes. These features suggest that the coagulation mechanism is involved and, indeed, although many patients die, recovery has been reported after anticoagulant therapy (Donadio & Holley, 1974).

There is a striking similarity between postpartum acute renal failure and the development of haemolytic uraemic syndrome in women taking oral contraceptives. This latter complication of oestrogen consumption was described by Tobon (1972). However, women who develop either one

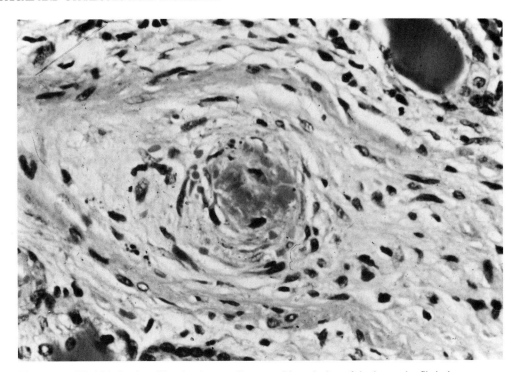

Fig. 56.10   Florid intimal proliferation in a small artery with occlusion of the lumen by fibrin in postpartum acute renal failure.

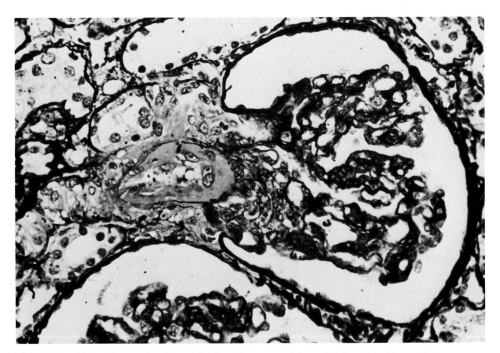

Fig. 56.11   Fibrinoid necrosis of the wall of an afferent arteriole and ischaemic collapse of the glomerular tuft in postpartum acute renal failure.

of these conditions do not show any increased susceptibility to the other. Yet women who develop the haemolytic uraemic syndrome after using the contraceptive pill have a greater chance of developing acute rejection following renal transplantation.

PRE-ECLAMPSIA AND HYPERTENSION

The term toxaemia of pregnancy has been used in an ill-defined way to describe the occurrence of hypertension, proteinuria and oedema in pregnancy. This syndrome has encompassed not only patients with pre-eclampsia/eclampsia but also patients with essential hypertension and hypertension secondary to other causes such as chronic renal disease. Since pre-eclampsia may be superimposed upon pre-existing hypertension or latent hypertension careful analysis is necessary to appreciate what is happening in an individual case (Lindheimer & Katz, 1977d).

Pre-eclampsia/eclampsia is a condition peculiar to pregnancy with characteristic morphological changes in glomeruli which can be revealed by renal biopsy. The severity of the glomerular lesions tends to roughly parallel the degree of proteinuria found clinically (Sheehan, 1980). Pre-eclampsia is uncommon before 20 weeks' gestation, unless associated with a hydatidiform mole or multiple pregnancy, and does not usually develop before 30 weeks' gestation. It is about seven times more frequent in first as compared with subsequent pregnancies. Other predisposing factors are essential hypertension, diabetes, fetal hydrops and extremes of reproductive age. The dramatic resolution of the syndrome following delivery tends to implicate the feto-placental unit in its aetiology although its marked association with first pregnancies has not been adequately explained.

In practice one does not normally have the assistance of the renal biopsy appearances in making the diagnosis of pre-eclampsia and therefore one is relying upon the interpretation of blood pressure readings and the assessment of proteinuria and oedema. Before analysing further the significance of various combinations of hypertension, oedema and proteinuria it is important to appreciate that accurate assessment of each of these three parameters can be difficult, particularly in deciding between the upper limits of normality and the first indication of pathological change. This area of uncertainty has no doubt contributed significantly to the confusion which surrounds the subject of pre-eclampsia.

The measurement of blood pressure is normally achieved by an indirect, non-invasive technique which is recognized as providing an estimation rather than an accurate reading. This makes the establishment of a normal value difficult, particularly when other factors such as age, smoking habits, family size, occupation, anxiety and discomfort are all known to be able to affect individual blood pressure readings. Furthermore pregnancy itself induces a relative fall in blood pressure estimations to an average of about 70 mmHg diastolic by the sixteenth week of gestation with a subsequent rise to an average of about 80 mmHg by the thirty-sixth week of gestation. Clinically the figure of 140/90 has been regarded as abnormal but perinatal mortality figures (Friedman, 1976) suggest that there is a sudden increase in mortality at blood pressure levels in excess of 125/75 throughout the period of observation in pregnancy.

Some degree of dependent oedema is almost universal in pregnancy and therefore pitting oedema in the legs can not be assumed to be due to pre-eclampsia. Oedema of the hands and face is much more likely to have a significant pathological basis.

The assessment of proteinuria may be roughly performed by a dipstick method or more accurately estimated as grams per 24 h specimen or grams per litre. It is usual practice to ignore small degrees of proteinuria (i.e. less than 300 mg/24 h). A false high reading for proteinuria may occur as a result of contamination of the urine by vaginal discharge or bleeding and could theoretically be due to orthostatic proteinuria, violent exercise or exposure to severe cold. With these caveats a level of proteinuria in excess of 300 mg/24 h is usually taken to be indicative of either pre-eclampsia or possibly some other glomerular disorder.

In practice, however, the clinical diagnosis of pre-eclampsia has often been made on the sole criterion of an elevated blood pressure in late pregnancy and early puerperium which falls to normal levels within 10 days of delivery. This syndrome is sometimes termed gestational hypertension and may prove to be due to either pre-eclampsia, latent essential hypertension revealed by pregnancy, or hypertension, either essential or of renal origin, that has abated during the middle trimester of pregnancy. Consequently the diagnosis of pre-eclampsia is insecure in the absence of further evidence such as significant proteinuria (i.e. > 300 mg/24 h) or renal biopsy, the latter rarely being available.

It had been noted by Sheehan (1980) that the classical morphological findings of pre-eclampsia are almost never seen in the absence of proteinuria, lending support to the value of proteinuria as a clinical sign of pre-eclampsia.

Since many of the follow-up studies of patients with pre-eclampsia are confused by the inclusion of cases of gestational hypertension, the conclusions with regard to the long-term consequences must be drawn with care (Chesley, 1980). Certainly such studies appear to show an increase in chronic hypertensive vascular disease in patients with 'pre-eclampsia'. However, when one begins to separate off the cases with gestational hypertension alone the incidence of development of chronic hypertensive disease falls correspondingly. Gestational hypertension tends to be much more common in heavy obese females and increases sharply with age, which is also true of essential hypertension. Conversely the perinatal mortality is not increased in women with gestational hypertension nor are the infants small for gestational age as occurs with pre-eclampsia. Thus gestational hypertension appears to represent latent essential hypertension unmasked by pregnancy. Indeed women with normotensive pregnancies have a much reduced chance of developing chronic hypertensive vascular disease than might be expected by comparison with matched unselected females. Thus pregnancy appears to be a useful screening test for chronic hypertension.

Although moderate proteinuria is a cardinal feature of pre-eclampsia, occasionally massive proteinuria with a full nephrotic syndrome may develop, as described in a series of patients by Roy First et al (1978).

Pathogenesis of pre-eclampsia

Innumerable theories have been propounded on the pathogenesis of pre-eclampsia, ranging from hormonal effects and the renin-angiotensin system through dietary excesses and deficiencies to more recent ideas carried along on the various cascade systems of haemostasis, kinins and prostaglandins (MacGillivray, 1981). However, none of these theories provides an explanation for the well-established high incidence of pre-eclampsia in first pregnancies. Even an abortion appears to provide protection against the development of pre-eclampsia in a subsequent pregnancy.

Logic would seem to dictate that a system with the capacity to modify its functions with time, such as the specific immune system, must be involved. Indeed it is generally accepted that a degree of immune tolerance is required in normal pregnancy to prevent rejection of the fetus and placenta. If immune tolerance were incompletely developed at the time of a first pregnancy then damage to the placental tissue would be expected and this could induce those changes we recognize as pre-eclampsia.

The fact that pre-eclampsia has a familial tendency (Chesley, 1980; Cooper et al, 1993) and also a racial predilection suggests that there may be a genetic abnormality which could be responsible for some women exhibiting impaired tolerance to the feto-placental unit, and thus being susceptible to the development of pre-eclampsia. Some caution needs to be observed in accepting that pre-eclampsia has a genetic basis since the clinical diagnosis of pre-eclampsia may include cases of essential hypertension which does have an inheritable basis.

The observation that twin pregnancies are particularly prone to induce pre-eclampsia, regardless of whether they are mono- or dizygotic, suggests that the phenomenon involves suppression or adaptation of a mechanism (i.e. tolerance) rather than an increased maternal-fetal incompatibility (Campbell et al, 1977). This idea is supported by the increased incidence of pre-eclampsia in association with other conditions where an enlarged placental mass develops, namely hydatidiform mole, triploidy, erythroblastosis fetalis and diabetes.

There seems to be no doubt that intravascular coagulation can be identified in many cases of pre-eclampsia, although this may well prove to be the consequence rather than the cause of pre-eclampsia. Many studies show that fibrin degradation products are elevated and when maternal tissues are available for examination some degree of intravascular thrombosis can be identified, particularly in severe disease. Certainly the changes seen in renal glomeruli (see below) are entirely consistent with a chronic low-grade fibrin deposition. Whether the final mechanisms which result in the pre-eclampsia syndrome depend on stimulation of the kinin system, a deficiency in prostacyclin production (Lewis, 1982) or the renin-angiotensin system is not established although all these systems are under scrutiny. Experimentally, placental ischaemia in the rabbit can induce a syndrome resembling eclampsia (Abitbol et al, 1976). Currently the most logical explanation for pre-eclampsia would seem to be that the relatively underdeveloped uterine vasculature releases thromboplastins and/or other substances which induce vascular spasm affecting the renal glomeruli in particular. Occasional relaxation of spasm may then allow coagulation to occur around damaged endothelial cells. It is of interest that Clark et al (1992) have shown that endothelin levels are elevated in pre-eclampsia and may contribute to renal vasoconstriction.

Renal changes in pre-eclampsia

The descriptive label of glomerular capillary endotheliosis was proposed by Spargo et al (1959) and is generally agreed to be the most characteristic lesion of pre-eclampsia. It describes an enlargement of the glomerular tuft (Fig. 56.12) due mainly to an increase in endothelial cell cytoplasm (Fig. 56.13). There is little overall increase in cellularity although there is a moderate widening of the mesangial areas. The endothelial cell cytoplasm shows a remarkable degree of swelling and vacuolation which encroaches considerably on the lumens of glomerular capillaries. Certainly the impression is that the endothelial cells have been damaged by vascular spasm or some agent or toxin, resulting in a markedly increased water content together with a variable degree of fatty change. The glomerular capillaries in pre-eclampsia usually appear bloodless in histological sections. However, this cannot be true in vivo or urine would not be produced at all. The most probable explanation of this observation is that as the intravascular pressure falls the blood in glomerular capillaries is expelled by the reflux of filtrate back from the urinary space and proximal tubule, and by the contraction of the glomerular tuft itself. The fatty change affecting the endothelial cells is variable both in degree and in the type of lipid present (Fig. 56.14). Neutral fat, phospholipid and cholesterol esters may be identified.

The mesangial cells, although not increased in number, show a marked expansion of their cytoplasmic processes, some of which also show fatty change. It is the cytoplasmic increase which explains the widening of mesangial areas described above, and may be associated with an increased production of mesangial matrix material. In the more advanced cases of pre-eclampsia the mesangial cell processes may begin to grow round the capillary loops in the subendothelial region (Figs 56.15–56.17). This phenomenon is known as mesangial cell interposition and may lead to the laying down of a basement membrane-like

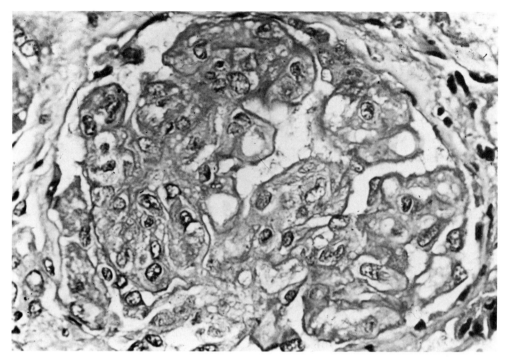

Fig. 56.12 Glomerular capillary endotheliosis due to swelling of endothelial cells in pre-eclampsia. The capillary lumens are largely obliterated.

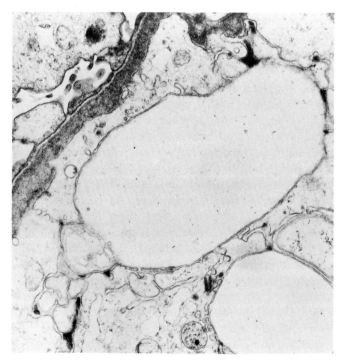

Fig. 56.13 Electronmicrograph showing swollen pale endothelial cell cytoplasm limited (top left) by a relatively normal glomerular capillary basement membrane in pre-eclampsia.

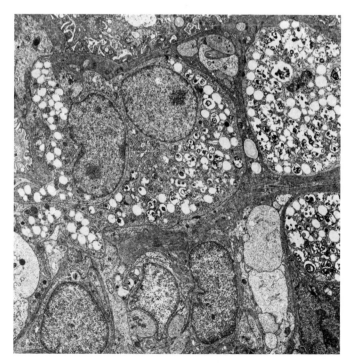

Fig. 56.14 Electronmicrograph showing swollen and vacuolated endothelial cells with numerous myelin bodies (residual bodies) from a case of pre-eclampsia.

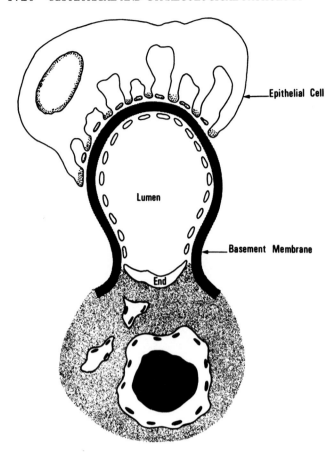

Fig. 56.15 Diagram of normal glomerular capillary loop with a mesangial or stalk cell at the base surrounded by mesangial matrix material. End = endothelial cell cytoplasm.

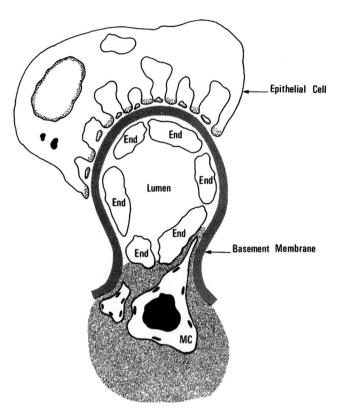

Fig. 56.16 Diagram to show the early changes of pre-eclampsia with endothelial cytoplasmic swelling and early mesangial cell interposition. End = endothelial cell cytoplasm; MC = mesangial cell.

material of mesangial matrix type in the subendothelial space of the glomerular capillary wall (Fig. 56.18). The effect of this is to produce a double-contour effect in part or all of the glomerular capillary loop when stained with methenamine silver (Fig. 56.19).

The subendothelial space is expanded initially by a pale amorphous substance (Fig. 56.20) which gives a positive reaction with antisera to fibrinogen and has been referred to as fibrinoid (Kincaid-Smith, 1991). Only occasionally are fibrin tactoids identified by electronmicroscopy, however. The subendothelial space may also contain occasional electron-dense deposits similar to those seen in immune complex disease. Immunofluorescent studies have given variable results but the general trend is for IgM and fibrin to be consistently identified (Tribe et al, 1979) while other immunoglobulins and complement components are infrequent or unimpressive (Fig. 56.21). Foidart et al (1983) have shown that the material deposited in the subendothelial zone of the capillary loops consists of structural basement membrane components as well as plasma-derived proteins, and suggest that this may be mediated by prostaglandin secretion.

Despite the remarkable changes occurring in the endothelial cells and subendothelial space, the original glomerular basement membrane remains surprisingly intact in morphological terms although it is presumably sufficiently altered in biochemical terms to permit significant proteinuria.

The epithelial cells are altered to the extent that they may contain large hyaline cytoplasmic droplets and villous proliferation of the cytoplasmic membrane. However, the most significant feature is the relative normality of the epithelial foot processes despite proteinuria which may be of severe proportions (Fig. 56.18). This strongly suggests that the concept that proteinuria is the direct result of foot process loss, as has been proposed in minimal change nephropathy and other glomerular disorders, is incorrect.

In up to 50% of cases of pre-eclampsia Seymour et al (1976) found adhesions between the glomerular tuft and the glomerular capsule. These were most likely to be identified at the site of origin of the proximal convoluted tubule from Bowman's capsule. In contrast to the other glomerular abnormalities seen in pre-eclampsia which resolve rapidly after parturition, the tuft adhesions have been shown to persist for many months or years as a permanent record of the episode of 'glomerular capillary endotheliosis' (Heaton & Turner, 1985).

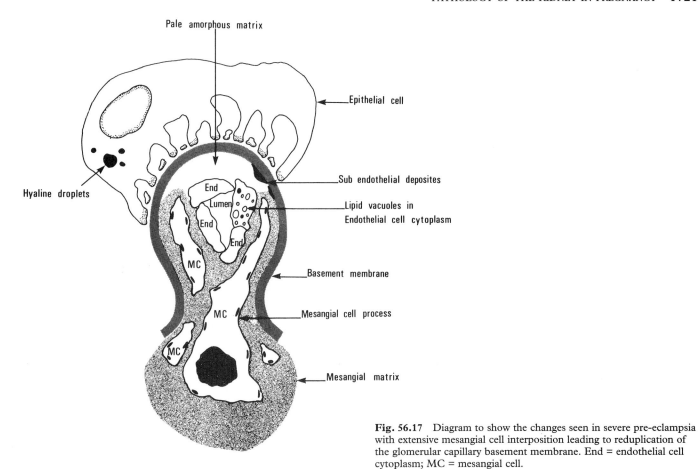

Fig. 56.17   Diagram to show the changes seen in severe pre-eclampsia with extensive mesangial cell interposition leading to reduplication of the glomerular capillary basement membrane. End = endothelial cell cytoplasm; MC = mesangial cell.

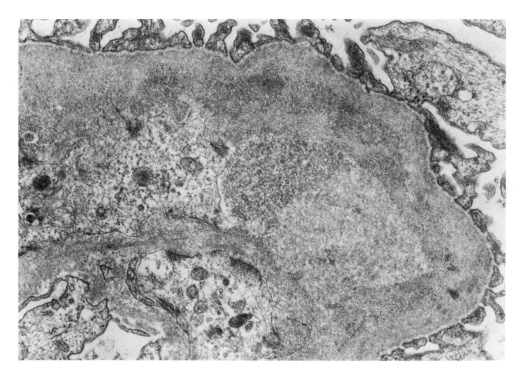

Fig. 56.18   Electronmicrograph showing normal foot processes at top and reduplicated glomerular capillary basement membrane adjacent to the residual capillary lumen (at bottom left) in pre-eclampsia.

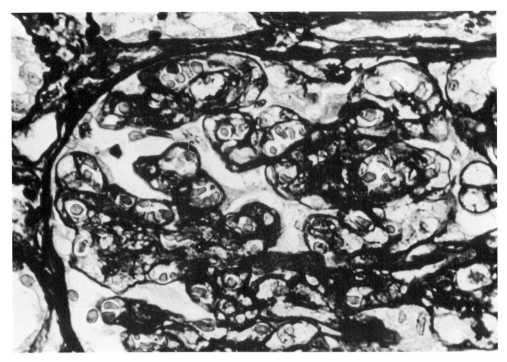

Fig. 56.19   Glomerulus with many capillary loops showing reduplication in pre-eclampsia.

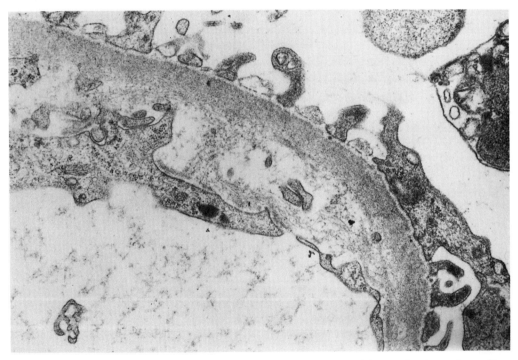

Fig. 56.20   Electronmicrograph with widening and pallor of the subendothelial zone of a glomerular capillary loop in pre-eclampsia.

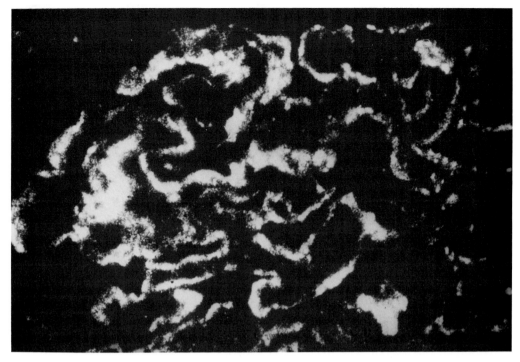

Fig. 56.21 Immunofluorescence photograph of glomerular IgM deposition in pre-eclampsia. (Provided by Dr. C. Tribe.)

A variety of vascular changes have been described in the kidneys of patients with eclampsia (Sheehan, 1980), including thickening of the media of arterioles, prominence of the juxtaglomerular apparatus, presence of 'elastic beads' in arterioles and fat in the walls of arterioles. However, none of these features is specific to pre-eclampsia and all may be seen in benign nephrosclerosis associated with hypertension.

The tubules are relatively unaffected by pre-eclampsia, showing only occasional non-specific features such as hyaline droplets and fatty change in occasional tubules. Even in eclampsia the tubular changes are relatively unimpressive being limited to some flattening of the epithelium of proximal tubules. Fully developed ischaemic necrosis of tubules is rare in eclampsia.

RENAL DISEASES CO-EXISTING WITH PREGNANCY

Some patients will enter pregnancy with pre-existing renal disease which may either be known or unsuspected. Alternatively the patient may acquire some form of renal disease coincidentally during the course of pregnancy. In either case if nephron loss has occurred it is likely to be masked, as far as conventional tests of renal function are concerned, by the considerable functional reserve which the healthy kidney possesses. Indeed, even when 75% of the renal mass has been destroyed the serum creatinine levels may be only slightly elevated.

In normal pregnancy the glomerular filtration rate rises by some 35%. Although few studies have been attempted on patients with renal disease in pregnancy, it would appear that a similar increase occurs in patients with mild to moderate renal impairment. Increases in creatinine clearance and reductions in serum creatinine have been noted in pregnancy by Bear (1976b) and Whalley et al (1975).

Bear (1976a) recommended that a serum creatinine level in excess of 1.7 mg/100 ml should generally be regarded as a contraindication to pregnancy, although some patients with higher levels as well as some patients with renal transplants have been delivered successfully.

Glomerular diseases which may co-exist with pregnancy

The most obvious presenting symptom of glomerular disease is proteinuria which, if severe, may be associated with a full nephrotic syndrome (proteinuria in excess of 3.5 g/100 ml, oedema, albuminuria and hypercholesterolaemia). Obviously the difficulty here is to differentiate between pre-eclampsia and other types of glomerular disorder and this may only be possible if a renal biopsy is performed. Hill et al (1988) have shown a high correlation between pre-existing renal pathology and the endotheliosis lesions of pre-eclampsia, suggesting that the pre-existing renal pathology increases the chances of developing pre-eclampsia in pregnancy.

Membranous glomerulonephritis

This form of chronic glomerular disease characterized by uniform thickening of glomerular capillary basement membranes is due to the accumulation of immunoglobulins and complement components (Figs 56.22 and 56.23).

These substances pass from the capillary lumen through the capillary wall and complex with each other to form 'in situ' aggregates of electron-dense material beneath the foot processes of the epithelial cells. In only a few cases can antigens be identified in these electron-dense 'deposits'.

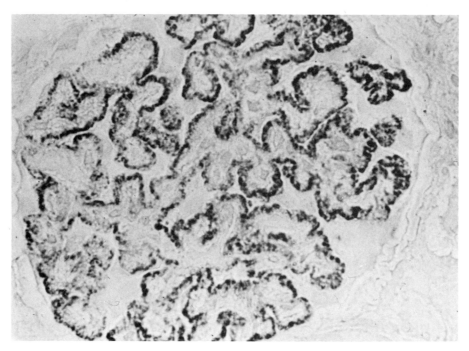

Fig. 56.22 Peripheral granular deposition of IgM in a glomerulus from a patient with membraneous glomerulonephritis. Immunoperoxidase technique.

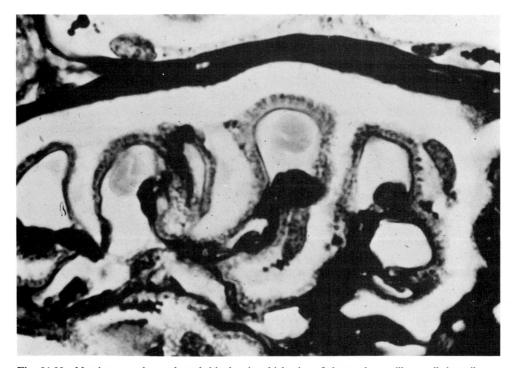

Fig. 56.23 Membranous glomerulonephritis showing thickening of glomerular capillary walls by spiky projections of the basement membrane interposed between immune deposits.

The prognosis is difficult to determine in an individual case since 75% progress to chronic renal failure over a period of 5–10 years while 25% remit spontaneously during that time. Although steroids have been suggested as a therapeutic agent, the evidence for their value is insubstantial. In progressive cases the glomeruli become increasingly sclerosed resulting in extensive loss of nephrons.

When patients with membranous nephropathy enter pregnancy with normal renal function the prognosis for a successful outcome is good in some series although proteinuria may be increased during pregnancy (Katz et al, 1980). Packham et al (1987) showed increased fetal loss in their series and in some instances worsening of maternal renal function.

Minimal change glomerulonephropathy

Minimal change glomerulonephropathy may develop during the course of pregnancy and be characterized by heavy proteinuria and glomeruli which appear normal by lightmicroscopy (Fig. 56.24). Electronmicroscopy demonstrates loss of the foot processes of the epithelial cells. The aetiology of this condition is unknown although it has sometimes been associated with a type 1 hypersensitivity reaction. The likely mechanism is a circulating factor which destroys or obliterates the glomerular polyanionic components thereby allowing polyanionic substances like serum albumin to pass freely into the urinary space.

Treatment with steroids is usually successful in this condition which has no tendency to progress to renal failure. There is, however, a tendency for proteinuria to be increased during pregnancy and for the infants to be small for gestational age (Katz et al, 1980).

Primary focal and segmental sclerosis and hyalinosis

It has already been mentioned above that segmental sclerosing lesions may develop as a complication of pre-eclampsia. However, some patients enter pregnancy with what for want of a better term is called focal and segmental sclerosis and hyalinosis. Classically this insidious condition presents with persistent proteinuria which fails to respond to steroid therapy. There may also be microscopic haematuria or even a full nephrotic syndrome. The segmental lesions tend to be progressive, leading eventually to hypertension and chronic renal failure. Packham et al (1988a) have shown that when these patients become pregnant both fetal loss and maternal complications are significantly increased.

Mesangiocapillary glomerulonephritis

Mesangiocapillary glomerulonephritis usually presents in adolescence or early adult life. It is always associated with a nephrotic syndrome and there may be some evidence of haematuria during acute exacerbations. The prognosis

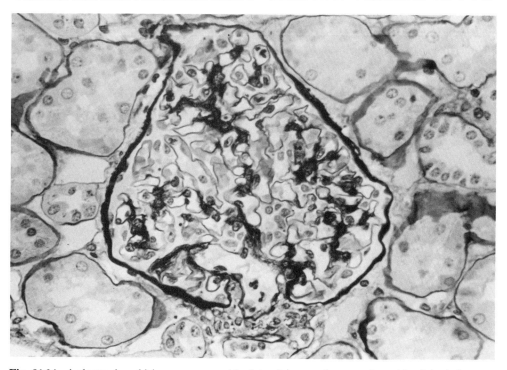

Fig. 56.24 A glomerulus which appears normal by lightmicroscopy from a patient with minimal change disease.

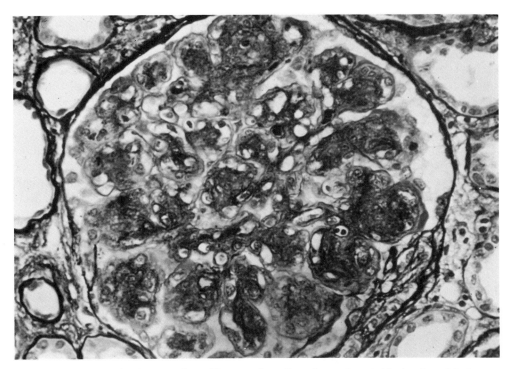

Fig. 56.25 A glomerulus from a patient with mesangiocapillary glomerulonephritis showing a lobular pattern due to marked mesangial cell proliferation.

is uniformly poor with universal progression to chronic renal failure over a period of 5–10 years. Lightmicroscopy shows that there are major abnormalities both in the capillary walls and in the mesangial regions of all glomeruli (Fig. 56.25). There is a tendency of the serum C3 levels to be low in this condition and a fraction called C3 nephritic factor may also be identified in the serum. In the most usual type of mesangiocapillary glomerulonephritis (type I) there are large subendothelial and mesangial deposits of C3 (Fig. 56.26) which seem to stimulate mesangial cell proliferation and subsequent interpositional growth around capillary walls. The capillary lumens become progressively occluded and finally this leads to glomerular sclerosis and nephron loss. There exists a less common type of mesangiocapillary glomerulonephritis called linear-dense deposit disease (type II) in which C3 is deposited within tubular basement membranes, Bowman's capsular basement membranes and the glomerular capillary basement membrane. Despite these differences in the morphological aspects the presentation, clinical features and prognosis are very similar to type I mesangiocapillary disease.

Cameron et al (1983) have shown that in patients with type I MCGN 20 pregnancies resulted in eight live births, five spontaneous abortions and seven induced abortions. In five patients with type II MCGN there were nine pregnancies which resulted in five live births and four induced abortions. Those women who became pregnant and whose pregnancies were allowed to continue were those who still had good renal function and were without hypertension. No deterioration in their renal function was demonstrated during pregnancy. However, if pregnancy had been continued in those patients with hypertension and compromised renal function, it is quite possible that a decline in renal function might be seen, as has been described for other forms of glomerulonephritis (Fairley et al, 1973).

Lupus nephritis

The term lupus nephritis includes a spectrum of glomerular changes from mild mesangial proliferation through increasing degrees of segmental proliferation and necrosis (Fig. 56.27) to a severe diffuse proliferative glomerulonephritis with extensive cellular crescent formation. In addition a greater or lesser degree of membranous pattern of glomerulonephritis may also be superimposed. In contrast to the types of glomerular disorders previously described, where the degree of glomerular abnormality was fairly uniform in a given case, lupus nephritis is characterized by considerable variation of involvement between the glomeruli, such that some may appear only mildly abnormal with a small amount of mesangial proliferation, whilst their neighbours may show severe necrotizing lesions with cellular crescent formation. As a consequence of the variety of immunological reactions which occur in systemic

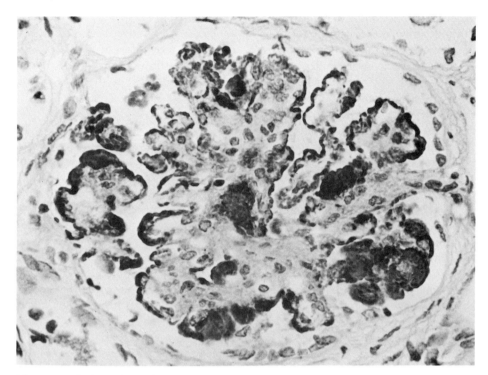

Fig. 56.26 A glomerulus stained to show C3 deposition in a patient with mesangiocapillary glomerulonephritis. Immunoperoxidase technique.

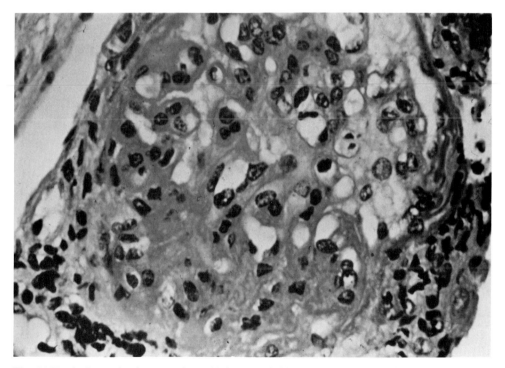

Fig. 56.27 A glomerulus from a patient with lupus nephritis showing cellular proliferation and sclerosis, particularly at the bottom left corner.

lupus a wide range of immunoglobulins and complement components are deposited within the glomeruli and may be identified using immunocytochemical techniques. They are also demonstrable as electron-dense deposits by electronmicroscopy and may occupy subepithelial, sub-endothelial or mesangial positions within the glomeruli. Similar but less obvious deposits may also be present along the tubular basement membranes associated with an interstitial nephritis. Although it is possible to suggest a diagnosis of lupus nephritis from the variable glomerular involvement and variety of immune reactants present in deposits at multiple sites the definitive diagnosis depends on satisfying the criteria of the American Rheumatology Society (Cohen et al, 1971). Since systemic lupus occurs primarily in women during the child-bearing years, the chances of lupus nephritis co-existing with pregnancy must be considered both in patients with pre-existing disease who wish to have children and in pregnancy when systemic lupus may be first diagnosed.

According to an extensive survey by Hayslett & Lynn (1980) the onset of systemic lupus erythematosus during pregnancy causes significant maternal morbidity and fetal loss to the order of 37%. In contrast, patients with known systemic lupus who have been in clinical remission for six months prior to conception have a favourable prognosis for a normal pregnancy and live birth. When the disease has been active during the six months prior to conception the possibility of further exacerbations is likely and the chances of a successful outcome are reduced by about

25%. Overall it appears that steroids are valuable in the suppression of active disease and do not induce developmental abnormalities in the fetus. Buyon (1990) suggests that by monitoring the levels of autoantibodies in the mother the damage to the fetus can be minimized.

Mesangial IgA disease

This is a relatively benign form of glomerular disease which is common in childhood and usually associated with haematuria precipitated by upper respiratory tract infections. Some cases do not present until early adult life and are then more likely to be associated with proteinuria and the development of hypertension. Lightmicroscopy shows mesangial proliferation within the glomerular tufts associated with mesangial deposits of IgA and C3 (Fig. 56.28). In a few glomeruli there may also be segmental proliferation with or without sclerosis. Kincaid-Smith et al (1980) have shown a very high incidence of segmental lesions in mesangial IgA disease following pregnancy and suggest that at least some of these lesions have been acquired as a consequence of pregnancy. They point out that intravascular coagulation is a well-recognized feature of pregnancy and acute thrombotic lesions within a glomerular capillary could explain the development of a segmental sclerosis of the tuft. They also showed that hypertension prior to pregnancy was a poor prognostic feature for fetal survival in their series. Packham et al (1988b) showed that maternal renal function declined in

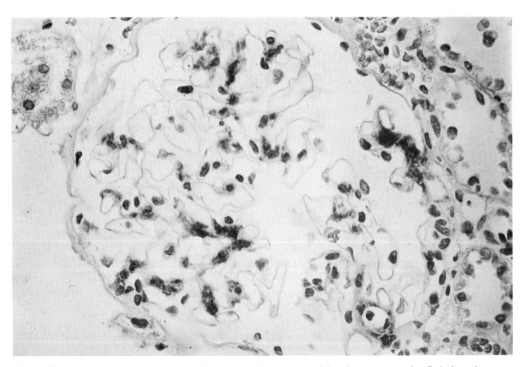

Fig. 56.28 A glomerulus with dark granular staining in the mesangial regions representing IgA deposits. Immunoperoxidase technique.

pregnancy in 26% of cases of a series of 116 pregnancies associated with IgA disease.

Scleroderma

Fortunately scleroderma with renal involvement is an uncommon association with pregnancy but the few reports which do exist demonstrate a disastrous outcome, with maternal death in most cases. As has already been mentioned, the renal vascular lesions of idiopathic postpartum acute renal failure are very similar to those of renal scleroderma with subintimal fibrosis of an extreme degree in arterial walls and fibrinoid necrosis of arterioles (Figs 56.29 and 56.30).

Acute post-infectious glomerulonephritis

The incidence of acute post-infectious glomerulonephritis has fallen to a very low level in recent years and seems to be particularly low in pregnancy, with even those cases suspected clinically proving to be acute exacerbations of more chronic forms of glomerulonephritis when renal biopsy is performed (Bear, 1976b).

Diabetic glomerulopathy

Diabetic glomerulopathy is an important complication of juvenile diabetes and the average time for it to occur is 17 years after the onset of the disease. Therefore some diabetic females will have developed the typical changes of diabetic glomerulopathy by the time they become pregnant. It certainly seems to be true that both pre-eclampsia and leg oedema are more frequent in diabetic women but there are conflicting views as to whether or not pregnancy has an adverse effect on diabetic glomerulopathy. Certainly, in patients who are only mildly affected, pregnancy appears to be well tolerated (Kitzmiller et al, 1981).

In diabetic glomerulopathy there is an excess production of the mucopolysaccharide type of material of which both the glomerular capillary walls and mesangial matrix are formed. The result of this over-production is a uniform thickening of the glomerular basement membranes (so-called diffuse glomerulosclerosis) and an increase in mesangial matrix material (so-called nodular glomerulosclerosis). Usually both patterns co-exist and occasional mesangial nodules may assume a considerable size, when they correspond to the description 'Kimmelstiel–Wilson nodules' (Fig. 56.31). Hyaline deposits due to the insudation of plasma proteins are usually particularly prominent in the walls of afferent arterioles in diabetic kidneys and this phenomenon is also seen in hypertensive vascular disease (Fig. 56.32). However, the presence of hyaline deposits in the walls of efferent arterioles is diagnostic of diabetic nephropathy. Degenerative changes may also be seen in larger vessels but these do not differ in character from those which result from hypertensive disease. It is

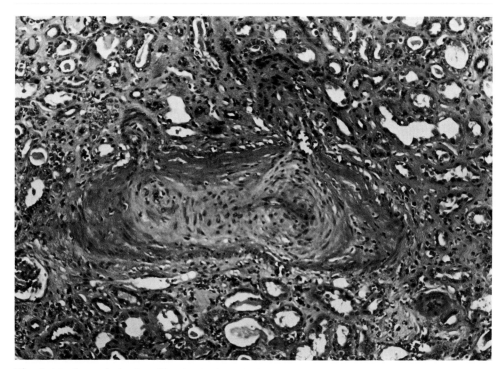

Fig. 56.29 Severe intimal proliferation in the wall of a small renal artery from a patient with scleroderma.

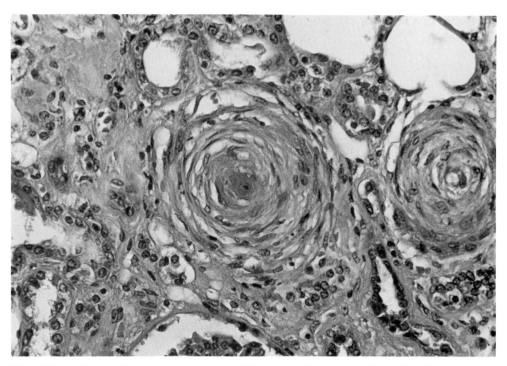

Fig. 56.30 Intimal proliferation and obstruction of the lumen of a renal arteriole by fibrin in a patient with scleroderma.

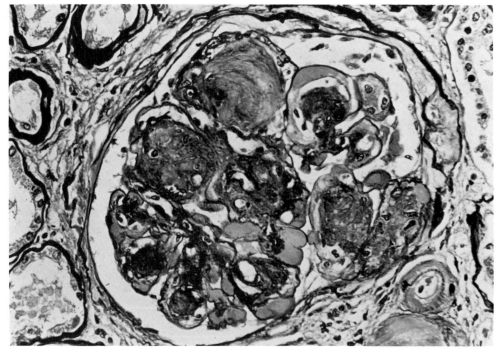

Fig. 56.31 Diabetic glomerulosclerosis with marked proliferation of the mesangial matrix leading to Kimmelstiel–Wilson nodule formation.

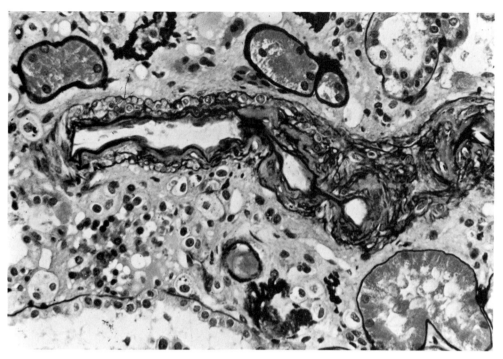

Fig. 56.32 A renal arteriole with irregular thickening of its wall on the right-hand side due to the insudation of hyaline material.

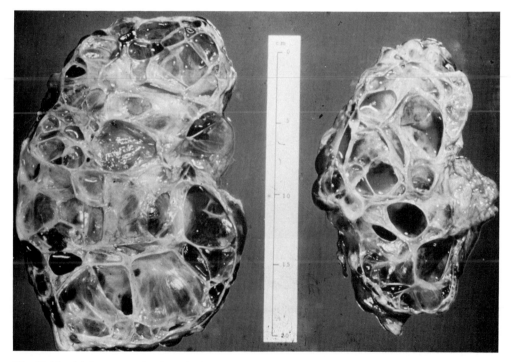

Fig. 56.33 Adult-type renal polycystic disease with extensive replacement of renal parenchyma by cysts of variable size.

now fortunately rare for a patient with diabetes to present with uncontrolled hyperglycaemia. In such a case extensive vacuolation of the renal tubular epithelial cells due to intracytoplasmic glycogen accumulation is described.

Non-glomerular renal diseases co-existing with pregnancy

Adult polycystic renal disease

Adult polycystic renal disease is almost always bilateral and may be discovered during the course of pregnancy. It is an autosomal dominant condition with massive enlargement of the kidneys by cysts of variable size into which haemorrhage may occur. The normal renal parenchyma is progressively destroyed leading eventually to chronic renal failure (Fig. 56.33). Provided the patient does not have hypertension and has reasonably normal renal function by conventional testing the pregnancy will normally proceed satisfactorily to term (Lindheimer & Katz, 1977c). The

presence, however, of two massively enlarged kidneys as well as the enlarged uterus within the abdomen may result in difficulty with respiration.

Pelvic ectopic kidney

The presence of a congenital ectopic kidney within the pelvic cavity may cause difficulty with a normal vaginal delivery and a caesarean section may therefore be required. It should also be noted that a pelvic ectopic kidney may represent a solitary kidney.

Urolithiasis

Urolithiasis is the commonest cause of severe abdominal pain in pregnancy and most of the stones which do occur contain calcium. There does seem to be an increased tendency for urinary tract infection to supervene in such cases (Coe et al, 1978).

REFERENCES

Abitbol M M, Gallo G R, Pirani C L et al 1976 Production of experimental toxemia in the pregnant rabbit. American Journal of Obstetrics and Gynecology 124: 460.

Bear R 1976a Pregnancy and lupus nephritis. Obstetrics and Gynecology 47: 715–719.

Bear R A 1976b Pregnancy in patients with renal disease. Obstetrics and Gynecology 48: 13–18.

Bonnar J 1976 Coagulation disorders. Journal of Clinical Pathology 29(suppl) 10: 35–41.

Brezis M, Rosen S, Silva P, Epstein F H 1984 Renal ischaemia: a new perspective. Kidney International 26: 375–383.

Buyon J P 1990 Systemic lupus erythematosus and the maternal-fetal dyad. Baillières Clinical Rheumatology 4: 85–103.

Cameron J S, Turner D R, Heaton J et al 1983 Idiopathic mesangiocapillary glomerulonephritis: comparison of Type I and II in children and adults and long term prognosis. American Journal of Medicine 74: 175–192.

Campbell D M, MacGillivray I, Thompson B 1977 Twin zygosity and pre-eclampsia. Lancet ii: 97.

Chesley L C 1980 Hypertension in pregnancy: definition, familial factor and remote prognosis. Kidney International 18: 234–240.

Clark B A, Halvorson L, Sachs B, Epstein F H 1992 Plasma endothelin levels in pre-eclampsia, elevation and correlation with uric acid levels and renal impairment. American Journal of Obstetrics and Gynecology 166: 962–968.

Coe F C, Parks J H, Lindheimer M D 1978 Nephrolithiasis during pregnancy. New England Journal of Medicine 298: 324–326.

Cohen A S, Reynolds W E, Franklin E C 1971 Preliminary criteria for the classification of systemic lupus erythematosus. Bulletin of Rheumatological Diseases 21: 643–648.

Cooper D W, Brennecke S P, Wilton A N 1993 Genetics of preeclampsia. Hypertension in Pregnancy 12: 1–23.

Donadio J V, Holley K E 1974 Post-partum acute renal failure: recovery after heparin therapy. American Journal of Obstetrics and Gynecology 118: 510–519.

Emmanuel D S, Lindheimer M D 1976 Recovery after prolonged anuria following septic abortion. Obstetrics and Gynecology 47: 36s–39s.

Eschenbach D A 1976 Urinary tract infections. In: Russell Ramon de Alvarez (ed) The kidney in pregnancy. Wiley, New York, ch 4, p 75.

Fairley K F 1970 The routine determination of the site of infection in the investigation of patients with urinary tract infection. In: Kincaid-Smith P, Fairley K F (eds) Renal infection and renal scarring. Mercedes, Melbourne, p 107.

Fairley K F, Whitworth J A, Kincaid-Smith P 1973 Glomerulonephritis and pregnancy. In: Kincaid-Smith P, Matthew T H, Becker E L (eds) Glomerulonephritis. Wiley, New York, p 997.

Felding C F 1968 Pregnancy following renal diseases. Clinical Obstetrics and Gynecology 11: 579–592.

Foidart J M, Nochy D, Nasgens B et al 1983 Accumulation of several basement membrane proteins in glomeruli of patients with pre-eclampsia and other hypertensive syndromes of pregnancy. Possible role of renal prostaglandins. Laboratory Investigation 49: 250–259.

Friedman E A 1976 Effect of blood pressure on perinatal mortality. In: Friedman E A (ed) Blood pressure edema and proteinuria in pregnancy. A R Liss, New York.

Grünfeld J P, Goneval D, Bournérais F 1980 Acute renal failure in pregnancy. Kidney International 18: 179.

Hayslett J P, Lynn R I 1980 Effect of pregnancy in patients with lupus nephropathy. Kidney International 18: 207–220.

Heaton J M, Turner D R 1985 Persistent renal damage following preeclampsia: a renal biopsy study of 13 patients. Journal of Pathology 147: 121–126.

Heptinstall R H 1992 Pathology of the kidney, 4th edn. Little Brown, Boston, ch 18, p 1289.

Hill P A, Zimmerman M, Fairley K F, Kincaid-Smith P, Ryan G B 1988 Pre-eclampsia: a clinico-pathological study of 23 cases. Clinical and Experimental Hypertension, Part B — Hypertension in Pregnancy 7: 343–358.

Hollenberg H K, Adams D F, Oken D E et al 1970 Acute renal failure due to nephrotoxins: renal hemodynamic and angiographic studies in man. New England Journal of Medicine 282: 1329–1336.

Katz A I, Davison J M, Hayslett J P, Singson E, Lindheimer M D 1980 Pregnancy in women with renal disease. Kidney International 18: 192–206.

Kincaid-Smith P 1983 Reflux nephropathy. British Medical Journal 286: 2002–2003.

Kincaid-Smith P 1991 The renal lesion of pre-eclampsia revisited. American Journal of Kidney Disease 17: 144–148.

Kincaid-Smith P S, Whitworth J A, Fairley K F 1980 Mesangial IgA nephropathy in pregnancy. Clinical and Experimental Hypertension 2: 821–838.

Kitzmiller J L, Brown E R, Phillippe M et al 1981 Diabetic nephropathy and perinatal outcome. American Journal of Obstetrics and Gynecology 141: 741–751.

Kleiner G J, Greston W M 1976 Current concepts of defibrination in the pregnant woman. Journal of Reproductive Medicine 17: 309–317.

Kleinknecht D, Grünfeld J P, Gomes P C 1973 Diagnostic procedures and long-term prognosis in bilateral renal cortical necrosis. Kidney International 4: 390–400.

Kunelis C T, Peters J L, Edmondson H A 1965 Fatty liver of pregnancy and its relationship to tetracycline therapy. American Journal of Medicine 38: 359–377.

Leading Article 1985 Urinary tract infection during pregnancy. Lancet 2: 190.

Lewis P 1982 The role of prostacyclin in pre-eclampsia. British Journal of Hospital Medicine 28: 393–395.

Lindheimer M D, Katz A I 1977a Kidney function and disease in pregnancy. Lea & Febiger, Philadelphia, ch 4, p 114.

Lindheimer M D, Katz A I 1977b Kidney function and disease in pregnancy. Lea & Febiger, Philadelphia, ch 5, p 168.

Lindheimer M D, Katz A I 1977c Kidney function and disease in pregnancy. Lea & Febiger, Philadelphia, ch 5, p 171.

Lindheimer M D, Katz A I 1977d Kidney function and disease in pregnancy. Lea & Febiger, Philadelphia, ch 6, p 193.

MacGillivray I 1981 Raised blood pressure in pregnancy: aetiology of pre-eclampsia. British Journal of Hospital Medicine 26: 110–119.

Morrin P A F, Handa S P, Valberg L S 1967 Acute renal failure in association with fatty liver of pregnancy. Recovery after fourteen days of complete anuria. American Journal of Medicine 42: 844–851.

Norden C W, Tuttle E P 1965 Impairment of urinary concentrating ability in pregnant women with asymptomatic bacteriuria. In: Kass E H (ed) Progress in pyelonephritis. Davis, Philadelphia, p 73.

Packham D K, North R A, Fairley K F, Whitworth J A, Kincaid-Smith P 1987 Membranous glomerulonephritis and pregnancy. Clinical Nephrology 28: 56–64.

Packham D K, North R A, Fairley K F, Hale B U, Whitworth J A, Kincaid-Smith P 1988a Pregnancy in women with primary focal and segmental hyalinosis and sclerosis. Clinical Nephrology 29: 185–192.

Packham D K, North R A, Fairley K F, Whitworth J A, Kincaid-Smith P 1988b IgA glomerulonephritis in pregnancy. Clinical Nephrology 30: 15–21.

Ransley P G, Risdon R A 1978 Reflux and renal scarring. British Journal of Radiology 51 (suppl 14): 1–35.

Reeves D S, Brumfitt W 1968 Localisation of urinary tract infection. In: O'Grady F, Brumfitt W (eds) Urinary tract infection. Oxford University Press, London, p 53.

Robson J A, Martin A M, Ruckley V et al 1968 Irreversible postpartum renal failure: a new syndrome. Quarterly Journal of Medicine 37: 423–455.

Roy First M, Ooi B S, Jao V, Pollak V E 1978 Pre-eclampsia with the nephrotic syndrome. Kidney International 13: 166–177.

Scheer R L, Jones D B 1967 Malignant nephrosclerosis in women postpartum. Journal of the American Medical Association 201: 600–604.

Seymour E Q, Petrucco O M, Clarkson A R et al 1976 Morphological and immunological evidence of coagulopathy in renal complications of pregnancy. In: Lindheimer M D, Katz A I, Zuspan F P (eds) Hypertension in pregnancy. Wiley, New York, p 139.

Sheehan H L 1980 Renal morphology in pre-eclampsia. Kidney International 18: 241–252.

Sheehan H L, Moore H C 1952 Renal cortical necrosis and the kidney of concealed accidental haemorrhage. Blackwell, Oxford.

Sims E A H, Krantz K E 1958 Serial studies of renal function during pregnancy and the puerperium in normal women. Journal of Clinical Investigation 37: 1764–1774.

Slater D N, Hague W M 1984 Renal morphological changes in idiopathic acute fatty liver of pregnancy. Histopathology 8: 567–581.

Spargo B, McCartney C P, Winemiller R 1959 Glomerular capillary endotheliosis in toxemia of pregnancy. Archives of Pathology 68: 593–599.

Sulavik S B 1975 Pulmonary disease. In: Burrow G B, Ferris T F (eds) Medical complications during pregnancy. Saunders, Philadelphia, p 549.

Thomas V, Shelkov A, Forland M 1974 Antibody-coated bacteria in urine and site of urinary tract infection. New England Journal of Medicine 290: 588–590.

Tobon H 1972 Malignant hypertension, uremia and hemolytic anemia in a patient on oral contraceptives. Obstetrics and Gynecology 40: 681–685.

Tribe C R, Smart G E, Davies D R, Mackenzie J C 1979 A renal biopsy study in toxaemia of pregnancy. Journal of Clinical Pathology 32: 681–692.

Turney J H, Marshall D H, Brownjohn A M, Ellis C M, Parsons F M 1990 The evolution of acute renal failure 1956–1988. Quarterly Journal of Medicine 74: 83–104.

Wagoner R D Holley K E, Johson W J 1968 Accelerated nephrosclerosis and post-partum acute renal failure in normotensive patients. Annals of Internal Medicine 69: 237–248.

Whalley P 1967 Bacteriuria of pregnancy. American Journal of Obstetrics and Gynecology 97: 723–738.

Whalley P J, Cunningham F G, Martin F G 1975 Transient renal dysfunction associated with acute pyelonephritis of pregnancy. Obstetrics and Gynecology 46: 174–177.

57. Pathology of the liver and gallbladder in pregnancy

Roderick N. M. MacSween

INTRODUCTION

This chapter deals with the changes which occur in liver function during normal pregnancy, liver diseases which are peculiar to pregnancy, liver disease developing concurrently with and complicating pregnancy, and established liver diseases complicated by pregnancy. Bile composition and gallbladder function in pregnancy are briefly reviewed with particular reference to cholelithiasis.

LIVER FUNCTION DURING NORMAL PREGNANCY

In general the liver functions normally in pregnancy and hepatic function is not markedly impaired (McNair & Jaynes, 1960; Hytten & Leitch, 1971; Seymour & Chadwick, 1979). There is no evidence of any increase in liver size. Spider naevi and palmar erythema, stigmata of chronic liver disease, may appear in late pregnancy but disappear soon after parturition. Total blood volume and cardiac output are increased by some 50%: total hepatic blood flow, however, remains unchanged (Munnell & Taylor, 1947) such that in the third trimester there is a relative decrease of 25–30% in the proportion of the cardiac output which passes through the liver (Robson et al, 1990). Consequently drugs that are cleared by the liver in a blood-flow dependent manner have a reduced clearance rate in pregnancy (Rustgi et al, 1993). Liver biopsy and electronmicroscopic studies have shown no significant alterations, the changes comprising some variation in liver cell size, a mild chronic inflammatory cell infiltrate in the portal tracts, variable changes in glycogen and fat content and some increase in smooth and rough endoplasmic reticulum and increased numbers of peroxisomes (Ingerslev & Teilum, 1945; Antia et al, 1958; Perez et al, 1971).

Standard liver function tests do show changes in the course of pregnancy and these are summarized in Table 57.1 (Haemmerli, 1966; Seymour & Chadwick, 1979; Krejs & Haemmerli, 1982; Krejs, 1983). The serum bilirubin and urinary bile pigments increase occasionally but

Table 57.1 Liver function tests in normal pregnancy

Remain within normal range
Serum aminotransferases
Serum γ-glutamyl transpeptidase
Serum 5-nucleotidase
Prothrombin time
Progressive increase
Serum alkaline phosphatase — × 2–4
Serum cholesterol — × 2
Serum fibrinogen — × 1/2
Bromsulphthalein dye retention — × 5
Progressive decrease
Serum albumin — × 1/3
Serum immunoglobulins — slight
Minor change and variable
Serum bilirubin

Note: all changes maximal at term except for albumin and fibrinogen which fall in the first trimester

the changes are erratic and not dependent on the stage of gestation. Bromsulphthalein (BSP) excretion tests (Combes et al, 1963) showed an increased uptake from the plasma and increased storage in the liver in the last trimester, with reduced active secretion into bile such that the maximal secretory rate (Tm) was reduced by 25%. These indices, however, quickly return to normal after delivery and the changes are thought to be due mainly to oestrogens (Kern et al, 1978). Changes in bile flow and in bile composition in pregnancy are discussed in the section on gallbladder function and gallstones in pregnancy.

The serum alkaline phosphatase shows a progressive increase and in the third trimester the levels are two to four times normal. The crude increase is largely due to placental alkaline phosphatase which constitutes 50% of the serum content at term; the bone iso-enzyme is also increased. However, the hepatic iso-enzyme also shows an increase in the last trimester, a change which suggests that pregnancy normally exerts a cholestatic effect. The serum levels of alkaline phosphatase may remain elevated for four to six weeks postpartum (Krejs, 1983).

Total serum protein concentration falls by 10 g/l in the first half of pregnancy and remains fairly constant thereafter. The reduction is due to haemodilution and mainly affects the albumin level with a small decrease in immunoglobulin levels. The albumin level is reduced by 35% at term. In contrast, fibrinogen levels are significantly increased from mid-term; α and β globulins, caeruloplasmin, transferrin and a number of other carrier proteins are slightly increased in the third trimester. These serum protein changes may persist for six to 12 weeks after delivery (Krejs, 1983). There is a slight increase in the level of unconjugated bile acids and there is a reduction in the enterohepatic circulation of bile acids.

Serum lipids of all classes increase through to term. The greatest changes affect triglycerides and cholesterol, which increase by 300% and 60% respectively, while phospholipids increase by 5% (Svanborg & Vikrot, 1965).

Liver function tests that remain normal in pregnancy

Disturbances of these are of most diagnostic help in suspected hepatic dysfunctions. The important indices are the serum aminotransferases, serum γ-glutamyl transpeptidase, serum 5-nucleotidase and the prothrombin time.

LIVER DISEASES PECULIAR TO PREGNANCY

Intrahepatic cholestasis of pregnancy

First described by Ahlfeld in 1883 (Ikonen, 1964), the classical accounts of the syndrome are those of Svanborg (1954) and Thorling (1955) from Sweden. More recently, Reyes and his colleagues from Chile have reported large series of cases and have reviewed this syndrome (Reyes et al, 1976, 1978; Reyes, 1982, 1992; Reyes & Simon, 1993). The syndrome has been variously referred to as hepatitis of pregnancy, jaundice of late pregnancy, recurrent jaundice of pregnancy, cholestatic jaundice of pregnancy and intrahepatic cholestasis of pregnancy, the description which is now favoured.

Whereas in most countries intrahepatic cholestasis of pregnancy occurs rarely, with a prevalence of between 1 in 1000 and 1 in 10 000 pregnancies (Haemmerli, 1966; Reyes, 1982), there is a 10–20-fold greater prevalence in Scandinavian countries, Poland, Chile and Bolivia (Reyes, 1982, 1992). In Chile it occurs in approximately 14% of full-term pregnancies, a figure which is peculiarly high and considerably greater than in some neighbouring South American countries (Reyes, 1982, 1992). In Chile and Bolivia the prevalence varies in different ethnic groups; it was over 20% in Chileans of Indian descent, and in Bolivia the prevalence of 8% in whites was a little less than half that found in indigenous Indians or people of Indian extraction (Reyes, 1992). There is a very low incidence in Oriental countries and among Negro populations. The prevalence of the syndrome has also showed changes with time and in Chile it fell between 1970 and 1980 but it has risen again since the mid 1980s (Reyes, 1992). A seasonal variation in incidence was reported in Finland with a higher incidence in winter (Laatikainen & Ikonen, 1975).

The classical clinical picture comprises pruritus developing in the third trimester of pregnancy, followed one to two weeks later by mild jaundice of an obstructive pattern with pale stools and dark urine. The pruritus varies in intensity, is worse at night and can be severe and incapacitating. Jaundice may not develop in some cases, and it is now generally accepted that so-called pruritus gravidarum is one end of the clinical spectrum and that a distinction between it and intrahepatic cholestasis of pregnancy is unnecessary; the biochemical abnormalities in the two conditions are similar but tend to be greater in the icteric patient (Reyes, 1982). The pruritus and jaundice persist until term and then quickly resolve in all cases, the pruritus remitting in 24–48 hours and seldom persisting more than one week after delivery, the jaundice in one to two weeks but occasionally persisting for a month. This rapid resolution postpartum is a diagnostic feature; persistence of pruritus or biochemical abnormalities for more than three months should raise the suspicion of some other cholestatic liver disorder.

The clinical pattern described is seen in 70% of cases, but in the remainder the picture is variable; pruritus may occur between weeks 25 and 29 or, exceptionally, earlier, but only very rarely in the first trimester. The jaundice may not develop for some weeks after the pruritus or may not occur at all; there is no correlation between the severity of the pruritus and the presence of, or the degree of, icterus. The syndrome also shows individual variability, some patients having recurrent cholestasis in each pregnancy, others having one or more asymptomatic pregnancies before the first cholestatic episode, and still others having pruritus and/or cholestasis in an unpredictable sequence in consecutive pregnancies (Furhoff, 1974; Reyes, 1982). Only rarely, however, does a woman who has had jaundice in one pregnancy have subsequent pregnancies in which a cholestatic syndrome does not develop, although this may show variation in its time of onset and in its severity (Reyes, 1982). The syndrome is more frequent when the pregnancy is multiple; in addition, in nulliparous women who developed intrahepatic cholestasis with a twin pregnancy, it did not recur with subsequent single pregnancies but only with twin pregnancies (Gonzales et al, 1989). Vanjak et al (1991) reported a single case in which there was an association between intrahepatic cholestasis of pregnancy and acute fatty liver of pregnancy (Vanjak et al, 1991). Co-existence of these two disorders has also been reported from Chile (Reyes et al, 1994) but the association was considered to be fortuitous. The patients generally feel well, although there is often an increased incidence of 'morning sickness' in early pregnancy (Johnson et al, 1975a). The liver and spleen are not usually palpable.

Liver function tests show a cholestatic pattern: the serum bilirubin does not usually exceed 85 µmol/l and fluctuates from week to week; the alkaline phosphatase is increased above the levels seen in normal pregnancy, may be by five to tenfold normal, and may persist at a high level or even increase for six to ten weeks after delivery (Haemmerli & Wyss, 1967); serum 5-nucleotidase is increased two to threefold; the aminotransferases may increase up to 250 U/l and, while considerably greater increases up to 1000 U/l have been reported, such levels should make one suspect acute hepatitis; the prothrombin time may be prolonged in cases with protracted jaundice but is quickly corrected by vitamin K administration.

Serum lipids, cholesterol, triglycerides and phospholipids are higher than in normal pregnancy (Johnson, 1975; Johnson et al, 1975b). The increase in serum triglycerides is greater than in other cholestatic syndromes (Johnson, 1975). In addition, there is evidence of altered lecithin metabolism in the liver, an abnormality which may be primary, which persists after delivery (Samsioe et al 1975, 1977) and which may be a factor predisposing to the twofold increased frequency of gallstones which occurs in women with intrahepatic cholestasis of pregnancy (Thorling, 1955). There is evidence of altered glucose metabolism with higher post-prandial and post-loading glucose levels than occur in matched pregnant controls (Wojcicka-Jagodzinska et al, 1989).

Serum total bile acids show increases up to 100-fold normal with a proportionately greater increase in cholic acid, in both serum and gallbladder bile, as compared with chenodeoxycholic and deoxycholic acid, and in comparison with that which occurs in normal pregnancy (Laatikainen & Ikonen, 1977; Laatikainen et al, 1978). The increases in serum bile acids have been shown to precede the onset of jaundice (Reyes, 1982). The levels return to normal within a few days of delivery. The bile acids are considered to be responsible for the pruritus.

Histological features

These are non-specific. There is a mild, often inconspicuous, cholestasis with perivenular hepatocellular and canalicular bile retention. This may be focal in the liver, suggesting a heterogeneous acinar response to the aetiological factor. Mild reactive Kupffer cell hyperplasia is evident but there is no liver cell necrosis and the portal tracts are healthy. Ultrastructural studies have also shown non-specific changes comprising liver cell swelling and loss of canalicular microvilli, features common to bile retention from any cause (Haemmerli, 1966; Adlercreutz et al, 1967; Kater & Mistilis, 1967). The changes revert to nor-

mal after delivery. The syndrome is thus one in which, as Haemmerli (1966) succinctly pointed out, 'cholestasis is clinically marked, biochemically moderate and histologically minimal'.

Pathogenetic mechanisms

The precise mechanisms of the cholestasis are not clear (Schorr-Lesnick et al, 1991a; Reyes, 1992; Reyes & Simon, 1993). No common environmental factors have been identified but the geographical variation in incidence suggests that genetic predisposition may be important. The studies of Reyes and his colleagues in Chile showing differences in incidence between descendants of different aboriginal groups also point to the importance of genetic factors (Reyes, 1982, 1992; Reyes & Simon, 1993). Familial aggregation of cases (Reyes et al, 1978; Reyes, 1982) and retrospective studies showing familial aggregation of intrahepatic cholestasis of pregnancy and contraceptive steroid induced cholestasis (Dalen & Westerholm, 1974) further support this concept. However, no specific genetic or phenotypic markers have been identified (Reyes, 1982); no particular associations with HLA antigens have been established although HLA B8 and BW16 seem to be more frequent in affected individuals (Schorr-Lesnick et al, 1991a).

There is much evidence in favour of the postulate that there is an unusual or hypersensitive reaction to oestrogens and/or progestagens (Reyes & Simon, 1993). Reduced biliary excretion of oestrogens (Adlercreutz et al, 1974) has been reported, and steroids not normally found in serum have been described in patients with intrahepatic cholestasis of pregnancy (Adlercreutz & Tenhunen, 1970). Low serum selenium and glutathione peroxidase activity has been demonstrated (Kauppila et al, 1987); the authors postulated that this provided indirect evidence that the capacity of the liver to metabolize oestrogen oxidation products was reduced. However, these various changes could well be secondary to the cholestasis and no specific cholestatic-producing metabolite has been identified.

The observations that women with intrahepatic cholestasis of pregnancy develop pruritus and abnormal liver function tests following oestrogen administration (Kreek et al, 1967a,b; Kreek & Sleisenger, 1970; Kreek, 1987) and that a history of 'pill-induced' cholestasis is frequently found in patients with intrahepatic cholestasis of pregnancy (Dalen & Westerholm, 1974; Kreek, 1987) strongly suggests that there is an increased sensitivity to steroid hormones in these patients. Following administration of low doses of oestrogens bromsulphthalein clearance tests were impaired in multiparous women with a past history of intrahepatic cholestasis of pregnancy, and in nulliparous women and males from families with a history of intrahepatic cholestasis of pregnancy, when compared with multiparous women with previous normal pregnancies (Reyes et al, 1981). These observations suggest a familial predisposition in intrahepatic cholestasis of pregnancy characterized by an exaggerated response to oestrogens; this exaggerated response, however, is independent of pregnancy itself (Vore, 1987). However, not all women with previous cholestasis in pregnancy show such an exaggerated response to oestrogen administration (Rannevik et al, 1972), so that its precise rôle is uncertain and other, possibly exogenous factors, as yet unknown, must be involved (Vore, 1987; Reyes, 1992).

The mechanism of action of oestrogens in producing the cholestasis is not fully understood (Reyes & Simon, 1993). Postulated effects include alteration in bile salt and electrolyte transport at the sinusoidal domains, decreased plasma membrane fluidity with a resultant change in lipid composition, again at the sinusoidal domain, and decreased bile flow and transport with increased permeability of the biliary tree.

Fetal and maternal effects

Despite an earlier assertion to the contrary (Haemmerli & Wyss, 1967), several studies have demonstrated high rates of fetal distress during labour and an increased risk of prematurity and fetal death (Kater & Mistilis, 1967; Reid et al, 1976; Furhoff & Hellstrom, 1973; Reyes, 1982). The prematurity rate and stillbirths may be as high as 54% and 9% respectively (Reyes, 1982). A positive correlation was shown between prematurity and the time of onset of pruritus but there was no correlation with the degree of hyperbilirubinaemia (Reyes, 1982). Reyes et al (1987) could not demonstrate a direct relationship between steatorrhoea or maternal nutritional impairment and fetal prognosis. The effects on the fetus may be due to bile acids or other metabolites which cross the placenta (Laatikainen, 1975). Non-specific degenerative changes in the placenta may contribute to this transfer (Laatikainen & Ikonen, 1977). Careful antenatal care is required and induction of labour may be indicated after 37 weeks (Reid et al, 1976).

The mother may suffer considerable morbidity because of the severity of the pruritus. Steatorrhoea occurs due to reduced bile secretions and may affect maternal nutrition (Reyes, 1982; Reyes et al, 1987). Vomiting tends to be more frequent and may be prolonged (Johnson et al, 1975a). There is an increased risk of postpartum haemorrhage, probably related to vitamin K deficiency. There is no evidence of any long-term effects on hepatic function (Furhoff & Hellstrom, 1974). There is, however, an increased frequency of gallstones, both on early follow-up and on follow-up after 15 years (Furhoff, 1974; Furhoff & Hellstrom, 1974; Glasinovic et al, 1989), the overall prevalence being twice or more that found in a similar normal population. The effects of normal pregnancy on gallbladder function are discussed elsewhere in this chapter. However, it is noteworthy that the fasting volume of the gallbladder may show an even greater increase in pregnancy complicated by intrahepatic cholestasis (Ylostalo et al, 1981).

Acute fatty liver of pregnancy

Although cases had clearly occurred previously (Stander & Cadden, 1934) it was Sheehan (1940) who first recognized the distinctive pathological features of obstetric acute yellow atrophy of the liver and differentiated this condition from acute yellow atrophy complicating viral and toxic hepatitis. His classical description of the histological findings in what is now referred to as acute fatty liver of pregnancy has not been improved upon.

The clinical features are reviewed in papers by Ober & Le Compte (1955), Moore (1956), Breen et al (1970), Davies et al (1980), Varner & Rinderknechts (1980), Burroughs et al (1982), Hague et al (1983), Pockros et al (1984), Rolfes & Ishak (1985), Riely (1987), Burroughs (1991), Schorr-Lesnick et al (1991a), Mabie (1992) and Reyes et al (1994). The prevalence is approximately 1 in 13 000. There is no racial variation in incidence (Pockros et al, 1984). Patients present in the last trimester of pregnancy, the large majority after the 35th week but some as early as 30 weeks and occasional cases postpartum. Primigravidae are more affected than multiparae, frequently there is a twin pregnancy, and male births are more common than female. Following a prodromal illness of three to seven days with general malaise but no marked fever, there is nausea, severe vomiting, frequently of altered blood and sometimes with frank haematemesis, associated with upper abdominal pain and tenderness; polydipsia with or without polyuria is a frequent feature; jaundice develops and then there is usually rapid progression to fulminant liver failure with fever, encephalopathy and coma. Many cases have hypertension and proteinuria suggesting toxaemia of pregnancy, a differential diagnosis which has to be considered (Burroughs et al, 1982; Rolfes & Ishak, 1986a,b). There is usually a marked neutrophil leucocytosis and haematological and biochemical evidence of disseminated intravascular coagulation is present with an increased prothrombin and partial thromboplastin time (Liebman et al, 1983; Pockros et al, 1984; Riely, 1987). This disturbance of coagulation accounts for many of the fatal complications of the disease; it is worth noting that it may even worsen after delivery (Pockros et al, 1984). The presence of circulating normoblasts, noted by Sheehan (1961), has been emphasized by Burroughs et al (1982) who noted them in blood films from 10 of 11 cases; they also found giant platelets. Ultrasonography showing increased echogenicity (Campillo et al, 1986) and computed tomography (Mabie et al, 1989) showing decreased attenuation are useful non-invasive methods of confirming fatty infiltration in the liver.

Biochemically, the hyperbilirubinaemia is moderate,

usually less than 150 μmol/l, but rarely it may exceed 350 μmol/l with peak levels occurring postpartum; the alkaline phosphatase is slightly greater than in normal pregnancy; the aminotransferases are variably raised, 100–1000 U/l (the aspartate aminotransferase being higher) and fall quickly after delivery; the prothrombin time is usually prolonged two to four times the normal; hypoglycaemia is often severe and may contribute to early coma; there is marked elevation in serum ammonia but, in contrast to fulminant viral or drug-induced hepatitis, there is a generalized fall in serum amino acids although glutamine, alanine and lysine levels may be raised (Burroughs et al, 1982); hyperuricaemia regularly occurs in the early stages and may, in part, be due to reduced renal clearance; serum immunoglobulin levels are not increased and this contrasts with the findings in acute viral hepatitis; serum amylase and lipase may be elevated because of an associated pancreatitis (Riely, 1987).

Histological features

Sheehan's description (1940) reads: '. . . there was a gross fatty change affecting the entire lobule except a sharply defined rim of normal cells around the portal tracts. The affected cells were bloated by a fine foam of tiny white vacuoles throughout the cytoplasm so that they resembled the cells of suprarenal cortex. The nuclei were normal and there was an entire absence of necrobiotic change'. These features are shown in Figures 57.1–57.3. The degree of fat accumulation may not be readily appreciated in paraffin-embedded sections and in suspected cases an oil Red-O staining of frozen sections is indicated (Fig. 57.2). In some cases the fatty change may be diffuse without periportal sparing (Burroughs et al, 1982). Canalicular and hepatocellular bilirubinostasis are present. There is Kupffer cell hyperplasia and aggregates of ceroid-laden macrophages are conspicuous. There is usually only a very

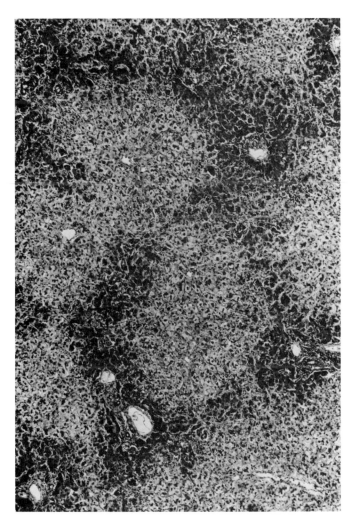

Fig. 57.1 Acute fatty liver of pregnancy: the darker staining periportal areas (zone 1 of the acinus) contrast with the paler fat-containing areas surrounding the hepatic veins and involving zones 2 and 3 of the acinus. Masson trichrome × 40.

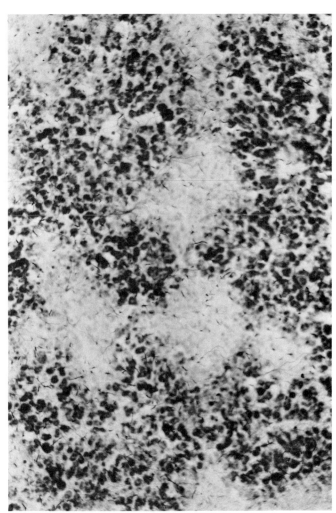

Fig. 57.2 Acute fatty liver of pregnancy: the distribution and the extent of lipid deposition is better appreciated on an oil Red-O stained frozen section. × 45.

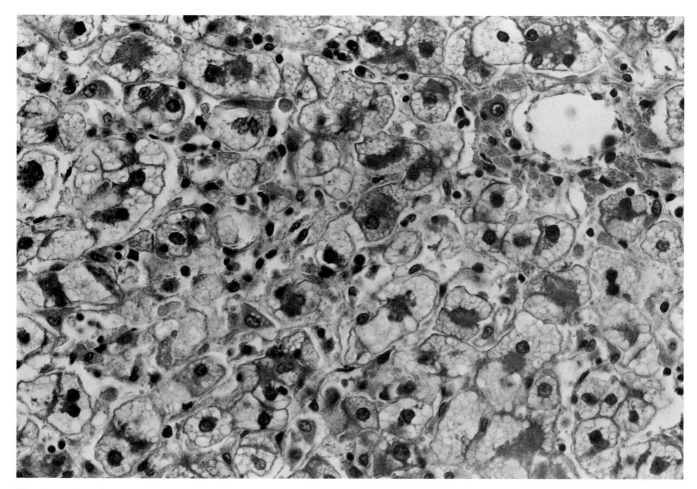

Fig. 57.3   Acute fatty liver of pregnancy: the liver cells in the perivenular area are swollen and their cytoplasm contains numerous small fat vesicles which surround the nucleus. There is a very light mononuclear cell infiltrate and some Kupffer cell hyperplasia. Masson trichrome × 860.

mild inflammatory cell reaction (Fig. 57.3), characterized by a mononuclear cell infiltrate in the parenchyma and portal tracts, sometimes with numbers of eosinophils and occasional plasma cells. Extramedullary haemopoiesis is often present. Intrasinusoidal fibrin deposits have also been noted and may occasionally be associated with small haemorrhages (Burroughs et al, 1982).

Cell necrosis is not a conspicuous feature on the haematoxylin and eosin stain. However, a reticulin stain (Fig. 57.4) does show evidence of liver cell loss indicating hepatocytolysis (Burroughs et al, 1982; Malatjalian & Badley, 1983). At autopsy the liver is usually small and, as Burroughs and his colleagues (1982) have pointed out, the reduced liver weight in the presence of fat accumulation does indicate substantial liver cell loss. A pattern of mid-zonal necrosis was noted in one case by Joske and his colleagues (1968). Biopsies in survivors have demonstrated progressive disappearance of the fat from the periportal to the perivenular zone (Duma et al, 1965) and, in the author's experience, this occurs within a few days of parturition.

Ultrastructural studies (Weber et al, 1979; Burroughs et al, 1982) have shown that the fat is not membrane bound: there is dilatation of the rough endoplasmic reticulum and some cells show cytoplasmic degeneration with autophagic vacuoles (Figs 57.5 and 57.6). The mitochondria show considerable variation in size, with many of giant and elongated appearance. A honeycomb appearance of the smooth endoplasmic reticulum has also been reported (Duma et al, 1965).

Maternal and fetal effects

The maternal and fetal mortality rates have been considered to be very high, in the order of 75–85% (Hatfield et al, 1972; Varner & Rinderknechts, 1980). However, in the series reported by Burroughs et al (1982), the maternal mortality was 33% and the fetal mortality 66%, and they drew attention to the wide range in the severity of the illness. Pockros and his colleagues (1984) reported a maternal mortality of 2/18 (11%) and a fetal mortality of 5/20 (25%), an improved survival which they attributed

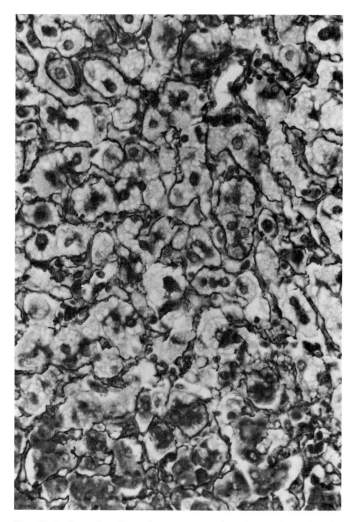

Fig. 57.4 Acute fatty liver of pregnancy: perivenular condensation of the reticulin framework as shown here indicates that there has been earlier hepatocytolysis. Gordon & Sweet's reticulin × 430.

to improved supportive therapy. Milder, non-fatal forms of the disease also occur (Bernuau et al, 1982; Pockros et al, 1984; Tsuki et al, 1984; Ebert et al, 1984; Hou et al, 1984; Riely 1984) and this will become increasingly recognized in patients who manifest milder symptomatology and biochemical abnormalities in the last trimester of pregnancy. Liver transplantation has been carried out in two cases (Ockner et al, 1990; Amon et al, 1993).

Maternal death is usually due to extrahepatic manifestations, massive gastrointestinal haemorrhage, usually from the oesophagus and/or stomach, disseminated intravascular coagulation or renal failure. Fatty infiltration of renal tubular epithelium has been reported (Slater & Hague, 1984). Pancreatitis may occur, sometimes with peripancreatic bleeding (Riely, 1987). In mothers who recover there is no evidence of any residual chronic liver disease and subsequent uncomplicated pregnancy is well documented (Duma et al, 1965; Breen et al, 1972;

Mackenna et al, 1977; Davies et al, 1980; Jenkins & Darling, 1980; Burroughs et al, 1982; Riely, 1984). There are now, however, three case reports of recurrent acute fatty liver of pregnancy (Barton et al, 1990; Schoeman et al, 1991; Reyes et al, 1994). The case reported by Schoeman and his colleagues is of interest because both infants, delivered by caesarean section, subsequently died at 6½ and 6 months of age. At autopsy they were found to have widespread fatty infiltration of liver, heart, kidney and skeletal muscle, thought to be due to an ill-defined disorder of long chain fatty acid oxidation.

Fetal death is due to stillbirth or prematurity and mild fatty change has been noted in the livers of stillborn infants (Haemmerli, 1966). Surviving infants have no abnormalities. There is a high incidence of male births (Burroughs et al, 1982).

Pathogenetic mechanisms

The aetiology of acute fatty liver of pregnancy is not known. There is no evidence of a genetic or metabolic defect and this would be improbable in view of the occurrence of subsequent normal pregnancies. Sherlock (1983) drew attention to the fact that a similar histological feature of microvesicular steatosis occurs in a number of other conditions:

a. Intravenous administration of tetracycline (Kunelis, 1965; Peters et al, 1967) and this has been reported in pregnant and non-pregnant women.

b. Sodium valproate toxicity (Gerber et al, 1979; Zimmerman & Ishak, 1982).

c. Reye's syndrome, the salient features of which are reviewed by Mowat (1983). It predominantly affects children, follows a mild, unremarkable, viral-like illness and is characterized by vomiting, coma and hypoglycaemia, raised aminotransferases and diffuse hepatic changes with inconspicuous necrosis. Circumstantial evidence of an association with salicylates has been produced.

d. Vomiting disease of Jamaica (Hill, 1952; Tanaka et al, 1976) which also affects children and is due to a toxic metabolite, hypolycin A, derived from Ackee apples.

Other microvesicular fat diseases involving the liver include congenital defects of urea cycle enzymes, Wolman's disease, cholesterol ester storage disease, Labrea hepatitis and alcoholic liver disease (for review see Burroughs, 1991 and Mabie, 1992).

Whether there is a final common pathway by which some of these different conditions produce a microvesicular steatosis in the liver is uncertain. On the basis of the effects of tetracycline and a similar effect of ethionine in experimental animals, it has been suggested that there is interference with lipoprotein metabolism, in particular inhibition of apoprotein synthesis with consequent reduced

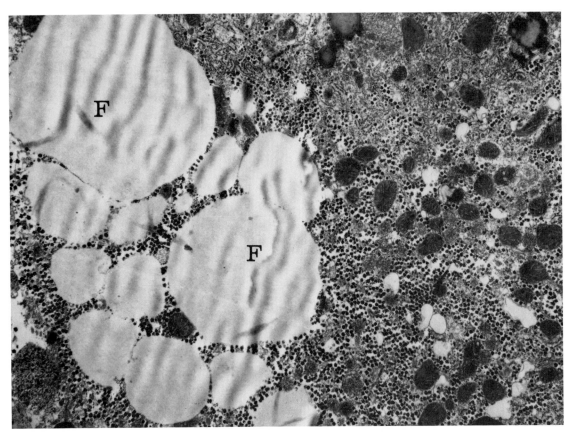

Fig. 57.5 Acute fatty liver of pregnancy: electronmicrograph showing non-membrane bound fat vacuoles (F) containing slightly osmophilic material. × 9000. (Reprinted with permission from Burroughs et al, 1982.)

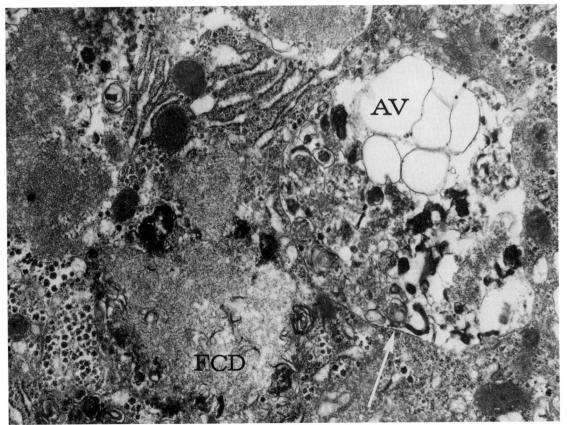

Fig. 57.6 Acute fatty liver of pregnancy: electronmicrograph showing fibrillar material in an area of focal cytoplasmic degeneration (FCD) and a single-membrane-bound autophagic vacuole (AV). × 22 500. (Reprinted with permission from Burroughs et al, 1982.)

removal of lipid from the liver. Studies on the nature of the fat accumulation in acute fatty liver of pregnancy showed that it comprises free fatty acids (Eisele et al, 1975) but the amounts present may be less than reported by these authors (Ockner et al, 1990). In contrast, in Reye's syndrome and other types of fatty liver, triglycerides accumulate. If this is confirmed then it would suggest that fatty liver of pregnancy is a distinctive lesion and pathogenetically unrelated to the other disorders which it morphologically resembles. On the basis of a clinical response to carnitine replacement Feller et al (1983) postulated that the syndrome may be due to carnitine loss enhanced by a period of undernutrition in late pregnancy. Acute fatty liver of pregnancy often occurs in patients with signs of toxaemia of pregnancy leading to the suggestion that it is part of the spectrum of pre-eclampsia (Riely, 1987; Burroughs, 1991). Minakami et al (1988), using the oil Red-O stain, reported microvesicular steatosis in all 41 liver biopsies in cases of pre-eclampsia, although only 11 had visible fat using haematoxylin and eosin and other conventional stains. Rolfes & Ishak (1986a,b), however, were of the opinion that there was no histological similarity between acute fatty liver and the liver changes in pre-eclampsia and eclampsia (see below).

Mitochondrial injury or an inherited or acquired deficiency of mitochondrial beta-oxidation pathway of fatty acids could also lead to microvesicular fat accumulation. Treem et al (1994) reported a patient with acute fatty liver of pregnancy whose child developed hypoglycaemia, coma and hepatic steatosis at 4 months of age. The child was shown to have defective fatty acid oxidation with long-chain 3-hydroxyacyl-coenzyme A dehydrogenase deficiency. The mother was subsequently shown to be heterozygous for this mitochondrial enzyme deficiency. Decreased mitochondrial oxidation of fatty acids has been demonstrated during late-term pregnancy in mice (Grimbert et al, 1993) and a syndrome similar to acute fatty liver of pregnancy occurs in sheep. Known as twin-lamb disease, it develops in the later stages of pregnancy, remits with parturition and is characterized by a severe fatty liver and fat accumulation in proximal renal tubules (Ferris et al, 1969). Further investigation of these animal models may shed some light on the obscure pathogenesis of acute fatty liver of pregnancy in the human.

The liver in toxaemia of pregnancy

The pathogenesis of toxaemia of pregnancy is discussed elsewhere in this text. Here we are concerned only with the pathological effects of toxaemia on the liver. In pre-eclampsia, minor non-specific hepatic changes have been noted with some hepatocellular pleomorphism and some reactive Kupffer cell hyperplasia (Antia et al, 1958). If jaundice occurs in the early stages it is haemolytic in type and in Sheehan's experience (1940, 1961) this affected 10% of fatal cases of toxaemia. Haemmerli (1966), in his review of 456 cases of jaundice in pregnancy, attributed 21 to toxaemia, an incidence of just under 5%. The jaundice is usually mild with serum bilirubin levels of less than 100 μmol/l, although in occasional cases the jaundice may be severe and first bring the patient to clinical notice (Killam et al, 1975; Long et al, 1977). In addition to the increase in bilirubin the alkaline phosphatase is also elevated and aminotransferase levels may be in the range of 500–1000 U/l.

The overall incidence of liver dysfunction in toxaemia of pregnancy has been reported as less than 50% (Haemmerli, 1966). Clinically, the patient with toxaemia may complain of some upper abdominal pain, the liver may be enlarged and is often tender. In Barron's experience (1992) pre-eclampsia is the commonest cause of hepatic tenderness and abnormal liver function tests in pregnancy and, in his view, hepatic involvement in pre-eclampsia always indicates severe maternal disease. Splenomegaly and frank evidence of acute liver failure do not occur.

The peculiar liver lesion which characterizes fatal cases of toxaemia of pregnancy comprises periportal intrasinusoidal fibrin deposition with irregular areas of liver cell necrosis and with a minimal inflammatory reaction (Figs 57.7 and 57.8). The hepatic arteries and arterioles in the immediately adjacent segment of the portal tract show plasmatic vasculosis with seepage of fibrin into their walls (Fig. 57.8). It seems likely that it is damage to these vessels which is responsible for the leakage of fibrin into the periportal parenchyma. Sheehan (1940) suggested that these changes were due to arteriolar spasm. More recently Rolfes & Ishak (1986a,b) also proposed that there is segmental vasospasm and vasodilation of hepatic arterioles with consequent damage to endothelial cells. It seems likely that the changes are similar to those occurring in other organs in severe toxaemia and that the initial injury is to the endothelial cell with consequent activation of intravascular coagulation. Sheehan (1940) found these periportal lesions in 90% of fatal cases, and he thought they developed in the last one to two days of life. However, Antia et al (1958) found the lesions in only five of 15 cases. In fatal cases with circulatory shock, due for example to hepatic rupture, perivenular ischaemic necrosis will also be present affecting zones three and two of the acinus.

In a study in which liver biopsies were carried out on 12 women with toxaemia (seven of whom had elevated serum aspartate aminotransferase and lactic dehydrogenase levels), 10 biopsies showed only minor changes on light-microscopy and in two there were focal areas of eosinophilic/fibrinoid necrosis (Arias & Marchilla-Jimenez, 1976). Using a direct immunofluorescence method, generalized and diffuse sinusoidal staining was demonstrated in all 12 biopsies with an anti-serum to fibrinogen, and, in

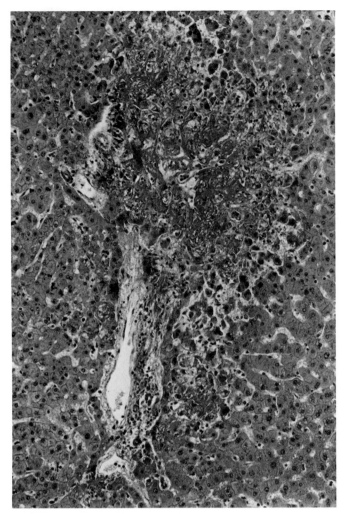

Fig. 57.7 Toxaemia of pregnancy: an irregular flame-shaped area of necrosis with fibrin deposition involving part of the periportal area. MSB × 110.

areas of necrosis, IgG, IgM and the C3 component of complement were also demonstrable. IgM and C3 deposition was also present in hepatic arterioles; no such deposits were demonstrated in biopsies from normal pregnant women. If these findings are confirmed they would suggest that in pre-eclampsia intrasinusoidal fibrin/fibrinogen deposition commonly occurs in the liver, similar to the changes which affect renal glomeruli (Vassalli et al, 1963).

The HELLP syndrome

Weinstein (1982) described 29 cases of severe pre-eclampsia/eclampsia complicated by haemolysis (H), elevated liver enzymes (EL) and a low platelet (LP) count. He suggested that this constituted a syndrome separate from severe pre-eclampsia. There has been considerable controversy and confusion, however, as to whether HELLP is a variant of pre-eclampsia/eclampsia or whether it represents a mild form of disseminated intravascular coagula-

tion — DIC (MacKenna et al, 1983; Weinstein, 1985; Sibai et al 1986; Martin et al, 1990; Sibai, 1990; Schorr-Lesnick et al, 1991b; Barton & Sibai, 1992). Barton & Sibai (1992) have defined the criteria for the HELLP syndrome: (i) haemolysis with an abnormal peripheral blood smear in which burr cells, schistocytes and spherocytes are present; (ii) a bilirubin level of > 25 μmol/l; (iii) serum aminotransferase levels greater than 70 U/l and lactate dehydrogenase levels greater than 600 U/l; (iv) a platelet count less than 100 000/mm³.

It is estimated that 2–12% of patients with toxaemia of pregnancy develop the HELLP syndrome. It occurs predominantly in multiparous women over 25 years old. Some cases occur a few hours to six days postpartum, (Barton & Sibai, 1992). Patients present with nausea or vomiting, epigastric or right upper quadrant pain, and headache. There may be oedema and the diastolic blood pressure is usually greater than 100 mmHg. Maternal complications include placental abruption, acute renal failure and hepatic rupture, with a maternal mortality rate of 3%. Recurrence of the syndrome has been reported in only one instance (Sibai et al, 1986). There is an increased incidence of intrauterine growth retardation and prematurity, and infants of affected mothers may have thrombocytopenia with DIC; the overall perinatal mortality rate is around 35%.

The liver biopsy shows features of a non-specific reactive hepatitis with a mild portal tract chronic inflammatory cell infiltrate. However, in some cases periportal or focal parenchymal necrosis with a fibrin exudate has been reported, similar to that described in eclampsia. Intrahepatic haemorrhage and subcapsular haematomas with rupture may occur (Barton & Sibai, 1992).

Spontaneous rupture of the liver

First reported by Abercrombie from Cape Town in 1844 (Golan & White, 1979), over 100 cases have now been recorded in the literature with a number of large series from South Africa. The topic has recently been reviewed by Neerhof et al (1989) and Smith et al (1991). The rupture occurs most commonly in association with toxaemia in the last trimester of pregnancy but in 15–20% of cases there is no associated hypertension; it sometimes occurs immediately postpartum; it more commonly affects multiparous women in their late twenties or early thirties but has been reported over an age range of 20–41; it predominantly involves the right lobe (Severino et al, 1970; Bis & Waxman, 1976; Hibbard, 1976; Golan & White, 1979). Isolated cases have been associated with a haemangioma (Yen, 1964), an amoebic abscess (Yen, 1964), liver cell carcinoma (Roddie, 1957; Bis & Waxman, 1976) and, more recently, with contraceptive steroid-related liver cell adenomas (Hibbard, 1976; Kent et al, 1978).

There is usually a history of trauma, often minor

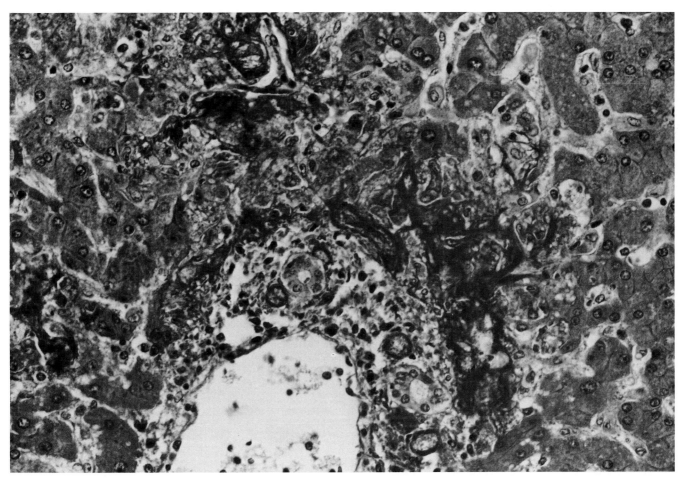

Fig. 57.8   Toxaemia of pregnancy: intrasinusoidal fibrin deposition and related liver cell necrosis is present in the periportal area; note also the dark staining of the peribiliary arterioles due to plasmatic vasculosis with escape of fibrin into their walls. Masson trichrome × 525.

however. The clinical presentation is acute with profound shock, sometimes out of proportion to the amount of blood which is found in the peritoneal cavity (Golan & White, 1979). In some cases upper abdominal pain, hepatic tenderness, nausea and vomiting have been present for some days. In a patient with toxaemia, clinical awareness of the risk of rupture may allow an early diagnosis to be made ultrasonically or by CT scanning, and may improve the prognosis (Sommer et al, 1979; Greca et al, 1984; Smith et al, 1991). The management of cases is surgical and requires emergency laparotomy with hepatic artery ligation, hepatic artery embolization or lobectomy (Loevinger et al, 1985; Terasaki et al, 1990). The maternal mortality rate is high (60–70%) with a correspondingly high fetal loss (Severino et al, 1970; Golan & White, 1979).

The rupture is thought to occur from subcapsular haematomas, which may be found without peritoneal haemorrhage and which may be continuous with haemorrhage within the liver substance (Lavery & Bowes, 1971; Sheehan & Lynch, 1973). In a case examined by the author focal intrahepatic haemorrhages were present together with larger areas of haemorrhage immediately subcapsular. These areas of haemorrhage were sharply circumscribed (Fig. 57.9) and within them the periportal areas showed appearances closely resembling those described in toxaemia of pregnancy (Fig. 57.10). The aetiology of the condition is uncertain. The increased vascular reactivity in toxaemia of pregnancy (Chesley, 1966) could, as Sheehan postulated, predispose to focal haemorrhagic liver infarction (Sheehan & Lynch, 1973). Likewise, the disseminated intravascular coagulation which accompanies toxaemia of pregnancy could lead to focal parenchymal haemorrhage which, in some cases, becomes confluent, proceeding to intrahepatic and subcapsular haematomas which subsequently rupture.

Miscellaneous group

Hyperemesis gravidarum

This condition, occurring in the first trimester of preg-

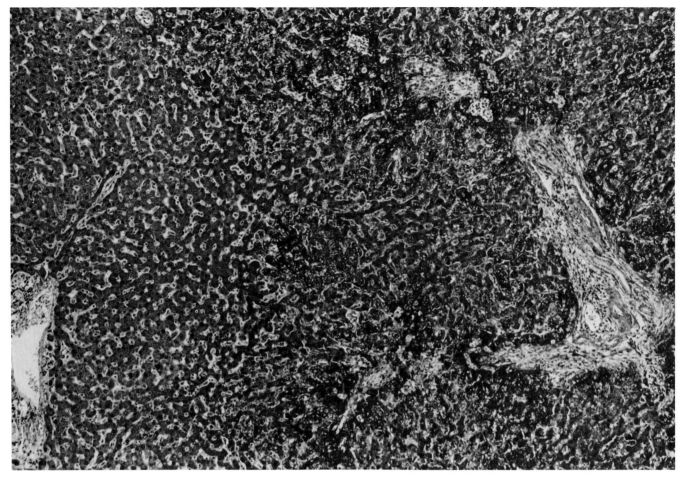

Fig. 57.9 Spontaneous rupture of the liver at 27 weeks' gestation in a patient with mild toxaemia: there is a fairly sharp delineation between normal liver (left) and the area showing haemorrhage and extensive sinusoidal fibrin deposition. MSB × 70.

nancy, accounted for jaundice in 27 (6%) of Haemmerli's review (1966) of 456 cases of pregnancy-associated jaundice. The majority of patients with hyperemesis gravidarum do not develop jaundice and when it occurs the degree is mild (Wallstedt et al, 1990; Abell & Riely, 1992). Histological examination of the liver in a small number of cases showed only non-specific changes (Sheehan, 1940; Adams et al, 1968; Richards et al, 1970). There may be a slight increase in aminotransferases; Wallstedt et al (1990) found elevated levels in 6 of 12 patients, with some having levels higher than 800 U/l.

Other causes of jaundice

Jaundice may occur in pregnancy in association with other medical conditions in which there is no distinct hepatic injury. These include megaloblastic anaemia of pregnancy, acute pyelonephritis and hydatidiform mole (Haemmerli, 1966). The management of these patients is that of their primary disease.

Liver pregnancy

This is very rare but in eight of a series of 236 extrauterine pregnancies placental attachment to the liver was recorded (Cornell & Lash, 1933). More recently, single case reports have been published (Murley, 1956; Meare et al, 1965; Kirby, 1969; Hietala et al, 1983; Mitchell & Teare, 1984; De Almeida Barbosa et al, 1991). In the report by Meare et al (1965) the pregnancy went to term but with eventual maternal and fetal death (see also Ch. 34).

LIVER DISEASES DEVELOPING CONCURRENTLY WITH PREGNANCY

Acute vital hepatitis

Viral hepatitis is the commonest cause of jaundice in pregnancy (Haemmerli, 1966) but there is some geographical variation in incidence and severity. In general, pregnant women are not more susceptible to viral hepatitis than the population at large. Infection may occur at any stage of

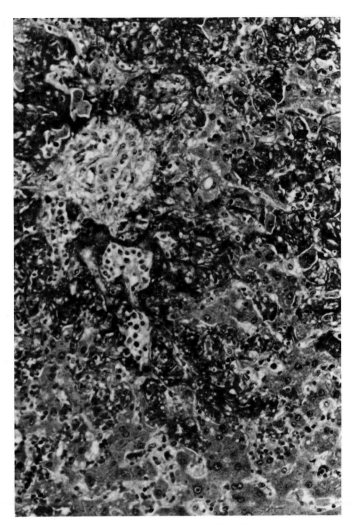

Fig. 57.10 From the same patient as Fig. 57.9. There is periportal haemorrhage, liver cell necrosis and fibrin deposition. There is a mild acute inflammatory cell reaction. MSB × 200.

pregnancy. The course of viral hepatitis is not affected by pregnancy and, with some exceptions discussed below, the outcome is the same as in the general population. Viral hepatitis, however, may affect the pregnancy and may have important effects on the fetus and the newborn. The epidemiological, clinical, biochemical and pathological features of viral hepatitis are dealt with in standard hepatological texts and the reader is referred to these (McIntyre et al, 1991; Millward-Sadler, 1992; Sherlock & Dooley, 1992). For an overview of viral hepatitis in pregnancy the reader is referred to Mishra & Seef (1992) and Rustgi et al (1993).

Hepatitis A

There are some reports of prematurity and stillbirths when infection occurs in the last trimester but there is no evidence that it causes congenital defects (Meadow, 1968;

Waterson, 1979). Transmitted hepatitis A as a cause of neonatal hepatitis is very uncommon, if it occurs at all (Schwer & Moosa, 1978; Tong et al, 1981; Williams & Ede, 1981; Mishra & Seef, 1992).

Hepatitis B

Infection in the third trimester produces an increased risk of prematurity, sometimes with an increased fetal mortality (Steven, 1981). There is no increase in congenital malformations and earlier reports of an increased risk of Down's syndrome have been refuted (Siegel, 1973; Madden et al, 1976).

The important aspect of maternal hepatitis B virus (HBV) infection is the risk of vertical transmission, both in mothers with acute infection and in mothers who have chronic HBV infection. Acute infection in the last trimester is particularly associated with vertical transmission, whereas this is not the case when maternal infection occurs earlier, unless the mother becomes a chronic carrier (Cossart, 1977; Isenberg, 1977). The incidence of chronic carriers of HBV shows considerable geographical variation and the risk of vertical transmission from affected mothers is also markedly different. The differences in transmission rate are related to differences in the HBeAg status of the mother although there may also be differences in racial susceptibility.

In western countries the transmission rate is less than 20% whereas in Asia and Africa the rate is more than 50% (Stevens et al, 1975, 1979; Derso et al, 1978). These differences also correlate with the 'e' antigen status of the mother. HBeAg positivity indicates active viral replication. In some studies vertical transmission was reported in all infants of HBeAg positive mothers (Okada et al, 1976) but the figure is now thought to be around 90% (Stevens et al, 1979); when the mother is HBeAb positive the figure is about 25% (Mowat, 1984). HBV infection can occur by horizontal transmission in the first year of life (Botha et al, 1984). An interesting and unexplained observation is an increased male : female ratio of children born to chronic HBV carriers (Drew et al, 1978).

Infection is acquired by inoculation at the time of birth when the infant is in direct contact with the infected maternal blood and amniotic fluid. Breast milk also contains viral antigens, but evidence of transmission via this route is equivocal. Caesarean section does not prevent transmission to the infant. More than 95% of those who become infected as neonates develop a chronic carrier state and develop chronic hepatitis (Thomas et al, 1988). In 2% of neonates there may be an acute hepatitis with rare cases of fulminant hepatitis. The precise mechanisms involved in the induction of tolerance to the virus in the neonate are unclear. Thomas et al (1988) postulated that HBeAg, which is one of the targets for a cellular immune response against HBV, crosses the placenta and induces tolerance. Maternal IgG against HBcAg also crosses the placenta and this antibody may block recognition of virus-infected cells by cytotoxic T cells.

Infants born to HBV carrier mothers should be treated with combined passive and active immunization. Recommended regimes include the administration of 0.5 ml of hyperimmune anti-HBs within 48 hours of birth, followed by active immunization with the first dose of HBs vaccine in the first week and repeated at one month and six months (Mishra & Seef, 1992). It is likely that in the future attempts will be made to introduce universal childhood vaccination (Centers for Disease Control, 1991).

Hepatitis D

Transmission of HDV from mother to infant is extremely rare and can only occur with simultaneous transmission of HBV (Zanetti et al, 1982).

Hepatitis C

Neonatal transmission of HCV can occur (Lee et al, 1990; Giovannini et al, 1990; Wejstal et al, 1990; Thaler et al, 1991) but evidence for long-term persistence of the infection and progression to chronic hepatitis has not yet been produced (Bach & Bodenheimer, 1992).

Hepatitis E

Hepatitis E, also known as enterically transmitted non-A, non-B hepatitis, has only recently been isolated (Reyes et al, 1990), and it is currently being actively investigated (Krawczynski, 1993; Reyes, 1993). It is transmitted in a similar way to hepatitis A and was the presumed agent in a number of epidemics peculiarly characterized by a high incidence in pregnancy with a case fatality rate of up to 20% (Melnick, 1957; Wong et al, 1980; Khuroo et al, 1981; Hla-Myint et al, 1985; Tsega et al, 1992). A few cases have been reported in America among Pakistani immigrants (De Cock et al, 1987).

Khuroo and his colleagues (1981) noted a higher incidence in pregnancy, eight times that in non-pregnant women; hepatitis was more than twice as common in the second and third trimesters, and fulminant hepatitis, occurring exclusively in the third trimester, affected 22% of pregnant women whereas only 3% of males and no non-pregnant females developed this complication. Transmission to the fetus has not been demonstrated. The reasons for these variations in HEV infection in pregnancy in developing countries are not clear. The effects of maternal nutrition have to be considered, and the suppressed immunity in pregnancy might predispose to a more virulent infection, although this does not apply to other viral infections. There are reports of a high incidence of dissemi-

nated intravascular coagulation in association with the disease (Krawczynski, 1993).

Herpes simplex hepatitis

This is a very rare infection in adults and usually occurs in immunocompromised patients. It may occur early in the last trimester of pregnancy. The first case in pregnancy was reported by Flewett et al (1969). Eight cases, four of whom died, were reviewed by Chase et al (1987). A further case, with maternal and fetal survival, was reported by Jacques & Qureshi (1992). The patients usually have no cutaneous manifestations of the herpes infection but the obstetrician should be aware of the possibility of this diagnosis when hepatic dysfunction occurs in the last trimester. Treatment with acyclovir is indicated. Neonatal herpes hepatitis due to transmission from the mother is well recognized.

Other infectious diseases

Amoebic abscess

A small number of cases of hepatic amoebiasis in pregnancy have been reported, sometimes with rupture of an abscess (Wagner et al, 1975; Cowan & Houlton, 1978; Mitchell & Teare, 1984b). In endemic areas an apparent increased susceptibility to amoebiasis in the pregnant patient has been attributed to impaired immune responsiveness (Abioye et al, 1972).

Pyogenic abscess

Pyogenic abscess in pregnancy has been reported in one case (Kopernick et al, 1988).

Echinococcal cysts

These may become symptomatic during pregnancy due to pressure effects (Kain & Keystone, 1988) and may require surgical intervention (Crow et al, 1990).

Leptospirosis

Leptospirosis in pregnancy has been reported and behaved similarly to the disease in non-pregnant females (Burroughs, 1991).

Malaria

Malaria may cause a hepatitic picture but of a mild degree (Arya & Prasad, 1988).

Drug- and toxin-induced hepatic injury

It is appropriate here only to discuss briefly drug-induced liver injury and the interested reader is referred to appropriate standard texts (Zimmerman & Ishak, 1987). The pregnant woman is liable to both intrinsic and idiosyncratic drug injury. However, because of increasing awareness of the possible direct effects or teratogenic effects on the fetus considerably greater care is being exercised in the administration of most drugs during pregnancy.

In some cases the toxic effects of certain drugs have been peculiarly but not exclusively associated with pregnancy, e.g. tetracycline (Kunelis et al, 1965; and see section on Acute fatty liver of pregnancy, p. 1738). In others the toxic effects may be exaggerated if they develop during pregnancy, e.g. chlorpromazine-induced cholestasis may be prolonged. In the presence of alcoholic liver disease fertility is reduced and fetal loss, in some series, has been greatest in cirrhosis of alcoholic aetiology complicating pregnancies. The fetal alcohol syndrome is now well recognized (Pratt, 1982) as a complication of alcohol ingestion during pregnancy and there are reports of hepatic abnormalities in affected infants (Habbick et al, 1979). Overdose from paracetamol, used as an analgesic of pregnancy, has been reported but without effect on the fetal liver (Ludmir, 1986; Kurzel, 1990).

Hepatic tumours

Hepatic adenomas (Kent et al, 1978) and focal nodular hyperplasia (Knowles et al, 1978) have been reported in pregnancy, though the latter lesion is not now thought to be associated with or dependent on steroids (Kerlin et al, 1983). Rupture with bleeding from adenomas may occur during pregnancy and in the puerperium (Hayes et al, 1977; Kent et al, 1977; Rooks et al, 1979). Indeed, pregnancy may result in increased growth and vascularity of these tumours and, in the presence of persisting lesions, pregnancy should possibly be postponed (Kent et al, 1978). The risk of a new lesion developing during pregnancy in someone who has had a pill-associated adenoma is not known, but an uneventful pregnancy following resection is recorded (Check et al, 1978).

Primary liver cell carcinoma and cholangiocarcinoma have been reported during pregnancy, and rupture of the liver has complicated liver cell carcinoma (Roddie, 1957; Purtilo et al, 1975). It is worth noting that human chorionic gonadotrophins may be demonstrated in 14% of patients with hepatocellular carcinoma (Braunstein et al, 1973). In addition alphafetoprotein levels are normally increased in late pregnancy, up to × 20 normal levels (< 20 ng/100 ml): still greater increases occur in the event of intrauterine fetal death (Adinolfi et al, 1975). However, levels above 200 ng/100 ml are diagnostic of primary liver carcinoma.

Hepatic haemangiomas are usually incidental tumours but there have been two recent reports in which these lesions were associated with high-output cardiac failure during pregnancy (Gong et al, 1988; Livneh et al, 1988).

Miscellaneous group

Budd–Chiari syndrome

It is of historical interest that in Chiari's first patient the clinical picture developed following childbirth (Chiari, 1899). There is a small number of reports of the syndrome in association with pregnancy and these have been reviewed by Rosenthal et al (1972), Tiliacos et al (1978), Khuroo & Datta (1980), and Artigas et al (1982). The syndrome usually develops postpartum and generally there is thrombosis of the major hepatic veins, usually without involvement of the inferior vena cava. The aetiology is not clear, although it has been postulated that it is due to a hypercoagulable state in pregnancy, possibly the effect of oestrogens. This would also afford an explanation for the reported association of the syndrome with the use of contraceptive steroids.

There is usually a poor prognosis; in Khuroo & Datta's series of 16 patients (1980) eight died within one year despite portacaval shunting. However, Vons et al (1984) reported three uneventful pregnancies in two women with this syndrome. The use of anticoagulants is of limited, if any, benefit. The histological changes in the liver (Bras & Brandt, 1987) are common to the syndrome irrespective of its aetiology. They comprise severe sinusoidal congestion, atrophy and necrosis of perivenular liver cells, replacement fibrosis and some periportal nodular regeneration in long-standing cases. Veno-occlusive disease, associated with pyrrolizidine alkaloids ingested in Jamaican bush tea, has been reported in one infant, presumably due to placental transfer (Roulet et al, 1988).

Spontaneous rupture of the splenic artery (see also Ch. 58)

Spontaneous rupture of the splenic artery in pregnancy is not uncommon and O'Grady and his colleagues reviewed 91 cases in 1977, 69% ruptured in the third trimester and 19% during labour or in the puerperium (Macfarlane & Thorbjarnarson, 1966). No recurring risk factor for spontaneous rupture has been noted in the cases associated with pregnancy; in a non-pregnant population portal hypertension, in particular, grand multiparity and trauma have been associated (Barrett & Caldwell, 1981). In reporting their own case Barrett & Caldwell (1981) noted that in only three pregnancy-associated cases of rupture was there documented evidence of portal hypertension.

Spontaneous rupture of the bile duct

Spontaneous rupture of the bile duct was reported by Lemay et al (1980) at 25 weeks' gestation and with a subsequent normal delivery at term. In common with the other 11 reported cases in non-pregnant patients, theirs was also associated with cholelithiasis. Choledochal cysts may first come to clinical notice during pregnancy, local kinking of the cyst presumably interfering with bile flow and resulting in cholangitis (Hopkins et al, 1990). There are two case reports of rupture of a choledochal cyst in pregnancy (Friend, 1958; Saunders & Jackson, 1969).

PREGNANCY IN PRE-EXISTING LIVER DISEASE

In patients with pre-existing liver disease the more advanced the disease, the greater is the likelihood of infertility. However, when pregnancy occurs the liver disease, in most instances, is not aggravated but if the liver disease is advanced complications may arise for the mother and there is likely to be increased fetal loss. The topic has been extensively reviewed by Varma (1987) and Lee (1992).

Chronic hepatitis

Chronic active hepatitis represents a morphological pattern of liver disease and may be seen in chronic viral hepatitis (HBV and HCV) in the autoimmune ('lupoid') form, in association with metabolic disorders such as Wilson's disease and alpha-1-antitrypsin deficiency and in association with certain drugs such as methyl dopa (Zimmerman & Ishak, 1987).

Chronic viral hepatitis

In chronic HBV and HCV infection there does not appear to be a worsening of the disease in the mother (Lee, 1992). The risk of vertical transmission of the viruses has been discussed above.

Chronic autoimmune hepatitis

Fertility has been estimated to be reduced to 50% of that in a control population and the reduction is probably in proportion to the severity of the chronic active hepatitis (Steven et al, 1979). In a report of seven patients with mild activity, so-called chronic persistent hepatitis, ten pregnancies were reported in a follow-up of three to eight years (Infeld et al, 1979). Four of these patients had a regular menstrual cycle with evidence of normal ovulation. Four elective abortions were performed for non-medical reasons. The six other pregnancies proceeded normally with no complications to mother or child.

In a series of 16 patients reviewed by Steven et al (1979) 30 pregnancies occurred. Of these, four were terminated on medical grounds, there were three spontaneous abortions and four perinatal deaths, with prematurity and reduced birth weight — an overall fetal loss of 30%; one infant had pyloric stenosis. A relapse of the liver disease occurred in only two patients and hepatic complications were minimal. Steven and his colleagues (1979) compared their findings with 36 pregnancies previously reported in the literature and in which five maternal deaths and six perinatal deaths occurred; it is reasonable to point out, however, that in some of these earlier reports, cirrhosis co-existed with the chronic active hepatitis and the liver disease was therefore probably more severe. In general, however, it would appear that when pregnancy does occur in chronic autoimmune hepatitis, it will progress uneventfully but there is an increased risk of fetal loss. In the management of the chronic hepatitis patient corticosteroids and azathioprine are the drugs of choice; during pregnancy the former may be continued but, in view of the possible risk of teratogenesis, the latter should be discontinued (Steven et al, 1979).

Cirrhosis and portal hypertension

Pregnancy in patients with cirrhosis is uncommon but by no means rare. Cirrhosis may often lead to amenorrhoea and sub-fertility but the true extent of this and the reasons for it are not clear. Furthermore, there may be a considerable variation in the interrelationship between pregnancy and cirrhosis and these may in part relate to the aetiology of the cirrhosis and in part to the degree of hepatic decompensation.

Whelton & Sherlock (1968) in their report of 16 pregnancies in 13 women, and from their review of 47 women with 54 pregnancies, concluded that the maternal prognosis was that of the underlying liver disease and was not different from that of a woman with cirrhosis who had not become pregnant; there was one maternal death in their series and one patient required an emergency portacaval shunt because of variceal bleeding at the fifth month; in four patients with primary biliary cirrhosis jaundice deepened in the third trimester and, although the bilirubin remained elevated after delivery, the prognosis was not altered; fetal wastage was high, only seven normal births resulting; there were three premature stillbirths, four spontaneous abortions and one neonatal death of a malformed infant. In Huchzermeyer's review (1971) of 21 personal cases and 74 earlier accounts, 15 maternal deaths were recorded, due mainly to bleeding from oesophageal varices in the last trimester or postpartum; perinatal deaths occurred in 10 of 71 full-term pregnancies.

Cheng (1977) compared two groups of patients, those with cirrhosis — 117 pregnancies in 92 patients — and those with non-cirrhotic portal hypertension due to extrahepatic portal obstruction — 32 pregnancies in 22 patients. These two groups in turn were subdivided into those with no portacaval shunt, those with a shunt and those in whom a shunt was performed during pregnancy. There was an increased incidence of spontaneous abortion in cirrhotic women without a shunt. In the two main groups termination of pregnancy between 21 and 37 weeks was calculated at 21% and 19% respectively. There was also a high perinatal mortality rate (18% and 12% respectively), due mainly to a high rate of stillbirths.

There was no significant increase in general complications (toxaemia, anaemia, etc.) between the two groups. However, postpartum haemorrhage was 8% in the cirrhotic patients, compared with none in the non-cirrhotic group, the highest incidence (26%) being seen in those who had had a previous shunt operation. Of 13 maternal deaths one occurred in the non-cirrhotic group, and of the 12 in the cirrhotic group, three occurred during the pregnancy, one during labour and eight in the puerperium. Bleeding from oesophageal varices occurred in 20% of cirrhotics but was much more common in the non-cirrhotic group at 44%; its occurrence was unpredictable in relation to the stage of pregnancy. Once bleeding occurred, however, the mortality rate was much greater in the cirrhotic group than in the non-cirrhotic group, 62% compared with 14%.

There are also reports of pregnancy in primary biliary cirrhosis (Ahrens et al, 1950; Whelton and Sherlock, 1968). In the largest series ten pregnancies were reported in nine patients with primary biliary cirrhosis (Nir et al, 1989). Jaundice and the degree of cholestasis tended to worsen in the late stages of the pregnancy but this was not invariable.

In cirrhotic patients changes in liver function tests during pregnancy are unpredictable (Cheng, 1977). In the majority of patients there may be no change but some deterioration may occur in about 40%; in successive pregnancies, however, the pattern may be inconsistent. Vaginal delivery is possible in most cases and caesarean section is indicated only for obstetric reasons. Injection sclerotherapy is now regarded as the elective treatment for oesophageal varices in pregnancy (Schreyer et al, 1982; Homburg et al, 1988; Salena & Sivak, 1988). Emergency portacaval shunting can also be carried out.

Metabolic liver diseases

Wilson's disease

Pregnancy in Wilson's disease has been reported in a large number of cases and this topic is reviewed by Scheinberg & Sternlieb (1975), Albukerk (1976), Walshe (1977, 1986) and Dupont et al (1990). Secondary amenorrhoea, reduced fertility and an increased incidence of spontaneous abortion occur and, in common with other manifestations of Wilson's disease, are all improved by the use of penicillamine. Pregnancy per se may improve the neurological manifestations although relapse has been recorded (Walshe, 1977); it is uncertain whether this is due to the increased levels of serum caeruloplasmin which occur during pregnancy. In advanced liver disease with portal hypertension pregnancy may aggravate the hepatic insufficiency. Penicillamine has not been shown to have teratogenic effects and may be continued throughout pregnancy, but if discontinued it should be restated in the event of any deterioration in the patient's condition or immediately after delivery. There are no apparent ill-effects on the fetus. Discontinuation of penicillamine during pregnancy was associated with fulminant fatal hepatitis postpartum in one patient who had had two previous successful pregnancies (Shimono et al, 1990). Trientine may also be used during pregnancy (Walshe, 1986).

Hereditary hepatic porphyria

The effects of pregnancy on various disturbances of porphyrin metabolism have been reviewed by Brodie and his colleagues (1976, 1977). The perinatal mortality is increased to 8% in the acute intermittent form and to 15% in hereditary coproporphyria. While frequent attacks of both forms occurred during pregnancy and in the puerperium these workers could not confirm a previous report of increased maternal mortality (Hunter, 1971).

Miscellaneous group

Hyperbilirubinaemia syndromes

Unconjugated bilirubin may cross the placenta, and Cotton et al (1981) reported kernicterus in one infant delivered by caesarean section in a case of fulminant liver failure due to cirrhosis.

Dubin–Johnson syndrome. This rare and benign form of hereditary idiopathic chronic intermittent conjugated hyperbilirubinaemia may first come to clinical notice when the patient is using oral contraceptives or during pregnancy, especially in the third trimester (Arias, 1961; Cohen et al, 1972; Dizoglio & Cardillo, 1973). Familial studies suggest an autosomal recessive pattern of inheritance (Wolkoff et al, 1973; Edwards, 1975). The liver shows a characteristic dark-green discolouration due to excess accumulation of a melanin-like pigment in parenchymal cells (Dubin & Johnson, 1954; Dubin, 1958; Essner & Novikoff, 1960). The pigment is in lysosomes, probably as a secondary storage effect (Muscatello et al, 1967), although some lysosomal enzyme abnormalities have been described (Seymour et al, 1977). Bromsulphthalein testing produced a virtually diagnostic pattern with a secondary rise in serum dye levels at 90 and 120 minutes (Shani et al, 1970). Urinary coproporphyrin excretion is abnormal, 90% being of the type I isomer whereas normally 75% is type III isomer (Kondo et al, 1976). Affected patients should be warned of the aggravating effects of pregnancy and contraceptive steroids. Abortion rates are said to be increased (Krejs, 1983).

Other familial syndromes. Gilbert's syndrome is probably not affected by pregnancy (Krejs, 1983). In Rotor's syndrome, similar to the Dubin–Johnson syndrome but without hepatic accumulation of pigment (Wolpert et al, 1977), jaundice has been reported to improve following pregnancy (Haverback & Wirtschafter, 1960).

Haemolytic disorders. A cholestatic syndrome and focal liver cell necrosis accompanied, morphologically, by agglutination of red cells in hepatic sinusoids may occur in sickle-cell crisis (Rosenblate et al, 1970; Bras & Brandt, 1987). This may develop in pregnancy with resolution after parturition (Haemmerli, 1966).

PREGNANCY AND LIVER TRANSPLANTATION

Liver transplantation has been carried out during pregnancy, in two cases of fulminant hepatitis B infection (Fair et al, 1990; Laifer et al, 1990) and in two cases of acute fatty liver of pregnancy (Ockner et al, 1990; Amon et al, 1993). The hepatitis B cases both required retransplantation within a few days. A live baby was born to one mother (Fair et al, 1990), caesarean section being carried out because of growth retardation, but in the case reported by Laifer et al (1990) the baby, also delivered by caesarean section, died. The patient treated for acute fatty liver was alive and well 18 months post transplant (Ockner et al, 1990).

Following liver transplantation for whatever cause normal menses return in a few weeks (Cundy et al, 1990), and successful pregnancies have been reported in many instances (see review by Burroughs, 1991). Pregnancy does not appear to predispose to graft rejection. There is a higher incidence of prematurity because of obstetrical indications for early delivery, and this is carried out by caesarean section in the majority of cases. Immunosuppressive regimes have to be modified during pregnancy and azathioprine, in particular, is usually stopped because of the potential (but as yet unproven) risk of teratogenicity.

BILE COMPOSITION, GALLBLADDER FUNCTION AND CHOLELITHIASIS

Gallstones are universally commoner in women than in men, are commoner in premenopausal than in postmenopausal women, and show an increased incidence in parous women, in women using oral contraceptives and in women whose pregnancy has been complicated by intrahepatic cholestasis of pregnancy (Bennion & Grundy, 1978; Kern, 1978; Barbara et al, 1987; Valdivieso et al, 1993). There is also evidence that there may be subpopulations of women, notably women aged less than 30, who may be susceptible to gallstone formation as a result either of oral contraceptives or pregnancy (Scragg et al, 1984). A similar increased risk may be seen in teenagers. These observations have indicated that hormonal factors may be important in cholelithiasis and have suggested that investigations of biliary and gallbladder function during pregnancy and in women using the contraceptive pill might indicate some pathogenetic mechanisms (Everson, 1993).

A progressive fall in bile flow, principally the bile acid independent fraction, has been demonstrated during pregnancy in the hamster (Reyes & Kern, 1979). Little is known, however, about the effects of pregnancy on bile flow in the human. Profound changes in bile lipid and bile acid composition occur at different stages of pregnancy. In the second and third trimester the lithogenic or cholesterol saturation index of fasting hepatic and gallbladder bile is significantly increased (Kern et al, 1981; Valdivieso et al, 1993). Whereas during normal ovulatory cycles no significant changes in the bile lipids were found, Kern et al (1982) confirmed the observations of Bennion et al (1976) that contraceptive steroids produced a significant increase in lithogenic index. The effect is thought to be due to oestrogens (Kern et al, 1982; Everson et al, 1991) although some studies have suggested that progestagens are responsible (Down et al, 1983). In pregnancy the increase in lithogenic index is the result of an increase in cholesterol secretion relative to phospholipid and bile acid secretion (Kern et al, 1981), the mean hourly rate of biliary lipid secretion remaining unchanged.

In the same studies Kern and his colleagues (1981, 1982) studied bile acid composition. There was an increase in the total bile acid pool size in the first trimester, but this was less marked in the latter two-thirds of pregnancy. The pool size for both cholic acid (CA) and chenodeoxycholic acid (CDCA) was also increased in the first trimester but thereafter only the pool size of CA was maintained. A progressive reduction of CDCA synthesis occurred as pregnancy progressed so that the CA:CDCA ratio in bile progressively increased (Kern et al, 1981), an effect which contraceptive steroids also produce (Bennion et al, 1976; Kern et al, 1982). The frequency of enterohepatic cycling of the bile acid pool was reduced by a third in pregnancy, in part due to a slowing of intestinal transit time and also due to changes in gallbladder function.

In pregnancy, fasting gallbladder volume is increased and emptying is incomplete due to a slower rate of emptying with a corresponding increase in residual volume; these changes increase progressively only during the first two trimesters and there is a return to normal postpartum (Braverman et al, 1980, 1988; Everson et al, 1982). In a recent study from Chile, ultrasonic examination of the gallbladder in 980 women immediately postpartum demonstrated gallstones in 12.2% compared with 1.3% in a control nulliparous group (Valdivieso et al, 1993). Disappearance of small gallstones, also demonstrated in this study, was thought to be due to the bile becoming unsaturated soon after delivery. An increase in fasting gallbladder volume was found in most women who had been on contraceptive steroids for many years but the rate of emptying was reduced only during an intraduodenal amino acid infusion; no changes in gallbladder function were demonstrable between different phases of normal ovulatory cycles (Everson et al, 1982).

The implications of these findings are that, in pregnancy, bile retention in the gallbladder is greatest at a time when gallbladder bile is most lithogenic. The precise interplay between oestrogens and progestagens in mediating the changes in bile composition and the functional changes in the gallbladder remain to be established (Everson, 1993). Progesterone receptors with high specific binding are present in the human gallbladder (Singletary et al, 1986) and there is circumstantial evidence that they may play a rôle in regulating its contractility (Daignault et al, 1988; Hould et al, 1988). The sluggish gallbladder of pregnancy (Cohen, 1980) may facilitate cholesterol precipitation, but whether the right conditions are effected simply by the demonstrated changes in bile composition remains to be proven (Holzbach, 1983). Studies on gallbladder function in other at-risk groups are now indicated.

Biliary obstruction by gallstones in pregnancy is rare, causing jaundice in only 27 of 450 cases in Haemmerli's series (1966). Cholecystitis, however, may occur but the incidence of cholecystectomy in the United States during pregnancy is less than 0.1% (Seymour & Chadwick, 1979).

REFERENCES

Abell T L, Riely C A 1992 Hyperemesis gravidarum. Gastroenterology Clinics of North America 21: 835–849.

Abioye A A, Lewis E A, McFarlane H 1972 Clinical evaluation of serum immunoglobulin in amoebiasis. Immunology 23: 937–946.

Adams R H, Gordon J, Combes B 1968 Hyperemesis gravidarum. I. Evidence of hepatic dysfunction. Obstetrics and Gynecology 31: 659–664.

Adinolfi A, Adinolfi M, Lessoff M H 1975 Alpha-feto-protein during development and in disease. Journal of Medical Genetics 12: 138–151.

Adlercreutz H, Tenhunen R 1970 Some aspects of the interaction between natural and synthetic female sex hormones and the liver. American Journal of Medicine 49: 630–648.

Adlercreutz H, Svanborg A, Anberg A 1967 Recurrent jaundice in pregnancy. II. A study of the estrogens and their conjugation in late pregnancy. American Journal of Medicine 42: 341–347.

Adlercreutz H, Tikkanen M J, Wichmann K et al 1974 Recurrent jaundice in pregnancy. IV. Quantitative determination of urinary and biliary estrogens, including studies in pruritus gravidarum. Journal of Clinical Endocrinology and Metabolism 38: 51–57.

Ahrens E H, Payne M A, Kunkel H G et al 1950 Primary biliary cirrhosis. Medicine 29: 299–364.

Albukerk J N 1976 The pregnant woman with Wilson's disease. New England Journal of Medicine 294: 670–671.

Amon E, Allen S R, Petrie R H et al 1993 Acute fatty liver of pregnancy associated with preeclampsia; management of hepatic failure with postpartum liver transplantation. American Journal of Perinatology 8: 278–279.

Antia F P, Bharadwaj T P, Watsa M C, Master J 1958 Liver in normal pregnancy, pre-eclampsia and eclampsia. Lancet 2: 776–778.

Arias F, Marchilla-Jimenez R 1976 Hepatic fibrinogen deposits in pre-eclampsia: immunofluorescent evidence. New England Journal of Medicine 295: 578–582.

Arias I M 1961 Studies of chronic familial non-haemolytic jaundice with conjugated bilirubin in the serum with and without an unidentified pigment in the liver cells. American Journal of Medicine 31: 510–518.

Artigas J M G, Estabanez J S, Faure M R A 1982 Pregnancy and the Budd-Chiari syndrome. Digestive Diseases and Sciences 27: 89–90.

Arya T V, Prasad R N 1988 Malarial hepatitis. Journal of the Association of Physicians of India 36: 294–295.

Bach N, Bodenheimer H C Jr 1992 Transmission of hepatitis C: sexual, vertical or exclusively blood-borne? Hepatology 16: 1492–1499.

Barbara L, Sama C, Morselli Labate A M et al 1987 A population study on the prevalence of gallstone disease: the Sirmione study. Hepatology 7: 913–917.

Barrett J M, Caldwell B H 1981 Association of portal hypertension and ruptured splenic artery aneurysm in pregnancy. Obstetrics and Gynecology 57: 255–257.

Barron W M 1992 The syndrome of pre-eclampsia. Gastroenterology Clinics of North America 21: 851–872.

Barton J R, Sibai B M 1992 Care of the pregnancy complicated by HELLP syndrome. Gastroenterology Clinics of North America 21: 937–950.

Barton J R, Sibai B M, Mabie W C et al 1990 Recurrent acute fatty liver of pregnancy. American Journal of Obstetrics and Gynecology 163: 534–538.

Bennion L J, Grundy M 1978 Risk factors for the development of cholelithiasis in man. New England Journal of Medicine 299: 1161–1167, 1221–1227.

Bennion L J, Ginsberg R L, Garnick M B, Bennett P 1976 Effects of oral contraceptives on the gallbladder bile of normal women. New England Journal of Medicine 294: 189–192.

Bernuau J, Degott C, Nouel O, Rueff B, Benhamou J P 1982 Non-fatal acute fatty liver of pregnancy. Gut 24: 340–344.

Bis K A, Waxman B 1976 Rupture of the liver associated with pregnancy: a review of the literature and report of two cases. Obstetrical and Gynecological Survey 31: 763–773.

Botha J F, Ritchie M J J, Dusheiko G M et al 1984 Hepatitis B virus carrier state in black children in Ovamboland: role of perinatal and horizontal infection. Lancet 1: 1210–1212.

Bras G, Brandt K-H 1987 Vascular disorders. In: MacSween R N M, Anthony P P, Scheuer P J (eds) Pathology of the liver, 2nd edn. Churchill Livingstone, Edinburgh, pp 315–334.

Braunstein G D, Vogel C L, Vaitukaitis J L, Ross G T 1973 Ectopic production of human chorionic gonadotrophin in Ugandan patients with hepatocellular carcinoma. Cancer 32: 223–226.

Braverman D Z, Johnson M L, Kern F Jr 1980 Effects of pregnancy and contraceptive steroids on gallbladder function. New England Journal of Medicine 302: 362–364.

Braverman D Z, Herbet D, Goldstein R et al 1988 Postpartum restoration of pregnancy-induced cholecystoparesis and prolonged intestinal transit time. Journal of Clinical Gastroenterology 10: 642–646.

Breen K J, Perkins K W, Mistilis S P, Shearman R 1970 Idiopathic acute fatty liver of pregnancy. Gut 11: 822–825.

Breen K J, Perkins K W, Schenker S, Dunkerley R C, Moore H C 1972 Uncomplicated subsequent pregnancy after idiopathic fatty liver of pregnancy. Obstetrics and Gynecology 40: 813–815.

Brodie M J, Beattie A D, Moore M R, Goldberg A 1976 Pregnancy and hereditary hepatic porphyria. In: Doss M (ed) Porphyrins in human diseases. Karger, Basel, pp 251–254.

Brodie M J, Moore M R, Thompson G G, Goldberg A, Low R A L 1977 Pregnancy and the acute porphyrias. British Journal of Obstetrics and Gynaecology 84: 726–731.

Burroughs A K 1991 Liver disease and pregnancy. In: McIntyre N, Benhamou J P, Bircher J, Rizzetto M, Rodes J (eds) Oxford textbook of clinical hepatology, vol 2. Oxford University Press, Oxford, pp 1319–1332.

Burroughs A K, Seong N H, Dojcinov D M et al 1982 Idiopathic acute fatty liver of pregnancy in 12 patients. Quarterly Journal of Medicine 205: 481–497.

Campillo B, Bernau J, Witz M-O et al 1986 Ultrasonography in acute fatty liver of pregnancy. Annals of Internal Medicine 105: 383–384.

Centers for Disease Control 1991 Hepatitis B virus: a comprehensive strategy for eliminating transmission in the United States through universal childhood vaccination. MMWR 40: 1–25.

Chase R A, Pottage J C Jr, Haber M A et al 1987 Herpes simplex viral hepatitis in adults: two cases and a review of the literature. Review of Infectious Diseases 9: 329–333.

Check J H, King L C, Rakoff A E 1978 Uncomplicated pregnancy following oral contraceptive-induced liver hepatoma. Obstetrics and Gynecology 52: 28s–29s.

Cheng Y-S 1977 Pregnancy in liver cirrhosis and/or portal hypertension. American Journal of Obstetrics and Gynecology 128: 812–822.

Chesley L C 1966 Vascular reactivity in normal and toxemic pregnancy. Clinical Obstetrics and Gynecology 9: 871–881.

Chiari H 1899 Uber die selbstandige Phlebitis obliterans der Hauptstamme der Venae hepaticae als Todesursache. Beitrage zur pathologischen Anatomie und zur allgemeinen Pathologie 26: 1–18.

Cohen L, Lewis C, Arias I M 1972 Pregnancy, oral contraceptives and chronic familial jaundice with predominantly conjugated hyper-bilirubinemia (Dubin-Johnson syndrome). Gastroenterology 62: 1182–1190.

Cohen S 1980 The sluggish gallbladder of pregnancy. New England Journal of Medicine 302: 397–398.

Combes E, Shibata H, Adams R, Mitchell B D, Tramell V 1963 Alteration in sulfabromophthalein sodium removal mechanisms from blood during normal pregnancy. Journal of Clinical Investigation 42: 1431–1436.

Cornell E L, Lash A F 1933 Abdominal pregnancy. International Abstracts of Surgery 8: 98–104.

Cossart Y E 1977 The outcome of hepatitis B virus infection in pregnancy. Postgraduate Medical Journal 53: 610–613.

Cotton D B, Brock B J, Schifrin B S 1981 Cirrhosis and fetal hyperbilirubinemia. Obstetrics and Gynecology 57: 25s–27s.

Cowan D B, Houlton C C 1978 Rupture of an amoebic liver abscess in pregnancy: a case report. South African Medical Journal 53: 460–461.

Crow J P, Larry M, Vento E G et al 1990 Echinococcal disease of the liver in pregnancy. HPB Surgery 2: 115–151.

Cundy T F, O'Grady J G, Williams R 1990 Recovery of menstruation and pregnancy after liver transplantation. Gut 31: 337–338.

Daignault P G, Fazekas A G, Rosenthall L et al 1988 Relationship between gallbladder contraction and progesterone receptors in patients with gallstones. American Journal of Surgery 155: 147–151.

Dalen E, Westerholm B 1974 Occurrence of hepatic impairment in women jaundiced by oral contraceptives and in their mothers and sisters. Acta Medica Scandinavica 195: 459–463.

Davies M H, Wilkinson S P, Hanid M A et al 1980 Acute liver disease with encephalopathy and renal failure in late pregnancy and the early puerperium: a study of fourteen patients. British Journal of Obstetrics and Gynaecology 87: 1105–1114.

De Almeida Barbosa A Jr, Rodriguez de Freitas L A, Andrade Mota M 1991 Primary pregnancy in the liver: a case report. Pathology Research and Practice 187: 329–331.

De Cock K M, Bradley D W, Sanford W L et al 1987 Epidemic non-A, non-B hepatitis in patients from Pakistan. Annals of Internal Medicine 106: 227–230.

Derso A, Boxall E H, Tarlow M J, Flewett T H 1978 Transmission of HBsAg from mother to infant in four ethnic groups. British Medical Journal 1: 949–952.

Dizoglio J A, Cardillo E 1973 The Dubin-Johnson syndrome and pregnancy. Obstetrics and Gynecology 42: 560–563.

Down R H L, Whiting M J, Watts J McK, Jones W 1983 Effect of synthetic oestrogens and progestagens in oral contraceptives on bile lipid composition. Gut 24: 253–259.

Drew J S, London W T, Lustbader E D et al 1978 Hepatitis B virus and sex ratio of offspring. Science 201: 687–692.

Dubin I N 1958 Chronic idiopathic jaundice: a review of fifty cases. American Journal of Medicine 24: 268–292.

Dubin I N, Johnson F B 1954 Chronic idiopathic jaundice with unidentified pigment in liver cells: a new clinicopathological entity with a report of 12 cases. Medicine 33: 155–197.

Duma R J, Dowling E A, Alexander H J, Sibrons D, Dempsey H 1965 Acute fatty liver of pregnancy: report of surviving patient studied with serial liver biopsies. Annals of Internal Medicine 63: 851–858.

Dupont P, Irion O, Breguin F 1990 Pregnancy in a patient with treated Wilson's disease: a case report. American Journal of Obstetrics and Gynecology 163: 1527–1528.

Ebert E C, Sun E A, Wright S H et al 1984 Does early diagnosis and delivery in acute fatty liver of pregnancy lead to improvement in maternal and infant survival? Digestive Diseases and Science 29: 453–455.

Edwards R H 1975 Inheritance of the Dubin-Johnson-Sprinz syndrome. Gastroenterology 68: 734–749.

Eisele J W, Barker E A, Smuckler E A 1975 Lipid content of the liver of fatty metamorphosis of pregnancy. American Journal of Pathology 81: 545–555.

Essner E, Novikoff A B 1960 Human hepatocellular pigment and lysosomes. Journal of Ultrastructural Research 3: 374–391.

Everson G T 1993 Pregnancy and gallstones. Hepatology 17: 159–161.

Everson G T, McKinley C, Lawson M, Johnson M, Kern F Jr 1982 Gallbladder function in the human female: effect of the ovulatory cycle, pregnancy, and contraceptive steroids. Gastroenterology 82: 711–719.

Everson G T, McKinley C, Kern F Jr 1991 Mechanisms of gallstone formation in women: effects of exogenous estrogen (premarin) and dietary cholesterol on hepatic lipid metabolism. Journal of Clinical Investigation 87: 237–246.

Fair J, Klein A G, Feng T, Merritt W T, Burdick J F 1990 Intrapartum orthotopic liver transplantation with successful outcome of pregnancy. Transplantation 50: 534–535.

Feller A, Ugarte G, Pino M E, Oberti C, Pisano R 1983 Acute fatty liver of pregnancy (AFLP): a possible disorder of carnitine (Ct) metabolism. Gastroenterology 84: 1150 (abstract).

Ferris T F, Herdson P B, Dunnill M S, Lee M R 1969 Toxemia of pregnancy in sheep: a clinical, physiological and pathological study. Journal of Clinical Investigation 48: 1643–1655.

Flewett T H, Parker R G F, Philip W M 1969 Acute hepatitis due to herpes simplex hepatitis in an adult. Journal of Clinical Pathology 22: 60–66.

Friend W D 1958 Rupture of choledochal cyst during confinement. British Journal of Surgery 46: 155.

Furhoff A K 1974 Itching in pregnancy: a 15 year follow up study. Acta Medica Scandinavica 196: 403–410.

Furhoff A K, Hellstrom K 1973 Jaundice in pregnancy: a follow up study of the series of women originally reported by L Thorling. I. The pregnancies. Acta Medica Scandinavica 193: 259–266.

Furhoff A K, Hellstrom K 1974 Jaundice in pregnancy: a follow up study of the series of women originally reported by L Thorling. II. Present health of the women. Acta Medica Scandinavica 196: 181–189.

Gerber N, Dickinson R G, Harland R C et al 1979 Reye-like syndrome associated with valproic acid therapy. Journal of Pediatrics 95: 142–144.

Giovannini M, Tagger A, Ribero M L et al 1990 Maternal-infant transmission of hepatitis C virus and HIV infections: a possible interaction. Lancet 335: 1116.

Glasinovic J C, Mage R M, Ferreiro O et al 1989 Cholelithiasis in a Chilean female population: prevalence and associated risk factors. Gastroenterology 96: A 601.

Golan A, White R G 1979 Spontaneous rupture of the liver associated with pregnancy: a report of 5 cases. South African Medical Journal 56: 133–136.

Gong B, Baken L A, Julian T M et al 1988 High output heart failure due to hepatic arteriovenous fistula during pregnancy: a case report. Obstetrics and Gynecology 72: 440–442.

Gonzales M C, Reyes H, Arrese M et al 1989 Intrahepatic cholestasis of pregnancy in twin pregnancies. Journal of Hepatology 9: 84–90.

Greca F H, Coelho J C U, Filho O D B, Wallbach A 1984 Ultrasonographic diagnosis of spontaneous rupture of the liver in pregnancy. Journal of Clinical Ultrasound 12: 515–516.

Grimbert S, Fromentz B, Fisch C et al 1993 Decreased mitochondrial oxidation of fatty acids in pregnant mice: possible relevance to development of acute fatty liver of pregnancy. Hepatology 17: 628–637.

Habbick B F, Casey R, Zaleski W A, Murphy F 1979 Liver abnormalities in three patients with fetal alcohol syndrome. Lancet 1: 580–581.

Haemmerli U P 1966 Jaundice during pregnancy with special reference on recurrent jaundice during pregnancy and its differential diagnosis. Acta Medica Scandinavica (suppl) 444: 1–111.

Haemmerli U P, Wyss H I 1967 Recurrent intrahepatic cholestasis of pregnancy: report of six cases and review of the literature. Medicine 46: 299–321.

Hague W M, Fenton D W, Duncan S L B, Slater D N 1983 Acute fatty liver of pregnancy: a review of the literature and six further cases. Journal of the Royal Society of Medicine 76: 752–761.

Hatfield A K, Stein J H, Greenberger N J, Abernethy R W, Ferris T F 1972 Idiopathic acute fatty liver of pregnancy: death from extrahepatic manifestations. American Journal of Digestive Disease 17: 167–178.

Haverback B J, Wirtschafter S K 1960 Familial nonhemolytic jaundice with normal liver histology and conjugated bilirubin. New England Journal of Medicine 262: 113–117.

Hayes D, Lamki H, Hunter I W E 1977 Hepatic cell adenoma presenting with intraperitoneal haemorrhage in the puerperium. British Medical Journal 12: 1394.

Hibbard L T 1976 Spontaneous rupture of the liver in pregnancy: a report of eight cases. American Journal of Obstetrics and Gynecology 126: 324–328.

Hietala S-O, Anderson M, Emdin S O 1983 Ectopic pregnancy in the liver: report of a case and angiographic findings. Acta Chirurgica Scandinavica 149: 633–635.

Hill K R 1952 The vomiting sickness of Jamaica. West Indian Medical Journal 1: 243–264.

Hla-Myint, Myint-Myint Soe, Tun-Khin et al 1985 A clinical and epidemiological study of an epidemic of non-A non-B hepatitis in Rangoon. American Journal of Tropical Medicine and Hygiene 34: 1183–1189.

Holzbach R T 1983 Gallbladder stasis: consequence of long-term parenteral hyperalimentation and risk factor for cholelithiasis. Gastroenterology 84: 1055–1058.

Homburg R, Bayer I, Lurie B 1988 Bleeding esophageal varices in pregnancy: a report of two cases. Journal of Reproductive Medicine 33: 784–786.

Hopkins N F, Benjamin I S, Thompson M H et al 1990 Complications of choledochal cysts. Annals of the Royal College of Surgeons of England 74: 229–235.

Hou S H, Levin S, Ahola S et al 1984 Acute fatty liver of pregnancy: survival with early Cesarean section. Digestive Diseases and Science 29: 449–452.

Hould F S, Fried G M, Fazekas A G et al 1988 Progesterone receptors regulate gallbladder motility. Journal of Surgical Research 45: 505–512.

Huchzermeyer H 1971 Schwangerschaft bei Leberzirrhose und chronischer Hepatitis. Acta Hepatosplenologica 18: 294–305.

Hunter D J S 1971 Acute intermittent porphyria and pregnancy. Journal of Obstetrics and Gynaecology of the British Commonwealth 78: 746–750.

Hytten F E, Leitch I 1971 The physiology of human pregnancy, 2nd edn. Blackwell Scientific Publications, Oxford.

Ikonen E 1964 Jaundice in late pregnancy. Acta Obstetricia and Gynecologica Scandinavica 43: suppl 5.

Infeld D S, Borkowf H I, Varma R R 1979 Chronic persistent hepatitis and pregnancy. Gastroenterology 77: 524–527.

Ingerslev M, Teilum G 1945 Biopsy studies on the liver in pregnancy. II. Liver biopsy on normal pregnant women. Acta Obstetricia et Gynecologica Scandinavica 25: 352–360.

Isenberg J N 1977 The infant and hepatitis B virus infection. Advances in Paediatrics 24: 445–498.

Jacques S M, Qureshi F 1992 Herpes simplex virus hepatitis in pregnancy: a clinicopathologic study of three cases. Human Pathology 13: 183–187.

Jenkins W F, Darling M R 1980 Idiopathic acute fatty liver of pregnancy: subsequent uncomplicated pregnancy. Journal of Obstetrics and Gynaecology 1: 100–101.

Johnson P 1975 Studies on cholestasis of pregnancy. IV. Serum lipids and lipoprotein in relation to duration of symptoms and severity of the disease and fatty acid composition of lecithin in relation to duration of symptoms. Acta Obstetricia et Gynecologica Scandinavica 54: 307–313.

Johnson P, Samsioe G, Gustafson A 1975a Studies in cholestasis of pregnancy. I. Clinical aspects and liver function tests. Acta Obstetricia et Gynecologica Scandinavica 54: 77–84.

Johnson P, Samsioe G, Gustafson A 1975b Studies on cholestasis of

pregnancy. II. Serum lipids and lipoproteins. Acta Obstetricia et Gynecologica Scandinavica 54: 105–111.

Joske R A, McCully D J, Mastaglia F L 1968 Acute fatty liver of pregnancy. Gut 9: 489–493.

Kain K C, Keystone J S 1988 Recurrent hydatid disease during pregnancy. American Journal of Obstetrics and Gynecology 159: 1216–1219.

Kater R M H, Mistilis S P 1967 Obstetric cholestasis and pruritus of pregnancy. Medical Journal of Australia 54: 638–640.

Kauppila A, Korpela H, Makila U-M, Yrjanheikki E 1987 Low selenium concentration and glutathione peroxidase activity in intrahepatic cholestasis of pregnancy. British Medical Journal 294: 150–152.

Kent D R, Nissen E D, Nisen S E, Chambers C 1977 Maternal death resulting from rupture of liver adenoma associated with oral contraceptives. Obstetrics and Gynecology (suppl) 50: 5s–6s.

Kent D R, Nissen S E, Ziehm D J 1978 Effect of pregnancy on liver tumor associated with oral contraceptives. Obstetrics and Gynecology 55: 148–151.

Kerlin P, Davis G L, McGill D B et al 1983 Hepatic adenoma and focal nodular hyperplasia: clinical, pathologic and radiologic features. Gastroenterology 84: 994–1002.

Kern F Jr 1978 Cholesterol gallstones. Gastroenterology 75: 514–517.

Kern F Jr, Erfling W, Simon F R, Dahl R, Mallory A, Starzl T E 1978 Effect of estrogen on the liver. Gastroenterology 75: 512–522.

Kern F Jr, Everson G T, De Mark B et al 1981 Biliary lipids, bile acids, and gallbladder function in the human female: effects of pregnancy and the ovulatory cycle. Journal of Clinical Investigation 68: 1229–1242.

Kern F Jr, Everson G T, De Mark B et al 1982 Biliary lipids, bile acids and gallbladder function in the human female: effects of contraceptive steroids. Journal of Laboratory and Clinical Medicine 99: 798–805.

Khuroo M S, Datta D V 1980 Budd-Chiari syndrome following pregnancy: report of 16 cases with roentgenologic, hemodynamic and histologic studies of the hepatic outflow tract. American Journal of Medicine 68: 113–121.

Khuroo M S, Teli M R, Skidmore S, Sofi M A, Khuroo M I 1981 Incidence and severity of viral hepatitis in pregnancy. American Journal of Medicine 70: 252–255.

Killam A P, Dillard S H, Patton R C, Pedersen P R 1975 Pregnancy-induced hypertension complicated by acute liver disease and disseminated intravascular coagulation. American Journal of Obstetrics and Gynecology 123: 823–828.

Kirby N G 1969 Primary hepatic pregnancy. British Medical Journal 1: 296.

Knowles D M, Casarella W J, Johnson P M, Wolff M 1978 The clinical, radiologic and pathologic characterisation of benign hepatic neoplasms: alleged associations with oral contraceptives. Medicine 57: 223–237.

Kondo T, Kuchiba K, Shimizu Y 1976 Coproporphyrin isomers in Dubin-Johnson syndrome. Gastroenterology 70: 1117–1120.

Kopernik G, Mazor M, Leiberman J R et al 1988 Pyogenic liver abscess in pregnancy. Israeli Journal of Medical Science 24: 245–246.

Krawczynski K 1993 Hepatitis E. Hepatology 17: 932–941.

Kreek M J 1987 Female sex steroids and cholestasis. Seminars in Liver Disease 7: 8–23.

Kreek M J, Sleisenger H E 1970 Estrogen induced cholestasis due to endogenous and exogenous hormones. Scandinavian Journal of Gastroenterology (suppl) 7: 122–131.

Kreek M J, Sleisenger M H, Jeffries G H 1967a Recurrent cholestatic jaundice of pregnancy with demonstrated estrogen sensitivity. American Journal of Medicine 43: 795–798.

Kreek M J, Wester E, Sleisenger M H et al 1967b Idiopathic cholestasis of pregnancy: the response to challenge with the synthetic estrogen, ethinyl estradiol. New England Journal of Medicine 277: 1391–1395.

Krejs G J 1983 Jaundice during pregnancy. Seminars in Liver Disease 3: 73–82.

Krejs G J, Haemmerli U P 1982 Jaundice during pregnancy. In: Schiff L, Schiff E R (eds) Diseases of the liver, 5th edn. Lippincott, Philadelphia, pp 1561–1580.

Kunelis C T, Peters J L, Edmondson H A 1965 Fatty liver of pregnancy and its relationship to tetracycline therapy. American Journal of Medicine 38: 359–377.

Kurzel R B 1990 Can acetaminophen excess result in maternal and fetal toxicity. Southern Medical Journal 83: 953–955.

Laatikainen T 1975 Fetal bile acid levels in pregnancies complicated by maternal intrahepatic cholestasis. American Journal of Obstetrics and Gynecology 122: 852–856.

Laatikainen T, Ikonen E 1975 Fetal prognosis in obstetric hepatosis. Annales Chirurgiae et Gynaecologiae Fenniae 64: 155–164.

Laatikainen T, Ikonen E 1977 Serum bile acids in cholestasis of pregnancy. Obstetrics and Gynecology 50: 313–318.

Laatikainen T, Lehtonen P, Hesso A 1978 Biliary bile acids in uncomplicated pregnancy and in cholestasis of pregnancy. Clinica Chimica Acta 85: 145–150.

Laifer S A, Darby M J, Scantlebury V P et al 1990 Pregnancy and liver transplantation. Obstetrics and Gynecology 76: 1083.

Lavery D W, Bowes R M 1971 Subcapsular haematoma of the liver in pregnancy: report of four cases. South African Medical Journal 45: 603–605.

Lee S D, Chan C Y, Wang Y J et al 1990 Mother to infant transmission of hepatitis C virus infection. Journal of Medical Virology 30: 178–180.

Lee W M 1992 Pregnancy in patients with chronic liver disease. Gastroenterology Clinics of North America 21: 889–903.

Lemay M, Granger L, Verschelden G et al 1980 Spontaneous rupture of the common bile duct during pregnancy. Canadian Medical Association Journal 122: 14–15.

Liebman H A, McGehee W G, Patak M J, Fienstein D I 1983 Severe depression of antithrombin III associated with disseminated intravascular coagulation in women with fatty liver of pregnancy. Annals of Internal Medicine 98: 330–333.

Livneh A, Langevitz P, Morag B 1988 Functionally reversible hepatic arteriovenous fistulas during pregnancy in patients with hereditary hemorrhagic telangiectasia. Southern Medical Journal 81: 1047–1049.

Loevinger E H, Vujic I, Lee W M, Anderson M C 1985 Hepatic rupture associated with pregnancy: treatment with transcatheter embolotherapy. Obstetrics and Gynecology 65: 281–284.

Long R G, Scheuer P J, Sherlock S 1977 Pre-eclampsia presenting with deep jaundice. Journal of Clinical Pathology 30: 212–215.

Ludmir J 1986 Maternal acetaminophen overdose at 15 weeks gestation. Obstetrics and Gynecology 67: 750–751.

Mabie W C 1992 Acute fatty liver of pregnancy. Gastroenterology Clinics of North America 21: 951–960.

Mabie W C, Dacus J V, Sibai B M et al 1989 Computed tomography in acute fatty liver of pregnancy. American Journal of Obstetrics and Gynecology 158: 142–145.

Macfarlane J, Thorbjarnarson B 1966 Rupture of splenic artery aneurysm during pregnancy. American Journal of Obstetrics and Gynecology 95: 1025–1037.

Mackenna J, Pupkin M, Crenshaw L, MacLeod M, Parker R 1977 Acute fatty metamorphosis of liver. American Journal of Obstetrics and Gynecology 127: 400–404.

Mackenna J, Dover N L, Brame R G 1983 Preeclampsia associated with hemolysis, elevated liver enzymes, and low platelets — an obstetric emergency? Obstetrics and Gynecology 62: 751–754.

McIntyre N, Benhamou J-P, Bircher J, Rizetto M, Rodes J 1991 Oxford textbook of clinical hepatology. Oxford University Press, Oxford.

McNair R D, Jaynes R V 1960 Alterations in liver function during normal pregnancy. American Journal of Obstetrics and Gynecology 80: 500–507.

Madden D L, Matthew E B, Dietzmann D E et al 1976 Hepatitis and Down's syndrome. American Journal of Mental Deficiency 80: 401–406.

Malatjalian D A, Badley B W D 1983 Acute fatty liver of pregnancy: light and electron microscopic studies. Gastroenterology 84: 1384 (abstract).

Martin J N Jr, Files J C, Black P G et al 1990 Plasma exchange for preeclampsia: I. Postpartum use for persistently severe preeclampsia-eclampsia with HELLP syndrome. American Journal of Obstetrics and Gynecology 162: 126–137.

Meadow S R 1968 Infectious hepatitis and stillbirth. British Medical Journal 1: 426.

Meare Y, Ekna J B, Raolison S 1965 Un cas de grossesse a implantation hepatique avec enfant vivant. Semaine des Hospitaux de Paris 41: 1430–1433.

Melnick J L 1957 A waterborne urban epidemic of hepatitis. In: Hartman F W, Lo Grippo G A, Mateer J G, Barron J (eds) Hepatitis frontiers. Little Brown, Boston, pp 211–225.

Millward-Sadler G H (ed) 1992 Wright's liver and biliary disease, 3rd edn. Bailliere-Tindall, London.

Minakami H, Oka N, Sato T et al 1988 Preeclampsia: a microvesicular fat disease of the liver? American Journal of Obstetrics and Gynecology 159: 1043–1047.

Mishra L, Seef L B 1992 Viral hepatitis, A through E complicating pregnancy. Gastroenterology Clinics of North America 21: 883–887.

Mitchell R W, Teare A J 1984a Primary hepatic pregnancy: a case report and review. South African Medical Journal 65: 200–202.

Mitchell R W, Teare A J 1984b Amoebic liver abscess in pregnancy: case report. British Journal of Obstetrics and Gynaecology 91: 393–395.

Moore H C 1956 Acute fatty liver of pregnancy. British Journal of Obstetrics and Gynaecology 63: 189–198.

Mowat A P 1983 Reye's syndrome: 20 years on (editorial). British Medical Journal 286: 1999–2001.

Mowat A P 1984 Pediatric liver disease. In: Arias I M, Frenkel M, Wilson J H P (eds) The liver annual 4. Elsevier, Amsterdam, pp 322–344.

Munnell E W, Taylor H C 1947 Liver blood flow in pregnancy — hepatic vein catheterisation. Journal of Clinical Investigation 26: 952–956.

Murley A H G 1956 Liver pregnancies. Lancet i: 994–995.

Muscatello U, Mussini I, Agnolucci M T 1967 The Dubin Johnson syndrome: an electron microscopic study of the liver cell. Acta Hepatosplenologica 14: 162–170.

Neerhof M G, Zelman W, Sullivan T 1989 Hepatic rupture in pregnancy: a review. Obstetrical and Gynecological Survey 44: 407–409.

Nir A, Sorokin Y, Abramovici H et al 1989 Pregnancy and primary biliary cirrhosis. International Journal of Gynaecology and Obstetrics 28: 279–282.

Ober W B, Le Compte P M 1955 Acute fatty metamorphosis of the liver associated with pregnancy: a distinctive lesion. American Journal of Medicine 19: 743–758.

Ockner S A, Brunt E M, Cohn S M et al 1990 Fulminant hepatic failure caused by acute fatty liver of pregnancy treated by orthotopic liver transplantation. Hepatology 11: 59–64.

O'Grady J, Day E, Toole A, Paust J C 1977 Splenic artery aneurysm rupture in pregnancy: a review and case report. Obstetrics and Gynecology 50: 627–630.

Okada K, Kamiyama I, Inomata M, Imai M, Miyakawa Y 1976 e antigen and anti-e in the serum of asymptomatic carrier mothers as indicators of positive and negative transmission of hepatitis B virus to their infants. New England Journal of Medicine, 294: 746–749.

Perez V, Gorodisch S, Casavilla F, Maruffo C 1971 Ultrastructure of human liver at the end of normal pregnancy. American Journal of Obstetrics and Gynecology 110: 428–430.

Peters R L, Edmondson H A, Mikkelsen W P, Tatter D 1967 Tetracycline induced fatty liver in non-pregnant patients. American Journal of Surgery 113: 622–628.

Pockros P J, Peters R L, Reynolds T B 1984 Idiopathic fatty liver of pregnancy: findings of ten cases. Medicine 63: 1–11.

Pratt O E 1982 Alcohol and the developing fetus. British Medical Bulletin 38: 48–52.

Purtilo D T, Clark J V, Williams R 1975 Primary hepatic malignancy in pregnant women. American Journal of Obstetrics and Gynecology 121: 41–44.

Rannevik G, Jeppsson S, Kullander S 1972 Effect of oral contraceptives on the liver in women with recurrent cholestasis (hepatosis) during previous pregnancies. British Journal of Obstetrics and Gynaecology 79: 1128–1136.

Reid R, Ivey K J, Rencoret R H, Storey B 1976 Fetal complications of obstetric cholestasis. British Medical Journal 1: 870–872.

Reyes G R 1993 Hepatitis E virus (HEV): molecular biology and emerging epidemiology. In: Boyer J L, Ockner R K (eds) Progress in liver diseases. WB Saunders, Philadelphia, pp 203–213.

Reyes G R, Purdie M A, Kim J P 1990 Isolation of a cDNA from the virus responsible for enterically transmitted non-A, non-B hepatitis. Science 247: 1335–1339.

Reyes H 1982 The enigma of intrahepatic cholestasis of pregnancy: lessons from Chile. Hepatology 1: 87–96.

Reyes H 1992 The spectrum of liver and gastrointestinal disease seen in cholestasis of pregnancy. Gastroenterology Clinics of North America 21: 905–921.

Reyes H, Kern F Jr 1979 Effect of pregnancy on bile flow and biliary lipids in the hamster. Gastroenterology 76: 144–150.

Reyes H, Simon F R 1993 Intrahepatic cholestasis of pregnancy: an estrogen related disease. Seminars in Liver Disease 13: 289–301.

Reyes H, Ribalta J, Gonzalez-Cerou M 1976 Idiopathic cholestasis of pregnancy in a large kindred. Gut 17: 709–713.

Reyes H, Gonzalez M C, Ribalta J et al 1978 Prevalence of intrahepatic cholestasis of pregnancy in Chile. Annals of Internal Medicine 88: 487–493.

Reyes H, Ribalta J, Gonzalez M C, Segovia N, Oberhauser O 1981 Sulfobromophthalein clearance tests before and after ethinyl estradiol administration in women and men with familial history of intrahepatic cholestasis of pregnancy. Gastroenterology 81: 226–331.

Reyes H, Rodrigan M E, Gonzalez M C 1987 Steatorrhoea in patients with intrahepatic cholestasis of pregnancy. Gastroenterology 93: 584–590.

Reyes H, Sandovat L, Wainstein A et al 1994 Acute fatty liver of pregnancy: a clinical study of 12 episodes in 11 patients. Gut 35: 101–106.

Richards R L, Willocks J, Dow T G B 1970 Jaundice in pregnancy. Scottish Medical Journal 15: 52–57.

Riely C A 1984 Acute fatty liver of pregnancy (editorial). Digestive Diseases and Science 29: 456–457.

Riely C A 1987 Acute fatty liver of pregnancy. Seminars in Liver Disease 7: 47–54.

Robson S C, Mutch E, Boys R J, Woodhouse K W 1990 Apparent liver blood flow during pregnancy: a serial study using indocyanine green clearance. British Journal of Obstetrics and Gynaecology 97: 720–724.

Roddie T W 1957 Haemorrhage from primary carcinoma of the liver complicating pregnancy. British Medical Journal 1: 31–39.

Rolfes D B, Ishak K G 1985 Acute fatty liver of pregnancy: a clinicopathologic study of 35 cases. Hepatology 5: 1149–1158.

Rolfes D B, Ishak K G 1986a Liver disease in toxemia of pregnancy. American Journal of Gastroenterology 81: 1138–1144.

Rolfes D B, Ishak K G 1986b Liver disease in pregnancy. Histopathology 10: 555–570.

Rooks J B, Ory H W, Ishak K G et al 1979 Epidemiology of hepatocellular adenoma: the role of oral contraceptive use. Journal of the American Medical Association 242: 644–648.

Rosenblate H J, Eisenstein R, Holmes A W 1970 The liver in sickle cell anemia: a clinical-pathologic study. Archives of Pathology 90: 235–245.

Rosenthal T, Shani M, Deutsch V, Samra H 1972 The Budd-Chiari syndrome after pregnancy: report of two cases and a review of the literature. American Journal of Obstetrics and Gynecology 113: 789–792.

Roulet M, Laurini R, Rivier L et al 1988 Hepatic veno-occlusive disease in newborn infant of a woman drinking herbal tea. Journal of Pediatrics 112: 433–436.

Rustgi V K, Fagiuoli S, Van Thiel D H 1993 The liver in pregnancy. In: Rustgi V K, Van Thiel D H (eds) The liver in systemic disease. Raven Press, New York, pp 267–283.

Salena B J, Sivak M V Jr 1988 Pregnancy and esophageal varices. Gastrointestinal Endoscopy 34: 492–493.

Samsioe G, Svendsen P, Johnson P, Gustafson A 1975 Studies in cholestasis of pregnancy. V. Gallbladder disease, liver function tests, serum lipids and fatty acid composition of serum lecithin in the non-pregnant state. Acta Obstetricia et Gynecologica Scandinavica 54: 417–423.

Samsioe G, Johnson P, Gustafson A 1977 Studies in cholestasis of pregnancy. VI. Fatty acid composition of glycero-phospholipids

before and after delivery. Acta Obstetricia et Gynecologica Scandinavica 56: 31–35.

Saunders P, Jackson B T 1969 Rupture of choledochus cyst in pregnancy. British Medical Journal 3: 573–574.

Scheinberg I H, Sternlieb I 1975 Pregnancy in penicillamine-treated patients with Wilson's disease. New England Journal of Medicine 293: 1300–1302.

Schoeman M N, Batey R G, Wilcken B 1991 Recurrent acute fatty liver of pregnancy associated with a fatty-acid oxidation defect in the offspring. Gastroenterology 100: 544–548.

Schorr-Lesnick B, Lebovics E, Dworkin B, Rosenthal W S 1991a Liver diseases unique to pregnancy. American Journal of Gastroenterology 86: 659–670.

Schorr-Lesnick B, Dworkin B, Rosenthal W S 1991b Haemolysis, elevated liver enzymes and low platelets in pregnancy (HELLP syndrome). Digestive Diseases and Science 36: 1649–1652.

Schreyer P, Caspi E, El-Hindi J M, Eshchar J 1982 Cirrhosis — pregnancy and delivery: a review. Obstetrical and Gynecological Survey 37: 304–312.

Schwer M, Moosa A 1978 The effects of hepatitis A and B in pregnancy on mother and fetus. South African Medical Journal 54: 1092–1095.

Scragg R K R, McMichael A J, Seamark R F 1984 Oral contraceptives, pregnancy and endogenous oestrogen in gall stone disease — a case-control study. British Medical Journal 288: 1795–1799.

Severino L J, Freedman W L, Makeshkumar A P 1970 Spontaneous subcapsular hematoma of liver during pregnancy. New York State Journal of Medicine 70: 2818–2821.

Seymour C A, Chadwick V S 1979 Liver and gastrointestinal function in pregnancy. Postgraduate Medical Journal 55: 343–352.

Seymour C A, Neale G, Peters T J 1977 Lysosomal changes in liver tissue from patients with Dubin-Johnson-Sprinz syndrome. Clinical Science and Molecular Medicine 52: 241–248.

Shani M, Gilon E, Ben-Ezzer J, Sheba C 1970 Sulfobromophthalein tolerance test in patients with Dubin-Johnson syndrome and their relatives. Gastroenterology 59: 842–847.

Sheehan H L 1940 The pathology of acute yellow atrophy and delayed chloroform poisoning. Journal of Obstetrics and Gynaecology of the British Empire 47: 49–62.

Sheehan H L 1961 Jaundice in pregnancy. American Journal of Obstetrics and Gynecology 81: 427–440.

Sheehan H L, Lynch J B 1973 Pathology of toxaemia of pregnancy. Churchill Livingstone, Edinburgh.

Sherlock S 1983 Acute fatty liver of pregnancy and the microvesicular fat diseases. Gut 24: 265–269.

Sherlock S, Dooley J 1992 Diseases of the liver and biliary system, 9th edn. Blackwell Scientific Publications, London.

Shimono N, Ishibashi H, Ikematsu H et al 1990 Fulminant hepatic failure during perinatal period in a pregnant woman with Wilson's disease. Hepatogastroenterology 37 (suppl 2): 122.

Sibai B M 1990 The HELLP syndrome (hemolysis, elevated liver enzymes, and low platelets): much ado about nothing? American Journal of Obstetrics and Gynecology 162: 311–316.

Sibai B M, Taslimi M M, El-Nazer A et al 1986 Maternal-perinatal outcome associated with the syndrome of hemolysis, elevated liver enzymes, and low platelets in severe preeclampsia-eclampsia. American Journal of Obstetrics and Gynecology 155: 501–509.

Siegel M 1973 Congenital malformations following chickenpox, measles, mumps and hepatitis. Journal of the American Medical Association 226: 1521–1524.

Singletary B K, Van Thiel D H, Eagon P K 1986 Estrogen and progesterone receptors in human gallbladder. Hepatology 6: 574–578.

Slater D N, Hague W M 1984 Renal morphological changes in idiopathic acute fatty liver of pregnancy. Histopathology 8: 567–581.

Smith L G, Moise K J, Dildy G A, Carpenter R J 1991 Spontaneous rupture of liver during pregnancy: current therapy. Obstetrics and Gynecology 77: 171–175.

Sommer D G, Greenway G D, Bookstein J J, Orloff M P 1979 Hepatic rupture with toxemia of pregnancy: angiographic diagnosis. American Journal of Radiology 132: 455–456.

Stander H J, Cadden J F 1934 Acute yellow atrophy of the liver in pregnancy. American Journal of Obstetrics and Gynecology 28: 61–69.

Steven M M 1981 Pregnancy and liver disease. Gut 22: 592–614.

Steven M M, Buckley J D, Mackay I R 1979 Pregnancy in chronic active hepatitis. Quarterly Journal of Medicine 48: 519–531.

Stevens C E, Beasley R P, Tsui J, Lee W C 1975 Vertical transmission of hepatitis B antigen in Taiwan. New England Journal of Medicine 292: 771–774.

Stevens C E, Neurath R A, Beasley R P, Smuzness W 1979 HBeAg and anti Hbe detection by radioimmunoassay: correlation with vertical transmission of hepatitis B virus in Taiwan. Journal of Medical Virology 3: 237–241.

Svanborg A 1954 A study of recurrent jaundice in pregnancy. Acta Obstetricia et Gynecologica Scandinavica 33: 434–444.

Svanborg A, Vikrot O 1965 Plasma lipid fractions, including individual phospholipids at various stages of pregnancy. Acta Medica Scandinavica 178: 615–630.

Tanaka K, Keen E A, Johnson B 1976 Jamaican vomiting disease: biochemical investigation of two cases. New England Journal of Medicine 295: 461–467.

Terasaki K K, Quinn M F, Lundell C J, Finck E J, Pentecost M J 1990 Spontaneous hepatic hemorrhage in pre-eclampsia: treatment with hepatic arterial embolization. Radiology 174: 1039–1041.

Thaler M M, Park C K, Landers D V et al 1991 Vertical transmission of hepatitis C virus. Lancet 338: 17–18.

Thomas H C, Jacyna M, Waters J, Main J 1988 Virus-host interaction in chronic hepatitis B virus infection. Seminars in Liver Disease 8: 342–349.

Thorling L 1955 Jaundice in pregnancy: a clinical study. Acta Medica Scandinavica (suppl) 151: 302.

Tiliacos M, Tsantoulas D, Tsoulias A et al 1978 The Budd-Chiari syndrome in pregnancy. Postgraduate Medical Journal 54: 686–691.

Tong M J, Thursby M, Takela J et al 1981 Studies on the maternal-infant transmissions of the viruses which cause acute hepatitis. Gastroenterology 80: 999–1004.

Treem W R, Rinaldo P, Hale D E et al 1994 Acute fatty liver of pregnancy and long-chain 3-hydroxyacyl-coenzyme A dehydrogenase deficiency. Hepatology 19: 339–345.

Tsega E, Hansson B G, Krawczynski E, Nordenfeld E 1992 Acute sporadic viral hepatitis in Ethiopia: causes, risk factors and effects on pregnancy. Clinical and Infectious Diseases 14: 961–965.

Tsuki Y, Sakamoto S, Fujimoto Y et al 1984 Two cases of idiopathic acute fatty liver of pregnancy with a milder clinical course. Acta Hepatologica Japonica 25: 666–673.

Valdiviesco V, Covarrubias C, Siegel F, Cruz F 1993 Pregnancy and cholelithiasis: pathogenesis and natural course of gallstones diagnosed in early puerperium. Hepatology 17: 1–4.

Vanjak D, Moreau R, Roche-Sicot J, Soulier A, Sicot C 1991 Intrahepatic cholestasis of pregnancy and acute fatty liver of pregnancy. Gastroenterology 100: 1123–1125.

Varma R 1987 Course and prognosis of pregnancy in women with liver disease. Seminars in Liver Disease 7: 59–66.

Varner M, Rinderknechts N 1980 Acute fatty metamorphosis of pregnancy: a maternal mortality and literature review. Journal of Reproductive Medicine 24: 177–180.

Vassalli P, Morris R H, McCluskey R T 1963 The pathogenic role of fibrin deposition in the glomerular lesions of toxemia of pregnancy. Journal of Experimental Medicine 118: 467–477.

Vons C, Smadja C, Franco D et al 1984 Successful pregnancy after Budd-Chiari syndrome. Lancet i: 975.

Vore M 1987 Estrogen cholestasis: membranes, metabolites or receptors. Gastroenterology 93: 643–649.

Wagner V P, Smale L E, Lischke J H 1975 Amebic abscess of the liver and spleen in pregnancy and the puerperium. Obstetrics and Gynecology 45: 562–565.

Wallstedt A, Riely C A, Shaver D et al 1990 Prevalence and characteristics of liver dysfunction in hyperemesis gravidarum. Clinical Research 38: 970–976.

Walshe J M 1977 Pregnancy in Wilson's disease. Quarterly Journal of Medicine 46: 73–83.

Walshe J M 1986 The management of pregnancy in Wilson's disease treated with trientine. Quarterly Journal of Medicine 58: 81–87.

Waterson A P 1979 Virus infections (other than rubella) during pregnancy. British Medical Journal 2: 564–566.

Weber F L, Snodgrass P J, Powell D E et al 1979 Abnormalities of hepatic mitochondrial urea-cycle enzyme activities and hepatic ultrastructure in acute fatty liver of pregnancy. Journal of Laboratory and Clinical Medicine 94: 27–41.

Weinstein L 1982 Syndrome of hemolysis, elevated liver enzymes, and low platelet count: a severe consequence of hypertension in pregnancy. American Journal of Obstetrics and Gynecology 142: 159–167.

Weinstein L 1985 Preeclampsia/eclampsia with hemolysis, elevated liver enzymes, and thrombocytopenia. Obstetrics and Gynecology 66: 657–660.

Wejstal R, Hermodsson S, Iwarson S, Norkrans G 1990 Mother to infant transmission of hepatitis C virus infection. Journal of Medical Virology 30: 178–180.

Whelton M J, Sherlock S 1968 Pregnancy in patients with hepatic cirrhosis: management and outcome. Lancet 2: 995–999.

Williams R, Ede R J 1981 Hepatitis in pregnancy (editorial). British Medical Journal 283: 1074–1075.

Wojcicka-Jagodzinska J, Kuczyriska-Sicinska J, Czaykowski K, Smolarczyk R 1989 Carbohydrate metabolism in the course of intrahepatic cholestasis of pregnancy. American Journal of Obstetrics and Gynecology 161: 959–964.

Wolkoff A W, Cohen L E, Arias I M 1973 Inheritance of the Dubin-Johnson syndrome. New England Journal of Medicine 288: 113–117.

Wolpert E, Pascasio F M, Wolkoff A W, Arias I M 1977 Abnormal sulphobromophthalein metabolism in Rotor's syndrome and obligate heterozygotes. New England Journal of Medicine 296: 1099–1101.

Wong D C, Purcell R H, Sreenivasan M A, Prasad S R, Pavri K M 1980 Epidemic and endemic hepatitis in India: evidence for a non A, non B hepatitis virus aetiology. Lancet ii: 876–879.

Yen S C 1964 Spontaneous rupture of liver during pregnancy. Obstetrics and Gynecology 23: 783–787.

Ylostalo P, Kirkinen P H, Heikkinen J et al 1981 Gallbladder volume in cholestasis of pregnancy. New England Journal of Medicine 304: 359.

Zanetti A R, Ferroni P, Magliano E M et al 1982 Perinatal transmission of the hepatitis B virus and of the HBV associated delta agent from mothers to offspring in northern Italy. Journal of Medical Virology 9: 139–148.

Zimmerman H J, Ishak K G 1982 Valproate-induced hepatic injury: analysis of 23 fatal cases. Hepatology 2: 591–597.

Zimmerman H J, Ishak K G 1987 Hepatic injury due to drugs and toxins. In: MacSween R N M, Anthony P P, Scheuer P J (eds) Pathology of the liver, 2nd edn. Churchill Livingstone, Edinburgh, pp 335–386.

58. Pathology of the cardiovascular system in pregnancy

Eckhardt G. J. Olsen   H. Fox

INTRODUCTION

With the continuing excellence of antenatal care in the developed countries, patients with known cardiac disease are so carefully supervised during pregnancy, labour and the puerperium that maternal deaths directly attributable to cardiac disorder rarely occur nowadays. Conversely, if pre-existing cardiac abnormalities are severe, either conception does not occur or termination of pregnancy is advised. It is therefore not surprising that material for the pathological study of the heart in pregnancy is now scarce.

This was not, however, the case in the past and one only has to refer to older texts of pathology to learn that, prior to the practice of antiseptic surgery, puerperal sepsis occurred in one in six women who were admitted to maternity hospitals, many of whom died as a result of bacterial septicaemia. The heart was not uncommonly involved in such a septicaemia with a resulting endocarditis or myocarditis. An example of this is shown in Figure 58.1, which shows a staphylococcal abscess in the walls of the left ventricle (Fig. 58.2). Such cases are happily now extremely rare.

This chapter will describe the involvement of the heart during pregnancy and the puerperium. The pathologist clearly needs to know the effects of pregnancy on the normal heart and may well be required to give an opinion not only as to whether pregnancy has contributed to the death of a cardiac patient but also as to whether cardiac disease has played a rôle in an obstetric death. The discussion will therefore be under three principal headings:

1. The effect of pregnancy on the normal heart
2. The effect of pregnancy on previously present cardiac disease
3. Cardiovascular disease arising during pregnancy or the puerperium.

Inevitably the effects of pregnancy on the heart are closely linked with physiological and clinical manifestations and these will therefore also be included in the various sections whenever appropriate.

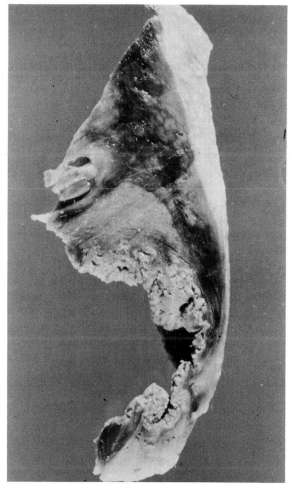

Fig. 58.1 An abscess in the left ventricular wall is illustrated which was due to staphylococcal septicaemia and myocarditis following delivery. (From Olsen, 1980a. By permission of Macmillan Publishers Ltd.)

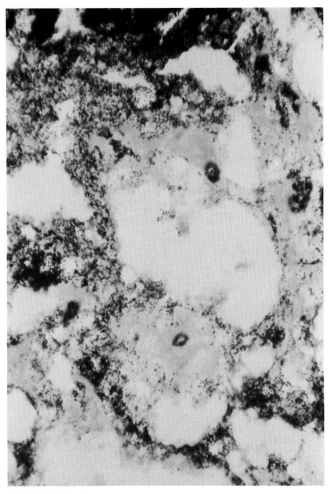

Fig. 58.2 Photomicrograph of the abscess illustrated in Fig. 58.1. The large number of staphylococci are clearly seen. Gram stain × 600.

THE EFFECT OF PREGNANCY ON THE NORMAL HEART

Heart size

Heart weight can be related either to body weight or to height. Zeek (1942) constructed a table of normal values according to height (Table 58.1) and these figures provide an approximate guide to normal heart weights. Because, however, epicardial fat is commonly not removed when weighing the heart and because variable lengths of the great vessels are often included in the heart weight, values of 30 grams above or below the weights stated in the table are acceptable as being within the normal range. For more accurate assessment of heart weight, particularly in cases of mild hypertrophy, separate recordings of ventricular and septal weights, after removal of the atria, atrioventricular rings, valves, epicardial fat and coronary arteries, are essential. The free walls of the right and left ventricles and the septum are separately weighed and the ratio is calculated (Fulton et al, 1952).

Table 58.1 Heart weights in relationship to height (from Zeek, 1942)

Height	Heart weight (in grams)
150 cm	215–275
152 cm	221–281
155 cm	224–284
160 cm	233–293
165 cm	242–302
170 cm	251–311
175 cm	260–320
180 cm	269–329
183 cm	274–334
185 cm	277–337
191 cm	286–346

Table 58.2 Normal wall thickness in the heart

Atrial walls 2–2.5 mm thick
Right ventricle (at the conus) 2–3 mm thick
Left ventricle 12–15 mm thick

Wall measurements are also helpful in the assessment of normal hearts (Table 58.2) but become unreliable if hypertrophy is accompanied by dilatation.

The haemodynamic changes of pregnancy (vide infra) have no lasting effect on the myocardium.

Haemodynamic changes

Circulatory changes begin in the first trimester of pregnancy and these physiological adaptions become clearly manifest by mid-gestation. The blood volume expands by 30–40%, this increase commencing in the first trimester and reaching a sustained plateau at the 30th week of gestation. Cardiac output also increases by up to 40% above that found in normal non-pregnant women, reaching a peak at mid-gestation and declining slightly during the last eight weeks of pregnancy. Initially the increased cardiac output is achieved by an increased stroke volume but heart rate increases progressively throughout pregnancy, to reach a peak of 95 at term, and stroke volume gradually returns to normal levels (Ueland & Metcalfe, 1975).

During labour and delivery there is a further increase in cardiac output with each contraction: there is also a transient rise in arterial blood pressure with each contraction and this is associated with a reflex bradycardia. Immediately following a vaginal delivery cardiac output increases by as much as 60% over pre-delivery levels, falling gradually to non-pregnant levels over the next two weeks.

These haemodynamic changes place no undue stress on the patient with a normal heart but may lead to cardiac decompensation if the functional capacity of the heart is impaired by pre-existing disease.

Changes in blood coagulation system

Platelet adhesiveness does not alter during pregnancy or labour but increases slightly after delivery, this alteration persisting for about 72 hours (Shaper, 1968). Fibrinolytic activity is depressed during pregnancy but assumes normal levels at delivery, this change occurring even before the umbilical cord is clamped (Shaper et al, 1965; Shaper, 1966). An initial rise above normal levels occurs for about 30 minutes with a subsequent return to sustained normal levels.

EFFECT OF PREGNANCY ON PREVIOUSLY PRESENT CARDIAC DISEASE

It is difficult to assess the true incidence of pre-existing heart disease complicating pregnancy as reports in the literature are often either studies of single cases or of large series emanating from specialized referral centres. Despite these limitations it is generally thought that about 1% of pregnant women will be suffering from some form of acquired or congenital heart lesion (Ehrenfeld et al, 1964). Ueland (1978) has pointed out that over the last few decades there has been a decrease in the incidence of heart disease in pregnancy: thus during the years 1940–1950 the incidence was between 2.3% and 3.3% whilst between 1960 and 1970 this incidence had fallen to between 0.57% and 1.5%.

Congenital and developmental heart disease

Wooley et al (1961) studied the course of 204 pregnancies in 103 women with congenital heart disease; in 80 of these patients the diagnosis had been confirmed by catheterization studies whilst in the remaining 23 patients the diagnosis was a purely clinical one. In the 80 fully confirmed cases the following congenital lesions were present:

atrial septal defect	31
patent ductus arteriosus	27
pulmonary stenosis	5
tetralogy of Fallot	5
coarctation of aorta	4
Ebstein's anomaly	3
aortic valve lesion	3
unclassified	2

In this series there was a spontaneous abortion rate of 17%, this being comparable to that found in an unselected control group of pregnant women. There was a correlation between fetal loss and maternal pulmonary hypertension, and 41 of the 48 abortions occurred in the 54 patients with atrial or ventricular septal defects. There was, however, only one maternal death in this series and this was due to staphylococcal endocarditis following dental extraction during pregnancy. Naeye et al (1967)

also concluded that the maternal mortality rate for women with congenital heart disease was about 1% and these studies indicate that many women with congenital cardiac lesions can sustain multiple pregnancies without untoward incident: further, the favourable results noted in unoperated women suggest that pregnancy is not, in itself, an indication for corrective cardiac surgery.

Coarctation of the aorta

This is defined as a significant narrowing of some part of the aorta, most commonly in the region of the ductus arteriosus. The classification of Edwards (1960) is recommended (Table 58.3) for precise anatomical categorization. The coarctation may be string-like, flask-shaped or resemble an hour glass (Cleland et al, 1956) and histologically there is thickening of the aortic media at the site of coarctation which may be associated with fibroelastic intimal thickening. The aortic media proximal to the coarctation shows an increase in elastic fibres whilst distal to the constriction there is a marked decrease in the medial content of such fibres.

Though views differ, it is generally held that pregnancy increases the risk of complications in patients with a coarctation, these complications including heart failure, rupture of the aorta, cerebral haemorrhage during labour and, very occasionally, aortic dissection. In one series of 53 cases no ill effects were noted in 36, but in 11 patients symptoms worsened and six maternal deaths occurred (Benham, 1949). A maternal mortality of 10% was noted in Pritchard's (1953) series of 79 cases and this compares with Goodwin's (1958) report of a 9.3% mortality in 123 cases. In Goodwin's series rupture of the aorta was

Table 58.3 Classification of coarctation

Group I:	Coarctation distal to ductus arteriosus (adult type) (A) with closed ductus (B) with patent ductus
Group II:	Coarctation proximal to ductus arteriosus (infantile type) (A) with closed ductus (B) with patent ductus
Group III:	Coarctation with anomalies of subclavian arteries or aortic arches (A) atresia or stenosis of left subclavian artery (B) stenosis of right subclavian artery (C) anomalous origin of right subclavian artery (1) distal to coarctation; (2) proximal to coarctation (D) double aortic arch with stenosis of right and coarctation of the left arch
Group IV:	Coarctation in unusual locations (A) proximal to left subclavian artery: (1) with normal branches; (2) with anomalous origin of the right subclavian artery (B) multiple sites (C) lower thoracic or abdominal; the latter (D'Abreu et al, 1959) may be subdivided into: (1) suprarenal; (2) interrenal; (3) infrarenal

the commonest cause of death but he did not think that pregnancy specifically increased the risk of this particular complication.

These findings have led some to recommend either surgical correction of the coarctation during pregnancy or caesarean section at term, particularly if there is a rise in blood pressure towards the end of pregnancy or during labour (Rosenthal, 1955). Others suggest that pregnancy should be allowed to proceed to term with shortening of the second stage of a vaginal delivery and resection of the anomaly after delivery (Goodwin, 1958; Ramin et al, 1989). Deal & Wooley (1973) felt that no general recommendation could be made for patients with a coarctation, each woman having to be managed on an individual basis.

Mortensen & Ellsworth (1965) compared the complications encountered in women with an untreated coarctation with those occurring in patients who had undergone corrective surgery before becoming pregnant (Table 58.4) and showed clearly that women with a corrected coarctation generally have fully normal pregnancies.

Left to right shunts

Left to right shunting occurs through an atrial septal defect, a ventricular septal defect or a patent ductus arteriosus, these being collectively the commonest congenital anomalies of the heart encountered in gravid women. As, during pregnancy, there is normally no significant alteration in the degree of shunting, the gravid state is well tolerated in patients with uncomplicated left to right shunts and there is no excess of maternal mortality (McAnulty et al, 1982; Clarke, 1991; Hess & Hess, 1992). If, however, the shunt becomes reversed during pregnancy the patient is placed at serious risk of congestive cardiac failure and death. Shunt reversal tends usually to occur in the immediately postpartum period and is due to a sudden rise in pulmonary pressure. It has been suggested that this is due to haemodynamic changes in the pulmonary circulation but Naeye et al (1967) found extensive thrombosis of the pulmonary vessels in autopsies on four fatal cases of postpartum shunt reversal.

Right to left shunts

Eisenmenger's syndrome. This term applies to the

Table 58.4 Complications during pregnancy in patients with and without surgical correction of aortic coarctation

	No operation	Coarctation repaired
Number of patients	9	8
Number of pregnancies	32	21
Normal pregnancies	3	18
Living babies	13	19
Obstetric complications	22	2
Cardiovascular or renal complications	16	1

development of high pulmonary vascular resistance in a patient with a previous left to right shunt, this occurring when pulmonary hypertension complicates a patent ductus arteriosus, ventricular septal defect or atrial septal defect. This association poses an extremely serious threat to a pregnant woman. Jones & Howitt (1965) reported a maternal mortality rate of 27.33% in women with this syndrome whilst in a later review of 70 pregnancies in 44 women with Eisenmenger's syndrome there was a maternal death rate of 52% (Gleicher et al, 1979): the mortality was higher in those patient with a ventricular septal defect (60%) than in those with either an atrial septal defect or a patent ductus arteriosus (44% and 41.7% respectively). Maarek-Charbit & Corone (1986) reviewed 42 pregnancies in women with Eisenmenger's syndrome and noted a 36% maternal mortality. Death occurs most commonly at, or soon after, delivery and is due to increased right to left shunting, either because of a fall in systemic pressure subsequent to blood loss or because of a rise in pulmonary pressure as a result either of haemodynamic changes or pulmonary embolism.

Fallot's tetralogy. This condition is defined as a ventricular septal defect with obstruction of the right ventricular outflow and a right to left shunt at rest or on effort. Four characteristic anatomical changes are seen in combination: a large ventricular septal defect, obstruction of pulmonary blood flow (which can occur at the infundibulum, at the pulmonary valve or above the pulmonary valve), overriding of the ventricular septal defect by the aorta and right ventricular hypertrophy.

This is the most common form of cyanotic congenital heart disease and when associated with pregnancy carries a high risk of cardiac failure or sudden death, the maternal mortality rate being between 4% and 12% (Mendelson, 1951; Meyer et al, 1964; Jones & Howitt, 1965; Ueland, 1978). Currently, however, unoperated patients are seldom encountered during pregnancy and it is clear that surgical correction of Fallot's tetralogy allows for a fully normal pregnancy. Singh et al (1982) reported 40 uneventful pregnancies in 27 women with a corrected tetralogy, there being no cardiac complications or maternal deaths.

Aortic stenosis

Isolated stenosis of the aortic valve is almost always congenital and accounts for just over 1% of all congenital heart disease. Several forms, such as 'dome-shaped deformity' or 'uni-commissural dome stenosis' have been described (Olsen, 1980a) whilst stenosis may also occur in cases of bicuspid aortic valves. This condition is rare in pregnancy but Arias & Pineda (1978) reported one example and reviewed 38 pregnancies in previously described cases. These patients were particularly prone to cardiac failure and death during pregnancy and had a maternal mortality rate of 17.4%, demise occurring particularly during labour and delivery. More recently, Easterling et al (1988) reviewed 5 cases of aortic stenosis during pregnancy: there were no maternal or fetal deaths. There is no advantage to pregnancy termination in women with aortic stenosis for this procedure is also associated with a high mortality rate (Ramin et al, 1989).

Isolated pulmonary stenosis

Pregnant women with this congenital valvular abnormality run a high risk of congestive cardiac failure: death is, however, uncommon and Knapp & Arditi (1968) reviewed 75 cases of pulmonary stenosis in pregnant women in whom there were no deaths. Patients previously treated by surgery or balloon valvuloplasty have trouble-free pregnancies (Pitkin, 1990).

Ebstein's anomaly

This abnormality is characterized by varying degrees of displacement of the posterior and septal leaflets of the tricuspid valve into the right ventricle and is accompanied by right ventricular and atrial changes. This anomaly accounts for less than 1% of congenital heart disease and has been rarely noted in pregnancy: Littler (1970) has, however, described a successful pregnancy in a woman with this defect.

Developmental abnormalities

A number of conditions are rather arbitrarily designated as 'developmental' rather than 'congenital'.

Mitral valve prolapse. This is an entity common in otherwise normal women of child-bearing age, its incidence in this group being variously estimated as between 4 and 28% (Markiewicz et al, 1976; Procacci et al, 1976; Boudoulas & Wooley, 1988). Most individuals are asymptomatic but a minority suffer chest pain, arrhythmias, palpitations or effort intolerance (Alpert et al, 1991; Alpert, 1993). Rupture of a chordae tendinae, congestive cardiac failure, infective endocarditis, cerebral embolism or sudden death may occur (Olsen, 1980a; Kolibash, 1988; Marks et al, 1989; Alpert, 1993). Clinically, there is typically a mid-systolic click followed by a late systolic murmur (Barlow et al, 1968) whilst morphologically there is a mucoid change of the valve leaflets, affecting predominantly the posterior leaflet of the mitral valve which is enlarged, sometimes considerably so. The pathogenesis of this abnormality is obscure but suggested aetiological factors include an inborn excessive prominence of the zona spongiosa (Olsen & Al-Rufaie, 1980), a biochemical abnormality (Davies et al, 1981) and an anatomical abnormality of the chordae tendinae (Becker & DeWit, 1979).

The effects of pregnancy on this lesion have been rarely described but Rayburn & Fontana (1981) have reviewed 42 pregnancies in 25 patients with a mitral valve prolapse: there were no cardiac complications, no increased risk of obstetrical complications and no maternal deaths.

Marfan's syndrome. This hereditary connective tissue disorder is characterized pathologically by aneurysmal dilatation of the root of the aorta and/or the ascending part of the aorta, accompanied by thinning of the aortic wall. This disorder also commonly affects the valve leaflets which are often thin, translucent and show a bluish tinge. Twenty five per cent of patients have a clinically detectable aortic regurgitation and if aortic insufficiency has been present for some time there is secondary valve thickening and, often, severe hypertrophy and dilatation of the left ventricle. Histologically, two features are seen in the aortic wall, the formation of medial mucoid pools and fragmentation of the medial elastic tissue (Fig. 58.3a & b): rarely, the mucoid pools attain cystic size (Keene et al, 1971: Olsen, 1975a). In the valve leaflets the zona spongiosa is particularly prominent whilst if there has been long-standing aortic regurgitation the aortic valve will be thickened by a superimposition of fibroelastic tissue. It should be noted that these pathological changes are sometimes found in patients with no other stigmata of Marfan's syndrome, the term 'Marfan forme fruste' being applied to such cases (Olsen, 1975a, b).

Complications of Marfan's syndrome include aortic dissection and rupture and there is a general belief that the incidence of these complications is increased during pregnancy, a maternal mortality of 50% being quoted for gravid women with this disorder (Ueland, 1978). Pyeritz (1981) reviewed all the 32 cases of previously reported Marfan's syndrome and confirmed this high mortality rate, 16 of the patients having died; he reported, however, a personal series of 105 pregnancies in women with Marfan's syndrome in which there was only one maternal death, this being in a woman who was in congestive cardiac failure before pregnancy supervened. Pyeritz concluded that whilst pregnancy in a woman with aortic root dilatation or aortic regurgitation was highly dangerous, those women without aortic root dilatation or aortic regurgitation usually did well in pregnancy and were not at increased risk of death.

Congenital heart block. Patients with this condition complicating pregnancy usually survive pregnancy with no untoward incident, though some will need temporary pacing (Eddy & Frankenfeld, 1977; Dalvi et al, 1992).

Acquired cardiovascular disease

Rheumatic heart disease

In the past the ratio of rheumatic to congenital heart disease in pregnancy was 20:1; in recent years, however, the incidence of rheumatic heart disease declined to the

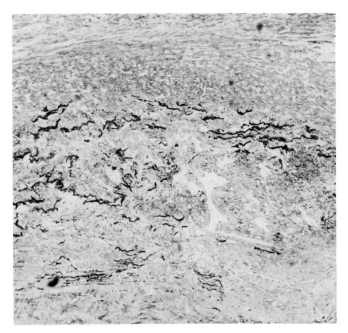

Fig. 58.3a The wall of the aorta in Marfan's disease. Extensive fragmentation of the medial elastic components is seen in all areas and is not confined to the region of mucoid pools. Miller's elastic van Gieson × 60.

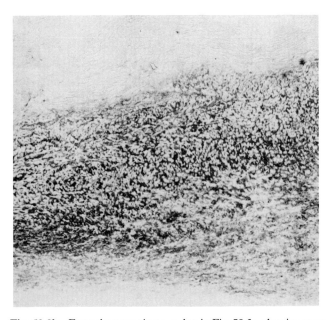

Fig. 58.3b From the same tissue as that in Fig. 58.3a, showing areas of acid mucopolysaccharides. Alcian Blue × 60.

extent that this ratio was only 3:1 (Ueland, 1978). Today this ratio is probably approaching unity (Shime et al, 1987).

The pathology of this disease, with its typical triad of valve thickening and commissural fusion together with chordal shortening and thickening, is well known, though predominantly commissural (Fig. 58.4) or largely chordal

forms are less well recognized. Histologically, the valve leaflets are thickened by fibroelastic tissue and there is a chronic inflammatory cell infiltration of variable intensity: an increased valvular vascularity, characterized particularly by the presence of thick-walled capillaries (Fig. 58.5), is a notable feature and is the only reliable criterion for distinguishing rheumatic from congenital valve disease.

In 75% of cases in which rheumatic heart disease complicates pregnancy the sole, or predominant, lesion is mitral stenosis. Women with this condition are at risk of developing pulmonary oedema, congestive heart failure, atrial fibrillation, acute circulatory failure and pulmonary thromboembolism, though the incidence of such complications has declined in recent years (Szekely et al, 1973). The overall mortality rate for women with mitral stenosis is now well under 1% (O'Driscoll et al, 1962; Ueland, 1978) though patients with either atrial fibrillation or pulmonary oedema have a mortality rate in the range of 17–20% (Ueland, 1984). In theory, the woman with mitral stenosis is at most risk towards the end of the second trimester and during the immediately postpartum period. The latter of these assumptions appears to be correct for nearly half of the obstetric deaths due to mitral stenosis occur during the puerperium, almost invariably because of acute pulmonary oedema. Of those patients dying during pregnancy relatively few die at the end of the second trimester, nearly 75% succumbing after the 32nd week of gestation. Mitral valvulotomy is sometimes required during pregnancy and the operation does not appear to carry any additional hazard when performed on gravid women (Knapp & Arditi, 1968; Esteves et al, 1991). Percutaneous balloon valvulotomy is also a safe procedure during pregnancy and is now probably the technique of choice (Glantz et al, 1993). Patients with aortic stenosis of rheumatic origin are thought to be at considerable risk during pregnancy: any sudden drop in cardiac output, due to hypovolaemia, may lead to sudden death and a maternal mortality rate in the region of 17% has been noted (Arias & Pineda, 1978). Women with mitral regurgitation, aortic regurgitation or with tricuspid valve disease usually tolerate pregnancy well (McAnulty et al, 1982; Clarke, 1991).

Infective endocarditis

This condition may, of course, develop in pregnancy as a complication of either congenital or rheumatic valvular disease. Payne et al (1982) described such a case and reviewed the 21 other cases of bacterial endocarditis occurring in gravid women which had been reported since 1957. Medical treatment is as successful in the pregnant patient as it is in the non-gravid woman but nevertheless the overall maternal mortality rate is approximately 20–25% (Cox & Leveno, 1989).

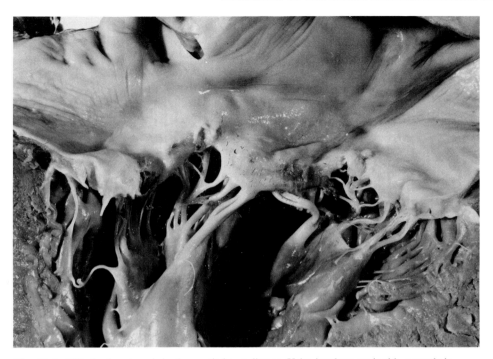

Fig. 58.4 Mitral valve stenosis in rheumatic heart disease. Valve involvement in this example is mainly commissural. The valve leaflets and some chordae are thickened but the latter are not shortened. A thrombus on the anterior leaflet can be seen.

Prosthetic heart valves

The success attained in treating both acquired and congenital heart disease by artificial valve replacement has resulted in an increasing number of women with valve prostheses becoming pregnant. As experience with such cases has accumulated it has become clear that most patients with a prosthetic valve have a haemodynamic reserve that is more than adequate for a safe pregnancy (Oakley & Doherty, 1976; Lutz et al, 1978; Chen et al, 1982; Oakley, 1983; Uetsuka et al, 1990; Badduke et al, 1991; Lee et al, 1994). A real danger is, however, presented to these women by the increased risk of thromboembolism whilst gravid and this makes it necessary for patients with a mechanical valve, but not those with bioprosthetic or homograft valves, to receive anticoagulants throughout pregnancy (McColgin et al, 1989; Clarke, 1991). Anticoagulants reduce considerably the risk to the mother but do, unfortunately, pose some dangers to the fetus. Coumarin derivatives, if taken in early pregnancy, are teratogenic and associated with a high incidence of abortion whilst their use at any stage of gestation carries a risk of central nervous system defects in the fetus, probably because of cerebral microhaemorrhages. The use of heparin is also associated with a high incidence of abortion, premature labour and stillbirth and is not fully effective in preventing valve thrombosis (Oakley, 1983).

Conditions of unknown aetiology

Hypertrophic cardiomyopathy. This condition, also known as idiopathic hypertrophic subaortic stenosis, belongs to the group of heart muscle diseases of unknown cause. It is recognized microscopically by asymmetric, often severe, hypertrophy of the interventricular septum and is characterized histologically by severe hypertrophy and disarray of the myocardial fibres. The myocardial nuclei are often of a bizarre shape and frequently surrounded by a clear glycogen-containing zone. Ultrastructurally, there is extensive disarray of myocardial fibrils with many abnormal inter- and intrafibrillar connections (Olsen, 1980b).

Pregnancy is potentially dangerous in this condition but Oakley et al (1979) have analysed a series of 54 pregnancies in 23 patients in which there were no maternal or fetal deaths, a result only achieved by careful management during the gestational period.

Takayasu's disease. This condition affects particularly women aged between 15 and 40 and predominantly involves the aorta and its main branches. The walls of the affected arteries are thicker than normal despite aneurysmal dilatation. Histologically, intimal thickening is uniform and severe, consisting of loosely arranged connective tissue which is rich in acid mucopolysaccharides but devoid of elastic tissue. There is destruction and fibrous replacement of the media with almost total loss of

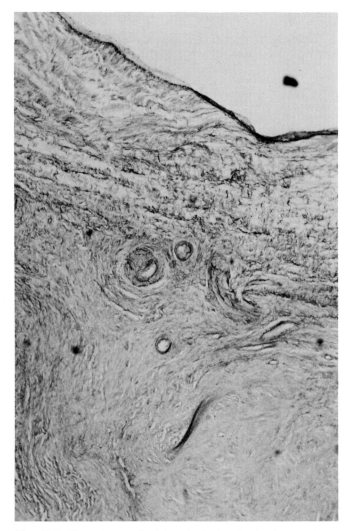

Fig. 58.5 Photomicrograph of the mitral valve showing increased vascularity. The capillary-sized vessels are invested with a thick muscular coat. From a patient with rheumatic heart disease who underwent valve replacement following successful pregnancy. Miller's elastic van Gieson × 64.

medial elastic tissue. The adventitia is often thickened to an extreme degree, anchoring the affected vessels to neighbouring structures (Olsen, 1980a).

Ishikawa & Matsuura (1982) and Jonge et al (1983) supplemented an earlier review by Hauth et al (1977) of Takayasu's disease complicating pregnancy. Ishikawa & Matsuura, working in Japan, described a personally studied series of 33 pregnancies in 27 patients and reviewed reports of 50 pregnancies in 46 patients. In general, the course of the disease does not appear to be influenced by pregnancy, some patients improving and others worsening during the gestational period. There is, however, a tendency for these patients to have an unusually marked elevation of arterial blood pressure during labour and immediately after delivery and this may cause cardiovascular embarrassment.

Primary pulmonary hypertension. Females, usually during their reproductive years, develop this disease much more commonly than do males and Shepherd et al (1957) have suggested that non-fatal amniotic fluid embolism during parturition may be an aetiological factor: no definite correlation with pregnancy has, however, been established. The haemodynamic changes of pregnancy throw a severe stress on the heart in this condition and the maternal mortality rate in pregnant patients with primary pulmonary hypertension is in the region of 50% (McCaffrey & Dunn, 1964; McAnulty et al, 1981); death may be due to congestive cardiac failure or to acute circulatory collapse.

CARDIOVASCULAR DISEASE ARISING DURING PREGNANCY OR THE PUERPERIUM

Myocardial infarction

During pregnancy total serum cholesterol values rise and the distribution between alpha and beta lipoproteins assumes a pattern similar to that found in men with ischaemic heart disease (Oliver & Boyd, 1955). Despite these changes myocardial infarction is rare during pregnancy: only 26 cases had been reported by 1960 (Watson et al, 1960), this figure rising to 30 by 1967 (Fletcher et al, 1967) to 39 by 1970 and to 70 by 1985 (Hankins et al, 1985). Despite the fact that total plasma lipids reach a peak during the latter part of pregnancy, myocardial infarction is almost equally divided between the first and second half of pregnancy.

In some cases infarction appears to be due either to coronary artery spasm, possibly consequent upon release of renin from ischaemic chorionic tissue (Sasse et al, 1975), or to thrombosis of a non-atheromatous coronary artery (Ciraulo & Markowitz, 1979): in one case infarction was attributed to an isolated arteritis of the coronary vessels (Ahronheim, 1977). Whatever the cause the infarction is usually anterior and commonly transmural (Nolan & Hankins, 1989). Myocardial infarction may easily be missed during pregnancy, chest pain being misdiagnosed as abdominal in origin and electrocardiographic changes being difficult to interpret because of elevation of the diaphragm. Nevertheless the prognosis is generally good, certainly in the first two trimesters, though the mortality rate in third-trimester infarctions can be as high as 45% (Nolan & Hankins, 1989). There is no reason to believe that the sequential healing process in the damaged myocardium differs in any way from that in the general non-pregnant population.

One particular, apparently highly lethal, form of myocardial infarction, fortunately rare, occurs during the first two weeks after delivery and tends particularly to affect primiparous women in their late twenties who have suffered during pregnancy from pregnancy-induced hypertension. Forty five percent of patients with this condition either die or suffer a cardiac arrest (Beary et al, 1979).

Arterial aneurysms

There is a particular tendency for the pregnant woman to suffer rupture of an arterial aneurysm. This propensity has been attributed partly to the haemodynamic changes which characterize the gravid state and partly to hormone-induced changes, such as intimal hyperplasia and altered organization of the media, in the arteries during pregnancy (Barrett et al, 1982). Some doubt has, however, recently been expressed as to whether pregnancy per se is a true risk factor for aneurysm formation, it being suggested that complicating hypertension may be of considerable importance (Wooley & Sparks, 1992).

Fifty per cent of women aged less than 40 who develop a dissecting aortic aneurysm are pregnant at the time this catastrophe occurs (Mandel et al, 1954). Advancing maternal age appears to be a significant risk factor during pregnancy but multiparity is not (Konishi et al, 1980): dissection occurs most commonly during the third trimester (49% of cases), the first two days of the puerperium (19% of cases) or labour (13%). Only 19% of aortic dissections occur during the first two trimesters (Konishi et al, 1980). The dissection is usually in the ascending aorta and has, in the past, been associated with a mortality rate in excess of 90%. There are, however, grounds for believing that the current aggressive surgical approach to a dissecting aortic aneurysm has much improved this gloomy prognosis (Barrett et al, 1982).

More than 100 examples of rupture of a splenic artery aneurysm during pregnancy have been described (O'Grady et al, 1977; Holdsworth & Gunn, 1992; Angelakis et al, 1993) and up to 50% of ruptured splenic artery aneurysms occur in pregnancy, predominantly during the first trimester (Vassalotti & Schaller, 1967; Barrett et al, 1982; Trastek et al, 1985; Holdsworth & Gunn, 1992). The maternal mortality from rupture in pregnancy is about 70% and the fetal mortality is as high as 95% (Trastek et al, 1985; Holdsworth & Gunn, 1992).

Seventeen cases of pregnancy-associated dissecting aneurysm of the coronary arteries have been recorded (Shaver et al, 1978; Barrett et al, 1982), all involving the anterior descending branch of the left coronary artery: in 15 cases the dissection occurred during the puerperium and only two patients survived. Most of the affected women have been relatively elderly and of moderately high parity. There have been 14 instances of ruptured renal artery aneurysm associated with pregnancy (Saleh & McLeod, 1977; Barrett et al, 1982) nearly all of which occurred antepartum: only four of the 14 patients survived. Four cases of pregnancy-related rupture of an ovar-

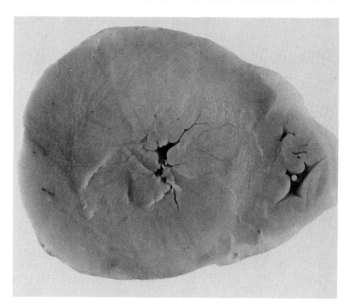

Fig. 58.6 Cross section of the ventricles in hypertensive heart disease, showing concentric hypertrophy of the left ventricle.

ian artery aneurysm have also been recorded, all rupturing in the immediate postpartum period (Barrett et al, 1982). Rupture of a cerebral artery aneurysm during pregnancy is discussed in Chapter 60.

Hypertensive disease of pregnancy

Death due to eclampsia is now very rare in western countries and demise due to cardiac failure in this condition is excessively rare. There has, in the past, been some debate as to the existence or otherwise of a specific 'toxaemic cardiomyopathy' (Benchimol et al, 1959) but it is now agreed that cardiac failure in pre-eclampsia or eclampsia is solely, and directly, attributable to hypertension. In fatal cases, the typical changes of hypertensive heart disease are found with concentric hypertrophy of the left ventricular wall (Fig. 58.6), often to a striking degree: there is not usually any marked dilatation. Histologically, the myocardial fibres are hypertrophied but in normal alignment: focal fibrous replacement may be noted (Fig. 58.7). Ultrastructurally, there is an increase in the number of myocardial mitochondria (Fig. 58.8), above the normal of one per two sarcomeres, together with folding of the nuclear membrane, enlargement of the Golgi apparatus and hypertrophy of the T tubular system. The amount of glycogen is increased and intramitochondrial glycogen deposits may be encountered (Maron & Ferrans, 1975; Olsen, 1980a).

Peripartal heart disease

The development of unexplained heart failure in late preg-

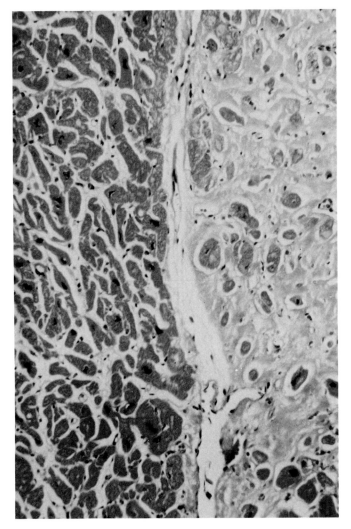

Fig. 58.7 Photomicrograph of the myocardium in hypertension showing fibre hypertrophy. There is an increase in diameter of the cardiocytes as well as nuclear changes of hypertrophy. A focus of replacement fibrosis is clearly seen. H & E × 60.

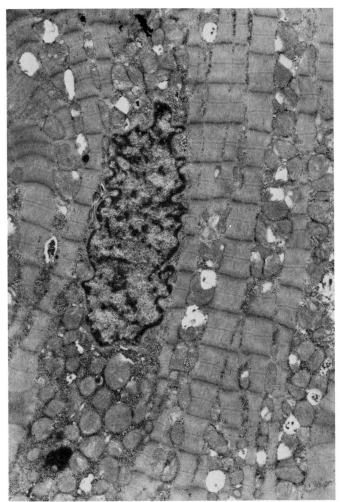

Fig. 58.8 Electronmicrograph of hypertrophy due to hypertension. The wall of the nucleus is slightly folded. An increase of mitochondria of up to 3 per 2 sarcomeres (normal 1 mitochondrion per 2 sarcomeres) between the myofibrils in parallel alignment can be observed. An increase in glycogen, best seen between the mitochondria in the perinuclear areas, is also present. Lead citrate and uranyl acetate × 8024.

nancy has been recognized for over a century (Meadows, 1960). Because of the differing times of onset of this condition it has been variously called 'peripartum cardiac failure' or 'peripartum cardiomyopathy': the WHO/ISFC Task Force recommended the term 'peripartal heart disease'. The condition is of world-wide distribution, having been reported in North America, Europe, South America, the Far East, the Caribbean and Australia (Meadows, 1960; Goodwin 1975; Aroney et al, 1986; Bassaw et al, 1992; Hsieh et al, 1992).

Peripartal heart disease may be defined as the development of heart failure occurring for the first time either in the last trimester of pregnancy or during the first three months after delivery in the absence of any determinable cause for the cardiac failure, such as eclampsia, hypertension or rheumatic heart disease (Hughes et al, 1970;

Demakis & Rahimtoola, 1971). Recently, the WHO Expert Committee on Cardiomyopathies has recommended that this definition should be extended to include the first six months after delivery. The incidence of this condition is difficult to ascertain and estimates have varied between 1 in 1300 to 1 in 4000 pregnancies (Woolford, 1952; Meadows, 1957; Vielle, 1984), the condition occurring most commonly in older, multiparous black women (Vielle, 1984). Data recording the incidence of this disease should, however, be treated with considerable scepticsm for Cunningham et al (1986) found that the clinical diagnosis could only be sustained in 7 of 28 patients who had been dubbed as suffering from peripartal heart disease.

Typically, patients present with left heart failure late in pregnancy or during the puerperium: dyspnoea, tachycar-

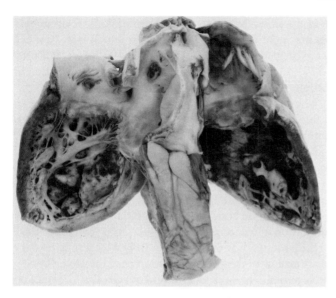

Fig. 58.9   Peripartal heart disease. The ventricular cavities have been displayed. Despite hypertrophy the myocardial walls are normal in thickness. This is due to severe dilatation masking the degree of hypertrophy that is present. Note the intracavitary thrombus. From a 27-year-old Nigerian woman who, following the onset of symptoms three weeks after a second uneventful pregnancy, died three months later. (By courtesy of Dr. J. F. Geddes from the Department of Histopathology, Royal Free Hospital, London.)

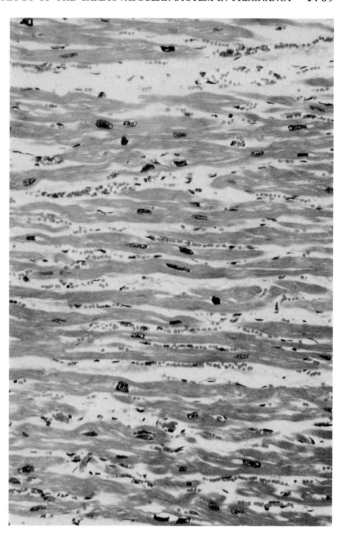

Fig. 58.10   From a patient with peripartal heart disease. The tissue had been obtained by means of the King's bioptome. The myocardial fibres are in parallel alignment, nuclear changes of hypertrophy (vesicular or pyknotic changes or blunting of the nuclear poles) are present but the diameter of cardiocytes is normal. This dissociation is due to stretching of the fibres. H & E × 160.

dia, oedema, embolism or pulmonary oedema make up the clinical picture whilst angina-like pain is not uncommon (Gilchrist, 1963; Lee & Cotton, 1989). Physical signs include a soft mitral systolic murmur, a third heart sound and cardiomegaly whilst an electrocardiogram shows evidence of left ventricular hypertrophy and non-specific S-T changes.

In fatal cases there is a uniform pathological appearance. The heart weight is considerably increased, up to twice its normal size, and there is dilatation of all the chambers. Because of this latter change the myocardial wall measurements may be normal despite the hypertrophy (Fig. 58.9). The myocardium appears pale and flabby whilst the endocardium is thickened: mural thrombi are commonly present, particularly in the apical region of the ventricles. The coronary arteries are usually normal.

Histologically, the myocardial fibres are in normal alignment and the nuclear abnormalities typical of hypertrophy, such as pyknosis or vesicular change, are seen: because of attenuation the diameter of the myocardial fibres is usually normal (Fig. 58.10). Varying degrees of fibrosis are usually present and there is an increase in interstitial connective tissue. The small intramural vessels are normal whilst the thickened endocardium shows a prominent smooth muscle component.

With the advent of the bioptome, histochemical and electronmicroscopic studies have been made possible in peripartal cardiomyopathy. Histochemical studies have shown a patchy decrease in myocardial glycogen and suc-

cinic dehydrogenase whilst ultrastructural studies have shown only the typical features of hypertrophy together with a number of non-specific degenerative changes.

The overall pathological picture is therefore totally non-specific and identical to that which has been described in dilated (congestive) cardiomyopathy (Olsen, 1972, 1980a). This resemblance further extends to the frequent finding, common to both conditions, of a significant increase in the number of chronic inflammatory cells in the interstitium of the myocardium together with fraying of adjacent myocardial fibres (Balchum et al, 1956; Meadows, 1960).

The aetiology, or aetiologies, of peripartal heart disease are unknown and it is still not clear whether this is a condition which is aetiologically linked to pregnancy or whether the gravid state simply unmasks pre-existent subclinical heart muscle disease which is made overt by the physiological stress imposed by pregnancy. This latter view is, however, unlikely for the prognosis in dilated cardiomyopathy is usually poor whilst most women with peripartal heart disease recover.

Suggested aetiological factors have included:

1. Malnutrition. Most women with peripartal heart disease come from a poor socio-economic background and thiamine deficiency has been suggested as a possible aetiological factor (Blegen, 1965). Walsh et al (1965) have also stressed the importance of malnutrition in this condition whilst Seftel & Susser (1961) have drawn attention to an association with prolonged lactation.

2. Alcohol. Gouley et al (1937) and Stuart (1968) have maintained that there is an association between the development of peripartal heart disease and excess alcohol consumption.

3. Pre-eclampsia. Hypertensive heart disease in late pregnancy may mimic peripartal heart disease but the view that peripartal heart disease is aetiologically linked with pre-eclampsia (Benchimol et al, 1959) is unlikely to be true if only because proteinuria is not found in patients with this condition.

4. Infection. The presence of an inflammatory cell infiltrate in this form of cardiac muscle disease has suggested to some that the lesion is essentially a myocarditis (Sainani et al, 1968; Koide et al, 1972; Melvin et al, 1982) and Coxsackie virus has been implicated as a possible aetiological agent.

5. Autoimmunity. It has been postulated that in dilated cardiomyopathy the cellular infiltrate of the myocardium is the hallmark of an immunologically mediated myocarditis (Olsen, 1983) and, extrapolating from this, it seems not unreasonable to suggest that this may also apply to some cases of peripartal heart disease.

6. Local customs. There is a high incidence of peripartal heart disease amongst women in the Hausa tribe of Nigeria. Here local customs result in the pregnant woman being placed in a high temperature and being given a special type of gruel, rich in sodium, to eat. These practices, believed to improve lactation, increase extracellular fluid and plasma volume and lead to an increased workload for the heart.

Despite this plethora of theories, peripartal heart disease remains a condition of unknown aetiology though it is possible that metabolic, immunological or infective agents serve as conditioning factors which may be necessary for its development (Goodwin, 1975; Lee & Cotton, 1989). Genetic or ethnic factors may play a rôle (Leading Article, 1976) but have not so far been identified.

The outcome of peripartal heart disease is variable. Some patients die suddenly and unexpectedly whilst heart failure may persist in others, this condition usually terminating in death (Demakis & Rahimtoola, 1971). The average duration of life in such cases is 4.7 years (Demakis et al, 1971) and subsequent pregnancies during this period are associated with progressive deterioration. These patients should be considered as candidates for cardiac transplantation (Lee & Cotton, 1989; Hess & Hess, 1992). Most patients, however, recover fully with a return of their heart size to normal: the condition may, however, recur in such patients in subsequent, and successive, pregnancies.

Idiopathic pericarditis

Pericarditis, of unknown origin, occurring during pregnancy has been described by Adams (1959) and Kraus et al (1978). The latter authors reported three cases: in two of their patients the disease was present before pregnancy whilst in the third woman the disease developed during pregnancy. All three pregnancies proceeded to term and resulted in healthy babies.

Idiopathic myocarditis

There have been a few reports of this condition complicating pregnancy (Mendelson, 1951; Faruque, 1965; Hibbard, 1975). The disease tends to occur during the third trimester and is associated with a very high maternal mortality.

Pregnancy after cardiac transplantation

There have now been several reports of successful pregnancies in women who have had a previous cardiac transplantation (Key et al, 1989; Camann et al, 1991; Darbois et al, 1991; Kirk, 1991; Carvalho et al, 1992).

The cardiovascular changes associated with pregnancy appear to be well tolerated by the transplanted heart.

REFERENCES

Adams C W 1959 Postviral myopericarditis associated with the influenza virus: report of 8 cases. American Journal of Cardiology 4: 56–67.

Ahronheim J H 1977 Isolated coronary periarteritis: report of a case of unexpected death in a young pregnant woman. American Journal of Cardiology 40: 287–290.

Alpert M A 1993 Mitral valve prolapse: mostly benign. British Medical Journal 306: 943–944.

Alpert M A, Mukerju V, Sabeti M, Russell J, Beitman B D 1991 Mitral valve prolapse, panic disorder and chest pain. Medical Clinics of North America 75: 1119–1133.

Angelakis E J, Bair W E, Barone J E, Lincer M 1993 Splenic artery aneurysm rupture during pregnancy. Obstetrical and Gynecological Survey 48: 145–148.

Arias F, Pineda J 1978 Aortic stenosis and pregnancy. Journal of Reproductive Medicine 20: 229–232.

Aroney C, Khafagi F, Boyle C, Bett N 1986 Peripartum cardiomyopathy: echocardiographic features in five cases. American Journal of Obstetrics and Gynecology 155: 103–106.

Badduke B R, Jamieson W R, Miyagishima R T et al 1991 Pregnancy and childbearing in a population with biologic valvular prostheses. Journal of Thoracic and Cardiovascular Surgery 102: 179–186.

Balchum O J, McCord M C, Blount S G Jr 1956 The clinical and hemodynamic pattern in non-specific myocarditis; a comparison with other entities also impairing myocardial efficiency. American Heart Journal 52: 430–443.

Barlow J B, Bosman C K, Pocock W A, Marchand P 1968 Late systolic murmur and non-ejection ('mid-late') systolic clicks: an analysis of 90 patients. British Heart Journal 30: 203–218.

Barrett J M, Hooydonk J E van, Boehm F H 1982 Pregnancy-related rupture of arterial aneurysms. Obstetrical and Gynecological Survey 37: 557–566.

Bassaw B, Ariyanayagam D C, Roopnarinesingh S 1992 Peripartum cardiomyopathy and arterial embolism. West Indian Medical Journal 41: 79–80.

Beary J F, Summer W F, Bulkley B H 1979 Post partum myocardial infarcts: a rare occurrence of uncertain etiology. American Journal of Cardiology 43: 158–161.

Becker A E, DeWit A P M 1979 Mitral valve apparatus: a spectrum of normality relevant to mitral valve prolapse. British Heart Journal 42: 680–689.

Benham G H H 1949 Pregnancy and coarctation of the aorta. Journal of Obstetrics and Gynaecology of the British Empire 56: 606–618.

Benchimol A B, Carneiro R V, Schlesinger P 1959 Postpartum heart disease. British Heart Journal 21: 89–100.

Blegen S D 1965 Post partum congestive heart failure. Acta Medica Scandinavica 178: 515–524.

Boudoulas H, Wooley C F 1988 Mitral valve prolapse: prevalence. In: Boudoulas H, Wooley C F (eds) Mitral valve prolapse and the mitral valve prolapse syndrome. Fortuna, Mount Kisco, NY, pp 161–170.

Camann W F, Jarcho J A, Mintz K J, Greene M F 1991 Uncomplicated vaginal delivery 14 months after cardiac transplantation. American Heart Journal 121: 939–941.

Carvalho A C, Almeida D, Cohen M 1992 Successful pregnancy, delivery and puerperium in a heart transplant patient with previous peripartum cardiomyopathy. European Heart Journal 13: 1589–1591.

Chen W W C, Chan C S, Lee P K, Wang R Y C, Wong V C W 1982 Pregnancy in patients with prosthetic heart valves: an experience with 45 pregnancies. Quarterly Journal of Medicine 203: 358–365.

Ciraulo D A, Markovitz A 1979 Myocardial infarction in pregnancy associated with a coronary artery thrombus. Archives of Internal Medicine 139: 1046–1047.

Clarke S L 1991 Cardiac disease in pregnancy. Obstetrics and Gynecology Clinics of North America 18: 237–256.

Cleland W P, Counihan T B, Goodwin J F, Steiner R E 1956 Coarctation of the aorta. British Medical Journal 2: 379–390.

Cox S M, Leveno K J 1989 Pregnancy complicated by bacterial endocarditis. Clinical Obstetrics and Gynecology 32: 48–53.

Cunningham F G, Pritchard J A, Hankins G D V et al 1986 Peripartum heart failure: idiopathic cardiomyopathy or compounding cardiovascular events. Obstetrics and Gynecology 67: 157–167.

Dalvi D B, Chaudhuri A, Kulkarni H L, Kale P A 1992 Therapeutic guidelines for congenital complete heart block presenting in pregnancy. Obstetrics and Gynecology 79: 802–804.

Darbois Y, Seebacher J, Vauthier-Brouzes O et al 1991 Transplantations cardiaques: repercussions sur la fecondite feminine. Bulletin de l'Academie National de la Medecine 175: 531–540.

Davies M J, Parker D J, Bonella D 1981 Collagen synthesis in floppy mitral valve. Abstract, Proceedings of the British Cardiac Society. British Heart Journal 45: 345.

Deal K, Wooley C F 1973 Coarctation of aorta and pregnancy. Annals of Internal Medicine 78: 706–710.

Demakis J G, Rahimtoola S H 1971 Peripartum cardiomyopathy. Circulation 44: 964–968.

Demakis J G, Rahimtoola S H, Sutton G C, Meadows W R, Szanto P B, Tobin J R, Gunnar R M 1971 Natural course of peripartum cardiomyopathy. Circulation 44: 1053–1061.

Easterling T R, Chadwick H S, Otto C M, Benedetti C J 1988 Aortic stenosis in pregnancy. Obstetrics and Gynecology 72: 113–118.

Eddy W A, Frankenfeld R H 1977 Congenital complete heart block in pregnancy. American Journal of Obstetrics and Gynecology 128: 223–225.

Edwards J E 1960 In: Gould S E (ed) Pathology of the heart, 2nd edn. Thomas, Springfield, Ill, p 449.

Ehrenfeld E N, Brezizinsky I A, Braon K, Sadowsky E, Sadowski A 1964 Heart disease in pregnancy. Obstetrics and Gynecology 23: 363–371.

Esteves C A, Ramos A I, Braga S L et al 1991 Effectiveness of percutaneous balloon mitral valvotomy during pregnancy. American Journal of Cardiology 68: 930–934.

Faruque A A 1965 Acute fulminating puerperal myocarditis. British Heart Journal 27: 139–143.

Fletcher E, Knox E W, Morton P 1967 Acute myocardial infarction in pregnancy. British Medical Journal 3: 586–588.

Fulton R M, Hutchinson E C, Jones A M 1952 Ventricular weight in cardiac hypertrophy. British Heart Journal 14: 413–420.

Gilchrist A R 1963 Cardiological problems in younger women: including that of pregnancy and the puerperium. British Medical Journal 1: 209–216.

Glantz J C, Pomerantz R M, Cunningham M J, Woods J R 1993 Percutaneous balloon valvulotomy of severe mitral stenosis during pregnancy: a review of the therapeutic options. Obstetrical and Gynecological Survey 48: 503–508.

Gleicher N, Midwall I, Hoenberger D, Jaffin H 1979 Eisenmenger's syndrome and pregnancy. Obstetrical and Gynecological Survey 34: 721–741.

Goodwin J F 1958 Pregnancy and coarctation of the aorta. Lancet 1: 16–20.

Goodwin J F 1975 Peripartal heart disease. Clinical Obstetrics and Gynecology 18: 125–131.

Gouley B A, McMillan T M, Bellet S 1937 Idiopathic myocardial degeneration associated with pregnancy and especially the puerperium. American Journal of Medical Sciences 194: 185–199.

Hankins G D V, Wendel D G, Leveno K J, Stoneham J 1985 Myocardial infarction in pregnancy: a review. Obstetrics and Gynecology 65: 139–146.

Hauth J C, Cunningham G J, Young B K 1977 Takayasu's syndrome in pregnancy. Obstetrics and Gynecology 59: 373–374.

Hess D B, Hess L W 1992 Management of cardiovascular disease in pregnancy. Obstetrics and Gynecology Clinics of North America 19: 679–695.

Hibbard L T 1975 Maternal mortality due to cardiac disease. Clinical Obstetrics and Gynecology 18: 27–36.

Holdsworth R J, Gunn A 1992 Ruptured splenic artery aneurysm in pregnancy: a review. British Journal of Obstetrics and Gynaecology 99: 595–597.

Hsieh C C, Chiang C W, Hsieh T T, Soong Y K 1992 Peripartum cardiomyopathy. Japanese Heart Journal 33: 343–349.

Hughes R A C, Kapur P, Sutton G C, Honey M 1970 A case of fatal postpartum cardiomyopathy. British Heart Journal 32: 272–276.

Ishikawa K, Matsuura S 1982 Occlusive thromboaortopathy (Takayasu's disease) and pregnancy: clinical course and management of 33 pregnancies and deliveries. American Journal of Cardiology 50: 1293–1300.

Jones A M, Howitt G 1965 Eisenmenger syndrome in pregnancy. British Medical Journal 1: 1627–1631.

Jonge M J M de, Knipscheer R J J L, Weigel H M 1983 Takayasu's or pulseless disease in pregnancy. European Journal of Obstetrics, Gynecology and Reproductive Biology 14: 241–249.

Keene R J, Steiner R E, Olsen E G J, Oakley C 1971 Aortic root aneurysm — radiographic and pathologic features. Clinical Radiology 22: 330–340.

Key T C, Resnik R, Dittrich H C, Reisner L S 1989 Successful pregnancy after cardiac transplantation. American Journal of Obstetrics and Gynecology 160: 367–371.

Kirk E P 1991 Organ transplantation and pregnancy: a case report and review. American Journal of Obstetrics and Gynecology 164: 1629–1634.

Knapp R C, Arditi L I 1968 Closed mitral valvulotomy in pregnancy. Clinical Obstetrics and Gynecology 11: 928–991.

Koide T, Saito Y, Sakamoto T, Murao S 1972 Peripartal cardiomyopathy in Japan. Japanese Heart Journal 13: 488–501.

Kolibash A J Jr 1988 Natural history of mitral valve prolapse. In: Boudoulas H, Wooley C F (eds) Mitral valve prolapse and the mitral valve prolapse syndrome. Futura, Mount Kisco, NY, pp 257–275.

Konishi Y, Tatsuta N, Kumada K et al 1980 Dissecting aneurysm during pregnancy and the puerperium. Japanese Circulation Journal 44: 726–733.

Kraus Z Y, Naparstek E, Eliakim M 1978 Idiopathic pericarditis and pregnancy. Australian and New Zealand Journal of Obstetrics and Gynaecology 18: 86–89.

Leading Article 1976 'Peripartum cardiac failure'. British Medical Journal 1: 302–303.

Lee C N, Wu C C, Lin P Y, Hsieh F J, Chen H Y 1994 Pregnancy following cardiac prosthetic valve replacement. Obstetrics and Gynecology 83: 353–356.

Lee W, Cotton D B 1989 Peripartum cardiomyopathy: current concepts and clinical management. Clinical Obstetrics and Gynecology 32: 54–67.

Littler W A 1970 Successful pregnancy in a patient with Ebstein's anomaly. British Heart Journal 32: 711–713.

Lutz O J, Noller K L, Spittell J A, Danielson G K, Fish C R 1978 Pregnancy and its complications following cardiac valve prostheses. American Journal of Obstetrics and Gynecology 131: 460–468.

McAnulty J H, Metcalfe J, Ueland K 1981 General guidelines in the management of cardiac disease. Clinical Obstetrics and Gynecology 24: 773–788.

McAnulty J H, Metcalfe J, Ueland K 1982 Cardiovascular disease. In: Burrow G N, Ferris T F (eds) Medical complications during pregnancy. Saunders, Philadelphia, pp 145–168.

McCaffrey R M, Dunn L J 1964 Primary pulmonary hypertension in pregnancy. Obstetrical and Gynecological Survey 19: 567–591.

McColgin S W, Martin J N, Morrison J C 1989 Pregnant women with prosthetic heart valves. Clinical Obstetrics and Gynecology 32: 76–88.

Mandel W, Evans E W, Walford R L 1954 Dissecting aortic aneurysm during pregnancy. New England Journal of Medicine 251: 1059–1061.

Maarek-Charbit M, Corone P 1986 Consultation de medicine: Hospital de la Pitie. Arch Maladies Coeur 79: 733–740.

Markiewizc W, Stoner J, London E, Hunt S A, Popp R L 1976 Mitral valve prolapse in one hundred presumably healthy young females. Circulation 53: 464–473.

Marks A R, Choong C U, Sanfillipo S J 1989 Identification of high risk and low risk subgroups of patients with mitral valve prolapse. New England Journal of Medicine 320: 1032.

Maron B J, Ferrans V J 1975 Intramitochondrial glycogen deposits in hypertrophied human myocardium. Journal of Molecular and Cellular Cardiology 7: 697–702.

Meadows W R 1957 Idiopathic myocardial failure in the last trimester of pregnancy and puerperium. Circulation 15: 903–914.

Meadows W R 1960 Postpartum heart disease. American Journal of Cardiology 6: 788–802.

Melvin K R, Richardson P J, Olsen B G J, Daly K, Jackson G 1982 Peripartum cardiomyopathy due to myocarditis. New England Journal of Medicine 307: 731–734.

Mendelson C L 1951 Acute isolated myocarditis in pregnancy. American Journal of Obstetrics and Gynecology 61: 1341–1347.

Meyer E C, Tulsky A S, Sigmann P, Silber E N 1964 Pregnancy in the presence of tetralogy of Fallot: observations on the patients. American Journal of Cardiology 14: 874–879.

Mortensen J D, Ellsworth H S 1965 Coarctation of the aorta and pregnancy. Journal of the American Medical Association 191: 596–598.

Naeye R, Hagstrom J W C, Talmadge B A 1967 Postpartum death with maternal congenital heart disease. Circulation 36: 304–312.

Nolan T E, Hankins G D V 1989 Myocardial infarction in pregnancy. Clinical Obstetrics and Gynecology 32: 68–75.

Oakley C 1983 Pregnancy in patients with prosthetic heart valves. British Medical Journal 286: 1680–1682.

Oakley C, Doherty P 1976 Pregnancy in patients after valve replacement. British Heart Journal 38: 1140–1148.

Oakley G D G, McGarry K, Limb D G, Oakley C M 1979 Management of pregnancy in patients with hypertrophic cardiomyopathy. British Medical Journal 1: 1749–1750.

O'Driscoll M K, Coyle C F V, Drury M I 1962 Rheumatic heart disease complicating pregnancy: the remote prospect. British Medical Journal 2: 767–768.

O'Grady J P, Day E J, Toole A L, Paust J C 1977 Splenic artery aneurysm rupture in pregnancy. Obstetrics and Gynecology 50: 627–630.

Oliver M F, Boyd C S 1955 Plasma lipid and serum lipoprotein patterns during pregnancy and the puerperium. Clinical Science 14: 15–23.

Olsen E G J 1972 Cardiomyopathies. In: Edwards J E, Brest A N (eds) Cardiovascular clinics. Clinical-pathologic correlations 1. Davis, Philadelphia, pp 239–261.

Olsen E G J 1975a Cardiovascular system. In: Harrison C V, Weinbren K (eds) Recent advances in pathology, vol 9. Churchill Livingstone, London, p 1.

Olsen E G J 1975b Marfan's disease. Pathologica et Microbiologica 43: 120–123.

Olsen E G J 1980a The pathology of the heart, 2nd edn. Macmillan Press, Basingstoke.

Olsen E G J 1980b The pathology of idiopathic hypertrophic subaortic stenosis (hypertrophic cardiomyopathy): a critical review. American Heart Journal 100: 553–562.

Olsen E G J 1983 Myocarditis — a case of mistaken identity. British Heart Journal 50: 303–311.

Olsen E G J, Al-Rufaie H K 1980 The floppy mitral valve: study on pathogenesis. British Heart Journal 44: 674–683.

Payne D C, Fishburne J I, Rufty A J, Johnston F R 1982 Bacterial endocarditis in pregnancy. Obstetrics and Gynecology 60: 247–250.

Pitkin R M 1990 Pregnancy and congenital heart disease. Annals of Internal Medicine 112: 445–454.

Pritchard J A 1953 Coarctation of the aorta and pregnancy. Obstetrical and Gynecological Survey 8: 775–791.

Procacci P M, Savran S V, Schreiter S L, Bryson A L 1976 Prevalence of clinical mitral-valve prolapse in 1169 young women. New England Journal of Medicine 294: 1086–1088.

Pyeritz R E 1981 Maternal and fetal complications of pregnancy in the Marfan syndrome. American Journal of Medicine 71: 784–790.

Ramin S M, Maberry M C, Gilstrap L C 1989 Congenital heart disease. Clinical Obstetrics and Gynecology 32: 41–47.

Rayburn W F, Fontana M E 1981 Mitral valve prolapse and pregnancy. American Journal of Obstetrics and Gynecology 141: 9–11.

Rosenthal L 1955 Coarctation of the aorta and pregnancy: report of 5 cases. British Medical Journal 1: 16–18.

Sainani G S, Krompotic E, Slodki S J 1968 Adult heart disease due to coxsackie virus B infection. Medicine 47: 133–147.

Saleh Y Z, McLeod F N 1977 Ruptured renal artery aneurysm in pregnancy: case report. British Journal of Obstetrics and Gynaecology 84: 391–393.

Sasse L, Wagner R, Murry F E 1975 Transmural myocardial infarction during pregnancy. American Journal of Cardiology 35: 448–452.

Seftel H, Susser M 1961 Maternity and myocardial failure in African women. British Heart Journal 23: 43–52.

Shaper A G 1966 Fibrinolytic activity in pregnancy, during parturition and the puerperium. Lancet 2: 874–876.

Shaper A G 1968 Platelet function. Lancet 1: 642–643.

Shaper A G, Macintosh D M, Kyobe J 1965 Fibrinolysis and plasminogen levels in pregnancy and the puerperium. Lancet 2: 706–708.

Shaver P J, Carrig T F, Baker W P 1978 Postpartum coronary artery disease. British Heart Journal 40: 83–86.

Shepherd J T, Edwards J E, Burchell H B, Swan H J G, Wood E H 1957 Clinical, physiological and pathological considerations in patients with idiopathic pulmonary hypertension. British Heart Journal 19: 70–82.

Shime J, Mocarski E J M, Hastings D et al 1987 Congenital heart disease in pregnancy: short and long term implications. American Journal of Obstetrics and Gynecology 156: 313–322.

Singh H, Bolton P J, Oakley C M 1982 Pregnancy after surgical correction of tetralogy of Fallot. British Medical Journal 285: 168–170.

Stuart K L 1968 Cardiomyopathy of pregnancy and puerperium. Quarterly Journal of Medicine 37: 463–478.

Szekely P, Turner R, Snaith L 1973 Pregnancy and the changing pattern of rheumatic heart disease. British Heart Journal 35: 1293–1303.

Trastek V F, Pairolero P C, Bernatz P E 1985 Splenic artery aneurysms. World Journal of Surgery 9: 378–383.

Ueland K 1978 Cardiovascular diseases complicating pregnancy. Clinical Obstetrics and Gynecology 21: 429–442.

Ueland K 1984 Cardiac diseases. In: Creasy R K, Resnik R (eds) Maternal fetal medicine. W B Saunders, Philadelphia, p 691.

Ueland K, Metcalfe J 1975 Circulatory changes in pregnancy. Clinical Obstetrics and Gynecology 18: 41–50.

Uetsuka Y, Higashidate N, Aosaki M et al 1990 Fifteen year experience with 24 pregnancies associated with prosthetic valve replacement. Journal of Cardiology 20: 929–935.

Vassalotti S B, Schaller J A 1967 Spontaneous rupture of splenic artery aneurysm during pregnancy: report of first known antepartum rupture with maternal and fetal survival. Obstetrics and Gynecology 30: 264–268.

Vielle J C 1984 Peripartum cardiomyopathies: a review. American Journal of Obstetrics and Gynecology 148: 805–818.

Walsh J J, Bench G E, Black H C, Ferrans V J, Hibbs 1965 Idiopathic myocardiopathies of the puerperium (postpartal heart disease). Circulation 32: 19–31.

Watson H, Emslie-Smith D, Herring J, Hill I G W 1960 Myocardial infarction during pregnancy and puerperium. Lancet 2: 523–526.

WHO/ISFC 1980 Report of the WHO-ISFC Task Force on the definition and classification of cardiomyopathies. British Heart Journal 44: 672–673.

Wooley C F, Sparks E H 1992 Congenital heart disease, heritable cardiovascular disease, and pregnancy. Progress in Cardiovascular Diseases 35: 41–60.

Wooley R F, Hugh V R, Ryan J M 1961 Pregnancy and congenital heart disease (abstract). Circulation 24: 1075.

Woolford R M 1952 Postpartum myocardiosis. Ohio State Journal of Medicine 48: 924–930.

Zeek P M 1942 Heart weight I. The weight of the normal heart. Archives of Pathology 34: 820–832.

59. Pathology of the nervous system in pregnancy

Helen Reid   P. O. Yates

INTRODUCTION

There are few, if any, diseases of the nervous system that are uniquely related to pregnancy, but there are a number that seem to be initiated or brought to light at this time, and others, previously known to be present, where management of the disease may have to be varied during the duration of pregnancy. In cases of maternal death it is important to examine the brain (Dawson, 1988). If the case history is suggestive of any disease of the spinal cord, peripheral nerves or muscle these should also be examined, the spinal cord should be removed and appropriate samples of peripheral nerve and muscle taken.

By far the most common disease of the central nervous system (CNS) is the abnormality of mood which a majority of women suffer as postpartum depression and which is perhaps due to a relative inhibition of prolactin release. It is often associated with a delay in lactation and may be cured by small doses of chlorpromazine which stimulate prolactin release. Ten per cent of women need much more prolonged treatment, having perhaps an underlying depressive diathesis.

Pregnancy certainly precipitates a puerperal psychosis in one out of every 250 women but almost all have a previous history of delusional states and in many the condition recurs outside pregnancy. Its incidence is probably much the same now as when reported by Bates (1848) early in the last century. Both steroid and polypeptide hormone systems have important regulatory actions on neurone function in the brain. The needs of pregnancy require, of course, quite a different action by these substances on other tissues of the body and often the hormones are present in unusually large amounts. Minor changes in permeability of the blood-brain barrier, which appear to be quite common in pregnancy, will allow leakage into the brain of uncontrolled quantities of these hormonal modulators of neurone transmission. It is, therefore, not surprising that mental disorder may appear at this time.

CHOREA GRAVIDARUM

A disease which is now rare in this country, but which may still remain a problem in countries where rheumatic fever is common, is chorea gravidarum. This condition is essentially a recrudescence of the Sydenham's chorea associated with active rheumatic disease and also found in women who have damaged basal ganglia as a result of hypoxic encephalopathy.

Chorea presents as an acute or subacute development of involuntary jerking movements of the face and extremities associated with hypotonia of the limbs and hyperreflexia. Most initial episodes occur during first pregnancies (80%), with up to a fifth of the women experiencing recurrences in subsequent pregnancies (Schipper, 1988). Symptoms become less after 1–2 months of onset and rarely persist beyond the puerperium.

Chorea has also been reported as appearing in some women two or three months after starting hormonal contraceptive pills, this appearing to be independent of the type and dose of oral contraceptive ingested (Schipper, 1988), although the oestrogen component may be important in the development of the movement disorder (Barber et al 1976).

Oestrogen may induce chorea in susceptible persons by enhancing dopaminergic neurotransmitters in the striatum (van Hartesveldt & Joyce, 1986): dopamine agonists exacerbate pre-existing chorea and induce involuntary movements in asymptomatic non-pregnant patients with a history of rheumatic fever. Therefore, when chorea does develop during pregnancy, it is not necessary to assume that pregnancy has provoked an exacerbation of rheumatic disease: it has simply revealed an underlying weakness of basal ganglia function. As it is a self-limiting condition usually no therapy is required.

VASCULAR DISORDERS

The dangers of the encephalopathy associated with pre-eclampsia and eclampsia are well known: these and intra-cranial haemorrhage (Dorfman, 1990; Simolke et al, 1991) are important causes of maternal death.

However, there are other vascular lesions which have been reported in pregnancy and although each condition individually accounts for a few cases only, taken together this is an important group as these other vascular lesions do cause a certain amount of morbidity and mortality.

Even so, eclampsia remains an important cause of maternal death. In one survey of 163 pregnancy-related deaths (Department of Health, 1989) 25 were due to pre-eclampsia and eclampsia, 11 occurred with pre-eclampsia and 14 with eclampsia; also in this survey there were the same number of deaths (25) due to pulmonary emboli.

The other vascular lesions that occur in or are associated with pregnancy are thromboembolism, atherosclerosis, migraine, coagulopathy, vasculitis and cerebral vasospasm (Weibers, 1985; Geraghty et al, 1991; Simolke et al, 1991). Pregnancy has been said to increase the risk of stroke by about 3–13 times. In a study from Glasgow (Jennett & Cross, 1967) of 65 female subjects aged 15–45 years with ischaemic stroke 35% were pregnant or puerperal at the time of the stroke: an increase of 3–4 times the prevalence rate in non-pregnant women. These workers thought that cerebrovascular accidents in their cases were arterial rather than venous in nature; however this is not now the general experience of strokes in pregnancy (Weibers & Whisnant, 1985; Srinivasan, 1988). In one centre in India only 8 out of 150 patients with cerebrovascular accidents had an arterial occlusion (Srinivasan, 1988); far more had venous sinus thrombosis. At the same centre there were 8000–9000 deliveries per year, out of whom 400 had pregnancy-induced hypertension and 50 had puerperal cerebral venous thrombosis (Srinivasan, 1988).

Encephalopathy of pre-eclampsia and eclampsia of pregnancy

Pre-eclampsia is characterized by a rapidly rising blood pressure, proteinuria and, in severe cases, generalized oedema; eclampsia is diagnosed when epileptiform fits supervene. Fully developed eclampsia is rare, but it is still one of the commonest causes of death related to pregnancy in the British Isles (Department of Health, 1989) and one of the major causes of death related to pregnancy in the western world.

Eclampsia occurs in around 1 per 2000 deliveries (Douglas & Redman, 1992). As well as the mortality rate associated with pre-eclampsia and eclampsia there can also be severe morbidity due to cerebral haemorrhages, cortical blindness, renal failure, disseminated intravascular coagulation, pulmonary oedema and psychosis.

Although pre-eclampsia/eclampsia is a condition spe-cifically linked with pregnancy, it shows much the same pathological changes in the brain as are to be found with the similar neurological picture that may accompany any rapidly developing or episodic hypertension, for example, with an amine-secreting phaeochromocytoma or a phase of primary or secondary malignant hypertension (Benedetti & Quilligan, 1980).

Pathologically the CNS changes occurring in eclampsia have been well described. Sheehan & Lynch (1973) found five major groups of cerebrovascular phenomena in eclampsia; these were:

1. petechial haemorrhages in patches in the cerebral cortex
2. multiple small areas of ischaemic softening, scattered throughout the brain, usually non-haemorrhagic
3. small areas of haemorrhage in subcortical white matter, usually localized to the upper part of the hemispheres
4. a single large haemorrhage in the white matter
5. haemorrhage in basal ganglia or pons, often with rupture into the ventricles.

Not all of these lesions are present in every case that comes to post mortem; for instance, intracerebral haemorrhage has been found only in 10–60% of fatal cases (Beck & Menezes, 1981).

In a further small study only one out of seven cases had a large haemorrhage within the brain (Richards et al, 1988). These workers reported a neuropathological study of seven patients who died, five with eclampsia and two with pre-eclampsia. They found that hypoxic-ischaemic damage and fibrinoid necrosis of the walls of small vessels were the most important neuropathological lesions. However, as oedema was not demonstrated histologically or on CT scan in pre-eclampsia they thought it unlikely that oedema formation was responsible for the prodromal signs and symptoms of eclampsia. They also thought it unlikely that oedema triggers the occurrence of seizures. The authors suggested that both the vasculopathy and hypoxic-ischaemic damage are involved in the pathogenesis of the oedema formation. The vasculopathy is acute vessel wall damage with plasmatic vasculosis and fibrinoid necrosis. In only one case were there fibrin thrombi occluding damaged vessels. Three of the cases had perivascular microhaemorrhages similar to those shown in Figure 59.1.

These lesions are also seen in hypertensive encephalopathy of other aetiology in which there is a breakdown of the blood-brain barrier. The blood-brain barrier is constituted by the endothelial cells of cerebral capillaries, which have different characteristics to most endothelial cells elsewhere in the body. They have tight junctions between them and there are few pinocytotic vesicles within the endothelial cytoplasm and little if any pinocytotic transport through their cytoplasm. They are cells with a

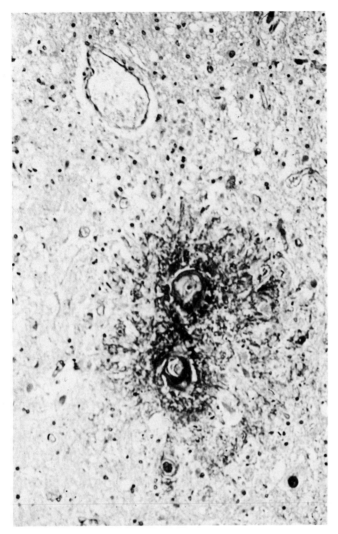

Fig. 59.1 Branches of a small artery showing necrosis of their walls and escape of fibrin into surrounding brain.

very high metabolic activity as indicated by the presence of an unusually large number of mitochondria in their cytoplasm; these are probably important in the number of processes whereby the endothelial cells can control solute fluxes across the capillary wall (Miller & Adams, 1992). These features of the endothelial cells act as the blood-brain barrier. In an animal model there are cerebral endo-thelial plasma membrane alterations in acute hypertension and this may lead to increased cerebrovascular permeabil-ity to proteins (Nag, 1986). The basement membrane outside these endothelial cells has an important filtering function and beyond this again there is a sheath of cyto-plasmic foot processes of astrocytes which have a further selective function in the two-way tissue transport system; the brain is almost unique in having no lymphatic drain-age and any resulting accumulation of extracellular solutes and fluid may be disturbing to the nutrition and function of nerve cells.

Cerebral venous thrombosis

It is difficult to ascertain the true incidence of this condi-tion as it occurs in the puerperium 1–4 weeks after child-birth and only occasional cases have been reported during pregnancy (Kalbag & Woolf, 1967): it is then usually a concomitant of septic abortion and thromboembolism (Fishman et al, 1957). Srinivasan (1988) found that cer-ebral venous thrombosis had a frequency of 4–5 per 100 obstetric admissions in his centre in India, which suggests a much greater frequency than in western countries where the incidence is 1 in 2500 to 1 in 10 000 deliveries.

In western countries, where antibiotics are more readily available, it is now unusual to have a septic cause for central venous thrombosis. A major factor is more likely to be a hypercoagulable state from various abnormalities of the blood, such as an increase in platelets, factors VII and IX, and fibrinogen or decreased fibrinolysis predis-posed to by dehydration, anaemia, cyanotic heart disease, polycythaemia vera, leukaemia or sickle cell disease. Other rarer causes are remote effects of carcinoma, Behçet's and Cogan's syndromes, cryofibrinogenaemias or the oral contraceptive pill (Srinivasan, 1988).

In puerperal venous thrombosis there are reports of increased plasma fibrinogen with high erythrocyte sedi-mentation rate, decreased fibrinolytic activity, increased platelet adhesive index and increased levels of beta-lipo-proteins and triglycerides with normal cholesterol values (Srinivasan, 1984). Congenital disorders known to cause thrombophilia are deficiencies of antithrombin III, protein C, protein S and certain types of dysfibrinogenaemia as well as homocystinuria (Schutta et al, 1991). Schutta and colleagues also suggested that a deficiency of plasminogen might predispose to thrombosis by slowing the rate of fibrinolysis; this has been found in some patients with thrombosis. Another condition which has been associated with deep venous thrombosis and, in some cases cerebral venous thrombosis, is the primary antiphospholipid syn-drome associated with an antiphospholipid antibody of IgG type 2 and 4 (Harris, 1992). This syndrome is also associated with repeated fetal loss. These patients seem to have a systemic autoimmune disorder that overlaps with systemic lupus erythematosus (SLE). Some patients do have SLE but others only have the antiphospholipid anti-bodies and the venous thrombi (Asherson et al, 1989; Brey et al, 1990; Brey & Coull, 1992) associated some-times with cerebral ischaemic damage (Montalban et al, 1991).

The anatomy of the superior sagittal sinus may also have a rôle to play in the formation of thrombi within it; the lumen has an inverted triangular shape and the arach-noid granulations project into the upper lateral angles and the cortical cerebral veins drain into its inferior angle. The lumen also contains fibrous trabeculae which favour thrombosis. If the upper half of the superior sagittal sinus is blocked, preventing the cerebrospinal fluid clearing function of the granulations, intracranial pressure increases without focal deficits, a condition known as pseudotumour cerebri. If the draining veins are blocked as well focal seizures and neurological defects occur.

In venous stasis collateral drainage opens up and if the thrombosis is slight and slow in forming there is less damage as the venous blood is drained through the collateral branches.

The condition often presents clinically as an epileptic fit which is soon followed by headache, drowsiness, vomiting and hemiplegia (Carroll et al, 1966; Chopra & Banerjee, 1989). The weakness and sensory disturbances can be unilateral or bilateral and involve the legs rather selectively. Confusion and psychotic symptoms can predominate and therefore puerperal psychosis needs to be excluded as do co-existing peripheral thrombosis, meningitis, postpartum eclampsia and space-occupying lesions. The radiological investigation of choice is magnetic resonance imaging (MRI) but if this is not available a CT scan should be followed by angiographic studies. CSF examination is rarely of diagnostic use and as, in many of the cases of venous sinus thrombosis, there is oedema of the brain the procurement of CSF by lumbar puncture is inadvisable for it may cause the death of the patient through brain movement and cerebellar coning.

It is the superior sagittal sinus and its draining veins which are commonly involved in the puerperium. However, occasional cases of thrombosis of the vein of Galen and its tributaries and associated straight sinus have been reported (Banerjee et al, 1979). Bitemporal lobe infarc-tion with occlusion of the veins of Labbe and the lateral sinuses is rare (Chopra & Banerjee, 1989).

Pathology of superior sagittal sinus thrombosis

The brain is swollen and there is usually thrombosis of the cerebral veins as well as the superior sagittal sinus. In the latter the thrombus present in the sinus is usually older than that in the draining cerebral veins. There may be some degree of lateral brain shift and tentorial herniation or even cerebellar coning if the oedema is extensive. The cerebral veins that are thrombosed can be unilaterally or bilaterally involved, but more often they are involved unilaterally (Gettlefinger & Kokman, 1977). There is discolouration of the cerebral gyri adjacent to the veins which are thrombosed; the brain surface is mottled and grey. Subarachnoid haemorrhage can be seen, within which are the cord-like rigid thrombosed veins. In these cases, on sectioning the brain, there is haemorrhagic infarction in the areas drained by the thrombosed veins (Fig. 59.2). As the patients die shortly after the onset of symptoms the infarcts are recent. Often the haemorrhagic infarcts have a central haematoma with softening of the surrounding brain with punctate haemorrhages. In those without a central haematoma there is softening of the brain with punctate haemorrhages.

Microscopically, in the early stages oedema is only seen with perineuronal and perioligodendrocytic haloes in the grey and white matter respectively; degeneration of the neurones in the affected area is also seen. In the slightly older lesions there is haemorrhagic necrosis. Thrombosis is present in veins of all sizes and there are multiple satel-

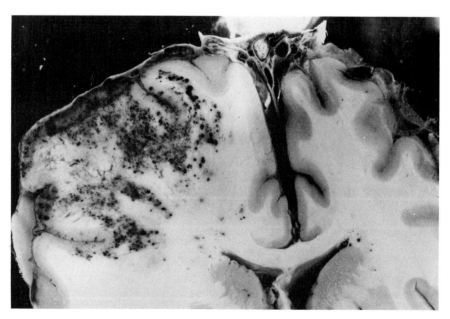

Fig. 59.2 Haemorrhagic infarction of one frontal lobe with thrombosis of surface veins and superior longitudinal sinus.

lite foci of ring or ball haemorrhages. Some of the venous walls show necrosis and there is polymorphonuclear leucocyte diapedesis. The affected neurones are shrunken and deeply staining (eosinophilic on H & E staining). Polymorphonuclear leucocytes and macrophages are present in small numbers; however if there are many polymorphonuclear leucocytes a septic cause should be looked for. Reactive astrocytes and haemosiderin deposition are not usually evident. If there is a longer survival before the patient succumbs, the brain shows cavitation, focal cortical atrophy and organized thrombi.

Pathology of thrombosis in other venous sinuses

In the less common thrombosis of the straight sinus and vein of Galen there are bilateral haemorrhagic infarcts of the thalami, basal ganglia and corpus callosum (Banerjee et al, 1979) or bilateral ischaemic necrosis with subcortical oedema (Milandre et al, 1990).

Microscopically the older thrombi are in the smaller branches of the terminal veins with newer thrombus formation in the great vein of Galen and torcular. There is diapedesis of polymorphonuclear leucocytes, necrosis of parenchyma and confluent haemorrhages around the thrombosed vessels.

Outcome of venous thrombosis

The overall mortality is 25% but if the affected women also have pulmonary embolism the morbidity and mortality rates are higher (Srinivasan, 1988). The outlook is usually good in the survivors, many recovering without significant neurological deficit (Weibers, 1985). The prognosis is better than that in arterial stroke (Chopra & Banerjee, 1989). However, the mortality rate in cases where there is deep cerebral venous sinus thrombosis, rather than in the superficial sagittal sinus, is worse — nine fatalities out of 15 cases in one series (Milandre et al, 1990).

Benign raised intracranial pressure

Minor non-fatal venous and sinus obstructions may be the basis for the condition known as benign raised intracranial pressure or pseudotumour cerebri, which sometimes presents in pregnancy but also occurs in women of fertile age at other times of raised oestrogen levels (Caroscio & Pellmar, 1979). The clinical presentation is one of raised intracranial pressure, without focal neurological signs, which usually subsides at the end of the pregnancy. Papilloedema, although transient, may cause a permanent loss of central vision. Occasionally the patient may show little clinical evidence of raised pressure but may have enlarged ventricles on CT scan and suffer a moderate degree of dementia. The condition is treatable by surgical procedures to provide alternative CSF drainage.

This condition is not, of course, confined to pregnancy and is seen as a sequel to head injury and to middle ear infections with related thrombosis of the lateral sinus and may be referred to as otitic hydrocephalus. Two mechanisms seem to be at work in pregnancy — the one already described above being a reduction of CSF absorption into partially occluded and thickened venous sinuses, the other being swelling of the brain due to hormonal related fluid imbalance (Powell, 1972).

Arterial obstruction

It was thought in the past that cerebrovascular accidents due to arterial causes were more common among pregnant women, especially during the second or third trimester, than in non-pregnant women of similar age. This is probably not so today; Weibers & Whisnant (1985) could only find one case of cerebral infarction in 26 099 live births during 1955–1979 in Rochester, USA.

Although specific arterial diseases such as giant cell arteritis and Moyamoya arteritis have been described as a cause, they are rare (Karasawa et al, 1980). Fibromuscular dysplasia has also been described (Ezra et al, 1989).

Rheumatic heart disease with atrial and valvular lesions remains in some parts of the world as a fairly common source of emboli. Such emboli often lodge in quite peripheral cerebral arteries producing small strokes and often only minor residual disability. It must be remembered that the cerebral arterial tree has enormous anastomotic potential, both extracranially and on the brain surface. Thus, if an occlusion is confined to the common or internal carotid artery, there is often no neurological disability in this age group because of the good state of other collateral vessels. However, if the thrombus arises in or extends to the middle cerebral artery, thus losing the benefit of the cross circulation from the circle of Willis, then hemiplegia, and sometimes death, is the outcome.

In these cases the infarct is usually found in the parietal and temporal lobes in the area supplied by the middle cerebral artery. It is usually an area of softening, with surrounding oedema; brain shift may also be present. The infarct shows varying degrees of liquefactive necrosis depending on how long the patient survived after the vessel was occluded. The infarct is usually pale and rarely haemorrhagic.

Intracerebral haemorrhage

The normal pathological mechanisms for the production of cerebrovascular disorders are not common in women of fertile age. Major intracerebral haemorrhage associated with essential hypertension is rare in this age group. Other factors associated with non-traumatic intracerebral bleeding in pregnancy are haematological disorders such as disseminated intravascular coagulation, often in association with placental abruption, leukaemia, thrombocytopenia, or carcinoma (Barno & Freeman, 1976). Anticoagulant therapy (Hirsh et al, 1972) is an obvious problem.

Rupture of berry aneurysms and haemorrhage from vascular malformations, although not common, are important because they can be accurately diagnosed and treatment given (Weibers, 1988).

Berry aneurysm of the circle of Willis

Subarachnoid haemorrhage from rupture of an aneurysm of the circle of Willis is an unduly frequent event during the gestational period and occurs in about one in 3000 pregnancies, 4% actually occurring during labour. Robinson et al (1972) thought they ruptured mainly after 26 weeks of gestation; however Dias & Sekhar (1990) thought they ruptured throughout gestation but that there was an increased incidence of rupture with advancing gestational age. There seems to be some special hormonal relationship here for there is an increase in the incidence of rupture of other aneurysms during gestation (see Ch. 58). It may be relevant that, of the vascular deaths reported in a large British survey of women taking hormonal contraceptive pills, one of the significant increases was in subarachnoid haemorrhage from a cerebral aneurysm (Beral & Kay, 1977). Similar findings were reported from the Framingham study (Sacco et al, 1984).

Although these aneurysms, occurring at the junctional points of the circle of Willis (Fig. 59.3), are often referred to as congenital aneurysms, only a few are ever found in childhood; indeed the commonest age for presentation is 50–60 years. Seventy per cent of normal people have the congenital defect in the vessel wall at the branching of the vessels of the circle which has long been considered to be the basis for the disease. It seems, therefore, that other factors must be of major importance in those cases that produce an aneurysm which ruptures and, indeed, there is a type III collagen defect in at least some of these patients (Pope et al, 1980). An innate difficulty with the healing of minor faults in the connective tissue of blood vessels together with the hormonal related changes in general collagenous tissues must combine in pregnancy to predispose to the rupture of aneurysms.

Dias & Sekhar (1990) in their review of 154 women who had intracranial haemorrhage from aneurysms and arteriovenous malformations found 77% due to aneurysms and 23% due to arteriovenous malformations. The average maternal age for ruptured aneurysms was 29.4 years, slightly older than that for arteriovenous malformations (26.7 years). Of all the aneurysms causing the first intracerebral haemorrhage 23% were diagnosed in the nulliparous group and the mean parity was two.

The sites of the aneurysms are similar to those reported in the non-gravid population: in the internal carotid artery (37%), posterior communicating artery (23%), anterior

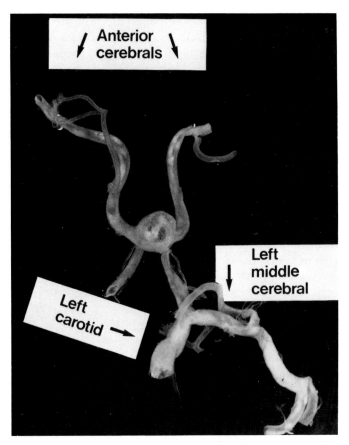

Fig. 59.3 Part of a dissected circle of Willis showing an aneurysmal sac arising at the junction of the left anterior cerebral and anterior communicating arteries.

communicating/anterior cerebral artery (23%), middle cerebral artery (23%) and vertebrobasilar system (10%).

Pathology

In those dying suddenly from ruptured aneurysms there is marked subarachnoid haemorrhage, particularly over the area of the aneurysm, and there may be no other neuropathological findings. The aneurysm should be looked for at the time of the post mortem, by dissecting the haematoma in the subarachnoid space off the circle of Willis and identifying it. Also the presence of other aneurysms should be excluded; in 17% of all aneurysmal cases more than one aneurysm is present. If an aneurysm is not found the vessels may be injected with water to see if there is a perforation where an aneurysm has been, and this is best done at the time of post mortem examination. The aneurysms are usually 1 cm or less in diameter; occasionally aneurysms as large as 2 cm are found.

In those women with a longer survival after onset of symptoms there can be large intracerebral and intraventricular haemorrhages with evidence of brain shift. In other cases there may be evidence of brain shift and subarachnoid haemorrhage but with no further haemorrhage in other sites. The problem then may be due to arterial spasm leading to infarction of the brain with surrounding oedema. Oxyhaemoglobin is probably the principal pathological agent in causing vasospasm (Macdonald & Weir, 1991).

In the Dias & Sekhar (1990) series the overall maternal mortality was 35% for aneurysms; these authors advocated surgical management of aneurysms in the pregnant woman and also suggested that with surgery for aneurysms the fetus would benefit, but pointed out that the physiological changes of pregnancy need to be taken into account in the neurosurgical management of the patient and that obstetrical and neonatological advice along with close monitoring would be needed.

Vascular malformations

These include arteriovenous malformations in which there are increased vessels per unit area with arterialized veins and thick-walled arteries and vascular hamartomas or angiomas. Not all arteriovenous malformations are associated with haemorrhages for some present with epilepsy and may never lead to intracerebral haemorrhage. Out of the various series of intracerebral haemorrhage in pregnant women 21–48% of cases are due to arteriovenous malformations (Dias & Sekhar, 1990). Most arteriovenous malformations are present in the parietal region with fewer found in the occipital lobes followed by the frontal and temporal lobes (Dias & Sekhar, 1990). Haemorrhage from an arteriovenous malformation tends to occur at a younger age than that due to a ruptured berry aneurysm. The haemorrhage can be subarachnoid, intracerebral or intraventricular. More commonly it is intracerebral with overlying subarachnoid haemorrhage; on

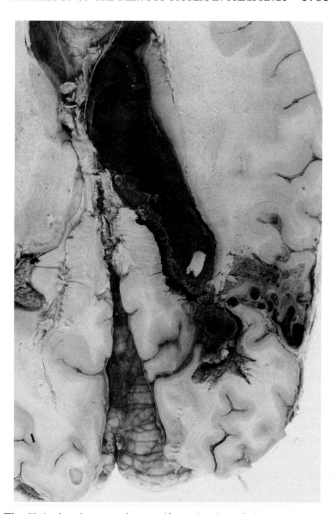

Fig. 59.4 Arteriovenous shunt malformation (so-called angioma) extending from the arachnoid surface of the occipital lobe to the wall of the ventricle. A large blood clot occupies the lateral ventricle.

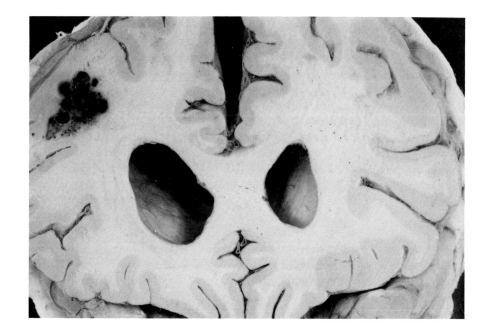

Fig. 59.5 Thin-walled venous angioma beneath cerebral cortex having no major arterial connection. There is some atrophy of white matter with dilatation of the lateral ventricle.

careful examination of the brain enlarged surface veins may be seen. The abnormal vessels of the arteriovenous malformation can be obvious in the larger malformations (Fig. 59.4); smaller ones may only be seen on histological examination. Haemorrhage from arteriovenous malformations in pregnancy may carry a higher risk than in the nongravid population and they may not benefit from surgical treatment (Dias & Sekhar, 1990). In another survey (Horton et al, 1990) of a group of 451 women who received proton beam therapy for their arteriovenous malformation there were 540 pregnancies resulting in 438 live births and 102 abortions, with 17 pregnancies complicated by a cerebral haemorrhage. They did not find that pregnancy significantly increased the rate of first cerebral haemorrhage from an arteriovenous malformation. Haemorrhage from an arteriovenous malformation occurs during gestation and not usually in the puerperium.

The other lesions which are a known cause of migrainous or epileptic attacks are capillary or venous angiomas (Fig. 59.5) but they have a low blood flow and never bleed significantly.

The argument is put forward by some that certain of the circulating steroids in pregnancy tend to cause a relaxation of smooth muscle; certainly elastic tissues are more extendable. This might be the explanation for the first appearance, commonly in pregnancy, of an arteriovenous lesion of the spinal cord, loosely called an angioma, but resembling more a venous varix (Arseni & Simionescu, 1959) (Fig. 59.6). This condition, once established with circulatory stasis and ischaemia, may persist after pregnancy as a varying degree of dysfunction of the lower spinal cord segments.

MIGRAINE

For most women who suffer from migraine, pregnancy brings temporary relief; in a few it appears for the first time and for about one in five it worsens. Hemiplegic migraine has been reported in pregnancy (Mandel, 1988). It is thought to be due to an abnormal response of vessels, in that they dilate to 5-HT (Pearce, 1991). However, there are cases where the headache appears to be related to known aneurysms or arteriovenous malformations of the brain and where the attacks are more frequent and severe at certain points in the menstrual cycle. One would expect such a minority of cases to worsen during pregnancy even if subarachnoid haemorrhage does not occur. Obviously ergotamine therapy is contraindicated at this time.

WERNICKE'S ENCEPHALOPATHY

Women who develop hyperemesis gravidarum must be considered to be in danger of acute deficiency of B vitamins, especially thiamine. If this is not provided by, say,

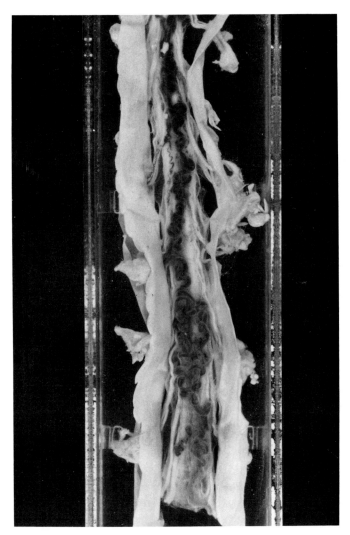

Fig. 59.6 Thoracolumbar spinal cord showing a subarachnoid venous varix.

50 mg intramuscularly at intervals, then there is a great danger of the abrupt onset of Wernicke's encephalopathy. This disease is not, of course, peculiar to pregnancy for it occurs in other cases of persistent vomiting such as pyloric stenosis or alcoholism. In Wernicke's encephalopathy transketolase activity is low; this is a thiamine-dependent enzyme in the pentose phosphate pathway. The most reliable test for thiamine deficiency is the thiamine pyrophosphate effect, where there is an increase in activity of transketolase when thiamine pyrophosphate is added to a preparation of the patient's red cells (Bergin & Harvey, 1992). There is evidence that those patients who develop Wernicke's encephalopathy have a form of transketolase that binds thiamine less avidly than that of controls (Blass & Gibson, 1977).

The lesions are most obvious in the corpora mamillaria and adjacent parts of the wall of the third ventricle, the floor of the fourth ventricle and the midbrain. There appears to be a local breakdown of the adhesion between

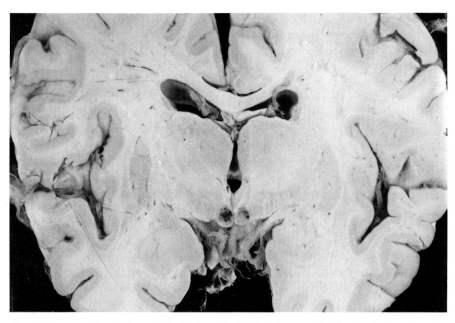

Fig. 59.7 Coronal slice through the brain at the level of the mamillary bodies. These show the characteristic focal petechial haemorrhagic lesions of Wernicke's encephalopathy.

capillary and arteriolar endothelial cells and a loss of the blood-brain barrier to an extent where seepage of plasma and even small haemorrhages occur; there is also loss of neurones (Fig. 59.7).

Because of the site of the damage, there will be some clinical evidence of damage to brain stem nuclei with, for example, extraocular palsies; damage to mamillary bodies will lead to confusion and, if treatment is not given early and urgently, a persistent loss of recent memory leading to Korsakoff's psychosis. Other evidence of B vitamin deficiency may be seen with the hyperaesthesia and calf tenderness of polyneuropathy or the dyspnoea, palpitations and cardiac failure of beri beri.

CENTRAL PONTINE MYELINOLYSIS

Another rare complication of hyperemesis gravidarum is central pontine myelinolysis (Castillo et al, 1989). This seems to follow a rapid correction of severe hyponatraemia. Bergin & Harvey (1992) reported a case of hyperemesis gravidarum where there was both central pontine myelinolysis and Wernicke's encephalopathy. Pathologically there is extensive demyelination in the pons and other areas of white matter; there is no inflammatory cell infiltrate and little gliosis. The condition can lead to coma and death.

TRAUMA

The commonest cause of death in young adults is trauma, and this can, unfortunately, happen to pregnant women;

the head may be injured alone or with other parts of the body. Head injuries in pregnant women are no different from head injuries generally; they can be minor, moderate or severe and the outcome depends upon their severity. In severe cases there can be damage to the scalp, skull and brain. If there is a temporal fracture the middle meningeal artery can be torn. This may lead to extradural haematoma, which classically has a lucid interval (clinically, the patient is conscious immediately after the traumatic episode but after some hours goes into coma and if not treated early enough may die because of the damage and oedema produced in the underlying compressed brain). Other lesions are subdural haematomas, produced by tearing of vessels and brain tissue, and subarachnoid haemorrhage which is found in patches, more so over the superolateral aspects of the cerebrum rather than in relation to the circle of Willis as in ruptured berry aneurysms. Brain contusions and lacerations are usually present in fatal cases. If the accident victim remains unconscious afterwards it is likely that there is diffuse axonal injury where tracts have been torn, leading to axon bulb formation after 24 hours of survival. The proximal ends of the axons swell and the distal portions, along with their myelin sheaths, undergo Wallerian degeneration. The brain in fatal cases can show evidence of oedema and brain shift; also in a substantial number of cases there is hypoxic/anoxic brain damage due to a hypoxic/anoxic episode at the time of the injury or shortly afterwards before adequate ventilation was commenced. This hypoxia/anoxia worsens the prognosis as it exacerbates the brain damage caused by the injury.

In one study the fetal outcome related mainly to direct fetal injury and to maternal haemodynamic insult (Drost et al, 1990); four fetuses were lost and one neonate died, because of the injuries received. There was only one maternal death in this series out of 318 cases.

INFECTIONS

Infections of the central nervous system do not seem as important in western countries as in the developing world where tuberculosis is common and tuberculous meningitis still occurs in pregnancy. Bacterial leptomeningitis could occur but there are no factors in pregnancy to increase its incidence in western countries.

A bacterial infection, listeria, is associated with repeated abortions but it is a rare cause of infection of the CNS in the mother. *Listeria monocytogenes* is a Gram-positive rod and infection is often transmitted to adults by contaminated food, e.g. coleslaw, unpasteurized milk, raw milk and products made from unpasteurized milk, poultry, shellfish and processed meats. It is transmitted to the fetus by blood-borne spread or passage through the birth canal. Low rates of carriage are present in the general population; however, the relationship between carriage and the disease is not clear (Lamont & Postlethwaite, 1986; Wenger & Broome, 1991). When it has occurred in adults a variety of lesions have been found in the CNS; mortality may be up to 30% (Nieman & Lorber, 1980). There may be meningitis, cerebritis or, more rarely, abscess formation; very occasionally there can be miliary focal granulomas in the meninges, but this is more common in infants. Listeria may produce suppuration of the brain substance in the absence of meningeal involvement.

At post mortem in adults with listeria meningitis the brain shows thickened meninges which contain both polymorphs and macrophages in varying numbers. There have also been reports of infection localized to the brain stem (Kennard et al, 1979). Multiple small abscesses in the pons and medulla have been reported (Howard et al, 1981) and in such cases the brain stem is swollen and softened. The abscesses in the brain stem contain polymorphs and Gram-positive bacilli, found intra- and extracellularly. Fibrinoid material in concentric layers in small vessels with perivascular cuffing has also been described.

ACQUIRED IMMUNODEFICIENCY SYNDROME (AIDS)

There is an increasing incidence of positivity to human immunodeficiency virus (HIV) and this can be present in pregnancy, with infected infants being born. Brains from such cases should be handled as set out in the recommendations (Advisory Committee for Dangerous Pathogens, 1990) for full precautions against infection by dangerous pathogens. The virus infects cells that carry on their surface CD4 antigen, part of which acts as a receptor for entry of HIV into these cells. The T lymphocytes of CD4 type (helper T cells) have the greatest CD4 surface antigen and therefore HIV easily infects these cells; the virus can also infect B lymphocytes, monocytes and macrophages. The pathology of HIV infection can be divided into pre-AIDS and AIDS (acquired immunodeficiency syndrome). In pre-AIDS there is a latent period of relative well-being, which is of variable length, a few months to years during which episodes of self-limiting Guillain–Barré-like acute or relapsing demyelinating peripheral neuropathy, mononeuritis multiplex or cranial neuropathies occur. In pre-AIDS, particularly in those who are drug misusers, there is a low-grade meningoencephalitis with increased numbers of mononuclear cells in the pia arachnoid and underlying brain tissue.

In the terminal stages of clinical AIDS there is progressive disease of the CNS in which, clinically, there is a varying combination of apathy, progressive behavioural or mental deterioration, ataxia, tremor and other involuntary movements (Price et al, 1988). The mental deterioration is similar to that seen in subcortical dementia. The pathological changes of encephalopathy, in the absence of opportunistic infections or lymphoma, are of a relatively normal brain macroscopically but variable microscopic changes; these may be widespread but require adequate sampling of the brain. The changes can be non-specific and are found in the central white matter and the deep grey matter with the cerebral cortex being relatively spared (Gray et al, 1988). These non-specific findings are diffuse or focal macrophage and microglial cell infiltration and reactive astrocytosis, which can be seen in cerebral and cerebellar white matter. The microglial cell infiltrates may be found in well-defined nodules in the grey or white matter. Perivascular cuffing by a few lymphocytes may be present as well. Prominent vacuolation of white matter is found in some cases, and most show pallor of the myelin. In some, but not all of the cases, 25–69% in different reported series, there are multinucleated giant cells in the perivascular spaces, particularly in cerebral white matter, basal ganglia and thalamus. These giant cells are thought to be derived from blood-derived monocytes and usually have 2–10 nuclei: HIV can be isolated from them (Esiri & Kennedy, 1992).

In those cases with focal neurological symptoms there can also be opportunistic infection or even lymphoma in the brain. The commonest opportunistic infections are cytomegalovirus, cryptococcosis and toxoplasmosis. Other viral infections reported in AIDS brains are the JC virus which causes progressive multifocal leucoencephalopathy, herpes simplex and varicella-zoster.

The lymphoma can be primary or systemic and occasional cases of metastatic Kaposi's sarcoma have been reported. Subarachnoid and intracerebral haemorrhage have also been reported as a result of thrombocytopenia, which is due to an autoimmune mechanism in AIDS. Cerebral infarction also occurs.

EPILEPSY

True, non-eclamptic, epilepsy is a fairly common disease with a prevalence of about one in 200 of the general population: the annual incidence of onset in the third and fourth decades, the fertile-years, is about one in 2000. As epilepsy is not uncommon, some women who already have epilepsy will become pregnant and some will have their onset of epilepsy during pregnancy. General information regarding the course of epilepsy during pregnancy and the type of epilepsy give no clear pointers on which to base predictions for the course of epileptic attacks during a single pregnancy (Gjerde et al, 1988; Holmes, 1988). There is no definite evidence that pregnancy worsens epilepsy. Bardy (1987) reported a series of cases where there was an increased frequency of seizures in 32% of cases, a decrease in 14% and no change in 23%, with 31% being seizure free during 24 months. Knight & Rhind (1975) reported that 5% of women are improved in that they have fewer attacks during pregnancy. Rarely has there been reported a true gestational epilepsy recurring only in successive pregnancies (Teare, 1980).

This variable picture is what might be expected when the many and various possible causes of such seizures are considered. There does not appear to be any prognostic help to be derived from the patient's age or previous history of precipitating factors.

The increases reported are mostly in the first trimester and are thought to be due in part to fluid retention, some women showing a considerable weight gain before the increase in the number of fits, and in part to poor drug control (Dimsdale, 1959). For various reasons, including an increase of hydroxylating enzyme activity in the liver and vomiting, the dose of phenytoin or phenobarbitone required to control a known tendency to epilepsy needs to be increased during pregnancy and reduced in the puerperium (Swainman, 1980; Leppik & Rask, 1988). Factors such as maternal sleep deprivation, stress and inadequate anticonvulsant levels could be of greater importance than hormonal epileptogenesis.

Unfortunately, the maternal and fetal demand for folate increases at the same time as a larger dose of phenytoin is reducing (as a side effect) the absorption rate of folic acid from the gut (Dahlke & Mertens-Roesler, 1967). Furthermore, increase of microsomal enzyme activity in liver cells may cause a more rapid folate metabolism and thus exaggerate a relative absorption deficiency (Bayliss et al, 1971). It is, perhaps, this effect on folate that makes the problem of drug teratogenicity of great importance in the control of epilepsy during pregnancy. There is quite a lot of evidence that in cases where the mother is treated with anti-epileptic drugs there is an especially large increase in the occurrence of cleft palate and in congenital heart disease (in both conditions about 10 times the expected number) (Fredrick, 1973; Annegers et al, 1974; Kallen, 1986). These defects are probably multifactorial though some may be due to low blood folate levels (Dansky et al, 1987). It is, however, quite clear that epileptic fits themselves will damage the fetus through the associated severe anoxia. The balance of risk in each case probably depends on the likely frequency of attacks. What is known is that if the pregnancies are carefully monitored throughout there is a good outcome for mother and fetus in most cases (Patterson, 1989). Pregnancy can be a time when epilepsy first occurs and is not related to eclampsia; in these instances the gravid patient requires a complete examination to exclude an identifiable and treatable cause for the epilepsy. A personally encountered patient with an astrocytoma had her first fits towards the end of pregnancy at the age of 31 years. Her attacks were of three types: (a) grand mal; (b) momentary unconsciousness with running eyes and nose; (c) ataxia with falling to the ground but no loss of consciousness. She continued to have these attacks for 18 years until her death because of a large astrocytoma in one temporal lobe and the basal ganglia. The tumour had shown very little other evidence of its presence by way of noticeable neurological deficits until a few months before death (Fig. 59.8).

Fatalities due to epilepsy in pregnancy are rare. The brain in patients dying acutely in status epilepticus may show oedema and brain shift but little else. In some cases there is no microscopic change but in others hippocampal sclerosis is seen, where the pyramidal neurones in Sommer's sector are lost with replacement gliosis and shrinkage of the hippocampus. This can be unilateral or bilateral. Neuronal loss may be seen in the cortex and Purkinje cell loss from the cerebellum. The brain should also be examined for the presence of neoplasms and evidence of old trauma with thinning of the cortical ribbon in areas of old contusions, particularly in the inferior aspects of the frontal and temporal lobes; these can also show yellow discolouration from the breakdown products of haemosiderin.

MULTIPLE SCLEROSIS

Multiple sclerosis is the most common disabling neurological disease of young people in the West, with a prevalence of up to one in 2000, varying greatly in different parts of the world with a gradual increase towards higher latitudes. Many women of fertile age will wish to be advised on whether the course of their disease will be affected by pregnancy. Statistically there is about two and a half times as great a relapse rate for such women but most relapses appear in the three months after delivery (Schapira et al, 1966; Birk et al, 1988). In one series (Birk et al, 1988) only 10% had worsening of their symptoms

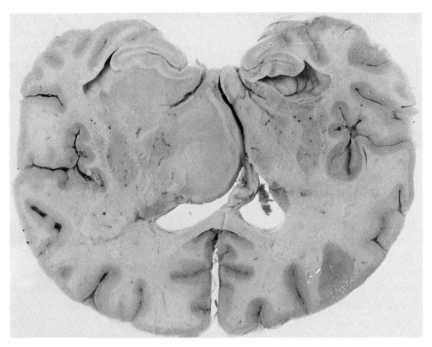

Fig. 59.8 Diffuse glioma infiltrating and expanding the basal ganglia and part of the temporal lobe on one side.

during pregnancy: these authors also concluded that multiple sclerosis had no adverse effect on pregnancy, labour or delivery.

In pregnant women with multiple sclerosis there are protective soluble factors that cause the disease to be less active in pregnancy and this may be the underlying reason for the reduction in the onset of multiple sclerosis in pregnancy (Birk et al, 1988): these protective factors are pregnancy-associated plasma protein and alpha-2-pregnancy-associated glycoprotein; fetal alphafetoprotein may also play some part in reducing the number of relapses of multiple sclerosis in pregnancy.

The pathology of multiple sclerosis varies depending on the length of time for which it has been present. In the established case the classic plaques of multiple sclerosis are seen throughout the CNS. Many are sited periventricularly around the lateral ventricles and are visible as well-defined grey lesions; sometimes they are seen at the surface of the pons and within the optic nerves. Microscopically there is loss of myelin and oligodendrocytes with gliosis; axons are reduced in number, subsequent to the loss of the myelin sheaths around the axons. At the margins of the plaque there is not such a sharp line between myelinated and non-myelinated axons and in some lesions increased numbers of oligodendrocytes and lymphocytes are found here as well. When there is disease activity, macrophages and reactive astrocytes may also be found at the edges of plaques.

In the earlier stages of multiple sclerosis the lesions are pink or yellow, soft and associated more with sites around small veins. Microscopically there is marked hypercellu-

larity with macrophages and reactive astrocytes; myelin sheaths in these hypercellular areas show disintegration. Axons and nerve cells are preserved.

The aetiology is unknown, however it is thought to be related to a hypersensitivity reaction to viral-damaged brain tissue after unidentified viruses have penetrated the blood-brain barrier. The macrophage infiltration in the earlier stages is thought to be important and there is damage to the myelin first with subsequent death of its associated oligodendrocyte. As some oligodendrocytes are known to proliferate at the edges of plaques remyelination does occur.

It is easier to correlate the plaques in the optic nerves and tracts as well as those in the brain stem and spinal cord to the clinical symptoms but much more difficult to correlate those in the rest of the cerebrum. Nerve conduction is slowed in demyelinated axons running through plaques, but such nerve processes, clothed only by astrocytes, may be very vulnerable to the disorders of the blood-brain barrier that have already been discussed. It may, therefore, be that clinical relapses in pregnancy are not necessarily evidence of the development of new lesions.

NEOPLASMS

Another situation in which it is difficult to assess the part that pregnancy plays in initiating or worsening the prognosis is intracranial neoplasms. The commonest primary brain tumour in adults is the astrocytoma; this is a group of neoplasms arising from the astrocytic cells in the CNS which in the World Health Organization classification of brain tumors (1993) includes: pilocytic astrocytomas (commoner in children), fibrillary astrocytoma, anaplastic astrocytoma and glioblastoma multiforme. In women, during the fertile period, the commonest primary brain tumours occur in the cerebral hemispheres and are usually the fibrillary astrocytomas; oligodendrogliomas can also occur but are not as frequent. Glioblastoma multiforme is rarer in this age group — the peak incidence is 55–60 years and on average the survival after histological diagnosis is 9 months whereas fibrillary astrocytomas have on average a 48-month survival. Also fibrillary astrocytomas invariably undergo a rapid growth phase later on, as demonstrated in the previous case history. The potential doubling time for glioblastoma multiforme is around 11–12 days (Hoshino et al, 1979) but as it is much slower in fibrillary astrocytomas these tumours are probably present before conception; this is not so in the more rapidly growing glioblastoma. As well as the primary brain tumours, tumours arising from the meninges, meningiomas, the cranial nerves, usually the vestibular portion of the eighth cranial nerve, and the anterior pituitary gland can occur in the fertile years.

As it is such a dramatic event when occurring in pregnancy there have been many case reports describing intracranial neoplasms diagnosed in pregnancy, suggesting that pregnancy is associated with the growth of intracranial neoplasms. However in one epidemiological study in Germany (Haas et al, 1986) there were reduced numbers of primary brain tumours and meningiomas in observed to expected ratios and these were statistically significant. Others agree that there is no higher incidence of primary brain tumour in pregnancy (Roelvink et al, 1987; Simon, 1988; Russell & Rubinstein, 1989). Haas and co-workers (1986) did find an increase, though not statistically significant, in the number of intracranial schwannomas in their series.

It is known and well recognized that intracranial meningiomas and schwannomas can show accelerated growth during pregnancy (Michelsen & New, 1968). The growth of meningiomas may be related to the presence of progesterone receptors on the tumour cells (Tilzer et al, 1982).

Haas and co-workers (1986) thought that the reduced incidence of astrocytomas in pregnancy could be due to the fact that those developing such a tumour may, because of disturbed hypothalamic function, have less chance of pregnancy due to reduced fertility, disturbances of ovulation, conception and implantation: these authors also suggested that even when pregnancy did start abnormal embryonic development with early loss would affect their epidemiological figures.

Choriocarcinomas related to pregnancy have a high propensity for brain metastases, but this occurs in the postpartum period (Gurwitt et al, 1975; Ishizuka et al, 1983). In such cases intracranial metastases may result in death and they may need surgical extirpation as well as chemotherapy and radiotherapy. Primary intracranial choriocarcinoma has also been recorded in women; by 1982, 61 such cases had been reported (Russell & Rubinstein, 1989).

PITUITARY

As well as the brain suffering from ischaemia during pregnancy there can also be ischaemia to the pituitary gland, particularly after postpartum haemorrhage, and this can lead to Sheehan's syndrome (Sheehan & Davis, 1982) with panhypopituitarism. With the ischaemia there is necrosis of the anterior pituitary gland which shrinks to produce an empty sella on radiological examination. In the empty sella syndrome the diaphragma sella is depressed and the suprasellar space is enlarged. Usually a rim of pituitary tissue is found in the fossa. There has also been a report of spontaneous resolution of Cushing's syndrome after pregnancy as a fortuitous result of pituitary necrosis (Aron et al, 1990).

CRANIAL AND PERIPHERAL NERVE LESIONS

The changes in tissue fluid content which characterize pregnancy have their effect also on the peripheral nervous system, which includes the cranial as well as the peripheral nerves. This is apparent in patients who have type I neurofibromatosis. This autosomal dominantly inherited condition with variable penetrance shows the abnormal gene on chromosome 17. Neurofibromas are tumours but whether they are true neoplasms is still not widely accepted. They are oedematous and collagenous lesions of nerve sheath with increased numbers of axons and dystrophy of Schwann cells.

Further gelatinous enlargement by the accumulation of extracellular fluid makes the abnormal dermal nerve plexuses in neurofibromatosis more obvious in pregnancy but these subside later and there is no evidence of any permanent change (Swapp & Main, 1973).

More commonly in pregnancy various entrapment neuropathies are reported (Massey & Cefalo, 1979). Bell's palsy is thought to be due to a swollen facial nerve negotiating the long bony facial canal and occurs over three times more often than expected (about 45/100 000 births), mostly in the last few weeks of pregnancy (Hilsinger et al, 1975).

Meralgia paraesthetica is due to bruising of the lateral cutaneous nerve of the thigh as it passes through the deep fascia. The carpal tunnel syndrome with tingling, numbness and pain in the median nerve distribution of hand and fingers may be a problem in as many as 20% of pregnant women (Gould & Wissinger, 1978) in that it often disturbs sleep and provokes the unwise use of analgesic and hypnotic drugs. There are many women whose first attack of sciatica occurred in pregnancy, often during labour, when ligamentous laxity allows rupture of the intervertebral disc.

As well as the above single entrapment neuropathies there are cases of autoimmune neuropathy (acute inflammatory demyelinating polyneuropathy or Guillain–Barré syndrome), which does not appear to be altered in its frequency or severity in pregnancy (McCombe et al, 1987). It causes a rapid onset of weakness and areflexia with few sensory symptoms. Cerebrospinal fluid shows an increase in protein with no increase in cells. About 60% of cases follow acute infectious illness. The nerves show myelin stripping by macrophages and considerable perivascular lymphocytic cuffing in the epineurium. It is treated by supportive measures: however, as respiratory failure and cardiac arrhythmias occur, all patients need adequate and careful monitoring. Most get better; only occasionally is plasmapheresis required as it is thought to be caused by a humoral factor (Harrison et al, 1984).

There is a chronic inflammatory demyelinating polyradiculoneuropathy which is known to occur during pregnancy, and the relapse rate is significantly increased in parous women; the relapses tend to occur during the third trimester and postpartum (McCombe et al, 1987). It can recur in following pregnancies (Jones & Berry, 1981). In this condition there is paraesthesia, weakness, hyporeflexia or areflexia and sensory impairment. The pathological changes in the nerves are similar to those seen in Guillain–Barré syndrome, without, however, such a high degree of inflammatory cell infiltrate in the nerves.

Trigeminal neuropathy can occur, although only occasionally, in pregnancy (Massey, 1988). However isolated mental nerve neuropathy even during pregnancy should always cause serious concern because of the association of numb chin with malignancy (Massey et al, 1981).

MYASTHENIA GRAVIS

Myasthenia gravis is a disease which most commonly presents in women of child-bearing age and so the strains of pregnancy may produce the first evidence of the condition. There is no reason to believe that the incidence is any greater at this time, but it appears to be the case that deterioration may occur in about 45% of cases, particularly during the postpartum period. Conversely, nearly a third of patients undergo a remission of their symptoms during pregnancy (Plauche, 1979). A weakness and easy fatiguability of proximal muscles and difficulty with respiration are obvious disadvantages during labour which should, therefore, be shortened by a low forceps delivery (Scott, 1976). Approximately 4% of pregnant women with myasthenia gravis die, usually as a result of entering either a myasthenic, or, less commonly, a cholinergic crisis (Plauche, 1979).

The pathological basis of this disease lies not in the nervous system but in the acetylcholine receptor protein on the surface of muscle fibres with which motor axons relate. These receptors are damaged or rendered ineffective because of the production of autoantibodies to this protein. This abnormal antibody production may be reduced following removal of the enlarged thymus or thymoma which is found in 70% of sufferers.

Apart from the obstetrical management of these patients a significant problem exists for the 12–20% of children born to such women who show transient neonatal myasthenia gravis (Plauche, 1979) due to the transplacental passage of anti-acetylcholine receptor antibodies.

Symptoms of hypotonia, inability to suck or respiratory difficulty usually improve during the first two days but in some infants they may persist for weeks, suggesting either a transplacental passage of maternal lymphocytes and the continued production of antibody or a continued supply of antibodies through breast milk. A small dose of anticholinesterase drugs would help to differentiate these cases from the floppy babies who have suffered hind-brain ischaemia following birth trauma to the neck.

MUSCLES

Another autoimmune disease is polymyositis, which may have a subacute or chronic course of muscle weakness, predominantly proximal and usually symmetrical. In the florid forms there can be tenderness and pain of the affected muscles with swelling. The serum creatine kinase is raised and muscle biopsy shows mononuclear (lymphocytic) infiltration of muscle fibres with degeneration and regeneration, but these areas can be patchy and therefore not present in the muscle tissue sampled.

In pregnancy polymyositis does occur, but it is rare and should be treated cautiously with steroids (Parry & Heiman-Patterson, 1988).

REFERENCES

Advisory Committee for Dangerous Pathogens 1990 HIV: the causative agent of AIDS and related conditions. 2nd revised guidelines. Department of Health, London.

Annegers J F, Elverback L R, Hauser W A 1974 Do anti-convulsants have a teratogenic effect? Archives of Neurology (Chicago) 31: 364–365.

Aron D C, Schnall A M, Sheeler L R 1990 Spontaneous resolution of Cushing's syndrome after pregnancy. American Journal of Obstetrics and Gynecology 162: 472–474.

Arseni C, Simionescu M D 1959 Vertebral haemangiomata. Acta Psychiatrica et Neurologica Scandinavica 34: 1.

Asherson R A, Khamastha M A, Ordi-Ros J et al 1989 The "primary" antiphospholipid syndrome: major clinical and serological features. Medicine 68: 366–374.

Banerjee A K, Gulati D R, Chhuttani P N 1979 Primary internal cerebral vein thrombosis in a young adult. Neurology India 27: 135–139.

Barber P, Arnold A, Evans G 1976 Recurrent hormone-dependent chorea: effects of estrogens and progesterone. Clinical Endocrinology 5: 23–29.

Bardy A H 1987 Incidence of seizures during pregnancy, labor and puerperium in epileptic women: a prospective study. Acta Neurologica Scandinavica 75: 356–360.

Barno A, Freeman D W 1976 Maternal deaths due to spontaneous subarachnoid hemorrhage. American Journal of Obstetrics and Gynecology 125: 384–392.

Bates J 1848 Remarks on the statistics, pathology and treatment of puerperal insanity. London Medical Gazette 42: 990–992.

Bayliss E M, Crowley J M, Preece J M 1971 Influence of folic acid on blood phenytoin levels. Lancet i: 62–63.

Beck D W, Menezes A H 1981 Intracerebral hemorrhage in a patient with eclampsia. Journal of the American Medical Association 246: 1442–1443.

Benedetti T J, Quilligan E J 1980 Cerebral edema in severe pregnancy induced hypertension. American Journal of Obstetrics and Gynecology 137: 860–862.

Beral V, Kay C R 1977 Mortality among oral contraceptive users. Lancet ii: 727–731.

Bergin P S, Harvey P 1992 Wernicke's encephalopathy and central pontine myelinolysis associated with hyperemesis gravidarum. British Medical Journal 305: 517–518.

Birk K, Smeltzer S C, Rudick R 1988 Pregnancy and multiple sclerosis. Seminars in Neurology 8: 205–213.

Blass J, Gibson G 1977 Abnormality of a thiamine-requiring enzyme in patients with Wernicke-Korshoff syndrome. New England Journal of Medicine 297: 1367–1370.

Brey R L, Coull B M 1992 Antiphospholipid antibodies: origin, specificity and mechanisms of action. Stroke 23 (suppl 1): 115–118.

Brey R L, Hart R G, Sherman C G, Tegeler C H 1990 Antiphospholipid antibodies and cerebral ischaemia in young people. Neurology 40: 1190–1196.

Caroscio J T, Pellmar M 1978 Pseudotumor cerebri: occurrence during the third trimester of pregnancy. Mount Sinai Journal of Medicine (New York) 45: 539–541.

Carroll J D, Leak D, Lee H A 1966 Cerebral thrombophlebitis in pregnancy and the puerperium. Quarterly Journal of Medicine 35: 347–368.

Castillo R A, Ray R A, Vaghmai F 1989 Central pontine myelinolysis and pregnancy. Obstetrics and Gynecology. 73: 459–461.

Chopra J S, Banerjee A K 1989 Primary intracranial sinovenous occlusions in youth and pregnancy. In: Toole J F (ed) Handbook of clinical neurology, vol 10 (54). Vascular diseases, part II. pp 425–452.

Dahlke M B, Mertens-Roesler E 1967 Malabsorption of folic acid due to diphenylhydantoin. Blood 30: 341–351.

Dansky L V, Andermann E, Rosenblatt D, Sherwin A L, Andermann F 1987 Anticonvulsants, folate levels and pregnancy outcome: a prospective study. Annals of Neurology 21: 176–182.

Dawson I 1988 The confidential enquiry into maternal deaths: its role and importance for pathologists. Journal of Clinical Pathology 41: 820–825.

Department of Health 1989 Report on confidential enquiries into maternal deaths in England and Wales 1982–84. Her Majesty's Stationery Office, London.

Dias M S, Sekhar L N 1990 Intracranial hemorrhage from aneurysms and arteriovenous malformations during pregnancy and the puerperium. Neurosurgery 27: 855–866.

Dimsdale H 1959 The epileptic in relation to pregnancy. British Medical Journal 2: 1147–1150.

Dorfman S F 1990 Maternal mortality in New York city, 1981–1983 . Obstetrics and Gynecology 76: 317–323.

Douglas K A, and Redman C W G 1992 Eclampsia in the United Kingdom: the 'BEST' way forward. British Journal of Obstetrics and Gynaecology 99: 355–356.

Drost T F, Rosemurgy A S, Sherman H F, Scott L H, Williams J K 1990 Major trauma in pregnant women: maternal/fetal outcome. Journal of Trauma 30: 574–578.

Esiri M M, Kennedy P G E 1992 Virus diseases. In: Adams J H, Duchern L W (eds) Greefield's Neuropathology, 5th edn. Edward Arnold, London, pp 370–378.

Ezra Y, Kidron D, Beyth Y 1989 Fibromuscular dysplasia of the carotid arteries complicating pregnancy. Obstetrics and Gynecology 73: 840–843.

Fishman R A, Cowen D, Silbermann M 1957 Intracranial venous thrombosis during the first trimester of pregnancy. Neurology 7: 217–219.

Fredrick J 1973 Epilepsy and pregnancy: a report from the Oxford record linkage study. British Medical Journal 2: 442–444.

Geraghty J J, Hoch D B, Robert M E, Vinters H V 1991 Fatal puerperal cerebral vasospasm and stroke in a young woman. Neurology 41: 1145–1147.

Gettlefinger D M, Kokman E 1977 Superior sagittal sinus thrombosis. Archives of Neurology (Chicago) 32: 2–4.

Gjerde I O, Strandjord R E, Ulstein M 1988 The course of epilepsy during pregnancy: a study of 78 cases. Acta Neurologica Scandinavica 78: 198–205.

Gould J S, Wissinger H A 1978 Carpal tunnel syndrome in pregnancy. Southern Medical Journal 71: 144–145.

Gray F, Gherardi R, Scaravilli F 1988 The neuropathology of the acquired immune deficiency syndrome, AIDS; a review. Brain 111: 245–266.

Gurwitt L J, Long J M, Clark R E 1975 Cerebral metastatic choriocarcinoma: a postpartum cause of "stroke". Obstetrics and Gynecology 45: 583–588.

Haas J F, Janisch W, Staneczek W 1986 Newly diagnosed primary intracranial neoplasms in pregnant women: a population-based assessment. Journal of Neurology, Neurosurgery and Psychiatry 49: 874–880.

Harris E N 1992 Serological detection of antiphospholipid antibodies. Stroke 23 (suppl 1): I3–I6.

Harrison B M, Hansen L A, Pollard J D, McLeod J G 1984 Demyelination induced by serum from patients with Guillain-Barre syndrome. Annals of Neurology 15: 163–170.

Hilsinger R L, Adour K K, Doty H E 1975 Idiopathic facial paralysis, pregnancy and the menstrual cycle. Annals of Otology, Rhinology and Laryngology 84: 433–442.

Hirsh J, Cade J F, Gallus A S 1972 Anticoagulants in pregnancy: a review of indications and complications (Editorial). American Heart Journal 83: 301–305.

Holmes G L 1988 Effects of menstruation and pregnancy on epilepsy. Seminars in Neurology 8: 234–239.

Hotton J C, Chambers W A, Lyons S L, Adams R D, Kjellberg R N 1990 Pregnancy and the risk of hemorrhage from cerebral arteriovenous malformations. Neurosurgery 26: 867–872.

Hoshino T, Wilson C B, Muraoka I 1979 The strathmokimetic (mitostatic) effect of vincristine and vinblastine on human gliomas. Acta Neuropathologica 47: 21–25.

Howard A J, Kennard C, Eykyn S, Higgs I 1981 Listerial infections of the CNS in the previous healthy adult. Infection 9: 1067–1072.

Ishizuka T, Tomoda Y, Kaseki S, Goto S, Hara T, Kobayashi T 1983 Intracranial metastasis of choriocarcinoma: a clinicopathologic study. Cancer 52: 1896–1903.

Jennett W B, Cross J N 1967 Influence of pregnancy and oral contraception on the incidence of strokes in women of childbearing age. Lancet 1: 1019–1023.

Jones M W, Berry K 1981 Chronic relapsing polyneuritis associated with pregnancy. Annals of Neurology 9: 413.

Kalbag R M, Woolf A L 1967 Cerebral venous thrombosis. Oxford University Press, London, pp 101–134.

Kallen B 1986 A register study of maternal epilepsy and delivery outcome with special reference to drug use. Acta Neurologica Scandinavica 73: 253–259.

Karasawa J, Kikuchi H, Furuse S 1980 Subependymal hematoma in Moyamoya disease. Surgical Neurology 13: 118–120.

Kennard C, Howard A J, Scholtz C, Swash M 1979 Infection of the brain stem by L. monocytogenes. Journal of Neurology, Neurosurgery and Psychiatry 42: 931–933.

Kleihues P, Burger P C, Scheithauer B W 1993 Histological typing of the central nervous system. World Health Organization International Histological Classification of Tumours. Springer-verlag, Berlin.

Knight A H, Rhind E G 1975 Epilepsy and pregnancy: a study of 153 cases in 59 patients. Epilepsia 16: 99–110.

Lamont R J, Postlethwaite R 1986 Carriage of Listeria monocytogenes and related species in pregnant and non-pregnant women in Aberdeen, Scotland. Journal of Infection 13: 187–193.

Leppik I E, Rask C A 1988 Pharmacokinetics of antiepileptic drugs during pregnancy. Seminars in Neurology 8: 240–246.

Mandel S 1988 Hemiplegic migraine in pregnancy. Headache 28: 414–416.

Mabie W C, Ratts T E, Sibai B M 1989 The central hemodynamics of severe pre-eclampsia. American Journal of Obstetrics and Gynecology 161: 1443–1448.

Macdonald R L, Weir B K A 1991 A review of hemoglobin and the pathogenesis of cerebral vasospasm. Stroke 22: 971–982.

Massey E W 1988 Mononeuropathies in pregnancy. Seminars in Neurology 8: 193–196.

Massey E W, Cefalo R C 1979 Neuropathies of pregnancy. Obstetrical and Gynecological Survey 34: 489–492.

Massey E W, Moore J, Schold C 1981 Mental neuropathy from systemic cancer. Neurology 31: 1277–1281.

McCombe P A, McManis P G, Frith J A, Pollard J D, McLeod J G 1987 Chronic inflammatory demyelinating polyradiculoneuropathy associated with pregnancy. Annals of Neurology 21: 102–104.

Michelsen J J, New P F J 1968 Brain tumour and pregnancy. Journal of Neurology, Neurosurgery and Psychiatry 32: 305–307.

Milandre L, Pellissier J F, Vincentelli F, Khalil R 1990 Deep cerebral venous system thrombosis in adults. European Neurology 30: 93–97.

Miller J D, Adams J H 1992 The pathophysiology of raised intracranial pressure. In: Adams J H, Duchen L W (eds) Greenfield's Neuropathology, 5th edn. Edward Arnold, London, pp 90–92.

Montalban J, Codina A, Ordi J, Vilardell M, Khamashta M A, Hughes G R V 1991 Antiphospholipid antibodies in cerebral ischaemia. Stroke 22: 750–753.

Nag S 1986 Cerebral endothelial plasma membrane alteration in acute hypertension. Acta Neuropathologica (Berlin) 70: 38–43.

Nieman R E, Lorber B 1980 Listeriosis in adults: a changing pattern: report of eight cases and review of the literature, 1968–1978. Review of Infectious Diseases 2: 207–227.

Parry G J, Heiman-Patterson T D 1988 Pregnancy and autoimmune neuromuscular disease. Seminars in Neurology 8: 197–204.

Patterson R M 1989 Seizure disorders in pregnancy. Medical Clinics of North America 73: 661–665.

Pearce J M S 1991 Sumaptriptan in migraine. British Medical Journal 303: 1491.

Plauche W C 1979 Myasthenia gravis in pregnancy: an update. American Journal of Obstetrics and Gynecology 135: 691–695.

Pope F M, Nicholls A C, Narsisi P, Bartlett J, Neil-Dwyer G, Dhoshi B 1980 Some patients with cerebral aneurysms are deficient in Type III collagen. Lancet i: 973–975.

Powell J L 1972 Pseudotumor cerebri and pregnancy. Obstetrics and Gynecology 40: 713–718.

Price R W, Brew B, Sidtis J, Rosenblum M, Scheck A C, Cleary P 1988 The brain in AIDS: central nervous system HIV-1 infection and AIDS dementia complex. Science 239: 586–591.

Richards A, Graham D, Bullock R 1988 Clinicopathological study of neurological complications due to hypertensive disorders of pregnancy. Journal of Neurology, Neurosurgery and Psychiatry 51: 416–421.

Robinson J L, Hall C J, Sedzimar C M 1972 Sub-arachnoid haemorrhage in pregnancy. Journal of Neurosurgery 36: 27–33.

Roelvink N C A, Kamphorst W, van Alphen H A M, Rao B R 1987 Pregnancy-related primary brain and spinal tumors. Archives of Neurology 44: 209–215.

Russell D S, Rubinstein L J 1989 Pathology of tumours of the nervous system, 5th edn. Edward Arnold, London, pp 750–753.

Sacco R, Wolf P, Bharucha N 1984 Subarachnoid and intracerebral hemorrhage: natural history, prognosis and precursive factors in the Framingham Study. Neurology 34: 847–854.

Schapira K, Poskanzer D C, Newell D J, Miller H 1966 Marriage, pregnancy and multiple sclerosis. Brain 89: 419–428.

Schipper H M 1988 Sex hormones in stroke, chorea and anticonvulsant therapy. Seminars in Neurology 8: 181–186.

Schutta H S, Williams E C, Baranski B G, Sutula T P 1991 Cerebral venous thrombosis with plasminogen deficiency. Stroke 22: 401–405.

Scott J S 1976 Immunology of human reproduction. Academic Press, London, pp 229–288.

Sheehan H L, Davis J C 1982 Post-partum hypopituitarism. Charles C Thomas, Springfield, Illinois.

Sheehan H L, Lynch J B 1973 Pathology of toxaemia of pregnancy. Williams & Wilkins, Baltimore, pp 524–584.

Simolke G A, Cox S M, Cunningham F G 1991 Cerebrovascular accidents complicating pregnancy and the puerperium. Obstetrics and Gynecology 78: 37–42.

Simon R H 1988 Brain tumors in pregnancy. Seminars in Neurology 8: 214–221.

Srinivasan K 1984 Ischemic cerebrovascular disease in the young, two common causes in India. Stroke 15: 733–735.

Srinivasan K 1988 Puerperal cerebral venous and arterial thrombosis. Seminars in Neurology 8: 222–225.

Swainman K F 1980 Antiepileptic drugs, the developing nervous system and the pregnant woman with epilepsy. Journal of the American Medical Association 244: 1477.

Swapp G H, Main R A 1973. Neurofibromatosis in pregnancy. British Journal of Dermatology 80: 431–435.

Teare A J 1980 True gestational epilepsy. South African Medical Journal 57: 546–547.

Tilzer L L, Plapp F V, Evans J P, Stone D, Alward K 1982 Steroid receptor proteins in human meningiomas. Cancer 49: 633–636.

Van Hartesveldt C, Joyce J 1986 Effects of estrogen on the basal ganglia. Neuroscience Biobehaviour Review 10: 1–14.

Weibers D O 1985 Ischemic cerebrovascular complications of pregnancy. Archives of Neurology 42: 1106–1113.

Weibers D O, Whisnant J P 1985 The incidence of stroke among pregnant women in Rochester, Minn, 1955 through 1979. Journal of the American Medical Association 254: 3055–3057.

Weibers D O, 1988 Subarachnoid hemorrhage in pregnancy. Seminars in Neurology 8: 226–229.

Wenger J D, Broome C V 1991 Bacterial meningitis: epidemiology. In: Lambert H P (ed) Infections of the central nervous system. Handbook of Infectious Diseases. Editors Kass E H, Weller T H, Woolff S M, Tyrrell D A p 27.

60. Pathology of multiple pregnancy

A. H. Cameron   Virginia J. Baldwin

INTRODUCTION

Twins occur in less than 2% of pregnancies in man. They are therefore exceptional and for this reason alone they merit special consideration. The vast majority of twin pregnancies are uncomplicated and so twinning must not be regarded as pathological. With higher orders of multiple births there is a major risk of prematurity, stillbirth and neonatal death which excludes them from the range of normality.

Study of twin pregnancies may shed some light on the increased incidence of malformations compared with that in singletons and the same applies to the rates of prematurity and chorioamnionitis. Some pathological states, such as the twin-transfusion syndrome and the acardiac malformation, are confined to twins and are of particular interest.

Examination of twins has much to contribute to the assessment of the relative rôles played by nature and nurture in normal and abnormal development during intrauterine life and postnatally. In such studies it is often assumed that the intrauterine environment is identical for a given pair of twins and that twins of similar appearance with a common placenta are genetically identical. Contrariwise, separate placentas are commonly taken to indicate dizygosity. None of these assumptions is reliable.

ZYGOSITY AND PLACENTATION

Twins derived from one fertilized egg — monozygotic — are classically considered genetically identical, but rare exceptions are well documented. The commonest discordance is in the sex chromosomes, usually absence of one X chromosome in one twin, most obvious with male twins where one becomes monosomy X with Ullrich–Turner syndrome (Perlman et al, 1990). Other patterns of numerical sex chromosome and autosome discordance (Dallpiccola et al, 1985) and discordance of chromosomal structure (Juberg et al, 1981) are less common. Cytogenetically discordant monozygotic twin pairs may arise

from either post-zygotic non-disjunction or anaphase lag, followed or accompanied by twinning, and are sometimes known as heterokaryonts. Clear confirmation of monozygosity in phenotypically and cytogenetically discordant twins is essential to diagnose heterokaryonts, and tissue as well as blood must be sampled for chromosome analysis to differentiate them from blood chimeras due to vascular anastomoses.

The placenta in monozygotic twins is usually single and monochorionic but there may be two separate placentas or a fused placenta with two chorionic sacs. If division occurs within three days of fertilization then monozygotic twins will develop two chorionic sacs which, like dizygotic placentas, may be separate or fused. If division occurs on days four to eight, after the formation of the chorion, then the placenta will be single and monochorionic with two amniotic sacs. Division after the formation of the amnion results in a monoamniotic sac and division after initiation of the primitive streak at about 12 days will result in conjoined twins (Fig. 60.1).

Dizygotic or two-egg twins always have dichorionic placentas and these may be separate or fused.

Figure 60.1 shows that monochorionic placentas always indicate monozygotic twins while dichorionic placentas, whether fused or separate, may be either monozygotic or dizygotic.

A third type of twinning, intermediate between monozygotic and dizygotic, has been postulated for some time, but could be confirmed only when sophisticated DNA technology became available. Dispermic monovular twinning refers to the fertilization of the oocyte and its first or second polar body by separate sperm. Fertilization of the diploid first polar body leads to a triploid twin (Bieber et al, 1981) while fertilization of the haploid second polar body, also called the tertiary oocyte, leads to a diploid twin (Boklage, 1987). The incidence of polar body twinning is not known because it requires detailed molecular analysis to determine the parent of origin of the components of the genetic material of the twins, and may be suspected only when the normal boy and normal girl are

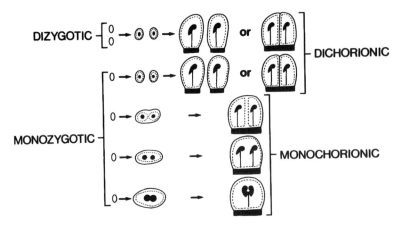

Fig. 60.1   Diagram of zygosity related to placentation.

contained in a proven monochorionic placenta (Baldwin, 1993).

Determination of zygosity

From the preceding observations it will be clear that examination of the placenta is of prime importance. If it is monochorionic then the twins are monozygotic: this is so in about 20% of twin pregnancies. A further 35% or so are of different sex; they will have dichorionic placentas and are dizygotic. This leaves about 45% who are of the same sex and have dichorionic placentas.

In practice, the 48% who are concordant for sex and have dichorionic placentas can be differentiated further only by careful genotyping. Table 60.1 shows the breakdown of 668 pairs of twins in Birmingham (Cameron, 1968). It will be seen that most of those of like sex with dichorionic placentas were shown by genotyping to be dizygotic but 8% of the total sample were dichorionic and monozygotic.

Genotyping

Although general physical appearances are usually reliable, they can be misleading. Monozygotic twins may lose their similarity if one of them should suffer from trauma, infection or malnutrition, for example, either during intrauterine development or postnatally. It is perfectly obvious that monozygotic twins are no longer identical if one is

run over by a motor car but a similar effect can be produced, for example, by relative ischaemia of the placental site or by neonatal infections such as meningitis. The twins remain monozygotic but are no longer identical.

In the newborn baby physical appearances may be particularly difficult to assess. Genetically determined differences may not yet have had time to develop and there may be misleading apparent differences due to moulding of the skull or other obstetrical factors.

Sex is a most reliable marker but examination of chromosomes is not required unless there are clinical grounds for suspecting some anomaly. Dermatoglyphic patterns are helpful on occasions (Smith & Penrose, 1955; Reed et al, 1978) but palm and finger prints are time-consuming to take and particularly difficult in the newborn.

The most readily available method is to examine an extensive battery of blood groups, red cell enzymes, and histocompatibility antigens. The wider the profile, the greater chance there is of detecting the dizygotics (Fisher et al, 1982; Cameron et al, 1983), although a sequential test system based on relative gene frequencies of the different blood group antigens in the population in question may be more efficient than a random search (Das Chaddhuri, 1991). Blood for this purpose should be taken from all newborn twins of the same sex.

Chromosomal polymorphisms using banding techniques may detect dizygosity, but direct analysis of chromosomal nucleic acid is the definitive tool to determine the degree of genetic identity. Current DNA technology requires only one small sample that does not have to be fresh, and the specificity far exceeds any other test system available, but because of its cost it probably should be reserved for carefully selected cases (Hill & Jeffreys, 1985; Kovacs et al, 1988; Azuma et al, 1989).

Organization

If something more than the investigation of occasional

Table 60.1   Analysis of 688 twin pairs

Different sex	35%	Dizygotic
Monochorionic	20%	Monozygotic
Same sex, dichorionic	45%	
	↓	
	Genotyping	
	↓	
Dizygotic 37%		Monozygotic 8%

clinical problems of twins is required then some sort of organization is required. The ideal is to provide a reliable data base which can be used not only for the investigation of individual clinical cases but also for wider purposes, ranging from the study of intrauterine growth to the genetic implications of malformations and other disturbances (Altshuler, 1982). Quite apart from academic and clinical considerations, the parents naturally want to know whether the twins are 'identical' or not.

Where local considerations are suitable, arrangements can easily be made for the examination of the placenta and for genotyping of the blood. This should be organized on a service basis, and it is important to enlist the cooperation of those involved — the midwives, obstetricians and paediatricians as well as laboratory staff.

The placentas from all twin and multiple pregnancies in the region should be sent to a single laboratory for examination. They should be sent fresh inside two plastic bags to prevent leakage of blood. The cords must be labelled at the time of delivery to identify twins I and II. Those that cannot be dispatched on the same day can be stored in the refrigerator but they should not be put in fixative. The laboratory is most conveniently part of a pathology department but it could well be within an obstetric department. The facilities required for examination are not elaborate but it is essential that there is a permanent member of staff with appropriate experience and interest.

Cord blood in appropriately labelled tubes should accompany all placentas from twins of the same sex. Again, they should be inside two plastic bags to avoid leakage. In the laboratory, the blood from monochorionic twins will be discarded and the remainder referred to the blood transfusion laboratory for genotyping. Alternatively the bloods may be referred directly to the BTS but the above suggestion cuts down the BTS work by about 30% and also allows the laboratory to check that appropriate blood samples have been taken. Arrangements with a specialized laboratory will be required if enzymatic genotyping is to be undertaken.

After the necessary examinations have been made a composite report should be issued which should include the observations on the placenta, the genotyping and an assessment of zygosity. The mother will have been discharged from hospital and so it should be arranged that the report is available to the obstetrician for the postnatal consultation and to the physician caring for the twins. It is essential that a copy of the report is readily available in the laboratory for future enquiries. The data is conveniently handled by computerization.

Examination of the placenta

The examination should be done by staff who have been properly trained; a number of descriptions of the appropriate procedures have been published (Benirschke &

Driscoll, 1967; Strong & Corney, 1967; Cameron, 1968; Fox, 1978; Shanklin & Perrin, 1984; Benirschke & Kaufmann, 1990; Baldwin, 1993). The aims are:

1. to establish the number of chorionic sacs
2. to investigate any possible vascular communications
3. to assess the size of the two placental components
4. to note any pathological features.

If the placentas are separate then there are obviously two chorionic sacs. Not uncommonly, separate placentas have adherent membranes and these are again dichorionic. Placentas with fused chorionic plates must be examined with care. It is sometimes difficult to identify the septum as the membranes may be partly torn or stripped. One must be confident that there is no septum before accepting the placentas as monoamniotic. The initial procedure is to identify the insertion of the two cords and this should indicate the two amniotic cavities. The intervening septum may be eccentric and not correspond to the junction of the two placentas. A monochorionic placenta has a diamniotic septum which is thin and transparent; careful teasing with forceps shows that it consists of two fine layers of membrane, both of which are continuous with the amnion covering the surface of the placenta. When these are stripped off there is no vestige remaining of the septum. By contrast, a dichorionic placenta has a dichorionic diamniotic septum which is thicker and more opaque. A layer of amnion can be stripped off either side leaving the central chorionic layer intact. It is impossible to strip the latter from the surface of the placenta as the two are continuous (Fig. 60.2). It is always wise to take a block for microscopy from the septum before attempting to separate its component layers.

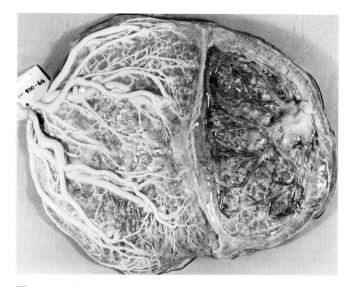

Fig. 60.2 A dichorionic placenta. The amnions have been stripped away but the chorionic element of the septum remains. The vessels of one cord have been injected with barium mixture and there are no anastomoses.

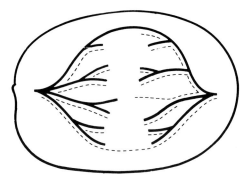

Fig. 60.3 Diagram of placental anastomoses. At the top an artery–artery communication is indicated by the solid line and at the bottom a vein–vein communication is indicated by the dotted line. Centrally, an unaccompanied artery from the left approaches an unaccompanied vein from the right; this is an indication of a probable artery–capillary–vein anastomosis.

Vascular communications can be found between the twins in the majority of monochorionic placentas but are almost never seen in dichorionic placentas. In the Birmingham survey, anastomoses were demonstrated in two of 53 dichorionic monozygotic placentas but in none of the 481 which were dichorionic and dizygotic (Cameron, 1968). Their importance lies not in their relation to zygosity but in their relation to fetal morbidity and mortality, as will be discussed later. They should be looked for in all fused placentas.

The surface vessels of the placenta resemble those of the retina in that the arteries cross over the underlying veins. There are two main types of communication —

those on the surface and those in the deep capillary circulation (Fig. 60.3). For their demonstration it is a necessary preliminary to flush thoroughly with warm saline solution the vessels of both placentas by cannulae inserted into the cord vessels. For dichorionic placentas, which are unlikely to show any anastomoses, it is then sufficient to infuse the vessels of one cord with a thin watery medium such as milk or Indian ink. This will exclude either type and none of the injected medium will pass to the other side.

Monochorionic placentas require more detailed examination. The vessels fanning out from either side towards the intermediate territory should be closely inspected. Normally the arteries and veins accompany each other but if an unaccompanied artery from one side approaches an unaccompanied vein from the opposite side, then there is probably an artery–capillary–vein (A–C–V) communication through the deep circulation. This should be confirmed by injection with a watery medium into the artery or vein, having first ligated the vessel proximal to the injection site. It is necessary to maintain a firm injection force for a minute or so. The medium will first fill the injected vessel and then, after a distinct interval, it will reappear in the vessel of the opposite side (Fig. 60.4). Some monochorionic placentas have two or three A–C–V anastomoses; in others none are demonstrable.

Surface communications are more obvious. They show direct continuity between arteries, or less commonly veins, of the two sides (A–A and V–V). Again they may be multiple or absent; some are very fine, others have a wide calibre throughout. Care must be taken not to miss anas-

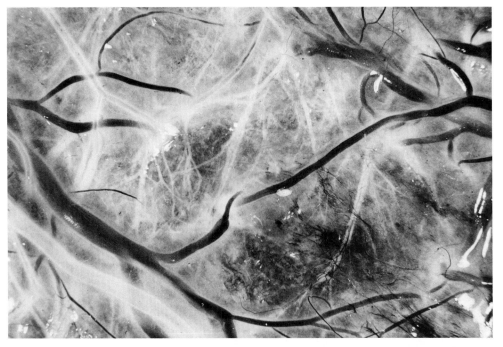

Fig. 60.4 An artery–capillary–vein anastomosis. The artery on the right has been injected with Indian ink and lies superficial to a vein. The ink has reappeared in a vein on the left which is crossed by an artery. The anastomosis is towards the centre where the two vessels approximate.

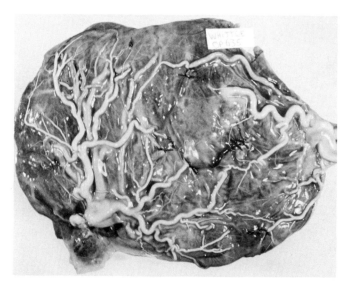

Fig. 60.5   Three artery–artery anastomoses shown by barium injection.

tomoses which course through the membranes adjacent to the margin of the placentas. These communications are best demonstrated by the injection of a thicker medium which does not pass through capillaries (Fig. 60.5). A solution of barium sulphate in gelatin, suitably coloured for arteries and veins, is useful (see Appendix).

In a busy pathology service that receives twin placentas frequently, adequate injection studies can be performed with a 50 cc syringe and air as the injected medium using needle sizes appropriate to the vessel diameters (Baldwin, 1993). The injection is made close to the suspected site of anastomosis, with back flow blocked by forceps. Careful documentation of the details of any anastomosis identified must be part of the written report, supplemented by a drawing if the relationships are complex. This information may be essential to explain untoward outcomes of mono-chorionic twins, especially if there was prenatal inter-vention in cases of twin transfusion (Baldwin, 1993).

The size of the placentas is best estimated by weight as surface area does not allow for variation in thickness. The placentas are weighed fresh and for the separate placentas nothing further is required. The dichorionic fused placen-tas should be divided along the junctional zone with a knife and the two parts weighed again. It is important to recognize that the junctional zone may not correspond to the line of the septum. This division and re-weighing is most conveniently done after fixation of the injected pla-centas: the junctional zone is indicated by the distribution of the injected media. The monochorionic placentas are divided and re-weighed in the same manner, the division passing through the middle of any common territory as defined by A–C–V anastomoses.

Twin placentas are liable to show the same range of pathological changes as singletons, and these should be

looked for and recorded. Some are particularly relevant to twins. For example, amnion nodosum is seen in the donor of a twin-transfusion syndrome and this should be borne in mind during the initial examination before stripping the membranes. Similarly, meconium staining may be seen and this should correspond with clinical observations and may serve as an extra check on the identification of the cords. The numbers of arteries in the cords should be noted as one is often absent in acardiac twins. It is also important to note the macroscopic degree of engorgement of the two placentas and to take a block prior to injections to check this microscopically.

TWIN-TRANSFUSION SYNDROME

The twin-transfusion syndrome occurs when there is un-balanced blood flow across intertwin placental chorionic vascular anastomoses. About a third of monochorionic placentas with intertwin anastomoses will have features of twin-transfusion syndrome (Boyd & Hamilton, 1970; Galea et al, 1982). These can occur acutely or chronically, or in combination.

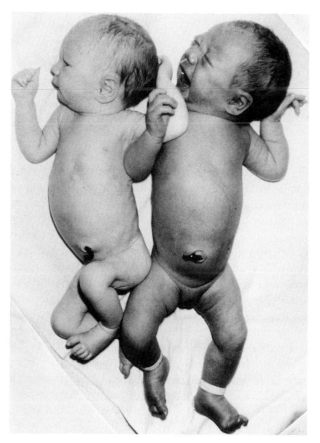

Fig. 60.6   Twin-transfusion syndrome. The larger twin is still more plethoric after exchange transfusions. At birth: twin I 3.6 kg, Hb 152%; twin II 2.2 kg, Hb 92%.

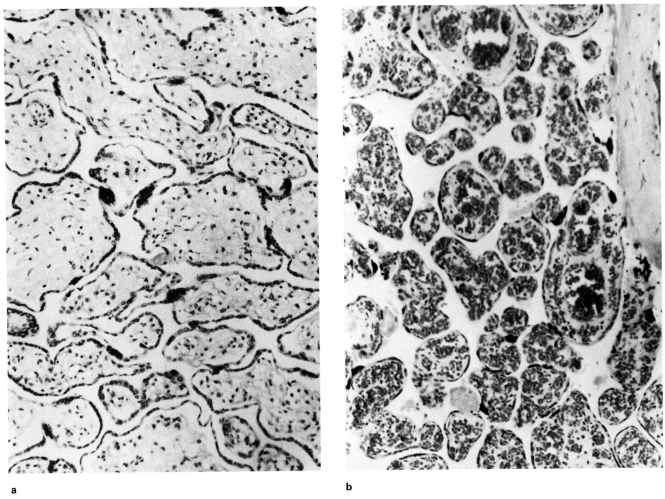

a   b

Fig. 60.7   Twin-transfusion syndrome. The donor placenta (**a**) has large villi like those in erythroblastosis. Those of the recipient (**b**) are intensely engorged. Hb at birth 67% and 170%.

The commonest pattern is a chronic imbalance resulting in a small, pale, anaemic donor twin with oligohydramnios, and a large, plethoric, polycythaemic recipient twin with polyhydramnios. This type of transfusion syndrome is more likely to occur when there are one or more A–C–V communications which are not accompanied by A–A or V–V anastomoses. Such associated communications would tend to compensate for the otherwise one-way transfer of blood. The syndrome varies in degree and mild cases may be undetected. Moderately affected twins require prompt attention at birth if they are to survive. More severely affected fetuses are often stillborn, or one or both may die in utero in early to mid pregnancy, and this syndrome is an important cause of the increased mortality of monochorionic monozygotic twins (Benirschke & Kim, 1973). The discordant growth, colour, and red cell volume values are evident in living neonates with a chronic transfusion syndrome (Fig. 60.6). The associated placenta will be monochorionic with appropriate vascular anastomoses, and often differential villous morphology

(Fig. 60.7). It is important to note that not all twins of different size or colour have suffered from a transfusion syndrome. Marked differences in size are quite common even when the placentas are separate and there is no haematological abnormality to suggest a transfusion effect (Fig. 60.8). On the other hand, a pair of twins may show marked differences of colour when one of them has lost blood into a retroplacental haematoma for example, or when there have been differences in the handling of the babies and clamping of the cord at delivery (Fig. 60.9).

The findings at necropsy of twins with chronic twin transfusion include the growth and colour differentials, with parallal changes in viscera. Donor organs are smaller and recipient organs are heavier than expected for fetal age and often fetal size. The greatest difference is in heart weights (Fig. 60.10), up to a factor of four between the twins, and this discrepancy may be the first identifiable feature of chronic transfusion (Boyd & Hamilton, 1970; Barr & Pridjian, 1991). A number of additional visceral lesions have been reported (Baldwin, 1993) including foci

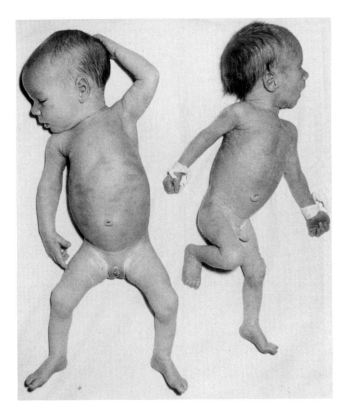

a

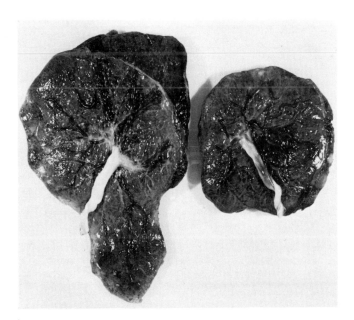

b

Fig. 60.8 **a** Unequal twins with **b** unequal placentas. Twin I, male, 1.7 kg, placenta 265 g; twin II, female, 3.1 kg, placenta 365 g.

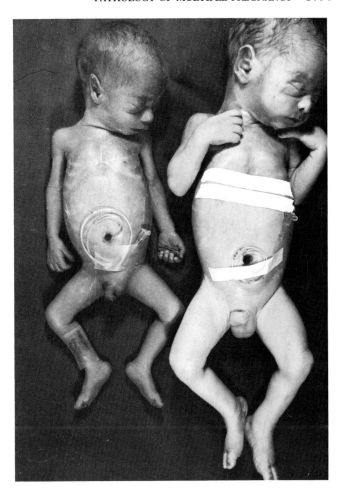

Fig. 60.9 Unequal twins of different colour. Twin I, male, 0.96 kg, died at four days with congenital heart disease; twin II, male, 1.8 kg, died at two days with hyaline membrane disease. The placenta was dichorionic.

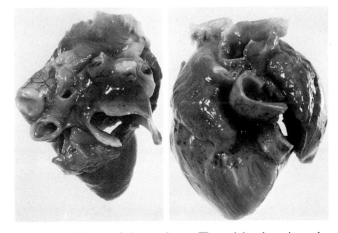

Fig. 60.10 Twin-transfusion syndrome. The recipient heart is much the larger. Twin I died at one hour, heart weight 13 g; twin II died at 11 days, heart weight 7 g.

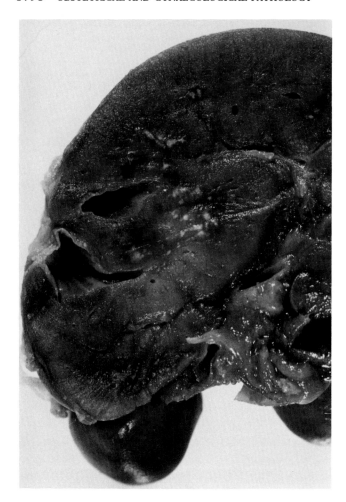

Fig. 60.11 Twin-transfusion syndrome. Foci of calcification on the cut surface of the liver of the recipient twin. Same case as Fig. 60.10.

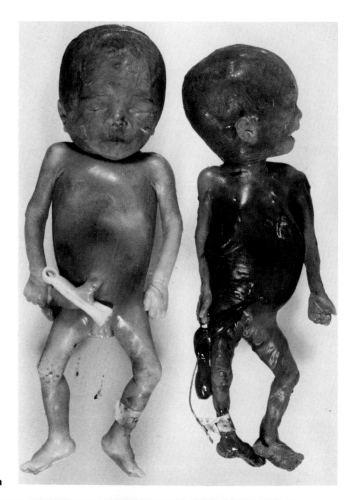

a

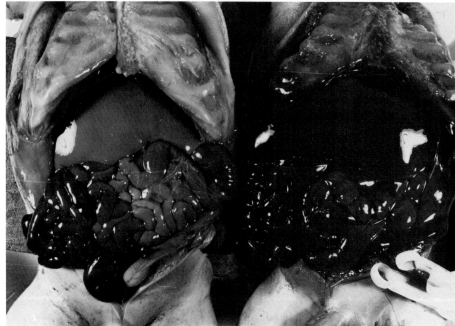

b

Fig. 60.12 Twin transfusion following intrauterine death. **a** Twin I, 662 g, pale, early maceration; twin II, 390 g, plethoric, moderately macerated. Spontaneous abortion at 20 weeks. **b** Internal appearances: twin I, pale, 2071 g; twin II, plethoric, 1891 g.

of necrosis, haemorrhage, fibrosis, haemosiderin, calcification (Fig. 60.11) and erythroblastosis in the donor.

Surface anastomoses may be responsible for an acute transfusion syndrome. It is strange that this is seldom detected clinically in spite of the common occurrence of wide surface anastomoses. Here there is no significant difference in the size of the twins to indicate a chronic undernutrition of the donor but there is a similar difference in colour. This is demonstrably due to an acute transfusion during labour. The cord bloods show no significant differences in the haematocrit, red cell count or haemoglobin level but examination after a few hours will show striking anaemia of the donor and hyperaemia of the recipient. Such infants may show cardiorespiratory distress at birth and require urgent correction of the blood volume.

An acute transfusion may occur as a complication of chronic transfusion, when there is intrauterine death of the donor, if the vascular anatomy is appropriate (Bendon & Siddigi, 1989). This can lead to a somewhat confusing presentation with the larger twin pale and the smaller twin plethoric (Fig. 60.12). In one series, 45% of autopsy cases of chronic transfusion were interpreted as having been complicated by a terminal reversed acute transfusion (Baldwin, 1993).

Much has been written about the potential complications resulting from the presence of intertwin anastomoses when one twin dies in utero. The survivor has been considered to be at risk for ischaemic complications, most importantly of the brain, with permanent impairment. Coagulation-inducing substances from the dead twin across the anastomoses have been incriminated, but concordant shock with death of one twin and a damaged survivor seems more likely (Norman, 1982).

FETAL GROWTH

As discussed above, there are usually marked differences in fetal growth as a result of the classic twin-transfusion syndrome. This is presumably due to a chronic state of hypoxaemia and undernutrition of the donor whilst the opposite applied to the recipient.

The effects of transfusion are excluded when dichorionic twins are considered but these also often show marked differences in size. It is possible that some such differences may be attributable to different genetic constitutions, but this possible effect is eliminated if monozygotic dichorionic twins are considered. There are often significant differences in size of monozygotic dichorionic twins, and it is reasonable to attribute such differences to local factors affecting the blood supply of the placenta, i.e. an environmental as opposed to a genetic effect. A consecutive sample of the Birmingham twins was examined with this in mind (Cameron, 1980). The sample consisted of 100 dichorionic dizygotic pairs and 100 dichorionic

Table 60.2 Analysis of 200 dichorionic placentas (1976–1979). In 31 of 47 unequal monochorionic placentas the smaller twin had the smaller placenta. There were similar findings in the dichorionic placentas (30 of 44).

	Monozygotic	Dizygotic
Total	100	100
Unequal placentas	47	44
Unequal related twins	31	30

monozygotic pairs (Table 60.2). A similar number of both sets (44 and 47) had placentas of significantly different size (greater than 10% difference). A similar number (30 and 31) of both sets showed a positive correlation with the birth weights (more than 10% difference).

This was taken to imply that the majority of twins of different size are different because they have larger placentas and are therefore better nourished. In the sizeable minority showing no such positive correlation, differences in the placental size may affect the blood supply to the placenta. A few cases of apparent discrepancy may possibly have been due to incorrect labelling of the cords but this is unlikely.

In addition to discordant placental size, other placental findings are important to unequal fetal growth. Developmental anomalies of placentation, especially anomalies of the umbilical cord vessels or insertion, and unilateral placental parenchymal disease are important in some cases. This is another reason why accurate identification of the cords at the time of delivery, and clinico-pathological correlation of the findings in each twin is essential (Boyd & Hamilton, 1970; Bleker et al, 1988; Baldwin, 1993).

Growth impairment and discordant growth is commoner with twins than singletons, and has a major impact on survival (O'Brien et al, 1986; Guaschino et al, 1987). The recovery potential probably relates to the degree and cause of growth impairment as reported follow-up studies provide conflicting results (Wilson, 1979; Altschuler, 1982; Ylitalo et al, 1988).

ACARDIAC MALFORMATIONS

Acardiac fetuses occur in about 1:500 twin deliveries, and although there are basic similarities of form, the anatomical details are infinitely varied (Potter & Craig, 1975; Sato et al, 1984). The twins are monochorionic and monozygotic and the co-twin is usually not malformed (Fig. 60.13). The affected twin may consist of an amorphous mass with thick myxoematous skin but usually there is a vertebral axis with some attempt at limb formation (Fig. 60.14). The lower half of the body is better developed than the upper. There is usually no proper head but there may be rudimentary facial features. Internally, there is usually a poorly developed base of skull, the heart is either absent or rudimentary and the viscera may be partly represented.

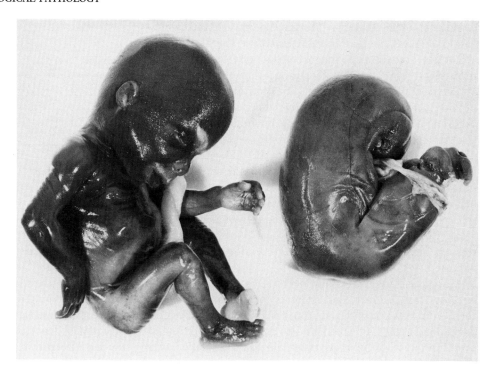

Fig. 60.13 Acardiac twin with normal co-twin. Spontaneous abortion at 20 weeks.

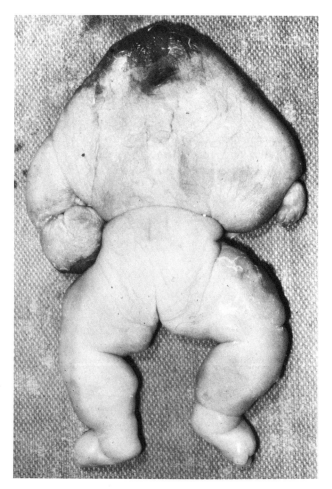

Fig. 60.14 Acardiac twin. There is no head and the upper limbs are poorly formed. The skin shows myxoematous thickening.

Although the form of the abnormal twin is highly variable, the one common feature in all cases is that it has no placental circulation of its own. The development of the abnormal twin is severely disturbed in early embryogenesis, and it is able to survive only by anastomosing its umbilical vessels to umbilical or chorionic vessels of its normal co-twin. This direct artery to artery and vein to vein anastomosis causes a reversal of blood flow in the anomalous twin. This twin-reversed arterial perfusion (TRAP) leads to additional degenerative lesions in the abnormally perfused twin (van Allen et al, 1983). Although the perfusing or pump twin is usually developmentally normal, it is at risk for high output cardiac failure.

FETUS PAPYRACEOUS

Death in utero usually results in a macerated fetus with much bloody fluid in the serous cavities. When there is intrauterine death of one of a pair of twins there are two possibilities. If there are placental anastomoses then the live twin may bleed into the dead twin; this may be fatal and constitute an acute post mortem twin-transfusion syndrome.

If there are no placental anastomoses, then the pregnancy is likely to continue. During this further time in utero, the body fluids and amniotic fluid of the dead twin will be resorbed, and the fetus becomes compressed by the surviving co-twin. The dead twin's portion of the placentation delivered with the survivor consists of a firm, pale and sclerotic mass with avascular villi embedded in fibrin. It may be present as a separate mass or residual

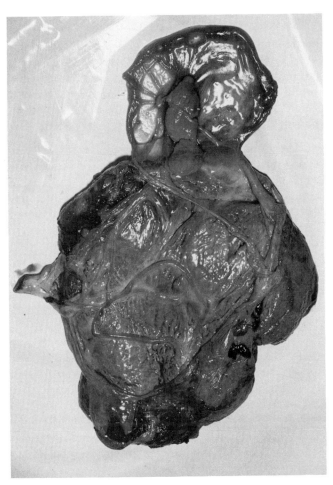

Fig. 60.15 Fetus papyraceous. An unsuspected finding in the placenta of an apparent singleton.

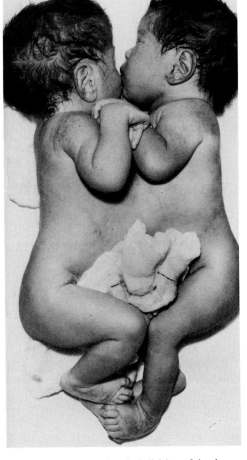

Fig. 60.16 Conjoined twins. Surgical division of the thoracopagus was unsuccessful. The twins shared a common liver and both had severe cardiovascular malformations.

portion of a single disc, depending on the original pattern of placentation (Potter & Craig, 1975). There may have been no clinical suggestion of the death of a twin, and the fetal remnant may be noticed first by the pathologist on careful examination of an apparently singleton placenta (Fig. 60.15). For this reason, the reported incidence of 1:12 000 live births (Livnat et al, 1978) is likely to be an underestimate.

The cause of death of these fetuses that will become papyraceous is not known in most cases, although anomalous insertions of the umbilical cord are more frequent and they are often described as growth retarded (Kindred, 1944; Desgranges et al, 1982).

CONJOINED TWINS

Conjoined twins are malformations initiated in the germinal disc after the formation of the amniotic cavity. Some may arise from partial fusion of otherwise separate discs, others are due to incomplete fission of a single disc. The twins may be united in either the sagittal plane with the duplicated parts facing in the same direction or in the coronal plane with the twins facing either towards or away from each other (Fig. 60.16). The former range from an apparent singleton with severe hypertelorism to a double-headed monster with duplication of the upper half of the trunk; the two components are usually symmetrical. Fusion in the coronal plane varies similarly in degree. The commonest forms are the face-to-face twins joined in the sternal region (thoracopagus) or umbilical area (xiphopagus) and the back-to-back twins joined in the lumbo-sacral regions (pygopagus); here there may be a marked degree of asymmetry, as in the so-called parasitic twin attached to the lumbar region (Fig. 60.17). The parasitic twin usually has a recognizable limb or digit and is to be distinguished from the sacro-coccygeal teratoma. The range of abnormalities is well illustrated by Potter & Craig (1975).

Conjoined twins usually show extensive sharing of common viscera and only the minor degree of thoracopa-

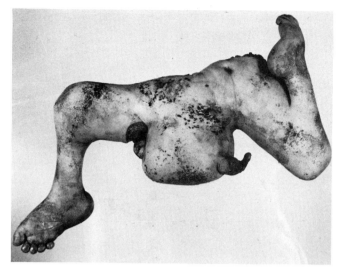

Fig. 60.17 Conjoined twin. A 'parasitic fetus' successfully removed from the lumbo-sarcal region of a well-formed co-twin.

gus/xiphopagus and the parasitic twins are amenable to successful surgical separation (Filler, 1986). The vast majority of conjoined twins are female (Benirschke et al, 1978).

CHIMERISM

The co-existence of two different cell lines in one individual may be due to mosaicism or chimerism. The former is due to changes in some cells of the zygote after fertilization; these may be gene mutations or chromosomal abnormalities resulting from non-disjunction (Kastern & Kryspin-Sorensen, 1988; Cote & Gyftodimou, 1991). In chimerism the two (or more) cell lines are derived from two different zygotes.

There is currently much interest in the field of experimental chimerism by cell transfer of embryos derived from agricultural stock but the relevance of chimerism to human twins is largely confined to abnormalities found in routine blood grouping (Benirschke & Kaufmann, 1990). Blood chimeras must arise through vascular anastomoses between the twins at some point of their development. Adequately documented anastomoses between twins who are each in their own chorionic sac are extremely rare, implying that blood chimeras must be monovular twins with a single chorion, possibly due to dispermic monovular twinning. Whole body chimerism may be detected if there is a mixture of sex chromosomes with accompanying gonadal abnormality (Benirschke et al, 1972). The origin of whole body chimerism is not understood but in some cases may result from zygote fusion after fertilization of eggs from a binovular follicle (Benirschke, 1972).

MORTALITY IN TWINS

The perinatal mortality rate in twins is about four times that in singletons, but the reported rates of 14–17% perinatal mortality of twins overall do not consider early fetal mortality (Benirschke & Kim, 1973). The results of several surveys are reviewed by Baldwin (1993) with the following highlights:

1. Ultrasound studies suggest that up to 78% of twins diagnosed in the first trimester are delivered as singletons (Landy et al, 1986).

2. Embryonic deaths and macerated fetuses often have lethal malformations, and anomalies of monochorionic monozygotic twinning, including twin-transfusion syndrome, are important causes of fetal death of both twins at all stages of pregnancy.

3. Ascending infection (chorioamnionitis) is an important cause of fresh stillbirth, and complications of prematurity are the main cause of perinatal and later neonatal mortality.

4. Up to one-quarter of perinatal twin deaths are attributed to problems associated with monozygosity, with mortality rates of monozygotic twins up to three times the rate of singletons (Myrianthopoulos, 1975; Leroy, 1976). Most of this monozygotic mortality is due to complications of monochorionic placentation and related anomalies — cord entanglements with monoamniotic twins, disturbances of twinning, and intertwin vascular anastomoses (Benirschke, 1961).

5. The perinatal mortality of monoamniotic twins is 5–6 times as high as that of diamniotic twins, not only because of increased prematurity but also because of major malformations such as conjoined twins and cord entanglements (Lumme & Saarikoski, 1986). The occurrence and true clinical significance of cord entanglements is probably less than generally assumed: the reported occurrence ranges from 5.5% (Wharton et al, 1968) to 66% (Benirschke, 1961) with mortality rates of 42% (Baldwin, 1993) to 100% of affected twin sets (Wharton et al, 1968).

6. Infancy and childhood mortality of twins is greater for sets with complications of prematurity or severe malformations. The sudden unexpected infant death rate in twins is approximately twice that in singletons (Kleinman et al, 1991); second-born twins are at four times the risk of first-born twins (Getts, 1981), but the concordance rate is no greater in monozygotic twins than that in dizygotic twins (Krauss & Borhani, 1972; Peterson et al, 1980).

RESEARCH POTENTIAL OF TWINS

The 'nature' versus 'nurture' concept as the basis for studies of twins has been applied to everything from attributes of personality to the incidence of cancer. While some

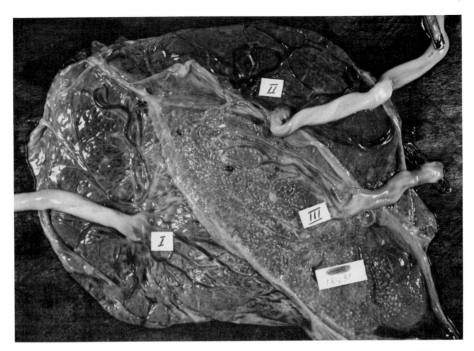

Fig. 60.18 Triplet placenta. There are three chorionic sacs and the blood groups were different. Placenta III shows amnion nodosum due to Potter's syndrome. There were no placental anastomoses.

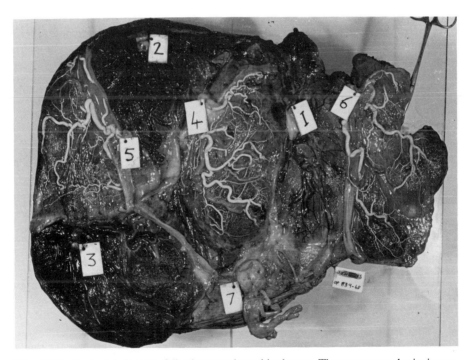

Fig. 60.19 Septuplet placenta, following gonadotrophin therapy. There are seven chorionic sacs with a fetus papyraceus in sac 7. Cords I, II and III have been injected with Indian ink and cords IV, V and VI with barium. There are no anastomoses. The six liveborn babies were shown to be different from each other by a combination of blood groups, enzyme types and sex. (Reproduced by kind permission from the Journal of Obstetrics and Gynaecology of the British Commonwealth 1969; 76: 692.)

insights have been gained, there are aspects to many of these studies that impair the value of their interpretations and represent constraints for future studies. These problems include inadequate information on zygosity and postzygotic genetic variations, loss of data due to increased monozygotic mortality, failure to consider differential 'environmental' influences in utero due to placental anatomy in particular and to the effects of labour and delivery (Emery, 1976; Baldwin, 1993). Increased rates of malformations are observed in twins, but this appears to be due to an excess load in monozygotic twins, although the importance of chorionicity is rarely assessed (Cameron et al, 1983). Many malformations are of low concordance, even in monozygotic twins, but without details of placentation and in-depth genetic studies it is difficult to assess the significance of this observation to concepts of pathogenesis of the anomalies as they relate to twins (Edwards, 1968; Hay & Wehrung, 1970; Baldwin, 1993). Adequate documentation of the placenta/placentas of twins must be the cornerstone of any study of the incidence of morbidity in twins.

The placenta is the only fetal organ which is freely available for investigation and the application of enzyme chemistry to placental tissue of twins gave early impetus to linkage studies and chromosome mapping (Corney & Robson, 1975). Edwards (1968) has also drawn attention to the potential for immunological research offered by the fused dichorionic dizygotic placenta in particular. Here there is close apposition not only of fetal and maternal tissues but also of unlike fetal tissues.

TRIPLET OR HIGHER MULTIPLE PREGNANCY

Multiple pregnancy may be monozygous or multizygous (Fig. 60.18). There may also be a combination of monozygous twins with a third or fourth fetus derived from separate ova. Those pregnancies that follow gonadotrophin or clomiphene therapy are usually multizygous. The same principles apply to the determination of zygosity and the examination of the placenta. The perinatal morbidity and mortality increases with the higher multiples, largely due to the risks of prematurity. Cameron et al (1969) described the findings in a septuplet pregnancy and pleaded for more adequate examination of the placenta in multiple pregnancy (Fig. 60.19). The newer DNA technology can be applied to clarify the patterns of higher multiple pregnancy.

APPENDIX

Injection medium for surface anastomoses

150 ml micropaque
 5 g gelatin
50 ml water
10 ml Tartrazine or Prussian Blue

Mix the micropaque and dye, then add the gelatin dissolved in warm water and mix well.

REFERENCES

Altshuler G 1982 Developmental aspects of twins, twinning and chimerism. In: Rosenberg H S, Bernstein J (eds) Perspectives in pediatric pathology. Masson, New York, ch 4.

Azuma C, Kamiura S, Nobunaga T et al 1989 Zygosity determination of multiple pregnancy by deoxyribonucleic acid fingerprints. American Journal of Obstetrics and Gynecology 160: 734–736.

Baldwin V J 1993 Pathology of multiple pregnancy. Springer-Verlag, New York.

Barr M, Pridjian G 1991 Growth effects in twins: clinical implications. Teratology (abstract) 43: 424.

Bendon R W, Siddigi T 1989 Clinical pathology conference: acute twin-to-twin in utero transfusion. Pediatric Pathology 9: 591–598.

Benirschke K 1961 Twin placenta in perinatal mortality. New York State Journal of Medicine 61: 1499–1508.

Benirschke K 1972 Origin and significance of twinning. Clinical Obstetrics and Gynecology 15: 220–235.

Benirschke K, Driscoll S G 1967 The pathology of the human placenta. Springer-Verlag, Berlin.

Benirschke K, Kaufmann P 1990 Pathology of the human placenta, 2nd edn. Springer-Verlag, New York.

Benirschke K, Kim C K 1973 Multiple pregnancy. New England Journal of Medicine 288: 1276–1284 and 1329–1336.

Benirschke K, Naftolin F, Gittes R, Khudr G, Yen S S C, Allen F H 1972 True hermaphroditism and chimerism. American Journal of Obstetrics and Gynecology 113: 449–458.

Benirschke K, Temple W W, Bloor C M 1978 Conjoined twins: nosology and congenital malformations. Birth Defects 14(6A): 179.

Bieber F R, Nance W E, Morton C C et al 1981 Genetic studies of an acardiac monster: evidence of polar body twinning in man. Science 213: 775–777.

Bleker O P, Oosting J, Hemrika D J 1988 On the cause of retardation of fetal growth in multiple gestations. Acta Geneticae Medicae Gemellologiae 37: 41–46.

Boklage C E 1987 Twinning, nonrighthandedness, and fusion malformations: evidence for heritable causal elements held in common. American Journal of Medical Genetics 28: 67–84.

Boyd J D, Hamilton W J 1970 The human placenta. Heffer, Cambridge.

Cameron A H 1968 The Birmingham twin survey. Proceedings of the Royal Society of Medicine 61: 229–234.

Cameron A H 1980 Unpublished observations.

Cameron A H, Robson E B, Wade-Evans T, Wingham J 1969 Septuplet conception: placental and zygosity studies. Journal of Obstetrics and Gynaecology of the British Commonwealth 76: 692–698.

Cameron A H, Edwards J H, Derom R, Thiery M, Bolaert R 1983 The value of twin surveys in the study of malformations. European Journal of Obstetrics, Gynecology and Reproductive Biology 14: 347–356.

Corney G, Robson E B 1975 Types of twinning and determination of zygosity. In: MacGillivray I, Nylander P P S, Corney G (eds) Human multiple reproduction. Saunders, London.

Cote G B, Gyftodimou J 1991 Twinning and mitotic-crossing over: some possibilities and their implications. American Journal of Human Genetics 49: 120–130.

Dallpiccola B, Stomeo C, Ferranti G, Di Lecce A, Purpura M 1985 Discordant sex in one of three monozygotic triplets. Journal of Medical Genetics 22: 6–11.

Das Chaddhuri A B 1991 Efficient sequential search of genetic systems for diagnosis of twin zygosity. Acta Geneticae Medicae Gemellologiae 40: 159–164.

Desgranges M F, DeMuylder X, Moutquin J M, Lazaro-Lopez F, Leduc B 1982 Perinatal profile of twin pregnancies: a retrospective review of 11 years (1969–1979) at Hopital Notre Dame Montreal, Canada. Acta Geneticae Medicae Gemellologiae 31: 157–163.

Edwards J H 1968 The value of twins in genetic studies. Proceedings of the Royal Society of Medicine 61: 227–229.

Emery A E H (ed) 1976 Twin studies, their use and limitations. In: Methodology in medical genetics. Churchill Livingstone, Edinburgh, ch 7.

Filler R M 1986 Conjoined twins and their separation. Seminars in Perinatology 10: 82–91.

Fisher R A, Sheppard D M, Lawler S D 1982 Twin pregnancy with complete hydatidiform mole (46,XX) and fetus (46,XY): genetic origin proved by analysis of chromosome polymorphism. British Medical Journal 284: 1218–1220.

Fox H 1978 Pathology of the placenta. WB Saunders, London.

Galea P, Scott J M, Goel K M 1982 Feto-fetal transfusion syndrome. Archives of Diseases in Childhood 57: 781–794.

Getts A 1981 SIDS: increased risk for second born twins. American Journal of Public Health 71: 317–318.

Guaschino S, Spinillo A, Stola E, Pesando P C 1987 Growth retardation, size at birth, and perinatal mortality in twin pregnancy. International Journal of Gynaecology and Obstetrics 25: 399–403.

Hay S, Wehrung D A 1970 Congenital malformations in twins. American Journal of Human Genetics 22: 662–678.

Hill A V S, Jeffreys A J 1985 Use of mini-satellite DNA probes for determination of twin zygosity at birth. Lancet 2: 1394–1395.

Juberg R C, Stallard R, Straughen W J, Avotri K J, Washington J W 1981 Clinicopathological conference: a newborn monozygotic twin with abnormal facial appearance and respiratory insufficiency. American Journal of Medical Genetics 10: 193–200.

Kastern W, Kryspin-Sorensen I 1988 Penetrance and low concordance in monozygotic twins in disease: are they the results of alterations in somatic genomes? Molecular Reproduction and Development 1: 63–75.

Kindred J E 1944 Twin pregnancies with one blighted. American Journal of Obstetrics and Gynecology 48: 642–682.

Kleinman J C, Fowler M G, Kessel S S 1991 Comparison of infant mortality among twins and singletons: United States 1960 and 1983. American Journal of Epidemiology 133: 133–143.

Kovacs B, Shahbahrami B, Platt L D, Comings D E 1988 Molecular prenatal determination of twin zygosity. Obstetrics and Gynecology 72: 954–956.

Kraus J F, Borhani N C 1972 Post-neonatal sudden unexplained death in California: a cohort study. American Journal of Epidemiology 95: 497–510.

Landy H J, Weiner S, Corson S L, Batzer F R, Bolognese R J 1986 The "vanishing twin"; ultrasonic assessment of fetal disappearance in the first trimester. American Journal of Obstetrics and Gynecology 155: 14–19.

Leroy F 1976 Major fetal hazards in multiple pregnancy. Acta Geneticae Medicae Gemellologiae 25: 299–306.

Lumme R H, Saarikoski S V 1986 Monoamniotic twin pregnancy. Acta Geneticae Medicae et Gemellologiae 35: 99–105.

Livnat E J, Burd L, Cadkin A, Keh P, Ward A B 1978 Fetus papyraceus in twin pregnancy. Obstetrics and Gynecology 51 supplement 1: 41s–45s.

Myrianthopoulos N C 1975 Congenital malformations in twins: epidemiologic survey. Birth defects. Original Articles Series XI(8): 1–39.

Norman M G 1982 Mechanisms of brain damage in twins. Canadian Journal of Neurological Sciences 9: 339–344.

O'Brien W F, Knuppel R A, Scerbo J C, Rattan P K 1986 Birth weight in twins: an analysis of discordancy and growth retardation. Obstetrics and Gynecology 67: 483–486.

Perlman E J, Stetten G, Tuck-Muller C M, Farber R A, Neuman W L, Blakemore K J, Hutchins G M 1990 Sexual discordance in monozygotic twins. American Journal of Medical Genetics 37: 551–557.

Peterson D R, Chinn N M, Fisher L D 1980 The sudden infant death syndrome: repetition in families. Journal of Pediatrics 97: 265–267.

Potter E L, Craig J M 1975 Pathology of the fetus and the infant. Year Book Medical Publishers, Chicago.

Reed T, Uchida I A, Norton J A, Christian J C 1978 Comparisons of dermatoglyphic patterns in monochorionic and dichorionic monozygotic twins. American Journal of Human Genetics 30: 383–391.

Sato T, Kaneko K, Konuma S, Sato I, Tamada T 1984 Acardiac anomalies: review of 88 cases in Japan. Asia-Oceana Journal of Obstetrics and Gynecology 10: 45–52.

Shanklin D R, Perrin E V D K 1984 Multiple gestation. In: Perrin E V D K (ed) Pathology of the placenta. Churchill-Livingstone, New York, ch 7.

Smith S M, Penrose L S 1955 Monozygotic and dizygotic twin diagnosis. Annals of Human Genetics London 19: 273–289.

Strong S J, Corney G 1967 The placenta in twin pregnancy. Pergamon Press, Oxford.

Van Allen M I, Smith D W, Shepard T H 1983 Twin reversed arterial perfusion (TRAP) sequence: a study of 14 twin pregnancies with acardius. Seminars in Perinatology 7: 285–293.

Wharton B, Edwards J H, Cameron A H 1968 Mono-amniotic twins. Journal of Obstetrics and Gynaecology of the British Commonwealth 75: 158–163.

Wilson R S 1979 Twin growth: initial defect, recovery, and trends in concordance from birth to nine years. Annals of Human Biology 6: 205–220.

Ylitalo V, Kero P, Erkkola R 1988 Neurological outcome of twins dissimilar in size at birth. Early Human Development 17: 245–255.

61. Immunopathology of pregnancy

Judith N. Bulmer   Peter M. Johnson

INTRODUCTION

The human fetus inherits 'transplantation' antigens from its father and thus forms a partial allograft with its mother. Nevertheless, in normal circumstances the feto-placental unit is able to survive within the uterus to full term with no apparent detrimental effect to either mother or fetus. The immunobiological system which has evolved to allow successful outbred reproduction in humans and other animal species is still not fully understood. However, evidence is accumulating that deficiencies in the immunological inter-relationships between mother and fetus which underpin normal pregnancy may play a rôle in the pathogenesis of a range of pregnancy disorders.

IMMUNOBIOLOGY OF TROPHOBLAST

Introduction

Human placentation is haemochorial in type with close apposition between maternal and fetal circulations. The chorionic villi forming the placenta are covered by an inner cytotrophoblast and an outer syncytiotrophoblast layer which forms an extensive fetal tissue interface with potentially immunocompetent leucocytes in maternal blood circulating in the intervillous space. An additional fundamental feature of normal human pregnancy is invasion of uterine decidua, myometrium and arteries by 'extravillous' trophoblast. During the first few weeks of pregnancy columns of cytotrophoblast cells proliferate from the chorionic villi and spread laterally to form the cytotrophoblast shell from which extravillous cytotrophoblast invades maternal uterine tissues. Cytotrophoblast migrates up uterine spiral arteries in two waves, reaching the terminal segments of radial arteries in the myometrium at 16–20 weeks' gestation (Pijnenborg et al, 1980); thus, arterial invasion by 'endovascular' trophoblast mediates the structural alterations required to accommodate the tenfold increase in uterine blood supply required to nourish the feto-placental unit. Mononuclear 'interstitial' trophoblast infiltrates through decidua and myometrium, some cells fusing to form multinucleate syncytial giant cells (Boyd & Hamilton, 1970; Pijnenborg et al, 1980). Extraembryonic fetal trophoblast cells thus have direct contact with maternal blood and cells within the uterus.

Invasion of maternal uterine tissues by fetal trophoblast is essential for normal feto-placental development and is tightly controlled, terminating in the inner third of the myometrium. Deficient trophoblast invasion has been noted in pre-eclampsia, intrauterine growth retardation and spontaneous abortion, whilst abnormally deep invasion is a feature of placenta accreta (Robertson et al, 1986; Bulmer, 1992). The control of trophoblast proliferation, differentiation and invasive potential may be inherent properties of trophoblast or regulated by maternal decidua, both of which suggest important rôles for characteristic molecules (antigens) expressed by villous and extravillous trophoblast populations.

Because of the paucity of material available for study there have been comparatively few immunological studies of the human blastocyst and the implantation process, although in vitro models of implantation are being developed. However, to date, most studies of the immunobiology of human pregnancy have focused on the postimplantation period when both normal and pathological tissues are available for investigation.

Expression of HLA antigens by villous trophoblast

Human leucocyte antigens (HLA), part of the major histocompatibility complex (MHC), are cell surface glycoprotein molecules which are of fundamental importance in presenting antigens to be recognized by T lymphocytes; they are highly polymorphic (alloantigenic) and also serve as the focus of histoincompatible transplantation rejection responses. Both villous syncytiotrophoblast and extravillous trophoblast are in direct contact with maternal immune cells in blood and decidua (see below) and have adapted various strategies to facilitate evasion of recognition and cytotoxic attack by the maternal immune

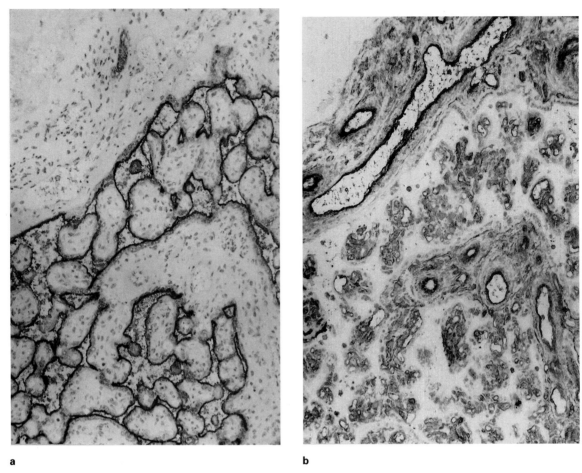

a   b

Fig. 61.1 Serial sections of term placenta labelled for: **a** placental alkaline phosphatase; and **b** class I MHC molecules. Villous trophoblast is reactive for PLAP but negative for class I MHC molecules while the villous stroma is class I MHC-positive. × 100.

system. Villous syncytiotrophoblast and cytotrophoblast unusually do not express any class I (HLA-A, B, C) or class II (HLA-DR, DR, DQ) MHC alloantigens (Fig. 61.1). There is also no class I or II MHC molecule expression by the human preimplantation embryo (Roberts et al, 1992). Fetal cells within the chorionic villous stroma, however, do express class I MHC antigens (representing the tissue type of the fetus) and, as gestation proceeds, increasing numbers of Hofbauer cells in the villous stroma also express class II MHC antigens (Sunderland et al, 1981; Sutton et al, 1983; Bulmer et al, 1988a). Villous trophoblast is inert to upregulation of MHC antigens by exogenous cytokines such as interferon-γ (IFNγ) (Hunt et al, 1987) and trophoblastic expression of classical MHC alloantigens appears to be regulated at the transcriptional level (Boucrat et al, 1993).

The absence of MHC antigens on villous trophoblast must play a central rôle in protecting this major and extensive fetal tissue interface from cytotoxic T cells or alloantibodies in maternal blood in the surrounding inter-villous spaces. Lack of MHC antigens also explains the well-recognized phenomenon that syncytial trophoblast

fragments can detach from the placenta, enter the venous circulation and may survive entrapped within the pulmo-nary vasculature for months, apparently without provok-ing a maternal immune response (Attwood & Park, 1961). Villous trophoblast therefore forms a complete HLA-negative fetal cell layer separating maternal immuno-competent cells in the intervillous spaces from the class I and II MHC-positive non-trophoblastic fetal cells in the villous stroma.

Expression of HLA antigens by extravillous trophoblast

Immunohistochemical studies with monoclonal antibodies (mAbs) directed against monomorphic determinants of class I MHC molecules provided the first evidence that, in contrast with villous trophoblast, extravillous trophoblast does strongly express a class I MHC antigen (Fig. 61.2). Later studies with a wider antibody panel indicated the unusual nature of this antigen compared with HLA-A and B molecules (Hsi et al, 1984; Redman et al, 1984; Wells et al, 1984). Serological, biochemical and molecular

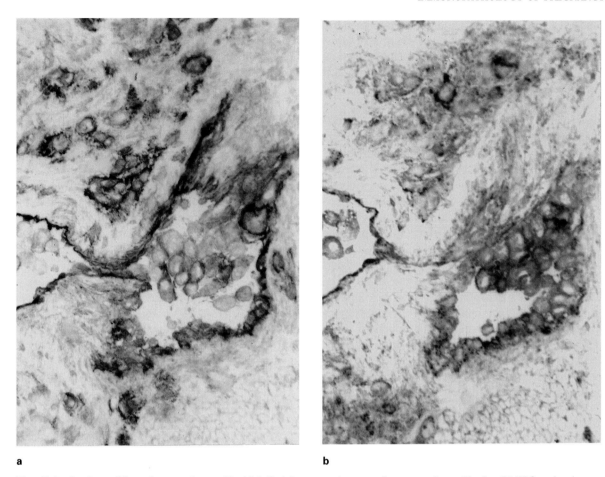

a   b

Fig. 61.2 Sections of first-trimester placental bed labelled for: **a** membrane co-factor protein; and **b** class I MHC molecules. Endovascular trophoblast express MCP and a class I MHC molecule, HLA-G. × 250.

investigations have now shown that the invasive extra-villous trophoblast cells selectively express the HLA-G non-classical class I MHC antigen and generally fail to express classical class I or II MHC antigens (Ellis et al, 1990; Kovats et al, 1990).

The HLA-G gene encodes a class I MHC 39 kD heavy chain transmembrane molecule with a truncated cytoplasmic tail, which associates with β2 microglobulin at the cell surface. It is closely homologous both structurally and genetically with other class I MHC molecules. HLA-G protein expression has not been identified on adult human tissues. HLA-G transcripts without protein expression have been reported in villous cytotrophoblast, possibly delineating preinvasive cells within the chorionic villi (Yelavarthi et al, 1991).

The selective expression of HLA-G by extravillous trophoblast suggests a specialized function in pregnancy. HLA-G might act as a fetal recognition molecule between cells in the placental bed, regulating either trophoblast invasion or immune responses by decidual leucocytes. HLA-G may mediate cell–cell adhesion via the CD8 suppressor/cytotoxic T cell molecule (Sanders et al, 1991), although CD8-positive T cells account for only a minor

population of leucocytes in decidua when most trophoblastic invasion occurs (see below). Unusual natural killer-type (NK) cells are abundant in early pregnancy decidua and it has been suggested that HLA-G could fundamentally protect the otherwise HLA-negative invasive trophoblast from maternal NK cell attack as a passive pauci-polymorphic cell surface class I MHC molecule: to date, studies with isolated decidual lymphocyte clones have given partial support to this concept (Chumbley et al, 1994; Deniz et al, 1994). Further elucidation of the rôle of HLA-G in normal pregnancy may eventually enhance understanding of pregnancy disorders associated with abnormal trophoblast invasion.

Expression of cell surface complement regulatory molecules by placental trophoblast

Complement regulatory protein molecules, decay accelerating factor (DAF; CD55), membrane co-factor protein (MCP; CD46) and CD59 (membrane attack complex inhibitory factor), are expressed by placental trophoblast throughout gestation. MCP acts as a cell surface co-factor for the enzymatic activity of factor I that inactivates C3b and C4b and is identical to cell surface antigens formerly designated as trophoblast-leucocyte cross-reactive or common (TLX) antigens (Bulmer & Johnson, 1985a; Purcell et al, 1990; Hsi et al, 1991; Holmes et al, 1992). MCP epitopes are expressed by a variety of nucleated cell types including both villous syncytio- and cytotrophoblast.

DAF also controls activation of complement component 3 (C3) by dissociation of the molecular components of C3 convertase produced by both the classical and alternative pathways of activation, as well as C4 convertase activity. DAF is expressed by villous syncytiotrophoblast and extravillous trophoblast, but not by villous cytotrophoblast (Holmes et al, 1990). The third cell surface complement regulatory protein, CD59, which is an inhibitor of the membrane attack complex, has been detected on all villous and extravillous trophoblast populations (Meri et al, 1991; Holmes et al, 1992). Expression of all three complement regulators by trophoblast is quantitively high compared with adult lymphoid cells or erythrocytes (Holmes et al, 1992). In adult tissues, complement regulators protect host cell surfaces from deposition of autologous C3b and C5b-9. Strong expression of these complement regulatory molecules by trophoblast at the maternofetal interface would fundamentally regulate any potential complement-mediated damage which could arise by maternal antibody attack or subclinical persistent complement activation consequent to haemostatic alterations due to local tissue damage and remodelling following trophoblast invasion.

Trophoblast proteinases and anti-proteinases

Proteolytic enzymes degrade extracellular matrix and basement membranes. The invasive capacity of malignant cells has been linked to increased production of metalloproteinases, lysosomal cathepsins and plasminogen activators (reviewed by Mullins & Rohrlich, 1983). The enzyme content of human trophoblast was examined initially by enzyme histochemistry (reviewed by Contractor, 1983) and later by immunohistochemistry. Alpha$_2$-macroglobulin (α_2M), which inhibits various endoproteases, binds to a surface protease on isolated syncytiotrophoblast microvillous plasma membrane (StMPM) vesicle preparations (Johnson et al, 1985). An absence of α_2M was noted in invasive hydatidiform mole and choriocarcinoma (Saksela et al, 1981); α_2M may thus play a rôle in regulating the invasive and degradative potential of trophoblast.

Both α_1-antiprotease and α_1-antichymotrypsin have been localized by immunohistochemistry to villous syncytiotrophoblast and endovascular trophoblast in normal and ectopic pregnancies but rarely in interstitial trophoblast (Braunhut et al, 1984; Earl et al, 1989). Plasminogen activator inhibitors (PAI) 1 and 2 have also been demonstrated in trophoblast both in vivo and in vitro with PAI 1 predominating in invasive cytotrophoblast (Feinberg et al,

1989). Expression of these enzymes and inhibitors may define trophoblast populations with differing proliferative and invasive potential.

Carbohydrate content of trophoblast populations

Lectins are proteins or glycoproteins derived from various biological sources which bind to carbohydrates of specific structure and configuration. Lectin histochemistry has been used to document cell surface carbohydrate alterations associated with cell transformation and differentiation and has distinguished trophoblast populations with differing proliferative and invasive potential. Binding of wheat germ agglutinin (WGA) to all trophoblast populations except the placental bed giant cells, which accumulate in the myometrium at the limit of trophoblast invasion, may reflect their decreased invasive capacity. Similarly, increased reactivity with Griffonia simplicifonica (GSII) of extravillous compared with villous trophoblast may define potentially invasive trophoblast (Lalani et al, 1987; Thrower et al, 1991). Analysis of blood group carbohydrate antigens has also defined subpopulations of villous and extravillous trophoblast (King & Loke, 1988). More sophisticated studies of carbohydrate structure may ultimately facilitate definition of factors controlling trophoblast invasion and proliferation.

Trophoblast differentiation antigens

Syncytiotrophoblast forms the major interface between maternal blood and fetal stromal and blood cells. At least fifty associated protein subunits have been identified by biochemical analysis of isolated human term placental StMPM preparations (Whyte et al, 1985). Identification of trophoblast-specific cell surface molecules is of interest for not only investigation of biological function but also their potential for prenatal diagnosis and contraceptive vaccines. Murine trophoblast-reactive mAbs have been developed by immunization with first-trimester and term StMPM vesicles and with isolated extravillous trophoblast. Using this approach, interesting trophoblast antigens have been characterized but, to date, antibodies with absolute specificity for trophoblast remain elusive (Anderson et al, 1987; Hsi & Johnson, 1992).

Throughout normal gestation, placental trophoblast cells are shed into the intervillous space and travel via the peripheral circulation to the pulmonary vasculature where they may become trapped yet persist without adverse reaction. Trophoblast-reactive antibodies have been used to detect and subsequently extract (Goodfellow & Taylor, 1982; Mueller et al, 1990) trophoblast cells from maternal peripheral venous blood with a view to their use as a minimally invasive procedure for obtaining fetal cells for prenatal diagnosis of genetic disorders. Positive selection with magnetic beads has yielded small numbers of trophoblast cells (Mueller et al, 1990) which would at present be inadequate for diagnosis of single gene recessive disorders rather than major polyploidys. Retrieval of trophoblast cells from the lower uterine segment in the first trimester of pregnancy may provide a useful alternative approach (Griffith-Jones et al, 1992; Adinolfi et al, 1993).

Oncotrophoblast antigens

Various fetal antigens are expressed also by adult tumour cells, notably alpha-fetoprotein (AFP) and carcinoembryonic antigen (CEA). Similarly, trophoblast-restricted antigens may be expressed by tumour cells but not by normal adult somatic tissues: these have been termed 'oncotrophoblast' antigens (Johnson, 1991), of which the heat-stable placental alkaline phosphatase iso-enzyme (PLAP) has been most thoroughly investigated. PLAP is expressed on the surface of villous syncytiotrophoblast (see Fig. 61.1) and some extravillous trophoblast in the second and third trimesters of pregnancy (Bulmer & Johnson, 1985a) and also by various human tumours, including ovarian and breast carcinomas and seminomas (McLaughlin et al, 1982; Sunderland et al, 1984; McDicken et al, 1985). The rôle of PLAP is unknown, although it may act as a cell surface regulator of growth and differentiation in both trophoblast and tumour cells. Although PLAP exhibits genetically-defined protein polymorphism, maternal immunity in pregnancy to paternally inherited PLAP has not been described: the continuous and initially low level of shedding of PLAP-positive syncytiotrophoblast cells and microvilli into maternal venous blood could induce immunological tolerance in the mother, as could exposure to PLAP in the seminal plasma (McLaughlin et al, 1986).

Endogenous retrovirus

Human placental syncytiotrophoblast normally expresses substantial amounts of intracellular assembled type C endogenous retroviral particles, particularly in early pregnancy (reviewed in Johnson et al, 1990). Retroviral particles have been noted in both normal and pathological placentas by electronmicroscopy, reverse transcriptase estimation, detection of antibody against retroviral protein antigens and detection of retroviral p30 antigen in syncytiotrophoblast (Kalter et al, 1973; Dalton et al, 1974; Nelson et al, 1978; Suni et al, 1984; Wahlström et al, 1984). The biological rôle of endogenous placental retrovirus is unknown: suggested normal functions include control of basic intracellular processes by retroviral proteins or LTR sequences, syncytiotrophoblast gene amplification by reverse transcriptase activity and a rôle for retroviral *env* genes in cell fusion and syncytialization (Johnson et al, 1990). Similarly, absence of endogenous retroviral sequences may be associated with pregnancy pathology such as gestational trophoblastic neoplasia.

Cell adhesion molecules

Adhesion molecules mediate cell–cell and cell–matrix interactions and play fundamental and important rôles in cell migration during embryogenesis, lymphocyte homing to specific sites and in the immune response. Varied expression of adhesion molecules may participate in regulation of the proliferative and invasive capacities of trophoblast subpopulations. One class of adhesion molecules is the integrins, which are dimeric proteins with many varied forms. Various β_1 integrins have been localized to villous and/or extravillous trophoblast with differing expression in first-trimester and term placental tissues (Korhonen et al, 1991; Damsky et al, 1992). Ligands include laminin, fibronectin and type IV collagen which can be produced by decidual cells (Aplin et al, 1988; Loke et al, 1989). Loss of $\alpha_6\beta_4$ integrin may be a marker for the invasive extravillous trophoblast populations (Aplin, 1993); and E-cadherin, a calcium-dependent intercellular adhesion molecule, is lost during the differentiation of cytotrophoblast to syncytiotrophoblast (Coutifaris et al, 1991). Differential expression of adhesion molecules and their ligands by trophoblast and decidua could play a rôle in regulating invasion by placental trophoblast into maternal uterine tissues: altered trophoblast integrin expression has been reported in pre-eclampsia (see below).

OTHER FETAL CELL TYPES IN THE PLACENTA

Hofbauer cells

Hofbauer cells are mononuclear phagocytes present in chorionic villous stroma and amniotic mesenchyme throughout gestation (Fox & Kharkongor, 1969; Nehemiah et al, 1981). Dilation of villous stromal vessels and stretching of amnion in third-trimester placentas causes distortion of Hofbauer cells. Their irregular 'dendritic' morphology, together with strong expression of class II MHC molecules, led to suggestions that Hofbauer cells may have an immunological rôle, functioning as potent fetal accessory cells; subsequent enzyme and immunohistochemical studies, however, indicated their macrophage nature (Jenkins et al, 1983; Sutton et al, 1983; Bulmer & Johnson, 1984; Sutton et al, 1986).

Hofbauer cells in amniotic mesenchyme and chorionic villous stroma have a similar phenotype, expressing CD45, CD14, CD4 and class II MHC molecules (Bulmer et al, 1988a) (Fig. 61.3). Some complement receptors and Fcγ receptors have been detected in cell suspensions and tissue sections (Bulmer & Johnson, 1984; Wainwright & Holmes, 1993; Saji et al, 1994).

The in vivo rôle of Hofbauer cells is not known. They are capable of both immune and non-immune phagocytosis and their lysosomal enzyme activity supports a phagocytic rôle (Wood, 1980; Loke et al, 1982; Bulmer & Johnson, 1984; Earl et al, 1989). However, their position

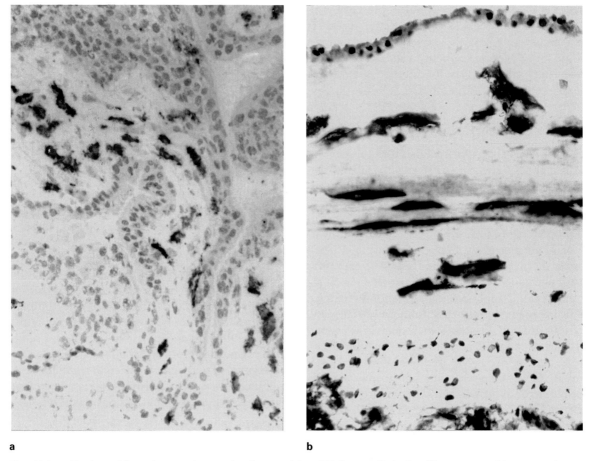

a   b

Fig. 61.3 **a** Sections of first-trimester placenta showing reactivity of Hofbauer cells in the villous stroma with a macrophage marker (anti-Leu-M3; CD14). **b** Term amniochorion labelled for class II MHC molecules. Attenuated macrophages in the amniotic mesenchyme are strongly class II MHC-positive. **a** × 100; **b** × 250.

at the extraembryonic interface of fetal tissue with the mother raises the possibility of a rôle in normal placental immunobiology. Macrophages purified from normal term placentas are able to suppress both mixed lymphocyte reactions and cell-mediated cytotoxicity (Uren & Boyle, 1990). Placental macrophages are also a potential source of cytokines, particularly IL1 (see below).

Endothelial cells

Fetal endothelial cells in the placenta are relatively unstudied: they express Fcγ receptors and also produce various cytokines (see below). Interestingly, several mAbs raised against trophoblast cross-react with fetal stem vessel endothelial cells, perhaps reflecting adaptation of both syncytiotrophoblast and endovascular cytotrophoblast to serve as a vascular lining layer (Anderson et al, 1987). Expression of class II MHC molecules by fetal endothelial cells varies even between placentas of similar gestational age. The expression of molecules implicated in the adhesion of malarial parasites to endothelial cells by placental

endothelial cells may play a rôle in the preferential sequestration of malarial parasites in the placenta during pregnancy (see below).

Intervillous spaces

Villous trophoblast is continually bathed in maternal blood circulating in the intervillous spaces. Thus, maternal lymphocytes and monocytes are in direct contact with fetal trophoblast and, in areas of trophoblast damage, with Hofbauer cells in the villous stroma. Despite their proximity to fetal cells, maternal leucocytes in intervillous space blood remain relatively unstudied, although T cells, monocytes, polymorphs and scanty B cells have been localized by immunohistochemistry. Mononuclear cells purified from intervillous space blood proliferate in response to various antigens and mitogens, the response differing between primiparae and multiparae (Rasheed et al, 1992, 1993). These cells merit further study, particularly with regard to cytokine production which could contribute to local immunosuppression.

CHARACTERIZATION AND FUNCTION OF DECIDUAL CELLS

Introduction

Human female genital tract mucosa is exposed to foreign antigens in both pregnant and non-pregnant states and has an integral mucosal immune system. Vagina, cervix, and Fallopian tubes appear to be protected by 'classical' mucosal immunity with intraepithelial T lymphocytes, mucosal T cells, macrophages and plasma cells and secretory IgA immunity (Brandtzaeg et al, 1993; Kutteh & Mestecky, 1994). The endometrium, however, lacks such a system, plasma cells not normally being detected. Nevertheless, the uterine cavity does not lack IgA since this descends from the Fallopian tubes.

Despite the paucity of plasma cells and the lack of a classical mucosal immune system, human endometrium contains abundant potentially immunocompetent cells. Leucocytes account for around 8% of stromal cells in proliferative and early secretory endometrium, increase in number dramatically in the late secretory phase and account for 30–40% of stromal cells in the first trimester of pregnancy (Bulmer et al, 1991a), forming aggregates around spiral arteries and adjacent to glands. Endometrial stromal leucocytes fall into three major groups: T lymphocytes, macrophages and phenotypically unusual granulated lymphocytes (Fig. 61.4). In a study of precisely timed endometrial biopsies stromal leucocytes around the time of implantation comprised 41% granulated lymphocytes, 32% T cells and 28% macrophages (Klentzeris et al, 1992). B lymphocytes, classical CD16-positive natural killer (NK) cells and polymorphs are scanty in normal endometrium.

T lymphocytes

CD3-positive T cells account for a minor proportion (15–20%) of leucocytes in first-trimester decidua, where they are scattered throughout decidua basalis and parietalis; they are more prominent in the second half of pregnancy when the number of granulated lymphocytes has declined. Approximately 75% of decidual T cells express CD8, contrasting with peripheral blood in which CD4-positive cells predominate. Selective concentration of T cells bearing the more infrequent $\gamma\delta$ T-cell receptor (TCR) heterodimer has been reported in murine endometrium and decidua (Heyborne et al, 1992; Croy et al, 1993) but expression of $\alpha\beta$ and $\gamma\delta$ TCR heterodimers by human endometrial T cells is disputed. Dietl et al (1990) failed to detect either $\alpha\beta$ or $\gamma\delta$ TCR on T cells in first-trimester human decidua. Others, however, detected β chain expression by most T cells in endometrium and decidua (Yeh et al, 1990; Bulmer et al, 1991b), implying expression of the $\alpha\beta$ TCR heterodimer, although expression

may be downregulated compared with T cells in peripheral blood (Morii et al, 1993). Christmas et al (1990, 1991) produced $\gamma\delta$ T-cell clones from first-trimester human decidua, thus confirming their presence, albeit in small numbers. No specific gene usage was noted for human reproductive tract $\gamma\delta$ T cells, despite consistent reports of preferential localization of Vγ6 cells in mouse female reproductive tract (Carding et al, 1990; Itohara et al, 1990; Nandi & Allison, 1991).

Decidual T cells are likely to function in intrauterine host defence mechanisms but, as the minor decidual leucocyte population, they have been relatively neglected in in vitro studies. CD8-positive T cells in human decidua could function as immunosuppressive cells. There is, however, little variation in absolute numbers of endometrial T cells during the menstrual cycle or in early pregnancy, an increase being anticipated should the cells have a specific function in pregnancy (Bulmer et al, 1991a; Klentzeris et al, 1992). Szekeres-Bartho et al (1989) detected progesterone receptor on peripheral blood CD8-positive T cells during pregnancy; however, there is no evidence of hormone dependence by T cells in endometrium, and progesterone receptors have not been detected by immunohistochemistry (Tabibzadeh & Satyaswaroop, 1989).

Endometrial T cells would also be expected to secrete cytokines. Various receptors for T-cell cytokine products are present on trophoblast and other uteroplacental cells. The 'immunotropism' hypothesis proposed that T-cell cytokine production is essential for normal placental growth and development. This hypothesis has subsequently been modified to suggest that T_H2 cytokines such as IL6 and IL10 which control the humoral arm of the immune response are preferentially produced during pregnancy, T_H1 cytokines such as IL2, IFNγ and TNFβ which influence cell-mediated responses being detrimental (Wegmann et al, 1993).

Macrophages

Macrophages account for 35–40% of stromal leucocytes in first-trimester human decidua and predominate at term when the numbers of granulated lymphocytes have declined. They are scattered throughout the decidua and, in the decidua basalis, may be very closely associated with extravillous trophoblast (Bulmer et al, 1988b). In non-pregnant endometrium, macrophages increase in number premenstrually and again in early pregnancy. Most decidual macrophages are class II MHC-positive (Bulmer et al, 1988a) and possess $\alpha_1$antiprotease, $\alpha_1$antichymotrypsin, non-specific esterase and acid phosphatase activity (Bulmer & Johnson, 1984; Earl et al, 1989).

In vitro studies of decidual macrophages have led to suggestions for in vivo rôles. Antigen-presenting cells,

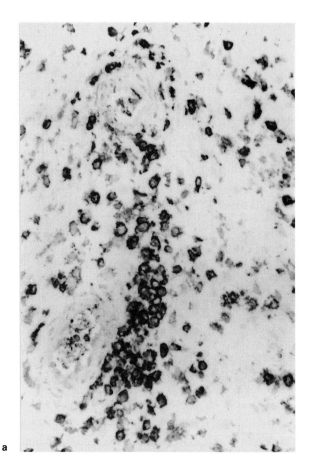

a

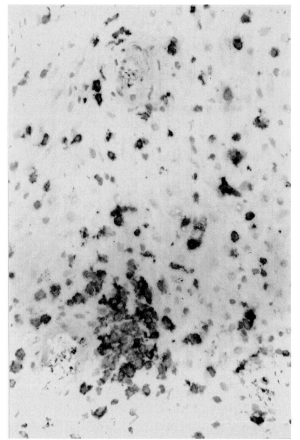

b

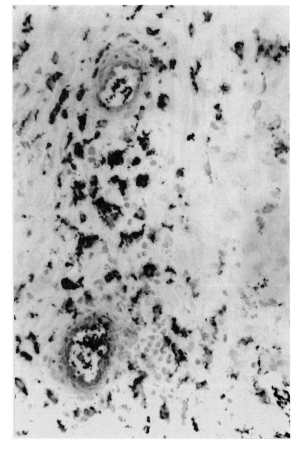

c

Fig. 61.4 Serial sections of first-trimester decidua labelled for: **a** CD45 (all leucocytes); **b** CD2 (T cells and some NK cells); **c** CD14 (macrophages). Note leucocytic aggregate around vessel composed of CD2+ eGL and CD14+ macrophages. × 160.

which can activate suppressor T cells, have been detected in first-trimester human decidua (Dorman & Searle, 1988; Oksenberg et al, 1988) but have not been thoroughly characterized apart from strong expression of class II MHC molecules. Macrophages are prime candidates for such a rôle, although occasional CD1-positive cells, which may possess potent accessory cell function, have been detected by immunohistochemistry in both non-pregnant endometrium and early pregnancy decidua (Bulmer & Sunderland, 1984; Kamat & Isaacson, 1987).

An immunosuppressive rôle, mediated by secretion of prostaglandin E_2 (PGE_2), has also been proposed and may block the lytic activity of cells in decidua with potential anti-trophoblast activity (Parhar et al, 1989). However, several other cell types have been implicated as suppressor cells in human decidua, including lymphocytes, epithelial cells and decidualized stromal cells, and their relative contributions and importance are not clear. Macrophages can also produce a range of cytokines, including M-CSF, G-CSF and TNFα. Decidual macrophages may therefore play a rôle in the complex cytokine networks which appear to operate within uteroplacental tissues (see below).

Their enzyme content suggests that decidual macrophages also have phagocytic potential. Invasion of uterine tissues by trophoblast is likely to produce tissue debris requiring removal by phagocytosis. Other potential non-specific macrophage functions include innate protection of host tissues against microbial infection. Nevertheless, expression by decidual macrophages of a molecule associated with downregulatory stages of inflammation has been considered to support an immunological non-inflammatory rôle (Mues et al, 1989).

Granulated lymphocytes

The largest leucocyte population in first-trimester human decidua comprises phenotypically unusual granulated lymphocytes, which account for up to 75% of the stromal leucocytes. Although present in proliferative and early secretory endometrium, endometrial granulated lymphocytes (eGL) dramatically increase in number in the late secretory phase and again in the first trimester of pregnancy (Bulmer et al, 1991a; Klentzeris et al, 1992). In the second half of pregnancy, they decline in number and appear to be present only in small numbers at term. Immunohistochemical studies of paraffin-embedded sections (Fig. 61.5) and cell suspensions have established that these cells are analogous to 'endometrial stromal granulocytes' (Körnchenzellen, K cells) which were formerly considered to be relaxin-producing stromal-derived cells (Bulmer et al, 1987a; Dallenbach-Hellweg, 1987).

Granulated lymphocytes in human endometrium and decidua have an unusual cell surface antigenic phenotype. They express CD56, a marker of natural killer (NK) cells, at a much higher density than on peripheral blood NK cells, but lack most other NK-cell markers such as CD16, CD11b and CD57 (Bulmer et al, 1991a; King et al, 1991). They lack the T-cell surface molecules CD3, CD4 and CD8 but some express CD2, a cell adhesion molecule expressed by T cells and some NK cells. Most are CD38-positive and CD69-positive, also reflecting some similarity to NK cells (Nishikawa et al, 1991) and a few express the β7 integrin mucosal lymphocyte antigen, HML1 (CD103) (Burrows et al, 1993). Although negative for the p55 high affinity chain of the IL2 receptor (CD25), eGL do express the low affinity p75 chain (Bulmer & Johnson, 1986; Starkey, 1991). Expression of CD69 and various β1 and β2 integrins may reflect in situ activation of eGL (Dietl et al, 1992; Burrows et al, 1993).

The eGL phenotype resembles a small population of peripheral blood large granular lymphocytes which are present at a higher percentage in the peripheral blood of women of reproductive age and may represent a differentiation stage of NK cells. However, eGL differ from these

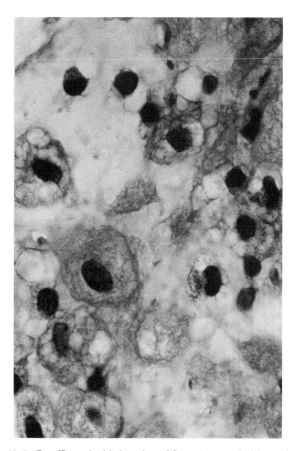

Fig. 61.5 Paraffin-embedded section of first-trimester decidua stained with phloxine tartrazine showing endometrial granulated lymphocytes. × 1000.

peripheral blood cells by exhibiting NK-cell activity in vitro, by their granularity and by their poor response to IL2 (Lanier et al, 1986; Nagler et al, 1989; Ritson & Bulmer, 1989; King et al, 1991).

The increase in eGL numbers in the late secretory phase appears to be due to local proliferation rather than to influx from the circulation (Pace et al, 1989; Klentzeris et al, 1992). Their prominence in the late luteal phase and early pregnancy suggests hormonal regulation, but eGL do not express either progesterone or oestrogen receptors (Tabibzadeh & Satyaswaroop, 1989; Morrison, 1992). eGL are consistently closely associated with decidualized stromal cells even at ectopic implantation sites; progesterone may regulate eGL proliferation and differentiation indirectly via receptors on other cells.

In both late secretory phase endometrium and early pregnancy decidua, eGL form aggregates adjacent to glands and vessels in the stratum functionalis. Adhesion molecules may play a rôle in determining the distribution of eGL within endometrium (Fig. 61.6). Approximately 50% of eGL express CD2, the LFA-2 adhesion molecule whose counter-receptor, LFA-3, is expressed by endometrial endothelial and epithelial cells. A similar proportion of eGL express the β2 integrin LFA-1, whose ligand

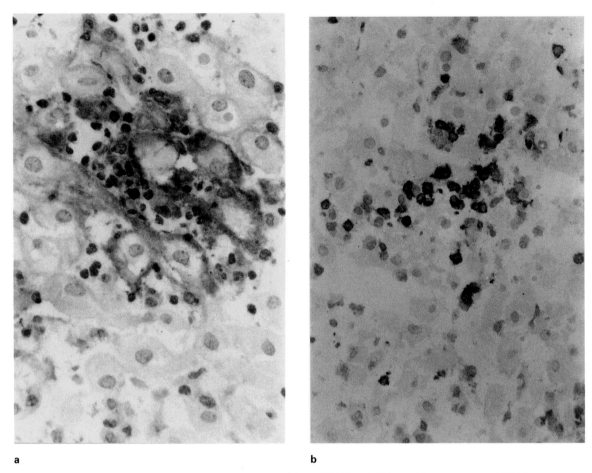

a   b

Fig. 61.6   Sections of normal first-trimester decidua labelled for: **a** ICAM-1; **b** CD11a. Note aggregate of CD11a+ lymphocytes associated with ICAM-1+ decidual stromal cells. × 400.

ICAM-1 is expressed by endometrial endothelial cells and by scattered stromal cells associated with lymphoid aggregates. Other adhesion molecules are expressed by a varying proportion of lymphocytes in endometrium and decidua (Bulmer et al, 1991b; Dietl et al, 1992; Burrows et al, 1993; Marzusch et al, 1993). Adhesion molecules play a rôle in lymphocyte homing and regulation of the immune response and are upregulated by various cytokines. Adhesion molecules may thus influence the distribution and function of eGL in normal and pathological pregnancy.

The function of eGL in normal human pregnancy is not known. Similar cells have been detected in primate endometrium during pregnancy and the granulated metrial gland (GMG) cells which accumulate in rat, mouse and hamster decidua basalis and metrial gland in the second half of pregnancy are considered to be analogous to human eGL (Peel, 1991). Granulated lymphocytes have also been detected in sheep endometrium in pregnancy (Lee et al, 1988; Gogolin-Ewens et al, 1989), a species with epitheliochorial placentation. Their distribution in secretory endometrium and early pregnancy decidua, and the

presence of intrauterine granulated cells in other species, suggests a fundamental rôle for eGL in normal pregnancy. Their antigenic phenotype and cytoplasmic granularity has raised the possibility that eGL are NK cells. CD56-positive granulated lymphocytes enriched from first-trimester human decidua by various techniques have consistently exhibited NK-type cytolytic activity (King et al, 1989; Manaseki & Searle, 1989; Ritson & Bulmer, 1989; Ferry et al, 1990) and IL2-activated eGL can lyse cultured trophoblast and choriocarcinoma cell lines (King & Loke, 1990; Ferry et al, 1991). Chromium release assays are a relatively insensitive measure of cytotoxic activity. Using time-lapse video recording of co-cultures, direct killing by mouse and rat GMG cells of occasional labyrinthine trophoblast without prior cytokine activation has been observed (Stewart & Mukhtar, 1988; Peel & Adam, 1991). Lysis of normal trophoblast by human eGL without IL2 activation may thus occur below the detection limits of the chromium release assay and close associations between eGL and normal trophoblast have been observed using scanning electronmicroscopy (Bulmer et al, 1991b).

Demonstration of trophoblast lysis after IL2 activation led to the suggestion that eGL may control trophoblast invasion into uterine tissues by detection and lysis of abnormally invasive cells (King & Loke, 1991). However, histological examination of placental bed tissues provides no evidence of direct killing of extravillous trophoblast cells in vivo. Furthermore, trophoblast invasion normally extends into the myometrium, a site at which eGL are absent. The lytic activity of eGL has also been questioned: Christmas et al (1990) produced clones of CD3-negative granulated lymphocytes from first-trimester human decidua and detected strong NK-cell activity only in CD16-positive clones, raising the possibility that the lytic activity of purified decidual CD56-positive eGL reported in other studies is due to the presence of small numbers of 'classic' CD16-positive NK cells originating from contaminating blood.

Several decidual cell types have been implicated as functionally suppressor-type cells in vitro but their relative in vivo importance remains to be determined. The description of a non-T non-B granulated lymphoid suppressor cell in mouse decidua which acts by secretion of a TGFβ_2-like molecule (Clark et al, 1990) raised speculation that eGL in human decidua may play a similar rôle. In vitro studies suggest that eGL may mediate a component of decidual suppressor activity but that other cells also make a substantial contribution (Bulmer et al, 1991c).

Cytokines appear to play a fundamental rôle in pregnancy, although the precise in vivo rôle of the complex cytokine networks in human uteroplacental tissues remains to be unravelled. NK cells can secrete various cytokines and eGL may fulfil their specialized rôle in pregnancy by secretion of these soluble polypeptides. TGFβ_2 may mediate immunosuppression in mouse decidua and deficient TGFβ_2-containing cells have been reported in human decidua in first-trimester pregnancies destined to abort (Clark et al, 1992), although the cell responsible for TGFβ_2 production has not been characterized. CD3-negative eGL clones produce TGFβ detected by bioassay as well as TNFα and IFNγ (Christmas et al, 1990), and freshly isolated CD56-positive decidual lymphocytes produce G-CSF, GM-CSF, M-CSF, TNFα and IFNγ and LIF (Saito et al, 1993).

In common with their proposed rat analogues, the GMG cells, eGL were thought to secrete relaxin which would facilitate trophoblast invasion of decidua (Dallenbach-Hellweg, 1987). Concerns about antibody specificity and failure to detect biological relaxin activity in the rat metrial gland (Larkin, 1974) cast doubt on this conclusion. Since both B and T lymphocytes are scanty in normal decidua, particularly in early pregnancy, together with macrophages, the granulated lymphocytes may provide the important immediate non-specific defence mechanism essential for the integrity of the extraembryonic membranes within their uterine host. The placenta may be exposed to various infectious agents including viruses, bacteria and parasites; local intrauterine immunosuppression may also increase susceptibility to infection of both mother and fetus.

Intraepithelial lymphocytes

Intraepithelial lymphocytes (IEL) in human endometrium and decidua have received less attention than their counterparts in the gastrointestinal tract. Macrophages, T cells and CD56-positive eGL can all occur in an intraepithelial position in endometrium, their relative numbers varying according to menstrual cycle stage. CD56-positive IEL increase in number during the menstrual cycle and, in early pregnancy, account for approximately 50% of the IEL population. CD3-positive, CD8-positive T cells account for the remaining IEL population and a substantial proportion of these are also granulated (Pace et al, 1991). Most intraepithelial T cells express the $\alpha\beta$ TCR heterodimer, the number of $\gamma\delta$ cells showing no enrichment (Bulmer et al, 1991b). The small number of IEL in endometrium compared with the stromal lymphocyte population has ensured their low profile in research studies to date.

Endometrial epithelial cells

Alterations in the phenotype of endometrial surface epithelium around the time of implantation have been documented in experimental animals. Lectin binding profiles differ between proliferative and secretory endometrium and early pregnancy decidua. Such changes in epithelial glycoconjugates may favour implantation: patients with primary unexplained infertility have altered surface and glandular epithelial glycoconjugate profiles in luteal phase endometrium compared with normal fertile women (Klentzeris et al, 1991).

Several characteristic antigens are shared by trophoblast and endometrial epithelial cells (Anderson et al, 1987). In pregnancy, endometrial glands substantially decrease or lose expression of class I MHC molecules and a minority may express class II MHC molecules (Johnson & Bulmer, 1984; Bulmer & Johnson, 1985b). Aggregates of eGL or, to a lesser extent, T cells are often related to endometrial glands, possibly reflecting their susceptibility to immune-mediated attack (Bulmer & Johnson, 1985b; Tabibzadeh, 1990).

Endometrial epithelial cells are a potent source of cytokines under hormonal regulation during pregnancy. Production of M-CSF and TNFα (Chen et al, 1991; Daiter et al, 1992) by epithelial cells in first-trimester human decidua has been documented. Secretion of pregnancy proteins, including PP14 which has been implicated as a potent decidual immunosuppressive molecule (Pockley et al, 1988) has also been documented. Production of cytokines and/or pregnancy proteins may account for reports of immunosuppressive activity by endometrial epithelial cells in vitro (Johnson et al, 1987).

Endometrial stromal cells

In addition to the endocrine and nutritional rôles of decidual cells, immunological functions have been proposed. Secretion of extracellular matrix components by decidual cells may regulate trophoblast invasion. The distribution in endometrium of fibronectin, laminin and type IV collagen differs during the menstrual cycle and early pregnancy (Aplin et al, 1988; Loke et al, 1989). Interactions with $\beta1$ integrins differentially expressed by various trophoblast populations (Korhonen et al, 1991; Damsky et al, 1992; Aplin, 1993) may govern the rate and extent of trophoblast invasion of uterine tissues.

Decidualized stromal cells may also have immunosuppressive activity. In common with decidual macrophages, decidual stromal cells have been implicated in PGE_2 production, causing in vitro suppression of potential anti-trophoblast activity which can be abrogated with anti-PGE_2 antibody or indomethacin (Parhar et al, 1988, 1989). Others, however, claim that epithelial cells are the predominant site of PGE_2 production in human decidua (Smith & Kelly, 1987). Decidual cells may mediate immunosuppression by other mechanisms. Decidual cells purified on a density gradient produce a 43–67 kD soluble suppressor factor which inhibits lymphoproliferation, IL2 receptor expression and IL2 production (Matsui et al, 1989). In common with other cells implicated in decidual immunosuppression, the in vivo rôle of decidual stromal cells in local immunoregulation in pregnancy remains uncertain.

Decidual stromal cells also produce cytokines, growth factors and pregnancy proteins. Production of IL1, TNFα, M-CSF, IL6 and TGFβ has been reported (Chen et al, 1991; Graham et al, 1992); and various growth factor receptors, including EGF receptor and IGF binding protein, have been localized to decidual cells (Bulmer et al, 1990; Bell, 1991).

MATERNAL SYSTEMIC IMMUNE RESPONSES IN PREGNANCY

Although considerable speculation has centred on the concept that active maternal immune recognition of her semi-allogeneic pregnancy leads to protective and beneficial immune and cytokine responses, substantive confirmatory data are scarce. Trophoblast lacks all polymorphic classical class I and class II MHC molecules and cannot be killed by cytotoxic T cells; trophoblast also resists complement-mediated and NK-cell attack. Despite some reports of maternal serum anti-trophoblast responses

(Davies & Browne, 1985), there is little convincing evidence for conventional antibody or cellular responses directed specifically against trophoblast in normal pregnancy (Hole et al, 1987).

Anti-HLA antibodies

Multiparous sera often contain antibodies to MHC and non-MHC cell surface antigens. Production of antibodies to paternal MHC antigens expressed by the fetus varies between species: in rats, alloantibodies are detected only in certain strain combinations and may have a genetic basis (Bell & Billington, 1983), whilst virtually all mares are antibody-positive on foaling (Antczak et al, 1984). In humans, sensitization to paternal MHC antigens occurs at a rate of less than 15% for each term pregnancy; maternal antibodies arise after exposure to fetal leucocytes in extra-embryonic tissues or by transfer of blood at parturition (Johnson, 1989). In many multiparous sera, antibodies are directed against broadly shared alloantigens, may occasionally react only with activated T cells and may not be ascribable to classical MHC specificities (Johnson & Stern, 1986; Konoeda et al, 1986).

Antibodies to class II MHC molecules which could block antigen presentation are infrequent, arising late in gestation when class II MHC molecules show strong expression by macrophages in placenta and membranes (Sutton et al, 1983; Bulmer et al, 1988a). Neither deleterious or advantageous effects have been demonstrated for anti-HLA antibodies induced by pregnancy (Johnson, 1989).

'Blocking factors'

Antibodies to other leucocyte cell surface structures have been detected in maternal sera and placental eluates, including anti-idiotypic antibodies reactive with maternal T-cell receptors for paternal MHC, non-cytotoxic antibodies which block B-cell Fc receptors and antibodies which inhibit T-cell function in the mixed lymphocyte reaction and other in vitro assays of lymphocyte function (Johnson & Stern, 1986; Johnson, 1989). Pregnancy sera also contain pregnancy-associated proteins and steroid hormones, some of which can inhibit T-lymphocyte function in vitro (Stimson, 1983). However, although some infections are commoner or reactivated during pregnancy, extrauterine immune competence is generally not seriously compromised during pregnancy (Billington, 1988). Thus, the in vivo importance of these 'blocking antibody' phenomena detected in vitro is obscure. Assays and results are often erratic and, at least in some cases, related to the purity of the substance tested. They are most likely to represent a consequence of pregnancy rather than being of fundamental biological importance for its maintenance. The non-essential role of 'blocking antibodies' is demonstrated by successful pregnancies occurring in agammaglobulinaemic women who suffer no increase in pregnancy failure above that related to their susceptibility to infection.

Cellular immunity

Altered numbers of B cells, T cells, NK cells and T-cell subset ratios during pregnancy have been reported with variations between non-pregnant and pregnant populations and between the three trimesters of pregnancy. Data, however, are variable and no consensus exists to date. Nevertheless, as stated above, systemic cellular immunity cannot be severely compromised during pregnancy since, apart from a few specific examples (see below), infections requiring cell-mediated immune responses are not generally commoner in pregnant women.

Cytotoxic T cells specific for paternally inherited fetal MHC antigens occur rarely in maternal peripheral blood during pregnancy (Sargent & Wilkins, 1988). Despite numerous studies over several years, there is little consistent evidence for non-specific suppression of systemic cell-mediated responses. Impaired proliferative responses to various micro-organisms and purified antigens, such as cytomegalovirus (Gehrz et al, 1981), malaria and candida (Rasheed et al, 1993), could be due to hormonal changes in pregnancy. Higher hormone levels may also explain differing responses in primiparous compared with multiparous women (Rasheed et al, 1993). Future studies of systemic immunity in pregnancy focusing on differences between parity groups and on defined cell populations may be worthwhile, although studies of local uteroplacental immunoregulation are likely to be more fruitful.

CYTOKINE NETWORKS WITHIN UTEROPLACENTAL TISSUES

Cytokines are soluble polypeptide molecules with a wide variety of activities. They are secreted by cells, act locally and have a short half life. An individual cytokine may have diverse effects on different cell types, an extreme example being IL1 which has over one hundred documented cellular effects.

Evidence is accumulating that cytokines play an important rôle in normal pregnancy (Hunt, 1989; Mitchell et al, 1993). Receptors for several cytokines are expressed by placental trophoblast, and cytokine production has been documented in both decidua and placenta, reflecting both paracrine and autocrine growth regulation. As well as their effects on placental growth and differentiation, cytokines may also contribute to local immunoregulation. Cytokines can also have detrimental effects on trophoblast and could play a rôle in pregnancy loss by a direct effect on trophoblast or by activation of cytotoxic cells. A rôle for cytokines in premature labour has also been proposed

(Romero et al, 1991). Abnormal serum or urine levels of cytokines or their soluble receptors in abnormalities of pregnancy such as premature labour, pre-eclampsia or intrauterine growth retardation may have predictive diagnostic value. Cytokines may well prove to be the fundamental regulatory molecules in normal pregnancy. However, at present, despite ever-increasing localization of cytokines, their receptors and inhibitory molecules in uteroplacental tissues, their in vivo rôle is unknown. Complex cytokine networks will be difficult to unravel and in vitro studies will be of limited use. Levels of serum, amniotic fluid or urinary cytokine or receptor may, however, prove valid predictive or diagnostic tests before their precise mechanism of action is established.

PRENATAL TRANSFER OF ANTIBODY AND CELLS FROM MOTHER TO FETUS

Maternal IgG of all four subclasses is transferred selectively into the fetal circulation after recognition by transporting Fcγ receptors (FcγR) on the apical surface of placental syncytiotrophoblast from the 20th gestational week onwards (Johnson, 1992). Selective transfer of IgG to the fetal circulation provides transient passive immunity following parturition, prior to the development of full immunocompetence during the first few months of life. Characterization of the FcγR on villous syncytiotrophoblast has been elusive; recent data suggest a relationship to leucocyte FcγRIIb or FcγRIII structures, or a contribution from placental alkaline phosphatase (Wainwright & Holmes, 1993; Nilsson et al, 1994; Saji et al, 1994).

Apart from the beneficial transfer of IgG anti-microbial antibody, deleterious IgG autoantibodies and anti-fetal alloantibodies could also potentially be transferred from the maternal to the fetal circulation. Most are trapped before reacting the fetal circulation by the placental 'sink' or 'sponge'. Early immunofluorescence studies drew attention to extensive IgG and complement deposits in the villous stroma of term placentas (Faulk & Johnson, 1977; Johnson et al, 1977). Maternal IgG antibodies specific for a fetal HLA allele will not reach the fetal circulation, having been bound efficiently by macrophages, fibroblasts and endothelial cells in the villous stroma. Maternal IgG antibodies to other fetal antigens expressed in the placenta will be similarly sequestered by binding to the appropriate antigen or by forming a soluble immune complex and binding to high-avidity FcγR expressed by villous stromal macrophages and fetal stem vessel endothelium (Johnson & Brown, 1981). Some adverse IgG antibodies may, however, escape the placental 'sink'. For example, anti-rhesus (D) and anti-platelet IgG antibodies encounter their respective antigens on fetal erythrocytes and platelets, respectively, in vessels. Lysis of erythrocytes and platelets will thus occur prior to trapping of immune complexes on placental FcγR-positive endothelium. Maternal IgG organ-specific autoantibodies directed against antigens absent from the placenta are also not retained. For example, transient neonatal hyperthyroidism may follow transplacental passage of maternal anti-thyroid IgG auto-antibodies which reach and directly act on the fetal thyroid, persisting into the neonatal period (Scott, 1976).

Transplacental trafficking of lymphocytes from mother to fetus has been difficult to evaluate. Chimerism has been detected in some children with severe combined immunodeficiency. Labelling techniques indicate that, while small numbers of maternal erythrocytes may enter the fetal circulation, leucocytes are generally excluded (Hunziker et al, 1984).

IMMUNOBIOLOGY OF PATHOLOGICAL PREGNANCY

The in vivo rôles of the various endometrial leucocyte populations and of the distinct trophoblast subpopulations remain to be established; in vitro studies have provided clues to function, but investigation of pathological pregnancy may cast light on in vivo importance.

Spontaneous abortion

It is an attractive hypothesis that spontaneous abortion may, in some cases, be explained by immune rejection of the semi-allogeneic feto-placental unit: unfortunately, there is little concrete evidence to support such a proposal. Reports of successful immunotherapy for recurrent miscarriage by infusion with paternal or third party leucocytes stimulated interest in the concept of immune-mediated pregnancy loss. To date virtually no supportive data have emerged and recent reports have cast doubt on the success of immunotherapy, the success rates for placebo groups being similar to those for treatment groups (Hill, 1990; Fraser et al, 1993). Furthermore, in a prospective study of women after three or more consecutive miscarriages the rate of successful subsequent pregnancy without treatment was similar to that of both placebo and treatment groups in immunotherapy trials (Regan et al, 1989). Psychotherapy may yield an even higher rate of successful pregnancy (Stray-Pedersen & Stray-Pedersen, 1988).

Investigation of spontaneous abortion is complex. Patients are heterogeneous, even at a given gestational age, encompassing genetic and medical causes as well as unexplained miscarriage. Clinical selection procedures at any individual centre will also vary. Patients suffering recurrent (three or more consecutive) miscarriages are more homogeneous but nevertheless will include diverse causes. Specimens suitable for histological and immunohistochemical studies are difficult to obtain: abortion may occur at home with resultant loss of tissue; and embryo death may occur days or weeks before clinical presenta-

tion, with development of secondary decidual inflammation and consequent uncertainty whether decidual leucocytes are the cause or effect of pregnancy loss.

Khong et al (1987) suggested that defective haemochorial placentation may explain some cases of spontaneous abortion. Deficient trophoblast invasion of spiral arteries was noted in two of seven first-trimester and five of five second-trimester spontaneous abortions. Deficient trophoblast invasion is well recognized in pre-eclampsia and intrauterine growth retardation (see below): the observations in spontaneous abortion raise the possibility of a common defect in placentation with differing clinical presentations.

Studies in murine pregnancy have, however, provided evidence that decidual leucocytes play a rôle in pregnancy loss. The CBA/J × DBA/2 murine mating combination produces a high rate of spontaneous pregnancy resorption which is increased by enhancement of NK-cell activity and decreased by an anti-NK-cell antibody. The implantation site of these resorbing pregnancies is infiltrated by NK cells (de Fougerolles & Baines, 1987; Gendron & Baines, 1988). Furthermore, the implantation site of resorbing pregnancies in the functionally T- and B-cell deficient SCID mouse is infiltrated by granulocytes, macrophages and large granular lymphocytes (Crepeau & Croy, 1988). These animal models suggest that non-specific immune cells may be implicated in pregnancy loss, rather than a specific attack against fetal alloantigens. Murine trophoblast is not normally susceptible to lysis by NK or cytotoxic T cells, although it can be killed by lymphokine-activated killer (LAK) cells generated by incubation of NK cells in high doses of IL2 (Head, 1989). Failure of local intrauterine suppression of IL2 could lead to generation of LAK cells capable of direct attack on the placental trophoblast. Altered decidual immunosuppression could lead to generation of LAK cells from resident decidual granulated lymphocytes or, alternatively, 'classic' NK cells may infiltrate from peripheral blood.

Studies of decidual leucocytes in human spontaneous abortion are scanty. Human trophoblast cells resist NK-cell lysis but are susceptible to LAK cells (King & Loke, 1990; Ferry et al, 1991). Nebel (1987) noted dense mononuclear cell infiltrates in deep decidua and around blood vessels in tissues from abortions occurring 22–30 days after embryo transfer on an in vitro fertilization programme but this cellular infiltrate was not characterized. Michel et al (1989) suggested that decidual lymphocytes with granules >1 μm diameter are a feature of normal pregnancy, whereas lymphocytes with granules <1 μm diameter occur in pregnancies destined to abort. Defective decidual immunosuppression was also noted in aborting pregnancies; suppression was attributed to decidual lymphocytes with large granules (Michel et al, 1990).

Abnormal uteroplacental cytokine profiles could also play a rôle in pregnancy loss. TNFα has been implicated in the CBA/J × DBA/2 mouse resorption model and systemic treatment of pregnant mice with anti-GM-CSF may be followed by resorption (Chaouat et al, 1990; Gendron et al, 1990). Deficient decidual TGFβ$_2$-containing cells have also been reported in aborting human pregnancies (Clark et al, 1992).

Thus, evidence from experimental animals and the few studies of human miscarriage reported to date, suggests that decidual leucocytes participate in pregnancy loss either by NK cell-type cytolytic mechanisms or by alterations in the local cytokine profile. Considerable scope for future studies remains, although patient heterogeneity and retrieval of suitable tissues without confounding secondary inflammation remain problematic.

Ectopic pregnancy

Ectopic pregnancy has an incidence of 1 in 100 conceptions in Europe and North America. Implantation is usually in the Fallopian tube and placental development and trophoblast invasion proceed normally until haemorrhage, pain or rupture necessitates surgical removal. Tubal abnormalities are often considered to account for tubal implantation, delaying passage of the fertilized ovum along the Fallopian tube. However, the Fallopian tube often appears normal and increased tubal receptivity or embryonic/extraembryonic factors may also play a rôle.

There are no major discrepancies in the expression of trophoblast and HLA antigens, trophoblast hormone products, fibronectin and laminin between normal intrauterine and ectopic tubal pregnancy (Earl et al, 1985, 1986, 1989). Absence of pregnancy-associated plasma protein A (PAPP-A) in villous syncytiotrophoblast in ectopic tubal pregnancy may reflect compromised PAPP-A synthesis, decreased serum levels having potential diagnostic value (Sinosich et al, 1983; Chemnitz et al, 1984).

Although common, decidualization of the tubal mucosa in ectopic pregnancy is often focal and incomplete (Pauerstein et al, 1986). Analysis of tubal leucocytes in ectopic pregnancy may be complicated by preceding chronic salpingitis or secondary inflammation. Immunohistochemical studies of the ectopic implantation site have revealed a majority population of class II MHC-positive macrophages, together with CD8-positive T cells and variable numbers of B cells and granulocytes (Earl et al, 1987a). eGL are detectable at the ectopic implantation site only in areas of mucosal decidualization (Bulmer et al, 1987b).

Uterine endometrium undergoes decidualization in ectopic pregnancy, acquiring a similar leucocyte content to that documented in intrauterine pregnancy (Bulmer et al, 1987b). Any essential rôle for eGL, either by regulation of maternal immune responses against the fetoplacental unit or by control of trophoblast growth and differentiation, would require secretion of a soluble factor capable of acting at a distant site. The lack of eGL at the ectopic implantation site with associated, often transmural, trophoblast invasion has been considered to support a fundamental rôle of granulated lymphocytes in the control of trophoblast invasion (King & Loke, 1991).

Adhesion molecules and their ligands may play a rôle in normal intrauterine implantation and trophoblast invasion. Tubal adhesion molecules in ectopic pregnancy have not yet been examined: inappropriate expression of these molecules could lead to implantation at an ectopic site. Endometrial epithelium in normal intrauterine pregnancy appears to lose or substantially decrease expression of class I MHC molecules and expresses class II MHC antigens less frequently than in non-pregnant endometrium (Johnson & Bulmer, 1984; Bulmer & Johnson, 1985b). Fallopian tube epithelium retains expression of class I MHC molecules in pregnancy and also expresses HLA-DR, DP and DQ. However, the consistent expression of class II MHC molecules by tubal epithelium in early and term intrauterine pregnancy suggests hormonal regulation in ectopic pregnancy rather than upregulation due to associated inflammation (Bulmer & Earl, 1987).

Pre-eclampsia

Several observations have suggested that pre-eclampsia, or pregnancy-induced hypertension, is due to a disordered maternofetal relationship. A placenta is a prerequisite for development of pre-eclampsia, which can occur without a fetus in hydatidiform mole and is cured by delivery of the placenta. Pre-eclampsia correlates with placental mass, the incidence being higher in molar pregnancy, twin pregnancy and hydrops fetalis (Fox, 1978).

Immunopathology noted in the chorionic villi of the delivered placenta in pre-eclampsia is likely to be secondary to immunopathology in the placental bed. Villous deposits of complement are increased in pre-eclampsia, particularly in severe disease, and may reflect immune-mediated damage (Sinha et al, 1984). Placentas in pre-eclampsia contain connective tissue components absent from normal placentas and the relative concentrations of fibronectin and type IV collagen in chorionic villi may be altered (Vardi & Halbrecht, 1974; Risteli et al, 1984). Early expression of the Ca1 antigen may reflect premature villous maturation (Bishop et al, 1988).

However, the main pathogenetic lesion is an inadequate maternal vascular response to pregnancy. In pre-eclampsia, physiological vascular changes are restricted to the decidua, the myometrial segments of the spiral arteries retaining their musculo-elastic wall and hence their ability to respond to vasomotor influences (Robertson et al, 1986). Indeed, Khong et al (1986) reported absence of physiological changes throughout the entire length of the spiral arteries in some cases of pre-eclampsia, these abnormalities being detectable by examination of the maternal-facing surface of the delivered placenta in either traditional sagittal slices or 'en face' blocks (Khong & Chambers, 1992). Detection of endovascular trophoblast in pre-eclampsia in the third trimester also suggests a failure in the normal maternofetal relationship since uteroplacental arteries have normally re-endothelialized by this stage of pregnancy.

Maternal vascular changes are abnormal and inadequate in pre-eclampsia with an apparent failure of the normal well-controlled maternofetal physiological relationship. Since the mechanisms underpinning the normal trophoblast invasion of maternal uterine tissues and vessels are unknown, the pathogenesis of the abnormality in pre-eclampsia remains obscure. Khong (1987) noted no significant differences in decidual leucocytes between normal and pre-eclamptic pregnancies, although the data were qualitative rather than quantitative. Tatarova et al (1989) quantitated 'endometrial stromal granulocytes' (eGL) in both decidua basalis and decidua parietalis and reported a progressive increase in eGL in mild and severe pre-eclampsia compared with normal pregnancy. These results require independent confirmation in a large study but raise the possibility that decidual leucocytes play a rôle in the defective trophoblastic vascular invasion. Adhesion molecules and their ligands are likely to play a rôle in normal controlled trophoblast invasion and hence could be involved in the pathogenesis of pre-eclampsia. Although these mechanisms remain obscure, Zhou et al (1993) have reported altered expression of adhesion molecules on trophoblast in pre-eclampsia compared with controls. However, it should be remembered that in pre-eclampsia the pathogenetic lesion arises early in the second trimester when immunopathological examination of the placental bed is not possible and well before the clinical syndrome becomes apparent.

'Acute atherosis' of spiral arteries in pre-eclampsia is characterized by fibrinoid necrosis and lipophage infiltration of the vessel wall with a perivascular mononuclear inflammatory cell infiltrate and is best observed in decidua parietalis. Acute atherosis was considered pathognomonic of pre-eclampsia, but similar changes have subsequently been reported in intrauterine growth retardation (IUGR), normotensive diabetes mellitus and systemic lupus erythematosus (SLE) (Sheppard & Bonnar, 1981; Robertson et al, 1986). Vascular morphology in acute atherosis resembles allograft rejection, raising the possibility of an immune pathogenesis. Complement (C3), IgG and fibrin have been localized to placental bed vessels in pre-eclampsia with decidual vascular C3 deposits detected only in association with IgG in one study (Kitzmiller & Benirschke, 1973; Hustin et al, 1983). However, the significance of C3 and Ig deposits in placental bed vessels in pre-eclampsia is doubtful since fibrin, C3 and other complement components have been detected in normal pregnancy. C3 and IgM associated with fibrinoid necrosis

and acute atherosis in pre-eclampsia, stable chronic hypertension and normotensive diabetes mellitus may reflect local intravascular coagulation and fibrinogenesis rather than an immune reaction (Kitzmiller et al, 1981; Weir, 1981; Wells et al, 1987).

In common with other pregnancy disorders, the pathogenetic lesions in pre-eclampsia may occur months before clinical presentation. Lichtig et al (1985) noted C3 deposits and morphological features of atherosis in spiral arteries in placental bed tissues from therapeutic terminations of apparently healthy pregnancies: changes were more frequent in primigravidae and could represent early pre-eclamptic lesions, detectable before clinical presentation. Deported trophoblast elements released from the placental site into maternal peripheral blood are more numerous in pre-eclampsia compared with normal pregnancy (Chua et al, 1991). Methods for separation of trace trophoblastic elements from maternal blood could ultimately allow quantitation of deported trophoblast and provide a predictive technique for the early diagnosis of pre-eclampsia.

Intrauterine growth retardation (IUGR)

Established causes of IUGR or small-for-gestational age (SGA) infants include maternal cigarette smoking, fetal infection and congenital malformation but most cases are unexplained and form a heterogeneous group. Concepts for an immunopathological aetiology are focused on detection of chronic villitis of unknown aetiology and/or acute atherosis in placental bed vessels in a proportion of cases. Acute atherosis was initially considered specific for pre-eclampsia arising *de novo* or superimposed on essential hypertension, renal disease, diabetes mellitus or SLE, but has subsequently been detected in severe IUGR regardless of blood pressure elevation. Dispute remains, however, regarding whether acute atherosis lesions in IUGR are confined to decidua basalis or extend into intramyometrial segments as in pre-eclampsia (Sheppard & Bonnar, 1976, 1981; De Wolf et al, 1980; Althabe et al, 1985; Labarrere et al, 1985; Robertson et al, 1986). IgM, C3 and C1q deposits have been detected in acute atherosis lesions in IUGR associated with normal blood pressure, hypertension and SLE, although in normotensive IUGR only minute IgG and C3 deposits were noted in vessels unaffected by acute atherosis (Hustin et al, 1983; Labarrere et al, 1985).

Inadequate physiological changes in uteroplacental arteries have also been reported in IUGR associated with normal blood pressure, both in intramyometrial segments and sometimes throughout the entire length of the spiral artery (Brosens et al, 1977; De Wolf et al, 1980; Gerretson et al, 1983; Khong et al, 1986). However, retarded intrauterine growth cannot be explained by the inadequate physiological changes in uteroplacental arteries leading to a deficient blood supply to the feto-placental unit, since similar changes have been observed in preeclampsia not complicated by IUGR.

Chronic villitis of unknown aetiology (VUE) has been reported in up to 24% of cases of SGA infants (Altshuler et al, 1975). Russell (1980) detected VUE in 7–8% of all delivered placentas and noted correlation between its severity and the degree of IUGR. Labarrere et al (1982) subsequently noted focal chronic villitis in 26% of control placentas compared with 86% of those associated with SGA infants. The pathogenesis of VUE is not known: infection from uterine sources has been suggested but no infective agent has been isolated. Others have favoured the hypothesis that VUE results from maternal immune attack against extraembryonic fetal tissues. An infiltrate of histiocytes, T lymphocytes, fibroblasts, polymorphs and plasma cells can be seen to disrupt the villous stroma and inflammatory lesions may also be detected in the intervillous spaces (Labarrere et al, 1990). It remains to be fully established whether the inflammatory cells are of maternal or fetal origin, a vital factor in determining the pathogenesis of this condition, although a recent in situ hybridization study has suggested that maternal T cells may cross the maternofetal barrier in VUE, suggesting an immune aetiology (Redline & Patterson, 1993).

VUE can be associated with acute atherosis and defective physiological vascular changes in pregnancies complicated by sustained chronic hypertension and preeclampsia not associated with IUGR. VUE has also been reported in recurrent IUGR and pregnancy failure (Russell et al, 1980; Labarrere & Althabe, 1987). It has been suggested that villitis may represent a fetal response within chorionic villi to a maternal immune attack which has led to abnormal placentation with defective physiological vascular changes (Labarrere & Althabe, 1985). IUGR has thus been linked with two lesions which may have an immune pathogenesis, namely defective physiological vascular changes and chronic villitis of unknown aetiology.

Systemic lupus erythematosus

Systemic lupus erythematosus (SLE) is associated with a high incidence of spontaneous abortion, prematurity and perinatal death. Despite little evidence, poor fetal outcome has been attributed to trophoblast damage, and immune complex deposition has been proposed as the cause of such injury (Theofilopoulos et al, 1981). Placentas from SLE patients showed pronounced granular deposits of IgG, C3 and fibrinogen on the trophoblast basement membrane, and anti-nuclear and anti-DNA autoantibodies have been eluted from some placentas. However, the significance of these observations is uncertain since similar IgG and C3 deposits occur in normal pregnancy (Faulk & Johnson, 1977). VUE is also common in SLE

(Labarrere et al, 1986). Retroviral particles have been described in delivered placentas from SLE patients but are also present in normal trophoblast where their significance is uncertain (Johnson et al, 1990).

Extensive placental infarcts in SLE have been attributed to necrotizing decidual vasculopathy. Uteroplacental arteries may show fibrinoid necrosis with a mononuclear or polymorphonuclear inflammatory cell infiltrate; acute atherosis with deposits of IgM, C3 and Clq has also been reported, as have defective physiological vascular changes (Abramowsky et al, 1980; Labarrere et al, 1986).

Both maternal uteroplacental arterial lesions and VUE have been noted in other autoimmune diseases; however, placental vascular damage appears to be more severe in SLE and has been related to poor fetal outcome (Labarrere et al, 1986).

Diabetes mellitus

Morphological changes documented in the placentas of diabetic women include cytotrophoblast hyperplasia, focal syncytial necrosis and trophoblast basement membrane thickening, all of which represent a response to placental damage. The pathogenesis of trophoblast injury is uncertain, with no evidence for hypoxia or immune complex deposition. Factors other than hyperglycaemia must play a rôle, since similar placental pathology occurs in both well-controlled gestational diabetes and overt diabetes, albeit more prominently and consistently in the latter, as well as in patients treated with subcutaneous insulin infusion to ensure normoglycaemia (Fox & Jones, 1983; Laurini et al, 1987).

Placentation in diabetes mellitus usually proceeds normally (Robertson, 1979) but acute atherosis and fibrinoid necrosis of spiral arteries has been reported: arterial lesions, often associated with IgM and C3 deposits, were noted in decidua basalis and parietalis in one-third of 41 normotensive diabetic patients (Kitzmiller et al, 1981). Uteroplacental vascular lesions in pre-eclampsia, IUGR, SLE, other autoimmune diseases and diabetes mellitus are similar, although they are unlikely to share a common pathogenetic mechanism.

Subinvolution of the uteroplacental arteries

Physiological vascular changes in normal pregnancy have been thoroughly documented but the precise sequence of events which occur during involution of the placental bed following delivery are less well known. Uteroplacental arteries undergo thrombosis and organization, the placental site subsequently shrinks and the endometrium regenerates. Subinvolution of the uteroplacental arteries is a well-recognized cause of postpartum haemorrhage, abrupt haemorrhage occurring one week to several months after delivery, with the highest incidence in the second postpartum week. Reported aetiological factors are multiparity and early ambulation, and subinvolution may recur in subsequent pregnancies. Regression of the uterine musculature and vasculature occurs at sites distant from the placental bed but there is failure of obliteration of the large uteroplacental arteries underlying the placental site (Lee et al, 1986).

Histological and immunohistochemical studies of both curettage and hysterectomy tissues from cases of subinvolution have led to the suggestion that this condition may also involve a disordered relationship between maternal cells and extraembryonic fetal cells in the placental bed (Andrew et al, 1989, 1992). Subinvoluted vessels contain thrombus, may lack an endothelial lining, and degenerate interstitial and endovascular trophoblast can persist, in contrast with the normal re-endothelialization of uteroplacental arteries in the third trimester. In common with other studies of complement components and immunoglobulins in placental bed tissues throughout gestation, deposits of C1q, C3d, C4, C9, IgG, IgA and IgM have been detected in normally involuted vessels but were virtually absent in subinvoluted vessels (Fig. 61.7). This

unusual condition may represent a further example of disordered maternofetal immune interactions and merits further consideration.

Placenta accreta

The histological diagnosis of placenta accreta can be made when placental chorionic villi oppose directly onto myometrium with no intervening decidua. Decidual deficiency may be patchy resulting in focal placental adherence, and penetration into the myometrium may not be uniform. The frequency of placenta accreta shows geographical variation and its cause is unknown, although previous surgical manipulation causing deficient endometrium such as curettage or caesarian section has been implicated.

Deficiency of decidua could lead to disruption of the normal maternofetal relationship in the placental bed resulting in undue trophoblastic invasion. In a detailed morphological study of placenta accreta (Khong & Robertson, 1987), decidua parietalis was readily identified and focal accreta sites were detected adjacent to morphologically

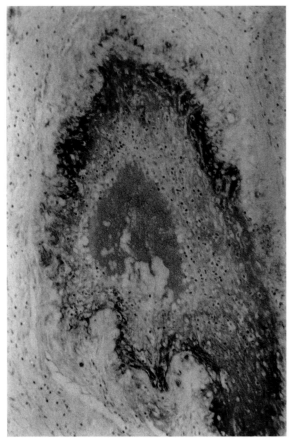

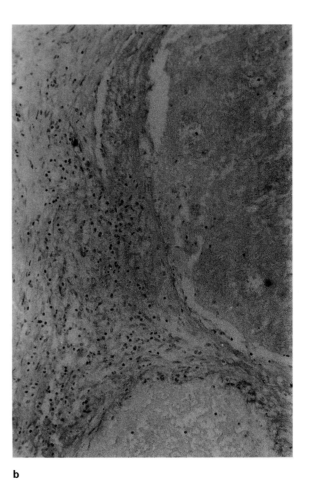

a

b

Fig. 61.7 Paraffin sections of placental bed tissues stained using an immunoperoxidase technique for C1q. **a** shows intense reactivity for C1q in a normally involuted uteroplacental artery while **b** shows lack of reactivity for C1q in subinvoluted vessels. × 100.

normal decidua basalis. Mononuclear and binucleate trophoblast accumulated at the junction of chorionic villi and myometrium while multinucleate trophoblast characteristic of normal third-trimester placental bed was absent. Physiological changes were absent in some spiral arteries but in others extended more deeply than normal, reaching the arcuate system. Features such as hyalinization of myometrium, abnormal extravillous trophoblast and the presence of a mononuclear inflammatory cell infiltrate in interstitial tissues have been considered to reflect varying degrees of destruction of maternal and fetal tissues resulting from loss of the normal balanced interaction between trophoblast and decidua. Excessive migration of extravillous trophoblast in some arteries could reflect a compensatory mechanism for inadequate invasion in others.

The proposal that the morphological features of placenta accreta suggest a disordered maternofetal relationship is compatible with the concept that decidua plays a rôle in the control of trophoblast invasion, deficiency allowing excessive invasion. As far as can be determined from paraffin-embedded tissues, the antigenic phenotype of trophoblast in placenta accreta is similar to that in normal pregnancy (Earl et al, 1987b). Cell populations in residual decidual tissue have not been characterized. Nevertheless, trophoblast invasion in normal pregnancy must be controlled by mechanisms outwith decidua since both interstitial and vascular trophoblast extends into myometrium. Although there have been reports of placenta accreta in early pregnancy (Hutton et al, 1983), the usual postpartum clinical presentation causes practical problems for investigation of pathogenetic mechanisms.

Maternal infection

Placental infection can arise via blood or from endometrium and takes the form of a villitis. Although the histological features of various placental infections have been described, immunopathological investigations are limited. Studies of pregnant mice with listeriosis led to the suggestion that the lack of T cells and macrophages in mouse decidua basalis increases the susceptibility of uteroplacental tissues to infection (Redline & Lu, 1989). Human decidua basalis does not show a comparable T-cell and macrophage deficiency, but the susceptibility of human uteroplacental tissues to infection remains uncertain. Reports of altered systemic immunity during pregnancy are inconsistent and whether pregnant women are at any increased risk of infection is disputed (Brabin, 1985; Hart, 1988). Control data from age-matched non-pregnant women over a given time period in a given geographical location are difficult to obtain, although two large surveys of viral infections in pregnant women do not show an unduly high incidence (Hart, 1988).

There are, however, case histories and early studies which lend support to the concept that virulence of some infections may increase during pregnancy, examples including influenza, cholera, measles, scarlet fever, varicella, diphtheria, gonorrhoea, giardiasis and babesiosis. Other studies have reported a high case fatality rate from certain infections during pregnancy, including hepatitis, amoebic colitis, typhoid, smallpox, coccidioidomycosis, *Plasmodium falciparum* malaria, poliomyelitis, influenza, tuberculosis and pneumonia, although the evidence has been disputed: for example, a severe form of hepatitis observed in pregnant women in the tropics has been related to inadequate maternal nutrition rather than to pregnancy (Brabin, 1985).

Although data concerning the incidence of primary infections during pregnancy compared with non-pregnant controls are sparse, more information is available for recurrent infections. Reactivation of cytomegalovirus (CMV) during pregnancy has been reported, with intrauterine infection occurring in up to 10% of serologically immune women. Excretion of CMV in urine, saliva and cervical secretions continues despite specific antibody and can be detected in 10% of pregnant and non-pregnant women. CMV excretion is suppressed in early pregnancy and rises later in gestation to 'normal' levels. Lymphocyte responses to CMV appear to be depressed during the third trimester of pregnancy (Gehrz et al, 1981). Transformation responses to other agents, including *Candida albicans, Chlamydia trachomatis*, tetanus toxoid and mumps virus, are also depressed in pregnancy compared with the same individuals postpartum and with non-pregnant controls (Brunham et al, 1983).

The effects of gestational age and parity on maternal susceptibility to infection and its effect on the fetus are also unclear. Only a small proportion of infants infected in utero with CMV are clinically ill at birth and infants born to mothers who experience hepatitis early in pregnancy are similarly not infected. The outcome on the infant of maternal infections during pregnancy appears dependent on the timing of infection which, in turn, may affect maternal antibody production. The effect of parity has not been systematically investigated, although infection during pregnancy may increase maternal immunity: a study of over 12 000 UK women showed that CMV seropositivity during pregnancy correlated with increasing parity (Tookey et al, 1992). Placental CMV infection causes a lymphocytic villitis composed predominantly of T cells but sometimes including plasma cells. Hyperplasia of Hofbauer cells in the villous stroma has also been noted (Schwartz et al, 1992). Parvovirus infection of the placenta also causes hyperplasia of Hofbauer cells, which show a significant increase in proliferation compared with normal placentas (Backe et al, 1993).

The frequency of infections during pregnancy merits further investigation. Reactivation of hepatitis B infection has been reported (Rawal et al, 1991) and human papillomavirus DNA has been detected more frequently during pregnancy, although this has been disputed in a recent study of 375 women which used the polymerase chain reaction (Kemp et al, 1992). Recent interest has, however, focused on two infections which cause morbidity and mortality during pregnancy, both for the mother and her infant. Malaria is frequent during pregnancy, even in hyperendemic areas where adults would normally be immune. Human immunodeficiency virus (HIV) can be transmitted from mother to fetus via the placenta resulting in active HIV infection in a significant proportion of offspring.

Malaria infection

Plasmodium falciparum malaria is 4–12 times commoner in pregnant women than in their non-pregnant counterparts. This increased susceptibility has been observed in both hyperendemic and mesoendemic areas and is most prominent in primigravidae, resistance being increasingly regained with multiparity (McGregor et al, 1983; Nosten et al, 1991). Maternal malaria in hyperendemic areas is rarely associated with severe systemic disease but, in mesoendemic areas, can lead to maternal death. Parasites are more numerous and persistent in placental blood compared with the peripheral circulation. Transplacental transmission and congenital malaria is rare but in both hyperendemic and mesoendemic areas maternal *P. falciparum* infection is associated with a high incidence of IUGR and hence with increased neonatal morbidity and mortality.

The reduced birth weight associated with maternal malaria infection has been attributed to placental damage, the classic histological appearance of placental malaria being that of a dense lymphocytic and monocytic infiltrate within the intervillous spaces. There is, however, a spectrum of histological changes ranging from detection of parasites with comparatively little pigment deposition, through the classical picture, to placentas containing malaria pigment deposits only: these appearances may represent progression from an active infection to active-chronic and finally to past-chronic phases (Bulmer et al, 1993a,b).

Evidence of placental damage includes cytotrophoblast prominence, trophoblast basement membrane thickening and fibrinoid necrosis (Fox, 1978; Bulmer et al, 1993b), but the explanation for the decreased birth weight remains uncertain. It has been suggested that the dense mononuclear cell infiltrate in the intervillous spaces may block transplacental nutrient transfer. Immune-mediated placental damage has also been proposed and is supported by the relationship of fibrinoid necrosis of villi to decreased birth weight (Bulmer et al, 1993b) and the detection of increased villous deposition of C1q, C3, C4, C9, fibrinogen and plasminogen (Galbraith et al, 1980). The rôle of cytokines should also be considered. TNFα is important

in the pathogenesis of cerebral malaria. Production of TNFα by maternal monocytes in the intervillous spaces could lead to placental damage by binding to specific TNFα receptors on the villous syncytiotrophoblast (Eades et al, 1988; Hampson et al, 1993). Cytokine networks may also explain the observation that birth weight is reduced even in mesoendemic areas after prompt treatment of malaria in pregnancy (Nosten et al, 1991).

Plasmodium falciparum appears to be selectively retained in the placenta. *P. falciparum* adheres to endothelium via specific adhesion molecules but adherence of parasites to villous syncytiotrophoblast in the delivered placenta has not been demonstrated by electronmicroscopy (Bray & Sinden, 1979). Expression of molecules known to act as malarial adhesion molecules by villous syncytiotrophoblast has not been described, although two of these, ICAM-1 and CD36, can be detected on villous stromal cells, fetal endothelial cells, decidual cells and vessels (Bulmer, Rasheed and Morrison, unpublished) (Fig. 61.8). The vitronectin receptor (CD51/CD61) has also been implicated as an adhesion molecule in malaria and has been localized to syncytiotrophoblast brush border (Vanderpuye et al, 1991). Specific retention of parasites must occur since the rapid blood flow through the intervillous spaces would not favour parasite accumulation.

The high incidence of *P. falciparum* malaria in primigravidae may be due to differing responses of intervillous space lymphocytes: proliferative responses of mononuclear cells separated from the placental intervillous space are lower than those of peripheral blood lymphocytes, and responses to both malaria and candida antigens are significantly lower in primiparae compared with multiparae (Rasheed et al, 1993). Although there may be fundamental immunological differences between first and subsequent pregnancies, these may be accounted for by increased cortisol levels in primiparae. Further studies of infected placental and placental bed tissues may enhance understanding of the pathogenesis and effects of malaria in pregnancy.

Human immunodeficiency virus

Prospective studies have shown that approximately 7–40% of infants born to HIV type 1 seropositive mothers in developed countries become infected with HIV, in some cases early in gestation (Centers for Disease Control, 1990; European Collaborative Study, 1991). Vertical transmission is thought to be transplacental but the exact mechanism is not clear. HIV has been isolated in culture of placentas from seropositive women and HIV core p24 antigens have been localized in Hofbauer cells (Martin et al, 1992; Mattern et al, 1992). Localization of HIV antigens to trophoblast is disputed: despite localization of viral antigen in intermediate trophoblast (Martin et al, 1992) and gp41 by in situ hybridization in first-trimester

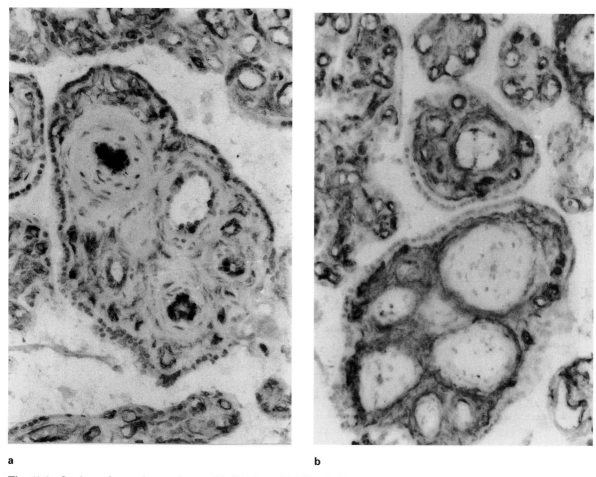

a   b

Fig. 61.8 Sections of normal term placenta labelled for: **a** ICAM-1; **b** CD36. Both these malarial adhesion molecules are expressed by stromal cells and/or endothelial cells in the villous stroma but are not expressed by villous syncytiotrophoblast. × 250.

villous trophoblast (Lewis et al, 1990), cross-reactivity of anti-gp120/160, p25 and p17 HIV antibodies with normal non-infected trophoblast has been reported (Lyden et al, 1993). The confounding effect of normal endogenous type C retroviral particle expression in normal non-infected placentas should also be considered.

The transmission route of HIV across the placenta is also disputed. Hofbauer cells express CD4 throughout gestation (Goldstein et al, 1988) and hence could function as a reservoir of placental HIV. David et al (1992) reported weak expression of CD4 on syncytiotrophoblast, apparently with specific reactivity of trophoblast cells with antibodies to gp120 and gp60 viral envelope protein. Purified placental cells could also be directly infected by HIV in vitro with inhibition by soluble CD4. However, subsequent studies have strongly disputed the expression of CD4 by trophoblast (Lairmore et al, 1993) and infection via Hofbauer cells appears most likely. HIV could also infect human placenta by binding of HIV-anti-HIV IgG immune complexes to syncytiotrophoblast Fcγ receptor. Considerable research is still required to determine

the precise mechanisms of transplacental transmission of HIV with a view to prevention of this major health problem.

Gestational trophoblastic disease

The pathology and genetics of gestational trophoblastic disease (GTD) are discussed elsewhere. Complete hydatidiform moles are diploid and androgenetic and hence fully allogeneic with their maternal host, as are a proportion of choriocarcinomas. It may be anticipated, therefore, that the maternal immune system would play a rôle in eliminating these. However, the protective mechanisms mediated by trophoblast and decidua in normal pregnancy may also operate in molar pregnancy. Although ABO blood group antigens influence the outcome in patients with trophoblastic disease the HLA system does not appear to influence the risk of initial development of a trophoblastic lesion (Bagshawe, 1976; Lawler, 1978). In a large study of patients with GTD, patients with choriocarcinoma had more HLA-compatible offspring than expected and, compared with normal pregnancy, anti-HLA antibodies were detected in a greater proportion of patients with molar pregnancies, in higher titres and persisted for longer (Lawler, 1978).

The mechanisms underlying the excessive trophoblast proliferation in complete and partial molar pregnancy are unknown. The distribution of trophoblast antigens (Fig. 61.9) is very similar to that in normal pregnancy of comparable gestational age. Placental alkaline phosphatase (PLAP) can be detected only in a minority of hydatidiform moles reflecting their evacuation during the first trimester (Berkowitz et al, 1986; Bulmer et al, 1988c). PLAP is normally undetectable in choriocarcinoma: since a proportion of choriocarcinomas follow normal term delivery and arise in the villous placenta (Fox & Laurini, 1988), trophoblast in choriocarcinoma may revert to a less mature phenotype. Further comparison of trophoblast antigens in choriocarcinomas following normal term delivery, molar pregnancy and non-molar abortion would be worthwhile.

Labelling of the villi with a mAb to a characteristic trophoblast antigen, NDOG1, persists later in gestation in molar pregnancy, possibly reflecting failure of development of molar villi. Diffuse extracellular NDOG1 reactivity at the advancing edge of choriocarcinomas is thought to reflect the rôle of hyaluronic acid in disruption of cell matrices and facilitation of invasion (Sunderland et al,

1985a; Bulmer et al, 1988c). Choriocarcinomas show similar antigenic heterogeneity to normal trophoblast and most trophoblast phenotypes identified in normal placentas are also present in choriocarcinomas. Expression of low molecular weight cytokeratins by all normal and neoplastic trophoblast populations may facilitate diagnosis, particularly in the rare placental site trophoblastic tumour (PSTT) which is composed of mononuclear trophoblast. Immunolocalization of placental hormone products may also aid diagnosis: PSTT has a high hPL content and is unreactive with syncytiotrophoblast markers, reflecting its origin from extravillous trophoblast (Kurman et al, 1984; Bulmer et al, 1988c).

Phenotypic differences between molar trophoblast and choriocarcinoma reflect differing behaviour. α_2-macroglobulin and pregnancy protein 4 (PP4) are protease inhibitors which may influence the invasive capacity of trophoblast: both have been detected in normal and molar pregnancy by immunohistochemistry but not in invasive mole and choriocarcinoma (Seppala et al, 1979; Saksela et al, 1981). Differential reactivity for sperm and stage-specific embryonic antigens between choriocarcinomas and hydatidiform moles has also been reported and may reflect more aggressive behaviour (Berkowitz et al, 1985a,b).

Expression of HLA antigens by villous and extravillous trophoblast in hydatidiform mole is similar to that in nor-

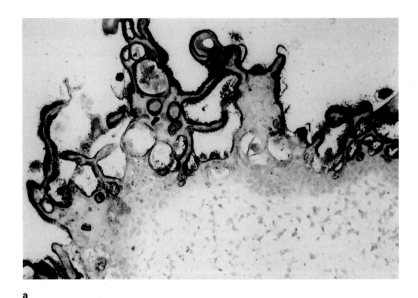

a

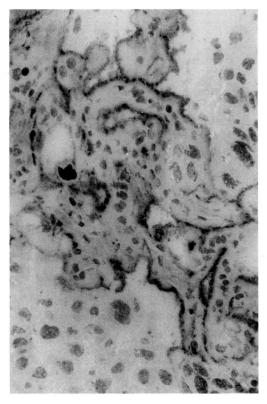

b

Fig. 61.9 a Sections of complete mole stained with a trophoblast-reactive monoclonal antibody NDOG1 showing intense reactivity with villous syncytiotrophoblast. **b** Sections of invasive mole reacted for placental alkaline phosphatase showing focal reactivity with syncytiotrophoblast. **a** × 79; **b** × 180.

mal placentas, with expression by extravillous trophoblast of a restricted polymorphic class I HLA molecule, presumed to be HLA-G (Fisher & Lawler, 1984; Sunderland et al, 1985b; Bulmer et al, 1988c). The class I MHC-positive chorionic villous stroma may represent the site of sensitization to paternal antigens (Lawler & Fisher, 1987). Expression of HLA antigens is comparable in partial, complete and invasive moles (Sasagawa et al, 1987; Bulmer et al, 1988c). Choriocarcinomas also show broadly similar expression of HLA antigens with class I MHC-negative syncytial elements and cytotrophoblast expressing an unusual class I MHC molecule (Sunderland et al, 1985c); and HLA-G has been identified in choriocarcinoma cell lines (Ellis, 1990). Choriocarcinoma is considered to arise from villous trophoblast: HLA-G positive cells could, therefore, reflect an extravillous origin or, more likely, differentiation to an extravillous phenotype following malignant transformation. Class II MHC molecules have not been detected on normal or molar trophoblast or choriocarcinoma cells by immunohistochemistry (Sunderland et al, 1985b,c; Bulmer et al, 1988c) but the GCH-1 choriocarcinoma line can transcribe both α and β class II MHC genes (Takahashi et al, 1987). The MHC antigen expression of PSTT has not yet been reported.

Cytokines, growth factors and their receptors have not been studied in detail in GTD. EGF receptors have been detected on molar trophoblast and the oncogenes c-myc and c-ras have been localized in molar pregnancy and in BeWo cells (Sarkar et al, 1986; Bulmer et al, 1990). The distribution of cytokines and their receptors in GTD has not been well documented but various cytokines exert stimulatory or inhibitory effects on choriocarcinoma cell lines and receptors for GM-CSF and IFNγ have been identified (Berkowitz et al, 1988; Fulop et al, 1992; Sasaki et al, 1992).

There have been few studies of maternal decidua in molar pregnancy. In contrast with normal pregnancy, Berkowitz et al (1982) did not detect complement or immunoglobulin at the implantation site in 10 molar pregnancies. Kabawat et al (1985) reported a fourfold increase in T cells in decidua basalis compared with normal pregnancy, with CD4-positive cells predominating. Endometrial granulated lymphocytes can be identified in paraffin sections of molar pregnancy decidua and CD56-positive cells are present in frozen sections (Bulmer et al, 1988c). Macrophages also form a major leucocytic component at the molar implantation site and are often closely associated with extravillous trophoblast.

Decidua in normal pregnancy produces a wide variety of cytokines which may play a rôle in the control of placental growth and differentiation. Evaluation of possible decidual influences on abnormal trophoblast proliferation in hydatidiform moles will require careful comparison of decidual leucocyte populations and cytokine production between normal and molar pregnancies.

CONCLUSION

Considerable advances have been made over recent years in our understanding of immunobiological mechanisms in both normal and pathological pregnancy. Elucidation of the immunological strategies which have evolved to allow successful development of the feto-placental unit in normal gestation will allow evaluation of the rôle of immune mechanisms in the pathogenesis of pregnancy disorders.

REFERENCES

Abramowsky C R, Vegas M E, Swinehart G, Gyves M T 1980 Decidual vasculopathy of the placenta in lupus erythematosus. New England Journal of Medicine 303: 668–672.
Adinolfi M, Davies A, Sharif S, Soothill P, Rodeck C 1993 Detection of trisomy 18 and Y-derived sequences in fetal nucleated cells obtained by transcervical flushing. Lancet 342: 403–404.
Althabe O, Labarrere C, Telenta M 1985 Maternal vascular lesions in placentae of small-for-gestational-age infants. Placenta 6: 265–276.
Altshuler G, Russell P, Ermocilla R 1975 The placental pathology of small-for-gestational age infants. American Journal of Obstetrics and Gynecology 121: 351–359.
Anderson D J, Johnson P M, Alexander N J, Jones W R, Griffin P D 1987 Monoclonal antibodies to human trophoblast and sperm antigens: report of two WHO-sponsored workshops, 30 June 1986, Toronto. Journal of Reproductive Immunology 10: 231–257.
Andrew A, Bulmer J N, Wells M, Morrison L, Buckley C H 1989 Subinvolution of the uteroplacental arteries in the human placental bed. Histopathology 15: 395–405.
Andrew A, Bulmer J N, Morrison L, Wells M, Buckley C H 1991 Subinvolution of the uteroplacental arteries: an immunohistochemical study. International Journal of Gynecological Pathology 10: 238–251.
Antczak D F, Miller J M, Remick L H 1984 Lymphocyte alloantigens of the horse. II. Antibodies to ELA antigens produced during equine pregnancy. Journal of Reproductive Immunology 6: 283–297.

Aplin J D 1993 Expression of integrin $\alpha6\beta4$ in human trophoblast and its loss from extravillous cells. Placenta 14: 203–215.
Aplin J D, Ayad S, Charlton A K 1988 An immunohistochemical study of human endometrial extracellular matrix during the menstrual cycle and the first trimester of pregnancy. Cell and Tissue Research 253: 231–240.
Attwood H D, Park W W 1961 Embolism to the lungs by trophoblast. Journal of Obstetrics and Gynaecology of the British Commonwealth 68: 611–617.
Backe E, Schwartz D, Zhang W, Panigel M, Lee F, Nahmias A 1993 Double immunolabelling to detect the proliferation of Hofbauer cells in normal and parvovirus infected placentas. Placenta 14: A3.
Bagshawe K D 1976 Risk and prognostic factors in trophoblastic neoplasia. Cancer 38: 1373–1385.
Bell S C 1991 The insulin-like growth factor binding proteins — the endometrium and decidua. Annals of the New York Academy of Sciences 622: 120–137.
Bell S C, Billington W D 1983 Anti-fetal alloantibody in the pregnant female. Immunological Reviews 75: 5–30.
Berkowitz R S, Mostoufi-Zadeh M, Kabawat S E, Goldstein D P, Driscoll S G 1982 Immunopathologic study of the implantation site in molar pregnancy. American Journal of Obstetrics and Gynecology 144: 925–930.
Berkowitz R S, Alberti O, Hunter N J, Goldstein D P, Anderson D J

1985a Localization of stage-specific embryonic antigens in hydatidiform mole, normal placenta and gestational choriocarcinoma. Gynecologic Oncology 20: 71–77.

Berkowitz R S, Alexander N J, Goldstein D P, Anderson D J 1985b Reactivity of anti-human sperm monoclonal antibodies with normal placenta, hydatidiform mole and gestational choriocarcinoma. Gynecologic Oncology 22: 334–340.

Berkowitz R S, Umpierre S A, Johnson P M, McIntyre J A, Anderson D J 1986 Expression of trophoblast-leukocyte common antigens and placental-type alkaline phosphatase in complete molar pregnancy. American Journal of Obstetrics and Gynecology 155: 443–446.

Berkowitz R S, Hill J A, Kurtz C B, Anderson D J 1988 Effects of products of activated leukocytes (lymphokines and monokines) on the growth of malignant trophoblast cells in vitro. American Journal of Obstetrics and Gynecology 158: 199–203.

Billington W D 1988 Maternal-fetal interactions in normal human pregnancy. Baillière's Clinical Immunology and Allergy 2: 527–549.

Bishop P W, Fox H, Morris J A, Malam J 1988 The expression of CA (Oxford) antigen by placental trophoblast in pre-eclampsia and hypertension. Journal of Pathology 154: 103A–104A.

Boucrat J, Hawley S, Robertson K, Bernard D, Loke Y W, Bouteiller P L 1993 Differential nuclear expression of enhancer A DNA-binding proteins in human first trimester trophoblast cells. Journal of Immunology 150: 3882–3894.

Boyd J D, Hamilton W J 1970 The human placenta. Heffer, Cambridge.

Brabin B J 1985 Epidemiology of infection in pregnancy. Reviews of Infectious Diseases 7: 579–603.

Brandtzaeg P, Christiansen E, Muller F, Purvis K 1993 Humoral immune response patterns of human mucosae, including the reproductive tracts. In: Griffin P D, Johnson P M (eds) Local immunity in reproductive tract tissues. Oxford University Press, Oxford, pp 97–130.

Braunhut S J, Blanc W A, Ramanarayanan M, Marboe C, Mesa-Tejada R 1984 Immunocytochemical localization of lysozyme and alpha-1-antichymotrypsin in the term human placenta: an attempt to characterize the Hofbauer cell. Journal of Histochemistry and Cytochemistry 32: 1204–1210.

Bray R S, Sinden R E 1979 The sequestration of Plasmodium falciparum infected erythrocytes in the placenta. Transactions of the Royal Society of Tropical Medicine and Hygiene 73: 716–719.

Brosens I, Dixon H G, Robertson W B 1977 Fetal growth retardation and the arteries of the placental bed. British Journal of Obstetrics and Gynaecology 84: 656–663.

Brunham R C, Martin D H, Hubbart T W et al 1983 Depression of the lymphocyte transformation response to microbial antigens and phytohemagglutinin during pregnancy. Journal of Clinical Investigation 72: 1629–1638.

Bulmer J N 1992 Immune aspects of pathology of the placental bed contributing to pregnancy pathology. Baillière's Clinical Obstetrics and Gynaecology 6: 461–488.

Bulmer J N, Earl U 1987 The expression of class II MHC gene products by fallopian tube epithelium in pregnancy and throughout the menstrual cycle. Immunology 61: 207–213.

Bulmer J N, Johnson P M 1984 Macrophage populations in the human placenta and amniochorion. Clinical and Experimental Immunology 57: 393–403.

Bulmer J N, Johnson P M 1985a Antigen expression by trophoblast populations in the human placenta and their possible immunobiological relevance. Placenta 6: 127–149.

Bulmer J N, Johnson P M 1985b Immunohistological characterization of the decidual leucocytic infiltrate related to endometrial gland epithelium in early human pregnancy. Immunology 55: 35–44.

Bulmer J N, Johnson P M 1986 The T lymphocyte population in first-trimester human decidua does not express the interleukin-2 receptor. Immunology 58: 685–687.

Bulmer J N, Sunderland C A 1984 Immunohistological identification of lymphoid populations in the early human placental bed. Immunology 52: 349–357.

Bulmer J N, Hollings D, Ritson A 1987a Immunocytochemical evidence that endometrial stromal granulocytes are granulated lymphocytes. Journal of Pathology 153: 281–288.

Bulmer J N, Ritson A, Earl U, Hollings D 1987b Immunocompetent

cells in human decidua. In: Chaouat G (ed) Reproductive immunology: materno-fetal relationship. Inserm, Paris, pp 89–100.

Bulmer J N, Morrison L, Smith J C 1988a Expression of Class II MHC gene products by macrophages in human uteroplacental tissues. Immunology 63: 707–714.

Bulmer J N, Smith J, Morrison L, Wells M 1988b Maternal and fetal cellular relationships in the human placental basal plate. Placenta 9: 237–246.

Bulmer J N, Johnson P M, Sasagawa M, Takeuchi S 1988c Immunohistochemical studies of fetal trophoblast and maternal decidua in hydatidiform mole and choriocarcinoma. Placenta 9: 183–200.

Bulmer J N, Thrower S, Wells M 1990 Expression of epidermal growth factor receptor and transferrin receptor by human trophoblast populations. American Journal of Reproductive Immunology 21: 87–93.

Bulmer J N, Morrison L, Longfellow M, Ritson A, Pace D 1991a Granulated lymphocytes in human endometrium: histochemical and immunohistochemical studies. Human Reproduction 6: 791–798.

Bulmer J N, Morrison L, Longfellow M, Ritson A 1991b Leucocytes in human decidua: investigations of surface markers and function. In: Chaouat G (ed) Materno-fetal relationship: molecular and cell biology. John Libbey Eurotext, Paris, pp 189–196.

Bulmer J N, Longfellow M, Ritson A 1991c Leukocytes and resident blood cells in endometrium. Annals of the New York Academy of Sciences 622: 57–68.

Bulmer J N, Rasheed F N, Francis N, Morrison L, Greenwood B M 1993a Placental malaria. I. Pathological classification. Histopathology 22: 211–218.

Bulmer J N, Rasheed F N, Morrison L, Francis N, Greenwood B M 1993b Placental malaria. II. A semiquantitative investigation of the pathological features. Histopathology 22: 219–225.

Burrows T D, King A, Loke Y W 1993 Expression of adhesion molecules by human decidual large granular lymphocytes. Cellular Immunology 147: 81–94.

Carding S R, Kyes S, Jenkinson E J, Kingston R, Bottomly K, Owen J J T, Hayday A C 1990 Developmentally regulated fetal thymic and extrathymic T-cell receptor γδ gene expression. Genes and Development 4: 1304–1315.

Centers for Disease Control 1990 HIV prevalence estimates and AIDS case projections for the United States. Morbidity and Mortality Weekly Report 39 RR 16: 1–31.

Chaouat G, Menu E, Clark D, Dy M, Minkowski M, Wegmann T G 1990 Control of fetal survival in CBA × DBA/2 mice by lymphokine therapy. Journal of Reproduction and Fertility 89: 447–458.

Chemnitz J, Tornehave D, Teisner B, Poulsen H K, Westergaard J G 1984 The localization of pregnancy proteins (hPL, SP1 and PAPP-A) in intra- and extrauterine pregnancies. Placenta 5: 489–494.

Chen H-L, Yang Y, Hu X-L, Yelavarthi K K, Fishback J L, Hunt J S 1991 Tumor necrosis factor alpha mRNA and protein are present in human placental and uterine cells at early and late stages of gestation. American Journal of Pathology 139: 327–335.

Christmas S E 1991 T-cell receptor gene expression by human γδ T cell clones from peripheral blood and reproductive tissues in relation to non-MHC-restricted cytotoxic function. Scandinavian Journal of Immunology 33: 627–637.

Christmas S E, Bulmer J N, Meager A, Johnson P M 1990 Phenotypic and functional analysis of human CD3– decidual leucocyte clones. Immunology 71: 182–189.

Chua S, Wilkins T, Sargent I, Redman C 1991 Trophoblast deportation in pre-eclamptic pregnancy. British Journal of Obstetrics and Gynaecology 98: 973–979.

Chumbley G, King A, Robertson K, Holmes N, Loke Y W 1994 Resistance of HLA-G and HLA-A2 transfectants to lysis by decidual NK cells. Cellular Immunology 155: 312–322.

Clark D A, Flanders K C, Banwatt D et al 1990 Murine pregnancy decidua produces a unique immunosuppressive molecule related to transforming growth factor β-2. Journal of Immunology 144: 3008–3014.

Clark D A, Lea R G, Underwood J et al 1992 A subset of recurrent first trimester-aborting women show subnormal TGF-β2 suppressor activity at the implantation site associated with miscarriage. Journal of Immunology and Immunopharmacology XII: 82.

Contractor S F 1983 Metabolic and enzymatic activity of human trophoblast. In: Loke Y W, Whyte A (eds) Biology of trophoblast. Elsevier, Amsterdam, pp 236–316.

Coutifaris C, Kao L-C, Schdev H M, Chin U, Babalola G O, Blaschuk O W, Strauss J F III 1991 E-cadherin expression during the differentiation of human trophoblasts. Development 113: 767–777.

Crepeau M A, Croy B A 1988 Evidence that specific cellular immunity cannot account for death of *mus caroli* embryos transferred to *mus musculus* with severe combined immune deficiency disease. Transplantation 45: 1104–1110.

Croy B A, Stewart C M, McBey B-A, Kiso Y 1993 An immunohistologic analysis of murine uterine T cells between birth and puberty. Journal of Reproductive Immunology 23: 223–233.

Daiter E, Pampfer S, Yeung Y G, Barad D, Stanley E R, Pollard J W 1992 Expression of colony-stimulating factor-1 in the human uterus and placenta. Journal of Clinical Endocrinology and Metabolism 74: 850–858.

Dallenbach-Hellweg G 1987 The normal histology of the endometrium. In: Histopathology of the endometrium. Springer-Verlag, Berlin, pp 25–92.

Dalton A J, Hellman A, Kalter S S, Helmke R J 1974 Ultrastructural comparison of placental virus with several type-C oncogenic viruses. Journal of the National Cancer Institute 52: 987–989.

Damsky C H, Fitzgerald M L, Fisher S J 1992 Distribution patterns of extracellular matrix components and adhesion receptors are intricately modulated during first trimester cytotrophoblast differentiation along the invasive pathway in vivo. Journal of Clinical Investigation 89: 210–222.

David F J E, Autran B, Tran H C et al 1992 Human trophoblast cells express CD4 and are permissive for productive infection with HIV-1. Clinical and Experimental Immunology 88: 10–16.

Davies M, Browne C M 1985 Pregnancy-associated nonspecific immunosuppression: mechanism for the activation of the immunosuppessive factors. American Journal of Reproductive Immunology and Microbiology 9: 84–90.

De Fougerolles A R, Baines M G 1987 Modulation of the natural killer cell activity in pregnant mice alters the spontaneous abortion rate. Journal of Reproductive Immunology 11: 147–153.

Deniz G, Christmas S E, Brew R, Johnson P M 1994 Phenotypic and functional cellular differences between human CD3– decidual and peripheral blood lymphocytes. Journal of Immunology 152: 4255–4261.

De Wolf F, Brosens I, Renaer M 1980 Fetal growth retardation and the maternal arterial supply of the human placenta in the absence of sustained hypertension. British Journal of Obstetrics and Gynaecology 87: 678–685.

Dietl J, Horny H P, Ruck P et al 1990 Intradecidual T lymphocytes lack immunohistochemically detectable T-cell receptors. American Journal of Reproductive Immunology 24: 33–36.

Dietl J, Ruck P, Marzusch K, Horny H-P, Kaiserling E, Handgretinger R 1992 Uterine granular lymphocytes are activated natural killer cells expressing VLA-1. Immunology Today 13: 236.

Dorman P J, Searle R F 1988 Alloantigen presenting capacity of human decidual tissue. Journal of Reproductive Immunology 13: 101–112.

Eades D K, Cornelius P, Pekala P H 1988 Characterization of the tumour necrosis factor receptor in human placenta. Placenta 9: 247–251.

Earl U, Wells M, Bulmer J N 1985 The expression of major histocompatibility complex antigens by trophoblast in ectopic tubal pregnancy. Journal of Reproductive Immunology 8: 13–24.

Earl U, Wells M, Bulmer J N 1986 Immunohistochemical characterization of trophoblast membrane antigens and secretory products in ectopic tubal pregnancy. International Journal of Gynecological Pathology 5: 132–142.

Earl U, Lunny D P, Bulmer J N 1987a Leucocyte populations in ectopic tubal pregnancy. Journal of Clinical Pathology 40: 901–915.

Earl U, Bulmer J N, Briones A 1987b Placenta accreta: an immunohistological study of trophoblast populations. Placenta 8: 273–282.

Earl U, Morrison L, Gray C, Bulmer J N 1989 Proteinase and proteinase-inhibitor localization in the human placenta. International Journal of Gynecological Pathology 8: 114–124.

Ellis S 1990 HLA G: at the interface. American Journal of Reproductive Immunology 23: 84–86.

Ellis S A, Palmer M S, McMichael A J 1990 Human trophoblast and the choriocarcinoma cell line BeWo express a truncated HLA class I molecule. Journal of Immunology 144: 731–735.

European Collaborative Study 1991 Children born to women with HIV-1 infection: natural history and risk of transmission. Lancet 337: 253–260.

Faulk W P, Johnson P M 1977 Immunological studies of human placentae: identification and distribution of proteins in mature chorionic villi. Clinical and Experimental Immunology 27: 365–375.

Feinberg R F, Kao L-C, Hamiowitz J E et al 1989 Plasminogen activator inhibitor types 1 and 2 in human trophoblasts. Laboratory Investigation 61: 20–26.

Ferry B L, Starkey P M, Sargent I L, Watt G M O, Jackson M, Redman C W G 1990 Cell populations in the human early pregnancy decidua: natural killer activity and response to interleukin-2 of CD56-positive large granular lymphocytes. Immunology 70: 446–452.

Ferry B L, Sargent I I, Starkey P M, Redman C W G 1991 Cytotoxic activity against trophoblast and choriocarcinoma cells of large granular lymphocytes from human early pregnancy decidua. Cellular Immunology 132: 140–149.

Fisher R A, Lawler S D 1984 The expression of major histocompatibility antigens in the chorionic villi of molar placentae. Placenta 5: 237–242.

Fox H 1978 Pathology of the placenta. W.B. Saunders, London.

Fox H, Jones C J P 1983 Pathology of trophoblast. In: Loke Y W, Whyte A (eds) Biology of trophoblast. Elsevier, Amsterdam, pp 137–185.

Fox H, Kharkongor N F 1969 Enzyme histochemistry of the Hofbauer cells of the human placenta. Journal of Obstetrics and Gynaecology of the British Commonwealth 76: 918–921.

Fox H, Laurini R N 1988 Intraplacental choriocarcinoma: a report of two cases. Journal of Clinical Pathology 41: 1085–1088.

Fraser E J, Grimes D A, Schultz K F 1993 Immunization as a therapy for recurrent spontaneous abortion: a review and meta-analysis. Obstetrics and Gynecology 82: 854–859.

Fulop V, Steller M A, Berkowitz R S, Anderson D J 1992 Interferon-γ receptors on human gestational choriocarcinoma cell lines: quantitative and functional studies. American Journal of Obstetrics and Gynecology 167: 524–530.

Galbraith R M, Fox H, Hsi B-L, Galbraith G M P, Bray R S, Faulk W P 1980 The human materno-foetal relationship in malaria. II. Histological, ultrastructural and immunopathological studies of the placenta. Transactions of the Royal Society of Tropical Medicine and Hygiene 74: 61–72.

Gehrz R C, Christianson W R, Linner K M, Conroy M M, McCue S A, Balfour H H 1981 A longitudinal analysis of lymphocyte proliferative responses to mitogens and antigens during human pregnancy. American Journal of Obstetrics and Gynecology 140: 665–670.

Gendron R L, Baines M G 1988 Infiltrating decidual natural killer cells are associated with spontaneous abortion in mice. Cellular Immunology 113: 261–267.

Gendron R L, Nestel F B, Lapp W S, Baines M G 1990 Lipopolysaccharide-induced fetal resorption in mice is associated with the intrauterine production of tumour necrosis factor-alpha. Journal of Reproduction and Fertility 90: 395–402.

Gerretsen G, Huisjes H J, Hardonk M J, Elema J D 1983 Trophoblast alterations in the placental bed in relation to physiological changes in spiral arteries. British Journal of Obstetrics and Gynaecology 90: 34–39.

Gogolin-Ewens K J, Lee C S, Mercer W R, Brandon M R 1989 Site-directed differences in the immune response to the fetus. Immunology 66: 312–317.

Goldstein J, Braverman M, Salafia C, Buckley P 1988 The phenotype of human placental macrophages and its variation with gestational age. American Journal of Pathology 133: 648–659.

Goodfellow C F, Taylor P V 1982 Extraction and identification of trophoblast cells in peripheral blood during pregnancy. British Journal of Obstetrics and Gynaecology 89: 65–68.

Graham C H, Lysiak J J, McRae K R, Lala P K 1992 Localization of transforming growth factor-β at the human fetal-maternal interface: role in trophoblast growth and differentiation. Biology of Reproduction 46: 562–571.

Griffith-Jones M D, Miller D, Lilford R J, Bulmer J N, Scott J 1992 First trimester trans-cervical cell retrieval (TraCeR) for atraumatic retrieval of trophoblast for the prenatal diagnosis of single gene defects in the fetus. British Journal of Obstetrics and Gynaecology 99: 508–511.

Hampson J, McLaughlin P J, Johnson P M 1993 Low-affinity receptors for tumour necrosis factor-α, interferon-γ and granulocyte-macrophage colony-stimulating factor are expressed on human placental syncytiotrophoblast. Immunology 79: 485–490.

Hart C A 1988 Pregnancy and host resistance. Baillière's Clinical Immunology and Allergy 2: 735–757.

Head J R 1989 Can trophoblast be killed by cytotoxic cells? In vitro evidence and in vivo possibilities. American Journal of Reproductive Immunology 15: 12–18.

Heyborne K D, Cranfill R L, Carding S R, Born W K, O'Brien R L 1992 Characterization of γδ T lymphocytes at the maternal-fetal interface. Journal of Immunology 149: 2872–2878.

Hill J A 1990 Immunological mechanisms of pregnancy maintenance and failure: a critique of theories and therapy. American Journal of Reproductive Immunology 22: 33–42.

Hole N, Cheng H M, Johnson P M 1987 Antibody reactivity against human trophoblast membrane antigens in the context of normal pregnancy and unexplained recurrent miscarriage. Colloque INSERM 154: 213–224.

Holmes C H, Simpson K L, Wainwright S H et al 1990 Preferential expression of the complement regulatory protein decay accelerating factor at the fetomaternal interface during human pregnancy. Journal of Immunology 144: 3099–3105.

Holmes C H, Simpson K L, Okada H et al 1992 Complement regulatory proteins at the feto-maternal interface during human placental development: distribution of CD59 by comparison with membrane cofactor protein (CD46) and decay accelerating factor (CD55). European Journal of Immunology 22: 1579–1585.

Hsi B-L, Johnson P M 1992 Monoclonal antibodies to human trophoblast: a workshop report. Trophoblast Research 6: 125–134.

Hsi B-L, Yeh C-J G, Faulk W P 1984 Class I antigens of the major histocompatibility complex on cytotrophoblast of human chorion laeve. Immunology 52: 621–629.

Hsi B-L, Hunt J S, Atkinson J P 1991 Differential expression of complement regulatory proteins on subpopulations of human trophoblast cells. Journal of Reproductive Immunology 19: 209–223.

Hunt J S 1989 Cytokine networks in the uteroplacental unit: macrophages as pivotal regulatory cells. Journal of Reproductive Immunology 16: 1–17.

Hunt J S, Andrews G K, Wood G W 1987 Normal trophoblasts resist induction of class I HLA. Journal of Immunology 138: 2481–2487.

Hunziker R D, Gambel P, Wegmann T G 1984 Placenta as a selective barrier to cellular traffic. Journal of Immunology 133: 667–671.

Hustin J, Foidart J M, Lambotte R 1983 Maternal vascular lesions in pre-eclampsia and intrauterine growth retardation: light microscopy and immunofluorescence. Placenta 4: 489–498.

Hutton L, Yang S S, Bernstein J 1983 Placenta accreta: a 26-year clinicopathologic review (1956–1981). New York State Journal of Medicine 83: 857–866.

Itohara S, Farr A G, Lafaille J J et al 1990 Homing of γδ thymocyte subset with homogeneous T-cell receptors to mucosal epithelia. Nature 343: 754–757.

Jenkins D M, O'Neill M, Johnson P M 1983 HLA-DR positive cells in the human amniochorion. Immunology Letters 6: 65–67.

Johnson P M 1989 Immunology of pregnancy. In: Turnbull A C, Chamberlain G V P (eds) Obstetrics. Churchill Livingstone, Edinburgh, pp 173–187.

Johnson P M 1991 Trophoblast membrane antigens for contragestational vaccine development. In: Runnebaum B, Rabe T, Kiesel L (eds) Female contraception and male fertility regulation. Parthenon Press, Carnforth, pp 115–122.

Johnson P M 1992 Immunology of human extraembryonic fetal membranes. In: Coulam C B, McIntyre J A, Faulk W P (eds) Immunological obstetrics. W W Norton, Philadelphia, pp 177–188.

Johnson P M, Brown P J 1981 Fcγ receptors in the human placenta. Placenta 2: 355–370.

Johnson P M, Bulmer J N 1984 Uterine gland epithelium in human pregnancy often lacks detectable maternal MHC antigens but does express fetal trophoblast antigens. Journal of Immunology 132: 1608–1610.

Johnson P M, Stern P L 1986 Antigen expression at human materno-fetal interfaces. Progress in Immunology 6: 1056–1059.

Johnson P M, Natvig J B, Ystehede U A, Faulk W P 1977 Immunological studies of human placentae: the distribution and character of immunoglobulins in chorionic villi. Clinical and Experimental Immunology 30: 145–153.

Johnson P M, Arnaud P, Werner P, Galbraith R M 1985 Native α₂-macroglobulin binds to a surface component of human placental trophoblast. Placenta 6: 323–328.

Johnson P M, Risk J M, Bulmer J N, Niewola Z, Kimber I 1987 Antigen expression at human materno-fetal interfaces. In: Wegmann T G, Gill T J III (eds) Maternal immunoregulation and fetal survival. Oxford University Press, New York, pp 181–196.

Johnson P M, Lyden T W, Mwenda J M 1990 Endogenous retroviral expression in the human placenta. American Journal of Reproductive Immunology 23: 115–120.

Kabawat S E, Mostoufi-Zadeh M, Berkowitz R S, Driscoll S G, Goldstein D P, Bhan A K 1985 Implantation site in complete molar pregnancy: a study of immunologically competent cells with monoclonal antibodies. American Journal of Obstetrics and Gynecology 152: 97–99.

Kalter S S, Helmke R J, Heberling R L et al 1973 C-type retrovirus particles in normal human placentas. Journal of the National Cancer Institute 50: 1081–1084.

Kamat B R, Isaacson P G 1987 The immunocytochemical distribution of leukocytic subpopulations in human endometrium. American Journal of Pathology 127: 66–73.

Kemp E A, Hakenewerth A M, Laurent S L, Gravitt P E, Stoerker J 1992 Human papillomavirus prevalence in pregnancy. Obstetrics and Gynecology 79: 649–656.

Khong T Y 1987 Immunohistologic study of the leukocytic infiltrate in maternal uterine tissues in normal and pre-eclamptic pregnancies at term. American Journal of Reproductive Immunology and Microbiology 15: 1–8.

Khong T Y, Chambers H M 1992 Alternative method of sampling placentas for the assessment of uteroplacental vasculature. Journal of Clinical Pathology 45: 925–927.

Khong T Y, Robertson W B 1987 Placenta creta and placenta praevia creta. Placenta 8: 399–409.

Khong T Y, De Wolf F, Robertson W B, Brosens I 1986 Inadequate maternal vascular response to placentation in pregnancies complicated by pre-eclampsia and by small-for-gestational age infants. British Journal of Obstetrics and Gynaecology 93: 1049–1059.

Khong T Y, Liddell H S, Robertson W B 1987 Defective haemochorial placentation as a cause of miscarriage: a preliminary study. British Journal of Obstetrics and Gynaecology 94: 649–655.

King A, Loke Y W 1988 Differential expression of blood-group-related carbohydrate antigens by trophoblast subpopulations. Placenta 9: 513–521.

King A, Loke Y W 1990 Human trophoblast and JEG choriocarcinoma cells are sensitive to lysis by IL2-stimulated decidual NK cells. Cellular Immunology 129: 435–448.

King A, Loke Y W 1991 On the nature and function of human uterine granular lymphocytes. Immunology Today 12: 432–435.

King A, Birkby C, Loke Y W 1989 Early human decidual cells exhibit NK activity against the K562 cell line but not against first trimester trophoblast. Cellular Immunology 118: 337–344.

King A, Wooding N B P, Carter N P, Loke Y W 1991 CD3⁻ leukocytes present in the human uterus during early placentation: phenotypic and morphologic characterization of the CD56⁺⁺ population. Developmental Immunology 1: 169–190.

Kitzmiller J L, Benirschke K 1973 Immunofluorescent study of placental bed vessels in pre-eclampsia of pregnancy. American Journal of Obstetrics and Gynecology 115: 248–251.

Kitzmiller J L, Watt N, Driscoll S G 1981 Decidual arteriopathy in hypertension and diabetes in pregnancy: immunofluorescent studies. American Journal of Obstetrics and Gynecology 141: 773–779.

Klentzeris L D, Bulmer J N, Li T-C, Morrison L, Warren A, Cooke I D 1991 Lectin binding of endometrium in women with unexplained infertility. Fertility and Sterility 56: 660–667.

Klentzeris L D, Bulmer J N, Warren A, Morrison L, Li T-C, Cooke I D 1992 Endometrial lymphoid tissue in the timed endometrial biopsy: morphometric and immunohistochemical aspects. American Journal of Obstetrics and Gynecology 167: 667–674.

Konoeda Y, Terasaki P I, Wakisaka A, Park M S, Mickey M R 1986 Public determinants of HLA indicated by pregnancy antibodies. Transplantation 41: 253–259.

Korhonen M, Ylanne J, Laitinen L, Cooper H M, Quaranta V, Virtanen I 1991 Distribution of the α1–α6 integrin subunits in human developing and term placenta. Laboratory Investigation 65: 347–356.

Kovats S, Main E K, Librach C, Stubblebine M, Fisher S J, DeMars R 1990 A class I antigen, HLA-G, expressed in human trophoblasts. Science 248: 220–223.

Kurman R J, Young R H, Norris H J et al 1984 Immunocytochemical localization of placental lactogen and chorionic gonadotrophin in the normal placenta and trophoblastic tumors, with emphasis on intermediate trophoblast and the placental site trophoblastic tumor. International Journal of Gynecological Pathology 3: 101–121.

Kutteh W H, Mestecky J 1994 Secretory immunity in the female reproductive tract. American Journal of Reproductive Immunology 31: 10–16.

Labarrere C, Althabe O 1985 Chronic villitis of unknown etiology and maternal arterial lesions in preeclamptic pregnancies. European Journal of Obstetrics, Gynecology and Reproductive Biology 20: 1–11.

Labarrere C, Althabe O 1987 Chronic villitis of unknown aetiology in recurrent intrauterine fetal growth retardation. Placenta 8: 167–173.

Labarrere C, Althabe O, Telenta M 1982 Chronic villitis of unknown aetiology in placentae of idiopathic small for gestational age infants. Placenta 3: 309–318.

Labarrere C, Alonso J, Manni J, Domenichini E, Althabe O 1985 Immunohistochemical findings in acute atherosis associated with intrauterine growth retardation. American Journal of Reproductive Immunology and Microbiology 7: 149–155.

Labarrere C A, Catoggio L J, Mullen E G, Althabe O H 1986 Placental lesions in maternal autoimmune diseases. American Journal of Reproductive Immunology and Microbiology 12: 78–86.

Labarrere C A, McIntyre J A, Faulk W P 1990 Immunohistologic evidence that villitis in human normal term placentas is an immunologic lesion. American Journal of Obstetrics and Gynecology 162: 515–522.

Lairmore M D, Cuthbert P S, Utley L L et al 1993 Cellular localization of CD4 in the human placenta. Journal of Immunology 151: 1673–1681.

Lalani E-N M A, Bulmer J N, Wells M 1987 Peroxidase-labelled lectin binding of human extravillous trophoblast. Placenta 8: 15–26.

Lanier L L, Le A M, Civin C I, Loken M R, Phillips J H 1986 The relationship of CD16 (leu 11) and leu 19 (NKH1) antigen expression on human peripheral blood NK cells and cytotoxic T lymphocytes. Journal of Immunology 136: 4480–4486.

Larkin L H 1974 Bioassay of rat metrial gland extracts for relaxin using the mouse interpubic ligament technique. Endocrinology 94: 567–570.

Laurini R N, Visser G H A, Van Ballegooie E, Schoots C J F 1987 Morphological findings in placentae of insulin-dependent diabetic patients treated with continuous subcutaneous insulin infusion. Placenta 8: 153–165.

Lawler S D 1978 HLA and trophoblastic tumours. British Medical Bulletin 34: 305–308.

Lawler S D, Fisher R A 1987 Immunogenicity of hydatidiform mole. Placenta 8: 195–199.

Lee C S, Gogolin-Ewens K, Brandon M R 1988 Identification of a unique lymphocyte subpopulation in the sheep uterus. Immunology 63: 157–164.

Lee E T C, Marley N J E, Bevan J R 1986 A rare late complication of first trimester induced abortion requiring hysterectomy —

subinvolution of the placental bed. British Journal of Obstetrics and Gynaecology 93: 777–781.

Lewis S H, Reynolds-Kohler C, Fox H E, Nelson J A 1990 HIV-1 trophoblastic and villous Hofbauer cells, and haematological precursors in eight-week fetuses. Lancet 335: 565–568.

Lichtig C, Deutsch M, Brandes J 1985 Immunofluorescent studies of the endometrial arteries in the first trimester of pregnancy. American Journal of Clinical Pathology 83: 633–636.

Loke Y W, Eremin P, Ashby J, Day S 1982 Characterization of the phagocytic cells isolated from the human placenta. Journal of the Reticuloendothelial Society 31: 317–324.

Loke Y W, Gardner L, Burland K, King A 1989 Laminin in human trophoblast-decidua interaction. Human Reproduction 4: 457–463.

Lyden T W, Johnson P M, Mwenda J M, Rote N S 1993 Immunolocalization of HIV-1 cross-reactive placental proteins in the normal non-infected human decidua and basal plate. Placenta 14: A46.

McDicken I W, McLaughlin P J, Tromans P M, Luesley D M, Johnson P M 1985 Detection of placental-type alkaline phosphatase in ovarian cancer. British Journal of Cancer 52: 59–64.

McGregor I A, Wilson M E, Billewicz W Z 1983 Malaria infection of the placenta in The Gambia, West Africa; its incidence and relationship to stillbirth, birthweight and placental weight. Transactions of the Royal Society of Tropical Medicine and Hygiene 77: 232–244.

McLaughlin P J, Cheng M H, Slade M B, Johnson P M 1982 Expression on cultured human tumour cells of placental trophoblast membrane antigens and placental alkaline phosphatase defined by monoclonal antibodies. International Journal of Cancer 30: 21–26.

McLaughlin P J, Lewis-Jones D I, Hutchinson G E, Johnson P M 1986 Placental-type alkaline phosphatase in human seminal plasma from fertile and infertile males. Fertility and Sterility 46: 934–937.

Manaseki S, Searle R F 1989 Natural killer (NK) cell activity of first trimester human decidua. Cellular Immunology 121: 166–173.

Martin A W, Brady K, Smith S I et al 1992 Immunohistochemical localization of human immunodeficiency virus p24 antigen in placental tissue. Human Pathology 23: 411–414.

Marzusch K, Ruck P, Geiselhart A et al 1993 Distribution of cell adhesion molecules on CD56++, CD3–, CD16– large granular lymphocytes and endothelial cells in first-trimester human decidua. Human Reproduction 8: 1203–1208.

Matsui S, Yoshimura N, Oka T 1989 Characterization and analysis of soluble suppressor factor from early human decidual cells. Transplantation 47: 678–683.

Mattern C F, Murray K, Jensen A, Farzagden H, Pang J, Modlin J F 1992 Localization of human immunodeficiency virus core antigen in term human placentas. Pediatrics 89: 207–209.

Meri S, Waldmann H, Lachmann P J 1991 Distribution of protectin (CD59), a complement membrane attack inhibitor, in normal human tissues. Laboratory Investigation 65: 532–537.

Michel M, Underwood J, Clark D A, Mowbray J, Beard R W 1989 Histologic and immunologic study of uterine biopsy tissue of women with incipient abortion. American Journal of Obstetrics and Gynecology 161: 409–414.

Michel M Z, Khong T Y, Clark D A, Beard R W 1990 A morphological and immunological study of human placental bed biopsies in miscarriages. British Journal of Obstetrics and Gynaecology 97: 984–988.

Mitchell M D, Trautman M S, Dudley D J 1993 Cytokine networking in the placenta. Placenta 14: 249–275.

Morii T, Nishikawa K, Saito S et al 1993 T-cell receptors are expressed but down-regulated on intradecidual T lymphocytes. American Journal of Reproductive Immunology 29: 1–4.

Morrison L 1992 Studies of the granules, phenotypic heterogeneity and distribution of endometrial granulated lymphocytes. MPhil Thesis, University of Leeds.

Mueller U W, Hawes C S, Wright A E et al 1990 Isolation of fetal trophoblast cells from peripheral blood of pregnant women. Lancet 336: 197–200.

Mues B, Langer D, Zwadlo G, Sorg C 1989 Phenotypic characterization of macrophages in human term placentae. Immunology 67: 303–307.

Mullins D E, Rohrlich S T 1983 The role of proteinases in cellular invasiveness. Biochimica et Biophysica Acta 695: 177–214.

Nagler A, Lanier L L, Cwirla S, Phillips J H 1989 Comparative studies of human FcRIII-positive and negative natural killer cells. Journal of Immunology 143: 3183–3191.

Nandi D, Allison J P 1991 Phenotypic analysis and γδ-T cell receptor repertoire of murine T cells associated with the vaginal epithelium. Journal of Immunology 147: 1773–1778.

Nebel L 1987 Clinical and experimental observations on malimplantation following IVF-ET. Colloque INSERM 154: 303–312.

Nehemiah J L, Schnitzer J A, Schulman H, Novikoff A B 1981 Human chorionic trophoblasts, decidual cells, and macrophages: a histochemical and electron microscopic study. American Journal of Obstetrics and Gynecology 140: 261–268.

Nelson J, Leong J A C, Levy J A 1978 Normal human placentas contain RNA-directed DNA polymerase activity like that in viruses. Proceedings of the National Academy of Science USA 65: 6263–6267.

Nilsson B M, Holm S, Stigbrand T I 1994 The human placental immunoglobulin G receptor and immunoglobulin G transport. American Journal of Obstetrics and Gynecology 171: 258–263.

Nishikawa K, Saito S, Morii T et al 1991 Accumulation of CD16– CD56+ natural killer cells with high affinity interleukin-2 receptors in human early pregnancy decidua. International Immunology 3: 743–750.

Nosten F, Kuile F T, Maelankirri L, Decludt B, White N J 1991 Malaria in pregnancy in an area of unstable endemicity. Transactions of the Royal Society of Tropical Medicine and Hygiene 84: 424–429.

Oksenberg J K, Mor-Yosef S, Ezra Y, Brautbar C 1988 Antigen presenting cells in human decidual tissue: III. Role of accessory cells in the activation of suppressor cells. American Journal of Reproductive Immunology and Microbiology 16: 151–155.

Pace D, Morrison L, Bulmer J N 1989 Proliferative activity in endometrial stromal granulocytes throughout menstrual cycle and early pregnancy. Journal of Clinical Pathology 42: 35–39.

Pace D P, Longfellow M, Bulmer J N 1991 Intraepithelial lymphocytes in human endometrium. Journal of Reproduction and Fertility 91: 165–174.

Parhar R S, Kennedy T G, Lala P K 1988 Suppression of lymphocyte alloreactivity by early gestational human decidua. I. Characterization of suppressor cells and suppressor molecules. Cellular Immunology 116: 392–410.

Parhar R S, Yagel S, Lala P K 1989 PGE2-mediated immunosuppression by first trimester human decidual cells blocks activation of maternal leukocytes in the decidua with potential anti-trophoblast activity. Cellular Immunology 120: 61–74.

Pauerstein C J, Croxatto H B, Eddy C A, Ramzy I, Walters M D 1986 Anatomy and pathology of tubal pregnancy. Obstetrics and Gynecology 67: 301–308.

Peel S 1991 Granulated metrial gland cells. Advances in Anatomy, Embryology and Cell Biology 115: 1–112.

Peel S, Adam E 1991 The killing of rat placental cells by rat and mouse granulated metrial gland cells in vitro. Placenta 12: 161–171.

Pijnenborg R, Dixon G, Robertson W B, Brosens I 1980 Trophoblast invasion of human decidua from 8–18 weeks of pregnancy. Placenta 1: 3–19.

Pockley A G, Mowles E A, Stoker R J, Westwood O M R, Chapman M G, Bolton A E 1988 Suppression of in vitro lymphocyte reactivity to phytohemagglutinin by placental protein 14. Journal of Reproductive Immunology 13: 31–39.

Purcell D F J, McKenzie I F C, Lublin D M et al 1990 The human cell-surface glycoproteins HuLy-m5, membrane co-factor protein (MCP) of the complement system, and trophoblast leucocyte-common (TLX) antigen, are CD46. Immunology 70: 155–161.

Rasheed F N, Bulmer J N, Morrison L et al 1992 Isolation of maternal mononuclear cells from placentas for use in in vitro functional assays. Journal of Immunological Methods 146: 185–193.

Rasheed F N, Bulmer J N, Dunn D T et al 1993 Suppressed peripheral and placental blood lymphoproliferative responses in first pregnancies: relevance to malaria. American Journal of Tropical Medicine and Hygiene 48: 154–160.

Rawal B K, Parida S, Watkins R P F, Ghosh P, Smith H 1991 Symptomatic reactivation of hepatitis B in pregnancy. Lancet 337: 364.

Redline R W, Lu C Y 1989 Localization of fetal major histocompatibility complex antigens and maternal leukocytes in murine placenta. Laboratory Investigation 61: 27–36.

Redline R W, Patterson P 1993 Villitis of unknown etiology is associated with major infiltration of fetal tissue by maternal inflammatory cells. American Journal of Pathology 143: 473–479.

Redman C W G, McMichael A J, Stirrat G M, Sunderland C A, Ting A 1984 Class I MHC antigens on human extravillous trophoblast. Immunology 52: 457–468.

Regan L, Braude P R, Trembath P L 1989 Influence of past reproductive performance on risk of spontaneous abortion. British Medical Journal 299: 541–545.

Risteli J, Foidart J M, Risteli L, Boniver J, Goffinet G 1984 The basement membrane proteins laminin and type IV collagen in isolated villi in pre-eclampsia. Placenta 5: 541–550.

Ritson A, Bulmer J N 1989 Isolation and functional studies of granulated lymphocytes in first trimester human decidua. Clinical and Experimental Immunology 77: 263–268.

Roberts J M, Taylor C T, Melling G C, Kingsland C R, Johnson P M 1992 Expression of the CD46 antigen, and absence of class I MHC antigen, on the human oocyte and preimplantation blastocyst. Immunology 75: 202–205.

Robertson W B 1979 Uteroplacental bloodflow in maternal diabetes. In: Sutherland H W, Stowers J M (eds) Carbohydrate metabolism in pregnancy and the newborn. Springer-Verlag, Berlin, pp 63–75.

Robertson W B, Khong T Y, Brosens I, De Wolf F, Sheppard B L, Bonnar J 1986 The placental bed biopsy: review from three European centers. American Journal of Obstetrics and Gynecology 155: 401–412.

Romero R, Avila C, Brekus C A, Morotti R 1991 The role of systemic and intrauterine infection in preterm parturition. Annals of the New York Academy of Sciences 622: 355–375.

Russell P 1980 Inflammatory lesions of the human placenta III: The histopathology of villitis of unknown aetiology. Placenta 1: 227–244.

Russell P, Atkinson K, Krishnan L 1980 Recurrent reproductive failure due to severe placental villitis of unknown etiology. Journal of Reproductive Medicine 24: 93–98.

Saito S, Nishikawa K, Mori T, Enomoto M, Narita N, Motoyoshi K 1993 Cytokine production by CD16–CD56bright natural killer cells in the human early pregnancy decidua. International Immunology 5: 559–563.

Saji F, Koyama M, Matsuzaki N 1994 Human placental Fc receptors. Placenta 15: 453–466.

Saksela O, Wahlstrom T, Lehtovirta P, Seppala M, Veheri A 1981 Presence of α2-macroglobulin in normal but not in malignant human syncytiotrophoblast. Cancer Research 41: 2507–2513.

Sanders S K, Giblin P A, Kavathas P 1991 Cell-cell adhesion mediated by CD8 and human histocompatibility leukocyte antigen G, a nonclassical major histocompatibility complex class I molecule on cytotrophoblasts. Journal of Experimental Medicine 174: 737–740.

Sargent I L, Wilkins T 1988 Maternal immune responses to the fetus in early pregnancy and recurrent miscarriage. Lancet 2: 1099–1100.

Sarkar S, Kacinski B M, Kohorn E I, Merino M J, Carter D, Blakemore K J 1986 Demonstration of myc and ras oncogene expression by hybridization in situ in hydatidiform mole and choriocarcinoma. American Journal of Obstetrics and Gynecology 154: 390–393.

Sasagawa M, Ohmomo Y, Kanazawa K, Takeuchi S 1987 HLA expression by trophoblast of invasive moles. Placenta 8: 111–118.

Sasaki K, Chiba S, Mano H, Yazaki Y, Hirai H 1992 Identification of a soluble GM-CSF binding protein in the supernatant of a human choriocarcinoma cell line. Biochemical and Biophysical Research Communications 183: 252–257.

Schwartz D A, Khan R, Stoll B 1992 Characterization of the fetal inflammatory response to cytomegalovirus placentitis. Archives of Pathology and Laboratory Medicine 116: 21–27.

Scott J S 1976 Pregnancy: nature's experimental system: transient manifestations of immunological disease in the child. Lancet i: 704–706.

Seppala M, Wahlstrom T, Bohn H 1979 Circulating levels and tissue localization of placental protein 5 (PP5) in pregnancy and trophoblastic disease: absence of PP5 expression in the malignant trophoblast. International Journal of Cancer 24: 6–10.

Sheppard B L, Bonnar J 1976 The ultrastructure of the arterial supply of the human placenta in pregnancy complicated by growth retardation. British Journal of Obstetrics and Gynaecology 83: 948–959.

Sheppard B L, Bonnar J 1981 An ultrastructural study of uteroplacental spiral arteries in hypertensive and normotensive pregnancy and fetal growth retardation. British Journal of Obstetrics and Gynaecology 88: 695–705.

Sinha D, Wells M, Faulk W P 1984 Immunological studies of human placentae: complement components in pre-eclamptic chorionic villi. Clinical and Experimental Immunology 56: 175–184.

Sinosich M J, Smith D H, Grudzinskas J G et al 1983 The prediction of pregnancy failure by measurement of pregnancy-associated plasma protein A (PAPP-A) following in-vitro fertilization and embryo transfer. Fertility and Sterility 40: 539–541.

Smith S K, Kelly R W 1987 The effect of estradiol-17β and actinomycin D on the release of PGF and PGE from separated cells of human endometrium. Prostaglandins 34: 553–561.

Starkey P M 1991 Expression on cells of early human pregnancy decidua of the p75 IL-2 and p145 IL-4 receptor proteins. Immunology 73: 64–70.

Stewart I, Mukhtar D D Y 1988 The killing of mouse trophoblast cells by granulated metrial gland cells in vitro. Placenta 9: 417–425.

Stimson W H 1983 The influence of pregnancy-associated serum proteins and steroids on the maternal immune response. In: Wegmann T G, Gill T J III (eds) Immunology of reproduction. Oxford University Press, New York, pp 281–301.

Stray-Pedersen B, Stray-Pedersen S 1988 Recurrent abortion: the role of psychotherapy. In: Beard R W, Ship F (eds) Early pregnancy loss: mechanisms and treatment. Springer-Verlag, New York, pp 433–440.

Sunderland C A, Naiem M, Mason D Y, Redman C W G, Stirrat G M 1981 The expression of major histocompatibility antigens by human chorionic villi. Journal of Reproductive Immunology 3: 323–331.

Sunderland C A, Davies J O, Stirrat G M 1984 Immunohistology of normal and ovarian cancer tissue with a monoclonal antibody to placental alkaline phosphatase. Cancer Research 44: 4496–4502.

Sunderland C A, Bulmer J N, Luscombe M, Redman C W G, Stirrat G M 1985a Immunohistological and biochemical evidence for a role for hyaluronic acid in the growth and development of the placenta. Journal of Reproductive Immunology 8: 197–212.

Sunderland C A, Redman C W G, Stirrat G M 1985b Characterization and localization of HLA antigens on hydatidiform mole. American Journal of Obstetrics and Gynecology 151: 130–135.

Sunderland C A, Sasagawa M, Kanazawa K, Stirrat G M, Takeuchi S 1985c An immunohistological study of HLA antigen expression by gestational choriocarcinoma. British Journal of Cancer 51: 809–814.

Suni J, Narvanen A, Wahlström T et al 1984 Human placental syncytiotrophoblastic M_r 75,000 polypeptide defined by antibodies to a synthetic peptide based on a cloned human endogenous retroviral DNA sequence. Proceedings of the National Academy of Science USA 81: 6197–6201.

Sutton L, Mason D Y, Redman C W G 1983 HLA-DR positive cells in the human placenta. Immunology 49: 103–113.

Sutton L, Gadd M, Mason D Y, Redman C W G 1986 Cells bearing class II MHC antigens in the human placenta and amniochorion. Immunology 58: 23–29.

Szekeres-Bartho J, Reznikoff-Etievant M F, Varga P, Pichon M-F, Varga Z, Chaouat G 1989 Lymphocytic progesterone receptors in normal and pathological human pregnancy. Journal of Reproductive Immunology 16: 239–247.

Tabibzadeh S 1990 Evidence of T-cell activation and potential cytokine action in human endometrium. Journal of Clinical Endocrinology and Metabolism 71: 645–649.

Tabibzadeh S, Satyaswaroop P G 1989 Sex steroid receptors in lymphoid cells of human endometrium. American Journal of Clinical Pathology 91: 656–663.

Takahashi H, Adachi S, Yoshiya N, Suzuki T, Kanazawa K, Takeuchi S 1987 Expression of HLA-DR molecules in human gestational choriocarcinoma cell lines and malignant cell lines. Placenta 8: 293–298.

Tatarova N A, Susloparov L A, Bistrova D A, Mikhailov V M 1989 Changes in the cellular stroma of decidual tissue in physiologically developing pregnancy and rising toxicosis. Archiv Anatomii Gistologii I Embriologii (Leningrad) 97: 76–82.

Theofilopoulos A N, Gleicher N, Pereira A B, Dixon F J 1981 The biology of immune complexes and their possible role in pregnancy. American Journal of Reproductive Immunology 1: 92–105.

Thrower S, Bulmer J N, Wells M 1991 Lectin binding of human trophoblast in normal and pathological human pregnancy. International Journal of Gynecological Pathology 10: 238–251.

Tookey P A, Ades A E, Peckham C S 1992 Cytomegalovirus prevalence in pregnant women: the influence of parity. Archives of Disease in Childhood 67: 779–783.

Uren S J, Boyle W 1990 Class II MHC antigen-positive macrophages from human placentae suppress strong MLR and CML reactions. Cellular Immunology 125: 235–246.

Vanderpuye O A, Labarrere C A, McIntyre J A 1991 A vitronectin-receptor-related molecule in human placental brush border membranes. Journal of Biochemistry 280: 9–17.

Vardi I, Halbrecht I 1974 Toxemia of pregnancy: 1. Antigens associated with toxemia of pregnancy in placental connective tissue. American Journal of Obstetrics and Gynecology 118: 552–558.

Wahlström T, Nieminen P, Narvanen A et al 1984 Monoclonal antibody defining a human syncytiotrophoblastic polypeptide immunologically related to mammalian retrovirus structural protein p30. Placenta 5: 465–474.

Wainwright S D, Holmes C H 1993 Distribution of Fc receptors on trophoblast during human development: an immunohistochemical and immunoblotting study. Immunology 80: 343–351.

Wegmann T G, Lin H, Guilbert L, Mossman T R 1993 Bidirectional cytokine interactions in the maternal-fetal relationship: is successful pregnancy a T_H2 phenomenon? Immunology Today 14: 353–356.

Weir P E 1981 Immunofluorescent studies of the uteroplacental arteries in normal pregnancy. British Journal of Obstetrics and Gynaecology 88: 301–307.

Wells M, Hsi B-L, Faulk W P 1984 Class I antigens of the major histocompatibility complex on cytotrophoblast of the human placental basal plate. American Journal of Reproductive Immunology 6: 167–174.

Wells M, Bennett J, Bulmer J N, Jackson P, Holgate C 1987 Complement component deposition in uteroplacental (spiral) arteries in normal human pregnancy. Journal of Reproductive Immunology 12: 125–135.

Whyte A, Ragge N, Loke Y W, Thiry L 1985 Human syncytiotrophoblast membrane protein defined using a heterologous antiserum. Clinical and Experimental Immunology 59: 227–234.

Wood G W 1980 Mononuclear phagocytes in the human placenta. Placenta 1: 113–123.

Yeh C J G, Bulmer J N, Hsi B-L, Tian W T, Rittershaus C, Ip S H 1990 T cell receptor γ/δ complex, not associated with CD3, is identified in human endometrial glandular epithelium. Placenta 11: 253–261.

Yelavarthi K K, Fishback J L, Hunt J S 1991 Analysis of HLA-G mRNA in human placental and extraplacental membrane cells by in situ hybridization. Journal of Immunology 146: 2847–2854.

Zhou Y, Damsky C H, Chiu K, Roberts J M, Fisher S J 1993 Pre-eclampsia is associated with abnormal expression of adhesion molecules by invasive cytotrophoblasts. Journal of Clinical Investigation 91: 950–960.

62. Pathology of maternal death

H. Fox

INTRODUCTION

The World Health Organization defines a maternal death as 'the death of a woman while pregnant or within 42 days of termination of pregnancy, irrespective of the duration or site of the pregnancy, from any cause related to or aggravated by the pregnancy or its management but not from accidental or incidental causes'. The Report on Confidential Enquiries into Maternal Deaths in the United Kingdom 1988–1990 (1994) has added to this definition a category of 'late maternal death' which applies to deaths occurring between 43 days and one year after delivery or abortion, this being necessary because of the currently frequent prolongation of existence by life-support systems.

There can be no doubt that, in western countries, maternal deaths have now declined to a very low rate, though it is difficult to obtain exact figures. This is due to a number of factors which include the use of different denominators (such as the number of women of reproductive age, the number of live births, the number of pregnancies), poor denominator data, a failure to identify maternal deaths because of coding errors, failure to include late maternal deaths, the inclusion of fortuitous deaths and the exclusion of deaths occurring in early pregnancy. Bouvier-Colle et al (1991) found that in France there was an under-reporting of 56% in the official statistics and that in other countries in western Europe and the USA the underestimation of maternal deaths ranged from 17–63%. Clearly, therefore, official data and international comparisons have to be regarded with some scepticism but within these restraints the current maternal death rate in the United Kingdom is 7 per 100 000 births (Report on Confidential Enquiries into Maternal Deaths in the United Kingdom 1988–1990, 1994), the comparable rates for other countries being 8.8 in the Netherlands, 9.1 in the United States, 30 in all developed countries, 270 in Latin America, 420 in Asia and 640 in Africa (Hogberg, 1985; Editorial, 1987; Schuitemaker et al, 1991; Grimes, 1994).

In England and Wales the number of maternal deaths per million of the female population aged 15–44 years has fallen from 9.0 in 1973–75 to 4.1 in 1988–90 whilst the maternal mortality rate per 100 000 pregnancies fell from 11 in 1973–75 to 7 in 1988–90.

Because maternal deaths are now so uncommon in most western countries few pathologists will have more than an extremely limited experience of conducting autopsies on such cases. Pathologists required to undertake such a postmortem examination will, however, find a very useful guide in the reviews of this topic by Rushton & Dawson (1982), Shanklin et al (1991) and Toner (1992); in these, the authors point out that there is no special mystique to autopsies on maternal deaths, stress the importance of taking adequate material for histological examination and review the more important causes of death associated with pregnancy.

CLASSIFICATION OF MATERNAL DEATHS

Maternal deaths can be classified into three broad groups:

1. *Direct maternal deaths.* These are defined as 'those resulting from obstetric complications of the pregnant state (pregnancy, labour and puerperium), from interventions, omissions, incorrect treatment or from a chain of events resulting from any of the above'.

2. *Indirect maternal deaths.* Deaths in this category are defined as 'those resulting from previous existing disease, or from disease which developed during pregnancy and which was not due to direct obstetric causes, but was aggravated by the physiologic effects of pregnancy'.

3. *Fortuitous maternal deaths.* This group is formed of 'deaths which occur during pregnancy or the puerperium from causes not related to the pregnancy or its complications or its management'.

It should be noted that this classification is dependent upon accurate establishment of the cause of death, usually by autopsy study. In some countries, however, accurate data of this type can not be obtained and the category of *pregnancy-related death* applies to 'the death of a woman while pregnant or within 42 days of termination of pregnancy, irrespective of the cause of death', this categorization being intended for those cases in which the cause of death can not be identified with precision.

The latest Report on Confidential Inquiries into Maternal Deaths in the United Kingdom (1994) covers the years 1988–90 and during this period there were complete details of 325 maternal deaths, of which 48 were late deaths. Of the 277 deaths occurring during pregnancy or within 42 days of termination of the pregnancy 145 (52.3%) were classed as direct, 93 (33.7%) as indirect and 39 (14%) as fortuitous. In this chapter only direct maternal deaths are considered. A majority of indirect maternal deaths are due to cardiovascular, hepatic, renal or neurological disorders and the pathology of these conditions is discussed in Chapters 56–59. Occasional indirect deaths are related to endocrine disorders, auto-immune diseases, blood dyscrasia and gastrointestinal disease: the interrelationships between medical conditions of this type and pregnancy are detailed in several comprehensive volumes (Burrow & Ferris, 1982; de Swiet, 1989; Reece et al, 1992).

Little point would be served by considering fortuitous maternal deaths. The pregnant woman can fall prey to any of the ills that beset humanity and many of these diseases neither influence the pregnancy nor are themselves influenced by the gravid state. Suffice it to say that trauma is the commonest cause of fortuitous maternal death, both in the United Kingdom (Confidential Report, 1994) and in the USA (Fildes et al, 1992), and that malignant disease is the second commonest.

DIRECT OBSTETRIC DEATHS

The main causes of direct maternal death in the United Kingdom during the years 1988–90 are detailed in Table 62.1: in many instances, of course, multiple factors were present which may have contributed to the demise of a particular woman but the Table indicates the single factor which was thought to play the predominant rôle.

A comparison of the figures for 1988–90 with those in previous Confidential Reports shows that there has been

Table 62.1 Main causes of direct maternal death in England and Wales 1988–90

Thromboembolism	33
Hypertensive diseases of pregnancy	27
Haemorrhage	22
Sepsis	17
Amniotic fluid embolism	11
Ectopic pregnancy	8
Anaesthetic-associated	4
Abortion	3
Ruptured uterus	2

a marked increase in deaths due to haemorrhage, ectopic pregnancy and sepsis since the early 1980s but a slight decrease in deaths from thromboembolic disease.

The figures for maternal deaths in the United Kingdom represent the most detailed analysis of maternal mortality in any western country; there are, almost certainly, minor differences in the pattern of disorders contributing to maternal mortality in other western countries but nevertheless the figures for England and Wales are probably roughly representative for contemporary industrialized (or post-industrialized) western countries. They are, however, far from being representative of the pattern encountered in lesser developed countries where there is a particularly high mortality rate from haemorrhage and sepsis (Duley, 1992).

Specific causes of direct maternal death

Pulmonary thromboembolism

Approximately one-third of fatal cases of obstetric pulmonary thromboembolism occur during pregnancy and about two-thirds during the puerperium. About half of the puerperal deaths from this cause take place during the first two weeks after delivery (particularly during the first seven days) but nearly half occur between two and six weeks after delivery: occasional cases of fatal embolism are encountered more than six weeks after delivery.

Factors predisposing to thromboembolism during pregnancy and the puerperium include advancing age, increasing parity, obesity, a history of previous thromboembolism and delivery by caesarean section (Tindall, 1971; Ruckley, 1992); some patients with a history of previous thromboembolic disease may have deficiencies of antithrombin III, protein C or protein S. Two groups of women thought to be at particular risk are those undergoing a surgical procedure, such as tubal ligation, during the puerperium and those in whom lactation has been suppressed by the administration of oestrogens (Daniel et al, 1967; Jeffcoate et al, 1968).

The pathological findings in obstetric cases of fatal pulmonary thromboembolism do not differ from those of this catastrophe in the non-pregnant patient. It is, however, mandatory that not only the leg be carefully examined for evidence of thrombosis but that attention also be directed towards the pelvic and ovarian veins.

Haemorrhage

Maternal death from haemorrhage is usually due to abruptio placentae, placenta praevia, postpartum bleeding or ruptured ectopic pregnancy; less common causes include a tear of the uterine wall, a tear of the cervix or a laceration of the vagina (Chamberlain, 1992). In most autopsies on fatal cases of obstetric haemorrhage the pathological findings are quite straightforward, but in performing such an autopsy several points should be kept in mind:

1. In cases of known or suspected placenta praevia in which the placenta is still in situ the uterus and vagina should be removed as a single block and the uterus subsequently opened from the fundus, this allowing for a clear demonstration of a placenta covering the lower uterine segment or internal cervical os. If the fetus and placenta have been delivered the lower uterine segment should be carefully examined histologically for evidence of a placental site reaction.

2. In women thought to have died from abruptio placentae it is necessary to confirm the presence of retroplacental bleeding. If the placenta has been delivered it should be examined for either adherent thrombus or a depressed empty crater on the maternal surface. If the placenta is still within the uterus the blood may have tracked from the retroplacental area to extend widely into the myometrium, this producing one variety of the so-called 'Couvelaire uterus'.

3. In cases of postpartum bleeding with retained placenta the placental implantation site should be examined histologically for evidence of placenta accreta.

4. Postpartum bleeding after the placenta has been delivered is usually due to uterine atony (Watson, 1980; Varner, 1991; Chamberlain, 1992) and the presence of small retained fragments of placental tissue should not be afforded undue significance.

5. Postpartum bleeding may be due to a coagulopathy. In most cases this is a consequence of a particular complication of pregnancy but occasionally postpartum bleeding is a manifestation of von Willebrand's disease or thrombocytopenic purpura (Watson, 1980).

6. Relatively minor degree of postpartum blood loss per vaginam may be associated with large pelvic haematomas (Pieri, 1958; Flegner, 1971); these not uncommonly prove fatal because the internal nature of the haemorrhage results in late diagnosis.

7. Unrecognized amniotic fluid embolism may be responsible for severe postpartum bleeding. Careful histological study of the pulmonary vessels for evidence of amniotic fluid embolism is therefore essential in all cases of fatal postpartum haemorrhage.

8. Disseminated intravascular coagulation may complicate abruptio placentae and thus accentuate the severity of the haemorrhage. Histological evidence of intravascular fibrin deposition should therefore be sought for in all cases of fatal abruption.

Sepsis

Sepsis may complicate abortion, vaginal delivery or caesarean section. Until relatively recently postabortal sepsis accounted for most obstetric deaths attributable to infection; the incidence of septic abortion has, however, fallen dramatically in England and Wales during the last few decades and there is now an approximately equal distribution of septic obstetric deaths between abortions, vaginal deliveries and caesarean sections. In the United States, however, maternal deaths from sepsis occur twice as commonly after caesarean section as they do after vaginal delivery (Eschenbach & Wager, 1980).

In many cases of maternal death from sepsis the autopsy findings are quite straightforward and include septic endometritis, myometrial abscesses, purulent salpingitis, pelvic peritonitis and septicaemia.

Several particular forms of obstetric sepsis do, however, merit further comment:

1. *Puerperal sepsis.* This, in its classical form, is now a rare complication of pregnancy in the western world though occasional cases of streptococcal puerperal sepsis are still encountered (Charles & Larsen, 1989). More commonly, when infection complicates a vaginal delivery, sepsis is due to organisms which ascend from the birth canal: in many such cases there has been a prolonged rupture of the membranes and chorioamnionitis (Stevenson, 1969) and it is therefore necessary in all cases of fatal puerperal sepsis to examine the placenta and membranes for evidence of an inflammatory process. When diagnosing a puerperal endometritis it is prudent to bear in mind that an apparently physiological leucocytic infiltration of the decidua occurs after most uncomplicated deliveries.

Although many cases of fatal puerperal sepsis are a result of infection with Gram-negative bacteria a minority are due to Clostridia: these organisms can produce a gas gangrene of the uterus and their entry into the bloodstream results in an acute haemolytic anaemia with jaundice, haemoglobinuria and renal failure.

2. *Purulent pelvic phlebitis.* This condition has a high mortality and is found in a significant proportion of women who die from puerperal infection. It is not related to phlebitis or phlebothrombosis of the leg veins or to bland thrombosis of the pelvic veins but is due to direct bacterial invasion of the pelvic venous plexuses. The bacteria damage the venous intima and this results in thrombosis (Collins et al, 1951): the thrombi subsequently become colonized by bacteria and undergo partial liquefaction. The infection spreads directly along the venous wall and also along the perivenous lymphatics and can cause a rapidly spreading purulent phlebitis and a pelvic cellulitis. The infected pelvic veins are filled with a mixture of partially liquefied thrombus, tissue debris and inflammatory cells and there is a tendency for showers of small septic emboli to be thrown off to produce multiple metastatic abscesses (Collins et al, 1951). Many emboli lodge in the pulmonary vasculature and, because they are small and multiple, produce a purulent pneumonitis rather than a typical pulmonary infarct.

Clinically, purulent pelvic phlebitis often develops between seven and 21 days after delivery, either in a woman who until then has appeared to be having a normal puerperium or in one who has persistent post-delivery infection. There is a sudden onset of chills, tachycardia and a swinging pyrexia, these symptoms soon being followed by respiratory complaints due to the multiple pulmonary emboli. Some patients present, however, with an acute onset of lower abdominal pain between two and five days after delivery (Eschenbach & Wager, 1980).

3. *Superficial fascial necrosis.* This is an extremely dangerous complication of an episiotomy wound infection; the infecting organisms are usually either haemolytic streptococci or anaerobic bacteria whilst some cases are infected by both these groups of organisms. The superficial fascia in the region in which an episiotomy incision is made is continuous with that of the abdominal wall, buttocks and legs: hence infection and necrosis of the superficial fascia may extend to any, or all, of these sites, a situation associated with severe toxic symptoms and terminating, not uncommonly, in death (Golde & Ledger, 1977; Ewing et al, 1979; Shy & Eschenbach, 1979). The involved areas are markedly oedematous and the overlying skin is discoloured and sometimes gangrenous. The necrotic fascia appears dull and grey.

4. *Septic shock.* This may complicate puerperal sepsis, gestational pyelonephritis or septic abortion. It is due to the entry of Gram-negative organisms into the bloodstream with subsequent release of endotoxins: these endotoxic substances are thought to be polysaccharide-lipid-protein complexes which are derived from the bacterial cell wall. The pregnant uterus offers extremely favourable conditions for the development of septic shock in so far as the dilated uterine veins and sinuses afford a readily accessible portal of entry for organisms into the maternal circulation.

The pathophysiology of septic shock is not yet fully understood but two important mechanisms appear to be implicated. Firstly, there is generalized vasoconstriction and impaired regional tissue perfusion, this being possibly due to the release of biogenic amines and kinins. Secondly, disseminated intravascular coagulation develops.

Clinically, septic shock is characterized by high fever and shock: in the early stages the patient is alert and flushed but later develops cold, clammy skin, mental confusion and progressive cardiac insufficiency.

At autopsy in such cases the principal findings are pelvic sepsis, fibrin thrombi in the renal glomerular capillaries, bilateral adrenal haemorrhage (a frequent but far from constant feature) and centrilobular hepatic necrosis (McCally & Vasicka, 1962). In cases which have followed a vaginal delivery there is usually a chorioamnionitis, and Studdiford & Douglas (1956) have described a characteristic placental bacteraemia in which clumps of organisms are seen in the intervillous space.

Some patients appear to recover from the acute episode of shock but then develop progressive respiratory distress, this being due to the development of the adult respiratory

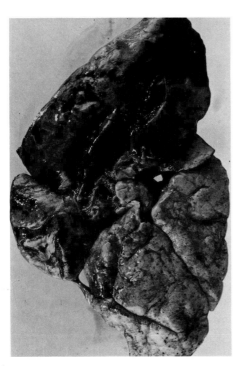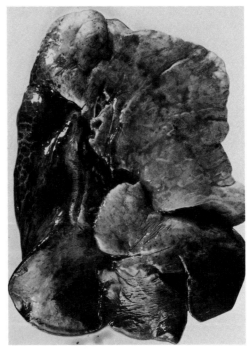

Fig. 62.1 Post mortem appearances of the lungs in a case of septic shock. There are irregular areas of congestion and collapse. (From Corrin & Spencer, 1981, courtesy of Professor B. Corrin.)

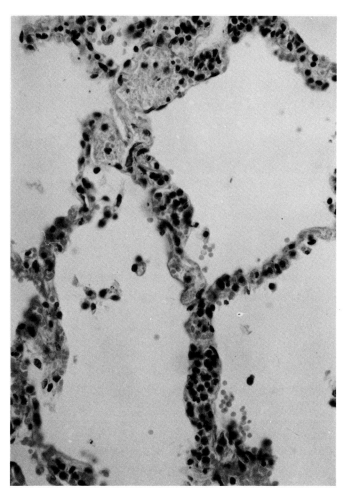

Fig. 62.2 Lungs in a case of septic shock. There is marked sequestration of polymorphs within the pulmonary capillaries. H & E × 324. (From Corrin & Spencer, 1981, courtesy of Professor B. Corrin.)

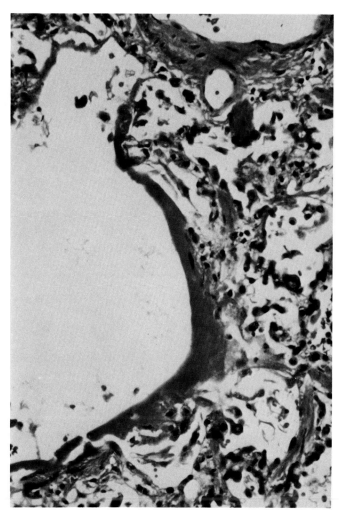

Fig. 62.3 Hyaline membrane formation in the lung following shock. × 52. (Courtesy of Dr. P. Hasleton and the Editor of *Histopathology*.)

distress syndrome (Hasleton, 1983; Weiner-Kronish et al, 1990). In fatal cases (Fig. 62.1) the lungs are heavy and show focal areas of airlessness and cerise discolouration (Corrin & Spencer, 1981). Histologically there is, in the acute stage, intense congestion of the pulmonary capillaries, focal alveolar collapse and patchy oedema. The pulmonary capillaries contain sequestrated polymorphonuclear leucocytes (Fig. 62.2) and platelets, often in association with microthrombi. In the later stages of the adult respiratory distress syndrome there is diffuse alveolar damage with hyaline membrane formation (Fig. 62.3) and pulmonary oedema. If the patient survives this phase there is a subsequent proliferation of alveolar and bronchiolar epithelium together with interstitial fibrosis. The pathogenesis of these pulmonary changes is far from being fully understood but it is postulated that the sequestration of red blood cells within the pulmonary capillaries leads to the release of free radicals (with subsequent lipid peroxidation) and to lysosomal degranulation (Corrin & Spencer, 1981).

Hypertensive disease of pregnancy

Many of the pathological changes found in pre-eclampsia and eclampsia have been described in Chapters 48, 56, 57 and 59 but it is appropriate to summarize here, in very brief form, the salient findings in fatal cases (Sheehan & Lynch, 1973; Govan, 1976; Fox, 1987):

1. Petechial haemorrhages may be found in the cerebral cortex, cerebellum and pons. Massive intracerebral haemorrhage is not uncommon and is a major cause of death in this disease.

2. Subcapsular haemorrhages and areas of infarction are often seen in the liver, these usually being most prominent in the right lobe (Fig. 62.4): occasionally there may be subcapsular rupture of the liver with a haemoperitoneum. Histologically the liver shows periportal necrosis and haemorrhage.

3. Subendocardial haemorrhages are found in the heart, particularly on the left side of the interventricular septum (Fig. 62.5).

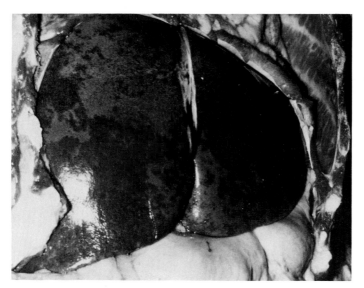

Fig. 62.4 Subcapsular haemorrhage in the liver of a patient dying from eclampsia.

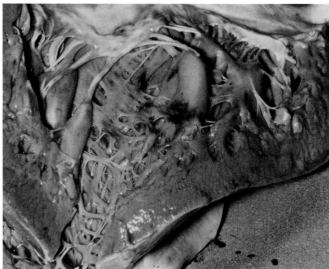

Fig. 62.5 Subendocardial haemorrhages in a fatal case of eclampsia.

4. In the lungs there is characteristically a bilateral haemorrhagic pneumonia.

5. The kidneys show glomerular abnormalities and the lower nephron is often obstructed by protein casts. Bilateral renal cortical necrosis may be found.

6. Acute ulceration of the stomach, oesophagus and duodenum is not uncommon.

7. Haemorrhages are frequently seen within the splenic pulp. The lymphoid tissue around branches of the arterial vessels within the spleen is often necrotic.

8. Streak haemorrhages are frequently seen in the adrenal cortex. Very occasionally there is massive bilateral intra-adrenal haemorrhage.

In the HELLP syndrome pre-eclampsia is associated with a haemolytic anaemia, elevated liver enzymes and low platelet counts (Weinstein, 1982). This condition usually resolves but a rebound thrombocytosis may develop and can predispose to thrombosis, a fatal case of carotid artery occlusion having been recorded under these circumstances (Katz & Cefalo, 1989).

Amniotic fluid embolism

It has traditionally been thought that during a normal pregnancy, labour and delivery there is no escape of liquor into the maternal circulation but that in a few patients an infusion of amniotic fluid occurs which results in a syndrome combining acute cardiopulmonary failure with a haemorrhagic tendency due to a coagulation defect. In recent years, however, this belief has been challenged by the suggestion that amniotic fluid may routinely enter the venous circulation and that the clinical picture of amniotic fluid embolism could be due to infusion of abnormal

amniotic fluid into the maternal circulation rather than to amniotic fluid per se (Clark, 1990, 1991). This view is based on the fact that studies of pregnant women undergoing pulmonary artery catheterization have shown that squames can commonly be detected in the maternal pulmonary arterial circulation (Plauche, 1983; Clark et al, 1986; Lee et al, 1986): this finding does not, however, in itself prove that amniotic fluid routinely enters the circulation for squames are introduced during venepuncture and hence this contention still awaits proof.

The portal of entry of amniotic fluid into the maternal circulation is not always clear though in a proportion of cases a definite uterine laceration, which presumably affords a site of ingress, is found. Attwood (1972) has emphasized that small lower segment tears, either incomplete or complete with an intact but ballooned broad ligament, are more likely to be associated with a fatal amniotic fluid embolism than are large uterine lacerations. Amniotic fluid infusion occurs through a small lower segment tear if the membranes have ruptured and the head, in crowning, forms a plug behind which each uterine contraction pumps fluid into the maternal bloodstream. When, by contrast, there is a large uterine laceration, amniotic fluid tends to leak principally into the peritoneal cavity whilst uterine contractions cease. It has been suggested that in those cases in which no uterine tear is apparent the route of entry may be through the small lacerations which normally occur in the endocervical veins during cervical dilatation (Anderson, 1967).

The cardiopulmonary failure in the amniotic fluid embolism syndrome has for many years been attributed to severe pulmonary hypertension with acute cor pulmonale, the pulmonary hypertension being variously attributed to mechanical obstruction of the pulmonary vasculature, reflex vasoconstriction of the pulmonary vessels, an anaphylactoid reaction or the presence of a vasoactive substance in the emboli. There is no real evidence that anaphylaxis plays any rôle in the production of this syndrome (Morgan, 1979) but experimental studies, using a variety of techniques on a variety of animals under a variety of circumstances and yielding a variety of results (Steiner & Lushbaugh, 1941; Cron et al, 1952; Hunter et al, 1956; Halmagyi et al, 1962; Attwood & Downing, 1963; Stolte et al, 1967; MacMillan, 1968; Reis et al, 1969; Rodgers et al, 1969, 1971; Adamsons et al, 1971; Kitzmiller & Lucas, 1972; Reeves et al, 1974), have on balance tended to suggest that a vasoactive substance plays a key rôle in the haemodynamic changes. Trypsin has been proposed as a candidate for this rôle (Attwood, 1972) but a more plausible suggestion is that the prostaglandin $PGF_{2\alpha}$, a substance present in amniotic fluid in significant amounts only during labour, precipitates the haemodynamic changes. Thus, Kitzmiller & Lucas (1972) showed that the vascular changes observed in amniotic fluid embolism could be reproduced in cats only by the injection of fluid from women who were actually in labour and noted that these changes could be replicated by injection of $PGF_{2\alpha}$. Reeves et al (1974) noted that the haemodynamic effects of amniotic fluid injection could be prevented by aspirin, a potent inhibitor of prostaglandin synthesis. Clark (1990) has proposed that leucotrienes, also a metabolite of arachidonic acid, may be involved as a vasoactive agent.

The classical concept of an acute cor pulmonale being fully responsible for the clinical features of the amniotic fluid embolism syndrome has, however, not been confirmed by haemodynamic studies in humans. These have, without exception, shown little or no increase in pulmonary arterial pressure (Dolyniuk et al, 1983; Clark et al, 1985, 1988; Girard et al, 1986; Noble & St Amand, 1993; Koegler et al, 1994) but have yielded conflicting results about left ventricular output, some finding depression of left ventricular function (Clark et al, 1985, 1988) and others demonstrating a normal (Koegler et al, 1994) or increased (Noble & St Amand, 1993) left ventricular output. It has been suggested that the failure to detect an elevated pulmonary arterial pressure may be because the pulmonary arterial vasoconstriction is short lived (less than 30 minutes) and has been dissipated before catheter studies could be undertaken and further claimed that, despite its transient nature, the pulmonary vasoconstriction produces severe hypoxia which damages the myocardium of the left ventricle (Clark et al, 1985; Clark, 1990, 1991). This view is given some credence by the finding that, in a woman who developed the clinical features of an amniotic fluid embolism whilst having her arterial oxygen saturation continuously measured, there was a drop in oxygen saturation from 98–100% to 70% within 30 seconds (Fava & Galizia, 1993).

There is disagreement as to the nature of the coagula-

tion defect which is a prominent feature of the clinical syndrome of amniotic fluid embolism. Attwood (1972) has pointed out that fibrin thrombi are very rarely seen in autopsies on women dying from amniotic fluid embolism but nevertheless most believe that the bleeding diathesis is due to disseminated intravascular coagulation, resulting from the presence within the emboli of a thromboplastic substance (Beller, 1974). Amniotic fluid can activate factor X and has a thromboplastin-like effect when added to normal plasma, properties suggesting that the fluid may contain tissue factor, a primary biological initiator of coagulation. Lockwood et al (1991) have indeed confirmed that tissue factor is present in amniotic fluid, that the presence of this substance accounts for virtually all the procoagulant activity of the fluid and that the quantity of this substance in the fluid increases progressively with increasing gestational age.

It is widely believed that advancing age, high parity, a large fetus, tumultuous labour, intrauterine fetal death and the use of uterine stimulants all predispose to the amniotic fluid embolism syndrome (Peterson & Taylor, 1970; Courtney, 1970; Gregory & Clayton, 1973). Morgan (1979), in his review of 272 reported cases of amniotic fluid embolism, was unable to confirm that there was any true association with the use of uterine stimulants, large babies or intrauterine fetal death. A tumultuous or hypertonic labour, though associated with an unduly high incidence of the amniotic fluid embolism syndrome, is by no means an essential prerequisite for this complication which may also occur during the course of an entirely normal labour, in women being delivered by caesarean section and in women who have not yet gone into labour. Amniotic fluid embolism syndrome can also complicate intrauterine injection of hypertonic saline for abortifacient purposes (Goldstein, 1968), intra-amniotic glucose infusion (Lee & Frampton, 1964), amniocentesis (Krause, 1969) and therapeutic saline amnioinfusion (Dragich et al, 1991; Dibble & Elliott, 1992; Maher et al, 1994). Surgical induction of abortion can be complicated by amniotic fluid embolism and, indeed, it has been claimed that approximately 12% of all deaths following legal abortion are attributable to this cause (Guidotti et al, 1981).

Clinically, the onset of symptoms in the amniotic fluid embolism syndrome is usually abrupt. There is a sudden onset of dyspnoea, cyanosis and shock: convulsions are not uncommon and are sometimes the presenting feature. Frequently the patient dies within a few minutes but if she survives this acute episode a haemorrhagic tendency soon supervenes and this often leads to severe, sometimes catastrophic, uterine bleeding. The mortality rate is thought to be very high, in the region of 90% (Morgan, 1979): the true death rate is, however, almost impossible to determine, largely because of the paradoxical situation that the mere fact of survival is commonly regarded as proof that an individual did not have amniotic fluid embolism (Benson, 1993) and because of the belief that the diagnosis can only be proven at autopsy. It is certainly true that absolute proof of the diagnosis does rest upon the autopsy findings but the clinical features are sufficiently striking and have a sufficient degree of specificity to allow for a clinical diagnosis (Clark, 1990, 1991). It was at one time hoped that the detection of squamous cells in pulmonary artery blood would allow for the confirmation of the diagnosis during life (Dolyniuk et al, 1983) but, as already remarked, squames can be found in the pulmonary blood of perfectly healthy pregnant women (Clark et al, 1986).

At autopsy the macroscopic findings in a case of amniotic fluid embolism syndrome are usually non-specific: the lungs are usually oedematous and show patchy atelectasis with marked dilatation of the right side of the heart and acute congestion of the liver. Occasionally a macroscopic diagnosis can be achieved by allowing blood from the pul-

monary arteries to collect within the pericardial sac after removal of the heart: vernix, lanugo hairs and greenish staining due to meconium may be seen (Attwood, 1972). Essentially, however, the diagnosis of amniotic fluid embolism rests upon the histological demonstration of amniotic fluid debris in the pulmonary vasculature. Four points require to be stressed:

1. Multiple blocks of lung tissue should be taken for histological examination.

2. If amniotic fluid debris is not detected in the pulmonary vasculature the diagnosis of amniotic fluid embolism can not be substantiated.

3. Although fetal squames have been detected in the blood of healthy women it would be unwise to assume that amniotic fluid debris in the pulmonary vasculature is a physiological event.

4. Trophoblastic emboli are not uncommonly found in

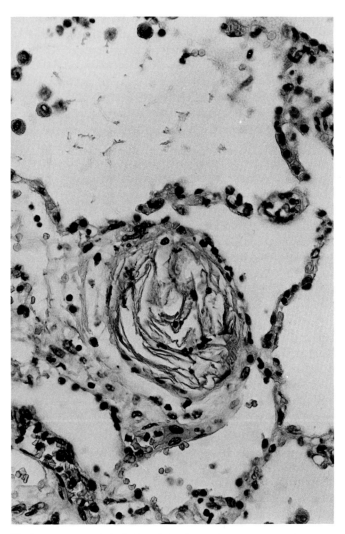

Fig. 62.6 An amniotic fluid embolus in a pulmonary vessel. This consists almost entirely of squames. H & E × 81. (Courtesy of Dr. D. I. Rushton, Birmingham.)

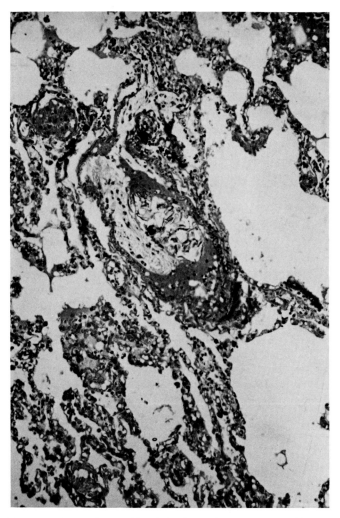

Fig. 62.7 An amniotic fluid embolus in a pulmonary vessel. This consists of a mixture of squames, mucus and meconium. Alcian Blue phloxine × 72.

the lung: these are evidence of a physiological process and are not indicative of amniotic fluid embolism.

The particulate matter that may be found in the pulmonary vessels includes epithelial squames (Fig. 62.6) from the fetal skin, lanugo hairs, fat from the vernix caseosa, bile and mucin (Figs 62.7 and 62.8), the latter two constituents being derived from fetal meconium passed into the liquor. Attwood (1972) has stressed the inadequacy of the haematoxylin and eosin stain for detecting amniotic debris; a better staining method for the demonstration of the various components of the emboli is the Alcian Blue phloxine technique which stains mucin green and squames red (Attwood, 1958). The best technique for detecting squames in amniotic fluid emboli (Fig. 62.9) is, however, to use an anti-keratin antibody (Garland & Thompson, 1983).

Using the Attwood stain, Peterson & Taylor (1970) studied 40 patients who had died of amniotic fluid embo-lism and found that although squames could be demonstrated in the pulmonary vessels in 80% of cases they were the major constituent of the emboli in only 20%: in the other 80% mucin was the most prominent particulate matter. Mucin was found principally in the small pulmonary arteries whilst squames tended to be more commonly seen in the arterioles and capillaries. Amniotic emboli may be found in capillaries in many organs outside the lungs but are usually few and small and of apparently little clinical importance.

The histological diagnosis of amniotic fluid embolism is usually straightforward but confusion may occasionally arise between epithelial squames and endothelial cells which have been shed from the walls of the pulmonary vessels; these latter cells are, however, usually nucleated (as compared to the generally anuclear squames) and do not take up the Alcian Blue phloxine stain (Attwood, 1972).

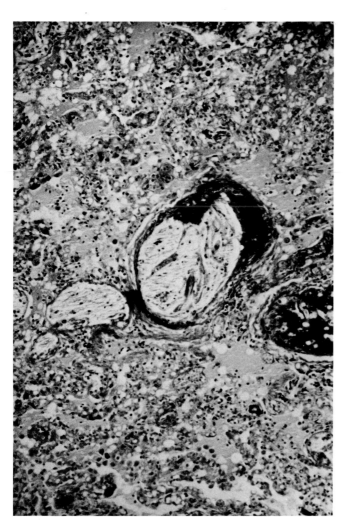

Fig. 62.8 An amniotic fluid embolus in a pulmonary vessel. This consists almost entirely of mucus and meconium. Alcian Blue phloxine × 72.

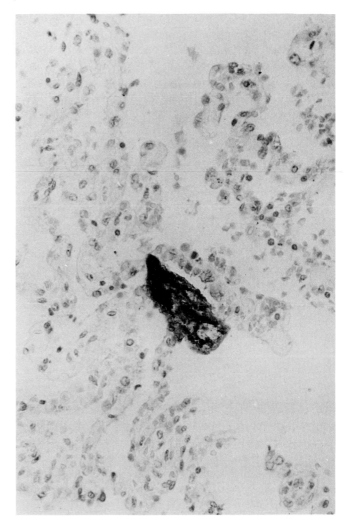

Fig. 62.9 Squames in an amniotic fluid embolus in a pulmonary vessel: these have been stained with an immunoperoxidase-linked anti-keratin antibody. × 126. (Courtesy of Dr. I. W. C. Garland, Aberdeen.)

Air embolism

The pregnant uterus is particularly vulnerable to air embolism because of the large venous sinuses that are exposed at placental separation. Air embolism may complicate an abortion, particularly an illegal abortion (Bryans, 1963; Fox, 1967), internal version, manual exploration of the uterus, replacement of an inverted uterus or manual removal of the placenta: it has been suggested that air embolism following intrauterine manipulations is due to air within the uterus becoming trapped by the operator's arm which occludes the vagina, any sudden increase in intrauterine pressure then tending to force the air into the venous sinuses (Nelson, 1960). Air entry into the maternal circulation may, very exceptionally, occur during an otherwise normal labour, vaginal delivery or caesarean section. Air embolism can also occur during pregnancy, well before the onset of labour (Ragan, 1981); this event may appear to develop spontaneously but is usually due to orogenital sexual activity (Bray et al, 1983). The practice of blowing into the vagina is one which is devoid of danger in the non-pregnant woman; however, the capacity of the vagina is considerably increased during pregnancy and under these circumstances this somewhat unusual sexual manoeuvre carries a serious risk of air embolism.

Air embolism during the puerperium is thought to be particularly associated with the performance by the patient of knee–chest exercises; the vagina has, during the puerperium, a capacity of about 1000 ml and this quantity of air may be trapped intravaginally by approximation of the thighs whilst in the knee–chest position and subsequently forced into the uterine veins when the patient returns her legs to the horizontal position.

The clinical picture of an air embolism is dependent upon the amount of air entering the maternal circulation but it is generally accepted that entry of 500–600 ml of air is usually fatal. In such cases there is a sudden onset of cyanosis, shock and acute cor pulmonale with a rapid progression to convulsions, coma and death. At autopsy, the cardinal finding is of dark, frothy, bubble-studded blood in the right side of the heart and also, often, in the inferior vena cava and in the uterine veins.

Acute uterine inversion

This is an uncommon complication of the puerperium occurring in about 1 in 6400 deliveries (Shah-Hosseini & Evrard, 1989); it may follow attempted manual removal of the placenta, particularly in cases of placenta accreta, but can also occur spontaneously and without warning (Kitchin et al, 1975; Watson et al, 1980). A patient with this complication tends to suffer severe haemorrhage and shock and a mortality rate of between 13% and 18% has traditionally been quoted (Bell et al, 1953; Bunke & Hofmeister, 1965; Moldavsky, 1967). The more recent trend towards prompt replacement of the uterus has dramatically reduced this death rate (Watson et al, 1980; Shah-Hosseini & Evrard, 1989; Phillippe et al, 1991; Rasmussen, 1992).

Acute uterine torsion

This is an extremely rare, but potentially fatal, catastrophe in pregnancy (Piot et al, 1973; Smith, 1975; Visser et al, 1983). Dextrorotation of the gravid uterus is common but axial rotation amounts to torsion if it exceeds 45°. Torsion usually occurs during labour, may lead to uterine rupture and is of unknown pathogenesis.

Rupture of the uterus

The incidence of uterine rupture during pregnancy is not known with any degree of certainty but it has been estimated that in western countries this catastrophe complicates about 1 in 2000 to 2500 pregnancies (Garnet, 1964; Schrinsky & Benson, 1978). In other parts of the world uterine rupture is, however, much more common occurring, for example, in 1 in 546 deliveries in a black South African population (Mokgokong & Marivate, 1976), in 1 in 425 deliveries in Kenya (Lema et al, 1991), in 1 in 119 deliveries in Conakry/Guinea (Balde et al, 1990) and in 1 in 97 pregnancies in a rural Turkish population (Kafkas & Taper, 1991).

Uterine rupture may be classified as traumatic, spontaneous or scar-associated and in most series between 30% and 60% have been due to rupture of a uterine scar. In the vast majority of these patients the scar has been due to a previous caesarean section but scars resulting from a previous myomectomy, including laparoscopic myomectomy (Harris, 1992), or cornual resection may also undergo rupture. Rupture has also occurred at the site of a previous invasive mole (Kaczmarek et al, 1994), following reimplantation into the uterus of the Fallopian tubes (Brandt & Larsen, 1989) and after surgical treatment of Asherman's syndrome (Deaton et al, 1989).

The scar of a previous classical caesarean section is much more susceptible to rupture than is that following a lower segment section, Garnet (1964) estimating that a classical scar is ten times more likely to rupture than is a lower segment scar. This does not imply, however, that most cases of scar rupture seen today follow a classical section for this operation is now performed so infrequently that the vast majority of scar ruptures occur in women who have had a lower segment section. It is important when dealing with a scar rupture to differentiate between a true rupture, which is usually associated with severe haemorrhage and can lead to maternal death, and simple dehiscence of the scar. In the latter condition the peritoneum overlying the scar is intact and separates the membranes, which bulge through the gaping edges of the dehiscent scar, from the peritoneal cavity: dehiscence is rarely associated with bleeding and is not a cause of maternal death (Yussman & Haynes, 1970). The absolute risk of uterine rupture following a lower segment section is extremely low, being in the range of 0.2–1.4% (Meehan et al, 1989; Farmer et al, 1991; Jones et al, 1991; Lurie et al, 1992).

The commonest causes of traumatic uterine rupture in western countries are probably internal version and forceful delivery through an incompletely dilated cervix (O'Driscoll, 1966): other precipitating factors include instrumentation whilst performing an illegal abortion, failed forceps delivery, shoulder dystocia, cephalopelvic disproportion and transverse lie (Schrinsky & Benson, 1978). Obstructed labour is by far the commonest cause in developing countries.

Spontaneous rupture should, by definition, occur in a normal uterus during a normal pregnancy or labour but, by convention, this diagnostic term is extended to include rupture of a congenitally abnormal uterus, rupture of a cornual pregnancy and rupture complicating placenta accreta. In the absence of these latter factors the cause of spontaneous uterine rupture is largely unknown. The rôle of oxytocic stimulation has been much debated for, whilst a proportion of cases of uterine rupture do follow administration of oxytocin (Golan et al, 1980), it has been doubted if use of this substance in a normal labour carries any risk of this complication, rupture only becoming a real possibility if oxytocin is administered in an already complicated labour. There has, however, been an increasing number of reports of uterine rupture following vaginal administration of prostaglandin E_2 for induction of labour (Sawyer et al, 1981; Larue et al, 1991; Maymon et al, 1992; Prasad & Ratnam, 1992; Azem et al, 1993), though the absolute risk of this complication is low. There are anecdotal reports of an association between cocaine usage and spontaneous uterine rupture (Gonsoulin et al, 1990; Trive et al, 1994) whilst rupture has occurred, probably coincidentally, in a woman exposed prenatally to DES (Adams et al, 1989).

Rupture of a lower segment section scar usually occurs during labour whilst rupture of a classical scar may occur at any time during pregnancy. Rupture of a myomectomy scar has been noted as early as the 16th week of pregnancy (Report on Confidential Enquiries into Maternal Deaths in England and Wales 1976–1978, 1982). Clearly, traumatic rupture usually occurs during labour and whilst most cases of spontaneous rupture also occur during labour (Milon et al, 1983), rupture of this type can occur at any stage of gestation (Taylor & Canning, 1979), the earliest recorded case being at the 19th week of pregnancy (de Wane & McCubbin, 1981).

The death rate associated with uterine rupture has been variously estimated as between 6.5% and 10% (Golan et al, 1980) though in most western centres the currently expected mortality rate would be much lower than this; in developing countries the mortality rate is in the range of 7.5–21% (Balde et al, 1990; Konje et al, 1990). There is general agreement that the mortality rate is highest in cases of spontaneous uterine rupture and lowest in scar ruptures (Schrinsky & Benson, 1978): this view may, however, be misleading in so far as many cases classed as scar ruptures are, in fact, examples of scar dehiscence, a condition not associated with maternal death.

Anaesthetic deaths

Anaesthesia-related deaths in pregnant women do not, in general, differ in any specific manner from those occurring during, or after, general surgical procedures. Obstetrical patients are, however, unduly prone to pulmonary aspiration of gastric contents, partly because of the increased intragastric pressure resulting from compression of the abdominal contents by the gravid uterus and partly because of the progesterone-induced relaxation of the gastro-oesophageal sphincter (Baggish & Hooper, 1974; Cohen, 1982). The clinical and pathological features of pulmonary aspiration depend very considerably on whether liquid or solid material is aspirated, the former being the more common.

Acid fluid aspiration. The clinical features resulting from aspiration of acid gastric juice into the lungs were first described by Mendelson (1946) and his name is usually applied to this syndrome. Aspiration may occur silently and, whilst quite severe symptoms may result from inhalation of relatively trivial quantities of fluid, it is generally estimated that a serious hazard to the patient is only presented when the volume of the aspirate exceeds 25 ml (Cohen, 1982). The pulmonary reaction to the highly acid gastric juice may develop immediately after aspiration or may be delayed for two to five hours, becoming apparent at a time when the patient is making an apparently satisfactory recovery from anaesthesia. There is a rapid onset of tachypnoea, cyanosis, tachycardia, hypotension and bronchospasm; this latter symptom may be an inconspicuous feature but can be sufficiently marked as to mimic an acute asthmatic attack. Most patients recover but a few progress to convulsions, coma and death.

Aspirated fluid damages the pulmonary vascular epithelium with consequent intra-alveolar haemorrhage and pulmonary oedema: the surfactant-producing cells are destroyed and there is an intra-alveolar exudate of oedema fluid, erythrocytes, polymorphonuclear leucocytes and fibrin, often with the formation of hyaline membranes. These changes result in alveolar collapse and consolidation which initiates a significant degree of shunting and hypoxia (Cohen, 1982). In fatal cases the lungs are heavy, congested and oedematous: there may be subpleural haemorrhages and serosanguineous fluid in the pleural cavities. The heart is dilated and may show subpericardial haemorrhages whilst the abdominal viscera are deeply congested (McCormick, 1967). Histologically, the alveolar changes described above will be present and there may also be extensive necrosis and desquamation of the bronchial epithelium.

These pulmonary changes are widely thought to be directly due to the acid nature of the inhaled liquid (Bartlett & Gorbach, 1975; Stewardson & Nyhus, 1977) and indeed the effects of aspiration of gastric juice have been likened to an acute chemical burn (Stewardson & Nyhus, 1977; Cohen, 1982). This view has been largely based upon experimental studies in which it has been shown that the severity of the lung lesions is related to the pH of the fluid and that pulmonary oedema is inevitable only if the pH of the aspirate is below 2.5 (Teabeaut, 1952; Awe et al, 1966; Wynne & Modell, 1977). Alexander (1968) has, however, maintained that the development of pulmonary oedema is independent of the pH of the inhaled liquid, suggesting that fluid alone can damage the alveolar capillary membrane and that acidity only potentiates the exudative reaction. Support has been given to this contention by Schwartz et al (1980) who showed that instillation of gastric juice at a pH of 5.9 into the lungs of dogs produced changes which were just as severe as those resulting from the use of fluid at a pH of 1.8.

Faecal fluid aspiration.   In patients with prolonged labour there is depression of intestinal peristalsis, increased intra-abdominal pressure and delayed emptying of the stomach: the gastric contents thus come to resemble those found in intestinal obstruction and not only have a high pH but may also contain numerous organisms (McCormick, 1967). Aspiration of this material may produce acute respiratory distress which can be accompanied by profound hypotension, the latter probably being due to toxic shock resulting from entry of bacteria into the circulation from the lungs.

Aspiration of solid material.   This, depending on the size and consistency of the inhaled particles, may cause variable degrees of airway obstruction: if the particulate matter is sufficiently large the patient may asphyxiate whilst collapse of a lobe or a segment may occur. Smaller particles appear to accentuate the effects of inhaled fluid and elicit an acute peribronchial inflammatory reaction which later becomes granulomatous in nature.

Pneumomediastinum

During labour the intense Valsalva manoeuvre associated with 'bearing down' causes a marked, transient elevation of pulmonary intra-alveolar pressure which may result in rupture of marginally situated alveoli with subsequent tracking of air, along perivascular tissue planes, towards the hilum and into the mediastinum (Bard & Hassini, 1975; Brandfass & Martinez, 1976). In most such cases the air is resorbed over a few days whilst in others escape of air from the mediastinum into the subcutaneous tissues relieves the build-up of pressure. Occasionally, however, a tension-pneumomediastinum develops and this may prove fatal.

Hyperemesis gravidarum

Death during pregnancy from hyperemesis gravidarum is now exceedingly rare. Sheehan (1939), at a time when this condition was more commonly fatal, studied the pathological changes in 19 autopsied cases and was unable to find any that could not be directly attributed to prolonged vomiting and starvation. The most consistent abnormalities were cardiac atrophy, centrilobular fatty change in the liver and fatty change in the renal tubules. A less common finding was a Wernicke's encephalopathy whilst rarely there may be bilateral retinal haemorrhages and degenerative changes in the peripheral nerves (Fairweather, 1968).

Salt poisoning

A number of deaths have followed injection of hypertonic saline into the gravid uterus for the induction of abortion. The autopsy findings in such cases are characteristic and consist of symmetrical haemorrhagic infarction of the brain, involving particularly the region of the amygdaloid nuclei and a Y-shaped area in the pons (Cameron et al, 1969). It is thought that these lesions are due to a sudden change in plasma osmolarity, either because of accidental intraperitoneal or intravenous injection of saline or by leakage of salt solution through tears in the amnion into the maternal tissues.

Water intoxication

Administration of oxytocin is occasionally followed by severe fluid retention and water intoxication. In a woman dying from this complication Lilien (1968) found only pulmonary and cerebral oedema at autopsy.

Ectopic pregnancy

This important cause of maternal death is considered in Chapter 34.

REFERENCES

Adams D M, Druzin M L, Cederqvist L L 1989 Intrapartum uterine rupture. Obstetrics and Gynecology 73: 471–473.

Adamsons K, Mueller-Heubach E, Myers R E 1971 The innocuousness of amniotic fluid infusion in the pregnant rhesus monkey. American Journal of Obstetrics and Gynecology 109: 977–984.

Alexander I G S 1968 The ultrastructure of the pulmonary alveolar vessels in Mendelson's (acid pulmonary aspiration) syndrome. British Journal of Anaesthesia 40: 408–414.

Anderson D G 1967 Amniotic fluid embolisms: a re-evaluation. American Journal of Obstetrics and Gynecology 98: 336–346.

Attwood H D 1958 The histological diagnosis of amniotic fluid embolism. Journal of Pathology and Bacteriology 76: 211–215.

Attwood H D 1972 Amniotic fluid embolism. In: Sommers S C (ed) Pathology annual. Appleton-Century-Crofts, New York, pp 145–172.

Attwood H D, Downing S E 1965 Experimental amniotic fluid and meconium embolism. Surgery, Gynecology and Obstetrics 120: 255–262.

Awe W B, Fletcher W S, Jacob S W 1966 The pathophysiology of aspiration pneumonitis. Surgery 60: 232–239.

Azem F, Jaffa A, Lessing J B, Peyser M R 1993 Uterine rupture with the use of a low-dose vaginal PGE2 tablet. Acta Obstetricia et Gynecologica Scandinavica 72: 316–317.

Baggish M S, Hooper S 1977 Aspiration as a cause of maternal death. Obstetrics and Gynecology 43: 327–336.

Balde M D, Breitbach G P, Bastert G 1990 Uterine rupture — an analysis of 81 cases in Conakry/Guinea. International Journal of Gynaecology and Obstetrics 32: 223–227.

Bard R, Hassini N 1975 Pneumomediastinum complicating pregnancy. Respiration 32: 185–188.

Bartlett J G, Gorbach S L 1975 The triple threat of aspiration pneumonia. Chest 65: 580–586.

Bell E J, Wilson G F, Wilson L A 1953 Puerperal inversion of the uterus. American Journal of Obstetrics and Gynecology 66: 767–777.

Beller F K 1974 Disseminated intravascular coagulation and consumption coagulopathy in obstetrics. Obstetrics and Gynecology Annual 3: 267–281.

Benson M D 1993 Non-fatal amniotic fluid embolism: three possible cases and a new clinical definition. Archives of Family Medicine 2: 989–994.

Bouvier-Colle M-H, Varnoux N, Costes P, Hatton F 1991 Reasons for the underreporting of maternal mortality in France as indicated by a survey of all deaths among women of childbearing age. International Journal of Epidemiology 20: 717–721.

Brandfass R T, Martinez D M 1976 Mediastinal and subcutaneous emphysema in labor. Southern Medical Journal 69: 1554–1555.

Brandt C A, Larsen B 1989 Uterine rupture after re-implantation of fallopian tubes. Acta Obstetricia et Gynecologica Scandinavica 68: 281–282.

Bray P, Myers R A M, Cowley R A 1983 Orogenital sex as a cause of non-fatal air embolism in pregnancy. Obstetrics and Gynecology 61: 553–557.

Bryans F E 1963 Vascular accidents in maternal mortality. Clinical Obstetrics and Gynecology 6: 861–873.

Bunke J W, Hofmeister F J 1965 Uterine inversion — obstetrical entity or oddity? American Journal of Obstetrics and Gynecology 91: 934–939.

Burrow G N, Ferris T F (eds) 1982 Medical complications during pregnancy, 2nd edn. Saunders, Philadelphia.

Cameron J M, Morgan A G, Robinson A E, Urich H 1969 Brain damage following therapeutic abortion by amniotic fluid replacement: an experimental approach. Journal of Obstetrics and Gynaecology of the British Commonwealth 76: 168–175.

Chamberlain G V P 1992 The clinical aspects of massive haemorrhage. In: Patel N (ed) Maternal mortality — the way forward. Royal College of Obstetricians and Gynaecologists, London, pp 54–62.

Charles D, Larsen B 1989 Puerperal sepsis. In: Turnbull A, Chamberlain G (eds) Obstetrics. Churchill Livingstone, Edinburgh, pp 917–932.

Clark S L 1990 New concepts of amniotic fluid embolism: a review. Obstetrical and Gynecological Survey 45: 360–368.

Clark S L 1991 Amniotic fluid embolism. Critical Care Clinics 7: 877–882.

Clark S L, Montz P J, Phelan J P 1985 Hemodynamic alterations associated with amniotic fluid embolism: a reappraisal. American Journal of Obstetrics and Gynecology 151: 617–621.

Clark S L, Pavlova Z, Greenspoon J et al 1986 Squamous cells in the maternal pulmonary circulation. American Journal of Obstetrics and Gynecology 154: 104–106.

Clark S L, Cotton D B, Gonik B et al 1988 Central hemodynamic alterations in amniotic fluid embolism. American Journal of Obstetrics and Gynecology 158: 1124–1126.

Cohen S E 1982 The aspiration syndrome. Clinics in Obstetrics and Gynaecology 9: 235–254.

Collins C G, MacCallum E A, Nelson E W, Weinstein B B, Collins J H 1951 Suppurative pelvic thrombophlebitis. I. Incidence, pathology and etiology. Surgery 30: 298–310.

Corrin B, Spencer H 1981 Some aspects of pulmonary pathology. In: Anthony P P, MacSween R N M (eds) Recent advances in histopathology 11. Churchill Livingstone, Edinburgh, pp 83–98.

Courtney L D 1970 Amniotic fluid embolism. British Medical Journal 1: 545.

Cron R S, Kilkenney G S, Wirthwein C, Evrard J R 1952 Amniotic fluid embolism. American Journal of Obstetrics and Gynecology 64: 1360–1363.

Daniel D G, Campbell H, Turnbull A C 1967 Puerperal thromboembolism and suppression of lactation. Lancet 2: 287–289.

Deaton J L, Maier D, Andreoli J 1989 Spontaneous uterine rupture during pregnancy after treatment of Asherman's syndrome. American Journal of Obstetrics and Gynecology 160: 1053–1054.

De Swiet M 1989 Medical disorders in obstetric practice, 2nd edn. Blackwell Scientific, Oxford.

De Wane J C, McCubbin J H 1981 Spontaneous rupture of an unscarred uterus at 19 weeks gestation. American Journal of Obstetrics and Gynecology 141: 222–224.

Dibble L A, Elliott J P 1992 Possible amniotic fluid embolism associated with amnioinfusion. Journal of Maternal and Fetal Medicine 1: 263–266.

Dolyniuk M, Oriel E, Vania H, Karlman R, Tomich P 1983 Rapid diagnosis of amniotic fluid embolism. Obstetrics and Gynecology 61: 28s–30s.

Dragich D A, Ross A F, Chestnut D H, Wenstrom K D 1991 Respiratory failure associated with amnioinfusion during labor. Anesthesia and Analgesia 72: 549–551.

Duley I 1992 Maternal mortality associated with hypertensive disorders of pregnancy in Africa, Asia, Latin America and the Caribbean. British Journal of Obstetrics and Gynaecology 99: 547–553.

Editorial 1987 Maternal health in Subsaharan Africa. Lancet i: 255–257.

Eschenbach D A, Wager G P 1980 Puerperal infections. Clinical Obstetrics and Gynecology 23: 1003–1037.

Ewing T C, Smale L E, Elliott F A 1979 Maternal deaths associated with postpartum vulvar edema. American Journal of Obstetrics and Gynecology 134: 173–177.

Fairweather D V I 1968 Nausea and vomiting in pregnancy. American Journal of Obstetrics and Gynecology 102: 135–175.

Farmer R M, Kirschbaum T, Potter D et al 1991 Uterine rupture during trial of labor after previous cesarean section. American Journal of Obstetrics and Gynecology 163: 996–1001.

Fava S, Galizia A C 1993 Amniotic fluid embolism. British Journal of Obstetrics and Gynaecology 100: 1049–1050.

Fildes J, Reed L, Jones N et al 1992 Trauma: the leading cause of maternal death. Journal of Trauma 32: 643–645.

Flegner J R H 1971 Postpartum broad ligament haematomas. Journal of Obstetrics and Gynaecology of the British Commonwealth 78: 184–189.

Fox H 1987 Histopathology of pre-eclampsia and eclampsia. In: Sharp F, Symonds M E (eds) Hypertension in pregnancy. Perinatology Press, Ithaca, N.Y., pp 119–130.

Fox L P 1967 Abortion deaths in California. American Journal of Obstetrics and Gynecology 98: 645–651.

Garland I W C, Thompson W D 1983 Diagnosis of amniotic fluid embolism using an antiserum to human keratin. Journal of Clinical Pathology 36: 625–627.

Garnet J D 1964 Uterine rupture during pregnancy: an analysis of 133 patients. Obstetrics and Gynecology 23: 898–905.

Golan A, Sandbank O, Rubin A 1980 Rupture of the pregnant uterus. Obstetrics and Gynecology 56: 549–554.

Golde S, Ledger W J 1977 Necrotizing fascitis in postpartum patients: a report of four cases. Obstetrics and Gynecology 50: 670–673.

Goldstein P J 1968 Amniotic fluid embolism complicating intrauterine saline abortion. American Journal of Obstetrics and Gynecology 101: 858–859.

Gonsoulin W, Borge D, Moise K J 1990 Rupture of unscarred uterus in association with cocaine abuse. American Journal of Obstetrics and Gynecology 163: 526–527.

Govan A D T 1976 The histology of eclamptic lesions. Journal of Clinical Pathology 29: Supplement (Royal College of Pathologists) 10: 63–69.

Gregory M G, Clayton E M 1973 Amniotic fluid embolism. Obstetrics and Gynecology 42: 236–244.

Grimes D A 1994 The morbidity and mortality of pregnancy: still risky business. American Journal of Obstetrics and Gynecology 170: 1489–1494.

Guidotti R J, Grimes D A, Cates W 1981 Fatal amniotic fluid embolism during surgically induced abortion, United States, 1972 to 1978. American Journal of Obstetrics and Gynecology 141: 257–261.

Halmagyi D F J, Starzecki B, Shearman R P 1962 Experimental amniotic fluid embolism. American Journal of Obstetrics and Gynecology 84: 251–256.

Harris W J 1992 Uterine dehiscence following laparoscopic myomectomy. Obstetrics and Gynecology 80: 545–546.

Hasleton P S 1983 Adult respiratory distress syndrome — a review. Histopathology 7: 307–332.

Hogberg U 1985 Maternal mortality — a worldwide problem. International Journal of Gynaecology and Obstetrics 23: 463–470.

Hunter R M, Scott J C, Schneider J P, Krieger J A 1956 Experimental amniotic fluid infusion: a preliminary report. American Journal of Obstetrics and Gynecology 72: 75–78.

Jeffcoate T N A, Miller J, Roos R F, Tindall V R 1968 Puerperal thromboembolism in relation to the inhibition of lactation by oestrogen therapy. British Medical Journal 4: 19–25.

Jones R O, Nagashima A W, Hartnett-Goodman M M, Goodlin R C 1991 Rupture of low transverse cesarean scars during trial of labor. Obstetrics and Gynecology 77: 815–817.

Kaczmarek J C, Kates R, Rau F et al 1994 Intrapartum uterine rupture in a primiparous patient previously treated for invasive mole. Obstetrics and Gynecology 83: 842–844.

Kafkas S, Taper C E 1991 Ruptured uterus. International Journal of Gynaecology and Obstetrics 34: 41–44.

Katz V L, Cefalo R C 1989 Maternal death from carotid artery thrombosis associated with the syndrome of hemolysis, elevated liver function and low platelets. American Journal of Perinatology 6: 360–362.

Kitchin J D, Thiacarajah S, May H V, Thornton W N 1975 Puerperal inversion of the uterus. American Journal of Obstetrics and Gynecology 123: 51–56.

Kitzmiller J L, Lucas W E 1972 Studies on a model of amniotic fluid embolism. Obstetrics and Gynecology 39: 626–627.

Koegler A, Sauder P, Marolf A, Jaeger A 1994 Amniotic fluid embolism: a case report with non-cardiogenic pulmonary edema. Intensive Care Medicine 20: 45–46.

Konje J C, Odukoya O A, Ladipo A O 1990 Ruptured uterus in Ibadan — a twelve year review. International Journal of Gynaecology and Obstetrics 32: 207–213.

Krause W 1969 Erfahrungen mit der transabdominalen Amniozentese. Zentralblatt fur Gynakologie 91: 1561–1566.

Larue L, Marpeau L, Percque M et al 1991 Rupture d'un uterus sain lors d'une interruption de grossesse par prostaglandines au deuxieme trimestre. Journal de Gynecologie et Obstetrique et de la Biologie de Reproduction 20: 269–272.

Lee H A, Frampton J 1964 Case of intra-amniotic glucose induction followed by non-fatal amniotic fluid embolism and acute renal failure. American Journal of Gynecology 90: 554–555.

Lee W, Ginsburg K A, Cotton D B et al 1986 Squamous and trophoblastic cells in the maternal pulmonary circulation identified by invasive hemodynamic monitoring during the peripartum period. American Journal of Obstetrics and Gynecology 155: 999–1002.

Lema V M, Ojwang S B, Wanjala S H 1991 Rupture of the gravid uterus: a review. East African Medical Journal 68: 430–441.

Lilien A A 1968 Oxytocin-induced water intoxication: a report of a maternal death. Obstetrics and Gynecology 32: 171–173.

Lockwood C J, Bach R, Guha A et al 1991 Amniotic fluid contains tissue factor, a potent initiator of coagulation. American Journal of Obstetrics and Gynecology 165: 1335–1341.

Lurie S, Hagay Z, Goldschmitt R, Insler V 1992 Routine previous cesarean scar exploration following successful vaginal delivery: is it necessary? European Journal of Obstetrics and Gynecology, and Reproductive Biology 45: 185–196.

McCally M, Vasicka A 1962 Generalized Schwartzman reaction and hypofibrinogenemia in septic abortion: report of a case. Obstetrics and Gynecology 19: 359–364.

McCormick P W 1967 Pulmonary aspiration in obstetrics. Hospital Medicine 2: 163–171.

Macmillan D 1968 Experimental amniotic fluid embolism. Journal of Obstetrics and Gynaecology of the British Commonwealth 75: 849–852.

Maher J E, Wenstrom K D, Hauth J C, Meis P J 1994 Amniotic fluid embolism after saline amnioinfusion: two cases and review of the literature. Obstetrics and Gynecology 83: 851–854.

Maymon R, Haimovich L, Shulman A et al 1992 Third trimester uterine rupture after prostaglandin E2 use for labor induction. Journal of Reproductive Medicine 37: 449–452.

Meehan F P, Burke G, Kehoe J T 1989 Update on delivery following prior cesarian section: a 15 year review 1972–1987. International Journal of Gynaecology and Obstetrics 30: 205–212.

Mendelson C L 1946 The aspiration of stomach contents into the lungs during obstetric anesthesia. American Journal of Obstetrics and Gynecology 52: 191–204.

Milon D, Chevrant-Breton O, Tekam S, Peton J, Saint-Marc C, Giraud J R 1983 Rupture of the uterus during labor without apparent cause. European Journal of Obstetrics, Gynecology and Reproductive Biology 15: 1–4.

Mokgokong E T, Marivate M 1976 Treatment of the ruptured uterus. South African Medical Journal 50: 1621–1624.

Moldavsky L F 1967 Management of inversion of the uterus: report of four cases. Obstetrics and Gynecology 29: 488–494.

Morgan M 1979 Amniotic fluid embolism. Anaesthesia 34: 20–32.

Nelson P K 1960 Pulmonary gas embolism in pregnancy and the puerperium. Obstetrical and Gynecological Survey 15: 449–481.

Noble W H, St Amand J 1993 Amniotic fluid embolism. Canadian Journal of Anaesthesia 40: 871–880.

O'Driscoll R 1966 Rupture of the uterus. Proceedings of the Royal Society of Medicine 59: 65–66.

Peterson E W, Taylor H B 1970 Amniotic fluid embolism: an analysis of forty cases. Obstetrics and Gynecology 35: 787–793.

Philippe H J, Goffinet F, Jacquemard F et al 1991 Les traitments des inversions uterines obstetricales: a propos de trois observations. Journal de Gynecologie et Obstetrique et Biologie de la Reproduction 20: 843–849.

Pieri R I 1958 Pelvic hematomas associated with pregnancy. Obstetrics and Gynecology 12: 244–258.

Piot D, Gluck M, Oxorn H 1973 Torsion of the gravid uterus. Canadian Medical Association Journal 109: 1010–1011.

Plauche W C 1983 Amniotic fluid embolism. American Journal of Obstetrics and Gynecology 147: 982–985.

Prasad R N, Ratnam S S 1992 Uterine rupture after induction of labour for intrauterine death using the prostaglandin E2 analogue sulprostone. Australian and New Zealand Journal of Obstetrics and Gynaecology 32: 282–283.

Ragan W D 1981 Antepartum air embolism. Journal of the Indiana State Medical Association 74: 30–32.

Rasmussen O B 1992 Puerperal inversion of the uterus. Acta Obstetricia et Gynecologica Scandinavica 71: 558–559.

Reece E A, Hobbins J C, Mahoney M J, Petrie R H 1992 Medicine of the fetus and mother. Lippincott, Philadelphia.

Reeves T, Daoud F S, Estriole M, Stone W H, McGary D 1974 Pulmonary pressor effects of small amounts of bovine amniotic fluid. Respiration Physiology 20: 231.

Reis R L, Pierce W S, Behrendt D M 1969 Hemodynamic effects of amniotic fluid embolism. Surgery, Gynecology and Obstetrics 129: 45–48.

Report on Confidential Enquiries into Maternal Deaths in England and Wales 1976–1978. 1982 Her Majesty's Stationery Office, London.

Report on Confidential Enquiries into Maternal Deaths in the United Kingdom 1988–1990. 1994 Her Majesty's Stationery Office, London.

Rodgers B M, Staroscik R N, Reis R L 1969 Amniotic fluid embolism: effects of myocardial contractility and systemic and pulmonary vascular resistance. Surgical Forum 20: 203–205.

Rodgers B M, Staroscik R N, Reis R L 1971 Effects of amniotic fluid on cardiac contractility and vascular resistance. American Journal of Physiology 220: 1979–1982.

Ruckley C A 1992 Diagnosis and management of thromboembolic disease during pregnancy and the puerperium. In: Patel N (ed) Maternal mortality — the way forward. Royal College of Obstetricians and Gynaecologists, London, pp 41–50.

Rushton D I, Dawson I M P 1982 The maternal autopsy. Journal of Clinical Pathology 35: 909–921.

Sawyer M M, Lipshitz J, Anderson G D, Dilts P V 1981 Third trimester uterine rupture associated with vaginal prostaglandin E$_2$. American Journal of Obstetrics and Gynecology 140: 710–711.

Schrinsky D C, Benson R C 1978 Rupture of the pregnant uterus: a review. Obstetrical and Gynecological Survey 33: 217–232.

Schuitemaker N W, Gravenhorst J B, Van Geijn H P et al 1991 Maternal mortality and its prevention. European Journal of Obstetrics and Gynecology and Reproductive Biology 42 (suppl): s31–s35.

Schwartz O J, Wynne J W, Gibbs C P, Hood C I, Kuck E J 1980 The pulmonary consequences of aspiration of gastric contents at pH values greater than 2.5. American Review of Respiratory Disease 121: 119–126.

Shah-Hosseini M, Evrard J R 1989 Puerperal uterine inversion. Obstetrics and Gynecology 73: 367–370.

Shanklin D R, Sommers S C, Brown D A et al 1991 The pathology of maternal death. American Journal of Obstetrics and Gynecology 165: 1126–1155.

Sheehan H L 1939 Pathology of hyperemesis and vomiting in late pregnancy. Journal of Obstetrics and Gynaecology of the British Empire 46: 685–699.

Sheehan H L, Lynch J B 1973 Pathology of toxaemia of pregnancy. Churchill Livingstone, Edinburgh.

Shy K K, Eschenbach D A 1979 Fatal perineal cellulitis from an episiotomy site. Obstetrics and Gynecology 54: 292–298.

Smith C A 1975 Pathologic uterine torsion: a catastrophic event in late pregnancy. American Journal of Obstetrics and Gynecology 123: 32–33.

Steiner P E, Lushbaugh C C 1941 Maternal pulmonary embolism by amniotic fluid as a cause of obstetric shock and unexpected death in obstetrics. Journal of the American Medical Association 117: 1245–1254.

Stevenson C A 1969 Maternal death from puerperal sepsis following vaginal surgery: a 17 year study in Michigan (1950–1966). American Journal of Obstetrics and Gynecology 104: 699–710.

Stewardson R H, Nyhus L M 1977 Pulmonary aspiration — an update. Archives of Surgery 112: 1192–1197.

Stolte L, van Kessel H, Seelen J, Eskes T, Wagatsuma T 1967 Failure to produce the syndrome of amniotic fluid embolism by infusion of amniotic fluid and meconium into monkeys. American Journal of Obstetrics and Gynecology 98: 694–697.

Studdiford W E, Douglas G W 1956 Placental bacteremia: a significant finding in septic abortion accompanied by vascular collapse. American Journal of Obstetrics and Gynecology 71: 842–858.

Taylor P J, Canning D C 1979 Spontaneous rupture of primigravid uterus. Journal of Reproductive Medicine 22: 168–170.

Teabeaut J R 1952 Aspiration of gastric contents — an experimental study. American Journal of Pathology 28: 50–67.

Tindall V R 1971 The aetiology and pathology of pulmonary embolism. In: Macdonald R R (ed) Scientific basis of obstetrics and gynaecology, 1st edn. Churchill Livingstone, London, pp 385–414.

Toner P G 1992 The role of the histopathologist in maternal death. In: Patel N (ed) Maternal mortality — the way forward. Royal College of Obstetricians and Gynaecologists, London, pp 79–83.

Trive B K, Bristwo R E, Hsu C D et al 1994 Uterine rupture associated with recent antepartum cocaine abuse. Obstetrics and Gynecology 83: 840–841.

Varner M 1991 Postpartum hemorrhage. Critical Care Clinics 7: 883–897.

Visser A A, Giesteira M V K, Heyns A, Marais C 1983 Torsion of the gravid uterus: case reports. British Journal of Obstetrics and Gynaecology 90: 89–97.

Watson P 1980 Postpartum hemorrhage and shock. Clinical Obstetrics and Gynecology 23: 985–1001.

Watson P, Besch N, Bowes W A 1980 Management of acute and subacute puerperal inversion of the uterus. Obstetrics and Gynecology 55: 12–16.

Weiner-Kronish J P, Gropper M A, Matthay M A 1990 The adult respiratory distress syndrome: definition and prognosis, pathogenesis and treatment. British Journal of Anaesthesia 65: 107–129.

Weinstein L 1982 Syndrome of hemolysis, elevated liver enzymes, and low platelet count: a severe consequence of hypertension in pregnancy. American Journal of Obstetrics and Gynecology 142: 159–167.

Wynne J W, Modell J H 1977 Respiratory aspiration of stomach contents. Annals of Internal Medicine 87: 466–474.

Yussman M A, Haynes D M 1970 Rupture of the gravid uterus: a 12 year study. Obstetrics and Gynecology 36: 115–120.

Index